D0620888

PSYCHIATRIC &
MENTAL HEALTH NURSING
for CANADIAN PRACTICE

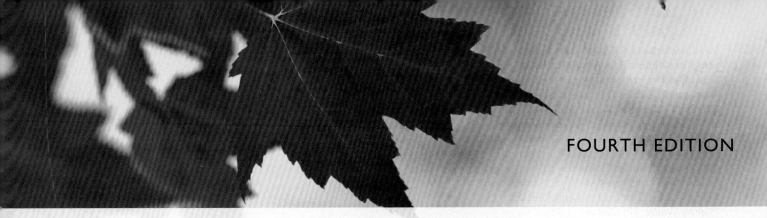

FOURTH EDITION

PSYCHIATRIC & MENTAL HEALTH NURSING
for CANADIAN PRACTICE

Wendy Austin, PhD, MEd (Counselling), BScN, RN

Professor Emeritus
Faculty of Nursing
The Dossetor Health Ethics Centre
University of Alberta
Edmonton, Alberta

Diane Kunyk, PhD, MSc, BScN, RN

Associate Professor
Faculty of Nursing
Adjunct Professor
The Dossetor Health Ethics Centre
University of Alberta
Edmonton, Alberta

Cindy Peternelj-Taylor, MSc, BScN, RN, DF-IAFN

Professor
College of Nursing
University of Saskatchewan
Saskatoon, Saskatchewan

Mary Ann Boyd, PhD, DNS, BC, APRN

Professor Emeritus
Southern Illinois University Edwardsville
Edwardsville, Illinois

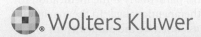

Philadelphia • Baltimore • New York • London
Buenos Aires • Hong Kong • Sydney • Tokyo

Vice President and Publisher: Julie K. Stegman
Senior Acquisitions Editor: Natasha McIntyre
Director of Product Development: Jennifer Forestieri
Development Editors: Dan Reilly, Greg Nicholl
Editorial Coordinator: Kerry McShane
Senior Marketing Manager: Sarah Schuessler
Editorial Assistant: Leo Gray
Senior Designer: Joan Wendt
Art Director: Jennifer Clements
Senior Production Project Manager: Alicia Jackson
Manufacturing Coordinator: Karin Duffield
Prepress Vendor: SPi Global

Fourth Edition

Copyright © 2019 Wolters Kluwer

© 2015 Wolters Kluwer. Copyright © 2010 Lippincott Williams & Wilkins. Copyright © 2008 Wolters Kluwer Health | Lippincott Williams & Wilkins. All rights reserved. This book is protected by copyright. No part of this book may be reproduced or transmitted in any form or by any means, including as photocopies or scanned-in or other electronic copies, or utilized by any information storage and retrieval system without written permission from the copyright owner, except for brief quotations embodied in critical articles and reviews. Materials appearing in this book prepared by individuals as part of their official duties as U.S. government employees are not covered by the above-mentioned copyright. To request permission, please contact Wolters Kluwer at Two Commerce Square, 2001 Market Street, Philadelphia, PA 19103, via email at permissions@lww.com, or via our website at lww.com (products and services). 2/2018

9 8 7 6 5 4 3 2 1

Printed in China

Library of Congress Cataloging-in-Publication Data
Names: Austin, Wendy, 1947- author. | Kunyk, Diane, 1957- author. | Peternelj-Taylor, Cindy, author. | Boyd, M. (Mary Ann), author.
Title: Psychiatric & mental health nursing for Canadian practice / Wendy Austin, Diane Kunyk, Cindy Peternelj-Taylor, Mary Ann Boyd.
Other titles: Psychiatric and mental health nursing for Canadian practice
Description: Fourth edition. | Philadelphia : Wolters Kluwer, [2019] | Includes bibliographical references and index.
Identifiers: LCCN 2017049374 | ISBN 9781496384874
Subjects: | MESH: Psychiatric Nursing—methods | Mental Disorders—nursing | Canada
Classification: LCC RC440 | NLM WY 160 | DDC 616.89/0231—dc23 LC record available at https://lccn.loc.gov/2017049374

This work is provided "as is," and the publisher disclaims any and all warranties, express or implied, including any warranties as to accuracy, comprehensiveness, or currency of the content of this work.

This work is no substitute for individual patient assessment based upon healthcare professionals' examination of each patient and consideration of, among other things, age, weight, gender, current or prior medical conditions, medication history, laboratory data and other factors unique to the patient. The publisher does not provide medical advice or guidance and this work is merely a reference tool. Healthcare professionals, and not the publisher, are solely responsible for the use of this work including all medical judgments and for any resulting diagnosis and treatments.

Given continuous, rapid advances in medical science and health information, independent professional verification of medical diagnoses, indications, appropriate pharmaceutical selections and dosages, and treatment options should be made and healthcare professionals should consult a variety of sources. When prescribing medication, healthcare professionals are advised to consult the product information sheet (the manufacturer's package insert) accompanying each drug to verify, among other things, conditions of use, warnings and side effects and identify any changes in dosage schedule or contraindications, particularly if the medication to be administered is new, infrequently used or has a narrow therapeutic range. To the maximum extent permitted under applicable law, no responsibility is assumed by the publisher for any injury and/or damage to persons or property, as a matter of products liability, negligence law or otherwise, or from any reference to or use by any person of this work.

LWW.com

CCS0218

This book is dedicated to our students who continually challenge us to be the best that we can be as nurses and educators. Our hope is that this textbook will contribute to your readiness for practice as you engage persons with mental health problems and disorders, regardless of the practice setting in which you encounter them. We trust that you will meet them with empathy, compassion, and respect, supporting their and their family's dignity and voice.

We gratefully acknowledge the loving support and patience of our families across this project. Their recognition of its value to the education of Canadian nurses was much appreciated by us.

Wendy, Diane, and Cindy

Canadian Contributors

Current Edition

Wendy Austin, PhD, MEd (Counselling), BScN, RN
Professor Emeritus
Faculty of Nursing
Dossetor Health Ethics Centre
University of Alberta
Edmonton, Alberta

Amy Bombay, PhD, MA
Assistant Professor
Department of Psychiatry, Faculty of Medicine
School of Nursing, Faculty of Health
Dalhousie University
Halifax, Nova Scotia

Geertje Boschma, PhD, MSN, MA, BSN, RN
Professor
School of Nursing
University of British Columbia
Vancouver, British Columbia

Diana Clarke, PhD, RN
Adjunct Professor
Rady Faculty of Health Sciences
University of Manitoba
Winnipeg, Manitoba

Anne Marie Creamer, PhD, MSN, RN
Nurse Practitioner, Primary Health Care
Saint Joseph's Community Health Centre
Horizon Health Network
Saint John, New Brunswick

Christine Davis, MEd, MN, BScN, CPMHN(C)
Professor
St. Lawrence College Collaborative BScN
Laurentian University
Brockville, Ontario

Charl Els, MBChB, MMedPsych, FCPsych, ABAM, MROCC
Clinical Professor
Department of Psychiatry
University of Alberta
Edmonton, Alberta

Carol Ewashen, PhD, MN, BN, RN
Associate Professor
Faculty of Nursing
University of Calgary
Calgary, Alberta

Lorelei Faulkner-Gibson, MN, BSN, RN
Clinical Nursing Educator
BCMHAS—Children's & Women's Mental Health Program
Children's & Women's Hospital Site
Vancouver, British Columbia

Dorothy Forbes, PhD, MN, BSN, RN
Professor Emeritus
Faculty of Nursing
Edmonton, Alberta

Cheryl Forchuk, PhD, RN, O Ont, FCAHS
Beryl and Richard Ivey Research Chair
Aging, Mental Health, Rehabilitation and Recovery
Lawson Health Research Institute
Western University
London, Ontario

Marlee Groening, MSN, RN
Clinical Nurse Specialist
Segal Intensive Tertiary Rehabilitation and British Columbia Psychosis Program
Tertiary Mental Health
Vancouver Coastal Health
Vancouver, British Columbia

Emily Jenkins, PhD, MPH, RN
Assistant Professor
School of Nursing
University of British Columbia
Vancouver, British Columbia

Arlene Kent-Wilkinson, PhD, MN, BSN, RN, CPMHN(C)
Associate Professor
College of Nursing
University of Saskatchewan
Saskatoon, Saskatchewan

Diane Kunyk, PhD, MSc, BScN, RN
Associate Professor
Faculty of Nursing
Adjunct Professor
Dossetor Health Ethics Centre
University of Alberta
Edmonton, Alberta

Gerri Lasiuk, PhD, MN, BSN, BA(Psych), RPN, RN, CFMHN(C)
Associate Professor
College of Nursing
University of Saskatchewan
Regina, Saskatchewan

Duncan Stewart MacLennan, MN
Faculty Lecturer
Faculty of Nursing
University of Alberta
Edmonton, Alberta

Shelley Marchinko, MN, RN
Instructor
College of Nursing
University of Manitoba
Winnipeg, Manitoba

Elizabeth A. McCay, PhD, RN
Professor
Daphne Cockwell School of Nursing
Ryerson University
Toronto, Ontario

Elaine Santa Mina, PhD, RN
Associate Professor
Daphne Cockwell School of Nursing
Ryerson University
Toronto, Ontario

Sharon L. Moore, PhD, RN, R Psych
Professor
Faculty of Health Disciplines
Athabasca University
Athabasca, Alberta

Lynn Musto, PhD, RPN, RN
Assistant Professor
School of Nursing
Trinity Western University
Langley, British Columbia

Tanya Park, PhD, RN
Assistant Professor
Faculty of Nursing
University of Alberta
Edmonton, Alberta

Cindy Peternelj-Taylor, MSc, RN, DF-IAFN
Professor
College of Nursing
University of Saskatchewan
Saskatoon, Saskatchewan

Carol Rupcich, MN, RN
Mental Health Therapist
Women's Mental Health Clinic
Foothills Medical Centre
Alberta Health Services
Calgary, Alberta

Nicole Snow, PhD, RN, CPMHN(C)
Assistant Professor
School of Nursing
Memorial University
St. John's, Newfoundland and Labrador

Kathryn Weaver, PhD, RN
Professor
University of New Brunswick
Fredericton, New Brunswick

Kimberly Wong, MBA, BSN, RN, CPMHN(C)
Senior Practice Lead, Child and Youth Mental Health
BC Children's Hospital
Vancouver, British Columbia

Phillip Woods, PhD, RPN
Professor
College of Nursing
University of Saskatchewan
Saskatoon, Saskatchewan

Previous Editions

Freida S. Chavez, MHSc, BScN, RN, CHE
Senior Lecturer
Faculty of Nursing
University of Toronto
Toronto, Ontario

Julia Gajewski-Noel, MN, BA, RN
Certificate in Mental Health Nursing
Senior Teaching Associate—Retired
Faculty of Nursing
University of New Brunswick
Fredericton, New Brunswick

Ruth Gallop, PhD, RN
Professor Emerita
Faculty of Nursing
University of Toronto
Toronto, Ontario

Mary Haase, PhD, BScN, RPN, RN
Faculty Member
BScN Program
MacEwan University
Edmonton, Alberta

Brad Hagen, PhD (Nsg), RN, R Psych
Associate Professor
Faculty School of Health Sciences
University of Lethbridge
Lethbridge, Alberta

Sandy Harper-Jaques, MN, RN, RMFT
Clinical Nurse Specialist
Adult Mental Health
CHR South Calgary Health Centre
Calgary, Alberta

Marion Healey-Ogden, PhD, MEd, MA, BSN, RN, RCC
Assistant Professor
Faculty of Nursing
Thompson Rivers University
Kamloops, British Columbia

L. Elizabeth Hood, PhD, MSN, RN
Clinical Nurse Specialist (Mental Health)
Regional Mental Health Program
Alberta Hospital Edmonton
Edmonton, Alberta

Jean Robinson Hughes, PhD, RN
Associate Professor
School of Nursing
Dalhousie University
Halifax, Nova Scotia

Annette M. Lane, PhD, RN
Assistant Professor
Faculty of Nursing
University of Calgary
Calgary, Alberta

Lori Houger Limacher, PhD, RN, RMFT
Private Practice
Calgary, Alberta

Ginette Pagé, PhD, RN
Clinical Nurse Specialist, Consultant in Nursing
Private Practice
Dunham, Québec

Hélène Provencher, PhD, RN
Professor
Faculty of Nursing
Laval University
Québec City, Québec

Tracey Tully, PhD, RN
Clinical Nurse Specialist
Sunnybrook and Women's College Health Sciences Centre
Toronto, Ontario

Stephen VanSlyke, MN, BN, RN
Senior Teaching Associate
Faculty of Nursing
University of New Brunswick
Fredericton, New Brunswick

Olive Yonge, PhD, RN, R Psych
Professor
Faculty of Nursing
Vice Provost (Academic Programs)
University of Alberta
Edmonton, Alberta

American Contributors to Previous Editions

Marjorie Baier, PhD, RN
Associate Professor
School of Nursing
Southern Illinois University Edwardsville
Edwardsville, Illinois

Doris E. Bell, PhD, BC, APRN
Professor of Nursing
Southern Illinois University Edwardsville
Edwardsville, Illinois

Ann R. Bland, PhD, BC, APRN
Associate Professor
Department of Baccalaureate and Graduate
   Nursing
Eastern Kentucky University
Richmond, Kentucky

Andrea C. Bostrom, PhD, BC, APRN, RN
Associate Professor and Dean of Academic Programs
Kirkhof College of Nursing
Grand Valley State University
Allendale, Michigan

Mary R. Boyd, PhD, RN
Associate Professor
College of Nursing
University of South Carolina
Columbia, South Carolina

Stephanie Burgess, PhD, APN-BC
Clinical Professor and Associate Dean for Nursing
   Practice
College of Nursing
University of South Carolina
Columbia, South Carolina

Rita Canfield, DNSc, MSN, RN
School of Nursing
Southern Illinois University Edwardsville
Edwardsville, Illinois

Jeanne A. Clement, EdD, BC, APRN, FAAN
Associate Professor and Director of Graduate Specialty
   Program in Psychiatric-Mental Health Nursing
College of Nursing
The Ohio State University
Columbus, Ohio

Harvey Davis, PhD, RN, CARN, PHN
Associate Professor
School of Nursing
San Francisco State University
San Francisco, California

Catherine Gray Deering, PhD, BC, APRN, BC, RN
Professor
Clayton State College
Morrow, Georgia

Peggy El-Mallakh, PhD, RN
Post-Doctoral Scholar
Chandler Medical Center
College of Nursing
University of Kentucky
Lexington, Kentucky

Barbara G. Faltz
Clinical Nurse Specialist
Addiction Treatment Services, Veterans Administration
Palo Alto Healthcare System
Palo Alto, California

Judith E. Forker, PhD, BC, APRN
Associate Dean for Academic Affairs
School of Nursing
Adelphi University
Garden City, New York

Denise M. Gibson, MSN, BC, APRN
Instructor
Southern Illinois University School of Nursing
   Edwardsville
Edwardsville, Illinois

Vanya Hamrin, MS, BC, APRN, RN
Assistant Professor
School of Nursing
Yale University
New Haven, Connecticut

Beverly Gilliam Hart, PhD, RN
Associate Professor of Baccalaureate and Graduate
    Nursing
Eastern Kentucky University
Richmond, Kentucky

Emily J. Hauenstein, PhD, BC, APRN, LCP
Professor
School of Nursing
University of Virginia
Charlottesville, Virginia

Nancy Anne Hilliker, MA, ANP, RN, CS
Nurse Practitioner
Barnes-Jewish Hospital
St. Louis, Missouri

Gail L. Kongable, MSN, RN, FNP
Associate Professor
Neurological Surgery
University of Virginia Health Systems
Charlottesville, Virginia

Kathy Lee, MS, BC, APRN, RN
Associate Professor and Psychiatric Mental Health
    Nurse Practitioner
School of Nursing—SNSN
Oregon Health & Science University
Center for Women's Health
Portland, Oregon

Susan McCabe, EdD, BC, APRN
Associate Professor
College of Nursing
East Tennessee State University
Johnson City, Tennessee

**Ruth Beckmann Murray, EdD, MSN, N-NAP,
  FAAN**
Professor Emerita
School of Nursing
Doisy College of Health Sciences
St. Louis University
St. Louis, Missouri

Robert B. Noud, MS, BC, APRN
Adjunct Faculty Staff
University of Missouri St. Louis
St. Louis University Hospital
St. Louis, Missouri

Maryellen C. Pachler, MSN, APRN
Child Psychiatric Nurse Practitioner
Child Study Center
School of Medicine
Yale University
New Haven, Connecticut

Nan Roberts, MS, BC, APRN
Director of Clinical Trials
Advent Research Institute
St. Peters, Missouri

Lawrence Scahill, PhD, MSN, FAAN
Professor of Nursing and Child Psychiatry
Child Study Center
Yale University
New Haven, Connecticut

Victoria Soltis-Jarrett, PhD, APRN-BC
Clinical Associate Professor and MSN Coordinator,
    Psychiatric Mental Health
Family Psychiatric Nurse Practitioner and Clinical
    Nurse Specialist
School of Nursing
University of North Carolina at Chapel Hill
Chapel Hill, North Carolina

Mickey Stanley, PhD, RN
Associate Professor
School of Nursing
Southern Illinois University Edwardsville
Edwardsville, Illinois

Roberta Stock, MS, BC, APRN
Advanced Practice Nurse
Comtrea, Inc.
Festus, Missouri

Sandra P. Thomas, PhD, RN, FAAN
Professor and Director, PhD Program
College of Nursing
The University of Tennessee
Knoxville, Tennessee

Barbara Jones Warren, PhD, BC, APRN
Associate Clinical Professor
College of Nursing
The Ohio State University
Executive Nurse
Ohio Department of Mental Health
Columbus, Ohio

Jane White, PhD, DNSc, BC, APRN
Vera E. Bender Professor of Nursing
Associate Dean for Research and Graduate Programs
Adelphi University
Garden City, New York

Lorraine D. Williams, PhD, BC, APRN, RN
Associate Professor
School of Nursing
Southern Illinois University Edwardsville
Edwardsville, Illinois

Rhonda Kay Wilson, MS, BSN, RN
Quality Manager
Chester Mental Health Center
Chester, Illinois

Richard Yakimo, PhD, BC, APRN
Assistant Professor
School of Nursing
Southern Illinois University Edwardsville
Edwardsville, Illinois

Reviewers

Pamela Adams, PhD, MScN, BN, JD
Professor and Coordinator
University of New Brunswick/Humber College
Toronto, Ontario

Nancy Clark, PhD, RN
Assistant Professor
School of Nursing
University of Victoria
Victoria, British Columbia

Nancy Fleming, MA(Ed), RN, HBScN
Professor and Coordinator
Lakehead University Confederation College BSCN
    Nursing Program
Confederation College
Thunder Bay, Ontario

Jim Hunter, MSN, RN
Faculty
School of Health Sciences
British Columbia Institute of Technology
Burnaby, British Columbia

Judy Osborne, MEd, BN, RN
Clinical Faculty
School of Health and Wellness
Fleming College
Peterborough, Ontario

Susan Power, RPN, MALT
Professor
Chair of the Admissions & Progressions Committee,
    BPN Program
Faculty of Health
Kwantlen Polytechnic University
Langley, British Columbia

Crystal Schauerte, MScN, BScN
Professor and Coordinator
School of Health and Community Studies
Algonquin College
Ottawa, Ontario

Wilma Schroeder, BN, RN, MMFT
Clinical Course Leader
Faculty of Nursing
Red River College
Winnipeg, Manitoba

Linda Terblanche, PhD
Associate Professor
School of Nursing
Trinity Western University
Langley, British Columbia

Mary Jean Thompson, MHS, MPC, BN, RN
Nursing Faculty
Division of Science and Health
Medicine Hat College
Medicine Hat, Alberta

Ann-Marie Urban, PhD, RPN, RN
Assistant Professor
Faculty of Nursing
University of Regina
Regina, Saskatchewan

Wendy Wheeler, MN, RN
Nursing Instructor
School of Health Sciences
Red Deer College
Red Deer, Alberta

Preface

In the fourth edition of *Psychiatric & Mental Health Nursing for Canadian Practice*, we are pleased to continue our efforts to present a Canadian perspective on psychiatric and mental health (PMH) nursing. We have included in this edition the 2015 *Entry-to-Practice Mental Health and Addiction Competencies for Undergraduate Nursing Education in Canada* to emphasize the expectation in Canada that all nurses have preparation to care for persons and families who have lived experience of mental health problems and disorders. There is recognition, as well, that there may be a need to consult with nurses with specialist training in PMH nursing. Increasingly, there is acknowledgement that physical and mental health are not separate entities. Chapter 9 in this textbook, *Biologic Basis of Practice*, should convince even skeptics of that reality. We continue to approach our understanding of PMH care with the advancements that are occurring in line with our national mental health strategy under the guidance of the Mental Health Commission of Canada (MHCC). The evolution of a recovery orientation to care has been such an advancement. Nurses and other health care professionals have a broader perspective on what constitutes recovery and a focus on strengths, resources, and rights, which are shaped by culturally safe practices. Trauma-informed care is essential to good practice, as well. That we must approach all persons in our care with a knowledge of trauma and its effects and consciously incorporate the principles of safety and choice is recognized across Canadian health care services. The implications for nursing care of *historical trauma* are presented in this edition. Chapter 3, *The Context of Mental Health Care: Cultural, Socioeconomic, and Geographic*, addresses the historical trauma of Aboriginal peoples in Canada. In this chapter, we respond to the Truth and Reconciliation Commission of Canada's call to action to educate nursing students regarding the history and legacy of residential schools by focusing on its significant and ongoing impact on mental health. Further understanding of trauma is to be found in Chapter 17, *Trauma- and Stress-Related Disorders, Crisis and Disaster*. This edition presents, too, the latest in the nursing care of the most prevalent of all mental disorders, although a preventable one:

addiction. Its burden on our society remains uncertain. As we go to press, opioid use is at epidemic proportions, causing unprecedented loss of life and our governments are working to create wise and comprehensive law for the regulation of marijuana use.

As in the previous editions, the terminology used to identify individual recipients of nursing care has been left to the preference of the chapter contributors. There are many pedagogical features of the textbook that we highlight here.

FEATURES

- Chapters open with **Learning Objectives**, **Key Terms**, and **Key Concepts** that cue students to the material they will encounter.
- **Research for Best Practice boxes** focus on specific studies, primarily Canadian, which contribute to improving nursing practice in PMH care. The selected studies reflect the broad range of research methods used to inform practice.
- The **In-a-Life feature** illustrates the way the topic of the chapter has shaped or been played out in a particular person's life.
- **Therapeutic Dialogue boxes** encourage the comparison of therapeutic and nontherapeutic communication by giving relevant examples of both.
- **Drug Profile boxes** present a profile of specific psychotropic medications, commonly prescribe in the treatment of mental disorders.
- **Psychoeducation Checklists** identify content areas for the education of persons with specific disorders and their families
- **Summary of Key Points** encapsulates core chapter content to facilitate assimilation and review.
- **Web Links** connect to sites of relevance to the chapter content, including key documents, professional practice organizations, national and international institutions and groups, such as the Government of Canada, the International Council of Nurses, and the World Health Organization.

TEACHING AND LEARNING RESOURCES

To facilitate mastery of this text's content, a comprehensive teaching and learning package has been developed to assist faculty and students.

Resources for Instructors

Tools to assist you with teaching your course are available upon adoption of this text at http://thePoint.lww.com/Austin4e

- A **Test Generator** lets you put together exclusive new tests from a bank containing hundreds of questions to help you in assessing your students' understanding of the material. Test questions link to chapter learning objectives.
- **PowerPoint Presentations** provide an easy way for you to integrate the textbook with your students' classroom experience, either via slide shows or handouts. Multiple-choice and true/false questions are integrated into the presentations to promote class participation and allow you to use i-clicker technology.
- An **Image Bank** lets you use the photographs and illustrations from this textbook in your PowerPoint slides or as you see fit in your course.
- **Case Studies** with related questions (and suggested answers) give students an opportunity to apply their knowledge to a client case similar to one they might encounter in practice.
- Plus **Practice and Learn Activities** and **Answers to the Movie Viewing Guides.**

Resources for Students

An exciting set of free resources is available to help students review material and become even more familiar with vital concepts. Students can access all these resources at http://thePoint.lww.com/Austin4e using the codes printed in the front of their textbooks.

- **NCLEX-Style Review Questions** for each chapter help students review important concepts and practice for NCLEX.
- **Lippincott Theory to Practice Video Series: Psychiatric–Mental Health Nursing** includes videos of true-to-life patients displaying mental health disorders, allowing students to gain experience and a deeper understanding of mental health patients. The video series allows viewing of complete patient interviews and also gives the opportunity to view snippets of those interviews, for closer analysis or classroom discussion. Theory to Practice topics such as Depression, Eating Disorders, and Addiction make up some of the innovative videos to help students in their course and beyond.
- **Movie Viewing Guides** have suggestions of movies, documentaries, videos, TED talks, biographies, and novels relevant to the chapter, as well as "viewing points" to consider for each resource.
- **Critical Thinking Challenges** are grounded in chapter content and aimed at stimulating both analytical and reflective thinking on the part of students.
- **Clinical Simulation Tutorials and Case Studies** on schizophrenia, depression, and the acutely manic phase that walk students through case studies and put them in real-life situations.
- **Journal Articles** provided for each chapter offer access to current research available in Wolters Kluwer journals.
- Plus **Media Reviews, Learning Objectives,** and **Drug Monographs.**

Contents

UNIT

6

Mental Health Across the Lifespan   715

UNIT

7

Care of Persons With Additional Vulnerabilities   865

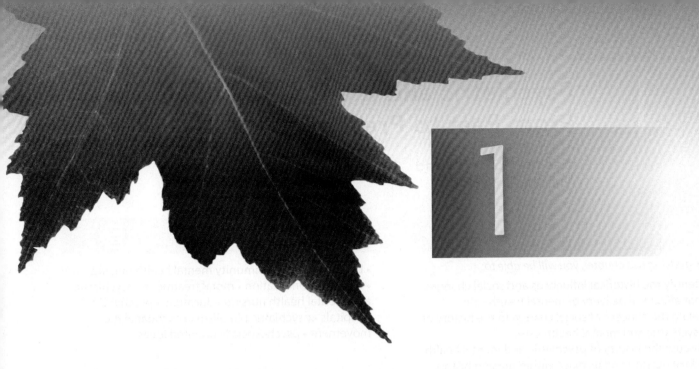

1

Contemporary Canadian Mental Health Care

1 Psychiatric and Mental Health Nursing: From Past to Present

Geertje Boschma and Marlee Groening

LEARNING OBJECTIVES

After studying this chapter, you will be able to:

- Identify the historical influences and social changes that affect the delivery of mental health care.
- Relate the concept of social change to the history of psychiatric and mental health care.
- Discuss the history of psychiatric and mental health (PMH) nursing and its place within nursing history.
- Analyze the theoretical arguments that shaped the development of contemporary scientific thought about PMH nursing practice.
- Summarize the impact of current social, economic, and political forces on the delivery of mental health services.

KEY TERMS

- biologic view • community mental health nursing • deinstitutionalization • moral treatment • psychiatric and mental health nursing education • psychiatric hospitals • psychiatric pluralism • psychoanalytic movement • psychosocially oriented ideas

KEY CONCEPTS

- historical context • social change

Until the 19th century, mentally ill people mainly were kept at home and cared for by their families. Sometimes, their legal guardians boarded them with other families for a fee, as part of a broader poor relief system. Only the most seriously afflicted people, whose behaviour was severely disturbing or who were considered a danger to themselves, their families, or other citizens, were locked in, often in prison or poorhouses. Indigent mentally ill people were grouped with old, sick, orphaned, or convicted people, and the circumstances in these scanty public facilities were most basic and often harsh. For those who could afford it, privately maintained institutions emerged as well (Boschma, 2003; Shorter, 1997).

EARLY FORMS OF INSTITUTIONAL CARE

Around the turn of the 15th century—the beginning of the European Renaissance—some towns in Europe established small-scale asylums as charitable enterprises, each one initially housing about 10 people. Most often, they were civilian, charitable initiatives in which neither the church nor doctors were involved. London's Bethlehem Hospital (famously known as "Bedlam") (Fig. 1.1), founded in 1371, and the Reinier van Arkel asylum, founded in 1442 in the Dutch town of Den Bosch, are early examples of the insane asylums or "mad houses" that would over the next centuries spread throughout Europe and, in the wake of colonialism, other parts of the world. These asylums were managed as large households, like other guesthouses or poorhouses, and administered by a board of noted citizens, with a steward and matron, often a married couple, taking charge of day-to-day management with the assistance of a few servants. With the social and economic changes of the 18th and 19th centuries, these homes grew into larger institutions (Boschma, 2003).

Religious orders, often under the protection or authority of the church, also involved themselves with charitable work and poor relief. Roman Catholic orders, for example, reemerged in 17th-century France during the Counter-Reformation, and many of them managed the care in small-scale, premodern hospitals. The orders themselves sometimes owned the houses. Influential cases in point were the male order of the Congregation of Lazarists and the female congregation of the Sisters of Mercy (or Daughters of Charity), founded by Vincent de Paul in 1625 and 1633, respectively (Jones, 1989). These orders produced early models for nursing work as a socially respectable endeavour at a time when medical care had barely developed and was scarcely available (Nelson, 1999, 2001; Porter, 1993). In the Americas, one of the first institutions that took in mentally ill people was San Hipólito in Mexico City, which opened in

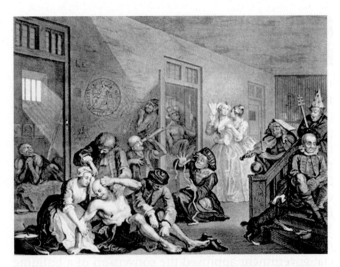

Figure 1.1. Interior of Bethlehem Asylum ("Bedlam"), London, as depicted by William Hogarth in his series *A Rake's Progress.* (From U.S. National Library of Medicine. Images from the history of medicine. National Institutes of Health, Department of Health and Human Services.)

1589 as a hospital for the insane, under the auspices of the Roman Catholic Church. It was run by the brothers of the order of La Caridad y San Hipólito, who, vowing poverty and charity, relied on alms to support themselves and worked as attendants in the institution (Leiby, 1992). The earliest forms of institutional treatment in Canada date back to the 19th century.

Diverse beliefs and approaches to deal with mental illness or attempts to treat it have been employed and must be understood in their historical context. Spiritual, biologic, and social explanations commonly were intertwined in popular perceptions of causes of mental illness. Evil spirits, sin, demonic possession, fears, contagious environments, or brain disturbances have figured in explanations of mental disorders and accordingly shaped people's responses, community resources, and medical treatment. History reflects that, generally, social fears and tolerance for what is deemed deviant behaviour are related to social stability and availability of resources. In periods of relative social stability, individuals with mental disorders often have a better chance to live safely within their communities. During periods of rapid social change and instability, there are more general anxieties and fears, and subsequently, more intolerance and ill treatment of people with mental disorders. As industrialization and urbanization increased during the 18th and 19th centuries, the rising middle class became concerned about a growing number of poor and deviant people who were not able to work and sustain themselves. At the same time, under the influence of ideas associated with the Enlightenment, medical and social ideas about mental illness changed, and medical concern with the treatment of mental illness increased. The insight gained ground that, rather than being afflicted by loss of reason or evil spirits, mentally

ill people were rational beings with a human nature common to all human beings and should be treated humanely. The idea of a moral, pedagogical treatment thus emerged that allegedly would help the suffering restore their innate capacity for self-control (Boschma, 2003; D'Antonio, 2006).

KEY CONCEPT

Social change, the structural and cultural evolution of society, is constant but often erratic. Psychiatric and mental health care has evolved within a **historical context** of social, economic, and political influences and cannot be separated from such realities.

A REVOLUTIONARY IDEA: HUMANE TREATMENT

By the height of the French Revolution in 1792, **moral treatment** became an influential idea that altered the care of the mentally ill and gave rise to important initiatives in which reform-minded physicians had an influential role. During this time, Philippe Pinel (1745–1826) was appointed physician to Bicetre, a hospital for men, which had a very poor reputation. Pinel, influenced by Enlightenment ideas, believed that the insane were sick patients who needed humane treatment, and he ordered the removal of the chains, stopped the abuses of drugging and bloodletting, and introduced more appropriate medical care. Three years later, the same standards were extended to Salpetrière, the asylum for female patients. At about the same time in England, William Tuke (1732 to 1822), a Quaker tea merchant in York and a member of the Society of Friends, raised funds for a retreat for mentally ill members of his Quaker community. The York Retreat, which opened in 1796, became another influential example for reform initiatives, introducing a regimen of humane, moral treatment, a pedagogical approach of kind supervision, proper medical treatment, and meaningful activities and distractions. Those reformers believed that a purposefully designed asylum provided a proper environment to indeed cure the mentally ill (D'Antonio, 2006). Based on these influential examples, throughout the Western world, purposefully designed asylums were established to provide sympathetic care in quiet, pleasant surroundings with some form of useful occupation such as weaving or farming. In the United States, the Quaker Friends Asylum was proposed in 1811 and opened 6 years later in Frankford, Pennsylvania (now Philadelphia), to become the second asylum in the United States. The humane and supportive rehabilitative attitude of the Quakers was seen as an extremely important influence in changing techniques of caring for those with mental disorders (D'Antonio, 2006).

IN-A-LIFE

Boarding Mentally Ill People With Families (12th to 19th Centuries)

THE GEEL LUNATIC COLONY, BELGIUM

The Legend of Saint Dymphna

According to legend, Dymphna, an Irish princess, came to Geel in the 6th century. Her father, the king of Ireland, disappointed that she was not a son, had left her and her mother in the care of a priest who converted them to Christianity. After Dymphna's mother died, the king became filled with grief and wanted another woman just like his former wife. His advisors decided that only his own daughter could match the queen. However, when her pagan father wanted to marry Dymphna, she fled out of fear with her priest and came to Geel. When the Irish king eventually found Dymphna and the priest, he beheaded both. In some sources, the legend tells that several lunatics witnessing this frightful scene suddenly became cured. Symbolic for her resistance to the spirit of evil, Dymphna became patron of lunatics, and the site of her death a place of miraculous healing. Some sources tell how the Saint Dymphna Guesthouse and chapel were built at this place, becoming a place of pilgrimage.

A Powerful Example of Family Care in Geel, Belgium

Since the Middle Ages (1286), the Saint Dymphna Guesthouse and chapel have existed in Geel, Belgium, eventually with a separate sick room for lunatic pilgrims. Chronically mentally ill patients who came to the Guesthouse as pilgrims seeking healing were often boarded out to families, and the Geel Lunatic Colony came into being. In the 19th century, the place became a formal institution with a strong emphasis on boarding outpatients with foster families, which became a model for many countries to follow. The legend of Saint Dymphna illustrates mythical and religious beliefs, explanations, and practices that have lost their meaning today. However, the cultural heritage of the Geel Colony demonstrates how powerful past ideas and beliefs can be in structuring creative and humane solutions to the care of mentally ill people.

Compiled from Parry-Jones, W. L. L. (1981). The model of the Geel Lunatic Colony and its influence on the nineteenth-century asylum system in Britain. In A. Scull (Ed.), *Madhouses, mad-doctors, and madmen. The social history of psychiatry in the Victorian Era* (pp. 201–217). London, UK: The Athlone Press; Boschma, G. (2003). *The rise of mental health nursing: A history of psychiatric care in Dutch asylum, 1890–1920.* Amsterdam, NL: Amsterdam University Press; and Goldstein, J. L., & Godemont, M. M. L. (2003). The legend and lessons of Geel: A 1500-year-old legend, a 21st-century model. *Community Mental Health Journal, 39*(5), 441–458.

THE 19TH AND EARLY 20TH CENTURIES: AN ERA OF ASYLUM BUILDING

In Canada, New Brunswick was the first of the old British North American provinces to open a mental institution. In 1835, a committee was appointed to prepare a petition to the provincial legislature proposing the establishment of a provincial lunatic asylum. Until then, counties had carried the responsibility under the Poor Laws system, to confine indigent insane families who were no longer able to be managed in local jails, or in poorhouses. As the population increased in the early 1800s, so did the number of mentally ill people in need of publicly provided care. In that same year, the provincial government approved the conversion of a building in Saint John, formerly a hospital for cholera patients, to a Provincial Lunatic Asylum until a new facility could be built. By 1848, this new facility was ready for use (Fig. 1.2) (Hurd, 1973/1916–17; Sussman, 1998).

During the latter half of the 19th century and beginning of the 20th century, each Canadian province established an asylum (Table 1.1). Involuntary confinement and institutional care became the dominant treatment modality for mentally ill people, replacing older forms of familial care and Poor Law–based approaches (Moran, 2000; Moran & Wright, 2006). In-depth historical analyses of admission patterns, one of the Ontario-based Homewood Retreat, for example, showed that gender differences were reflective of the social situation of the time (Warsh, 1989). Another analysis of the British Columbia

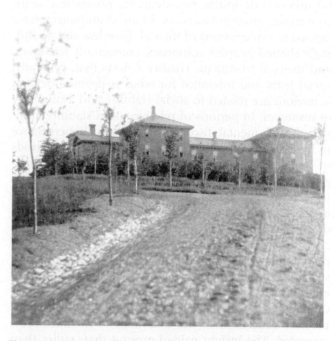

Figure 1.2. Canada's first hospital for mentally ill people, Saint John, New Brunswick, ca. 1885. (From Provincial Archives of New Brunswick, Saint John Stereographs—P86-67.)

Table 1.1	The First Asylums in British North America and Canada	
Province	**Date**	**Notes**
Quebec	1845	• Beauport, or the Quebec Lunatic Asylum, was opened. • A small dwelling for 12 mentally ill women was erected by Bishop St. Vallier.
	1714	• The Hotel Dieu cared for indigents, the crippled, and "idiots."
New Brunswick	1848	• The Provincial Lunatic Asylum was erected.
	1835	• Canada's first mental hospital opened in a small wooden building, a former cholera hospital, and was used as a temporary asylum.
Ontario	1850	• The Provincial Lunatic Asylum in Toronto admitted patients.
	1841	• Mentally ill people were placed in county jails until 1841, after which the Old York Jail served as a temporary asylum.
Newfoundland	1854	• An asylum for mentally ill patients was erected and admitted its first patients.
Nova Scotia	1857	• The first patients were admitted to the Provincial Hospital for the Insane.
British Columbia	1872	• A remodelled provincial general hospital (the old Royal Hospital) was opened as the Asylum for the Insane in British Columbia.
Prince Edward Island	1877	• The Prince Edward Island Hospital for the Insane was built.
Manitoba	1886	• The Selkirk Lunatic Asylum was opened.
Saskatchewan	1914	• The Saskatchewan Provincial Hospital admitted the first patients.
Alberta	1911	• The Provincial Asylum for the Insane opened in Ponoka.
Yukon and Northwest Territories		• These districts had no asylums in the early 20th century. The Royal North West Mounted Police assisted in transporting mentally ill patients to asylums in neighbouring provinces.

Adapted from Sussman, S. (1998). The first asylums in Canada: A response to neglectful community care and current trends. *Canadian Journal of Psychiatry, 43*, 260–264; Hurd, H. M. (Ed.). (1973, originally printed 1916–1917). *The institutional care of the insane in the United States and Canada* (Vol. IV). New York, NY: Arno Press.

psychiatric system revealed that many Aboriginal patients died soon after being admitted to the asylum, often from tuberculosis (Menzies & Palys, 2006).

The Legal Basis for Mental Health Care

Following the terms established by the British North America Act of 1867, the organization of mental health care in Canada became provincially based, and each province developed its own legislation to deal with problems created by mental illness. In the late 19th century,

all provinces passed legislation, most often called an Insanity Act, to provide a legal basis to publicly supported confinement of mentally ill persons. In the course of the 20th century, the legislation has been updated several times and eventually renamed a provincial Mental Health Act, reflecting changing views and a stronger medical influence on the care and treatment of people with mental illness. In the beginning of institutional psychiatric care in Canada, all patients admitted to public institutions were certified patients. Today, patients are being admitted to an institutional facility on either a voluntary or a certified basis. A carefully designed legal process has to be followed for patients admitted as certified patients under the terms of a mental health act, although criteria may differ between provinces. In several provinces, the use of community treatment orders is a new development under the mental health act (see Chapter 3 for the current legal context of mental health care).

A Social Reformer: Dorothea Lynde Dix

An ardent advocate for this new form of state-supported, public care was Dorothea Lynde Dix (1802–1887). Her crusade for more humane treatment generated much of the reform of mental health care systems in North America in the 19th century (Fig. 1.3). Almost 40 years of age, Dix, a retired school teacher living in Massachusetts, was solicited by a young theology student to help in preparing a Sunday school class for women inmates at the East Cambridge jail. Dix herself led the class and was shocked by living conditions in the jail. She was particularly struck by the treatment of inmates with mental disorders. It was the dead of winter, and the jail was providing no heat. When she questioned the jailer about this, his answer was that "the insane need no heat." The prevailing myth was that the insane were insensible to extremes of temperature. Dix's outrage initiated a long struggle in care reform (Lightner, 1999).

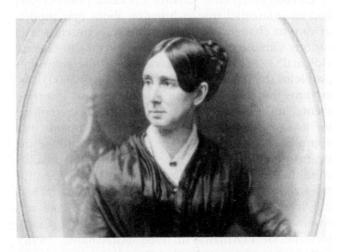

Figure 1.3. Dorothea Lynde Dix. (From U.S. National Library of Medicine Digital Collections. National Institutes of Health, Department of Health and Human Services.)

Influenced by a wider social reform movement that had a strong cultural influence throughout the Western world, drawing men and women into a wide range of reform activities, Dix followed the pattern of new women's activism that were also employed by social reformers such as Elizabeth Fry in prison reform and Josephine Butler in protecting women against prostitution (Van Drenth & De Haan, 1999). Dix diligently investigated the conditions of jails and the plight of mentally ill people while promoting the building of mental hospitals. In Canada, she was instrumental in advocating for mental institutions in Halifax and St. John's (Hurd, 1973/ 1916–17; Lightner, 1999). Dix eventually expanded her work into Great Britain and other parts of Europe.

Life Within Early Institutions

Despite the good intentions of early reformers, the approach inside the institution was one of custodial care and practical management, and treatment rarely occurred. The major concern was the management of a large number of people, many of whom exhibited disruptive behaviours. Patient numbers grew rapidly after provinces became legally responsible for financing care of the mentally ill. Institutions soon experienced severe overcrowding and had little more to offer than food, clothing, pleasant surroundings, and perhaps some means of employment and exercise. Limited resources made life in these institutions difficult. Although they were typically under the direction of a medical superintendent, overcrowding and resource shortages created rowdy, dangerous, and often unbearable situations. Quiet patients were involved in work as institutions grew into self-contained communities that produced their own food and made their own clothing. Day-to-day care was in the hands of lay personnel who shared with patients the routines of eating, sleeping, and working. Once admitted, many patients were cut off from society.

Ontario psychiatrist Charles K. Clarke (1857–1924) had an influential role in bringing about new models of care to change this situation. As superintendent of various Ontario psychiatric hospitals (e.g., Rockwood Hospital, 1881–1905), he was aware of the enormous problems that asylums experienced (Brown, 2000). The asylums under his direction saw continuous improvements, including the introduction of nurse training for asylum personnel. To find better treatments and approaches, he advocated for an urban centre for the treatment of acute mental illness under the best possible conditions and supported by university-based scientific research, which was eventually established in 1925 as the Toronto Psychiatric Hospital. Clarke's name was commemorated when the hospital became the Clarke Institute of Psychiatry in 1966 (Greenland, 1996). Following a merger with other Ontario institutions, the Clarke Institute would become part of the Centre for Addiction and Mental Health.

The deplorable state of large mental institutions soon gave rise to public commotion. In 1908, the American Clifford Beers (1876–1943) published an autobiography, *A Mind That Found Itself*, depicting his 3-year experience in three different types of hospitals: a private for-profit hospital, a private nonprofit hospital, and a state institution. He reported that in each facility, he had been beaten, choked, and imprisoned for long periods in dark, dank, padded cells and for many days had been confined in a straitjacket. He became an ardent advocate of the reform of psychiatric care. Beers' cause was supported by a prominent neuropathologist, Adolf Meyer (1866–1950), who suggested the term "mental hygiene" for bringing about improvement of people's mental health in a manner similar to other public health initiatives. By 1909, Beers had helped form a National Committee for Mental Hygiene, through whose efforts there developed child guidance clinics, prison clinics, and industrial mental health approaches. Beers and Meyer found a close Canadian ally in Clarence Hincks, a leading Toronto psychiatrist who was instrumental in founding the Canadian National Committee for Mental Hygiene (CNCMH) in 1918, together with his colleague Charles Clarke.

The appalling situation of Canadian provincial mental hospitals triggered particular political concern following World War I, when returning veterans suffering from shell shock had to rely on existing psychiatric facilities in their home provinces. A new belief gained ground in scientific approaches and reliance on expert knowledge in the prevention of mental illness. These views were intertwined with class-based concern about an alleged weak-mindedness among lower social classes and the need for betterment of the human race, influenced by eugenic ideas of the time (Dyck, 2013). This context of change provided a climate for expanding professionalism of many groups, including psychiatrists, psychologists, and nurses. The CNCMH clearly promoted improvement of mental hospitals. Introducing a trained nursing staff was part of this strategy. Voluntary admission controlled by physicians was supported, thus advancing the view that mental illness was similar to any physical illness.

Development of Psychiatric and Mental Health Nursing

Early Developments

As part of psychiatric reform, the CNCMH promoted the introduction of training schools for mental nurses, later called psychiatric nurses, similar to nurse training schools in general hospitals (Boschma, Yonge, & Mychajlunow, 2005; Tipliski, 2004). During his tenure as superintendent of Rockwood Mental Hospital (1881–1905), Charles Clarke was instrumental in establishing one of the first nurse training schools for female personnel at this hospital and then at the Provincial Hospital in Toronto (Brown, 2000). Well-educated women with a sense of order and compassion had been essential in the introduction of training schools in general hospitals. In their efforts to model **psychiatric hospitals** after the general hospitals, psychiatrists took that ideal and geared the training of mental nurses toward women. The trained nurses provided them with the assistance they needed for new therapies and enhanced the hospital's reputation (Boschma, 2003; Brown, 2000; Connor, 1996), as it was thought that women had the right moral, feminine characteristics for good patient care. Whereas in general hospitals, the care of male patients was put in the hands of female nurses assisted by male orderlies, in psychiatry this shift was less easily made, owing to the nature of difficult patient behaviour. Male attendants retained a prominent place in the care of the mentally ill, but their training obtained a lower status, or, in the Ontario mental hospitals, they initially did not receive any training at all (Tipliski, 2002). See Box 1.1 for historical highlights.

Regional Influences

In western Canada, which had a stronger orientation to British traditions of institutional care, the introduction of mental nurse training schools did not occur until the 1930s, by which time men were also being trained. In Alberta, for example, in 1932, the Department of Health hired psychiatrist Charles A. Barager, initially as acting superintendent and soon as commissioner of mental health service, to implement reform. Barager came from Manitoba, where he had introduced a nurse training school as superintendent at the Brandon Asylum (Dooley, 2004). He had a strong belief in the ability of female compassion: "The nursing of mental patients requires women of finer personality, of wider sympathies, greater self-control and higher intelligence than even the nursing of those who are physically ill" (Tipliski, 2002, p. 95).

Barager's term in Alberta was short lived (he died in 1936), but the training for nurses and attendants that he initiated in the Alberta Hospital at Ponoka had a lasting influence. Despite opposition to his ideas from the Registered Nurses Association in Alberta, which had controlled the registration of nurses since 1916, he was able to secure approval for a new diploma in mental nursing through the Alberta Department of Health. He also established arrangements with general hospitals so that, after 2 years of training in the mental hospital, female nurse students could undertake an additional 18 months of training at a general hospital and take licensing exams for registered nurses, after which they would return to the mental hospital. For male attendants, a 3-year certificate course was implemented, leading to a diploma in mental nursing. Male graduates did not obtain registered nursing status, reflective of the gendered context in which mental nurse training emerged. Skilled nursing was essential for new therapies, such as electroshock and insulin coma therapy introduced in the 1940s. Alberta Hospital at Ponoka also had a large infirmary with many frail and sick elderly patients (Boschma et al., 2005).

BOX 1.1 Highlights From Psychiatric Mental Health Nursing History

1888 The first mental nurse training school established at Kingston's Rockwood Asylum

1918 Foundation of the Canadian National Committee of Mental Hygiene

1920 First psychiatric nursing text published, *Nursing Mental Diseases*, by Harriet Bailey

1922 First Registration of Nurses Act passed in Ontario including nurse training schools at the mental hospitals

1930s Mental hospitals in western Canada established schools for mental nurses and attendants

1950 Psychiatric Nurses Association of Canada (PNAC) founded

1952 Publication of Hildegard E. Peplau's *Interpersonal Relations in Nursing*

1963 *Perspectives in Psychiatric Care* and *Journal of Psychiatric Nursing* first issued

1979 PNAC working paper on Standards of Practice for Psychiatric Nurses published

1986 The Canadian Nurses Association establishes a national certification program for specialty nursing practice

1988 Canadian Federation of Mental Health Nurses (CFMHN) founded

1995 CFMHN *Standards of Psychiatric and Mental Health Nursing Practice* published

2006 CFMHN *Standards for Psychiatric-Mental Health Nursing*, 3rd edition published

2014 CFMHN *Standards for Psychiatric-Mental Health Nursing*, 4th edition, provides direction to all nurses and to the public on acceptable practices of psychiatric–mental health nurses (http://cfmhn.ca/professionalPractices).

2015 *Canadian Association for Schools of Nursing (CASN) and Canadian Federation of Mental Health Nurses (CFMHN)* jointly developed Entry-to-Practice Mental Health and Addiction Competencies for Undergraduate Nursing Education in Canada.

This climate of change created many new opportunities for working- and middle-class men and women to pursue careers as psychiatric nurses, and nurses began to articulate nursing knowledge in nursing textbooks. The first psychiatric and mental health (PMH) nursing textbook that appeared in North America was *Nursing Mental Diseases*, written by Bailey (1920). The content of the book reflected an understanding of mental disorders of the times and set forth nursing care in terms of appropriate procedures.

■ MODERN THINKING

As PMH nursing began to develop as a profession in the early 20th century, it incorporated new perspectives on mental illness that were emerging, particularly ideas on prevention as well as biologic views on mental illness. These new theories would profoundly shape the future of mental health care for all practitioners. Chapter 8 examines the underlying ideologies, but it is important to understand their development within the social and historical context to appreciate fully their impact on treatment approaches.

Evolution of Scientific Thought

In the early 1900s, there were two opposing views of mental illness: the belief that mental disorders had biologic origins and the belief that the problems were attributed to environmental and social stresses. **Psychosocially oriented ideas** proposed that mental disorders resulted from environmental and social deprivation. Moral treatment grew out of this idea, and the notion of prevention advocated by the mental hygiene movement also reflected a psychosocial orientation. The **biologic view** held that mental illnesses had a biologic cause and could be treated with physical interventions. Biologic approaches and physical treatments such as bed rest; wet packs, which entailed wrapping patients in wet sheets; and prolonged baths became popular around 1900 as part of the rise of scientific psychiatry. They were grounded in the idea that overstrained nerves should obtain rest. Such treatments turned out to be largely ineffective.

Meyer and Psychiatric Pluralism

Adolf Meyer bridged the ideologic gap between the two approaches by introducing the concept of **psychiatric pluralism**, an integration of human biologic functions with the environment. He focused on investigating how organic functions related to the person and how the person, constituted of these organs, related to the environment (Neill, 1980). Unfortunately, this included the surgical treatment of psychosis by one of his disciples, Henry Cotton, who believed infection caused insanity and attempted to cure patients by removing sites of sepsis such as the teeth, tonsils, and colon (Scull, 2005). Meyer's ideas had little chance to evolve and flourish as the emerging psychoanalytic theories would

soon dominate the psychiatric world in North America for a long time to come. It was not until after World War II, when a new emphasis on community-based care evolved, that environmental views and psychosocial approaches gained renewed prominence with the application of psychosocial rehabilitation models for people living with severe and persistent mental illness (Shepherd, Boardman, & Slade, 2008).

Freud and Psychoanalytic Theory

Sigmund Freud (1856–1939) and the **psychoanalytic movement** of the early 1900s promised a radically new approach to PMH care. Trained as a neuropathologist, Freud developed a personality theory based on unconscious motivations for behaviour, or drives. Using a new technique, psychoanalysis, he delved into the patient's feelings and emotions regarding past experiences, particularly early childhood and adolescent memories, to explain the basis of aberrant behaviour. He showed that symptoms of hysteria could be produced and made to disappear while patients were in a subconscious state of hypnosis.

According to the Freudian model, normal development occurred in stages, with the first three—oral, anal, and genital—being the most important. The infant progressed through the oral stage, experiencing the world through symbolic oral ingestion; into the anal stage, in which the toddler developed a sense of autonomy through withholding; and on to the genital stage, in which a beginning sense of sexuality emerged within the framework of the oedipal relationship. Freud posited that any interference in this normal development, such as psychological trauma, would give rise to neurosis or psychosis.

Primary causes of mental illnesses were now viewed as psychological, and any physical manifestations or social influences were considered secondary (Malamud, 1944). Psychoanalysts believed that mental illnesses originated from disturbed personality development and faulty parenting. They categorized mental illnesses either as a psychosis (severe) or as a neurosis (less severe). A psychosis impaired daily functioning because of breaks in contact with reality. A neurosis was less severe, but individuals were often distressed about their problems. The terms psychosis and neurosis entered common, everyday language and added credibility to Freud's conceptualization of mental disorders. Freud's ideas would soon represent the forefront of psychiatric thought, and they shaped society's view of mental health care. Freudian ideology dominated psychiatry well into the 1970s. Intensive psychoanalysis, aimed at repairing the trauma of the original psychological injury, was the treatment of choice. Psychoanalysis was costly and time consuming and required lengthy training; few could perform it, and as a result, thousands of patients in state institutions with severe mental illnesses were essentially ignored.

Integration of Biologic Theories into Psychosocial Treatment

Until the 1940s, the biologic understanding of mental illness did not result in effective treatment. Early somatic treatments based on these views often were unsuccessful because of the lack of understanding and knowledge of the biologic basis of mental disorders. As discussed, the use of hydrotherapy, or baths, was an established procedure in mental institutions. The use of warm baths and, in some instances, ice cold baths were thought to produce calming effects for patients with mental disorders. Still, baths often ended up as a form of restraint rather than as a therapeutic practice and the physiologic responses were poorly understood. During the 1930s and 1940s, other biologic treatments emerged, which sparked new hope that they would result in effective treatment, such as insulin coma therapy and electroconvulsive therapy (ECT) (Kneeland & Warren, 2002; Shorter & Healy, 2007). Yet, often, these biologic procedures were applied either indiscriminately or inappropriately with substantial side effects including psychosurgery and ECT (see Chapter 13). ECT, the application of a short (1 to 2 seconds) electrical current to the brain in order to generate a convulsion for an allegedly healing effect, was first used around 1940. Unlike the original procedure, contemporary ECT is modified by being applied under anaesthesia. Psychosurgical treatment, direct surgical intervention in lobes of the brain, also called lobotomy, began to be applied as of the late 1940s. Results from such brain therapies were mixed, and by the 1970s, the use of lobotomy became increasingly controversial; the use of ECT as treatment across a broad range of disorders was also questioned, but in its modified form, it now is widely used for the treatment of depression (Boschma, 2015; Kneeland & Warren, 2002; Pressman, 2002). Recent insights resulting from brain research and new technologic advancements such as electromagnetic brain-stimulating techniques have generated a renewed interest in biologic treatments, offering new possibilities for treatment of depression and other neurophysiologic disorders (George, 2003). Thanks to modern technology and improved methods, neurosurgical techniques, such as deep brain stimulation, as well as ECT and transcranial magnetic stimulation can now be applied more humanely with positive therapeutic outcomes for some psychiatric disorders (George, 2003; Rai, Kivisalu, Rabheru, & Kang, 2010; Sadowsky, 2006).

Support for the biologic approaches received an important boost in the early 1950s as successful symptom management with psychopharmacologic agents became a more widespread possibility. Psychopharmacology revolutionized the treatment of mental illness and led to an increased number of patients discharged into the community, and the eventual focus on the brain became a key to understanding psychiatric disorders. Chlorpromazine was an early neuroleptic drug that became widely used. Profound behavioural changes observed as a result of this medication in long-term mentally ill patients created an enormous enthusiasm about the potential of new medications. Understanding of the working of these drugs was in infancy, however, and their side effects soon became serious drawbacks. As knowledge increased and the management of side effects improved, psychopharmacotherapeutics obtained a central place in the treatment of mental illness. The introduction of lithium in the early 1970s brought a lasting change in the treatment of bipolar disorder, as did antidepressants in the treatment of mood disorders (LaJeunesse, 2000). Nurses obtained an essential role in administering medications, monitoring their effects, and teaching patients about their effects.

New Trends in Post–World War II Mental Health Care

Following the experiences of World War II, insight grew among governments, as well as health professionals, that psychiatric services had to be placed on a new footing. By the end of the 1940s, patients in overcrowded and isolated psychiatric hospitals outnumbered the number of patients in other health care facilities, including general hospitals. Increased federal funding for health services and training of health care personnel created new opportunities. The implementation of universal health insurance for hospital care and medical services during the 1950s and 1960s, based on a 50/50 cost sharing between federal and provincial governments, generated funding for the establishment of psychiatric departments in general hospitals, shifting the focus of services away from large provincial institutions (Ostry, 2009).

The Canadian Mental Health Association (CMHA), renamed from the earlier CNCMH, had an instrumental role in policy development for integrated services in general hospitals and the community. In its influential 1963 report, *More for the Mind*, the CMHA argued that mental illness had to be dealt with in ways similar to those of physical illness, and it argued for the application of multiple perspectives—medical, social, and familial—in multidisciplinary services and community treatment. A critical social movement also emerged, protesting the poor circumstances in large mental hospitals and the lack of patient rights. Psychiatry became the target of fierce debate and antipsychiatric critique in the 1970s (Crossley, 2006). Power relationships and the dominance of the medical model were questioned, and an emerging patient movement obtained a new voice and presence in mental health. Canada saw its first patient-led community mental health initiative with the foundation of the Mental Patient Association of Vancouver in 1971, a unique organization that transformed Canada's psychiatric landscape (MPA Founders Collective, 2013) (Fig. 1.4). The MPA formed as a patient driven, grassroots response to deinstitutionalization and tragic gaps

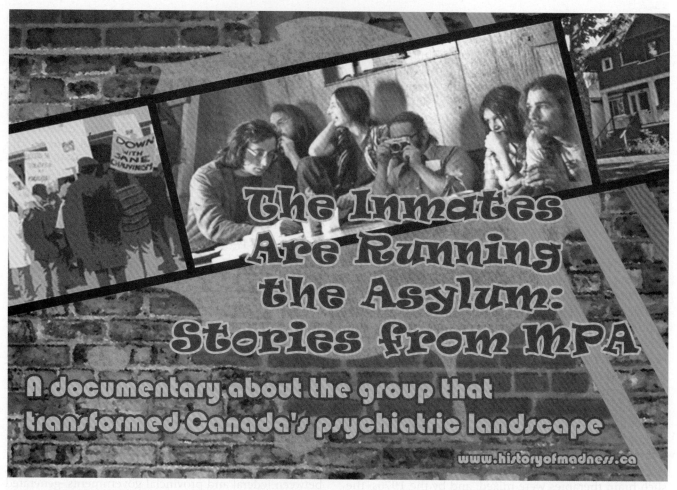

Figure 1.4. Postcard announcing the documentary film "The inmates are running the asylum: Stories from the MPA (2013) on Vancouver's MPA (Mental Patient Association)." (Courtesy of Megan Davies.) MPA formed in 1971 as a grassroots response to deinstitutionalization and tragic gaps in community mental health, a patient-driven initiative inverting traditional mental health hierarchies (MPA Founders Collective, 2013). For full documentary, see: http://historyofmadness.ca/the-inmates-are-running-the-asylum/

in community mental health, inverting traditional mental health hierarchies (MPA Founders Collective, 2013). Improving support and resources for people with mental illness within the community became a key mental health target (Fingard & Rutherford, 2011).

A shift in 20th century mental health policy resulted in **deinstitutionalization**, the downsizing of the large provincial psychiatric hospitals, and a new orientation on community-based services to support people with mental illness within their own communities (Boschma, 2011; Dyck, 2011). Services and treatments diversified. Biologic approaches, such as use of psychopharmacology and safer application of ECT, were complemented by new rehabilitative services, the use of group therapy and other psychotherapies, as well as the provision of day treatment. In the 1950s, mental hospitals began to reduce their size and, over the course of the next decades, many closed, or changed their focus—a process that in Canada would last until the end of the 20th century. In British Columbia, for example, the provincial

mental hospital Riverview closed its doors permanently in 2012 (Hall, 2012). During the second half of the 20th century, funding for mental health care became part of the larger health care system, with a stronger emphasis on general hospital–based psychiatry and community-based care. Nurses had an essential role in this transformation in the emerging field of **community mental health nursing** (Boschma, 2012).

In the late 1970s, the federal government modified the funding structure for health care, reducing its share in the cost. Provinces developed different models and strategies to fund specialized services such as alcohol and substance abuse treatment programs, which following World War II were pressing mental health care needs. To address the needs of different population groups, subspecialties also emerged, such as child psychiatry, forensic, and geriatric services. The perception of health care as a human right enhanced consumer and volunteer involvement, as well as public education on mental illness, and it increased the demand for patient autonomy.

Continued Evolution of Psychiatric and Mental Health Nursing

The new multidisciplinary approaches and services generated a pressing need for more and better trained mental health care personnel, including nurses. The changes created a context for new developments in **PMH nursing education**. Organized responses of provincial professional nurses' organizations, as well as efforts of hospital administrators and psychiatrists to continue staffing psychiatric hospitals through hospital-based nurse training programs, resulted in a diverse pattern of PMH nurse education. As of the 1950s, Canada entertained two models of education for PMH nursing, resulting in the preparation of two different professional nursing groups for nursing care in mental health services. Regional influences played a large role in the generation of the two models. On the one hand, general hospital–based schools of nursing, especially in eastern Canada, began to integrate psychiatric nursing into their curriculum. In Ontario, for example, under the influence of the mental hygiene movement, as of the 1930s, general hospital training schools began to include care of mentally ill patients into their training. Student nurses attended the provincial psychiatric hospitals for a brief period of training, called an affiliation program. Conversely, mental nurse trainees, mostly women, from the psychiatric hospital–based nurse training programs opted for an affiliation to the general hospital, resulting in both groups' obtaining the title of registered nurse. After World War II, the provincial government and the provincial association of registered nurses in Ontario formalized this pattern into a permanent structure. Gradually, the psychiatric hospital–based programs decreased in number and size, and the registered nurse became the main nursing care provider in mental health services (Tipliski, 2004).

In the less densely populated western Canadian provinces, the pattern emerged of general hospital nurse trainees choosing affiliation experiences at the psychiatric hospitals, but the bulk of nursing care in the provincial hospitals continued to be provided by nurses and attendants graduated from psychiatric hospital–based nurse training programs (Hicks, 2011). As noted previously of Alberta Hospital in Ponoka, some western provinces established an affiliation program for female mental nurse trainees, and its graduates obtained the title of registered nurse. The program was limited in size, however, and many women worked in the institution as untrained attendants until the 1960s. Male trainees received a diploma in mental nursing. In British Columbia, a training school for mental nurses, later called psychiatric nurses, was established in 1930 at Essondale, which eventually became Riverview Hospital (Fig. 1.5).

In the western provinces, the government had less control over nurse training than in neighbouring Ontario. Provincial associations of registered nurses

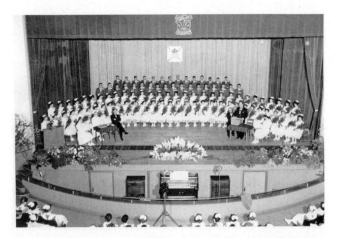

Figure 1.5. Graduation ceremony, School of Psychiatric Nursing, Essondale (Riverview Hospital), ca. 1950s. (From Historical collection, Riverview Hospital Historical Society, Coquitlam, BC.)

in western provinces failed to support affiliation for psychiatric hospital–based nurse trainees, while medical superintendents of psychiatric hospitals retained much of their influence over psychiatric nurse education (Boschma et al., 2005; Tipliski, 2004).

Around 1950, attendants in the province of Saskatchewan took the lead in obtaining political support for a different pattern of nurse education that would lead to a separate Psychiatric Nurses Act and subsequent training acts independent of provincial registered nurse practice acts. In Saskatchewan, registered nurses had never successfully integrated into the mental hospitals. Although the psychiatric training program that had existed for Saskatchewan asylum attendants since the 1930s was expanded after World War II to address the new need for psychiatric expertise, it never resulted in registration as a nurse. Dissatisfied with their exclusion from any professionally recognized nursing title, provincial hospital attendants, who in Saskatchewan had obtained the right to unionize after the election of the new Co-operative Commonwealth Federation government in 1944, became instrumental in generating union support, as well as backing from the new government, for legislation of a separate psychiatric nurses act, which passed Parliament in 1948. In 1950, the Psychiatric Nurses Association of Canada was formed. Their action resulted in a distinct professional group of psychiatric nurses (Hicks, 2011; Tipliski, 2004). During the 1950s, all four western Canadian provinces passed acts that entitled graduates of western Canadian psychiatric hospital–based nurse training programs to receive the title of psychiatric nurse. The two separate models of psychiatric nursing education still exist today and have over past decades been integrated into the regular education system, resulting in baccalaureate education programs in generic and psychiatric nursing education.

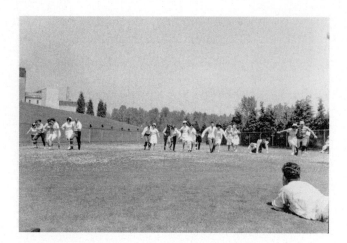

Figure 1.6. Sports Day on Riverview Hospital grounds, nurses, and patients, 1966. (From Historical collection, Riverview Hospital Historical Society, Coquitlam, BC.)

THE LATE 20TH AND EARLY 21ST CENTURY

In the post–World War II era, nurses continued their work in facilitating the therapeutic climate within psychiatric hospitals (Fig. 1.6). The shift to community mental health and deinstitutionalization generated many new functions for PMH nurses (Boschma et al., 2005). Nurses obtained a central role in supporting large numbers of discharged patients in their transition to living in the community. In the psychiatric hospitals and general hospital units, nurses obtained new therapeutic roles in group therapies, and their work in community mental health services expanded (Boschma, 2012). New theoretical models became available that emphasized building therapeutic nurse–patient relationships and holistic nursing approaches. Hildegard Peplau, who in recent scholarship has been considered the most important psychiatric nurse of the 20th century, proved to be a strong leader in the development of these new frameworks for psychiatric nursing (Boschma et al., 2005; Calaway, 2002).

Expansion of Holistic Nursing Care

In 1952, Peplau published the landmark work *Interpersonal Relations in Nursing*. It introduced PMH nursing practice to the concepts of interpersonal relations and the importance of the therapeutic relationship. In fact, the nurse–patient relationship was defined as the very essence of PMH nursing and supported a holistic perspective on patient care (see Chapters 5, 6, and 7). These new frameworks underscored a new professional and disciplinary independence for nurses.

By 1963, two US-based nursing journals, the *Journal of Psychiatric Nursing* (now the *Journal of Psychosocial Nursing and Mental Health Services*) and *Perspectives in Psychiatric Care*, as well as the *Canadian Journal of Psychiatric Nursing* (1975–1990), focused on psychiatric nursing. Also, the *Canadian Journal for Nursing Research* began to publish PMH nursing research. During the 1980s, the Canadian

Federation of Mental Health Nurses (CFMHN) formed as an interest group of the Canadian Nurses Association with a view to promoting the interests of mental health nurses and bringing matters of mental health nursing interest and psychiatric patient care to the attention of the public at large. In 1995, this group published the Canadian Standards of Psychiatric and Mental Health Nursing Practice. Based on the influential work of Patricia Benner (1984), the standards were written within a framework of "domains of practice." This promoted a holistic perspective on nursing care, with PMH nurses practicing in a variety of settings with a variety of clientele. The emphasis was on activities ranging from health promotion to health restoration. The standards reflected the belief that PMH nursing should be research driven, continually incorporating new findings into nursing practice. Relying on these standards, the Canadian Nurses Association created the opportunity to become certified in mental health nursing as part of their larger certification program of specialty nursing areas established during the 1980s. The CFMHN updated its standards in 2006 and again in 2014 to incorporate the most recent perspectives on PMH care. The 2006 revisions to the standards were unique in that input was sought for the first time from mental health care consumers (Beal et al., 2007). In 2015, CFMHN joined the Canadian Association for Schools of Nursing to jointly develop entry-to-practice mental health and addiction competencies for undergraduate nursing education in Canada for the first time. These provide guidance for both practice and education (see Chapter 5).

Contemporary Issues

During the 1980s, wrinkles in the social fabric of mental health care emerged. The mixed results of deinstitutionalization became apparent and generated a series of government-commissioned reports in all provinces to improve mental health services. Enormous variation existed among provinces in the extent and timing in which they implemented deinstitutionalization policies. People with mental disorders were discharged into communities that were often ill prepared to offer community support programs, housing, or vocational opportunities. Communities were sometimes hesitant in accepting people with persistent mental illness in their midst, and stigma remained attached to mental health services (Hector, 2001; Sealy & Whitehead, 2004). The 1981 Charter of Rights and Freedoms reflected a public statement intended to counter such responses (Greenland, Griffin, & Hoffman, 2001).

Self-help groups and family and consumer organizations, such as the Schizophrenia Society of Canada and the Mood Disorder Society of Canada, have become active participants in mental health care services during the past decades. Outreach and mobile crisis response teams emerged to address problems people with severe mental illness experienced in the community. A new category of "revolving door" patients signified that long-term, severe mental illness remained a persistent problem, with patients continuously moving in and out of the acute care system. Also, the interconnected issues of severe mental illness, substance dependency, and inadequate community resources and housing have resulted in a growing number of homeless people with mental illness, as well as a large population of mentally ill winding up in the criminal justice systems. Within these groups, the specific mental health needs of women remain poorly addressed, while the threat of suicide is increasingly recognized as a severe mental health concern for women and men, with men diagnosed with depression experiencing higher suicide rates than women (Gagnon & Oliffe, 2015).

Public awareness is growing that diverse cultural populations have distinctive mental health needs and experience inequity in the social and mental health pressures placed upon them. Aboriginal mental health is a critical issue in Canada because Aboriginal communities experience disproportionate rates of both physical and mental illness (Varcoe, Browne, & Einboden, 2015). Enhancing historical understanding of the health issues and inequities affecting aboriginal peoples is central to the work of the Truth and Reconciliation Commission, established in 2008, to address and acknowledge the detrimental impact and consequences of Canada's residential school system imposed upon Aboriginal families until 1984 (The Truth and Reconciliation Commission of Canada, 2015). Closely intertwined with the residential school system were Canada's Indian Hospitals, established for treatment of tuberculosis among aboriginal people, the effects of which, because of the very nature of the colonial structure of the Indian Health Services, have been similarly detrimental (Meijer Drees, 2013). An unbalanced health care system that has not been adaptive to the specific health needs of Aboriginal peoples, therefore, is in need of urgent attention (see Chapter 3). Healing efforts to include voices and stories of Aboriginal people and to acknowledge their experiences in ways that foster awareness and provide nurses with tools to strengthen their professional ability in Aboriginal health care are a key and much needed focus in current health research (MacNaughton, 2015). Today, mental health services are still fragmented and not sufficiently developed to meet the needs of diverse populations. Millions of adults and children are disabled by mental illness every year. When compared with all other diseases, mental illness ranks first in terms of causing disability in North America and Western Europe (Hart Wasekeesikaw, 2006; Morrow, 2002; World Health Organization, 2001).

The New Era of Health Care Reform

Both public and private expenditures for health care services have increased in North America. Still, financial and social barriers continue to affect the overall funding for mental health service. Large networks of public and private organizations share responsibility for mental health care, with the state remaining as the major decision maker for resource allocation. The emphasis is on reducing expensive institutional care and increasing the resources devoted to community-based care for mentally ill people. By the 1990s, new federal initiatives in mental health policy were urgently needed to address systemic issues of fragmentation. In 1998, the Canadian Alliance on Mental Illness and Mental Health (CAMIMH) was formed as a conjoint initiative of the Canadian Psychiatric Association, the CMHA, the Mood Disorder Association of Canada, the National Network for Mental Health, and the Schizophrenia Society of Canada. Consumers and service providers jointly began to lobby the federal government to come to an action plan and a new national agenda for mental health care (Beauséjour, 2001). Two years later, the CAMIMH joined the Canadian Collaborative Mental Health Initiative, which was formed to focus specifically on the improvement of mental health care in the primary health care setting. Consumers and caregivers were actively involved in this collaborative initiative (see Chapters 7 and 11).

In 2002, the CAMIMH published its first report, a collation of the latest Canadian data on mental illness, with assistance from Health Canada (2002). Among other aspects of mental health care, the report revealed that 86% of hospitalizations for mental illness in Canada occurred in general hospitals. This profound change from traditional institutional care to general hospital care underscored the need for additional and improved acute and community-based mental health services. A senate-commissioned review of the Canadian health care system resulted in a call for better service: *Out of the Shadows at Last: Transforming Mental Health, Mental Illness and Addiction Services in Canada* (Kirby & Keon, 2006). The report highlighted the need to counter fragmentation and to address the disparate services provided across the provinces and between rural and urban regions, complicated by unique regional multicultural needs. Stories of Canadians suffering from mental illness illustrated the complex issues of stigmatization and discrimination. The report also drew attention to the determinants affecting health, health care, housing, employment, social welfare, as well as the justice system for Canadians with mental health concerns (Kirby & Keon, 2006). The lack of a nationwide mental health strategy and the inconsistency between provincial jurisdictions that determine mental health policies and service delivery were key findings. Some critics of the report noticed a lack of emphasis on "preventative determinants" and a lack of recognition of the depth of disability caused by mental illness (Arboleda-Flórez, 2005), while some women's advocate groups challenged the report's "silence" on the disparities between mental health and addiction services for men and women (Canadian Women's Health Network, 2006). The findings and recommendations from the CAMIMH and Kirby reports became the impetus for the establishment in 2007 of the Mental Health Commission of Canada.

BOX 1.2 Changing Directions, Changing Lives: The Mental Health Strategy for Canada (May 2012)

Six key strategic directions to address the mental health needs for Canadians.

- *Promote* mental health across the lifespan in homes, schools, and workplaces, and *prevent* mental illness and suicide wherever possible.
- Foster *recovery* and well-being for people of all ages living with mental health problems and illnesses, and uphold their *rights*.
- Provide *access* to the appropriate combination of services, treatments, and supports, when and where people need them.

- Reduce *disparities* in risk factors and access to mental health services, and strengthen the response to the needs of *diverse* communities and Northerners.
- Work with *First Nations, Inuit, and Métis* to address their mental health needs, acknowledging their distinct circumstances, rights, and cultures.
- Mobilize *leadership*, improve knowledge, and foster *collaboration* at all levels.

From Mental Health Commission of Canada. (2012). *Changing directions, changing lives: The mental health strategy for Canada.* Retrieved from http://strategy.mentalhealthcommission.ca/pdf/strategy-text-en.pdf

---

Developing a National Mental Health Strategy

Canada's national health strategy was first adopted in 1984 through the Canada Health Act, which set out the values, principles, and guidelines for health care. While to some degree mental health care principles are ensconced in the overall Act, there continued to be significant gaps and inconsistencies in mental health care across the country, and Canada continued to be the only one of the eight wealthiest nations without a national mental health strategy (Kirby, 2009).

To address these gaps, Health Canada funded the Mental Health Commission of Canada, a 10-year initiative, established outside the federal health mandate, but with a structure that mirrored inclusiveness with regard to membership and stakeholder participation (Goldbloom & Bradley, 2012). The MHCC was originally assigned three primary objectives: to develop a mental health strategy for Canada, begin an antistigma campaign, and create a knowledge exchange centre to promote research and build capacity and opportunities in evidence-based mental health strategies. In 2012, the Commission issued a comprehensive national mental

health strategy with six strategic directions (Box 1.2). It further initiated several research projects to enhance evidence-based practice of which two are highlighted here: the *At Home/Chez Soi* initiative, a mental health research project examining housing for mentally ill individuals in five large urban settings and a Mental Health First Aid project, involving provision of training to the public on how to identify the early signs and symptoms of mental illness and suitable interventions for the unique needs of youth or adults (Hwang, Stergiopoulos, O'Campo, & Gozdzik, 2012). An issue of concern of the *At Home/Chez Soi* project, ending in 2013, was that financial support to consolidate their novel approaches was not guaranteed (Goldbloom & Bradley, 2012). Affordable, low-cost housing for people living with mental illness remains a key health issue and a persistent point of policy debate (Nelles & Spence, 2013).

Many insights have been gained through the MHCC initiatives, and its contributions are ongoing. In 2016, the MHCC released its strategic plan for 2017–2022, going beyond its original 10-year mandate and addressing three key strategic priority areas to meet mental health needs of Canadians (Box 1.3).

BOX 1.3 The MHCC's 2017–2022 Strategic Plan: Strategic Objectives and Priorities

- Strategic Objective 1: **Leadership, Partnership, and Capacity Building**
  - Increasing the effectiveness of Canada's mental health system by convening stakeholders, developing and influencing sound public policy, and inspiring collective action.
- Strategic Objective 2: **Promotion and Advancing of *The Mental Health Strategy for Canada***
  - Encouraging actions that advance *the Strategy*.

- Strategic Objective 3: **Knowledge Mobilization**
  - Developing and sharing effective and innovative knowledge.

From Mental Health Commission of Canada. (2016). Retrieved from http://www.mentalhealthcommission.ca/English/mhcc-strategic-plan-2017-2022

A series of fundamental and persistent challenges stay on the policy agenda, however, forming key focus areas requiring attention of policy makers and health professionals, including needs of youth and seniors, housing, stigma, suicide prevention among all age groups, and workplace issues. Also, mental health of immigrants and refugees has moved up on the mental health policy agenda in recent years (see Chapter 3) (Agic, McKenzie, Tuck, & Antwi, 2016). While mental illness is no longer invisible, we still need to work on ways to provide permanent and persistent support for the most vulnerable populations. These challenges are not unique to Canada. They have been recognized at a global level by the World Health Organization. Accepted by the World Health Assembly in May 2013, the Comprehensive Mental Health Action Plan 2013–2020 has four major objectives:

- Strengthen effective leadership and governance for mental health.
- Provide comprehensive, integrated, and responsive mental health and social care services in community-based settings.
- Implement strategies for promotion and prevention in mental health.
- Strengthen information systems, evidence, and research for mental health.

This plan continues to promote and guide a transformative worldwide mental health agenda (WHO, 2013).

The challenge before Canadian nurses at this time is to strive to address these national and global goals. We must work with a view to include mental health around the world while working within existing constraints to provide cost-effective services. To address pressing mental health care needs in the 21st century, nurses must continue to participate in devising and implementing a continuum of mental health services that provides access for all and to develop appropriate partnerships with other health professionals and consumer groups.

SUMMARY OF KEY POINTS

- Throughout history, attitudes and treatment toward those with mental disorders have drastically changed as a result of the changing socioeconomic backdrop of our society and the development of new theories and study by key individuals and groups.
- During the 1800s, as mental illness began to be viewed as an illness, more humane and moral treatments began to develop.
- Social reformers such as Dorothea Dix, Charles Clarke, Clifford Beers, and Clarence Hincks dedicated their efforts to raising society's awareness and advocating public responsibility for the proper treatment of persons with mental illness. At the turn

of the 19th century, mental hospitals started implementing Schools of Nursing to build psychiatric nursing capacity and quality within the hospitals.

- Theoretic arguments characterized the evolution of scientific thought and psychiatric practice. Gradually, the importance of the biologic aspect of mental disorders was recognized while psychosocial approaches were also developed. After the 1950s, the discipline of nursing began to add to the theoretical basis of mental health practice, adding holistic and interpersonal frameworks of psychiatric nursing.
- Although the need for PMH nursing was recognized near the end of the 19th century, initially, there was resistance to training attendants for the care of the insane. At the initiative of Charles Clarke, medical superintendent of Rockwood Hospital (1881–1905), the first Training School for Mental Nurses was established in 1888.
- All provinces gradually adapted to education for PMH nurses. By the 1930s, all provinces had established training schools for asylum attendants and nurses. In the era following World War II, provinces started to downsize mental hospitals in a process of deinstitutionalization and a shift to community-based care. Two models of education for psychiatric nurses emerged, leading to two distinct professional groups.
- Key federal and provincial initiatives generated political support and funding for mental health services, but these remain inadequate to many pressing mental health issues.
- The establishment of the Mental Health Commission of Canada in 2007 has generated a series of projects to fill the gap of a lack of a national mental health strategy and is moving beyond its initial 10-year mandate to address ongoing mental health issues affecting Canadians.

 Web Links

athome.nfb.ca/#/athome/home The National Film Board of Canada presents this clever interactive Web documentary on the radical research project that is revealing the true cost of homelessness in Canada.

cpa.ca/docs/File/Practice/strategy-text-en.pdf In 2012, the government of Canada presented "Changing directions, changing lives: The mental health strategy for Canada" a culmination of the policy work conducted by the Mental Health Commission of Canada established in 2007. It provides direction for mental health services at a national level.

cna-aiic.ca/en/on-the-issues/national-expert-commission The Canadian Nurses Association (CNA) published the 2012 CNA National Experts Commission report *A Nursing Call to Action: The Health of Our Nation, The Future of Our Health System* (with a discussion of mental health and disabilities on page 10) to inform health policy from a nursing point of view.

cna-aiic.ca/~/media/cna/page-content/pdf-en/ps85_mental_health_e.pdf?la=en CNA's statement on mental health can be found here. It is another policy tool.

parl.gc.ca/content/sen/committee/381/soci/rep/report1/repintnov04vol1part3-e.htm This site gives an historical overview of mental health service delivery and addiction treatment in Canada to support committee work of the Parliament of Canada and to inform the public.

cfmhn.ca/professionalPractices The Web site of the Canadian Federation of Mental Health Nurses lists the Canadian standards of mental health nursing.

rpnc.ca/history This Web site gives background on the foundations of the Registered Psychiatric Nurses Associations existing in western Canadian provinces. It also lists national regulations for Registered Psychiatric Nurses.

cmha.ca/about-cmha/history-of-cmha/#.V4kkM9IrKM8 The history of the Canadian Mental Health Association highlights this organization's long-standing role in mental health policy.

ntrc.ca/about.php Upon completion of the Truth and Reconciliation Commission's reports in 2015 the work of the TRC has been transferred to the National Centre for Truth and Reconciliation at the University of Manitoba—this site provides important background information and historical context to the work of the TRC. Final Report, Volume 5, deals specifically with the legacy of Canada's residential schools and its impact on Aboriginal health.

historyofmadness.ca This public Canadian Web site offers digital archive and resources, educational tools, and historical research findings on the history of mental health care, created to enhance critical thinking, heritage preservation, and historical research in the fields of psychiatric medicine and mental health. The site has a special section "More for the Mind" on histories of mental health for the class room.

References

Agic, B., McKenzie, K., Tuck, A., & Antwi, M. (2016). *Supporting the mental health of refugees to Canada. Report of the Mental Health Commission.* Ottawa, ON: Mental Health Commission of Canada.

Arboleda-Flórez, J. (2005). The epidemiology of mental illness in Canada. *Canadian Public Policy: Analyse de Politique, 31*(s1), 13–16.

Bailey, H. (1920). *Nursing mental diseases.* New York, NY: Macmillan.

Beal, G., Chan, A., Chapman, S., Edgar, J., McInnis-Perry, G., Osborne, M., & Mina, E. S. (2007). Consumer input into standards revisions: Changing practice. *Journal of Psychiatric and Mental Health Nursing, 14,* 13–20.

Beauséjour, P. (2001). Advocacy and misadventures in Canadian Psychiatry. In Q. Rae-Grant (Ed.), *Psychiatry in Canada: 50 years, 1951–2000* (pp. 137–148). Ottawa, ON: Canadian Psychiatric Association.

Beers, C. (1908). *A mind that found itself.* New York, NY: Longmans, Green, & Co.

Benner, P. (1984). *From novice to expert: Excellence and power in clinical nursing practice.* Menlo Park, CA: Addison-Wesley.

Boschma, G. (2003). *The rise of mental health nursing: A history of psychiatric care in Dutch asylum, 1890–1920.* Amsterdam, The Netherlands: Amsterdam University Press.

Boschma, G. (2011). Deinstitutionalization reconsidered: Geographic and demographic changes in mental health care in British Columbia and Alberta, 1950–1980. *Histoire Sociale/Social History, 44*(88), 223–256.

Boschma, G. (2012). Community mental health nursing in Alberta, Canada: An oral history. *Nursing History Review, 20,* 103–135.

Boschma, G. (2015). Beyond the cuckoo's nest: Nurses, electro-convulsive therapy and Dutch general hospital psychiatry. In G. Fealy, C. Hallett, & S. Malchau Dietz (Eds.), *Histories of nursing practice* (pp. 100–122). Manchester, UK: Manchester University Press.

Boschma, G., Yonge, O., & Mychajlunow, L. (2005). Gender and professional identity in psychiatric nursing practice in Alberta, Canada, 1930–1975. *Nursing Inquiry, 12*(4), 243–255.

Brown, W. H. (2000). Dr. C. K. Clarke and the Training School for Nurses. In E. Hudson (Ed.), *The provincial asylum in Toronto: Reflections on social and architectural history* (pp. 167–180). Toronto, ON: Toronto Region Architectural Conservancy.

Calaway, B. J. (2002). *Hildegard Peplau: Psychiatric nurse of the century.* New York, NY: Springer.

Canadian Association for Schools of Nursing & Canadian Federation of Mental Health Nurses (2015). *Entry-to-practice mental health and addiction competencies for undergraduate nursing education in Canada.* Ottawa, ON.

Canadian Women's Health Network. (2006). *Women, mental health, mental illness and addiction in Canada. Response to out of the shadows at last.* Retrieved from http://www.cwhn.ca/resources/cwhm/mentalHealth.html

Connor, P. J. (1996). "Neither courage nor perseverance enough": Attendants at the Asylum for the Insane, Kingston, 1877–1905. *Ontario History, 88*(4), 251–272.

Crossley, M. L. (2006). *Contesting psychiatry: Social movements in mental health.* New York, NY: Routledge.

D'Antonio, P. (2006). *Founding friends: Families, staff, and patients at the Friends Asylum in early nineteenth century Philadelphia.* Bethlehem, PA: Lehigh University Press.

Dooley, C. (2004). "They gave their care, but we gave loving care": Defining and defending boundaries of skill and craft in the nursing service of a Manitoba Mental Hospital during the Great Depression. *Canadian Bulletin of Medical History, 21*(2), 229–251.

Dyck, E. (2011). Dismantling the asylum and charting new pathways into the community: Mental health care in twentieth-century Canada. *Histoire Sociale/Social History, 44*(88), 181–196.

Dyck, E. (2013). *Facing eugenics: Reproduction, sterilization, and the politics of choice.* Toronto, ON: University of Toronto Press.

Fingard, J., & Rutherford, J. (2011). Deinstitutionalization and vocational rehabilitation for mental health consumers in Nova Scotia since the 1950s. *Histoire Sociale/Social History, 44*(88), 385–408.

Gagnon, M., & Oliffe, J. L. (2015). Male depression suicide: What NPs should know. *The Nurse Practitioner, 40*(11), 50–55.

George, M. S. (2003). Stimulating the brain: The emerging new science of electrical brain stimulation. *Scientific American, 289*(3), 66–73.

Goldbloom, D., & Bradley, L. (2012). The Mental Health Commission of Canada: The first five years. *Mental Health Review Journal, 17*(4), 221–228.

Goldstein, J. L., & Godemont, M. M. L. (2003). The legend and lessons of Geel: A 1500-year-old legend, a 21st-century model. *Community Mental Health Journal, 39*(5), 441–458.

Greenland, C. (1996). Origins of the Toronto Psychiatric Hospital. In E. Shorter (Ed.), *TPH: History and memories of the Toronto Psychiatric Hospital* (pp. 1925–1966). Toronto, ON: Wall & Emerson.

Greenland, C., Griffin, J., & Hoffman, B. F. (2001). Psychiatry in Canada from 1951–2000. In Q. Rae-Grant (Ed.), *Psychiatry in Canada: 50 years, 1951–2001* (pp. 1–16). Ottawa, ON: Canadian Psychiatric Association.

Hall, N. (2012). *Closure of Riverview Hospital marks end of era in mental health treatment.* Vancouver Sun. Retrieved from http://www.vancouversun.com/index.html

Hart Wasekeesikaw, F. (2006). Challenges for the new millennium: Nursing in First Nations. In M. McIntyre, E. Thomlinson, & C. McDonald (Eds.), *Realities of Canadian nursing: Professional, practice and power issues* (pp. 415–433). Philadelphia, PA: Lippincott Williams & Wilkins.

Health Canada. (2002). *A report on mental illnesses in Canada.* Ottawa, ON: Author.

Hector, I. (2001). Changing funding patterns and the effect on mental health care in Canada. In Q. Rae-Grant (Ed.), *Psychiatry in Canada: 50 years, 1951–2001* (pp. 59–76). Ottawa, ON: Canadian Psychiatric Association.

Hicks, B. (2011). Gender, politics, and regionalism: Factors in the evolution of registered psychiatric nursing in Manitoba, 1920–1960. *Nursing History Review, 19,* 103–126.

Hurd, H. M. (Ed.). (1973, originally printed 1916–17). *The institutional care of the insane in the United States and Canada* (Vol. IV). New York, NY: Arno Press.

Hwang, S. W., Stergiopoulos, V., O'Campo, P., & Gozdzik, A. (2012). Ending homelessness among people with mental illness: The At Home/Chez Soi randomized trial of a Housing First intervention in Toronto. *BMC Public Health, 12*(1), 787–802.

Jones, C. (1989). *The charitable imperative: Hospitals and nursing in ancien régime and revolutionary France.* London, UK: Routledge.

Kirby, M. (2009). *Key note address.* Halifax, NS: Mental Health Commission of Canada National Child and Youth Mental Health Day.

Kirby, M. J. L., & Keon, W. J. (2006). Out of the shadows at last: Transforming mental health, mental illness and addiction services in Canada. Retrieved from Parliament of Canada website: http://www.parl.gc.ca/39/1/parlbus/commbus/senate/com-e/soci-e/rep-e/rep02may06-e.htm

Kneeland, T. W., & Warren, C. A. B. (2002). *Pushbutton psychiatry: A history of electroshock in America.* Westport, CT: Praeger.

LaJeunesse, R. A. (2000). *Political asylums.* Edmonton, AB: Muttart Foundation.

Leiby, J. S. (1992). San Hipólito's treatment of the mentally ill in Mexico City, 1589–1650. *The Historian, 54*(3), 491–498.

Lightner, D. L. (Ed.). (1999). *Asylum, prison, and poorhouse: The writings and reform work of Dorothea Dix in Illinois.* Carbondale and Edwardsville, IL: Southern Illinois University Press.

MacNaughton, A. (2015). Tuberculosis (TB) storytelling: Improving community nursing TB program delivery. Master's Thesis (Nursing), University of British Columbia (Posted on UBC Circle: https://open.library.ubc.ca/cIRcle/collections/ubctheses/24/items/1.0223067).

Malamud, W. (1944). The history of psychiatric therapies. In J. K. Hall, G. Zilboorg, & H. Bunker (Eds.), *One hundred years of American psychiatry* (pp. 273–323). New York, NY: Columbia University Press.

Meijer Drees, L. (2013). *Healing histories: Stories from Canada's Indian Hospitals.* Edmonton, AB: The University of Alberta Press.

Menzies, R., & Palys, T. (2006). Turbulent spirits: Aboriginal patients in the British Columbia psychiatric system, 1879–1950. In J. E. Moran & D. Wright (Eds.), *Mental health and Canadian society: Historical perspectives* (pp. 149–175). Montreal and Kingston, BC: McGill-Queen's University Press.

Moran, J. E. (2000). *Committed to the state asylum: Insanity and society in nineteenth-century Quebec and Ontario.* Montreal and Kingston, BC: McGill-Queen's University Press.

Moran, J. E., & Wright, D. (Eds.). (2006). *Mental health and Canadian society: Historical perspectives.* Montreal and Kingston, BC: McGill-Queen's University Press.

MPA Founders Collective. (2013). "The inmates are running the asylum: Stories from the MPA [Mental Patient Association]": A documentary about the group that transformed Canada's psychiatric landscape. DVD, 36-minutes. Producer: Megan Davies, Co-Producer: Marina Morrow, Associate Co-Producer: Geertje Boschma. © History of Madness Productions 2013. Available at: http://historyofmadness.ca/the-inmates-are-running-the-asylum/

Morrow, M. (2002). *Violence and trauma in the lives of women with serious mental illness: Current practices in service provision in British Columbia.* Vancouver, BC: Centre of Excellence for Women's Health.

Neill, J. (1980). Adolf Meyer and American psychiatry today. *American Journal of Psychiatry, 137*(4), 460–464.

Nelles, H., & Spence A. (2013). *Blended financing for impact: The opportunities for social finance in supportive housing. Report commissioned by the Mental Health Commission of Canada and stakeholders.* Retrieved from http://www.marsdd.com/wp-content/uploads/2013/03/MaRS_BlendedFinancingforImpact_2013.pdf

Nelson, S. (1999). Entering the professional domain: The making of the modern nurse in 17th century France. *Nursing History Review, 7,* 171–187.

Nelson, S. (2001). *Say little, do much: Nursing, nuns, and hospitals in the nineteenth century.* Philadelphia, PA: University of Pennsylvania Press.

Ostry, A. (2009). The foundations of national public hospital insurance. *Canadian Bulletin of Medical History, 26*(2), 261–282.

Parry-Jones, W. L. L. (1981). The model of the Geel Lunatic Colony and its influence on the nineteenth-century asylum system in Britain. In A. Scull (Ed.), *Madhouses, mad-doctors, and madmen. The social history of psychiatry in the Victorian Era* (pp. 201–217). London, UK: The Athlone Press.

Peplau, H. (1952). *Interpersonal relations in nursing.* New York, NY: Putnam.

Porter, R. (1993). *Disease, medicine and society in England 1550–1860.* Houndmills, UK: Macmillan Education.

Pressman, J. D. (2002). *Psychosurgery and the limits of medicine.* Cambridge, MA: Cambridge University Press.

Rai, S., Kivisalu, T., Rabheru, K., & Kang, N. (2010). Electroconvulsive therapy clinical database: A standardized approach in tertiary care psychiatry. *Journal of Electro-Convulsion-Therapy (ECT), 26*(4), 304–309.

Sadowsky, J. (2006). Beyond the metaphor of the pendulum: Electroconvulsive therapy, psychoanalysis, and the styles of American psychiatry. *Journal of the History of Medicine, 61,* 1–25.

Scull, A. (2005). *Madhouse: A tragic tale of megalomania and modern medicine.* New Haven, CT: Yale University Press.

Sealy, P., & Whitehead, P. C. (2004). Forty years of deinstitutionalization of psychiatric services in Canada: An empirical assessment. *Canadian Journal of Psychiatry, 49,* 249–257.

Shepherd, G., Boardman, J., & Slade, M. (2008). *Making recovery a reality.* Retrieved from http://www.centreformentalhealth.org.uk/publications/making_recovery_a_reality.aspx?ID=578

Shorter, E. (1997). *A history of psychiatry: From the era of the asylum to the age of Prozac.* New York, NY: John Wiley & Sons.

Shorter, E., & Healy, D. (Eds.). (2007). *Shock therapy: A history of electroconvulsive treatment in mental illness.* Toronto, ON: University of Toronto Press.

Sussman, S. (1998). The first asylums in Canada: A response to neglectful community care and current trends. *Canadian Journal of Psychiatry, 43,* 260–264.

The Truth and Reconciliation Committee of Canada. (2015). *Honoring the truth, reconciling for the future: Summary of the final report of the Truth and Reconciliation Commission of Canada.* Retrieved from www.trc.ca

Tipliski, V. M. (2002). Parting at the crossroads: The development of education for psychiatric nursing in three Canadian provinces, 1909–1955. Ph.D. thesis, University of Manitoba, Winnipeg, MB.

Tipliski, V. M. (2004). Parting at the crossroads: The emergence of education for psychiatric nursing in three Canadian provinces, 1909–1955. *Canadian Bulletin of Medical History, 21*(2), 253–279.

Van Drenth, A., & De Haan, F. (1999). *The rise of caring power: Elizabeth Fry and Josephine Butler in Britain and the Netherlands.* Amsterdam, NL: Amsterdam University Press.

Varcoe, C. M., Browne, A. J., & Einboden, R. (2015). *Prince George: Sociohistorical, geographical, political and economic context profile.* Vancouver & Prince George, BC: EQUIP Healthcare: Research to equip primary healthcare for equity, in partnership with Central Interior Native Health Society, University of British Columbia. Posted on UBC Circle: https://circle.ubc.ca/bitstream/handle/2429/52327/EQUIP_Report_PrinceGeorge_Sociohistorical_Context_2015.pdf?sequence=1

Warsh, C. K. (1989). *Moments of unreason: The practice of Canadian psychiatry and the Homewood Retreat, 1883–1923.* Montreal and Kingston, BC: McGill-Queen's University Press.

World Health Organization. (2001). The world health report: Mental health 2001. In *Mental health: New understanding, new hope.* Geneva, IL: Author.

World Health Organization. (2013). *Comprehensive mental health action plan 2013–2020.* Retrieved from http://www.who.int/mental_health/action_plan_2013/en/

Mental Health, Mental Disorder, Recovery, and Well-Being

Wendy Austin

Adapted from the chapter "Mental Health and Mental Illness" by Marion Healey Ogden

LEARNING OBJECTIVES

After studying this chapter, you will be able to:

- Recognize the integral relationship between mental and physical health.
- Define mental health and mental illness.
- Explain the concepts of recovery and well-being.
- Discuss Canada's national mental health strategy.
- Describe the diagnosis and classification of mental disorders with the criteria of the *Diagnostic and Statistical Manual of Mental Disorders* (5th ed.).
- Define mental health literacy and the role of mental health first aid.
- Identify the role of research in psychiatric and mental health nursing.

KEY TERMS

- Canadian Index of Wellbeing (CIW) • Classification and Measurement System of Functional Health (CLAMES) • gender differences • mental health literacy • social progress

KEY CONCEPTS

- mental health • mental disorder • recovery • well-being

This chapter presents and explores concepts foundational to psychiatric and mental health (PMH) nursing practice. While these key concepts may appear to be straightforward and even obvious at first glance, their meaning continues to evolve. For instance, nurses, other health care professionals, and the public have for some time viewed "recovery" as the restoration of health. However, as a cornerstone of Canada's strategy on mental health and the World Health Organization's (WHO) mental health action plan, the concept embraces more. Recovery is envisioned as gaining hope and purpose; understanding one's abilities, disabilities, rights and resources; and living a meaningful, satisfying life even with mental health problems or illnesses (Mental Health Commission of Canada [MHCC], 2009, 2015; WHO, 2013). It is important that nurses have a deep understanding of these basic terms, as such knowledge will implicitly and explicitly shape their practice.

■ MENTAL HEALTH

Mental health, as defined by the Mental Health Commission of Canada (MHCC, 2013), is "a state of well-being in which the individual realizes his or her own potential, can cope with the normal stresses of life, can work productively and fruitfully, and is able to make a contribution to his or her own community" (p. 3).

Mental health is not the polar opposite of mental illness. In fact, one can experience mental health while one is living with a severe mental disorder. Imagine mental health and mental illness as existing on two separate and simultaneously occurring continua (Epp, 1988). Optimal mental health and minimal mental health represent the extremes on one continuum, while maximal mental disorder and absence of mental disorder represent the extremes on the other continuum (Fig. 2.1). It is possible that a person with a mental disorder can experience optimal mental health (quadrant A), and a person without a mental disorder can experience minimal mental health (quadrant D). This situation is similar to that of a person with diabetes who, using diet, exercise, and medication, is healthy and symptom free, and a person without a diagnosable medical condition who, eating a diet of "fast food," avoiding exercise, and smoking a pack of cigarettes daily, can be unhealthy. Both the level of mental health and the severity of a person's mental disorder can vary over his or her lifetime.

Mental health and physical health are integrated, not distinct. The separation of the mental and physical aspects of health is highly problematic. As the first Director-General of WHO, the Canadian psychiatrist Brock Chisholm stipulated, there is no true physical health without mental health (Kolappa, Henderson, & Kishore, 2013). The WHO's Mental Health Action Plan

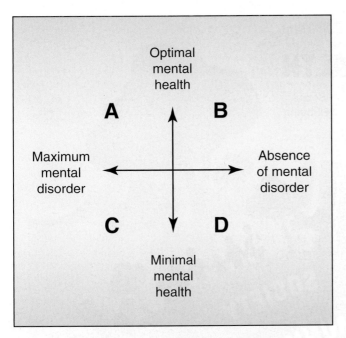

Figure 2.1. Diagram of mental health and mental disorder continua. (Adapted from Epp, J. (1988). *Mental health for Canadians: Striking a balance* (Cat. H39-128/1988E). Ottawa, ON: Supply and Services Canada.)

2013–2020 (WHO, 2013) calls for integrated, holistic approaches to prevention, promotion, care, rehabilitation, and support aimed at both mental and physical health care needs. The International Council of Nurses' (ICN) (2008) position is that all nurses must have knowledge and skills to respond to mental health needs, including their own. Canadian nurses recognize that they play a crucial role in enacting Canada's mental health strategy.

KEY CONCEPT

Mental health is a state of well-being in which the individual realizes self-potential, copes with life stresses, and is able to work productively and contribute to his or her society. It is integral to general health and can be possessed and enhanced, including in the presence of mental illness.

Information regarding Canadians' mental health and its determinants is important to the achievement and monitoring of Canada's mental health strategy. The *Positive Mental Health Surveillance Indicator Framework*, developed by The Public Health Agency of Canada, structures such information using five indicators of positive mental health and 25 risk and protective factors across individual, family, community, and society domains (Orpana, Vachon, Dykxhoorn, McRae, & Jayaraman, 2016). See Figure 2.2.

WELL-BEING

Mental health is considered a state of well-being, but what does "well-being" mean? The Oxford English Dictionary (OED Online, 2014) defines well-being as "the state of being healthy, happy, or prosperous; physical, psychological, or moral welfare." A Canadian phenomenological study suggests that well-being is not purposeful but that it lies on the journey through life events and is experienced when the individual is self-forgetful about how she or he is supposed to live and, instead, engages in living well. It is experienced as coming home to self where the notion of home is critical (Healey-Ogden & Austin, 2011). It is noteworthy that one of the exemplars of well-being in this study was terminally ill.

Canadian Index of Wellbeing

The **Canadian Index of Wellbeing (CIW)** is used as a measure of the quality of life in Canada. With data primarily from Statistics Canada, the CIW is calculated using 64 indicators across eight interconnected quality-of-life domains: community vitality, democratic engagement, education, environment, healthy populations, leisure and culture, living standards, and time use (CIW, 2016). The 2016 CIW report states that, from 1994 to 2014, Canada's Gross Domestic Product (GDP) grew by 38% but wellbeing only improved by 9.9%. The gap between the richest and the poorest in our society continues to grow, a cause for concern as poor health and well-being outcomes, even for the wealthy, are associated with societies with greater inequality.

Using measures like the CIW to examine our national status is important. The GDP provides a measurement of national income, but growth in the GDP is affected by all goods and service activities (including smoking, hiring more police when crime is on the upswing, over-harvesting our forests, increasing use of fossil fuels): it is like a giant calculator with an addition but no subtraction button. The CIW allows a broader depth of understanding that, when used with GDP, will allow Canadians to move towards a society with a quality of life that all may enjoy.

Social Progress Index

In 2016, based on the Social Progress Index (SPI), Canada was ranked the world's second most socially advanced country; Finland was first and the United States of America (USA), 19th (Porter, Stern with Green, 2016). The SPI measures national progress in delivering social and environmental value. It was created to complement the GDP index to give a more holistic picture of a country's overall performance. For example, Canada's GDP ranks tenth globally, while the USA ranks first. **Social progress** is defined as "the capacity of a society to

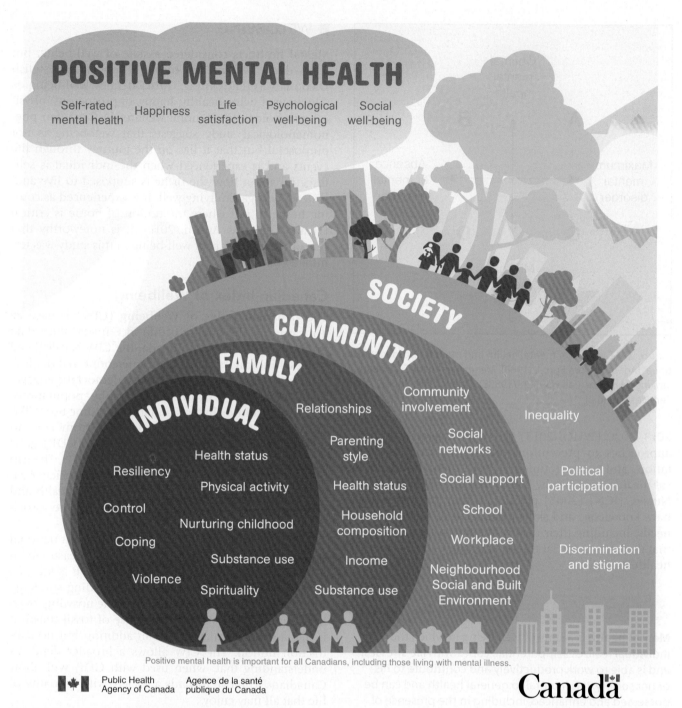

Figure 2.2. Positive Mental Health Surveillance Framework. (©All Rights Reserved. *Monitoring positive mental health and its determinants in Canada: the development of the Positive Mental Health Surveillance Indicator Framework.* Public Health Agency of Canada, 2016. Reproduced with permission from the Minister of Health, 2016.)

meet the basic human needs of its citizens, establish the building blocks that allow citizens and communities to enhance and sustain the quality of their lives, and create the conditions for all individuals to meet their full potential" (Porter & Stern with Green, p. 12). The SPI represents components of basic human needs (i.e., nutrition and basic medical care, water and sanitation, shelter, personal safety), foundations of well-being (i.e., access

to basic knowledge, access to information and communication, health and wellness, environmental quality), and opportunity (i.e., personal rights, personal freedom and choice, tolerance and inclusion, access to advance education). Canada leads the world on "opportunity," being first in "access to advanced education," and continues to perform strongly compared to countries with similar GDPs on "tolerance and inclusion" due to tolerance towards religious minorities and immigrants (Porter & Stern with Green). Challenges appear to lie in the areas of environmental quality, access to information and communications, and health and wellness.

KEY CONCEPT

Well-being is an individual's sense of being content and happy with life and life situation; a sense of flourishing.

■ MENTAL ILLNESS

Each year, one in five Canadians will be living with a mental health problem or illness; this translates to nearly 7 million people. The annual cost of mental health problems and disorders is estimated at $50 billion (MHCC, 2013). Mental disorder is the medical term for mental illness and refers to a diagnosable health condition based on an accepted classification system with criteria related to alterations in mood and affect, behaviour, and thinking and cognition. These alterations are beyond the parameters of psychological states such as sadness and grief that may be encountered in a life. Cultural definitions of responses must be considered. When a particular culture sees certain behaviours as normal, its members will not view the behaviour as a symptom of a mental disorder. For example, it is common in some religious groups to "speak in tongues." To an observer, it may appear that the individuals are experiencing hallucinations (see Chapter 10), a psychiatric symptom, but this behaviour is usual for this group within a particular setting.

KEY CONCEPT

Mental disorders are health conditions characterized by alteration in a variety of factors that include mood and affect, behaviour, and thinking and cognition. The disorders are associated with various degrees of distress and impaired functioning.

Diagnosing Mental Disorders

Classification systems for medical diagnoses identify the criteria required for a particular condition to be diagnosed and provide a common language for health care professionals to use. The two most accepted psychiatric classifications are the Mental and Behavioural Disorders Section of the WHO's *International Statistical Classification of Diseases and Related Health Problems (ICD)*, 10th edition (*ICD-10*) (WHO, 2010), and the American Psychiatric Association's (2013) *Diagnostic and Statistical Manual of Mental Disorders* (*DSM*). In North

America, the *DSM* classification is most commonly used. Its fifth edition, the *DSM-5*, includes the equivalent *ICD-10* Codes for reference. ICD-11 is in development; a 2018 release date is foreseen. The differences between these systems are not grounded in scientific disagreements but rather differences in historical and committee processes (APA, 2013).

The DSM-5

The *DSM-5* has three sections: (I) an introduction and explanation of its use, including a caution regarding its forensic use; (II) the diagnostic criteria and codes; and (III) emerging measures (assessment) and models (e.g., cultural formulation), an alternative model for personality disorders, and conditions for further study (e.g., Internet gaming disorder). For clinical utility, the *DSM-5* is organized along development and life span lines (e.g., diagnoses reflecting developmental processes appearing early in life are at the beginning). Mental disorders are delineated in a way such that cultural, social, and familial norms and values can be recognized as influencing the expression and experience of symptoms, signs, and behaviours addressed in the criteria (APA, 2013). See Box 2.1 for *DSM-5* diagnostic categories and

BOX 2.1 *DSM-5* Diagnostic Categories

Neurodevelopmental Disorders

Schizophrenia Spectrum and Other Psychotic Disorders

Bipolar and Related Disorders

Depressive Disorders

Anxiety Disorders

Obsessive–Compulsive and Related Disorders

Trauma- and Stressor-Related Disorders

Dissociative Disorders

Somatic Symptom and Related Disorders

Feeding and Eating Disorders

Sleep–Wake Disorders

Sexual Dysfunctions

Gender Dysphoria

Disruptive, Impulse Control, and Conduct Disorders

Substance-Related and Addictive Disorders

Neurocognitive Disorders

Personality Disorders

Paraphilic Disorders

Other Mental Disorders

Medication-Induced Movement Disorders

Other Adverse Effects of Medication

Source: American Psychiatric Association. (2013). *Diagnostic and statistical manual of mental disorders* (5th ed.). Arlington, VA: Author.

BOX 2.2 *DSM-5* and Other Conditions That May Be a Focus of Clinical Attention or May Affect Diagnosis, Course, Prognosis, or Treatment

Relationship Problems

Abuse and Neglect

Educational and Occupational Problems

Housing and Economic Problems

Other Problems Related to Social Environment (e.g., phase of life problem, problems related to living alone)

Problems Related to Crime or Interaction With the Legal System

Other Health Service Encounters for Counselling and Medical Advice

Problems Related to Other Psychosocial, Personal, and Environmental Circumstances (e.g., unwanted pregnancy, experience with war, victim of torture)

Other Circumstances of Personal History (e.g., self-harm, nonadherence to medical treatment)

Source: American Psychiatric Association. (2013). *Diagnostic and statistical manual of mental disorders* (5th ed.). Arlington, VA: Author.

Box 2.2 for other conditions that may be a focus of clinical attention or may affect diagnosis, course, prognosis, or treatment.

Gender Differences and the DSM-5

The *DSM-5* notes gender differences (or the lack thereof) for several disorders. **Gender differences** are defined in the *DSM-5* as "variations that result from biological sex as well as an individual's self-representation that includes the psychological, behavioral, and social consequences of one's perceived gender" (APA, 2013, p. 15). The variations may result from only biologic sex differences, self-representation of gender, or both. Gender influences illnesses in several ways, including risk for a disorder, symptom presentation, and willingness to endorse symptoms (which impacts willingness to seek help for them). Events related to reproductive life cycle (e.g., postpartum period) affect risk and symptom expression.

Culture and the DSM-5

The *DSM-5* uses three concepts to point to ways culture influences the illness experience, including symptom presentation, help-seeking behaviours, expectations of and response to treatment, and adaptation to living with the illness (APA, 2013). These concepts are *cultural syndrome, cultural idiom of distress,* and *cultural explanation or perceived cause* (APA, 2013, p. 14). See Chapter 3 for a discussion of culture and mental illness, including culture and the *DSM-5*.

"Saving Normal"

In his book, *Saving Normal: An Insider's Revolt Against Out-of-Control Psychiatric Diagnosis, DSM-5, Big Pharma, and the Medicalization of Ordinary Life,* Allen Frances (2013), the Chair of the *DSM-IV* Task Force, expressed serious reservations about the *DSM-5*. He wants to "save normal" in that he finds aspects of everyday life are being transformed into illness. For instance, he suggests that grief is becoming "medicalized," reducing the dignity of grief's pain, interfering with processing the loss, and reducing the use of rituals that can console. The grieving person, he argues, may be put at risk if prescribed unnecessary medication. Frances is concerned that "Big Pharma's" marketing of their products means that "psychiatric illness" also gets marketed. Shyness readily becomes "social phobia"; ardent interest in something (e.g., chocolate, the Internet) becomes an addiction. He is concerned that psychiatry stay within appropriate bounds.

Diagnosis as Labelling

Receiving a diagnosis can be a relief for an individual and his or her family if it allows for better understanding of symptoms, signs, and behaviour and means that treatment can begin (Hayne, 2001). As a way of labelling a particular person's illness, however, diagnosis can have negative consequences, such as the loss of personal identity if the labelled person becomes viewed as the disease and experiences stigma associated with mental illness. To avoid labelling a person, refer to individuals using person-first language. For example, refer to someone with diabetes mellitus as a "person with diabetes" rather than as a "diabetic." Likewise, someone with a mental disorder should be referred to as a "person with schizophrenia" or as a "person living with bipolar disorder" rather than as "schizophrenic" or as "bipolar." Understanding labelling processes can facilitate conceptualization and implementation of stigma reduction strategies (Yang et al., 2012). It is particularly important that nurses and other health care professionals avoid the pitfalls of negative labelling and stigmatization (Kirby & Keon, 2006).

Health States and Mental Illness

An overview of how living with a specific mental illness can affect everyday quality of life is available from the Health Analysis Division of Statistics Canada: *Health State Descriptions for Canadians: Mental Illnesses* (Langlois, Samokhvalov, Rehm, Spence, & Connor Gorber, 2012). This document is part of a series describing health states related to the diseases classified in Canadian Population Health Impact of diseases research. Using the **Classification and Measurement System of Functional Health (CLAMES)** in which 11 attributes (each with 4 to 5 levels) are used to indicate daily functioning, aspects

BOX 2.3 Attributes of the Classification and Measurement System of Functional Health (CLAMES)

Core	Supplementary
Pain or discomfort	Anxiety
Physical functioning	Speech
Emotional state	Hearing
Fatigue	Vision
Memory and thinking	Use of hands and fingers
Social relationships	

From Langlois, K. A., Samokhvalov, A. V., Rehm, J., Spence, S. T., & Connor Gorber, S. K. (2012). *Health state descriptions for Canadians: Mental illnesses.* Statistics Canada, catalogue no. 82-619 MIE2005002. Ottawa, ON: Statistics Canada.

of living with a particular disorder are described (see Box 2.3). As well, there is a brief review of the disorder, including prevalence and treatment. For example, living with agoraphobia at moderate and severe levels is portrayed.

Mental Health Literacy

The Canadian Alliance on Mental Illness and Mental Health (CAMIMH) was funded by the Public Health Agency of Canada to examine Canadians' **mental health literacy**, defined as "the knowledge and skills that enable people to access, understand, and apply information for mental health" (CAMIMH, 2008, p. 2). Unfortunately, it was found that stigma and discrimination are negatively influencing Canadian' responses to people with mental illnesses, especially serious mental illnesses. Also affected is Canadians' willingness to disclose having a mental illness, especially in the workplace.

Mental Health First Aid

A resource of the MHCC, Mental Health First Aid (MHFA) Canada, is aimed at improving mental health literacy through providing the awareness, knowledge, and skills to help people cope with potential or developing mental health problems in themselves or others. It focuses on the signs and symptoms of mental health problems and disorders, ways to provide initial comfort and support, and guidance as to seeking appropriate professional assistance (see Web Links).

■ RECOVERY

Recovery, viewed as an active process unique to each individual, is a cornerstone of Canada's approach to

mental health care (Kirby & Keon, 2006). Conceptually, this process is broader than clinical recovery (i.e., remission or cure) and, although persons with mental illness certainly can experience clinical recovery, recovery is viewed as being about having a satisfying and hopeful life, even with mental health problems or illness. A recovery orientation for nurses and other health care professionals means that engagement with those in their care involves a focus on those persons' strengths, resources, and rights and is shaped by culturally safe and competent practices. This orientation requires a less medically centred approach and a wider perspective on what constitutes positive outcome measures (see Chapter 8).

KEY CONCEPT

Recovery related to mental illness means "gaining and retaining hope, understanding of one's abilities and disabilities, engagement in an active life, personal autonomy, social identity, meaning and purpose in life and a positive sense of self." It is not synonymous with "cure" (WHO, 2013, p. 39).

■ THE MENTAL HEALTH OF CANADIANS

Nurses need to be engaged in the national strategy that guides Canada's approach to addressing the mental health of Canadians. The six key directions of the strategy (see Chapter 1, Box 1.2) involve promoting mental health across the life span, including in the workplace; fostering recovery and well-being for those living with mental health problems and illnesses and upholding their rights; providing appropriate services and reducing disparities in access to them; working with First Nations, Inuit, and Métis people to address their needs; and mobilizing collaboration and leadership at all levels. The MHCC plays a catalytic role in the strategy's enactment, promoting positive change through knowledge exchange. An example of a successful initiative is *At Home/Chez Soi*, based on the principles of "Housing First (HF)" that require immediate access (without readiness conditions) to permanent housing along with community-based supports for homeless persons with mental illness and which emphasize consumer choice and self-determination, recovery orientation, individualized and person-driven supports, and social and community integration (Goering et al., 2014). The project showed that this approach can work in Canadian cities of different sizes and ethnoracial and cultural composition, that it rapidly ends homelessness, and that it is a sound investment (Goering et al., 2014). The MHCC has a toolkit for communities interested in implementing HF projects.

BOX 2.4 Research for Best Practice

BEING BOTH NURSE AND PATIENT WITH A MENTAL ILLNESS

Peterson, A. L. (2016). Finding identity and meaning as a nurse with a mental illness. Archives in Psychiatric Nursing, 30(5), 558–562.

Focus: The author critically reflects upon her identity as nurse–patient while connecting and analyzing the personal and the cultural aspects of this experience.

Method: Autoethnography is a form of ethnographic research in which a critical focus is taken on the social and cultural aspects of a personal experience, as well as the inward, personal aspects. The resulting text can be in various forms such as personal or photographic essays, poetry, or a novel. In this study, the narrative form is that of a nursing journal article. Readers of autoethnographic texts bring their own experiences/contexts to it, and there is an expectation that they should aim to actively engage with the text, cognitively and emotionally. Texts of shared personal insights can inspire self-awareness and deepen cultural understandings of readers.

Findings: An excerpt reveals the dual identity experienced as the nurse author became ill: *I'd been coming up with various excuses for what was wrong with me and why I didn't feel like myself, but eventually I concluded, with careful clinical reflection, that I met the diagnostic criteria for major depressive disorder. If anything, I felt relieved that what was happening to me fit with a familiar label. Still, though, I opted not to seek help, thinking that because I was a mental health nurse, I should be able to take care of myself; if I couldn't, that would mean I was a bad nurse (p. 559).* For this nurse, it was the biologic model of mental illness that primarily shaped her perspective on her illness. She could differentiate between her ill and well self and between the disease process and sociocultural responses to her illness. As an in-patient, she responded to co-patients in ways informed by nursing. Discharged, she was conflicted re: sharing insights about a former co-patient's current condition with his care team.

Implications: Nurses with an illness attain a new identity as patient, but also as nurse–patient, and their understanding of the meaning of illness can evolve. Critical reflection may enable them to find new meanings about their experience and sharing their insights with other nurses may promote increased understanding of the patient experience and that of the nurse–patient.

■ RESEARCH-BASED CARE

In the urgent quest to improve the lives of Canadians living with a mental health problem or illness, research will be a major tool. Nurses are challenged to generate evidence for best care interventions, to use methods of inquiry that allow a better understanding of the experiences of mental health, mental illness, recovery and well-being, and to translate new knowledge into better care. For instance, the science related to decreasing the use of seclusion and restraint or that which underscored the need to determine an individual's trauma-related experiences when diagnosing, as well as research showing the efficacy of new approaches to mental health community services, are transforming care in positive ways. In most chapters of this textbook, "Research for Best Practice" is featured. As well as noting the implications research findings have for practice, attention should be paid to the various research methods that are being utilized, from randomized controlled trials (RCTs) to philosophical inquiry. In this chapter, an autoethnographic study of a mental health nurse's experience as nurse–patient is featured (see Box 2.4).

The need to improve mental health care is a global one, requiring shared efforts, as indicated by the fourth global target of the WHO Action Plan (2013): "to strengthen information systems, evidence, and research for mental health" (p. 22).

SUMMARY OF KEY POINTS

- Four complex concepts are the cornerstone of Canada's mental health strategy and fundamental to psychiatric and mental health nursing practice: mental health, well-being, mental illness, and recovery.
- "There is no health without mental health." Mental health needs to be integrated into general health in all areas of practice and around the world.
- ICN takes the position that all registered nurses must have the knowledge and skills to respond to mental health needs, including their own.
- Measures used to explore well-being include the CIW and the SPI.
- The medical term for mental illness is mental disorder. In Canada, the *DSM* is the most commonly used classification of mental disorders. Its fifth edition was released in 2013, the *DSM-5*. The Mental and Behavioural Disorders section of the ICD classification of the WHO is an alternative system that can also be used.

- Diagnosis can be used in a way that increases negative labelling of persons living with mental health problems or illnesses. It is important not to use language such as "She is a schizophrenic," but rather say "She has schizophrenia."
- Health Canada describes health states related to specific diseases using the CLAMES, which indicates daily functioning attributes of living with that disease or disorder.
- Nurses need to play a role in increasing the mental health literacy of Canadians.
- The six strategic directions of our national mental health strategy guide the Canadian approach to mental health and mental health care.

Web Links

athome.nfb.ca/#/athome At this interactive Web site of the MHCC and the National Film Board, "At Home: In Search of a Cure for a 21ˢᵗ Century Crisis," evocatively presents the At Home/Chez Soi initiative of the MHCC and the evidence it provides for a new way to address the homelessness affecting many Canadians with mental illness.

camimh.ca This site of the Canadian Alliance on Mental Illness and Mental Health offers many resources, including its 2016 *Mental Health Now!* policy document that calls on governments in Canada to improve mental health care through such actions as increased funding, acceleration of mental health innovation, development of pan-Canadian mental health indicators to monitor mental health system performance, and investment in social infrastructure.

hc-sc.gc.ca Health Canada provides information on primary health care, health care systems, mental health and wellness, and the health of indigenous Canadians.

mentalhealthcommission.ca For current information on the enactment of our national mental health strategy and the work of the MHCC, including its reports, go to this site.

mhfa.ca At this site of the MHCC's Mental Health First Aid initiative, an interactive map can be found that indicates MHFA training opportunities across Canada.

partnersformh.ca Partners for Mental Health is a Canadian charitable organization that aims at supporting the enactment of the national mental health strategy. It highlights issues; supports research, events, and policies; and encourages public action for change.

phac-aspc.gc.ca The Public Health Agency of Canada's Web site provides links to mental health reports and best practices. The 2016 statistics from the Positive Mental Health Surveillance Indicator Framework can be found here.

socialprogressimperative.org/data/spi The SPI data set is available here.

uwaterloo.ca/canadian-index-wellbeing/resources Information and resources on the CIW can be found at this University of Waterloo site.

who.int/topics/mental_health.en/ WHO's mental health resources/links are found here.

WHO.int/mental_health/mindbank MiNDbank where comprehensive information regarding national and international mental health resources can be found. This resource is one means of supporting the enactment of best practice standards and human rights.

References

American Psychological Association (APA). (2013). *Diagnostic and statistical manual of mental disorders* (5th ed.). Arlington, VA: Author.

Canadian Alliance on Mental Illness and Mental Health (CAMIMH). (2008). *National integrated framework for enhancing mental health literacy in Canada: Final report*. Retrieved from www.camimh.ca

Canadian Index of Wellbeing. (2016). *How are Canadians really doing? The 2016 Canadian Index of Wellbeing report*. Waterloo, ON: Canadian Index of Wellbeing & University of Waterloo.

Epp, J. (1988). *Mental health for Canadians: Striking a balance* (Cat. H39-128/1988E). Ottawa, ON: Supply and Services Canada.

Frances, A. (2013). *Saving normal: An insider's revolt against out-of-control psychiatric diagnosis, DSM-5, Big Pharma, and the medicalization of ordinary life*. New York, NY: HarperCollins.

Goering, P., Veldhuizen, S., Watson, A., Adair, C., Kopp, B., Latimer, E., … Aubry, T. (2014). *National At Home/Chez Soi final report*. Calgary, AB: MHCC.

Hayne, Y. M. (2001). *To be diagnosed: The experience of presenting with chronic mental illness* (unpublished doctoral thesis). University of Alberta, Canada.

Healey-Ogden, M., & Austin, W. (2011). Uncovering the lived experience of well-being. *Qualitative Health Research, 21,* 85–98. doi: 10.1177/1049732310379113

International Council of Nurses. (2008). *Position statement: Mental health*. Retrieved from http://www.icn.ch/publications/position-statements/

Kirby, M. J., & Keon, W. J. (2006). *Out of the shadows at last: Highlights and recommendations*. Ottawa, ON: The Standing Committee on Social Affairs, Science and Technology.

Kolappa, K., Henderson, D., & Kishore, S. P. (2013). No physical health without mental health: Lessons unlearned? *Bulletin of the World Health Organization, 91*(1), 3–3A.

Langlois, K. A., Samokhvalov, A. V., Rehm, J., Spence, S. T., & Connor Gorber, S. K. (2012). *Health state descriptions for Canadians: Mental illnesses*. Statistics Canada, catalogue no. 82-619. MIE2005002. Ottawa, ON: Statistics Canada.

Mental Health Commission of Canada. (2009). *Toward recovery & well-being: A framework for a Mental Health Strategy for Canada*. Retrieved from http://www.mentalhealthcommission.ca/English/document/241/toward-recovery-and-well-being

Mental Health Commission of Canada. (2013). *Making the case for investing in mental health in Canada*. Retrieved from http://www.mentalhealthcommission.ca/English/node/5020

Mental Health Commission of Canada. (2015). *Guidelines for recovery-oriented practice. Hope. Dignity. Inclusion*. Ottawa, ON: Author.

OED Online. (2014). "well-being, n". Oxford University Press. Retrieved from http://www.oed.com.login.ezproxy.library.ualberta.ca/view/Entry/227050?redirectedFrom=well-being

Orpana, H., Vachon, J., Dykxhoorn, J., McRae, L., & Jayaraman, G. (2016). Monitoring positive mental health and its determinants in Canada: The development of the Positive Mental Health Surveillance Indicator Framework. *Health Promotion and Chronic Disease Prevention in Canada: Research, Policy and Practice, 36*(1), 1–10.

Peterson, A. L. (2016). Finding identity and meaning as a nurse with a mental illness. *Archives in Psychiatric Nursing, 30*(5), 558–562. doi: 10.1016/j.apnu.2016.04.003

Porter, M. E., & Stern, S., with Green, M. (2016). *Social Progress Index*. Retrieved from http://www.socialprogressimperative.org/global-index/

World Health Organization. (2010). *International Statistical Classification of Diseases and Related Health Problems (10th rev.) (ICD-10)*. Geneva, Switzerland: Author.

World Health Organization. (2013). *Mental health action plan 2013–2020*. Geneva, Switzerland: Author.

Yang, L. H., Lo, G., WonPat-Borja, A. J., Singla, D. R., Link, B. G., & Phillips, M. R. (2012). Effects of labeling and interpersonal conflict upon attitudes towards schizophrenia: Implications for reducing mental illness stigma in urban China. *Social Psychiatry and Psychiatric Epidemiology, 47*(9), 1459–1473.

3 The Context of Mental Health Care: Cultural, Socioeconomic, and Geographic

Arlene Kent-Wilkinson
and Wendy Austin

LEARNING OBJECTIVES

After studying this chapter, you will be able to:

- Identify cultural, socioeconomic, and geographical challenges to the provision of mental health care across Canada.
- Explore the cultural roots of mental illness and its relationship to beliefs of religion and spirituality.
- Relate the concepts of cultural identity, cultural competence, and cultural safety to the role of the nurse in mental health care.
- Consider the unique culture of Aboriginal people in Canada and their health beliefs.
- Describe factors related to the pre- and postmigration mental health of immigrants and refugees to Canada.
- Identify the influence of socioeconomic factors on the mental health of Canadians.
- Describe the mental health care delivery issues related to providing services in Canada's many geographic areas.

KEY TERMS

- aboriginal • assimilation • colonialism • cultural diversity • cultural humility • cultural identity • ethnocentrism • health disparity • historical trauma • indigenous • prejudice • religion • residential school syndrome • spirituality • stereotyping • telehealth

KEY CONCEPTS

- cultural competence • cultural safety • culture • discrimination • diversity • poverty • stigma

Health, including the mental health, of any human population is the product of a complex web of cultural, environmental, historical, physiologic, psychological, spiritual, and socioeconomic factors. This chapter examines cultural, socioeconomic, and geographical contexts of mental health in Canada. Culture will be examined with regard to cultural identity and diversity, as well as the cultural roots of spirituality and religion. The unique culture of Canada's **Aboriginal** people (also known as **indigenous** people) will be a focus, as will be the factors that influence the mental wellness of immigrants and refugees to Canada. Socioeconomic factors that influence mental health and the geographic context of mental health care will be explored. The role and the responsibility of the nurse in meaningfully addressing the contexts shaping Canadian mental health care will be emphasized.

CULTURAL CONTEXT OF MENTAL HEALTH CARE

Culture is the "learned values, beliefs, norms and way of life that influence an individual's thinking, decisions and actions in certain ways" (Canadian Nurses Association [CNA], 2017, p. 21; College of Nurses of Ontario [CNO], 2009, p. 3). Culture reflects the basic values and biases through which we interpret the world around us and make decisions about our own behaviour and our relationships with others. Our culture shapes our perceptions and attitudes, from our personal space comfort zones to our attitudes toward mental health and mental illness. Culture is reflected in an individual's symptom expression, the meaning ascribed to illness and treatment choices (National Collaborating Centre for Aboriginal Health [NCCAH], 2016). A challenge to all individuals is to gain insight into their own culturally learned ideas and values and to guard against an assumption that these are the correct and proper ones for everyone. This assumption is termed **ethnocentrism**.

KEY CONCEPT

Culture is the "learned values, beliefs, norms and way of life that influence an individual's thinking, decisions and actions in certain ways" (CNA, 2017, p. 21; CNO, 2009, p. 3).

Cultural Diversity in Canada

Canada is a culturally diverse nation. Other than Aboriginal peoples, most Canadians are descendants of immigrants or are immigrants themselves. According to the National Household Survey of 2011, more than one-fifth of Canadians are foreign-born, the highest rate of all the G8 countries (Statistics Canada, 2016a, 2016b). Canada is among the most multicultural of Western nations. The city of Toronto, with over half of its population born outside of the country, has officially been named "the most diverse city in the world" (The Culture Trip, 2017). It is home to 230 different nationalities with over 140 languages spoken (BlogTO, 2016).

Diversity is "the variation between people in terms of a range of factors such as ethnicity, national origin, race, gender, gender identity, gender expression, ability, age, physical characteristics, religion, values and beliefs, sexual orientation, socio-economic class or life experiences" (CNA, 2017, p. 21). Overall, Canadians have a positive view of immigration and cultural diversity, considering both as assets to Canada. The 2016 Social Progress Index placed Canada second among 133 nations, citing among other aspects tolerance for minority communities (Cecco, 2016; Social Progress Imperative, 2016).

KEY CONCEPT

Diversity is variation among people in terms of factors such as ethnicity, natural origin, race, gender identity, gender expression, ability, age, physical characteristics, religion, values and beliefs, sexual orientation, socioeconomic class or life experiences (CNA, 2017, p. 21; RNAO, 2007) and considered an asset to our society by Canadians.

Canadian Multiculturalism Policy

In 1971, Canada became the first country to adopt a policy of multiculturalism as an official government policy (Canadian Museum of Immigration at Pier 21, 2017). *The Canadian Multiculturalism Policy, 1971,* advocated support for the maintenance and development of heritage cultures and the reduction of barriers to full and equitable participation of all Canadians in the life of the larger society (Government of Canada, 2017a). The *Multiculturalism Policy of Canada, 1971,* affirmed the rights, dignity, and value of all Canadians regardless of ethnic, linguistic, or religious background. The policy confirmed the rights of Aboriginal people in Canada and recognized Canada's two official languages, as well as the need to preserve and enhance the use of other languages. Canada's multicultural policy has encouraged broad immigration.

Cultural Roots of Mental Health and Illness

The experience of mental illness is influenced by culture. Symptoms of a disorder that are prominent in one culture may be insignificant or absent in another and may be interpreted as normal in a third. Some mental disorders may be a recent development in response to cultural change. For example, posttraumatic stress disorder (PTSD) can be manifested in the plight of refugees coming to a new country and to the effects of government policies of colonization (i.e., residential school syndrome) resulting in intergenerational trauma, as will be discussed later in the chapter.

Cultural Identity

Culture is strongly linked to identity; the suppression or marginalization of one's **cultural identity** has a negative impact on self-worth. However, if a culture is valued and supported, individuals and communities self-identifying with that culture will experience a sense of belonging and value. Shared cultural beliefs, practices, and language create social cohesion in communities, which can positively influence the health of individuals. Culture is the foundation of both individual and collective identity, and its erosion can adversely affect mental health and well-being, leading to depression, anxiety, substance abuse, and even suicide (Kirmayer, Brass, & Tait, 2000; NCCAH, 2016). When cultural practices and language are denied to communities, as historically occurred with many Aboriginal communities in Canada, social cohesion and health are negatively affected (Brascoupé & Waters, 2009).

Cultural Beliefs About Health

Every culture has a conception of what constitutes health and illness and how illness should be treated. It is crucial to understand how the relationship between culture and health influences health behaviours in your patients. The "healthy immigrant effect" identifies that the health of new immigrants is generally better than that of the Canadian born but tends to decline as years lived in Canada increase (Statistics Canada, 2015). There are many factors contributing to this, one being the loss of social connections in one's home country. Transnational ties occur when immigrants can maintain connection with their country of origin (Statistics Canada). This bond helps to maintain social connections and cultural identity. In the context of Aboriginal populations, moving off reserve and into urban areas can make the maintaining of traditional cultural ties difficult, thereby affecting cultural identity and social connections.

Cultural beliefs influence the ways both health professionals and patients view health, illnesses/diseases and their causes, treatment options, how and where they seek help, and their views about dying and death (Mayhew, 2016). It influences beliefs about the choice to engage in health-promoting behaviours, whether to seek advice about concerns from a traditional healer or a medical doctor, as well as whether to follow treatment options (Canadian Medical Protective Association, 2014).

Beliefs about mental illness are intimately linked with concepts of religion, social values, norms, and ideals of human relationships. These shared beliefs determine the nature of traditional medicine and provide the framework for interpreting symptoms and guiding action in response to them. Western medicine and psychiatry are premised on the belief that mental illness is caused by biologic and experiential events; many other cultures ascribe a metaphysical or spiritual cause as well.

Traditional medical practices of Aboriginal people are closely related to other aspects of the culture, especially their **spirituality**. Getting in touch with one's own spirituality is identified as a key to recovery or healing. There is a holistic approach taken and, although spiritual rites have been modified throughout the years, they continue to be practiced. Spirituality is linked to a sense of life purpose and personal identity and is seen as a key element for finding one's place in the world. To most Aboriginal people, the concept of spirituality refers to a sense of direction: it is not a religion but a way of life. The Royal Commission of Aboriginal Peoples (1996) noted spirituality as a critical component of health for Aboriginal people because it permeates every aspect of life. Health to Aboriginal people is ultimately the achievement of equilibrium, whereby a state of harmony connects to health and disharmony to illness.

Cultural Beliefs and the Mental Health of Immigrants and Refugees to Canada

Perceptions of health and well-being and of mental health differ across and within societies. For example, some immigrants may not be familiar with Western ideas about mental health and mental illness nor with Western-style health services. They may use informal support systems, such as family and friends, rather than formal services to deal with mental health problems (Chaze, Thomson, George, & Guruge, 2015). Mental illness may be conceptualized differently by immigrant groups. Research has shown, for instance, that some South and East Asian immigrant women conceptualize mental health as "peace with oneself and a tenable and maintainable goal in life" and mental illness as "a bad spirit" residing within oneself (Chiu, Ganesan, Clark, & Morrow, 2005, p. 645). Depression may not be a term familiar to some groups as it was not used in their prior communities, nor did people there seek out medical help for symptoms we identify here as "depression" (Chaze et al., 2015).

Thus, cultural beliefs and practices can be barriers to identifying symptoms of mental illness and to mental health service utilization (Chaze et al., 2015). It can affect the adoption of preventive and health promotion measures such as vaccination, birth control, and prenatal care and influence health-related choices (Mayhew, 2016). Just as linguistic accommodation through interpreters is important to safe care, cultural brokers may assist in the provision of services to diverse ethnoracial clients (Kirmayer, Dandeneau, Marshall, Phillip, & Williamson, 2011). Assessment of each patient's cultural beliefs related to health can be essential. Ensuring cultural safety for patients is critical to overall safe nursing care and necessary to improving patient outcomes (NCCAH, 2013).

Immigrants and refugees have different migrant trajectories. Immigrants usually made a choice to move to another country, even if economic, family, and other factors played a role in that decision. Refugees fled their country of origin due to a natural disaster, war, or persecution. As well as the trauma that forced their migration, refugees may have lived for months or years in crowded refugee camps, uncertain of any future home. Research with refugees, in recipient countries, reveals that prolonged detention, insecure residency status, restricted access to services, and inability to access work or education exacerbate the effects of depression and PTSD related to past trauma (Silove, Ventevoge, & Rees, 2017). For PTSD among refugees, the strongest predictor is exposure to torture; for depression, it is number of traumas (Silove et al., 2017).

While premigration factors influencing mental health may differ for immigrants and refugees, postmigration determinants of mental health are similar. A scoping review of Canadian studies (all situated in Ontario and Quebec) from 1990 to 2013 regarding the mental health of immigrant and refugee youth found that determinants of mental health among immigrants and refugees have been identified as "individual (e.g., age, gender, language fluency, ethnicity, knowledge of the health care system); familial (e.g., family (in)stability, socio-economic status, intergenerational conflict); institutional (e.g., availability (or lack) of access to appropriate care and services, (non)acceptance of foreign credentials); and societal (e.g., discrimination, racism, poverty)" (Guruge & Butt, 2015, p. e72–e73). The authors of this review note that, for the mental health of youth, family involvement was important; the first year in Canada was a critical period; and schools are a strategic point for services. See Box 3.1 for research regarding refugee health and help-seeking behaviours. The MHCC (2016) is working to support the mental health of refugees who have come to Canada.

Diagnostic Cultural Formulations

The American Psychiatric Association (APA) *Diagnostic and Statistical Manual of Mental Disorders* (DSM) did

BOX 3.1 Research for Best Practice

HEALTH AND CANADIAN REFUGEES WHO FLED COLLECTIVE VIOLENCE

Mabaya, G., & Ray, S. I. (2014). The meaning of health and help-seeking behaviours among refugees who have experienced collective violence prior to emigration: A Canadian perspective. Canadian Journal of Community Mental Health, 33(3), 71–85. doi:10.7870/cjcmh-2014-024

Question: What is the meaning of health and help-seeking behaviours to refugees in Canada who left their home countries due to collective violence?

Findings: The experience of collective continued to affect their current lives. Prior to migration, participants had been "under constant threat of imminent death"; there was no help to seek. Feeling fearful, helpless, empty, and even worthless, these refugees described constant suffering. Being in Canada has brought hope and peace and a renewed sense of life, with health equated, for some, with lack of suffering (p. 77). They live, however, "with

an invisible wound of trauma" and remain silent about their past. Most have not sought help for their emotional wounds, except for one couple in which one was a social worker who knew to seek psychological help (p. 80). Health care in Canada was viewed as a privilege, good and fair if not perfect. Based on the mistrust of health care practitioners in their home countries, trust was an issue.

Implications: The ongoing trauma of collective violence needs to be understood by Canadian health care practitioners as do the difficulties that these individuals have in seeking help. A focus on establishing trust through patience and empathy by being attentive to individual stories when they are shared will be crucial. Specialized mental health services for this population would be an asset.

---

not specifically address culture until its fourth edition (*DSM-IV*) (APA, 1994). After exploring different ways of facilitating the application of a cultural perspective to the process of clinical interviewing, a cultural formulation outline was adopted. In 2013, the APA published the *DSM-5* (APA, 2013a). The fifth edition explicitly seeks to provide culturally appropriate diagnosis by incorporating cultural sensitivity throughout the manual. In the introduction of the DSM-5, mental disorders are defined "in relation to cultural, social, and familial norms and values. Culture provides interpretive frameworks that shape the experience and expression of the symptoms, signs, and behaviors that are criteria for diagnosis" (APA, 2013b, p. 13). The DSM-5 provides criteria reflecting cross-cultural variation, outlines cultural concepts of distress, and offers an interview tool. The criteria are designed to be as universally valid across different cultures as possible. For example, "offending others" has been added to the criteria for social anxiety disorder to better reflect the appearance of social anxiety disorder in Japan, where avoiding harm to others is of greater concern than avoiding harm to oneself (APA, 2013b).

Because symptoms manifest and are understood differently across cultures, clinicians must attend to relevant aspects of a patient's context when making a diagnosis. For instance, depending on the patient's culture, panic attacks may manifest as uncontrollable crying and headaches or as difficulty breathing. Clinicians' awareness of cultural, ethnic, and linguistic differences allows for more accurate diagnoses and more effective treatment.

■ RELIGION AS A CULTURAL SYSTEM

Culture, spirituality, and religion are central and interconnecting components of human societies (Chaze et al., 2015). **Religion** (from the Latin *religare*, to bind) can be defined as an organized set of beliefs providing answers to questions about life through sacred texts, rituals, and practices usually experienced within a community (Blanch, 2007; Chaze et al., 2015). Spirituality as "meaning making" helps individuals to achieve personal understanding of life and their circumstances (Ameling & Povilonis, 2001, p. 16). Prior to the advent of modern medicine, when praying and offerings to the divine were often all that could be done, illness and recovery were inescapably linked with spirituality or faith (Skip Knox, 2004).

Religions in Canada

Canada aims to be a nation of tolerance, respect, and religious harmony with support for religious pluralism important to our political culture. Statistics Canada's 2011 National Household Survey revealed that the majority of Canadians were Christians, although this number has been decreasing since 2001; those with no religious affiliation formed the second largest and youngest group; Muslims came third with the greatest increase in numbers. The numbers of persons identifying as Hindu, Sikh, and Buddhist are increasing, as well, with Jewish numbers slightly decreasing (Statistics Canada, 2016d). The Christian religion in Canada is divided into eight subgroups (Anglican, Baptist, Catholic [7 denominations], Christian Orthodox [13 denominations], Lutheran, Pentecostal, Presbyterian, United Church, and "Other Christian" [45 denominations]), with 19 religions listed under "Other," including traditional (Aboriginal) spiritual (Canadian Magazine of Immigration, 2016). The religious, as well as the racial, ethnic, and linguistic, diversity of the Canadian population continues to grow, presenting unique challenges to social institutions and governments.

Religious Beliefs and Approaches to Mental Illness

The Canadian Mental Health Strategy (Mental Health Commission of Canada [MHCC], 2012) recognizes the vulnerability of immigrants, refugees, and racialized groups in relation to mental health and mental health service utilization; improving services to them is a priority. A challenge is to understand the role of religion, culture, and spirituality in a person's life without stereotyping them. Religious and spiritual beliefs can play a role in coping with illness, improving quality of life, and sustaining recovery. Activities and worshipping practices such as praying, spiritual reading, meditation, and repeating God's names are described by some immigrants as spiritual resources for mental health care (Chiu et al., 2005). If one believes, however, that mental health symptoms are wholly spiritual in nature, help will not be sought in health services. For instance, a 2017 study by Okpalauwaekwe, Mela, and Oji found that some people from Nigeria attribute mental illnesses to supernatural causes or believe that the person is being punished for bad deeds. Such beliefs have them seeking help from traditional healers or religious groups rather than physicians. If depression is understood from within a religious context, individuals may seek solace in prayer; fortunately, they may also take strength from their faith to seek other forms of help, including health care (Chaze et al., 2015). It is important that information regarding mental health and mental health services are available to new immigrants in an accessible form so that lack of knowledge about them is not a factor.

Although religion and spirituality may be important components of health and healing for immigrants, they may encounter in Canada a health care system that is science-based and not sufficiently acknowledging the spiritual aspects of care. A review of evidence-based literature concluded that many health practitioners are reluctant to incorporate spirituality into their practice because of the historical belief that it is antithetical to science. Other reasons include the ambiguity of their understandings of spirituality and lack of training in implementing spirituality in patient care. As well, health practitioners can allow their own religious beliefs impact their provision of care (Chaze et al., 2015). (See Chapter 11 for interventions in the spiritual domain.)

■ ABORIGINAL PEOPLE IN CANADA

According to the 2011 Canadian census, 1,400,685 people in Canada (4.3% of the total population) self-identify as First Nation, Métis, or Inuit; there are nearly 600 recognized First Nation governments or bands in Canada (Statistics Canada, 2016c). Although often treated as a single group, there are many Indigenous cultures in Canada, each having a unique heritage, language, set of cultural practices, and spiritual beliefs. See Box 3.2 for definitions of the three groups of Aboriginal people in Canada: First Nations, Inuit, and Métis.

Cultural Diversity Among Aboriginal People of Canada

The cultural and linguistic differences among Aboriginal groups are greater than the differences that divide European nations. In addition to intergroup social, cultural, and environmental differences, there is an enormous diversity of values, lifestyles, and perspectives within any community or urban Aboriginal population.

Colonialism, Assimilation, and Historical (Intergenerational) Trauma

Colonialism is the institutionalized, political domination of one nation over another, including when one nation overthrows another for the purpose of domination (Paquette, Beauregard, & Gunter, 2017). It involves direct political administration by the colonial power, control of all economic relationships, and a systematic attempt to transform the culture. Colonialism involves the exploitation or subjugation of people by a larger or wealthier power (Peters, 2017).

Before confederation and up through the first half of the 20th century, the strategy of the government of Canada toward First Nations was a colonial one. **Assimilation** was the government policy to "Canadianize" Aboriginal people to the extent that they would abandon their own culture and adopt the dominant culture (i.e., French or British Canadian) and religion (i.e., Catholic or Protestant) (Thira, 2005). Aboriginal populations have been subjected to **historical trauma**, which is the cumulative effect of maltreatment across generations and which results in the reproduction of maladaptive social and cultural patterns with each generation (see Chapter 17).

Effects of Colonialism

Colonialism in Canada had significant negative mental health effects for Aboriginal people, as well as causing intergenerational trauma (Roy, 2014). These mental health issues include "depression, alcoholism, suicide, and violence" (Kirmayer, Macdonald, & Brass, 2000). Fetal alcohol spectrum disorder and **residential school syndrome**, a form of PTSD with a significant cultural

---

BOX 3.2 Definitions: Aboriginal Peoples of Canada

Aboriginal peoples is a collective name for all the original peoples of Canada and their descendants. Section 35 of the Constitution Act of 1982 specifies that Aboriginal peoples in Canada consist of three groups: Indian (First Nations), Inuit, and Métis. *Indigenous peoples* is used, as well, as a collective name for all original peoples of Canada and their descendants.

First Nation(s). The term First Nations came into common usage in the early 1980s to replace band or Indian, which some people found offensive (see Indian). Despite its widespread use, there is no legal definition for this term in Canada. Some communities have adopted First Nation to replace the term band. Many people prefer to be called First Nations or First Nations people instead of Indians.

Indian. The term Indian collectively describes all the Indigenous peoples in Canada who are not Inuit or Métis. Indian peoples are one of three peoples recognized as aboriginal in the Constitution Act of 1982 along with Inuit and Métis. Three categories apply to Indians in Canada: Status, Nonstatus, and Treaty. *Status Indians* are those entitled to have their names included on the Indian Register, an official list maintained by the federal government based on certain criteria. Only Status Indians are recognized as Indians under the *Indian Act* and entitled to certain rights and benefits under the law. *Nonstatus Indians* are people who consider themselves Indians or members of a First Nation but whom the government of Canada does not recognize as Indians under the *Indian Act*, because they either are unable to prove their Indian status or have lost their status rights.

Nonstatus Indians are not entitled to the same rights and benefits available to Status Indians. *Treaty Indians* are descendants of Indians who signed treaties with Canada and who have a contemporary connection with a treaty band.

Inuit. The Inuit are Aboriginal people in Northern Canada, who live above the tree line in Nunavut, the Northwest Territories, Northern Quebec, and Labrador. The word Inuit means *people* in the Inuit language—*Inuktitut.* The singular of Inuit is Inuk. Inuit are a circumpolar people, inhabiting regions in Russia, Alaska, Canada and Greenland, united by a common culture and language. There are approximately 55,000 Inuit living in Canada.

Métis refers to people of mixed First Nation and European ancestry, distinct from First Nations and having their own unique culture. The word Métis is French for "mixed blood." Section 35 of the *Constitution Act* of 1982 recognizes Métis as one of the three aboriginal peoples of Canada. Historically, the term Métis applied to the children of French fur traders and Cree women in the prairies, of English and Scottish traders and Dene women in the North, and of British and Inuit in Newfoundland and Labrador.

National Aboriginal Health Organization. (2012). Defining Aboriginal peoples within Canada: NAHO terminology guidelines. *Journal of Aboriginal Health (JAH) & International Journal of Indigenous Health (IJIH).* Retrieved from https://journals.uvic.ca/journalinfo/ijih/IJIHDefiningIndigenousPeoplesWithinCanada.pdf

Her Majesty the Queen in Right of Canada, represented by the Minister of Citizenship and Immigration Canada. (2012). *Discover Canada: The Rights and Responsibilities of Citizenship.* Retrieved from http://www.cic.gc.ca/english/pdf/pub/discover.pdf

---

component and impacting children (Douglas, 2013), affect Aboriginal communities.

A case study of 95 Aboriginal survivors of residential schools, who had undergone a clinical assessment and for whom there were mental health profiles, revealed that all but two had a mental disorder, the most common being PTSD, substance abuse disorder, and major depression. All had experienced sexual abuse (Corrado & Cohen, 2010). Further trauma is perpetuated today in the form of suicide and family violence, which then significantly contribute to substance abuse and major depression. Substance abuse is a major health issue. Alcohol-related Aboriginal deaths are almost double that of the nonaboriginal Canadian population; drug-related overdose rates are two to five times higher (Russell, Firestone, Kelly, Mushquash, & Fischer, 2016). Further, perceptions of negative media coverage of events related to substance abuse have reinforced racism and nega-

tive stereotypes (Richmond & Cook, 2016). Perpetual trauma has left many communities in social and mental distress, where anger, hopelessness, lack of purpose, and pessimism has become the norm. Suicides have become the way to "communicate distress and escape when these seem to be few other options" (Health Canada, 2013, p. 8). These detrimental effects of colonialism on Aboriginal populations are not unique to Canada but are experienced by many Indigenous people around the globe.

Residential Schools

From first contact, the European missionaries sought to convert local Aboriginal people and save their souls. The Indian Residential School (IRS) system arose out this history. In 1874, the federal government began to develop and administer the IRS (Health Canada, 2013). The schools were located in every province and territory except Newfoundland (where the entire Aboriginal population had been decimated), New Brunswick, and Prince Edward Island. Approximately 150,000 children, some as young as four, were taken to these schools between 1896 and 1996, when the last one (on the Gordon Reserve in Saskatchewan) was closed (Joseph, 2014). (Most of the federally run residential schools were closed by the mid-1970s.) An estimated 80,000 people alive today attended an IRS in Canada (Health Canada).

The loss of their cultural identity, including seasonal ceremonies, storytelling, rituals, and health beliefs, and of knowledge of their languages affected the children's relationships with their own families and communities. They were to assimilate into the mainstream culture and its dominant religions and ways of life (Kuhl, 2017). The effects of this racist-based forced assimilation has had lasting and profound effects on Aboriginal people that persist to present day (McNally & Martin, 2017; Truth and Reconciliation Commission of Canada, 2015). That many of the children experienced physical, psychological, and/or sexual abuse greatly deepened this traumatic legacy (Health Canada, 2013). It can be linked to the high suicide rates, mental illness, inadequate parenting skills, and sexual/physical violence to be found in some communities (Kumar & Nahwegahbow, 2016).

Effects on Mental Health and Addiction

The IRS is recognized as a contributing factor to the poorer health status seen in many Aboriginal populations today. Survivors face various health problems such as poorer general and self-rated health, increased rates of chronic and infectious diseases, and mental and emotional well-being including mental distress, depression, addictive behaviours and substance misuse, stress, and suicidal behaviours (Wilk, Maltby, & Cooke, 2017). Research indicates that exposure to the IRS system along with a history of abuse is associated with suicidal thoughts and behaviours (Elias et al., 2012). In fact, researchers using data from the 2012 Aboriginal Peoples Survey (APS) examined the relationship of IRS attendance of a previous generation family member and the current health of off-reserve First Nations, Métis, and Inuit Canadians in terms of five outcomes: self-perceived health, mental health, distress, suicidal ideation, and suicide attempt. All outcomes were directly affected: lower self-perceived physical and mental health and higher risk for distress and suicidal thoughts and behaviours, with the odds of a suicide attempt within the past 12 months twice as high for those with familial attendance in the IRS (Hackett, Feeny, & Tompa, 2016). Suicide has been, at times, an emergency-level public health issue for a community (Rutherford, 2016). Suicide rates are twice as high in Aboriginal populations than in nonaboriginal populations (McQuaid et al., 2017).

A growing concern is gang activity among Aboriginal youth (Preston, Carr-Stewart, & Bruno, 2012). Group membership can bring young people a sense of belongingness and purpose. Although gangs can promote such feelings, their members are more susceptible to making poor life decisions (Kyoung, Landais, Kolahdooz, & Sharma, 2015). Research suggests such gang formation, too, has its roots in the legacy of aggressive assimilation and colonization, as well as the challenges of adapting to contemporary society, and a lack of positive coping mechanisms (Mercredi, 2015).

National Efforts to Make Amends and Support Recovery from the IRS System

In 1996, the Canadian government published the report of the *Royal Commission on Aboriginal Peoples (RCAP): People to people, nation to nation* (Government of Canada, 2010) with recommendations about a wide range of social and economic issues. As less than 1% of health care workers in Canada are of Aboriginal ancestry, affecting the provision of health services to this population, it was recommended this number be increased. Federal and provincial initiatives were implemented.

In 1998, the Indian Affairs Minister, Jane Stewart, apologized to Aboriginal people in Canada for the IRS system, announcing a $350-million healing fund (O'Hara & Treble, 2000). The fund's mandate was to "encourage and support Aboriginal people in building and supporting sustainable healing processes that address the legacy of physical and sexual abuse in the residential school system, including intergenerational impacts" (Waldram, Herring, & Young, 2006, p. 19). The 2002 report of the Commission on the Future of Health Care in Canada, the Romanow Report, addressed the necessity for health care and policy improvements for Aboriginal populations, including importance of transferring responsibilities to Aboriginal people for the management and delivery of their health care.

Then, in September 2007, the largest class action settlement in Canadian history, the IRSs Settlement Agreement, came into effect, recognizing the damage inflicted by the IRS system and establishing a multibillion-dollar fund to help former students in their recovery. It has five main components: Common Experience Payment, Independent Assessment Process, the Truth and Reconciliation Commission (TRC), Commemoration, and Health and Healing Services (Government of Canada, 2016). Health Canada (2013) and Aboriginal Affairs and Northern Development Canada (2013) have developed a series of services to support IRS survivors and their families.

In 2008, the government of Canada apologized to Indigenous people for the harmful effects of assimilation policies that resulted in the IRS system (King, Smith, & Gracey, 2009). In 2009, the TRC (2015) began a 5-year process of gathering and preserving information from former students and their families about the effects of

IRS system to ensure Canadian society recognized what happened and its long-term impact and to support reconciliation with Aboriginal people. The TRC records are housed at the University of Manitoba.

Aboriginal Health Care in Canada

Diversity of social, economic, and political circumstances among Aboriginal communities means that there are many different approaches to health and healing. Many people are raised to believe that the body is governed by four elements comprising the spiritual, emotional, mental, and physical. Traditionally, Aboriginal people have a holistic view of health, based on ways of knowing and being, wherein mental health is considered a part.

Aboriginal Mental Health

To be ill, including mentally ill, is to be out of balance in one of these elements (Douglas, 2013). The holistic view of health goes beyond the four identified elements to include the value of the collective group over the individual, an approach contrary to individualistic Western thinking (Little Bear, 2012). Notions of sanity and insanity and of personality disorders are not defined. These differences in views may present challenges to Aboriginal people accessing care and in caregiver's delivery of care, including system barriers such as institutional policy.

A literature review of Indigenous knowledge (Marsh, Coholic, Cote-Meek, & Najavits, 2015) reveals that most Indigenous scholars propose that the wellness of an Aboriginal community can only be adequately measured from within an Indigenous knowledge framework that is holistic, inclusive, and respectful of the balance between the spiritual, emotional, physical, and social realms of life. Treatment interventions need to honour the historical context and history of Aboriginal people. Cultural identity, community involvement, and empowerment are seen as important to health outcomes.

The Indian Act, 1876

The Indian Act of 1876 is the only national-level legislative act for First Nations still in effect. It ascribes health and health care of Aboriginal people to the federal government, while nonaboriginal health care is under provincial purview (Richmond & Cook, 2016). [It also established the IRS system.] It formalized the reserve system, assigning financial responsibility and power over band administration, education, and health care to the federal government (Boksa, Joober, & Kirmayer, 2015).

Health Services to Aboriginal Populations

During the time of early settlement and once the Indian Act of 1876 was signed, the Canadian government felt a moral and obligatory responsibility to the health of those considered Status Indian (Dempsey & Gottesman,

2011; Reading, 2015). It was reinforced with an increase in diseases and a belief that assimilation (from the Latin *assimilationem*, "similarity"; taking into the community) was the only way to guarantee good health (Reading, 2015), along with the signing of Treaty 6 in which the government guaranteed "to provide medicine" (Douglas, 2013, p. 84). The responsibility of Aboriginal health services has been shuffled through different departments since 1904: from the "Department of Indian Affairs" to the "Medical Services Branch," which changed names in 2000 to the "First Nations and Inuit Health Branch" (Government of Canada, 2007). The NCCAH (2011a) suggested that due to the lack of clarity within the Indian Act, in combination with the British North America Act, which assigned health to provincial control and Indian Affairs to federal control, the health of Aboriginal people at times falls between cracks in health services.

Indigenization of Curricula

Curriculum changes in schools to teach younger generations about the IRS system have been introduced, using resource guides prepared by First Nations educators, to ensure that all generations understand the historical context of residential schools and to develop students' awareness about the reconciliation process (First Nations Education Steering Committee, 2017). This is a response, in part, to a call from the TRC, which called, too, upon Canadian medical and nursing schools to have a required course on Aboriginal health issues. Such a course should include the history and legacy of residential schools and Indigenous teachings and practices. The *United Nations Declaration on the Rights of Indigenous People*, as well as other treaties and documents pertaining to Aboriginal rights, need to be in the curriculum, as do skills in intercultural competency, conflict resolution, human rights, and antiracism. Although nursing curricula have had some Indigenous content, including elective courses on Aboriginal health (Kent-Wilkinson, 2017), for the TRC call to be answered, more must be achieved.

Trauma-Informed Care in Services

Trauma-informed care (TIC) has evolved in Canadian health services as a means of establishing a safe environment for all patients, impacted by historical violence such as residential schooling (Browne & Baker, 2016; see Chapter 17).

Mental Health Strategy for Canada

Canada's first national mental health strategy, Changing Directions, Changing Lives: Mental Health Strategy for Canada, 2012 (MHCC, 2012), identifies six strategic directions, including one focused on Aboriginal mental health, with First Nations, Métis, and Inuit people each identified as separate priorities. Aboriginal rural, urban, and remote challenges and social determinants of health issues are prioritized.

Strength-Based Approach

Government policies related to Aboriginal populations have too often used a deficit- or problem-focused approach (Paraschak & Thompson, 2013). Such an approach identifies barriers to good health without identifying strengths. Aboriginal people, however, culturally focus on strengths, bringing resilience to the forefront (Graham & Martin, 2016). Ensuring a strength-based focus is taken with Aboriginal patients is important to the provision of culturally safe care (Douglas, 2013).

STEREOTYPING, PREJUDICE, DISCRIMINATION, AND STIGMA

It can be challenging for one cultural group to understand the values, beliefs, and patterns of accepted behaviour of a different cultural group. This can be especially true regarding mental illness. Some cultures view mental health disorders as a condition for which the ill person must be punished or ostracized from society; other cultures believe that family and community members are key to the care and treatment of persons with mental illness.

The effects of mental illness reach beyond the individual with the illness; mental health conditions, including addictions, also impact families, communities, and health care systems. Mental illness indirectly affects all Canadians through family members, friends, and colleagues. Families may become casualties under the stress of caring for acutely mentally ill relatives, especially within a rejecting community. Thus, the concepts of stereotyping, prejudice, discrimination, and stigma are important in understanding the lives of people with mental disorders, their families, and cultural groups. They are important to this "global, multifaceted problem" (Gronholm, Henderson, Deb, & Thornicroft, 2017, p. 1341).

Stereotyping

Stereotyping is expecting individuals to act in a characteristic manner that conforms, most often, to a negative perception of their cultural group. It occurs because of lack of exposure to sufficient members of the group in question. Media representations of people with mental illness (e.g., movies, television, magazines, and newspapers) help perpetuate negative stereotypes of those with this type of medical disorder. When stereotyping occurs by health care practitioners, patients and families are put at risk. Not only will they not be culturally safe, but their care will be put in jeopardy. Stereotyping associated with Aboriginal culture can create barriers to access, resulting in poor health outcomes. For example, in Winnipeg, a man died in an emergency room as the hospital failed to provide him with medical care, assuming he was drunk or homeless rather than in need of medical care (Puxley,

2014). (See Critical Thinking Challenges on thePoint for the Media Case Study, *Stereotyping, Discrimination, Stigma: Alcohol and Aboriginal Peoples*.)

Prejudice

Prejudice is a hostile attitude toward others simply because they belong to a group that is considered to have objectionable characteristics. Everyone has some biases and prejudices, but health care personnel need to acknowledge and examine their biases in preparation for safe, competent, compassionate, and ethical care for all patients and families. If they do not address their biases in a meaningful way, their ability to form trusting, healing relationships will be affected.

Discrimination

Discrimination is the negative differential treatment of others because they are members of a certain group or identified as being negatively different. Discrimination can include ignoring, derogatory name-calling, denying services, and threatening. Discrimination arises from a lack of understanding and appreciation of differences among people, but it can be overcome.

Nurses, too, can experience subtle discrimination from patients and families; patients may express a desire to have a nurse "more like them" assigned to their care. Alberta Pasco's (2004) study of Filipino Canadians' experience of hospital care found that her participants initially desired nurses who were "one of us" (*hindi ibang tao*). However, non-Filipino nurses became "one of us" as the patient came to know the nurse as a caring person who was kind, respectful, and trustworthy.

KEY CONCEPT

Discrimination is negative differential treatment of others because they are members of a certain group or identified as being negatively different.

Stigma

Stigma is negative, discriminatory, and rejecting attitudes and behaviour toward a characteristic or element exhibited by an individual or group. It can occur at three levels: self, public, and structural (MHCC, 2013a). The stigma of mental illness is evident across history (see Chapter 1) and still exists as a significant and problematic issue. Self-stigma occurs when a person with a mental health illness internalizes the negative views of others and feels ashamed about their illness. This not only seriously diminishes their sense of self-worth but can prevent them from seeking help. Public stigma is influenced by cultural misbeliefs about those with mental illness: they will never recover; they are dangerous, unpredictable, and violent; they should not be around other people; they are flawed as human beings. Such stigma is oppressive and alienating. It can act as a barrier in all aspects of life: housing, education, employment, and health care. The stigma of mental illness can affect families of persons with mental illness, as well. Their status in their community can be affected; they may be assigned blame for the illness of their family member. It can affect health professionals who choose to practice in psychiatric and mental health settings (Harrison & Hauck, 2017). Such a career choice can be silently queried: Lack of "real" skills? Personal psychological problems? It is evident in its effects upon recruitment and retention to this clinical area. Stigma occurring at the institutional level is evident when persons with mental illness are denied their basic rights. Bias against mental illness can also affect funding for health services and research. (See the *Movies and Other Things* feature on the-Point for the brief but poignant video, *We need to end the stigma about mental illness: You are not alone.*)

KEY CONCEPT

Stigma is negative, discriminatory, and rejecting attitudes and behaviour toward a characteristic or element exhibited by an individual or group. It can occur at three levels: self, public, and structural.

Reducing Stigma and Discrimination

The government of Canada's report, *Out of the Shadows at Last, 2006,* indicated that the stigma of mental illness pervades all levels of Canadian society (Standing Senate Committee on Social Affairs, Science and Technology, 2006). In response, the *Opening Minds* program was initiated by the MHCC in 2009 with the goal of changing Canadians' behaviours and attitudes toward mental illness and making the acknowledgment of having a mental health problem or disorder and the seeking mental health care more socially acceptable (MHCC, 2009, 2013a). *Opening Minds* promotes contact-based education that involves individuals with lived experience of mental illness sharing their experiences of illness and recovery. When possible, it builds on existing programs, sharing resources such as toolkits, and aims to replicate successful programs and best practices (MHCC, 2013a). Interventions to reduce the discrimination and stigma of mental illness are being conducted within many countries and globally. See Box 3.3 for *a Research for Best Practice* study of such interventions.

Triple Stigma in Corrections in Canada

In 2012, the *Mental Health Strategy for Corrections in Canada* pointed out the double stigmatization of having a mental illness and being an offender (Correctional Services Canada, 2012). A triple stigmatization has been since identified in a Saskatchewan needs assessment of mental health services in corrections: having a mental

---

BOX 3.3 Research for Best Practice

INTERVENTIONS TO REDUCE DISCRIMINATION AND STIGMA

Gronholm, P. C., Henderson, C., Deb, T., & Thornicroft, G. (2017). Interventions to reduce discrimination and stigma: The state of the art. Social Psychiatry Psychiatric Epidemiology, 52(3), 249–258. doi:10.1007/s00127-017-1341-9

Question: What is the evidence that interventions to reduce stigma and discrimination have a lasting impact?

Method: Narrative synthesis of systematic reviews published since 2012. Antistigma interventions were categorized in terms of *education* (replacing myths about mental illness with knowledge), *education and contact* (direct or indirect interactions with persons with mental illness), *mental health literacy* (increase knowledge of programs, improve attitudes, and stimulate helping behaviours), and *rights-based programs* (legal rights of people with mental illness). Example of intervention: *See Me in Scotland,* Scotland's antistigma and discrimination program.

Results: There is evidence for small to moderate positive impacts of mass media campaigns and of

interventions for targeted groups in terms of stigma-related knowledge, attitudes, and intended behaviour in terms of desire for contact. However, there is limited evidence regarding positive impacts lasting over the long term. There is evidence that interventions based on contact among targeted groups improved attitudes, but not necessarily changes in knowledge.

Implications: Experienced and anticipated discrimination/stigma in combination have very negative effects on persons with mental illness: poor access to mental and physical health care, reduced life expectancy, exclusion from higher education, exclusion from employment, increased risk of contact with criminal justice systems, victimization, poverty, and homelessness. For many people, these consequences have been described as worse than the experience of the mental illness itself. There is urgent need for proven, lasting interventions, as well as better evaluation methods for them.

illness, being an offender, and being Aboriginal by racial descent (Kent-Wilkinson et al., 2012a, 2012b).

Role of Nursing and Nursing Education

Every nursing student brings with them to their new profession the attitudes and beliefs of their family and culture. It can initially be a challenge to live fully up to the demand that "Nurses do not discriminate on the basis of a person's race, ethnicity, culture, political and spiritual beliefs, social or marital status, gender, gender identity, gender expression, sexual orientation, age, health status, place of origin, lifestyle, mental or physical ability, socio-economic status, or any other attribute" (CNA, 2017, p. 15). As a student gains clinical practice and gains experience in the role of nurse, this challenge becomes more easily met.

This approach is advocated by the Canadian Association of Schools of Nursing (CASN) and the Canadian Federation of Mental Health Nurses (CFMHN) in their joint publication, *Entry-to-Practice Mental Health and Addiction Competencies for Undergraduate Nursing Education* (CASN & CFMHN, 2015), and by the CFMHN's 2016 position paper on *Mental Health and Addiction Curriculum in Undergraduate Nursing Education in Canada* (Kent-Wilkinson et al., 2016) that the most effective response to increasing knowledge of mental health and disorder and decreasing the stigma of mental illness is to ensure evidence-informed nursing education through a significant increase of psychiatric mental health theory and practice in undergraduate nursing curricula.

▌ CULTURAL COMPETENCE AND CULTURAL SAFETY

Cultural competency and cultural safety are critical components of undergraduate and postgraduate education of health care practitioners, providing a foundation for what will be a continuous learning process. Opportunities for students to share their own cultural backgrounds with each other and to interact with various cultural groups are strategies that support the development of competence (Repo, Vahlberg, Salminen, Papadopoulos, & Leino-Kilpi, 2017).

Cultural Competence

Cultural competence is considered an entry-to-practice competence that is evident in quality practice environments and improves health outcomes. For nurses, it is the application of respect, equity, and cultural sensitivity and the valuing of diversity to the knowledge, skills, and attitudes required to provide appropriate care in relation to cultural characteristics of their clients. It is both process and outcome oriented (Alexander, 2008). Obtaining cultural competence is an ongoing, lifelong process, not an end.

Cultural competence starts with an appreciation of diversity and its influence on relationships and situations (CNA, 2010). Practitioner need to recognize the attributes of their own culture and the way in which it shapes their own beliefs and behaviours. Then there is need to acknowledge their knowledge deficits regarding the cultures of others. The CNA (2010) suggests that this part of cultural competence involves understanding **cultural diversity** through an "atmosphere of respect" (p. 1). As awareness, knowledge, and skill evolve, cultural competence develops (Purnell, 2016).

Exposure and face-to-face encounters, along with keeping an open mind to the individual's experiences, can contribute to this development. For instance, nurses can become culturally competent when working in Aboriginal communities by being open to learning about their culture, beliefs, and practices. They may participate in cultural ceremonies when invited, learn a few words of the language, gain knowledge of traditional events, and attend conferences or classes that focus on Aboriginal culture.

Cultural competence is particularly important to understanding the way in which culture is influencing perceptions of health needs and ensuring this understanding influences nursing practice. Cultural competence also involves collaborative approach with other specialists (CNA, 2014). Nurses not only act as advocates but also strive to promote accessible and culturally friendly services in the areas of health promotion and education (MHCC, 2016). Being culturally competent is a strategy in addressing racial and ethnic health disparities in healthcare by ensuring services are culturally safe and meeting patients' needs (McCalman, Jongen, & Bainbridge, 2017).

KEY CONCEPT

Cultural competence is "a set of consistent behaviors, attitudes, and policies that enable a system, agency or individual to work within a cross cultural context or situation" (Watt, Abbott, & Reath, 2016).

Cultural humility is a concept that is helpful in confronting persistent colonial ideas in mental health care. Cultural humility is defined as: "A lifelong commitment to self-evaluation and self-critique to redress power imbalances and to develop and maintain mutually respectful dynamic partnerships based on mutual trust" (Minkler & Wallerstein, 2008, p. 100). Cultural humility is a process of self-reflection and discovery to build honest and trustworthy relationships (Yeager & Bauer-Wu, 2013).

Cultural Safety

Cultural safety is both a process and an outcome whose goal is greater equity. Cultural safety focuses on root causes of "power imbalances and inequitable social relationships in health care" (Browne et al., 2009, p. 168) and promotes integrity, social justice, and respect (McGough, Wynaden, & Wright, 2017). It is composed of three components: cultural awareness, cultural sensitivity, and cultural competence (CNA, 2010; Registered Nurses Association of Ontario, 2007). Cultural competence cannot fully address health care inequities. Cultural safety, however, goes beyond cultural awareness and sensitivity to examining power differentials in health care services (Richardson, Yarwood, & Richardson, 2016); it addresses the causes of inequities (CNA, 2010). For example, research in British Columbia, involving ethnographic interviews with four Aboriginal organizations and one health authority, as well as a critical review of policies, determined that cultural safety was undermined by dominant approaches to decision-making and funding that were shaped by social history and politics. This study supported the shift to delivery models that are "by Indigenouts for Indigenous" (Josewski, 2012).

Aboriginal people commonly have had negative experiences within Canada's health care system, shaped by their marginalization from the development of dominant care systems (Hole, Evans, Berg, & Smith, 2015). Providing culturally safe care to patients and families in our multicultural society is necessary to the fostering health and wellness in our communities.

KEY CONCEPT

Cultural safety grows from an analysis of power imbalances and institutional discrimination, related to health and health care, in order that the root causes of health inequities can be addressed. It is composed of three components: cultural awareness, cultural sensitivity, and cultural competence (CNA, 2010; RNAO, 2007).

Health care practitioners, the institution, and the patient are all key players in the creation and maintenance of cultural safety as a reciprocal process. Each accommodates the other's values and culture within the clinical setting (Douglas, 2013). Many health care organizations are insufficiently equipped to provide cultural safety, given that it requires engagement with communities, including Aboriginal people, immigrants, and refugees. Such engagement allows a space to be created in which patients and families feel safe to be open and express their concerns.

Strategies a health care organization can implement include the provision of information and training sessions on cultural safety, individual practitioners (or a team) choosing to learn more about a specific cultural group (NCCAH, 2013), and the use of cultural brokers, persons knowledgeable about a culture, its language, and the health care organization, who offer guidance and assistance in patient care situations.

SOCIOECONOMIC CONTEXT OF MENTAL HEALTH CARE

Socioeconomic circumstances influence our health status. Factors such as income and social status, social support networks, education, employment and working conditions, physical environment, and available health services affect one's well-being. Poverty is no longer a problem of developing regions only; it is on the rise in developed countries (UN Development Programme [UNDP], 2016). Although Canada has consistently ranked in the top five on the UN Human Development Index, it has slipped to 10th place (UNDP, 2016). The well-being of Aboriginal people in Canada plays a role in this. In 2014, the report of the UN Special Rapporteur on the rights of Indigenous peoples regarding Canada noted that Canada has yet to close the well-being gap between Aboriginal people and other Canadians. Urgent action, he stated, was needed to address a housing crisis and to provide sufficient funding for education, health care, and child welfare; better coordination in the delivery of services was required (Anaya, 2014).

Poorer socioeconomic circumstances and social exclusion can increase the likelihood of adopting unhealthy or risky behaviours and create feelings of hopelessness and helplessness among those affected and vulnerable (Statistics Canada, 2013, para 12). Vulnerable groups are groups in society who are "systematically disadvantaged in a way that leads to a risk of emotional or physical harm; in health care, harms are related to diminished health and well-being" (Oberle & Raffin Bouchal, 2009, as cited in CNA, 2017, p. 27).

Social Determinants of Health

Social determinants of health are defined as "the conditions in which peoples are born, grow, live, work, and age, including the health system. These circumstances are shaped by the distribution of money, power and resources at global, national or local levels, which are themselves influenced by policy choices" (World Health Organization, 2017a, para 1). Healthy child development is among the most important determinants of health. Preconception to the age of six is a critical time for a child's brain development, as positive stimulation during these years influences learning, behaviour, and health into adulthood, as well as a child's sense of identity (Douglas, 2013; McIvor, 2009).

Poverty

Poverty is associated with the undermining of a range of key human attributes, including health. The poor are exposed to greater personal and environmental health risks, are less well nourished, have less information, and are less able to access health care; they thus have a higher risk of illness and disability. Conversely, illness can reduce household savings, lower learning ability, reduce productivity, and lead to a diminished quality of life, thereby perpetuating or even increasing poverty (World Health Organization, 2017b). The poorest of the poor around the world have the worst health. Within countries, the evidence shows that in general, the lower an individual's socioeconomic position, the worse their health (WHO, 2017a).

Poverty creates hopelessness (endpoverty.org, 2017). In the day-to-day lives of the very poor, poverty becomes a network of disadvantages. The result is generation after generation of people who lack access to education, health care, adequate housing, proper sanitation, and good nutrition. They are the most vulnerable to disasters, armed conflict, and systems of political and economic oppression, and they are powerless to improve their circumstances. These conditions often carry with them dysfunctional family and societal relationships, paralyzingly low self-esteem, mental health problems, and spiritual darkness.

KEY CONCEPT

Poverty is the lack of income and access to essential goods and services, housing, and employment required to meet the necessities of life relative to one's society.

Poverty and Mental Health

Poverty and mental health (as well as overall health) are linked such that "the lower an individual's socioeconomic status, the worse their health" and vice versa (WHO, 2017b). Understanding this relationship is key to addressing poverty, promoting mental health, and supporting the recovery of persons with mental illness. For persons who are poor and predisposed to developing a mental illness, a loss of income, employment, and housing can increase the chance of their becoming mentally ill or, if recovered, of relapsing. Further, developing a mental illness can seriously interrupt a person's education or career path, leading to fewer and less secure employment opportunities and, correspondingly, a lower income. As a result, a drift into poverty can occur, particularly for those with a recurrent mental illness. (See Chapter 2 re: homelessness and the mentally ill.)

Investment in Mental Health

The economic burden of mental health and addiction in Canada is estimated at $51 billion per year. This cost to the Canadian economy includes health care dollars spent, lost productivity, and reductions in health-related quality of life (MHCC, 2013b; Mood Disorders Society of Canada [MDSC], 2014). If one in five Canadians lives with a mental health or an addiction problem, then 20% of the health care budget is needed to address this reality. Nurses must be prepared to provide preventative mental health education to reduce the increasing costs associated with mental health conditions as well as to promote quality of life (Kent-Wilkinson et al., 2016).

Strong evidence for the value of mental health interventions comes from work with children and youth in such areas as conduct disorders, depression, parenting, and suicide awareness and prevention (Roberts & Grimes, 2011). Nurses prepared in mental health assessment and care of children and youth can thus serve as an investment in the mental health (Kent-Wilkinson et al., 2016; see Chapters 29 and 30). Work is being done to examine what is needed for the future. *Life and Economic Impact of Major Mental Illnesses in Canada* is an examination of the economic impact of major mental illnesses in Canada, beginning in 2011 and annually over the next three decades (Smetanin et al., 2011). In 2011, the direct cost of mental illness was $42.3 billion and, indirectly, $6.3 billion. By 2041, it is predicted that costs will be magnified due to an increase in the number of those with mental illness (due to population growth and aging). In 2016, *Mental Health Now! Advancing the Mental Health of Canadians: The Federal Role*, prepared by the Canadian Alliance on Mental Illness and Mental Health (CAMIMH, 2016), identified five recommendations to improve access to mental health care for Canadians: increase federal funding for access to mental health services to 25% of the total cost; create a Mental Health Innovation Fund to support mental health care innovation; measure and monitor mental health by creating pan-Canadian indicators; establish an expert advisory panel; and invest in social infrastructure. Such work, along with Canada's mental health strategy, is contributing to the improvement of mental health care.

Socioeconomic Influences on Aboriginal Mental Health

Aboriginal health in Canada is impacted by 13 determinants of health, but the social support determinant is one that affects both the individual and the community. The well-being of individuals can be shaped by relationships, and the caring and respect involved (Douglas, 2013). Relationships assist in safeguarding against both physical and mental illnesses, by providing "feelings of belonging and being cared for, loved, respected and valued" (NCCAH, 2012, p. 38). Many traditional Aboriginal societies have strong family and community supports, which can offer a sense of social inclusion and, therefore, improve recovery rates when illness does occur (Douglas, 2013). Aboriginal heritage and geographic location are also factors affecting this social support determinant, as there are many access inequities within this population that influence individual and community health. (See Box 3.4.)

Poverty and Aboriginal Mental Health

As poverty rates are high among Aboriginal populations, poor mental health is also common. Approximately "60% of First Nation children on reserves live in poverty" (Kirkup, 2016), while 40% of Aboriginal children living off reserves do so (NCCAH, 2010). Children who are born into poverty are at higher risk for negative outcomes of low birth weight, learning disabilities, mental health problems, burns and injuries, and other health conditions such as asthma, obesity, and iron deficiency anaemia (Conroy, Sandel, & Zuckerman, 2010). Poverty is linked, as well, to violence (Douglas, 2013). Children who are exposed to violence, especially from loved ones, and experience attachment issues are more likely to participate in acts of violence as adults, creating a cycle of violence (Macinnes, Macpherson, Austin, & Schwannauer, 2016). Children learn to internalize their environments, assume them as normal, and pass such experiences along to their own children (Douglas, 2013).

Disparities in Mental Health Outcomes

There are substantial differences among Aboriginal communities, including in relation to mental health issues. Suicide rates reported within Aboriginal populations, however, are, in general, double that of the rest of the Canadian population (Crawford, 2016). Suicide rates

are five to seven times higher for First Nations youth as for nonaboriginal youth; Inuit youth have rates among the highest in the world, at 11 times the national average (Health Canada, 2016). Aboriginal alcohol-related deaths are nearly twice that of nonaboriginal Canadians (43.7 vs. 23.6 per 100,000), with Aboriginal youth at two to six times at greater risk for alcohol-related problems than their nonaboriginal counterparts (Russell et al., 2016). Fetal alcohol spectrum disorders (FASD) in Aboriginal women is found to be about 16 times higher than in the general public (Popova, Lange, Probst, Parunashvili, & Rehn, 2017).

Factors that create **health disparity** between Aboriginal peoples and the general Canadian population include reduced and impeded access to health services. The lack of clarity on whom delivers health services and whom is responsible financially can be a barrier to accessing treatment (NCCAH, 2011a, 2011b, 2011c; Richmond & Cook, 2016). This barrier has led to limited health services, resulting for some in death (Douglas, 2013). Significant gaps still exist in primary care on reserves, despite significant financial investment in millions of dollars. Such gaps were made highly visible in the case of an Aboriginal boy that resulted in *Jordan's Principle*. Jordan River Anderson was a child with complex medical needs, who was hospitalized and unable to access home care due to a dispute between the federal and Manitoba governments over allocation of home care costs. Jordan died at age five, in hospital. Jordan's Principle, passed in December 2007, calls on the government of first contact to pay for services and seek reimbursement later so no child's health and well-being is tangled in red tape (Blackstock, 2012). The Canadian Human Rights Tribunal in 2016 ordered the federal government to implement the full scope of Jordan's Principle (Galloway, 2017). (See the Media Case Study, *Jordan's Principle*, in Critical Thinking Challenges on the Point.)

Other factors of health disparity include the negative impacts on healthy child development due to intergenerational trauma and the negative impacts of colonization on aboriginal cultural identity (Aguiar & Halseth, 2015; Douglas, 2013). The diverse nature of factors that create health disparities indicates that addressing health inequities cannot be achieved by the health sector alone but needs a collaborative, multisectoral approach (Reading & Halseth, 2013).

Role of Nursing and Health Care Professionals

Nurses are responsible to maintain "an awareness of major health concerns, such a *poverty*, inadequate shelters, food insecurity and violence, while working for *social justice* (individually and with others) and advocating for laws, policies and procedures that bring about equity" (CNA, 2017, p. 19). Social justice is defined as "the fair distribution of society's benefits and responsibilities and

---

BOX 3.4 Determinants of Health in Analyzing Aboriginal Health in Canada

1. Income and Social Status
2. Social Support Systems
3. Education and Literacy
4. Employment and Working Conditions
5. Social Environment
6. Personal Health Practices
7. Healthy Child Development
8. Biology and Genetic Endowment
9. Health Services
10. Gender
11. Culture
12. Physical Environment
13. Ecosystem Health

Douglas, V. (2013). *Introduction to Aboriginal health and health care in Canada: Bridging health and healing.* New York, NY: Springer Publishing Company.

their consequences. Social justice focuses on the relative position of one social group in relations to others in society as well as on the root causes of disparities and what can be done to eliminate them" (CNA, 2017, p. 26).

Mental illness puts a person at greater risk for poverty and homelessness, which, in turn, places serious constraints on regaining and maintaining health. While addressing poverty and homelessness is outside the realm of health care systems, nurses should be aware of their impact on mental health and be able to identify relevant policy changes that could be enacted in both public and private spheres (MHCC, 2012).

GEOGRAPHIC CONTEXT OF MENTAL HEALTH CARE

Although comprehensiveness, universality, portability, and accessibility are key components of the *Canada Health Act* (Government of Canada, 2017b), getting mental health services to rural and remote communities continues to be a challenge. Most mental health services are in urban areas, with access for people in the far North being very different from that of people living in the more highly populated areas of Canada. All age groups in rural and remote areas have limited access to health care, but the lack of resources is particularly problematic for children and older adults, who have specialized needs.

"Rural" is defined by Statistics Canada (2017a) as an area with a population of under 1,000 people and a population density of less than 400 inhabitants per square kilometre. The rural population of Canada has been declining since 1851, when nine in ten Canadians lived in rural areas (Statistics Canada, 2017b). Today, more than 80% of Canadians live in metropolitan areas, with over one in three Canadians living in Toronto, Montréal, or Vancouver (Statistics Canada, 2017c).

"Remoteness" involves a community's proximity to other places and services, such as health services, with proximity being measured by such metrics as travel time and travel cost (Alasia, Bédard, Bélanger, Guimond, & Penney, 2017). Figure 3.1 is a map of the geographic distribution of accessibility to health services in Canada. Many remote communities are home to aboriginal people. Health care services in remote communities have a strong focus on prevention; utilize smaller, integrated teams with a broad scope of practice; and look to visiting services for specialized treatment (Wakerman, Bourker, Humphreys, & Taylor, 2017). Being the second largest country in the world with a diverse population of under 36 million requires ongoing dedication and innovation in the provision of health care.

Availability, accessibility, acceptability, and quality of health services are key elements of the right to health (UN Committee on Economic, Social and Cultural Rights, 2000). (See Fig. 3.2.) These elements are useful in considering health services in rural and remote communities in Canada. This discussion focuses on the first three elements: availability, accessibility, and acceptability.

Availability

Nurses and nurse practitioners (NPs) play key roles in making health care available in rural and remote areas or in Canada's north, where the nursing station is often

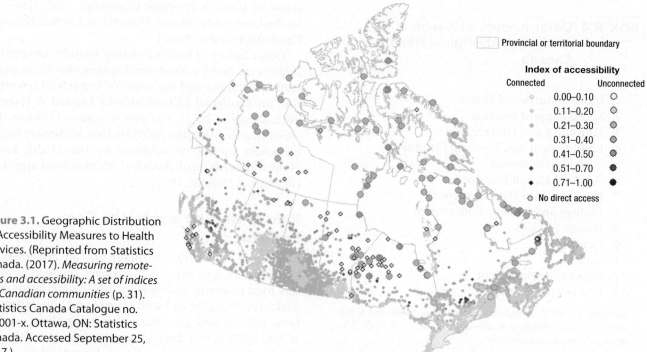

Figure 3.1. Geographic Distribution of Accessibility Measures to Health Services. (Reprinted from Statistics Canada. (2017). *Measuring remoteness and accessibility: A set of indices for Canadian communities* (p. 31). Statistics Canada Catalogue no. 18-001-x. Ottawa, ON: Statistics Canada. Accessed September 25, 2017.)

Provincial or territorial boundary

Index of accessibility

Connected		Unconnected
◇	0.00–0.10	○
◦	0.11–0.20	○
◦	0.21–0.30	○
●	0.31–0.40	○
●	0.41–0.50	○
●	0.51–0.70	●
●	0.71–1.00	●
◌	No direct access	

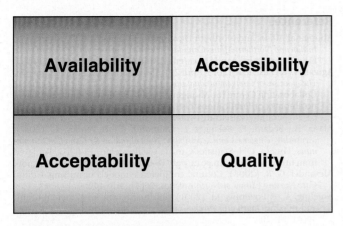

Figure 3.2. Elements of the right to health.

the first point of contact and nurses may be the only health care professionals and thus the primary health care providers. Nurses may be required to work outside their scope of practice in certain circumstances in order to provide essential services and need to have supportive mechanisms in place to authorize them to do so (Auditor General of Canada, 2015). They may act as advocates, collaborators, or mediators in encouraging the development of public policies and resources for their region.

For persons with mental health problems or mental illness, including addiction, a shared care approach to services may be used in which specialists support the integration of mental health services in primary care (Kates et al., 2011). The Canadian Collaborative Mental Health Initiative provides a "Rural and Isolated Toolkit" to support such collaboration (Haggarty, Ryan-Nicholls, & Jarva, 2010).

Accessibility

Transportation is a major barrier to the receipt of health services in rural areas. Costs of travel and accommodation for patients and families can be high, in dollars and energy. Services should be delivered in communities where possible, but the small population of some rural communities can be a deterrent. As well, specialized services are in large urban centres. Mobile service delivery and specialist circuits are options used to address this issue.

Persons with severe and persistent mental illness may be able to remain within their community if such approach is used, providing they have sufficient social support and continuing access to services. Local health care situations are shaped by their own unique social and structural factors, which need to be addressed if availability is to be optimized (Fitzpatrick, Perkins, Luland, Brown, & Corvan, 2017). Despite shared care approaches, access to care can be a serious problem. A Canadian needs assessment survey of rural/remote physicians regarding access to child and adolescent mental

health services revealed that there are issues with long waiting lists, a lack of child/adolescent psychiatrists, and the need of other disciplinary services (e.g., paediatricians, psychologists, and social workers). System issues, such as a need for a more systematized, transparent referral process, were also noted (Zayed et al., 2016).

Telehealth (e.g., telepsychiatry) is an effective tool that can reduce wait times and travel time and costs. Telehealth is the use of electronic information and communication technologies to support health care services over distance. It ranges from the retrieval of laboratory results or other health records posted on a network to the direct assessment and treatment of an individual by primary care providers to consultation with specialists through videoconferencing. In fact, in specialized care through telehealth, mental health is a top area of consultation (Caxaj, 2016).

Acceptability

In rural and remote areas, there may be a lack of information regarding mental health and psychiatric care. Help-seeking behaviours may be affected by an expectation that one should be self-reliant and independent. As well, social and cultural aspects of a community can increase risk for mental health stigma and diminish anonymity. First Nations people may be unable to find health services that they find culturally appropriate (Caxaj, 2016). The high staff turnover that tends to exist in health services in remote communities can impede the ability of practitioners to engage in the community and establish trusting relationships, essential to working within rural and remote communities (Davy, Hartfield, McArthur, Munn, & Brown, 2016).

While preparation for nursing in remote areas usually involves mandatory advanced life support training, adequate preparation for mental health care seems essential, as well. NPs, for instance, should be skilled in this area (Creamer & Austin, 2017). A survey study of NPs across Canada revealed that the majority of NPs would like more theoretical and/or clinical preparation in mental health. They rated their existing mental health educational preparation at a mean of 2.6 on a scale of 1 to 5, with "5" equaling "very well prepared" (Creamer, Mill, Austin, & O'Brien, 2014).

Geographic location remains a significant factor in the challenge to provide mental health services to all Canadians who require them. Technologic innovations can make a positive difference, but attention must continue to be paid to the social and cultural aspects of mental health care and to the sufficient preparation of health professionals in mental health care.

🍁 SUMMARY OF KEY POINTS

- *Culture* is defined as a way of life that manifests the learned beliefs, values, and accepted behaviours that are transmitted socially within a specific group.

- Religious beliefs are closely intertwined with beliefs about health and mental illness.
- There are many Indigenous cultures in Canada, with unique heritages, languages, cultural practices, and spiritual beliefs. Treatment interventions need to honour the historical context and history of Aboriginal people.
- Cultural identity, community involvement, and empowerment can be important to health outcomes.
- Stigmatization occurs as a result of prejudice, discrimination, and stereotyping. Cultural groups and people with mental illness are often stigmatized.
- Cultural safety consists of cultural awareness, cultural sensitivity, and cultural competence. It is an obligation of all Canadian nurses.
- Mental health services should be integrated as completely as possible into the helping systems currently accepted by the culture.
- Access to mental health treatment is particularly limited for those living in rural, remote, and northern areas or for those living in poverty.
- The four key elements of the right to health care are availability, accessibility, acceptability, and quality.

 Web Links

camimh.ca *The Canadian Alliance on Mental Illness and Mental Health (CAMIMH)* is Canada's largest mental health advocacy group. It is an alliance of mental health organizations composed of health care providers as well as of the mentally ill and their families.

cmha.ca *The Canadian Mental Health Association (CMHA)* is a national voluntary organization that promotes mental health and serves consumers and others through education, public awareness, research, advocacy, and direct services.

disabilityrightsintl.org/ *Disability Rights International (DRI)* is an advocacy organization dedicated to the recognition and enforcement of rights of people with mental disabilities.

mentalhealthcommission.ca *The Mental Health Commission of Canada (MHCC)* is a nonprofit organization created to focus national attention on mental health issues, to work to improve the mental health of Canadians, and to reduce the stigma associated with this disease.

www.shared-care.ca/ This website of the Canadian Collaborative Mental Health Initiative has toolkits that are useful to health care professionals.

statcan.gc.ca/daily-quotidien/130508/dq130508b-eng. htm?HPA The 2011 National Household Survey: Immigration, place of birth, citizenship, ethnic origin, visible minorities, language, and religion in Canada can be found at this site.

wfmh.org *The World Federation for Mental Health (WFMH)* is the only international, multidisciplinary, grassroots advocacy and education mental health organization.

who.int/about/en The World Health Organization (WHO) is the United Nations agency for health. The objective set out in its constitution is the attainment, by all peoples, of the highest possible level of health.

References

Aboriginal Affairs and Northern Development Canada. (2013). *A history of Indian and Northern Affairs Canada. Government of Canada.* Retrieved from http://www.aadnc-aandc.gc.ca/eng/1314977281262/1314977321448

Aguiar, W., & Halseth, R. (2015, April 29). *Aboriginal peoples and historic trauma: The processes of intergenerational transmission.* Prince George, BC: National Collaborating Centre for Aboriginal Health. Retrieved from http://www.nccah-ccnsa.ca/Publications/Lists/Publications/Attachments/142/2015-04-28-alexanderHalseth-RPT-IntergenTraumaHistory-EN-Web.pdf

Alasia, A., Bédard, F., Bélanger, J., Guimond, G., & Penney, C. (2017). *Measuring remoteness and accessibility: A set of indices for Canadian communities.* Ottawa, ON: Statistics Canada Catalogue no. 18-001-x. Retrieved from http://www.statcan.gc.ca/pub/18-001-x/18-001-x2017002-eng.pdf

Alexander, G. R. (2008). Cultural competence models in nursing. *Critical Care Nursing Clinics of North America, 20*(4), 415–442.

Ameling, A., & Povilonis, M. (2001). Spirituality, meaning, mental health and nursing. *Journal of Psychosocial Nursing and Mental Health Services, 39*(4), 14–20.

American Psychiatric Association. (1994). *Diagnostic and statistical manual of mental disorders* (DSM-IV, 4th ed.). Washington, DC: Author.

American Psychiatric Association. (2013a). *Cultural concepts in DSM-5.* Arlington, VA: American Psychiatric Publishing. Retrieved from http://www.psychiatry.org/File%20Library/Practice/DSM/DSM-5/Cultural-Concepts-in-DSM-5.pdf

American Psychiatric Association. (2013b). *Diagnostic and statistical manual of mental disorders* (DSM-5, 5th ed.). Arlington, VA: American Psychiatric Publishing.

Anaya, J. (2014, July 4). *Report of the Special Rapporteur on the rights of indigenous peoples.* New York, NY: Human Rights Council, UN General Assembly. Retrieved from http://unsr.jamesanaya.org/docs/countries/2014-report-canada-a-hrc-27-52-add-2-en.pdf

Auditor General of Canada. (2015, Spring). *Report 4: Access to health services for remote First Nations communities.* Retrieved from http://www.oag-bvg.gc.ca/internet/English/parl_oag_201504_04_e_40350.html#hd3a

Blackstock, C. (2012, August). Jordan's Principle: Canada's broken promise to First Nations children? *Pediatric Child Health, 17*(7), 368–370. Retrieved from https://www.ncbi.nlm.nih.gov/pmc/articles/PMC3448536/

Blanch, A. (2007). Integrating religion and spirituality in mental health: The promise and the challenge. *Psychiatric Rehabilitation Journal, 30*(4), 251–260.

BlogTO. (2016, May 15). *Toronto named the most diverse city on the world.* Retrieved from http://www.blogto.com/city/2016/05/toronto_named_most_diverse_city_in_the_world/

Boksa, P., Jooper, R., & Kirmayer, L. J. (2015). Mental wellness in Canada's Aboriginal communities: Striving toward reconciliation. *Journal of Psychiatry and Neuroscience, 40*(6), 363–365. doi:10.1503/jpn.150309

Brascoupé, S., & Waters, C. (2009). Cultural safety: Exploring the applicability of the concept of cultural safety to Aboriginal health and community wellness. *Journal of Aboriginal Health, 5*(2), 6–41.

Browne, S. M., & Baker, C. N. (2016). Measuring trauma-informed care: The attitudes related to trauma-informed care (ARTIC) Scale. *Trauma Psychology News, 12*(1). Retrieved from http://traumapsychnews.com/2016/03/measuring-trauma-informed-care-the-attitudes-related-to-trauma-informed-care-artic-scale/

Browne, A. J., Varcoe, C., Smye, V., Reimer-Kirkham, S., Lynam, M. J., & Wong, S. (2009). Cultural safety and the challenges of translating critically oriented knowledge in practice. *Nursing Philosophy, 10*(3), 167–179.

Canadian Alliance on Mental Health and Mental Illness. (2016, September 6). *Mental health now! Advancing the mental health of Canadians: The federal role.* Ottawa, ON: Author. Retrieved from http://www.camimh.ca/wp-content/uploads/2016/09/CAMIMH_MHN_EN_Final_small.pdf

Canadian Association of Schools of Nursing & Canadian Federation of Mental Health Nurses. (2015). *Entry-to-practice mental health and addiction competencies for undergraduate nursing education.* Ottawa, ON: Author. Retrieved from http://www.casn.ca/wpcontent/uploads/2015/11/Mental-health-Competencies_EN_FINAL-3-Oct-26-2015.pdf

Canadian Magazine of Immigration. (2016, November 26). *Religion in Canada.* Retrieved from http://canadaimmigrants.com/religions-in-canada/

Canadian Medical Protective Association. (2014). *When medicine and culture intersect.* Retrieved from https://www.cmpa-acpm.ca/en/advice-publications/browse-articles/2014/when-medicine-and-culture-intersect

Canadian Museum of Immigration at Pier 21. (2017). *Canadian multiculturalism policy, 1971.* Retrieved from http://www.pier21.ca/research/immigration-history/canadian-multiculturalism-policy-1971

Canadian Nurses Association. (2010). *Promoting cultural competence in nursing [Position statement].* Retrieved from http://www.cna-aiic.ca/~/

media/cna/page%20content/pdf%20en/2013/07/26/10/37/ps114_cultural_competence_2010_e.pdf

Canadian Nurse's Association. (2014). *Aboriginal health nursing and Aboriginal health: Charting policy direction for nursing in Canada.* Retrieved from https://www.cna-aiic.ca/~/media/cna/page-content/pdf-en/aboriginal-health-nursing-and-aboriginal-health_charting-policy-direction-for-nursing-in-canada.pdf?la=en

Canadian Nurses Association. (2017). *Code of ethics for registered nurses.* Ottawa, ON: Author. Retrieved from https://www.cna-aiic.ca/html/en/Code-of-Ethics-2017-Edition/index.html

Caxaj, C. S. (2016). A review of mental health approaches for rural communities: Complexities and opportunities in the Canadian context. *Canadian Journal of Community Mental Health, 35*(1), 29–45.

Cecco, L. (2016, June 29). Social progress index: Canada takes second spot on social progress ranking. *The Globe and Mail.* Retrieved from https://www.theglobeandmail.com/news/social-progress-index-canada-isalright/article30647376/

Chaze, F., Thomson, M. S., George, U., & Guruge, S. (2015). Role of cultural beliefs, religion, and spirituality in mental health and/or service utilization among immigrants in Canada: A scoping review. *Canadian Journal of Community Mental Health, 34*(3), 87–101. Retrieved from https://doi.org/10.7870/cjcmh-2015-015

Chiu, L., Ganesan, S., Clark, N., & Morrow, M. (2005). Spirituality and treatment choices by South and East Asian women with serious mental illness. *Transcultural Psychiatry, 42*(4), 630–656.

College of Nurses of Ontario. (2009). *Culturally sensitive care [Practice guideline].* Retrieved from http://www.cno.org/globalassets/docs/prac/41040_culturallysens.pdf

Conroy, K., Sandel, M., & Zuckerman, B. (2010). Poverty grown up: How childhood socioeconomic status impacts adult health. *Journal of Developmental & Behavioural Pediatrics, 31*(2), 154–160.

Corrado, R. R., & Cohen, I. M. (2010). Mental health profiles for a sample of British Columbia's Aboriginal survivors of the Canadian residential school system. In *Aboriginal Health Foundation's a compendium of Aboriginal healing foundation research* (pp. 5–6). Ottawa, ON: Aboriginal Health Foundation. Retrieved from http://www.ahf.ca/downloads/research-compendium.pdf

Correctional Service Canada. (2012). *Mental health strategy for corrections in Canada: A Federal-Provincial-Territorial Partnership.* Correctional Service Canada, Government of Canada. Retrieved from http://www.csc-scc.gc.ca/health/092/MH-strategy-eng.pdf

Crawford, A. (2016). Suicide among Indigenous Peoples in Canada The Canadian Encyclopedia. Retrieved from http://www.thecanadianencyclopedia.ca/en/article/suicide-among-indigenous-peoples-in-canada/

Creamer, A. M., & Austin, W. (2017). Canadian nurse practitioner core competencies identified: An opportunity to build mental health and illness skills and knowledge. *The Journal for Nurse Practitioners, 13*(5), e231–e236. Retrieved from http://dx.doi.org/10.1016/j.nurpra.2016.12.017

Creamer, A. M., Mill, J., Austin, W., & O'Brien, B. (2014). Canadian nurse practitioners' therapeutic commitment to persons with mental illness. *Canadian Journal of Nursing Research, 46*(4), 13–32. Retrieved from http://cjnr.archive.mcgill.ca/article/viewFile/2464/2458

Davy, C., Hartfield, S., McArthur, A., Munn, Z., & Brown, A. (2016). Access to primary health care services for Indigenous peoples: A framework synthesis. *International Journal for Equity in Health, 15,* 163. Retrieved from http://dx.doi.org/10.1186/s12939-016-0450-5

Dempsey, J., & Gottesman, D. R. (2011). Indigenous people: Government programs (Revised by Gretchen Albers). *The Canadian Encyclopedia.* Retrieved from http://www.thecanadianencyclopedia.ca/en/article/government-programs-concerning-aboriginal-people/

Douglas, V. (2013). *Introduction to Aboriginal health and health care in Canada: Bridging health and healing.* New York, NY: Springer Publishing Company.

Elias, B., Mignone, J., Hall, M., Hong, S. P., Hart, L., & Sareen, J. (2012). Trauma and suicide behaviour histories among a Canadian Indigenous population: An empirical exploration of the potential role of Canada's residential school system. *Social Science and Medicine, 74*(10), 1560–1569. doi:10.1016/j.socscimed.2012.01.026

endpoverty.org. (2017). *About poverty.* Oakton, VA: Author. Retrieved from http://endpoverty.org/effects-of-poverty/

Fitzpatrick, S. J., Perkins, D., Luland, T., Brown, D., & Corvan, E. (2017). The effect of context in rural mental health care: Understanding integrated services in a small town. *Health and Place, 45,* 70–76. doi:10.1016/j.healthplace.2017.03.004

First Nations Education Steering Committee. (2017). *Indian residential schools and reconciliation resources.* Retrieved from http://www.fnesc.ca/irsr/

Galloway, G. (2017). Ottawa still failing to provide adequate health care on reserves: Report. *The Globe and Mail.* Retrieved from https://www.theglobeandmail.com/news/politics/ottawa-still-failing-to-provide-adequate-health-care-on-reserves-report/article33746065/

Government of Canada. (2007, October 25). *History of providing health services to First Nations people and Inuit.* Retrieved from https://www.canada.ca/en/health-canada/corporate/about-health-canada/branches-agencies/first-nations-inuit-health-branch/history-providing-health-services-first-nations-people-inuit.html

Government of Canada. (2010). Highlights from the Report of the Royal Commission of Indigenous Peoples RCAP 1996: People to people, nation to nation. *Indigenous and Northern Affairs Canada.* Retrieved from http://www.aadnc-aandc.gc.ca/eng/1100100014597/1100100014637

Government of Canada. (2016). *Indian residential schools settlement agreement—Health support component.* Retrieved from https://www.aadnc-aandc.gc.ca/eng/1466537513207/1466537533821

Government of Canada. (2017a). Canadian multiculturalism act (R.S.C., 1985, c. 24, 4th Supp.). *Justice Laws Website.* Retrieved from http://laws-lois.justice.gc.ca/eng/acts/C-18.7/

Government of Canada. (2017b). Canada health act, 1984. (R.S.C., 1985, c. C-6). *Justice Laws Website.* Retrieved from http://laws-lois.justice.gc.ca/eng/acts/C-6/FullText.html

Graham, H., & Martin, S. (2016). Narrative descriptions of miyo-mahcihoyān (physical, emotional, mental, and spiritual well-being) from a contemporary Néhiyawak (Plains Cree) perspective. *International Journal of Mental Health Systems, 10,* 58. doi:10.1186/s13033-016-0086-2

Gronholm, P. C., Henderson, C., Deb, T., & Thornicroft, G. (2017). Interventions to reduce discrimination and stigma: The state of the art. *Social Psychiatry Psychiatric Epidemiology, 52*(3), 249–258. http://dx.doi.org/10.1007/s00127-017-1341-9

Guruge, S., & Butt, H. (2015). A scoping review of mental health issues and concerns among immigrant and refugee youth in Canada: Looking back, moving forward. *Canadian Journal of Public Health, 106*(2), e72–e78. doi:10.17269/CJPH.106.4588

Hackett, C., Feeny, D., & Tompa, E. (2016). Canada's residential school system: Measuring the intergenerational impact of familial attendance on health and mental health outcomes. *Journal of Epidemiology and Community health, 70*(11), 1096–1105.

Haggarty, J. M., Ryan-Nicholls, K. D., & Jarva, J. A. (2010). Mental health collaborative care: A synopsis of the Rural and Isolated Toolkit. *Rural and Remote Health, 10*(1314), 1–10. Retrieved from http://ww.rrh.org.au

Harrison, C. A., & Hauck, Y. H. (2017). Breaking down the stigma of mental health nursing: A qualitative study reflecting opinions from western Australian nurses. *Journal of Psychiatric and Mental Health Nursing, 24*(7), 513–522. doi:10.1111/jpn.12392

Health Canada. (2013). *Indian residential schools.* Retrieved from http://www.hc-sc.gc.ca/fniah-spnia/services/indiresident/index-eng.php

Health Canada. (2016). *First Nations and Inuit health: Suicide prevention.* Retrieved from http://www.hc-sc.gc.ca/fniah-spnia/promotion/suicide/index-eng.php

Her Majesty the Queen in Right of Canada, represented by the Minister of Citizenship and Immigration Canada. (2012). *Discover Canada: The Rights and Responsibilities of Citizenship.* Retrieved from http://www.cic.gc.ca/english/pdf/pub/discover.pdf

Hole, R., Evans, M., Berg, L. D., & Smith, M. L. (2015). Visibility and voice: Aboriginal people experience culturally safe and unsafe health care. *Qualitative Health Research, 25*(12), 1662–1674. http://dx.doi.org/10.1177/1049732314566325

Joseph, B. (2014). *What is residential school syndrome?.* Retrieved from https://www.ictinc.ca/blog/what-is-residential-school-syndrome

Josewski, V. (2012). Analysing 'cultural safety' in mental health policy reform: Lessons from British Columbia, Canada. *Critical Public Health, 22*(2), 223–234. doi:10.1080/09581596.2011.616878

Kates, N., Mazowita, G., Lemire, F., Jayabarathan, A., Bland, R., Selby, P.,... Audet, D. (2011). The evolution of collaborative mental health care in Canada: A shared vision for the future. *Canadian Journal of Psychiatry, 56*(5), I1–I10.

Kent-Wilkinson, A. (2017). Aboriginal timeline in Canada: Health and legislation. *College of Nursing, University of Saskatchewan.* Retrieved from http://www.usask.ca/nursing/aboriginaltimelines

Kent-Wilkinson, A., Blaney, L., Groening, M., Santa Mina, E., Rodrigue, C., & Hust, C. (2016). *CFMHN's 3rd position paper 2015: Mental health and addiction curriculum in undergraduate nursing education in Canada.* Prepared by members of the Canadian Federation of Mental Health Nurses' Education Committee. Toronto, ON: CFMHN.

Kent-Wilkinson, A., Sanders, S. L., Mela, M., Peternelj-Taylor, C., Adelugba, O., Luther, G., & Wormith, J. S. (2012a). *Needs assessment of forensic mental health services and programs for offenders in Saskatchewan: Executive summary.* Study conducted by Forensic Interdisciplinary Research: Saskatchewan Team (FIRST) Centre for Forensic Behavioural Sciences and Justice Studies. Saskatoon, SK: University of Saskatchewan. Retrieved from http://www.usask.ca/cfbsjs/documents/2.%20EXECUTIVE%20SUMMARY_Nov%2029,%202012.pdf

Kent-Wilkinson, A., Sanders, S. L., Mela, M., Peternelj-Taylor, C., Adelugba, O., Luther, G., & Wormith, J. S. (2012b). *Needs assessment of forensic mental health services and programs for offenders in Saskatchewan: Condensed Report.* Conducted by Forensic Interdisciplinary Research: Saskatchewan Team (FIRST). Centre for Forensic Behavioural Sciences and Justice Studies. Saskatoon, SK: University of Saskatchewan. Retrieved from http://www.usask.ca/cfbsjs/research/pdf/research_reports/3_Condensed_FINAL_REPORT_Dec_3_2012.pdf

King, M., Smith, A., & Gracey, M. (2009). Indigenous health part 2: The underlying causes of the health gap. *The Lancet, 374*(9683), 76–85.

Kirkup, K. (2016, May 17). 60% of First Nation children on reserve live in poverty, institute says. *The Canadian Press.* Retrieved from http://www.cbc.ca/news/indigenous/institute-says-60-percent-fn-children-on-reserve-live-in-poverty-1.3585105

Kirmayer, L., Dandeneau, S., Marshall, E., Phillips, M., & Williamson, K. (2011). Rethinking resilience from indigenous perspectives. *Canadian Journal of Psychiatry, 56*(2), 84–91. Retrieved from http://indigenous-psych.org/Interest%20Group/Kirmayer/2011_CJP_Resilience.pdf

Kirmayer, L. J., Brass, G. M., & Tait, C. L. (2000a). The mental health of Aboriginal peoples: Transformations of identity and community. *Canadian Journal of Psychiatry, 45*(7), 607–616.

Kirmayer, L. J., Macdonald, M. E., & Brass, G. M. (2000b, May 29). *The mental health of Indigenous peoples, 45*(7). Retrieved from https://www.mcgill.ca/tcpsych/files/tcpsych/Report10.pdf

Kuhl, J. L. (2017). Putting an end to the silence: Educating society about the Canadian residential school system. *Bridges: An Undergraduate Journal of Contemporary Connections, 2*(1). Retrieved from http://scholars.wlu.ca/cgi/viewcontent.cgi?article=1013&context=bridges_contemporary_connections

Kumar, M. B., & Nahwegahbow, A. (2016). Aboriginal peoples survey, 2012 past-year suicidal thoughts among off-reserve First Nations, Metis and Inuit adults aged 18 to 25: Prevalence and associated characteristics. *Statistics Canada.* Retrieved from http://www.statcan.gc.ca/pub/89-653-x/89-653-x2016011-eng.htm

Kyoung, J. Y., Landais, E., Kolahdooz, F., & Sharma, S. (2015). Framing health matters. Factors influencing the health and wellness of urban Aboriginal youths in Canada: Insights of in-service professionals, care providers, and stakeholders. *American Journal of Public Health, 105*(5), 881–890. http://dx.doi.org/10.2105/AJPH.2014.3024

Little Bear, L. (2012). Traditional knowledge and humanities: A perspective by a Blackfoot. *Journal of Chinese Philosophy, 39*(4), 518–527. http://dx.doi.org/10.1111/j.1540-6253.2012.01742.x

Mabaya, G., & Ray, S. I. (2014). The meaning of health and help-seeking behaviours among refugees who have experienced collective violence prior to emigration: A Canadian perspective. *Canadian Journal of Community Mental Health, 33*(3), 71–85. doi:10.7870/cjcmh-2014-024

Macinnes, M., Macpherson, G., Austin, J., & Schwannauer, M. (2016). Examining the effect of childhood trauma on psychological distress, risk of violence and engagement, in forensic mental health. *Psychiatry Research, 246,* 314–320.

Marsh, T. N., Coholic, D., Cote-Meek, S., & Najavits, L. M. (2015). Blending Aboriginal and Western healing methods to treat intergenerational trauma with substance use disorder in Aboriginal peoples who live in Northeastern Ontario, Canada. *Harm Reduction Journal, 12,* 14. http://dx.doi.org/10.1186/s12954-015-0046-1

Mayhew, M. (2016). How culture influences health. *Canadian Paediatric Society.* Retrieved from http://www.kidsnewtocanada.ca/culture/influence

McCalman, J., Jongen, C., & Bainbridge, R. (2017). Organizational systems' approaches to improving cultural competence in healthcare: A systematic scoping review of the literature. *International Journal for Equity in Health, 16,* 78. Retrieved from https://equityhealthj.biomedcentral.com/articles/10.1186/s12939-017-0571-5

McGough, S., Wynaden, D., & Wright, M. (2017). Experience of providing cultural safety in mental health to Aboriginal patients: A grounded theory study. *International Journal of Mental Health Nursing.* Retrieved from http://onlinelibrary.wiley.com/doi/10.1111/inm.12310/ful

McIvor, O. (2009). Language and culture as protective factors for a-risk communities. *Journal of Aboriginal Health, 5*(1), 6–25.

McNally, M., & Martin, D. (2017). First Nations, Inuit and Métis health. *Healthcare Management Forums, 3*(2), 117–122. Retrieved from http://journals.sagepub.com/doi/abs/10.1177/0840470416680445

McQuaid, R. J., Bombay, A., McInnis, O. P., Humeny, C., Matheson, K., & Anisman, H. (2017). Suicide ideation and attempts among First Nations peoples living on reserve in Canada: The intergenerational and cumulative effects of Indian residential schools. *The Canadian Journal of Psychiatry, 62*(6), 422–430. doi:10.1177/0706743717702075

Mental Health Commission of Canada. (2009, November). *Toward recovery and well-being.* Retrieved from https://www.mentalhealthcommission.ca/sites/default/files/FNIM_Toward_Recovery_and_Well_Being_ENG_0_1.pdf

Mental Health Commission of Canada. (2012). *Changing directions, changing lives: The mental health strategy for Canada.* Calgary, AB: Author.

Retrieved from http://strategy.mentalhealthcommission.ca/pdf/strategy-images-en.pdf

Mental Health Commission of Canada. (2013a). *Opening minds: Interim report.* Ottawa, ON: Author. Retrieved from http://www.mentalhealthcommission.ca/English/initiatives-and-projects/opening-minds/opening-minds-interim-report

Mental Health Commission of Canada. (2013b). *Why investing in mental health will contribute to Canada's economic prosperity and to the sustainability of our health care system.* Ottawa, ON: Author.

Mental Health Commission of Canada. (2016, January). *Supporting the Mental Health of Refugees to Canada.* Ottawa, ON: Author. Retrieved from https://ontario.cmha.ca/wp-content/files/2016/02/Refugee-Mental-Health-backgrounder.pdf

Mercredi, O. W. (2015). *Aboriginal initiatives: Aboriginal gangs a report to the Correctional Service of Canada on Aboriginal youth gang members in the federal corrections system.* Retrieved from http://www.csc-scc.gc.ca/aboriginal/5-eng.shtml

Minkler, M., & Wallerstein, N. (Eds.). (2008). *Community based participatory research for health: Process to outcomes* (2nd ed.). San Francisco, CA: Jossey Bass.

Mood Disorders Society of Canada. (2014). *Workplace mental health.* Guelph, ON: Author. Retrieved from http://www.mooddisorderscanada.ca/documents/WorkplaceHealth_En.pdf

National Aboriginal Health Organization. (2012). Defining Aboriginal peoples within Canada: NAHO terminology guidelines. *Journal of Aboriginal Health (JAH) & International Journal of Indigenous Health (IJIH).* Retrieved from https://journals.uvic.ca/journalinfo/ijih/IJIHDefiningIndigenousPeoplesWithinCanada.pdf

National Collaborating Centre for Aboriginal Health. (2010). *Poverty as a social determinant of First Nations, Inuit, and Métis health.* Retrieved from http://www.nccah-ccnsa.ca/docs/fact%20sheets/social%20determinates/NCCAH_fs_poverty_EN.pdf

National Collaborating Centre for Aboriginal Health. (2011a). *Setting the context: The Aboriginal health legislation and policy framework in Canada.* Prince George, BC: Author. Retrieved from http://www.nccah-ccnsa.ca/docs/Health%20Legislation%20and%20Policy_English.pdf

National Collaborating Centre for Aboriginal Health. (2011b). *Access to health services as a social determinant of First Nations, Inuit and Métis health.* Retrieved from http://www.nccah-ccnsa.ca/docs/fact%20sheets/social%20determinates/Access%20to%20Health%20Services_Eng%202010.pdf

National Collaborating Centre for Aboriginal Health. (2011c). Looking for Aboriginal health in legislation and policies, 1970 to 2008: The policy synthesis project. Prepared by J. Lavoie, L. Gervais, J. Toner, O. Bergeron, & G. Thomas for the *NCCAH.* Prince George, BC: Author. Retrieved from http://www.nccah-ccnsa.ca/Publications/Lists/Publications/Attachments/28/Looking%20for%20Aboriginal%20Health%20in%20Legislation%20and%20Polcies%20(English%20-%20Web).pdf

National Collaborating Center for Aboriginal Health. (2012). The state of knowledge of Aboriginal health: A review of Aboriginal public health in Canada. Retrieved from https://www.ccnsa-nccah.ca/docs/context/RPT-StateKnowledgeReview-EN.pdf

National Collaborating Center for Aboriginal Health. (2013). *Cultural safety in health care.* Retrieved from http://www.nccah-ccnsa.ca/368/Cultural_Safety_in_Healthcare.nccah

National Collaborating Centre for Aboriginal Health. (2016). *Culture and language as social determinants of First Nations, Inuit, and Metis health.* Retrieved from http://www.nccah-ccnsa.ca/Publications/Lists/Publications/Attachments/15/NCCAH-FS-CultureLanguage-SDOH-FNMI-EN.pdf

Oberle, K., & Raffin Bouchal, S. (2009). *Ethics in Canadian nursing practice: Navigating the journey.* Toronto, ON: Pearson.

O'Hara, J., & Treble, P. (2000, June 26). Abuse of trust: What happened behind the walls of residential church schools is a tragedy that has left native victims traumatized. *Maclean's, 6,* 16.

Okpalauwaekwe, U., Mela, M., & Oji, C. (2017). Knowledge of and attitude to mental illness in Nigeria: A scoping review. *Integrative Journal of Global Health, 1*(1). Retrieved from http://www.imedpub.com/articles/knowledge-of-and-attitude-to-mental-illnesses-in-nigeria-a-scoping-review.php?aid=18642

Paquette, J., Beauregard, D., & Gunter, C. (2017). Settlers colonialism and cultural policy: The colonial foundation and refoundation of Canadian cultural policy. *International Journal of Cultural Policy, 23*(3), 269–284. http://doi.org/10.1080/10286632.2015.1043294

Paraschak, V., & Thomson, K. (2013, October 18). Finding strength(s): Insights on Aboriginal physical cultural practices in Canada. *Sport in Society, 17*(8). Retrieved from http://www.tandfonline.com.cyber.usask.ca/doi/full/10.1080/17430437.2013.838353?scroll=top&needAccess=true

Pasco, A. (2004). Cross-cultural relationships between nurses and Filipino Canadian patients. *Journal of Nursing Scholarship, 36*(3), 239–246.

Peters, J. (2017). Impact: Colonialism in Canada. *CM: Canadian Review of Materials, 23*(30), 231.

Popova, S., Lange, S., Probst, C., Parunashvili, N., & Rehm, J. (2017). Prevalence of alcohol consumption during pregnancy and fetal alcohol spectrum disorders among the general and Aboriginal populations in Canada and the United States. *European Journal of Medical Genetics, 60*(1), 32–48.

Preston, J. P., Carr-Stewart, S., & Bruno, C. (2012). The growth of Aboriginal youth gangs in Canada. *Canadian Journal of Native Studies, 32*(2), 193–207. Retrieved from search.proquest.cm.libproxy.ureina:2048/docview/149836593/fulltextPDF/A8BCD0432CED422CPQ/1?accountid=13480

Purnell, L. (2016). Are we really measuring cultural competence? *Nursing Science Quarterly, 29*(2), 124–127.

Puxley, C. (2014, December 12). Man's death after 34-hour ER wait must be ruled homicide, family's lawyers tell inquest. *The Canadian Press.* Retrieved from http://news.nationalpost.com/news/canada/mans-death-after-34-hour-er-wait-must-be-ruled-homicide-familys-lawyers-tell-inquest

Reading, C. (2015). Structural determinants of Aboriginal peoples' health. In M. Greenwood, S. de Leeuw, N. M. Lindsay, & C. Reading (Eds.), *Determinants of Indigenous peoples' health in Canada* (pp. 3–15). Toronto, ON: Canadian Scholars' Press Inc.

Reading, J., & Halseth, R. (2013). *Pathways to improving well-being for Indigenous peoples: How living conditions decide health.* Prince George, BC: National Collaborating Centre for Aboriginal Health. Retrieved from http://www.nccah-ccnsa.ca/en/publications.aspx?sortcode=2.8.10&publication=102

Registered Nurses' Association of Ontario. (2007). *Embracing cultural diversity in health care: Developing cultural competence.* Toronto, ON: Author.

Repo, H., Vahlberg, T., Salminen, L., Papadopoulos, I., & Leino-Kilpi, H. (2017). The cultural competence of graduating nursing students. *Journal of Transcultural Nursing, 28*(1), 98–107. http://doi.org/10.1177/1043659616632046

Richardson, A., Yarwood, J., & Richardson, S. (2016, November 30). Expressions of cultural safety in public health nursing practice. *Nursing Inquiry, 24*(1). doi:10.1111/nin.12171

Richmond, C. A. M., & Cook, C. (2016). Creating conditions for Canadian Aboriginal health equity: The promise of healthy public policy. *Public Health Reviews, 37*(2). Retrieved from http://dx.doi.org.cyber.usask.ca/10.1186/s40985-016-0016-5

Roberts, G., & Grimes, K. (2011). *Return on investment: Mental health promotion and mental illness prevention.* Ottawa, ON: Canadian Institute for Health Information. Retrieved from http://tools.hhr-rhs.ca/index.php?option=com_mtree&task=viewlink&link_id=6080&lang=en

Roy, A. 2014). Intergenerational trauma and Aboriginal women: Implications for mental health during pregnancy. *First Peoples Child and Family Review, 9*(1). Retrieved from http://journals.sfu.ca/fpcfr/index.php/FPCFR/article/view/189

Royal Commission of Aboriginal Peoples. (1996). *Final report.* Ottawa, ON: Communication Group.

Russell, C., Firestone, M., Kelly, L., Mushquash, B., & Fischer, C. (2016). Prescription opioid prescribing, use/misuse, harms and treatment among Aboriginal people in Canada: A narrative review of available data and indicators. *Rural and Remote Health, 16*(4), 3974. Retrieved from http://www.rrh.org.au/articles/subviewnew.asp?ArticleID=3974

Rutherford, K. (2016, April 9). *Attawapiskat declares state of emergency over spate of suicide attempts.* Sudbury, ON: CBC News.

Silove, D., Ventevoge, P., Rees, S. (2017). The contemporary refugee crisis: An overview of mental health challenges. *World Psychiatry, 16*(2), 130–139.

Skip Knox, E. L. (2004). *History of western civilization.* Retrieved from http://history.boisestate.edu/westciv/plague/10.shtml

Smetanin, P., Stiff, D., Briante, C., Adair, C. E., Ahmad, S., & Khan, M. (2011). *The life and economic impact of major mental illnesses in Canada: 2011 to 2041.* RiskAnalytica, on behalf of the Mental Health Commission of Canada. Retrieved from https://www.mentalhealthcommission.ca/sites/default/files/MHCC_Report_Base_Case_FINAL_ENG_0_0.pdf

Social Progress Imperative. (2016). *Social progress index: Canada.* Retrieved from http://www.socialprogressindex.com/

Standing Senate Committee on Social Affairs, Science and Technology. (2006). *Out of the shadows at last: Transforming mental health, mental illness and addiction services in Canada.* Ottawa, ON: Author. Retrieved from http://www.parl.gc.ca/Content/SEN/Committee/391/soci/rep/pdf/rep02may06part1-e.pdf

Statistics Canada. (2013). *Canadian community health survey: Mental health, 2012.* Government of Canada. Ottawa, ON: Author. Retrieved from http://www.statcan.gc.ca/daily-quotidien/130918/dq130918a-eng.htm

Statistics Canada. (2015). *2011 National Household Survey (NHS). Survey guide.* Ottawa, ON: Author. Retrieved from http://www12.statcan.gc.ca/nhs-enm/2011/ref/nhs-enm_guide/index-eng.cfm

Statistics Canada. (2016a). *2011 National Household Survey. Data tables. Immigration and ethno-cultural diversity.* Ottawa, ON: Author. Retrieved from http://www12.statcan.gc.ca/nhs-enm/2011/dp-pd/dt-td/index-eng.cfm

Statistics Canada. (2016b). *Immigration and ethnocultural diversity in Canada. 2011 National Household Survey.* Ottawa, ON: Author. Retrieved from http://www12.statcan.gc.ca/nhs-enm/2011/as-sa/99-010-x/99-010-x2011001-eng.cfm

Statistics Canada. (2016c). *Aboriginal peoples in Canada: First Nations people, Métis and Inuit, 2011.* Retrieved from http://www12.statcan.gc.ca/nhs-enm/2011/as-sa/99-011-x/99-011-x2011001-eng.cfm

Statistics Canada. (2016d). *Religions in Canada. 2011 National Household Survey.* Ottawa, ON: Author. Retrieved from http://www12.statcan.gc.ca/nhs-enm/2011/as-sa/99-010-x/99-010-x2011001-eng.cfm#a6

Statistics Canada. (2017a). *Population centre and rural area classification 2016.* Retrieved from http://www23.statcan.gc.ca/imdb/p3VD.pl?Function=getVD&TVD=339235

Statistics Canada. (2017b). *Canadian demographics at a glance* (2nd ed.). Cat. No. 91-003-X. Retrieved from www.statcan.gc.ca/pub/91-003-x/91-003-x2014001-eng.pdf

Statistics Canada. (2017c). *Census Profile, 2016 Census.* Retrieved from http://www12.statcan.gc.ca/census-recensement/2016/dp-pd/prof/index.cfm?Lang=E

The Culture Trip. (2017, February 9). *Toronto named the most diverse city in the world by BBC Radio.* Retrieved from https://theculturetrip.com/north-america/canada/articles/toronto-named-most-diverse-city-in-the-world-by-bbc-radio/

Thira, D. (2005). *Beyond the four waves of colonization.* Retrieved from http://www.swaraj.org/fourwaves.htm

Truth and Reconciliation Commission of Canada. (2015). *Honoring the truth, reconciling for the future: Summary of the final report of the Truth and Reconciliation Commission.* Retrieved from http://www.trc.ca/websites/trcinstitution/File/2015/Honouring_the_Truth_Reconciling_for_the_Future_July_23_2015.pdf

UN Committee on Economic, Social and Cultural Rights. (2000, August 11). *General comment No. 14: The Right to the Highest Attainable Standard of Health (Art. 12 of Covenant).* Retrieved from http://www.refworld.org/docid/4538838d0.html

UN Development Programme. (2016). *Human Development Report, 2016: Human development for everyone.* Retrieved from http://hdr.undp.org/sites/default/files/2016_human_development_report.pdf

Wakerman, J., Bourke, L., Humphreys, J. S., & Taylor, J. (2017). Is remote health different to rural health? *Rural and Remote Health, 17*(3832), 1–8. Retrieved from http://www.rrh.org.au

Waldram, J. B., Herring, D. A., & Young, T. K. (2006). *Aboriginal health in Canada: Historical, cultural and epidemiological perspectives* (2nd ed.). Toronto, ON: University of Toronto Press.

Watt, K., Abbott, P., & Reath, J. (2016). Developing cultural competence in general practitioners: An integrative review of the literature. *BMC Family Practice, 17*(158). Retrieved from https://bmcfampract.biomedcentral.com/articles/10.1186/s12875-016-0560-6

Wilk, P., Maltby, A., & Cooke, M. (2017). Residential schools and the effects on Indigenous health and well-being in Canada-a scoping review. *Public Health Reviews, 38*, 8. http://dx.doi.org/10.1186/s40985-017-0055-6

World Health Organization. (2017a). *Social determinants of health.* Geneva, CH: Author. Retrieved from http://www.who.int/social_determinants/en/

World Health Organization. (2017b). *Poverty.* Geneva, CH: Author. Retrieved from http://www.who.int/topics/poverty/en/

Yeager, K. A., & Bauer-Wu, S. (2013). Cultural humility: Essential foundation for clinical researchers. *Applied Nursing Research, 26*(4), 251–256. http://doi.org/10.1016/j.apnr.2013.06.008

Zayed, R., Davidson, B., Nadeau, L., Callanan, T. S., Fleisher, W. Hope-Ross, L., ... Steele, M. (2016). Canadian rural/remote primary care physicians' perspectives on child/adolescent mental health care service delivery. *Journal of the Canadian Academy of Child and Adolescent Psychiatry, 25*(1), 24–34.

4 The Continuum of Canadian Mental Health Care

Diane Kunyk

Adapted from the chapter "The Continuum of Psychiatric and Mental Health Care" by Cheryl Pollard

LEARNING OBJECTIVES

After studying this chapter, you will be able to:

- Identify the different treatment settings and associated programs along the continuum of care.
- Discuss the role of the nurse along the continuum of care.
- Describe current health care trends in psychiatric and mental health services.
- Describe the importance of integrated services for people with mental illness or mental health concerns.

KEY TERMS

- case management • community-based residential services • consultation • crisis response • empowerment • illness prevention • integrated approach • intensive outpatient program • intensive residential services • mental health promotion • partnership • primary care primary health care • referral • reintegration • relapse • self-help • stabilization • supportive employment

KEY CONCEPTS

- collaborative mental health care • continuum of care

Health care systems need to have well-integrated psychiatric and mental health (PMH) care across the continuum, from health promotion to recovery and rehabilitation. Most mental illnesses are not caused by a single factor but are a result of a combination of factors. These causative factors relate to the complex interactions between biologic, social, psychological, and spiritual aspects of people's lives. Effective PMH care must be able to address people's needs across these areas. As a result, the continuum of PMH care includes a range of services.

Across all aspects of the Canadian health care system, health professionals, such as nurses, are expected to provide appropriate care to people with mental health concerns and/or mental illness. PMH services offer more specialized expertise in meeting the needs of people who have a mental illness. Resources that foster people's sense of self, social inclusion and belonging, and meaning and purpose, and that empower individuals to develop their capacity for well-being are important components of the PMH care continuum. Many of these resources are "outside" the formal health care system and are provided in the community by religious organizations, educational institutions, recreational associations, as well as family and peer groups.

■ PRIMARY HEALTH CARE APPROACH

Primary health care (not to be confused with "primary care") was adopted by the World Health Organization

(WHO) in 1978 as the basis for the delivery of health services (WHO, 2008a). It is an approach that encompasses five types of health care: promotive, preventive, curative, rehabilitative, and supportive/palliative. It is based on the principles of accessibility, public participation, health promotion, appropriate technology (i.e., adapted to the community's social, economic, and cultural developments), and intersectoral cooperation (necessary as health and well-being are linked to social and economic policies). Canadian nurses are expected to apply these principles in their practice across the continuum of care (Canadian Nurses Association [CNA], 2012). The Mental Health Commission of Canada (MHCC), in 2012, put forward recommendations for action that closely align with the principles of primary health care.

■ DEFINING THE CONTINUUM OF CARE

The continuum of care represents the complex, integrated system of services provided by health professionals in general and by those with specialized psychiatric and mental expertise, as well as the supports provided by informal providers and organizations within the community that help people to maintain and to restore their mental health and well-being.

The continuum of care begins with health promotion strategies for preventing people from experiencing mental health problems or becoming mentally ill, as well as improving the mental health status of the whole population. When people do experience a mental health problem or a mental illness, most of the services in Canada are situated in community settings. Inpatient care (hospitalization) may be periodically necessary, but it is typically of very short duration. There are also components of the continuum that are focused on the PMH care needs of specific patient populations, such as children and families, seniors, military personnel, people with brain injuries, people who are involved with the legal system, people with addictions, and people with developmental challenges. Such services are typically provided by specially trained mental health professionals.

The continuum of care extends beyond the services for acute events to support recovery. The MHCC (2012) defines the concept of recovery as "living a satisfying, hopeful, and contributing life, even when there are on-going limitations caused by mental health problems and illnesses" (p. 7). Recovery also includes the concept of well-being—an individual realizing his or her potential. In order to facilitate recovery and well-being for individuals, family, groups, or communities, the MHCC has concluded that care provision must be founded on core principles. These include hope and optimism, focused on the individual, occurring in the context of the individual's life, and responsive to diversity among individuals. Working with First Nations, Inuit and Métis, and transforming existing services and systems are also considered fundamental (MHCC, 2015).

The goal of PMH care is to deliver the right care (appropriate medical, nursing, psychological, social, and spiritual services), by the right person, to the right person and/or family members, at the right time and in the right place. By doing so, this continuum facilitates the stability, continuity, and comprehensiveness of service provision to an individual over their lifetime. Further components of the continuum of care range from supportive interventions by informal community support providers to professional service providers delivering clinical treatment in the community to professional services being provided in a hospital setting. Due to the complexity of the continuum of care, individuals and families may require assistance with the coordination of their care, services, and supports. The preconditions to continuity of care include such elements as easy access, availability of services, and adequate information about the service.

KEY CONCEPT

A **continuum of care** consists of an integrated health system of supports and services designed to maximize people's health and well-being across the lifespan that is provided by health professionals (some who offer specialized services, such as psychiatric mental health services), as well as by nonprofessional caregivers.

Coordination of Care

Coordination of care is the integration of appropriate services so that individualized person-centred care and treatment is provided. Appropriate services are those that are tailored to promote recovery and well-being of the individual and family (when appropriate) through holistic care that supports and develops an individual's strengths, addresses vulnerabilities, promotes cultural competency and safety, inspires hope, facilitates empowerment, and offers choice and responsibility. Patients' input and opinions need to be solicited, including what they require in terms of knowledge, skills, and support to make decisions as well as their ability to participate in their own care. Patient-centred care is that which establishes a **partnership** among practitioners, patients, and their families (when appropriate) to ensure that decisions respect patients' wants, needs and preferences. Although continuity in care is recognized as an important goal, the reality is that it often falls short of expectations, and the improvement of coordination care is a critical factor for patient satisfaction (Government of Alberta, 2015).

The move toward increasing professional coordination of services and social supports is considered to be a priority across the Canadian health care system (Canadian Foundation for Healthcare Improvement, 2014). There are many terms that are used to describe these types of coordinating services. They include the following: **case management**, service coordination, care management, care coordination, service navigation, and transition care services. Although the terms may be different, the services provided can be described as a collaborative, patient-driven process designed to support the patient's achievement of goals within a complex health, social, and fiscal environment. To meet patient goals, the coordinator of services for patients and families may need to liaise and develop collaborative and cooperative relationships among many different service partners, such as **primary care** services, public health, mental health, social services, housing, education, the workplace, and the criminal justice system, to name but a few.

See Box 4.1 for principle function of case management and Box 4.2 for dimensions of recovery-oriented practice.

The Nurse as Manager of Patient Services

Due to the often cyclical nature of serious mental illness, nurses serve in various pivotal functions across the continuum of care. These functions can involve both direct care and coordination of the care delivered by others. The role of manager of patient services (also referred to as case manager or care coordinator) does not refer to the client or patient but to service provision. When functioning in this position, the nurse must have commanding knowledge of the patient's and family's needs, areas of strengths, and the available community

---

BOX 4.1 Principle Functions of Case Management

- **Assessment**
  Case management includes conducting a comprehensive assessment of the patient's health needs.
- **Patient-centred**
  Case management is patient/caregiver centred, involves the patient in the decision-making process, and is sometimes driven or provided by the patient.
- **Navigation**
  Case management provides navigation through the wide spectrum of services to meet patient needs. It moves beyond the boundaries of programs and service sectors, and includes assisting patients with transitioning their care.
- **Collaboration/coordination**
  Case management strategies include developing and carrying out a care plan collaboratively with patients, their families, primary health care providers, and others. It builds upon clinical expertise and the collaborative relationships/formalized partnerships among health care professionals, patients, and their caregivers.
- **Health promotion/illness prevention**
  Case management strategies enhance health promotion, illness prevention, and risk mitigation through patient education and emphasis on enhancing patient self-care capacity. Case management incorporates the principles of population health and the broad determinants of health.

- **Quality of care**
  Case management incorporates evidence-based practice to promote quality of care, problem solving, and exploring options for improving care.
- **Communication**
  Case management requires facilitating effective communication and coordination between the patient, the patient's family, primary health care providers, and others to minimize fragmentation and maximize evidence-based care delivery.
- **Advocating**
  Case management advocates on behalf of patients to receive quality care, the health care team to be supported in providing quality services, and effective use of health resources. The case manager also promotes the patient to similarly self-advocate and to achieve independence.
- **Flexibility**
  Case management considers alternative plans, when necessary, to achieve desired outcomes.
- **Education**
  Case management provides patients and their families with the education and support that enables patients to understand their care needs, to make informed decisions, and to be confident in providing self-care.

Adapted from Alberta Health and Wellness. (2006). *System case management for continuing care clients: Prepared for Continuing Care Leaders Council.* Edmonton, AB: Author; and from Kathol, R., Perez, R., & Cohen, J. (2010). *The integrated case management manual* (p. 4). New York, NY: Springer Publishing Company.

---

resources. In order for nurses to be successful, they must practice with the philosophy that recovery is defined by the patient, not the service provider, and a belief that well-being is possible for all people living with a mental illness. The nurse must also have expertise in working with the family as a unit. The repertoire of required skills includes collaboration, teaching, management, leadership, followership, as well as group, critical thinking, and research skills. A nurse working as a case manager arguably has one of the most diverse roles within the psychiatric services continuum.

What is becoming increasingly apparent is the critical and important role that the nurse has in developing therapeutic relationships with patients. Contemporary models of mental health care strive to promote inclusion and empowerment and to recognize the preferences of individuals. This requires that relationships must be built with patients and their families in order to meet their needs and expectations. The nurse–patient relationship is not only foundational for including patients in their care planning but also influences patient engagement in

ongoing mental health care (Newman, O'Reilly, Lee, & Kennedy, 2015).

COMPREHENSIVE MENTAL HEALTH SYSTEM: CORE PROGRAMS AND SERVICES

Each Canadian province has slightly different services to promote mental health, prevent mental illness, and provide treatment services and/or community supports to people with a mental health problem or mental illness. All, however, should be based on a commitment to patient-centred care (CNA, 2012; MHCC, 2012).

Mental Health Promotion and Illness Prevention

Effective and efficient mental health service delivery systems have integrated **mental health promotion** and **illness prevention** into all aspects of the system. Mental

BOX 4.2 Six Dimensions of Recovery-Oriented Practice

1. **Creating a Culture and Language of Hope.** Recovery is possible and is essentially about hope. Hope stimulates recovery, and acquiring the capabilities to nurture hope is the starting point for building a mental health system geared to fostering recovery.

2. **Recovery Is Personal.** Each person is unique and has a right to determine, to the greatest extent possible, their own path to mental health and well-being. Recovery acknowledges the individual nature of each person's journey of wellness and their right to find their own way to living a life of value and purpose.

3. **Recovery Occurs in the Context of One's Life.** Most of a person's recovery journey occurs outside the mental health system. Therefore, fostering recovery necessitates understanding people within the context of their lives. Family, friends, neighbours, local community, schools, workplaces, and spiritual and cultural communities all influence mental health and well-being and have an important role in recovery.

4. **Responding to the Diverse Needs of Everyone Living in Canada.** Recovery-oriented practice is grounded in principles that encourage and enable respect for diversity and that are consistent with culturally safe, responsive, competent practice.

5. **Working with First Nations, Inuit and Métis.** There is common ground between recovery principles and shared Indigenous understandings of wellness that provides a rich opportunity for learning and strengthening mental health policy and practice.

6. **Recovery Is About Transforming Services and Systems.** Achieving a fully integrated recovery-oriented mental health system is an ongoing process. The commitment to recovery needs to find expression in everything a health organization does including ensuring support for a workforce that has the skills and resources required to deliver recovery-oriented practice.

Summary from Mental Health Commission of Canada. (2015). *Guidelines for recovery-oriented practice, Hope, Dignity, Inclusion* (pp. 15–17). Ottawa, ON: Author.

---

health promotion strategies are directed toward addressing the determinants of health that can impact the population's mental health. These strategies recognize and address the broader issues, which promote mental health which are largely dependent on intersectoral approaches. Several mental health promotion policies and programs have been mainstreamed into Canada's government and business sectors. A few examples of these include early childhood intervention programs, nutritional and psychosocial interventions for vulnerable populations, and community-based violence prevention that involves community policing initiatives.

See Box 4.3 for a summary of best practices related to mental health promotion.

Mental illness prevention strategies are designed to keep something from happening. This something may be the illness itself, the severity or duration of the illness, or a disability associated with the illness or disease. The WHO has identified three categories of prevention strategies that will reduce the risk of experiencing an illness: (1) universal prevention, targets the general population; (2) selective prevention, targets groups or individuals at higher risk for a specific illness than the general population; and (3) indicated prevention, targets people at

BOX 4.3 Best Practices

MENTAL HEALTH PROMOTION

- Early childhood interventions
- Support to children
- Socioeconomic empowerment of women
- Social support for elderly populations
- Programs targeted at vulnerable groups, including minorities, Indigenous peoples, migrants, and people affected by conflicts and disasters
- Mental health promotional activities in schools
- Mental health interventions at work

- Housing policies
- Violence prevention programs
- Community development programs
- Poverty reduction and social protection for the poor
- Antidiscrimination laws and campaigns
- Promotion of the rights, opportunities, and care of individuals with mental disorders

From World Health Organization. (2016). *Mental health: Strengthening our response.* Geneva, Switzerland: Author.

high risk for mental illness (WHO, 2002). An important example of illness prevention services is respite services for family caregivers of persons with a mental illness. The goals of respite programs are typically threefold:

- To validate and reinforce the necessity and value of informal caregiving within the continuum of care.
- To provide support and advocacy to informal caregivers.
- To prevent unnecessary long-term care placements and hospitalizations due to informal caregiver burnout. Respite services can be provided within the home, within a community living option (group home or supportive living setting), or may be provided within an inpatient setting.

Another example of a mental illness prevention strategy is the practice of providing critical incident stress debriefings. For example, if a volunteer fire crew responded to the scene of a very gruesome accident, the community mental health services may offer a critical incident stress debriefing. This intervention strategy is provided as a means to help the fire crew members avoid the potential onset of posttraumatic stress disorder.

Consumer Self-Help and Consumer/Survivor Initiatives

The knowledge and experiences of people living with mental illness are recognized and supported as part of a comprehensive mental health care system. In 2012, the MHCC identified six strategic directions to achieve its vision that "All people living in Canada have the opportunity to achieve the best possible mental health and well-being" (MHCC, 2012, p. 10). Half of these strategic directions require the direct involvement of people with or who have experienced a mental illness. For example, in order to uphold patient rights and foster recovery and well-being, patients and their families need to be actively involved in decisions about services (MHCC, 2012). The importance of input from patients goes beyond decisions about their own care; it extends to the broader health care system. Expanding the "leadership role of people living with mental health problems and illnesses, and their families, in setting mental health related policy" (MHCC, 2012, p. 19) will improve knowledge and foster collaboration, which will ultimately have significant positive effects on decision making within the mental health care system. The recognition of the importance of having people with mental health problems or mental illness making decisions about their care and about the health care system is due in part to the determination and advocacy of **self-help** groups and organizations of people who have experienced mental illness (Segal, Silverman, & Temkin, 2013), many of whom refer to themselves as "consumers." Some consider themselves "survivors"—not of their illness but of their health care experience.

Two out of three Canadians with mental illness do not get the help they need (MHCC, 2009). For example, most people who receive treatment for depression in primary care receive only a single session in a year (Bilsker, Goldner, & Anderson, 2012). Rather than a continuum of care, mental health services are mainly operated on a reactive, acute-care model. Addiction services are particularly underinvested with a greater proportion of mental health and addiction health system resources invested in providing care for mental health problems (Wild, Wolfe, Wang, & Ohinmaa, 2014).

One strategy that is used to extend assistance to people with mental health problems or mental illness is through consumer/survivor initiatives organizations (Lurie, 2012). These are self-help organizations operated exclusively by and for people with serious mental illness. Rather than being treatment services, they are self-help groups that promote the values of member **empowerment**, participation, social justice, and community. The work of these organizations is helping to decrease the stigma associated with mental illness and to make care more accessible. They have also been found to be as effective as traditional services for employment, living arrangements, and reducing hospital admissions (Doughty & Tse, 2011).

Crisis Response Systems and Psychiatric Emergency Services

Crisis intervention services are an important part of a comprehensive mental health system. An organized approach is required to treat individuals in crisis, including a mechanism for rapid access to care (24 hours a day, 7 days a week), telephone crisis services, mobile **crisis response**, access to crisis emergency residential services, or psychiatric emergency services in hospitals. Crisis response systems emphasize crisis supports that are flexible, portable, and person centred (Krupa, Stuart, Mathany, Smart, & Chen, 2010). This type of short-term intervention care focuses on deescalation, **stabilization**, symptom reduction, and prevention of **relapse** requiring inpatient services.

Crisis intervention units can be found in the emergency department of a general or psychiatric hospital or in crisis centres within a community mental health centre. Patients in crisis demonstrate severe symptoms of acute mental illness, including labile mood swings, suicidal ideation, or self-injurious behaviours. This treatment option therefore demands a high degree of nursing expertise. Patients in crisis usually require medications such as anxiolytics or benzodiazepines for symptom management. Key nursing roles include making an accurate assessment, delivering short-term therapeutic interventions, and administering medication. Nurses will also facilitate **referrals** for increased community services or support, for admission to the hospital, or for outpatient services. See Box 4.4 for research indicating that lack of housing can contribute to a mental health crisis and that identifying housing issues of the individual in crisis in the emergency department assessment is important.

BOX 4.4 **Research for Best Practices**

HOMELESSNESS AND HOUSING CRISES: INDIVIDUALS WITH MENTAL HEALTH ISSUES ACCESSING SERVICES

Forchuk, C., Reiss, J. P., Mitchell, B., Even, S., & Meier, A. (2015). Homelessness and housing crises among individuals accessing services within a Canadian emergency department. Journal of Psychiatric and Mental Health Nursing, 22, 354–359.

Background: Poverty and homelessness disproportionately affect those with mental health issues. Individuals who have mental health issues and are homeless or who are experiencing a housing crisis have been found to access emergency departments (ED) more frequently than those with stable housing.

Method: This mixed-method study collected (1) administrative data to determine the prevalence of ED patients with housing crises and (2) interviews with patients who visited the ED with mental health crises exacerbated by housing crises.

Findings: Housing was not the primary reason for accessing the emergency department, but all participants noted that housing was a contributing stressor. Homeless individuals are significantly more likely to access EDs with mental health concerns when compared with individuals with stable housing.

Implications: Crisis service providers and emergency department staff, especially nurses, can play an important role in screening for housing issues and connecting individuals to outside services. Routine screening for housing issues in the ED may help identify other issues that have contributed to the mental health crisis and the ED visit.

Crisis Stabilization

When the immediate crisis does not resolve quickly, the next step is crisis stabilization. The primary purpose of stabilization is to control precipitating symptoms through medications, behavioural interventions, and coordination with other agencies for appropriate aftercare. The major focus of nursing care in a short-term inpatient setting is symptom management and linkage to community resources. During stabilization, the major components of nursing care are ongoing assessment; short-term, focused interventions; and medication administration while monitoring efficacy and side effects. Nurses may also provide focused group psychotherapy designed to develop and strengthen patients' personal management strategies. See Box 4.5 for a summary of best practices related to crisis response services.

Psychosocial Emergency Preparedness and Response

A national priority is to be prepared for emergencies (e.g., transportation accidents, power outages, terrorist threats) and disasters (e.g., floods, fires, tornadoes, outbreaks of disease). Most emergencies, local in nature, are handled at that level; however, partnership is a key principle of Canada's emergency management directorate (Emergency Management Policy Directorate, 2011). The federal government, when assistance is requested or when an emergency involves more than one province or territory, mobilizes resources and coordinates federal response in the health sector through Public Safety Canada. Health Canada and the Public Health Agency of Canada play critical roles in emergency response to risks to public health. The psychosocial aspect of preparedness and response is recognized as an essential component (Health Canada, 2011).

In times of major emergencies and disasters, individuals, families, and entire communities face severe risks to psychosocial (as well as physical) well-being,

BOX 4.5 **Best Practices**

PSYCHIATRIC NURSES IN ADVANCED PRACTICE

Research Evidence

Psychiatric nurses in advanced practice perform multifaceted roles and provide mental health care services in various contexts. Not only are they able to obtain significant results in managing clients, psychiatric nurses are valuable in developing partnerships with nonmental health service providers.

Key Elements of Best Practice

Key elements of psychiatric nurses in advanced practice include the provision of:
- Psychosocial interventions
- Nurse-directed services in health care contexts
- Psychiatric nursing consultation services

From Fung, Y. L., Chan, Z., & Chien, W. T. (2014). Role performance of psychiatric nurses in advanced practice: A systematic review of the literature. *Journal of Psychiatric and Mental Health Nursing, 21*, 698–714. doi: 10.111/jpm.12128

and the mental health system can be overwhelmed. "The dominoes start falling backwards" was a metaphor used to describe the effects of the 2012 hurricane Sandy on New York City's mental health system ("Mental health considerations," 2013): the number of people requiring care increased dramatically, while services to treat them decreased or failed due to destruction and/or lack of personnel. Canada's psychosocial preparedness and response initiative offers services to help Canadians better prepare for disasters and emergencies (e.g., resiliency building) as well as consultation during disaster response.

Primary Care

Primary care refers to the first point of access to the health care system. Provincial health care planning has typically divided the delivery of the services for physical illness and mental illness. This has resulted in a system that fragments people's needs, which is both counterproductive and harmful. An **integrated approach** is required that assists people in managing illness, regardless of its origin. The integrated approach begins with ensuring that the services and supports that are delivered are done so in a patient-centred manner. This means that people are empowered: choice is promoted; they remain in control, and when possible, remain in their community. A patient-centred approach emphasizes the partnership that the person with mental illness has with the service providers. It does not shift responsibility on people to "get themselves together," "get over it," or "deal with it." This model does not place blame on the affected individual; rather, people with mental illness are true partners in their recovery. Although the extent of a person's involvement will depend on his or her particular circumstances, it is only through involvement in their own recovery that people who experience a mental illness can expect the best possible health and well-being.

Collaborative mental health care models have been established in response to specialist mental health service provider shortages, access issues, and the recognition that family physicians are the first point of contact for approximately 85% of people with mental illness (Kirby, 2008). These models have been described using a variety of terms: integrated care, shared care, collaborative care, and managed care, among others. In essence, collaborative care recognizes that primary care for mental health is essential, but to be fully effective, it must be supported by additional levels of care as no single service setting, or provider, can meet everyone's mental health needs (WHO, 2008a). See Box 4.6 for best practices related to the goals and potential activities of collaborative mental health care services. See Box 4.7 related to the benefits of integrating mental health into primary care.

KEY CONCEPT

Collaborative mental health care refers to "care that is provided from different specialties, disciplines, or sectors that work together to offer complementary services and mutual support. As in any effective partnership, common goals, clear and equitable decision making, and open and regular communication are key" (Kates et al., 2011, p. 2).

BOX 4.6 Best Practices

GOALS AND POTENTIAL ACTIVITIES OF COLLABORATIVE MENTAL HEALTH CARE SERVICES

Goals

- Improve access to a comprehensive range of high-quality and effective health care services.
- Improve outcomes for people who use the mental health system.
- Integrate community services across sectors.

Potential Activities

- Regular visits by a mental health care worker to a primary care setting.
- Unified programs that offer mental health and physical health care through one administration and financial entity.
- Regular telephone consultation between primary care and mental health providers.
- Integration of specialized care providers such as psychiatrists, psychologists, nurses, social workers, pharmacists, occupational therapists, and dietitians within primary care settings.
- Joint development of treatment plans by consumers and providers.
- Incorporation of mental health interventions into the management of general medical conditions (e.g., diabetes).
- Meeting the primary health care needs of individuals with severe and persistent mental illness
- Strategies to improve access to community mental health services.
- Development of more formal partnerships with specialized service providers.

From Kates, N., Mazowita, G., Lemire, F., Jayabarathan, A., Bland, R., Selby, P., & Audet, D. (2011). The evolution of collaborative mental health care in Canada: A shared vision for the future. *The Canadian Journal of Psychiatry*, 56(5), 1–10.

BOX 4.7 Benefits of Integrating Mental Health Into Primary Care

1. **The burden of mental disorders is great.** Mental disorders are prevalent in all societies. They create a substantial personal burden for affected individuals and their families, and they produce significant economic and social hardships that affect society as a whole.

2. **Mental and physical health problems are interwoven.** Many people suffer from both physical and mental health problems. Integrated primary care services help ensure that people are treated in a holistic manner, meeting the mental health needs of people with physical disorders, as well as the physical health needs of people with mental disorders.

3. **The treatment gap for mental disorders is enormous.** In all countries, there is a significant gap between the prevalence of mental disorders and the number of people receiving treatment and care. Primary care for mental health helps close this gap.

4. **Primary care for mental health enhances access.** Integrating mental health into primary care is the best way of ensuring that people get the mental health care they need. When mental health is integrated into primary care, people can access mental health services closer to their homes, thus keeping their families together and maintaining their daily activities. Primary care services also facilitate

community outreach and mental health promotion, as well as long-term monitoring and management of affected individuals.

5. **Primary care for mental health promotes respect of human rights.** Mental health services delivered in primary care minimize stigma and discrimination. This also removes the risk of human rights violations that occur in psychiatric hospitals.

6. **Primary care for mental health is affordable and cost-effective.** Primary mental health care services are less expensive than are psychiatric hospitals, for patients, communities, and governments alike. In addition, patients and families avoid indirect costs associated with seeking specialist care in distant locations. The treatment of common mental disorders is very cost-effective, and even small investments by governments can bring important benefits.

7. **Primary care for mental health generates good health outcomes.** The majority of people with mental health disorders treated in primary care have good outcomes, particularly when linked to a network of services at secondary level and in the community.

From World Health Organization. (2008b). *Integrating mental health into primary care: A global perspective.* Geneva, Switzerland: Author.

The other levels of care required to support primary care providers include secondary service components. These components include opportunities for **consultation** and support through referrals regarding patient care needs outside the primary care provider's current competency level, as well as supervision and support to facilitate further skill development and education of the primary care provider. Collaborative mental health care also extends to include formal and informal community supports for people with mental illness, such as housing, education, and recreational organizations. It has been demonstrated that people with mental illness who receive good community care services and support have better health and mental health outcomes, and better quality of life, than do those people who were treated in psychiatric hospitals (WHO, 2008a). However, there is a small proportion of the population that requires very specialized services. These are people who have treatment resistant or very complex presentations of illness, those who lack community support, and/or those requiring forensic services.

Outpatient Care

Outpatient care is a level of care that occurs outside of a hospital or institution. Outpatient services usually are less intensive and are provided to patients who do not require inpatient services. Many patients enroll in

outpatient services immediately upon discharge from an inpatient setting. Others are enrolled as a means of providing treatment services when hospitalization is not required. This promotes a continued connection with their community and community **reintegration**, medication management and monitoring, and symptom management. Patients and their families have the right to choose their home or community as the site for service provision. When remaining at home with their families and other supports, individuals with mental health concerns or mental illnesses are more socially integrated into society (Hair, Shortall, & Oldford, 2013). Outpatient services are provided by private practices, clinics, and community mental health centres.

Intensive Outpatient Programs

The primary focus of **intensive outpatient programs** is on stabilization and relapse prevention for highly vulnerable individuals who are able to function autonomously on a daily basis. People who meet these criteria have returned to their previous lifestyle although their quality of life is still impacted by their mental illness (e.g., interacting with family, resuming work, or returning to school). Participation in outpatient programs is a benefit to individuals who still require frequent monitoring and support within a therapeutic milieu that enables them to remain connected to the community. The duration of treatment and level of services rendered are based on the patient's immediate needs. Treatment duration usually is time limited, with sessions offered 3 to 4 hours per day and 2 to 3 days per week for 6 to 12 weeks. See Box 4.8 for best practices related to bridging the gaps in inpatient care and outpatient care.

Housing and Community Support

With the focus on community-based care, there has also been increasing attention to housing and community support. As people have transitioned from primarily receiving services as an inpatient for serious mental illness to receiving those services within their community, there has been increased demands on families, communities, local mental health workers, and other community agencies (Sealy, 2012). Consequently, as symptoms wax and wane over the course of a chronic mental illness, families, caregivers, and workers in non–health community agencies often experience caregiving fatigue. Despite the challenges for the caregivers, one of the largest hurdles to overcome for people living with a serious and chronic mental illness is finding appropriate housing to meet their immediate social, financial, and safety needs. Most individuals with severe forms of mental illness live in some form of supervised or supported community living situation, which ranges

from highly supervised congregate settings to independent apartments. Those who lack the resources to find housing suffer higher rates of substance abuse, physical illness, incarceration, and victimization (Jakubec, Tomazewski, Powel, & Osuji, 2012). In a study that looked at 500 homeless people in three different Canadian cities, 92.8% of the participants had a mental illness (Krausz et al., 2013).

Supported Housing

There has been a paradigm shift from reliance on the residential continuum to what is now known as supported housing. Supportive housing has site-based health and social services that are aimed at improving the health and residential stability of highly disadvantaged individuals (Hwang et al., 2011). **Community-based residential services** provide a place for people to reside during a 24-hour period or any portion of the day, on an ongoing basis. A residential facility can be publicly or privately owned. **Intensive residential services** are staffed for patient treatment. These services may include medical, nursing, psychosocial, vocational, recreational, or other support services. Combining residential care and mental health services, this treatment form offers rehabilitation and therapy to people with serious and persistent mental illnesses, including chronic schizophrenia, bipolar disorder, and unrelenting depression. These services may provide short-term treatment for

---

BOX 4.8 Best Practices

BRIDGING THE GAPS IN INPATIENT AND OUTPATIENT CARE

Research Evidence

Well-designed follow-up studies show the following:
- Barriers to mental health services impede access to care.
- Psychological barriers include fear of public rejection (stigmatization) and participant's judgments of the therapist.
- Physical barriers include travel barriers that are caused by restricted finances, physical abilities, geographical location, or personal responsibilities (work, school, child care).

Preliminary study results suggest that Web- and telephone-based interventions can address a number of barriers to mental health services that are traditionally delivered.

Key Elements of Best Practice

- Distance mental health delivery systems (Web- and telephone-based) can be used to overcome physical and psychological access barriers.

- Regardless of service delivery system, establishing an effective therapeutic relationship is critical to the success of therapy.
- People with mental health problems or illness continue to experience social alienation and stigma. Care providers, whether they are providing care in person or in another manner, must be aware of the potential fear of public rejection.
- The ability of the care provider to create an environment with a sense of social presence and belonging is critical to potential success of the interventions.

From Lingley-Pottie, P., McGrath, P., & Andreou, P. (2013). Barriers to mental health care: Perceived delivery system differences. *Advances in Nursing Science, 36*(1), 51–61. doi: 10.1097/ANS.0b013e31828077eb

stays from 24 hours to 3 or 6 months or long-term treatment for several months to years.

Nursing has an important role in the care of people who have severe and persistent mental illnesses and who require long-term stays at residential treatment facilities. Nurses provide PMH nursing care with a focus on psychoeducation, basic social skills training, aggression management, activities of daily living training, and group living. Education on symptom management, understanding mental illnesses, and medication management is essential to recovery. *The Canadian Standards for psychiatric-mental health nursing* guides the nurse in delivering patient care (Canadian Federation of Mental Health Nurses, 2014) (see Chapter 5).

Supportive Employment

A key component in a comprehensive mental health system is also the provision of supports for employment. Gruhl (2012) identifies that "how people with serious mental illness spend their time has been less emphasized in care programs than whether people are compliant with medication, asymptomatic and not in hospital" (p. 379). Employment is strongly linked to a person's sense of self-worth and personal environment. **Supportive employment** services assist individuals to find work; assess individuals' skills, attitudes, behaviours, and interest relevant to work; offer vocational rehabilitation or other training; and provide work opportunities. Supportive employment programs—individual placement and support services—are highly individualized and competitive. For example, in Ontario, funding has shifted from a fee-for-service to an outcomes-based funding model (Gewurtz, Cott, Rush, & Kirsh, 2012). Service providers deliver on-site support and job-coaching services on a one-to-one basis. They occur in real work settings and are used for patients with severe mental illnesses. The primary focus is to maintain attachment between the mentally ill person and the workforce (see Chapter 16).

Acute Inpatient Care

Acute inpatient hospitalization involves the most intensive treatment and is considered the most restrictive setting in the continuum. Inpatient treatment is reserved for acutely ill patients who, because of a mental illness, meet one or more of three criteria: high risk for harming oneself, high risk for harming others, or inability to care for one's basic needs. The delivery of inpatient care can occur in a psychiatric hospital or psychiatric unit within a general hospital. Admission to inpatient environments can be voluntary or involuntary (see Chapter 3). Provincial legislation (mental health acts) describes conditions that warrant hospitalization. Length of inpatient stay is kept as short as possible without harmful effects on patient outcomes.

 SUMMARY OF KEY POINTS

- The continuum of PMH care must be well integrated within the overall health care system and shaped by the principles of primary health care: accessibility, public participation, health promotion, appropriate technology, and intersectoral cooperation.
- The continuum of care is a comprehensive system of services and programs spanning the range from mental health promotion and illness prevention to very specialized services designed to match the needs of the individuals and populations with the appropriate care and treatment, which vary according to levels of service, structure, and intensity of care.
- The nurse's specific responsibilities vary according to the setting. In most settings, nurses function as members of an interprofessional team. Consumers of mental health services and their families should be considered as core members of that team.
- An integrated approach to delivering a patient-centred mental health care is required to ensure effective and efficient services.

 Web Links

cmha.ca The Canadian Mental Health Association advocates leadership by the federal and provincial governments to ensure equitable access to services and treatment across Canada.

hc-sc.gc.ca The Health Canada Web site provides current information about federal initiatives in mental health policy and practice.

www.mindyourmind.ca This is a Web site for youth and young adults and the professionals who work with them to access information about resources and tools related to mental health and mental illness. These resources are designed to reduce the stigma associated with mental illness and increase access and use of community support, both professional and peer based.

mind.org.uk This is the Web site of Mind, the leading mental health charity in England and Wales. Among its objectives is to inspire the development of quality services that reflect expressed need and diversity.

ACKNOWLEDGEMENT

The author thanks Michael Lee (RN, MN student) for his valuable critique and literature search.

References

Alberta Health and Wellness. (2006). *System case management for continuing care clients: Prepared for Continuing Care Leaders Council.* Edmonton, AB: Author.

Bilsker, D., Goldner, E., & Anderson, E. (2012). Supported self-management: A simple, effective way to improve depression care. *The Canadian Journal of Psychiatry, 57*(4), 203–209.

Canadian Federation of Mental Health Nurses. (2014). *Canadian standards of psychiatric and mental health nursing: Standards of practice* (4th ed.). Toronto, ON: Author. Retrieved from http://cfmhn.ca/professionalPractices?f=7458545122100118.pdf&n=212922-CFMHN-standards-rv-3a.pdf&inline=yes

Canadian Foundation for Healthcare Improvement. (2014). *Healthcare priorities in Canada: A backgrounder.* Retrieved from http://www.cfhi-fcass.ca/sf-docs/default-source/documents/harkness-healthcare-priorities-canada-backgrounder-e.pdf

Canadian Nurses Association. (2012). *Position statement on mental health services.* Ottawa, ON: Author.

Doughty, C., & Tse, S. (2011). Can consumer-led mental health services be equally effective? An integrative review of CLMH services in high-income countries. *Community Mental Health Journal, 47*(3), 252–266. doi: 10.1007/s10597-010-9321-5

Emergency Management Policy Directorate. (2011). *An emergency management framework for Canada* (2nd ed.). Ottawa, ON: Author. Retrieved from http://www.publicsafety.gc.ca/cnt/rsrcs/pblctns/mrgnc-mngmnt-frmwrk/index-eng.aspx

Forchuk, C., Reiss, J. P., Mitchell, B., Even, S., & Meier, A. (2015). Homelessness and housing crises among individuals accessing services within a Canadian emergency department. *Journal of Psychiatric and Mental Health Nursing, 22*, 354–359. doi: 10.1111/jpn.12212

Fung, Y. L., Chan, Z., & Chien, W. T. (2014). Role performance of psychiatric nurses in advanced practice: A systematic review of the literature. *Journal of Psychiatric and Mental Health Nursing, 21*, 698–714. doi: 10.111/jpm.12128

Gewurtz, R., Cott, C., Rush, B., & Kirsh, B. (2012). The shift to rapid job placement for people living with mental illness: An analysis of consequences. *Psychiatric Rehabilitation Journal, 35*(6), 428–434. doi: 10.1037/h0094575

Government of Alberta. (2015). *Valuing mental health: Report of the Alberta Mental Health Review Committee.* Retrieved from http://www.health.alberta.ca/documents/Alberta-Mental-Health-Review-2015.pdf

Gruhl, K. (2012). Transitions to work for persons with serious mental illness in northeastern Ontario, Canada: Examining barriers to employment. *Work, 41*(4), 379–389. doi: 10.3233/WOR-2012-1315

Hair, H., Shortall, R., & Oldford J. (2013). Where's help when we need it? Developing responsive and effective brief counseling services for children, adolescents, and their families. *Social Work in Mental Health, 11*(1), 16–33. doi: 10.1080/15332985.2012.716389

Health Canada. (2011). *Emergency preparedness.* Retrieved from http://www.hc-sc.gc.ca/hc-ps/ed-ud/prepar/index-eng.php

Hwang, S., Gogosis, E., Chambers, C., Dunn, J., Hoch, J., & Aubry, T. (2011). Health status, quality of life, residential stability, substance use, and health care utilization among adults applying to a supportive housing program. *Journal of Urban Health: Bulletin of the New York Academy of Medicine, 88*(6), 1079–1090. doi: 10.1007/s11524-011-9592-3

Jakubec, S., Tomaszewski, A., Powell, T., & Osuji, J. (2012). "More than the house": A Canadian perspective on housing stability. *Housing, Care and Support, 15*(3), 99–108. doi: 10.1108/14608791211268518

Kates, N., Mazowita, G., Lemire, F., Jayabarathan, A., Bland, R., Selby, P., & Audet, D. (2011). The evolution of collaborative mental health care in Canada: A shared vision for the future. *The Canadian Journal of Psychiatry, 56*(5), 1–10.

Kathol, R., Perez, R., & Cohen, J. (2010). *The integrated case management manual.* New York, NY: Springer Publishing Company.

Kirby, M. (2008). Mental health in Canada: Out of the shadows forever. *Canadian Medical Association Journal, 178*(10), 1320–1322.

Krausz, R., Clarkson, A., Strehlau, V., Torchalla, I., Li, K., & Schuetz, C. (2013). Mental disorder, service use, and barriers to care among 500 homeless people in 3 different urban settings. *Social Psychiatry and Psychiatric Epidemiology, 48*(8), 1235–1243. doi: 10.1007/s00127-012-0649-8

Krupa, T., Stuart, H., Mathany, A., Smart, J., & Chen, S. P. (2010). An evaluation of a community-based, integrated crisis-case management service. *Canadian Journal of Community Mental Health, 29*(5 Suppl), 125–137.

Lingley-Pottie, P., McGrath, P., & Andreou, P. (2013). Barriers to mental health care: Perceived delivery system differences. *Advances in Nursing Science, 36*(1) 51–61. doi: 10.1097/ANS0b013e31828077eb

Lurie, S. (2012). And now for something completely different ... Self management. *The Canadian Journal of Psychiatry, 57*(4), 201–202. Retrieved from http://publications.cpa-apc.org

Mental Health Commission of Canada. (2009). *Toward recovery and well-being: A framework for a mental health strategy for Canada.* Calgary, AB: Author.

Mental Health Commission of Canada. (2012). *Changing directions, changing lives: The mental health strategy for Canada.* Calgary, AB: Author.

Mental Health Commission of Canada. (2015). *Guidelines for recovery-oriented practice, Hope, Dignity, Inclusion.* Ottawa, ON: Author.

Mental health considerations: The unseen effects of disaster. (2013). *Environmental Health Perspectives, 121*(5), A159.

Newman, D., O'Reilly, P. L., Lee, S. H., & Kennedy, D. (2015). Mental health service users' experiences of mental health care: An integrative literature review. *Journal of Psychiatric and Mental Health Nursing, 22*, 171–182. doi: 10.1111/jpm.12202View

Sealy, P. (2012). The impact of the process of deinstitutionalization of mental health services in Canada: An increase in accessing of health professionals for mental health concerns. *Social Work in Public Health, 27*(3), 229–237. doi: 10.1080/19371911003748786

Segal, S., Silverman, C., & Temkin, T. (2013). Are all consumer-operated programs empowering self-help agencies? *Social Work in Mental Health, 11*(1), 1–15. doi: 10.1080/15332985.2012.718731

Wild, T. C., Wolfe, J., Wang, J., & Ohinmaa, A. (2014). *Gap analysis of public mental health and addictions programs (GAP-MAP): Final report.* Edmonton, AB: Government of Alberta. Retrieved from http://www.health.alberta.ca/documents/GAP-MAP-Report-2014.pdf

World Health Organization. (2002). *Prevention and promotion in mental health.* Geneva, Switzerland: Author.

World Health Organization. (2008a). *The world health report 2008: Primary health care—Now more than ever.* Geneva, Switzerland: Author.

World Health Organization. (2008b). *Integrating mental health into primary care: A global perspective.* Geneva, Switzerland: Author.

World Health Organization. (2016). *Mental health: Strengthening our response.* Geneva, Switzerland: Author.

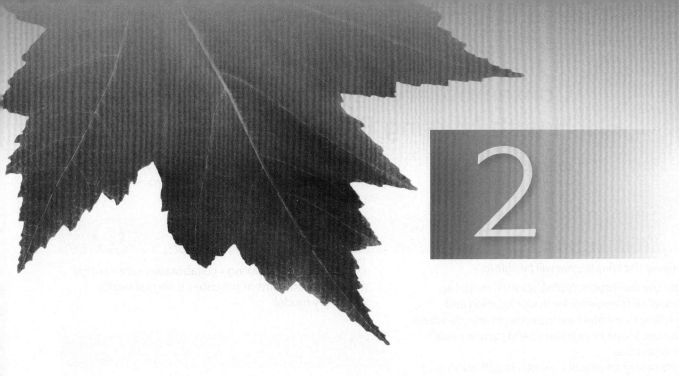

Foundations
of Psychiatric and Mental Health Nursing Practice

Wendy Austin

Adapted from the chapter "Contemporary
Psychiatric and Mental Health Nursing Practice" by
Wendy Austin and Margaret Osborne

LEARNING OBJECTIVES

After studying this chapter, you will be able to:

- Explain the bio/psycho/social/spiritual model as a conceptual framework for understanding and responding to mental health problems and disorders.
- Explain the scope of psychiatric and mental health nursing practice.
- Describe entry-to-practice mental health nursing competencies.
- Discuss the role of standards of practice for Canadian nurses.
- Specify five key components of psychiatric and mental health nursing.
- Discuss current challenges of psychiatric and mental health nursing.
- Identify national and international organizations with relevance to psychiatric and mental health nursing practice.

KEY TERMS

- clinical decision-making • collaborative care • critical pathways • domains of practice • e-Mental health • recovery model

KEY CONCEPTS

- bio/psycho/social/spiritual model • competency • standards of practice

This chapter introduces the bio/psycho/social/spiritual model as an approach to understanding human health that informs psychiatric and mental health (PMH) nursing practice. The scope of PMH nursing is explained, entry-to-practice competencies for mental health nursing outlined, and standards of practice explicitly describing the obligations of nurses in Canadian PMH care settings presented. The discussion of the challenges of PMH nursing sets the stage for the rest of the textbook through an overview of the dynamic nature of this aspect of nursing.

THE BIO/PSYCHO/SOCIAL/SPIRITUAL MODEL OF PMH NURSING

Contemporary PMH nursing uses theories from the biologic, psychological, and social sciences as a basis of practice, as well as knowledge of the spiritual aspects of human life. This holistic approach, referred to as the bio/psycho/social/spiritual model of PMH nursing, is necessary to guide understanding of the individual who is experiencing mental health problems or a mental disorder. Holism joins the biologic, psychological, social, and spiritual domains in an integrated, dynamic conceptualization of human health. The model provides a basis for the organization of nursing care and is used throughout this text for integrating theoretic knowledge and the nursing process (Fig. 5.1).

KEY CONCEPT

The **bio/psycho/social/spiritual model** consists of separate but interacting domains that can be understood independently but that are mutually interdependent with the other domains.

Biologic Domain

The *biologic* domain consists of the biologic theories related to mental disorders and problems as well as all of the biologic processes related to other health problems. For instance, there is evidence of neurobiologic changes in most mental disorders which informs our understanding of the causes and/or presentation of

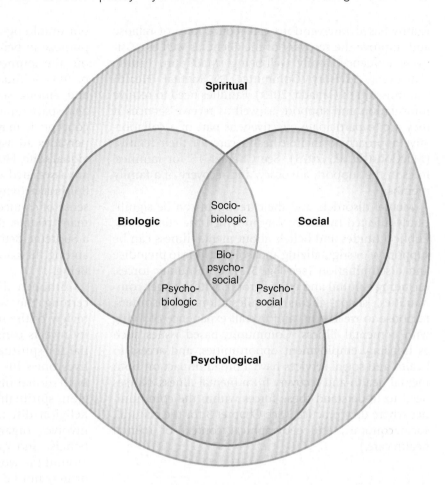

Figure 5.1. Bio/psycho/social/spiritual model. (Originally adapted from Abraham, I., Fox, J., & Cohen, B. (1992). Integrating the bio into the biopsychosocial: Understanding and treating biological phenomena in psychiatric–mental health nursing. *Archives of Psychiatric Nursing, 6*(5), 296–305.)

those disorders. Within this domain, theories and concepts shape interventions that focus on an individual's physical functioning, such as exercise, relaxation, sleep, and nutrition. Neurobiologic theories serve as a basis for understanding such biologic treatments as pharmacologic agents and electroconvulsive therapy (ECT) (see Chapter 12).

Psychological Domain

The *psychological* domain contains the theoretical basis of the psychological processes: thoughts, feelings, and behaviours (intrapersonal dynamics) that influence one's emotions, cognitions, and actions. The psychological and nursing sciences generate theories and research that are critical to understanding an individual's symptoms and responses to mental disorders. Although most mental disorders have been found to have a biologic component, they are often manifested in psychological symptoms. The person with a thought disorder may express atypical behaviour that needs to be interpreted within the context of the neurobiologic dysfunction of the mental disorder.

Many PMH nursing interventions are based on knowledge generated within this domain. Cognitive approaches, behavioural therapies, and client education are all based on the use of theories from the psychological

domain. These interventions are explained in Unit 3. PMH interventions are also based on the use of interpersonal communication techniques, which require nurses to develop awareness of their own, as well as their client's, internal thoughts, feelings, and behaviours. For nurses, exploring and understanding their own intrapersonal dynamics and motivation are critical to gaining understanding of their clients. Such understanding is necessary to the development of therapeutic relationships and to helping clients learn about their disorders and participate in their treatment and its management. Motivating clients to engage in learning activities best occurs within the context of a therapeutic relationship (see Chapter 6).

Social Domain

The *social* domain includes theories that account for the influence of social forces (including cultural forces) encompassing the client, family, and community. This knowledge base is generated from social and nursing sciences and delineates the connections within families and communities that affect the health and treatment of people with mental disorders. Understanding family factors, including origin, extended family, and other significant relationships, contributes to the total understanding and treatment of individual clients.

Family-based interventions can reduce rates of relapse and improve the recovery of the client, as well as positively influence family well-being (MacCourt, Family Caregivers Advisory Committee, & Mental Health Commission of Canada, 2013). Families need to receive information and support, as well as receive services if they are to participate effectively as part of a collaborative approach to mental health care for their relative (MacCourt et al., 2013). See Chapter 15 for families' roles in the support, advocacy, and recovery of a family member.

Mental disorders and their treatment can be significantly affected by the society in which the client lives. Public attitudes and beliefs about mental illness can be supportive or stigmatizing and isolating due to prejudice and discrimination (see Fig. 5.2). Community forces, including cultural and ethnic groups within larger communities, shape clients' manifestation of disorders, response to treatment, and overall experience of living with a mental illness. Community-based issues such as housing, employment opportunities, and access to health and social services have a broad impact on both mental health and recovery from mental illness. Nurses need to understand these forces within the communities where they practice. (See Chapter 3 for the cultural, socioeconomic, and geographical context of mental health care.)

Spiritual Domain

The spiritual domain encompasses the bio/psycho/social domains. Spirituality relates to the core of whom we are; one definition of spirituality is "the essence of our being, which permeates our living and infuses

our unfolding awareness of who and what we are, our purpose in being, and our inner resources; and shapes our life journey" (Dossey, Keegan, & Guzzetta, 2004, p. 91). Spirituality comprises the connections within and among self, others, and the universe over time and space. Spirituality is a complex, even mysterious, concept: it may be regarded as the driving force that pervades all aspects of and gives meaning to an individual's life. Hope, trust, reconciliation, and inspiration are associated with the spiritual domain (Barss, 2012). Spiritual activity involves introspection, reflection, and a sense of connectedness to others or to the universe. For many people, this connectedness focuses ultimately on a Supreme Being. God, Allah, Jehovah, and Creator are among the names that refer to a worshipped Supreme Being.

Although there remains a lack of agreement concerning the way spirituality should be defined, a review of the interprofessional literature on spirituality reveals common themes: everyone has the potential for spirituality and spiritual growth; the way one lives one's life is reflective of spirituality; spirituality is relational in nature; and there is a link among religion, spirituality, and moral norms (Catalano, 2015). Religion differs, however, from spirituality. Religion involves organized systems of rituals, patterns of beliefs, and groups of people usually congregating around the worship of a deity. A religious person may or may not be spiritual; a person's spirituality may or may not involve religion.

Spiritual growth may be stimulated by pivotal life events, including distressing ones like being diagnosed with a mental disorder. It can be very difficult, however, to transcend one's current reality and the suffering

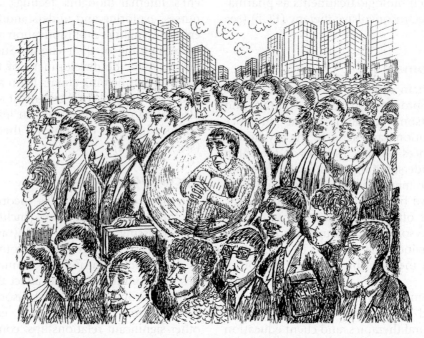

Figure 5.2. Drawing by Al Mier. (Used with permission for educational purposes.)

it may entail. Individuals living with a mental illness often struggle with loss of meaning and purpose and wonder, "Why has this happened to me?". They may be affected by religious or cultural beliefs that view mental illness as a form of punishment. The nurse can help individuals experiencing spiritual distress by supporting their efforts to find meaning in their circumstances, which may include meditation, contemplation, prayer, and other spiritual practices that may give comfort. The relationship of the body, mind, relation, and spirit in the content of human health is holistic, synergistic, and unifying. It is central to the process of recovery and well-being.

ENTRY-TO-PRACTICE MENTAL HEALTH COMPETENCIES

Nursing education is guided, in part, by the practice competencies expected of a credentialed nurse upon entry to practice. The competencies are identifiable, measurable descriptions of the knowledge, skills, and attitudes deemed essential to the particular nursing role (e.g., registered nurse, registered psychiatric nurse, licensed/registered practical nurse [LPNs/RPNs]). As students study and gain practice experiences, the entry-to-practice competencies of their future occupation are helpful guides. Those of Canadian registered nurses (RNs) and registered psychiatric nurses (RPNs) follow. The competency profiles for LPN/RPN are delineated by provincial and

territorial jurisdictions. These can be located through the Canadian Council for Practical Nurse Regulators (CCPNR) (see Web Links).

KEY CONCEPT

A **competency** is the capability of acting appropriately and effectively in a role. It involves the use of internal resources (e.g., knowledge, skills, attitudes) and external resources (e.g., policies, the interprofessional team, research).

CASN/CFMHN Entry-to-Practice Mental Health and Addiction Competencies

The competencies expected of all Canadian RNs upon entry to practice have been delineated by the Canadian Association of Schools of Nursing (CASN) in partnership with the Canadian Federation of Mental Health Nurses (CFMHN). *Entry-to-Practice Mental Health and Addiction Competencies for Undergraduate Nursing Education in Canada* (CASN with CFMHN, 2015) is a national framework that outlines essential knowledge, attitudes, and skills all RNs should possess as they begin to practice. The competencies are organized within domains (identified by provincial/territorial nursing regulatory bodies) along with achievement indicators. See Boxes 5.1 to 5.5.

BOX 5.1 CASN and CFMHN Entry-to-Practice Mental Health and Addiction Competencies for Undergraduate Nursing Education in Canada

DOMAIN 1 PROFESSIONAL RESPONSIBILITY AND ACCOUNTABILITY

COMPETENCY 1

The nurse provides care in accordance with professional and regulatory standards when promoting mental health and preventing or managing mental health conditions and/or addiction.

Indicators

1.1 Understands and applies mental health–related legislation, and upholds the rights and autonomy of persons with a mental health condition and/or addiction.

1.2 Therapeutically engages with persons experiencing a mental health condition and/or addiction, with dignity and respect.

1.3 Recognizes stigmatizing and discriminating attitudes regarding mental health conditions and

addiction in health care professionals and/or self, as well as the detrimental impact of such attitudes on health care outcomes and responds therapeutically.

1.4 Applies policies related to principles of health promotion and prevention of injury (i.e., least restraint) in caring for persons with a mental health condition and/or addiction.

1.5 Demonstrates knowledge related to the process of voluntary and involuntary care.

1.6 Protects clients, self, and others from harm in situations where a person with a mental health condition and/or addiction poses a safety risk while maintaining the client's dignity and human rights.

Canadian Association of Schools of Nursing with the Canadian Federation of Mental Health Nurses. (2015). *Entry to practice mental health and addiction competencies for undergraduate education in Canada*. Ottawa, ON: Canadian Association of Schools of Nursing. Used with permission.

> **BOX 5.2** CASN and CFMHN Entry-to-Practice Mental Health and Addiction Competencies for Undergraduate Nursing Education in Canada

DOMAIN 2 KNOWLEDGE-BASED PRACTICE

COMPETENCY 2

The nurse uses relational practice to conduct a person-focused mental health assessment, and develops a plan of care in collaboration with the person, family, and health team to promote recovery.

Indicators

Knowledge

2.1 Demonstrates an understanding of the concepts of mental health, developmental, and situational transitions and the spectrum of mental health conditions and addictions as they are manifested in individuals across the life span.

2.2 Demonstrates an understanding of how mental health comorbidities increase severity, levels of disability, and use of mental health services.

2.3 Describes key elements of relevant theories, including but not limited to stress, coping, adaptation, development, harm reduction, crisis intervention, recovery, loss, and grief, and articulates their implications for clinical practice.

2.4 Demonstrates knowledge of the possible effects of complementary therapies on mental health conditions and addiction.

2.5 Understands the complex interrelationship of physiology, pathophysiology, and mental health (e.g., neuroleptic malignant syndrome, delirium, hypertension, etc.).

2.6 Demonstrates knowledge of medications used to treat addiction and withdrawal, including opiate replacement medications.

Assessment

2.7 Conducts a mental status exam.

2.8 Uses a range of relational and therapeutic skills including listening, respect, empathy, reaffirmation, mutuality, and sensitivity in assessments and care planning for persons experiencing a mental health condition and/or addiction.

2.9 Demonstrates the ability to identify clients' emotional, cognitive, and behavioural states, as well as level of anxiety, crisis states, indices of aggression, self-harm, suicide, risk to others,

competency to care for self, and signs of substance abuse, addiction, and withdrawal.

Planning Care

2.10 Plans care in partnership with clients to promote mental health, prevent a mental health condition and addiction, minimize negative effects on physical health, manage or reduce symptoms of mental health conditions, and foster recovery and resilience.

2.11 Recognizes the role of social determinants of health on mental health outcomes and incorporates this when planning care of persons experiencing a mental health condition and/or addiction.

2.12 Uses a trauma-informed approach to plan care and recognizes the negative effects of violence, abuse, racism, discrimination, colonization, poverty, homelessness, and early childhood maltreatment (such as neglect) on mental health.

COMPETENCY 3

Provides and evaluates person-centred nursing care in partnership with persons experiencing a mental health condition and/or addiction, along the continuum of care and across the life span.

Indicators

3.1 Communicates therapeutically with persons and families who are experiencing a range of mental health conditions and/or addiction, abuse, bereavement, or crisis.

3.2 Uses self therapeutically in providing health-promoting, preventive, and supportive care for persons experiencing a mental health condition and/or addiction.

3.3 Engages clients in strengths-based care that promotes resilience.

3.4 Advocates for persons experiencing a mental health condition and/or addiction.

3.5 Demonstrates basic knowledge of psychobiology in relation to psychopharmacology and the therapeutic dose range, side effects, interactions, and adverse effects of psychotropic medications across the life span.

3.6 Engages individuals and families in learning about a mental health condition and/or addiction and its management.

BOX 5.2 CASN and CFMHN Entry-to-Practice Mental Health and Addiction Competencies for Undergraduate Nursing Education in Canada (*Continued*)

3.7 Provides care to persons experiencing a mental health condition and/or addiction that is recovery oriented and trauma informed and uses principles of harm reduction and addresses social determinants of health.

3.8 Administers medication used to treat a mental health condition and/or addiction safely; monitors clients for therapeutic effects, side effects, and adverse reactions to medications; and intervenes effectively when side effects and adverse effects of medications occur.

Canadian Association of Schools of Nursing with the Canadian Federation of Mental Health Nurses. (2015). *Entry to practice mental health and addiction competencies for undergraduate education in Canada.* Ottawa, ON: Canadian Association of Schools of Nursing. Used with permission.

BOX 5.3 CASN and CFMHN Entry-to-Practice Mental Health and Addiction Competencies for Undergraduate Nursing Education in Canada

DOMAIN 3 ETHICAL PRACTICE

COMPETENCY 4

Acts in accordance with the CNA Code of Ethics when working with persons experiencing a mental health condition and/or addiction

Indicators

4.1 Provides a safe and respectful environment to voluntary and involuntary clients seeking or receiving treatment for a mental health condition and/or addiction.

4.2 Assists persons with a mental health condition and/or addiction in making informed decisions about their health care and symptom management.

4.3 Demonstrates cultural competency and cultural safety when caring for diverse persons with a mental health condition and/or addiction.

Canadian Association of Schools of Nursing with the Canadian Federation of Mental Health Nurses. (2015). *Entry to practice mental health and addiction competencies for undergraduate education in Canada.* Ottawa, ON: Canadian Association of Schools of Nursing. Used with permission.

BOX 5.4 CASN and CFMHN Entry-to-Practice Mental Health and Addiction Competencies for Undergraduate Nursing Education in Canada

DOMAIN 4 SERVICE TO THE PUBLIC

COMPETENCY 5

The nurse works collaboratively with partners to promote mental health and advocate for improvements in health services for persons experiencing a mental health condition and/or addiction.

Indicators

5.1 Demonstrates knowledge of the health care system in order to contribute to the improvement of mental health and addiction services.

5.2 Recognizes the impact of the organizational culture on the provision of mental health care to persons experiencing mental health conditions and addiction, and acts to ensure appropriate services are delivered safely.

5.3 Facilitates and engages in collaborative, inter- and intraprofessional, and intersectoral practice when providing care for persons with a mental health condition and/or addiction.

Canadian Association of Schools of Nursing (CASN) with the Canadian Federation of Mental Health Nurses (CFMHN). (2015). *Entry to practice mental health and addiction competencies for undergraduate education in Canada.* Ottawa, ON: Canadian Association of Schools of Nursing. Used with permission.

BOX 5.5 CASN and CFMHN Entry-to-Practice Mental Health and Addiction Competencies for Undergraduate Nursing Education in Canada

DOMAIN 5 SELF-REGULATION

COMPETENCY 6

Develops and maintains competencies through self-reflection and new opportunities working with persons experiencing a mental health condition and/or addiction

Indicators

6.1 Evaluates one's individual practice and knowledge when providing care to persons with a mental health condition and/or addiction, and seeks help as required.

6.2 Identifies one's own morals, values, attitudes, beliefs, and experiences related to mental health

conditions and/or addiction and the effect these may have on care.

6.3 Identifies learning needs related mental health conditions and addiction.

6.4 Seeks new knowledge, skills, and supports related to mental health conditions and addiction.

6.5 Evaluates self-learning related to mental health conditions and addiction.

Canadian Association of Schools of Nursing (CASN) with the Canadian Federation of Mental Health Nurses (CFMHN). (2015). *Entry to practice mental health and addiction competencies for undergraduate education in Canada.* Ottawa, ON: Canadian Association of Schools of Nursing. Used with permission.

Registered Psychiatric Nursing Entry-to-Practice Competencies

The client-centred competency framework for RPNs was approved by the Registered Psychiatric Nurse Regulators of Canada (RPNRC) in 2014. There are seven categories with key and enabling competencies. The competencies are considered equal in importance

and are to be viewed as an integrated whole. Evolving these competencies and acquiring further ones occurs in practice and through orientation, continuing education, and professional development (RPNRC, 2014). Along with the approved standards of practice and code of ethics, the competencies delineate the safe, competent, and ethical practice expected of RPNs in Canada. See Boxes 5.6 to 5.12.

BOX 5.6 Registered Psychiatric Nurses Entry-to-Practice Competencies

COMPETENCY 1

THERAPEUTIC RELATIONSHIPS AND THERAPEUTIC USE OF SELF

Therapeutic use of self is the foundational instrument that registered psychiatric nurses use to establish therapeutic relationships with clients to deliver care and psychosocial interventions.

1.1 Apply therapeutic use of self to inform all areas of psychiatric nursing practice.

1.1.1 Utilize one's personality consciously and with full awareness in an attempt to establish relationships.

1.1.2 Assess and clarify the influences of one's personal beliefs, values, and life experiences on interactions.

1.1.3 Differentiate between a therapeutic relationship and a social, romantic, sexual relationship.

1.1.4 Recognize, identify, and validate the feelings of others.

1.1.5 Recognize and address the impact of transference and countertransference in the therapeutic relationship.

1.1.6 Demonstrate unconditional positive regard, empathy, and congruence in relationships.

1.1.7 Monitor the communication process and adapt communication strategies accordingly by using a variety of verbal and nonverbal communication skills.

1.1.8 Critique the effectiveness of therapeutic use of self on others.

1.1.9 Engage in personal and professional development activities to enhance the therapeutic use of self.

1.1.10 Engage in self-care activities to decrease the risk of secondary trauma and burnout.

1.2 Establish a therapeutic relationship with the client.

1.2.1 Develop a rapport and promote trust through mutual respect, genuineness, empathy, acceptance, and collaboration.

1.2.2 Establish and negotiate boundaries (e.g., role and service offered, length and frequency of meetings, responsibilities) to clarify the nature, content, and limits of the therapeutic relationship.

BOX 5.6 Registered Psychiatric Nurses Entry-to-Practice Competencies (*Continued*)

1.2.3 Engage with the client to explore goals, learning, and growth needs (e.g., problem identification, thought exploration, feelings, and behaviours).

1.2.4 Differentiate between therapeutic and nontherapeutic communication techniques.

1.2.5 Apply therapeutic communication strategies and techniques to reduce emotional distress, facilitate cognitive and behavioural change, and foster personal growth (e.g., active listening, clarifying, restating, reflecting, focusing, exploring, therapeutic use of silence).

1.3 Maintain the therapeutic relationship.

1.3.1 Engage in ongoing assessment, planning, implementation, and evaluation over the course of the psychiatric nurse–client relationship.

1.3.2 Apply strategies, techniques and resources to meet client goals (e.g., conflict resolution, crisis intervention, counselling, clinically appropriate use of self-disclosure).

1.3.3 Collaborate with the client to help achieve client-identified goals.

1.3.4 Adapt therapeutic strategies when encountering resistance and ambivalence.

1.3.5 Provide teaching and coaching around client goals and evaluate learning.

1.3.6 Dedicate time to maintain the relationship with the client.

1.3.7 Engage in systematic review of progress with the client.

1.3.8 Address the impact of transference and countertransference in the therapeutic relationship.

1.3.9 Engage in consultation to facilitate, support, and enhance the therapeutic use of self.

1.4 Terminate the therapeutic relationship.

1.4.1 Identify the end point of the therapeutic relationship.

1.4.2 Summarize the outcomes of the therapeutic relationship with the client.

1.4.3 Evaluate the therapeutic process and outcomes of the interventions.

1.4.4 Establish the boundaries of the posttherapeutic relationship.

1.4.5 Determine the need for follow-up and establish referral(s) accordingly.

Registered Psychiatric Nurse Regulators of Canada. (2014). *Registered psychiatric nurse-entry level competencies*. Edmonton, AB: Author. Used with permission.

BOX 5.7 Registered Psychiatric Nurses Entry-to-Practice Competencies

COMPETENCY 2
BODY OF KNOWLEDGE AND APPLICATION

Registered psychiatric nurses' practice is comprised of foundational nursing knowledge and specialized psychiatric nursing knowledge. RPNs integrate general nursing knowledge and knowledge from the sciences, humanities, research, ethics, spirituality, and relational practice with specialized knowledge drawn from the fields of psychiatry and mental health. RPNs use critical inquiry and apply a decision-making process in providing psychiatric nursing care for clients. There are two categories under this competency: evidence-informed knowledge and application of body of knowledge.

Evidence: Informed Knowledge

2.1 Demonstrate knowledge of the health sciences, including anatomy, physiology, microbiology, nutrition, pathophysiology, psychopharmacology, pharmacology, epidemiology, genetics, and prenatal and genetic influences on development.

2.2 Demonstrate knowledge of social sciences and humanities, including psychology, sociology, human growth and development, communication, statistics, research methodology, philosophy, ethics, spiritual care, determinants of health, and primary health care.

2.3 Demonstrate knowledge of nursing science: conceptual nursing models, nursing skills, procedures, and interventions.

2.4 Demonstrate knowledge of current and emerging health issues (e.g., end-of-life care, substance use, vulnerable or marginalized populations).

2.5 Demonstrate knowledge of community, global, and population health issues (e.g., immunization, disaster planning, pandemics).

2.6 Demonstrate knowledge of applicable informatics and emerging technologies.

(Continued)

BOX 5.7 Registered Psychiatric Nurses Entry-to-Practice Competencies *(Continued)*

2.7 Demonstrate evidence-informed knowledge of psychopathology across the life span.

2.7.1 Demonstrate knowledge of disorders of developmental health and mental health.

2.7.2 Demonstrate knowledge of resources and diagnostic tools (e.g., standardized assessment scales, the Diagnostic and Statistical Manual of Mental Disorders).

2.8 Demonstrate knowledge of the disorders of addiction, as well as relevant resources and diagnostic tools (e.g., standardized screening tools, detoxification, and withdrawal guidelines).

2.9 Demonstrate knowledge of therapeutic modalities (e.g., individual, family, and group therapy and counselling, psychopharmacology, visualization, consumer-led initiatives).

2.10 Demonstrate knowledge of how complementary therapies can impact treatment (e.g., naturopathy, acupuncture).

2.11 Demonstrate knowledge of conceptual models of psychiatric care (e.g., Trauma-Informed Care, Recovery Model, Psychosocial Rehabilitation).

2.12 Demonstrate evidence-informed knowledge of the impact of social, cultural, and family systems on health outcomes.

2.13 Demonstrate knowledge of interpersonal communication, therapeutic use of self, and therapeutic relationships.

2.14 Demonstrate knowledge of the dynamic of interpersonal abuse (e.g., child, spousal, or elder abuse).

2.15 Demonstrate knowledge of mental health legislation and other relevant legislation (e.g., privacy laws).

Application of Body of Knowledge

2.16 Conduct a comprehensive client assessment.

2.16.1 Select an evidence-informed framework applicable to the type of assessments required (e.g., biopsychosocial, cultural model, community assessment model, multigenerational family assessment).

2.16.2 Perform holistic assessment (e.g., physical, mental health, social, spiritual, developmental, and cultural).

2.16.3 Perform an in-depth psychiatric evaluation (e.g., suicide, history of violence, trauma, stress, mental status, self-perception, adaptation and coping, substance use and abuse).

2.16.4 Collaborate with the client to identify health strengths and goals.

2.17 Formulate a clinical judgement based on the assessment data (e.g., nursing diagnosis, psychiatric nursing diagnosis).

2.17.1 Identify psychiatric signs and symptoms that are commonly associated with psychiatric disorders, using current nomenclature (e.g., the Diagnostic and Statistical Manual of Mental Disorders).

2.17.2 Identify clinical indicators that may negatively impact the client's well-being (e.g., pain, hyperglycemia, hypertension).

2.17.3 Incorporate data from other sources (e.g., laboratory tests, collateral information).

2.17.4 Use critical thinking to analyze and synthesize data collected to arrive at a clinical judgement.

2.18 Collaborate with the client to develop a treatment plan to address identified problems, minimize the development of complications, and promote functions and quality of life.

2.18.1 Discuss interventions with the client to achieve client-directed goals and outcomes (e.g., promote health, prevent disorder and injury, foster rehabilitation, and provide palliation).

2.18.2 Plan care using treatment modalities such as psychotherapy and psychopharmacology.

2.18.3 Propose a plan for self-care that promotes client responsibility and independence to the maximum degree possible (e.g., relaxation techniques, stress management, coping skills, community resources, complementary and alternative therapies).

2.19 Implement a variety of psychiatric nursing interventions with the client, according to the plan of care.

2.19.1 Assess the ethical and legal implications of the interventions before providing care.

2.19.2 Perform required nursing interventions to address physical conditions, including, but not limited to, intravenous therapy and drainage tubes, skin and wound care, metabolic screening, and management of withdrawal symptoms.

2.19.3 Perform safe medication administration by a variety of methods (e.g., oral, parenteral).

2.19.4 Provide complex psychiatric nursing interventions (e.g., facilitating group process, conflict resolution, crisis interventions, individual, group and family counselling, assertiveness training, somatic therapies, pre- and post-ECT [electroconvulsive therapy] care, milieu therapy, and relaxation).

BOX 5.7 Registered Psychiatric Nurses Entry-to-Practice Competencies *(Continued)*

2.19.5 Provide ongoing health education and teaching to promote health and quality of life, minimize the development of complications, and maintain and restore health (e.g., social skills training, anger management, relapse prevention, assertiveness training, and communication techniques).

2.19.6 Coordinate appropriate referrals and liaise to promote access to resources that can optimize health outcomes.

2.20 **Use critical thinking and clinical judgement to determine the level of risk and coordinate effective interventions for psychiatric and nonpsychiatric emergencies.**

2.20.1 Intervene to minimize agitation, de-escalate agitated behaviour, and manage aggressive behaviour in the least restrictive manner.

2.20.2 Intervene to prevent self-harm or minimize injury related to self-harm.

2.20.3 Conduct an ongoing suicide risk assessment and select an intervention from a range of evidence-informed suicide prevention strategies (e.g., safety planning, crisis intervention, referral to alternative level of care).

2.20.4 Apply crisis intervention skills with clients experiencing acute emotional, physical, behavioural, and mental distress (e.g., loss, grief, victimization, trauma).

2.20.5 Recognize and intervene to stabilize clients experiencing medical emergencies (e.g., shock, hypoglycemia, management of neuroleptic malignant syndrome, cardiac events).

2.21 **Collaborate with the client to evaluate the effectiveness and appropriateness of the plan of care.**

2.21.1 Collect, analyze, and synthesize data to evaluate the outcomes from the plan of care.

2.21.2 Use a critical inquiry process to continuously monitor the effectiveness of client care in relation to anticipated outcomes.

2.21.3 Solicit the client's perception of the nursing care and other therapeutic interventions that were provided.

2.21.4 Modify and individualize the plan of care in collaboration with the client and according to evaluation findings.

Registered Psychiatric Nurse Regulators of Canada. (2014). *Registered psychiatric nurse entry-level competencies.* Edmonton, AB: Author. Used with permission.

BOX 5.8 Registered Psychiatric Nurses Entry-to-Practice Competencies

COMPETENCY 3

COLLABORATIVE PRACTICE

RPNs work in collaboration with team members, families, and other stakeholders to deliver comprehensive psychiatric nursing care in order to achieve the client's health goals.

3.1 **Establish and maintain professional relationships that foster continuity and client-centred care.**

3.1.1 Use interpersonal communication skills to establish and maintain a rapport among team members.

3.1.2 Share relevant information with team members, clients, and stakeholders in a timely manner.

3.1.3 Promote collaborative and informed shared decision-making.

3.2 **Partner effectively with team members in the delivery of client-centred care.**

3.2.1 Demonstrate knowledge of the roles, responsibilities, and perspectives of team members and stakeholders.

3.2.2 Inform stakeholders of the roles and responsibilities of psychiatric nursing and the perspectives of the RPN when required.

3.2.3 Engage participation of additional team members as required.

3.2.4 Accept leadership responsibility for coordinating care identified by the team.

3.3 **Share responsibility for resolving conflict with team members.**

3.3.1 Identify the issues that may contribute to the development of conflict.

3.3.2 Recognize actual or potential conflict situations.

3.3.3 Employ effective conflict resolution and reconciliation approaches and techniques.

3.3.4 Negotiate to mitigate barriers in order to optimize health care outcomes.

Registered Psychiatric Nurse Regulators of Canada. (2014). *Registered psychiatric nurse entry-level competencies.* Edmonton, AB: Author. Used with permission.

BOX 5.9 Registered Psychiatric Nurses Entry-to-Practice Competencies

COMPETENCY 4
ADVOCACY

Registered psychiatric nurses use their expertise and influence to support their clients to advance their health and well-being on an individual and community level.

4.1 Collaborate with clients to take action on issues that may impact their health and well-being.

4.1.1 Advocate for needed resources that enhance the client's quality-of-life services and social inclusion (e.g., housing, accessibility, treatment options, basic needs).

4.1.2 Inform clients of their rights and options (e.g., appeals, complaints).

4.1.3 Support the client's right to informed decision-making (e.g., treatment plan, treatment orders).

4.1.4 Support client autonomy and right to choice (e.g., right to live at risk).

4.1.5 Promote the least restrictive treatment and environment.

4.2 Promote awareness of mental health and addictions issues by providing accurate information and challenging negative attitudes and behaviour that contribute to stigma and discrimination.

4.3 Collaborate with others to take action on issues influencing mental health and addictions.

4.3.1 Demonstrate knowledge and understanding of demographic and sociopolitical environments.

4.3.2 Recognize the impact of mental illness and stigma on society and the individual.

4.3.3 Recognize attitudes and behaviours that contribute to stigma.

4.3.4 Provide education to the community about mental health and addictions.

4.3.5 Engage with stakeholders and the community to promote mental health and wellness.

4.3.6 Engage in addressing social justice issues at an individual or community level (e.g., poverty, marginalization).

Registered Psychiatric Nurse Regulators of Canada. (2014). *Registered psychiatric nurse entry-level competencies.* Edmonton, AB: Author. Used with permission.

BOX 5.10 Registered Psychiatric Nurses Entry-to-Practice Competencies

COMPETENCY 5
QUALITY CARE AND CLIENT SAFETY

Registered psychiatric nurses collaborate in developing, implementing, and evaluating policies, procedures, and activities that promote quality care and client safety.

5.1 Use reflective practice and evidence to guide psychiatric nursing practice.

5.1.1 Reflect on and critically analyze practice (e.g., journaling, supervision, peer review) to inform and change future practice.

5.1.2 Reflect on current evidence from various sources and determine relevance to client need and practice setting (e.g., published research, clinical practice guidelines, policies, decision-making tools).

5.1.3 Integrate evidence into practice decisions to maximize health outcomes.

5.1.4 Evaluate the effectiveness of the evidence in practice.

5.2 Engage in practices to promote physical, environmental, and psychological safety.

5.2.1 Recognize potential risks and hazards, including risk for suicide and violence.

5.2.2 Use recognized assessment tools to address potential risks and hazards (e.g., medication reconciliation, client falls assessment tool).

5.2.3 Implement interventions to address potential risks and hazards (e.g., protocols, clinical practice guidelines, decision-making tools).

5.2.4 Evaluate the effectiveness of the interventions in practice.

5.2.5 Report and document safety risks and hazards.

5.2.6 Identify and address occupational hazards related to working with unpredictable behaviours, such as violence and suicide (e.g., burnout, secondary traumatization).

5.3 Integrate cultural awareness, safety, and sensitivity into practice.

BOX 5.10 Registered Psychiatric Nurses Entry-to-Practice Competencies *(Continued)*

5.3.1 Evaluate personal beliefs, values, and attitudes related to own culture and others' culture.

5.3.2 Explore the client's cultural needs, beliefs, practices, and preferences.

5.3.3 Incorporate the client's cultural preferences and personal perspectives into the plan of care when applicable.

5.3.4 Adapt communication to the audience while considering social and cultural diversity based on the client's needs.

5.3.5 Engage in opportunities to learn about various cultures (e.g., talking to client, attending cultural events, and courses).

5.3.6 Incorporate knowledge of culture and how multiple identities (e.g., race, gender, ethnicity, sexual orientation, disability) shape one's life experience and contribute to health outcomes.

Registered Psychiatric Nurse Regulators of Canada. (2014). *Registered psychiatric nurse entry-level competencies.* Edmonton, AB: Author. Used with permission.

BOX 5.11 Registered Psychiatric Nurses Entry-to-Practice Competencies

COMPETENCY 6

HEALTH PROMOTION

Registered psychiatric nurses use their expertise to promote the physical and mental health of clients to prevent disease, illness, and injury.

6.1 Engage in health promotion and the prevention of disease, illness, and injury.

6.1.1 Integrate knowledge of the determinants of health, health disparities, and health inequities when assessing health promotion needs.

6.1.2 Develop and implement evidence-informed health promotion strategies and programs based on a range of theories and models (e.g., Stages of Change, Health Belief Model, Social Learning Theory).

6.1.3 Select and implement evidence-informed interventions to promote health and prevent disease, illness, and injury (e.g., health communication, health education, community action, immunization, harm reduction).

6.1.4 Engage clients to seek out or develop resources that promote health (e.g., support groups, exercise programs, spiritual organizations).

6.1.5 Contribute to the development of policies and standards that support health promotion, and prevent disease, illness, and injury (e.g., falls prevention, medication reconciliation, prevention and management of aggressive behaviour, cultural sensitivity).

6.1.6 Advocate for health-promoting health care systems and environments.

6.2 Engage in mental health promotion when collaborating with clients.

6.2.1 Integrate knowledge of determinants of health in the assessment process (e.g., social inclusion, discrimination, economic resources, violence).

6.2.2 Recognize the impact that the interrelationship of comorbid physical and mental health issues have on overall health (e.g., diabetes, cardiovascular disease, cancer, obesity).

6.2.3 Gather information about biologic, psychological, spiritual, social, and environmental risk and protective factors specific to mental health during the assessment process (e.g., metabolic status, exposure to violence, support systems).

6.2.4 Incorporate strategies into health care planning that strengthen protective factors and enhance resilience (e.g., principles of recovery, psychosocial rehabilitation, holistic care, cultural continuity).

6.2.5 Contribute to the development of policies and standards that support mental health promotion (e.g., preventing and minimizing restraint and seclusion, promoting client autonomy).

6.3 Engage in the prevention of mental illness, and substance-related and behavioural addictions, when collaborating with clients.

6.3.1 Use a variety of strategies to address stigma and discrimination around mental health and addictions issues (e.g., acting as a positive role model, reflective practice, engaging communities in dialogue, responding to media portrayal of mental illness, addressing stigmatizing and discriminatory language, promoting social change, participation, and inclusion).

6.3.2 Recognize and address the impact of societal factors that contribute to mental health and addictions issues (e.g., abuse, poverty, trauma).

(Continued)

BOX 5.11 Registered Psychiatric Nurses Entry-to-Practice Competencies *(Continued)*

6.3.3 Incorporate strategies into health care planning that reduce risk (e.g., smoking cessation, responsible substance use, strengthening community networks, violence prevention, healthy childhood development, stress management, increasing social capital, responsible gambling).

6.3.4 Incorporate trauma-informed philosophies and best practices into health care planning.

6.3.5 Assist clients to gain insight into the relationship between mental illness and addictions.

6.3.6 Integrate harm reduction philosophies and best practices into health care planning (e.g., methadone maintenance, needle exchange, safe sex, nicotine replacement therapy).

6.3.7 Engage and empower clients to seek out and/or develop resources that support relapse prevention (e.g., self-help groups, Alcoholics Anonymous, Narcotics Anonymous, Gamblers Anonymous).

6.3.8 Contribute to the development of policies and standards that support the prevention of mental illness and addictions (e.g., alcohol use during life stages, smoke-free environment, workplace health, suicide awareness).

6.4 Engage in suicide prevention when collaborating with clients.

6.4.1 Identify individuals, groups, communities, and special populations that are at risk for suicide.

6.4.2 Collaborate with communities in suicide prevention and postvention activities (e.g., skill building, antibullying programs, school-based education).

Registered Psychiatric Nurse Regulators of Canada. (2014). *Registered psychiatric nurse entry-level competencies.* Edmonton, AB: Author. Used with permission.

BOX 5.12 Registered Psychiatric Nurses Entry-to-Practice Competencies

COMPETENCY 7

ETHICAL, PROFESSIONAL, AND LEGAL RESPONSIBILITIES

Registered psychiatric nurses (RPNs) practice within legal requirements, demonstrate professionalism, and uphold professional codes of ethics, standards of practice, bylaws, and policies.

7.1 Practice in compliance with federal and provincial/territorial legislation and other legal requirements.

7.1.1 Demonstrate knowledge of the legislation governing psychiatric nursing practice.

7.1.2 Adhere to the psychiatric nursing code of ethics, standards of practice, and bylaws of the regulatory authority.

7.1.3 Practice within the jurisdiction's legislated scope of practice for psychiatric nurses and understand that the scope of practice may be influenced by limits and conditions imposed by the regulatory authority, employer policies, and the limits of individual competence.

7.1.4 Adhere to and apply the jurisdiction's mental health legislation.

7.1.5 Adhere to and apply other relevant legislation that has an impact on practice.

7.1.6 Protect client confidentiality and adhere to relevant legislation that governs the privacy, access, use, retention, and disclosure of personal information.

7.1.7 Adhere to legal requirements regarding client consent.

7.1.8 Adhere to any legislated duty to report, including the duty to report abuse or to report unprofessional or unsafe practice, or the risk of such.

7.1.9 Adhere to standards and policies regarding proper documentation, including being timely, accurate, clear, concise, and legible.

7.2 Assume responsibility for upholding the requirements of self-regulation in the interest of public protection.

7.2.1 Accept responsibility for own actions, decisions, and professional conduct.

7.2.2 Practice within own level of competence and use professional judgement when accepting responsibilities, including seeking out additional information or guidance when required.

7.2.3 Demonstrate an understanding of the regulatory purpose of own governing body and the significance of participating in professional activities of a regulatory nature.

7.2.4 Demonstrate an understanding of the significance of fitness to practice in the context of public protection, and strive to maintain a level of personal

---

BOX 5.12 Registered Psychiatric Nurses Entry-to-Practice Competencies *(Continued)*

health, mental health, and well-being in order to provide safe, competent, and ethical care.

7.2.5 Question orders, decisions, or actions that are unclear or inconsistent with positive client outcomes, best practices, health and safety standards, or client wishes.

7.2.6 Protect clients and take steps to prevent or minimize harm from unsafe practices.

7.2.7 Engage in a process of continuous learning and self-evaluation, including following the requirements of the regulatory authority's continuing competence program.

7.3 Demonstrate a professional presence and model professional behaviour.

7.3.1 Conduct oneself in a manner that promotes a positive image of the profession.

7.3.2 Respond professionally, regardless of the behaviour of others.

7.3.3 Articulate the role and responsibilities of an RPN.

7.3.4 Practise within agency policies and procedures, and exercise professional judgement when using these, or in the absence of agency policies and procedures.

7.3.5 Organize and prioritize own work and develop time management skills for meeting responsibilities.

7.3.6 Demonstrate initiative, curiosity, flexibility, creativity, and beginning self-confidence.

7.3.7 Demonstrate professional leadership (e.g., act as a role model, coach, and mentor to others; support knowledge transfer; engage in professional activities).

7.4 Uphold and promote the ethical values of the profession.

7.4.1 Conduct oneself in a manner that reflects honesty, integrity, reliability, and impartiality.

7.4.2 Avoid situations that could give rise to a conflict of interest and ensure that the vulnerabilities of others are not exploited for one's own interest.

7.4.3 Identify the effects of one's own values, biases, and assumptions on interactions with clients and other members of the health care team.

7.4.4 Recognize ethical dilemmas and implement steps toward a resolution.

7.4.5 Differentiate between personal and professional relationships and maintain the boundaries of the psychiatric nurse–client relationship (e.g., addressing power differentials, use of personal disclosure).

Registered Psychiatric Nurse Regulators of Canada. (2014). *Registered psychiatric nurse entry-level competencies*. Edmonton, AB: Author. Used with permission.

▮ STANDARDS OF PROFESSIONAL PRACTICE

As regulated health professions, nurses are given the authority to practice under provincial or territorial laws that set out governance, registration, and discipline requirements as a means of protecting the public. These laws require provincial or territorial nursing regulatory bodies to set, monitor, and enforce standards of practice that, along with a code of ethics (see Chapter 7), articulate a profession's values, knowledge, and skills. Such standards facilitate a profession's self-governance because they make explicit the profession's expectations of its members' competency and performance.

KEY CONCEPT

Standards of practice are used by self-regulating professional groups to identify their expected and achievable competencies and to make explicit their obligations to the public.

CFMHN Standards of Practice

PMH nursing has been a designated Canadian Nurses Association (CNA) specialty since 1995. The Canadian Federation of Mental Health Nurses (CFMHN) is the national association for the specialty and sets PMH nursing standards for RNs. The *Canadian Standards of Psychiatric–Mental Health Nursing* was developed by expert PMH nurses in 1996 (Austin, Gallop, Harris, & Spencer, 1996), revised in 1998, 2006, and most recently in 2014 (CFMHN, 2014). The Standards of Practice document is freely available at the CFMHN Web site (see Web Links). The standards are organized by a **domains of practice** framework (Benner, 1984), with competencies classified within seven domains (see Web Links).

It is acknowledged that nurses' achievement of competent practice is shaped by the nursing model they utilize as well as by the social, cultural, economic, and political factors that act on health care. Beliefs underlying the CFMHN standards include the belief that the therapeutic nurse–client relationship, based on trust and mutual respect, is at the core of PMH nursing practice and holistic, ethical, and culturally competent care.

Collaborative relationships with individuals, families, communities, and different populations, as well as with interprofessional colleagues, are highly valued. Key practice foci are the alleviation of stigma and discrimination, the protection of human rights, and the promotion of recovery and well-being for those living with mental illness. Advocacy for equitable access to health care resources, for practice environments that promote safe and positive work relationships, for research and its application to improvements in care and treatment, and for social action to promote political and social awareness that impacts health care policy, is considered part of the nursing role.

National certification in this specialty from the CNA can be achieved by RNs who have either a minimum of 3,900 hours in the specialty area over the past 5 years or who have completed a formal post–basic nursing course/program of at least 300 hours in the past 10 years and have 2,925 hours of practice in the specialty area. As well, verification by a supervisor/consultant that the practice experience was acquired and successful completion of the CNA's PMH nursing certification examination is required. Recertification is necessary every 5 years. RNs with certification in PMH nursing sign "CPMHN(C)," as well as "RN," after their name.

Registered Psychiatric Nurses Standards of Practice

In Western Canada (Manitoba, Saskatchewan, Alberta, and British Columbia) and the Yukon, the distinct profession of RPNs is regulated by separate provincial/territorial associations. For instance, the College of the Registered Psychiatric Nurses of Alberta (CRPNA, 2013) has provincial standards of practice that meet the conditions of Alberta's Health Professions Act, which stipulates that failure to meet the CRPNA standards constitutes unprofessional conduct. The Registered Psychiatric Nurse Regulators of Canada (RPNRC), a national association, approves the code of ethics and standards of practice of Canadian RPNs (see Web Links).

The CCPNR Standards of Practice

The CCPNR (2013), a federation of provincial and territorial members who are legislated as responsible to the public for safe practice of licensed and registered practical nurses, oversees and approves the standards of LPN/RPN practice in Canada (see Web Links).

▍ KEY COMPONENTS OF PMH NURSING PRACTICE

Clinical Decision-Making

Decision-making involves critical thinking and is at the core of clinical practice. **Clinical decision-making** focuses on choices made in clinical settings. In addition to complex decisions, such as collecting, processing, and organizing information and formulating nursing approaches, many moment-to-moment decisions are made, such as deciding whether a client should receive a PRN medication. The development and implementation of efficacious interventions involve critical analysis of client, family, and community data, as well as making decisions about care. Such decision-making should involve the client, family, and other significant stakeholders as much as ethically, legally, and logistically possible. Reflective thinking about the client's illness experience and personal response to the treatment and care situation is an important aspect of choosing interventions. The nurse needs to have a thorough understanding of the rationale and the theoretical underpinnings of the client's care plan.

Critical Pathways in Care Planning

Many health care facilities use **critical pathways** to ensure a quality level of care in a cost-effective way. These care paths are similar to individual treatment plans in that all the disciplines' interventions are included on one plan. Critical pathways, however, are designed for a hypothetical client who has typical symptoms and who follows an expected course of treatment. Care paths are not developed for each individual client. This unification of care can be helpful if it means that best practices shape the care received by all clients and if it facilitates the use of expert knowledge by all those providing care. It is not helpful if the unique needs and situation of each client and family are ignored, or if nurses are restrained in their provision of thoughtful, sensitive care. Care paths, which identify key interventions and related best practices for a typical client with a specific mental disorder, can be helpful study tools for students.

Recovery as the Framework for Mental Health Care

Recovery, defined as "a process in which people with mental health problems and illnesses are empowered and supported to engage actively in their own journey of well-being," has been placed at the centre of Canada's national mental health strategy (Mental Health Commission of Canada [MHCC], 2009, p. 122). The recovery process is envisioned as enabling individuals to have a meaningful, fulfilling life and is supported by the strengths of the individual, family, and community (see Chapter 8). The World Health Organization's (2013) "Mental Health Action Plan 2013–2020" acknowledges the importance of promoting and enhancing recovery, identifying the need for community-based mental health services "to encompass a recovery-based approach that puts the emphasis on supporting individuals with mental disorders and psychosocial disabilities to achieve their own aspirations and goals"(p. 14). In 2015, the MHCC released guidelines for recovery-oriented practice as a way to promote and advance the consistent application of recovery principles across clinical settings (MHCC, 2015).

This vision of "recovery" that is about quality of life, rather than the more narrow notion of clinical recovery, challenges nurses and other health professionals to reassess their practice. Reorientation to a recovery-centric model is an opportunity to identify ways to improve everyday practice. It may mean that a new perspective on what constitutes "evidence" for best care will be taken; or more active ways to engage family and community resources sought; or perhaps it will be greater vigilance regarding restrictive practices. Nursing associations (e.g., CFMHN, RPNC) are ensuring that a **recovery model** of practice informs practice standards. Standards are therefore excellent resources for identifying ways to enact a recovery framework in mental health care.

Trauma-Informed Care

Traumatic events experienced across the life span can have long-term, bio/psycho/social/spiritual consequences. Events that can be traumatic include abuse (physical, psychological, or sexual), assault, community violence, combat, torture, suicide of a significant other, neglect, natural or human-caused disasters, forced displacement, witnessing death, destruction, or suffering, and other similar occurrences. Persons with such experiences can become distressed or retraumatized in health care settings, with memories being triggered by physical assessments, by procedures, or by restrictive interventions such as the application of restraints (Reeves, 2015). It is important that treatment and care of any individual is carried out with awareness that the person may have a trauma history (see Chapter 17).

Universal trauma precautions, used with all clients, can ensure that this happens (Raja, Hasnain, Hoersch, Gove-Yin, & Rajagopalan, 2015). Precautions are based on the knowledge that in health care settings, trauma survivors need to have a sense of control, to utilize personal coping mechanisms (e.g., holding onto a particular object, such as a purse), and may have a fear of being physically exposed or touched. These precautions involve simple actions. Staff should wear clearly visible identification that specifies their names and roles, and they should introduce themselves to their clients and family members. When carrying out procedures, clients should be informed of the time and steps involved and asked if they have any questions, worries, or preferences regarding the process. It is important to determine if there is something that would make them more comfortable (Raja et al., 2015).

As well as understanding the potential impact of traumatic events and the ways in which traumatic memories may be triggered in health care settings, nurses need to recognize their own history of trauma (Reeves, 2015). This history may include experiences gained in the role of nurse, from vicarious knowledge of horrors revealed in clients' trauma disclosures, to their own witnessing of tragic incidents. Self-understanding and attention to one's own well-being are important to sustaining one's capacity for competent and compassionate care.

Collaborative Care

PMH care has a long tradition of using an interprofessional approach, with several disciplines working together in the provision of client care. Collaboration to ensure that interventions from the different disciplines are integrated in the delivery of care is essential. For instance, when a nurse and a psychologist simultaneously work with a client on changing a behaviour related to medication adherence, they need to work together to have congruent, integrated approaches and to share information regarding client needs and progress. An effective interprofessional approach in which close collaboration occurs with clients, families, and the care team is required across the continuum of mental health care (prevention to rehabilitation). A coordinator, "case manager," or "patient/client navigator" has been found to be an important aspect of effective **collaborative care** (Kates et al., 2011)—a role often held by a nurse (see Chapter 4).

A Canadian study, which explored new graduates' experiences of interprofessional collaboration, found that organizational environments where the nurses found relationships to be respectful and supportive and where they had opportunities for collaborative experiences and knowledge of others' roles and of how and when to collaborate fostered confidence in interprofessional work; a challenge was to balance self and others' expectations (Pfaff, Baxter, Jack, & Ploeg, 2014).

■ CHALLENGES OF PMH NURSING

The challenges of PMH nursing are shaped by new knowledge arising from research, new dimensions of health care generated by biotechnologic advances, and the reality that nursing practice is becoming more specialized and autonomous. This section discusses a few of the challenges.

Knowledge Development, Dissemination, and Application

Results of new research efforts continually redefine our knowledge base relative to mental disorders and their treatment. Consider the significant advances in neurobiologic knowledge. In the 1970s, the cause of schizophrenia was hypothesized to be overactivity of dopamine. Later, it was discovered that other neurotransmitters seemed to play a role as well. Such knowledge resulted in new medications becoming available with various side effect profiles, requiring nurses to redefine their monitoring and interventions related to medication administration. Advances in our understanding of genetics and epigenetics are occurring, bringing new knowledge but also new ethical issues. The presence of comorbid medical disorders is acknowledged as significant to the treatment of mental disorders. For example, hypertension, hypothyroidism, hyperthyroidism, and diabetes mellitus can each affect the disease trajectory of mental disorders. In some settings, the nurse may be the only health care provider who has a background in medical disorders, such as human immunodeficiency viral illness, acquired immunodeficiency syndrome, and other somatic health problems.

The challenge for nurses today is to stay abreast of the advances in holistic health care in order to provide safe, competent care to individuals with mental disorders. Nurses must strive to provide evidence-based nursing care, developing their knowledge on an ongoing basis. Accessing up-to-date information through journals, electronic databases, and continuing education programs is a recognized responsibility. Not only do nurses need to access current research studies but they also must evaluate the usefulness of the studies. For instance, one research project supporting a particular treatment approach may not be as meaningful as several statistically significant studies, assessed in systematic reviews. The results of qualitative research studies, although not generalizable, can have important implications for practice, for instance, insights that can deepen our understanding of client experiences. Resources such as the International Knowledge Exchange Network for Mental Health (IKEN-MH), evolving through the Mental Health Commission of Canada (MHCC), with a current focus on innovative practices and systematic evidence for the design and management of mental health services and the World Health Organization's MiNDbank are important to the improvement of care (see Web Links).

Health Care Delivery System Challenges

Continuing challenges for Canadian nurses include supporting the integration of mental health care within primary health care, articulating the influence of the determinants of health on mental health, and playing a strong, effective role in the enactment of Canada's national strategy for mental health.

Consumers of mental health services and their families are gaining voice and calling for meaningful changes in the delivery of services. Inequities in health care for marginalized populations, such as those living with a chronic mental illness, are being challenged, as are paternalistic approaches to the delivery of care. One source of this challenge is the Canadian Alliance on Mental Illness and Mental Health (CAMIMH). The CAMIMH, created in 1998, consists of consumers, their families, researchers, and care providers from numerous professions. Their mission is to influence national policy, to speak in a unified voice, and to focus strategically on mental health and mental illness. Active partnership

among users of services, nurses and other health providers, and the community at large is necessary to effect the positive changes initiated by our national strategy in mental health.

Overcoming Stigma and Discrimination

Overcoming the stigma and discrimination related to mental illness, a priority of the MHCC, needs to occur within health care systems. Not only do persons with mental health disorders and their families experience stigmatization due to some health care professionals' avoidance, discomfort, or even disdain, but professionals who practice in PMH settings may also experience stigma by association. Psychiatry has a dark history reflected in images of asylums with chained inmates (e.g., Bedlam), negative media portrayals (e.g., "One Flew Over the Cuckoo's Nest"), and lack of recognition of the scientific basis of contemporary psychiatric care. Mental health professionals may be seen as less skilled than their colleagues in other areas and be less respected (Bhugra et al., 2015). This can result in health science students, including those in nursing, not considering mental health care as a career choice.

e-Mental Health

e-Mental Health is the name given to mental health services and education delivered across distances using communication and information technologies. The MHCC's (2014) briefing paper, *E-Mental Health in Canada: Transforming the Mental Health System Using Technology*, notes that such services (which can be self-guided or partly self-guided) can be as effective as those provided face to face. As cost-effective alternatives to traditional mental health care, e-Mental health approaches are particularly useful across Canada's vast geography. Services range from information and advocacy to assessment, intervention, monitoring, and evaluation. The technologies involved include telephones, mobile devices, emailing, videoconferencing, social media, as well as Web-based and software programs.

An evolving, related area is that of gamification, which involves interactive (including online) computer games as an engaging means of offering education and training (Ricciardi & De Paolis, 2014). Often using simulation platforms, they are increasingly being developed for education in nursing and other health care professions. The College and Association of Nurses in Alberta, for example, explored the use of gamification as a way to teach RNs about jurisprudence and to confirm their competence in this registration requirement. Evaluation of the project revealed that nurses did learn about jurisprudence, felt engaged, and appreciated the ease of participation; 97% believed what they learned would influence their practice (Lemermeyer & Sadesky, 2016).

PMH NURSING IN A GLOBAL COMMUNITY

As members of a global community, Canadian nurses recognize their role in achieving "health for all." Mental health is a particularly disadvantaged aspect of health care around the world, so capacity building for mental health care is a pressing priority (Kakuma et al., 2011). Mental health care can be effectively delivered in primary care settings through collaboration among skilled, nonspecialist professionals, trained lay workers, consumer representatives, and caregivers when supported by mental health specialists in consultative roles for services and training (Kakuma et al., 2011). There is a great need, as well, to ensure that all delivery of mental health care upholds the dignity and human rights of those receiving it (Austin, 2017).

The International Society of Psychiatric–Mental Health Nurses (ISPN), an organization with student members, works to unite and strengthen the presence and voice of PMH nurses and to promote quality care for individuals and families with mental health problems. The World Federation for Mental Health (WFMH), an organization to which nurses belong, has as its mission, since its founding in 1948, the advancement of mental health promotion, prevention, and care among all people. It works with governments from more than 100 countries and nongovernment groups. WFMH sponsors World Mental Health Day, which occurs annually on October 10. Organizations are an important pathway for nurses' contribution to the improvement of mental health and mental health care across the globe.

SUMMARY OF KEY POINTS

- The bio/psycho/social/spiritual model focuses on separate but interdependent dimensions of biologic, psychological, social, and spiritual factors in the assessment and treatment of mental disorders. This comprehensive and holistic approach to mental disorders is the foundation for effective PMH nursing practice and is used as the basic organizational framework for this text.
- Entry-to-practice competencies outline the essential knowledge, skills, and attitudes required at the onset of a credentialed nursing role.
- Standards of practice set out the explicit responsibilities and competencies of a profession.
- PMH nurses collaborate with other disciplines and many times act as coordinators in the delivery of care.
- PMH nurses need to be aware of team dynamics and their impact on care. When nurses practice in interprofessional settings, there may be an overlapping of professional roles. Nurses are accountable for both discrete and shared functions that they perform in their practice.
- Challenges facing nurses practicing in PMH settings include knowledge development, dissemination, and application; e-Mental Health; addressing stigma and discrimination within health care systems; and working to make the health care system more collaborative and responsive to the mental health needs of Canadians.
- Provincial, national, and global organizations are important pathways for nurses' contributions to improving mental health and mental health care worldwide.

 Web Links

camimh.ca The Canadian Alliance on Mental Illness and Mental Health provides key reports, news, and information regarding mental illness and its treatment on its Web site.

ccmhi.ca Canadian Collaborative Mental Health Initiative, a consortium of 12 national organizations, including CNA, CFMHN, and RPNC, seeks to improve the delivery of mental health services within primary care through interdisciplinary collaboration. A series of papers and toolkits related to collaborative care can be found here.

ccpnr.ca This site of the Canadian Council for Practical Nurse Regulators offers links to the provincial and territorial regulators that have information on the competency profiles for LPNs/RPNs.

cfmhn.ca The Canadian Federation of Mental Health Nurses Web site has the complete standards of practice document.

cna-aiic.ca/ The Canadian Nurses Association Web site has information regarding credentialing as a PMH nurse.

cpa-apc.org The Canadian Psychiatric Association, a voluntary organization of psychiatrists, publishes the *Canadian Journal of Psychiatry* among other periodicals and information. Clinical practice guidelines and position and discussion papers are available here.

ispn-psych.org The International Society of Psychiatric–Mental Health Nurses Web site has links to their publications, including position statements and psychiatric nursing journals.

mentalhealthcommission.ca/English/initiatives/11859/iken-mh The MHCC's International Knowledge Exchange Network for Mental Health facilitates searching of focus areas, such as mental health and the law, First Nations, Inuit, and Métis, peer support.

porticonetwork.ca An e-Mental health resource, the *Portico Network* is a trustworthy Web site created by the Centre for Addiction and Mental Health in Toronto. It is an excellent resource, offering information re: disorders, treatment options, and primary care toolkits; opportunities for training or consultation; and links to partner sites. It is open to the public.

rpnc.ca The Registered Psychiatric Nurses of Canada Web site has their standards of practice and code of ethics document plus links to provincial RPN association Web sites.

who.int/mental_health/mindbank/en/ This WHO online platform provides access to international resources related to mental health, disability, and general health, including policies and law and service standards. Browsing by country and region is possible.

wfmh.com This World Federation for Mental Health site gives information about World Mental Health Day (October 10) and free access to the WFMH Bulletin.

References

Abraham, I., Fox, J., & Cohen, B. (1992). Integrating the bio into the bio-psychosocial: Understanding and treating biological phenomena in psychiatric–mental health nursing. *Archives of Psychiatric Nursing, 6*(5), 296–305. doi: 10.1016/0883-9471(92)90041-G

Austin, W. (2017). Global health ethics and mental health. In E. L. Yearwood & V. P. Hines-Martin (Eds.) *Routledge handbook of global mental health nursing* (pp. 71–90). New York, NY: Routledge.

Austin, W., Gallop, R., Harris, D., & Spencer, E. (1996). A domain of practice approach to the standards of psychiatric and mental health nursing. *Journal of Psychiatric and Mental Health Nursing, 3,* 111–115.

Barss, K. S. (2012). T.R.U.S.T.: An affirming model for inclusive spiritual care. *Journal of Holistic Nursing, 30*(1), 24–24. doi: 10.1177/0898010111418118

Benner, P. (1984). *From novice to expert: Excellence and power in clinical nursing practice.* Menlo Park, CA: Addison-Wesley.

Bhugra, D. Sartorius, N., Fiorillo, A., Evans-Lacko, S., Ventriglio, A., Hermans, M.H.M., … Gaebel, W. (2015). EPA guidance on how to improve the image of psychiatry and of the psychiatrist. *European Psychiatry, 30*(3), 423–430. doi: 10.1016/j.eurpsy.2015.02.003

Canadian Association of Schools of Nursing with Canadian Federation of Mental Health Nursing. (2015). *Entry to practice mental health and addiction competencies for undergraduate nursing education in Canada.* Retrieved from http://www.casn.ca/wp-content/uploads/2015/11/Mental-health-Competencies_EN_FINAL-3-Oct-26-2015.pdf

Canadian Federation of Mental Health Nurses. (2014). *The Canadian standards of psychiatric and mental health nursing* (4th ed.). Toronto, ON: Author. Retrieved from http://cfmhn.ca/

Catalano, J. T. (2015) *Nursing now: Today's issues, tomorrow's trends* (7th ed.). Philadelphia, PA: F. A. Davis Company.

College of Registered Psychiatric Nurses of Alberta (CRPNA). (2013). *Code of ethics and standards of psychiatric nursing practice.* Edmonton, AB: Author.

Dossey, B. M., Keegan, L., & Guzzetta, C. E., (2004). *Holistic nursing: A handbook for practice* (4th ed.). Frederick, MD: Aspen.

Kakuma, R., Minas, H., van Ginneken, N., Dal Paz, M. R., Desiraju, K., Morris, J. E., … Scheffler, R. M. (2011). Human resources of mental health care: current situation and strategies for action. *The Lancet, 378,* 1654–1663. doi: 10.1016/S0140-6736(11)61093-3

Kates, N., Mazowita, G., Lemire, F., Jayabarathan, A., Bland, R., Selby, P., … Audet, D. (2011). The evolution of collaborative mental health care in Canada: A shared vision for the future: Position paper of the Canadian Psychiatric Association & the College of Family Physicians of Canada. *The Canadian Journal of Psychiatry, 56*(5), 1–10.

Lemermeyer, G., & Sadesky, G. (2016). The gamification of jurisprudence: Innovation in registered nurse regulation. *Journal of Nursing Regulation, 7*(3), 1–7. doi: 10.1016/S2155-8256(16)32314-6

MacCourt, P., Family Caregivers Advisory Committee, Mental Health Commission of Canada. (2013). *National guidelines for a comprehensive service system to support family caregivers of adults with mental health problems and illnesses.* Calgary, AB: Mental Health Commission of Canada. Retrieved from http://www.mentalhealthcommission.ca

Mental Health Commission of Canada. (2009). *Toward recovery and well-being: A framework for a mental health strategy for Canada.* Ottawa, ON: Author.

Mental Health Commission of Canada. (2014). *E-Mental Health in Canada: Transforming the Mental Health System Using Technology.* Ottawa: Author. Retrieved from http://www.mentalhealthcommission.ca/English/document/27081/e-mental-health-canada-transforming-mental-health-system-using-technology

Mental Health Commission of Canada. (2015). *Guidelines for recovery-oriented practice. Hope. Dignity. Inclusion.* Ottawa, ON: Author.

Pfaff, K. A., Baxter, P. E., Jack, S. M. & Ploeg, J. (2014). Exploring new graduate nurse confidence in interprofessional collaboration: A mixed methods study. *International Journal of Nursing Studies, 51*(8), 1142–1152. doi: 10.1016/j.ijnurstu.2014.01.001

Raja, S., Hasnain, M. Hoersch, M., Gove-Yin, S., & Rajagopalan, C. (2015). Trauma-informed care in medicine: Current knowledge and future research directions. *Family Community Health, 38*(3), 216–226. doi: 10.1097/FCH.0000000000000071

Reeves, E. (2015). A synthesis of the literature in trauma-informed care. *Issues in Mental Health Nursing, 36*(9), 698–709. doi: 10.3109/01612840.2015.1025319

Registered Psychiatric Nurse Regulators of Canada. (2014). *Registered psychiatric nurse entry-level competencies.* Retrieved from http://www.rpnc.ca/sites/default/files/resources/pdfs/RPNRC-ENGLISH%20Compdoc%20%28Nov6-14%29.pdf

Ricciardi, F., & De Paolis, L. T. (2014). A comprehensive review of serious games in health professions. *International Journal of Computer Games Technology, 14,* Article ID 787968, 11 pages. doi: 10.1155/2014/787968

World Health Organization. (2013). *Comprehensive mental health action plan 2013–2020.* Retrieved from http://www.who.int/mental_health/action_plan_2013/en/

Communication and the Therapeutic Relationship

Cheryl Forchuk

LEARNING OBJECTIVES

After studying this chapter, you will be able to:

- Identify the importance of self-awareness in nursing practice.
- Develop a repertoire of verbal and nonverbal communication skills.
- Develop a process for selecting effective communication techniques.
- Explain how the nurse can establish a therapeutic relationship with clients by using rapport and empathy.
- Examine the physical, emotional, social, and spiritual boundaries of the nurse–client relationship.
- Discuss the significance of defence mechanisms.
- Explore each of the three phases of the nurse–client relationship: orientation, working, and resolution.
- Describe motivational interviewing (MI), including assumptions and techniques.
- Describe the transitional relationship model (TRM), including assumptions and components.

KEY TERMS

- active listening • boundaries • communication blocks • content themes • countertransference • defence mechanisms • empathic linkages • empathy • motivational interviewing • nontherapeutic • nonverbal communication • orientation phase • passive listening • process recording • rapport • resolution phase • self-disclosure • symbolism • telehealth • transference • validation • verbal communication • working phase

KEY CONCEPTS

- nurse–client relationship • self-awareness • therapeutic communication

---

Clients with mental health disorders may have special communication and relationship needs that require advanced therapeutic communication skills. In psychiatric and mental health (PMH) nursing, the nurse–client relationship is an important tool used to reach treatment goals. The purposes of this chapter are to (1) help the nurse develop self-awareness and communication techniques needed for a therapeutic nurse–client relationship, (2) examine the specific stages or steps involved in establishing the relationship, (3) explore the specific factors that make a nurse–client relationship successful and therapeutic, and, (4) differentiate therapeutic from nontherapeutic relationships.

■ SELF-AWARENESS

Self-awareness is the process of understanding one's own beliefs, thoughts, motivations, biases, and limitations and recognizing how they affect others. Without self-awareness, nurses will find it impossible to establish and maintain therapeutic relationships with clients. "Know thyself" is a basic tenet of PMH nursing (see Box 6.1).

To come to self-awareness, nurses can carry out self-examination. Self-examination involves reflecting on the personal meaning of the current nursing situation. This reflection can relate to similar past situations and issues related to personal values and beliefs. Self-examination can provoke anxiety and is rarely comfortable; it can occur alone or with help from others. Self-examination without the benefit of another's perspective can lead to a biased view of self. Conducting self-examination is best with a trusted individual who can give objective but realistic feedback. The development of self-awareness requires a willingness to be introspective and to examine personal beliefs, attitudes, and motivations.

KEY CONCEPT

Self-awareness is the process of understanding one's own beliefs, thoughts, motivations, biases, and limitations and recognizing how they affect self and others.

BOX 6.1 "Know Thyself"

Do you have any physical problems or illnesses?

Have you had significant traumatic life events (e.g., divorce, death of a significant person, abuse, disaster)?

Do your family or significant others have prejudiced or embarrassing beliefs and attitudes about groups different than yours?

Would sociocultural factors in your background contribute to being rejected by members of other cultures?

Do you have strong religious beliefs that shape your daily life?

If your answer to any of these questions is yes, how would these experiences and beliefs affect your ability to care for clients with these characteristics?

THE BIO/PSYCHO/SOCIAL/ SPIRITUAL SELF

Each nurse brings a bio/psycho/social/spiritual self to nursing practice. The client perceives the biologic dimension of the nurse in terms of physical characteristics: age, gender, body weight, height, ethnic or racial background, and any other observed physical characteristics. The nurse can have a certain genetic composition, illness, or unobservable physical disability that may influence the quality or delivery of nursing care. The nurse's psychological state also influences how he or she analyzes client information and selects treatment interventions. An emotional state or behaviour can inadvertently influence the therapeutic relationship. For example, a nurse who has just learned that her child is misusing drugs and who has a client with a history of drug use may inadvertently project a judgmental attitude toward her client, which would interfere with the formation of a therapeutic relationship. The nurse needs to examine underlying emotions, motivations, and beliefs and determine how these factors shape behaviour.

The nurse's social biases can be particularly problematic for the nurse–client relationship. Although the nurse may not verbalize these values to clients, some are readily evident in the nurse's behaviour and appearance, such as how the nurse acts or appears at work. The nurse's religious beliefs or feelings can also affect interactions. For instance, beliefs about divorce, abortion, or same sex relationships can affect how the nurse interacts with a client who is dealing with such issues.

UNDERSTANDING PERSONAL FEELINGS AND BELIEFS AND CHANGING BEHAVIOUR

Nurses must understand their own personal feelings and beliefs and try to avoid projecting them onto clients. This is not an easy task. For instance, due to ethnocentrism, our own sociocultural values may not be readily apparent. It takes effort to develop self-awareness, but it will enhance the nurse's objectivity and foster a nonjudgmental attitude, which is so important in building and maintaining trust throughout the nurse–client relationship. Soliciting feedback from colleagues and supervisors about how personal beliefs or thoughts are being projected onto others is a useful self-assessment technique. One of the reasons that ongoing clinical supervision is so important is that the supervisor really knows the nurse and is able to continually observe for inappropriate communication and question assumptions that the nurse may hold, as well as reinforce helpful behaviour.

Once a nurse has identified and analyzed personal beliefs and attitudes, prejudicial behaviours may change. The change process requires introspective analysis that may result in viewing the world differently. Through self-awareness and conscious effort, the nurse can change learned behaviours to engage effectively in therapeutic relationships with clients. Nevertheless, a nurse may realize that some attitudes are too ingrained to support a therapeutic relationship with a client with different beliefs. In such cases, the nurse should refer the client to someone who may be better able to be therapeutically helpful.

COMMUNICATION

Effective communication skills, including verbal and nonverbal techniques, are the building blocks for all successful relationships. The nurse–client relationship is built on therapeutic communication, the ongoing process of interaction through which meaning emerges (see Box 6.2). **Verbal communication**, which is principally achieved by spoken words, includes the underlying emotion, context, and connotation of what is actually said. **Nonverbal communication** includes gestures, expressions, and body language. Both the client and the nurse use verbal and nonverbal communication. **Empathic linkages** are the direct communication of feelings. To respond therapeutically in a nurse–client relationship, the nurse is responsible for assessing and interpreting all forms of client communication.

Therapeutic and social relationships are very different. In a therapeutic relationship, the nurse focuses on the client and client-related issues, even when engaging in social activities with that client. For example, a

BOX 6.2 Principles of Therapeutic Communication

1. The client should be the primary focus of the interaction.
2. A professional attitude sets the tone of the therapeutic relationship.
3. Use self-disclosure cautiously and only when the disclosure has a therapeutic purpose.
4. Avoid social relationships with clients.
5. Maintain client confidentiality.
6. Assess the client's intellectual competence to determine the level of understanding.
7. Implement interventions from a theoretic base.
8. Maintain a nonjudgmental attitude. Avoid making judgements about the client's behaviour and giving advice. By the time the client sees the nurse, he or she has had plenty of advice.
9. Guide the client to reinterpret his or her experiences rationally.
10. Track the client's verbal interaction through the use of clarifying statements. Avoid changing the subject unless the content change is in the client's best interest.

nurse may take a client shopping and out for lunch. Even though the nurse is engaged in a social activity, that trip should have a definite purpose, and conversation should focus only on the client. The nurse must not attempt to meet his or her own social or other needs during the activity.

KEY CONCEPT

Therapeutic communication is the ongoing process of interaction through which meaning emerges.

■ USING VERBAL COMMUNICATION

The process of verbal communication involves a sender, a message, and a receiver. The client is often the sender, and the nurse is often the receiver (Fig. 6.1), but communication always works two ways. The client formulates an idea, encodes a message (puts ideas into words), and then transmits the message with emotion. The client's words and their underlying emotional tone and connotation communicate his or her needs and emotional problems or issues. The nurse receives the message, decodes it (interprets the message, including its feelings,

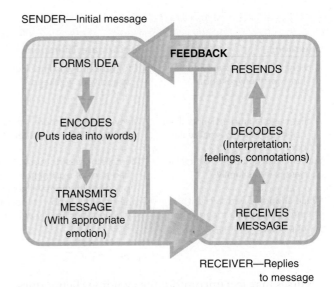

SENDER—Initial message

FORMS IDEA

ENCODES
(Puts idea into words)

TRANSMITS MESSAGE
(With appropriate emotion)

FEEDBACK

RESENDS

DECODES
(Interpretation: feelings, connotations)

RECEIVES MESSAGE

RECEIVER—Replies to message

Figure 6.1. The communication process. (Adapted from Boyd, M. (1995). Communication with clients, families, healthcare providers, and diverse cultures. In M. Strader & P. Decker (Eds.), *Role transition to client care management* (p. 431). Norwalk, CT: Appleton & Lange.)

connotation, and context), and then responds to the client. On the surface, this interaction is deceptively simple, but unseen complexities lie beneath. Is the message that the nurse receives consistent with the client's original idea? Did the nurse interpret the message as the client intended? Is the verbal message consistent with the nonverbal flourishes that accompany it? **Validation** is essential to ensure that the nurse has received the information accurately. (See section "Validation" later in this chapter for further discussion.)

Self-Disclosure

One of the most important principles of therapeutic communication for the nurse to follow is to focus the interaction on the client's concerns. **Self-disclosure**, telling the client personal information, generally is not a good idea since the conversation should focus on the client, not the nurse. If a client asks the nurse personal questions, the nurse should elicit the underlying reason for the request. The nurse can then determine how much, if any, personal information to disclose. In revealing personal information, the nurse should be purposeful and have identified therapeutic outcomes. For example, a male client struggling with the implications of marriage and fidelity asks a male nurse if he has ever had an extramarital affair. The nurse interprets the client's statement as seeking role-modelling behaviour for an adult man and judges self-disclosure in this instance to be therapeutic. He responds honestly that he does not engage in affairs and redirects the discussion back to the client's concerns.

Table 6.1	Self-Disclosure in Therapeutic Versus Social Relationships	
Situation	**Appropriate Therapeutic Response**	**Inappropriate Social Response With Rationale**
A client asks the nurse if she had fun over the weekend.	"The weekend was fine. How did you spend your weekend?"	"It was great. My boyfriend and I went to dinner and a movie." (This self-disclosure has no therapeutic purpose. The response focuses the conversation on the nurse, not on the client.)
A client asks a student nurse if she has ever been to a particular bar.	"Many people go there. I'm wondering if you have ever been there."	"Oh yes—all the time. It's a lot of fun." (Sharing information about outside activities is inappropriate.)
A client asks a nurse if mental illness is in his family.	"Mental illnesses do run in families. I've had a lot of experience caring for people with mental illnesses."	"My sister is being treated for depression." (This self-disclosure has no purpose, and the nurse is missing the meaning of the question.)
While shopping with a client, the nurse sees a friend, who approaches them.	To her friend: "I know it looks like I'm not working, but I really am. I'll see you later."	"Hi, Bob. This is Jane Doe, a client." (Introducing the client to the friend is very inappropriate and violates client confidentiality.)

Nurses may feel uncomfortable avoiding clients' questions for fear of seeming rude. Sometimes, they disclose too much personal information because they are trying to be nice. However, being nice is not necessarily therapeutic. As appropriate, redirecting the client, giving a neutral or vague answer, or saying "Let's talk about you" may be all that is necessary to limit self-disclosure. In some instances, nurses may need to tell the client directly that they will not share personal information (Table 6.1).

Verbal Communication Techniques

Nurses use many verbal techniques in establishing relationships and helping clients focus on their problems and goals. Asking a question, restating, and reflecting are examples of such techniques. These techniques may seem artificial at first, but with practice, they can be useful.

One of the most difficult but often most effective techniques is the use of silence during verbal interactions. By maintaining an open silence, the nurse allows the client to gather thoughts and to proceed at his or her own pace.

Listening is another valuable tool. Silence and listening differ in that silence consists of deliberate pauses to encourage the client to reflect and eventually respond. Listening is an ongoing activity by which the nurse attends to the client's verbal and nonverbal communication. The art of listening is developed through careful attention to the content and meaning of the client's speech. There are two types of listening: passive and active. **Passive listening** involves sitting quietly and letting the client talk. A passive listener allows the client to ramble and does not focus or guide the thought process. Passive listening does not foster a therapeutic relationship.

Through **active listening**, the nurse focuses on what the client is saying to interpret and respond to the message objectively. While listening, the nurse concentrates on the underlying meaning of what the client says. The nurse's verbal and nonverbal behaviours indicate active listening. The nurse usually responds indirectly,

using techniques such as open-ended statements, reflection (Table 6.2), and questions that elicit additional responses from the client. In active listening, the nurse should avoid changing the subject and instead follow the client's lead although at times, it is necessary to respond directly to help a client focus on a specific topic or to clarify content, thoughts, or beliefs.

Some verbal techniques, however, block interactions and inhibit therapeutic communication (Table 6.3). One of the biggest blocks to communication is giving advice, particularly that which others likely have already given. Giving advice is different from supporting a client through decision making. The therapeutic dialogue presented in Box 6.3 differentiates between advice (telling the client what to do or how to act) and therapeutic communication, by which the nurse and the client explore alternative ways of viewing the client's world. The client then can reach his or her own conclusions about the best approaches to use.

■ USING NONVERBAL COMMUNICATION

Gestures, facial expressions, and body language actually communicate more than do verbal messages. Under the best circumstances, body language mirrors or enhances verbal communication. However, if verbal and nonverbal messages are conflicting, the listener likely will believe the nonverbal message since it functions on a more basic level. For example, if a client says he feels fine but has a sad facial expression and is slumped in a chair away from others, a message of sadness will more likely be received than the client's words. The same is true of a nurse's behaviour. If a nurse tells a client she is happy to see him, but her facial expression communicates indifference, the client will receive the message that the nurse is indifferent. At times, people with mental health problems have difficulty verbally expressing themselves and interpreting the emotions of others. Nurses therefore need to continually assess the nonverbal communication needs of clients. Eye contact (or lack thereof),

Technique	Definition	Example	Use
Acceptance	Encouraging and receiving information in a nonjudgemental and interested manner	*Client*: I have done something terrible. *Nurse*: I would like to hear about it. It's OK to discuss it with me.	Used in establishing trust and developing empathy
Confrontation	Presenting the client with a different reality of the situation	*Client*: My best friend never calls me. She hates me. *Nurse*: I was in the room yesterday when she called.	Used cautiously to immediately redefine the client's reality However, it can alienate the client if used inappropriately. A nonjudgemental attitude is critical for confrontation to be effective.
Doubt	Expressing or voicing doubt when a client relates a situation	*Client*: My best friend hates me. She never calls me. *Nurse*: From what you have told me, that does not sound like her. When did she call you last?	Used carefully and only when the nurse feels confident about the details. It is used when the nurse wants to guide the client toward other explanations.
Interpretation	Putting into words what the client is implying or feeling	*Client*: I could not sleep because someone would come in my room and rape me. *Nurse*: It sounds like you were scared last night.	Used in helping the clients identify underlying thoughts or feelings
Observation	Stating to the client what the nurse is observing	*Nurse*: You are trembling and perspiring. When did this start?	Used when a client's behaviours (verbal or nonverbal) are obvious and unusual for that client
Open-ended statements	Introducing an idea and letting the client respond	*Nurse*: Trust means…. *Client*: That someone will keep you safe.	Used when helping the client explore feelings or gain insight
Reflection	Redirecting the idea back to the client	*Client*: Should I go home for the weekend? *Nurse*: Should you go home for the weekend?	Used when the client is asking for the nurse's approval or judgement. Use of reflection helps the nurse maintain a nonjudgemental approach.
Restatement	Repeating the main idea expressed; lets the client know what was heard	*Client*: I hate this place. I don't belong here. *Nurse*: You don't want to be here.	Used when trying to clarify what the client has said
Silence	Remaining quiet, but nonverbally expressing interest during an interaction	*Client*: I am angry!! *Nurse*: (Silence) *Client*: My wife had an affair.	Used when the client needs to express ideas but may not know quite how to do it. With silence, the client can focus on putting thoughts together.
Validation	Clarifying the nurse's understanding of the situation	*Nurse*: Let me see if I understand.	Used when the nurse is trying to understand a situation the client is trying to describe

posture, movement (e.g., shifting in chair, pacing), facial expressions, and gestures are nonverbal behaviours that communicate thoughts and feelings. A client with low self-esteem may be unable to maintain eye contact and thus may spend a great deal of time looking toward the floor. A client who is pacing and restless may be agitated or having a reaction to medication. A clenched fist may indicate that a person feels angry or hostile.

Nonverbal behaviour is culturally specific. The nurse must therefore be careful to understand his or her own cultural context as well as that of the client. For example, in some cultures (e.g., First Nation, Métis and Inuit peoples of Canada), it is considered disrespectful to look directly into another person's eyes. Other cultures may see a person who makes little eye contact as "hiding something" or having low self-esteem. Other examples of nonverbal communication that may vary considerably among cultures are whether one points with the finger, nose, or eyes and how much hand gesturing one uses.

Nurses should use positive body language, such as sitting at the same eye level as the client with a relaxed posture that projects interest and attention. Leaning slightly forward helps engage the client. Generally, the nurse should not cross his or her arms or legs during therapeutic communication because such postures erect

Table 6.3	Techniques That Inhibit Communication			
Technique	**Definition**	**Example**	**Problem**	
Advice	Telling a client what to do	*Client*: I can't sleep. It is too noisy. *Nurse*: Turn off the light and shut your door.	The nurse solves the client's problem, which may not be the appropriate solution and encourages dependency on the nurse.	
Agreement	Agreeing with a particular viewpoint of a client	*Client*: Abortions are sinful. *Nurse*: I agree.	The client is denied an opportunity to change his or her view now that the nurse agrees.	
Challenges	Disputing a client's beliefs with arguments, logical thinking, or direct order	*Client*: I'm a cowboy. *Nurse*: If you are a cowboy, what are you doing in the hospital?	The nurse belittles the client and decreases self-esteem. The client will avoid relating to the nurse who challenges.	
Disapproval	Judging a client's situation and behaviour	*Client*: I'm so sorry. I did not mean to kill my mother. *Nurse*: You should be. How could anyone kill their mother?	The nurse belittles the client. The client will avoid the nurse.	
Reassurance	Telling a client that everything will be OK	*Client*: Everyone thinks I'm bad. *Nurse*: You are a good person.	The nurse makes a statement that may not be true. The client is blocked from exploring feelings.	

BOX 6.3

THERAPEUTIC DIALOGUE

Giving Advice Versus Recommendations

Ms. J has just received a diagnosis of phobic disorder and been given a prescription for fluoxetine. She was referred to the home care agency because she does not want to take her medication. She is fearful of becoming suicidal. Two approaches are given below.

Ineffective Communication (Advice)

Nurse: Ms. J, the doctor has ordered the medication because it will help you.

Ms. J: I don't want to take the medication because I am afraid of becoming suicidal. I heard that some of this psychiatric medication does that. I haven't had any attacks for 2 weeks.

Nurse: This medication has rarely had that side effect. You should try it and see if you have any suicidal thoughts.

Ms. J: OK. (The nurse leaves and Ms. J does not take the medication. Within a week, Ms. J is taken to the emergency room with a panic attack.)

Effective Communication (Recommendations)

Nurse: Ms. J, how have you been doing?

Ms. J: So far, so good. I haven't had any attacks for 2 weeks.

Nurse: I understand that the doctor gave you a prescription for medication that may help with the panic attacks.

Ms. J: Yes, but I don't want to take it because I am afraid of becoming suicidal. I heard that some of this psychiatric medication does that.

Nurse: Have you ever had feelings of hurting yourself?

Ms. J: Not really.

Nurse: If you took the medication and had thoughts like that, what would you do?

Ms. J: I don't know.

Nurse: I think I see your dilemma. This medication may help your panic attacks, but the suicidal thoughts are a real fear. Is that it?

Ms. J: Yeah, that's it.

Nurse: Are there any circumstances under which you would be able to try the medication?

Ms. J: If I knew that, I would not have suicidal thoughts.

Nurse: I can't guarantee that, but I could call you every few days to see if you are having any of these thoughts and help you deal with them.

Ms. J: Oh, that will be OK.

(Ms. J successfully took the medication.)

Critical Thinking Challenge

- Contrast the communication in the first scenario with that in the second.
- What therapeutic communication techniques did the second nurse employ that may have contributed to a better outcome?
- Are there any cues in the first scenario that indicate that the client will not follow the nurse's advice? Explain.

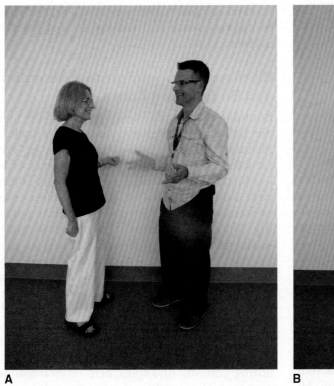 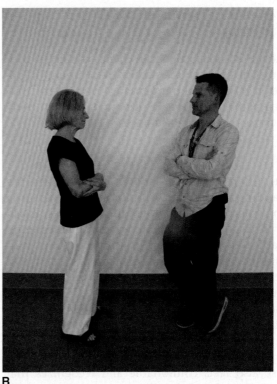

Figure 6.2. A and B: Open and closed body language.

barriers to interaction. Uncrossed arms and legs project openness and a willingness to engage in conversation (Fig. 6.2). Verbal responses should be consistent with nonverbal messages.

■ RECOGNIZING EMPATHIC LINKAGES

Empathic linkages are the communication of feelings (Peplau, 1952/1988). This form of communication commonly occurs with anxiety. The nurse may become aware of subjective feelings of anxiety. It may be difficult for the nurse to determine whether the anxiety is communicated interpersonally or whether the nurse is personally reacting to some of the content of what the client is communicating. However, being aware of one's own feelings and analyzing them is crucial to determining the source of the feelings.

■ SELECTING COMMUNICATION TECHNIQUES

In therapeutic communication, the nurse chooses the best words to say and uses nonverbal behaviours that are consistent with these words. If a client is angry and upset, should the nurse invite the client to sit down and discuss the problem, walk quietly with the client, or simply observe the client from a distance and not initiate conversation? Choosing the best response begins

with assessing and interpreting the meaning of the client's communication—both verbal and nonverbal.

Nurses should not necessarily take verbal messages literally, especially when a client is upset or angry. For example, a nurse enters the room of a newly admitted client who accusingly says, "You locked me up and threw away the key." The nurse could respond defensively that she had nothing to do with the client being admitted; however, that response would end in an argument and communication would be blocked. It would be more appropriate for the nurse to recognize that the client is communicating frustration at being in a locked psychiatric unit, and not take the accusation personally.

The nurse also needs to identify the desired client outcome. To do so, the nurse should engage the client with eye contact (if culturally appropriate) and quietly try to interpret the client's feelings. In the example just discussed, the desired outcome is for the client to clarify the hospitalization experience. The nurse responds by saying, "It must be frustrating to feel locked up." The nurse focuses on the client's feelings rather than the accusations, which reflects an understanding of the client's feelings. The client knows that the nurse accepts these feelings, which leads to further discussion. It may seem impossible to plan reactions for each situation, but with practice, the nurse will begin to respond consistently in a therapeutic way.

APPLYING COMMUNICATION CONCEPTS

When the nurse is interacting with clients, additional considerations can enhance the quality of communication. This section describes the importance of rapport, validation, empathy, and the role of boundaries and body space in nurse–client interactions.

Rapport

Rapport, interpersonal harmony characterized by understanding and respect, is important in developing a trusting, therapeutic relationship. Nurses establish rapport through interpersonal warmth, a nonjudgmental attitude, and a demonstration of understanding. A skilled nurse will establish rapport that will alleviate the client's anxiety in discussing personal problems.

People with mental health problems often feel alone and isolated. Establishing rapport helps lessen those feelings. When rapport develops, a client feels comfortable with the nurse and finds self-disclosure easier. The nurse also feels comfortable and recognizes that an interpersonal bond or alliance is developing. All these factors—comfort, sense of sharing, and decreased anxiety—are important in establishing and building the nurse–client relationship.

Validation

Validation is explicitly confirming with another person one's own thoughts or feelings with respect to a specific event or behaviour. To do so, the nurse must own his or her own thoughts or feelings by using "I" statements. Validating communication generally refers to observations, thoughts, or feelings and seeks explicit feedback. For example, a nurse who sees a client pacing the hallway before a planned family visit may question whether the client is anxious. Validation may occur with a statement such as, "I notice you pacing the hallway. I wonder if you are feeling anxious about the family visit?" The client may agree, "Yes. I keep worrying about what is going to happen!," or disagree, "No. I have been trying to get into the bathroom for the last 30 minutes, but my roommate is still in there!"

Empathy

The use of **empathy** in a therapeutic relationship is central to PMH nursing. Empathy is the ability to experience, in the present, a situation as another did at some time in the past. It is the ability to put oneself in another person's circumstances and feelings. The nurse does not need to have actually had the experience but has to be able to imagine the feelings associated with it. Empathic communication involves the nurse receiving information from the client with open, nonjudgmental acceptance and communicating this understanding of the experience and feelings so that the client feels understood.

Bio/Psycho/Social/Spiritual Boundaries and Body Space Zones

Boundaries are the defining limits of individuals, objects, or relationships. Boundaries mark territory, identifying what is "mine" from what is "not mine." Human beings have many different types of boundaries. Material boundaries, such as fences around property, artificially imposed territorial lines, and bodies of water, can define territory as well as provide security and order. Within the bio/psycho/social/spiritual model, personal boundaries have physical, psychological, social, and spiritual dimensions. Physical boundaries are those established in terms of physical closeness to others—whom we allow to touch us or how close we want others to stand near us. Psychological boundaries are established in terms of emotional distance from others—how much of our innermost feelings and thoughts we want to share. Social boundaries, such as norms, customs, and roles, help us establish our closeness and place within the family, culture, and community. Spiritual boundaries, related to such things as our understanding of the meaning of life, our religious values, and/or our sense of relationship with a greater power, shape our way of being in the world. Boundaries are not fixed, but dynamic. When boundaries are involuntarily transgressed, the individual can feel threatened and may respond to the perceived threat. The nurse must elicit permission before implementing interventions that invade personal boundaries.

Personal Boundaries

Every individual is surrounded by four different body zones. These were identified by Hall (1990) as the intimate zone (e.g., whispering and embracing), the personal zone (e.g., for close friends), the social zone (e.g., for acquaintances), and the public zone (usually for interacting with strangers). These zones provide varying degrees of protection against unwanted physical closeness during interactions. The breadth of each zone varies according to culture. Some cultures define the intimate zone narrowly and the personal zones widely. Friends in these cultures stand and sit close while interacting. While other cultures may define the intimate zone widely and are uncomfortable when others stand close to them, the variability of intimate and personal zones has implications for nursing. For a client to be comfortable with a nurse, the nurse needs to protect the intimate zone of that individual. The client usually will allow the nurse to enter the personal zone but will express discomfort if the nurse breaches the intimate zone. For the nurse, the difficulty lies in differentiating personal and intimate zones for each client.

The nurse's awareness of his or her own need for intimate and personal space is another prerequisite for therapeutic interactions with the client. It is important that a nurse feels comfortable while interacting with clients. Establishing a comfort zone may well entail fine-tuning the size of body zones. Recognizing this will help the nurse understand occasional, inexplicable reactions to the proximity of clients.

Professional Boundaries

For nurses, professional boundaries are also essential to consider in the context of the nurse–client relationship. Clients often enter such relationships at a very vulnerable point, and nurses need to be aware of professional boundaries to avoid exploitation of the client. For example, in a friendship, there is a two-way sharing of personal information and feelings, but as mentioned previously, the focus is on the client's needs, and the nurse generally does not share personal information or attempt to meet his or her own needs through the relationship. The client may seek a friendship or sexual relationship with the nurse (or vice versa), which would be a violation of the professional role. Although professional boundaries are about power, influence, and control, they are not clear and precise. Professional boundaries can become blurred and ambiguous, given the familiarity, trust, and emotional intensity often involved in therapeutic relationships. It is important to be vigilant about potential abuses of power present in all such relationships (Austin, Bergum, Nuttgens, & Peternelj-Taylor, 2006). The results of a self-administered survey study of over 900 Registered Nurses and Registered Psychiatric Nurses practicing in Alberta revealed that only one respondent reported having dated a current client (rarely); nine reported having dated a discharged client (rarely or sometimes), while six nurses reported having had a sexual relationship with a discharged client in the past (Campbell, Yonge, & Austin, 2005).

There are several indicators that a nurse–client relationship may be crossing professional boundaries. These include gift-giving by either party, a nurse spending inordinate time with a particular client, a nurse strenuously defending or explaining a client's behaviour in team meetings, a nurse's feeling he or she is the only one who truly understands the client, a nurse and client's keeping secrets, and a nurse's thinking frequently about a client outside of work (College of Nurses of Ontario, 2013; Forchuk et al., 2006; Gallop et al., 2002). Provincial regulatory bodies may have guidelines or firm rules, such as stipulating how long, following the termination of a therapeutic relationship, before one may engage in a romantic or sexual relationship. Within psychiatric disciplines, a romantic or sexual relationship with a former client is considered inappropriate, regardless of the length of time since the professional relationship was terminated. In nursing, the guidelines are generic and do not identify differences between specialties.

Nevertheless, the professional implications of a personal relationship following a nursing relationship that involved psychotherapy are serious and must be carefully considered. Guidelines are generally quite vague regarding when a friendship would be appropriate, but such relationships are not appropriate when the nurse is actively providing care to the client. An exceptional case could be a relationship that pre-existed that of nurse with client, for which another nurse is unavailable, such as in a nursing outpost (College of Nurses of Ontario, 2013). Similarly, relationships to meet the nurse's needs that are acquired through the nursing context, such as a relationship with a client's family member, also breach professional boundaries. It is important that the nurse be familiar with the standards of practice related to boundaries and therapeutic relationships of his or her provincial regulatory and professional associations. When concerns arise related to therapeutic boundaries, the nurse must seek clinical supervision or transfer care of the client immediately. The therapeutic dialogue presented in Box 6.4 illustrates how to respond

BOX 6.4

THERAPEUTIC DIALOGUE

Client Request for Nurses' Contact Information

How should a nurse respond when a client asks for his/her phone number or Facebook contact? Politely clarify that the relationship is professional, and the nurse will not share this information.

Context: The client located the nurse on Facebook and submitted a friend request. The nurse did not accept the friend request and did not message the client online to explain why.

At the next meeting with the client, the nurse brought up the Facebook request.

Nurse: "I noticed that you sent a friend request to me over Facebook."

Client: "Yes, I did. I was wondering why you didn't accept my friend request."

Nurse: "I did not accept it because what we have is a professional relationship, and it would not be appropriate for me to have social contact with clients outside of the therapeutic setting."

Client: "Oh. I was hoping to contact you if I had some questions after discharge."

Nurse: "Your discharge date is approaching. We have discussed community resources that are available, and follow-up appointments will continue with your physician. How are you feeling about discharge?"

to a client's request for the nurse's personal contact information.

Defence Mechanisms

Defence mechanisms (or coping mechanisms) are defined in the fifth edition of the *Diagnostic and Statistical Manual of Mental Disorders (DSM-5)* (APA, 2013) as "mechanisms that mediate the (client's) reaction to emotional conflicts and to external stressors. Some defense mechanisms (e.g., projection, splitting, acting out) are almost invariably maladaptive. Others (e.g., suppression, denial) may be either maladaptive or adaptive, depending on their severity, their inflexibility, and the context in which they occur" (American Psychiatric Association, 2013, p. 819). The concept of defence mechanisms originated with Freud's psychoanalytic theory and was conceived as the way the ego protected the individual from overwhelming anxiety (see Chapter 8). Healthy individuals use various defence mechanisms throughout their lives. A defence mechanism becomes pathologic when it is used so persistently that it becomes maladaptive. Suppression or denial, for instance, involves a process where anxiety-provoking information is not accepted (for suppression, this is conscious, and for denial, this is unconscious). These two defence mechanisms may be either maladaptive or adaptive depending on their severity and the context in which they occur. Other defence mechanisms such as projection (attributing one's own feelings onto another), splitting (self or others viewed as all bad or all good), and acting out (expressing unconscious feelings in actions rather than words), however, are almost invariably maladaptive.

As nurses develop therapeutic relationships, they will recognize their clients, and perhaps themselves, using defence mechanisms. As defence mechanisms are almost always used unconsciously, it will be difficult for a nurse to readily identify his or her own without reviewing the relationship with someone else. With experience, the nurse will evaluate the purpose of a defence mechanism and then determine whether it should be discussed with the client. For example, if a client is using humour to alleviate an emotionally intense situation, that may be very appropriate. On the other hand, if someone continually rationalizes antisocial behaviour, the use of the defence mechanism should be discussed.

■ ANALYZING INTERACTIONS

It is not unusual for people with mental health disorders to have difficulty communicating. For example, perceptual, cognitive, and information-processing deficits, typical of people with schizophrenia, can interfere with the person's ability to express ideas, understand concepts, and accurately perceive the environment. Because of the complexity of communication, mental health professionals monitor their interactions with clients using various methods, including audio recording, video recording, and **process recording** (writing a verbatim transcript of the interaction). A video or audio recording of an interaction provides the most accurate monitoring but is cumbersome to use. Process recording, one of the easiest methods to use, is adequate in most situations. Nurses should use it when first learning therapeutic communication and during times when communication becomes problematic. In a process recording, the nurse records, from memory, the verbatim interaction immediately after the communication (Box 6.5). The nurse then analyzes the content of the interaction in terms of the words and their meaning for both the client and the nurse. The analysis is especially important because the ability to communicate verbally is often compromised in people with mental disorders.

Words may not have the same meaning for the client as they do for the nurse. Clarification of meaning becomes especially important. The analysis can identify symbolic meanings, themes, and blocks in communication. **Symbolism**, the use of a word or phrase to represent an object, event, or feeling, is used universally. For example, automobiles are named for wild animals that represent speed, prowess, and beauty. In people with mental disorders, the use of words to symbolize events, objects, or feelings is often idiosyncratic, and they cannot explain their choices. For example, a person who is feeling scared and anxious may tell the nurse that bombs and guns are exploding. It is up to the nurse to make the connection between the bombs and guns and the client's feelings and then validate this with the client. Because of the client's cognitive limitations, the individual may express feelings only symbolically.

Some clients, for example, those with developmental disabilities or neurocognitive challenges, may have difficulty with abstract thinking and symbolism. Conversations may be interpreted literally. For example, in response to the question "What brings you to the hospital?" a client might reply, "The ambulance." In these situations, the nurse must be cautious to avoid using symbols or metaphors. Concrete language, that is, language reflecting what can be observed through the senses, will be more easily understood.

Verbal behaviour is also interpreted by analyzing **content themes**. Clients often express concerns or feelings repeatedly in several different ways. After a few sessions, a common theme emerges. Themes may emerge symbolically, as in the case with the client who constantly talks about the "guns and bombs." Alternatively, a theme may simply be identified as a recurrent thread of a story that a client retells at each session. For example, a client who always explained his early abandonment by his family led his nurse to hypothesize that he had an underlying fear of rejection. The nurse was then able to test whether there was an underlying fear and to develop strategies to help the client explore the fear (Box 6.6). It is important to involve clients in analyzing

BOX 6.5 Process Recording

Setting: The living room of Mr. S's home. His parents are in the room but cannot hear the conversation. Mr. S is sitting on the couch and the nurse is sitting on a chair. This is the nurse's first visit after Mr. S's discharge from the hospital.

Client	Nurse	Comments/Interpretation
	How are you doing, Mr. S?	*Plan:* Initially develop a sense of trust and initiate a therapeutic relationship.
I'm fine. It's good to be home. I really don't like the hospital.	You didn't like the hospital?	*Interpretation:* Mr. S does not want to return to the hospital.
		Use reflection to begin to understand his experience.
NO. The nurses lock you up. Are you a nurse?	Yes. I'm a nurse. I'm wondering if you think that I will lock you up.	*Interpretation:* Mr. S is wondering what my role is and whether I will put him back in the hospital.
You could tell my mom to put me back in the hospital.	Any treatment I recommend I will thoroughly discuss with you first. I am here to help you stay out of the hospital. I will not discuss anything with your mother unless you give me the permission to do so.	Use interpretation to clarify Mr. S's thinking.
		Mr. S is wondering about my relationship with his mother.
		Explain my role.

themes so that they may learn this skill. Within the therapeutic relationship, the person who does the work is the one who develops the competencies, so the nurse must be careful to share this opportunity with the client (Peplau, 1952/1988).

Communication blocks are identified by topic changes that either the nurse or the client makes. Topics are changed for various reasons. A client may change the topic from one that does not interest him or her to one that he or she finds more meaningful. However, an individual often changes the topic because he or she is

BOX 6.6 Themes and Interactions

Session 1	Client discusses the death of his mother at a young age.
Session 2	Client explains that his sister is now married and never visits him.
Session 3	Client says that his best friend in the hospital was discharged and he really misses her.
Session 4	Client cries about a lost kitten.

Interpretation: Theme of loss is pervasive in several sessions.

uncomfortable with a particular subject. Once a topic change is identified, the nurse or client hypothesizes the reason for it. If the nurse changes the topic, he or she needs to determine why. The nurse may find that he or she is uncomfortable with the topic or may not be listening to the client. Beginning mental health nurses who are uncomfortable with silences or trying to elicit specific information from the client often change topics.

The nurse must also record and interpret the client's nonverbal behaviour in light of the verbal behaviour. Is the client saying one thing verbally and another nonverbally? The nurse must consider the client's cultural background. Is the behaviour consistent with cultural norms? The nurse must also record and interpret the client's nonverbal behaviour in light of the verbal behaviour. Is the client saying one thing verbally and another nonverbally? Is the person's nonverbal behaviour inconsistent with what is normal behaviour for that person? Is it inconsistent with the person's cultural norms as previously expressed in his or her everyday life?

■ THE NURSE–CLIENT RELATIONSHIP

The nurse–client relationship is a dynamic process that changes with time. It can be viewed in steps or phases with characteristic behaviours for both the client and the nurse. This text uses an adaptation of Hildegard

Peplau's model that she introduced in her seminal work, *Interpersonal Relations in Nursing* (1952/1988). The nurse–client relationship is conceptualized in three overlapping phases that evolve with time: orientation phase, working phase, and resolution phase. Box 6.7 describes factors that facilitate and interfere with the development of the nurse–client relationship from the client perspective based on an international review of the literature in six Western countries.

The **orientation phase** is the phase during which the nurse and client get to know each other. During this phase, which can last from a few minutes to several months, the client develops a sense of trust in the nurse. The second phase is the **working phase**, in which the client uses the relationship to examine specific problems and learn new ways of approaching them. The final stage, the **resolution phase**, is the termination stage of the relationship and lasts from the time the problems are actually resolved to the close of the relationship. The relationship does not develop in a linear manner; rather, the relationship may be predominantly in one phase, but reflections of all phases can be seen in most nurse–client relationships.

KEY CONCEPT

The **nurse–client relationship** is a dynamic process that changes with time. It can be viewed in steps or phases with characteristic behaviours for both the client and the nurse.

Orientation Phase

The orientation phase begins when the nurse and client meet and ends when the client begins to identify problems to be examined within the relationship. During the orientation phase, the nurse discusses the client's expectations, explains the purpose of the relationship and its boundaries, and facilitates the development of the relationship. It is natural for the nurse and client to be more nervous during the first few sessions. The goal of the orientation phase is to develop trust and security within the nurse–client relationship. During this initial phase, the nurse listens intently to the client's history and perception of problems and begins to understand the client and identify themes. The use of empathy facilitates the development of a positive therapeutic relationship.

First Meeting

During the first meeting, it is important to outline both nursing and client responsibilities. The nurse is responsible for providing guidance throughout the therapeutic relationship, protecting confidential information, and maintaining professional boundaries. The client is responsible for attending agreed-upon sessions, interacting during the sessions, and participating in the nurse–client relationship. The nurse should also explain clearly to the client the role of the nurse as well as pragmatic issues, such as meeting times, handling of missed sessions, and the estimated length of the relationship. Issues related to recording information and how

---

BOX 6.7 **Research for Best Practice**

> #### CLIENT PERSPECTIVE OF FACTORS THAT FACILITATE AND INTERFERE WITH INTERPERSONAL RELATIONSHIPS WITH CARE PROVIDERS

Cutcliffe, J. R., Santos, J. C., Kozel, B., Taylor, P., & Lees, D. (2015). Raiders of the lost art: A review of published evaluations of inpatient mental health care experiences emanating from the United Kingdom, Portugal, Canada, Switzerland, Germany, and Australia. International Journal of Mental Health Nursing, *24(5), 375–385.*

Purpose: This review identifies from the client perspective key factors that can facilitate or interfere with the development of the therapeutic relationships with mental health/psychiatric nurses. The authors comment that evidence from the literature may not align with practices in the clinical environment.

Methods: The authors reviewed and contrasted published academic research findings and client surveys from six Western countries (United Kingdom, Portugal, Canada, Switzerland, Germany, and Australia).

Findings: This international review found common themes among client values that can facilitate relationships with care providers and influence outcomes in treatment, including nurses' demonstration of warmth, humanity, and genuineness; concern for dignity; displaying respect; providing emotional support; and inclusion in treatment. Factors that can inhibit the therapeutic alliance include nurses being unapproachable, overly "professional," and controlling; overreliance on medication; client underinvolvement in decision making; and insufficient formal or informal "talk therapy."

Implications for Practice: Client outcomes are influenced by the quality of the nurse–client relationship. Nurses must be aware of how clients perceive their behaviour to further the therapeutic alliance.

the nurse will work within the interprofessional team should also be made explicit.

It is not unusual for both the nurse and the client to feel anxious at the first meeting. The nurse should recognize the anxieties and attempt to alleviate them before the meeting. The client's behaviour during this first meeting may indicate to the nurse some of the client's problems in interpersonal relationships. For example, a client may talk nonstop for 15 minutes or may boast of sexual conquests. What the client chooses to tell or not to tell is significant. What a client first does or says may not accurately indicate his or her true feelings or the situation. In the beginning, clients may deny problems or choose not to discuss them as defence mechanisms or to prevent the nurse from getting to know them. The client is usually nervous and insecure during the first few sessions and may exhibit behaviour reflective of these emotions, such as rambling. Often by the third session, the client can better focus on a topic.

Confidentiality in Treatment

Ideally, nurses include people who are important to the client in planning and implementing care. The nurse and client should discuss the issue of confidentiality in the first session. The nurse should be clear about any information that is to be shared with anyone else. Usually, the nurse shares significant assessment data and client progress with a supervisors and interprofessional team members, including physicians. Most clients expect the nurse to communicate with other mental health professionals and are comfortable with this arrangement. Boundaries around what information can be shared with whom, and under what circumstances, are covered under provincial/territorial legislation, such as mental health acts and health information acts. Appropriate behaviour regarding confidentiality and social media are important to address. Nurses, including nursing students, are prohibited from discussing client information online, such as in personal blogs or on Facebook. It is therefore important that each nurse be aware of the legislation in the province or territory in which he or she is practising.

Testing the Relationship

This first part of the orientation phase, called the "honeymoon phase," is usually pleasant. However, the therapeutic team typically hits rough spots before completing this phase. The client begins to test the relationship to become convinced that the nurse will really accept him or her. Typical testing behaviours include forgetting a scheduled session or being late. Clients may also express anger at something a nurse says or accuse the nurse of breaking confidentiality. Another common pattern is for the client to introduce a relatively superficial issue first as if it is the major problem. Nurses must recognize that these behaviours are designed to test the relationship and establish its parameters, not to express rejection or

dissatisfaction with the nurse. Nursing students often feels personally rejected when clients engage in testing and may even become angry with the client. It is important for nurses and nursing students alike to understand the behaviour as testing and continue to be available to the client. With the adoption of consistent responses, these behaviours usually subside. Testing needs to be understood as a normal way that human beings develop trust.

Some issues specific to mental health clients can occur. For example, a client experiencing paranoia, by definition, is going to have difficulty establishing trust and may require a longer orientation phase. A client who is depressed may have difficulty expressing needs and may require periods of silence to feel comfortable in moving forward in the relationship.

Working Phase

When the client begins identifying problems to work on, the working phase of the relationship has started. Problem identification can yield a wide range of issues, such as managing symptoms of a mental disorder, coping with chronic pain, examining issues related to sexual abuse, and dealing with problematic interpersonal relationships. Through the relationship, the client begins to explore the identified problems and develop strategies to resolve them. By the time the working phase is reached, the client has developed enough trust that he or she can examine the identified problems within the security of the therapeutic relationship. In the working phase, the nurse can use various verbal and nonverbal techniques to help the client examine problems and support the client to plan strategies to address concerns.

Transference (unconscious assignment to others of the feelings and attitudes that the client originally associated with important figures) and **countertransference** (the provider's emotional reaction to the client based on personal unconscious needs and conflicts) become important issues in the working phase (refer to Box 6.8). For example, a client could be hostile to a nurse because of the underlying resentment of authority figures; the nurse, in turn, could respond defensively because of earlier experiences of anger. The client uses transference to examine problems. During this phase, the client is psychologically vulnerable and emotionally dependent on the nurse. The nurse needs to recognize countertransference and prevent it from eroding professional boundaries.

Many times, nurses are eager to implement rehabilitation plans. However, implementation of such plans require the clients' trust, and ability to identify what issues they wish to work on, within the context of the relationship. Nurses can facilitate the development of trust by displaying positive qualities that many clients value in the therapeutic relationship, such as respect,

BOX 6.8

THERAPEUTIC DIALOGUE

Countertransference in Nurse–Client Relationship

A client and nurse are having a formal talk therapy session. The nurse is grieving the recent loss of her father after a prolonged illness. The client is an adolescent who lives at home with his parents and is having challenges in the area of family relationships.

Client: "I am having problems with my dad again."

Nurse: "What sort of problems?"

Client: "He just won't leave me alone. When I'm in my room, he walks in whenever he wants and doesn't give me privacy."

Nurse: "That sounds like it is frustrating for you."

Client: "It is. I get so mad! I even threw a book at him once so he would get out."

Nurse: "Was he hurt?"

Client: "I didn't care."

Nurse: "Well, your dad will not be around forever. It is important to have a good relationship with your parents."

empathy, honesty, companionship, and friendliness (Moreno-Poyato et al., 2016).

Resolution Phase

The final stage of the nurse–client relationship is the resolution phase, which begins when the actual problems are resolved and ends with the termination of the relationship. During this phase, the client is redirected toward a life without this specific therapeutic relationship. The client connects with community resources, solidifies a newly found understanding, and practices new behaviours. The client takes responsibility for follow-up appointments and interacts with significant others in new ways. New problems are not addressed during this phase, except in terms of what was learned during the working stage. The nurse assists the client in strengthening relationships, making referrals, and recognizing and understanding signs of future relapse.

Termination begins on the first day of the relationship, when the nurse explains that this relationship is time limited and is established to help manage and resolve the client's problems. Because a therapeutic relationship is dependent, the nurse must constantly evaluate the client's level of dependence and continually support the client's move toward independence. Termination is usually stressful for the client who must sever ties with the nurse and who has shared thoughts and feelings and given guidance and support over many sessions. Depending on previous experiences with terminating relationships, some clients may not handle their emotions well during termination. Some may not show up for the last session to avoid their feelings of sadness and separation. Many clients will also display anger about the relationship ending. Clients may express anger toward the nurse or displace it onto others. One of the best ways to handle the anger is to help the client acknowledge it, to explain that anger is a normal emotion when a relationship is ending, and to reassure the client that it is acceptable to feel angry. The nurse should also reassure the client that anger subsides once the relationship is over.

Another typical termination behaviour is raising old problems that have already been resolved. The nurse may feel frustrated if clients in the termination phase present resolved problems as if they were new. The nurse may feel that the sessions were unsuccessful. In reality, clients are unconsciously attempting to prolong the relationship and avoid its ending. Nurses should avoid addressing these problems. Instead, they should reassure clients of having already covered those issues and learned methods to control them. They should explain that the client may be feeling anxious about the relationship ending and redirect the client to newly acquired skills and abilities in forming new relationships, including support groups and social groups. The final meeting should focus on the future (see Box 6.9). The nurse can reassure the client that the nurse will remember him or her, but the nurse should not agree to see the client outside the relationship. Many clients who have difficulty establishing relationships may similarly have difficulty letting go of supportive relationships. The ending of the therapeutic relationship is a significant opportunity for client learning, including the opportunity for healthy closure to relationships. The nurse needs to plan for and to support this learning.

■ NONTHERAPEUTIC RELATIONSHIPS

Although it is hoped that all nurse–client relationships will go through the phases as described in the previous section, this is not always the case. **Nontherapeutic** relationships also go through predictable phases (Forchuk et al., 2000). These relationships also start in the orientation phase. However, trust is not established, and the relationship moves to a *phase of grappling and struggling*. The nurse and client both feel very frustrated and keep varying their approach with each other in an attempt to establish a meaningful relationship. This is different from a prolonged orientation phase in that the efforts are not sustained; they vary constantly. The nurse may try having longer or shorter meetings, being more or less directive, and varying the therapeutic stance from warm

BOX 6.9

THERAPEUTIC DIALOGUE

The Last Meeting

Ineffective Approach

Nurse: Today is my last day.
Client: I need to talk to you about something important.
Nurse: What is it?
Client: I have been hearing voices again.
Nurse: Oh, how often?
Client: Every night. You are the only one I'm going to tell.
Nurse: I think you should tell the new nurse.
Client: She is too new. She won't understand. I feel so bad about your leaving. Is there any way you can stay?
Nurse: Well, I could check on you tomorrow.
Client: Oh, would you? I would really appreciate it if you would give me your new telephone number.
Nurse: I don't know what the number will be, but it will be listed in the telephone book.

Effective Approach

Nurse: Today is my last day.
Client: I need to talk to you about something important.
Nurse: We talked about that. Anything "important" needs to be shared with the new nurse.
Client: But, I want to tell you.
Nurse: Saying good-bye can be very hard.
Client: I will miss you.
Nurse: Your feelings are very normal when relationships are ending. I will remember you in a very special way.
Client: Can I please have your telephone number?
Nurse: No, I can't give that to you. It is important that we say good-bye today.
Client: OK. Good-bye. Good luck.
Nurse: Good-bye.

Critical Thinking Challenge

- What were some of the mistakes the nurse in the first scenario made?
- In the second scenario, how does therapeutic communication in the termination phase differ from effective communication in the working phase?

and friendly to aloof. Clients in this phase may try to talk about the past but then change to discussions of the here and now. They may try talking about their family and in the next meeting talk about their work goals. Both the client and the nurse grapple and struggle to come to a common ground, and both become increasingly frustrated with each other. Eventually, the frustration becomes so great that the pair gives up on each other and moves to a *phase of mutual withdrawal*. The nurse may schedule seeing this client at the end of the shift and "run out of time" so that the meeting never happens. The client will leave the unit or otherwise be unavailable during scheduled meeting times. If a meeting does occur, the nurse will try to keep it short, rationalizing, "What's the point—we just cover the same old ground anyway." The client will attempt to keep it superficial and stay on safe topics. "You can always ask about your medications—nurses love to health teach, you know." Obviously, no therapeutic progress can be made in such a relationship. The nurse may be hesitant to ask for a therapeutic transfer, assuming that a relationship would similarly fail with another nurse. However, each relationship is unique, and difficulties in one relationship do not predict difficulties in the next. Clinical supervision early on may assist the development of the relationship, but often, a therapeutic transfer to another nurse is required.

A narrative review by Moreno-Poyato and colleagues (2016) identified several factors that may interfere with the establishment of the therapeutic relationship from the perspectives of nurses and clients. For instance, nurses may face multiple barriers, including increasing administrative responsibilities, shortened length of inpatient stay, fear of causing harm, lack of experience individualizing client care, organizational structure and policy, and negative perceptions of the workplace environment. Clients, on the other hand, found that the amount of time allotted to interactions to be the most prominent factor impeding the relationship. Other limitations perceived by clients include inaccessible nursing staff, insufficient involvement in care, being treated as an object or a problem to solve, authoritarian or paternalistic staff, and a tense or unsafe atmosphere.

STRATEGIES WITHIN THE THERAPEUTIC RELATIONSHIP

Motivational Interviewing

One evidence-based strategy is **motivational interviewing** (MI). MI is a clinical method designed to facilitate change in client behaviour by engaging a client's own autonomous decision-making ability. Practitioners of MI seek to selectively elicit and reinforce the client's own arguments for change. Carried out in a collaborative manner, MI encourages the client to make his or her own decisions through directed counselling that addresses increasing preferred behaviours and decreasing nonpreferred behaviours. MI is inherently exploratory and adaptive.

MI involves at least two processes: increasing preferred behaviours and decreasing nonpreferred behaviours. Ambivalence is an expected part of the process of change, and resistance to change is to be expected. In the efforts to help patients, two critical components emerge that are iteratively assessed for their influence. These are *conviction* (importance) and *confidence*. Strategies for increasing the patient's conviction include asking questions regarding the relative importance of changing behaviour, examining the risks and benefits of the particular behaviour and of changing, exploring concerns about behaviour, having the "hypothetical look over the fence," and exploring possible next steps. Enhancing confidence also includes brainstorming solutions, focusing on successful past efforts, and serial reassessment and repetition of the process. Asking the patient open-ended questions, listening reflectively, issuing affirming and summarizing statements, and also eliciting self-motivational statements from patient are conducive to building motivation for change. These include problem recognition, expression of concern, the intention to change, and a sense of optimism. Refer to Box 6.10 for the principles of MI.

Some of the signals of successful MI are the following: the nurse is speaking slowly; the patient is doing much more of the talking than the nurse; the patient is actively talking about behaviour change; and finally, the nurse is listening very carefully and gently directing the interview at appropriate moments. The acronym FRAMES (*feedback, responsibility, advice, menu, empathy, self-efficacy*) was coined by Miller and Sanchez (1994) to summarize elements of brief interventions with patients using MI (refer to Box 6.11).

MI has been shown to produce statistically significant results when successfully employed, and a variety of external factors may affect long-term outcomes. Often, these external factors are interpersonal and social forces (Berg, Ross, & Tikkanen, 2011). The negative effect of these factors indicates that MI assumes that risky behaviours are largely under the control of individuals (Berg et al., 2011). Acknowledging this assumption helps to make clear why MI may not be effective for some clients.

Effective practice of MI requires ongoing instruction and feedback. Topics discussed in this chapter, such as self-awareness, empathic linkages, active listening, and avoidance of defence mechanisms, will all have to be

---

BOX 6.10 The Principles of Motivational Enhancement

1. **Avoid arguing:** Generally, the more the therapist tells a patient "You can't do this," the more likely he or she will respond, if unconsciously, with "I will." Resistance to change is influenced by how the therapist responds to the patient's ambivalence.

2. **Express empathy:** The attitude underlying empathy might also be called acceptance, and it is not the same as approval of harmful behaviour, but rather an unconditional acceptance of where the patient is at in terms of the behaviour. Through skilful reflective listening, the therapist can seek to understand the patient's feelings and perspectives without judging, criticizing, or blaming. Paradoxically, this kind of acceptance of people as they are appears to free them to change, whereas insistence on change and nonacceptance of "where they are at" in the process of change can have the effect of keeping people as they are. It is not helpful to view the patient as "problematic," "pathologic," "unwilling to change," or "incapable of change"; rather, the patient's situation is understood as one of being "stuck."

3. **Develop discrepancy:** Motivation for change is created when people perceive a discrepancy between their present behaviour and important personal goals. Thus, MI aims at developing discrepancy until it overrides attachment to the present behaviour. This is accomplished without coercion. It is the patient who gives voice to concerns and intentions to change.

4. **Roll with resistance:** When encountering resistance, the therapist acknowledges ambivalence as natural. The patient is invited to consider new information and perspectives. The responsibility for change is repeatedly handed back to the patient, but with the offer of help and support. It is not the therapist's role to generate all the solutions or to tell the patient what to do. Directive approaches may elicit "Yes, but..." responses from the patient, with little or no change following and often a disengagement and dropping out of treatment.

5. **Support self-efficacy:** This refers to the reinforcement of the patient's belief in his or her ability to carry out and succeed. Change is a stepwise approach, and each small step along the journey should be reinforced and supported. The therapist's expectations about a patient's chances for recovery can have a powerful impact on outcome.

Source: Miller, W. R., & Rollnick, S. (2002). *Motivational interviewing: Preparing people for change.* New York, NY: Guilford Press.

BOX 6.11 FRAMES: Effective Elements of Brief Intervention

FEEDBACK

Provide patients with personal feedback regarding their individual status, such as personal alcohol and other substance consumption relative to norms, information about elevated liver enzyme values, and so forth.

RESPONSIBILITY

Emphasize the individual's freedom of choice and personal responsibility for change. General themes are as follows:

1. It's up to you; you're free to decide to change or not.
2. No one else can decide for you or force you to change.
3. You're the one who has to do it if it's going to happen.

ADVICE

Include a clear recommendation or advice on the need for change, typically in a supportive and concerned, rather than in a judgmental, manner.

MENU

Provide a menu of treatment options, from which patients may pick those that seem more suitable or appealing.

EMPATHIC COUNSELLING

Show warmth, support, respect, and understanding in communication with patients.

SELF-EFFICACY

Reinforce self-efficacy or an optimistic feeling that he or she can change.

---

effectively employed to achieve MI's desired results. MI has been shown to be effective in a variety of clinical settings (Barnett, Sussman, Smith, Rohrbach, & Spruijt-Metz, 2012; Chen, Creedy, Lin, & Wollin, 2012; Cronk et al., 2012; Day, 2013). However, there are a broad range of techniques in which PMH nurses can be trained that significantly improve outcomes (Barwick, Bennett, Johnson, McGowan, & Moore, 2012). According to Miller and Moyers (2006, p. 3), these techniques are as follows:

- Openness to collaboration with clients' own expertise
- Proficiency in client-centred counselling, including accurate empathy
- Recognition of key aspects of client speech that guides the practice of MI
- Eliciting and strengthening client change talk
- Rolling with resistance
- Negotiating change plans
- Consolidating client commitment
- Switching flexibly between MI and other intervention styles

Transitional Relationship Model

The transitional relationship model (TRM) evolved from the transitional discharge model, originally developed to help people through the discharge process. An extension of Peplau's theory, TRM is based on the assumption that people heal in relationships and require both professional and therapeutic peer relationships. The TRM was developed to sustain therapeutic relationships throughout the client's transition from hospital to the community. There are two essential components to this model: professional support and peer support. The professional's role is to bridge the therapeutic relationship over the discharge (or other transition) process so that the therapeutic relationship with the client is not terminated until the client enters another professional relationship with a care provider (e.g., a nurse staying involved after discharge until a community relationship is established). The peer support component is essential during the transition from hospital to community. Peer supporters are generally trained and supported through a consumer–survivor group. In other words, people need both professionals and an experienced friend. Studies have found that this approach reduces the time in hospital (Forchuk, Martin, Chan, & Jensen, 2005) and reduces readmissions (Reynolds et al., 2004).

While TRM had previously been shown to be an effective model of discharge (Forchuk, Jewell, Schofield, Sircelj, & Valledor, 1998), the most recent evaluation in 36 tertiary care psychiatric wards examined the facilitators and barriers to successful implementation (Forchuk et al., 2013). The results of the study demonstrated that a complex relationship existed between a variety of factors necessary for successful implementation. Of the implementation strategies offered to wards, which included educational modules, on-ward champions, and documentation systems, the effectiveness of implementation varied as a result of the staff feeling overwhelmed, poor group dynamics, and unforeseen losses of on-ward champions. This suggests the need for careful introduction of TRMs in order to continually foster ongoing support, education, and communication.

BOX 6.12 Research for Best Practice

TELEPHONE VERSUS FACE-TO-FACE INTERVENTIONS: PERCEIVED DIFFERENCES IN THERAPEUTIC PROCESS AND TREATMENT BARRIERS

Lingley-Pottie, P., McGrath, P., & Andreou, P. (2013). Barriers to mental health care: Perceived delivery system differences. Advances in Nursing Science, 36(1), 51–61.

Question: Are there differences in perceived treatment barriers between participants' experiences with distance versus face-to-face therapy?

Methods: In this "within-subject" questionnaire study, 60 participants from the *Strongest Families* telephone intervention program (Halifax, Nova Scotia) who had previous experience with face-to-face professional counselling were sampled by convenience. In the program, families who have a child with behaviour difficulties receive educational materials (handbooks, videos) and 12 weekly telephone sessions with a trained, nonprofessional coach. The questionnaire queried perceived treatment barriers using the Treatment Barrier Index (TBI) and therapeutic processes (e.g., therapeutic alliance). Questionnaires were completed by telephone, from a face-to-face perspective, and from a distance treatment perspective.

Findings: Statistically significant differences were found between delivery system TBI scores: there were few barriers with distance treatment. Therapeutic process differences suggested enhanced therapeutic alliance and self-disclosure with distance treatment.

Implications for Practice: Increased access, convenience, and a sense of privacy (visual anonymity) are aspects of therapy using distance technologies that enhance the quality of the therapeutic experience for some individuals and families.

Technology and the Therapeutic Relationship

Traditionally, the nurse–client relationship has been face to face. However, changes to information and communication technologies, particularly in the past decade, have significantly changed how health professionals and their clients interact. **Telehealth** is the extension of health care service delivery across distance by use of information and communication technologies such as telephone, video, and the Internet. Telehealth in Canada has been particularly effective in improving access to health professionals by clients in rural locales (Geffen, Gordon, & Chien, 2011). In the instance of *telenursing*, telehealth can involve something as basic as a phone call between a nurse and client or something as complex as assisting with a remote surgical procedure. For the purposes of PMH nursing in particular, there are important things to consider about the communicative aspect of the therapeutic relationship in situations mediated by communication technology. Nonverbal communication, which makes up so much of an interaction between nurse and client, is lessened or largely absent; access to necessary technology may also be difficult for some clients; it can be difficult to ensure that health providers do not step outside the scope of their practice; and issues of privacy, security, and consent can be more complicated in these situations. In order to address the latter issues, many agencies presently do not allow e-mail communication. A system can be set up behind a secure hospital firewall (Forchuk et al., 2013), but access control is always a concern with sensitive information. It is important to be aware of agency policy and security before using any Web-based communication. Public platforms, such as Facebook, do not allow privacy, sufficient security, or confidentiality for use in health care communication. The Internet can be a useful tool for health teaching or for finding resources, but its increasing use in mediating relationships, including those between health care providers and clients, raises issues of personal autonomy and consent (e.g., how a client's data are stored, exchanged, and used), persistent threats to privacy and confidentiality, and other issues of risk management. Refer to Box 6.12 for a summary of a research study on differences between telephone and face-to-face interventions.

SUMMARY OF KEY POINTS

- To deal therapeutically with the emotions, feelings, and problems of clients, nurses must understand their own cultural values and beliefs and interpersonal strengths and limitations.
- The nurse–client relationship is built on therapeutic communication, including verbal and

nonverbal interactions between the nurse and client. Some communication skills include active listening, positive body language, appropriate verbal responses, and the ability of the nurse to interpret appropriately and analyze the client's verbal and nonverbal behaviours.

- Two of the most important communication concepts are empathy and rapport.
- Defence mechanisms, used by all individuals, can be adaptive or maladaptive depending on factors like context, inflexibility, and severity.
- In the nurse–client relationship, as in all types of relationships, certain physical, psychological, social, and spiritual boundaries and limitations need to be observed.
- The therapeutic nurse–client relationship consists of three major and overlapping stages or phases: the orientation phase, in which the client and nurse meet and establish the parameters of the relationship; the working phase, in which the client identifies and explores problems; and the resolution phase, in which the client learns to manage the problems and the relationship is terminated.
- The nontherapeutic relationship also consists of three major and overlapping phases: the orientation phase, the grappling and struggling phase, and the phase of mutual withdrawal.
- Strategies that can be used within therapeutic relationships include MI and TRM.

Web Links

www.nurseone.ca/~/media/nurseone/page-content/pdf-en/ps89_telehealth_e.pdf?la=en This link takes you to the 2007 Canadian Nurses Association position statement, *Telehealth: The role of the nurse*, addressing the nurse–patient relationship, client safety, security, confidentiality and privacy, and other pertinent issues.

www.crnbc.ca/Standards/PracticeStandards/Pages/boundaries.aspx At this site is practice standard (2016) of the College of Registered Nurses of British Columbia for *Boundaries in the Nurse-Patient Relationship*.

www.cno.org/globalassets/4-learnaboutstandardsandguidelines/prac/learn/modules/tncr/pdf/tncr-chapter3.pdf The College of Nurses of Ontario's *Practice standard: Therapeutic nurse-client relationship*, can be found here.

publish.uwo.ca/~cforchuk/peplau/Homepage of nurse theorist, *Hildegard Peplau*.

www.youtube.com/watch?v=J_EJQgKihvk&feature=youtu.be Video by L. Killam re: *Therapeutic Relationships in Nursing: The Profession's Perspective Part 1*. www.youtube.com/watch?v=wN9bf7L_9oY *Part 2* is here.

rnao.ca/bpg/guidelines/establishing-therapeutic-relationships The Registered Nurses Association of Ontario's guidelines, *Establishing therapeutic relationships* are here.

References

American Psychiatric Association. (2000). *Diagnostic and statistical manual of mental disorders* (4th ed., text revision). Washington, DC: Author.

American Psychiatric Association. (2013). *Diagnostic and statistical manual of mental disorders* (5th ed.). Washington, DC: Author.

Austin, W., Bergum, V., Nuttgens, S., & Peternelj-Taylor, C. (2006). A re-visioning of boundaries in professional helping relationships: Exploring other metaphors. *Ethics & Behavior, 16*(2), 77–94. doi:10.1207/s15327019eb1602_1

Barnett, E., Sussman, S., Smith, C., Rohrbach, L. A., & Spruijt-Metz, D. (2012). Motivational interviewing for adolescent substance use: A review of the literature. *Addictive Behaviors, 37*(12), 1325–1334. doi:10.1016/j.addbeh.2012.07.001

Barwick, M. A., Bennett, L. M., Johnson, S. N., McGowan, J., & Moore, J. E. (2012). Training health and mental health professionals in motivational interviewing: A systematic review. *Children & Youth Services Review, 34*(9), 1786–1795. doi:10.1016/j.childyouth.2012.05.012

Berg, R. C., Ross, M. W., & Tikkanen, R. (2011). The effectiveness of MI4MSM: How useful is motivational interviewing as an HIV risk prevention program for men who have sex with men? A systematic review. *AIDS Education & Prevention, 23*(6), 533–549. doi:10.1521/aeap.2011.23.6.533

Boyd, M. (1995). Communication with clients, families, healthcare providers, and diverse cultures. In M. Strader & P. Decker (Eds.), *Role transition to client care management* (p. 431). Norwalk, CT: Appleton & Lange.

Campbell, R. J., Yonge, O., & Austin, W. (2005). Intimacy boundaries between mental health nurses and psychiatric patients. *Journal of Psychosocial Nursing and Mental Health Services, 43*(5), 33–41.

Chen, S. M., Creedy, D., Lin, H. S., & Wollin, J. (2012). Effects of motivational interviewing intervention on self-management, psychological and glycemic outcomes in type 2 diabetes: A randomized controlled trial. *International Journal of Nursing Studies, 49*(6), 637–644. doi:10.1016/j.ijnurstu.2011.11.011

College of Nurses of Ontario. (2013). *Practice standard: Therapeutic nurse-client relationship* (rev. ed.). Toronto, ON: Author.

Cronk, N. J., Russell, C. L., Knowles, N., Matteson, M., Peace, L., & Ponferrada, L. (2012). Acceptability of motivational interviewing among hemodialysis clinic staff: A pilot study. *Nephrology Nursing Journal, 39*(5), 385–391.

Cutcliffe, J. R., Santos, J. C., Kozel, B., Taylor, P., & Lees, D. (2015). Raiders of the lost art: A review of published evaluations of inpatient mental health care experiences emanating from the United Kingdom, Portugal, Canada, Switzerland, Germany, and Australia. *International Journal of Mental Health Nursing, 24*(5), 375–385. doi:10.1111/inm.12159

Day, P. (2013). Using motivational interviewing with young people: A case study. *British Journal of School Nursing, 8*(2), 97–99. doi:10.12968/bjsn.2013.8.2.97

Forchuk, C., Carmichael, C., Golea, G., Johnston, N., Martin, M. L., Patterson, P., ... Bethune-Davies, P. (2006). *Nursing best practice guideline: Establishing therapeutic relationships* (rev. suppl.). Toronto, ON: Registered Nurses Association of Ontario.

Forchuk, C., Jewell, J., Schofield, R., Sircelj, M., & Valledor, T. (1998). From hospital to community: Bridging therapeutic relationships. *Journal of Psychiatric and Mental Health Nursing, 5,* 197–202.

Forchuk, C., Martin, M. L., Chan, Y. C., & Jensen, E. (2005). Therapeutic relationships: From psychiatric hospital to community. *Journal of Psychiatric and Mental Health Nursing, 12,* 556–564.

Forchuk, C., Martin, M. L., Jensen, E., Ouseley, S., Sealy, P., Beal, G., ... Sharkey, S. (2013). Integrating an evidence-based intervention into clinical practice: 'transitional relationship model'. *Journal of Psychiatric and Mental Health Nursing, 20*(7), 584–594. doi:10.1111/j.1365-2850.2012.01956.x

Forchuk, C., Westwell, J., Martin, M. L., Bamber-Azzapardi, W., Kosterewa-Tolman, D., & Hux, M. (2000). The developing nurse–client relationship: Nurses perspectives. *Journal of the American Psychiatric Nurses Association, 6*(1), 3–10. doi:10.1016/S1078-3903(00)90002-8

Gallop, R., Choiniere, J., Forchuk, C., Golea, G., Jonston, N., Levac, A. M., ... Wynn, F. (2002). *Nursing best practice guideline: Establishing therapeutic relationships*. Toronto, ON: Registered Nurses Association of Ontario.

Geffen, M., Gordon, D., & Chien, E. (2011). Telehealth benefits and adoption: Connecting people and providers across Canada. Report commissioned by Canada Health Infoway. Retrieved from https://www.infoway-inforoute.ca/en/component/edocman/resources/reports/333-telehealth-benefits-and-adoption-connecting-people-and-providers-full

Hall, E. T. (1990). *The hidden dimension*. New York, NY: Anchor Books.

Lingley-Pottie, P., McGrath, P., & Andreou, P. (2013). Barriers to mental health care: Perceived delivery system differences. *Advances in Nursing Science, 36*(1), 51–61. doi:10.1097/ANS.0b013e31828077eb.

Miller, W. R., & Moyers, T. (2006). Eight stages in learning motivational interviewing. *Journal of Teaching in the Addictions, 5*(1), 3–17. doi:10.1300/J188v05n01_02

Miller, W. R., & Rollnick, S. (2002). *Motivational interviewing: Preparing people for change.* New York, NY: Guilford Press.

Miller, W. R., & Sanchez, V. C. (1994). Motivating young adults for treatment and lifestyle change. In G. S. Howard & P. E. Nathan (Eds.), *Alcohol use and misuse by young adults.* Notre Dame, IN: University of Notre Dame Press.

Moreno-Poyato, A. R., Monteso-Curto, P., Delgado-Hito, P., Suarez-Perez, R., Acena-Dominguez, R., Carreras-Salvador, R., ... Roldan-Merino,

J. F. (2016). The therapeutic relationship in inpatient psychiatric care: A narrative review of the perspective of nurses and patients. *Archives of Psychiatric Nursing, 30*(6), 782–787. doi:10.1016/j.apnu.2016.03.001

Peplau, H. E. (1952/1988). *Interpersonal relations in nursing.* London, UK: MacMillan.

Reynolds W., Lauder W., Sharkey, S., Maciver S., Veitch T., & Cameron, D. (2004). The effect of a transitional discharge model for psychiatric patients. *Journal of Psychiatric and Mental Health Nursing, 11*(1), 82–88.

Wendy Austin and Arlene Kent-Wilkinson

Wendy Austin and
Arlene Kent-Wilkinson

LEARNING OBJECTIVES

After studying this chapter, you will be able to:

- Identify the ways in which mental health legislation protects and promotes the well-being of Canadians.
- Discuss the way that the *UN Charter* and international agreements provide a foundation for mental health legislation.
- Explain the key components of your provincial/territorial Mental Health Act, including the criteria and processes for voluntary and involuntary admission and for mandatory outpatient treatment.
- Discuss the determination of "competency."
- Identify the ways a substitute decision-maker can be chosen.
- Describe the role of the nurse in upholding the rights of persons whose care and treatment is regulated by mental health legislation.
- Explain the phrase, "not criminally responsible due to a mental disorder."
- Define ethics.
- Distinguish between the domains of ethics and law.
- Describe the nurse as a moral agent and the resources available to support this role.
- Identify the most common approaches to ethics that inform health ethics.
- Describe the components of an ethical practice environment.
- Distinguish between a moral dilemma and moral distress.
- Consider the components of an ethical decision-making framework.
- Identify and discuss eight ethical issues in psychiatric and mental health nursing.

KEY TERMS

- admission certificate • beneficence • best interests • capable wishes • casuistry • community treatment order • competence • conditional leave • conscientious objection • deontology • ethics of care • feminist ethics • formal patient • human rights • involuntary admission • justice • mandatory outpatient treatment • modified best interests • nonmaleficence • practical wisdom • principlism • relational ethics • renewal certificate • respect for autonomy • review panel • substitute decision-maker • utilitarianism • virtue

KEY CONCEPTS

- ethics • mental health act • moral agent • moral dilemma • moral distress

In this chapter, the legal and ethical aspects of mental health care practice are presented. Although both are essential to the creation and maintenance of a just society, the law and ethics are separate domains. In a perfect world, societal laws would be totally compatible with ethical behaviours in every situation. In the real world, however, this is not always the case. Citizens may need to work to change laws that they believe do not support ethical action. In serving and protecting the public, it is crucial that nurses know and understand the laws relevant to nursing and can enact their code of ethics in daily practice. Codes are aspirational in nature but also have a regulatory purpose and a role in ensuring that the Canadian public receives quality nursing care.

THE LAW AND PSYCHIATRIC AND MENTAL HEALTH CARE

Every society needs laws to achieve its objectives. Mental health legislation is a means to protect and promote the mental well-being of citizens. Such legislation codifies fundamental protection of the rights of persons with mental disorders and provides a mechanism for the care and treatment of those whose illness interferes with their ability to recognize their need for medical assistance and/or their ability to seek it. The absence of such protection would limit their right to the best available health care.

Human Rights and Mental Health Legislation

A fundamental basis for mental health legislation is **human rights**. Set out in normative documents, human rights are recognition of the dignity and worth of every human being. Rights are delineated in such documents as the *Canadian Charter of Rights and Freedoms* (1982) and the United Nations *Universal Declaration of Human Rights* (1948). Key rights and principles include equality and nondiscrimination, the right to privacy and individual autonomy, freedom from inhuman and degrading treatment, the principle of the least restrictive environment, and the rights to information and participation. The Canadian Nurses Association (CNA) has a position statement, *Registered Nurses, Health and Human Rights* (2011), that is a helpful reference for nurses. (See Web Links.)

In 2010, Canada ratified the United Nations' *Convention on the Rights of Persons With Disabilities* (CRPD, 2006). As a signatory of the Convention, Canada is committed to ensuring the promotion and protection of the human rights of all persons with disabilities. Disability in the CRPD is understood from a social perspective as arising from the way in which the environment interacts with a person's condition rather than the condition itself. It provides a basis for legislation, policies, and regulations for eliminating barriers to the societal participation of those with a mental illness. A resource provided by the World Health Organization (WHO) is MiNDbank, an online platform that brings together international and national policies, strategies, laws, and standards for mental health and disability and promotes dialogue, debate, and research for the purposes of achieving national reforms that conform to international human rights and best practice standards (see Web Links).

Significant Canadian and international rights documents are listed in Table 7.1. Principles for the protection of persons with mental illness and the improvement of mental health services adopted by the United Nations in 1991 (UN, 1991) are outlined in Box 7.1. Information regarding national and international advocacy organizations is found in the Web Links section at the end of this chapter.

Table 7.1 Canadian and International Rights Agreements Relevant to Mental Health

Year	Agreement
1948	Universal Declaration of Human Rights
1966	The International Covenant on Economic, Social, and Cultural Rights
1966	The International Covenant on Civil and Political Rights
1982	Canadian Charter of Rights and Freedoms
1984	Canada Health Act
1986	Canada Employment Equity Act
1990	Declaration of Caracas
1991	Principles of Protection of Persons With Mental Illness
2007	United Nations Declaration on the Rights of Indigenous Peoples

Mental Health Legislation in Canada

Legislation in Canada strongly influences the context of our mental health care. Each province and territory is guided by its own Mental Health Act, which provides a framework for the delivery of mental health services and establishes rules and procedures governing the commitment of persons suffering from mental disorders. Each Act permits certain infringements upon a person's rights and freedoms only to the extent necessary to ensure that the person receives required care and treatment. Procedural safeguards are outlined, which must be followed when such curtailment of a person's rights

---

BOX 7.1 Rights of Persons with Mental Illness

- Right to medical care (Principle 1.1)
- Right to be treated with humanity and respect (Principle 1.2)
- Equal protection right (Principle 1.4)
- Right to be cared for in the community (Principle 7)
- Right to provide informed consent before receiving any treatment (Principle 11)
- Right to privacy (Principle 13)
- Freedom of communication (Principle 13)
- Freedom of religion (Principle 13)
- Right to voluntary admission (Principles 15 and 16)
- Right to judicial guarantees (Principle 17)

From United Nations. (1991). Principles for the protection of persons with mental illness and the improvement of mental health care. Adopted by General Assembly resolution 46/119 of 17 December 1991, Office of the United Nations High Commissioner for Human Rights. Retrieved from http://www.unhchr.ch/html/menu3/b/68.htm

becomes temporarily necessary. Each act must be congruent with the rights stipulated under the *1982 Charter of Rights and Freedoms* (Butler & Phillips, 2013), and the resources to enforce the Act must be in place. Internet access information for the various mental health acts can be found in Table 7.2. A nonlegal element of the protection for persons whose rights are temporarily curtailed due to a mental disorder is the recovery-oriented approach to care expected of Canadian mental health services (Mental Health Commission of Canada, 2009; see Chapter 2).

Mental Health Acts within Canada can allow **involuntary admission** of a person to a designated facility. Although the language varies by province and territory, the conditions that must be met are usually that an examination by a physician (note: the Nunavut Mental Health Act uses the term "mental health practitioner" rather than "physician"; psychologists can play a role in the involuntary process in Nunavut) indicates that the person has a mental disorder, is likely to cause harm to self or others or to suffer substantial mental or physical deterioration or serious physical impairment, and is unsuitable for admission to a facility other than as a **formal patient**. An **admission certificate** allows the person to be conveyed to a mental health facility and to be detained and cared for during a 24-hour period. Within that time, the person must be assessed by a physician (usually staff of that facility). Two admission certificates are required for the person to remain a formal patient; otherwise, they must be released at the end of the 24-hour period. These two admission certificates are sufficient to detain the person as a formal patient for a period of 1 month. **Renewal certificates** can extend the formal patient designation for another month. There must be two renewal certificates completed, each by a physician (usually, one of the physicians must be a psychiatrist) following an independent examination of the person. See Figure 7.1 for a flowchart of formal patient certification in the province of Alberta.

The **competence** of the person to make decisions regarding treatment, and thus able to give consent, must be assessed. Competence, in this respect, means being able to be informed and to understand (at a basic level) matters relevant to the decision and to understand the consequences of the decision. Competence is not a fixed capacity; it changes over time. There are specific provisions within mental health acts regarding the evaluation of competency and what action may be taken if a person is deemed not competent.

When a person is unable to consent to treatment, consent from a **substitute decision-maker** may be sought. Depending on the jurisdiction, these substitute decision-makers can be state appointed, appointed by the person when competent, or be a guardian or relative. There are different criteria to guide substitute decision-making: **best interests** (e.g., treatment will make the person less

Table 7.2 Mental Health Acts	
Province/Territory	**Web Site Addresses of Mental Health Acts in Canada**
Alberta	Mental Health Act www.albertahealthservices.ca/mha.asp
British Columbia	Mental Health Act www2.gov.bc.ca/gov/content/health/managing-your-health/mental-health-substance-use/mental-health-act
Manitoba	Mental Health Act web2.gov.mb.ca/laws/statutes/ccsm/m110e.php
New Brunswick	Mental Health Act www.canlii.org/en/nb/laws/stat/rsnb-1973-c-m-10/latest/rsnb-1973-c-m-10.html
Newfoundland and Labrador	Mental Health Care and Treatment Act www.health.gov.nl.ca/health/mentalhealth/mentalhealthact.html
Northwest Territories	Mental Health Actwww.canlii.org/en/nu/laws/stat/rsnwt-nu-1988-c-m-10/latest/rsnwt-nu-1988-c-m-10.html
Nova Scotia	Mental Health Act nslegislature.ca/legc/bills/59th_1st/1st_read/b109.htm
Nunavut	Mental Health Act www.canlii.org/en/nu/laws/stat/rsnwt-nu-1988-c-m-10/latest/rsnwt-nu-1988-c-m-10.html?searchUrlHash=AAAA AQASTWVudGFsIEhlYWx0aCBBY3QgAAAAAAE
Ontario	Mental Health Act www.e-laws.gov.on.ca/html/statutes/english/elaws_statutes_90m07_e.htm
Prince Edward Island	Mental Health Act www.princeedwardisland.ca/sites/default/files/legislation/m-06_1.pdf
Quebec	Act Respecting the Protection of Persons Whose Mental State Presents a Danger to Themselves or to Others www.canlii.org/en/qc/laws/stat/cqlr-c-p-38.001/latest/cqlr-c-p-38.001.html
Saskatchewan	Mental Health Services Act www.publications.gov.sk.ca/details.cfm?p=626
Yukon	Mental Health Act www.gov.yk.ca/legislation/acts/mehe.pdf

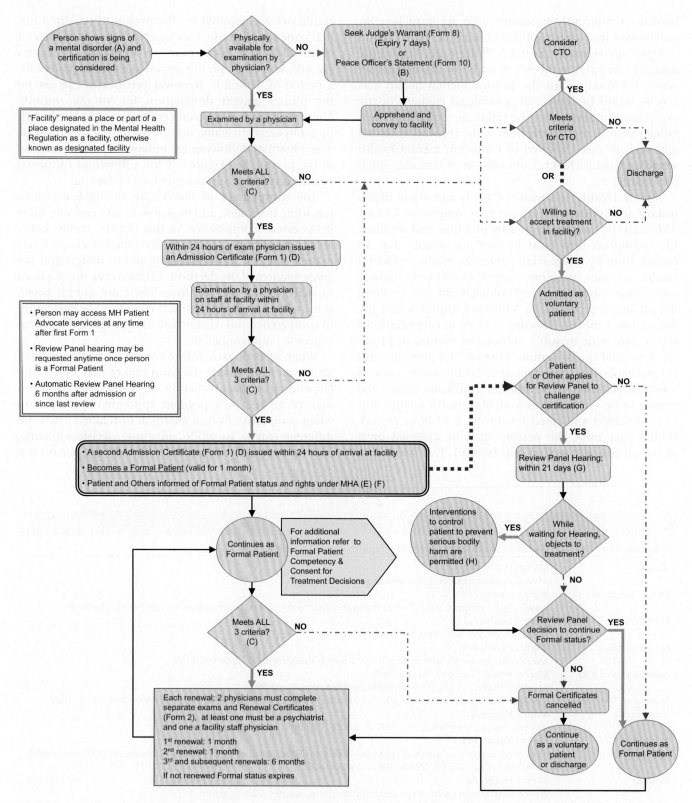

Figure 7.1. Process of Formal Patient Certification, Mental Health Act of Alberta. (Source: Alberta Health Services. (2010). Guide to the Mental Health Act and Community Treatment Order Legislation, p. 41. Author. Retrieved from www.albertahealthservices.ca/MHA.asp.)

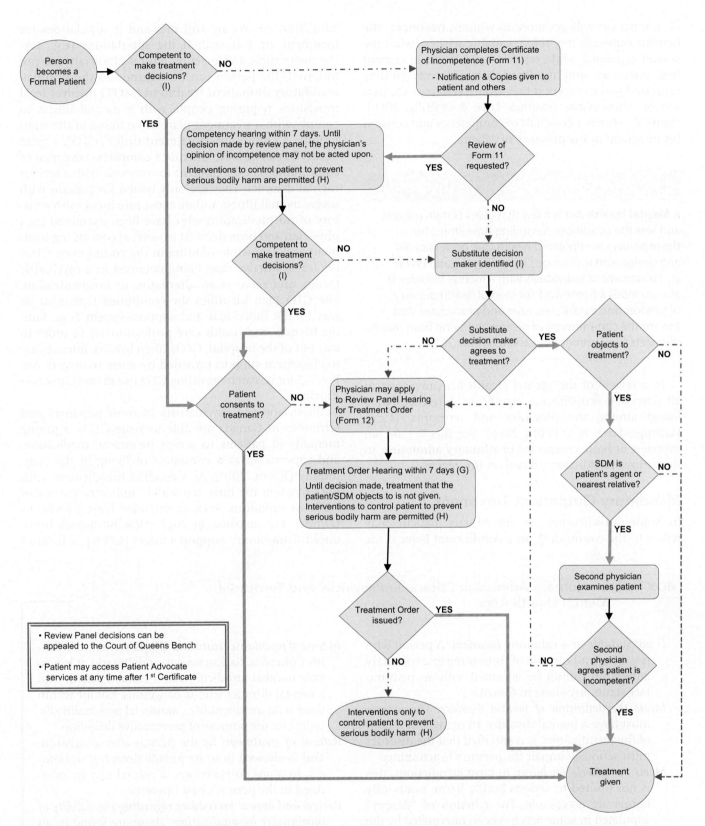

Figure 7.2. Process of Formal Patient Competency & Consent for Treatment Decisions, Mental Health Act of Alberta. (Source: Alberta Health Services. (2010). Guide to the Mental Health Act and Community Treatment Order Legislation, p. 41. Author. Retrieved from www.albertahealthservices.ca/MHA.asp.)

ill, the person will get more ill without treatment, the benefits outweigh any risks), **capable wishes** (what the person expressed while capable, even if not in current best interests), and **modified best interests** (follow expressed wishes except if they would endanger the person or others (Gray, Hastings, Love, & O'Reilly, 2016). Figure 7.2 shows a flowchart of competency and consent for treatment in the province of Alberta.

KEY CONCEPT

A **Mental Health Act** is a law that gives certain powers and sets the conditions (including time limits) for those powers to stipulated health care professionals and designated institutions regarding the admission and treatment of individuals with a mental disorder. It also provides a framework for mental health delivery of services and establishes rules and procedures that govern the commitment of persons suffering from mental disorders (Government of Saskatchewan, 2015).

In a review of the Mental Health Act provisions in all Canadian jurisdictions, significant differences were found among the provinces and territories (Gray, Hastings, Love, & O'Reilly, 2016). See Box 7.2 for an overview of basic criteria for **involuntary admission** in the various jurisdictions, based on this review.

Mandatory Outpatient Treatment

In some jurisdictions, an involuntary patient may return to the community on a **conditional leave** if the admission criteria are still met and if stipulations for treatment are followed. If the stipulations (e.g., taking medication and meeting with a physician) are not followed, the person can be returned to the hospital. **Mandatory outpatient treatment (MOT)** involves legal provisions requiring people with a mental illness to comply with a treatment plan while living in the community. A **community treatment order (CTO)**, a form of MOT, is an order to provide a comprehensive plan of community-based treatment to someone with a serious mental disorder. They are only issued for persons with severe mental illness and, in most provinces, with a history of hospitalization who have been examined by a physician and been deemed in need of continuing treatment and care while residing in the community. CTOs are less restrictive than being detained in a psychiatric facility and serve as an alternative to hospitalization. The CTO plan identifies the conditions that must be met by the individual and support system (e.g., family, friends, and health care professionals) in order to stay out of the hospital. CTOs often involve intense case management support provided by nurse managers. See Box 7.3 for research regarding CTO use in one Canadian province.

Physicians and psychiatrists in most provinces and territories in Canada are able to issue CTOs requiring mentally ill patients to accept treatment, medication, and supervision as a condition of living in the community (Rynor, 2010). All Canadian jurisdictions, with the exception the three territories, authorize the use of CTOs or variations, such as extended leave provisions (Rynor). For instance, in 2017, New Brunswick introduced Community Support Orders (CSOs), a form of

---

BOX 7.2 Involuntary Admission Criteria in Provincial and Territorial Mental Health Acts

Is not suitable as a voluntary inpatient: A person who is willing and capable of consenting to a voluntary admission cannot be admitted with an involuntary status anywhere in Canada.

Meets the definition of mental disorder: The person must have a mental disorder. In many, but not all of the jurisdictions, it is specified that the disorder must seriously impair the person's functioning.

Meets the criteria for harm: In most jurisdictions, this is not limited to serious bodily harm; nonbodily harms are acceptable. The criterion of "danger" stipulated in some acts has been interpreted by the courts to mean bodily harm.

Likely to suffer substantial mental or physical deterioration: This is included in some provinces (British Columbia, Saskatchewan, Manitoba, and Ontario) as an alternative to the harm criterion.

In need of psychiatric treatment: This is a criterion in British Columbia, Saskatchewan, and Ontario. It is possible in other jurisdictions to commit a person with a mental disorder who is dangerous, but for whom there is no treatment (e.g., antisocial personality disorder) for the purpose of preventative detention.

Refusal of treatment: By the person after admission: This is allowed in some jurisdictions but not others. In some jurisdictions, a refusal can be overruled in the person's best interests.

Review and appeal procedures regarding the validity of involuntary hospitalization: These are found in all jurisdictions.

Source: Gray, J. E., Hastings, T. J., Love, S., & O'Reilly, R. L. (2016). Clinically Significant Differences among Canadian Mental Health Acts: 2016. *Canadian Journal of Psychiatry, 61*(4), 222–226. doi:10.1177/0706743716632524

BOX 7.3 Research for Best Practice

EXPLORING COMMUNITY TREATMENT ORDERS IN AN EASTERN CANADIAN PROVINCE

Snow, N. (2015). Exploring community treatment orders: An institutional ethnographic study. Unpublished doctoral dissertation, University of Alberta, Edmonton, AB

Research Question: What is happening with the use of community treatment orders (CTOs) in an eastern Canadian province? This question was based on the perceived disconnect between what was *supposed to be happening* with CTO legislation and what was *actually happening* in practice.

Method: Institutional ethnography (IE) was used to explore everyday actualities and how they are socially organized to occur in the manner they do. People's ordinary behaviours are concerted by overarching social patterns (ruling relations) of which most are unaware. Individuals with experience related to CTOs such as families, frontline health professionals including nurses, administrators, and others were interviewed to elicit their descriptions of working with, developing, or enforcing the legislation. Relevant documents (e.g., included mental health legislation, CTO forms, policies, position statements) were mapped with the descriptions,

yielding insight into institutionally sanctioned ways of implementing CTOs and how these "butted against" the experiential knowledge of their everyday use.

Findings: Differences of opinion were found among the self-reported experiences of CTOs by families, nurses, physicians, and others, who are involved with CTOs. This lack of consensus is reflective of confusion in the process of enacting the legislation, the expectation that legislation can ensure consistency across the various situations where a CTO may be implemented, and the contradictory goals of legal practices and the practices of nurses and other health care professionals. CTO legislation is not focused on therapeutic interventions but is a means of policing the enforcement of mandated care. A major goal is reducing the risk of harm for members of the public by persons with exacerbation of their illness. Treatment compliance does not equal therapeutic engagement; legislating compliance is counterintuitive to the concept of recovery. In many instances, the care of individuals with severe mental illness is socially organized to fall upon family members to monitor and deliver, and this occurs with CTOs.

---

supervised community care ordered by a physician and agreed to by the patient (Government of New Brunswick, 2017). See Figure 7.3 for a flowchart of the CTO process in the province of Alberta.

Review Panels

All jurisdictions have a check on the involuntary aspects of mental health legislation. Usually a **review panel** (court or tribunal) chaired by a lawyer and composed of four or five persons with representative expertise (e.g., a lawyer, a psychiatrist, a physician, and a member of the public), the panel accepts applications for review by formal patients in designated facilities, persons subject to a CTO, and physicians of a formal patient. The panel will review whether formal patients are competent or should continue to be detained in the facility or have treatment decisions made for them. Usually, for formal patients who have been detained for 6 months through renewal certificates, some form of review is conducted by the panel without an application from the patient. Decisions of review panels may be appealed at the highest level of provincial court (Court of Queen's Bench).

Canadian Nurses' Responsibility Regarding Mental Health Legislation

It is the responsibility of nurses to understand the Mental Health Act of their province/territory. Nurses need to be able to explain the Act's basic provisions to people with mental illness and their families. In the province of Saskatchewan, their *Guide to Mental Health Service Act* outlines other functions of nurses, such as explaining patient and family rights, keeping track of certificate expiry dates, reporting to review panels, supervising CTOs and providing information to other clinicians and family members (Government of Saskatchewan, 2015, p. 125). These functions are similar to those expected of nurses in other provinces and territories.

In some jurisdictions, amendments to their Mental Health Acts have expanded the role of nurses when particular criteria are met. For example, in Saskatchewan, a nurse in a mental health centre may detain a voluntary patient requesting discharge if the nurse has reasonable grounds to believe that the patient now meets the criteria for involuntary status and needs to be examined by a physician. If this detention occurs, the medical examination

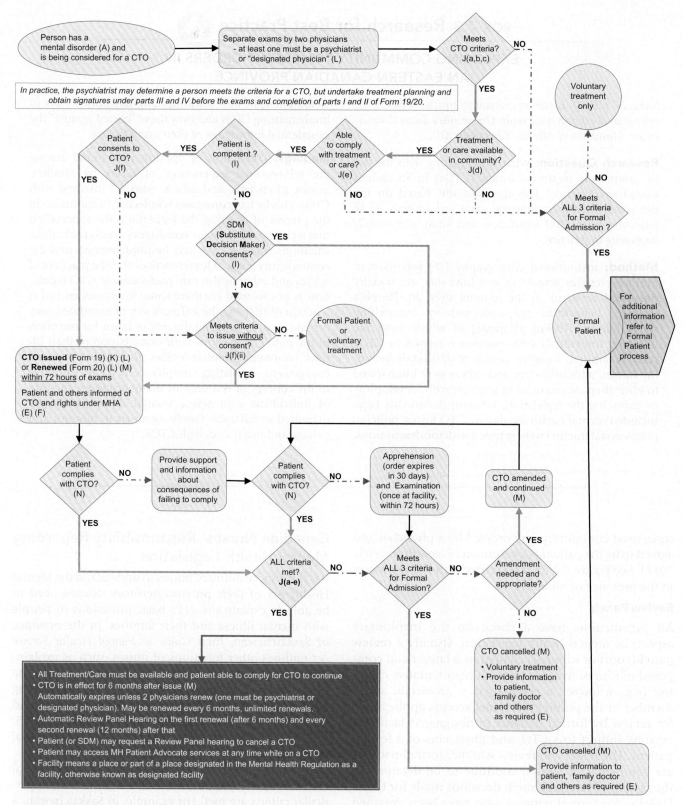

Figure 7.3. Community Treatment Orders (CTO). (Community Source: Alberta Health Services. (2010). Guide to the Mental Health Act and Community Treatment Order Legislation, p. 41. Author. Retrieved from www.albertahealthservices.ca/MHA.asp.)

must happen within 3 hours. As well, in this province, a nurse may be deemed a "prescribed health professional" in some circumstances and permitted to complete and issue a certificate that enables a person to be taken for examination by a physician with admitting privileges to a mental health centre. In every jurisdiction, nurses have an important advocacy role ensuring that the rights of persons coming under a mental health act are protected.

The Criminal Code and Mental Disorders

Separate from mental health legislation are the legal provisions that can require people to follow treatment as a condition of probation. The law allows for persons to be found *Not Criminally Responsible due to a Mental Disorder* for an offense if they are suffering from a mental disorder that makes them incapable of appreciating the nature of the act or knowing that what they did was wrong. In these cases, the offender with mental illness needs to comply with treatment monitored by the Criminal Code Review Boards (see Chapter 35).

Medical Assistance in Dying

In June 2016, an amendment to the Criminal Code made medical assistance in dying (MAID) legal in Canada provided all required conditions are met. MAID is defined as "(a) the administrating by a medical practitioner or nurse practitioner of a substance to a person, at their request, that causes their death; or (b) the prescribing or providing by a medical practitioner or nurse practitioner of a substance to a person, at their request, so that they may self-administer the substance and in doing so cause their own death" (An Act to Amend the Criminal Code, s. 241.1[a][b]).

To be eligible for MAID, an individual must have a medical condition, which meets four criteria. These are that:

a. "they have a serious and incurable illness, disease or disability;
b. they are in an advanced state of irreversible decline in capability;
c. illness, disease or disability or that state of decline causes them enduring physical or psychological suffering that is intolerable to them and that cannot be relieved under conditions that they consider acceptable; and
d. their natural death has become reasonably foreseeable, taking into account all of their medical circumstances, without a prognosis necessarily having been made as to the specific length of time that they have remaining" (An Act to Amend the Criminal Code, s. 241.1[a][b]).

The criteria that the illness is in an irreversible state of decline and that natural death is foreseeable have meant that persons for which mental illness is the sole underlying medical condition are not eligible. This has generated some controversy, and as this text goes to press, a change in the law is under advisement by the federal government. Those who argue for change point to the Charter rights of persons with mental illness. They contend, rightfully so, that mental illness can cause terrible suffering to the extent that life can seem not worth living. Those who support the law as it stands argue that the decline and suffering may be related more to lack of access to effective treatment than to the state of the disease. Mental health care, it can be argued, is significantly underfunded.

As well, the stigma of mental illness not only prevents people from seeking treatment but contributes greatly to the suffering associated with the illness. Persons with the label "mentally ill" are too readily excluded from society because of stigma. Just as access to good pain control and palliative care should have occurred before a request for MAID due to severe pain is made, access to good social support and quality of life measures needs to occur for persons with mental illness. John Maher, Canadian psychiatrist and editor in chief of the *Journal of Ethics in Mental Health* (2017, p. 1), asks, "How are people who already struggle with feeling like they are a burden on society or loved ones going to see this debate (on eligibility for MAID)? As fostering their autonomy or giving them a push towards death?" Dialogue among Canadians regarding this law and its potential change to our society will be important. It must be asked, does the law as it stands protect and promote the well-being of Canadians, a major purpose of legislation, or is a change necessary?

ETHICS AND PSYCHIATRIC AND MENTAL HEALTH NURSING CARE

Ethics is about how we should live; it is *"aiming at the 'good' with and for others in just institutions"* (Ricouer, 1992, p. 172, original italics). Ethics is about learning how to reach our potential as human beings, and so it is about values, relationships, principles, duties, rights, and responsibilities. In writing about ethics in *On Equilibrium*, Saul (2001) noted that, although we may think about ethics as something exotic or romantic, for heroes or saints, ethics is actually down to earth and practical: it needs to be an everyday part of our lives and built into our society.

Moral philosophy considers ways that individuals may approach decisions about how to act and how to be. The work of moral philosophers offers guidance in ethical actions. Although some philosophers differentiate ethics from morality, ethics and morals can be used as interchangeable terms (ethics comes from *ethos*, Greek for *custom; morals* comes from *mores*, Latin for *custom*) and are so used here.

KEY CONCEPT

Ethics is consideration of the way a person should act to live a good life with and for others. Moral philosophy offers ideas about how to decide this. Just institutions enable and support ethical actions.

Health Ethics

Somerville (2000) describes Canada as a secular society, with diverse religious groups: we have no common, external, absolute moral authority. She asks, how can we know, as a society, how to respond to new approaches to science, technology, and health care? Contemporary ethics is shaped by factors such as intense individualism (the individual coming before the common good), corporatism (dominance of business interests), unprecedented advances in science and technology, the power of the media, the increased use of law as a means to resolve disputes that are inherently about values, and a loss of a sense of the sacred. She proposes that two absolute values, *profound respect for life* and *commitment to the human spirit*, will allow us to make ethical societal choices.

Somerville (2000, p. xii) uses the metaphor of a canary to signify key issues that "test the ethical air in our societal mineshaft." As canaries once served to detect toxic gas in underground mines (i.e., sick or dead canaries warned miners that the air was unsafe), these issues warn us that the ethical tone of our society is putting us at risk. The way in which Canadians address the well-being of those living with mental illness is recognizable to those practicing in mental health care as an ethical canary.

It is an ethical responsibility for nurses to keep abreast of societal issues, at a local, national, or global level, and to respond to those that may be informed by nursing expertise. The Canadian Nurses Association's (CNA) Code of Ethics identifies ethical actions that nurses can do to address social issues that affect health and well-being (CNA, 2017).

The Ethical Nurse

Stating "I am a nurse" is a type of moral claim. Nurses have a fiduciary relationship with the public. (*Fiducial* comes from the Latin, *fidere*, to trust.) Nurses, as professionals, profess or claim that they will use their specialized knowledge and skills for the benefit of the public in a trustworthy way. Nurses are trusted to be ethical (Austin, 2006). In polls, nurses are consistently rated the most honest and ethical professionals (Gallup, 2016). Whenever nurses enact their professional responsibilities, they are active as moral agents. Being ethical as a nurse requires more than having moral courage in times of crises (although it may require this); it requires the everyday expression of a commitment to the well-being of those in their care (Levine, 1977).

KEY CONCEPT

A **moral agent** is a person engaged in determining or expressing a moral (ethical) choice.

■ CODES OF ETHICS FOR NURSES

To guide nurses in enacting their moral agency, codes of ethics have been developed by nursing associations. These are statements of the shared values and recognized duties and commitments of the profession. They set the ethical standards for practice and inform other disciplines and the public about the ethical commitments of nurses.

Although codes of ethics in nursing are for registered or licensed professionals, students are expected to be in compliance with their relevant code. Persons cared for by students should know the student status of the caregiver; students' caregiving should be congruent with their level of learning.

The Canadian Nurses Association's *Code of Ethics for Registered Nurses*

The Canadian Nurses Association's Code of Ethics for Registered Nurses (CNA, 2017) is framed by seven values with related ethical responsibilities: providing safe, compassionate, competent, and ethical care; promoting health and well-being; promoting and respecting informed decision-making; honouring dignity; maintaining privacy and confidentiality; promoting justice; and being accountable. The code document includes "ethical endeavours related to broad societal issues," ways that RNs may strive, on their own and collectively, to change systems and social structures to promote greater equity for all. There is a glossary of pertinent terms and an example of an ethical model to help with reflection and decision-making (the Oberle and Raffin model), as well as reference to other models. Delineated, too, are ways to apply the code in certain circumstances, for example, responding to incompetent, noncompassionate, unsafe, or unethical care and ethical consideration in relationships with nursing students.

Nurses' right to follow their conscience is identified in the code, with steps in declaring a conflict with conscience outlined. **Conscientious objection** is defined as "a situation in which a nurse informs their employer about a conflict of conscience and the need to refrain from providing care because a practice or procedure conflicts with the nurse's moral beliefs" (CNA, 2017, p. 21; CRNBC, 2017). It is important to recognize that the objection to a procedure or an aspect of care must be a moral concern and not due to fear, convenience, or prejudice and that the nurse must maintain the safety of the person receiving care until other nursing is available.

Ethics Guidelines for Registered Psychiatric Nurses

Registered psychiatric nurses (RPNs) in Canada are guided by codes of ethics designated by their provincial colleges or association. RPNs in Alberta, for instance, follow a provincial code of ethics (congruent with Alberta's Health Professions Act) with the principles of beneficence, nonmaleficence, integrity, fidelity, respect for autonomy, and justice (College of RPNs of Alberta, 2013). For RPNs in Manitoba and the Yukon (and congruent with their applicable health professions legislation), the values framing their code of ethics are "safe, competent, and ethical practice to ensure the protection of the public"; "respect for the inherent worth, right of choice, and dignity of persons"; "health, mental health, and well-being"; and "quality practice" (College of RPNs of Manitoba, 2017). The College of RPNs of British Columbia is guided by the RPNs of Canada's code (RPNC, 2010), upholding four core values: "safe, competent, and ethical practice"; "respect for the inherent worth, right of choice, and dignity of persons"; "health, mental health, and well-being"; and "quality practice" (p. 3). The values of the code of the RPN Association of Saskatchewan are "professional accountability, unconditional respect, wholistic health, and quality practice milieu." See Web Links for access to the various RPN codes of ethics.

■ APPROACHES TO ETHICS

There are several theoretical approaches to ethical knowledge that inform ethical action in health care. Some are based on moral philosophy and others on concepts such as human rights. A brief outline of the most common approaches follows. See Table 7.3 for a summary.

Virtue Ethics

Virtue ethics, emphasizing the character of the moral agent, was the earliest approach to ethics used in nursing (Fowler, 1997). A virtuous person is one who, without strict reliance on rules, is wise enough to perceive how to act well in a particular situation. Lists of the virtues vary, but they include compassion, courage, tolerance, prudence, honesty, humility, and trustworthiness. Aristotle (1996), the Greek philosopher whose works most inform virtue theory, believed that acquiring the virtues would assist a person to flourish as a human being. He found our moral upbringing to be important: we learn the virtues through our relationships. Observing compassion in others, for instance, can help us to develop a compassionate disposition. To acquire a virtue, it must become habitual; it is not enough, for instance, to be occasionally honest. Aristotle's concept of the virtue of *phronesis* or **practical wisdom** seems particularly relevant to nurses. It means having the sensitivity, imagination, and experience to do what is ethically fitting in difficult situations (Austin, 2007a).

In a profession with role-specific duties and responsibilities (evidenced by such things as a code of ethics),

Approach	Core Elements	Proponents	Critiques
Virtue ethics	Character of the moral agent Some virtues: honesty, courage, compassion, practical wisdom	Aristotle Alasdair MacIntyre	Exclusive focus on the agent
Deontology	Duty based Some acts are wrong in themselves. Universality Do not treat others as a means to an end (respect)	Immanuel Kant	Disregard of consequences Impartiality over relationship Emotion = irrationality
Utilitarianism	Consequence based Actions are right if they promote the best outcome (e.g., happiness, pleasure, satisfaction) for most people.	Jeremy Bentham John Stuart Mill	Utility as the only principle Majority rules
Principlism	Based on a set of principles compatible with most moral theories. Nonmaleficence, beneficence, respect for autonomy, justice	Tom Beauchamp James Childress	Too abstract Which has priority when principles compete?
Casuistry	Case based Use of paradigm cases to identify issues and courses of action for a new case	Albert Jonsen Stephen Toulmin	Keeps the status quo Can miss the broad issues
Ethics of care	Care based Connection/responsibility for others Emotional responsiveness	Carol Gilligan Nel Noddings	Creates a dichotomy between "care" (feminine) and "justice" (masculine) approaches to ethics Valorizes women as caregivers
Feminist ethics	Addresses power inequities, dominance, and oppression	Annette Baier Susan Sherwin	Lacks impartiality Lacks universal norms
Relational	Ethical action involves relationships. Context matters; emotion accepted Dialogue is supported. Aims for the "fitting" response	Vangie Bergum John Dossetor	Too relativistic Lacks impartiality Lacks universality
Human rights	Rights based (negative and positive) Every person is entitled to certain basic rights.	John Locke Thomas Paine United Nations	As a concept, it is "nonsense" Too legalistic Too individualistic

Table 7.3 Approaches to Ethics

a trait that supports the good of that practice acquires the status of a moral virtue. A professional's virtues, in that sense, are necessary to his or her role (Radden & Sadler, 2008). In *After Virtue*, MacIntyre (1984) raises a question worthy of reflection: What would a person (nurse) lack, who lacked the virtues?

Deontology

Deontology (from the Greek *deon* or *duty*) postulates duty or obligation as the basis of doing right. This is duty not as in following external orders but as self-imposed obligation. This approach is also termed *Kantian ethics* because the work of Kant (1996), an 18th-century philosopher, laid its foundation. Kant believed that we should use reason alone to determine how to act. Reason unhampered by emotions or desires allows us to determine the types of acts that are wrong in themselves, no matter how good their consequences might be. Kant stipulated that a criterion (a *categorical imperative*) for judging the reason (or "maxim") for one's actions is universality: one should act only on a choice that one can conceive of as a universal law. Is a lie acceptable if it saves someone from danger? No, because lying cannot be willed as a universal principle. If we lie to help a person in trouble, truth will be subverted and society corrupted. In Kantian ethics, the moral worth of a person's action is determined by the intent of the person, not the effects of the action. If you act rightly, you are not responsible for bad effects.

Kant stipulated a second imperative: act so that you treat others always as an end and never as a means. Kant argued that we must treat one another with dignity and respect; it is wrong to use other people for our own purposes. Informed consent is grounded on this belief. For instance, individuals should not be used as research subjects unless they understand what will happen and agree to it. Nor should we, according to Kantian ethics, place individuals at risk in research by depriving them of the best-known treatment in order to carry out a placebo-controlled study, even though this would provide the most valid evidence.

Kant's emphasis on the individual's rational capacity as the facilitator of moral action can be seen as highly relevant to psychiatric ethics, as it is the impairment of rational capacity alone that justifies coercive or involuntary psychiatric treatment (Robertson, Morris, & Walter, 2007). Kantian ethics supports the quest for universal ethical principles, such as the efforts of the United Nations Educational, Scientific, and Cultural Organization (UNESCO) (see "Human Rights" below). It upholds that, from a moral standpoint, all persons should be treated the same. A major problem, however, is its disregard for the role of consequences in ethical action. Consequences, however, are the sole focus of the next approach.

Utilitarianism

The principle of utility is the foundation of **utilitarianism**: actions are right in proportion to their tendency to promote happiness. What is right to do is what gives the best consequences (e.g., happiness, pleasure, preference, satisfaction) for the greater number of people. Bentham (1983) and Mill (2002), philosophers of the 18th and 19th centuries, originated this theory that uses a type of cost/benefit analysis to determine the moral worth of an action.

The principle of utility can also be applied to determining which moral rules to follow. This is termed rule utilitarianism and holds that once we decide on the best rules, we should follow them, even if in some situations happiness is not maximized. A rule utilitarian might determine that a good rule for a nurse is not to go against hospital policies except if it is necessary for the best interests of a patient. Covertly putting an antipsychotic medication in an acutely ill person's food, for instance, might be regarded as ethically acceptable in a special circumstance when such an action causes the least suffering to the ill person (Ipperciel, 2003). A Kantian would never approve of this, and despite ethical justification from a utilitarian perspective, such an act can result in a disciplinary or legal action.

Principlism

In the principles approach, it is believed that a few moral principles (ethical norms) can provide a basis for moral reasoning in health ethics (Beauchamp, 1994). Four *prima facie* (at first sight) principles are widely accepted: nonmaleficence, beneficence, respect for autonomy, and justice (Beauchamp & Childress, 2013). **Nonmaleficence** as a principle means that one should do no harm. **Beneficence** means that one should do, or attempt to do, good and make things better (promote benefit) for others when one can. **Respect for autonomy** (also considered as respect for persons) means an obligation to respect a person's right to be self-governing and his or her ability to make decisions. **Justice** is conceived as obligations of fairness in the distribution of benefits and risks. A criticism of **principlism** is that four principles cannot sufficiently capture moral norms (Walker, 2009). Another common criticism is that when principles compete, as they will in complex situations, there is no framework for settling the conflict.

The nature of mental illness creates situations in which respect for autonomy and beneficence conflict. How should one act when persons with a mental illness choose to act in ways that bring them harm? For instance, what if a person with schizophrenia is living homeless on the streets? Should respect for autonomy be upheld, or should there be an intervention to bring the person to shelter? Respect for autonomy is dependent on persons' competence to make their own informed decisions, and evaluating such competence can be difficult.

IN-A-LIFE

Jan Storch (1940–)

CANADIAN NURSE ETHICIST

Public Persona

Dr. Jan Storch's laudatory leadership in nursing ethics in Canada includes helping launch a centre of health ethics (at the University of Alberta) and a provincial health ethics network (in Alberta), being the President of the Canadian Bioethics Society (CBS) and the National Council on Ethics in Human Research, doing research in ethics, publishing widely (including two editions of the ethics text, *Toward a Moral Horizon*), and speaking passionately about ethics to diverse audiences. Her guidance of the 2008 centenary revision of CNA's *Code of Ethics* was the fourth time she has contributed to CNA in this way and she has been instrumental in the latest (2017) revision. She served as member and chair of the Research Ethics Board for Health Canada and the Public Health Agency of Canada for over a decade. Her own current research involves exploring the nature of nursing leadership and ways to create moral practice environments. More recently, Jan has researched and made presentations on MAID; her expertise has been sought by three national bodies preparing documents in this area. She has received awards as an outstanding nurse from the nursing associations of Alberta and British Columbia, a 1:100 CNA Centennial Award, a 1:100 College and Association of Registered Nurses of Alberta Centennial Award, a CBS Lifetime Achievement Award, and two honorary doctorates and has been recognized as a leading public intellectual.

Personal Realities

Jan Storch is a wife, mother, grandmother, nurse, and professor emeritus at the University of Victoria. Her deep commitment to ethical health care and to nurses' role in it is truly inspirational.

Casuistry or Case-Based Ethics

Casuistry (pronounced kăzh' ū-ĭ;-strē), from the Latin *casus* for *case*, is the use of case comparisons to facilitate moral reasoning and decision-making. It is a bottom-up approach in which one starts with the details of the present case and locates that case in a taxonomy of cases as a way to identify the pertinent ethical concerns and responses (Jonsen, 1991; Jonsen & Toulmin, 1988). The focus in casuistry is on agreement about cases, not necessarily principles or theories, and precedents are central to this approach. Past decisions about what was right or wrong in significant cases serve to inform decisions about the new case. (This is similar to what happens in legal judgements.) The nurse using this approach will need to decide how the "case" does and does not fit paradigmatic cases. Suggested steps to use in doing this follow (Strong, 2000):

1. Identify the main ethical values and concerns relevant to the case.
2. Identify the main alternative courses of action that can be taken.
3. Identify the casuistic factors (i.e., the morally relevant ways the cases of this type differ).
4. Compare the case with relevant paradigm cases that have been identified.

Casuistry seems congruent with the way nurses think in practice. When a clinical situation confronts us, we often think of similar situations that we have experienced, or we turn to paradigm cases to guide us. A criticism of casuistry is that there is a risk that one will miss the broad issues and that prevalent beliefs and practices will not be sufficiently questioned.

The Ethics of Care and Feminist Ethics

The **ethics of care** can be viewed as a feminine approach to ethics (Sherwin, 1992). Gilligan (1982), in researching moral development, found that females seemed to differ from males in their approach to ethical decision-making. Females focused on caring, connectedness, and responsibility rather than the deductive reasoning and abstract principles preferred by males. She argued that women are different from men in their approach to moral decisions, not inferior to them. (Aristotle and Kant both assumed that the moral agent was male.) The perspective of the world as a web of interdependent relationships in which our responsibility to one another is implicit is increasingly predominant in health ethics, as is the recognition that receptivity, relatedness, and responsiveness, as well as emotions, like compassion, are important components of ethical responses (Noddings, 1984; Sherwin, 1992).

Feminist ethics differs from the ethics of care in that it comes from a political perspective, offering insight into oppression (unjust, unwarranted use of power) and dominance in individual and societal-level relationships. Using understandings gained from the analysis of women's oppression, feminist ethicists illuminate negative power differentials that may be so inherent as to be invisible and remain unquestioned. Because feminist ethics combines political dimensions with the core values of care and commitment, it offers a constructive framework for challenging the oppression of people with mental illness.

Relational Ethics

Relational ethics is based on the assumption that all ethical actions are situated in relationship. Ideas of duty and utility, principles, and the character of the moral agent are accepted as important in informing action, but relationship is taken as foundational. Ethics is about how we treat one another, individually and within society, as well as how we resolve moral problems. Ethical situations are encompassed by complexity and uncertainty, and an understanding of the complexities, which shape life, needs to be cultivated.

Within this perspective, one strives to be responsive to the situation at hand in such a way that genuine dialogue is opened and mutual respect fostered among those involved. Feelings and emotions are viewed as a component of rational thinking and are explored, not ruled out as too subjective or confusing. Context matters. Not anything goes, but one's actions need not only to be shaped by ethical knowledge but also to be adapted to the specific circumstances of the situation. In relational ethics, one aims for the fitting response (Niebuhr, 1963). Questions can be raised within this approach (e.g., issues of power and control) that may not be raised in approaches that focus primarily on moral reasoning (Bergum & Dossetor, 2005). Refer, for example, to relational ethics perspectives on responses to nurses who have an addiction (Kunyk & Austin, 2012), on nurses' responsibilities during an epidemic (Austin, 2008), and on hope in palliative care (Olsman, Willems, & Leget, 2016). Core elements of relational ethics are mutual respect, engagement, embodied knowledge, attention to the interdependent environment, and uncertainty/vulnerability (Austin, Bergum, & Dossetor, 2003a; Bergum & Dossetor, 2005). A relational ethics decision-making framework is outlined in Box 7.4.

Human Rights

The idea of **human rights** dates back to 1215 and Britain's Magna Carta, to the natural rights language of the philosopher John Locke (Locke, 1689/2016) in the 17th century, and to Thomas Paine's *Rights of Man* (Paine, 1779/1996) in the 18th century. The central assumption of human rights is that all persons have certain claims or entitlements because of their humanness. Rights can be conceived as negative or positive. Negative rights are usually civil or political in nature, with the state or others required to refrain from obstructing these rights (e.g., freedom of speech, freedom to worship). Positive rights are obligations of the state or others to

---

BOX 7.4 A Relational Ethics Decision-Making Framework

KEY QUESTIONS

1. What is happening here?
2. What are the alternatives for ethical action?
3. What is the most fitting thing to do?
4. What happened as the result of our action?

QUESTION 1: WHAT IS HAPPENING HERE?

- What are the ethical questions? Their context?
- Who is involved? (Who are the moral agents?) What are their commitments to one another?
- What further information do we need?
- Are there legal, organizational, professional, cultural, religious, or any other aspects to consider? Are values in conflict?
- What resources do we have? Need?
- Patient and family resources (e.g., personal directive)?
- Health care resources (e.g., access to home care)?
- Ethics resources: principles, precedents, codes, policies, guidelines, ethicists/ethics committees, etc.?
- To what, in particular, do we need to attend?

QUESTION 2: WHAT ARE THE ALTERNATIVES FOR ETHICAL ACTION?

- What are the consequences for each alternative?
- What might constrain ethical action?

- What, if anything, makes me or others uncomfortable in regard to a potential action?
- Remember: refraining from making a decision is still a decision.

QUESTION 3: WHAT IS THE MOST FITTING THING TO DO?

- What is the best way to carry out the decision (or plan)?
- Who is affected? Who needs to be involved?
- How may disparate views be bridged?

TAKE ACTION

QUESTION 4: WHAT HAPPENED AS THE RESULT OF OUR ACTION?

- What concerns remain?
- Is anyone distressed about the result?
- Is further action desirable?
- Do we need to address systemic factors that gave rise to the situation?
- Would we act in the same way again?
- What did we learn?

Copyright: Wendy Austin, University of Alberta, Canada.

provide a right (e.g., right to health, right to education). These rights are typically social, cultural, or economic in nature.

Rights relating to health are included in many international documents, such as the United Nations' (UN) 1948 *Universal Declaration of Human Rights* (*UDHR*) and the UN's 1991 *Principles for the Protection of Persons with Mental Illness and for the Improvement of Mental Health Care. The Convention of the Rights of Persons with Disabilities* (2006) articulates the rights of persons with disabilities to an optimal quality of life, including appropriately competent and thoughtful care from health care professionals. It is human rights law that allows for international scrutiny of a nation's health policies and practices (Gostin, 2001).

"Health" as a human right means that every person has a right to the highest attainable level of health (including a standard of living that is adequate for health) and access to health care and social services as needed. There are tangible connections between health and human rights (Mann et al., 1999). First, *health policies and practices have an impact on human rights.* For instance, MOT for persons with a mental illness is an infringement on individual rights. This infringement can only be justified if it is in the person's best interests or for the necessary protection of the public. Second, *human rights violations impact health.* Torture, for instance, may have longlasting effects on an individual's mental health. The International Council of Nurses (ICN) not only supports the United Nation's *UDHR* but also stipulates in *Torture, Death Penalty and Participation by Nurses in Executions* (ICN, 1998) that nurses may not voluntarily participate in any deliberate infliction of physical or mental suffering. The World Psychiatric Association's (1996) *Madrid Declaration on Ethical Standards for Psychiatric Practice* stipulates the same for psychiatrists. Third, *health professionals have a responsibility to protect human rights by helping the public identify rights violations.* It is important to note that the WHO (2012) claims that some of the most serious human rights violations against persons with mental illness and substance abuse problems occur in health care settings.

ICN recognizes the call from the United Nations Human Rights Council (2017), which states that mental health is a priority and needs to be integrated with physical health, "professionally, politically and geographically" (p. 18). The report of the Special Rapporteur to the Council notes that power imbalances are a greater problem in mental health care than chemical imbalances and recommends that care be recovery and community based, promoting social inclusion, and that promotion and prevention be a focus. Further, the need for rights-based treatments and psychosocial support is emphasized.

A rights approach is not without its critics. It has been argued that such an approach is too legalistic and the law too slow and ineffective in addressing rights violations and that it is too individualistic, placing the individual in an antagonistic position against the community (Austin, 2001). In 2005, bioethics and human rights were brought together in the *Universal Declaration on Bioethics and Human Rights,* adopted by UNESCO. Among other things, its principles uphold respect for autonomy, the solidarity among human beings, and the need for sharing the benefits of scientific research and for protecting future generations and the planet itself.

■ ETHICAL PRACTICE ENVIRONMENTS

Health care environments need to be understood as moral communities where practice is grounded in compassion, empathy, and professionalism (Austin, 2012). For psychiatric and mental health (PMH) settings to be morally habitable, a "culture of questioning" must be actively nurtured (Austin, Bergum, & Nuttgens, 2004). This means that ethical questions are to be expected as an everyday aspect of practice, not perceived as challenging or troublesome. Consultation with a clinical ethicist or ethics committee should be viewed as an acceptable option, a common use of an ethics resource.

Interprofessional communication, collaboration, and conflicts are critical factors in the ethical climate of health care areas (Austin, 2007b). Research in PMH settings has revealed for some time that the desire to get along with colleagues can trump "doing the right thing" (Carpenter, 1991; Fisher, 1995) and that staff conflict influences the way an ethical situation is resolved (Forchuk, 1991). Institutional policies, demands, and supports also play a role. Institutional constraints on a nurse's ability to advocate for patients have been identified as a common contributor to nurses' moral distress (Rittenmeyer & Huffman, 2009). In a critical incident study of nurses' perceptions of what promotes an ethical climate, it was found that being able to meet the needs of patients and families "in a considerate way" and sharing responsibilities among a team were significant. These facilitated voicing care concerns amid a collegial environment (Silén, Kjellström, Christensson, Sidenvall, & Svantesson, 2012).

▌ MORAL DILEMMAS AND MORAL DISTRESS

A moral dilemma is a morally relevant conflict (Audi, 1995). It may be defined more narrowly as a situation in which one has an obligation to act but must choose between two incompatible alternatives. In health ethics, frameworks have been developed to facilitate the decision-making process. Decision-making frameworks are tools to guide ethical deliberation, based on particular or composite approaches (see Box 7.4).

A definition of moral distress, composed by incorporating elements from the work of experts (Austin, 2016), is:

the embodied response (e.g., frustration, anger, sleeplessness, headache, nausea, anxiety, anguish, etc.) of an individual to a moral problem for which the individual assumes some moral responsibility, makes a moral judgment about the appropriate ethical action to be taken but, due to real or perceived constraints, participates by act or omission in what they regard as moral wrongdoing (Jameton, 1984, 2013; Nathaniel, 2006; Wilkinson, 1987–1988).

Moral distress is a risk component of health care provision and its associated responsibility. It is not a sign of weakness, but rather an indication of one's sensitivity to the ethics of practice and a commitment to public trust (Austin, 2016). Studies of the moral distress experienced by nurses and other health care professionals in PMH settings have indicated that lack of resources, institutional demands, and unrealistic demands on the part of society that deviant behaviour be controlled are contributing factors (Austin, Bergum, & Goldberg, 2003b; Austin, Kagan, Rankel, & Bergum, 2008; Austin, Rankel, Kagan, Bergum, & Lemermeyer, 2005). Research indicates that when nurses experience moral distress, they either choose to continue giving voice to their ethical concerns or they withdraw—from ethically challenging situations, from their position, or entirely from the discipline of nursing (Pauly, Varcoe, & Storch, 2012). Opportunities for discussing and processing care situations that are ethically challenging (e.g., informal or formal debriefings, ethics consultation, ethics rounds, ethics committees) are important to the prevention and resolution of moral distress (Austin, 2017). Nursing leaders play a key role in supporting such opportunities, as well as in creating positive ethical climates where voicing ethical concerns is an expectation of members of interprofessional teams rather than viewed as problematic (Schick Makaroff, Storch, Pauly, & Newton, 2014). Nursing's approach to moral distress has evolved since it was first described in the 1980s; we now acknowledge the need for speaking up, dialogue, cooperation, and moral resilience (Jameton, 2017).

KEY CONCEPT

A **moral dilemma** is a conflict in which one feels a moral obligation to act but must choose between incompatible alternatives.

KEY CONCEPT

Moral distress is an embodied response that occurs when one acknowledges an ethical obligation, makes a moral choice regarding fitting ethical action, but is then unable to act on this moral choice because of internal or external constraints.

ETHICAL ISSUES IN PSYCHIATRIC AND MENTAL HEALTH CARE SETTINGS

It is not possible in this chapter to identify all the complex ethical issues of PMH settings; rather, selected significant ones are discussed. Although some issues may not be unique to this specialty area (e.g., confidentiality), all are shaped by the PMH context and by the potential vulnerability of individuals living with a stigmatized illness. Such vulnerability is increased for those who have a mental disorder that can sometimes affect their competency to give informed consent to treatment and who may thus receive treatment involuntarily.

Threats to Dignity

An important aspect of ethical nursing care involves safeguarding the dignity of patients, as violated dignity can lead to suffering and a loss of self-worth. Nurses in PMH settings, when asked about experiences that involved preserving patient dignity, described being genuinely "present" with patients (e.g., supporting a patient through emotions like anger) and being their advocate. Issues of dignity arising for patients in PMH settings have been identified through study of their experiences. For instance, patients with experience of a coercive intervention (e.g., seclusion, restraints, or rapid tranquillization) describe feeling powerless and/or hopeless as they felt neither sufficiently informed about nor involved in their treatment plan, including medications and being held within a hospital environment, which seemed prison-like (Chambers et al., 2014). It can be in the "small things" where dignity resides: awareness of patients as more than their illness, in choice and tone of language, and in gestures and courtesies associated with acts of daily living (Skorpen, Rehnsfeldt, & Thorsen, 2015). When nurses described their experiences of violations to the dignity of patients who had an involuntary PMH treatment status, they noted patients being ignored or not taken seriously, being physically "violated" through restraints, being betrayed by broken promises, and being exposed (e.g., medication given in front of others; personal history shared with the entire team). They identified the power differential between staff and patients as a potential source of loss of dignity, as was predefining patients by their diagnosis (Gustafsson, Wigerblad, & Lindwall, 2014).

Maureen Foy (2007), mother of a young woman with a severe and persistent mental illness, described her experience as a family member. One example she offered occurred when her daughter was admitted to a crisis unit in a Canadian general hospital:

> Over a period of two to three hours of waiting, the staff did not speak to us or look at us once. It was as though we were not there, we were invisible. There were no words of comfort or care. There was no information given and we were left to wonder on our own what or whom we were waiting

for.... Staff looked through us, around us, above us, below us, but they did not look at us. At a time of crisis and in a place where you go for help and maybe even care, this is hard to bear. This behaviour silences you (p. 1).

She notes that advancements in brain imaging, psychotropic drugs, and models of therapy are nothing if comfort and compassion are not shown to the persons needing care.

Nurses and other health care professionals must consistently ask: What is it like to use our mental health services? What is it like to be our patient or our patient's family member? The value of respect, integral to the support of dignity, is very evident in policy documents and the literature of PMH nursing, but too frequently, there is a disconnect between what is espoused and what occurs in practice; ongoing attentiveness to nursing actions that may convey disrespect is crucial to ethical practice (Cutcliffe & Travale, 2013).

Behaviour Control, Seclusion, and Restraint

Recovery-oriented, trauma-informed mental health care demands that the least intrusive and restrictive interventions are used in protecting and reducing risk to patients. This means that individual rights, dignity, and autonomy are respected and that there is "the least possible recourse" to measures (mechanical, chemical, environmental, or physical) to limit a person's activity or to control behaviour (MHCC, 2009, p. 121). Restrictive measures are to be used only when absolutely necessary and then with sensitivity and great caution. They can have serious relational consequences (see Chapter 11).

Coercion and control in PMH care are abiding ethical and clinical issues. The health care team must continually evaluate whether these measures equate with best practice when being considered as an intervention. Expressing moral doubt about such clinical interventions, however, can be difficult. It can delay rapid response to a crisis situation, can be viewed as professional inexperience or weakness, or can be taken as criticism of one's colleagues or leaders (Molewijk, Kok, Husum, Pedersen, & Aasland, 2017). Nevertheless, as coercion involves limiting the autonomy of an individual through institutional power, it seems important that the query, "Is this the right action?" gets raised (Molewijk et al., 2017). Ethical reflexivity and dialogue can help nurses and other team members to ensure that whatever form such measures take that they are clinically and morally justified. Institutional support for staff's ethical questioning, ongoing evaluation of its policies and practices, and training to increase of staff's competence in dealing with aggression, distress, and psychoses can lead to greater use of alternatives to coercion and control (Norvoll, Hem, & Pedersen, 2017). Ethical consultation, for instance, with a clinical ethicist, can help health care teams to engage in meaningful dialogue regarding the use of coercive measures and increase their capacity for dealing with such ethical issues (Austin, 2017). PMH settings should be well-designed healing places with sufficient numbers of competent, compassionate staff. When this is not so, it is an ethical issue.

Psychiatric Advance Directives

Psychiatric advance directives (PADs) are a legal resource for people to use for times when their decision-making ability is compromised by a mental illness (MHCC, 2009). Advance directives allow for designation of a surrogate decision-maker who can act on one's behalf when one is not competent to do so. It can delineate one's preferred choices to guide the surrogate and the health care team. As an individual with a bipolar disorder noted, "It will give me peace of mind to know that if I get to the point where I can't say anything, there is something in place that will represent myself" (Ambrosini, Bemme, Crocker, & Latimer, 2012, p. 4). PADs are a useful tool in communicating with physicians, avoiding side effects by identifying specific medications that an individual wishes to avoid, and preventing involuntary treatment. Research indicates that PADs not only give patients a sense of control and increase the use of treatments congruent with patient preferences but also lower the need for coercive interventions (Olsen, 2017). Nurses can support patients in their preparation of PADs and can actively and consistently foster autonomy through learning patient preferences and helping reduce constraints to independence.

Relational Engagement: "Boundaries"

Engagement in therapeutic relationships is an important aspect of most, if not all, PMH care, and complex ethical issues are situated in the boundaries of these relationships (see Chapter 6). Although "boundary," the term commonly used to describe the limits of therapeutic relationships, implies clear, firm borders that should not be crossed, actual practice can be more complicated. Gift giving is an example. Although accepting a gift from a patient can be seen as an initial step down the "slippery slope" toward a boundary violation and something to be always avoided, a particular situation may be more complex (Austin, Bergum, Nuttgens, & Peternelj-Taylor, 2006). Refusing a small, homemade gift from a grateful patient may be a hurtful act. Accepting a significant gift from a vulnerable patient, on the other hand, may be viewed as theft (Griffith, 2016). Nurses need to be thoughtful about the meaning of a gift and seek out knowledgeable advice from members of the team and clinical supervisors.

Not unlike refusal of a gift, declining a "friend invitation" on a social networking site such as Facebook can be a complex ethical issue and require similar thoughtful deliberation (Ginory, Sabatier, & Eth, 2012). In fact, "breaching patient confidentiality and privacy has become increasingly common for nurses and students since the advent of social media" (Smith & Knudson, 2016, p. 911). In a study of student nurses' unethical behaviour, use of social media was found to positively correlate with students' unethical behaviour (as did year of birth, with younger students having a greater degree of unethical behaviour) (Smith & Knudson, 2016).

The use of email for therapeutic communication and patient-centred care raises similar issues, as does other uses of health information technology, which soon may be commonplace, such as virtual home visits to patients (a form of telehealth) and patients' submission of health data (e.g., stress measures) through their smartphones. Internet security will be a dominant concern. Interacting online with patients is challenging and requires that professional boundaries be maintained, including the avoidance of dual relationships; nurses and health care staff need to monitor their online presence (Ginory et al., 2012).

One of the most serious types of boundary violation is the sexual harassment and abuse of patients. Despite policies of zero tolerance, abuse occurs and is known to be significantly underreported (Rodgers, 2004). Professionals who commit serious boundary violations at times argue that it was a mutual decision made with the patient. Given the power differentials in therapeutic relationships, this "defence" is unacceptable.

Transgressions of boundaries are most often discussed as *overinvolvement. Underinvolvement* can also be an ethical issue. Lack of time to engage with patients has been found to contribute to nurses' moral distress (Austin et al., 2003a). Countertransference experienced by the nurse may affect therapeutic availability if the nurse fails to address it appropriately (see Chapter 6). A negative response may be evoked as well, when a patient rejects care, is abusive, or is guilty of a morally reprehensible act, such as child abuse (Liaschenko, 1994). Liaschenko found that when nurses had difficulty connecting with a patient, they chose among three options: to emotionally distance themselves from the patient, to transfer the patient to another nurse, or to make a conscious effort to be respectful and provide good care. The nurses in this study recognized difficulties in "bridging the gap" to a patient as an ethical issue.

In order to engage ethically with patients, nurses must attend to their own personal and professional boundaries and must respect those of others. Education about boundaries is helpful, as are strategies such as clinical supervision and resources such as *Professional Boundaries for Registered Nurses: Guidelines for the Nurse–Client Relationship* (College and Association of Registered Nurses of Alberta, 2011) and the practice standard, *Boundaries in the Nurse Client Relationship* of the Colleges of Registered Licensed Practical Nurses, Registered Nurses, and Registered Psychiatric Nurses of British Columbia (2017).

Confidentiality and Privacy

Maintaining privacy and confidentiality is an ethical responsibility of nurses. See the ethical responsibilities related to upholding this value in the CNA Code of Ethics for Registered Nurses (2017, p. 14). Privacy is a basic human right, and individuals may not wish their personal information disclosed to others or for others to intrude upon their personal space. Legislation at the federal and provincial/territorial levels protects personal health information, and there are regulations that allow individuals to access and request correction of their personal information. Privacy laws in Canada include the *Privacy Act* (Justice Canada, 2014a), which limits the collection, use, and disclosure of personal information in federal government agencies, and the *Personal Information Protection and Electronic Documents Act* (PIPEDA) (Justice Canada, 2014b) with which all provinces and territories must comply. PIPEDA regulates personal information collection, use, and disclosure that occur in commercial activities (including personal health information), requiring that organizations obtain informed consent to use individuals' personal information, secure it, and provide them with access to their own information, which they may request to have corrected.

Canada has a Privacy Commissioner who advocates for privacy rights and is able to publicly report on the handling of personal information from public and private organizations, to investigate complaints, and to promote public awareness of privacy issues (Office of the Privacy Commissioner of Canada [OPCC], 2015). A priority concern of the OPCC is that information about our bodies is merging with information technology. Digital measurement of vital signs; collection of biometric data for recreational, forensic, and commercial purposes; implantable sensors that communicate internal status (e.g., blood pressure; glucose levels); biomedical electronics (e.g., implants that read brain activity; genetic testing); and automated medical records have brought us to a place where we have an incredible level of intimate information about our bodies and our health status. The risk to the privacy of our health information is similarly amplified (OPCC). Nurses will need to keep informed on the risks and ways to counter them as this most personal of private information increasingly exists in digital form.

Privacy can be particularly important in PMH settings, given the stigma and discrimination attached to mental disorders and to psychiatric care. Consent is a central factor in decisions related to privacy and confidentiality, and this factor becomes more complicated when the person involved has an illness that affects their ability to give consent. Overall, nurses safeguard the information learned in the context of their professional relationships, sharing it outside the health care team only with the patients' permission or as legally required.

Disclosure of information within the health care team occurs as necessary for treatment and care, but when patients confide information that is not relevant to the patient's health and well-being, this type of information is not shared. Patients and families need to be made aware that health information and care decisions are shared among the team. This is particularly important as there can be misconception that anything communicated to a health professional is protected as confidential, even within legal testimony. Such communication, however, cannot be presumed privileged in the way that attorney–client communication is held to be. As well, there are situations that legally require the reporting of information received in a patient care situation. Mandatory reporting of child abuse and abuse of adults in care are examples. (Refer to provincial and territorial legislation for reporting requirements.) Nurses are expected to intervene if others within the health care system fail to meet obligations regarding confidentiality and privacy (CNA, 2017).

Too strict observation of privacy and confidentiality rules can create problems if it means that families and other caregivers are excluded from knowledge that can help them protect and support persons with a mental disorder when they are at risk. A balance needs to be found between respecting the person's privacy and facilitating family assistance (MHCC, 2009). PADs are a way to address this potential problem.

Advances in Neurotechnology

Advances in neurotechnology are providing new insights into how the human brain functions as well as creating potential ways of changing it. Not only does this bring new threats to privacy as the uses being explored include detection of lying and prediction of violent or criminal behaviour but it brings possible threats to autonomy through invasive and noninvasive ways of influencing the brain (Ryberg, 2017). It has been queried whether use of such technologies can be a threat to personhood (Racine & Affleck, 2016). Neuroethics is the area of health ethics exploring such ethical issues.

Its work has relevance to mental health as the uses of neurotechnology have clinical implications in this field. There are implications, for instance, in manipulation of memory, which is being made possible through procedures such as transcranial magnetic stimulation, transcranial direct current stimulation, deep brain stimulation, and the use of pharmacologic agents (e.g., donepezil and propranolol). While this manipulation may have treatment benefits for such disorders as posttraumatic stress, anxiety dementia, and drug abuse (Agren, 2014; Cestari, Rossi-Arnaud, Saraulli, & Constanzi, 2014), there are fundamental ethical implications to be considered. Will using neurotechnology in such ways alter an individual's perception of "true self"? Will only pleasant memories be deemed acceptable? Will those unable to afford enhancements be at a great disadvantage in education and the workplace? In other words, what will such technology do to us? To date, there is limited evidence that treatments using such neurotechnology have caused loss of personal identity. There remains, however, a need for continued evaluation of the use of neurotechnology in selective alteration of memories, oversight to ensure research and clinical guidelines are followed (Racine & Affleck, 2016), and social dialogue and relevant policies developed as the science evolves (Robillard & Illes, 2016).

Advances in Genetics

Advances in genetics raise other concerns, given events in history. Eugenics (Greek for "wellborn") was once a worldwide movement, beginning at the onset of the 20th century, that aimed at improving the human race. In 1939, in Nazi Germany, a program was initiated that lead to the killing of thousands of "incurable" psychiatric patients deemed to have a life "not worth living" that weakened their society. Nurses actively participated in this program (Aly & Roth, 1984; Benedict & Kuhla, 1999; McFarland-Icke, 1999). For the most part, however, eugenics involved preventing the physically and mentally disabled from reproducing; sterilization was a favoured strategy.

With contemporary advances in genetic engineering, a new eugenics is evolving. Genetic testing may make possible prenatal selection and termination of a pregnancy when the foetus is at risk for a mental disorder. (It is doubtful, however, that direct linkages between a given gene and a psychiatric disorder exist; see Chapter 9.) Genetic profiles of individuals may lead to discrimination and to "genetic essentialism" (i.e., a person is defined by his or her genes). In considering the ethical acceptability of specific clinical genetic testing, questions should be asked, such as follows: What is the purpose of the test? How predictive is the test? How stigmatized is the condition being tested for? Do effective interventions exist for it? Will the testing affect third parties, such as family members? (Hoop, 2008). Increasingly, others' access to one's genetic information is a realistic concern. Private companies and researchers, hoping to develop new treatments, are seeking legal access to medical records from governments. Although data are anonymized in such cases, confidentiality remains at issue.

These concerns have increased with the current development of "personalized medicine." Described often as adapting treatment to the individual patient's needs and preferences, personalized medicine is, at its basics, medicine adapted to a person's genomic makeup. Its success is evident in oncology, most dramatically in the treatment of lung cancer. It has the potential to predict, for instance, a person's response to a specific treatment and vulnerability to adverse events (Perna & Nemeroff, 2017). This individualizing of treatment fits well with psychiatry's original approach (Perna & Nemeroff, 2017), and a journal, *Personalized Medicine in Psychiatry*, was created in 2017 to support dialogue and communication of research regarding this approach. To evolve the genetic evidence that is the basis of personalized medicine, significant genetic research needs to occur. Its risks and benefits will need to be continually assessed and monitored, but there is considerable promise for better care.

Social Justice

Conditions of fundamental equality and justice are important to optimal mental health. Justice, a principle of fair treatment of individuals and groups and of promotion of the common good within society, is a core value underpinning the CNA *Code of Ethics* (2017). It is acknowledged that broad societal issues affect health and well-being, and thus, nurses need to be cognizant of these issues, including at the global level, and to safeguard human rights, equity, and fairness in their practice, acting as advocates for positive change. Part II of the CNA Code describes examples of what nurses can do to address social inequities, including using the principles of primary health care for the benefit of patients and the public, working for social justice, advocating for policies and laws that support equity, and promoting environmental preservation and restoration (CNA, 2017). Although nursing codes of ethics, including that of ICN, indicate that nurses have a role in social justice, an international, qualitative study of nurses' perceptions of this role concluded that educational and organizational support for development of this role is lacking and that nursing advocacy needs to broaden to encompass social justice (Walter, 2017).

The social injustices related to mental illness due to stigma and discrimination exist worldwide. According to the WHO, financing for mental health remains poor with low- and middle-income countries spending less than 2 dollars (US) per capita on mental health, and although 1 in 10 persons has a mental disorder, only 1% of the global health workforce practice in mental health (WHO, 2015). This is so despite the recognition of mental, neurologic, and substance disorders as the leading cause of years lived with disability, based on Global Burden of Disease data (Whiteford et al., 2013).

Research Ethics

Research is vitally important to the improvement of the lives of persons with mental illness and their families, as well as in the determination of ways to prevent mental illness and foster mental health and well-being. However, it is vital that risks and benefits are identified, ensuring individuals are never exploited. Canada has delineated ethics policies for federal research funding agencies in the *Tri-Council Policy Statement: Ethical Conduct of Research Involving Humans* guided by the core

principles of respect for persons and concern for welfare and justice (Canadian Institutes of Health Research, Natural Sciences and Engineering Research Council of Canada, & Social Sciences and Humanities Research Council of Canada, 2014, p. 6).

Informed consent is key to the protection of research subjects. The Tri-Council policy requires that consent to participate in research must be voluntary, ongoing, and informed. A person who lacks capacity to make an informed decision is not necessarily deprived of the right to participate in research. Participation may occur if the person is involved in the decision-making process as much as possible, with consent given by an authorized third party that is based on the best interests of the person. In the area of psychiatry, however, there is some debate over whether the research participation of hospitalized persons who are currently deemed not competent to make decisions due to a mental disorder is ethical. The high level of vulnerability of such persons and their dependence on the health care system and its personnel, including for the term of their confinement, calls their involvement in research into question for some (Elliott & Lankin, 2016).

Informed consent in addiction research has also been queried. Research on cravings (intense desires for a drug) for the purpose of understanding their neurobiologic and cognitive bases may allow development of better treatment for addiction. However, substance-dependent research participants to give genuinely informed consent and to fully understand the risks may be diminished by potential access to their drug of addiction (Carter & Hall, 2013).

Study designs in psychiatric research that raise particular ethical concerns include (1) placebo-controlled studies that deprive participants in the placebo arm of the research of existing treatment, (2) washout studies in which subjects' medications are discontinued, and (3) challenge studies, such as pharmaceutical or psychological challenges administered under controlled conditions, usually with some deception, so that the subject's response may be observed, as these can cause adverse effects (DuVal, 2004). Many ethical issues arise, for instance, in clinical trials research in severe mood disorders. Such research is needed, however, given the lack of effective treatments. A review of the evidence regarding risks suggests that it is possible to conduct research in this area safely, even with drug withdrawals and placebo controls (Nugent, Miller, Henter, & Zarate, 2017). Ongoing attention to the balance of risks and benefits, however, remains essential.

In the history of psychiatric research in Canada, there is a strong reminder that vigilance in terms of ethics is necessary. In the 1950s and early 1960s, the "depatterning" experiments of Dr. Ewen Cameron at the Allen Memorial Institute, McGill University (partially funded by the U.S. Central Intelligence Agency), attempted to erase the memories of patients and insert new "positive" ideas. Without their consent, patients were "brainwashed," with many permanently losing their memories. Although Dr. Cameron was an international leader in psychiatric medicine with the reputation of being a humanitarian, his research caused great harm (Collins, 1988). Remembering that such serious violations of research ethics have occurred can act as a safeguard against future contraventions.

 SUMMARY OF KEY POINTS

- Ethics and law are separate domains. Nurses must be vigilant about the laws that affect their practice.
- Key issues can warn us about the ethical tone of our society; many of these issues are situated in health care. The way in which Canadians address the well-being of persons living with mental illness is one of these issues.
- Whenever nurses enact their professional responsibilities, they are active as moral agents. Nursing practice involves an attentiveness and responsiveness to their duties and commitments.
- Nurses' regulatory bodies support ethical practice through codes of ethics, position statements, and resources.
- There are theoretical approaches to ethical knowledge (based on moral philosophy and concepts such as human rights) that inform health ethics. These include virtue ethics, deontology, utilitarianism, principlism, casuistry, ethics of care, feminist ethics, relational ethics, and human rights.
- Practice environments need to be morally habitable and support ethical questioning and dialogue.
- Frameworks for ethical decision-making are available to assist in resolving moral dilemmas.
- Moral distress occurs when one is unable to act on an ethical judgement and/or fulfill one's ethical obligations as one believes one should.
- There are many complex ethical issues in PMH settings. These include issues related to threats to dignity, including behaviour control and restraint, relational engagement ("boundaries"), confidentiality and privacy, genetics, research ethics, and social justice.
- PADs are a tool intended to support the autonomy of patients. They have been found to facilitate therapeutic alliance and promote treatment integration.

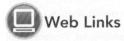 **Web Links**

Advocacy Organizations for Persons with Mental Illness and Their Families

camimh.ca Canadian Alliance on Mental Illness and Mental Health (CAMIMH)

cmha.ca Canadian Mental Health Association (CMHA)

disabiliyrightsintl.org Disability Rights International (DRI)

mdsc.ca Mood Disorders Society of Canada (MDSC)

mentalhealthcommission.ca Mental Health Commission of Canada (MHCC)

schizophrenia.ca Schizophrenia Society of Canada

wfmh.org World Federation for Mental Health (WFMH)

who.int/en World Health Organization (WHO)

Codes of Ethics for Nurses in Canada

cna-aiic.ca/_on-the-issues/best-nursing/nursing-ethics The CNA Web site gives access to their *Code of Ethics for Registered Nurses.*

www.crpnbc.ca/wp-content/uploads/2011/02/2010_Code_Standards.pdf *The Code of Ethics and Standards of Practice for Registered Psychiatric Nurses in Canada* used by RPNs in British Columbia.

www.crpnm.mb.ca/psychiatric-nursing/standards-and-code-of-ethics The College of Registered Psychiatric Nurses of Manitoba *Code of ethics.*

www.rpnas.com/about/code-of-ethics Registered Psychiatric Nurses Association of Saskatchewan *Code of ethics.*

Flowcharts

albertahealthservices.ca/MHA.asp On this site, flowcharts on Process of Formal Patient Certification (p. 41), Formal Patient: Competency & Consent for Treatment Decisions (p. 75), and Community Treatment Orders (p. 97) can be found from the Province of Alberta (2010) Guide to the Mental Health Act and Community Treatment Order Legislation.

Health Ethics Centres and Related Resources

bioethics.ca Canadian Bioethics Society

bioethics.georgetown.edu The Bioethics Research Library at Georgetown University

bioethics.medicine.dal.ca Dalhousie University, Department of Bioethics

ethics.ubc.ca The W. Maurice Young Centre for Applied Ethics, University of British Columbia

fabnet.org International Network of Feminist Approaches to Bioethics

mcgill.ca/biomedicalethicsunit McGill University Biomedical Ethics Unit

ualberta.ca/bioethics Dossetor Health Ethics Centre, University of Alberta

jcb.toronto.ca University of Toronto Joint Centre for Bioethics

Canadian Resources for Relevant to Legal and Ethical Aspects of Practice

cna-aiic.ca/~/media/cna/page-content/pdf-en/ps85_mental_health_e.pdf?la=en CNA position paper on *Mental Health Services.*

cna-aiic.ca/~/media/cna/page-content/pdfen/ps116_health_and_human_rights_2011_e.pdf?la=en CNA position paper on *Registered Nurses, Health and Human Rights.*

pre.ethics.gc.ca The Interagency Panel on Research Ethics Web site provides access to the *Tri-Council Policy Statement on*

Ethical Conduct for Research Involving Humans and links to other research ethics Web sites.

priv.gc.ca Office of the Privacy Commissioner of Canada.

United Nations

unesco.org/new/en/social-and-human-sciences/themes/bioethics UNESCO's bioethics site, where the UNESCO Declaration of Bioethics and Human Rights can be found, also provides access to the Global Ethics Observatory (GEObs) with worldwide databases in ethics (e.g., environmental ethics).

who.int/mental_health/mindbank/en The World Health Organization's MiNDbank is a repository of national and international resources related to mental health, addiction, disability, and human rights.

References

Agren, T., (2014). Human reconsolidation: A reactivation and update. *Brain Research Bulletin, 105,* 70–82. doi.org/10.1016/j.brainresbull.2013.12.010. Retrieved from www.sciencedirect.com/science/article/pii/S0361923013002062

Aly, G., & Roth, K. H. (1984). The legalization of mercy killings in medical and nursing institutions in Nazi Germany from 1938 to 1941. *International Journal of Law and Psychiatry, 7,* 145–163.

Ambrosini, D., Bemme, D., Crocker, A., & Latimer, E. (2012). Narratives of individuals concerning psychiatric advanced directives: Qualitative study. *Journal of Ethics in Mental Health, 6,* 1–9.

An Act to Amend the Criminal Code and to Make Related Amendments to Other Acts, S. C. 2016, c. 3. Retrieved from http://laws-lois.justice.gc.ca/PDF/2016_3.pdf

Aristotle. (1996). *Nicomachean ethics.* H. Rackham (Trans.). Ware, UK: Wordsworth Classics.

Audi, R. (Ed.). (1995). *The Cambridge dictionary of philosophy.* Cambridge, UK: Cambridge University Press.

Austin, W. (2001). Using the human rights paradigm in health ethics: The problems and the possibilities. *Nursing Ethics, 8*(13), 183–195.

Austin, W. (2006). Toward an understanding of trust. In J. Cutcliff & H. McKenna (Eds.), *The essential concepts of nursing* (pp. 317–330). London, UK: Churchill Livingstone.

Austin, W. (2007a). The Terminal: A tale of virtue. *Nursing Ethics, 14*(1), 54–61.

Austin, W. (2007b). The ethics of everyday practice: Healthcare environments as moral communities. *Advances in Nursing Science, 30*(1), 81–88.

Austin, W. (2008). Ethics in a time of contagion: A relational perspective. *Canadian Journal of Nursing Research, 40*(4), 10–24.

Austin, W. (2012). Moral distress and the contemporary plight of health professionals. *HEC Forum, 24*(1), 27–38.

Austin, W. (2016). Contemporary healthcare practice and the risk of moral distress. *Healthcare Management Forum, 29*(3):131–133. doi:10.1177/0840470416629163.

Austin, W. (2017). What is the role of ethics consultation in the moral habitability of health care environments? *AMA Journal of Ethics, 19*(6), 595–600.

Austin, W., Bergum, V., & Nuttgens, S. (2004). Addressing oppression in psychiatric care: A relational ethics perspective. *Ethical Human Psychology and Psychiatry, 6*(1), 69–78.

Austin, W., Bergum, V., Nuttgens, S., & Peternelj-Taylor, C. (2006). A re-visioning of boundaries in professional helping relationships: Exploring other metaphors. *Ethics & Behaviour, 16*(2), 77–94.

Austin, W., Kagan, L., Rankel, M., & Bergum, V. (2008). The balancing act: Psychiatrists' experience of moral distress. *Medicine, Health Care and Philosophy, 11,* 89–97.

Austin, W., Rankel, M., Kagan, L., Bergum, V., & Lemermeyer, G. (2005). To stay or to go, to speak or stay silent, to act or not to act: Moral distress as experienced by psychologists. *Ethics & Behavior, 15*(3), 197–212.

Austin, W., Bergum, V., & Dossetor, J. (2003a). Relational ethics: An action ethic as foundation for health care. In V. Tschudin (Ed.), *Approaches to ethics* (pp. 45–52). Woburn, MA: Butterworth-Heinemann.

Austin, W., Bergum, V., & Goldberg, L. (2003b). Unable to answer the call of our patients: Mental health nurses' experiences of moral distress. *Nursing Inquiry, 10*(3), 177–183.

Beauchamp, T. (1994). The "four principles" approach. In R. Gillon (Ed.), *Principles of health care ethics* (pp. 3–12). New York, NY: John Wiley & Sons.

Beauchamp, T., & Childress, J. (2013). *Principles of biomedical ethics* (7th ed.). New York, NY: Oxford University Press.

Benedict, S., & Kuhla, J. (1999). Nurses' participation in the euthanasia programs of Nazi Germany. *Western Journal of Nursing Research, 21*(2), 246–263.

Bentham, J. (1983). *Deontology together with a table on the springs of action and the article on utilitarianism.* Oxford, UK: Oxford University Press.

Bergum, V., & Dossetor, J. (2005). *Relational ethics: The full meaning of respect.* Hagerstown, MD: University Publishing Group.

Butler, M., & Phillips, K. (2013, August 15). *In Brief: Current issues in mental health in Canada: The federal role in legal and social affairs in mental health; Publication No, 2013-75-e.* Ottawa, ON: Library of the Parliament of Canada. Retrieved from lop.parl.ca/Content/LOP/ResearchPublications/2013-76-e.htm

Canadian Institutes of Health Research, Natural Sciences and Engineering Research Council of Canada, and Social Sciences and Humanities Research Council of Canada. (2014). *Tri-council policy statement: Ethical conduct for research involving humans.* Ottawa, ON: Authors. Retrieved from www.pre.ethics.gc.ca/pdf/eng/tcps2-2014/TCPS_2_FINAL_Web.pdf

Canadian Nurses Association (CNA). (2017). *Code of ethics for registered nurses.* Ottawa, ON: Author.

Carpenter, M. (1991). The process of ethical decision making in psychiatric nursing practice. *Issues in Mental Health Nursing, 12,* 179–191.

Carter, A., & Hall, W. (2013). Ethical implications of research on craving. *Addictive Behaviors, 38,* 1593–1599.

Cestari, V., Rossi-Arnaud, C., Saraulli, D., & Constanzi, M. (2014). The MAP(K) of fear: From memory consolidation to memory extinction. *Brain Research Bulletin, 105,* 8–16. doi:10.1016/j.brainresbull.2013.09. Retrieved from www.ncbi.nlm.nih.gov/pubmed/24080449

Chambers, M., Gallagher, A., Borschmann, R., Gillard, S., Turner, K., & Kantaris, X. (2014). The experience of detained mental health service users: Issues of dignity in care. *BMC Medical Ethics, 15*(50), 1–8. doi:10.1186/1472-6939-15-50

College and Association of Registered Nurses of Alberta. (2011). *Professional boundaries for registered nurses: Guidelines for the nurse–client relationship.* Edmonton, AB: Author.

College of Registered Nurses of British Columbia. (2017). *Duty to provide care [Practice standard].* Vancouver, BC: Author. Retrieved from https://www.crnbc.ca/Standards/Practice Standards/Pages/delegating/aspx

College of Registered Psychiatric Nurses (RPNs) of Alberta. (2013). *Code of ethics and standards of psychiatric nursing practice.* Edmonton, AB: Author.

College of Registered Psychiatric Nurses of Manitoba. (2017). *Code of ethics.* Winnipeg, MB: Author. Retrieved from www.crpnm.mb.ca/psychiatric-nursing/standards-and-code-of-ethics/

Colleges of Registered Licensed Practical Nurses, Registered Nurses, and Registered Psychiatric Nurses of British Columbia. (2017). *Practice standard: Boundaries in the nurse client relationship.* Vancouver, BC: Authors. Retrieved from www.crnbc.ca/Standards/PracticeStandards/Lists/GeneralResources/432NurseClientRelationshipsPracStd.pdf

Collins, A. (1988). *In the sleep room: The story of the CIA brainwashing experiments in Canada.* Toronto, ON: Lester & Orpen Dennys.

Cutcliffe, J. R., & Travale, R. (2013). Respect in mental health: Reconciling the rhetorical hyperbole with the practical reality. *Nursing Ethics, 20*(3), 273–284.

DuVal, G. (2004). Ethics in psychiatric research: Study design issues. *Canadian Journal of Psychiatry, 49*(1), 55–59.

Elliott, C., & Lankin, M. (2016). Restrict the recruitment of involuntarily committed patients for psychiatric research. *JAMA Psychiatry, 73*(4), 317–318.

Fisher, A. (1995). The ethical problems encountered in psychiatric nursing practice with dangerous mentally ill persons. *Scholarly Inquiry for Nursing Practice: An International Journal, 9*(2), 193–208.

Forchuk, C. (1991). Ethical problems encountered by mental health nurses. *Issues in Mental Health Nursing, 12,* 375–383.

Fowler, M. (1997). Nursing's ethics. In A. Davis, J. Liaschenko, M. Aroskar, & T. Drought (Eds.), *Ethical dilemmas and nursing practice* (pp. 17–34). Stamford, CT: Appleton & Lange.

Foy, M. (2007). Thoughts on the ethics of compassion. *Journal of Ethics in Mental Health, 2*(1), 1–2.

Gallup. (2016, December). Honesty/ethics in professions. Retrieved from http://www.gallup.com/poll/1654/honesty-ethics-professions.aspx

Gilligan, C. (1982). *In a different voice: Psychological theory and women's development.* Cambridge, MA: Harvard University Press.

Ginory, A., Sabatier, L. M., & Eth, S. (2012). Addressing therapeutic boundaries in social networking. *Psychiatry, 75*(1), 40–48.

Gostin, L. (2001). Beyond moral claims: A human rights approach in mental health. *Cambridge Quarterly of Healthcare Ethics, 10,* 264–274.

Government of New Brunswick. (2017, February 14). News Release/ Revised/Community support orders introduced to help those suffering from mental illness. Retrieved from www2.gnb.ca/content/gnb/en/ news/news_release.2017.02.0203.html

Government of Saskatchewan. (2015). *Mental Health Services Act of Saskatchewan M-13.1*. Regina, SK: Publications Centre. Retrieved from http://www.publications.gov.sk.ca/details.cfm?p=626

Gray, J. E., Hastings, T. J., Love, S., & O'Reilly, R. L. (2016). Clinically significant differences among Canadian Mental Health Acts: 2016. *Canadian Journal of Psychiatry, 61*(4), 222–226. doi:10.1177/0706743716632524

Griffith, R. (2016). When accepting a gift can be professional misconduct and theft. *British Journal of Community Nursing, 21*(7), 365–367.

Gustafsson, L-K., Wigerblad, Å, & Lindwall, L. (2014). Undignified care: Violation of patient dignity in involuntary psychiatric hospital care from a nurse's perspective. *Nursing Ethics, 21*(2), 176–186. doi:10.1177/0969733013490592

Hoop, J. (2008). Ethical considerations in psychiatric genetics. *Harvard Review of Psychiatry, 16*(6), 322–336.

International Council of Nurses. (1998). *Torture, death penalty and participation by nurses in executions*. Geneva, CH: Author. Retrieved from hrlibrary.umn.edu/instree/executions.html

Ipperciel, D. (2003). Dialogue and discussion in a moral context. *Nursing Philosophy, 4*, 211–224.

Jameton, A. (1984). *Nursing practice: The ethical issues*. Englewood Cliffs, NJ: Prentice Hall.

Jameton, A. (2013). A reflection on moral distress in nursing together with a current application of the concept. *Bioethical Inquiry, 10*, 297–308.

Jameton, A. (2017). What moral distress in nursing history could suggest about the future of health care. *AMA Journal of Ethics, 19*(6), 617–628.

Jonsen, A. (1991). Casuistry as methodology in clinical ethics. *Theoretical Medicine, 12*, 295–307.

Jonsen, A., & Toulmin, S. (1988). *The abuse of casuistry: A history of moral reasoning*. Berkeley, CA: University of California Press.

Justice Canada. (2014a). Privacy act, R.S.C. 1985, c. P-21. Retrieved from laws-lois.justice.gc.ca/PDF/P-21.pdf

Justice Canada. (2014b). Personal information protection and electronic documents act, S.C. 2000, c. 5. Retrieved from http://laws.justice.gc.ca/PDF/P-8.6.pdf

Kant, I. (1996). *Practical philosophy*. M. Gregor (Trans.). Cambridge, UK: Cambridge University Press.

Kunyk, D., & Austin, W. (2012). Nursing under the influence: A relational ethics perspective. *Nursing Ethics, 19*(3), 380–389.

Levine, M. (1977). Nursing ethics and the ethical nurse. *American Journal of Nursing, 77*(5), 845–849.

Liaschenko, J. (1994). Making a bridge: The moral work with patients we do not like. *Journal of Palliative Care, 10*(3), 83–89.

Locke, J. (1689/2016). *Second treatise of government, and a letter concerning toleration*. Oxford, UK: Oxford University Press.

MacIntyre, A. (1984). *After virtue* (2nd ed.). Notre Dame, IN: University of Notre Dame.

Maher, J. (2017). Editorial. What troubles me as a psychiatrist about the physician assisted suicide debate in Canada. *Journal of Ethics in Mental Health, 10*, 1–4. Retrieved from www.jemh.ca/issues/open/documents/JEMH%20vol%2010%20editorial.pdf

Mann, J., Gostin, L., Gruskin, S., Brennan, T., Lazzarini, Z., & Fineberg, H. (1999). Health and human rights. In J. Mann, S. Gruskin, M. Grodin, & G. Annas (Eds.). *Health and human rights: A reader* (pp. 7–20). New York, NY: Routledge.

McFarland-Icke. B. R. (1999). *Nurses in Nazi Germany: Moral choice in history*. Princeton, NJ: Princeton University Press.

Mental Health Commission of Canada (MHCC). (2009). *Toward recovery & well-being: A framework of a mental health strategy for Canada*. Calgary, AB: Authors.

Mill, J. S. (2002). *The basic writings of John Stuart Mill: On liberty, the subjection of women and utilitarianism*. New York, NY: Modern Library.

Molewijk, B., Kok, A., Husum, T., Pedersen, R., & Aasland, O. (2017). Staff's normative attitudes towards coercion: The role of moral doubt and professional context—A cross-sectional survey study. *BMC Medical Ethics, 18*(37), 1–14. doi:10.1186/s12910-017-0190-0

Nathaniel, A. (2006). Moral reckoning in nursing. *Western Journal of Nursing Research, 28*(4), 419–438.

Niebuhr, R. (1963). *The responsible self*. San Francisco, CA: Harper.

Noddings, N. (1984). *Caring: A feminine approach to ethics and moral education*. Berkeley, CA: University of California Press.

Norvoll, R., Hem, M. H., & Pedersen, R. (2017). The role of ethics in reducing and improving the quality of coercion in mental health care. *HEC Forum, 29*(1), 59–74.

Nugent, A. C., Miller, F. G., Henter, I. D., & Zarate, C. A. Jr. (2017). The ethics of clinical trials research in severe mood disorders. *Bioethics, 31*(6), 443–453. doi:10.1111/bioe.12349

Office of the Privacy Commissioner of Canada (OPCC). (2015). *Setting the priorities for the Office of the Privacy Commissioner: A conversation with stakeholders/summaries of privacy issues for discussion/the body as information*. Gatineau, QC: Author.

Olsen, D. (2017). Increasing the use of psychiatric advance directives. *Nursing Ethics, 24*(3), 265–267. doi:10.1177/09697330|7708881

Olsman, E., Willems, D., & Leget, C. (2016). Solicitude: Balancing compassion and empowerment in a relational ethics of hope—An empirical-ethical study in palliative care. *Medicine, Health Care and Philosophy, 19*(1), 11–20. doi:101007/s11019-015-9642-9

Paine, T. (1779/1996). *Rights of man*. Ware, UK: Wordsworth Editions.

Pauly, B. M., Varcoe, C., & Storch, J. (2012). Framing the issues: Moral distress in health care. *HEC Forum, 24*(1), 1–11.

Perna, G., & Nemcroff, C. B. (2017). Personalized medicine in psychiatry: Back to the future. *Personalized Medicine in Psychiatry, 1–2*, 1. doi:org/10.1016/j.pmip.2017.01.001

Racine, E., & Affleck, W. (2016). Changing memories: Between ethics and speculation. *AMA Journal of Ethics, 18*(12), 1241–1248.

Radden, J., & Sadler, J. (2008). Character virtues in psychiatric practice. *Harvard Review of Psychiatry, 16*(6), 373–380.

Registered Psychiatric Nurses of Canada (RPNC). (2010). *Code of ethics & standards of psychiatric nursing practice*. Edmonton, AB: Author.

Ricouer, P. (1992). *Oneself as another*. K. Blamey (Trans.). Chicago, IL: University of Chicago Press. (Original work published 1990).

Rittenmeyer, L., & Huffman, D. (2009). How professional nurses working in hospital environments experience moral distress: A systematic review. *JBI Library of Systematic Reviews, 7*(28), 1233–1290.

Robertson, M., Morris, K., & Walter, G. (2007). Overview of psychiatric ethics V: Utilitarianism and the ethics of duty. *Australasian Psychiatry, 15*(5), 402–410.

Robillard, J. M., & Illes, J. (2016). Manipulating memories: The ethics of yesterday's science fiction and today's reality. *AMA Journal of Ethics, 18*(12), 1225–1231.

Rodgers, S. (2004). Sexual abuse by health care professionals: The failure of reform in Ontario. *Health Law Journal, 12*, 71–102.

Ryberg, J. (2017). Neuroethics and brain privacy: Setting the stage. *Res Publica, 23*, 153–158. doi:10.1007/s111.58-016-9340-3

Rynor, B. (2010). Value of community treatment orders remains at issue. *Canadian Medical Association Journal, 182*(8), E337–E338.

Saul, J. R. (2001). *On equilibrium*. Toronto, ON: Penguin/Viking.

Schick Makaroff, K., Storch, J., Pauly, B., & Newton, L. (2014). Searching for ethical leadership in nursing. *Nursing Ethics, 21*(6) 642–658. doi:10.1177/0969733013513213

Sherwin, S. (1992). *No longer patient: Feminist ethics and health care*. Philadelphia, PA: Temple University Press.

Silén, M., Kjellström, S., Christensson, L., Sidenvall, B., & Svantesson, M. (2012). What actions promote a positive ethical climate? A critical incident study of nurses' perceptions. *Nursing Ethics, 19*(4), 501–512.

Skorpen, F., Rehnsfeldt, A., & Thorsen, A. A. (2015). The significance of small things for dignity in psychiatric care. *Nursing Ethics, 22*(7), 754–764.

Smith, G. C., & Knudson, T. K. (2016). Student nurses' unethical behavior, social media, and year of birth. *Nursing Ethics, 23*(8), 910–918. doi:10.1177/0969733015590009

Snow, N. (2015). *Exploring community treatment orders: An institutional ethnographic study*. Unpublished doctoral dissertation, University of Alberta, Edmonton, AB.

Somerville, M. (2000). *The ethical canary: Science, society and the human spirit*. Toronto, ON: Penguin Books.

Strong, C. (2000). Specified principlism: What is it, and does it really resolve cases better than casuistry? *Journal of Medicine and Philosophy, 25*(3), 323–341.

United Nations. (1991). Principles for the protection of persons with mental illness and the improvement of mental health care. Adopted by General Assembly resolution 46/119 of 17 December 1991, Office of the United Nations High Commissioner for Human Rights. Retrieved from www.unhchr.ch/html/menu3/b/68.htm

United Nations. (2006, December 13). *Convention on the rights of persons with disabilities and optional protocol*. New York, NY: Author. Retrieved from http://www.un.org/disabilities/documents/convention/convopt-prot-e.pdf

United Nations Human Rights Council. (2017, June 6–23). *Thirty-fifth session, Agenda item 3: Report of the Special Rapporteur on the right of everyone to the enjoyment of the highest attainable standard of physical and mental*

health. New York, NY: Author. Retrieved from www.icn.ch/images/
stories/documents/projects/nursing_policy/UN%20Mental%20
health%20report.pdf

Walker, T. (2009). What principlism misses. *Journal of Medical Ethics, 35*(4),
229–231.

Walter, R. R. (2017) Emancipatory nursing praxis: A theory of social justice
in nursing. *Advances in Nursing Science, 40*(3), 225–243. doi:10.1097/
ANS.0000000000000157

Whiteford, H., Degenhardt, L., Rehm, J., Baxter, A. J., Ferrari, A. J., Erskine,
H. E., … Vos, T. (2013). Global burden of disease attributable to men-
tal and substance use disorders: Findings from the Global Burden of
Disease Study 2010. *The Lancet, 382*, 1575–1586.

Wilkinson, J. M. (1987–1988). Moral distress in nursing practice:
Experience and effect. *Nursing Forum, 23*(1), 16–29.

World Health Organization. (2012). *Quality rights tool kit: Assessing and
improving quality and human rights in mental health and social care facilities*. Geneva, Switzerland: Author. Retrieved from http://www.who.int/
mental_health/publications/QualityRights_toolkit/en/

World Health Organization. (2015, July 14). Media release: Global health
workforce, financing remains low for mental health. Retrieved from www.
who.int/mediacentre/news/notes/2015/finances-mental-health/en/

World Psychiatric Association. (1996). Madrid declaration of ethical standards for psychiatric practice. Retrieved http://www.wpanet.org/detail.
php?section_id=5&content_id=48

CHAPTER 8

Theoretic Basis of Practice

Wendy Austin

Adapted from the chapters "Theoretic Basis of Psychiatric and Mental Health Nursing" by Ginette Pagé and by Mary Ann Boyd

LEARNING OBJECTIVES

After studying this chapter, you will be able to:

- Explain the need for theory-based psychiatric and mental health (PMH) nursing practice.
- Compare the key elements of theories that provide a basis for such practice.
- Describe the common nursing theories used in PMH nursing.
- Identify theories that contribute to understanding human beings and their mental health.

KEY TERMS

- anima • animus • archetype • behaviourism • change
- classical conditioning • cognition • collective unconscious • conscious • countertransference
- disinhibition • ego • elicitation • empathy • extrovert
- id • interpersonal relations • introvert • modelling • need
- object relations • operant behaviour • preconscious
- persona • reclamation • role • self-actualization • self-efficacy • self-system • shadow • superego • transaction
- transference • unconditional positive regard • unconscious

KEY CONCEPTS

- recovery • theory

This chapter presents an overview of some of the nursing and other theories that serve as the knowledge base for psychiatric and mental health (PMH) nursing practice. Many of the theories underlying this practice are evolving, and only some have research support to date. As acknowledged in the *Canadian Standards of Psychiatric-Mental Health Nursing* (2014), PMH nurses use knowledge from nursing, the health sciences, and related mental health disciplines in their practice. The chapter begins, then, with selected nursing theories and moves to some of the many theories that underlie our understanding of the biologic, psychological, social, and spiritual aspects of human knowledge and experience.

■ NURSING THEORIES

Nursing theories are essential in conceptualizing nursing practice. Some theories described here are commonly referred to as models, not as theories, and we have followed common practice. We are not, however, differentiating between a model and a theory, as this remains an area of some debate within nursing.

A nurse may choose to base his or her practice consistently on one nursing theory or may choose to use a specific theory depending on the care situation. For example, in nursing a person with schizophrenia who

has problems related to maintaining self-care, Dorothea Orem's deficit theory (1991) may be particularly useful. Peplau's model (1952) may be more helpful in addressing relationship issues. The theory or theories used by a nurse reveal the way that nurse conceives his or her practice.

KEY CONCEPT

A **theory** "is an imaginative grouping of knowledge, ideas, and experience that are represented symbolically and seek to illuminate a given phenomenon" (Watson, 1988, p. 1).

Theories as Maps

The study of theories in the health sciences can be experienced as an oppressive task by students unless the meaningful link between theory and practice is made evident (Georges, 2005). If it is recognized that theories are maps that orientate us to our care environments and guide our practice, their relevance becomes apparent. Like a map, a theory is an attempt to represent the real world and is only as useful as its correspondence to the terrain to be travelled. Just as maps need to be redrawn when the landscape changes, theories need to change with our knowledge of the human condition and the world.

The Visionary: Nightingale

Florence Nightingale, the founder of modern nursing, is recognized as the first nurse researcher and the pioneer of theory development in nursing. The patterns of knowing of contemporary nursing are to be found in her work begun in the 1800s (Clements & Averill, 2006). The respect for her legacy is apparent: International Nurses Day is celebrated on her birthday, May 12, and Canada's National Nursing Week occurs that same week. Nightingale's model emerged from her clinical work in hospitals and in the Crimean War, where unhealthy physical environments for the sick prevailed (Nightingale, 1859). This is the reason that the primary focus of her model, although not neglecting psychosocial and spiritual needs, is on improving environmental conditions. Nightingale's intent was to create healthy surroundings that help alleviate suffering and promote well-being. Health, for her, included the ability to use "every power we have." For example, she considered that giving false reassurance to sick people was an unacceptable behaviour. For Nightingale, the curative process was accomplished by nature alone: medicine and nursing do not cure. Nursing activities, therefore, were to put patients in the best state for nature to act upon them.

Interpersonal Relations Models

Interpersonal Relations: Hildegard Peplau

Hildegard Peplau introduced the first systematic framework for PMH nursing in her book *Interpersonal Relations in Nursing* (1952). A major contribution was her conceptualization of the nurse–patient relationship and its phases (see Chapter 6). Although her work continues to stimulate debate, she led PMH nursing out of the confinement of custodial care into a unique model for practice.

Peplau (1992) believed in the importance of **interpersonal relations**, which included interactions between person and family, parent and child, or patient and nurse. She emphasized empathic linkage, the ability to feel in oneself the feelings experienced by another person or people. The interpersonal transmission of anxiety or panic is the most common empathic linkage, but other feelings, such as anger, disgust, and envy, can also be communicated nonverbally to others. Peplau believed that if nurses pay attention to what they feel during a relationship with a patient, they can gain invaluable observations of feelings a patient is experiencing, even those the patient has not yet recognized. Peplau's theory has been identified as a useful framework for educating nursing students on communicating holistically with older adults (Deane, 2015).

The **self-system** is an important concept in Peplau's model. Peplau defined the self as an "antianxiety system" and a product of socialization. The self proceeds through personal development that is always open to revision but tends toward stability. For example, in parent–child relationships, patterns of approval, disapproval, and indifference are used by children to define themselves. If the verbal and nonverbal messages have been derogatory, children incorporate these messages and also view themselves negatively. The concept of **need** is also important to Peplau's model. Needs are primarily of biologic origin but are met within a sociocultural environment. When a biologic need is present, it gives rise to tension that is reduced and relieved by behaviours meeting that need. According to Peplau, nurses should strive to recognize patients' patterns and style of meeting their needs in relation to their health status and help them to identify available resources, such as food and interpersonal support.

Anxiety is an important concept for Peplau, who contended that unless anxiety is understood, professional practice is unsafe. There are various levels of anxiety (mild, moderate, severe, and panic levels), each having observable behavioural cues. These cues Peplau considered "relief behaviours." For example, some people may relieve their anxiety by yelling and swearing, whereas others seek relief by withdrawing. In both instances, anxiety, according to Peplau, is generated by an unmet self-system security need.

IN-A-LIFE

Hildegard Peplau (1909–1999)

PSYCHIATRIC NURSE OF THE CENTURY

Peplau became a nurse in 1931 in Pennsylvania. During World War II, she joined the Army Nurse Corps and worked in a neuropsychiatric clinic in London. She obtained a Master's Degree (1947) and a PhD (1953) from Columbia University. Peplau took the lead in the development of psychiatric nursing as a specialty at the Master's level and developed the theory of psychodynamic nursing. Peplau has numerous publications, with her most influential works being *Interpersonal Relations in Nursing* (1952), *Aspects of Psychiatric Nursing* (1957), and *Principles of Patient Counselling* (1964).

Her ideas regarding the centrality of relationship to nursing practice and the efficacy of the use of self as a nursing tool have had far-reaching effects. She envisioned nursing as a discipline independent from medicine and worked to ensure that this was so. Drawing on interdisciplinary knowledge from psychology, education, and pragmatic educational philosophy, she deeply influenced nursing's professional and scientific development. Her achievements occurred during a time when strong leadership from women was frowned upon, and she faced many conflicts and controversies throughout a 50-year career that included being President of the American Nurses Association and consultant to the World Health Organization in psychiatric nursing. She was named one of 50 Great Americans by Marquis' *Who's Who*. Hildegard Peplau was an honorary member of the Canadian Federation of Mental Health Nurses.

Source: Calaway, B. J. (2002). *Hildegard Peplau: Psychiatric nurse of the century*. New York, NY: Springer.

The Dynamic Nurse–Patient Relationship: Ida Jean Orlando

In 1954, Ida Jean Orlando studied the factors that enhanced or impeded the integration of mental health principles in the basic nursing curriculum. From this study, she published *The Dynamic Nurse–Patient Relationship* (1961). A nursing situation for Orlando (1961, 1972) involves the patient's behaviour, the nurse's reaction, and anything that does not relieve the distress of the patient, which Orlando understands as related to the individual's inability to meet or communicate his or her own needs. She focuses on the whole patient, rather than on disease or institutional demands. Her ideas continue to be useful today with research supporting her model (Olson & Hanchett, 1997). Orlando's model has been used, for example, as a framework for guiding nurses in addressing patient risk for falls, which can be higher on psychiatric units than on acute medical care areas due to patient experiences with cognitive disturbances and the side effects of some psychotropic medication (Abraham, 2011).

Existential and Humanistic Theoretic Perspectives

Seeking Life Meaning: Joyce Travelbee

Influenced by Peplau and Orlando, Joyce Travelbee provided an existential perspective on nursing based on the works of Viktor Frankl, an existential philosopher (see Spiritual Theories section in this chapter). Existentialists believe that humans seek meaning in their life and experiences. Travelbee believed that the nurse's spiritual values and philosophical beliefs about suffering would determine the extent to which the nurse could help ill people find meaning in their situation. She understood "suffering" as a feeling of displeasure

ranging from simple and transitory mental, physical, or spiritual discomfort to extreme anguish and beyond to the malignant phase of despair (Travelbee, 1971). Travelbee expanded the area of concern of mental illness to include long-term physical illnesses. Overall, her use of the interpersonal process as a nursing intervention (Travelbee, 1969) and her focus on suffering and illness helped to define areas of concern for nursing.

Humanbecoming: Rosemarie Rizzo Parse

Quality of life as perceived by a person and their family is the focus of the nurse within the humanbecoming model. When Parse (2007) was asked what the practice of nurses using this model would be like in 2050, she imagined that their repertoire would remain focused on enhancing quality of life and attending to human freedom and dignity. While the quality of life will be different in 2050, it will still be unique to the individual. The individual (not to be understood as reducible to qualities or traits) is perceived as open and free to ascribe meaning to life (through values and beliefs developed) and to bear responsibility for choices (Parse, 1987). Reality for an individual is cocreated with the environment. It is in the rhythm of moving closer and away from others where creativity and change (becoming different) occur (Leddy & Pepper, 1998). Three principles structure Parse's model:

- Meaning: "Structuring meaning is the imaging and valuing of language."
- Rhythmicity: "Configuring rhythmical patterns of relation is the revealing-concealing and enabling-limiting of connecting-separating."
- Transcendence: "Cotranscending with possible is the powering and originating of transforming." (Parse, 2007, p. 309)

Permeating these three principles are the postulates of *illimitability* (indivisible, unbounded knowing extending to infinity), *paradox* (rhythm expressed as pattern preference), *freedom* (contextually construed liberation), and *mystery* (the unexplainable). The language of humanbecoming can be challenging, but the vision of personhood that it offers can richly inform nursing practice. It can be applied, for instance, when caring for a family experiencing a stillbirth or loss of a newborn, guiding the nurse to support the family's exploration of paradoxical feelings (such as simultaneous guilt and powerlessness) rather than attempting to make them "feel better" (Wilson, 2016).

Primacy of Caring: Patricia Benner

Patricia Benner has developed a particular notion of nursing as a caring relationship. As a caring profession, nursing "is guided by the moral art and ethics of care and responsibility" (Benner & Wrubel, 1989, p. xi), and nursing practice is based upon "the lived experience of health and illness" (p. 8). Based upon Heidegger's phenomenologic philosophy, Benner describes the person as "a self-interpreting being ... (who) gets defined in the course of a life ... (and) has an effortless and nonreflective understanding of the self in the world" (p. 41). Well-being (the human experience of health or wholeness) is, as is being ill, a distinct way of being in the world. With a phenomenologic view, Benner believes the environment situates meaning. People enter situations with their own sets of meanings, habits, and perspectives, and their personal interpretations affect the way they respond in those situations. Benner and Wrubel's identification of the domains of nursing practice, as described in *The Primacy of Caring*, was used to frame the original Canadian standards of PMH nursing practice (Austin, Gallop, Harris, & Spencer, 1996).

Caring: Jean Watson

The science of caring was initiated by Jean Watson (1979) based on the belief that caring is the foundation of nursing. Watson (2005) recommends that specific theories of caring be developed in relation to specific human conditions and health and illness experiences. The science of caring is based on seven assumptions and ten "carative" factors (Barnhart, Bennett, Porter, & Sloan, 1994). One of the assumptions is that "effective caring promotes health and individual or family growth" (p. 153); one of the carative factors is that "a trusting relationship ... involves congruence, **empathy**, nonpossessive warmth, and effective communication" (p. 152). The model has evolved to address more specifically the spiritual dimension of the nurse's role, including helping the patient to grow spiritually (Watson, 1988). For Watson, spiritual well-being is the foundation of human health, and she suggests that a troubled soul can lead to illness and disease.

Watson's view is applicable to the care of those who seek help for mental illness. This model emphasizes the importance of sensitivity to self and others; the development of helping and trusting relations; the promotion of interpersonal teaching and learning; and provision for a supportive, protective, and corrective mental, physical, sociocultural, and spiritual environment. The application of Watson's caring model to the environmental transformation of a unit with a history of disengaged, dissatisfied nurses and poor clinical practice indicators was significantly successful in measurable ways, such as health system employee engagement scores (from 35th to 85th percentile) and specialty certification (from 6% to 64% of staff) (Summerell, 2015).

The Tidal Model of Mental Health Recovery and Reclamation: Philip Barker

Philip Barker's Tidal Model (Barker & Buchanan-Barker, 2005) incorporates Barker and colleagues' Model for Empowering Interactions. It emphasizes the centrality of the lived experience of the person in care and is based on the assumption that people are their life stories and that they generate meaning through such stories (Barker, 2001a). It is focused on helping people to recover their lives after an arrest in development, a breakdown, or a disruption in the flow of life. This **reclamation** of one's own life story is necessary to recovery. The nurse's role is envisioned as helping the persons seeking care to discover, identify, and address the problems or challenges affecting them at this point in life. Nurses are to foster the creation of a safe haven in which the persons can recuperate and recover. Recovery is clarified by each person in a particular way but is defined in this model generally as "getting going again" (Barker & Buchanan-Barker, 2010, p. 171).

Change (i.e., becoming different) is a core element in this model (hence the metaphor of the tide), and the nurse's role will be shaped by the changing needs of patients across the continuum of care (e.g., critical, transitional, or developmental care) and the provision of interdependent services (Barker, 2001b). Box 8.1 outlines the Tidal Model's "10 commitments" of care.

The Tidal Model considers the domains of self, world, and others. They are metaphorical settings for the unfolding of the person's story. The process of exploring the person's experience may begin within any of the domains (Barker & Buchanan-Barker, 2010). Tidal processes, used with much flexibility, assist in exploring the person's experience within each domain. A personal security plan is considered in the self domain to help the person to feel as safe as possible. A holistic assessment is an aspect of the world domain as a means of more deeply exploring the person's lifework and problems in living. Group work in various forms is part of the process in the others domain in order to encourage individuals to share aspects of themselves as persons rather than patients (Barker & Buchanan-Barker, 2010).

The first Canadian application of this model was at the Royal Ottawa Mental Health Centre. In their evaluation of its implementation, they found that stories were captured in the holistic assessments of patients and that risk incidents (e.g., restraint use) decreased (Brookes, Murata, & Tansey, 2008).

Systems Models

Health Promotion: The McGill Model of Nursing

This model was developed under the guidance of Dr. Moyra Allen by the students and faculty of McGill University School of Nursing. It distinguishes nursing

---

BOX 8.1 Ten Commitments of the Tidal Model

1. *Value the voice*: The person's own account of his or her story is the beginning and end point of the helping encounter. Records of care should represent the patient's own voice.

2. *Respect the language*: People develop their own unique way of telling their story. It is not necessary to "rewrite" the story in the language of psychiatry and psychiatric nursing.

3. *Develop genuine curiosity*: Those who seek to be of assistance to the person need to develop ways of expressing genuine interest in the story so that they might better understand the storyteller.

4. *Become the apprentice*: One is the authority on one's own life story. Professionals learn from the person what needs to be done, rather than leading.

5. *Use the available toolkit*: The person's story contains examples of "what has worked" or "what might work" for this person. These are the main tools to use in helping the person's recovery.

6. *Craft the step beyond*: The professional helper and the person work together to construct an appreciation of what needs to be done *now*. The

first step is the crucial step, revealing the power of change and pointing toward the ultimate goal of recovery.

7. *Give the gift of time*: There is no value in asking "How much time do we have?" The question is "How do we use this time?"

8. *Reveal personal wisdom*: One of the key tasks for the helper is to assist in revealing the person's life wisdom that will sustain and guide his or her recovery.

9. *Know that change is constant*: The professional helper needs to become aware of how change is happening and discover the way that knowledge may steer the person out of danger and distress and help remain on the journey to recovery.

10. *Be transparent*: Both the person and the professional embody the opportunity to become a team. The professional can support this by being transparent at all times, helping the person understand *what* is being done and *why*.

Source: Buchanan-Barker, P., & Barker, P. (2008). The Tidal Commitments: Extending the value base of mental health recovery. *Journal of Psychiatric and Mental Health Nursing, 15*, 93–100.

---

from other health disciplines but also identifies their complementary relationships (Allen, 1977). The model's four major concepts are health, family (person), collaboration, and learning (Gottlieb & Rowat, 1987). Health is considered the focus of the practice of nursing and is seen as coexisting with illness. Coping and development are health processes that facilitate functioning and satisfaction with life; family (person) is viewed as the unit of concern. The person is perceived through his or her web of significant relationships. Family and person are considered open systems in constant interaction with their environment. The environment is viewed "as the context within which health and healthy ways of living are learned" (p. 56). Collaboration and learning are essentials for the nurse to structure a learning environment to meet "the needs, goals, and problem-solving styles of the family (person) … based upon the family (person's) strengths and resources" (p. 51). This strength-based component (rather than a deficit focus) of the McGill model makes it particularly useful in assessment, planning, and intervention with families (Feeley & Gottlieb, 2000).

Goal Attainment: Imogene M. King

The theory of goal attainment developed by Imogene M. King is based on a model that includes three interacting systems: personal, interpersonal, and social (King, 1971). King believed that human beings interact with the environment and that the individual's perceptions influence reactions and interactions. For King, nursing involves caring for the human being, with the goal of health defined as adjusting to the stressors in both internal and external environments. She defines nursing as a "process of human interactions between nurse and patient whereby each perceives the other and the situation; and through communication, they set goals, explore means, and agree on means to achieve goals" (King, 1981, p. 144). The process is initiated to help the patient cope with a health problem that compromises the ability to maintain social roles, functions, and activities of daily living (King, 1992). In this theory, the person is goal oriented and purposeful, is reacting to stressors, and is viewed as an open system interacting with the environment. It is within an interpersonal system of nurse and client that the healing process is performed. Interaction is depicted in which the outcome is a **transaction**, defined as the transfer of value between two or more people. The transaction process is what occurs in nursing situations. In the past, King's theory has been applied to group therapy for inpatient juvenile offenders, maximum security state offenders, and community parolees (Laben, Dodd, & Snead, 1991) and as a nursing framework for individual psychotherapy (DeHowitt, 1992). It continues to be used: as example, to investigate the effectiveness of clinical pathways for a surgical procedure in terms of clinical quality, cost, and patient and staff satisfaction (Knowaja, 2006).

Systems and Stress: Betty Neuman

The purpose of Neuman's (1989) systems model is to guide the actions of the professional caregiver through the assessment and intervention processes by focusing on two major components: the nature of the relationship between the nurse and patient and the patient's response to stressors. The patient may be an individual, group (e.g., a family), or community. The nurse is an "intervener" who attempts to reduce an individual's encounter with stress and to strengthen the person's ability to deal with stressors. The patient is viewed as a collaborator in setting health care goals and determining interventions. Neuman was one of the first PMH nurses to include the concept of stressors in understanding nursing care.

The Neuman systems model has been applied in diverse settings, including community health, family therapy, renal nursing, perinatal nursing, and mental health nursing of older adults (DeWan & Ume-Nwagbo, 2006; Neuman, Newman, & Holder, 2000; Olowokere & Okanlawon, 2015; Partlak Günüşen, Üstün, & Gigliotti, 2009).

Self-Care: Dorothea Orem

Self-care is the focus of the general theory of nursing initiated by Dorothea Orem in the early 1960s. The theory has three main focuses: self-care, self-care deficit, and a theory of nursing systems (Orem, 1991). Self-care is defined as those activities performed independently by an individual to promote and maintain personal well-being throughout life. Self-care deficits occur when an individual has a deficit in attitude (motivation), knowledge, or skill that impedes the meeting of self-care needs. Nurses can help individuals meet self-care requisites through five approaches: acting or doing for, guiding, teaching, supporting, and providing an environment to promote the patient's ability to meet current or future demands. The nursing systems theory refers to a series of actions a nurse takes to meet patient self-care requirements, which vary from patients totally dependent on the nurse for care to those who need only some education and support. Orem's emphasis on promoting independence of the individual and on self-care activities is of particular importance to PMH nursing (Biggs, 2008). This emphasis fits well with recovery principles, and it has potential use in moving inpatient psychiatric cultures toward a recovery focus and in guiding research that explores patients' self-care agency to recovery outcomes (Seed

& Torkelson, 2012). See, for instance, Pickens' (2012) exploration of nursing strategies to enhance motivation of persons with schizophrenia to engage in self-care activities.

Adaptation: Callista Roy

Callista Roy's nursing model is often selected by nurses working in inpatient psychiatric units because they find its concepts particularly relevant to their practice. Roy's adaptation model (1974), originating in 1964, describes humans as living adaptive systems with two coping mechanisms: the regulator and the cognator. The regulator copes with physiologic stimuli and the cognator with psychosociocultural stimuli. Manifestations of the coping mechanisms can be assessed by four adaptive modes: physiologic needs, self-concept, role function, and interdependence. In this model, the nursing process has six steps: "assessment of behaviour, assessment of stimuli (focal, contextual, and residual), nursing diagnosis, goal setting, intervention, and evaluation" (Lutjens, 1991a, p. 10). Research informed by this model includes a study of the sharing of the experience of a traumatic event from both the storyteller's and the listener's perspectives (Cummins, 2011).

Unitary Human Beings: Martha Rogers

The central concept of nursing for Martha Rogers is energy fields, which are open systems (Rogers, 1970). With its principles of homeodynamics—integrality, resonancy, and helicy—her abstract system offers a perspective of change as continuous and evolutionary (Rogers, 1994). Health and nonhealth are considered value laden, with the purpose of nursing being the promotion of human betterment. Important concepts are accelerating change, paranormal phenomena, and rhythmic manifestation of change. Rogers' science enables us to see human phenomena differently (Lutjens, 1991b), including a psychiatric disorder (Thompson, 1990). Her influence on other nursing perspectives, such as Rosemarie Parse's health as humanbecoming, is evident. According to Lego (1973), the holistic, unitary human beings approach differentiates a nurse psychotherapist from other psychotherapists. An example of research based on Roger's theory is Coakley, Barron, and Annese (2016) study of the experience and impact of therapeutic touch (TT) treatments for nurse colleagues. TT, based on Roger's understanding of energy fields as interactive, involves the transfer of energy through the hands of one person to another for the purpose of healing. It was found that changes in the heart rate, blood pressure, cortisol levels, and perceived levels of comfort of nurse participants, whom provided and received TT, indicated that a sense of well-being was promoted.

■ BIOLOGIC THEORIES

Biologic theories are clearly important in understanding the manifestations of mental disorders and caring for people with these illnesses. This importance is growing as we gain further knowledge of the brain. Because this is so, there is a separate chapter, Chapter 9, on the biologic foundations of PMH nursing. This chapter addresses many of the important neurobiologic theories and introduces other new fields of study. Further knowledge about the biologic domain can be found in Chapter 12, which focuses on psychopharmacology and other biologic treatments. In Chapter 11, many of the biologically focused nursing interventions can be found.

■ PSYCHOLOGICAL THEORIES

Psychodynamic Theories

Psychodynamic theories explain human development processes, especially in early childhood, and their effects on thought and behaviour. The study of the unconscious is a key aspect of psychodynamic theory (Ellenberger, 1970). Many important concepts in PMH nursing began with the Austrian physician Sigmund Freud (1856–1939). Psychodynamic theories initially attempted to explain the cause of mental disorders, but etiologic explanations have not been consistently supported by empiric research. These theories, however, proved to be especially important in the development of therapeutic relationships, techniques, and interventions (Table 8.1).

Table 8.1 Psychological Theories: Psychodynamic and Humanistic

Theorist	Overview	Major Concepts	Applicability
Psychoanalytic			
Sigmund Freud (1856–1939)	Founder of psychoanalysis. Believed that the unconscious could be accessed through dreams and free association. Developed a personality theory and theory of infantile sexuality.	Id, ego, superego; Consciousness; Unconscious mental processes; Libido; Object relations; Anxiety and defence mechanisms; Free associations, transference, and countertransference	Individual therapy approach used for enhancement of personal maturity and personal growth
Anna Freud (1895–1982)	Application of ego psychology to psychoanalytic treatment and child analysis with emphasis on the adaptive function of defence mechanisms	Refinement of concepts of anxiety, defence mechanisms	Individual therapy, childhood psychoanalysis
Neo-Freudian			
Alfred Adler (1870–1937)	First defected from Freud; Founded the school of individual psychology	Inferiority	Added to the understanding of human motivation
Carl Gustav Jung (1875–1961)	After separating from Freud, founded the school of psychoanalytic psychology. Developed new therapeutic approaches.	Redefined libido; Introversion; Extroversion; Persona	Personalities are often assessed on the introversion and extroversion dimensions
Karen Horney (1885–1952)	Opposed Freud's theory of castration complex in women and his emphasis on the Oedipus complex. Argued that neurosis was influenced by the society in which one lived.	Situational neurosis; Character	Beginning of feminist analysis of psychoanalytic thought
Humanistic			
Abraham Maslow (1921–1970)	Concerned himself with healthy rather than sick people. Approached individuals from a holistic–dynamic viewpoint	Needs; Motivation	Used as a model to understand how people are motivated and needs that should be met
Frederick S. Perls (1893–1970)	Awareness of emotion, physical state, and repressed needs would enhance the ability to deal with emotional problems.	Reality; Here and now	Used as a therapeutic approach to resolve current life problems that are influenced by old, unresolved emotional problems
Carl Rogers (1902–1987)	Based theory on the view of human potential for goodness. Used the term *client* rather than *patient*. Stressed the relationship between the therapist and the client.	Empathy; Positive regard	Individual therapy approach that involves never giving advice and always clarifying client's feelings

Psychoanalytic Theory

Study of the Unconscious

In Sigmund Freud's psychoanalytic model, the human mind was conceptualized in terms of **conscious** mental processes (an awareness of events, thoughts, and feelings with the ability to recall them) and **unconscious** mental processes (thoughts and feelings that are outside awareness and are not remembered). Freud believed that the unconscious part of the human mind is only rarely recognized by the conscious part, as in remembered dreams. The term **preconscious** was used to describe unconscious material that is capable of entering consciousness. Uncovering unconscious material to help patients gain insight into unresolved issues was basic to the psychotherapy Freud developed.

Personality and Its Development

Freud's personality structure consists of three parts: the id, ego, and superego (Freud, 1927). According to Freud, the **id** is formed by unconscious desires, primitive instincts, and unstructured drives, including sexual and aggressive tendencies that arise from the body. The **ego** consists of the sum of certain mental mechanisms, such as perception, memory, and motor control, as well as specific defence mechanisms. The ego controls movement, perception, and contact with reality. The capacity to form mutually satisfying relationships is a fundamental function of the ego, which is not present at birth but is formed throughout a child's development. The **superego** is that part of the personality structure associated with ethics, standards, and self-criticism. A child's identification with important and esteemed people in early life, particularly parents, helps form the superego.

Object Relations and Identification

Freud introduced the concept of **object relations**, the psychological attachment to another person or object. He believed that the choice of a love object in adulthood and the nature of the relationship depend on the nature and quality of the child's object relationships during the early formative years. A child's first love object is the mother, who is the source of nourishment and the provider of pleasure. Gradually, as the child separates from the mother, the nature of this initial attachment influences any future relationships. The development of the child's capacity for relationships with others progresses from a state of narcissism to social relationships, first within the family and then within the larger community. Although the concept of object relations is fairly abstract, it can be understood in terms of a child who imitates her mother and then becomes like her mother in adulthood. This child has incorporated her mother as a love object, identifies with her, and becomes like her as an adult. This process becomes especially important in understanding an abused child who, under certain circumstances, becomes the adult abuser.

Anxiety and Defence Mechanisms

For Freud, anxiety was a specific state of unpleasantness accompanied by motor discharge along definite pathways, the reaction to danger of object loss. Defence mechanisms protected a person from unwanted anxiety. Although they are defined differently than in Freud's day, defence mechanisms still play an explanatory role in contemporary PMH practice. Defence mechanisms are discussed in Chapter 6.

Sexuality

According to Freud, the energy or psychic drive associated with the sexual instinct, called the *libido*, translated from Latin as "pleasure" or "lust," resides in the id. When sexual desire is controlled and not expressed, tension results and is transformed into anxiety (Freud, 1905). Freud believed that adult sexuality is an end product of a complex process of development that begins in early childhood and involves a variety of body functions or areas (oral, anal, and genital zones) that correspond to stages of relationships, especially with parents.

Psychoanalysis

Freud (1949) developed *psychoanalysis*, a therapeutic process of accessing the unconscious and with the mature adult mind resolving the conflicts that originated in childhood. As a system of psychotherapy, psychoanalysis attempted to reconstruct the personality by examining free associations (spontaneous, uncensored verbalizations of whatever comes to mind) and the interpretation of dreams (Freud, 1955). Freud believed that therapeutic relationships had their beginnings within the psychoanalytic framework.

Transference and Countertransference

Transference is the displacement of thoughts, feelings, and behaviours originally associated with significant others from childhood onto a person in a current therapeutic relationship (Moore & Fine, 1990). For example, a woman's feelings toward her parents as a child may be transferred to the therapist: if she were unconsciously angry with her parents, she may feel inexplicable anger and hostility toward her therapist. In psychoanalysis, the therapist uses transference as a therapeutic tool to help the patient understand emotional problems and their origin. It is considered an essential aspect of therapy. **Countertransference**, on the other hand, is defined as the direction of all the therapist's feelings and attitudes toward the patient. Feelings and perceptions caused by countertransference may interfere with the therapist's ability to understand the patient.

Neo-Freudian Models

Many of Freud's followers ultimately established their own forms of psychoanalysis. The various psychoanalytic schools have adopted other names because their doctrines deviated from Freudian theory.

Adler's Foundation for Individual Psychology

Alfred Adler was a Viennese psychiatrist, founder of the school of individual psychology, and an early colleague of Freud who disagreed with Freud's focus on instinctual determination. He focused instead on the social aspects of human existence. Adler believed mental health involves love, work, and community. For Adler (1963), the motivating force in human life is a striving for superiority. Seeking perfection and security while trying to avoid feelings of inferiority can lead the individual to adopt a life goal that is unrealistic and frequently expressed as an unreasoning desire for power and dominance (i.e., *inferiority complex*). Because inferiority is intolerable, the compensatory mechanisms set up by the mind may result in self-centred attitudes, overcompensation, and a retreat from life's problems.

Adler focused on growth, lifestyle, and becoming: humans are looking to realize their potential, to flourish within their community. Adlerian theory is based on principles of mutual respect, choice, responsibility, consequences, and belonging. It informs both psychotherapy (e.g., family therapy and Ellis' (1973) Rational Emotive Therapy) and education.

Jung's Analytical Psychology

One of Freud's earliest colleagues, Carl Gustav Jung, a Swiss psychoanalyst, created a model called *analytical psychology*. For Jung, humans were influenced not only by their past but also by their hopes for the future. He not only supported the idea of a personal unconscious but also proposed a second psychic system, inherited and universal to all humans, the **collective unconscious**. Within the collective unconscious are **archetypes**, symbols common to all cultures. Images such as "mother" or "hero" or "trickster," for instance, have forms common to every society (Jung, 1959). Jung described humans as having both feminine and masculine characteristics; therapy may help an individual develop more fully as a person by embracing both aspects of himself or herself. The feminine side of men is the **anima**; the masculine side of women is the **animus**. His concept of **persona** (the mask one wears in society, one's public self) is similar to Freud's superego (Jung, 1966). The **shadow** is Jung's image for the dark side of every person, the side we do not like to recognize or show to others. To evolve as an individual, one needs to become aware of and integrate the shadow into one's personality.

Jung believed in the existence of two psychological types: the **extrovert** (who finds meaning in the world) and the **introvert** (who finds meaning within). He also described four primary modes of orientation to the world: *thinking, feeling, intuition,* and *sensation*. Although he argued that each of these functions exists in an individual, certain preferences will dominate. Our unconscious is revealed often through our least developed mode. The Myers-Briggs Type Indicator test is based on Jung's personality theory.

Horney's Feminine Psychology

Karen Horney, a German American psychiatrist, challenged many of Freud's basic concepts and introduced principles of feminine psychology. Recognizing a male bias in psychoanalysis, Horney questioned the psychoanalytic belief that women felt disadvantaged because of their genital organs, and she rejected Freud's concept of "penis envy." She argued that there are significant cultural reasons for women to strive to obtain qualities or privileges that are defined by a society as masculine and that women truly were at a disadvantage in a paternalistic culture (Horney, 1939). She observed that men have a deep-seated dread of women that is revealed in analysis (Horney, 1932). Her primary concept was that of basic anxiety: early (childhood) feelings of helplessness and isolation which one strives to cope with and resolve. According to Horney, this anxiety underlies all of an individual's relationships and can help explain behaviour. Horney (1950) named the unrealistic expectations that one puts on oneself "tyranny of the should." With other Neo-Freudians, such as Eric Fromm, she introduced sociocultural dimensions of human behaviour into the psychoanalytical model.

Humanistic Theories

Humanistic theories were generated as a reaction against psychoanalytic premises of instinctual drives and are based on the views of human potential for goodness. Humanist therapists focus on one's ability to learn about oneself, acceptance of self, and exploration of personal capabilities. Within the therapeutic relationship, the patient begins to develop positive attitudes and views himself or herself as a person of worth. The focus is not on investigation of repressed memories but on learning to experience the world in a different way.

Rogers' Client-Centred Therapy

Carl Rogers, an American psychologist, developed new methods of client-centred therapy. Rogers (1980) defined empathy as the capacity to assume the internal reference of the client in order to perceive the world in the same way as the client. To use empathy in the therapeutic process, the counsellor must be nondirective but not passive. Thus, the counsellor's attitude and nonverbal communication are crucial. He advocated that the therapist develops **unconditional positive regard**, a nonjudgmental caring, for the client (Rogers, 1980) and believed that the therapist's emotional investment (i.e., true caring) in the client is essential to the therapeutic process. Genuineness on the part of the therapist, in contrast with the passivity of the psychoanalyst, is seen as key.

Gestalt Therapy

Another humanistic response to the psychoanalytic model was Gestalt therapy, developed by Frederick S. (Fritz) Perls. Perls believed that modern civilization inevitably produces neurotic anxiety because it forces people to repress natural desires and frustrates an inherent human tendency to adjust biologically and psychologically to the environment. For a person to be cured, unmet needs must be brought back to awareness. Perls rejected the notion that intellectual insight enabled people to change. His individual and group exercises aimed to enhance a person's awareness of emotions, physical state, and repressed needs as well as physical and psychological stimuli in the here-and-now environment (Perls, 1969).

Maslow's Hierarchy of Needs

Abraham Maslow developed a humanistic model that is used in PMH nursing today (Maslow, 1998). His major contributions were to the understanding of human needs and motivation (Maslow, 1970). He studied exemplary healthy individuals (e.g., Albert Einstein) whom he saw as self-actualizing and described their characteristics. For instance, he noted that they were creative, had a deep sense of kinship with others, and had a strong sense of ethics. People are self-actualized when they are making the most of their unique human potential. Maslow's view of human motivation was based on a hierarchy of needs, ranging from lower-level survival needs, such as air, water, basic food, and shelter, to higher-level needs, such as those for belonging and esteem and, finally, for **self-actualization**. One must meet lower-level needs before moving to the higher-level ones (see Fig. 8.1). According to Maslow's model, values such as truth, beauty, and justice are aspects of our metaneeds, and their persistent deprivation can lead to spiritual–existential ailments often expressed as apathy, boredom, hopelessness, and

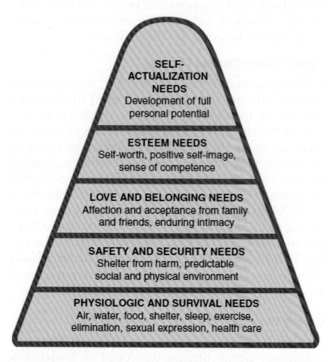

Figure 8.1. Maslow's hierarchy of needs.

powerlessness (Hoffman, 1996). Maslow's model offers a framework for assessment.

Applicability of Psychodynamic Theories to PMH Nursing

Several concepts in psychodynamic models are core elements in PMH nursing practice, such as interpersonal relationships, needs, anxiety, defence mechanisms, transference, and countertransference. Many of these concepts are further developed within nursing theories. A key psychodynamic concept, the therapeutic relationship, is recognized as a core of PMH nursing intervention.

Behavioural Theories

Behavioural theories, with roots in the discipline of psychology, offer important explanatory models for PMH nursing in terms of the way in which people act and learn (Table 8.2).

Early Stimulus–Response Theories

Pavlovian Theory

One of the earliest behavioural theorists was Ivan P. Pavlov, who was studying the gastric functioning of dogs when he noticed that stomach secretions of dogs were stimulated by triggers other than food, such as the sight and smell of food. He became interested in this anticipatory secretion. Through his experiments, he was able to stimulate secretions with a variety of other laboratory nonphysiologic stimuli. Thus, a clear connection was made between thought processes and physiologic responses.

In Pavlov's model, there is an unconditioned stimulus (not dependent on previous training) that elicits an unconditioned (i.e., specific) response. In his experiments, meat was the unconditioned stimulus, and salivation was the unconditioned response. Pavlov would then select other stimuli, such as a bell, a ticking metronome, and a triangle drawn on a large cue card, presenting this conditioned stimulus just before the meat, the unconditioned stimulus. If the conditioned stimulus was repeatedly presented before the meat, eventually salivation was elicited by the conditioned stimulus. This phenomenon was called **classical** (Pavlovian) **conditioning** (Pavlov, 1927/1960).

John B. Watson and the Behaviourist Revolution

At about the same time Pavlov was working in Russia, John B. Watson initiated the psychological revolution known as **behaviourism** in the United States. He developed two principles: frequency and recency. The principle of frequency states that the more often a given response is made to a given stimulus, the more likely the response to that stimulus will be repeated. The principle of recency states that the more recently a given response to a particular stimulus is made, the more likely it will be repeated. Watson's major contribution

Table 8.2 Psychological Theories: Behavioural, Cognitive, and Developmental

Theorist	Overview	Major Concepts	Applicability
Stimulus–Response Theories			
Ivan P. Pavlov (1849–1936)	Classical conditioning	Unconditioned stimuli Unconditioned response Conditioned stimuli	Important in understanding learning of automatic responses such as habitual behaviours
John B. Watson (1878–1958)	Introduced behaviourism, believed that learning was classical conditioning called *reflexes*; rejected distinction between the mind and the body	Principle of frequency Principle of recency	Focuses on the relationship between the mind and the body
Reinforcement Theories			
B. F. Skinner (1904–1990)	Developed an understanding of the importance of reinforcement and differentiated types and schedules	Operant behaviour Respondent behaviour Continuous reinforcement Intermittent reinforcement	Important in behaviour modification
Edward L. Thorndike (1874–1949)	Believed in the importance of effects that followed behaviour	Reinforcement	Important in behaviour modification programs
Cognitive Theories			
Albert Bandura (b. 1925)	Developed social cognitive theory, a model for understanding how behaviour is learned from others	Modelling Disinhibition Elicitation Self-efficacy	Important in helping patients learn appropriate behaviours
Aaron Beck (b. 1921)	Conceptualized distorted cognitions as a basis for depression.	Cognitions Beliefs	Important in cognitive therapy
Kurt Lewin (1890–1947)	Developed field theory, a system for understanding learning, motivation, personality, and social behaviour	Life space Positive valences Negative valences	Important in understanding motivation for changing behaviour
Edward Chace Tolman (1886–1959)	Introduced the concept of cognitions; believed that human beings act on beliefs and attitudes and strive toward goals	Cognition	Important in identifying the person's beliefs
Developmental Theories			
Erik Erikson (1902–1994)	Viewed psychosocial development as influenced by environment and occurring in stages, each one having a task to resolve	Eight stages Trust vs. mistrust Autonomy vs. shame/doubt Initiative vs. guilt Industry vs. inferiority Identity vs. role diffusion Intimacy vs. isolation Generativity vs. stagnation Ego integrity vs. despair	Allows unresolved developmental tasks to be identified
Jean Piaget (1896–1980)	Viewed intelligence as adaptation to the environment. Understood cognitive development in children to be like embryonic development: increasing differentiation in structure	Children learn particular concepts only when they have reached the appropriate stage of development	Important in assessment of children Useful in age-appropriate health education for children
Carol Gilligan (1936–)	Gender differences in moral development	Found a tendency for females to be more focused in relationships and issues of care in resolving moral problems, while males tend to apply abstract principles such as justice	Important in the evolution of gender studies

was the rejection of the distinction between body and mind and his emphasis on the study of objective behaviour (Watson & Rayner, 1917).

Reinforcement Theories

Edward L. Thorndike

A pioneer in experimental animal psychology, Edwin L. Thorndike, studied the problem-solving behaviour of cats to determine whether animals solved problems by reasoning or instinct. He found that neither choice was completely correct; animals gradually learn the correct response by "stamping in" the stimulus–response connection. The major difference between Thorndike and behaviourists such as Watson was that Thorndike believed in the importance of the effects that followed the response or the reinforcement of the behaviour.

He was the first reinforcement theorist, and his view of learning became the dominant view in learning theory (Thorndike, 1916, c.1906).

B. F. Skinner

One of the most influential behaviourists, B. F. Skinner, recognized two different kinds of learning, each involving a separate kind of behaviour. *Respondent behaviour*, or the end result of **classical conditioning**, is elicited by specific stimuli. Given the stimulus, the response occurs automatically. The other kind of learning is referred to as **operant behaviour**. In this type of learning, the distinctive characteristic is the consequence of a particular behavioural response not a specific stimulus. The learning of operant behaviour is also known as *conditioning*, but it is different from the conditioning of reflexes. If a behaviour occurs and is followed by reinforcement, it is probable that the behaviour will recur. For example, if a child climbs on a chair, reaches the faucet, and is able to get a drink of water successfully, it is more likely that the child will repeat the behaviour (Skinner, 1935). Skinner wrote a book about a utopian community based on the principles of behaviourism that he titled *Walden II* (Skinner, 1976).

Cognitive Theories

The initial behavioural studies focused attention on human actions without attention to the internal thinking process. As complex behaviour was examined and could not be accounted for by strictly behavioural explanations, thought processes became new subjects for study. Cognitive theories, an outgrowth of different theoretic perspectives including the behavioural and the psychodynamic, attempted to link internal thought processes with human behaviour.

Albert Bandura's Social Cognitive Theory

Acquiring behaviours by learning from other people is the basis of social cognitive theory developed by the psychologist Albert Bandura, born in Mundare, Alberta. Bandura developed his ideas after being concerned about violence on television contributing to aggression in children. He believes that important behaviours are learned by internalizing behaviours of others. His initial contribution was identifying the process of **modelling**: pervasive imitation or one person trying to be like another. According to Bandura, the model may not need to be a real person but could be a character in history or generalized to an ideal person (Bandura, 1977).

The concept of **disinhibition** is important to Bandura's model and refers to the situation in which someone has learned not to make a response; then, in a given situation, when another is making the inhibited response, the individual becomes disinhibited and also makes the response. Thus, the response that was "inhibited" now becomes disinhibited through a process of imitation. For example, during severe dieting, an individual may have learned to resist eating large amounts of food. However, when at a party with a friend who eagerly fills a plate at a buffet, the person also eats large amounts of food.

In the instance of disinhibition, the desire to eat is already there, and the individual indulges that desire. However, in another instance called **elicitation**, there is no desire present, but when one person starts an activity, others want to do the same. An example of this occurs when a child is playing with a toy and the other children now want to play with the same toy even though they showed no interest in it before that time.

An important concept of Bandura's model is **self-efficacy**, a person's sense of his or her ability to deal effectively with the environment which he develops in his work, *Self-Efficacy: The Exercise of Control* (1997). Efficacy beliefs influence how people feel, think, motivate themselves, and behave. The stronger the self-efficacy, the higher the goals people set for themselves and the firmer their commitment to them. Social cognitive theory extends to understanding collective efficacy and the way in which people strive to shape and control their lives.

Aaron T. Beck: Thinking and Feeling

American psychiatrist Aaron T. Beck of the University of Pennsylvania devoted his career to understanding the relationship between **cognition** and mental health. For Beck, cognitions are verbal or pictorial events in the stream of consciousness. He realized the importance of cognitions when treating people with depression, finding that the depression improved when patients began thinking differently. He believed that people with depression had faulty information-processing systems that led to biased cognitions. These faulty beliefs cause errors in judgment that become habitual errors in thinking. When individuals incorrectly interpret life situations, they judge themselves too harshly and jump to inaccurate conclusions. Individuals may, for example, truly believe that they have no friends and therefore no one cares. On examination, the evidence for the beliefs is faulty. For instance, it may be that there has been no contact with anyone because of moving from one city to another or because calls are not returned nor invitations accepted. Thus, distorted beliefs are the basis of the cognitions. Beck, Thase, and Wright (2003) developed cognitive therapy, a successful approach for the treatment of depressive disorders (Chapter 22). Beck (2011) continues to develop cognitive–behavioural therapy. See Chapter 13 for an overview of cognitive–behavioural techniques.

Applicability of Cognitive and Behavioural Theories to PMH Nursing

Interventions based on cognitive and behavioural theories are important in nursing. For example, patient education interventions are usually based on learning principles derived from these theories, and the teaching of new coping skills for patients in their recovery is usually based on them. Changing an entrenched habit involves helping people to identify what motivates them, recognize cues that precede the behaviour they desire to change, and create new lifestyle habits. Examples of cognitive and behavioural interventions used on inpatient hospital units include privilege systems and token economies and the application of cognitive–behavioural interventions (see Chapter 13).

Developmental Theories

Developmental theories explain normal human growth and development and focus on change over time. Many are presented in terms of stages based on the assumption that normal development proceeds stage-by-stage longitudinally. Human development, however, does not necessarily unfold sequentially and in the same way for each person.

Erik Erikson: Psychosocial Development

Erik Erikson's psychosocial developmental model, an expansion of Freud's psychosexual development theory, is commonly used in nursing. Each of Erikson's eight stages is associated with a specific task that can be successfully or unsuccessfully resolved. The model is organized according to developmental conflicts by age: basic trust versus mistrust, autonomy versus shame and doubt, initiative versus guilt, industry versus inferiority, identity versus role diffusion, intimacy versus isolation, generativity versus stagnation, and ego integrity versus despair. Erikson's wife, Joan Serson Erickson, extended his theory to include old age as a ninth stage, gerotranscendence (Erikson & Erikson, 1997). Gerotranscendence theory focused on the continued growth in dimensions such as spirituality and inner strength (see Chapter 31).

Within Erickson's theory, successful resolution of a crisis leads to essential strength and virtues. For example, a positive outcome of the trust versus mistrust crisis is the development of a basic sense of trust. If the crisis is unsuccessfully resolved, the infant moves into the next stage without a sense of trust. According to this model, a child who is mistrustful will have difficulty completing the next crisis successfully and, instead of developing a sense of autonomy, will more likely be full of shame and doubt (Erikson, 1963). One of Erikson's major contributions was the recognition of the turbulence of adolescent development. Erikson wrote extensively about adolescence, youth, and identity formation. When adolescence begins, childhood ways must be given up, and body changes must be reconciled with the individual's social position, previous history, and identifications. An identity is formed. This task of reconciling how young people see themselves and how society perceives them can become overwhelming and lead to role confusion and alienation (Erikson, 1968).

Research has explored developmental stages of this model with mixed results. For instance, in an early study, male college students who measured low on identity also scored low on intimacy ratings (Orlofsky, Marcia, & Lesser, 1973), lending support to the idea that identity precedes intimacy. Yet in another study, intimacy was found to begin developing early in adolescence, prior to the development of identity (Ochse & Plug, 1986). Studying fathers with young children, Christiansen and Palkovitz (1998) found that *generativity* (defined as the need or drive to produce, create, or effect a change) was associated with a paternal identity, psychosocial identity, and psychosocial intimacy. In a longitudinal study testing Erikson's model, 86 men were assessed at 21 years of age and then at 52 years. Fifty-six percent of the men achieved generativity, which was associated with work achievement, close friendships, successful marriage, altruistic behaviours, and mental health. Favourable predictors in young adulthood included a warm family environment and good peer relationships (Westermeyer, 2004). Research also suggests that gender influences development. One study found generativity to be associated with well-being in both males and females. In males, however, generativity seems related to the urge for self-protection, self-assertion, self-expansion, and mastery, while in women, the antecedents may be the desire for contact, connection, and union (Ackerman, Zuroff, & Moskowitz, 2000). A Canadian study that investigated grandparents' role in the socialization of children within the family queried whether midlife generativity would predict parents' descriptions of grandparenting problems. It did: generative fathers were more optimistic that problems with grandparents would be solved; both generative mothers and fathers showed higher levels of forgiveness of grandparents (Pratt, Norris, Cressman, Lawford, & Hebblethwaite, 2008).

Jean Piaget: Learning in Children

One of the most influential people in child psychology was Jean Piaget, who was the first to make a systematic study of cognitive development (Piaget, 1936). Piaget viewed intelligence as an adaptation to the environment. He proposed that cognitive growth is like embryologic growth: an organized structure increasingly differentiates over time. He determined that readiness is an important consideration in children's learning. According to Piaget, a particular concept should be taught to children only when they have reached an appropriate stage of development. Piaget developed a system that explains how knowledge develops and changes. Each stage of cognitive development represents a particular structure with major characteristics (Piaget, 1957). Piaget tested his theory through observation of his own children; the theory was never subjected to formal testing.

The major strength of his model was its recognition of the central role of cognition in development and the discovery of surprising features of young children's thinking. For nursing, Piaget's model provides a framework in which to define different levels of thinking and use the data in the assessment and intervention processes.

Carol Gilligan: Gender Differentiation

Psychologist Carol Gilligan studied the ways males and females approached moral problems and identified differences (Gilligan, 1982). She wrote about these differences in moral development in her 1982 landmark work, *In a Different Voice: Psychological Theory and Women's Development.* While males tended to approach moral problems by applying abstract rules such as those related to justice, the females in her study were more likely to be concerned with preserving the relationships of those involved and with responsibilities related to care. For Gilligan, attachment within relationships is the important factor for successful female development. Thus, traditional models of development that advocate separation as a primary goal of human development, such as Erikson's, disadvantage women. They can be viewed as impaired by the importance placed on attachments. According to Gilligan, female development does not follow a progression of stages but is based on experiences within relationships. This may be the case for males, as well, in their development of a strong sense of self (Nelson, 1996).

The scientific merit of Gilligan's work has been challenged by many critics, including feminist scholars, but it has had a significant impact on the development of gender studies (Graham, 2012).

Applicability of Developmental Theories to PMH Nursing

Developmental theories are used in understanding childhood and adolescent experiences and their manifestations as adult problems. When working with children, nurses can use developmental models to help gauge development and mood. However, because most of the models are based on the assumptions of the linear progression of stages and have not been adequately tested, applicability has limitations. In addition, these models were based on a relatively small number of children who typically were raised in a Western middle-class environment. Most do not account for gender differences and diversity in lifestyles and cultures.

■ SOCIAL THEORIES

Numerous social theories underlie PMH nursing practice, and the nursing profession itself serves a specific societal function. This section represents a sampling of important social theories that nurses may use. This discussion is not exhaustive and should be viewed by the student as including only some of the theoretic perspectives that may be applicable.

Family Dynamics

Family dynamics are the patterned interpersonal and social interactions that occur within the family structure over the life of a family. Family dynamics models are based on systems theory describing a phenomenon in terms of a set of interrelated parts, in which the change of one part affects the total functioning of the system. A system can be "open" and interacting in the environment or "closed," completely self-contained, and not influenced by the environment. The family is viewed organizationally as an open system in which one member's actions influence the functioning of the total system. Most of the theoretic explanations have emerged from treatment case studies, rather than from systematic development of theory based on generalizable research. Consequently, the limitation of available research should be considered when these models are used to understand family interactions and plan patient care (see Chapter 15).

Applicability of Family Theories to PMH Nursing

Family theories are especially useful to nurses who are assessing family dynamics and planning interventions (Wright & Leahey, 2013). Family systems models are used to help nurses form collaborative relationships with patients and families dealing with health problems. While only nurses with specialized training in family therapy will be engaged in it, understanding family dynamics is important in every nurse's practice, and family theories must inform nurses' family interventions (see Chapter 15). The mental health problems or mental illness of a family member will have important implications for the entire family system.

Role Theories

A **role** describes an individual's social position and function within an environment. Anthropologic theories explain members' roles that relate to a specific society. For example, the universal role of healer may be assumed by a nurse in one culture and a spiritual leader in another. Societal expectations, social status, and rights are attached to these roles. Psychological theories, which are concerned about roles from a different perspective, focus on the individual and the self. The responsibilities of a parent are often in conflict with the personal needs for time alone. All of the Neo-Freudian and humanist models that have been discussed focus on reciprocal social relationships or interactions that determine how the mind develops.

Applicability of Role Theories to PMH Nursing

Role theories emphasize the importance of social interaction in either the individual's choice of a particular role or society's recognition of it. Several nursing models have role as a major concept, including King (1971), Roy (1974), and Peplau (1952). PMH nursing uses role concepts in understanding group interaction and the role of the patient in the family and community (see Chapters 14 and 15). In addition, milieu therapy approaches discussed in later chapters are based on the patient's assumption of a role within the psychiatric care environment.

Sociocultural Perspectives

Gender and culture are now recognized as significant in determining human behaviour, including the manifestation of mental health problems and illness, as well as in shaping our understanding of health and disease. Critical and emancipatory scholarship is furthering our understanding of the way power differences can stigmatize and marginalize minority groups and can take institutionalized form. Canadian society is addressing these issues in our national mental health strategy that stresses the importance of health care services that are gender and culturally sensitive.

Gender

There is no foundational figure in the application of feminist approaches to psychotherapy, but rather many scholars who used feminist theory to inform and advance practice (Truscott, 2010).

From Horney's (1932) *Feminine Psychology* to Chesler's (1972) *Women and Madness* to Brown's (2010) *Feminist Therapy*, feminist therapists have been challenging societal, political, and medical conventions that frame gender in oppressive and discriminatory ways. They have reintroduced validity to concepts such as emotions and embodied knowledge that were previously deemed irrational and thus dysfunctional. Throughout the development of feminist approaches to therapy, a constant has been that the constructs of gender, power, and powerlessness inform the therapy process; feminist therapy is not just for women (Brown, 2010).

Since the 1970s, gender identity and sexual orientation studies have been bringing together scholarship from areas such as biology, psychology, sociology, science, philosophy, political science, and ethics to further understanding and knowledge of lesbian, gay, bisexual, transgender, and intersex (LGBTI) identities. Such knowledge is important to the competent and ethical practice of nurses and other health professionals, but significant gaps remain. Research indicates, for instance, that nurses lack knowledge regarding the nursing needs of transgendered persons and experience uncertainty regarding how to interact with them and their families (Carabez, Eliason, & Martinson, 2016). Further, nursing curricula needs to better address LGBTI health (Carabez et al., 2015). There is a pressing need for nursing research, scholarship, and education to advance our understanding in this area.

Culture

Likewise, postcolonial theories and Marxist approaches have been introduced and call on nurses to attend to the ways that the various notions of race and class function in our understanding of psychiatric illness and mental health, respectively. "The social and moral mandate of nursing is now seen to include illumination of the experiences of those marginalized within society and within health care" (Kirkham & Anderson, 2002, p. 2).

Madeleine Leininger: Transcultural Health Care

Concern about the impact of culture on the treatment of children with psychiatric and emotional problems led Madeleine Leininger, a nurse anthropologist, to develop a new field called transcultural nursing, which is directed toward holistic, congruent, and beneficent care. She used concepts from anthropology and nursing (from such theorists as Henderson, 1966; Rogers, 1970; Watson, 1979) to depict universal and diverse dimensions of human caring. Because caring is an integral part of being human, as well as a learned behaviour, caring is culturally based (Leininger, 1991, 1999). Care is considered the essence of nursing, and caring manifestations include compassion, presence, and enabling (Leininger, 1993). Leininger developed a model to depict her theory symbolically. The model depicts the "world view, religion, kinship, cultural values, economics, technology, language, ethnohistory, and environmental factors that are predicted to explain and influence culture care" (p. 27).

Applicability of Sociocultural Theories to PMH Nursing

Sociocultural theories are important to PMH nursing practice as the sociocultural aspect is integral to mental health. Adequate nursing assessments and interventions are not possible without consideration of the role of the individual within the family and within society and the significance of familial and cultural norms. Understanding cultural values is crucial to meaningful interactions with persons, families, and communities (see Chapter 3). Health care systems have their own cultures, as well, and it is necessary for nurses to ensure that the care environment is safe and conducive to healing and recovery (see Chapter 11). Sociocultural theories inform many group interventions (see Chapter 14).

■ SPIRITUAL THEORIES

Frankl's Logotherapy

Viktor Frankl was an Austrian psychiatrist who survived being a prisoner in Nazi concentration camps during World War II. In his book *Man's Search for Meaning*, he describes the way he discovered the importance of meaning to human existence (Frankl, 1992). Frankl wrote that each of us needs to find a reason to live. Life, otherwise, can seem empty. An existentialist therapy, logotherapy is focused on helping a person find meaning in life. Based on his experience, Frankl concluded that love was the greatest salvation. Even when one's only option is to endure suffering, contemplation of a beloved enables suffering to be endured in an honourable way (Frankl, 1992).

Yalom's Existential Psychotherapy

Influenced by Frankl's work, Irving Yalom grounds his existential psychotherapy upon what he considers central or ultimate life concerns: death, freedom, isolation, and meaninglessness. As each person attempts to confront these concerns, conflicts may arise. In his theory, Yalom (1980) describes how life concerns play a role in psychopathology and psychotherapy. For instance, "fear of death plays a major role in our internal experience; it haunts as does nothing else" (p. 27). A childhood developmental task is to deal with this fear. Often, however, we use denial to keep awareness of death at bay. Ineffective modes of facing our mortality can result in psychopathology; psychotherapy, therefore, may need to be aimed at death awareness. Yalom does not claim the existential orientation is *the* paradigm from which to understand all behaviour: the human being is too complex for this to be possible. However, existential psychotherapy is a useful, systematic approach for addressing many people's clinical situation or symptoms (Box 8.2).

Applicability of Spiritual Theories to PMH Nursing

As well as directly influencing nurse theorists such as Travelbee, these theoretic perspectives allow nurses to explore the way the search for meaning in life and death shapes human development, experience, and understanding.

RECOVERY AS A FRAMEWORK FOR MENTAL HEALTH CARE

In the Canadian Senate report *Out of the Shadows at Last: Transforming Mental Health, Mental Illness and Addiction Services in Canada,* recovery is placed at the centre of mental health reform. It is acknowledged that recovery is an active process rather than an end point and that each individual's path to recovery is unique (Kirby & Keon, 2006, p. 5). When the framework for such a transformation of the health care system was presented

---

BOX 8.2 Research for Best Practice

RESPONDING TO THE EXISTENTIAL SUFFERING OF PATIENTS WITH SEVERE, PERSISTENT MENTAL ILLNESS (SPMI)

Moonen, C., Lemiengre, J., & Gastmans, C. (2016). *Dealing with existential suffering of patients with severe, persistent mental illness: Experiences of psychiatric nurses in Flanders (Belgium).* Archives of Psychiatric Nursing, 30(2), 219–225.

Background: The existential suffering of persons living with a SPMI can be directly related to their illness, its symptoms and treatment, and/or indirectly to the stigma, loneliness, and loss of autonomy and self-esteem associated with SPMI.

Research Question: How do nurses deal with patients with SPMI who experience hopeless existential suffering?

Method: A qualitative research design informed by grounded theory was used. Semistructured interviews were completed with 15 nurses who were asked to describe a concrete trajectory of care with which the nurse was involved for a patient with a SPMI experiencing existential suffering. Twenty cases were described by participants.

Findings: A process-related development of nursing care was identified with four pillars or nonsequential phases. Observing/meeting the patient initiated the process but also continued as the relationship evolved. Evaluating status of the patient and getting to know the patient was part of this phase, usually involving questioning

by the nurse as expressing themselves can be difficult for persons with SPMI. The next pillar was focused on acknowledgment of the person by the nurse as a full individual beyond the status of patient. Genuinely seeing and listening to the person was augmented in small ways (e.g., learning preferences such as favourite TV show). Recognition of the patient's suffering by taking it seriously and expressing empathy occurred. Development of a caring relationship built upon trust followed. Respectful care of the patient across physical, mental, relational, social, and spiritual domains was given. Such a relationship supports patients in expressing distress and suffering and in exploring ways to find meaning and purpose in their lives. Concluding the relationship was the final pillar for nurses whose patients left hospital or were transferred. One nurse's patient died by suicide. Other nurses described continuing the relationship. Contextual factors (institutional, team, individual) influenced the process by stimulating or restricting it.

Implications for Nursing: The existential suffering of patients with SPMI can go unacknowledged in mental health care. Nurses can support such patients through the development of a caring, trust-based relationship and by being aware of the universal need of all humans to find purpose and meaning in their lives.

(Mental Health Commission of Canada, 2009), recovery was conceived of as broader than *clinical* recovery (remission or cure). While persons with mental illness do experience clinical recovery, recovery is better understood as living a satisfying and hopeful life, even with mental health problems or illness.

Recovery

A recovery orientation is a significant shift from the medically centred approach to mental health care. Persons with mental illness and their families are to be engaged in such a way that strengths, resources, and rights are acknowledged. Health professionals are to practice in culturally safe ways that respond meaningfully to diversity; address complex mental health needs in the least restrictive ways possible; and broaden the types of evidence they use to evaluate individual improvements in health and well-being. Like other health professionals, nurses will need to assess, and perhaps adapt, their current theoretical perspectives in regard to the centrality of recovery.

KEY CONCEPT

Recovery is "a process in which people living with mental health problems and illnesses are empowered and supported to be actively engaged in their own journey of well-being. The recovery process builds on individual, family, cultural, and community strengths and enables people to enjoy a meaningful life in their community while striving to achieve their full potential" (Mental Health Commission of Canada, 2009, p. 122).

SUMMARY OF KEY POINTS

- Nursing theories form the conceptual basis for nursing practice and are useful in a variety of PMH settings.
- The Tidal Model and its focus on the person's experience and on recovery are increasingly used as an approach to care in PMH settings.
- The traditional psychodynamic framework helped form the basis of early nursing interpersonal interventions, including the development of therapeutic relationships and the use of such concepts as transference, countertransference, empathy, and object relations.
- The cognitive and behavioural theories are often used in strategies that help patients change behaviour and thinking.
- Sociocultural theories remain important in understanding and interacting with patients as members of families, cultures, and society.

- Spiritual theories offer a way to consider the human search for meaning in life and how a patient's view of life can affect his or her health and well-being.
- The recovery orientation recommended by Canada's mental health strategy is an important paradigm shift in the approach to mental health care.

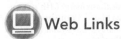 Web Links

www.ebscohost.com/academic/lgbt-life-with-full-text This database indexes leading books, articles, magazines, and newspapers related to LGBT topics.

www.florence-nightingale.co.uk/ This is the site of the Florence Nightingale Museum.

www.feministvoices.com/carol-gilligan/ This site, Psychology's Feminist Voices, provides a brief overview of Carol Gilligan and a video-taped interview with her.

www.freud.org.uk This is the Web site of the Freud Museum in London. It has pictures, publications, and links to other relevant sites.

www.humanbecoming.org The International Consortium of Parse Scholars' Web site has an overview of the humanbecoming theory and related research.

www.jungianstudies.org This is the site of the International Association of Jungian Studies which will be of interest to those wanting to learn more about his work.

www.mcgill.ca/nursing/about/model/ This site offers information about the McGill model and its origins and examples of its application in nursing practice.

nursingtheories.weebly.com/ Most of the major nursing theories are delineated at this Web site.

www.societyofrogerianscholars.org/publications.html *Visions: The Journal of Rogerian Nursing Science* can be found at this Web site.

www.tidal-model.com/ *The* evolution of the Tidal Model and its core concepts are presented.

References

Abraham, S. (2011). Fall prevention conceptual framework. *Health Care Manager, 30*(2), 179–184.

Ackerman, S., Zuroff, D. C., & Moskowitz, D. S. (2000). Generativity in midlife and young adults: Links to agency, communion, and subjective well-being. *International Journal of Aging and Human Development, 5*(1), 17–41.

Adler, A. (1963). *The practice and theory of individual psychotherapy.* Paterson, NJ: Littlefield, Adams.

Allen, M. (1977). Comparative theories of the expanded role in nursing and its implications for nursing practice: A working paper. *Nursing Papers/Perspectives en Nursing, 9,* 38–45.

Austin, W., Gallop, R., Harris, D., & Spencer, E. (1996). A domains of practice approach to the standards of psychiatric and mental health nursing practice. *Journal of Psychiatric and Mental Health Nursing, 3,* 111–115.

Bandura, A. (1977). *Social learning theory.* Englewood Cliffs, NJ: Prentice-Hall.

Bandura, A. (1997). *Self-efficacy: The exercise of control.* New York, NY: W. H. Freeman and Company.

Barker, P. (2001a). The Tidal Model: The lived-experience in person-centred mental health nursing care. *Nursing Philosophy, 2,* 213–223.

Barker, P. (2001b). The Tidal Model: Developing a person-centred approach to psychiatric and mental health nursing. *Perspectives in Psychiatric Care, 37,* 79–87.

Barker, P., & Buchanan-Barker, P. (2005). *The Tidal Model: A guide for mental health professionals.* London, UK: Brunner-Routledge.

Barker, P., & Buchanan-Barker, P. (2010). The Tidal Model of mental health recovery and reclamation: Application in acute care settings. *Issues in Mental Health Nursing, 31,* 171–180.

Barnhart, D. A., Bennett, P. M., Porter, B. D., & Sloan, R. S. (1994). Jean Watson: Philosophy and science of caring. In A. Marriner-Tomey (Ed.), *Nursing theorists and their work* (3rd ed., pp. 148–162). St. Louis, MO: Mosby.

Beck, J. (2011). *Cognitive behavior therapy: Basics and beyond.* New York, NY: Guilford Press.

Beck, A. T., Thase, M. D., & Wright, J. H. (2003). Cognitive therapy. In R. E. Hales & S. C. Ydofsky (Eds.), *Textbook of clinical psychiatry* (4th ed., pp. 1245–1283). Washington, DC: American Psychiatric Publishers, Inc.

Benner, P., & Wrubel, J. (1989). *The primacy of caring: Stress and coping in health and illness.* Menlo Park, CA: Addison-Wesley.

Biggs, A. (2008). Orem's self-care deficit nursing theory: Update on the state of the art and science. *Nursing Science Quarterly, 21*(3), 200–206.

Brookes, N., Murata, L., & Tansey, M. (2008). Tidal waves: Implementing a new model of mental health recovery and reclamation. *Canadian Nurse, 104*(8), 23–27.

Brown, L. (2010). *Feminist therapy.* Washington, DC: American Psychiatric Association.

Buchanan-Barker, P., & Barker, P. (2008). The Tidal commitments: Extending the value base of mental health recovery. *Journal of Psychiatric and Mental Health Nursing, 15,* 93–100.

Calaway, B. J. (2002). *Hildegard Peplau: Psychiatric nurse of the century.* New York, NY: Springer.

Canadian Federation of Mental Health Nurses (CFMHN). (2014). *The Canadian standards of psychiatric and mental health nursing* (4th ed.). Toronto, ON: Author.

Carabez, R., Eliason, M. J., & Martinson, M. (2016). Nurses' knowledge about transgender patient care: A qualitative study. *Advances in Nursing Science, 39*(3), 257–271.

Carabez, R., Pelligrini, M., Mankovitz, A., Eliason, M., Ciano, M., & Scott, M. (2015). "Never in all my years...": Nurses' education about LGBT Health. *Journal of Professional Nursing, 31*(4), 323–329.

Chesler, P. (1972). *Women and madness.* Garden City, NY: Doubleday.

Christiansen, S. L., & Palkovitz, R. (1998). Exploring Erikson's psychosocial theory and development: Generativity and its relationship to paternal identity, intimacy, and involvement in childcare. *Journal of Men's Studies, 7*(1), 133–156.

Clements, P., & Averill, J. (2006). Finding patterns of knowing in the work of Florence Nightingale. *Nursing Outlook, 54,* 268–274.

Coakley, A. B., Barron, A. M., & Annese, C. D. (2016). Exploring the experience and impact of therapeutic touch treatments for nurse colleagues. *Visions: The Journal of Rogerian Nursing Science, 22*(1), Manuscript 1, 13 pages.

Cummins, J. (2011). Sharing a traumatic event. The experience of the listener and the storyteller within the dyad. *Nursing Research, 60*(6), 386–392.

Deane, W. H. (2015). Incorporating Peplau's theory of interpersonal relations to promote holistic communication between older adults and nursing students. *Journal of Holistic Nursing, 34*(1), 35–41.

DeHowitt, M. (1992). King's conceptual model and individual psychotherapy. *Perspectives in Psychiatric Care, 28*(4), 11–14.

DeWan, S. A., & Ume-Nwagbo, P. N. (2006). Using the Neuman systems model for best practices. *Nursing Science Quarterly, 19*(1), 31–35.

Ellenberger, H. (1970). *The discovery of the unconscious: The history and evolution of dynamic psychiatry.* London, UK: Lane, Penguin Press.

Ellis, A. (1973). *Humanistic psychotherapy: The rational-emotive approach.* New York, NY: McGraw-Hill.

Erikson, E. (1963). *Childhood and society* (2nd ed.). New York, NY: Norton.

Erikson, E. (1968). *Identity: Youth and crisis.* New York, NY: Norton.

Erikson, E., & Erikson, J. (1997). *The lifecycle completed, extended version.* New York, NY: Norton.

Feeley, N., & Gottlieb, L. (2000). Nursing approaches for working with family strengths and resources. *Journal of Family Nursing, 6*(1), 9–24.

Frankl, V. (1992). *Man's search for meaning: An introduction to logotherapy* (4th ed.). Boston, MA: Beacon Press.

Freud, S. (1905). Three essays on the theory of sexuality (1953). In J. Strachey, A. Freud, A. Strachey, & A. Tyson (Eds.). *The standard edition of the complete psychological works of Sigmund Freud* (pp. 135–248). London, UK: Hogarth Press.

Freud, S. (1927). The ego and the id (1957). In E. Jones (Ed.). *The international psycho-analytical library* (No. 12). London, UK: Hogarth Press.

Freud, S. (1949). *An outline of psychoanalysis.* New York, NY: Norton.

Freud, S. (1955). *The interpretation of dreams.* London, UK: Hogarth Press.

Georges, J. (2005). Linking nursing theory and practice: A critical-feminist approach. *Advances in Nursing Science, 28*(1), 30–57.

Gilligan, C. (1982). *In a different voice: Psychological theory and women's development.* Cambridge, MA: Harvard University Press.

Gottlieb, L., & Rowat, K. (1987). The McGill model of nursing: A practice-derived model. *Advances in Nursing Science, 9*(4), 51–61.

Graham, R. (2012). Carol Gilligan's persistent "voice": Thirty years after the feminist classic "In a Different Voice" shook up psychology, do its claims hold up at all? In The Boston Globe. Retrieved from http://www.bostonglobe.com/

Henderson, V. (1966). *The nature of nursing: A definition and its implications for practice, research, and education.* New York, NY: Macmillan.

Hoffman, E. (Ed.). (1996). *Future visions: The unpublished papers of Abraham Maslow.* Newbury Park, CA: Sage Publications, Inc.

Horney, K. (1932). *Feminine psychology.* New York, NY: Norton.

Horney, K. (1939). *New ways in psychoanalysis.* New York, NY: Norton.

Horney, K. (1950). *Neurosis and human growth.* New York, NY: Norton.

Jung, C. G. (1959). *The basic writings of C. G. Jung.* New York, NY: Modern Library.

Jung, C. G. (1966). On the psychology of the unconscious: The personal and the collective unconscious. In C. Jung (Ed.), *Collected works of C. G. Jung* (2nd ed., Vol. 7, pp. 64–79). Princeton, NJ: Princeton University Press.

King, I. M. (1971). *Toward a theory for nursing: General concepts of human behavior.* New York, NY: John Wiley and Sons.

King, I. M. (1981). *A theory for nursing: Systems, concepts, process.* New York, NY: John Wiley and Sons.

King, I. M. (1992). King's theory of goal attainment. *Nursing Science Quarterly, 5*(1), 19–26.

Kirby, M. J. L., & Keon, W. J. (2006). Out of the shadows at last: Transforming mental health, mental illness and addiction services in Canada. Retrieved from Parliament of Canada website: http://www.parl.gc.ca/39/1/parlbus/commbus/senate/com-e/soci-e/rep-e/rep-02may06-e.htm

Kirkham, S. R., & Anderson, J. M. (2002). Postcolonial nursing scholarship: From epistemology to method. *Advances in Nursing Science, 25*(1), 1–17.

Knowaja, K. (2006). Utilization of King's interacting systems framework and theory of goal attainment with new multidisciplinary model: Clinical pathway. *Australian Journal of Advanced Nursing, 24*(2), 44–49.

Laben, J., Dodd, D., & Snead, L. (1991). King's theory of goal attainment applied in group therapy for inpatient juvenile sexual offenders, maximum security state offenders, and community parolees, using visual aids. *Issues in Mental Health Nursing, 12*(1), 51–64.

Leddy, S., & Pepper, J. M. (1998). *Conceptual basis of professional nursing* (4th ed.). Philadelphia, PA: Lippincott.

Lego, S. (1973). Nurse psychotherapists: How are we different? *Perspectives in Psychiatric Care, 11,* 144–147.

Leininger, M. (1991). *Culture care diversity and universality: A theory of nursing.* New York, NY: National League for Nursing.

Leininger, M. (1993). Assumptive premises of the theory. In C. Reynolds & M. Leininger (Eds.), *Madeleine Leininger: Cultural care diversity and universality theory. Notes on nursing theories* (Vol. 8, pp. 15–30). Newbury Park, CA: Sage Publications, Inc.

Leininger, M. (1999). What is transcultural nursing and culturally competent care? *Journal of Transcultural Nursing, 10*(1), 9.

Lutjens, L. R. (1991a). *Callista Roy: An adaptation model.* Newbury Park, CA: Sage Publications, Inc.

Lutjens, L. R. (1991b). *Martha Rogers: The science of unitary human beings.* Newbury Park, CA: Sage Publications, Inc.

Maslow, A. (1970). *Motivation and personality* (rev. ed.). New York, NY: Harper & Brothers.

Maslow, A. (1998). *Toward a psychology of being* (3rd ed.). New York, NY: John Wiley & Sons.

Mental Health Commission of Canada. (2009). *Toward recovery and well-being: A framework for a mental health strategy for Canada.* Ottawa, ON: Author.

Moonen, C., Lemiengre, J., & Gastmans, C. (2016). Dealing with existential suffering of patients with severe, persistent mental illness: Experiences of psychiatric nurses in Flanders (Belgium). *Archives of Psychiatric Nursing, 30*(2), 219–225.

Moore, B., & Fine, B. (Eds.). (1990). *Psychoanalytic terms and concepts.* New Haven, CT: American Psychoanalytic Association and Yale University Press.

Nelson, M. (1996). Separation versus connection, the gender controversy: Implications for counseling women. *Journal of Counseling and Development, 74*(4), 339–344.

Neuman, B. (1989). *The Neuman systems model* (2nd ed.). East Norwalk, CT: Appleton & Lange.

Neuman, B., Newman, D. M. L., & Holder, P. (2000). Leadership and scholarship integration: Using the Neuman system model for 21st-century professional nursing practice. *Nursing Science Quarterly, 13*(1), 60–63.

Nightingale, F. (1859). *Notes on nursing: What it is and what it is not.* London, UK: Harrison, Bookseller to the Queen.

Ochse, R., & Plug, C. (1986). Cross-cultural investigation of the validity of Erikson's theory of personality development. *Journal of Personality and Social Psychology, 50*(6), 1240–1252.

Olowokere, A. E., & Okanlawon, F. A. (2015). Application of Neuman system model to psychosocial support of vulnerable school children. *West African Journal of Nursing, 26*(1), 14–25.

Olson, J. & Hanchett, E. (1997). Nurse-expressed empathy, patient outcomes, and the development of a middle-range theory. *Image: The Journal of Nursing Scholarship, 29*(1), 71–76.

Orem, D. (1991). *Nursing concepts of practice* (4th ed.). St. Louis, MO: Mosby–Year Book.

Orlando, I. J. (1961). *The dynamic nurse–patient relationship.* New York, NY: G. P. Putnam's Sons.

Orlando, I. J. (1972). *The discipline and teaching of nursing process.* New York, NY: G. P. Putnam's Sons.

Orlofsky, J., Marcia, J., & Lesser, I. (1973). Ego identity status and the intimacy versus isolation crisis of young adulthood. *Journal of Personality and Social Psychology, 27*(2), 211–219.

Parse, R. R. (1987). *Nursing science: Major paradigms, theories, and critiques.* Philadelphia, PA: Saunders.

Parse, R. R. (2007). The humanbecoming school of thought in 2050. *Nursing Science Quarterly, 20*, 308–311.

Partlak Günüşen, N., Üstün, B., & Gigliotti, E. (2009). Conceptualization of burnout from the perspective of the Neuman systems model. *Nursing Science Quarterly, 22*(3), 200–204.

Pavlov, I. P. (1927/1960). *Conditioned reflexes.* New York, NY: Dover Publications.

Peplau, H. (1952). *Interpersonal relations in nursing.* New York, NY: G. P. Putnam & Sons.

Peplau, H. (1992). Interpersonal relations: A theoretical framework for application in nursing practice. *Nursing Science Quarterly, 5*(1), 13–18.

Perls, F. (1969). *In and out of the garbage pail.* Lafayette, CA: Real People Press.

Piaget, J. (1936). *Origins of intelligence in the child.* London, UK: Routledge & Kegan Paul.

Piaget, J. (1957). *Construction of reality in the child.* London, UK: Kegan Paul.

Pickens, J. (2012). Development of self-care agency through enhancement of motivation in people with schizophrenia. *Self-Care, Dependent-Care & Nursing, 19*(1), 47–52.

Pratt, M., Norris, J., Cressman, K. Lawford, H., & Hebblethwaite, S. (2008). Parents' stories of grandparenting concerns in the three-generational family: Generativity, optimism, and forgiveness. *Journal of Personality, 76*(3), 581–604.

Rogers, C. (1980). *A way of being.* Boston, MA: Houghton Mifflin.

Rogers, M. E. (1970). *An introduction to the theoretical basis of nursing.* Philadelphia, PA: F.A. Davis.

Rogers, M. E. (1994). The science of unitary human beings: Current perspectives. *Nursing Science Quarterly, 7*(1), 33–35.

Roy, C. (1974). The Roy adaptation model. In J. P. Riehl & C. Roy (Eds.), *Conceptual models for nursing practice* (pp. 135–144). New York, NY: Appleton-Century-Crofts.

Seed, M. & Torkelson, D. (2012). Beginning the recovery journey in acute psychiatric care: Using concepts from Orem's self-care deficit nursing theory. *Issues in Mental Health Nursing, 33*, 394–398.

Skinner, B. F. (1935). The generic nature of the concepts of stimulus and response. *Journal of General Psychology, 12*, 40–65.

Skinner, B. F. (1976). *Walden II.* New York, NY: Macmillan.

Summerell, P. (2015). P. Jean Watson's caritas processes: A model for transforming the nursing practice environment. *Critical Care Nurse, 35*(2), e66–e67.

Thompson, J. E. (1990). Finding the borderline's border: Can Martha Rogers help? *Perspectives in Psychiatric Care, 26*(4), 7–10.

Thorndike, E. L. (1916, c.1906). *The principles of teaching, based on psychology.* New York, NY: A. G. Seiler.

Travelbee, J. (1969). *Intervention in psychiatric nursing: Process in the one-to-one relationship.* Philadelphia, PA: F.A. Davis.

Travelbee, J. (1971). *Interpersonal aspects of nursing* (2nd ed.). Philadelphia, PA: F.A. Davis.

Truscott, D. (2010). *Becoming an effective psychotherapist: Adopting a theory of psychotherapy that is right for you and your client.* Washington, DC: American Psychological Association.

Watson, J. (1979). *Nursing: The philosophy and science of caring* (2nd ed.). Boston, MA: Little, Brown.

Watson, J. (1988). *Nursing: Human science and human care: A theory of nursing.* New York, NY: National League for Nursing.

Watson, J. (2005). *Caring science as sacred science.* Philadelphia, PA: F.A. Davis.

Watson, J. B., & Rayner, R. (1917). Emotional reactions and psychological experimentation. *American Journal of Psychology, 28*, 163–174.

Westermeyer, J. (2004). Predictors and characteristics of Erikson's Life Cycle Model among men: A 32-year longitudinal study. *International Journal of Aging and Human Development, 58*(1), 29–48.

Wilson, D. R. (2016). Parse's nursing theory and its application to families experiencing empty arms. *International Journal of Childbirth Education, 31*(2), 29–33.

Wright, L. & Leahey, M. (2013). *Nurses and families: A guide to family assessment and intervention* (6th ed.). Philadelphia, PA: F.A. Davis.

Yalom, I. D. (1980). *Existential psychotherapy.* New York, NY: Basic Books.

Adapted from the chapter "The Biologic Foundations of Psychiatric Nursing" by Susan McCabe and Mary Ann Boyd

LEARNING OBJECTIVES

After studying this chapter, you will be able to:

- Identify ways in which the brain changes across the life span and affects behaviour.
- Describe the association between biologic functioning and symptoms of psychiatric disorders.
- Describe the approaches researchers have used to study the central nervous system and the significance of each approach.
- Locate the brain structures primarily involved in psychiatric disorders and describe the primary functions of these structures.
- Assess symptoms of common psychiatric disorders in terms of central nervous system functioning.
- Describe the mechanisms of neuronal transmission.
- Identify the location and function of neurotransmitters significant to hypotheses regarding major mental disorders.
- Discuss the basic utilization of new knowledge gained from fields of study, including psychoendocrinology, psychoimmunology, and chronobiology.
- Discuss the role of genetics in the development of psychiatric disorders.

KEY TERMS

- amino acids • animal models • autonomic nervous system • basal ganglia • biogenic amines • biologic markers • chronobiology • cortex • epigenetics • frontal, parietal, temporal, and occipital lobes • genome • hippocampus • limbic system • neurohormones • neuropeptides • polymorphism • psychoendocrinology • psychoneuroimmunology • receptors • risk factors • symptom expression • synapse • zeitgebers

KEY CONCEPTS

- neurotransmitters • plasticity

All behaviours recognized as human result from actions that originate in the brain and its dense interconnection of neural networks. Modern research has increased understanding of how the complex circuitry of the brain interacts with the external environment, memories, and experiences. Through the spinal column and peripheral nerves, along with other systems, such as the endocrine and immune systems, the brain constantly receives and processes information. As the brain shifts and sorts through the amazing amount of information it processes every hour, it decides on actions and initiates behaviours that allow each person to act in entirely unique and very human ways. As we age, our brain changes and, in turn, impacts our behaviour. See Table 9.1 for examples.

■ FOUNDATIONAL CONCEPTS

This chapter is a review of the basic information necessary for understanding neuroscience as it relates to the

role of the psychiatric and mental health (PMH) nurse. The review includes basic central nervous system (CNS) structures and functions, basic mechanisms of neurotransmission, general functions of the major neurotransmitters, basic structure and function of the endocrine system, genetic research, circadian rhythms, neuroimaging techniques, and biologic tests. This chapter was written with the assumption that the reader has a basic knowledge of human biology, anatomy, and pathophysiology. The chapter is not intended as a full presentation of neuroanatomy and physiology but rather as an overview of the structures and functions most critical to the role of the PMH nurse.

The Biologic Basis of Behaviour, Emotions, and Cognition

As our understanding of the brain grows, evidence accumulates that most human behaviours, thoughts, and

Table 9.1   Brain Changes Across the Life Span

Developmental Period	Some Brain Changes	Some Behavioural Changes
Gestational	By 3rd week gestation: formation of liquid-filled neural tube. First month: neuron production occurring at a maximum of 250,000 per minute. Around 14 week, neurons begin to migrate to form different brain areas, yet around 20 week, half of the cells are pruned. By birth, 100 billion neurons developed. Neural connections are immature but developing.	At birth, babies can hear, smell, see, and respond to touch. Prenatal stress, drugs, alcohol, and smoking impact brain development.
Early childhood to preschool	Rapid increase in synapses with strengthening in connections of those frequently used. Elimination of unused connections. Number of white matter neurons in the motor nervous system increases.	There is increasing range of more complex actions (e.g., lifting head to crawling to running).
School age	Growth to peak volume in some parts of the temporal lobes. Between 5 and 11 years, neural connections increase, especially in frontal, parietal, and temporal lobes associated with language and cognition.	The capacity to manage social situations increases. Many language and cognition milestones are reached between 5 and 11 years of age.
Adolescence	Continuing frontal lobe development. Areas involved in reward, motivation, and emotion developing. Unused connections are pruned.	Abstract reasoning develops. Intensity and urgency of emotions are heightened.
Young adulthood	Frontal lobe development involved in goal-directed behaviour matures. White matter connections increasing.	Mastery of impulse control and planning abilities occurs, and the ability to integrate information improves.
Pregnancy	Grey matter reductions in areas of social cognition lasting at least 2 years after birth. Hippocampus loses volume.	Promotes maternal attachment
Middle age	White matter connections strengthen. Temporal lobe white matter increases.	Abstract reasoning, math and special reasoning, and verbal abilities increase. Optimism and social appropriateness increase.
Menopause	Estrogen impacts neuron and synapse development; prefrontal cortex and hippocampus especially impacted.	Variable, but modest verbal memory loss. If ovaries removed surgically, more severe consequences
Old age	Some structures and areas shrink and less white matter.	Complex mental processes may be negatively affected. Speed of processing decreases. Vocabulary and experience-based knowledge remain strong.

Adapted from Rojahn, S. (2013). *Tracking brain connections in utero.* Retrieved from https://www.technologyreview.com/s/511551/tracking-brain-connections-in-utero/; Northeastern University. (2010). *Traumatic brain injury resource for survivors and caregivers.* Retrieved from http://www.northeastern.edu/nutraumaticbraininjury/braintbi-anatomy/brain-changes-over-the-lifespan/; Hara, Y., Waters, E., McEwen, B., & Morrison, J. (2015). Estrogen effects on cognitive and synaptic health over the lifecourse. *Physiological Reviews, 95,* 785–807. doi:10:1152/physrev.00036.2014; Sanders, L. (2016). Pregnancy linked to long-term changes in mom's brain: Loss of gray matter may aid in caring for baby. *Science News.* Retrieved from https://www.sciencenews.org/article/pregnancy-linked-long-term-changes-moms-brain

emotions have a biologic basis. Whether it is responding angrily to someone, impulsively making a purchase, or struggling to make a decision, behaviours are in large part rooted in the neurocircuitry of the brain. So when common psychiatric symptoms manifest as abnormal behaviours (e.g., seeing things that are not there, attempting suicide, talking in odd or unusual ways), we look to the brain. **Symptom expression** is a term referring to the behavioural symptoms seen in mental illness and the link to the neurobiologic basis of the symptom. Because symptoms of psychiatric illness are expressed mainly as behavioural disturbance and because behavioural symptoms are linked to anomalies in brain functioning, nurses need to understand disease symptoms in relation to brain function.

Just as a breathing problem is often a symptom of a respiratory disorder, psychiatric symptoms are often indicators of CNS problems. Understanding this fundamental concept makes it much easier to understand the scientific rationale for many of the nursing care and treatment decisions presented in this book.

As you read this chapter, think about what you know about the symptoms of mental illness. Nurses must be able to make the connection among (1) patients' psychiatric symptoms, (2) the probable alterations in brain functioning linked to those symptoms, and (3) the rationale for treatment and care practices. Knowledge of the CNS is an inescapable aspect of modern PMH nursing.

IN-A-LIFE

Sidney Crosby and a Life-Changing Concussion

PUBLIC PERSONA

Called "the best player in the world," Sidney Crosby has played in the National Hockey League since he was 18 years old. In January 2011, while playing for the Pittsburgh Penguins, he was struck on the head during a game. Later he described feeling "off, headaches, a little sick." Shortly after this, he was sidelined for the rest of the season because of a concussion. At the time of the injury, he was leading the NHL in scoring.

REALITIES

Concussions are common sports injuries, but they are not evident on x-rays, magnetic resonance imagings (MRIs), or computed tomography (CT) scans. They occur when the person is hit on the head or face or through a whiplash injury. When this happens, the brain strikes the inside of the skull and is bruised where it hits the skull and on the opposite side where it bounces back. As a result, the person may suffer physical, cognitive, or emotional symptoms after the injury. In some cases, the symptoms can last for years. In 2010–2011, there were 2,766 hospitalizations in Canada for concussion-related injuries (Morrish & Carey, 2013). June has been declared Brain Injury Awareness Month in Canada. Sidney Crosby, after missing 2 years of play, is back in the game.

Sources: Graves, W. (2013, January 15). *Sidney Crosby says he's free of concussion symptoms.* Associated Press. Retrieved from http://www.cbc.ca/sports/hockey/nhl/sidney-crosby-says-he-s-free-of-concussion-symptoms-1.1400543
Morrish, J., & Carey, S. (2013). *Concussions in Canada. Canada Injury Compass, Spring 2013.* Toronto, Canada: Parachute.
Wyshynski, G. (2011). *Sidney Crosby talks concussion, "irresponsible" blind side hits and when Penguins knew about injury.* Retrieved from http://ca.sports.yahoo.com/nhl/blog/puck_daddy/post/Sidney-Crosby-talks-concussion-irresponsible-?urn=nhl-305051

Genetics

It has been noted for decades that family members of individuals who have one of the major mental disorders, such as schizophrenia, bipolar disorder, or panic disorder, have an increased risk for the same disorder. In fact, the 1823 archives of London's Bethlehem Royal Hospital (Bedlam) noted that physicians needed to identify whether there was a hereditary component to the person's illness (McGuffin & Southwick, 2003). **Animal models** have greatly increased the ability of researchers to understand the influence of genetics on symptom expression in psychiatric disorders, and many of the common psychiatric disorders that nurses encounter have a known genetic component. As genetic knowledge increases, treatments that work at the genetic level are being developed (Oedegaard et al., 2016).

Genetic *processes* control how humans develop from a single-cell egg into an adult human. Genes control the regrowth of hair and skin cells, the growth and connection of nervous system cells, and our biologic reaction to stress, among other processes. Genes make humans dynamic organisms, capable of growth, change, and development. The Human Genome Project, completed in 2003, mapped the complete set of human genes, or **H**, carried by all of us and transmitted to our offspring. There are about 30,000 genes in the human **genome**, with the brain accounting for only about 1% of the body's DNA. The completed human genome provided researchers with a map of the exact sequence of the 3 billion nucleotide bases that make up human organisms. If printed out, the entire human genome sequence would fill one thousand 1,000-page telephone books. Now that it is completed, the genome map is used to study the function of specific genes and their disease-inducing capacity when they malfunction. One of the things to come from the Human Genome Project is a catalogue of common human genetic variations, called the HapMap.

A gene comprises short segments of DNA and is packed with the "instructions" for making proteins that have a specific function. At a cellular level, the genes themselves do not directly control how the nerves function. Rather the genes control the proteins that regulate neural functioning. It is not an unchangeable state fixed at some point in neuronal development. Individual nerve cells may respond to neurochemical changes outside the cell, producing different proteins for adaptation to the new environment. This dynamic nature of gene function highlights the manner in which the body and the environment interact and how environmental factors influence gene expression. The diathesis–stress model holds that the diathesis (derived from a Greek word for "disposition" or "vulnerability") or biologic risk(s) interacts with environmental stressors and, depending on how successful the compensatory mechanisms work, a mental illness may or may not develop (Stahl, 2008).

When genes are absent or malfunction, protein production is altered, and bodily functions are disrupted. A gene or part of a gene can be altered, and when this change occurs commonly and has an effect on human behaviour, it is called a **polymorphism** (Quigley, 2015). For example, recent research has demonstrated that individuals with schizophrenia are at risk for 22q11.2 deletion syndrome, a genetic subtype of schizophrenia in which there is a deletion on part of chromosome 22 (Merico et al., 2015). This deletion has been linked with a number of abnormalities, including craniofacial and cardiovascular alterations and behavioural and learning problems.

Population Genetics

The study of molecular genetics in psychiatric disorders is quite new. Because the exact genetic bases of psychiatric disorders remain unclear and animal models are hard to produce for some disorders, much of what we know about the genetics of these disorders comes from studies that trace given disorders within groups of people. This technique, called *population genetics*, involves the analysis of genetic transmission of a trait within families and populations to determine risks and patterns of transmission. The risk of a given disorder occurring in the general population can then be compared with the risk within families and between groups of relatives. These studies rely on the initial identification of an individual who has the disorder and include the following principal methods:

- Family studies, which analyze the occurrence of a disorder in first-degree relatives (biologic parents, siblings, and children), second-degree relatives (grandparents, uncles, aunts, nieces, nephews, and grandchildren), and so on.
- Twin studies, which analyze the presence or absence of the disorder in pairs of twins. The *concordance rate* is the measure of similarity of occurrence in individuals with similar genetic makeup.
- Adoption studies, which compare the risk for the illness developing in offspring raised in different environments. The strongest inferences may be drawn from studies that involve children separated from their parents at birth.

Few traits are completely heritable. Colour blindness and blood type are examples of traits that exist because of heredity alone. Monozygotic twins have identical genetic contributions; therefore, both would have colour blindness or the same blood type if they expressed that gene. This is 100% concordance. If a disorder was completely unrelated to genetics, then monozygotic twins would have the same concordance rates as dizygotic (fraternal) twins, who share roughly the same proportion of genes that ordinary siblings do—50%. If there is a genetic contribution with environmental influence, the concordance rates would be less than 100% for monozygotic twins but significantly greater than for dizygotic twins. Such is the case with several psychiatric disorders. Although no conclusive evidence exists for a complete genetic cause of most psychiatric disorders, significant evidence suggests that strong genetic contributions exist for most (Pirooznia et al., 2012). It is likely that psychiatric disorders are *polygenic*. This means that more than one gene is involved in producing a psychiatric disorder and that the disorder develops from genes interacting, which produces a risk factor, and environmental influences that lead to the expression of the illness. The environmental factors may include stress, infections, poor nutrition, catastrophic loss, complications during pregnancy, and exposure to toxins. Thus,

genetic compositions convey vulnerability, or a risk for the illness, but the right set of environmental factors must be present for the disease to develop in the at-risk individual. Additionally, specific genes may convey risk for more than one disorder (Agius & Aquilina, 2014).

Using the human genome map and databases containing human samples of DNA sequences, markers for genetic variations associated with particular illnesses can be identified. Research studies using these tools are called genome-wide association studies. For example, APOE 4, a genetic polymorphism, is found in approximately 15% of the population and is linked to increased risk for atherosclerosis and Alzheimer's disease. The next step in making this research applicable is to find out whether one treatment works better in those with different genetic profiles. However, these studies remain controversial, and it is important to keep in mind that mental illnesses are not determined by one polymorphism but rather by a complex interaction between the environment and multiple genes.

When considering information regarding risks for genetic transmission of psychiatric disorders, it is important to remember several key points:

- Psychiatric disorders have been described and labelled quite differently across generations, and errors in diagnosis may occur.
- Similar psychiatric symptoms may have considerably different causes, just as symptoms such as chest pain may occur in relation to many different causes.
- Genes that are present may not always cause the appearance of the trait.
- One gene alteration may cause different symptoms in different people.
- Several genes work together in an individual to produce a given trait or disorder.
- A biologic cause is not necessarily only genetic in origin. Environmental influences alter the body's functioning and often mediate or worsen genetic risk factors.

As public awareness of genetic evidence grows, it is likely that nurses will be faced with patients or family members requesting genetic testing or needing information regarding their likelihood of risk for a psychiatric disorder. As a result, PMH nurses increasingly will need greater understanding of the role genetics play in mental illness.

Epigenetics

Epigenetics (*epi* meaning "above") is the study of the mechanisms by which genetic inheritance is modified without any change in an organism's genetic (DNA) sequence. It is not a new field—the term was coined in 1942 by Conrad Waddington (1957)—but 21st-century science has been making significant advances in this area, indicating that in the ancient nature versus nurture debate, it is not "either/or" but about interaction. Stem cell and other research are revealing that cell development is highly flexible and plastic (Shah & Allegrucci, 2013).

It has been known for some time that all cells in an individual organism have the identical genetic makeup (genotype) but can function in radically different ways (e.g., as a heart cell, a skin cell, a brain cell, etc.). As influences (environmental, lifestyle) on the genotype occur prenatally and across the life span, cell genes are distinctively expressed (phenotype) (Marques & Fleming Outeiro, 2013). An individual's *epigenome* is made up of chemicals that change or mark his or her genome (complete set of DNA) in a way that directs genetic expression (how gene information is used) (National Human Genome Research Institute, 2013). Epigenetic phenomena are related to chromatin structure and organization, chromatin being the protein–DNA complex that makes up the nucleus of a cell. The epigenome marks (turns on or off) the genome through a variety of processes such as DNA methylation and histone acetylation, which may down-regulate or up-regulate gene expression, respectively, or histone methylation and phosphorylation, which may activate or repress protein transcription; gene expression can also be silenced by RNA, a nucleic acid (Tafet & Nemeroff, 2016).

Epigenetic changes are necessary to development and health, but some may trigger disease (National Institute on Aging, 2011). It was in 1983 that evidence of a link between epigenetic changes and disease was first noted: persons with colorectal cancer were found to have less DNA methylation in their diseased tissue than in their normal tissue (Simmons, 2008).

Epigenetics is a key research area in the quest to understand health, aging, and disease (Kundu, 2013). In terms of Canadian genomic research, Genome Canada and the Canadian Institutes of Health Research (CIHR) are supporting projects that will demonstrate how genomics-based research can contribute to a more evidence-based approach to health (GenomeCanada, 2017). One American genome-wide association study involved researchers looking for variants in the genome among individuals with a particular health concern or trait and working to identify genes directly associated with aging (National Institute on Aging, 2011). An example of such research relevant to psychiatry and mental health is a study by Labonté et al. (2013) in which it was discovered that there were DNA methylation changes in the hippocampal DNA of persons who had completed suicide. It is possible to imagine that sometime in the future, genome sequencing might become routine in patient diagnosis (Marx, 2015). One can imagine, as well, the ethical issues that will arise with such "routine."

Risk Factors

The concept of genetic susceptibility suggests that an individual may be at increased risk for a psychiatric disorder. Research into risk factors is an important avenue of study. Just as knowledge of risk factors for diabetes and heart disease led to the development of preventive interventions, learning more about risk factors for psychiatric disorders will lead to preventive care practices. Specific risk factors for psychiatric disorders are just beginning to be understood, and some of the environmental influences listed previously may be examples of risk factors. These events, circumstances, or demographic features are more likely to occur in individuals who experience a particular psychiatric disorder. In the absence of one specific gene for major psychiatric disorders, risk factor assessment may be a logical alternative for predicting who is more likely to experience psychiatric disorders or certain conditions such as aggression or suicidality. This is a growing area of PMH nursing; nurses are playing an important role in mental health promotion and illness prevention.

CURRENT RESEARCH APPROACHES AND ADVANCES

Neuroscience researchers have applied several approaches to the study of the CNS structure and function. These approaches occur with both human research and animal models. The approaches, highlighted in Table 9.2, include the following:

- Comparative
- Developmental
- Chemoarchitectural
- Cytoarchitectural
- Functional

These different approaches to studying the CNS have significantly increased our understanding of its normal functioning and how a disease affects behaviour and contributes to the development of psychiatric disorders. Research shows that areas of the brain, and the groups of nerve cells that constitute that area, often work together as functional units. A hierarchy of function exists in which primary sensory input is used in an increasingly more complex and integrated manner across areas of the brain. In addition, some areas of the brain, such as those that control basic levels of alertness and attention, must work correctly for information to be received, understood, and used by higher levels of the brain to organize a response. The brain's functional units work together to control or contribute to specific behaviours or emotions.

The *integrated approach* to brain development is the term used to describe the interactive working of brain areas and function. Understanding the work as an integration of parts allows us to understand that specific areas of the brain control specific functions. For example, there is a speech area in the brain, a mood area, an appetite area, and so on. Understanding the functions of areas of the brain allows nurses to assess a patient's

Table 9.2	Approaches to the Study of Neuroanatomy	
Approach	**Purpose**	**Potential Limitations**
Comparative	Explores and compares behaviour across animal nervous systems, from a simple primitive cordlike structure in some species to the large complex structure of the human brain	Difficult to correlate animal behaviour to human, especially emotional New brain structures do not necessarily correlate to new behaviour.
Developmental	Studies nervous system structure within an individual or species of animal across different stages of development	Impossible to follow one human being's neuronal development Individual variation in development complicates comparisons of individuals across a specific point of time in development.
Chemoarchitectural	Identifies differences in location of neurochemicals such as neurotransmitters throughout the brain	Boundaries between regional changes are subtle and may vary across individuals.
Cytoarchitectural	Identifies differences or variations in cell type, structure, and density throughout the brain, mapping these variations by location	Boundaries between regional changes are subtle and may vary across individuals.
Functional	Identifies location of predominant control over various behavioural functions within the brain Studies often conducted on the basis of dysfunction from a localized injury to the brain	Several regions or structures within the brain may contribute to one behaviour, making predominant control difficult to assign. Controversy exists in correlating normal brain function to damaged brain tissue.

symptoms largely as the expression of a problem in a specific brain area. Just as a person with an irregular heartbeat is experiencing disruption in normal cardiac function, a person who fails to eat because of depression is experiencing a disruption in the brain's normal appetite and mood function.

Neuroplasticity is an important concept when describing brain function. The changes in neural environment can come from internal sources such as a change in electrolytes or from external sources such as exercise, toxins, and viruses. With neuroplasticity, nerve signals may be rerouted, cells may learn new functions and gain sensitivity, the number of cells may increase or decrease, or some nerve tissue may to some extent be regenerated. Neuroplasticity contributes to understanding how function may be restored over time after

brain damage occurs or how an individual may react over time to psychotherapy or a continuous pharmacotherapy regimen.

There are several behavioural principles that may impact brain plasticity (see Table 9.3). For example, brains are most plastic during infancy and early childhood, when large adaptive learning tasks should normally occur. With age, brains become less plastic, which explains why it is easier to learn a second language at the age of 5 years than at 55 years. Brains are still capable of change though; when nurses teach mindful attention to breathing, they are promoting positive brain change, likely in the amygdala–dorsal prefrontal cortex pathways (Doll et al., 2016). Understanding these principles provides a framework for nurses coaching new emotional, cognitive, and behavioural skills.

Table 9.3	Principles of Experience-Derived Brain Plasticity
Principle	**Example**
1. Use it or lose it	Brain circuits not used in task performance over time can decay.
2. Use it and improve it	Through extended training, brain plasticity can be induced.
3. Learning something new	Repeating something already learned does not induce plasticity but learning something new will.
4. Repeat, repeat, repeat	Repeating a new or relearned skill may be needed to induce long-term changes.
5. Be intense but not too intense	Training too intensely can worsen things; balance is needed.
6. Brain age matters	Plasticity occurs more easily in a younger brain.
7. Timing matters	Certain types of plasticity change follow a pattern.
8. A little can go a long way	Plasticity in one set of neurons can promote ongoing development in the same or other areas of the brain.
9. Make it important	Motivation and attention are important mediators.
10. Plasticity in one form can block a different plasticity within the same circuit	Developing brain circuits to do one skill may block learning another.

Adapted from Kleim, J., & Jones, T. (2008). Principles of experience-dependent neural plasticity: Implications for rehabilitation after brain damage. *Journal of Speech, Language, and Hearing Research, 51,* S225–S239.

KEY CONCEPT

Plasticity is the ability of the brain to change its structure and function in response to internal and external pressures (Kleim & Jones, 2008).

Neuroimaging

Since the 1980s, technologic advances in neuroimaging techniques have been a major aid to the current understanding of how the human brain functions. As knowledge grows, neuroimaging techniques are moving from research to routine clinical use, requiring nurses to understand this technology. Two basic neuroimaging methods are structural and functional neuroimaging. See Table 9.4 for methods of neuroimaging.

Structural Neuroimaging

Structural neuroimaging techniques were the first form of neuroimaging that allowed visualization of brain structures. Structural images show what normal structures of the brain look like and allow clinicians to identify tissue abnormalities, changes, or damages. Commonly used structural neuroimaging techniques include computed tomography (CT) scanning and magnetic resonance imaging (MRI). Although these techniques are useful in identifying what the brain looks like, they do not reveal anything about how the brain works.

Table 9.4   Methods of Neuroimaging

Method	Description	Considerations
Structural Imaging		
Computed tomography (CT), also called computed axial tomography (CAT)	Uses x-ray technology to measure tissue density; is readily available; can be completed quickly, and less costly; may be used for screening, but many disease states are not clearly seen; use of contrast medium improves resolution	Contrast medium may produce allergic reactions; individuals with increased risk for contrast media complications include those with: History of previous reactions Cardiac disease Hypertension Diabetes Sickle cell disease Contraindications for use of contrast: Iodine/shellfish allergies Renal disease Pregnancy
Magnetic resonance imaging (MRI)	Uses a magnetic field to magnetize hydrogen atoms in soft tissue, changing their alignment—this creates a tiny electric signal, which can be received to produce an image; produces greater resolution than a CT, diagnosing more subtle pathologic changes.	Patients may experience headaches, dizziness, and nausea; symptoms of anxiety, claustrophobia, or psychosis can increase; contraindicated when patients have aneurysm clips, internal electrical, magnetic, or mechanical devices such as pacemakers, metallic surgical clips, sutures, or dental work, which distort the image; claustrophobia.
Functional Neuroimaging		
Positron emission tomography (PET)	Uses positron emitting isotopes (very short-lived radioactive entities such as oxygen-15) to image brain functioning; isotopes are incorporated into specific molecules to study cerebral metabolism, cerebral blood flow, and specific neurochemicals.	Images appear blurry, lacking anatomic detail, but have been extremely useful in research to study distribution of neuroreceptors and the action of pharmacologic agents; invasive procedure, use of radioactivity limits the number of scans done with a single individual.
Single-photon emission computed tomography (SPECT)	Like PET, SPECT uses radioisotopes that produce only one photon; data are collected as a three-dimensional volume, and two-dimensional images can be constructed on any plane; less expensive than PET technology.	Less resolution and sensitivity than the PET, but inhalation methods may be used, allowing for some repeated studies; useful in drug dependency research.
Functional magnetic resonance imaging (fMRI)	Combines spatial resolution of MRI with the ability to image neural activity; is able to show sequential, movie-type images of blood flow in the brain as it is happening; shows whether brain activity occurs simultaneously or sequentially in different areas of the brain while engaged in selected activities	Requires no radiation and can be completely noninvasive; individual can be imaged many times, in different clinical states, before or after treatments; removes many of the ethical constraints when studying children and adolescents with psychiatric disorders.
Magnetic resonance spectroscopy (MRS)	Uses the same imaging equipment as the fMRI; by altering scanning parameters, signals represent specific chemicals in the brain.	Noninvasive, repeatable, may be ideal for longitudinal studies, but has limited spatial resolution, especially with molecules that occur in low concentrations.

Computed Tomography

CT (also referred to as computed axial tomography or CAT) scanning first allowed scientists and clinicians to see structures inside the brain without more invasive and potentially dangerous methods. CT scans still use an x-ray beam passed through the head in serial slices. High-speed computers measure the decreased strength in the x-ray beam that results from absorption, and the computer assigns a shade of gray that reflects that change. The degree of energy absorbed by a tissue is proportionally related to its density. For example, cerebrospinal fluid (CSF) absorbs the least, so it appears the darkest, whereas bone absorbs the most and appears light. The computer then develops a 3D x-ray image. This technique is good at detecting skull fractures and injuries or abnormalities such as a subdermal hematoma requiring surgery. White matter and gray matter are more difficult to discriminate with CT technology.

CT scans can be done with or without contrast material. Contrast materials are used to increase the visibility of certain tissues or blood vessels. If a contrast agent is used, an iodinated or other material is intravenously administered to enhance the CT image. Although CT scanning is a relatively safe, noninvasive procedure, the contrast material may have some adverse effects in some patients. Some patients receiving contrast materials report a metallic taste in the mouth, and some experience mild nausea, rashes, or joint pain. In rare instances, severe allergic responses, including anaphylaxis, may develop, so nurses must closely monitor patients who have received contrast materials. In addition, because the CT equipment itself may frighten the patient, the nurse should educate the patient about the scan. Some patients may need to be accompanied by a nurse during the procedure for ongoing reassurance. Radiation exposure by a CT scan is approximately 400 times that of a standard chest x-ray (Miglioretti & Simth-Bindman, 2011).

Magnetic Resonance Imaging

MRI is performed by placing a patient into a long tube that contains powerful magnets. The magnetic field causes hydrogen-containing molecules (primarily water) to line up and move in symmetric ways around their axes. The magnetic field is then interrupted in pulses, causing the molecules to turn 90 or 180 degrees. Electromagnetic energy is released when the molecules return to their original position. The energy released is related to the density of the tissue and is detected by the MRI device, resulting in a scan measurement of the density of the examined tissue. The MRI can produce three-dimensional images extremely clearly, allowing for gross discrimination of white and gray matters, detection of subacute haemorrhages, and rough areas of white matter damage. Sometimes, contrast material is used.

MRI scans produce more information than CT images, but MRI scans are more complicated and costly.

In addition, MRI scans cannot be used for all patients. Because MRI uses magnet energy, individuals with pacemakers, metal plates, bone replacements, aneurysm clips, or other metal in their body cannot undergo the procedure; pregnant women also cannot have MRI scans. The loud noise of the equipment and the very narrow tube in which the patient must lie still can trigger claustrophobic responses in some people. Adequate preparation of the patient by the nurse should eliminate any surprises. Assistance with shallow breathing techniques, mental distractions, or other anxiety-reducing strategies may help. Many MRI facilities are equipped with music to mask the whirring of the equipment and provide a distraction through the lengthy testing period. Some tubes are now being made of clear plastic to decrease the claustrophobic sensation.

Diffusion Tensor Magnetic Resonance Imaging

This special type of MRI produces information on white matter not presently available through any other techniques (Fig. 9.1). It cannot show what is happening to individual neurons, but it can identify what is happening at the fibre bundle level. The images are based on microscopic movement of water protons in tissues (Shenton et al., 2012). Water moves freely in CSF but is more restricted by other structures such as axons and myelin sheaths. Water can move more freely in a direction parallel to the axon but less freely perpendicular to the axon. Therefore, the directions of the axons will determine the direction of the water diffusion. If, for example, diffusion in the white matter is found to be less restricted than expected, it can mean that the myelin sheaths or axons are damaged or less dense. Diffusion tensor imaging (DTI) cannot identify the cause of the diffusion changes. This technology is being used to investigate white matter changes in schizophrenia, dementia, and other psychiatric illnesses. Ongoing developments in this technique

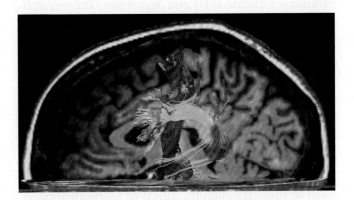

Figure 9.1. Diffusion tensor imaging (DTI). DTI is specifically useful is evaluating white matter tracts because of the highly directional diffusion in normal white matter bundles. Diffusion tractography can be used to visualize specific white matter tracts. Here, a sagittal 3D view shows corticospinal tracts (*blue*) and superior longitudinal fasciculus (*green*) tracts in a normal subject.

will allow scientists to visualize and measure damage in fibre tracts connecting different brain regions.

Functional Neuroimaging

Although structural imaging identifies what the brain looks like, the scans do not show how the brain is working. Functional neuroimaging techniques measure physiologic activities, providing insight into how the brain works. These methods let researchers study such activities as cerebral blood flow, neuroreceptor location and function, and distribution patterns of specific chemicals within the brain. Single-photon emission computed tomography (SPECT) and positron emission tomography (PET) are the primary methods used to observe metabolic functioning. Both procedures require administering radioactive substances that emit charged particles, which are then measured by scanning equipment. SPECT and PET differ in the type of isotopes used, the method of measuring isotope uptake, and therefore the equipment used. Because these procedures measure function, the patient is usually asked to perform specific tasks during the test. The commonly used Wisconsin Card Sorting Test (WCST) requires the individual to sort cards with different numbers, colours, and shapes into piles based on specified rules. This task requires the use of the brain's frontal lobe, an important area for concept formation and decision making and an area that often is disrupted in many psychiatric disorders.

CAUTION: Pregnant health care workers should avoid caring for patients who have had a nuclear scan for 24 hours after the scan. Caregivers need to check their institution's guide for other safety precautions when caring for patients who have been exposed to nuclear material.

Single-Photon Emission Computed Tomography

SPECT is helpful in measuring regional cerebral blood flow. In one study, SPECT scans were used to study decreases in blood flow in the brains of individuals with Parkinson's disease (PD) and depression. The researchers were able to identify brain areas that were perfused differently in the depressed persons compared to the brains of those who had PD but were not depressed (Kim et al., 2016). SPECT scans are also used to confirm changes in cerebral blood flow caused by certain drugs. For example, caffeine and nicotine cause a generalized decrease in cerebral blood flow. At present, this technique is used more in academic settings. It is less expensive than the PET exam. New compounds have been developed recently to visualize the numbers or density of **receptors** in various areas of the brain, which may assist in understanding the effects of psychopharmacologic medications and neuroplastic changes in brain tissue over time.

Positron Emission Tomography

PET uses a radioactively charged particle (most commonly glucose) to measure that particle's activity in various brain regions. Because cells use glucose as fuel for cellular action, the higher the rate of glucose use detected by the PET scan, the higher the rate of metabolic activity in different areas of the brain. Abnormalities in glucose consumption, indicating more or less cellular activity, are found in Alzheimer's disease, seizures, strokes, malignancies, and a number of psychiatric disorders. Scanning may be performed while the individual is at rest or performing a cognitive task. PET scans are often used to measure regional cerebral blood flow and neurotransmitter system functions.

Bridging the Structure–Function Gap

As structural and functional neuroimaging techniques advance, attempts are being made to develop imaging procedures that detail structure and function at the same time. Magnetic resonance spectroscopy (MRS) and functional magnetic resonance imaging (fMRI) are examples. The fMRI is useful for showing structure while localizing function and providing high-resolution images. Like other forms of neuroimaging, the fMRI is noninvasive, but it requires no radioactive agent, making it economical and safer than PET and SPECT (Hennig, Speck, Koch, & Weiller, 2003).

MRS uses the same machinery as fMRI and provides precise and clear images of neuronal membranes as well as measures of metabolic cellular function (Currie et al., 2013). In addition to these procedures, magnetoencephalography (MEG) is being used. MEG testing records magnetic fields generated by neuronal activity. These results are paired with a technique that images anatomical information such as MRI, to provide both the structural and functional information. Table 9.3 summarizes these neuroimaging methods. These neuroimaging procedures are becoming useful in clinical practice.

Transcranial magnetic stimulation (TMS) is an investigational, research, and treatment tool that painlessly delivers an alternating current through a metal coil placed around the scalp. The current causes a magnetic field to be generated, and this induces an electrical current that changes firing along neurons. Depending on where and at what frequency the treatment is applied, areas of the brain may be inhibited or excited. It has been found to provide mixed results in the treatment of depression. Adverse effects can include skin burns and lesions, and in some, depression may switch to mania (Holtzheimer, 2013). TMS has been used to investigate plasticity, medication effects, and nervous propagation along nerves. Additionally, it has been used in rehabilitation and operative settings.

NEUROANATOMY OF THE CENTRAL NERVOUS SYSTEM

With advances in brain science comes greater understanding of the biologic basis of mental illnesses.

Therefore, nurses must increasingly be aware of the anatomic intricacy of the CNS as a foundation for modern psychiatric nursing assessments and interventions.

Although this section discusses each functioning area of the brain separately, each area is intricately connected and functions interactively with the others. The CNS contains the brain, brainstem, and spinal cord, whereas the total human nervous system includes the peripheral nervous system (PNS) as well. The PNS consists of the neurons that connect the CNS to the muscles, organs, and other systems in the periphery of the body. Whatever affects the CNS may also affect the PNS, and vice versa.

Cerebrum

The largest part of the human brain, the cerebrum, fills the entire upper portion of the cranium. The **cortex**, or outermost surface of the cerebrum, makes up about 80% of the human brain. The cortex is several millimetres thick and is composed of cell bodies mixed with capillary blood vessels. This mixture makes the cortex grey-brown, hence the term *grey matter*. The cortex contains a number of bumps and grooves in a fully developed adult brain, as shown in Figure 9.2. This "wrinkling" allows for a large amount of surface area to be confined in the limited space of the skull. The increased surface area allows for more potential connections between cells within the cortex. The grooves are called fissures if they extend deep into the brain and *sulci* if they are shallower. The bumps or convolutions are called gyri. Together, they provide many of the landmarks for the subdivisions of the cortex. The longest and deepest groove, the longitudinal fissure, separates the cerebrum into left and right hemispheres. Although these two divisions are nearly symmetric, there is some variation in the location and size of the sulci and gyri in each hemisphere. Substantial variation in these convolutions is found in the cortex of different individuals.

Left and Right Hemispheres

The cerebrum can be roughly divided into two halves, or hemispheres. Each hemisphere controls functioning mainly on the opposite side of the body. For about 95% of people, the left hemisphere is dominant, whereas about 5% of individuals have mixed dominance. The right hemisphere provides input into receptive nonverbal communication, spatial orientation, and recognition; intonation of speech and aspects of music; facial recognition and facial expression of emotion; and nonverbal learning and memory. In general, the left hemisphere is more involved with verbal language function, including areas for both receptive and expressive speech control. In addition, the left hemisphere provides strong contributions to temporal order and sequencing, numeric symbols, and verbal learning and memory. However, the intact brain may not be neatly organized with one side being the dominant because the degree of lateralization differs across individuals. The two hemispheres are connected by the corpus callosum, a bundle of neuronal tissue that allows information to be exchanged quickly between the right and left hemispheres. An intact corpus

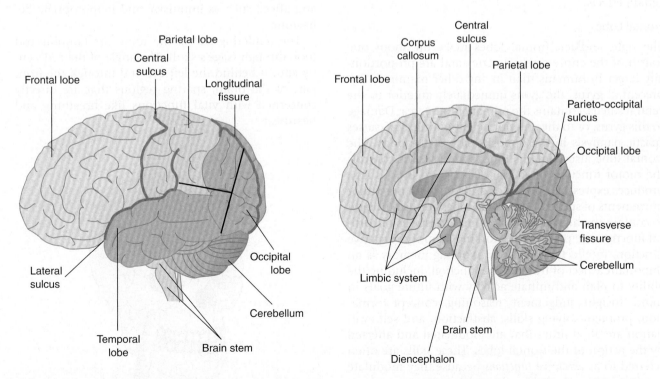

Figure 9.2. Lateral and medial surfaces of the brain. **Left:** the left lateral surface of the brain. **Right:** the medial surface of the right half of a sagittally hemisected brain.

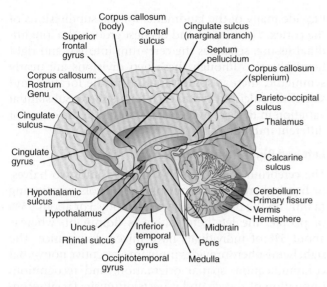

Figure 9.3. Gyri and sulci of the cortex.

callosum is required for the hemispheres to function in a smooth and coordinated manner.

Lobes of the Brain

The lateral surface of each hemisphere is further divided into four lobes: the **frontal, parietal, temporal, and occipital lobes** (Fig. 9.3). The lobes work in coordinated ways, but each is responsible for specific functions. Knowledge of these unique functions is helpful for understanding how damage to these areas produces the symptoms of mental illness and how medications that affect the functioning of these lobes can produce certain effects.

Frontal Lobes

The right and left frontal lobes make up about one fourth of the entire cerebral cortex and are proportionally larger in humans than in any other mammal. The precentral gyrus, the gyrus immediately anterior to the central sulcus, contains the primary motor area. Damage to this gyrus, or to the anterior neighbouring gyri, causes spastic paralysis in the opposite side of the body. The frontal lobe also contains Broca's area, which controls the motor function of speech. Damage to Broca's area produces expressive aphasia or difficulty with the motor movements of speech. The frontal lobes are also thought to contain the highest or most complex aspects of cortical functioning: personality, working memory, executive function, intellect, and speech. Working memory is an important aspect of frontal lobe function, including the ability to plan and initiate activity with future goals in mind. Insight, judgement, reasoning, concept formation, problem-solving skills, abstraction, and self-evaluation are all abilities that are modulated and affected by the action of the frontal lobes. These skills are often referred to as *executive functions* because they modulate more primitive impulses through numerous connections to other areas of the cerebrum.

When normal frontal lobe functioning is altered, executive functioning is decreased, and modulation of impulses can be lost, leading to changes in mood and personality. The importance of the frontal lobe and its role in the development of symptoms common to psychiatric disorders are emphasized in later chapters that discuss disorders such as schizophrenia, attention deficit hyperactivity disorder, and dementia. Box 9.1 describes how altered frontal lobe function can affect mood and personality.

BOX 9.1 Frontal Lobe Syndrome

In the 1860s, Phineas Gage became a famous example of frontal lobe dysfunction. Mr. Gage was a New England railroad worker who had a thick iron-tamping rod propelled through his frontal lobes by an explosion. He survived but suffered significant changes in his personality. Mr. Gage, who had previously been a capable and calm supervisor, began to show impatience, labile mood, disrespect for others, and frequent use of profanity after his injury (Harlow, 1868). Similar conditions are often called *frontal lobe syndrome*. Symptoms vary widely among individuals. In general, after damage to the dorsolateral (upper and outer) areas of the frontal lobes, the symptoms include a lack of drive and spontaneity. With damage to the most anterior aspects of the frontal lobes, the symptoms tend to involve more changes in mood and affect, such as impulsive and inappropriate behaviour.

The rendering shows the route the tamping rod took through Gage's skull. The angle of the rod's entry shot it behind the left eye and through the front part of the brain, sparing regions that are directly concerned with vital functions like breathing and heartbeat.

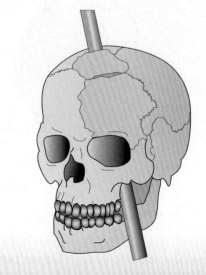

Parietal Lobes

The postcentral gyrus, immediately behind the central sulcus, contains the primary somatosensory area (Fig. 9.2). The posterior areas of the parietal lobe appear to coordinate visual and somatosensory information. Damage to this area produces complex sensory deficits, including neglect of contralateral sensory stimuli and spatial relationships. The parietal lobes contribute to the ability to recognize objects by touch, calculate, write, recognize fingers of the opposite hands, draw, and organize spatial directions, such as how to travel to familiar places. They are important for speech and maintaining focused attention.

Temporal Lobes

The temporal lobes contain the primary auditory and olfactory areas. Wernicke's area, located at the posterior aspect of the superior temporal gyrus, is primarily responsible for receptive speech. The temporal lobes also integrate sensory and visual information involved in the control of written and verbal language skills, as well as visual recognition. The **hippocampus**, an important structure discussed in its own section later in this chapter, lies in the internal aspects of each temporal lobe and contributes to memory. Other internal structures of this lobe are involved in the modulation of mood and emotion.

Occipital Lobes

The primary visual area is located in the most posterior aspect of the occipital lobes. Damage to this area results in a condition called *cortical blindness*. In other words, the retina and optic nerve remain intact, but the individual cannot see. The occipital lobes are involved in many aspects of visual integration of information, including colour vision, object and facial recognition, and the ability to perceive objects in motion and judge distance.

Association Cortex

Although not a lobe, the association cortex is an important area that allows the lobes to work in an integrated manner. Areas of one lobe of the cortex often share functions with an area of the adjacent lobe. When these neighbouring nerve fibres are related to the same sensory modality, they are often referred to as *association* areas. For example, an area in the inferior parietal, posterior temporal, and anterior occipital lobes integrates visual, somatosensory, and auditory information to provide the abilities required for basic academic skills. These areas, along with numerous connections beneath the cortex, are part of the mechanisms that allow the human brain to work as an integrated whole.

Subcortical Structures

Beneath the cortex are layers of tissue composed of the axons of cell bodies. The axonal tissue forms pathways that are surrounded by glia, a fatty or lipid substance, which has a white appearance and gives these layers of neuron axons their name—*white matter*. Structures inside the hemispheres, beneath the cortex, are considered subcortical. Many of these structures, essential in the regulation of emotions and behaviours, play important roles in our understanding of mental disorders. Figure 9.4 provides a coronal section view of the grey matter, white matter, and important subcortical structures.

Basal Ganglia

The **basal ganglia** are subcortical grey matter areas in both the right and left hemispheres that contain interconnected cell bodies or nuclei. These nuclei include the caudate nucleus, putamen, globus pallidus, claustrum, subthalamus, and substantia nigra. The basal ganglia are involved with motor functions and in association with both the learning and programming of behaviours or activities that are repetitive and that over time become automatic. The basal ganglia have many connections with the cerebral cortex, thalamus, midbrain structures, and spinal cord. Damage to portions of these nuclei may produce changes in posture or muscle tone. In addition, damage may produce abnormal movements, such as twitches or tremors. Parkinson's disease is the most common disorder of the basal ganglia. They can be adversely affected by some of the medications used to treat psychiatric disorders, leading to side effects and other motor-related problems.

Pituitary

The pituitary gland, often called the *master gland*, has two distinct parts, the anterior pituitary and the posterior pituitary. Located just below the hypothalamus, the anterior pituitary consists of glandular epithelial tissue and is connected to the hypothalamus by a vascular link. In contrast, the posterior pituitary is composed of neural tissue and is connected to the hypothalamus by a neural pathway. When stimulated, the posterior pituitary releases oxytocin or vasopressin (also known as antidiuretic hormone), two small peptide hormones that are produced in the hypothalamus. The anterior pituitary produces and releases seven different hormones—growth hormone (GH), thyroid-stimulating hormone (TSH), adrenocorticotropin hormone (ACTH), follicle-stimulating hormone (FSH), luteinizing hormone (LH), melatonin-stimulating hormone, and prolactin—when stimulated by a corresponding hormone from the hypothalamus (e.g., corticotrophin-releasing hormone stimulates secretion of ACTH). Together with the pituitary gland, the hypothalamus functions as one of the primary regulators of many aspects of the endocrine system. Its functions are involved in the control of visceral activities, such as body temperature, arterial blood pressure, hunger, thirst, fluid balance, gastric motility, and gastric secretions.

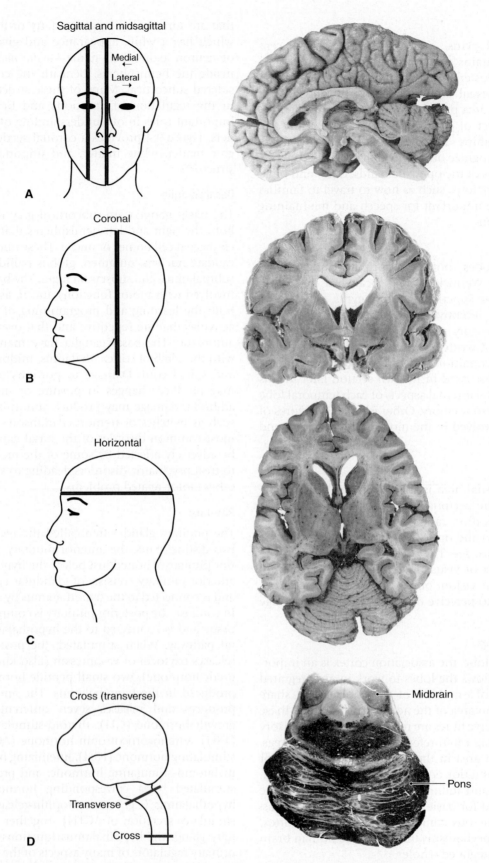

Figure 9.4. Three standard planes for visualizing brain structure: **(A)** sagittal, **(B)** coronal, and **(C)** horizontal cuts are made by physically slicing or rendered using imaging techniques. The transverse or crosscut **(D)** gives a view of subcortical structures. (Reprinted with permission from Bhatnagar, S. (2013). *Neuroscience for the study of communicative disorders*. Philadelphia, PA: Lippincott Williams & Wilkins.)

Of note, increased release of prolactin can result from blockade of naturally occurring dopamine by various medications, including antipsychotics, antidepressants, opiates, and cocaine. This can result in galactorrhea, menstrual irregularities in women, erectile dysfunction in men, and loss of libido and infertility in both men and women.

Limbic System

The **limbic system** is essential to understanding the many hypotheses related to psychiatric disorders and emotional behaviour in general. Basic emotions, needs, drives, and instinct begin and are modulated in the limbic system. Hate, love, anger, aggression, and caring are basic emotions that originate within the limbic system. Not only does the limbic system function as the seat of emotions but also, because emotions are often generated based on our personal experiences, the limbic system is involved with aspects of memory. Hypothesized changes in the limbic system play a significant role in many theories of major mental disorders, including schizophrenia, depression, and anxiety disorders (see Chapters 20 to 23). The limbic system is called a "system" because it comprises several small structures that work in a highly organized way. These structures include the hippocampus, thalamus, hypothalamus, amygdala, and limbic midbrain nuclei. See Figure 9.5 for identification and location of the structures within the limbic system and their relationship to other common CNS structures.

Hippocampus. The hippocampus is involved in forming and storing memories, especially the emotions attached to a memory. Our emotional response to memories and our association with other related memories are functions of how information is stored within the hippocampus. While most neurons are formed from before birth, the neurons in the hippocampus continue to

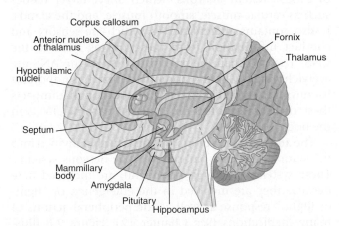

Figure 9.5. The structures of the limbic system are integrally involved in memory and emotional behaviour. Theories link changes in the limbic system to many major mental disorders, including schizophrenia, depression, and anxiety disorders.

form throughout life. Although memory storage is not limited to one area of the brain, destruction of the left hippocampus impairs verbal memory, and damage to the right hippocampus results in difficulty with recognition and recall of complex visual and auditory patterns. The main body of the hippocampus extends into the temporal lobe. Deterioration of the nerves of the hippocampus and other related temporal lobe structures found in Alzheimer's disease produces the disorder's hallmark symptoms of memory dysfunction.

Thalamus. The thalamus is composed of several distinct subnuclei, each with its own specialized connections to many regions in the cerebral cortex. Sometimes called the "relay-switching centre of the brain," the thalamus functions as a regulatory structure to relay all sensory information, except smell, sent to the CNS from the PNS. The thalamus also relays memory, emotions, cognitions, behaviours, and motor functions. It regulates by filtering incoming information and determining what to pass on or what not to pass on to the cortex. In this fashion, the thalamus prevents the cortex from becoming overloaded with sensory stimulus. The thalamus is thought to play a part in controlling electrical activity in the cortex. Parts of the thalamus are involved in alertness, awareness, and memory. Injury to the anterior medial thalamus can cause alterations in autonomic functions, mood, and the sleep–wake cycle.

Hypothalamus. Basic human activities, such as sleep–rest patterns, body temperature, and physical drives (e.g., hunger and sex), are regulated by the hypothalamus, which rests deep within the brain. In emotional situations, the hypothalamus perceives changes and stimulates a visceral response through the autonomic nervous system, such as an increase in heart rate when we feel angry. Dysfunction of this structure, whether from disorders or because of the adverse effects of drugs used to treat mental illness, produces common psychiatric symptoms, such as appetite and sleep problems.

Nerve cells within the hypothalamus secrete hormones such as antidiuretic hormone, which when sent to the kidneys accelerates the reabsorption of water, and oxytocin, which acts on smooth muscles to promote contractions, particularly within the walls of the uterus. Because cells within the nervous system produce these hormones, they are often referred to as **neurohormones** and form a communication mechanism through the bloodstream to control organs that are not directly connected to nervous system structures.

Deregulation of the hypothalamus can be manifested in symptoms of certain psychiatric disorders.

Amygdala. The amygdala is directly connected to more primitive centres of the brain involving the sense of smell. It has numerous connections to the hypothalamus and lies adjacent to the hippocampus. The amygdala provides an emotional component to memory and is involved in modulating aggression, fear, anxiety, and sexuality. Impulsive acts of aggression and violence have been linked to dysregulation of the amygdala, and erratic firing of the nerve cells in the amygdala is a focus of investigation in bipolar mood disorders (see Chapter 22). The amygdala is also the part of the brain most affected by psychoactive drugs.

Limbic Midbrain Nuclei. The limbic midbrain nuclei are a collection of neurons (including the ventral tegmental area and the locus coeruleus) that appear to play a role in the biologic basis of addiction. Sometimes referred to as the pleasure centre or reward centre of the brain, the limbic midbrain nuclei function to chemically reinforce certain behaviours, ensuring their repetition. Emotions such as feeling satisfied with good food, the pleasure of nurturing, and the enjoyment of sexual activity originate in the limbic midbrain nuclei. The reinforcement of activities such as nutrition, procreation, and nurturing young are all primitive aspects of ensuring the survival of a species. When functioning in abnormal ways, the limbic midbrain nuclei can begin to reinforce unhealthy or risky behaviours, such as drug abuse. Exploration of this area of the brain is in its infancy but offers potential insight into addictions and their treatment.

Other Central Nervous System Structures

The extrapyramidal motor system is a bundle of nerve fibres connecting the thalamus to the basal ganglia and cerebral cortex. Muscle tone, common reflexes, and automatic voluntary motor functioning, such as walking, are controlled by this nerve tract. Dysfunction of this motor tract can produce hypertonicity in muscle groups. In Parkinson's disease, the cells that compose the extrapyramidal motor system are severely affected, producing many involuntary motor movements. A number of medications, which are discussed in Chapter 12, also affect this system.

The pineal body is a pinecone-shaped organ, measuring just 5 to 8 mm in length and 3 to 5 mm in width. It is located above and medial to the thalamus. Because the pineal gland easily calcifies, it can be visualized by neuroimaging and often is a medial landmark. Its functions remain somewhat of a mystery, despite long knowledge of its existence. It contains secretory cells that release the neurohormone melatonin and other substances. These hormones are thought to have a number of regulatory functions within the endocrine system. Darkness and hypoglycemia increase the release of melatonin. Melatonin has been associated with sleep and emotional disorders. In addition, it has been postulated that melatonin has a role in modulating immune function.

The *locus coeruleus* is a tiny cluster of norepinephrine-containing neurons that fan out and innervate almost every part of the brain, including most of the cortex, the thalamus and hypothalamus, the cerebellum, and the spinal cord. Just one neuron from the coeruleus can connect to more than 250,000 other neurons. Although it is very small, because of its wide-ranging neuronal connections, this tiny structure has influence in the regulation of attention, time perception, sleep–rest cycles, arousal, learning, pain, and mood, and it seems most involved with information processing of new, unexpected, and novel experiences. Some think its function/dysfunction may explain why individuals become addicted to substances and seek risky behaviours, despite awareness of negative consequences.

The brainstem, located beneath the thalamus, is composed of the midbrain, pons, and medulla and has important life-sustaining functions. Nuclei of numerous neural pathways to the cerebrum are located in the brainstem. They are significantly involved in mediating symptoms of emotional dysfunction. These nuclei are also the primary source of several neurochemicals, such as serotonin, that are commonly associated with psychiatric disorders. Table 9.5 summarizes some of the key-related nuclei.

The cerebellum is in the posterior aspect of the skull, beneath the cerebral hemispheres. This large structure controls movements and postural adjustments. To regulate postural balance and positioning, the cerebellum receives information from all parts of the body, including muscles, joints, skin, and visceral organs, as well as from many parts of the CNS.

Closely associated with the spinal cord, but not lying entirely within its column, is the autonomic nervous system, a subdivision of the PNS. It was originally given this name for being independent of conscious thought, that is, automatic. However, it does not necessarily function as autonomously as the name indicates. This system contains efferent (nerves moving away from the CNS) or motor system neurons, which affect target tissues such as cardiac muscle, smooth muscle, and the glands. It also contains afferent nerves, which are sensory and conduct information from these organs back to the CNS. The two main neurotransmitters of the ANS are acetylcholine (ACh) and norepinephrine. It is important for nurses to recognize that any medication that impacts these neurotransmitters can have far-reaching effects in the body.

The **autonomic nervous system** is further divided into the sympathetic and parasympathetic nervous systems. These systems, although peripheral, are included here because they are involved in the emergency, or "fight-or-flight," response as well as the peripheral actions of many medications (see Chapter 12). Figure 9.6 illustrates the innervations of various target organs by the autonomic nervous system. Table 9.6 identifies the actions of the sympathetic and parasympathetic nervous systems on various target organs.

Table 9.5   Classic and Putative Neurotransmitters, Their Distribution and Proposed Functions

Neurotransmitter	Cell Bodies	Projections	Proposed Function
Acetylcholine Dietary precursor: choline	Basal forebrain Pons Other areas	Diffuse throughout the cortex, hippocampus Peripheral nervous system	Important role in learning and memory Some role in wakefulness and basic attention Peripherally activates muscles and is the major neurochemical in the autonomic system
Monoamines Dopamine Dietary precursor: tyrosine	Substantia nigra Ventral tegmental area Arcuate nucleus Retina olfactory bulb	Striatum (basal ganglia) Limbic system and cerebral cortex Pituitary	Involved in involuntary motor movements Some role in mood states, pleasure components in reward systems, and complex behaviour such as judgement, reasoning, and insight
Norepinephrine Dietary precursor: tyrosine	Locus coeruleus Lateral tegmental area and others throughout the pons and medulla	Very widespread throughout the cortex, thalamus, cerebellum, brainstem, and spinal cord Basal forebrain, thalamus, hypothalamus	Proposed role in learning and memory, attributing value in reward systems; fluctuates in sleep and wakefulness Major component of the sympathetic nervous system responses, including "fight or flight"
Serotonin Dietary precursor: tryptophan	Raphe nuclei Others in the pons and medulla	Widespread throughout the cortex, thalamus, cerebellum, brainstem, and spinal cord	Proposed role in the control of appetite, sleep, mood states, hallucinations, pain perception, and vomiting
Histamine Dietary precursor: histidine	Hypothalamus	Cerebral cortex Limbic system Hypothalamus Found in all mast cells	Control of gastric secretions, smooth muscle control, cardiac stimulation, stimulation of sensory nerve endings, and alertness
Amino Acids GABA	Derived from glutamate without localized cell bodies	Found in cells and projections throughout the CNS, especially in intrinsic feedback loops and interneurons of the cerebrum Also in the extrapyramidal motor system and cerebellum	Fast inhibitory response postsynaptically, inhibits the excitability of the neurons and therefore contributes to seizure, agitation, and anxiety control
Glycine	Primarily the spinal cord and brainstem	Limited projection, but especially in the auditory system and olfactory bulb Also found in the spinal cord, medulla, midbrain, cerebellum, and cortex	Inhibitory Decreases the excitability of spinal motor neurons but not cortical
Glutamate	Diffuse	Diffuse, but especially in the sensory organs	Excitatory Responsible for the bulk of information flow
Neuropeptides Endogenous opioids, (e.g., endorphins, enkephalins)	A large family of neuropeptides, which has three distinct subgroups, all of which are manufactured widely throughout the CNS	Widely distributed within and outside the CNS	Suppresses pain, modulates mood and stress Likely involvement in reward systems and addiction Also may regulate pituitary hormone release Implicated in the pathophysiology of diseases of the basal ganglia
Melatonin One of its precursors: serotonin	Pineal body	Widely distributed within and outside the CNS	Secreted in dark and suppressed light, helps regulate the sleep–wake cycle as well as other biologic rhythms
Substance P	Widespread, significant in the raphe system and spinal cord	Spinal cord, cortex, brainstem, and especially sensory neurons associated with pain perception	Involved in pain transmission, movement, and mood regulation
Cholecystokinin	Predominates in the ventral tegmental area of the midbrain	Frontal cortex where it is often colocalized with dopamine Widely distributed within and outside the CNS	Primary intestinal hormone involved in satiety, also has some involvement in the control of anxiety and panic

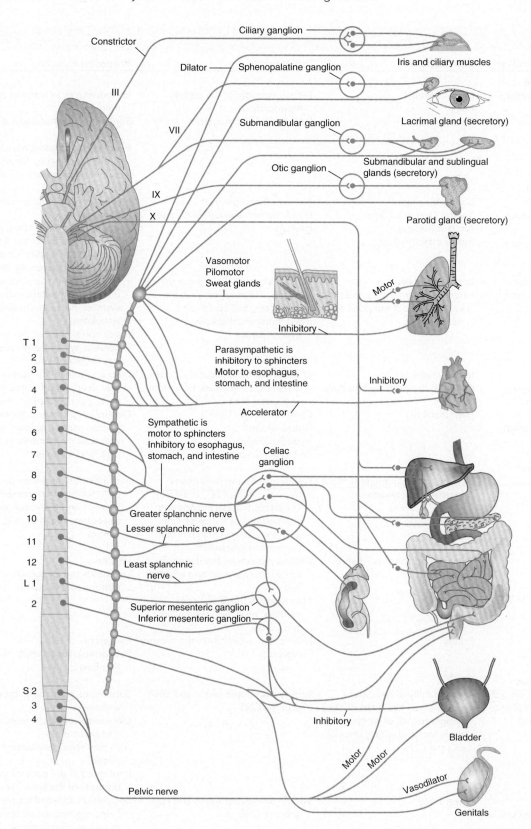

Figure 9.6. Diagram of the autonomic nervous system. Note that many organs are innervated by both sympathetic and parasympathetic nerves. (Adapted from Schaffe, E. E., & Lytle, I. M. (1980). *Basic physiology and anatomy*. Philadelphia, PA: J.B. Lippincott.)

Table 9.6   Peripheral Organ Response in the Autonomic Nervous System

Effector Organ	Sympathetic Response	Parasympathetic Response (Acetylcholine)
Eye		
• Iris sphincter muscle	Preganglionic neurons—acetylcholine	Constriction to normal
• Ciliary muscle	Postganglionic neurons—mostly norepinephrine	Accommodation for near vision
	Dilation	
	Relaxation	
Heart		
• Sinoatrial node	Increased rate	Decrease rate to normal
• Atria	Increased contractility	Decrease in contractility
• Atrioventricular node	Increased contractility	
	Decrease in conduction velocity	
Blood vessels	Depending on type of sympathetic receptor, stimulation can cause constriction or dilation.	Dilation of vessels supplying penis and clitoris only
Lungs		
• Bronchial muscles	Relaxation	Constriction to normal
• Bronchial glands		Secretion
Gastrointestinal Tract		
• Motility and tone	Relaxation (decreased peristalsis)	Increased (for normal peristalsis)
• Sphincters	Contraction	Relaxation
• Secretion glands	Decrease secretion	Stimulation
Urinary Bladder		
• Detrusor muscle	Relaxation	Contraction
• Trigone and sphincter	Contraction	Relaxation
Uterus	Contraction (pregnant)	Variable
	Relaxation (nonpregnant)	
Skin		
• Pilomotor muscles	Contraction	No effect
• Sweat glands	Increased secretion	No effect
Glands		
• Salivary	Stimulation of small volume of thick saliva	Stimulation of large volume of watery saliva
• Sweat	Increased secretion	None
• Adrenal medulla	Stimulation of epinephrine and norepinephrine secretion	None
• Endocrine pancreas	Inhibition of insulin secretion; stimulation of glucagon secretion	Stimulation of insulin and glucagon secretion

NEUROPHYSIOLOGY OF THE CENTRAL NERVOUS SYSTEM

At their most basic level, the human brain and connecting nervous system are composed of billions of cells (Fig. 9.7). There are two main types of brain cells: glia and neurons.

Glial Cells

There are three types of glial cells: astrocytes, oligodendrocytes, and microglial cells. There is five times the number of astrocytes in the brain as neurons. Astrocytes are involved in regulating blood flow in the brain and forming the blood–brain barrier and "scaffolding" of the CNS (Sofroniew & Vinters, 2010). Controlled intracellular calcium concentrations are involved in astrocyte-to-astrocyte communication and astrocyte-to-neuron communication. Astrocytes do not initiate or pass electrical potentials along their processes. Astrocyte dysfunction may be related to anxiety, addiction behaviours, depression, and schizophrenia, and future treatments

may target these cells. Other studies are looking at the link between astrocyte dysfunction and other CNS conditions, including Alzheimer's, Parkinson's, neuropathic pain, and migraine.

Oligodendrites produce the myelin sheath, which speeds electrical conduction over the axons. In multiple sclerosis, the myelin sheath is damaged by an immune attack and conduction of the action potential fails. Microglia are the immune cells of the brain, constantly scanning for threats like damaged cells and infection.

Neurons and Nerve Impulses

About 100 billion cells are nerve cells, or neurons, responsible for receiving, organizing, and transmitting information. Neurons come in many sizes, shapes, and lengths. These factors and where they are located in the brain determine how they function (Fig. 9.8). Each neuron has a cell body, or soma, which holds the nucleus containing most of the cell's genetic information. The soma also includes other organelles, such as ribosomes

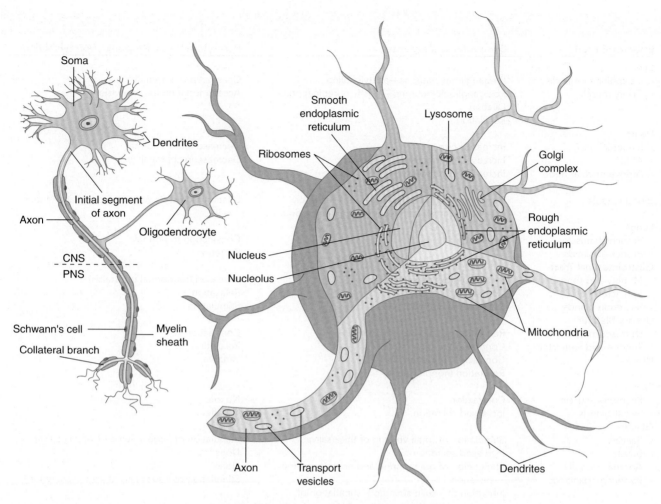

Figure 9.7. Cell body and organelles of an axon.

and endoplasmic reticulum, both of which carry out protein synthesis; the Golgi apparatus, which contains enzymes to modify the proteins for specific functions; vesicles, which transport and store proteins; and lysosomes, responsible for degradation of these proteins. Located throughout the neuron, mitochondria, containing enzymes and often called the "cell's engine," are the site of many energy-producing chemical reactions. These cell structures provide the basis for secreting numerous chemicals by which neurons communicate.

It is not just the vast number of neurons that accounts for the complexities of the brain but also the enormous number of neurochemical interconnections and interactions between neurons. A single motor neuron in the spinal cord may receive signals from more than 10,000 sources of interconnection with other nerves. Although most neurons have only one axon, which varies in length and conducts impulses away from the soma, each has numerous dendrites, receiving signals from other neurons. Because axons may branch as they terminate, they also have multiple contacts with other neurons.

Nerve signals are prompted to fire by a variety of chemical or physical stimuli. This firing produces an electrical impulse. The cell's membrane is a double layer of phospholipid molecules with embedded proteins. Some of these proteins provide water-filled channels through which inorganic ions may pass. Each of the common ions—sodium, potassium, calcium, and chloride—has its own specific molecular channel. These channels are voltage gated and thus open or close in response to changes in the electrical potential across the membrane. At rest, the cell membrane is polarized with a positive charge on the outside and about a 270-mV charge on the inside, owing to the resting distribution of sodium and potassium ions. As potassium passively diffuses across the membrane, the sodium pump uses energy to move sodium from the inside of the cell against a concentration gradient to maintain this distribution. An action potential, or nerve impulse, is generated as the membrane is depolarized and a threshold value is reached, which triggers the opening of the voltage-gated sodium channels, allowing sodium to surge into the cell. The inside of the cell briefly becomes positively charged

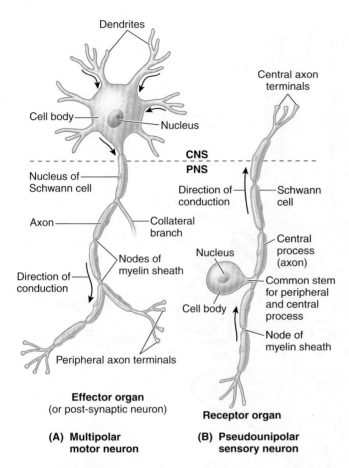

Figure 9.8. The two most common neurons are the **(A)** motor and **(B)** sensory neuron. (Reprinted with permission from Moore, K. L., Agur, A. M. R., & Dalley, A. F. (2014). *Clinically oriented anatomy.* Philadelphia, PA: Lippincott Williams & Wilkins.)

and the outside negatively charged. Once initiated, the action potential becomes self-propagating, opening nearby sodium channels. This electrical communication moves into the soma from the dendrites or down the axon by this mechanism.

Synaptic Transmission

For one neuron to communicate with another, the electrical process must change to a chemical communication. The synaptic cleft, a junction between one nerve and another, is the space where the electrical intracellular signal becomes a chemical extracellular signal. Various substances are recognized as the chemical messengers between neurons.

Neurotransmitters are small molecules that directly and indirectly control the opening or closing of ion channels. Neuromodulators are chemical messengers that make the target cell membrane or postsynaptic membrane more or less susceptible to the effects of the primary neurotransmitter. Some of these neurochemicals are synthesized quickly from dietary precursors, such as tyrosine or tryptophan, or enzymes inside the cytoplasm of the neuron, but most synthesis occurs in

the ends of the axons, called *terminals*, or the neuron itself. Some neurochemicals can reduce the membrane potential and enhance the transmission of the signal between neurons. These chemicals are called *excitatory neurotransmitters*. Other neurochemicals have the opposite effect, slowing down nerve impulses, and these substances are called *inhibitory neurotransmitters*.

As the electrical action potential reaches the terminals, calcium ion channels are opened, causing an influx of Ca^{++} ions into the neuron. This increase in calcium stimulates the release of neurotransmitters into the **synapse**. Rapid signalling between neurons requires a ready supply of neurotransmitters. These neurotransmitters are stored in small vesicles grouped near the cell membrane at the terminals. Because nerve terminals do not have the ability to manufacture proteins, the transmitters that fill these vesicles are small molecules, such as the bioamines (dopamine and norepinephrine) or the **amino acids** (glutamate or γ-aminobutyric acid [GABA]). Actions of these small molecules are discussed in the neurotransmitters section later in this chapter. When stimulated, the vesicles containing the neurotransmitter fuse with the cell membrane, and the neurotransmitter is released into the synapse (Fig. 9.9). The neurotransmitter then crosses the synaptic cleft to a receptor site on the postsynaptic neuron and stimulates adjacent neurons. This is the process of neuronal communication.

Embedded in the postsynaptic membrane are a number of proteins that act as receptors for the released neurotransmitters. The "lock-and-key" analogy has often been used to describe the fit of a given neurotransmitter to its receptor site. Each neurotransmitter has a specific receptor, or protein, for which it and only it will fit. The target cell, when stimulated by the neurotransmitter, will respond by evoking its own action potential and either producing some action common to that cell or acting as a relay to keep the messages moving throughout the CNS. This pattern of the electrical signal from one neuron, converted to chemical signal at the synaptic cleft, picked up by an adjacent neuron, again converted to an electrical action potential and then to a chemical signal, occurs billions of times a day in billions of different brain cells. It is this electrical–chemical communication process that allows the structures of the brain to function together in a coordinated and organized manner.

When the neurotransmitter has completed its interaction with the postsynaptic receptor and stimulated that cell, its work is done and it needs to be removed. It can be removed by natural diffusion away from the area of high neurotransmitter concentration at the receptors by being broken down by enzymes in the synaptic cleft or through reuptake through highly specific mechanisms into the presynaptic terminal.

Many psychopharmacologic agents, particularly antidepressants, act by blocking the reuptake of the neurotransmitters, thereby increasing the available

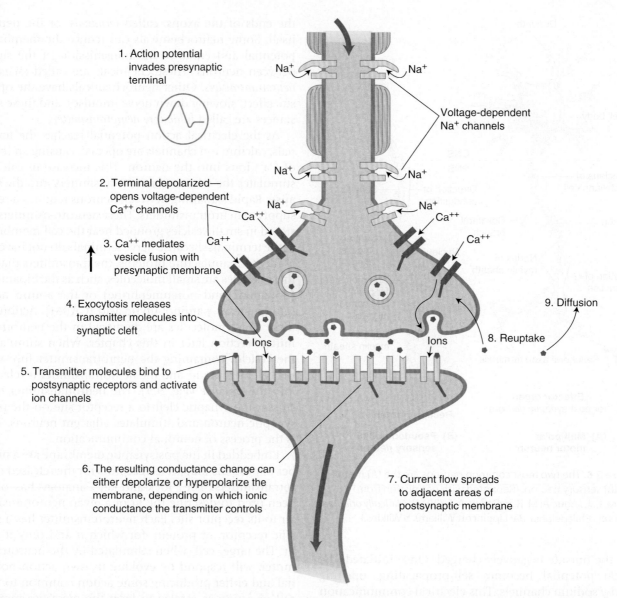

1. Action potential invades presynaptic terminal

Na⁺   Na⁺

Voltage-dependent Na⁺ channels

Na⁺   Na⁺

2. Terminal depolarized—opens voltage-dependent Ca⁺⁺ channels

Na⁺   Na⁺
Ca⁺⁺   Ca⁺⁺
Ca⁺⁺   Ca⁺⁺

3. Ca⁺⁺ mediates vesicle fusion with presynaptic membrane

9. Diffusion

4. Exocytosis releases transmitter molecules into synaptic cleft

Ions   Ions   8. Reuptake

5. Transmitter molecules bind to postsynaptic receptors and activate ion channels

6. The resulting conductance change can either depolarize or hyperpolarize the membrane, depending on which ionic conductance the transmitter controls

7. Current flow spreads to adjacent areas of postsynaptic membrane

Figure 9.9. Synaptic transmission. The most significant events that occur during synaptic transmission: (*1*) the action potential reaches the presynaptic terminal; (*2*) membrane depolarization causes Ca⁺⁺ terminals to open; (*3*) Ca⁺⁺ mediates fusion of the vesicles with the presynaptic membrane; (*4*) transmitter molecules are released into the synaptic cleft, by exocytosis; (*5*) transmitter molecules bind to postsynaptic receptors and activate ion channels; (*6*) conductance changes cause an excitatory or inhibitory postsynaptic potential (excitatory and inhibitory processes are alternately referred to as depolarization and hyperpolarization), depending on the specific transmitter; (*7*) current flow spreads along the postsynaptic membrane; and (*8*) transmitter remaining in the synaptic cleft returns to the presynaptic terminal by reuptake or (*9*) diffuses into the extracellular fluid. (Adapted and reproduced from Schauf, C., Moffett, D., & Moffett, S. (1990). *Human physiology*. St. Louis, MO: Times Mirror/Mosby, with permission.)

amount of chemical messenger. Presynaptic binding sites for neurotransmitters may serve not only as reuptake mechanisms but also as autoreceptors to perform various regulatory functions on the flow of neurotransmitters into the synapse. When these presynaptic autoreceptors are saturated, the neuron slows down or stops releasing neurotransmitters. The neurotransmitters taken back into the presynaptic neuron may be stored in vesicles for rerelease, or they may be broken down by enzymes, such as monoamine oxidase, and removed entirely.

The primary steps in synaptic transmission are summarized in Figure 9.9. The preceding discussion contains only the basic mechanisms of neuronal communication. Many other factors that modulate or contribute to the communication between neurons are only beginning to be discovered. Examples include peptides that are released into the synapse and thought to behave like neurotransmitters or that also can appear in combination with another neurotransmitter. These peptides, known as *cotransmitters*, are believed to have a modulatory effect on the primary neurotransmitter.

KEY CONCEPT

Neurotransmitters are small molecules that directly and indirectly control the opening or closing of ion channels.

Receptor Activity

Both presynaptic and postsynaptic receptors have the capacity to change, developing either a greater than usual response to the neurotransmitter, known as *supersensitivity*, or a less than usual response, called *subsensitivity*. These changes represent the concept of neuroplasticity of brain tissue, which was discussed earlier in the chapter. The change in sensitivity of the receptor is most commonly caused by the effect of a drug on a receptor site or by disease that affects the normal functioning of a receptor site. Drugs can affect the sensitivity of the receptor by altering the strength of attraction or affinity of a receptor for the neurotransmitter, by changing the efficiency with which the receptor activity translates the message inside the receiving cell, or by decreasing over time the number of receptors.

These mechanisms may account for the long-term, sometimes severely adverse, effects of psychopharmacologic drugs, the loss of effectiveness of a given medication, or the loss of effectiveness of a medication after repeated use in treating recurring episodes of a psychiatric disorder. A disease may cause a change in the normal number or function of receptors, thereby altering their sensitivity (Stahl, 2008). It has been hypothesized that depression is caused by a reduction in the normal number of certain receptors, leading to an abnormality in their sensitivity to neurotransmitters such as serotonin and norepinephrine. A decreased response to continued stimulation of these receptors is usually referred to as desensitization or *refractoriness*. This suspected subsensitivity is referred to as *down-regulation* of the receptors.

Receptor Subtypes

The nervous system uses many different neurochemicals for communication, and each specific chemical messenger requires a specific receptor on which the chemical can act. More than 100 different chemical messengers have been identified, with new ones being uncovered frequently as research on the functioning of the brain becomes more and more precise. In addition to the sheer number of receptors needed to accommodate these chemicals, the neurotransmitters may produce different effects at different synaptic sites. The ability of a neurotransmitter to produce different actions is, in part, because of the specialization of its receptors. The different receptors for each neurochemical messenger are referred to as *receptor subtypes* for the chemical. Each major neurotransmitter has several different subtypes of receptors, allowing the neurotransmitter to have different effects in different areas of the brain. For example, dopamine, a common

neurotransmitter discussed in the next section, has five different subtypes of receptors that have been identified. Numbers usually name the receptor subtypes. In the example of dopamine, the various subtypes of receptors are called D_1, D_2, D_3, and so on. Knowledge of the different subtypes helps in understanding both the effects and side effects of medications used to treat mental disorders.

Neurotransmitters

Many substances have been identified as possible chemical messengers, but not all chemical messengers are neurotransmitters. Classic neurotransmitters are those that meet certain criteria agreed on by neuroscientists. The traditional criteria include the following:

- The chemical is synthesized inside the neuron.
- The chemical is present in the presynaptic terminals.
- The chemical is released into the synaptic cleft and causes a particular effect on the postsynaptic receptors.
- An exogenous form of the chemical administered as a drug causes identical action.
- The chemical is removed from the synaptic cleft by a specific mechanism.

Neurotransmitters can be grouped into categories that reflect chemical similarities of the neurotransmitter. Common practice classifies certain chemicals as neurotransmitters even though their ability to meet the strict traditional definition may be incomplete. For the purposes of this section, the classification of neurotransmitters will use this common system of classifying neurotransmitters. Common categories of neurotransmitters include the following:

- Cholinergic neurotransmitters
- Biogenic amine neurotransmitters (sometimes called *monoamines* or *bioamines*)
- Amino acid neurotransmitters
- Neuropeptide neurotransmitters

Neurotransmitters are also classified by whether their action causes physiologic activity to occur or to stop occurring. All of the neurotransmitters commonly involved in the development of mental illness or affected by the drugs used to treat these illnesses are excitatory except one, GABA, which is inhibitory. The significance of this concept is discussed in the section about amino acids. Neurotransmitters are found wherever there are neurons, and neurons are contained in both the CNS and PNS. Because psychiatric mental disorders occur in the CNS, the following sections discuss neurotransmitters from the perspective of the CNS.

Cholinergic

Acetylcholine (ACh) is a primary cholinergic neurotransmitter. Found in the greatest concentration in the

PNS, ACh provides the basic synaptic communication for the parasympathetic neurons and part of the sympathetic neurons, which send information to the CNS. Understanding both the action of ACh and the receptor subtypes for this neurotransmitter assists nurses in understanding the complex side effects of common medications used to treat mental disorders.

Cholinergic neurons, so named because they contain ACh, follow diffuse projections throughout the cerebral cortex and limbic system, arising primarily from cell bodies in the base of the frontal lobes. Pathways from this region also project throughout the hippocampus (Fig. 9.10). These connections suggest that ACh is involved in higher intellectual functioning and memory. Individuals who have Alzheimer's disease or Down's syndrome often exhibit patterns of cholinergic neuron loss in regions innervated by these pathways (such as the hippocampus), which may contribute to their memory difficulties and other cognitive deficits. Some cholinergic neurons are afferent to these areas bringing information from the limbic system, highlighting the role that ACh plays in communicating emotional state to the cerebral cortex. ACh is an excitatory neurotransmitter, meaning that when released into a synapse, it causes the postsynaptic neuron to initiate some action.

The subtypes of ACh receptors are divided into two groups: the muscarinic receptors and the nicotinic receptors. Many psychiatric medications are anticholinergic agents, which block the effects of the muscarinic ACh receptors. This blocking effect of ACh causes common side effects, such as dry mouth, blurred vision, constipation, urinary retention, and tachycardia, which are seen in many psychotropic medications. Excessive blockade of ACh can cause confusion and delirium, especially in older patients, as discussed in Chapter 32. Table 9.5 lists the effects of ACh on various organs in the parasympathetic system. Awareness of what organs are impacted by different medications that impact ACh and other neurotransmitters will help nurses link medications with their effects.

Biogenic Amines

The **biogenic amines** (bioamines) consist of small molecules manufactured in the neuron that contain an amine group. These include dopamine, norepinephrine, and epinephrine, which are all synthesized from the amino acid tyrosine; serotonin, which is synthesized from tryptophan; and histamine, manufactured from histidine. Of all the neurotransmitters, the biogenic amines are most central to current hypotheses of psychiatric disorders and hence are described individually in more detail.

Dopamine

Dopamine is an excitatory neurotransmitter found in distinct regions of the CNS, and it is involved in cognitive, motor, and neuroendocrine functions. Dopamine levels are decreased in Parkinson's disease, and abnormal dopaminergic activity has been associated with schizophrenia (see Chapter 20). Dopamine is also the neurotransmitter that stimulates the body's natural "feel good" reward pathways, producing pleasant euphoric sensation under certain conditions. Abnormalities of dopamine use within the reward system pathways are suspected to be a critical aspect of the development of drug and other addictions. The dopamine pathways are distinct neuronal areas within the CNS in which the neurotransmitter dopamine predominates. Three major dopaminergic pathways have been identified.

The mesocortical and mesolimbic pathways originate in the ventral tegmental area and project into the medial aspects of the cortex (mesocortical) and the medial aspects of the limbic system inside the temporal lobes, including the hippocampus and amygdala (mesolimbic). Sometimes, they are considered to be one pathway and at other times two separate pathways. The mesocortical pathway has major effects on cognition, including such functions as judgement, reasoning, insight, social conscience, motivation, the ability to generalize learning, and reward systems in the human brain. It contributes to some of the highest seats of cortical functioning. The mesocortical system may be linked to the negative symptoms of schizophrenia. The mesocortical pathway also strongly influences emotions and has projections that affect memory and auditory reception. Abnormalities in the mesolimbic system may be linked with positive symptoms of schizophrenia.

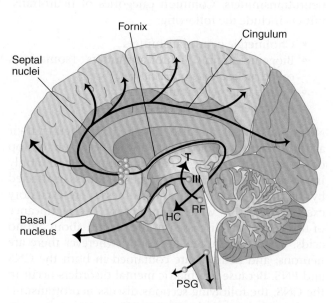

Figure 9.10. Cholinergic pathways. HC, hippocampal formation; PSG, parasympathetic ganglion cell; RF, reticular formation; T, thalamus. (Adapted from Nolte, J., & Angevine, J. (1995). *The human brain: In photographs and diagrams.* St. Louis, MO: Mosby.)

Another major dopaminergic pathway begins in the substantia nigra and projects into the basal ganglia, parts of which are known as the *striatum*. This pathway, called the *nigrostriatal pathway*, influences the extrapyramidal motor system, which serves the voluntary motor system and allows involuntary motor movements. Destruction of dopaminergic neurons in this pathway has been associated with Parkinson's disease.

The last dopamine pathway originates from projections of the mesolimbic pathway and continues into the hypothalamus, which then projects into the pituitary gland. Therefore, this pathway, called the *tuberoinfundibular pathway*, has an impact on endocrine function and other functions, such as metabolism, hunger, thirst, sexual function, circadian rhythms, digestion, and temperature control. Figure 9.11 illustrates the dopaminergic pathways.

As noted previously, scientists have identified at least five subtypes of dopamine receptors in the CNS. These subtypes are distributed differently throughout the brain. For example, the D_1 subtype receptor and its related receptor subtype, D_5, predominate in areas that affect memory and emotions, such as the cortex, hippocampus, and amygdala. They have not been detected in the substantia nigra. D_2 receptors are richly distributed throughout the neurons in the extrapyramidal motor

system, whereas D_4 receptors are richly distributed in the frontal cortex, with few in the nigrostriatal system. Antipsychotic medications, discussed in Chapter 12, act by blocking the effects of dopamine at the receptor sites.

Many of the medications that are most effective on the acute symptoms of psychosis have a strong attraction or affinity for D_2 receptors and a weaker but modest correlation with D_1 receptors. Because D_2 receptors predominate in the nigrostriatal pathway, medications that have a weaker blockade of D_2 will have fewer extrapyramidal motor system effects. Side effects and adverse effects from the involuntary motor system are at times extremely debilitating to individuals. Based on the assumption that these dopamine receptor subtypes have different functions in the CNS, new medications are being designed to affect more predominantly one subtype than another, presumably avoiding effects on systems containing other subtypes and thus avoiding potential side effects of the medication. Researchers are attempting to develop new antipsychotic medications that avoid or minimize the effects on D_2 and therefore diminish the occurrence of extrapyramidal effects.

Norepinephrine

Norepinephrine was first demonstrated to be the primary neurotransmitter of the PNS in 1946. Whereas it is commonly found in the PNS, norepinephrine is also critical to CNS functioning. Norepinephrine is an excitatory neurochemical that plays a major role in generating and maintaining mood states. Decreased norepinephrine has been associated with depression, and excessive norepinephrine has been associated with manic symptoms. Because norepinephrine is so heavily concentrated in the terminal sites of sympathetic nerves, it can be released quickly to ready the individual for a fight-or-flight response to threats in the environment. For this reason, norepinephrine is thought to play a role in the physical symptoms of anxiety.

Nerve tracts and pathways containing predominantly norepinephrine are called *noradrenergic* and are less clearly delineated than the dopamine pathways. In the CNS, noradrenergic neurons originate in the locus coeruleus, where more than half of the noradrenergic cell bodies are located. Because the locus coeruleus is one of the major timekeepers of the human body, norepinephrine is involved in sleep and wakefulness. From the locus coeruleus, noradrenergic pathways ascend into the neocortex, spread diffusely (Fig. 9.12), and enhance the ability of neurons to respond to whatever input they may be receiving. In addition, norepinephrine appears to be involved in the process of reinforcement, which facilitates learning. Noradrenergic pathways innervate the hypothalamus and thus are involved to some degree in endocrine function. Anxiety disorders and depression are examples of psychiatric illnesses in which dysfunction of the noradrenergic neurons may be involved.

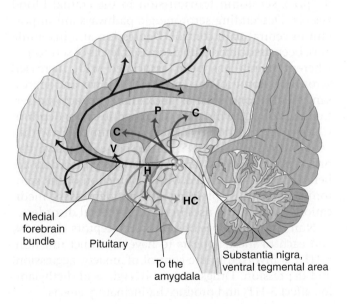

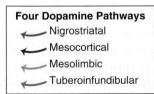

Four Dopamine Pathways
Nigrostriatal
Mesocortical
Mesolimbic
Tuberoinfundibular

Figure 9.11. Dopaminergic pathways. C, caudate nucleus; H, hypothalamus; HC, hippocampal formation; P, putamen; V, ventral striatum. (Adapted from Nolte, J., & Angevine, J. (1995). *The human brain: In photographs and diagrams.* St. Louis, MO: Mosby.)

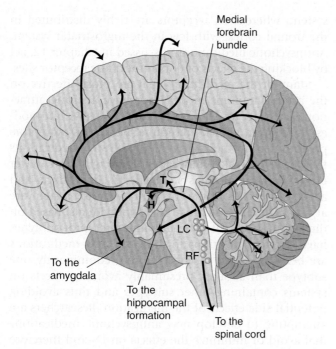

Figure 9.12. Noradrenergic pathways. H, hypothalamus; LC, locus coeruleus; RF, reticular formation; T, thalamus. (Adapted from Nolte, J., & Angevine, J. (1995). *The human brain: In photographs and diagrams*. St. Louis, MO: Mosby.)

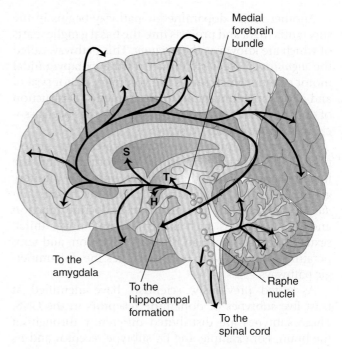

Figure 9.13. Serotonergic pathways. H, hypothalamus; S, septal nuclei; T, thalamus. (Adapted from Nolte, J., & Angevine, J. (1995). *The human brain: In photographs and diagrams*. St. Louis, MO: Mosby.)

Epinephrine

Epinephrine is very similar to norepinephrine chemically; however, in contrast to norepinephrine, only very small amounts of epinephrine are produced and released in the brain. Relatively few neurons in the brain use epinephrine as a neurotransmitter, and those are located in the caudal pons and the medulla. Epinephrine is found in much higher concentrations in the rest of the body, where it is secreted directly from the adrenal gland into the blood circulation.

Serotonin

Serotonin (also called 5-hydroxytryptamine or 5-HT) is primarily an excitatory neurotransmitter that is diffusely distributed within the cerebral cortex, limbic system, and basal ganglia of the CNS. Serotonergic neurons also project into the hypothalamus and cerebellum. Figure 9.13 illustrates serotonergic pathways. Serotonin plays a role in emotions, cognition, sensory perceptions, and essential biologic functions, such as sleep and appetite. During the rapid eye movement (REM) phase of sleep, or the dream state, serotonin concentrations decrease, and muscles subsequently relax. Serotonin is also involved in the control of food intake, hormone secretion, sexual behaviour, thermoregulation, and cardiovascular regulation. Some serotonergic fibres reach the cranial blood vessels within the brain and the pia mater, where they have a vasoconstrictive effect. The potency of some new medications for migraine headaches is related to their ability

to block serotonin transmission in the cranial blood vessels. Descending serotonergic pathways are important in central pain control. Depression and insomnia have been associated with decreased levels of serotonin, whereas mania has been associated with increased serotonin. Some of the most well-known antidepressant medications, such as fluoxetine (Prozac) and sertraline (Zoloft), which are discussed in more depth in Chapter 12, function by raising serotonin levels within certain areas of the CNS. Obsessive–compulsive disorder, panic disorder, and other anxiety disorders are believed to be associated with dysfunction of the serotonin pathways, explaining why antidepressant medications have several uses in treating mental disorders.

Numerous subtypes of serotonin receptors also exist, and each of these appears to have a distinct function. $5\text{-}HT_{1a}$ is involved in the control of anxiety, aggression, and depression. Drugs such as lysergic acid diethylamide affect $5\text{-}HT_2$ and produce hallucinatory effects.

Histamine

Histamine neurons originate predominantly in the hypothalamus and project to all major structures in the cerebrum, brainstem, and spinal cord. Exerting an influence in autonomic and neuroendocrine function, it is associated with many activities, including arousal, cognition, learning and memory, sleep, appetite, and seizures. Many psychiatric medications can block the effects of histamine postsynaptically and produce side effects such as sedation, weight gain, and hypotension.

Amino Acids

Amino acids are the building blocks of proteins and have many roles in intraneuronal metabolism. In addition, amino acids can function as neurotransmitters in as many as 60% to 70% of the synaptic sites in the brain. Amino acids are the most prevalent neurotransmitters. Virtually, all of the neurons in the CNS are activated by excitatory amino acids, such as glutamate, and inhibited by inhibitory amino acids, such as GABA and glycine. Many of these amino acids coexist with other neurotransmitters.

γ-Aminobutyric Acid

GABA is the primary inhibitory neurotransmitter for the CNS. The pathways of GABA exist almost exclusively in the CNS, with the largest GABA concentrations in the hypothalamus, hippocampus, basal ganglia, spinal cord, and cerebellum. GABA functions in an inhibitory role in control of spinal reflexes and cerebellar reflexes. It has a major role in the control of neuronal excitability through the brain. In addition, GABA has an inhibitory influence on the activity of the dopaminergic nigrostriatal projections. GABA also has interconnections with other neurotransmitters. For example, dopamine inhibits cholinergic neurons, and GABA provides feedback and balance.

Decreased GABA activity is involved in the development of seizure disorders. Three specific subtype receptors have been identified for GABA: A, B, and C. Alcohol, certain anaesthetics, benzodiazepine antianxiety drugs, and sedative–hypnotic barbiturate drugs work because of their affinity for GABA$_A$ receptor sites. Interest in the beneficial effects of these drugs has led to increased interest in GABA receptor sites. Nurses frequently see alcohol used to self-treat anxiety; understanding how alcohol impacts the GABA receptors will help explain this behaviour. Recent military engagements have highlighted the risk for posttraumatic stress disorder with and without depressive and substance use disorders among veterans. One recent American study found polymorphisms in a GABA transporter mechanism that places veterans at risk for these disorders (Bountress et al., 2017). In the future, nurses may be called to participate in testing that may help identify those at risk and engage in prevention and treatment efforts.

Glutamate

Glutamate, the most widely distributed excitatory neurotransmitter, is the main transmitter in the associational areas of the cortex. Glutamate can be found in a number of pathways from the cortex to the thalamus, pons, striatum, and spinal cord. In addition, glutamate pathways have a number of connections with the hippocampus. Some glutamate receptors may play a role in the long-lasting enhancement of synaptic activity. In the hippocampus, this enhancement may have a role in learning and memory. Too much glutamate is harmful to neurons, and considerable interest has emerged regarding its neurotoxic effects.

Conditions that produce an excess of endogenous glutamate can cause neurotoxicity by overexcitation of the neuronal tissue. This process, called excitotoxicity, increases the sensitivity of glutamate receptors, produces overactivation of the receptors, and is increasingly being understood as a critical piece of the cascade of events involved in physical symptoms of alcohol withdrawal in dependent individuals. Excitotoxicity is also believed to be part of the pathology of conditions such as ischemia, hypoxia, hypoglycemia, and hepatic failure. Dysfunction of the glutamate system may be involved in depression, drug addiction, psychosis, fragile X syndrome, and Parkinson's disease (Ouellet-Plamondon & George, 2012).

Neuropeptides

Peptides are short chains of amino acids. **Neuropeptides** exist in the CNS and have a number of important roles as neurotransmitters, neuromodulators, or neurohormones. Neuropeptides were first thought to be pituitary hormones, such as adrenocorticotropin, oxytocin, and vasopressin, or hypothalamic-releasing hormones, such as corticotropin-releasing hormone and thyrotropin-releasing hormone (TRH). However, when an endogenous morphine-like substance was discovered in the 1970s, the term endorphin, or endogenous morphine, was introduced. Although amino acids and monoamine neurotransmitters can be produced directly from dietary precursors in any part of the neuron, neuropeptides are, almost without exception, synthesized from messenger RNA in the cell body. To date, two types of neuropeptides have been identified: opioid and nonopioid. Opioid neuropeptides, such as endorphins, enkephalins, and dynorphins, act in endocrine functioning and pain suppression. Nonopioid neuropeptides, such as substance P and somatostatin, play roles in pain transmission and endocrine functioning.

There are considerable variations in the distribution of individual neuropeptides, but some areas are especially rich in cell bodies containing neuropeptides. These areas include the amygdala, striatum, hypothalamus, raphe nuclei, brainstem, and spinal cord. Many of the interneurons of the cerebral cortex contain neuropeptides, but there are considerably fewer in the thalamus and almost none in the cerebellum.

■ OTHER

The endocannabinoid (EC) system (named after the marijuana plant, cannabis, and its active ingredient delta-9-tetrahydrocannabinol [THC]) is a lipid signalling system that seems to be found almost everywhere in the body (Griffing & Thai, 2015). The EC system consists of four subtypes of receptors, two of which, cannabinoids 1 and 2 (CB 1 and CB 2), are reported on most frequently; two primary EC molecules (anandamide and 2-AG); and enzymes that synthesize and degrade the ECs. The EC system communicates its messages in a different way: it works backward. When the postsynaptic neuron is activated, ECs, which are made on demand from fat cells in the neuron, are released from the cell and travel backward to the presynaptic neuron where they attach to cannabinoid receptors.

THC causes pharmacologic actions similar to anandamide and 2-AG, which are present in small amounts in the brain. CB1-R receptors are abundant in the brain, specifically the mesocorticolimbic system, the spinal cord, and the peripheral neurons. CB1-R receptors are particularly concentrated on both GABA–releasing neurons (inhibitory neurons) and glutamate-releasing neurons (excitatory). However, because the receptors are all over the body, ECs have many effects, impacting memory, mood, brain reward systems, drug addiction, and metabolic processes, such as lipolysis, glucose metabolism, the immune system and energy balance. Interestingly, CB1R gene polymorphisms have been described, but their effects are not well understood. Some are associated with anxiety and depression.

The complexities of neuronal transmission are enormous. Nurses have a significant role in assessing symptoms and administering and monitoring medications for patients with psychiatric disorders. Knowledge of neurotransmitters is essential because even a single dose of a drug affecting this system may cause relief of symptoms or have adverse effects. The actions of psychopharmacologic agents and related nursing responsibilities are discussed more fully in Chapter 12. In addition, many nursing interventions designed to effect changes in such functions as sleep, diet, stress management, exercise, and mood modulation affect these neurotransmitters and neuropeptides, directly or indirectly. More research is needed to understand the bio/psycho/social/spiritual aspects of nursing care.

■ NEW FIELDS OF STUDY

As the complexity of the nervous system and its interrelationship with other body systems and the environment have become more fully understood, new fields of study have emerged. From the discussion of neuroanatomy and neurotransmitters, it is logical to deduce that understanding the endocrine system and its interrelationship with the nervous system is essential. Although it has long been observed that individuals under stress have compromised immune systems and are more likely to acquire common diseases, only recently have changes in the immune system been linked to some psychiatric illnesses (Capuron & Miller, 2011; Tafet & Nemeroff, 2016). In addition, as biologic rhythms have become

more fully understood and defined, new information suggests that dysfunction of these rhythms may not only result from a psychiatric illness but also contribute to its development. Therefore, the following sections provide a brief overview of psychoendocrinology, psychoneuroimmunology, and chronobiology.

Psychoendocrinology

Psychoendocrinology examines the relationships among the nervous system, endocrine system, and behaviour. Messages are conveyed within the endocrine system mainly by hormones, and neurohormones are those substances excreted by special neurons within the nervous system. Neurohormones are cellular substances and are secreted into the bloodstream and transported to a site where they exert their effect. Of the several types of hormones, peptides are the most common hormones in the CNS.

The hypothalamus sends and receives information through the pituitary, which then communicates with structures in the peripheral aspects of the body. Figure 9.14 presents an example of the communication of the anterior pituitary with a number of organs and structures. Axes, the structures within which the neurohormones are providing messages, are the most often

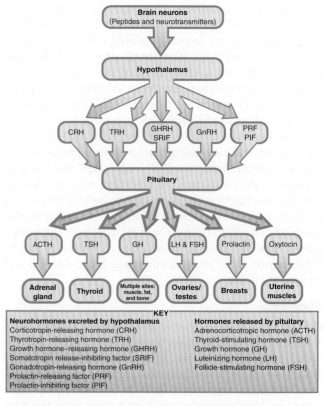

Figure 9.14. Hypothalamic and pituitary communication system. The neurohormonal communication system between the hypothalamus and the pituitary exerts effects on many organs and systems.

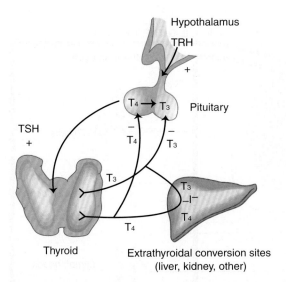

Figure 9.15. Hypothalamic–pituitary–thyroid axis. The regulation of thyroid-stimulating hormone (TSH or thyrotropin) secretion by the anterior pituitary. Positive effects of thyrotropin-releasing hormone (TRH) from the hypothalamus and negative effects of circulating triiodothyronine (T_3) and T_3 from intrapituitary conversion of thyroxine (T_4).

studied aspect of the neuroendocrine system. These axes always involve a feedback mechanism. For example, the hypothalamic–pituitary–thyroid axis regulates the release of thyroid hormone by the thyroid gland using TRH hormone from the hypothalamus to the pituitary and TSH from the pituitary to the thyroid. Figure 9.15 illustrates the hypothalamic–pituitary–thyroid axis. The hypothalamic–pituitary–gonadal axis regulates estrogen and testosterone secretion through LH and FSH.

Interest in psychoendocrinology is heightened by various endocrine disorders that produce psychiatric symptoms. Addison's disease (hypoadrenalism) produces depression, apathy, fatigue, and occasionally psychosis. Hypothyroidism produces depression and some anxiety. Administration of steroids can cause depression, hypomania, irritability, and, in some cases, psychosis. Some psychiatric disorders have been associated with endocrine system dysfunction. For example, some individuals with mood disorders show evidence of dysregulation in the adrenal, thyroid, and GH axes.

Psychoneuroimmunology

Psychoneuroimmunology is the study of immunology as it relates to emotions and behaviour. The immune system protects the body from foreign pathogens. Overactivity of the immune system can occur in autoimmune diseases such as systemic lupus erythematosus, allergies, or anaphylaxis. Too little activity may result from cancer and serious infections, as is the case with AIDS. Evidence suggests that communication between the nervous system and the immune system is bidirectional. Specific immune system dysfunctions may result

from damage to the hypothalamus, hippocampus, or pituitary and may produce symptoms of psychiatric disorders. Negative events and emotions influence catecholamines (norepinephrine and epinephrine), ACTH, cortisol, GH, and prolactin (Christensen, 2008). Each of these hormones can affect the immune function. Figure 9.16 illustrates the interaction between stress and the immune system. This figure also demonstrates the true bio/psycho/social/spiritual nature of the complex interrelationship of the nervous system, the endocrine system, the immune system, and environmental or emotional stress.

Immune dysregulation may also be involved in the development of psychiatric disorders. This can occur by allowing neurotoxins to affect the brain, damaging the neuroendocrine tissue or damaging tissues in the brain at locations such as the receptor sites. Some antidepressants have been thought to have antiviral effects. Symptoms of diseases such as depression may follow an occurrence of serious infection, and prenatal exposure to infectious organisms may be associated with the development of schizophrenia. Stress and conditioning have specific effects on the suppression of immune function.

Cytokines are hormone-like proteins that control the intensity and duration of the body's immune response. An example of a cytokine is interferon alpha, a medication used in the treatment of cancer and hepatitis. Unfortunately, up to 45% of people treated with interferon develop major depression (Capuron & Miller, 2011). Depression and anxiety are linked to cytokines that promote inflammation (Tafet & Nemeroff, 2016). Although there is still much to learn about the relationship of psychiatric disorders and the immune system, it is clear that nurses must develop and implement interventions designed to enhance immune function in psychiatric patients.

Chronobiology

Chronobiology involves the study and measure of time structures or biologic rhythms. Some rhythms have a circadian cycle, or 24-hour cycle, whereas others, such as the menstrual cycle, operate in different periods. Rhythms exist in the human body to control endocrine secretions, sleep–wake cycles, body temperature, neurotransmitter synthesis, and more. These cycles may become deregulated and may begin earlier than usual, known as a phase advance, or later than usual, known as a phase delay.

Zeitgebers are specific events that function as time givers or synchronizers and that set biologic rhythms. Light is the most common example of an external zeitgeber. The suprachiasmatic nucleus of the hypothalamus is an example of an internal zeitgeber. Some theorists think that psychiatric disorders may result from one or more biologic rhythm dysfunctions. For example, depression may in part be a phase advance disorder, including

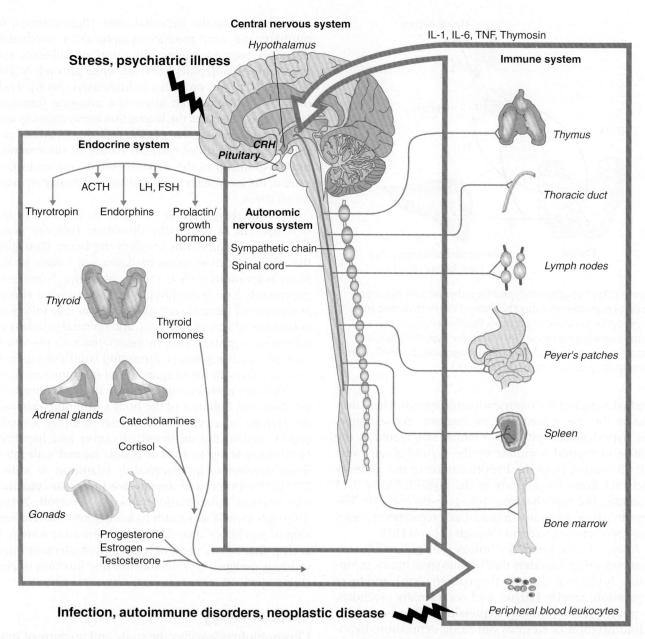

Figure 9.16. Examples of the interaction between stress or psychiatric illness and the immune system through the endocrine system. ACTH, adrenocorticotropic hormone; CRH, corticotropin-releasing hormone; FSH, follicle-stimulating hormone; IL, interleukin; LH, luteinizing hormone; TNF, tumour necrosis factor.

early-morning awakening and decreased time of onset of REM sleep. Seasonal affective disorder may be the result of shortened exposure to light during the winter months. Exposure to specific artificial light often relieves symptoms of fatigue, overeating, hypersomnia, and depression.

■ DIAGNOSTIC APPROACHES

Now that researchers understand more about neural transmission, brain functioning, and psychopharmacology, focus is shifting to applying the knowledge in order to find **biologic markers** for the psychiatric disorders previously thought to have only a psychological

component. Biologic markers are diagnostic test findings that occur only in the presence of the psychiatric disorder and include such findings as laboratory and other diagnostic test results and neuropathologic changes noticeable in assessment. These markers increase diagnostic certainty and reliability and may have predictive value, allowing for the possibility of preventive interventions to forestall or avoid the onset of illness.

In addition, biologic markers could assist in developing evidence-based care practices. If markers can be used reliably, they would help identify the most effective treatments and determine the expected prognosis for given conditions. The PMH nurse should be aware of the most current information on biologic markers so that information, limitations, and results can be discussed knowledgeably with the patient.

Laboratory Tests and Neurophysiologic Procedures

For many years, laboratory tests have been used in the attempt to measure levels of neurotransmitters and other CNS substances in the bloodstream. Many of the metabolites of neurotransmitters can be found in the urine and CSF as well. However, these measures have had only limited utility in elucidating what is happening in the brain. Levels of neurotransmitters and metabolites in the bloodstream or urine do not necessarily equate with levels in the CNS. In addition, availability of the neurotransmitter or metabolite does not predict the availability of the neurotransmitter in the synapse, where it must act or directly relate to the receptor sensitivity. However, in addition to neuroimaging procedures like MRIs, studies of fresh brain tissue removed in neurosurgery and postmortem studies have helped localize neurotransmitters, their function, and pharmacologic properties. These studies have provided clues but are not conclusive and therefore are not routinely used.

Although no commonly used laboratory tests exist that directly confirm a mental disorder, laboratory tests are still an active part of care and assessment of psychiatric patients. Many physical conditions mimic the symptoms of mental illness, and many of the medications used to treat psychiatric illness can produce health problems. For these reasons, the routine care of patients with psychiatric disorders includes the use of laboratory tests such as complete blood counts, thyroid studies, electrolytes, hepatic enzymes, and other evaluative tests. Nurses need to be familiar with these procedures and assist patients in understanding the use and implications of such tests.

Electroencephalography

Developed in the 1920s by Hans Berger, an electroencephalograph (EEG) measures electrical activity in the uppermost layers of the cortex. Electrodes are placed on 8 to 20 sites upon the patient's scalp. The EEG machine is equipped with graph paper and recording pens that trace the electrical impulses generated over each electrode. Until the use of CT scanning in the 1970s, the EEG was the only method for identifying brain abnormalities. It remains the simplest and least invasive method for identifying some disorders.

An EEG may be used in psychiatry to differentiate possible causes of a patient's symptoms. For example, some types of seizure disorders, such as temporal lobe epilepsy, head injuries, or tumours, may present with predominantly psychiatric symptoms. In addition, metabolic dysfunction, delirium, dementia, altered levels of consciousness, hallucinations, and dissociative states may require EEG evaluation.

Normal patterns seen on EEGs are called alpha, beta, theta, and delta waves; the rhythms may vary depending on the age of the person. Factors that may interfere with obtaining accurate results include being unable to remain still or cooperate during the test, being hypoglycemic or hypothermic, and hair that is dirty, oily, or treated with hair products. Spikes and wave pattern changes are indications of brain abnormalities. Spikes may be the focal point from which a seizure occurs. However, abnormal activity often is not discovered on a routine EEG while the individual is awake. For this reason, additional methods are sometimes used. Nasopharyngeal leads may be used to get physically closer to the limbic regions. The patient may be exposed to a flashing strobe light while the examiner looks for activity that is not in phase with the flashing light or may be asked to hyperventilate for 3 minutes to induce abnormal activity if it exists. Sleep deprivation may also be used. This involves keeping the patient awake throughout the night before the EEG evaluation. The patient may then be drowsy and fall asleep during the procedure.

Abnormalities are more likely to occur when the patient is asleep. Sleep may also be induced using medication; however, EEG wave patterns can be affected by medications such as anticonvulsants and anxiolytics, as well as by other substances that act as sedatives or stimulants. For example, the benzodiazepine class of drugs increases the rapid and fast beta activity and lithium increases theta activity. In addition to reassuring, preparing, and educating the patient for the examination, the nurse should carefully assess the history of substance use and report this information to the examiner. If a sleep deprivation EEG is to be done, caffeine or other stimulants that might help the patient stay awake should be withheld because they may change the EEG patterns.

Polysomnography

Polysomnography is a special procedure that involves recording the EEG throughout a night of sleep. See Chapter 28 for a discussion of sleep studies.

Other Neurophysiologic Methods

Evoked potentials (EPs), also called event-related potentials, use the same basic principles as an EEG. They measure changes in electrical activity in the visual, somatosensory, and auditory pathways in response to a given stimulus. Electrodes placed on the scalp measure a large waveform that stands out after the administration of repetitive stimuli, such as a click or flash of light. There are several different types of EPs to be measured, depending on the sensory area affected by the stimulus, the cognitive task required, or the region monitored, any of which can change the length of time until the wave occurrence. EPs are used extensively in psychiatric research. In clinical practice, EPs are used primarily in the assessment of demyelinating disorders, such as multiple sclerosis.

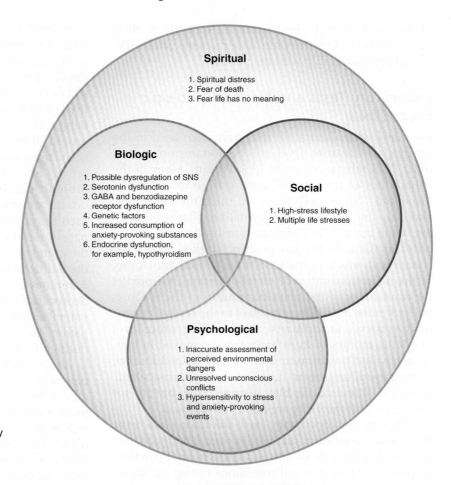

Spiritual

1. Spiritual distress
2. Fear of death
3. Fear life has no meaning

Biologic

1. Possible dysregulation of SNS
2. Serotonin dysfunction
3. GABA and benzodiazepine receptor dysfunction
4. Genetic factors
5. Increased consumption of anxiety-provoking substances
6. Endocrine dysfunction, for example, hypothyroidism

Social

1. High-stress lifestyle
2. Multiple life stresses

Psychological

1. Inaccurate assessment of perceived environmental dangers
2. Unresolved unconscious conflicts
3. Hypersensitivity to stress and anxiety-provoking events

Figure 9.17. Bio/psycho/social/spiritual etiologies for patients with generalized anxiety disorders. GABA, γ-aminobutyric acid; SNS, sympathetic nervous system.

INTEGRATION OF THE BIOLOGIC, PSYCHOLOGIC, SOCIAL, AND SPIRITUAL DOMAINS

Basic knowledge in the neurosciences has become essential content for the practising nurse. In a truly holistic bio/psycho/social/spiritual model, all psychological and social influences are seen as interacting with the complex human biologic system. For example, treatment of generalized anxiety disorder would involve addressing etiologies in each of these areas (see Fig. 9.17). As research continues to increase our understanding of the biologic dimension of psychiatric disorders and mental health, nursing care will focus on human biology in increasingly sophisticated ways. Nurses must integrate this information into all aspects of nursing management, including:

- Assessment—genetic, physical, and environmental factors that contribute to the symptoms of psychiatric disorders; biologic rhythm changes; cognitive abilities that may affect or complicate interventions; and **risk factors** that may predict development of psychiatric symptoms or disorders
- Diagnosis—difficulties related to diet, exercise, or sleep that may change the individual's biology; quality of life difficulties based on biologic

changes; and knowledge deficits concerning the biologic basis of psychiatric disorders or treatment
- Interventions—designed to modify biologic changes and physical functioning, designed to enhance biologic treatments, or modified to consider cognitive dysfunction related to psychiatric disorders

SUMMARY OF KEY POINTS

- Neuroscientists now view behaviour and cognitive function as results of complex interactions within the CNS and its plasticity or its ability to adapt and change in both structure and function.
- Each hemisphere of the brain is divided into four lobes. The frontal lobe controls motor speech function, personality, and working memory—often called the executive functions that govern one's ability to plan and initiate action. The parietal lobe controls sensory functions. The temporal lobe contains the primary auditory and olfactory areas. The occipital lobe controls visual integration of information.
- The structures of the limbic system are integrally involved in memory and emotional behaviour. Dysfunction of the limbic system has been linked with major mental disorders, including schizophrenia, depression, and anxiety disorders.

- Neurons communicate with each other through synaptic transmission. Neurotransmitters excite or inhibit a response at the receptor sites and have been linked to certain mental disorders. These neurotransmitters include ACh, dopamine, norepinephrine, serotonin, GABA, and glutamate.
- Psychoendocrinology examines the relationship between the nervous system and endocrine system and the effects of neurohormones excreted by special neurons to communicate with the endocrine system in effecting behaviour. Psychoneuroimmunology focuses on the nervous system as regulating immune function, which may play a significant role in effecting psychological states and psychiatric disorders. Chronobiology focuses on the study and measure of time structures or biologic rhythms occurring in the body and associates dysregulation of these cycles as contributing factors to the development of psychiatric disorders.
- Biologic markers are physical indicators of disturbances within the CNS that differentiate one disease process from another, such as biochemical changes or neuropathologic changes. These biologic markers can be measured by several methods of testing, including electroencephalography, polysomnography, EPs, CT scanning, MRI, PET, and SPECT. The nurse must be familiar with each of these.

Web Links

thebrain.mcgill.ca/ McGill University hosts this excellent presentation of "the brain from top to bottom," with the latest research informing explanations of the brain's anatomy and physiology, its relationship with mind and behaviour, and brain disorders from biologic, psychological, and social perspectives.

loni.usc.edu/ This is the site of the Laboratory of Neuro Imaging (LONI) at the University of Southern California. LONI is dedicated to the development of comprehensive brain mapping in order to improve understanding of the brain.

braintour.harvard.edu/click-watch-learn Several fascinating video talks about the brain are available at this site.

ted.com At this site, you can access many educational, entertaining talks on the brain, such as "Jocelyne Bloch: The brain may be able to repair itself—with help" and "Rebecca Brachman: Could a drug prevent depression and PTSD?"

www.brain-map.org/ The Allen Institute for Brain Science has a site that posts many interesting interactive tools describing current areas of brain research.

References

Agius, M., & Aquilina, F. F. (2014). Comorbidities and psychotic illness. Part 1: Philosophy and clinical consequences. *Psychiatria Danubina, 26*(Suppl 1), 246–249.

Bhatnagar, S. (2013). *Neuroscience for the study of communicative disorders.* Philadelphia, PA: Lippincott Williams & Wilkins.

Bountress, K. E., Wei, W., Sheerin, C., Chung, D., Amstadter, A. B., Mandel, H., & Wang, Z. (2017). Relationships between GAT1 and PTSD, depression, and substance use disorder. *Brain Sciences, 7*(1), 6. MDPI AG. Retrieved from http://dx.doi.org/10.3390/brainsci7010006

Capuron, L., & Miller, A. (2011). Immune system to brain signaling: Neuropsychopharmacological implications. *Pharmacology and Therapeutics, 130*, 226–238.

Christensen, J. (2008). Stress and disease. In M. Feldman & J. Christensen (Eds.), *Behavioral medicine: A guide for clinical practice* (3rd ed.). New York: McGraw-Hill.

Currie, S., Hadjivassiliou, M., Crave, I., Wilkinson, I., Griffiths, P., & Hoggard, N. (2013). Magnetic resonance spectroscopy of the brain. *Postgraduate Medical Journal, 89*, 94–106.

Doll, A., Hölzel, B. K., Mulej Bratec, S., Boucard, C. C., Xie, X., Wohlschläger, A. M., & Sorg, C. (2016). Mindful attention to breath regulates emotions via increased amygdala-prefrontal cortex connectivity. *Neuroimage, 134*, 305–313. doi: 10.1016/j.neuroimage.2016.03.041

GenomeCanada. (2017). *New funding opportunity—2017 Large-scale applied research project competition: Genomics and precision health.* Retrieved from https://www.genomecanada.ca/en/news-and-events/news-releases/new-funding-opportunity-2017-large-scale-applied-research-project

Graves, W. (2013, January 15). *Sidney Crosby says he's free of concussion symptoms.* Associated Press. Retrieved from http://www.cbc.ca/sports/hockey/nhl/sidney-crosby-says-he-s-free-of-concussion-symptoms-1.1400543

Griffing, G., & Thai, A. (2015). Endocannabinoids. *Medscape.* Retrieved from http://emedicine.medscape.com/article/1361971-overview#a1

Harlow, J. M. (1868). Recovery after severe injury to the head. *Publication of the Massachusetts Medical Society, 2*, 327.

Hennig, J., Speck, O., Koch, M. A., & Weiller, C. (2003). Functional magnetic resonance imaging: A review of methodological aspects and clinical applications. *Journal of Magnetic Resonance Imaging, 18*(1), 1–15.

Holtzheimer, P. E. (2013). *Unipolar depression in adults: Treatment with transcranial magnetic stimulation (TMS).* Retrieved from http://www.uptodate.com/index

Kim, Y., Jeong, H. S., Song, I., Chung, Y., Namgung, E., & Kim, Y. (2016). Brain perfusion alterations in depressed patients with Parkinson's disease. *Annals of Nuclear Medicine, 30*(10), 731–737.

Kleim, J., & Jones, T. A. (2008). Principles of experience-dependent neuroplasticity: Implications for rehabilitation after brain damage. *Journal of Speech, Language, and Hearing Research, 51*, S225–S239.

Kundu, T. K. (Ed.). (2013). *Epigenetics: Development and disease.* New York: Springer.

Labonté, B., Suderman, M., Maussion, G., Lopez, J. P., Navarro-Sánchez, L., Yerko, V. G., … Turecki, G. (2013). Genome-wide methylation changes in the brains of suicide completers. *American Journal of Psychiatry, 170*(5), 511–520.

Marques, S., & Fleming Outeiro, T. (2013). Epigenetics in Parkinson's and Alzheimer's diseases. In T. K. Kundu (Ed.), *Epigenetics: Development and disease* (pp. 507–525). New York: Springer.

Marx, V. (2015). The DNA of a nation. *Nature, 524*(7566), 503–505. doi: 10.1038/524503a

McGuffin, P., & Southwick, L. (2003). Fifty years of the double helix and its impact on psychiatry. *Australian and New Zealand Journal of Psychiatry, 37*, 657–661.

Merico, D., Zarrei, M., Costain, G., Ogura, L., Alipanahi, B., Gazzellone, M. J., … Bassett, A. S. (2015). Whole-genome sequencing suggests schizophrenia risk mechanisms in humans with 22q11.2 deletion syndrome. *G3 (Bethesda, Md.), 5*(11), 2453–2461. doi: 10.1534/g3.115.021345

Miglioretti, D., & Simth-Bindman, R. (2011). Overuse of computed tomography and associated risks. *American Family Physician, 83*, 1252–1254.

Moore, K. L., Agur, A. M. R., & Dalley, A. F. (2014). *Clinically oriented anatomy.* Philadelphia, PA: Lippincott Williams & Wilkins.

Morrish, J., & Carey, S. (2013). *Concussions in Canada. Canada Injury Compass, Spring 2013.* Toronto, Canada: Parachute.

National Human Genome Research Institute. (2013). *Fact sheets: Epigenomics.* National Institutes of Health. Retrieved from http://www.genome.gov/27532724

National Institute on Aging. (2011; updated April 2013). *Biology of aging: Research today for a healthier tomorrow.* US Department of Health and Human Services. Retrieved from http://www.nia.nih.gov/health/publication/biology-aging

Nolte, J., & Angevine, J. (1995). *The human brain: In photographs and diagrams.* St. Louis, MO: Mosby.

Oedegaard, K. J., Alda, M., Anand, A., Andreassen, O. A., Balaraman, Y., Berrettini, W. H., … Kelsoe, J. R. (2016). The pharmacogenomics of bipolar disorder study (PGBD): Identification of genes for lithium response in a prospective sample. *BMC Psychiatry, 16*, 129. doi: 10.1186/s12888-016-0732-x

Ouellet-Plamondon, C., & George, T. (2012). *Glutamate and psychiatry in 2012: Up, up and away!* Retrieved from http://www.psychiatrictimes.com/bipolar-disorder/glutamate-and-psychiatry-2012%E2%80%94-and-away

Pirooznia, M., Seifuddin, F., Judy, J., Mahon, P. B., Potash, J. B., & Zandi, P. P. (2012). Data mining approaches for genome-wide association of mood disorders. *Psychiatric Genetics, 22*(2), 55–61. doi: 10.1097/YPG.0b013e32834dc40d

Quigley, P. (2015). Mapping the human genome: Implications for practice. *Nursing, 45*(9), 26–34. doi:10.1097/01.NURSE.0000470413.71567.fd

Schaffe, E. E., & Lytle, I. M. (1980). *Basic physiology and anatomy.* Philadelphia, PA: J.B. Lippincott.

Schauf, C., Moffett, D., & Moffett, S. (1990). *Human physiology.* St. Louis, MO: Times Mirror/Mosby.

Shah, M., & Allegrucci, C. (2013). Stem cell plasticity in development and cancer: Epigenetic origin of cancer stem cells. In T. K. Kandu (Ed.). *Epigenetics: Development and disease* (pp. 545–565). New York: Springer.

Shenton, M., Hamoda, H., Schneiderman, J., Bouiz, S., Pasternak, O., Rathi, Y., ... Zafonte, R. (2012). A review of magnetic resonance imaging and diffusion tensor imaging findings in mild traumatic brain injury. *Brain Imaging and Behavior, 6,* 137–192.

Simmons, D. (2008). *Epigenetic influence and disease.* Retrieved from http://www.nature.com/scitable/topicpage/epigenetic-influences-and-disease-895

Sofroniew, M., & Vinters, H. (2010). Astrocytes: Biology and pathology. *Acta Neuropathologica, 119,* 7–35.

Stahl, S. (2008). *Stahl's essential psychopharmacology: Neuroscientific basis and practical applications* (3rd ed.). New York: Cambridge University Press.

Tafet, G. E., & Nemeroff, C. B. (2016). The links between stress and depression: Psychoneuroendocrinological, genetic, and environmental interactions. *Journal of Neuropsychiatry and Clinical Neurosciences, 28*(2), 77–88. doi: 10.1176/appi.neuropsych.15030053

Waddington, C. (1957). *The strategy of the genes: A discussion of some aspects of theoretical biology.* London, UK: Allen & Unwin.

Wyshynski, G. (2011). *Sidney Crosby talks concussion, "irresponsible" blindside hits and when Penguins knew about injury.* Retrieved from http://ca.sports.yahoo.com/nhl/blog/puck_daddy/post/Sidney-Crosby-talks-concussion-irresponsible-?urn=nhl-305051

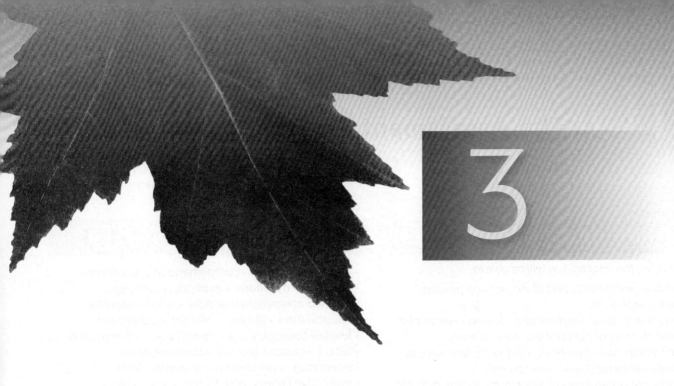

3

Interventions in Psychiatric and Mental Health Nursing Practice

10 The Assessment Process

Gerri Lasiuk

Adapted from the chapter "The Assessment Process" by Gerri Lasiuk and Kathleen Hegadoren

LEARNING OBJECTIVES

After studying this chapter, you will be able to:

- Identify assessment as part of the nursing process.
- Define assessment.
- Differentiate comprehensive and focused assessments.
- Explain the role of observation, interviewing, examination, and consultation in the performance of psychiatric/mental health assessment.
- Identify important areas of assessment for the biologic, psychological, and social domains of a psychiatric/mental health nursing assessment.
- Discuss the synthesis of the bio/psycho/social/spiritual assessment data.

KEY TERMS

- affect • cisgender • comprehensive assessment
- delusion • dysphoric • euphoric • euthymic
- focused assessment • gender • gender identity
- hallucination • illusion • insight • judgement
- level of consciousness • mental status examination
- mood • nursing process • objective data
- orientation • perception • promotive factors
- protective factors • risk factors • sex • sexual orientation • subjective data • thought content
- thought process • trans affirmative practices
- transgender • transsexual

KEY CONCEPTS

- assessment • mental status examination

The **nursing process** is a systematic and dynamic approach to collecting and analyzing client information and is the first step in the provision of nursing care. The four essential components of the nursing process are assessment, planning, implementation, and evaluation. This chapter deals with assessment—activities involved with the collection, validation, analysis, synthesis, and documentation of information concerning clients' responses to health and illness.

■ ASSESSMENT AS A PROCESS

Standard II of the *Canadian Standards of Psychiatric and Mental Health Nursing* states:

Effective assessment, diagnosis, and monitoring are central to the nurse's role and depend upon theory as well as upon understanding the meaning of the health or illness experience from the perspective of the client. The nurse explains the assessment process to the client and provides feedback. Knowledge is integrated with the nurse's conceptual model of nursing practice, which provides a framework for processing client data and for developing client-focused plans of care. The nurse makes professional judgements based upon

evidence and recognizes and includes the client as a valued partner (Canadian Federation of Mental Health Nurses [CFMHNs], 2014, p. 7).

This statement underscores the importance of assessment as the basis for developing a plan of care.

Assessment is not a one-time activity; it is an ongoing, purposeful, systematic, and dynamic process in nurses' relationships with individuals in their care. As per the Canadian Federation of Mental Health Nurses (2014), effective assessment requires that the nurse:

1. Collaborates with clients and with other members of the health care team to gather holistic, client-centred assessments through observation, engagement, examination, interview (using respectful, recovery focussed language), and consultation while attending to confidentiality and pertinent legal statutes
2. Assesses, documents, and analyzes data to identify health status, potential for wellness, health care deficits, potential for risk to self and others; alterations in thought content and/or process, affect behaviour, communication and decision-making abilities; substance use and dependency; and history of trauma and/or abuse (emotional, physical, neglect, sexual, or verbal)

3. Formulates and documents a plan of care in collaboration with the client, family, and mental health team that supports recovery and reintegration/social inclusion in the community through discharge planning and provision for ongoing support, all while recognizing variability in the client's ability to participate in the process

4. Refines and expands client assessment information by assessing and documenting significant change(s) in the client's status and by comparing new data with the baseline assessment and client goals

5. Assesses and anticipates potential needs and risks continuously, collaborating with the client to examine his/her environment for risk factors such as self-care, housing, nutrition, economic support, psychological state, and social interactions

6. Determines the most appropriate and available therapeutic modality that meets the client's needs, and assists the client to access necessary resources. (p. 8).

KEY CONCEPT

Assessment is a purposeful, systematic, and dynamic process in nurses' relationships with individuals in their care. It involves the collection, validation, analysis, synthesis, organization, and documentation of client health–illness information.

■ TYPES OF ASSESSMENT

Depending on the client's needs and the context of care, an assessment may be comprehensive or focused. A **comprehensive assessment** includes a complete health history (Table 10.1) and physical examination; considers the psychological, emotional, social, spiritual, ethnic, and cultural dimensions of health; attends to the client's health–illness experience; and endeavours to understand their lived experience. The purpose of a comprehensive assessment is to develop a holistic understanding of the individual's problems and needs as well as his or her strengths and resources. It is performed in collaboration with the client and other members of the treatment team and is the basis for establishing baseline health–illness information necessary to establish a diagnosis, identify treatment goals, and develop a plan of care.

Because of its broad scope, and the time it takes to develop rapport, a comprehensive assessment may take days or even weeks to complete. Members of the health care team collect information from several sources, including individual clients and their families, other health care providers, social service and justice personnel, educators, employers, and existing client records.

All this is done while attending to issues of confidentiality and relevant legal statutes.

A **focused assessment** is the collection of specific information about a specific need, problem, or situation and may involve evaluation of such things as medication effects, risk for self-harm/suicide, knowledge deficits, or the adequacy of supports and resources. As the name suggests, focused assessments are briefer, narrower in scope, and more present oriented than are comprehensive assessments. Focused assessments may also be used to screen individuals who are at high risk for particular problems or disorders. In these instances, nurses often employ standardized assessment tools (e.g., Glasgow Coma Scale [GCS], Mini-Mental Status Examination [MMSE], or Hamilton Rating Scale for Depression [HAM-D]).

The type of assessment required in a given situation depends on two key factors: the immediate needs of the client and the practice setting. Efforts to perform a comprehensive assessment during a psychiatric emergency (e.g., when an individual is floridly psychotic or actively suicidal) can be both dangerous and futile. The quality and trustworthiness of the information collected in these circumstances are biased by the client's symptoms and by the high emotionality of the situation. The priority in such situations is to perform a focused assessment that provides the treatment team with sufficient information to address the client's symptoms and to ensure the safety of all involved.

The type of assessment nurses perform is also largely determined by the setting in which they work. The mandate of a psychiatric and mental health (PMH) facility or program determines the type of service it offers, which in turn dictates the nature of the assessment required. During a first admission to a psychiatric unit, for example, an individual is likely to undergo a comprehensive assessment. In contrast, nurses working with a telehealth line or with a mobile mental health crisis team will collect only the information required to address the immediate problem or crisis.

Assessment Techniques

PMH assessments involve observation of the individual at different times of the day and in different circumstances, interviews with the individual and family members, consultation with other health care providers, and analyses and synthesis of findings from physical and mental examinations into a care plan.

Observation

Although verbal communication is vital to the assessment process, nonverbal cues also communicate important information about the client's health–illness experience (see Chapter 6). Nurses use all five senses and integrate assessment into all their encounters

Table 10.1   Health History and Significance to Psychiatric and Mental Health Problems

Data	Considerations/Significance
Source of Information	Ideally, the client is the primary source of information; consultation with secondary sources is necessary with minors or when the client is unable to provide information.
	Note the apparent reliability and consistency of the information provided.
Identification/Biographic Information	Legal name/nicknames/aliases, date and place of birth, gender, address, telephone numbers, relationship status, next of kin, ethnicity, religious/spiritual affiliation, employer, education, and provincial/territorial health insurance number
	Because this information is relatively nonthreatening, it is a safe place to begin an assessment. It also provides important clues about an individual's current living situation.
Primary Reason for Seeking Care	Record this verbatim because it speaks to the client and family perceptions of and insight into existing problems, judgement, and goals for treatment.
Past Health	
Past illness, injury, and/or hospitalization	Note positive history of childhood diseases, especially viral infection, which have been linked to some psychiatric disorders (e.g., schizophrenia).
	Inquire about surgeries and trauma, particularly those resulting in concussion or loss of consciousness.
	Ask about parental alcohol and drug use (especially during pregnancy), birth trauma, lengthy/repeated separation from parents/caregivers because of hospitalization, a pattern of injury suggestive of childhood abuse/neglect, and surgeries.
Chronic illnesses	Chronic illnesses (e.g., diabetes and thyroid dysfunction), even when well controlled, may affect mental status.
	Highlight known allergies, type of reaction, usual treatment, and effectiveness of treatment.
Family Health History	Record the name, age, and current health status of close relatives (spouse/partner, children, parents, siblings, grandparents, and aunts/uncles). If a family member is deceased, note the date and cause of death and indications of unresolved grief/loss.
	Inquire specifically about diseases/disorders that "run in the family," particularly psychiatric disorders and addictions. A genogram is a useful tool for recording this information.
	Many psychiatric disorders are genetically linked, so a family health history provides information about the client's risk factors. It also provides clues about social roles, the availability of social support, and family resources/stressors.
	Coping strategies, both effective and ineffective, are learned early in life from our family of origin. A family health history can help to identify these.
Developmental Considerations	Note achievement of important developmental milestones as well as social and educational difficulties. This information may be indicative of attentional or interpersonal deficits, behavioural problems, a chaotic family environment, acquired brain injury, or childhood mental illness.
	Ask about early parental death or separation because these may be associated with alterations in attachment and later relationship difficulties.
	The Canadian government's practice of removing Indigenous children to residential schools traumatized children, fragmented families, decimated cultures/languages, and contributed to serious social and psychological problems that still reverberate among First Nations people.
Immunization/HIV/Hepatitis Status	Individuals with severe and persistent mental illness often live in severe poverty and lack knowledge and resources for health promotion. In addition, many have lifestyles that put them at risk for serious communicable diseases.
Psychological Trauma	Ask: "Have you ever experienced or witnessed anything that threatened your life or safety or the life or safety of a loved one?" If yes, probe for details.
	Psychological trauma associated with natural disasters, motor vehicle crashes, combat, abuse/assault (physical or sexual), and childhood neglect is associated with a number of PMH problems (e.g., particularly posttraumatic stress disorder, other anxiety disorders, and depression).
Current Health Status	Provides information about medical conditions that affect mental status, global functioning, and quality of life.
	A systematic approach to performing a health history ensures thoroughness, helps the clinician to organize/cluster the data, and cues the informant's memory.
	Analyze significant symptoms (see Box 10.4).
Integument	Ask about problems/changes in the skin, hair, and nails. Note the presences of scars, piercings/body art, lesions/sores, rashes, discolouration, itching, or unusual sensations.
	Piercings and body art are expressions of one's personal aesthetic, which is part of self-concept. They may also indicate identification with particular social groups.
Sensory systems	Note sensory deficits and the presence of prescription lenses, contact lenses, hearing aids, and dentures.
	Uncorrected sensory deficits can affect an individual's day-to-day function and ability to communicate.
	Record the report of unusual perceptions or sensations because these may be related to perceptual or thought disturbances.
Respiratory	Note problems/disease, recurrent infections, cough, sputum, shortness of breath, noisy respirations, and smoking history.

Table 10.1   Health History and Significance to Psychiatric and Mental Health Problems *(Continued)*

Data	Considerations/Significance
Cardiovascular/haematologic	Inquire about history of cardiac disease/problems, palpitations, arrhythmias, murmurs, dizzy spells, coldness/blueness/swelling of extremities, and leg pain while walking. Individuals who experience panic episodes often present at emergency departments because their signs and symptoms mimic heart attack. Inquire about anaemia, bleeding disorders, fatigue, blood transfusions, bruising, and cancers. Monitoring of some long-term neuroleptic medication use (e.g., lithium and clozapine) requires regular blood tests.
Gastrointestinal	Ask about changes in appetite, weight, and bowel patterns; nausea, vomiting, indigestion, and gastroesophageal reflux disease; antacid and laxative use; history of disease (e.g., ulcers, irritable bowel syndrome, and cancer); and rectal discharge/bleeding. Alterations in gastrointestinal function are implicated in some mental disorders and as a side effect of many psychotropic medications. For example, a person who is depressed may not have an appetite or not have the energy to prepare food. Others may respond to distressing emotions by eating more than usual. As well, the anticholinergic effects of antipsychotic medication can cause constipation, whereas lithium carbonate can cause diarrhoea.
Genitourinary	Note pain/burning on urination, frequency, urgency, dribbling/incontinence, hesitancy, colour of urine, history of urinary tract infection/kidney disease, and frequent nighttime urination. Anticholinergic effects of antipsychotic medication can cause urinary hesitancy and/or retention.
Reproductive/breasts	Ask females about menarche; usual pattern of menses (frequency, duration, colour/amount of bleeding, and recent changes), obstetrical history (pregnancies, live births, miscarriages, abortions), infertility, dysmenorrhoea (pain, excessive bleeding), past or current infection/disease (e.g., sexually transmitted infections, sores/lesions, and unusual discharge or odour), date of last Pap smear, sexual orientation, sexual activity (including level of sexual desire, change in frequency of sexual activity, satisfaction with sexual relationships, painful intercourse), and contraceptive use. Ask males about number of children, infertility, past or current infection/disease (e.g., sexually transmitted infections, sores/lesions, and penile/rectal discharge), date of last testicular and prostate examinations, sexual orientation; sexual activity (including level of sexual desire, change in frequency of sexual activity, satisfaction with sexual relationships, painful intercourse, erectile/ejaculatory problems), and contraceptive use. Ask both men and women about past disease, changes in breasts or nipples (e.g., masses/lumps, pain, and discharge), and breast self-examination. Note the date of female clients' last mammogram. Attitudes, beliefs, and expressions of sexuality provide important information about an individual's self-concept, gender identification, quality of relationships, and overall satisfaction with life. Changes in level of desire and frequency of sexual activity are common in many psychiatric disorders, including depression, anxiety, and mania. Side effects of selective serotonin reuptake inhibitors are decreased sexual desire and erectile/ejaculatory dysfunction. Suicide rates among gay and lesbian youth are higher than the national average.
Musculoskeletal	Note problems with mobility, limited range of motion, pain or weakness, joint problems, disease/injury (e.g., osteoporosis), use of prosthetics, and impairments to activities of daily living.
Endocrine	Ask about disease/illness (e.g., diabetes, hypothyroidism/hyperthyroidism, and goitre); changes in height, weight, hair and skin, appetite, and energy level; excessive thirst; frequent urination; weakness; heat/cold intolerance; and current hormone therapy. Diseases of the endocrine system can imitate symptoms associated with psychiatric disorders (e.g., depression, anxiety, mania, eating disorders, and dementia).
Neurologic	Ask about head trauma, alterations in consciousness, seizures, headaches, changes in cognition and memory, and sensory and motor disturbances (numbness, tingling, loss of sensation, tremors, lack of coordination, balance problems, and pain). As well, inquire about alterations in personality, speech, or ability to manage activities of daily living. Neurologic signs and symptoms are associated with many psychiatric disorders as well as with side effects/toxicity of some neuroleptic medications (e.g., neuroleptic malignant syndrome [NMS], serotonin syndrome, and lithium toxicity).
Current Medications (including over-the-counter preparations and herbal remedies)	Specify the name of the medication, purpose, usual dose, frequency, effectiveness, side effects, prescriber, and the length of time the client has been taking it. This information helps to assess the client's health-promoting behaviours and potential knowledge deficits. Individuals with serious and persistent mental illness often take several different medications, which puts them at risk for drug–drug and drug–food interactions.
Health/Lifestyle Health promotion/maintenance	Ask individuals to evaluate their overall health and to describe what they do on a daily, weekly, and yearly basis to promote and maintain their health. Note the dates of their last physical examination, visit to a dentist, and eye examination.

(Continued)

Table 10.1   Health History and Significance to Psychiatric and Mental Health Problems *(Continued)*

Data	Considerations/Significance
Nutritional patterns	Ask about usual eating patterns and whether there have been any recent changes. Changes in eating patterns are associated with many affective states and psychiatric disorders.
	Particularly note dissatisfaction with weight and shape as well as activities aimed at weight loss. Body dissatisfaction is a factor in eating disorders and contributes to self-concept. It is particularly common among girls/women, elite athletes, and those with occupations that emphasize physical appearance (e.g., modelling and dancing).
	Psychiatric symptoms, neuroleptic medication, and poverty can all affect nutritional status.
	The weight gain associated with many neuroleptic medications increases individuals' risk for type II diabetes.
Sleep/rest patterns	Changes in sleep patterns can be a response to stress or symptoms of a psychiatric disorder.
	Probe a positive response about alterations in usual sleep patterns. Ask about *sleep onset* (latency between going to bed and falling asleep), *sleep maintenance* (frequency of wakening during the night and ease of falling back to sleep), and *early morning wakening* (consistently waking up before one needs to be up). Also, ask about whether the individual generally feels rested/refreshed.
	Alterations in sleep patterns are common in many psychiatric disorders (e.g., depression, mania, and schizophrenia). For many individuals with serious and persistent mental illness, sleep disturbances are early signs of relapse.
Activity/exercise	Ask about usual activity level and type and amount of exercise.
	Involvement in social activities and hobbies enhances health and reduces stress. Withdrawal from these things may be early signs of illness.
	Two of the negative symptoms of schizophrenia are anhedonia (decreased ability to experience pleasure) and avolition (lack of motivational drive and energy). These explain why many individuals with schizophrenia sleep excessively.
	Alterations in usual activities are associated with many mental disorders including depression, mania, schizophrenia, and some eating disorders.
Tobacco, alcohol and non-prescription drug use, and problem gambling	*Alcohol.* Ask about age at first use, preferred type (beer, wine, or spirits), usual pattern of drinking, and any recent changes to that pattern. It is also important to explore whether the individual or those close to the individual believe that alcohol is a problem in the individual's life. If yes, probe for details.
	Many people use alcohol to self-medicate—that is, to cope with stress, unpleasant emotions, sleep disturbances, and so forth.
	Nonprescription drugs. Ask about the age of first use, drug(s) of choice, dose, route, and frequency of nonprescription drug use. Probe for information about the effects of drug use (physical, psychological, emotional, social, legal, and economic).
	Problem gambling. Ask at what age it began, game(s) of choice, frequency, and average amount of money lost per month. Probe for information about the consequences (physical, psychological, emotional, social, legal, and economic).

with clients. Attention to nuances of dress, behaviour, facial expression, gestures, and interactions with others (particularly when the individual is not aware of being observed) provide important information that may not otherwise be revealed through conversation. For example, as well as observing hygiene and personal grooming, the nurse considers whether the client's dress is appropriate to the season and situation. Other important observations include behavioural evidence of perceptual disturbances or disordered thoughts (e.g., listening or talking to unseen others) and apparent inconsistencies between what an individual reports and what the nurse observes.

Examination

A comprehensive health assessment includes a health history, a physical examination, and diagnostic testing. This is particularly important in the provision of holistic PMH care because, compared with the general population, individuals who live with serious mental illness are at greater risk for developing a range of chronic physical conditions and have a shorter life expectancy (Correll, Detraux, De Lepeleire, & De Hert, 2015; De Hert et al., 2011). The converse is also true. For example, approximately 25% to 50% of Canadians who live with a chronic illness will also suffer from depression (HealthPartners/Partinaire Santé, 2015).

Persons living with mental illness can develop physical health problems as a result of the illness itself and/or as a consequence of treatment. Mental illnesses may disrupt hormone systems and sleep–wake cycles, while psychotropic medications have side effects such as weight gain to cardiac arrhythmias (Leucht, Burkard, Henderson, Maj, & Sartorius, 2007), all of which can contribute to increased vulnerability to a range of physical conditions. Other risk factors that contribute to the development of physical illnesses include smoking, alcohol and drug use, obesity, poverty, and self-care deficits. It is also important to note that medical conditions can mask, imitate, or worsen psychiatric symptoms. The situation is further complicated because some mental illnesses cause an individual to misattribute physical sensations, making it difficult to recognize and describe his or her symptoms. For example, those who have panic attacks can attribute their symptoms to a myocardial infarction or heart attack.

The **mental status examination** (MSE) is one type of focused assessment used to systematically assess an individual's psychological, emotional, social, and neurologic functioning. Although the components of the MSE are standard across clinical settings, the findings are highly subjective and rely heavily on the clinician's knowledge, communication skills, interpretation, and judgement. For this reason, it is important for clinicians to be self-reflective and to collaborate with colleagues to develop an unbiased understanding of the client's experience.

Interview

An assessment interview is a semistructured conversation aimed at building rapport, obtaining facts, clarifying perceptions and meanings, validating observations, and comparing understandings. Skillful interviewing is much more than asking an individual questions about signs and symptoms; it is both an art and a science and takes practice to develop (Box 10.1). Effective interviewers train themselves to be fully present in the situation and are genuinely warm and respectful and approach clients as collaborators working toward the same ends. Above all, competent interviewers engage in what Rogers (1975) referred to as empathic listening, which he describes as:

> ...being sensitive, moment by moment, to the changing felt meanings which flow in the other person and to the fear or rage or tenderness or confusion or whatever he or she is experiencing. It means temporarily living in the other's life, moving about in it delicately without making judgments (p. 4).

Because many psychiatric symptoms are beyond an individual's awareness, nurses may also interview family and friends to obtain client-related information. That being said, Canadian privacy legislation imposes obligations on government departments and public agencies, including health-serving facilities, to respect privacy rights and to limit the collection, use, and disclosure of personal information. Today, every province and territory have privacy laws, and it is the responsibility of every nurse to know the limits of information sharing under that legislation (Office of the Privacy Commission of Canada, 2012).

It is often the case that novice interviewers are so overwhelmed by their own anxieties about interviewing that they focus on their own experience and on asking

---

BOX 10.1 Factors That Facilitate Effective Interviewing

- As much as possible, **negotiate the terms of the interview with all the participants** (e.g., choose a mutually agreeable time and place; clearly state your purpose; and continually invite the clients to express their thoughts, feelings, wants, and needs). This conveys respect, invites a collaborative alliance, and fosters rapport.
- **The environment.** Choose a private and comfortable setting that is free from interruption.
- **Realistic time management.** Be clear at the outset how much time you have available for an interview and make a realistic plan about what you can achieve.
- **Be attentive to your nonverbal communication.** Sit at the same level as the client and maintain an open body posture. If you make notes, inform the client at the beginning of the interview; keep your notes brief so you can attend to the conversation.
- **Avoid jargon** and choose language that is clear, simple, and developmentally and culturally appropriate. Repeatedly check with the clients to ensure that they understand what you are saying.
- **Begin with a less sensitive topic and move toward sensitive issues as rapport develops**.
- Leave some time at the end of the encounter for **closure and future planning**. This involves monitoring the available time and notifying the client when the interview is coming to an end.

---

questions to elicit needed information. When this happens, the client's needs and the relational nature of the interaction are forgotten. Box 10.2 identifies some interviewer behaviours that can impede effective interviewing.

Collaboration

A growing body of evidence stresses the importance of interprofessional collaboration in all health care settings. In a review of the evidence, the World Health Organization (2010) identified the following benefits of interprofessional practice: reduced lengths of hospital stay, improved quality of life for patients/clients and families, improved access to care, enhanced patient/client safety, and improved recruitment and retention of health care professionals. The shift toward primary health care brings with it an emphasis on teams of health professionals who are accountable for providing comprehensive services to clients. Collaborative practice among nurses, physicians, and

---

BOX 10.2 Barriers to Effective Interviewing

- **Lack of clarity about the purpose and parameters of the interview** is like embarking on a journey without a clear destination. A statement such as "Mrs. Woods, my name is Kate Donovan. I am a nurse on this unit and I would like to spend the next hour or so getting to know more about you and completing your admission assessment. Is that okay with you?" conveys respect, informs the client of your intent, and begins the process of negotiating a contract for the encounter.
- **Asking too many closed-ended questions.** Closed-ended questions invite brief responses and are most useful for eliciting specific facts, like those needed in a focused assessment. Heavy reliance on them tends to orient the interview around the interviewer's desire for information and prevents clients from introducing or expanding on topics of importance to them.
- **Avoiding silence.** Often in response to their own discomfort or anxiety, interviewers rush to fill all silences with words. Pauses in the conversation allow both the client and the interviewer time to reflect on their experience in the moment, to formulate or elaborate on their responses, to switch speakers, or to turn the conversation to a new topic.

- **Asking complex questions.** A complex question is really several questions presented as one, as in "Why did you come to the hospital today, who brought you, and how did you get here?" These types of questions are confusing to the respondent, who often does not know which to answer first. Successful interviewers ask one question at a time, listen carefully to the answer, and probe for more detail if it is not clear.
- **Making assumptions.** Effective interviewers are those who understand that each individual experiences and understands the world in his or her own unique way. The failure to clarify and validate what the client means results in misunderstanding and inaccuracies.
- **Avoiding or ignoring expressions of emotion.** Emotions are rich communications. They provide insight into the meaning an individual assigns to an experience or event. Minimizing or ignoring an expression of emotion sends a powerful message. For example, "There are parts of you that I do not acknowledge," or "Your emotions are frightening or unimportant." Competent practitioners need to maintain a high level of self-awareness in order to remain grounded in their own experience so that they can bear witness to others.

---

other practitioners result in better health, improved access to services, more efficient use of resources, and higher levels of satisfaction for both consumers and health professionals.

PMH teams typically include clients and their families, nurses, physicians, psychologists, social workers, pharmacists, occupational therapists, and recreational therapists. Depending on the treatment setting and the client's particular needs, other professionals (e.g., teachers, clergy or spiritual leaders, other medical specialists) may be regular contributors to the team or participate on an ad hoc basis. In some settings, one member of the team may be assigned to be the client's primary therapist or case manager and takes on the role of coordinating team activities to address the client's needs. Teams meet together frequently to share information, to develop and evaluate treatment goals, and to provide ongoing support.

In most North American PMH treatment facilities, the interdisciplinary team works to develop a psychiatric diagnosis based on the *Diagnostic and Statistical Manual of Mental Health Disorders*, 5th edition (*DSM-5*) (American Psychiatric Association, 2013). The *DSM-5* provides a common language and standard criteria for the classification of mental disorders.

BIO/PSYCHO/SOCIAL/SPIRITUAL PSYCHIATRIC/MENTAL HEALTH NURSING ASSESSMENT

A bio/psycho/social/spiritual PMH nursing assessment begins with the assumption that humans are whole, integrated beings who live in constant and reciprocal relationship with their physical and social environments (Fig. 10.1). The bio/psycho/social/spiritual model presented in Chapter 5 provides a framework for assessing the physical, psychological, emotional, social, and spiritual dimensions of health. Whereas the goal of medical assessment is the diagnosis and treatment of disease and illness, nursing assessment aims to develop a holistic understanding of the individual's lived health–illness experience. In addition to identifying health problems and deficits, it attends to strengths and resources and evaluates how these affect the individual's quality of life and activities of daily living.

Types and Sources of Information

Client information or data fall into two broad categories: objective and subjective. **Objective data** (signs) are directly observable and measurable. The physical examination, vital signs, and diagnostic tests all yield objective

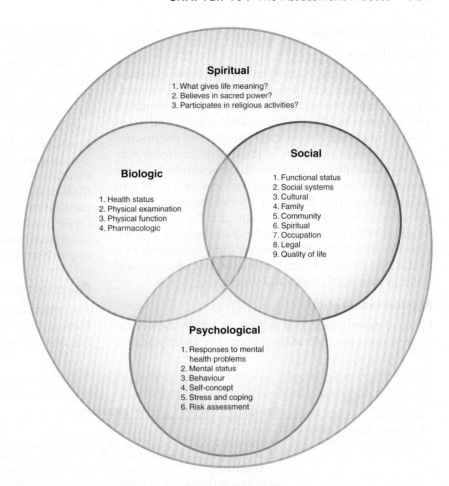

Spiritual
1. What gives life meaning?
2. Believes in sacred power?
3. Participates in religious activities?

Biologic
1. Health status
2. Physical examination
3. Physical function
4. Pharmacologic

Social
1. Functional status
2. Social systems
3. Cultural
4. Family
5. Community
6. Spiritual
7. Occupation
8. Legal
9. Quality of life

Psychological
1. Responses to mental health problems
2. Mental status
3. Behaviour
4. Self-concept
5. Stress and coping
6. Risk assessment

Figure 10.1. Bio/psycho/social/spiritual nursing assessment.

data. In contrast, **subjective data** (symptoms) are neither directly observable nor measurable. Subjective data are what the client and others report about their observations, beliefs, emotions, perceptions, experiences, and motivations. A health history provides this type of data. Subjective information provides a window into an individual's lifetime experiences and the meanings attached to those experiences. These are influenced by personal history and developmental stage, past learning, ethnicity and culture, and spirituality and offer insight into the sense an individual makes of the world. It is critical for nurses to remember that individuals act and react to the *meanings they assign* to events and experiences, rather than to the events or experiences themselves.

Both objective and subjective data are generated from *primary* or *secondary* sources. Individual clients are the primary sources of information about themselves. Secondary data, on the other hand, come from all other sources, including family, other health care providers, written reports, and client records.

Documentation

Health care records are important vehicles for communication as well as being legal documents. The type of information collected and how it is documented are regulated by the program or facility in which the nurse practices. In turn, programs and facilities develop documentation policies and procedures to comply with provincial and territorial legislation.

Generally speaking, there are two common approaches to documentation: *source-oriented* and *problem-oriented* documentations. In source-oriented documentation, each discipline is assigned a section of the client record (e.g., nurses' notes or physicians' notes). Although this approach identifies the discipline of the person making the entry, it tends to fragment the data, which is antithetical to holistic care. In problem-oriented documentation, everyone involved with the care of an individual makes entries in the same section of the record. This not only facilitates interprofessional collaboration but also keeps team members oriented toward the client's identified goals, needs, and problems.

Information may be entered in the client record in several ways, including fillable forms, flow sheets, checklists, and narrative notes. Electronic health records are becoming more common because they are more efficient, save time, and facilitate sharing of client information. In many settings, practitioners use the SOAP (subjective data, objective data, assessment, and plan implementation/evaluation), DAR (data, action, and plan), or PIE (problem, implementation, and evaluation) methods to organize their notes. Another approach to documentation is *charting by exception*, which involves documenting only those client health–illness responses that deviate from well-articulated standards.

Biologic Domain

Health History

The health history establishes a subjective database about the client's current and past health–illness experience, identifies strengths and resources, suggests actual and potential health problems and deficits, and is an opportunity to build rapport. Depending on the practice setting, different members of the health care team may take responsibility for sections of the health history. For example, the social worker may perform the family and social assessments, the occupational therapist undertakes the occupational assessment, and the recreational therapist often assesses the individual's exercise and leisure activities. Table 10.1 outlines the components of a health history and relates the significance of important findings to mental health and illness.

Physical Examination

Physical examination is a process by which a clinician collects objective information about the client's health.

Components include anthropomorphic measurements (e.g., height and weight), vital signs, an examination of all body systems, and diagnostic testing appropriate to the individual's age, level of risk, and sex. The physical examination aids in diagnosing disease or illness, establishes a baseline for evaluating change, and provides an opportunity to validate information provided in the health history. With respect to laboratory studies, particular attention is paid to any abnormalities of hepatic, renal, or urinary function because these systems metabolize or excrete many psychiatric medications. In addition, abnormal white blood cell (WBC) and electrolyte levels are noted. See Table 10.2 for selected haematologic measures and their relevance to psychiatric disorders.

Psychological Domain

The psychological domain includes manifestations of PMH problems/disorders; mental status; stress and coping; and risk assessment.

Table 10.2 Selected Haematologic Measures and Their Relevance to Psychiatric Disorders		
Test	**Result**	**Implications**
Complete Blood Count (CBC)		
Leucocyte count (WBC)	Leucopenia (↓ WBC)	May be a side effect of phenothiazines, clozapine, or carbamazepine
	Agranulocytosis (↓ granulocytic WBC)	Risk is 10–20 times greater with clozapine than with other antipsychotics. Lithium causes a benign mild to moderate increase (11,000–17,000/µL).
	Leucocytosis (↑ WBC)	NMS can be associated with increases of 15,000–30,000/mm^3 in about 40% of cases.
WBC differential	"Shift to the left"—from segmented neutrophils to band forms	This shift suggests a bacterial infection but has been reported in about 40% of cases of NMS.
Red blood cell (RBC) count	Polycythaemia (↑ RBC)	Primary form (true polycythaemia) is associated with several disease states; requires further evaluation.
		Secondary form is compensation for decreased oxygenation (e.g., chronic obstructive pulmonary disease).
		Blood is more viscous, which is exacerbated by being dehydrated.
	↓ RBCs	Associated with some types of anaemia; requires further evaluation
Haematocrit (Hct)	↑ Hct	Associated with dehydration
	↓ Hct	Associated with anaemia; may be related to alterations in mental status, including asthenia, depression, and psychosis
		20% of women of childbearing age in North America have iron deficiency anaemia.
Haemoglobin (Hgb)	↓ Hgb	Indicative of anaemia; evaluation of cause requires review of erythrocyte indices.
Erythrocyte indices, such as red cell distribution width (RDW)	↑ RDW	Finding suggests a combined anaemia resulting from both vitamin B$_{12}$ and folic acid deficiencies and iron deficiency, as found in chronic alcoholism.
		Oral contraceptives also decrease vitamin B$_{12}$.
Other Haematologic Measures		
Vitamin B$_{12}$	Deficiency	May be associated with neuropsychiatric symptoms such as psychosis, paranoia, fatigue, agitation, marked personality change, dementia, and delirium
Folate	Deficiency	Associated with alcohol use and with medications such as phenytoin, oral contraceptives, and estrogens
Platelet count	Thrombocytopenia (↓ platelets)	Associated with use of some psychiatric medications, such as carbamazepine, phenothiazines, or clozapine and with other nonpsychiatric medications; may also cause thrombocytopenia
		Also, associated with some disease states; requires further evaluation

Table 10.2   Selected Haematologic Measures and Their Relevance to Psychiatric Disorders *(Continued)*

Test	Result	Implications
Serum Electrolytes		
Sodium	Hyponatremia (serum sodium)	Associated with significant alterations in mental status. May be related to Addison's disease, the syndrome of inappropriate secretion of antidiuretic hormone, polydipsia, and carbamazepine use
Potassium	Hypokalaemia (↓ serum potassium)	Associated with weakness, fatigue, electrocardiogram changes, paralytic ileus, and muscle paresis
		Common in individuals exhibiting bulimic behaviour, psychogenic vomiting, misuse of diuretics, and/or excessive laxative use. Hypokalaemia may be life threatening.
Chloride	Elevation	Chloride tends to increase to compensate for lower bicarbonate.
	Decrease	Associated with binging and purging behaviour
Bicarbonate	Elevation	Associated with binging and purging, disordered eating, excessive laxative use, and/or psychogenic vomiting
	Decrease	May develop in individuals who hyperventilate (e.g., panic disorder)
Renal Function Tests		
Blood urea nitrogen	Elevation	Associated with alterations in mental status (e.g., lethargy and delirium), dehydration, and medications excreted by the kidney, such as lithium and amantadine
Serum creatinine	Elevation	Indicative of decreased renal function; typically does elevate until 50% of nephrons in the kidney are damaged
Serum Enzymes		
Amylase	Elevation	Associated with the binging and purging behaviour in eating disorders; tends to decline when these behaviours stop
	Alanine aminotransferase (ALT) > aspartate aminotransferase (AST)	This disparity is common in acute forms of viral and drug-induced hepatic dysfunction.
ALT (formerly serum glutamic pyruvic transaminase)	Elevation	Mild elevations are common with use of sodium valproate.
AST (formerly serum glutamic oxaloacetic transaminase)	AST > ALT	Severe elevations are associated with chronic hepatic disease and myocardial infarction.
Creatinine phosphokinase	Elevations of the isoenzyme related to muscle tissue	Associated with muscle tissue injury
		Level is elevated in NMS and by repeated intramuscular injections (e.g., depot antipsychotics).
Thyroid Function		
Serum triiodothyronine (T₃)	Decrease	Associated with hypothyroidism and other non–thyroid-related diseases
		Individuals with depression may convert less T₄ to T₃ peripherally, but not out of the normal range.
		Medications such as lithium and sodium valproate may suppress thyroid function, but clinical significance is unknown.
	Elevation	Indicative of hyperthyroidism; T₃ toxicosis is associated with alterations in mood, anxiety, and symptoms of mania.
Serum thyroxine (T₄)	Elevation	Indicative of hyperthyroidism
Thyroid-stimulating hormone	Elevation	Associated with hypothyroidism, which shares features of depression with the additional physical signs of cold intolerance, dry skin, hair loss, bradycardia, and so forth
		Lithium may also cause elevations.
	Decrease	Considered nondiagnostic; may be associated with hyperthyroidism, pituitary hypothyroidism, or even euthyroid status

Responses to Mental Health Problems

In broad terms, PMH disorders are manifest as "clinically significant patterns of behaviour or emotions that are associated with some level of distress, suffering, or impairment in one or more areas such as school, work, social and family interactions, or the ability to live independently" (Canadian Psychiatric Association, n.d.). The identification and understanding of PMH conditions vary through history and across cultures. Current thinking is that mental health–illness exists on a continuum such that mental health and mental illness can coexist simultaneously within the same person. A recent systematic review of studies conducted around the world reported that in one in five respondents (17.6%) met criteria for a mental disorder in the previous year and 29.2% experienced a common mental disorder at some time during their lives (Steel et al., 2014). Like other illnesses, PMH disorders affect individuals and their families in many different ways. An important part of assessing the psychological domain is to explore the individual's experience of illness. Many have specific fears about losing their jobs, about their families, or about their personal safety. It is also important to identify the person's strategies for managing the illness and the effectiveness of those strategies. A simple question such as "How do you deal with your voices when you are with other people?" may initiate a discussion about an experience or symptom.

Mental Status Examination

The MSE (Box 10.3) is a systematic assessment of an individual's appearance, affect, behaviour, and cognitive function. It provides "a snapshot" of the person's subjective report and experiences and the examiner's observations and impressions at the time of the interview. It is performed by health practitioners across several disciplines and clinical settings to evaluate developmental, neurologic, and psychiatric disorders.

The MSE is not to be confused with the Mini-Mental State Examination (MMSE; Folstein, Folstein, & McHugh, 1975), which is a screening tool used to evaluate cognitive impairment.

BOX 10.3 Components of the Mental Status Examination

1. General observations
   a. Appearance
   b. Psychomotor behaviour
   c. Attitude toward interviewer
2. Mood
3. Affect
4. Speech
5. Perception
6. Thought
   a. Content
   b. Process/form
7. Sensorium
   a. Level of consciousness
   b. Orientation (person, place, time)
   c. Memory (immediate retention and recall; recent, short term, and long term)
   d. Attention and concentration
   e. Comprehension and abstract reasoning
8. Insight
9. Judgement

KEY CONCEPT

The **mental status examination** is a systematic assessment of an individual's appearance, affect, behaviour, and cognitive processes. It provides "a snapshot" of the person's subjective report and experiences and the examiner's observations and impressions at the time of the interview. It is performed by health practitioners across several disciplines and clinical settings to evaluate developmental, neurologic, and psychiatric disorders.

General Observations

This section of the MSE provides a brief narrative summary of the examiner's observations and impressions of the individual at the time of the interview. Although an individual's health history remains relatively stable, his or her mental status is variable over time. (For a video demonstration of elements of an MSE, see http://aitlvideo.uc.edu/aitl/MSE/MSEkm.swf)

Appearance

Describe the individual's general appearance and presentation. Note manner and appropriateness of dress, personal hygiene, odours, pupil size, and obvious identifying characteristics, such as tattoos and piercings. Physical signs such as skin tone (e.g., duskiness, pallor, or flushing), nutritional status, and energy level (e.g., catatonia, lethargy, or restlessness) provide clues to the person's general level of health–illness.

Psychomotor behaviour/activity

Observe and note the individual's behaviour during the interview, including posture, gait, motor coordination, facial expression, mannerisms, gestures, and activity. Pay particular attention to cues to the person's emotional state (e.g., muscle tension, purposeless repetitive movements, and restlessness).

Attitude toward interviewer

The individual's attitude toward the interviewer and the interview process may be described as accommodating, cooperative, open, friendly, apathetic, bored, guarded, suspicious, hostile, or evasive. The following is an example of how the interviewer may describe the individual:

Mr. D. is a tall, thin, Caucasian man, who looks older than his stated age of 47 years. He is unshaven, his hair is uncombed, and he has a strong body odour. His clothing is stained and dishevelled but appropriate to the season. He reports feeling "jumpy," and he declined to sit during the interview, opting instead to pace around the interview room. His posture is erect and his movements are quick, purposeful, and well coordinated; he displays no unusual mannerisms. Mr. D. was cooperative with the interview process, although his verbal responses were brief and he did not maintain eye contact.

Mood and Affect

In everyday usage, the terms mood and affect are used interchangeably. In the context of an MSE, however, these words refer to specific phenomena. **Mood** refers to a pervasive and sustained emotion and is what the person reports about his or her prevailing emotional state. Although mood does vary with internal and external changes, it tends to be stable over time and reflects the person's disposition or worldview. Mood can be assessed by asking a simple, open-ended question like, "How have you been feeling over the past while?" Whatever the person answers, the interviewer should probe to find whether this is typical or is a response to some recent life event. A person who is generally positive and content will remain so even when bad things happen. He or she will tend to view adversity as a temporary period of unpleasantness in a basically happy life. In contrast, an individual whose mood tends to be negative or depressed views life through dark-coloured glasses. He or she experiences life as difficult and sees happiness as fleeting.

Mood may be sustained for days or weeks, or it may fluctuate during the course of a day. For example, some individuals who are depressed have a diurnal variation in their mood; they experience their lowest mood in the morning, but as the day progresses, their mood lifts, and they feel somewhat better in the evening. Terms used to describe mood include **euthymic** (normal), **euphoric** (elated), and **dysphoric** (depressed, disquieted, restless).

Affect refers to immediately expressed or observed emotion that is inferred by the examiner from facial expressions, vocalizations, and behaviour. During the assessment, an individual's affect may change as he or she talks about an immediate experience or recent life events. Affect is described in terms of its range, intensity, appropriateness, and stability. Affective range can be full or constricted. Individuals who express several emotions that are consistent with their stated feelings and the content of their speech are saying are described as having a full range of affect that is congruent with the situation. On the other hand, a person who speaks of the recent, tragic death of a loved one in a monotone voice with little outward expression of his or her internal feeling state is described as having constricted affect. In evaluating the appropriateness of a particular response, the nurse must consider both the meaning of the event to the individual and cultural norms. Descriptions of intensity attempt to quantify an affective response. Intensity may be characterized as heightened, blunted, or flat. The phrase blunted affect describes limited emotional expression, whereas flat affect is its near absence. The person whose affect is flat speaks in a monotone voice and has little or no facial expression. Stability of affect can be described as mobile (normal) or labile. If a person displays a wide range of strong emotions in a relatively short period of time, his or her affect is described as being labile.

Speech

Patterns and characteristics of speech provide clues about the individual's thoughts, emotions, and cognitive processes. They also convey information about the person's understanding of the situation and ability to read and respond to social cues. Speech is described in terms of its quantity, rate and fluency of production, and quality. In assessing speech quantity, the individual may be described as talkative, verbose, or expansive or as having paucity or poverty of speech. Rate of speech may be slow, hesitant, fast, or pressured, whereas fluency refers to the apparent ease with which speech is produced. Pressured speech is speech that is rapid and increased in amount and difficult to understand; it is often associated with mania. Aphasic disturbances are problems of speech output and may be neurologic, cognitive, or emotional in origin. Speech quality refers to its characteristics, such as monotone, whispered, slurred, mumbled, staccato, or loud. During conversation, the interviewer also notes speech impediments (e.g., stuttering), response latency (the length of time it takes for the individual to respond to a question or comment), and repetition, rhyming, or unusual use of words.

Perception

Perception is the complex series of mental events involved with taking in of sensory information from the environment and the processing of that information into mental representations. Two perceptual disturbances commonly associated with mental illness are hallucinations and illusions. **Hallucinations** are false sensory perceptions not associated with external stimuli and are not shared by others. Although auditory hallucinations are the most common, hallucinations may be experienced in any of the five major sensory modalities: auditory, visual, tactile, olfactory, or gustatory. Most people are familiar with hypnagogic hallucinations—false sensory perceptions that occur while falling asleep; these are not associated with mental disorder. Of more concern are command hallucinations, the false perception of commands or orders that an individual feels obligated to obey. For example, a person may hear voices telling him or her to harm or kill oneself or someone else. **Illusions** are the misperception or misrepresentation of real sensory stimuli (e.g., misidentifying the wind as a voice calling one's name or thinking that a label on a piece of clothing is an insect).

Thought

Because thought is not directly observable, it is indirectly assessed through language in terms of its content and process (form). **Thought content** refers to the subject matter occupying a person's thoughts; **thought process** is the manner in which thoughts are formed and expressed. Some individuals are very forthcoming about the content of their thoughts, whereas others are more reticent to talk about them. Assessing thought requires the clinician to carefully attend to and explore unusual

---

BOX 10.4 Alterations in Thought Content

Delusion—a false, fixed belief, based on an incorrect inference about reality. It is not shared by others and is inconsistent with the individual's intelligence or cultural background and cannot be corrected by reasoning.

Delusions of control—the belief that one's thoughts, feelings, or will are being controlled by outside forces. The following are some specific examples of delusions of control:

- **Thought insertion**—the belief that thoughts or ideas are being inserted into one's mind by someone or something external to one's self.
- **Thought broadcasting**—the belief that one's thoughts are obvious to others or are being broadcast to the world.
- **Ideas of reference**—the belief that other people, objects, and events are related to or have a special significance for one's self (e.g., a person on television is talking to or about him or her).

Paranoid delusions—an irrational distrust of others and/or the belief that others are harassing, cheating, threatening, or intending one harm.

Bizarre delusion—an absurd or totally implausible belief (e.g., light waves from space communicate special messages to an individual).

Somatic delusion—a false belief involving the body or bodily functions.

Delusion of grandeur—an exaggerated belief of one's importance or power.

Religious delusion—the belief that one is an agent of or specially favoured by a greater being.

Depersonalization—the belief that one's self or one's body is strange or unreal.

Magical thinking—the belief that one's thoughts, words, or actions have the power to cause or prevent things to happen; similar to Jean Piaget's notion of preoperational thinking in young children.

Erotomania—the belief that someone (often a public figure) unknown to the individual is in love with them or involved in a relationship with them.

Nihilism—the belief that one is dead or nonexistent.

Obsession—a repetitive thought, emotion, or impulse.

Phobia—a persistent, exaggerated, and irrational fear.

BOX 10.5 Alterations in Thought Process

Loosening of association—the lack of a logical relationship between thoughts and ideas; conversation shifts from one topic to another in a completely unrelated manner, making it confusing and difficult to follow.

Circumstantiality—the individual takes a long time to make a point because his or her conversation is indirect and contains excessive and unnecessary detail.

Tangentiality—similar to circumstantiality, except that the speaker does not return to a central point or answer the question posed.

Thought blocking—an abrupt pause or interruption in one's train of thoughts, after which the individual cannot recall what he or she was saying.

Neologisms—the creation of new words.

Flight of ideas—rapid, continuous verbalization, with frequent shifting from one topic to another.

Word salad—an incoherent mixture of words and phrases.

Perseveration—a persisting response to a stimulus even after a new stimulus has been presented.

Clang association—the use of words or phrases that have similar sounds but are not associated in meaning; may include rhyming or puns.

Echolalia—the persistent echoing or repetition of words or phrases said by others.

Verbigeration—the meaningless repetition of incoherent words or sentences; typically associated with psychotic states and cognitive impairment.

Pressured speech—speech that is increased in rate and volume and is often emphatic and difficult to interrupt; typically associated with mania or hypomania.

or recurring themes in the individual's conversation. Box 10.4 lists some common disturbances of thought content, and Box 10.5 lists some common disturbances of thought process.

Sensorium

This portion of the MSE assesses brain function and cognitive abilities.

Level of consciousness

Evaluating **level of consciousness** (LOC) assesses arousal or wakefulness. If the individual is nonresponsive, the nurse applies increasing levels of stimulation (e.g., verbal, tactile, and painful) to elicit a response. The GCS (Teasdale & Jennett, 1974) is often used to assess LOC. Terms commonly used to describe LOC include alert, awake, lethargic, somnolent, stuporous, or comatose.

Orientation

Orientation is a cognitive function involving awareness of the dimensions of time, person, and place. Alterations in orientation can be caused by a number of factors including injury, drugs, brain lesions, and dementia. The examiner determines orientation by asking questions about time, place, and person because impairments tend to exist in this order (i.e., a sense of time is impaired before a sense of place). Begin with specific questions about the date, time of day, location of the interview, and name of the interviewer and move to more general questions if necessary. For example, if the client knows the year, but not the exact date, the nurse can ask the season.

Memory

Memory function is traditionally divided into four spheres: immediate retention and recall; recent memory; short-term memory; and remote or long-term memory. To check immediate retention and recall, the nurse gives the person three unrelated words to remember and asks him or her to recite them immediately and at 5- and 15-minute intervals during the interview. To test recent memory, the nurse asks questions about events of the past few hours or days. Short-term memory involves things that occurred within the past few weeks or months. The nurse assesses remote or long-term memory by asking about events of years ago. If they are personal events and the answers seem incorrect, the nurse may check them with a family member.

Attention and concentration

To test attention and concentration, the nurse asks the individual to count backward, aloud, from 100 by increments of 7 (e.g., 93, 86, 79, and so on) or to start with 20 and subtract 3. The nurse must decide which is most appropriate for the patient/client considering education and understanding; subtracting 3s from 20 is the easier

of the two tasks. Another way to test these areas is to ask the person to spell a simple word, such as house, backward.

Insight and Judgement

Insight and judgement are related concepts that involve the ability to examine ideas, conceptualize facts, solve problems, and think abstractly. **Insight** describes a person's understanding of a set of circumstances. It reflects awareness of his or her own thoughts and feelings and an ability to compare them with the thoughts and feelings of others. For example, persons with impaired insight may not believe that they have mental illness. They may have delusions and hallucinations or be hospitalized for bizarre and sometimes dangerous behaviour but do not grasp that this is unusual or abnormal.

Judgement is the ability to reach a logical decision about a situation and to choose a reasonable course of action after examining and analyzing various possibilities. Throughout the interview, the nurse evaluates the person's problem-solving abilities and capacity to learn from past experience. For example, a nurse might conclude that an individual who repeatedly chooses partners who are abusive demonstrates poor judgement in selecting partners. Another way to assess judgement is to give a simple scenario and ask the person to identify the best response. An example of such a scenario is, "What would you do if you found a bag of money outside a bank on a busy street?" If the client responds, "run with it," his or her judgement is questionable.

Stress and Coping Patterns

Everyone lives with some degree of stress in their life (see Chapter 17 for a full discussion). For vulnerable individuals, however, stress may contribute to the development of PMH disorders. Identification of major stressors in an individual's life helps the nurse to develop and support the use of successful coping behaviours in the future. The nurse should identify the individual's current stressors and coping strategies and evaluate the effectiveness of the latter. This information is vital to the overall plan of care because it highlights both problem areas and resources.

Assessing Risk and Protective Factors

An individual's mental health–illness is influenced by the complex interaction of individual characteristics or attributes, socioeconomic circumstances, and environmental factors (World Health Organization, 2012) (Table 10.3). Assessment takes into account both the presence and balance of risk factors, protective factors, and promotive factors. **Risk factors** are characteristics, conditions, situations, and events that increase the individual's vulnerability to threats to safety or well-being. Throughout this text, assessment of risk factors focuses

Table 10.3 Overview of Risks to Mental Health Over the Life Course

Setting	Home/Family	School	Social Media	Work	Community
Culture	Low socioeconomic status	Adverse learning environment	Discrimination/social inequities		
Community	Poor housing/living conditions	Difficulties at school	Bullying	Unemployment	Neighbourhood violence/crime
Family	Substance use in pregnancy Trauma or maltreatment Family conflict/violence Parental mental illness	Peer pressure		Job stress or insecurity	Poor civic amenities Debt/poverty
Person	Gender	Antisocial or criminal behaviour	Bereavement		
	Insecure attachment Malnutrition Low self-esteem Psychoactive drug use				Elder abuse

Physical ill health

→

Prenatal period	Childhood	Adolescence	Adulthood	Older adulthood

Adapted from Kieling, C., Baker-Henningham, H., Belfer, M., Conti, G., Ertem, I., Omigbodun, O., … Rahman, A. (2011). Child and adolescent mental health worldwide: Evidence for action. *Lancet, 378*(9801), 1515–1525.

on risks to safety, risks for developing PMH disorders, and risks for increasing, or exacerbating, symptoms and impairment in individuals with an existing psychiatric disorder. **Protective factors** are attributes or conditions of an individual, family, and/or community when present reduces, mitigates, or eliminates risk. **Promotive factors** are conditions or attributes of individuals, families, and/or communities that actively enhance well-being. Taken together, protective and promotive factors increase the probability of positive, adaptive, and healthy outcomes, even in the face of risk and adversity.

Assessing safety is a priority and a part of every encounter with clients. Examples include the risk for deliberate self-harm or suicide; risk for violence toward others; and risk for adverse events, such as falls, seizures, allergic reactions, or elopement. Nurses must assess these risk factors on a priority basis. For example, they must assess the risk for violence or suicide and take measures to prevent injury, such as implementing environmental constraints, before addressing other assessment factors.

Suicide/Self-Harm

Suicide is "an intentional, self-inflicted act that results in death" (Emmanuel et al., 2015, p. 2). In contrast, "self-harm, while purposeful, is often repetitive behaviour that involves the infliction of harm to one's body without suicidal intent" (Emmanuel et al., 2015, p. 2) and is often used as a method to relieve psychological distress.

A suicide risk assessment involving gathering specific details regarding:

Suicidal ideation—thoughts about deliberate self-harm or of self-inflicted death

Threats of suicide—a verbal or behavioural indication (direct or indirect) that an individual is planning to end his or her life

Suicide attempt—action taken with the intent of ending one's life

Self-harm—Thoughts of or deliberate self-injurious behaviours not intended to end one's life (e.g., carving, cutting, scratching, or burning one's skin; pulling one's hair; ingestion of toxic substances; or hitting oneself)

To ascertain this information, the nurse asks specific questions such as the following (see Chapter 19 for a full discussion):

- Have you ever tried to harm or kill yourself? If the answer is "yes," probe for details about precipitating circumstances, means, and outcome. If the individual has thought about suicide but not acted on these thoughts, determine why not.
- Do you have a plan for how you might kill yourself? If the answer is "yes," ask for details (e.g., when and by what means).
- Do you have the things you need to carry out this plan?
- Have you made preparations for your death (e.g., writing a good-bye note, putting finances in order, and/or giving away possessions)?
- What does the future hold for you? Probe for indications of hopelessness, a sense of helplessness, a loss of enjoyment in life, guilt or shame, anger, or impaired judgement.

From this assessment, the nurse and other members of the team determine the individual's level of risk for self-harm and intervene as necessary. Most PMH programs and facilities use rating scales to quantify an individual's risk for self-harm. Those deemed to be at high risk are usually hospitalized and constantly observed.

Assaultive or Homicidal Ideation

A safety assessment also includes an evaluation of the level of threat an individual poses to others. Of particular importance are delusions or hallucinations that involve harming or killing others. Questions to ask to ascertain assaultive or homicidal ideation are as follows:

- Do you intend to harm someone? If yes, whom?
- Do you have a plan for how you might do this? If yes, what are the details of the plan?
- Do you have the things that you need to carry out your plan? (If the plan requires a weapon, is it readily available?)

Social Domain

A comprehensive assessment also attends to social dimensions of an individual's life. Much of this information is elicited during the health history and the MSE, and it includes information about the individual's current living situation, the individual's family of origin, and the existence and quality of significant relationships (see Chapter 15). The treatment team also assesses work, education, and social and leisure activities. As well, the team observes the individual's interactions with those around him or her. This component of the assessment helps to identify important strengths and resources as well as problems and deficits.

Assessing Gender Identity

Important determinants of health that are often overlooked in a compressive health assessment relate to sex and gender. **Sex** refers to biologic and physiologic features associated with being male, female, or intersex (a group of conditions in which there is discrepancy between the external genitals and the internal genitals). On the other hand, **gender** denotes socially constructed characteristics (e.g., sex-based norms and roles). **Gender identity** is "... one's self identification along a male/female or man/woman continuum, regardless of the composition of the physical body" (Carabez, Eliason, & Martinson, 2016, p. 257). It is different from **sexual orientation**: a person's sexual and emotional attraction to another person and the behaviour and/or social affiliation that may result from this attraction (American Psychological Association [APA], 2015, p. 862).

Until recently, it was widely believed that all humans belonged to one of two genders determined solely by their biologic sex (masculine men/males and feminine women/females). This concept is termed gender binary because it provides only two possibilities for gender (National LGBT Health Education Center, n.d.). Current evidence supports the notion that gender exists on a continuum whose endpoints are anchored by male/man and female/woman. These terms describe variations in gender:

Cisgender indicates someone whose sense of personal identity and gender aligns with that assigned at birth. (In Latin, "cis" means "on this side of" whereas "trans" means "the other side of".)

Transsexual, **transgender**, gender nonconforming, gender questioning, and nonbinary gender are general terms referring to persons whose gender identity that does not match the sex they were assigned at birth. They may self-identify as male, female, both, or neither. Persons who identify as nonbinary gender may be heterosexual or bisexual.

It is important for nurses to understand how gender norms and roles influence a person's vulnerability to various health conditions and diseases and physical and mental health over the lifespan. The complex interactions among these things influence a person's willingness and ability to access health services and their adherence with treatment. Estimates of the number of persons who identify as nonbinary gender range widely from 0.17 to 1,333 per 100,000 (Meier & Labuski, 2013) and are low due to the absence of gender identity-related questions on surveys and hospital/clinic admission forms used to identify these individuals (Conron, Landers, Reisner, & Sell, 2014). In the recent past, there have been efforts to remedy this, and there is a growing body of literature focusing on lesbian, gay, bisexual, and transgender (LGBT) health. Existing research reports widespread discrimination and stigma toward LGBT persons, which contributes to disparities in health disorders and risk behaviours, negative social influences, and poorer access to health care (for a review, see Carabez et al., 2016). Box 10.6 summarizes transaffirmative practices.

Functional Status

Understanding how an individual functions in his or her day-to-day life is a vital part of assessment. The *DSM-5* recommends clinicians use the *Cross-Cutting Symptom Measure* at the initial interview and over time to follow changes in status and treatment response (American Psychiatric Association, 2013). Level 1 of the adult version of this tool is a self-rated survey of 13 symptom domains for adults. For children and adolescents, level 1 has 12 domains to be rated by a parent/guardian. Level 2 of the tool allows for more in-depth assessment of some domains.

The *DSM-5* also provides a *Clinician-Rated Dimension of Psychosis Symptom Severity* scale in which clinicians

BOX 10.6 Transaffirmative Practices

Nurses across all health care settings will encounter persons who identify as nonbinary gender. Unfortunately, many health care providers are uninformed, uncomfortable, and even hostile toward these individuals (Kosenko, Rintamaki, Raney, & Maness, 2013; McCann, 2015; Poteat, German, & Kerrigan, 2013). This recognition has motivated health care systems and individual providers to develop **transaffirmative practices** (APA, 2015) (also called culturally competent trans care [Surreira, 2014] and affirmative care for patients with nonbinary gender identities [National LGBT Health Education Center, n.d.]) that are informed, knowledgeable, respectful, and responsive (APA, 2015; Coleman et al., 2012). Among other things, these affirmative practices include:

- Knowledge that sexual and gender diversity exist on a continuum and that gender identity may not align with sex assigned at birth
- Awareness of how one's attitudes toward and knowledge of gender identity affects the provision of safe and competent of care
- An understanding of how stigma and discrimination affect the health across the lifespan of trans and gender nonconforming persons
- A commitment to recognizing and eliminating systemic barriers to equitable services (e.g., do not assume gender binary, ask people how they prefer to be addressed [name and pronouns], gender inclusive washrooms; provide known local resources that specialize in transgender services)

rate the severity (0 to 4) of eight symptom domains (e.g., hallucinations, delusions, negative symptoms, etc.) experienced by the client over the past 7 days. The use of the *World Health Organization Disability Assessment Schedule 2.0* (WHODAS 2.0; Üstün, Kostanjsek, Chatterji, & Rehm, 2010), a self-administered tool, is recommended for assessing the difficulties experienced over the past 30 days due to health (including mental health) conditions. It explores six domains: understanding and communicating (cognition); moving and getting around (mobility); hygiene, dressing, eating, and staying alone (self-care); interacting with other people (getting along); domestic responsibilities, leisure, work, and school (life activities); and joining in community activities (participation). If the individual is unable to complete the questionnaire, a knowledgeable informant is asked to complete it. (See Web Links for the site where the WHODAS 2.0 can be found.)

Ethnic and Cultural Assessment

Ethnicity and culture profoundly affect an individual's worldview and frame the person's beliefs about life, death, health and illness, and roles and relationships. As part of a comprehensive assessment, the nurse must consider ethnic and cultural factors that influence health and illness (see Chapter 3). To understand these, the nurse should ask the following questions:

- Do you think of yourself as belonging to a particular ethnic or cultural group? If yes, which one(s)?
- What parts of your culture are most important to you? (Probe for details about values, beliefs, personal practices, social customs, behaviours, etc.)
- What does health mean to you?
- What does illness mean to you?
- How do you define good and evil?
- What things do you do to make yourself physically and mentally healthy?
- To whom do you turn when you feel physically or mentally ill?

The *DSM-5* offers a *Cultural Formulation Interview* schedule for clinicians' use in obtaining information about the way culture may be influencing important aspects of an individual's clinical presentation (American Psychiatric Association, 2013).

Spiritual Assessment

Nurses must be aware of their own spirituality and religious beliefs to ensure that it does not interfere with assessment of the client's spirituality. See Chapter 5 for a definition of spirituality. Examples of questions that may foster an understanding of an individual's spirituality include the following:

- What gives your life meaning?
- What brings joy to your life?
- Do you believe in God or a higher power?
- Do you participate in any religious activities? If yes, which ones?
- Do you feel connected with the world?

🍁 SUMMARY OF KEY POINTS

- Assessment is a purposeful, systematic, and dynamic process that is ongoing throughout the nurse's relationship with individuals in his or her care. It involves the collection, validation, analysis, synthesis, organization, and documentation of the client's health–illness information.
- A comprehensive assessment includes a health history and physical examination; considers the psychological, emotional, social, spiritual, ethnic, and cultural dimensions of health; attends to the meaning of the client's health–illness experience; and evaluates how all this affects the individual's daily living.

- A focused assessment is the collection of specific information about a particular need, problem, or situation. It is briefer, narrower in scope, and more present oriented than is a comprehensive assessment.
- Techniques of data collection include observation, interview, physical and mental examinations, and collaboration.
- Biologic assessment includes health history, physical examination, and diagnostic testing.
- Assessment of the psychological domain includes understanding the individual's response to mental health problems, MSE, evaluation of stress and coping, and risk assessment.
- The MSE is a systematic assessment of an individual's appearance, affect, behaviour, and cognitive function. It provides "a snapshot" of the person's subjective report and experiences and the examiner's observations and impressions at the time of the interview. It is performed by health practitioners across several disciplines and clinical settings to evaluate developmental, neurologic, and psychiatric disorders.
- Risk factors are those characteristics, conditions, situations, or events that increase the individual's vulnerability to threats to safety or well-being. Examples include the risk for self-harm or suicide, violence toward others, and the risk for adverse events, such as falls, seizures, allergic reactions, or elopement.
- Protective factors are attributes or conditions of an individual, family, and/or community that reduce, mitigate, or eliminate risk.
- Promotive factors are conditions or attributes of individuals, families, and/or communities that actively enhance well-being.
- The social assessment involves a family and relationship assessment, evaluation of functional status, and information about the individual's ethnicity and culture.
- Nurses must be aware of their own spiritual beliefs and ensure that those beliefs do not affect their spiritual assessment of their clients.

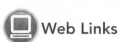 **Web Links**

aitlvideo.uc.edu/aitl/MSE/MSEkm.swf An explanation and video clips of various elements of a mental status examination.

http://cfmhn.ca/professionalPractices?f=7458545122100118.pdf&n=212922-CFMHN-standards-rv-3a.pdf&inline=yes A copy (pdf) of the Canadian Federation of Mental Health Nurses' Standards of Practice can be found at this link on their Web site.

library.med.utah.edu/neurologicexam/html/mentalstatus_normal.html This site describes a full neurologic examination, including the video clips of various components of the mental health status examination.

psychcentral.com/ocdquiz.htm This is a public service site that has several self-report mental health screening tests.

http://www.who.int/classifications/icf/whodasii/en/ This is the World Health Organization Web site where the WHODAS2.0, its manual, and the user agreement can be found.

References

American Psychiatric Association. (2013). *Diagnostic and statistical manual of mental disorders* (5th ed.). Washington, DC: Author.

American Psychological Association (APA). (2015). Guidelines for psychological practice with transgender and gender nonconforming people. *American Psychologist, 70*(9), 832–864. http://dx.doi.org/10.1037/a0039906

Canadian Federation of Mental Health Nurses. (2014). *Canadian standards of psychiatric and mental health nursing* (4th ed.). Toronto, ON: Author.

Canadian Psychiatric Association. (n.d.). *Mental illness and work.* Retrieved from https://ww1.cpa-apc.org/MIAW/pamphlets/Work.asp

Carabez, R. M., Eliason, M. J., & Martinson, M. (2016). Nurses' knowledge about transgender patient care: A qualitative study. *Advances in Nursing Science, 39*(3), 257–271. doi:10.1097/ANS.0000000000000128

Coleman, E., Bockting, W., Botzer, M., Cohen-Kettenis, P., DeCuypere, G., Feldman, J., … Zucker, K. (2012). Standards of care for the health of transsexual, transgender, and gender nonconforming people, version 7. *International Journal of Transgenderism, 13*(4), 165–232. http://dx.doi.org/10.1080/15532739.2011.700873

Conron, K. J., Landers, S. J., Reisner, S. L., & Sell, R. L. (2014). Sex and gender in the U.S. health surveillance system: A call to action. *American Journal of Public Health, 104*(6), 970–976. doi:10.2105/AJPH.2013.301831

Correll, C. U., Detraux, J., De Lepeleire, J., & De Hert, M. (2015). Effects of antipsychotics, antidepressants and mood stabilizers on risk for physical diseases in people with schizophrenia, depression and bipolar disorder. *World Psychiatry, 14*(2), 119–136.

De Hert, M., Correll, C. U., Bobes, J., Cetkovich-Bakmas, M., Cohen, D., Detraux, J., & Leucht, S. (2011). Physical illness in patients with severe mental disorders. I. Prevalence, impact of medications and disparities in health care. *World Psychiatry, 10*(1), 52–77.

Emanuel, L. L., Taylor, L, Hain, A., Combes, J. R., Hatlie, M. J., Karsh B., … Walton, M. (Eds.). (2015). *The Patient Safety Education Program—Canada (PSEP—Canada) Curriculum.* Retrieved from http://www.patientsafetyinstitute.ca/en/education/PatientSafetyEducationProgram/PatientSafetyEducationCurriculum/Documents/Module%2013a%20Preventing%20Suicide%20and%20Self-Harm.pdf

Folstein, M. F., Folstein, S. E., & McHugh, P. R. (1975). Mini-mental state. A practical method for grading the cognitive state of patients for the clinician. *Journal of Psychiatric Research, 12*(3), 189–198.

HealthPartners/Partenaire Santé. (2015). *Chronic disease and mental health report.* Retrieved from https://healthpartners.ca/sites/default/files/HealthPartners_Chronic_Disease_and_Mental_Health_Report_June17_2015.pdf

Kieling, C., Baker-Henningham, H., Belfer, M., Conti, G., Ertem, I., Omigbodun, O., Rahman, A. (2011). Child and adolescent mental health worldwide: Evidence for action. *Lancet, 378*(9801), 1515–1525.

Kosenko, K., Rintamaki, L., Raney, S., & Maness, K. (2013). Transgender patient perceptions of stigma in health care contexts. *Medical Care, 51*(9), 819–822. doi:10.1097/MLR.0b013e31829fa90d.51:819-822

Leucht, S., Burkard, T., Henderson, J., Maj, M., & Sartorius, N. S. (2007). Physical illness and schizophrenia: A review of the literature. *Acta Psychiatrica Scandinavica, 116*(5), 317–333.

McCann, E. (2015). People who are transgender: Mental health concerns. *Journal Psychiatric and Mental Health Nursing, 22*(1), 76–81. doi:10.1111/jpm.12190

Meier, S. C., & Labuski, C. M. (2013). The demographics of the transgender population. In A. K. Baumle (Ed.), *International handbook of the demography of sexuality* (pp. 289–327). New York, NY: Springer.

National LGBT Health Education Center. (n.d.). *Providing affirmative care for patients with non-binary gender identities.* Retrieved from http://www.lgbthealtheducation.org/wp-content/uploads/2016/11/Providing-Affirmative-Care-for-People-with-Non-Binary-Gender-Identities.pdf

Office of the Privacy Commission of Canada. (2012). *Privacy legislation in Canada.* Retrieved from http://www.priv.gc.ca/resource/fs-fi/02_05_d_15_e.asp

Poteat, T., German, D., & Kerrigan, D. (2013). Managing uncertainty: A grounded theory of stigma in transgender health care encounters. *Social Science and Medicine, 84*, 22–29. http://dx.doi.org/10.1016/j.socscimed.2013.02.019

Rogers, C. R. (1975). Empathic: An unappreciated way of being. *The Counseling Psychologist, 5*(2), 2–10. Retrieved from http://tcp.sagepub.com/cgi/reprint/5/2/2-a

Steel, Z., Marnane, C., Iranpour, C., Chey, T., Jackson, J. W., Patel, V., & Silove1, D. (2014). The global prevalence of common mental disorders: A systematic review and meta-analysis 1980–2013. *International Journal of Epidemiology, 43*(2), 476–493. doi: 10.1093/ije/dyu038

Surreira, C. (2014). *Culturally competent LGBT care* (Unpublished doctor of nursing practice capstone project). University of Massachusetts, Amherst, MA.

Teasdale, G., & Jennett B. (1974). Assessment of coma and impaired consciousness. A practical scale. *Lancet, 304*(7872), 81–84.

Üstün, T. B., Kostanjsek, N., Chatterji, S., & Rehm, J. (Eds.). (2010). *Measuring health and disability: Manual for WHO Disability Assessment Schedule (WHODAS 2.0)*. Geneva, IL: World Health Organization.

World Health Organization. (2010). *Framework for action on interprofessional education and collaborative practice*. Retrieved from http://www.who.int/hrh/resources/framework_action/en/

World Health Organization. (2012). *Risks to mental health: An overview of vulnerabilities and risk factors*. Retrieved from http://www.who.int/mental_health/mhgap/risks_to_mental_health_EN_27_08_12.pdf

11 Diagnosis, Interventions, and Outcomes in Psychiatric and Mental Health Nursing

Nicole Snow,
Christine Davis, and
Wendy Austin

LEARNING OBJECTIVES

After studying this chapter, you will be able to:

- Define the components of nursing diagnoses.
- Discuss the use of nursing diagnoses and outcomes in psychiatric and mental health care.
- Discuss the way clinical knowledge and judgement and a commitment to collaboration with clients and families determines the selection of nursing interventions.
- Explain the use of best practice guidelines for psychiatric and mental health care.
- Describe the application of nursing interventions for the biologic domain.
- Describe the application of nursing interventions for the psychological domain.
- Describe the application of nursing interventions for the social domain.
- Describe the application of nursing interventions for the spiritual domain.
- Discuss the relationship between client-centred care, client outcomes, and quality care.
- Demonstrate the process of developing individual outcome statements.

KEY TERMS

- automatic thinking • behaviour modification
- behaviour therapy • chemical restraint • cognitive interventions • conflict resolution • counselling
- cultural brokering • de-escalation • defining characteristics • diagnosis-specific outcomes
- discharge outcomes • distraction • guided imagery
- home visits • indicators • initial outcomes
- milieu therapy • observation • physical restraint
- psychoeducation • recovery orientation
- reminiscence • revised outcomes • seclusion
- simple relaxation techniques • spiritual care
- structured interaction • token economy

KEY CONCEPTS

- best practice guidelines • collaboration • person- and family-centred care • defining characteristics • nursing diagnosis • nursing interventions • outcomes

---

After completing an assessment of the individual who is to receive care, nurses generate appropriate nursing diagnoses based on the assessment data. The experienced nurse can readily cluster the assessment data to support one nursing diagnosis over another. Mutually agreed upon goals flow from nursing diagnoses and provide guidance in determining appropriate interventions. Initial outcomes are determined and then are monitored and evaluated throughout the care process. Measuring outcomes not only demonstrates clinical effectiveness but also helps to promote rational clinical decision making and is reflective of the nursing interventions.

Psychiatric and mental health (PMH) nursing interventions are nursing activities that promote mental health, prevent mental illness, assess dysfunction, assist clients to regain or improve their coping abilities, and/or prevent further disabilities. Based on clinical knowledge and judgement, and a commitment to collaboration and partnership with clients and their families, nursing interventions include any treatment that a nurse performs to enhance client outcomes. These interventions are direct (performed through interaction with the client) or indirect (performed away from but on behalf of the client) (Bulechek, Butcher, Dochterman, & Wagner, 2013). Interventions can be either nurse-initiated treatment, which is an autonomous action in response to a nursing diagnosis, or physician-initiated treatment, which is a response to a medical diagnosis as a result of a physician's order. The *Canadian Standards of Psychiatric-Mental Health Nursing* (Canadian Federation of Mental Health Nurses [CFMHN], 2014) describe the scope of PMH nursing practice, delineate nursing competencies, and guide the selection of interventions for implementation in the plan of care (see Web Links). This chapter describes the development of nursing diagnoses, person-centred care, and individual outcomes in nursing within the context of the Canadian health care system.

After many factors are considered, including a client's self-care activities, the selection of nursing approaches involves integrating biologic, psychological, social, and

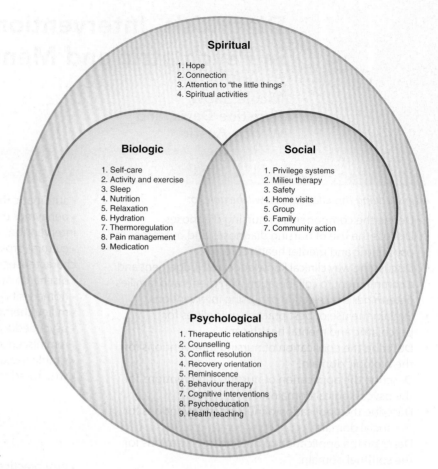

Figure 11.1. PMH nursing interventions.

spiritual interventions into a comprehensive plan of care with and for the client (Fig. 11.1). Nurses provide care in various roles. In some settings, such as an acute care hospital or the home, the nurse provides direct nursing care. In other settings, such as the community, the nurse may assume the role of case manager, who primarily coordinates care for all disciplines, including nursing. In this instance, the nurse may be responsible for all or part of direct nursing care as well as for ensuring that agreed-on care is appropriate for the client, even if other providers deliver it. The nurse may also be the leader or manager of a nursing unit and thus responsible for delegating the care to paraprofessional and nonprofessional providers; however, he or she remains accountable for the client's care. In all of these instances, the nurse, working in partnership with the client and/or the client's family, plans and initiates safe and appropriate interventions.

A COMMITMENT TO COLLABORATION AND PERSON-CENTREDNESS

The current trend in Canadian nursing practice is moving away from the nurse as an expert on a client's needs and towards a person- and family-centred approach, recognizing that individuals are unique (Registered Nurses Association of Ontario [RNAO], 2015), make meaning of their own lived experiences, and should participate as they can in all aspects of their care (Canadian

Collaborative Mental Health Initiative [CCMHI], 2006). This means that plans of care are created and provided with respect for the preferences, values, and particular needs of the person and implemented as much as possible in partnership with the person and his or her family. The nurse needs to be able to discuss with them the risks and benefits of proposed interventions.

In order to enhance mental health services in primary care, the CCMHI was formed in 2004. This is a consortium of 12 national organizations representing community services, consumer, family and self-help groups, dieticians, family physicians, nurses, occupational therapists, pharmacists, psychologists, psychiatrists, and social workers. Its work centres on the needs of individual users of services. This person-centred care involves individuals, families, and caregivers in all areas of care, from treatment choices to evaluation.

Canadian nurses are committed to working together with persons and their families, including those experiencing PMH issues. The *Canadian Collaborative Mental Health Care Charter* (CCMHI, 2006) was developed by national organizations of consumers and providers of mental health services (including the Canadian Nurses Association, the Registered Psychiatric Nurses of Canada, and the Canadian Federation of Mental Health Nurses). The charter identifies seven principles of collaborative clinical decisions and interventions: health promotion and prevention of mental health problems;

holistic promotion; collaboration; partnership; respect for diversity; information exchange; and resources.

KEY CONCEPT

A **person- and family-centred approach to care** places the person and his or her family members at the centre of health care, its practices, and services, in such a way that individuals are genuine partners with health care providers for their health (RNAO, 2015).

KEY CONCEPT

Collaboration is the process of working together towards common goals. Sharing knowledge and information can be an important aspect of the process.

EVOLUTION OF NURSING DIAGNOSIS AND INDIVIDUAL OUTCOMES

The concepts of nursing diagnosis and individual outcomes are not new. Florence Nightingale identified client/patient problems and analyzed client/patient outcomes during the Crimean War. Aydelotte (1962) published one of the first nursing studies involving client/patient outcomes. Lang and Clinton (1984) proposed nursing outcomes to include physical health status, mental health status, social and physical functioning, health attitude, knowledge and behaviour, use of professional health resources, and client/patient perception of the quality of nursing care. Marek (1989) identified 15 nursing outcome categories: physiologic measures; symptom control; frequency of service; home maintenance; psychosocial measures; well-being; functional status; goal attainment; patient behaviours; client/patient satisfaction; client/patient knowledge; rehospitalization; safety; cost; and resolution of nursing diagnoses. Further changes in health care provision and the nursing process in the 1990s resulted in efforts being focused on developing outcomes that could be used to evaluate nursing effectiveness. In 1998, the Nursing Outcomes Classification (NOC) taxonomy, with a structure similar to the Nursing Intervention Classification (NIC), was developed. The fifth edition has 7 domains, 32 classes, and 490 outcomes (Moorhead, Johnson, Maas, & Swanson, 2013). Although the importance of identifying intervention outcomes has been the subject of nursing research since the 1960s, escalating health care costs have forced the demonstration of measurable outcomes. Concerns about quality, cost, and use of limited resources have contributed to the current emphasis on both evidence-based practice and individual outcomes. With the expansion of nursing knowledge gained through measuring intervention effectiveness, the nursing discipline evolves.

In Canada in the early 2000s, the RNAO was funded by the Ontario Ministry of Health and Long-Term Care to develop, implement, evaluate, and revise Best Practice

---

BOX 11.1 Examples of RNAO Practice Guidelines

Assessment and care of adults at risk for suicidal ideation and behaviour

Care transitions

Crisis intervention

Delirium, dementia, and depression in older adults

Embracing cultural diversity in health care

Engaging clients who use substances

Enhancing healthy adolescent development

Establishing therapeutic relationships

Facilitating client-centred learning

Integrating smoking cessation into daily nursing practice

Interventions for postpartum depression

Person- and family-centred care

Preventing and addressing abuse and neglect of older adults

Promoting safety: alternative approaches to the use of restraints

Supporting clients on methadone maintenance treatment

Women abuse: Screening, identification, and initial response

Guidelines (BPGs) that would inform nursing practice in a number of areas and better ensure outcomes, thereby reducing costs (RNAO, 2012a, 2012b).

Box 11.1 provides examples of available RNAO guidelines. The purpose of BPGs is multifaceted: to deliver care that is effective and based on current evidence, to aid in seeking resolutions to clinical problems, to meet or exceed current quality standards in providing excellent care, to initiate use of innovations, to eliminate interventions that are not meeting best practice standards, and to foster clinical excellence through supportive work environments (RNAO, 2012a, 2012b).

The evidence-based practice movement, from which BPGs evolved, is not without its critics. Canadian nurse scholar and researcher David Holmes and colleagues argue that "ready-made" guidelines can serve to impede nurses' critical thinking and thus diminish the social, political, and ethical responsibilities of the discipline. Taking the BPGs of RNAO as a case study, they suggest further that BPGs facilitate the control and regulation of nursing practice by health care organizations (Holmes, Murray, Arron, & McCabe, 2008).

KEY CONCEPT

Best practice guidelines (BPGs), also termed clinical practice guidelines (CPGs), are broad or specific recommendations for health care based on the best current evidence.

■ DERIVING A NURSING DIAGNOSIS

Nursing diagnoses provide clearer identification of discipline-specific knowledge and practice (Carpenito, 2017a). As the basis for planning nursing interventions, these are used in diverse practice settings. Clusters of data lead the nurse to choose certain diagnoses over others. For example, when assessing an individual, the nurse observes that his or her responses are often self-negating (e.g., "I always mess things up," "I never get it right"). The nurse also observes that he or she seems indecisive and lacking in problem-solving abilities (e.g., "I can never decide what the right thing to do is, and when I do finally choose, it is always wrong"). Nonverbal and verbal information are used to identify **defining characteristics**. Observations of an individual sitting with her head down, making no eye contact, and dressed in dirty clothes are important data. Such observations support the hypothesis that the individual has a disturbance in self-esteem. Further assessment will help the nurse determine whether the self-esteem disturbance is chronic or situational.

Related factors are those that influence or change the individual's health status. They are grouped into four categories: pathophysiologic, biologic, or psychological (e.g., cognitive problems); treatment related (e.g., medications, diagnostic studies, and surgeries); situational (e.g., environmental, home, community, and person); and maturational (e.g., age-related influences on health) (Carpenito, 2017b). To continue with the assessment example, the nurse learns that the individual has lost three jobs within the past year, resulting in financial problems. These situation-related factors further support the nursing diagnosis of self-esteem disturbance.

KEY CONCEPT

"A **nursing diagnosis** is a clinical judgement about individual, family, or community responses to actual or potential problems/life processes" and involves selecting provides nursing interventions to achieve desired outcomes (Carpenito, 2017b, p. 9). See Box 11.2 for examples of nursing diagnoses pertinent to PMH nursing.

KEY CONCEPT

Defining characteristics are key signs and symptoms (clues) that relate to each other and that validate a nursing diagnosis. The nurse analyzes these clues to formulate a cluster of data, which helps in making a diagnosis or diagnoses that reflects the actual or potential health status or problems of the individual.

KEY CONCEPT

Outcomes are the individual's response to nursing care at a given point in time. An outcome is concise, stated in few words, and in neutral terms. Outcomes describe an individual's state, behaviour, or perception that is variable and can be measured (Table 11.1).

■ DEVELOPING INDIVIDUAL OUTCOMES

Outcomes should be individualized and linked to nursing diagnoses through the nursing process. By linking outcomes to the nursing diagnosis, it is possible to monitor nursing practice and facilitate clinical decision making and knowledge development (see Table 11.2). Outcomes can be defined as an individual's response to care that is the end result of a process, a treatment, or a nursing intervention and should be monitored and documented over time and across clinical settings. **Diagnosis-specific outcomes** show that the intervention resolved the problem or nursing diagnosis. At other times, the outcome is nonspecific (i.e., not diagnosis specific, meaning it does not show resolution of the diagnosis). In that case, the outcome is abstract or general. Outcomes may be used to evaluate interventions by other health care disciplines as well as nursing. For example, occupational therapy may contribute significantly to an individual's psychosocial adaptation.

The process of working toward these outcomes can be outlined in a systematic manner that identifies the required health care professionals and other supports

BOX 11.2 Examples of Nursing Diagnoses Pertinent to PMH Nursing

Anxiety
Anxiety, Death
Body Image, Disturbed
Coping, Ineffective
Family Processes, Dysfunctional
Hope, Readiness for Enhanced
Personal Identity, Disturbed
Mood Regulation, Impaired
Neglect, Self
Confusion, Acute; Chronic
Risk for Suicide
Self-Mutilation
Self-Care Deficit Syndrome
Self-Harm, Risk for
Spiritual Distress

Selected from list of nursing diagnoses in Carpenito, L. J. (2017b). *Handbook of nursing diagnosis* (15th ed.). Philadelphia, PA: Lippincott Williams & Wilkins.

Table 11.1 Example of Outcomes

Diagnosis	Outcome	Intervention
Spiritual distress	Will finding meaning and purpose in life, including in the illness experience	Have spiritual leader discuss restriction exemptions as they apply to those who are seriously ill or hospitalized. Provide reading materials about religious and spiritual restrictions and exemptions. Provide accurate information about health regimen, treatment plan, and medications. Chart results.
Related to conflict between religious or spiritual beliefs and prescribed health regime		Explain the nature and purpose of therapy. Discuss possible outcomes without therapy; be factual, be honest, but do not attempt to frighten or force person to accept treatment. Support client making informed decisions—even if decision conflicts with own values.

Indicators
a. Expresses decreased feelings of guilt and fear
b. Relates that supported in his or her decisions about health regimen
c. States that conflict has been eliminated or reduced

From Carpenito, L. J. (2017a). *Nursing diagnosis: Application to clinical practice* (15th ed.). Philadelphia, PA: Lippincott Williams & Wilkins.

and their actions. The Centre for Addictions and Mental Health (CAMH) is a Canadian leader in mental health treatment and research. It has identified a number of approaches (integrated pathways) to aid individuals in receiving treatment and support for their mental health concerns (CAMH, 2016). Integrated care pathways tend to have these characteristics:

- The focus is on the client's overall journey.
- Ensure clients receive the right care and treatment at the right time.
- Involve care decisions based on evidence.
- Effective teamwork among care providers (e.g., physician, nurse, psychologist, pharmacist, social worker).
- Empower and inform clients and their caregivers (CAMH, 2016, p. 3).

This process is mapped as *Admission > Assessment > Treatment (Medication and NonMedication Treatment) > Planning for Discharge > Discharge* (CAMH, 2016, p. 6). Once this process is under way, there is a need to identify what indicators will indicate outcome attainment.

Table 11.2 Example—Linkage of Nursing Diagnosis and Outcomes

Diagnosis	Outcome
1. Disturbed body image	Verbalize and demonstrate increased positive feelings
2. Chronic confusion	Asks for validation of reality
3. Risk for self-harm	Identify personal triggers for self-harm

From Carpenito, L. J. (2017b). *Handbook of nursing diagnosis* (15th ed.). Philadelphia, PA: Lippincott Williams & Wilkins.

Indicators answer the question "How close is the individual moving towards the outcome?" The indicator represents the dimensions of the outcome. Outcome indicators represent or describe individual status, behaviours, or perceptions evaluated during an individual's assessment. **Indicators** are a measurement of individual progress in relation to the individual's outcomes and can serve as intermediate outcomes in a clinical pathway or standardized care plan. In nursing care planning, outcomes can be **initial outcomes** (those written after the initial individual interview and assessment), **revised outcomes** (those written after each evaluation), or **discharge outcomes** (those outcomes to be met before discharge). Because of the decreased length of stay or days of service, discharge outcomes often are not met but are passed along to the community nurse. If these discharge outcomes continue to be relevant, they become initial outcomes in community or home care.

Documentation of Outcomes

Nurses are accountable for documentation of individual outcomes, nursing interventions, and any changes in diagnosis, care plan, or both. Individual responses to care are documented as changes in behaviour or knowledge and can include the degree of satisfaction with the health care provided (Kleinpell, 2003). Outcomes can be expressed in terms of the individual's actual responses (e.g., no longer reports hearing voices) or the status of a nursing diagnosis at a point in time after implementation of nursing interventions, such as "caregiver role strain resolved." This documentation is important for further research and quality of care studies.

Table 11.3	Results of Nursing Interventions	
Diagnosis	**Patient Outcome**	**Nursing Intervention**
Ineffective coping, related to ineffective problem-solving skills	The person will make decisions and follow through with appropriate actions to change provocative situations in the person's environment.	Assess causative and contributing factors. Establish rapport. Assess present coping status. Assess level of depression on functioning. Assist the client in developing appropriate problem-solving strategies. Teach problem-solving techniques. Teach self-monitoring tools. Facilitate emotional support from others. Initiate health teaching and referrals as indicated.
	Indicators a. Verbalize feelings related to emotional state. b. Focus on the present. c. Identify response patterns and the consequences of resulting behaviour. d. Identify personal strengths and accept support through the nursing relationship.	

From Carpenito, L. J. (2017). *Nursing diagnosis: Application to clinical practice* (15th ed., pp. 227–230). Philadelphia, PA: Lippincott Williams & Wilkins.

Purposes of Individual Outcomes

The primary purposes of developing individual outcomes are to ensure quality care and that the needs of the individual are being met. They provide guidelines for what is expected of the individual and direction for continuity of care that reflects current knowledge in the field of nursing. The measurement of individual outcomes helps to meet the goal of continuous quality improvement (see Table 11.3 for Expected Outcomes of Nursing Interventions).

Accountability is an important concept in health care. Nursing and other disciplines are being pressured within health service systems to justify their practice, to demonstrate to users of services that they deliver quality care, and to control health care costs. Measurement of outcomes can be used to determine quality of care during a single episode of illness and across the continuum of care and can assist in discharge planning. Outcomes also can be used to determine quality of care in different systems and between systems. Evaluation of individual outcomes can help validate nursing interventions by identifying which interventions are effective. Outcomes can also be a communication tool between nurses, and with case managers, caregivers, and policy makers. They can be used to conduct program evaluations and to develop research databases.

■ NURSING INTERVENTIONS

Nursing Interventions Classification (NIC) (Bulechek et al., 2013) is an extensive system of specific interventions, with discrete activities for each. The NIC system is based on data collected from surveys of nurses, who identified the interventions that were ultimately classified. The NIC taxonomy includes classes or groups of interventions categorized according to seven domains: physiologic basic; physiologic complex; behavioural; safety; family; health system; and community. The NIC taxonomy represents both basic and specialty advanced nursing practices. For example, both basic and specialist nurses use interventions such as reinforcing positive behaviour; however, the advanced practice psychiatric nurse may be the developer of the plan and use it as part of psychotherapy with the client. This text is strongly influenced by the framework of interventions identified in the *Canadian Standards of Psychiatric-Mental Health Nursing* (CFMHN, 2014) (see Chapter 5 and Web Links).

KEY CONCEPT

Nursing interventions are treatments or activities, based upon clinical judgment and knowledge, that are used by nurses to enhance patient or client outcomes (Bulechek et al., 2013).

Interventions for the Biologic Domain

Biologic interventions focus on physical functioning and are directed towards the client's self-care, activities and exercise, sleep, nutrition, relaxation, hydration, and thermoregulation as well as pain management and medication management. In the NIC taxonomy, these interventions are found within the physiologic basic and physiologic complex domains.

Promotion of Self-Care Activities

Self-care is the ability to perform activities of daily living (ADLs) successfully. Many clients with PMH problems can manage self-care activities such as bathing, dressing appropriately, selecting adequate nutrition, and sleeping regularly. (Although maintaining adequate nutrition and promoting normal sleep hygiene are considered self-care activities, they are discussed in separate sections because of their significance in mental health care.) Others, however, cannot manage such self-care activities, either because of their symptoms or as a result of the side effects of medications. Because nursing is concerned with maintaining the client's health and well-being, a focus on ADLs can become a nursing priority.

Orem's (1991) nursing model is based on the concept of self-care deficit (see Chapter 8). Deficits in self-care may be related to attitude (motivation), knowledge, or skill. The model identifies five nursing approaches to deficits in a client's self-care: acting or doing for; guiding; teaching; supporting; and providing an environment to promote the client's ability to meet current or future demands. The emphasis is on helping the individual develop independence. In the inpatient setting, the nurse works with the client so that basic self-care activities are completed. During acute phases of psychiatric disorders, the inability to attend to basic self-care tasks (e.g., getting dressed) is very common. Therefore, the ability to complete personal hygiene activities (e.g., dental care, grooming) is monitored, and clients are assisted in completing such activities. In a psychiatric facility, clients are encouraged and expected to develop independence in completing these basic self-care activities to the best of their ability. In the community, monitoring these basic self-care activities is always a part of the nursing visit or clinic appointment.

Activity and Exercise Interventions

The nurse must attend to the client's level of activity. Encouraging regular activity and exercise can improve general well-being and physical health. A healthy lifestyle that includes daily exercise can help clients deal with the weight gain and type II diabetes associated with many psychotropic medications. In some psychiatric disorders (e.g., schizophrenia and depression), people become sedentary and appear to lack the motivation to complete ADLs. This lack of motivation is part of the disorder and requires nursing intervention. In addition, side effects of medication that include sedation and lethargy can compound the problem (Toups et al., 2017). It is possible for exercise behaviour to become an abnormal focus of attention, such as for some individuals with anorexia nervosa.

When assuming the responsibility of a direct care provider, the nurse can help clients identify realistic activities and exercise goals. Some institutions have other professionals (e.g., recreational therapists) available for the implementation of exercise programs. As a case manager, the nurse should consider the activity needs of individuals when jointly setting goals. As a leader or manager of a psychiatric unit, the nurse can influence ward routines that promote activity and exercise.

Sleep Interventions

Many psychiatric disorders and medications are associated with sleep disturbances. Sleep is also disrupted in clients with dementia. These clients may have difficulty falling asleep or may frequently awaken during the night. In dementia of the Alzheimer type, individuals may reverse their sleeping patterns by napping during the day and staying awake at night. In addition, there is increasing concern regarding the use of electronic devices such as computers and smartphones or playing video games prior to bedtime. In a study by Vallance, Buman, Steninson, and Lynch (2015), there was a positive association between increased screen time (i.e., use of a computer or other electronic device) and difficulty falling asleep.

Nonpharmacologic interventions are always used first for sleep disturbances because of the side-effect risks associated with the use of sedatives and hypnotics (see Chapter 12). Sleep interventions to communicate to clients include the following:

- Go to bed only when tired or sleepy.
- Establish a consistent bedtime routine.
- Avoid stimulating foods, beverages, or medications.
- Avoid naps in the late afternoon or evening.
- Eat lightly before retiring and limit fluid intake.
- Use the bed only for sleep or intimacy.
- Avoid emotional stimulation before bedtime.
- Use behavioural and relaxation techniques.
- Limit distractions.
- Reduce exposure to electronic devices prior to bedtime.

For some clients, disrupted sleep can become chronic and problematic. Obtaining adequate sleep is vital for optimal daily functioning, and it is imperative that nurses assess for sleep disturbances and possible disorders, and intervene appropriately. More information about sleep disorders and the nursing process involved in caring for an individual with sleep disturbances is provided in Chapter 28.

Nutrition Interventions

Psychiatric disorders and medication side effects can affect eating behaviours. For varying reasons, some individuals eat too little, whereas others eat too much. For instance, homeless individuals with mental illness have difficulty maintaining adequate nutrition because of their deprived circumstances. Substance abuse also interferes with maintaining adequate nutrition, through either stimulation or suppression of appetite or through neglecting nutrition because of drug-seeking behaviour. Nutrition interventions should therefore be specific and relevant to the individual's circumstances and mental health. In addition, recommended daily allowances are important in the promotion of physical and mental health, and nurses should consider them when planning care. Resources for planning include Canada's Food Guide and/or Canada's Food Guide for First Nations, Inuit, and Métis (Minister of Health Canada, 2007a, 2007b) (see Web Links).

Some psychiatric symptoms involve changes in perceptions of food, appetite, and eating habits. If a client believes that food is poisonous, he or she may eat sparingly or not at all. Interventions are then necessary to address the suspiciousness as well as to encourage adequate intake of recommended daily allowances. It may be necessary to allow clients to examine foods, participate in preparation, and test the meal's safety by eating slowly or after everyone else.

Obesity can be a problem for individuals being treated for a mental disorder. Antipsychotics, antidepressants, and mood stabilizers are associated with weight gain, which is thought to be related to changes in metabolism and appetite caused by some of these medications. Many clients stop taking medications because of the weight gain. Excessive weight gain can be especially stressful to the individual's emotional well-being, as well as detrimental to physical health. However, nurses should encourage clients to avoid quick weight loss programs because they are not effective. Furthermore, hypoglycaemia can exacerbate a depressed mood and lead to suicidal thoughts. If weight gain is a problem, the best approach is to assist the client to monitor current intake and develop realistic strategies for changing eating patterns combined with a healthy lifestyle.

Relaxation Interventions

Relaxation promotes comfort, reduces anxiety, alleviates stress, eases pain, and prevents aggression. It can diminish the effects of hallucinations and delusions. The many different relaxation techniques used as mental health interventions range from simple deep breathing to biofeedback to hypnosis. Although some techniques such as biofeedback require additional training and, in some instances, certification, nurses can easily apply simple relaxation, distraction, and imagery techniques.

Simple relaxation techniques encourage and elicit relaxation to decrease undesirable signs and symptoms. **Distraction** is the purposeful focusing of attention away from undesirable sensations. Distraction techniques include counting, exercising, reading, listening to music, watching television, or playing (e.g., video games). The important factor is that the particular distraction works for the person. Other factors in choice of technique involve its appropriateness based on energy level, age, developmental level, and literacy. Individuals should try out and practice the distraction technique of their choice before they need to use it (Bulechek et al.,

2013). **Guided imagery** is the purposeful use of imagination to achieve relaxation or to direct attention away from undesirable sensations. It is especially useful in stress management. With this technique, clients imagine themselves doing something pleasurable and relaxing, such as lying on the beach or watching snow fall. They are encouraged (with permissive directions from the nurse, such as "If you wish…") to slowly experience the scene and to express how they feel and think about it. Slow, deep breathing is also encouraged (Bulechek et al., 2013). Guided imagery is an independent nursing intervention that can be used for such clients as those experiencing anxiety (Jallo, Cozens, Smith, & Simpson, 2013). However, as clients may experience unexpected, albeit therapeutic, reactions (e.g., crying) during guided imagery, students should not attempt this technique with clients unless supervised.

As a direct care provider, the nurse may teach the client relaxation exercises. As a case manager, nurses can include relaxation exercises in the plan of care. The unit leader can be responsible for ensuring that appropriately prepared staff members implement relaxation exercises. Relaxation techniques that involve physical touch (e.g., back rubs) must be used particularly carefully, if at all, for people with mental disorders. Touching and massaging are often not appropriate for clients who have a history of physical or sexual abuse. Such clients may find touch too stimulating or misinterpret it as being sexual or aggressive. It is important for the nurse to maintain open communication with and elicit feedback from the client when providing physical interventions.

Hydration Interventions

Assessing fluid status and monitoring fluid intake and output are often important interventions. Overhydration or underhydration can be a symptom of a psychiatric disorder. For example, some clients with psychotic disorders experience chronic fluid imbalance. For these individuals, a treatment protocol that includes a target weight procedure can help prevent both overhydration and water intoxication and promote self-control. The nurse functions as the direct care provider (e.g., teaching client), unit leader (e.g., delegating weighing of the client to staff), or coordinator of the protocol.

Many psychiatric medications affect fluid and electrolyte balance (see Chapter 12). For example, when taking lithium carbonate, clients must have adequate fluid intake, with special attention paid to serum sodium levels. When sodium levels drop through perspiration, lithium is used in place of sodium, which in turn leads to lithium toxicity (Malhi, Adams, & Berk, 2009). Many psychiatric medications cause dry mouth (Morrison, Meehan, & Stomski, 2015b), which in turn causes individuals to drink fluids excessively. Interventions that help clients understand the relationship of medications to fluid and electrolyte balance are important in their overall care.

Thermoregulation Interventions

Many psychiatric disorders can disturb the body's normal temperature regulation. Thus, clients cannot sense temperature increases or decreases and consequently cannot protect themselves from extremes of hot or cold. This problem is especially difficult for people who are homeless or live in substandard housing, such as some rooming houses. In addition, many psychiatric medications can also affect the ability to regulate body temperature.

Interventions include educating clients about the problem of thermoregulation, identifying potential extremes in temperatures, and developing strategies to protect the client from the adverse effects of temperature changes. For example, community nurses often engage in active outreach to at-risk clients during extreme weather alerts.

Pain Management

Emotional reactions are often manifested as pain. For instance, unexplained chronic pain can be a somatoform symptom (see Chapter 24). Chronic pain is particularly problematic when no cause for it is identified.

Nurses in PMH settings are more likely to provide care to clients experiencing chronic pain than acute pain. However, a single intervention is seldom successful for relieving chronic pain. In some instances, pain is managed by medication; in other instances, nonpharmacologic techniques are used, such as simple relaxation techniques, distraction, or imagery. Indeed, relaxation is one of the most widely used cognitive and behavioural approaches to pain. Psychoeducation, stress management techniques, and biofeedback are also used in pain management.

The key to managing pain is engaging the client in identifying how it is disrupting his or her personal, social, professional, and family life. Education focusing on the pain, the use of medications for treatment, and the development of cognitive skills are important pain management components. In some cases, redefining treatment success as improvement in functioning, rather than alleviation of pain, may be necessary. The interaction between stress and pain is important; that is, increased stress leads to increased pain (Brataas & Evensen, 2016). Individuals can better manage their pain when stress is reduced.

Medication Management

Nurses use many medication management interventions to help clients maintain therapeutic regimens. Medication management involves more than the actual administration of medications. Nurses assess medication effectiveness and side effects and consider interactions with other drugs, herbal remedies, or homeopathic preparations. In addition, nurses assess any factors that may affect the client's adherence to a medication regimen, such as concerns regarding weight gain or reproductive ability, attitude towards taking medication, or

cost issues. Education regarding medication must be made available to the client in appropriate ways, including information regarding the recognition and reporting of side effects. Suggesting strategies to assist the client in taking medication on time can be helpful (Morrison, Meehan, & Stomski, 2015a). Treatment with psychopharmacologic agents can be lengthy because of the chronic nature of many disorders. Medication management occurs in both acute and community care settings, and medication follow-up may include home visits as well as telephone calls. Many clients remain on medication regimens for years, never becoming medication free. Clients may require considerable support from health care professionals, including nurses, that is focused on their individual needs and the context (Kauppi, Hätönen, Adams, & Välimäki, 2015). Medication education is thus an ongoing intervention that requires careful documentation, monitoring, and engagement with the client.

Interventions for the Psychological Domain

Emphasis in the psychological domain is on emotion, behaviour, and cognition. The nurse–client relationship serves as the basis for interventions directed towards the psychological domain. Because the therapeutic relationship is discussed extensively in Chapter 6, it is not covered in this chapter. This section covers counselling, conflict resolution, recovery orientation, reminiscence, behaviour therapy, cognitive interventions, psychoeducation, health teaching, and spiritual interventions. Chapter 8 presents the theoretic basis for many of these interventions.

Nurses in the direct care role will use all of the psychological interventions to respond to the health care problems of their clients. Nurses in case manager roles will also frequently use interventions from the psychological domain in order to promote recovery and empower the client to make changes. The nurse manager oversees the use of the psychological interventions and evaluates the staff's ability to use the interventions and assess outcomes.

Counselling Interventions

Counselling interventions are specific, time-limited interactions between a nurse and a client, family, or group experiencing immediate or ongoing difficulties related to their health or well-being. Counselling is usually short-term and focuses on improving coping abilities, reinforcing healthy behaviours, fostering positive interactions, or preventing illnesses and disabilities. Counselling strategies are discussed throughout this text. Psychotherapy is generally a long-term approach aimed at improving or helping clients regain previous health status and functional abilities. Mental health specialists, such as advanced practice nurses, use psychotherapy.

Conflict Resolution

A conflict involves an individual's perceptions, emotions, and behaviours. In a conflict, a person believes that his or her own needs, interests, wants, or values are incompatible with someone else's (Boggs, 2016). The individual experiences fear, sadness, bitterness, anger, hopelessness, or some combination of these emotions in response to the perceived threat. Misunderstandings, poor communication, value or goal differences, personality issues, and stress can interplay to contribute to this conflict and impact its resolution (Boggs, 2016).

Conflict resolution is a specific type of intervention through which the nurse helps clients resolve disagreements or disputes with family, friends, or other individuals. Conflicts can be positive if individuals see the problem as solvable and providing an opportunity for growth and interpersonal understanding. The nurse may be in the position of actually resolving a family conflict or teaching family members how to resolve their own conflicts positively. In addition, because nurses are frequently in positions of leadership, they often need conflict resolution skills to settle employee conflicts.

Conflict Resolution Process

Calmness and objectivity are important in resolving any client or family conflict. The desired outcome of conflict resolution is a "win–win" situation in which each party feels positive about the outcome. The nurse will take the following steps in conflict resolution:

1. Identify conflict issues.
2. Know the nurse's own response to the conflict.
3. Separate the problem from the people involved.
4. Stay focused on the issue and the underlying motivations behind the position the other person took.
5. Identify available options.
6. Try to identify established standards to guide the decision-making process (Boggs, 2016).

It is important to be aware of what is causing the conflict. This can be difficult to discern at times, and open, honest, and respectful communication is necessary to facilitate this awareness. It is helpful when all parties involved are able to reflect on their reactions to the conflict and what triggers their emotional responses. It is best and most constructive when all involved are able to focus on the issue at hand and not be critical of the people involved. The focus needs to be on the here and now of the problem, without dwelling on issues that have occurred in the past. Once all parties understand the underlying reasons for the dispute, attention can be given to developing options on how to appropriately address it. As much as possible, this development should be a collaborative process with all parties contributing fairly to the outcome (Boggs, 2016).

Cultural Brokering in Client–System Conflicts

Clients may be marginalized within the health care system due to potentially stigmatizing factors, such as poverty, sexual orientation, lack of formal education, race, or ethnicity. Differences in cultural values and languages between clients and health care organizations can contribute to clients' feelings of powerlessness. For example, people who are new immigrants, who are homeless, or who need to make informed decisions under stressful conditions may be unable to navigate the health care system. The nurse can help through **cultural brokering** or the use of culturally appropriate strategies that aid in bridging or mediating between the client's culture and the health care system (Bulechek et al., 2013). The health care system can be understood as a culture in and of itself, with culture shock being a potential experience for clients and families new to it.

For the "nurse as broker" to be effective, he or she establishes and maintains a sense of connectedness or relationship with the client. In turn, the nurse also establishes and cultivates networks with other health care facilities and resources. Cultural sensitivity enables the nurse to be aware of and sensitive to the needs of clients from a variety of cultures. Cultural competence is necessary for the brokering process to be effective (see Chapter 3).

Recovery Orientation

Recovery-focused interventions are becoming more prevalent in PMH care. The Recovery Model comes out of the mental health consumer movement and the work of Dr. William Anthony (1993). Nurses apply this orientation to their everyday interactions with their clients. For example, in care of individuals with severe persistent mental illnesses such as schizophrenia or bipolar disorder, a **recovery orientation** means helping the person regain functioning or "get on with life," despite having ongoing symptoms of the psychiatric illness. Recovery may refer to what the client does, how the nurse functions, or how the mental health system is organized. In taking this approach, there is recognition that a cure is not necessary for a sense of recovery for the individual with mental illness. At present, cure may not be possible for some mental disorders (Mental Health Commission of Canada, 2015). The Mental Health Commission of Canada (MHCC) has created guidelines for utilizing a recovery-oriented approach to mental health and illness in the Canadian context. These guidelines flow from six integral dimensions of practicing with a recovery focus. These dimensions are as follows:

- Creating a culture and language of hope.
- Recovery is personal.
- Recovery occurs in the context of one's life.
- Responding to the diverse needs of everyone living in Canada.
- Working with First Nations, Inuit, and Métis.
- Recovery is about transforming services and systems (Mental Health Commission of Canada, 2015, pp. 15–17).

One approach to recovery, the Tidal Model, was created by nurses for use in mental health practice settings (Barker & Buchanan-Barker, 2010a, 2010b). The Tidal Model emphasizes the importance of a collaborative relationship between the nurse and the client. The client's perspectives and individual experiences are accepted and valued. Recovery is contingent on the health professional having a genuine interest in the client and his or her experiences. The process is open, transparent, and based on the mutual establishment of goals that both parties work together to achieve. It is recognized that recovery requires time and commitment from both the nurse and the client and that the process of change is enhanced through a genuine, nurturing therapeutic relationship (see Chapter 8 for more information on this model).

Reminiscence

Reminiscence, the thinking about or relating of past experiences, is used as a nursing intervention to enhance life review particularly for older adults. Reminiscence encourages clients, either in individual or in group settings, to discuss their past and review their lives. Through reminiscence, individuals can identify past coping strategies that can support them in current stressful situations. Clients can also use reminiscence to maintain self-esteem, stimulate thinking, and support the natural healing process of life review (Djukanovic, Carlsson, & Peterson, 2016). Activities that facilitate reminiscence include writing an account of past events, making a tape recording and playing it back, explaining pictures in family albums, drawing a family tree, and writing to old friends (see Chapter 31 for health promotion with the older person).

Behaviour Therapy

Behaviour therapy interventions focus on reinforcing or promoting desirable behaviours or altering undesirable ones. The basic premise is that because most behaviours are learned, new functional behaviours can also be learned. Behaviours—not internal psychic processes—are the targets of the interventions. The models of behavioural theorists serve as a basis for these interventions (see Chapter 8).

Behaviour Modification

Behaviour modification is a specific, systematized behaviour therapy technique that can be applied to individuals, groups, or systems. The aim of behaviour modification is to reinforce desired behaviours and extinguish undesired ones. Desired behaviour is rewarded to increase the likelihood that clients will repeat it and, over time, replace the problematic behaviour with it. Behaviour modification is used for various problematic behaviours, such as dysfunctional eating and addictions, and often is used in the care of children and adolescents.

Token Economy

Primarily used in rehabilitative inpatient settings or schools, a **token economy** applies behaviour modification techniques to multiple behaviours. In a token economy, clients are rewarded with points or tokens for demonstrating selected desired behaviours (Holmes & Murray, 2011). They can use these tokens to purchase meals, leave the unit, watch television, or wear street clothes, for example. In less restrictive environments, clients use tokens to purchase additional privileges, such as attending social events. Token economies can be helpful in creating a structured therapeutic environment for children with developmental delays or autism (Matson & Boisjoli, 2009), and the strategy has also been shown to work with hospitalized aggressive clients (Bisconer, Green, Mallon-Czajka, & Johnson, 2006). There has been a decline, however, in the use of token economies as a treatment approach since the 1980s. In some settings, such as forensic psychiatry, there is concern that the use of particular behaviour modification programs, such as token economies, does not respect the autonomy of the clients being served (Holmes & Murray, 2011).

Cognitive Interventions

Cognitive interventions are verbally structured interventions that reinforce and promote desirable, or alter undesirable, cognitive functioning. The belief underlying this approach is that thoughts guide emotional reactions, motivations, and behaviours. Cognitive interventions do not solve problems for clients but rather help clients develop new ways of viewing situations so that they can solve problems themselves (Beck Institute for Cognitive Behavior Therapy, 2017). Nurses may use several models as the basis for cognitive interventions, but all models assume that by changing the cognitive appraisal of a situation (view of the world) and by examining the meaning of events, clients can reinterpret situations. In turn, emotional changes will follow the cognitive changes, and, ultimately, behaviours will change.

Because people develop their thinking patterns throughout their lifetime, many thoughts become so automatic that they are outside individuals' awareness. Thus, a person may be unaware of the automatic thoughts that influence his or her actions or other thoughts. **Automatic thinking** is often subject to errors or tangible distortions of reality that contradict objective appraisals. For example, a client with depression may be convinced that no one cares about him when, in fact, his family and friends are deeply concerned. Illogical thinking, another thinking error, occurs when a person draws a faulty conclusion. For example, a college student is so devastated by failing an examination that she perceives it as catastrophic and that her college career is over.

To engage in cognitive treatment, the client must be capable of introspection and reflection about thoughts and fantasies. Cognitive interventions are used in a wide range of clinical situations, from short-term crises to persistent mental disorders. Cognitive interventions also include thought stopping, contracting, and cognitive restructuring. These specific interventions are discussed in Chapter 13.

Psychoeducation

Psychoeducation uses educational strategies to teach clients the skills they lack because of a psychiatric disorder. The goal of psychoeducation is a change in knowledge and behaviour. Nurses use psychoeducation to meet the educational needs of clients by adapting teaching strategies to their disorder-related issues. As clients gain skills, functioning improves. For example, some clients may need to learn how to maintain their morning hygiene. Others may need to understand their illness and cope with hearing voices that others do not hear.

Specific psychoeducation techniques are based on adult learning principles, such as beginning at the point the learner is currently at and building on his or her current experiences. Thus, the nurse assesses the client's current skills and readiness to learn. From there, the nurse individualizes a teaching plan for each client. He or she can conduct such teaching in a one-to-one situation or in a group format.

Psychoeducation is a continuous process of assessing, setting goals, developing learning activities, and evaluating for changes in knowledge and behaviour. Nurses use it with individuals, groups, families, and communities. Psychoeducation serves as a basis for psychosocial rehabilitation, a service-delivery approach for those with severe and persistent mental illness (see Chapters 20 and 21).

Health Teaching

With teaching–coaching, the nurse "attempts to understand the life experience of the client and uses this understanding to support and promote learning related to health and personal development" (CFMHN, 2014, p. 19). Based on the principles of teaching, health teaching involves collaborating with the client to determine learning needs and transmitting new information, "while considering the context of the client's life experiences. [The nurse] considers readiness, culture, literacy, language, preferred learning style, and resources available" (CFMHN, 2014, p. 9). According to the *Canadian Standards of Psychiatric-Mental Health Nursing*, "all interactions between the nurse and patient are potentially teaching/learning situations" (CFMHN, 2014, p. 9). Thus, in health teaching, the nurse attends holistically to potential health care problems. For example, if a person has diabetes mellitus and is taking insulin, the nurse provides health care teaching related to diabetes and the interaction of this problem with the mental disorder. Clients may need or want a family member or friend to be taught ways to assist and/or support them,

as well. For instance, in the preceding example, teaching a family member or a friend of the client about diabetes and its treatment, including the administration of insulin, might be an important component of the health education.

There are many learning aids and tools that can assist individuals to increase their health literacy and understanding of their personal health situation. These range from pamphlets, diagrams, and books to websites, apps, and video gaming (see Box 11.3 for research on the use of video games in nursing care). Nurses have a role in helping clients identify appropriate resources and need to be aware that credibility (e.g., Is the source of a website reliable?), cost (e.g., Does the client have a mobile phone and is this app affordable?), accessibility (e.g., Does the client have Internet access?), and ease of use (Is the client comfortable with video games?) will be factors in the effectiveness of a learning aid or tool.

Evaluation is a necessary aspect of teaching: has the client learned the knowledge and skills required to maintain his or her health? Evaluation is an ongoing process. While some information may be readily acquired, other knowledge and skills may need more time or teaching. Review of the material throughout the teaching–learning process is a good strategy, as is having the client "teach-back" what has been learned. Aids to retaining important information, such as written or audio materials that can be reviewed at home, are helpful (RNAO, 2012a, 2012b).

Nurses need to be vigilant in the teaching–coaching role that they do not conflate the client's learning style with their own preferred way to learn. The nurse must also be aware of his or her own feelings when providing client education about what might be considered sensitive or culturally taboo topics. For example, some psychiatric medications have sexual side effects that significantly contribute to medication noncompliance. Nurses need to develop skills and confidence to educate clients about this important concern as many clients are embarrassed to raise it with health care professionals (Quinn, Happell, & Browne, 2012) (see Fig. 11.2 for "EASE", a brief guide to health education with clients).

Interventions for the Social Domain

The social domain includes the individual's environment and its effect on his or her responses to mental disorders and distress. Interventions within the social domain are geared towards couples, families, friends, and large and small social groups, with special attention given to ethnicity and community interactions. In some instances, nurses design interventions that affect a client's environment, such as helping a family member decide to place a loved one in long-term care. In other instances, the nurse actually modifies the environment to promote positive behaviours through providing opportunities for clients to interact with others. For example, this can be

BOX 11.3 Research for Best Practice

USING VIDEO GAMES IN NURSING CARE

From Pater, P., Shattell, M. M., & Clary, M. (2015). Video games as nursing interventions. Issues in Mental Health Nursing, 36, *156–160.*

Purpose: To explore the research literature to identify whether or not gaming has potential as a therapeutic intervention.

Method: Using an integrative literature review method, the researchers searched CINAHL, MEDLINE, and ProQuest electronic databases for articles that met their inclusion criteria. These were that the researchers had "studied a video game in a healthcare setting; used live subjects (i.e., is not a simulation); used quantitative methods in an effort to show efficacy of treatments (outcomes); and reported outcomes" (p. 156).

Findings: Evidence of the use of video games in promoting health and health care interventions since the 1970s was noted. With gaming consoles increasingly prevalent in private homes and health care facilities, there has been an increased awareness in the potential associated with their therapeutic use. These uses include cognitive–behavioural therapy for depression, anxiety, and anger management and interventions with veterans. Effective video games had the potential to "educate, empower, and encourage" (p. 159). Limitations and concerns identified included a dearth of information regarding nurses' attitudes towards the use of video games for therapeutic purposes, as well as affordability (e.g., program, equipment, and training costs) and a lack of nursing knowledge regarding how to therapeutically implement the games.

Implications for Nursing: With increased developments in virtual technology becoming more accessible in gaming platforms, further advancements in gaming's therapeutic potential is possible. Nurses need to be aware of the availability of such resources and their therapeutic usefulness, as well as to increase their skill in identifying patients for which gaming may be particularly effective as an intervention.

Health Education with Clients: EASE

ENGAGE
Collaborative approach
Learn about client's life situation
Learn client priorities and preferences

ASSESS
Health literacy needs
Client's learning style
Availability of learning resources

STRATEGIZE & START
Create learning goals and plan with client
Select or develop learning tools
Enact plan
Encourage

EVALUATE
Ongoing
Review
Client "teaches-back"

Figure 11.2. Health education with clients: EASE.

accomplished through group or recreational activities for holidays or other special events, which clients can attend. Group and family interventions are discussed in Chapters 14 and 15, respectively.

Milieu Therapy

Milieu therapy provides a stable and coherent social organization to facilitate an individual's treatment. (The terms milieu therapy and *therapeutic environment* are often used interchangeably.) In milieu therapy, the design of the physical surroundings, structure of client activities, and promotion of a stable social structure and cultural setting enhance the setting's therapeutic potential. A therapeutic milieu facilitates client interactions and promotes personal growth. Although inpatient psychiatric units are increasingly used for intensive, short-term care of acutely and severely ill clients who are discharged as soon as possible to community care, milieu therapy remains important to these environments. In a phenomenologic study with clients hospitalized on an acute care psychiatric unit in Nova Scotia, the environment is revealed as an integral aspect of clients' illness and recovery experience. The anecdotes of the clients show that the milieu can create potential for destruction as well as healing. Clients could feel afraid and abandoned or connected and affirmed;

they considered relationships as central to the milieu (Thibeault, Trudeau, d'Entremont, & Brown, 2010).

Milieu therapy is the responsibility of the nurse in collaboration with the client and other health care providers. The basic concepts of milieu therapy include safety and security, validation, open communication, and structured interaction.

Safety and Security

The milieu should be a healing place in which clients feel safe, secure, and cared for while dealing with their illness. The physical surroundings are important in this process and should be clean and comfortable, with special attention paid to promoting a noninstitutionalized environment. Pictures on walls, comfortable furniture, and soothing colours help clients relax. Most facilities encourage clients and nursing staff to wear street clothes, which helps decrease the formalized nature of hospital settings and promotes nurse–client relationships. Research suggests that the absence of a therapeutic milieu can be experienced by clients and nurses in parallel ways (Shattell, Andes, & Thomas, 2008). For instance, nurses can feel caged in by an enclosed nursing station, while clients experience similar feelings by locked unit doors.

Therapeutic milieus emphasize client involvement in treatment decisions and operation of the unit. Too often, the stigma of mental illness can exist within institutional walls, and clients can be treated in a paternalistic manner. On most inpatient psychiatric units, clients participate in maintaining the quality of the physical surroundings, such as assuming responsibility for making their own beds, attending to their own belongings, and keeping an acceptable living area. Families are viewed as a part of the client's life; family involvement is encouraged. Thus, family members should feel welcomed and safe in the milieu, as well.

Validation

In a therapeutic environment, validation is another process that affirms a client's individuality. Clients should feel validated as persons of worth and deserving of respect. Staff–client interactions should constantly reaffirm the client's humanity and his or her human rights. The importance of the client's personal story, history, experience, and understanding of his or her illness must be recognized in all aspects of care.

Open Communication

In open communication, health and treatment information is shared with clients and families. Client self-disclosure is invited within the support of a nurse–client relationship, with attention paid to the parameters of confidentiality that exist within that therapeutic relationship. These parameters may change with the care situation. For instance, if the client is undergoing a forensic assessment, information disclosed may be shared with the justice system (e.g., law courts). The client needs to understand this

(see Chapter 35). Further, the environment is shaped to facilitate optimal interaction and resocialization. Support, attention, praise, and reassurance given to clients improve self-esteem and increase confidence. Client education is also a part of this support, including guidance regarding effective coping skills. Nurses and other team members should strive to role model effective communication when interacting with one another as well as with clients and families. The dynamics of team interactions can affect the milieu in both positive and negative ways.

Structured Interaction

Structured interaction is a purposeful interaction that is intended to help clients cope with particular behaviours or to learn better ways of interaction. For instance, the treatment team may assign structured interactions to specific clients as part of their treatment. Specific attitudes or approaches are assumed with individual clients or in response to particular client behaviour if beneficial to the client. These approaches include indulgence, flexibility, passive or active friendliness, matter-of-fact attitude, casualness, watchfulness, or kind firmness. For example, if and when a client becomes overexcited by daily events, the team may provide a matter-of-fact attitude when responding; or if a client's illness includes delusions that lead him or her to engage in risky behaviour, the team may intervene with an attitude of kind firmness.

Milieu treatments are based on the individual needs of the clients and include relaxation groups, discussion groups, and medication groups. Spontaneous and planned activities are possible on a short-term unit as well as in a long-term setting. In the community, it is possible to apply milieu therapy approaches in day treatment centres, group homes, and single dwellings.

Promotion of Client Safety on Psychiatric Units

A critical aspect of nursing in PMH settings is the promotion of client safety, especially in inpatient units. It is critical because clients may be so severely ill that they engage in behaviours harmful to themselves or others. Clients experiencing delusions and hallucinations, for instance, can be responding to perceptions not based in reality. They can react with fear or in self-defence to dangers only they perceive. Sensitivity to the client's world as she or he is living it underlies nursing interventions used to keep the client safe. Interventions begin with observation and de-escalation and may evolve to the use of containment strategies, such as seclusion or physical or chemical (medication) restraints for clients with an involuntary status. See Chapter 7 for a discussion of ethical issues related to the use of behaviour control and restraint.

Psychiatric units vary in their rate of incidences of client behaviours such as aggression, self-harm, medication refusal, and suicide attempts that put both clients and care team at risk and frequently result in application of containment measures with the client (Bowers, 2014). Key influences on these incidences have been identified as "the patient community, patient characteristics, the regulatory framework, the staff team, the physical environment and outside hospital" (Bowers, 2014, p. 501). Examples in these domains include the following:

- Patient community: discord among patients, as when property is damaged; the contagion of emotions such as anxiety and noise levels within the community
- Patient characteristics: symptoms and their severity (e.g., hallucinations, delusions); staffing levels for care and support
- Outside hospital: tension in family, loss of accommodation or relationship, or bad news
- Physical environment: clean, tidy, respectful atmosphere and opportunities for client choice
- Staff team: levels of staff anxiety and frustration, ideology of care, rules, consistency
- Regulatory framework: Legal status (e.g., involuntary admission); denial of an appeal

Recognition of these influences allows them to be addressed in ways that better promote client and staff safety (Bowers, 2014).

Observation

Like all hospitalized clients, individuals hospitalized on a psychiatric unit are observed by the nurses caring for them. **Observation** is the ongoing assessment of the client's status to identify and subvert any potential problem. The nature of mental disorders shapes the focus of the nurses' observations. In psychiatric settings, for instance, clients are ambulatory and thus more susceptible to environmental hazards. In addition, judgement and cognition impairment are symptoms of many psychiatric disorders. The reason for the client's admission may be, in fact, that they pose a danger to themselves or others. When nursing in PMH settings, observation involves thoughtful, knowledgeable regard of the persons and consistent, responsible monitoring for any potential harm to themselves or others.

The intensity of the observation of the client depends on the assessed level of risk. Clients may be simply asked to "check in" at different times of the day, whereas other clients may be observed every 15 minutes by an assigned staff member. Some clients, such as those seen at a high risk for suicide, may be constantly observed by a staff member assigned to only them. Mental health facilities have policies that specify levels of observation for clients at varying degrees of risk.

De-escalation

De-escalation is an interactive process of calming and redirecting a client who has an immediate potential for violence directed towards self or others. This intervention involves assessing the situation and preventing it from escalating to one in which injury occurs to the client or others. Once the nurse has assessed the situation,

he or she responds matter-of-factly to it, using various interventions that can include a request for the client and/or others to leave the situation, distraction, and conflict resolution. Psychiatric staff members are usually trained in responding to situations of aggression as a team and, thus, are often able to de-escalate such situations effectively (see Chapter 18 for information on the management of aggression and violence). Nurses can use various interventions in this situation, including distraction, conflict resolution, and cognitive interventions.

Seclusion

Seclusion is the "involuntary supervised isolation of a patient in a locked, nonstimulating room" (Van Der Merwe, Muir-Cochrane, Jones, Tziggili, & Bowers, 2013, p. 203). A client is placed in seclusion for purposes of safety or behavioural management. The nature and physical content of the seclusion room can vary. It generally has no furniture except a mattress and a blanket. The walls may be padded. The room must be environmentally safe, with no hanging devices, electrical outlets, or windows from which the client could jump. Once a client is placed in seclusion, he or she is observed at all times (i.e., continuous or constant observation).

Research regarding the experiences of using seclusion rooms has yielded conflicting data. Seclusion can be an extremely negative client experience (Van Der Merwe et al., 2013). Consequently, its use is seriously questioned, and many facilities have completely abandoned its practice. Clients have disputed the calming effects of seclusion and have perceived it as an instrument of power and control, and their outcomes may actually be worse if seclusion is used (Holmes, Kennedy, & Perron, 2004). However, clients have also reported the use of seclusion rooms in aiding them feel safe and protected (Larue et al., 2013). Mental health staff appear to identify the potential for negative client perceptions and experiences regarding seclusion rooms but tend to feel that it can also be beneficial for clients who need that high level of restriction (Van Der Merwe et al.). If units are adequately staffed and personnel are trained in dealing with assaultive clients, seclusion is rarely needed. If seclusion is used, it must follow the same guidelines as the use of restraints.

Restraint

Restraint is the most restrictive safety intervention and is only used in the most extreme circumstances and as a measure of last resort. Alternative approaches to the use of restraint include adjusting the environment in ways such as reducing stimulation, increasing or decreasing social interaction, providing access for the client to his or her preferred coping strategy, review of prescribed medication for potential change, use of appropriate distraction or relaxation techniques, and access to comfort zones or rooms (MacDaniel, Bramer, & Hogan, 2009;

RNAO, 2012a, 2012b). The Registered Nurses Association of Ontario's best practice guideline, "Promoting Safety: Alternative Approaches to the Use of Restraints," is an excellent resource (see Web Links).

In Canada, the laws for restricting the freedom of clients against their will are specific to each province. Provincial mental health acts govern the situations under which restraint may be used in their jurisdiction.

Chemical restraint is the use of medication to control clients or manage their behaviour. This is distinct from medication used to treat their psychiatric illness. A **physical restraint** is any human or mechanical method that restricts the freedom of movement or normal access to one's body, material, or equipment and cannot be easily removed (National Alliance on Mental Illness, 2008). Different types of physical restraints are available. Wrist restraints restrict arm movement. Four-point restraints are applied to the wrists and ankles in bed. When five-point restraints are used, all extremities are secured, and another restraint is placed across the chest (see Fig. 11.3).

In addition to following provincial law, the nurse must also adhere to hospital policies regarding restraint. A physician's order is necessary for restraint, and nurses should document all of the previously tried de-escalation interventions before the restraint was applied. Nurses should limit the use of restraints to times when an individual is judged to be a danger to self or others. As well, they should apply restraints only until the client has gained control over his or her behaviour. When a client is in physical restraints, the nurse should closely observe the client and protect him or her from self-injury. It is the nurse's responsibility to be aware of the institutional policies that govern this.

A review of qualitative evidence on nurses' decision making related to physical restraint suggests that nurse-based factors (e.g., perception of client's behaviour, willingness to take risks, own comfort level) and context-based factors (e.g., other team members, presence of family, the health care organization) can hinder

nurses from making "an ethically balanced" decision on restraint use (Goethals, Dierckx de Casterlé, & Gastmans, 2011, p. 1207).

Given the negative consequences to the client and the impact on the nurse–client relationship, it is essential that nurses treat the client with respect and dignity at all times during a psychiatric emergency that necessitates seclusion or restraint. Canadian nursing research (Larue et al., 2013) has identified factors influencing client perspectives regarding seclusion: behaviour of the health professional upon entering the seclusion room, such as demonstrating understanding, listening, and reassurance; the offer of help in regaining control; and explanation of the situation to the client, such as seclusion as a means of addressing the need for calm, sleep, and safety. Some client participants voiced concerns regarding lack of alternatives to seclusion being offered and recommended changes to the physical environment.

Every incident of seclusion or restraint should be followed up by a thorough debriefing. Postseclusion and/or restraint reviews involve discussion with clients regarding their experience, analysis by the care team of factors that influenced the decision to intervene and possible preventative strategies, and appraisal by the health care organization of potential influencing factors, such as staffing (Goulet & Larue, 2016; Holmes, Murray, & Knack, 2015). Education on the ethical, clinical, and legal issues related to restraint practices is very important (Kontio et al., 2009).

Home Visits

Clients usually have been hospitalized or have received treatment for acute psychiatric symptoms before being referred to a home care service. The goal of **home visits**, the delivery of nursing care in the client's living environment, is to maximize the client's functional ability within the nurse–client relationship and with the family or partner, as appropriate. The nurse who makes home visits needs to be able to work independently, is skilled in teaching clients and families, can administer and monitor medications, and uses community resources for the client's needs. Traditional home visits are regaining popularity, particularly when the client has concomitant psychiatric and physical illnesses.

Home visits can be especially useful when helping reluctant clients to enter therapy, conducting a comprehensive assessment, strengthening a support network, and maintaining clients in the community when their condition deteriorates. Home visits are also useful in helping individuals adhere to their medication regimen. The nurse, for instance, can gain a better understanding of the barriers to taking medication as prescribed and assists the client and family to address them. One major advantage of home visits is the opportunity to provide family members with information and education and to engage them in planning and interventions.

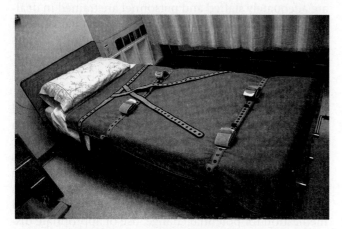

Figure 11.3. Bed with five-point restraints. (Courtesy of Alberta Hospitals, photographer Pat Morrison.)

Home visits also offer the nurse an opportunity to develop cultural sensitivity to families from a variety of backgrounds. Home-based interventions require the nurse to gain an understanding, as much as possible, of the family structure and interactions, including the roles various members play, how the family functions in terms of responsibilities, and the family life cycle (see Chapter 15). A family's cultural background influences all of these factors and is important to consider when planning interventions. The home visit also allows the nurse to identify clients who lack support from others in their daily lives.

The home visit process consists of three steps: the previsit phase, the home visit, and the postvisit phase. During previsit planning, the nurse sets goals for the home visit based on data received from other health care providers or the client. Any safety precautions that should be taken for the visit should be identified and acted upon. For instance, winter road conditions for a rural home visit or crime levels in an urban district to be visited may need to be considered. The nurse and the client agree on the time of the visit. While the nurse travels to the home, a general assessment can be made of the neighbourhood for access to services, socioeconomic factors, safety, and other factors relevant to the client's well-being within the community.

The actual visit can be divided into four parts. The first is the greeting phase, usually brief, in which the nurse begins to connect with the client and family members in their home setting. Greetings are important as they set the atmosphere for the visit and, on the part of the nurse, should be friendly but professional. In some cultures, the greeting phase may involve more formal interactions, such as taking food or tea with family members. The second phase establishes the focus of the visit. Sometimes, the purpose of the visit is medication administration, health teaching, or counselling. The client and family must be clear regarding the purpose. The implementation of the service is the next phase and should use most of the visit time. If the purpose of the visit is problem solving or decision making, the family's cultural values may determine the types of interaction and decision-making approaches. Closure is the last phase, the end of the home visit. It is a time to summarize and clarify important points. The nurse should also schedule any additional visits and reiterate client expectations between visits. Usually, the nurse is the only provider to see the client regularly. The nurse should acknowledge family members when leaving if they were not a part of the visit.

The postvisit phase includes documentation, reporting, and follow-up planning. This time is also when the nurse may meet with supervisors or colleagues and presents data from the home visit at the team meeting.

Community Action

Nurses have a unique opportunity to promote mental health awareness and support humane treatment for people with mental disorders including addiction. Activities range from being an advisor to support groups to participating in the political process through lobbying efforts and serving on community mental health boards. These unpaid activities are usually outside the realm of a particular job. However, an important role of professionals is to provide community service in addition to services through income-generating positions.

Interventions for the Spiritual Domain

Spiritual care cannot be readily separated from the bio/psycho/social components of care. It involves, rather, giving attention to all aspects of the individual's life and life circumstances and takes direction from his or her reality (Sawatzky & Pesut, 2005). In doing so, the nurse identifies spiritual needs and strives to help the individual meet these needs (Pesut, 2006). The integrative nature of spirituality, and therefore of spiritual care, can make it difficult to isolate and identify spiritual needs, document spiritual interventions, and stipulate outcomes. Although spirituality always has been a core aspect of nursing care, nurses can be hesitant to address this component of their practice. However, a Canadian study of nurses' experiences of spiritual nursing care found that there was a common dimension across all the nurses' descriptions: "[S]piritual nursing care is about developing caring relationships through fostering connections to promote spiritual comfort and well-being" (Carr, 2008, p. 690). An attitude of respect and concern for the client's comfort, dignity, and well-being and recognition of the client as a person with a past, present, and future were seen as core to connection, even with individuals who appeared not to want the connection or who could not communicate.

Four critical qualities for **spiritual care** emerged from the research data: *receptivity, humanity, competency,* and *positivity. Receptivity* involves being open to clients as a person and being genuinely present to them. It may mean simply "being with" (not just doing for) the client. *Humanity* is about being human, or put another way, being "real." It can be offering "the little things" that reveal thoughtful caring, such as knocking before entering the client's room, offering a favourite food to stimulate a client's poor appetite, or taking time to view family photos on display. *Competency* is enabling the client to know that she or he is in good hands. It reflects the integrative aspect of spiritual care that includes good bio/psycho/social care. *Positivity* describes the positive approach necessary to spiritual care. The nurse's attitude is one of hope and determination, of encouragement and good humour. *Positivity* is not about smiling all the time or insisting on only happy feelings being expressed. It is about fostering a positive spirit in others through one's own hopeful energy (Carr, 2008). These qualities of spiritual care underscore the importance of the nurse's own well-being and the therapeutic environment (see Chapter 6).

Times of illness and crisis can be opportunities for personal or spiritual growth for a person. The person may seek to connect or reconnect with others, with nature, with a power greater than him or herself (that may be named in various ways, such as God, the Creator, or Allah, or not named out of respect), or with some aspect of the sacred (Baldacchino & Draper, 2001). Nurses can support clients in their spiritual growth by listening to them as they describe their seeking; by responding to any requests for meeting with a religious leader/guide such as a minister, priest, rabbi, imam, lama, or elder; or by facilitating the use of religious ritual, such as a smudging ceremony for an Aboriginal client who requests it. Aspects of care for the spiritual domain relevant to particular disorders or age of human development may be found in this text in units *Care and Recovery for Persons with a Psychiatric Disorder* and *Mental Health Across the Lifespan*.

■ EVALUATION OF OUTCOMES

Evaluation of individual outcomes involves answering the following questions:

- What were the benefits for the individual?
- What was the individual's level of satisfaction?
- Was the outcome diagnosis specific or nonspecific?
- What was the cost-effectiveness of the intervention?

When measuring outcomes, nurses must consider the time frame. Identifying the intermediate outcome indicators that may be achieved in one setting versus the indicators that can be achieved in a second setting provides for a measurement of progression and enhances continuity of care. Nevertheless, not until the individual is discharged or moved to a community setting can it be known if indicators (for instance, "demonstration of confidence when alone at home," "demonstration of confidence in role skills (worker/mother)," "demonstration of self-advocacy behaviour") are achieved. Outcomes can be measured immediately after the nursing intervention or after time passes. However, outcomes based on health prevention and health promotion diagnoses can be challenging to measure and may need to occur after considerable time has passed.

❧ SUMMARY OF KEY POINTS

- Nurses should work collaboratively with clients and families in determining interventions.
- Nurses develop interventions from assessment data and may organize them around nursing diagnoses. The client's needs, values, and preferred outcomes and the *Canadian Standards of Psychiatric-Mental Health Nursing* (CFMHN, 2014) guide the selection of interventions.

- A client's ability to manage self-care activities can fluctuate with symptom severity. The Orem (1991) self-care model can be used to conceptualize client needs (related to attitude, knowledge, and skill) and choose appropriate interventions.
- The *Canadian Standards of Psychiatric-Mental Health Nursing* (CFMHN, 2014) supports the importance of outcome identification.
- Outcomes must be measurable and indicative of the individual's progress.
- More research is needed to identify individual outcomes as they relate to nursing diagnoses and interventions.
- Nursing diagnoses, nursing interventions, and individual outcomes are initially derived from the assessment data.
- Initial, revised, and discharge outcomes can be included in a nursing care plan.
- Outcome statements can cover the bio/psycho/social/spiritual domains.
- Nursing care, from assessment to outcome measurement, needs to be person and family centred. This means more than a recognition of the person's right to participate in health care decisions. It means genuine respect for the person's life experience and hopes for recovery.
- Interventions focusing on the biologic domain include activity and exercise; sleep, nutrition, relaxation, hydration, and thermoregulation interventions; pain management; and medication management. Nutritional interventions are used with most clients with psychiatric disorders. Medication management is a priority because of the long-term nature of the disorders and the importance of medication compliance.
- Interventions focusing on the psychological domain include counselling, behaviour therapy, cognitive interventions, psychoeducation, health teaching, and others. Implementation of these interventions requires a broad theoretic knowledge base.
- Interventions focusing on the social domain include group and family approaches, milieu therapy, safety interventions, home visits, and community action. On an inpatient psychiatric unit, the nurse uses milieu therapy to maximize the treatment effects of the client's environment.
- Interventions focusing on the spiritual domain involve a relationship and connection with the client that encompass the qualities of receptivity, humanity, competency, and positivity.

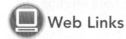 **Web Links**

canada.ca/en/health-canada/services/canada-food-guides.html Canada's food guides are available for download, free of charge, at this Health Canada site.

hc-sc.gc.ca/fn-an/food-guide-aliment/educ-comm/index-eng.php At this Health Canada website can be found the *Eat well and Be Active Educational Toolkit*, a resource you can use to help educate adults and children about eating healthy and being active.

cfmhn.ca/professionalPractices?f=7458545122100118.pdf&n=212922-CFMHN-standards-rv-3a.pdf&inline=yes The Canadian Federation of Mental Health Nurses' practice standards are freely available at this link.

nursingcenter.com The Lippincott Nursing Centre at this site has student resources, including articles and information about nursing topics, such as patient education. Membership is free.

rnao.ca/bpg/guidelines The best practice guidelines of the Registered Nurses Association of Ontario (RNAO) are found here and may be downloaded free of charge.

References

Anthony, W. A. (1993). Recovery from mental illness: The guiding vision of the mental health service system in the 1990's. *Psychosocial Rehabilitation Journal, 16*, 11–23.

Aydelotte, M. K. (1962). The use of individual welfare as a criterion measure. *Nursing Research, 11*, 10–14.

Baldacchino, D., & Draper, P. (2001). Spiritual coping strategies: A review of the nursing research literature. *Journal of Advanced Nursing, 34*(6), 833–841.

Barker, P. J., & Buchanan-Barker, P. (2010a). The Tidal Model of mental health recovery and reclamation: Application in acute care settings. *Issues in Mental Health Nursing, 31*, 171–180.

Barker, P. J., & Buchanan-Barker, P. (2010b). The Tidal Model of mental health recovery and reclamation: Application in acute care settings. *Issues in Mental Health Nursing, 31*, 171–180.

Beck Institute for Cognitive Behavior Therapy (2017). *What is cognitive behavior therapy?* Retrieved from https://www.beckinstitute.org/get-informed/what-is-cognitive-therapy/

Bisconer, S. W., Green, M., Mallon-Czajka, J., & Johnson, J. S. (2006). Managing aggression in a psychiatric hospital using a behaviour plan: A case study. *Journal of Psychiatric and Mental Health Nursing, 13*(5), 515–521.

Boggs, K. (2016). Resolving conflict between nurse and client. In E. Arnold & K. Boggs (Eds.), *Interpersonal relationships: Professional communication skills for nurses* (7th ed.). St. Louis, MO: Elsevier.

Bowers, L. (2014). Safewards: A new model of conflict and containment on psychiatric wards. *Journal of Psychiatric and Mental Health Nursing, 21*, 499–508.

Brataas, H. V., & Evensen, A. E. (2016). Life stories of people on sick leave from work because of mild mental illness, pain, and fatigue. *Work, 53*(2), 285–291.

Bulechek, G., Butcher, H., Dochterman, J., & Wagner, C. (Eds.) (2013). *Nursing interventions classification (NIC)* (6th ed.). St. Louis, MO: Elsevier.

Canadian Collaborative Mental Health Initiative (CCMHI). (2006). *Canadian Collaborative Mental Health Charter*. Mississauga, ON: Author.

Canadian Federation of Mental Health Nurses (CFMHN). (2014). *Canadian standards of psychiatric-mental health nursing* (4th ed.). Toronto, ON: Author.

Carpenito, L. J. (2017a). *Nursing diagnosis: Application to clinical practice* (15th ed.). Philadelphia, PA: Lippincott Williams & Wilkins.

Carpenito, L. J. (2017b). *Handbook of nursing diagnosis* (15th ed.). Philadelphia, PA: Lippincott Williams & Wilkins.

Carr, T. (2008). Mapping the processes and qualities of spiritual nursing care. *Qualitative Health Research, 18*(5), 686–700.

Centre for Addiction and Mental Health. (2016). *Integrated care pathways*. Retrieved from http://www.camh.ca/en/hospital/care_program_and_services/ICPs/Pages/default.aspx

Djukanovic, I., Carlsson, J., & Peterson, U. (2016). Group discussions with structured reminiscence and a problem-based method as an intervention to prevent depressive symptoms in older people. *Journal of Clinical Nursing, 25*(7/8), 992–1000.

Goethals, S., Dierckx de Casterlé, B., & Gastmans, C. (2011). Nurses' decision-making in cases of physical restraint: A synthesis of qualitative evidence. *Journal of Advanced Nursing, 68*(6), 1198–1210. doi: 10.1111/j.1365-2648.2011.05909.x

Goulet, M. H., & Larue, C. (2016). Post-seclusion and/or restraint review in psychiatry: A scoping review. *Archives of Psychiatric Nursing, 30*(1), 120–128.

Holmes, D., & Murray, S. J. (2011). Civilizing the "barbarian": A critical analysis of behavior modification programs in forensic psychiatric settings. *Journal of Nursing Management, 19*, 293–301.

Holmes, D., Kennedy, S. L., & Perron, A. (2004). The mentally ill and social exclusion: A critical examination of the use of seclusion from the patient's perspective. *Issues in Mental Health Nursing, 25*, 559–578.

Holmes, D., Murray, S. J., Arron, A., & McCabe, J. (2008). Nursing best practice guidelines: Reflecting on the obscene rise of the void. *Journal of Nursing Management, 16*, 394–403.

Holmes, D., Murray, S. J., & Knack, N. (2015). Experiencing seclusion in a forensic psychiatric setting: A phenomenological study. *Journal of Forensic Nursing, 11*(4), 200–213.

Jallo, N., Cozens, R., Smith, M., & Simpson, R. (2013). Effects of a guided imagery intervention on stress in hospitalized pregnant women: A pilot study. *Holistic Nursing Practice, 27*(3), 129–139.

Kauppi, K., Hätönen, H., Adams, C. E., & Välimäki, M. (2015). Perceptions of treatment adherence among people with mental health problem and health care professionals. *Journal of Advanced Nursing, 71*(4), 777–788.

Kleinpell, R. M. (2003). Measuring advanced practice nursing outcome, strategies and resources. *Critical Care Nurse, 23*, 6–10.

Kontio, R., Välimäki, M., Putkonen, H., Cocoman, A., Turpeinen, S., Kuosmanen, L., & Joffe, G. (2009). Nurses' and physicians' educational needs in seclusion and restraint practices. *Perspectives in Psychiatric Care, 45*(3), 198–207.

Lang, N. M., & Clinton, J. F. (1984). Assessment of quality of nursing care. *Annual Review of Nursing Research, 2*, 135–163.

Larue, C., Dumais, A., Boyer, R., Goulet, M. H., Bonin, J. P., & Baba, N. (2013). The experience of seclusion and restraint in psychiatric settings: Perspectives of patients. *Issues in Mental Health Nursing, 34*, 317–324.

MacDaniel, M., Van Bramer, J., & Hogan M. F. (2009). *Comfort rooms: A preventative tool used to reduce the use of restraint and seclusion in facilities that serve individuals with mental illness.* Retrieved from www.omh.ny.gov/omhweb/resources/publications/comfort_room/comfort_rooms.pdf

Malhi, G. S., Adams, D., & Berk, M. (2009). Is lithium in a class of its own? A brief profile of its clinical use. *Australian and New Zealand Journal of Psychiatry, 43*(12), 1096–1104.

Marek, K. D. (1989). Outcome measurement in nursing. *Journal of Nursing Quality Assurance, 4*(1), 1–9.

Matson, J. L., & Boisjoli, J. A. (2009). The token economy for children with intellectual disability and/or autism: A review. *Research in Developmental Disabilities, 30*(2), 240–248.

Mental Health Commission of Canada. (2015). *Guidelines for recovery-oriented practice, hope, dignity, inclusion.* Ottawa, ON: Author.

Minister of Health Canada. (2007a). *Eating well with Canada's Food Guide.* Ottawa, ON: Author. Retrieved from www.healthcanada.ca/foodguide

Minister of Health Canada. (2007b). *Eating well with Canada's Food Guide for First Nations, Inuit, and Métis.* Ottawa, ON: Author. Retrieved from www.healthcanada.ca/foodguide

Moorhead, S., Johnson, M., Maas, M., & Swanson, E. (2013). *Nursing Outcomes Classification (NOC): Measurement of health outcomes* (5th ed.). St. Louis, MO: Mosby.

Morrison, P., Meehan, T., & Stomski, N. J. (2015a). Australian case managers' perception of mental health consumers use of anti-psychotic medications and associated side-effects. *International Journal of Mental Health Nursing, 24*, 104–111.

Morrison, P., Meehan, T., & Stomski, N. J. (2015b). Living with antipsychotic medication side effects: The experience of Australian mental health consumers. *International Journal of Mental Health Nursing, 24*, 253–261.

National Alliance on Mental Illness. (2008). *Policy topics: What are restraints and seclusion?* Retrieved from http://www.nami.org/Template.cfm?Section=Issue_Spotlights&template=/ContentManagement/ContentDisplay.cfm&ContentID=7791

Orem, D. (1991). *Nursing concepts of practice* (4th ed.). St. Louis, MO: Year Book.

Pater, P., Shattell, M. M., & Clary, M. (2015). Video games as nursing interventions. *Issues in Mental Health Nursing, 36*, 156–160.

Pesut, B. (2006). Fundamental or foundational obligation? Problematizing the ethical call to spiritual care in nursing. *Advances in Nursing Science, 29*(2), 125–133.

Quinn, C., Happell, B., & Browne, G. (2012). Opportunity lost? Psychiatric medications and problems with sexual side function: A role for nurses in mental health. *Journal of Clinical Nursing, 21*(3/4), 415–423.

Registered Nurses Association of Ontario (RNAO). (2012a). *Toolkit: Implementation of best practice guidelines* (2nd ed.). Toronto, ON: Author. Retrieved from www.rnao.ca

Registered Nurses Association of Ontario (RNAO). (2012b). *Facilitating client centred learning.* Retrieved from www.rnao.ca

Registered Nurses Association of Ontario (RNAO). (2015). *Person- and family- centred care- 2015*. Toronto, ON: Author. Retrieved from www.rnao.ca

Sawatzky, R., & Pesut, B. (2005). Attributes of spiritual care in nursing practice. *Journal of Holistic Nursing, 23*(1), 19–33.

Shattell, M., Andes, M., & Thomas, S. (2008). How patients and nurses experience the acute care psychiatric environment. *Nursing Inquiry, 15*(3), 242–250.

Thibeault, C., Trudeau, K., d'Entremont, M., & Brown, T. (2010). Understanding the milieu experiences of patients on an acute inpatient psychiatric unit. *Archives of Psychiatric Nursing, 24*(4), 216–226.

Toups, M., Carmody, T., Greer, T., Rethorst, C., Grannemann, B., & Trivedi, M. H. (2017). Exercise as an effective treatment for positive valence symptoms in major depression. *Journal of Affective Disorders, 209,* 188–194.

Vallance, J. K., Buman, M. P., Stevinson, C., & Lynch, B. M. (2015). Associations of overall sedentary time and screen time with sleep disorders. *American Journal of Health Behaviour, 39*(1), 62–67.

Van Der Merwe, M., Muir-Cochrane, E., Jones, J., Tziggili, M., & Bowers, L. (2013). Improving seclusion practice: Implications of a review of staff and patient views. *Journal of Psychiatric and Mental Health Nursing, 20,* 203–215.

12 Psychopharmacology and Other Biologic Treatments

Duncan Stewart MacLennan

Adapted from the chapter "Psychopharmacology and Other Biologic Treatments" by Kathleen Hegadoren and Gerri Lasiuk

LEARNING OBJECTIVES

After studying this chapter, you will be able to:

- Explain psychotropic drug actions by describing the role of neurotransmitter chemicals and their receptor sites.
- Explain the three major mechanisms that explain the actions of psychotropic medications in the central nervous system.
- Define the three properties that determine the strength and effectiveness of a medication.
- Describe more specific mechanisms of action for each of the major classes of psychopharmacologic medication.
- Describe the major therapeutic effects as well as prevalent side effects of various classes of psychotropic medications.
- Suggest appropriate nursing methods to administer medications.
- Implement interventions to minimize side effects of psychopharmacologic medications.
- Differentiate acute and chronic medication-induced movement disorders.
- Identify aspects of patient teaching that nurses must implement for successful maintenance of patients using psychotropic medications.
- Analyze the potential benefits and risks associated with other forms of somatic treatments, including electroconvulsive therapy, light therapy, and nutrition therapy.
- Evaluate potential causes of nonadherence and implement interventions to improve adherence with treatment regimens.

KEY TERMS

- absorption • adherence • affinity • agonists • akathisia • antagonist • bioavailability • dystonia • efficacy • excretion • first-pass metabolism • half-life • intrinsic activity • kindling • metabolism • pharmacogenomics • phototherapy • potency • pseudoparkinsonism • selectivity • side effects • solubility • tardive dyskinesia • target symptoms • therapeutic index • tolerance • toxicity

KEY CONCEPTS

- psychopharmacology • receptors

In the early 1900s, Emil Kraeplin classified mental disorders based on clusters of observed symptoms, providing the basic tenets of the contemporary biologic approach to understanding and treating psychiatric disorders. However, this approach fell out of favour as psychoanalytic, psychodynamic, interpersonal, and other therapies flourished, and mental disorders were increasingly assumed to have primarily a psychological aetiology. In the 1950s, when it was discovered that the phenothiazine medications, such as chlorpromazine (Thorazine), relieved many of the symptoms of psychosis and that iproniazid, a medication for treating

tuberculosis, elevated mood, there was renewed interest in neurophysiology and biologic treatments for treating mental disorders.

This chapter reviews the major classes of psychopharmacologic drugs used in treating mental disorders, including antipsychotics, mood stabilizers, antidepressants, antianxiety medications, and stimulants, and provides a basis for understanding the specific biologic treatments of psychiatric disorders that are described more fully in later chapters.

The targets for psychiatric medications are predominantly located in the central nervous system (CNS).

This chapter focuses on understanding the impact of psychotropic medications on the basic unit of CNS functioning, the synapse, and on receptors embedded in neuronal cell membranes. This basic understanding allows the nurse to accept the role and responsibilities of administering medications, proactively monitoring and treating side effects, and educating the patient and family, which are all crucial to successful psychopharmacologic therapy. In addition to psychopharmacologic therapy, other biologic treatments are used. These therapies include electroconvulsive therapy (ECT), light therapy, and nutritional therapy and are discussed later in this chapter.

KEY CONCEPT

Psychopharmacology is a subspecialty of pharmacology that studies medications that affect behaviour through their actions in the CNS and that are used to treat psychiatric and neurodegenerative disorders. It is important to remember, however, that many drugs used to treat other conditions, such as pain syndromes, heart disease, and autoimmune disease, may also have powerful effects in the brain.

■ PHARMACODYNAMICS

A small amount of medication can have a significant and large effect on cell function. When tiny molecules of medication are compared with the vast amount of cells in the human body, the fraction seems disproportionate. Yet the drugs used to treat mental disorders often have profound effects on behaviour. To understand how this occurs, one needs to understand both *where* and *how* drugs work.

Targets of Drug Action: Where Drugs Act

Most drug molecules do not act on the entire cell surface, but rather at receptor sites, binding sites on enzymes, or transporters that remove neurotransmitter molecules from the synapse. Many psychopharmacologic drugs, especially older classes, act at multiple receptors. Newer agents are more specific to one type of receptor, but none act exclusively on one type of receptor. Understanding where receptors (and their subtypes), enzymes, and transporters are located within the body can be useful to explain the effects (including side effects) of specific drugs.

Consider diphenhydramine (Benadryl), a drug often used to treat allergic reactions, which works by interfering with histamine receptors (antagonist, discussed below). As it turns out, the histamine 1 (H1) receptor is located in smooth muscles, in endothelial cells, and *in the brain*. When a person takes this drug to counter the effects of an allergic reaction (in the body tissues outside of the brain), the drug also has an effect on H1 receptors

in the brain and causes sedation. Newer generation antihistamine drugs, such as loratadine (Claritin), will still have an effect on H1 receptors, but the drug molecules do not readily cross the blood–brain barrier. Little to no drug effect will occur at histamine receptors within the brain; thus, sedation is less likely to occur. The distribution of receptors in specific brain regions also plays a role in the side effect profile. For example, dopamine antagonists can produce dystonic movements because high concentrations of dopamine receptors are found in the region of the brain that controls fine motor movement.

Receptors are proteins that are embedded within the cell membrane and have binding sites for both naturally occurring chemicals (called *endogenous substances*) and drugs. Endogenous brain chemicals involved in neurotransmission, such as dopamine and serotonin, bind to specific groups of receptors. Administered drugs may compete with neurotransmitters for these receptors by mimicking or blocking the action of the neurotransmitter.

KEY CONCEPT

Receptors are associated with the work of German chemist Paul Erhlich, who in 1900 suggested that a receptive substance exists within the cell membrane. The biologic action of a drug depends on how its structure interacts with a specific receptor. Thus, a basic understanding of how receptors work is key to understanding how many drugs work in the body.

Receptors

Many drugs have been developed to act specifically at the receptor sites. When bound to the receptor, these drugs act as **agonists**—chemicals producing the same biologic action as the neurotransmitter itself—or as **antagonists**—chemicals blocking the biologic action of an agonist at a given receptor. Figure 12.1 illustrates the action of an agonist and an antagonist drug at a receptor site. A drug's ability to interact with a given receptor type may be judged by three properties: selectivity, affinity, and intrinsic activity.

Selectivity

The first property, called **selectivity**, is the ability of the drug to be specific for a particular receptor. If a drug is highly selective, it will interact only with its specific receptors in the areas of the body where these receptors occur and, therefore, not affect tissues and organs where its receptors do not occur. Using a "lock-and-key" analogy, only a specific, highly selective key will fit a given lock. The more selective a drug is, the more likely it will affect only the specific receptors for which it is meant. A less selective drug will more likely bind to receptors intended for other neurochemicals and cause more unintended effects, or side effects. As an example, dopamine 2 (D2) receptors are the location of interest in treating the positive symptoms

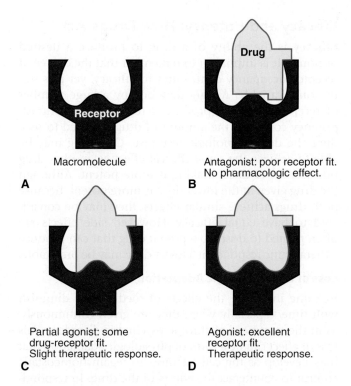

Figure 12.1. A–D: Agonist and antagonist drug–receptor interactions at receptor sites.

of schizophrenia. While haloperidol, an antipsychotic medication, does target these D2 receptors and reduces symptoms of schizophrenia, the drug will also interact (to varying degrees) with other receptors including H1 receptors, alpha 1 and 2 receptors, serotonin receptors, and other dopamine receptors. This lack of selectivity accounts for many side effects associated with this drug.

Affinity

The second property is that of **affinity**, which is the degree of attraction or strength of the bond between the drug and its receptor. Normally, these bonds are produced by relatively weak electrochemical attractions. Basic to the action of almost all CNS drugs within the body is their ability to bind to a receptor, produce a response, move off the receptor, and continue to repeat this binding/unbinding process until the drug is cleared from the body. There are some exceptions to this transient bond formation, such as is seen in a class of drugs that binds to an enzyme and is discussed in that section.

Intrinsic Activity

The final property of a drug's ability to interact with a given receptor is that of **intrinsic activity**, or the ability of the drug to produce a biologic response once it binds to a receptor. This is a measure of "how much response" a drug produces and ranges from maximal response (full agonist) to partial response (partial agonist) to no response (antagonist). Full agonists provide a maximal response, meaning that the biologic response from the receptor produced by the drug is the same as if it were

stimulated by naturally occurring endogenous molecules. Partial agonists, while only capable of producing a partial response, may also be used to "block" the complete response produced by endogenous molecules (or other drugs). Buprenorphine, an opioid agent, is a partial agonist and can be used to decrease symptoms (or prevent) of an opioid overdose. Drugs that act as agonists have all three properties: selectivity, affinity, and intrinsic activity. However, antagonists have only selectivity and affinity because they produce no biologic response by attaching to that receptor. In complex biologic systems, such as the brain, preventing an agonist from binding can yield multiple cellular and ultimately behavioural responses. An example of this is the antipsychotic class, all members of which are antagonists.

Ion Channels

Some drugs act directly on ion channels embedded in the nerve cell membrane. Examples include local anaesthetics that block the entry of sodium into the cell, preventing an action potential. The benzodiazepine drugs, frequently used in psychiatry as anticonvulsants and antianxiety and hypnotic drugs to help with sleep disturbances, are an example of drugs that affect a specific ion channel of the nerve cell membrane. The benzodiazepine molecule, such as diazepam (Valium), works by binding to a region of the gamma-aminobutyric acid (GABA) receptor–chloride channel complex. The binding site for these drugs is different from where GABA itself binds. When bound, these drugs increase the frequency and duration of chloride ion movement through GABA into the cell. This causes a decrease in the ability of that cell to conduct a nerve impulse. Thus, they are referred to as being indirect agonists or positive modulators of the $GABA_A$ channel.

Enzymes

Enzymes are complex proteins that catalyze specific biochemical reactions within cells and are the targets for some drugs used to treat mental disorders. For example, monoamine oxidase (MAO) is the enzyme required to break down most monoamine neurotransmitters, such as norepinephrine, serotonin, and dopamine, and can be inhibited by medications from a group of antidepressants called monoamine oxidase inhibitors (MAOIs). There are two types of MAO. MAO-A is more specific to norepinephrine and serotonin than it is for dopamine. This increase in available norepinephrine and serotonin is thought to initiate the cascade of cellular changes that ultimately relieve the symptoms of depression. MAO-B is more specific to dopamine and is used to treat Parkinson's disorder, a neurodegenerative disorder where dopamine neurons die off.

Instead of the on–off property in relation to drugs that bind to receptors, the older MAOIs form a strong covalent bond with the enzyme. This causes irreversible changes to the enzyme, and more enzymes will need to be produced in order for further breakdown of neurotransmitters to occur. This irreversibility may contribute to serious side effects and is a major reason these drugs are seldom used in contemporary practice. Although they have similar effects, some MAOIs (e.g., moclobemide) do not form covalent bonds and so are called reversible. In this case, the enzymes are not reversibly changed and are thus available to be used to break down neurotransmitters (such as serotonin and norepinephrine) during their unbound state. This flexibility significantly improves the drug safety profile for these novel MAOIs.

Carrier Proteins: Uptake Receptors

Neurotransmitters are small organic molecules that are released in response to a change in the polarity of the cell membrane (called an action potential), interact with receptors, and then are transported back into the neuronal cell by carrier proteins. These transporters have binding sites specific for the type of molecule to be transported. After a neurotransmitter, such as serotonin, has activated receptors in the synapse, its actions are terminated by these transporters that take serotonin back up into the presynaptic cell. Medications specific for this site may block or inhibit this transport and, therefore, increase the amount of the neurotransmitter in the synaptic space available for action on the receptors.

A primary action of most of the antidepressants is to increase the amount of neurotransmitters in the synapse by blocking their reuptake. Older antidepressants, like the tricyclic antidepressants (TCAs), block the reuptake of more than one neurotransmitter and have affinity for other receptors, which produces increased side effects. Some antidepressants, such as fluoxetine (Prozac) and sertraline (Zoloft), are more selective for serotonin, whereas reboxetine is more selective for norepinephrine. These medications are called selective serotonin reuptake inhibitors (SSRIs) and selective norepinephrine reuptake inhibitors (NSRIs), respectively. Newer antidepressants that are selective to both serotonin and norepinephrine are called SNRIs (e.g., venlafaxine [Effexor] and duloxetine [Cymbalta]). These more selective medications have reduced the number of side effects experienced by the patients. Figure 12.2 illustrates the reuptake blockade of serotonin by an SSRI.

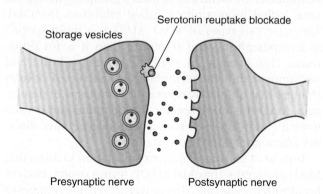

Figure 12.2. Reuptake blockade of a transporter for serotonin by an SSRI.

Efficacy and Potency: How Drugs Act

Efficacy is the ability of a drug to produce a desired response. It is important to remember that the degree of receptor occupancy contributes to efficacy, yet it is not the only variable. A drug may occupy a large number of receptors but not produce a response. In contrast, **potency** considers the amount of drug required to produce the desired biologic response. One drug may be able to achieve the same clinical effect as another drug but at a lower dose, making it more potent. Although the drug given at the lower dose is more potent, because both drugs achieve similar effects, they may be considered to have equal efficacy. However, side effects are often related to dose, so a potent drug that can produce a therapeutic response at a lower dose may be preferable.

Loss of Effect: Biologic Adaptation

In some instances, the effects of medications diminish with time, especially when they are given continuously, as in the treatment of chronic psychiatric disorders. This loss of effect can be a form of physiologic adaptation that may develop as the cell attempts to regain homeostatic control to counteract the effects of the drug. In responding to a prolonged drug exposure, an individual's body may increase (or decrease) the rate of receptor firing, the number of receptors on a cell's surface, or the amount of enzymes used to metabolize the drug. Cycling female hormones can also affect response to drugs. Progesterone and its metabolites bind to the same GABA receptor as do the benzodiazepines and can affect the efficacy of benzodiazepines at certain stages of the menstrual cycle. In this instance, drug effect may be dependent on menstrual phase. These are only a few reasons for decreased drug effectiveness (Box 12.1). **Tolerance** is a gradual decrease in the action of a drug at a given dose or concentration in the blood. This decrease may take days or weeks to develop and results in the loss of therapeutic effect of a drug. This loss of effect is often called *treatment refractoriness*.

Other forms of physiologic adaptation result in a gradual tolerance that may be helpful in the case of unpleasant side effects, such as drowsiness or nausea. For example, the SSRIs can cause nausea and gastrointestinal upset when first started, but these side effects are short-lived. With forewarning about these temporary

---

BOX 12.1 Mechanisms Causing Decrease in Medication Effects

- Change in receptor density or affinity
- Depletion of neurotransmitter stores
- Increased metabolism of the drug
- Physiologic adaptation
- Interaction with female hormones

side effects, patients are more likely to stay on the medication and not discontinue the drug regime on their own. This information is important for the nurse to communicate to patients experiencing such side effects so that they can be reassured that the effects will subside.

Target Symptoms and Side Effects

Psychiatric medications are indicated for specific symptoms, referred to as target symptoms. **Target symptoms** are those measurable specific symptoms expected to improve with medication use. The target symptoms for each class of medication are discussed more fully in later sections of this chapter. Because receptors for neurotransmitters such as serotonin are found in all regions of the brain and in the periphery, serotonin-related

drugs produce widespread effects in many body systems. For example, these drugs interact with receptors in the gastrointestinal tract and in facial motor nerves, causing gastrointestinal upset and bruxism (clenching and grinding of teeth). These unwanted effects of medications are called **side effects**.

Knowledge of a medication's affinity for receptors and subtypes of receptors may give some indication of the likelihood that specific target symptoms might improve and what side effects might be expected. Table 12.1 provides a brief summary of possible physiologic effects from drug actions on specific neurotransmitters. For example, antagonists with high affinity for acetylcholine receptors of the muscarinic subtype will be more likely to cause such side effects as dry mouth, blurred

Table 12.1 Pharmacodynamic Properties of Antidepressants		
Neurotransmitter/ Receptor Action	**Physiologic Effects**	**Examples of Drugs That Exhibit High Affinity**
Reuptake Inhibition Blockade		
Norepinephrine reuptake inhibition	Antidepressant action Potentiation of pressor effects of norepinephrine Side effects: tachycardia, tremors, insomnia, erectile and ejaculation dysfunction	desipramine reboxetine
Serotonin reuptake inhibition	Antidepressant action Antiobsessional effect Antianxiety effect Side effects: gastrointestinal distress, nausea, headache, nervousness, motor restlessness, and sexual side effects, including anorgasmia	fluoxetine paroxetine
Receptor Mediated		
Histamine (H_1) receptor antagonism	Side effects: sedation, drowsiness, hypotension, and weight gain	quetiapine imipramine clozapine olanzapine
Muscarinic Acetylcholine receptor antagonism	Side effects: anticholinergic (dry mouth, blurred vision, constipation, urinary hesitancy and retention, memory dysfunction) and sinus tachycardia	imipramine amitriptyline thioridazine clozapine
Norepinephrine receptor (α_1 receptor) antagonism	Potentiation of antihypertensive effect of prazosin and terazosin Side effects: postural hypotension, dizziness, reflex tachycardia, sedation	amitriptyline clomipramine clozapine amitriptyline
Norepinephrine receptor (α_2 receptor) antagonism	Increased sexual desire (yohimbine) Interactions with antihypertensive medications, blockade of the antihypertensive effects of clonidine Side effect: priapism	clomipramine clozapine trazodone yohimbine
Norepinephrine receptor (β_1 receptor) antagonism	Antihypertensive action (propranolol) Side effects: orthostatic hypotension, sedation, depression, sexual dysfunction (including impotence and decreased ejaculation)	propranolol
Serotonin receptor (5-HT_{1a}) agonist	Antidepressant action Antianxiety effect Possible control of aggression	trazodone risperidone ziprasidone
Serotonin receptor (5-HT_2) antagonism	Antipsychotic action Some antimigraine effect Decreased rhinitis Side effects: hypotension, ejaculatory problems, weight gain, metabolic disorders	risperidone clozapine olanzapine ziprasidone haloperidol
Dopamine receptor (D_2) antagonism	Antipsychotic action Side effects: extrapyramidal symptoms, such as tremor, rigidity (especially acute dystonia and parkinsonism); endocrine changes, including elevated prolactin levels	ziprasidone

vision, constipation, urinary hesitancy or retention, and nasal congestion. This information should serve only as a guide in predicting side effects because of considerable interindividual variability in drug responses, and not all underlying mechanisms have been elucidated. The nurse should use this information to focus assessment on these areas. If the symptoms are mild, simple nursing interventions suggested in Table 12.2 should be implemented. If symptoms persist or are severe, the prescriber should be notified immediately. Patients need to be encouraged to report side effects and to be aware that suggestions and solutions may be available to address the side effects. For example, changing from one drug to another within the same class of psychotropics can often decrease unwanted side effects.

Drug Toxicity

All drugs have the capacity to be harmful as well as helpful. **Toxicity** generally refers to the point at which concentrations of the drug in the body have gone beyond

Table 12.2 Managing Common Side Effects of Psychiatric Medications

Side Effect or Discomfort	Intervention
Blurred vision	Reassurance (generally subsides in 2–6 weeks)
Dry eyes	Warn ophthalmologist; no eye examination for new glasses for at least 3 weeks after a stable dose
	Artificial tears may be required; an increased use of wetting solutions for those wearing contact lenses
Dry mouth and lips	Frequent rinsing of the mouth, good oral hygiene, sucking sugarless candies, lozenges, lip balm, lemon juice, and glycerin mouth swabs
Constipation	High-fibre diet; encourage bran, fresh fruits, and vegetables
	Metamucil (must consume at least 16 oz of fluid with dose)
	Exercise, increase fluids
	Mild laxative
Urinary hesitancy or retention	Monitor frequently for difficulty with urination, changes in starting or stopping stream
	Notify prescriber if difficulty develops
	A cholinergic agonist, such as bethanechol, may be required
Nasal congestion	Nose drops, moisturizer
Sinus tachycardia	Assess for infection
	Monitor pulse for rate and irregularities
	Withhold medication and notify prescriber if resting rate exceeds 100 bpm
Decreased libido and ejaculatory inhibition	Consider change to another drug in same class or change class of drug
Postural hypotension	Frequent monitoring of lying-to-standing blood pressure during dosage adjustment period, immediate changes and accommodation, measure pulse in both positions
	Advise the patient to get up slowly, sit for at least 1 minute before standing (dangling legs over side of bed), and stand for 1 minute before walking or until light-headedness subsides
	Increase hydration, and avoid caffeine
	Notify prescriber if symptoms persist or significant blood pressure changes are present
Photosensitivity	Protective clothing
	Dark glasses
Dermatitis	Use of sun block; remember to cover *all* exposed areas
	Stop medication usage
	Consider medication change, may require a systemic antihistamine
	Initiate comfort measures to decrease itching
Impaired psychomotor functions	Advise the patient to avoid dangerous tasks, such as driving
	Avoid alcohol, which increases this impairment
Drowsiness or sedation	Encourage activity during the day to increase accommodation
	Avoid tasks that require mental alertness, such as driving
	May need to adjust dosing schedule or, if possible, give single daily dose at bedtime
	May need a cholinergic medication if sedation is the problem
	Avoid driving or operating potentially dangerous equipment
	May need change to less-sedating medication
	Provide quiet and decreased stimulation when sedation is the desired effect
Weight gain	Exercise and diet teaching; regular weighing
	Caloric control and regular monitoring of blood glucose levels
Oedema	Check fluid retention
	Reassurance
	May need a diuretic
Irregular menstruation	Reassurance (reversible)
Amenorrhea	May need to change class of drug
	Reassurance and counselling (does not indicate lack of ovulation)
	Instruct the patient to continue birth control measures
Vaginal dryness	Instruct in use of lubricants

the safe range and may become harmful or poisonous to the body. However, what is considered harmful? Side effects can be harmful but not toxic, and individuals vary widely in their responses to medications. **Therapeutic index**, a concept often used to discuss the toxicity of a drug, is a ratio between median toxic dose and median effective dose (the dose at which 50% of the population will experience drug toxicity and drug effectiveness, respectively). A high therapeutic index means that there is a large range between the dose at which the drug begins to take effect and a dose that would be toxic to the body. Drugs with a low therapeutic index have a narrow range and are often carefully monitored through blood levels. This concept has some limitations. The therapeutic index of a medication also may be greatly changed by the coadministration of other medications or drugs. For example, alcohol consumed with most CNS depressant drugs will have added depressant effects, greatly increasing the likelihood of toxicity or death.

Despite the limitations of the therapeutic index, it is a helpful guide for nurses, particularly when working with potentially suicidal individuals. Nurses must be aware of the potential for overdose and closely monitor the availability of drugs for these patients. In some cases, prescriptions may have to be dispensed daily or weekly until a suicidal crisis has passed to ensure that patients do not have access to lethal doses of drugs. The choice of drug can also help address toxicity. For example, the TCAs can be lethal in overdose, whereas SSRIs are not; SSRIs are thus the safer choice for higher-risk patients and adolescents.

PHARMACOKINETICS: HOW DRUGS MOVE THROUGH THE BODY

The field of pharmacokinetics (PK) describes how a drug moves throughout the body to get to its target receptors and then is eliminated. The four processes of PK are Absorption, Distribution, Metabolism, and Excretion (ADME). Overall, the goal in PK is to describe and predict the time course of drug concentrations throughout the body and factors that may interfere with these processes. Together with the principles of pharmacodynamics, this information can be helpful to the psychiatric nurse in ways such as facilitating or inhibiting drug effects and predicting behavioural response.

Absorption and Routes of Administration

Absorption

The first phase of PK is **absorption**, defined as the movement of the drug from the site of administration into the plasma. It is important to consider the impact of routes by which a drug is administered on the process of absorption. The primary routes available include oral (both tablet and liquid), sublingual, intramuscular (IM) (short- and long-acting agents), and intravenous (used

for rapid treatment of adverse reactions and rarely for the treatment of the primary psychiatric disorder). The nurse needs to know about the advantages and disadvantages of each route and the subsequent effects on absorption (Table 12.3).

Drugs taken orally are usually the most convenient for the patient; however, this route is also the most variable because absorption can be slowed or enhanced by a number of factors. Taking certain drugs orally with food or antacids may slow the rate of absorption or change the amount of the drug absorbed. For example, the β-receptor antagonist propranolol exhibits increased blood levels when taken with food. Antacids containing aluminum salts decrease the absorption of most antipsychotic drugs; thus, antacids must be given at least 1 hour before administration or 2 hours after.

Oral preparations absorbed from the gastrointestinal tract into the bloodstream first go to the liver through the portal vein. There, they may be metabolized in such a way that most of the drug is inactivated before it reaches the rest of the body—this is called **first-pass metabolism**. The consequence of first-pass metabolism is that the fraction of the drug reaching systemic circulation is reduced, sometimes substantially. First-pass metabolism explains why the dose of propranolol given intravenously is so much less than the oral dose. **Bioavailability** describes the amount of the drug that actually reaches systemic circulation. The route by which a drug is administered significantly affects bioavailability. With some oral drugs, the amount of drug entering the bloodstream is decreased by first-pass metabolism and bioavailability is lower.

Other factors affecting absorption should also be considered when administering drugs. Liver disease and dysfunction can decrease first-pass metabolism and result in increased drug levels and thus an increased risk for side effects. Gastric motility also affects how the drug is absorbed. Increasing age, many disease states, and concurrent medications can reduce gastrointestinal (GI) motility and slow absorption. Other factors, such as blood flow in the GI system, drug formulation, and chemical factors, may also interfere with absorption. Nurses must be aware of a patient's physical condition and use of medications or other substances that can interfere with drug absorption.

In full strength, many liquid preparations, especially antipsychotics, irritate the mucosal lining of the mouth, oesophagus, and stomach and must be adequately diluted. Nurses must be careful when diluting liquid medications because some liquid concentrate preparations are incompatible with certain juices or other liquids. If a drug is mixed with an incompatible liquid, a white or grainy precipitant usually forms, indicating that some of the drug has bound to the liquid and inactivated. Thus, the patient actually receives a lower dose of the medication than intended. Therefore, some medications should be given at least an hour apart.

Table 12.3   Selected Forms and Routes of Psychiatric Medications

Preparation and Route	Examples	Advantages	Disadvantages
Oral tablet	Basic preparation for most psycho-pharmacologic agents, including antidepressants, antipsychotics, mood stabilizers, anxiolytics, etc.	Convenience	Variable rate and extent of absorption, depending on the drug May be affected by the contents of the intestines May show first-pass metabolism effects May not be easily swallowed by some individuals
Oral liquid	Also known as concentrates Many antipsychotics, such as halo-peridol, chlorpromazine, thiorida-zine, risperidone The antidepressant fluoxetine Antihistamines, such as diphenhydramine Mood stabilizers, such as lithium citrate	Ease of incremental dosing Easily swallowed In some cases, more quickly absorbed	More difficult to measure accurately Depending on drug: • Possible interactions with other liquids, such as juice, forming precipitants • Possible irritation to mucosal lining of the mouth if not properly diluted
Rapid-dissolving tablet	Atypical antipsychotics, such as olanzapine and risperidone Handy for people who have trouble swallowing or for patients who let medication linger in the cheek for later expectoration Can be taken when water or other liquid is unavailable	Dissolves almost instanta-neously in the mouth	The patient needs to remember to have completely dry hands and to place tablet in the mouth immediately Tablet should not linger in the hand
Sublingual	Lorazepam	Rapid action, no first-pass metabolism	Increased risk for tolerance and psychological dependence
Intramuscular	Some antipsychotics, such as haloperidol, chlorpromazine, and risperidone Anxiolytics, such as lorazepam Anticholinergics, such as diphenhydr-amine and benztropine mesylate No antidepressants No mood stabilizers	More rapid acting than oral preparations No first-pass metabolism	Injection-site pain and irritation Some medications may have erratic absorption if heavy muscle tissue at the site of injection is not in use High-potency antipsychotics in this form may be more prone to adverse reactions, such as NMS
IM depot (or long acting)	Haloperidol decanoate, fluphen-azine decanoate, paliperidone palmitate	May be more convenient for some individuals who have difficulty following medication regimens	Significant pain at injection site
Intravenous	Anticholinergics, such as diphenhydr-amine, benztropine mesylate Diazepam used as an anticonvulsant	Rapid and complete availability to systemic circulation	Inflammation of tissue surrounding site Often inconvenient for the patient and uncomfortable Continuous dosage requires use of a constant-rate IV infusion

With new technologies come novel administration routes and drug forms, one of which is the rapid-dissolving oral pill. Manufacturers have different procedures for developing rapid-dissolving drugs, and these are patented with unique names. Common forms include the DuraSolv and Quick Tab technologies. Many drugs are available in rapid-dissolving form, including the atypical antipsychotic olanzapine (Zyprexa, Zydis), risperidone (Risperdal M-Tab), and mirtazapine (Remeron SolTab). Nurses need to be aware of the special administration and patient-teaching requirements of the rapid-dissolving drug forms. To take an orally disintegrating tablet, the nurse or patient should use dry hands to peel back the foil packaging, immediately take out the tablet, and place it into the mouth. The tablet will quickly dissolve and can be swallowed with saliva. No water is needed to swallow disintegrating tablets. This is advantageous when a patient cannot swallow well or is unwilling to swallow pills, or when water is not readily available.

Distribution

Even after a drug enters the bloodstream, several factors affect how it is distributed in the body. Distribution of a drug reflects how easy it is for a drug to pass out of the systemic circulation and move into other types of tissues, such as brain, abdominal organs, skin, or bone, where target receptors are found. Factors that affect medication distribution to specific tissues in the body include the

Table 12.4   Factors Affecting Distribution of a Drug

Factor	Effect on Drug Distribution
Size of the organ	Larger organs require more drug to reach a concentration level equivalent to other organs and tissues.
Blood flow to the organ	The most important contributor to distribution, the major organs have the highest blood flow (heart, lung, liver, brain, kidney) and thus have the greatest drug exposure.
Ionic characteristics	Small drugs with no molecular charge move easily across cell membranes by passive transfer rather than needing active transport and thus will be widely distributed.
Plasma protein binding	If a drug binds well to plasma proteins, particularly to albumin, it will stay in the body longer.
Anatomic barriers	Both the gastrointestinal tract and the brain are surrounded by layers of cells that control the passage or uptake of substances. Lipid-soluble substances are usually readily absorbed and pass the blood–brain barrier.

amount of blood flow or perfusion within the tissue; how lipophilic ("fat-loving") the drug is; plasma protein binding; and anatomic barriers, such as the blood–brain barrier, that the drug must cross. Highly perfused organs like the heart, liver, kidney, and brain are quickly and extensively exposed to any drug. Almost all psychotropic drugs are lipophilic, making it easier for the drug to passively cross epithelial cell membranes that line blood vessels and to cross the blood–brain barrier. Table 12.4 provides a summary of how some significant factors affect distribution. Two of these factors, ionic characteristics and protein binding, warrant additional discussion with regard to how they relate to psychiatric medications.

Ionic Characteristics of Drugs

Drugs in the bloodstream can be charged molecules (in the form of positive or negative ions) or can be uncharged. There are many charged components within cell membranes. Thus, drugs that have an electrical charge cannot passively cross through a cell membrane; instead, they must be transported by carrier proteins. Uncharged drugs (also called lipophilic or "fat-loving" drugs) can move easily across cell membranes. Most psychiatric drugs are very lipophilic and can move into major organ systems, as well as cross the blood–brain barrier. However, this characteristic means that psychopharmacologic agents can also cross the placenta. It also means that these agents can be taken into fat stores. Drugs stored in fatty tissue are only slowly released back into the systemic circulation for eventual elimination. This is why a lipophilic drug can be detected long after discontinuation in older women and overweight individuals. This effect may also account for unexpected drug–drug interactions when substitute drugs regimes are initiated quickly.

Protein Binding

Many drugs bind to large carrier proteins in the bloodstream, referred to as plasma protein binding. The degree to which a drug is bound to these plasma proteins affects the drug's ability to interact with receptors. Only unbound or "free" drugs can move across membranes to their target receptors. High protein binding prolongs the drug's duration of action, allowing for less frequent dosing. Many of the psychiatric drugs are more than 90% protein bound. Chronic disease and normal aging can decrease the amounts of plasma proteins, shifting the ratio of bound drug to free drug. For highly bound drugs like the classic antipsychotics, a decrease of only 10% of bound drug (e.g., from 90% to 80%) would translate into a doubling of free drug and significantly increase the risk for side effects.

Metabolism

The duration of drug action also depends on the body's ability to change or alter a drug chemically. **Metabolism**, also called biotransformation, is the process by which the drug is altered, usually by adding to the drug molecule or breaking the drug molecule into smaller pieces, both processes making the molecule or the pieces more polar. Through the processes of metabolism, lipid-soluble drugs become more polar or hydrophilic so that they may be excreted more readily.

There are two types of metabolic transformation that occur in drug metabolism: phase 1 reactions (mostly using CYP enzymes) produce metabolites, and phase 2 reactions (mostly through the addition of chemical side chains) produce conjugates. In phase 1 metabolism, active, inactive, or toxic metabolites are produced. The PK and pharmacodynamics of each metabolite may either be similar or very different from their parent compound. For instance, the antidepressant imipramine is metabolized to a pharmacologically active substance, desipramine, which also has antidepressant effects (desipramine is also available on its own as an antidepressant). Prozac (fluoxetine), an SSRI antidepressant, is metabolized in the liver and forms an active metabolite, norfluoxetine, which has a very long half-life. This is important when changing from fluoxetine to another antidepressant to avoid potential side effects from having two antidepressants still acting in the body. Metabolism may also change an inactive drug (called a prodrug) to an active one or an active drug to a toxic metabolite. Codeine is an example of a prodrug that must be metabolized before having analgesic properties. Acetaminophen is a safe drug used in normal doses but provides a classic example of a toxic drug metabolite. Acetaminophen is metabolized by CYP enzymes and produces a toxic metabolite. This toxic metabolite is then conjugated by glutathione (phase 2 reaction) to a nontoxic conjugate and eliminated through bile or urine. With an overdose, stores of glutathione are depleted; the levels of the toxic metabolite rise and cause liver cell death. Death can occur from acute liver failure.

The cytochrome P-450 superfamily of metabolic enzymes (or CYP450s) is responsible for most drug metabolism. The classification of the CYP450 superfamily uses a combination of numbers and letters to denote families, subfamilies, and individual enzymes. Most psychiatric drugs are metabolized by members of the 1A, 2D, and 3A subfamilies of CYP450 enzymes. The 3A family is the most abundant, constituting more than 60% of the liver enzyme weight. The metabolizing activity of some of the CYP450 enzymes can be altered by drugs and environmental chemicals. Some drugs, like phenobarbital, induce CYP450 activity. Drugs that induce enzyme activity are known as *CYP enzyme inducers*. This effect increases drug metabolism and thus decreases drug levels of any drug taken with phenobarbital. If the drug level fall below a therapeutic concentration, then the drug may be less effective. Other common substances, such as tobacco smoke, alcohol, and coal tar in charcoal-broiled foods, can induce specific CYP450 enzymes. Alternately, drugs can inhibit CYP450 activity (these are *CYP enzyme inhibitors*) and thus increase drug levels, potentially pushing drug concentrations into toxic ranges. Some of the SSRIs are potent inhibitors of CYP2D6. Grapefruit juice is an inhibitor of CYP3A enzymes. Not all SSRIs are equal in their potency to inhibit CYP2D6. Paroxetine (Paxil) is the most potent, producing more than 90% inhibition of this enzyme subfamily, whereas sertraline exhibits mild effects, with only 20% to 50% inhibition (Dalfen & Stewart, 2001). The newer SSRI citalopram has minimal inhibiting properties. CYP450 enzymes contribute to the enormous individual differences in the overall efficacy and the side effect profiles (Clarke, Karalliedde, Collignon, & Abeyratne, 2016).

The differences in CYP enzyme activity are often caused by genetic variations (Eap, 2016). DNA variants in the CYP450 system and the enzymes encoded by these genes have been investigated for several CYP enzymes in relation to specific ethnic and racial groups. For example, about 3% of Caucasians and more than 20% of Japanese are poor metabolizers of CYP2C19. About 2% of Chinese, but up to 10% of Caucasians, are poor metabolizers of CYP2D6 (Baker, Urichuk, & Coutts, 1998). The science of **pharmacogenomics** blends pharmacology with genetic knowledge and is concerned with understanding and determining an individual's specific CYP450 makeup and then individualizing medications to match the person's CYP450 profile. Scientists are beginning to connect DNA variants with individual responses to medical treatments, identify particular subgroups of patients, and develop drugs customized for those populations (Crettol, De Leon, Hiemke, & Eap, 2014).

Nurses should remain alert to the possibilities of drug–drug interactions when patients are receiving more than one medication, especially in older adults. Pharmacology texts and dedicated websites are helpful reference sources. In addition, if an individual receiving a medication experiences an unusual reaction or suddenly loses effect from a medication that had previously been working, the nurse should carefully assess other substances that the person has recently consumed, including prescription medications, nonprescription remedies, dietary supplements or changes, and substances of abuse (including alcohol and tobacco). The widespread use of herbal products has introduced another potential source of drug–drug interaction. A good example of this is St. John's wort, a botanical product used extensively in Europe for mild depression and emerging as a potential therapy for pain management (Galeotti, 2017). Drug–drug interactions have been reported for St. John's wort and alprazolam, amitriptyline, and cyclosporine (Izzo, Hoon-Kim, Radhakrishnan, & Williamson, 2016). There are also drug–endogenous product interactions. The most notable examples are estrogens and progesterone. Through a pharmacodynamic mechanism, progesterone can decrease the effectiveness of the benzodiazepines, but it can also affect drug concentrations as it is an inhibitor of CYP3A enzymes. Estrogens inhibit CYP1A2. During periods of high hormone levels (ovulation, luteal phase of the menstrual cycle, and pregnancy), these interactions may become clinically significant for women.

Excretion

Excretion refers to the elimination of drugs from the body either unchanged or as metabolites. Clearance refers to the total volume of blood, serum, or plasma from which a drug is completely removed from the bloodstream per unit of time. The driving force that determines the time required to eliminate a drug is usually the concentration of drug and the clearance rate. The elimination **half-life** ($t_{1/2}$) refers to the time required for plasma concentrations of the drug to be reduced by 50%. For example, 50% of a drug is cleared in one $t_{1/2}$. In the next $t_{1/2}$, 50% of the remaining concentration would be eliminated (leaving 25% of the original concentration), then after the third $t_{1/2}$, there would be 12.5% remaining. Thus, it usually takes four to seven half-lives for a drug to be completely eliminated from the body. Notable exceptions to this decrease by percent concentration include alcohol and acetylsalicylic acid, in which the specific enzymes responsible for metabolism limit the speed at which elimination can occur.

For this reason, elimination is at a set rate irrespective of concentration, which is why in the case of alcohol, it can be calculated how many drinks it takes per hour to reach a blood alcohol level of 0.5 (a common legal level indicative of impairment) and the time required to eliminate all alcohol from the system. In the case of acetylsalicylic acid overdose, increasing the renal clearance through changes in pH or increasing fluid volume will not affect the time required for elimination because it is determined by enzyme activity, not blood flow.

As indicated previously, the goal of most metabolic processes is to decrease the lipophilic nature of drugs by increasing their ionic characteristics. Drugs that are in a more ionic form in the bloodstream can be easily removed by the kidney and excreted through urine. However, many psychiatric medications are large molecules and thus can also be removed through bile and eliminated in faeces. Lithium, a mood stabilizer, is a notable exception, being eliminated exclusively through the kidney. Any impairment in renal function or renal disease, or even temporary dehydration (e.g., from flu symptoms or even strenuous exercise), may lead to severe toxic symptoms (Ott, Stegmayr, Salander Renberg, & Werneke, 2016). Biliary elimination can lead to "enteroportal recirculation," a process by which active drug or metabolites that were excreted in bile into the small intestine are reabsorbed into the portal circulation, go through the liver again, and end up back into the systemic circulation. A well-known example of this is oral contraceptives. Oral antibiotics change the intestinal environment, can decrease recirculation, and thus affect the contraceptive efficacy. This same process of reabsorption may also contribute to the plasma concentration of psychiatric drugs over time.

Dosing refers to the administration of medication over time so that a consistent drug concentration may be achieved or maintained without reaching toxic levels. In general, it is necessary to give a drug at intervals no greater than the half-life of the medication to avoid excessive fluctuation of concentration in the plasma between doses. With repeated dosing, a certain amount of the drug is accumulated in the body. This accumulation will reach a point where the quantity of drug entering the body is equal to that which is leaving the body. This is called *steady-state plasma concentration* or simply *steady state*. The rate of accumulation is determined by the half-life of the drug. Drugs generally reach steady state in four to five times the elimination half-life. However, because elimination or excretion rates may vary significantly, fluctuations may still occur, and dose schedules may need to be individualized.

The nurse should remember that although these principles can support best practice, they are not substitutes for ongoing individual assessment of indicators of treatment response or unwanted effects and recording individual perceptions about drug effects.

Individual Variations in Drug Effects

Many factors affect drug absorption, distribution, metabolism, and excretion. These factors may vary among individuals, depending on their age, genetics, and ethnicity. Nurses must be aware of and consider these individual variations in the effects of medications.

Age

PK is influenced by life cycle stages. For example, gastric absorption changes with age. Gastric pH in a newborn is 6 to 8 and decreases to 1 to 3 over the first 24 hours (the pH remains elevated in a premature infant) (Nicolas, Bouzom, Chanteux, & Ungell, 2017). This significantly affects drug absorption. Changes in drug absorption are also seen in older adults because of increased gastric pH, decreased gastric emptying, slowed gastric motility, and reduced splanchnic circulation. Normally, these changes do not significantly impair the oral absorption of a medication, but addition of common conditions, such as diarrhoea, may significantly alter and reduce absorption.

Renal function is also altered in both very young and older adult patients. Infants who are exposed in utero to medications that are excreted through the kidneys may experience toxic reactions to these medications because renal function in the newborn is only about 20% of that of an adult. In less than a week, renal function develops to adult levels, but in premature infants, the process may take longer. Renal function also declines with age. Creatinine clearance in a young adult is normally 100 to 120 mL per minute, but after the age of 40, this rate declines by about 10% per decade. Medical illnesses, such as diabetes and hypertension, may further the loss of renal function. When creatinine clearance falls below 30 to 60 mL per minute, the excretion of drugs by the kidneys is significantly impaired and potentially toxic levels may accumulate.

Metabolism changes across the lifespan, especially in infancy and childhood. At birth, many of the liver enzymes are not fully functional, whereas in early childhood, there is evidence of increased activity compared with adulthood. For example, CYP1A2 activity is reduced in the first 4 months but increased between ages 1 and 2 years; CYP2D6 activity is reduced until ages 3 to 5 years, and CYP3A4 is reduced in the 1st month of life but increased between ages 1 and 4 (Mahmood, 2016). Thus, paediatric pharmacotherapeutics cannot simply be based on relative dosing by weight. With age, blood flow to the liver and the mass of liver tissue both decrease. The activities of hepatic enzymes also slow with age. As a result, the ability of the liver to metabolize medications may show as much as a fourfold decrease between the ages of 20 and 70. Again, the use of multiple drugs in older adults adds to metabolic burden, potentially increasing drug levels of each individual drug.

Most psychiatric medications are bound to proteins. Albumin is one of the primary circulating proteins to which drugs bind. The production of albumin by the liver is lower in neonates, peaks in early childhood, and generally declines with age. In addition, a number of medical conditions change the ability of medications to bind to albumin. Malnutrition, cancer, and liver disease decrease the production of albumin, which translates to more unbound drug available to interact with target receptors and an increased risk for adverse or toxic effects.

Ethnicity and Genetic Makeup

It is clear that genetics plays a significant role in the metabolism of medications. Studies of identical and nonidentical twins show that much of the individual variability in elimination half-life of a given drug is genetically determined. Individuals of Asian descent have decreased activities of enzymes involved in the second stage of ethanol metabolism compared with Caucasians and thus produce higher concentrations of acetaldehyde, resulting in such adverse symptoms as flushing, palpitations, and headache. Asian research subjects have been found to be more susceptible to the effects of drugs such as mephenytoin than are Caucasian individuals, whereas individuals of African descent were less sensitive (Klotz, 2007). Several case reports indicate that Asians require one half to one third the dose of antipsychotic medications required by Caucasians and that they may be more sensitive to side effects because of higher blood levels (Zhou, 2003). Lower doses of antidepressant medications are also often required for individuals of Asian descent. Although many of these variations appear to be related to the cytochrome P450 genetic differences discussed earlier, more research is needed to understand fully the underlying mechanisms and to identify groups that may require different approaches to medication treatment. This work is underway.

■ PHASES OF DRUG TREATMENT

The nurse is involved in all the phases of medication treatment. Considerations in terms of assessment, treatment issues such as **adherence** (keeping with the therapeutic regimen), prevalence and severity of side effects, and expected time lines for symptom relief vary across the phases of treatment, but all involve potential nursing actions. These phases include initiation, stabilization, maintenance, and discontinuation of the medication. Nurses must be concerned with treatment phases as a guide for what may be expected as they administer medications and monitor individuals receiving medications across each of these phases. The following subsections discuss some of the knowledge required and the assessments and interventions to be performed by the nurse within each phase.

Initiation Phase

Before beginning to take medications, patients must undergo several assessments.

- A psychiatric evaluation, including past health history and previous medication treatment response, will clarify diagnosis and determine target symptoms for medication use.
- An open discussion regarding adherence issues, such as attitudes toward drug treatments, patient-specific goals for the drug therapy, any lifestyle issues that affect the structuring of a drug regimen (e.g., shift work, type of occupation and current job responsibilities, reproductive issues), and any health insurance issues related to prescription benefits (ability to afford the drug) will help to identify barriers to the patient's willingness and ability to manage the medication regimen.
- Physical examination and indicated laboratory tests, often including baseline tests such as complete blood count (CBC), liver and kidney function tests, electrolyte levels, urinalysis, and possibly thyroid function tests and electrocardiogram (ECG). This may be done to exclude physical health issues presenting as psychiatric concerns. These tests and other assessments (such as tools to measure depression) may be used to track progress of treatment and evaluate for potential drug complications.
- Any other current medications, including over-the-counter medications, herbal remedies and mixtures from health food stores, or naturopathic or homoeopathic visitations, and alcohol, tobacco, marihuana, and illicit drug use should be identified to prevent harmful drug interactions.

Nurses should perform their own premedication evaluations, including baseline physical assessments that focus on preexisting symptoms, such as gastrointestinal distress, sexual function/libido, or restrictions in range of motion that may later be confused with side effects. Comparing future symptoms to patients' baseline status may be useful in detecting the improvement or worsening of symptoms and potentially detect drug side effects (e.g. extrapyramidal symptoms). An assessment of cognitive functioning will assist the nurse in assessing whether memory aids or other supports are necessary to assist the individual in safely taking medications. Information from the psychosocial and lifestyle assessment should be reviewed in consultation with the prescriber and other members of the interprofessional team to develop a plan that is acceptable to the patient and will improve functioning, minimize side effects, and improve quality of life.

In all situations, recommendations and treatment alternatives should be developed and reviewed with input from the individual seeking treatment. Doing so will allow the patient to ask questions and receive complete information about drug effects and the most common side effects, thus allowing for fully informed consent, improved therapeutic relationships, and possibly therapeutic outcomes. Patients are often overwhelmed during the initial phases of treatment and may have symptoms that make it difficult for them to participate fully in treatment planning. Information is often forgotten or may need to be repeated and provided in written form for ongoing reference. Nurses must keep their detailed drug knowledge current to be able to answer questions and provide ongoing education.

When use of the medication is initiated, nurses should treat the first dose as if it were a "test" dose. They should observe the patient closely for sensitivity to the medication, such as changes in blood pressure, pulse, or temperature; changes in mental status; allergic reactions; dizziness; ataxia; or gastric distress. Other common side effects that may occur with even one dose of medication should also be closely monitored. A protocol for reporting side effects and determining which ones should trigger immediate urgent follow-up should be in place. In Canada, health professionals may report adverse drug reactions to Health Canada's MedEffect program online at www.healthcanada.gc.ca/medeffect

Stabilization Phase

During stabilization, the medication dosage is often adjusted to achieve the maximum amount of improvement with a minimum number of side effects. This process is sometimes referred to as *titration*. Nurses must continue to assess target symptoms, looking for change or improvement and side effects. If medications are being increased rapidly, such as in a hospital setting, nurses must closely monitor temperature, blood pressure, pulse, mental status, common side effects, and unusual adverse reactions.

On an outpatient basis, nurses must provide both verbal and written materials to individuals who are receiving the medication as to the expected outcome and potential side effects. This educational support should include factors that may influence the effectiveness of the medication, such as whether to take the medication with food, common interventions that may minimize side effects if they develop, and what side effects require immediate attention. Again, a plan is needed to clearly identify what to do if adverse reactions develop and what adverse reactions should prompt immediate attention. The plan should include emergency telephone numbers or available emergency treatment and should be reviewed frequently.

Therapeutic drug monitoring is important in this phase of treatment for drugs with a narrow therapeutic index, such as lithium, valproate, and carbamazepine. Nurses must be aware of when and how these levels are to be determined and assist patients in learning these procedures. Plasma levels of other psychiatric medications can be evaluated, for example, to rule them out as a potential source of treatment nonresponse related to increased metabolism.

Unfortunately, the first medication chosen often does not adequately improve the patient's target symptoms. This can be very discouraging, particularly in a population in which powerlessness and hopelessness are inherent in the disorder. This possibility must be discussed before initiating antidepressant drug therapy. Most of the time, a substitute drug from the same class or a drug from a new class will be given. Medications may also be changed when adverse reactions or seriously uncomfortable side effects occur or these effects substantially interfere with the individual's quality of life. Nurses should be familiar with the PK of both drugs to be able to monitor side effects and possible drug–drug interactions during this transition period.

At times, an individual may show only partial improvement from a medication, and the prescriber may try an augmentation strategy. *Augmentation* refers to the addition of another medication to enhance or potentiate the effects of the first medication. For example, a prescriber may add a mood stabilizer, such as lithium, to an antidepressant to improve the overall efficacy of the antidepressant. These strategies are often used in so-called treatment-resistant situations. *Treatment resistance* has various definitions, but most often, it means that after several medication trials, the individual has gained, at best, only partial improvement. Treatment-resistant symptoms often require multiple medications. Multiple medications may affect different physiologic processes and, in combination, provide overall synergistic or additive pharmacologic effects. Nurses must be familiar with the potential effects, side effects, drug interactions, and rationale for this type of complex treatment regimen.

Maintenance Phase

Once the individual's target symptoms have improved, medications may be continued to prevent relapse or reoccurrence. *Relapse* usually refers to reemerging symptoms in response to premature discontinuation of treatment, whereas *reoccurrence* refers to an entirely new episode that occurs over time after full remission was achieved. Higher risk for relapse in depression is associated with individuals who are older, have chronic episodes, have severe symptoms or psychotic symptoms, or have three or more previous or more frequent episodes. Other reasons for reemerging symptoms, despite continued use of medication, include the loss of drug efficacy, comorbid medical illness, psychosocial stressors, and concurrent use of prescription or nonprescription medications. Whatever the reason, patients must be educated about their target symptoms and have a plan of action if the symptoms return. The nurse has a central role in assisting individuals to monitor their own symptoms, manage psychosocial stressors, and avoid other factors that may cause the exacerbation of symptoms that were previously under control.

Some side effects or adverse reactions emerge only after the individual has been receiving the medication for an extended period. Specific examples are discussed in later sections of this chapter.

Discontinuation Phase

Many psychiatric medications require a tapered discontinuation. Tapering involves slowly reducing dosage while monitoring closely for reemergence of key symptoms, such as a drop in mood, increased anxiety, sleep disturbance, thought disorder, or decreased level of self-care. Some psychiatric disorders, such as mild depression or adjustment disorder, may respond to several months of treatment and not reoccur. Other disorders, such as bipolar disorder, chronic major depressive disorder, and schizophrenia, usually require continued medication treatment for extended periods of time and in fact may never be discontinued. A withdrawal syndrome, affecting up to 25% of individuals after abrupt cessation of the SSRIs, has been described and includes such symptoms as dizziness, restlessness, increased anxiety and mood lability, GI upset, and fatigue (Cosci, 2016). The restoration of the drug therapy relieves the symptoms within 24 hours. Untreated, the symptoms can last 1 to 3 weeks. Withdrawal effects and rebound effects (increased anxiety and/or sleep disturbance) have also been described for abrupt discontinuation of benzodiazepines.

Nurses must be aware of the potential for these symptoms, monitor them closely, and implement measures to minimize their effects. They should support individuals throughout this process, whether they can successfully stop taking the medication or must continue the treatment. Even if patients can successfully discontinue use of the medication without a return of symptoms, nurses may help implement preventive measures to avoid the reoccurrence of the psychiatric disorder. In the roles of advocate, patient educator, and provider of interpersonal support, nurses often have a central role in helping patients incorporate preventive mental health strategies into their daily routine.

◼ ANTIPSYCHOTIC MEDICATIONS

It is hard to imagine how psychiatric illnesses were treated before the development of psychopharmacologic medications. Antipsychotic medications were among the very first drugs ever used to treat psychiatric disorders. First synthesized by Paul Charpentier in 1950, chlorpromazine became the interest of Henri Lorit, a French surgeon, who was attempting to develop medications that controlled preoperative anxiety. Administered in intravenous doses of 50 to 100 mg, chlorpromazine produced drowsiness and indifference to surgical procedures. At Lorit's suggestion, a number of psychiatrists began to administer chlorpromazine to agitated psychotic patients. In 1952, Jean Delay and Pierre Deniker, two French psychiatrists, published the first report of chlorpromazine's calming effects with psychiatric patients (Granger, 1999). They soon discovered it was especially effective in relieving hallucinations and delusions associated with schizophrenia. As more psychiatrists began to prescribe the medication, the use of restraints and seclusion in psychiatric hospitals dropped sharply, ushering in a revolution in psychiatric treatment.

Since that time, numerous antipsychotic medications have been developed. Older, typical antipsychotic medications, available since 1954, are equally effective, inexpensive drugs that vary in the degree to which they cause certain groups of side effects. Table 12.5 provides a list of selected antipsychotics grouped by the nature of their chemical structure and indicating the likelihood of certain side effects. These medications treat the symptoms of psychosis, such as hallucinations, delusions, bizarre behaviour, disorganized thinking, and agitation.

Typical and Atypical Antipsychotics

Initially, the term *major tranquilizer* was applied to this group of medications. Later, major tranquilizers were known as *neuroleptics*, which more accurately describes the action of drugs such as chlorpromazine and haloperidol. Neuroleptic means "to clasp the neuron." The term reflects the common and often significant neurologic side effects produced by these types of drugs. The development of newer antipsychotic drugs that have less significant neurologic side effects has led to these older agents being used as secondary, not first-line, drugs. The term *typical antipsychotic* now identifies the older antipsychotic drugs with greater risk for neurologic side effects, and *atypical antipsychotic* identifies the newer generation of antipsychotic drugs with fewer adverse neurologic effects within the common dosing regimes.

Indications and Mechanisms of Action

Antipsychotic medications generally are indicated for treating acute psychosis or severe agitation. Possible target symptoms for antipsychotics include hallucinations, delusions, paranoia, agitation, assaultive behaviour, bizarre ideation, disorientation, social withdrawal, catatonia, blunted affect, thought blocking, insomnia, and anorexia when these symptoms are the result of an acute exacerbation of a psychotic disorder like schizophrenia, acute hypomania associated with bipolar disorder, a psychotic response to an acute change in health status (observed with severe burns or admission to an intensive care unit), or use of specific illicit drugs.

In general, the older, typical antipsychotics, such as haloperidol (Haldol), chlorpromazine, and thioridazine (Mellaril), are equally effective in relieving hallucinations,

Table 12.5   Side Effect Comparison of Selected Antipsychotic Medications

Drug Category Drug Name	Sedation	Extrapyramidal	Anticholinergic	Orthostatic Hypotension
Standard (Typical) Antipsychotics				
Phenothiazines				
chlorpromazine (Thorazine)	+4	+2	+3	+4
thioridazine (Mellaril)	+3	+1	+4	+4
mesoridazine (Serentil)	+3	+1	+4	+3
fluphenazine (Prolixin)	+1	+4	+1	+1
perphenazine (Trilafon)	+2	+3	+2	+2
trifluoperazine (Stelazine)	+1	+3	+1	+1
Thioxanthenes				
thiothixene (Navane)	+1	+4	+1	+1
Dibenzoxazepines				
loxapine (Loxitane)	+2	+3	+2	+3
Butyrophenones				
haloperidol (Haldol)	+1	+4	+1	+1
Dihydroindolones				
molindone (Moban)	+2	+3	+1	+1
Atypical Antipsychotics				
clozapine (Clozaril)	+4	+/0	+4	+4
risperidone (Risperdal)	+1	+/0	+/0	+1
olanzapine (Zyprexa)	+4	+/0	+2	+1
quetiapine fumarate (Seroquel)	+4	+/0	+/0	+3
ziprasidone HCl (Geodon)	+1	+/0	+1	+2
aripiprazole (Abilify)	+1	+/0	+/0	+1

delusions, and bizarre ideation, termed "positive" symptoms of schizophrenia. The "negative" symptoms—blunted affect, social withdrawal, lack of interest in usual activities, lack of motivation, poverty of speech, thought blocking, and inattention—do not respond as well to the typical antipsychotics and in some cases may even be worsened by such agents. Newer atypical antipsychotics, such as clozapine (Clozaril), risperidone (Risperdal), olanzapine (Zyprexa), quetiapine (Seroquel), and ziprasidone (Geodon), are more effective at improving negative symptoms. Although antipsychotic medications are the primary treatment for schizophrenia and related illnesses, such as schizoaffective disorder, schizophreniform disorder, and brief psychotic disorder, they are increasingly being used to treat other psychiatric and medical illnesses. Psychotic symptoms that occur during a major depressive episode, anxiety, or bipolar disorder can be treated with antipsychotics, primarily on a short-term basis.

Off-label uses of the drug have led to significant inappropriate prescribing of antipsychotic agents, particularly in the treatment of anxiety, dementia insomnia, and post-traumatic stress disorder (Painter et al., 2017). Although off-label prescribing may provide some symptom relief in the aforementioned cases, more research is needed to fully understand safety and drug efficacy. Nonetheless, haloperidol and olanzapine are both seemingly effective in treating drug-related psychosis, such as that caused by phencyclidine or crystal methamphetamine. Both typical and atypical antipsychotics have been used to treat delirium in intensive care settings (often termed ICU psychosis). ICU delirium is generally seen as a poor prognostic indicator for people

in intensive care settings and potentially complicated by antipsychotic related adverse drug reactions, which occur in about 20% of ICU patients. Newer drugs such as risperidone and ziprasidone, though underutilized, infrequently cause adverse drug reactions and should be used instead of drugs such as haloperidol or olanzapine (Hale, Kane-Gill, Groetzinger, & Smithburger, 2016; Marshall et al., 2016).

The typical antipsychotic drugs are generally effective in decreasing so-called positive target symptoms because they are potent postsynaptic dopamine antagonists. Chapter 20 discusses the link between dopamine and disorders such as schizophrenia and provides additional details about how lowering dopamine levels helps reduce target symptoms. The atypical antipsychotic medications differ from the typical antipsychotics in that they block serotonin receptors that reside on dopamine neurons as well as dopamine receptors. The differences between the mechanism of action of the typical and atypical antipsychotics help to explain their differences in efficacy in relation to both positive and negative symptoms and side effect profiles.

Pharmacokinetics

Antipsychotic medications administered orally have a variable rate of absorption complicated by the presence of food, antacids, smoking, and even the coadministration of anticholinergics, which slow gastric motility. Clinical effects begin to appear in about 30 to 60 minutes. Absorption after IM administration produces greater bioavailability but increases risk for side effects. It is important to remember that IM medications are absorbed more slowly when patients are immobile, such as when restrained for long periods of time, because erratic absorption may occur when muscles are not in use. For example, the patient's arm may be more mobile than are the buttocks. The deltoid has better blood perfusion, and thus medications are more readily absorbed. The nurse must also remember that plastic syringes may absorb some medications. This is true of the antipsychotics, and injectable medications should never be allowed to remain in the syringe longer than 15 minutes.

The metabolism of these drugs occurs almost entirely in the liver, where hepatic microsomal enzymes convert these highly lipid-soluble substances into water-soluble metabolites that can be excreted through the kidneys. Therefore, these medications are subjected to the effects of other drugs that induce or inhibit the cytochrome P-450 system described earlier. Table 12.6 summarizes many of the possible medication interactions with antipsychotics, including those resulting from changes in hepatic enzymes. Careful observance of concurrent medication use, including prescribed, over the counter, and substances of abuse, is required to avoid drug–drug interactions.

Excretion of these substances tends to be slow because the drugs can easily accumulate in fat stores. Most antipsychotics have a half-life of 24 hours or longer, but many also have active metabolites with longer half-lives. These two effects make it difficult to predict elimination time,

and metabolites of some of these agents may be found in the urine months later. After discontinuation, drug accumulated in body fat will diffuse back into plasma. Over the course of several days, the drug concentration in the plasma will move below the minimum concentration required to produce a drug effect. At this point, the drug benefit or adverse drug event will typically disappear. In combination with a longer drug half-life, the long elimination time does allow the medication to be given in once-daily dosing. This schedule increases adherence and reduces the impact of the peak occurrence of some side effects, such as sedation during the day.

High lipid **solubility**, accumulation of the drug in the body, and other factors have also made it difficult to correlate blood levels with therapeutic effects. Although these can be measured for a number of antipsychotics, their correlation with therapeutic response has been inconsistent. Haloperidol and clozapine correlate well and may be helpful in determining whether an adequate blood level has been reached and maintained during a trial of medication. Table 12.7 shows the therapeutic ranges available for some of the antipsychotic medications. Plasma levels may also be helpful in identifying absorption problems or metabolic differences (high or low metabolizer), determining adherence, and identifying adverse reactions from drug–drug interactions.

The potency of the antipsychotics also varies widely and is of specific concern when considering typical

Table 12.6	Chemical Interactions With Antipsychotic Medications
Agent	**Effect**
Alcohol	Phenothiazines potentiate CNS depressant effects
	Extrapyramidal reactions may occur
Barbiturates	Speed action of CYP enzymes so that antipsychotic is metabolized more quickly, reducing phenothiazine and haloperidol plasma levels; barbiturate levels may also be reduced by phenothiazines; potentiate CNS depressant effect
Tricyclic antidepressants	Can lead to severe anticholinergic side effects; some antipsychotics (especially phenothiazines or haloperidol) can raise the plasma level of the antidepressant, probably by inhibiting metabolism of the antidepressant
Hydrochlorothiazide and hydralazine	Can produce severe hypotension
Aluminum salts (antacids)	Impair gastrointestinal absorption of the phenothiazines, possibly reducing therapeutic effect
	Administer antacid at least 1 hour before or 2 hours after the phenothiazine
Tobacco	Heavy consumption requires larger doses of antipsychotic because of CYP enzyme induction. Similarly, when patients are restricting from smoking or quit, smaller doses may be required.
Charcoal (and charbroiled food)	Decreases absorption of phenothiazines
Anticholinergics	May reduce the therapeutic actions of the phenothiazines, increase anticholinergic side effects, lower serum haloperidol levels, worsen symptoms of schizophrenia, increase symptoms of tardive dyskinesia
Meperidine	May result in excessive sedation and hypotension when coadministered with phenothiazines
Fluoxetine	Case report of serious extrapyramidal symptoms when used in combination with haloperidol
Lithium	May induce disorientation, unconsciousness, extrapyramidal symptoms, or possibly the risk for NMS when combined with phenothiazines or haloperidol
Carbamazepine	Decreases haloperidol serum levels, decreasing its therapeutic effects
Phenytoin	Increase or decrease in phenytoin serum levels; thioridazine and haloperidol serum levels may be decreased
Methyldopa	May potentiate the antipsychotic effects of haloperidol or may produce psychosis
	Serious elevations in blood pressure may occur with methyldopa and trifluoperazine
General anaesthesia (barbiturates)	Antipsychotic may potentiate effect of anaesthetic; may increase the neuromuscular excitation or hypotension

Table 12.7 Antipsychotic Medications				
Generic (Trade) Drug Name	Usual Dosage Range (mg/day)	Half-Life (hours)	Therapeutic Blood Level	Approximate Equivalent Dosage (mg)
Standard (Typical) Antipsychotics				
Phenothiazines				
chlorpromazine (Thorazine)	50–1,200	2–30	30–100 mg/mL	100
thioridazine (Mellaril)	50–600	10–20	1–1.5 ng/mL	100
mesoridazine (Serentil)	50–400	24–48	Not available	50
fluphenazine (Prolixin)	2–20	4.5–15.3	0.2–0.3 ng/mL	2
perphenazine (Trilafon)	12–64	Unknown	0.8–12.0 ng/mL	10
trifluoperazine (Stelazine)	5–40	47–100	1–2.3 ng/mL	5
Thioxanthenes				
thiothixene (Navane)	5–60	34	2–20 ng/mL	4
Dibenzoxazepines				
loxapine (Loxitane)	20–250	19	Not available	15
Butyrophenones				
haloperidol (Haldol)	2–60	21–24	5–15 ng/mL	2
Dihydroindolones				
molindone (Moban)	50–400	1.5	Not available	10
Atypical Antipsychotics				
clozapine (Clozaril)	300–900	4–12	141–204 ng/mL	50
risperidone (Risperdal)	2–8	20	Not available	1
olanzapine (Zyprexa)	5–10	21–54	Not available	Not available
quetiapine fumarate (Seroquel)	150–750	7	Not available	Not available
ziprasidone HCl (Geodon)	40–160	7	Not available	Not available
aripiprazole (Abilify)	10–30	75–94	Not available	Not available

antipsychotic drugs. As Table 12.7 indicates, 100 mg chlorpromazine is roughly equivalent to 2 mg haloperidol and 5 mg trifluoperazine. Although drugs that are more potent are not inherently better than less potent drugs, differentiating low-potency versus high-potency antipsychotics may be helpful to estimate drug dosing if one antipsychotic drug is switched to another. Given that each antipsychotic agent has differing side effect profiles, a change in antipsychotic may be needed if patients are experiencing adverse drug effects.

Ultimately, selection of medication from the group of typical antipsychotics depends predominately on predicted side effects, prior history of treatment response, whether or not a depot preparation will be needed during maintenance, concurrent medications, and other medical conditions.

Drug Formulations: Long-Acting Preparations

In Canada, there are several different types of long-acting injectable antipsychotic agents. First-generation agents include haloperidol decanoate, flupenthixol decanoate, and zuclopenthixol decanoate. Second-generation agents include aripiprazole monohydrate (Abilify), aripiprazole lauroxil (Aristada), olanzapine pamoate (Zyprexa Relprevv), paliperidone palmitate (Invega Sustenna), and risperidone microsperes (Risperdal Consta). Note that two different formulations of aripiprazole exist, the dosing of each formulation differs. These antipsychotics may be administered by injection once every 2 to 4 weeks. After administration, the drug is slowly released from the injection site; therefore, these forms of the drugs are referred to as *depot preparations.*

Long-acting injectable medications maintain a fairly constant blood level between injections. Because they bypass problems with gastrointestinal absorption and first-pass metabolism, this method may enhance therapeutic outcomes for the patient by decreasing individual drug concentration variability due to kinetic differences. Depot injections, though controversial, are increasingly being used as a first-line agent to improve drug adherence and therapeutic outcomes (Breit & Hasler, 2016; Kenicer, Ellahi, Davies, Walker, & Cheyne, 2016). There are 43% more arrests or hospitalizations, due to psychotic symptoms, among those prescribed oral versus depot antipsychotic formulations. This points to significant concerns relating to drug adherence accruing among individuals with psychotic symptoms (Khan, Salaria, Ovais, & Ide, 2016). Box 12.2 describes research exploring mode of delivery and drug adherence.

Nurses should be aware that the injection site may become sore and inflamed if certain precautions are not taken. Although many depot formulations are available in prefilled syringes, a filtered needle is preferred for the long-term use of depot medications to avoid any aspiration of glass particulates (Preston & Hegadoren, 2004). Because the medication is meant to remain in the injection site, the needle should be dry, and a deep IM injection should be given by the Z-track method. (Note: Do not massage the injection site. Rotate sites and document in the patient's record.)

Both olanzapine and risperidone are also available in a quick-release formulation in Canada. Olanzapine is often used to treat acute agitation. In circumstances

BOX 12.2 Research for Best Practice

ANTIPSYCHOTIC DRUG ADHERENCE AMONG HOMELESS ADULTS IN VANCOUVER

From Rezansoff, S. N., Moniruzzaman, A., Fazel, S., Procyshyn, R., & Somers, J. M. (2016). Adherence to antipsychotic medication among homeless adults in Vancouver, Canada: A 15-year retrospective cohort study. Social Psychiatry and Psychiatric Epidemiology, 51(12), 1623–1632.

Question: What factors influence psychotropic drug adherence among people who are homeless?

Method: Patient-specific prescription details were drawn from a province-wide database of all dispensed prescriptions. The medication possession ration (MPR) was used to categorize the sample population as either having higher or lower levels of antipsychotic adherence. Sociodemographic and health status data were collected at the outset of the 15-year study. The effects of the baseline data on MPR over time were examined using both univariate and multivariate statistics.

Findings: Higher rates of adherence to antipsychotic medication were associated with connectedness to health services (hospitalization or primary medical services) and with long-acting antipsychotic prescriptions. Lower rates of adherence to antipsychotic medication were associated with diagnosis of a blood-borne infectious disease and homelessness of longer than 3 years.

Implications for Practice: Nurses must continue to advocate for meaningful public programs to reduce homelessness in Canada and to improve health service access to vulnerable populations with severe mental illness. Further, the use of long-acting injectable antipsychotic medications seems to be a plausible approach to improve drug adherence among people who are homeless.

---

where rapid sedation is needed and the patient is able and willing to take an oral medication, this formulation may be advantageous.

Side Effects, Adverse Reactions, and Toxicity

Various side effects and interactions can occur with antipsychotics (see Tables 12.6 and 12.7), with the typical antipsychotics producing more significant side effects than the atypical antipsychotics. The side effects vary largely based on their degree of affinity to different neurotransmitter receptors and their subtypes.

Cardiovascular Side Effects

Cardiovascular side effects, such as orthostatic hypotension, depend on the degree of blockade of α-adrenergic receptors. Low-potency typical antipsychotics, such as chlorpromazine and thioridazine, and the atypical antipsychotic clozapine have a high degree of affinity for α-adrenergic receptors and, therefore, produce considerable orthostatic hypotension. Other cardiovascular side effects from typical antipsychotics have been rare, but occasionally they cause ECG changes that have a benign or undetermined clinical effect. Thioridazine (Mellaril) and ziprasidone (Geodon) have both been associated with prolonged QT intervals and should be used cautiously in patients who have increased QT intervals or are taking other medications that may prolong the QT interval (Taylor, 2003).

Anticholinergic Side Effects

Anticholinergic side effects resulting from the blockade of muscarinic acetylcholine receptors are another common concern with the typical and some of the atypical antipsychotic drugs. Dry mouth, slowed gastric motility, constipation, urinary hesitancy or retention, vaginal dryness, blurred vision, dry eyes, nasal congestion, and confusion or decreased memory are examples of these side effects. Interventions for decreasing the impact of these side effects are outlined in Table 12.2. This group of side effects occurs with many of the medications used for psychiatric treatment. Sometimes a cholinergic medication, such as bethanechol, may reduce the peripheral effects but not the CNS effects. Using more than one medication with anticholinergic effects often increases the symptoms. Older adult patients are often more susceptible to a potential toxicity that results from high blockade of acetylcholine. This toxicity is called an *anticholinergic* crisis and is described, along with its treatment, in Chapter 20. The likelihood of anticholinergic side effects, along with sedation and extrapyramidal side effects, from antipsychotics is explored in Table 12.5.

Weight Gain

Weight gain has been associated with antipsychotic drugs since chlorpromazine was developed but is more frequently observed with the atypical drugs such as clozapine and olanzapine. The exact physiologic mechanisms that contribute to weight gain are unknown, but the most promising data include investigations of the histamine H(1), 5-HT(2A), 5-HT(2C), muscarinic M(3), and adrenergic receptors (Roerig, Steffen, & Mitchell, 2011). The weight gain related to antipsychotic medications is linked to an increased risk for type II diabetes, heart disease, and hyperlipidemia. Those at higher risk for developing metabolic or cardiovascular disorders are those individuals who show more rapid weight gain in the 1st week of drug treatment. A Quebec study (N = 19,582) showed that the risk for initiation of a pharmacologic treatment for diabetes or dyslipidemia is significantly higher with olanzapine than with risperidone (Moisan, Gregoire, Gaudet, & Cooper, 2005). The chronic health problems of diabetes and cardiovascular illness occur much more often in individuals with mental illness than in the general population, making it essential for nurses to assist patients in dealing effectively with issues of weight gain.

Endocrine and Sexual Side Effects

Endocrine and sexual side effects result primarily from the blockade of dopamine in the tuberoinfundibular pathways of the hypothalamus. As a result, prolactin level in the blood may increase with almost all the typical antipsychotics but less commonly with the atypical antipsychotics. Increased prolactin causes breast enlargement and rare but potential galactorrhoea (milk production and flow), decreased sexual drive, amenorrhoea, menstrual irregularities, and increased risk for tumour growth in preexisting breast cancers. Bromocriptine, a dopamine agonist, may alleviate these symptoms, but more likely, these symptoms necessitate a change in medication. Endocrine side effects can occur in males as well. Retrograde ejaculation (backward flow of semen) is rare, but it may be painful and can occur with all of the antipsychotics. A more common side effect is erectile dysfunction, including difficulty achieving and maintaining an erection. Anorgasmia, or the inability to achieve orgasm, may develop in women.

Blood Disorders

Blood dyscrasias are rare but have received renewed attention since the introduction of clozapine. Agranulocytosis is an acute reaction that causes the individual's white blood cell count to drop to very low levels, and concurrent neutropenia, a drop in neutrophils in the blood, develops. In the case of the antipsychotics, the medication suppresses the bone marrow precursors to these blood cells. The exact mechanism by which the drugs produce this effect is unknown. The most notable symptoms of this disorder include high fever, sore throat, and mouth sores. Although benign elevations in temperature have been reported in individuals taking clozapine, no fever should go uninvestigated. Untreated agranulocytosis can be life threatening. Although agranulocytosis can occur with any of the antipsychotics, the risk with clozapine is 10 to 20 times greater than with the other antipsychotics (Bilici, Tekelioglu, Efendioglu, Ovali, & Ulgen, 2003). Therefore, prescription of clozapine requires weekly blood samples for the first 6 months of treatment and then every 2 weeks after that for as long as the drug is taken. Drawing of these samples must continue for 4 weeks after clozapine use has been discontinued. If sore throat or fever develops, medications should be withheld until a leukocyte count can be obtained. Hospitalization, including reverse isolation to prevent infections, is usually required. Agranulocytosis is more likely to develop during the first 18 weeks of treatment.

Miscellaneous

Photosensitivity reactions to antipsychotics, including severe sunburns or rash, most commonly develop with the use of low-potency typical antipsychotics. Sunblock must be worn on all areas of exposed skin when taking these drugs. In addition, sun exposure may cause pigmentary deposits to develop, resulting in the discoloration of exposed areas, especially the neck and face. This discoloration may progress from a deep orange colour to a blue grey. Skin exposure should be limited and skin tone changes reported to the prescriber. Pigmentary deposits may also develop on the retina of the eye, especially with high doses of thioridazine, even for a few days. This condition is called *retinitis pigmentosa* and can lead to significant visual impairment. Therefore, thioridazine should never be administered in doses greater than 800 mg per day.

Antipsychotics may also lower a patient's seizure threshold. Patients with an undetected seizure disorder may experience seizures early in treatment. Those who have a preexisting condition should be monitored closely.

Neuroleptic malignant syndrome (NMS) and water intoxication are two serious complications that may result from antipsychotic medications. Characterized by rigidity and high fever, NMS is a rare condition but a medical emergency that may occur abruptly with even one dose of medication. Temperature must always be monitored when administering antipsychotics, especially high-potency medications. Water intoxication may develop gradually with long-term use. This condition is characterized by the patient's consumption of large quantities of fluid (polydipsia) and the resulting effects of sodium depletion (hyponatremia).

Medication-Related Movement Disorders

Medication-related movement disorders are a group of side effects or adverse reactions that are commonly caused by typical antipsychotic medications but less commonly with atypical antipsychotic drugs. These disorders of abnormal motor movements can be divided into two groups: acute extrapyramidal syndromes (EPSs), which are acute abnormal movements developing early in the course of treatment (sometimes after just one dose), and chronic syndromes, which develop from longer exposure to antipsychotic drugs. The atypical antipsychotic drugs are most likely to cause movement disorders.

Acute Extrapyramidal Syndromes

Acute EPSs occurs in as many as 90% of all patients receiving typical antipsychotic medications (Chouinard & Chouinard, 2008). These syndromes include **dystonia**, parkinsonism, and **akathisia** (an involuntary movement disorder). They develop early in treatment, sometimes from as little as one dose. Although the abnormal movements are treatable, they are at times dramatic and frightening, causing physical and emotional impairments that often prompt patients to stop taking their medication. Some milder forms of EPS may occur with classes of medication other than antipsychotics, including the SSRIs. The acute EPS often are mistaken for aspects of anxiety, rather than medication side effects. Nurses play a vital role in the early recognition and treatment of these syndromes. Early recognition can save the patient considerable discomfort, fear, and impairment. All nurses must be aware of these symptoms, notifying the prescriber as soon as possible and implementing selected medication changes and other interventions. Several medications can control acute EPS (Table 12.8).

Dystonia, sometimes referred to as an *acute dystonic reaction*, is impaired muscle tone that generally is the first extrapyramidal symptom to occur, usually within a few days of initiating use of an antipsychotic. Dystonia is characterized by involuntary muscle spasms, especially of the head and neck muscles. Patients usually first complain of a thick tongue, tight jaw, or stiff neck. The

syndrome can progress to a protruding tongue, oculogyric crisis (eyes rolled up in the head), torticollis (muscle stiffness in the neck, which draws the head to one side with chin pointing to the other), and laryngopharyngeal constriction. In severe cases, the spasms may progress to the intercostal muscles, producing more significant breathing difficulty for patients who already have respiratory impairment from asthma or emphysema.

Drug-induced parkinsonism is sometimes referred to as **pseudoparkinsonism** because its presentation is identical to Parkinson's disease without the same destruction of dopaminergic cells. These symptoms include the classic triad of rigidity, slowed movements (bradykinesia), and tremor. The rigid muscle stiffness is usually seen in the arms. Bradykinesia can be observed by the loss of spontaneous movements, such as the absence of the usual relaxed swing of the arms while walking. In addition, masklike faces or loss of facial expression and a decrease in the ability to initiate movements also are present. Usually, tremor is more pronounced at rest, but it can also be observed with intentional movements, such as eating. If the tremor becomes severe, it may interfere with the patient's ability to eat or maintain adequate fluid intake. Hypersalivation is possible

Table 12.8   Drug Therapies for Acute Medication-Related Movement Disorders

Agents	Typical Dosage Ranges	Routes Available	Common Side Effects
Anticholinergics			
benztropine (Cogentin)	2–6 mg/day	PO, IM, IV	Dry mouth, blurred vision, slowed gastric motility causing constipation, urinary retention, increased intraocular pressure; overdose produces toxic psychosis
trihexyphenidyl (Artane)	4–15 mg/day	PO	Same as benztropine, plus gastrointestinal distress Older adults are most prone to mental confusion and delirium.
biperiden (Akineton)	2–8 mg/day	PO	Fewer peripheral anticholinergic effects Euphoria and increased tremor may occur
Antihistamines			
diphenhydramine (Benadryl)	25–50 mg q.i.d. to 400 mg daily	PO, IM, IV	Sedation and confusion, especially in older adults
Dopamine Agonists			
amantadine (Symmetrel)	100–400 mg daily	PO	Indigestion, decreased concentration, dizziness, anxiety, ataxia, insomnia, lethargy, tremors, and slurred speech may occur on higher doses Tolerance may develop on fixed dose
β-Antagonist (Blockers)			
propranolol (Inderal)	10 mg t.i.d. to 120 mg daily	PO	Hypotension and bradycardia Must monitor pulse and blood pressure Do not stop abruptly as this may cause rebound tachycardia
Benzodiazepines			
lorazepam (Ativan)	1–2 mg IM 0.5–2 mg PO	PO, IM	All may cause drowsiness, lethargy, and general sedation or paradoxical agitation Confusion and disorientation in older adults
diazepam (Valium)	2–5 mg t.i.d.	PO, IV	Most side effects are rare and will disappear if dose is decreased
clonazepam (Rivotril)	1–4 mg/day	PO	Tolerance and withdrawal are potential problems

as well. Pseudoparkinsonism symptoms may occur on one or both sides of the body and develop abruptly or subtly, but usually within the first 30 days of treatment.

Akathisia is characterized by the inability to sit still. The person will pace, rock while sitting or standing, march in place, or cross and uncross the legs. All these repetitive motions have an intensity that is frequently beyond the explanation of the individual. In addition, akathisia may be present as a primarily subjective experience without obvious motor behaviour. This subjective experience includes feelings of anxiety, jitteriness, or the inability to relax, which the individual may or may not be able to communicate. It is extremely uncomfortable for a person experiencing akathisia to be forced to sit still or be confined. These symptoms are sometimes misdiagnosed as agitation or an increase in psychotic symptoms, but if the nurse administers an antipsychotic medication PRN (from the Latin pro re nata, which roughly translated means "as needed"), the symptoms will not abate and will often worsen. Differentiating akathisia from agitation may be aided by knowing the person's symptoms before the introduction of medication. Psychotic agitation does not usually begin abruptly after antipsychotic medication use has been started, whereas akathisia may occur after administration. In addition, the nurse may ask the patient if the experience is felt primarily in the muscles (akathisia) or in the mind or emotions (agitation).

Akathisia is the most difficult acute medication-related movement disorder to relieve. It does not usually respond well to anticholinergic medications and is uncommon in patients receiving atypical antipsychotics. It is thought that the pathology of akathisia may involve more than just the extrapyramidal motor system. It may include serotonin changes that also affect the dopamine system (Kulkarni & Naidu, 2003). A number of medications have been used to reduce symptoms, including β-adrenergic blockers, anticholinergics, antihistamines, and low-dose antianxiety agents (Pierre, 2005). The usual approach to treatment is to change to an atypical antipsychotic if possible. If not, reducing the dose of typical antipsychotic medication can be tried. During this time, nurses must closely assess for worsening of symptoms. β-Adrenergic blockers, such as propranolol (Inderal), given in doses of 30 to 120 mg per day, have been most successful (Miller & Fleischhacker, 2000). Nurses must monitor the patient's pulse and blood pressure because propranolol can cause hypotension and bradycardia. If the patient's pulse falls below 60 bpm, propranolol should not be given and the prescriber should be notified. Normal signs of hypoglycaemia may be blocked by propranolol; therefore, patients with diabetes must monitor their blood or urine glucose levels carefully, especially because they are under physical stress from the disorder.

A number of nursing interventions may reduce the impact of these syndromes. Individuals with acute EPS need frequent reassurance that this is not a worsening of their psychiatric condition but instead is a treatable side effect of the medication. They also need validation that what they are experiencing is real and that the nurse is concerned and will be responsive to changes in these symptoms. Physical and psychological stress appears to increase the symptoms and further frighten the patient; therefore, decreasing stressful situations becomes important. These symptoms are often physically exhausting for the patient, and nurses should ensure that the patient receives adequate rest and hydration.

Risk factors for acute EPS include previous episodes of EPS and use of high-dose injected antipsychotics for acute psychotic symptoms or agitation. Listen closely when patients say they are "allergic" or have had "bad reactions" to antipsychotic medications. Often, they are describing one of the medication-related movement disorders, particularly dystonia, rather than a rash or other allergic symptoms. About 90% of the individuals who have experienced EPS in the past will again have these symptoms if the use of an antipsychotic medication is restarted (Meyer, 2007). High-potency medications, such as haloperidol and fluphenazine, are more likely to cause EPS. Age and gender appear to be risk factors for specific syndromes. Acute dystonia occurs most often in young men, adolescents, and children; akathisia is more common in middle-aged women. Older adult patients are at the greatest risk for experiencing pseudoparkinsonism. Although the occurrence of EPS is decreasing as atypical medications are more commonly used, acute EPS remains a serious clinical concern. Risperidone in high doses carries with it the same risk of EPS as does the typical antipsychotics.

Chronic Syndromes

Chronic syndromes develop from the long-term use of antipsychotics. They are serious and afflict about 20% of the patients who receive typical antipsychotics for an extended period (Pierre, 2005). These conditions can be irreversible and cause significant impairment in self-image, social interactions, and occupational functioning. Early symptoms and mild forms may go unnoticed by the person experiencing them because they frequently remain beyond the individual's awareness. Therefore, nurses in contact with individuals who are taking antipsychotic medications for months or years must be vigilant in monitoring for symptoms of these typical chronic conditions.

First identified in 1957, **tardive dyskinesia** is the most well known of the chronic syndromes. It involves irregular, repetitive involuntary movements of the mouth, face, and tongue, including chewing, tongue protrusion, lip smacking, puckering of the lips, and rapid eye blinking. Abnormal finger movements are common as well. In some individuals, the trunk and extremities are also involved, and in rare cases, irregular breathing and swallowing lead to belching and grunting noises. These symptoms usually begin no earlier than after 6 months of treatment or when the medication is reduced or withdrawn. Once thought to be irreversible, considerable controversy now exists as to whether or not this is true.

Part of the difficulty in determining the irreversibility of tardive dyskinesia is that any movement disorder that persists after the discontinuation of antipsychotic medication has been described as tardive dyskinesia. Atypical forms are now receiving more attention because some researchers believe that they may have different underlying mechanisms of causation. Some of these forms of the disorder appear to remit spontaneously. Symptoms of what is now called *withdrawal tardive dyskinesia* appear when use of an antipsychotic medication is reduced or discontinued and remit spontaneously in 1 to 3 months. *Tardive dystonia* and *tardive akathisia* have also been described. Both appear in a manner similar to the acute syndromes but continue after the antipsychotic medication has been withdrawn. More research is needed to determine whether these syndromes are distinctly different in origin and outcome.

The risk for experiencing tardive dyskinesia increases with age. Although the prevalence of tardive dyskinesia averages 15% to 20%, the rate rises to 50% to 70% in older adults receiving antipsychotic medications (Tariot, Salzman, Yeung, Pultz, & Rak, 2000). Cumulative incidence of tardive dyskinesia appears to increase 5% per year of continued exposure to antipsychotic medications (Levy et al., 2002). Women are at higher risk than are men. Individuals with affective disorders, particularly depression, are at higher risk than are those who have schizophrenia. Any individual receiving antipsychotic medication may experience tardive dyskinesia; therefore, nurses must be particularly alert to individuals at higher risk. Risk factors are summarized in Box 12.3. The causes of tardive dyskinesia remain unclear. Lack of a consistent theory of aetiology for the chronic medication-related movement disorder syndromes has led to inconsistent and disappointing treatment approaches. No one medication relieves the symptoms. Dopamine agonists, such as bromocriptine, and many other drugs have been tried. Even dietary precursors of acetylcholine, such as lecithin, and nutritional therapies, such as vitamin E supplements, may prove to be beneficial.

BOX 12.3 Risk Factors for Tardive Dyskinesia

- Age older than 50 years
- Female
- Affective disorders, particularly depression
- Brain damage or dysfunction
- Increased duration of treatment
- Standard antipsychotic medication
- Use of acute higher doses of antipsychotic medication

The best approach to treatment remains avoiding the development of the chronic syndromes. Preventive measures include use of atypical antipsychotics, using the lowest possible dose of typical medication, minimizing use of PRN medication, and closely monitoring individuals in high-risk groups for development of the symptoms of tardive dyskinesia. All members of the mental health treatment team who have contact with individuals taking antipsychotics for longer than 3 months must be alert to the risk factors and earliest possible signs of chronic medication-related movement disorders.

Monitoring tools, such as the Abnormal Involuntary Movement Scale (AIMS; Simpson & Angus, 1970), should be used routinely to standardize assessment and provide the earliest possible recognition of the symptoms. Standardized assessments should be performed at a minimum of 3- to 6-month intervals. The earlier the symptoms are recognized, the more likely they will resolve if the medication can be changed or its use discontinued. Newer, atypical antipsychotic medications have a much lower risk for causing tardive dyskinesia and are increasingly being considered first-line medications for treating schizophrenia.

MOOD STABILIZERS (ANTIMANIA MEDICATIONS)

Mood stabilizers, or antimania medications, are psychopharmacologic agents used primarily for stabilizing mood, particularly those of mania in bipolar disorders. For a number of years, lithium was the only drug known to stabilize the symptoms of mania. Although it remains the gold standard of treatment for acute mania and maintenance of bipolar disorders, not all individuals experience a positive response to lithium, and increasingly, other drugs are being used. Valproic acid, lamotrigine, and atypical antipsychotic agents such as olanzapine and quetiapine are increasing being used either alone or in combination with lithium for improved efficacy in treatment-resistant cases. The combination of lithium and lamotrigine has demonstrated the highest efficacy in reducing suicidal symptoms and depressive relapse (Takeshima, 2017). Many other drugs, including other anticonvulsants, atypical antipsychotics, and adrenergic blocking agents in conjunction with antidepressants, are used frequently to prevent episodes of hypomania or depression (Brunoni, Moffa, Sampaio-Júnior, Gálvez, & Loo, 2017; Yatham & Kesavan, 2017). The first-line use of antidepressant agents to augment a drug response in bipolar depression is replaced with atypical antipsychotic agents (Post, 2016).

Lithium

Lithium, a naturally occurring element, was first discovered in the early 1800s. In 1949, Australian John Cade found that lithium reduced agitation in some patients experiencing psychosis, and in the 1950s, Schou (1978) published reports that lithium controlled and prevented the symptoms of mania. Since then, it has become a mainstay in psychopharmacology. Lithium is effective in only about 40% of patients with bipolar disorder; other agents may be coadministered to increase treatment efficacy among those with incomplete response to lithium alone (Bauer & Gitlin, 2016). Although lithium is not a perfect drug, a great deal is known regarding its use—it is inexpensive, it has restored stability to the lives of thousands of people, and it remains the gold standard of bipolar pharmacologic treatment.

Indications and Mechanisms of Action

The target symptoms for lithium are the symptoms of mania, such as rapid speech, jumping from topic to topic (flight of ideas), irritability, grandiose thinking, impulsiveness, and agitation. While lithium does seem to be effective in treating depressive disorders, caution is needed in interpreting these results. Specifically, depressive symptoms seen in hypomania may be mistakenly diagnosed as a depressive disorder—thus, lithium's efficacy in treating "depression" may be actually point to a misdiagnosis (Takeshima, 2017). It has also been shown to be helpful in reducing impulsivity and aggression in certain psychiatric patients.

Lithium has been effective in treating several nonpsychiatric disorders, such as cluster headaches. Because lithium stimulates leukocytosis, it often improves the neutrophil counts of patients who are undergoing chemotherapy or who have other conditions that cause neutropenia. In addition, lithium has been investigated as an antiviral agent because it appears to inhibit the replication of several DNA viruses, including herpes virus. Additional research is needed to fully understand the mechanisms of these effects.

Lithium is actively transported across cell membranes, altering sodium transport in both nerve and muscle cells. It replaces sodium in the sodium–potassium pump and is retained more readily than sodium inside the cell. Conditions that alter sodium content in the body, such as vomiting, diuresis, and diaphoresis, alter lithium retention. The results of lithium influx into the nerve cell lead to increased storage of catecholamines within the cell, reduced dopamine neurotransmission, increased norepinephrine reuptake, increased GABA activity, and increased serotonin receptor sensitivity (Bschor et al., 2003). The specific mechanisms by which lithium improves the symptoms of mania are complex, most likely involving the sum of all or part of these actions and more.

Pharmacokinetics

Lithium carbonate is available orally in capsule, tablet, and liquid forms. Slow-release preparations are also available. Lithium is readily absorbed in the gastric system and may be taken with food, which does not impair absorption. Peak blood levels are reached in 1 to 4 hours, and the medication is usually completely absorbed in 8 hours. Slow-release preparations are absorbed at a slower, more variable rate.

Lithium is not protein bound, and its distribution into the CNS across the blood–brain barrier is slow. The onset of action is usually 5 to 7 days and may take as long as 2 weeks. The elimination half-life is 8 to 12 hours, and 18 to 36 hours in individuals whose blood levels have reached steady state. Lithium is almost entirely excreted by the kidneys. Conditions of renal impairment or decreased renal function in older adults decrease lithium clearance and may lead to toxicity. Several medications affect renal function and therefore change lithium clearance. See Chapter 22 for a list of these and other medication interactions with lithium. About 80% of lithium is reabsorbed in the proximal tubule of the kidney along with water and sodium. In conditions that cause sodium depletion, such as dehydration caused by fever, strenuous exercise, hot weather, increased perspiration, and vomiting, the kidney attempts to conserve sodium. Because lithium is a salt, the kidney retains lithium as well, leading to increased blood levels and potential toxicity. Significantly increasing sodium intake causes lithium levels to fall.

Lithium is usually administered in doses of 300 mg two to three times daily. During the acute phases of mania, blood levels of 0.8 to 1.4 mEq/L are usually attained and maintained until symptoms are under control. During maintenance, the dosage is reduced, and dosages are adjusted to maintain blood levels of 0.4 to 1 mEq/L. As a drug with a narrow therapeutic range or index, blood levels are monitored frequently, usually every 3 to 5 days. These increases may be slower in older adults or patients who experience uncomfortable side effects. Blood levels should be monitored 12 hours after the last dose of medication. In the hospital setting, nurses should withhold the morning dose of lithium until the serum sample is drawn to avoid falsely elevated levels. Individuals who are at home should be instructed to have their blood drawn in the morning about 12 hours after their last dose and before they take their first dose of medication.

Lithium clears the body relatively quickly after the discontinuation of its use. It is important to remember that almost half of the individuals who discontinue lithium treatment abruptly experience a relapse of symptoms within a few weeks (Goodwin & Ghaemi, 2000; Kennedy et al., 2003). Some research suggests that discontinuation of the use of lithium for individuals whose symptoms have been stable may lead to lithium losing its effectiveness when use of the medication is restarted (Kennedy et al., 2003). Patients should be warned of the risks in abruptly discontinuing their medication and should be advised to consider the options carefully in consultation with their prescriber.

Side Effects, Adverse Reactions, and Toxicity

At lower therapeutic blood levels, side effects from lithium are relatively mild. These reactions correspond with peaks in plasma concentrations of the medication after administration, and most subside during the first few weeks of therapy. Frequently, individuals taking lithium complain of excessive thirst and an unpleasant metallic-like taste. Sugarless throat lozenges may be useful in minimizing this side effect. Other common side effects include an increased frequency of urination, fine head tremor, drowsiness, and mild diarrhoea. Weight gain occurs in about 20% of the individuals taking lithium. Nausea may be minimized by taking the medication with food or by use of a slow-release preparation. See Chapter 22 for a summary of selected nursing interventions to minimize the impact of common side effects associated with lithium treatment. Patients most frequently discontinued their own medication use because of concerns with mental slowness, poor concentration, and memory problems.

As blood levels of lithium increase, the side effects of lithium become more numerous and severe. Early signs of lithium toxicity include severe diarrhoea, vomiting, drowsiness, muscular weakness, and lack of coordination. Lithium should be withheld and the prescriber consulted if these symptoms develop. Lithium toxicity can easily be resolved in 24 to 48 hours by discontinuing the medication, but haemodialysis may be required in severe situations. See Chapter 22 for a summary of the side effects and symptoms of toxicity associated with various blood levels of lithium.

Monitoring of creatinine concentration, thyroid hormones, and CBC every 6 months during maintenance therapy helps to assess the occurrence of other potential adverse reactions. Kidney damage is considered an uncommon but potentially serious risk for long-term lithium treatment. This damage is usually reversible after discontinuation of the lithium use. A gradual rise in serum creatinine and decline in creatinine clearance indicate the development of renal dysfunction. Individuals with preexisting kidney dysfunction are susceptible to lithium toxicity.

Lithium may alter thyroid function, usually after 6 to 18 months of treatment. About 30% of the individuals taking lithium exhibit elevations in thyroid-stimulating hormone, but most do not show the suppression of circulating thyroid hormone. Thyroid dysfunction from lithium treatment is more common in women, and some individuals require the addition of thyroxine to their care. During maintenance, thyroid-stimulating hormone levels may be monitored. Nurses should observe for dry skin, constipation, bradycardia, hair loss, cold intolerance, and other symptoms of hypothyroidism. Other endocrine system effects result from hyperparathyroidism, which increases parathyroid hormone levels and calcium. Clinically, this change is not significant, but elevated calcium levels may cause mood changes, anxiety, lethargy, and sleep disturbances. These symptoms may erroneously be attributed to depression if hypocalcaemia is not investigated.

Lithium use must be avoided during pregnancy because it has been associated with birth defects, especially when administered during the first trimester. If lithium is given during the third trimester, toxicity may develop in a newborn, producing signs of hypotonia, cyanosis, bradykinesia, cardiac changes, gastrointestinal bleeding, and shock. Diabetes insipidus may persist for months. Lithium is also present in breast milk, and women should not breastfeed while taking lithium. Women expecting to become pregnant should be advised to consult with their physician before discontinuing the use of birth control methods.

Anticonvulsants

Anticonvulsant therapies are becoming increasingly popular in the treatment of bipolar depression (Molina, Durán, López-Muñoz, Álamo, & Toledo-Romero, 2016). While anticonvulsant drug also carry significant risk of adverse drug reactions such aplastic anaemia and agranulocytosis, the overall monitoring of these drugs are much simpler when compared to lithium (Post, 2016). The clinical advantage of using anticonvulsant drugs over lithium is not fully known. However, early research indicates that individuals taking lithium have better short- and long-term memory and executive function compared to those taking anticonvulsant drugs (Sabater et al., 2016). With the exception of gabapentin (Neurontin), the benefit of anticonvulsant use in bipolar disorder has been well established (Melvin, Carey, Goodman, Oldham, & Ranney, 2008). Other researchers have found an increased risk of suicide among individuals taking anticonvulsant drugs for the bipolar 1 disorders (Bellivier et al., 2017). Nonetheless, further research to clarify benefits of anticonvulsant use in bipolar depression is needed (Corrado & Walsh, 2016).

Indications and Mechanisms of Action

Anticonvulsant medications in general are primarily indicated for treating seizure disorders. Target symptoms for the use of anticonvulsants with bipolar disorder include all the symptoms of mania discussed earlier. However, anticonvulsants are often used for individuals who have not experienced response to lithium or who are identified as having rapid cycling. Studies have shown some common traits in these individuals. Those who do not experience response to lithium most often are those who have a dysphoric or mixed mania. These individuals experience an increase in physical activity during manic episodes without any elevation in mood. They often are referred to as *mixed states* because they have elements of both depression and mania. These individuals exhibit symptoms of high anxiety, agitation, and irritability, which are then target symptoms for the use of anticonvulsants. Empirical data show carbamazepine and valproic acid to be effective in mood stabilization.

The term *rapid cycling* is applied when individuals experience four or more episodes of either depression or mania during a 12-month period. This occurs more often in women than in men. These patients make up a group of individuals who experience poor response to lithium treatment. Mood instability is also a target symptom of anticonvulsant medications. The theory of the mechanism of action of the anticonvulsants involves the concept of kindling as it applies to mood disorders.

Kindling refers to the emergence of spontaneous firing of nerve cells in response to repeated subthreshold electrical stimulation. Once brain regions, such as the amygdala, have been "kindled," it takes considerably less stimulation to initiate a seizure. In the case of mood disorders, it is hypothesized that "kindled" brain regions include the areas associated with emotional regulation. The stimulation of these regions by increasingly minor stressors or other environmental factors produces mood swings instead of a seizure.

Anticonvulsants have "antikindling" properties and decrease the sensitization of affected cells, making them less easy to stimulate. In general, the anticonvulsant mood stabilizers have many actions, but it is their effects on ion channels, reducing repetitive firing of action potentials in the nerves, that most directly decreases manic symptoms. In addition, drugs such as carbamazepine affect the release and reuptake of several neurotransmitters, including norepinephrine, GABA, dopamine, and glutamate. They also change several second messenger systems. No single mechanism has yet accounted for the anticonvulsants' ability to stabilize mood. Divalproex sodium also has been shown to have numerous neurotransmission effects. The most widely held theory of how it stabilizes mood swings relates to its effects on GABA. As the major inhibitory neurotransmitter in the CNS, increased levels of GABA and improved responsiveness of the neurons to GABA lead to the control of epileptic activity. Divalproex sodium increases levels of GABA in the CNS by activating its synthesis, inhibiting the catabolism (destructive metabolism) of GABA, increasing its release, and increasing receptor density (Solomon, Keitner, & Ryan, 1998). Other foci for research into the underlying mechanisms involved in mood stabilization are specific intracellular signalling pathways, in particular involving calcium signalling and inositol monophosphate (Dubovsky, Thomas, Hijazi, & Murphy, 1994).

Pharmacokinetics

Carbamazepine is an unusual drug and is absorbed in a somewhat variable manner. The liquid suspension is absorbed more quickly than the tablet form, but food does not appear to interfere with absorption. Peak plasma levels occur in 2 to 6 hours. Because high doses influence peak plasma levels and increase the risk for side effects, carbamazepine should be given in divided doses two or three times a day. The suspension, which has higher peak plasma levels and lower trough levels, must be given more frequently than the tablet form.

Valproic acid is more rapidly absorbed, but the enteric coating of divalproex sodium adds a delay of as long as 1 hour. Peak serum levels occur in about 1 to 4 hours. The liquid form (sodium valproate) is absorbed more rapidly and peaks in 15 minutes to 2 hours (Loscher, 2002). Food appears to slow absorption but does not lower bioavailability of the drug. Valproate is a good example of the importance of considering *bioequivalence*, a term referring to the abilities of two formulations of the same drug to induce a therapeutic response of similar magnitude and duration (Zintzaras, 2005). For example, divalproex, an enteric-coated formulation, has a half-life of 12 to 16 hours; is not affected by food intake and achieves more consistent plasma levels than valproic acid, which has a shorter half-life (8 hours); should not be taken with food; and produces gastrointestinal irritation in about 40% of patients.

Carbamazepine and valproic acid are highly protein bound; therefore, patients who are older, medically ill, or malnourished may experience the effects of increased unbound levels of both drugs. When given with other drugs that are competing for the same protein-binding sites, higher levels of unbound drug may occur. In both cases, these individuals risk more side effects and fluctuations in medication plasma levels. Newer agents for the treatment of bipolar affective disorder, such as gabapentin, have little protein binding and therefore are not subject to some of these effects. Carbamazepine and valproic acid also cross easily into the CNS and move into the placenta as well. Both are associated with an increased risk for birth defects, including spina bifida, and carbamazepine accumulates in foetal tissue. Carbamazepine and valproic acid are metabolized by the cytochrome P-450 system of microsomal hepatic enzymes. However, one of the metabolites of carbamazepine is potentially toxic. When other concurrent medications inhibit the enzymes that break down this toxic metabolite, severe adverse reactions are often the result (e.g., decreased prothrombin times and hepatotoxicity; Kalapos, 2002). Medications that inhibit this breakdown include erythromycin, verapamil, and cimetidine (now available in nonprescription form).

Carbamazepine activates its own metabolism through induction of the P-450 microsomal hepatic enzymes. Patients receiving carbamazepine may experience a precipitant drop in therapeutic blood levels and a relapse in symptoms, requiring a dosage increase for as long as 2 to 3 months after steady state has been achieved. Although valproic acid is also affected by other medications that stimulate the P-450 system, it does not enhance its own metabolism. Both carbamazepine and valproic acid are available in slow-release, extended-action forms, allowing for decreased daily dosing and improved adherence.

Nurses need to educate patients about potential drug interactions, especially with nonprescription medications. Nurses can also inform other health care practitioners who may be prescribing medication that these patients are taking carbamazepine. It is important to note that oral contraceptives may become ineffective, and female patients should be advised to use other methods of birth control.

Side Effects, Adverse Reactions, and Toxicity

The most common side effects of carbamazepine are dizziness, drowsiness, tremor, visual disturbance, nausea, and vomiting. These side effects may be minimized by initiating treatment in low doses. Patients should be advised that these symptoms will diminish, but care should be taken when changing positions or performing tasks that require visual alertness. Giving the drug with food may diminish nausea. Valproic acid also causes gastrointestinal disturbances, tremor, and lethargy. In addition, it can produce weight gain and alopecia (hair loss). These symptoms are transient and should diminish with the course of treatment. Dietary supplements of zinc and selenium may be helpful to patients experiencing hair loss. Constipation and urinary retention occur in some individuals. Nurses should monitor urinary output and assist patients to increase fluid consumption to decrease constipation.

Transient elevations in liver enzymes occur with both carbamazepine and valproic acid, but rarely do symptoms of hepatic injury occur. If the patient reports abnormal pain or shows signs of jaundice, the prescriber should be notified immediately. Several blood dyscrasias are associated with carbamazepine, including aplastic anaemia, agranulocytosis, and leucopenia. Patients should be advised to report fever, sore throat, rash, petechiae, or bruising immediately. In addition, advise patients of the importance of completing routine blood tests throughout treatment (including complete blood cell count and liver function tests).

Both valproic acid and carbamazepine may be lethal if high doses are ingested. Toxic symptoms appear in 1 to 3 hours and include neuromuscular disturbances, dizziness, stupor, agitation, disorientation, nystagmus, urinary retention, nausea and vomiting, tachycardia, hypotension or hypertension, cardiovascular shock, coma, and respiratory depression. Carbamazepine appears to be more lethal at lower doses, but valproic acid is absorbed rapidly, and gastric lavage may be ineffective, depending on time from ingestion.

Of the newer anticonvulsant drugs, lamotrigine (Lamictal) in rare cases produces severe, life-threatening rashes that usually occur within 2 to 8 weeks of treatment. This risk is highest in children. The use of lamotrigine should be immediately discontinued if a rash is noted. Topamax (topiramate) carries an increased risk for kidney stone formation. It can also cause a decrease

in serum digoxin levels and may decrease effectiveness of oral birth control agents. In addition, ongoing ophthalmologic monitoring is required because of reports of acute myopia with secondary glaucoma. In some women, these anticonvulsants may decrease the effectiveness of oral birth control agents. Because of the potentially significant adverse reactions that the anticonvulsants can produce, careful patient teaching and monitoring are required.

■ ANTIDEPRESSANT MEDICATIONS

Researchers in the 1950s who were investigating other drugs related to the phenothiazines for the treatment of psychosis discovered that imipramine, a related compound, relieved the symptoms of depression. Imipramine was the first of a number of medications that contained a three-ring structure in their chemical makeup and produced improvement in depression. These medications became known as TCAs. Table 12.9 lists other related TCAs still in use today.

Concurrent with the discovery of TCAs, an antibiotic, iproniazid, used in treating tuberculosis, was found to alleviate the symptoms of depression. Iproniazid increased the monoamine neurotransmitters by inhibiting MAO, the enzyme that breaks down these neurotransmitters inside the nerve cell. Iproniazid is no longer used, but related, more effective drugs, phenelzine and tranylcypromine, make up a subgroup of antidepressants called the MAOIs. The Canadian clinical guidelines for the treatment of depressive disorders developed by the CANMAT Depression Working Group (Kennedy et al., 2016) as first-line treatment recommendations for a major depressive episode (based on level I evidence and little evidence of differences in efficacy or tolerability) include SSRIs, SNRIs, agomelatine, mirtazapine, vortioxetine, and bupropion. Box 12.4 describes factors influencing choice of antidepressants. These classes and specific drugs are described below.

TCAs, MAOIs, and More

Throughout the 1960s and 1970s, the TCAs and MAOIs were the primary medications for treating depression. Research continued to develop new agents with increased effectiveness, while decreasing the side effects and potential lethal effects. In the 1980s, several medications that were significantly different in chemical structure were introduced. Bupropion (Wellbutrin), introduced in 1987, had actions that were significantly different from those of previous antidepressants, but concern about the risk for seizures and other side effects limited initial excitement about its use. In 1988, the release of fluoxetine (Prozac) received much public attention and resulted in an increased awareness of depression and its treatment. Fluoxetine was the first of a class of drugs

Table 12.9 Antidepressant Medications

Generic (Trade) Drug Name	Usual Dosage Range (mg/day)	Half-Life (hours)	Therapeutic Blood Level (ng/mL)
Tricyclic			
amitriptyline (Elavil)	50–300	31–46	110–250
clomipramine (Anafranil)	25–250	19–37	80–100
doxepin (Sinequan)	25–300	8–24	100–200
imipramine (Tofranil)	30–300	11–25	200–350
amoxapine (Asendin)	50–600	8	200–500
desipramine (Norpramin)	25–300	12–24	125–300
nortriptyline (Aventyl)	30–100	18–44	50–150
protriptyline (Vivactil)	15–60	67–89	100–200
Selective Serotonin Reuptake Inhibitors			
fluoxetine (Prozac)	20–80	2–9 days	72–300
sertraline (Zoloft)	50–200	24	Not available
paroxetine (Paxil)	10–50	10–24	Not available
fluvoxamine (Luvox)	50–300	17–22	Not available
citalopram (Celexa)	20–50	35	Not available
escitalopram (Lexapro)	10–20	27–32	Not available
Norepinephrine Selective Reuptake Inhibitors			
reboxetine	12	12	Not available
Norepinephrine and Serotonin Selective Reuptake Inhibitors			
venlafaxine	75–375	5–11	100–500
duloxetine	60–80	9–19	Not available
Other Antidepressant Medications			
trazodone (Desyrel)	150–600	4–9	650–1,600
nefazodone (Serzone)	100–600	2–4	Not available
bupropion (Wellbutrin)	200–450	8–24	10–29
mirtazapine (Remeron)	15–45	20–40	Not available
Monoamine Oxidase Inhibitors			
moclobemide (Manerix)	300–600	6–10	Not available
phenelzine (Nardil)	15–90	24 (effect lasts 3–10 days)	Not available
tranylcypromine (Parnate)	10–60	24 (effect lasts 3–10 days)	Not available

that acted "selectively" on one neurotransmitter, in this case serotonin. Other similarly selective medications, sertraline (Zoloft), paroxetine (Paxil), and fluvoxamine (Luvox), soon followed and together make up the SSRIs. The newest SSRIs include citalopram (Celexa) and escitalopram oxalate (Cipralex). Reboxetine is the only norepinephrine selective reuptake inhibitor available in Canada. Two available drugs, venlafaxine (Effexor) and duloxetine (Cymbalta), are selective to both serotonin

---

BOX 12.4 Factors Influencing Choice of Antidepressants

- Prior medication response
- Drug interactions and contraindications
- Medication responses in family members
- Concurrent medical and psychiatric disorders
- Patient preference
- Age of the patient
- Cost of medication

---

and norepinephrine. Agomelatine is a newer drug with targets at the melatonin and serotonin receptors. Vortioxetine is also a new SSRI-type drug with additional agonist or partial agonist at multiple serotonin receptor subtypes and antagonist to 5-HT7. The TCAs are now considered as second-line treatments and the MAOIs as third-line treatments (Kennedy et al., 2016).

Indications and Mechanisms of Action

The TCAs have multiple effects on a variety of receptors in the CNS, including reuptake inhibition at serotonin and norepinephrine transporters; down-regulation of specific serotonin and noradrenergic receptors; and blockade of cholinergic, adrenergic, and histamine receptors. On the other hand, the MAOIs are more specific in their actions. They inhibit MAO, an enzyme that breaks down monoamines, such as serotonin, thereby increasing synaptic neurotransmission, resulting in clinical improvement.

The primary indication for antidepressant medications is depression, thus the name "antidepressant." Symptoms such as loss of interest in the person's usual activities (anhedonia), depressed mood, lethargy or decreased energy, insomnia, decreased concentration, loss of appetite, and suicidal ideation usually respond (see Chapter 22 for a more complete discussion of the symptoms of depression). Antidepressants are also used to treat other symptoms and disorders, and increasingly the name antidepressant is somewhat misleading.

Antidepressants are prescribed to treat the whole range of anxiety disorders (see Chapter 23). Antidepressants are also used to treat eating disorders (see Chapter 25), depression in bipolar disorders, dysthymia, chronic pain disorders, and premenstrual syndrome. More sedating antidepressants are sometimes used in small doses to address sleep disturbances. Trazodone, amitriptyline, mirtazapine, and other agents have been used alone or as adjunctive interventions for sleep disturbance. Antidepressants are also used for other sleep disorders, such as sleep apnoea. Symptoms of some psychiatric disorders of childhood (see Chapter 30), such as attention deficit hyperactivity disorder (ADHD), enuresis (bed-wetting), and school phobia, often respond to antidepressant medication.

At times, the symptoms of depression present in an "atypical" manner, which is called *atypical depression*. Individuals with atypical depression have a mixture of anxiety and depression, increased appetite and sleep rather than the typical insomnia and loss of appetite, mood reactivity rather than consistent low mood, worsening of the symptoms in the evening, and oversensitivity to such interpersonal feelings as rejection. These target symptoms of atypical depression are more often seen in women and respond better to the MAOIs, such as phenelzine (Nardil), or to the mixed action antidepressants (those that have both direct neurotransmitter receptor action and reuptake properties), such as trazodone or nefazodone (Kennedy et al., 2016).

Pharmacokinetics

All of the antidepressant medications are well absorbed from the gastrointestinal system; however, some individual variations exist. For example, food slightly increases the amount of trazodone absorbed but decreases its maximum blood concentrations and lengthens the time to peak effects from 1 hour on an empty stomach to 2 hours with food. Food also increases the maximum concentrations of sertraline in the bloodstream and decreases the time to peak plasma levels, whereas fluoxetine and fluvoxamine are unaffected, although food may delay the absorption of fluoxetine. Food has little effect on the TCAs.

Nurses should review pharmacokinetic information as it applies to each individual medication. They must consider how this information will affect the patient's use of the medication given the target symptoms for which the drug is intended. For example, if trazodone is being used on a continuous dose schedule

for its antidepressant effect, the effects of food probably matter very little. However, if trazodone is being used in a small dose at bedtime to assist a patient to sleep, an empty stomach becomes important because food would lengthen the time of onset of clinical effects, in this case, sleep.

The TCAs undergo considerable first-pass metabolism but reach peak plasma concentrations in 2 to 4 hours. The TCAs are highly bound to plasma proteins, which make the association between blood levels and therapeutic clinical effects difficult. However, some plasma ranges have been established. Table 12.9 includes the available ranges for therapeutic blood levels of the TCAs. In addition, times to steady-state plasma levels have wide variations, and the effective dose of medication must be individualized. Other antidepressants are also highly protein bound, which means that drugs that compete for these binding sites may cause fluctuations in blood levels of the antidepressants. Venlafaxine has the lowest protein binding; therefore, drug interactions of this type are not expected with this medication. Blood level changes caused by the presence of other drugs competing with binding sites are not expected.

The onset of action also varies considerably, depending on specific symptoms. For example, an improvement in sleep often occurs earlier than effects on overall mood or anhedonia. Complete relief of symptoms may take several weeks. Full enzyme inhibition with the MAOIs may take as long as 2 weeks, but the energizing effects may be seen within a few days. The variable onset of action may add to their sense of discouragement and powerlessness.

Although antidepressants are primarily excreted by the kidneys, their routes of metabolism vary. Most of the TCAs have active metabolites that act in much the same manner as the parent drug. Therefore, in determining the rate of elimination, one must consider the half-lives of these metabolites. Most of these antidepressants may be given in a once-daily single dose. If the medication causes sedation, this dose should be given at bedtime. Fluoxetine cause more activation of energy and must be given in the morning. Venlafaxine, nefazodone, and bupropion are examples of antidepressants whose shorter half-life periods and other factors require administration two or three times per day. Extended-release venlafaxine formulation has allowed daily dosing with this drug. Fluoxetine and its active metabolite have particularly long half-lives, remaining present for as long as 5 to 6 weeks. This may affect a number of decisions. For example, women who wish to have children and are taking fluoxetine ideally should discontinue use of the agent at least 6 weeks before attempting to conceive. They should be advised to consult their prescriber before making this decision. Due to this long half-life, fluoxetine would also not be a good choice for intermittent use for premenstrual dysphoric disorder. Table 12.9 provides information about the average elimination half-lives of most of the antidepressants.

Most of the antidepressants are metabolized by the P-450 enzyme system so that drugs that induce this system tend to decrease blood levels of the antidepressants, and inhibitors of this system increase antidepressant blood levels. This effect varies according to the subfamily that is induced. For example, fluvoxamine (Luvox) substantially inhibits CYP1A2. Thus, other drugs that are metabolized by the system experience slower metabolism. These include such medications as amitriptyline, clomipramine, imipramine, clozapine, propranolol, theophylline, and caffeine (Armstrong, Cozza, & Oesterheld, 2002). Paroxetine, fluoxetine, and duloxetine are very potent inhibitors of CYP2D6, as well as being substrates for this CYP enzyme.

Side Effects, Adverse Reactions, and Toxicity

Side effects of the antidepressant medications vary considerably. Because the TCAs act at several types of receptors, in addition to serotonin and norepinephrine receptors, these drugs have many unwanted effects. Conversely, the SSRIs are more selective for serotonin and have comparatively fewer and better tolerated side effects. Attention to a patient's ability to tolerate side effects is critical because uncomfortable side effects are the primary reason patients discontinue medication treatment. With the TCAs, sedation, orthostatic hypotension, and anticholinergic side effects are the most common sources of discomfort for patients receiving these medications. See Chapter 22 for a comparison of side effects of antidepressant medications.

Receptor affinities may be helpful in predicting which side effects are most likely to occur with a given medication. Table 12.1 provides a summary of major receptor targets for common antidepressants. Using this table in conjunction with Chapter 22, nurses may be able to predict which side effects will be most common with each medication. Interventions to assist in minimizing these side effects are listed in Table 12.2.

Sexual dysfunction is a relatively common side effect, especially with the SSRIs. Erectile and ejaculation disturbances occur in men and anorgasmia in women. This side effect is often difficult to assess if the nurse has not obtained a sexual history before the initiation of use of the medication. Anorgasmia is particularly common with the SSRIs and often goes unreported, frequently because nurses and other health care providers do not ask. Bupropion and nefazodone (Serzone) appear to be least likely to cause sexual disturbance. In addition, when sexual dysfunction is related to the medication, several treatment options are available. These include a change in dose or type of antidepressant or, less frequently, using other medications to treat this side effect. Nurses must take responsibility for

discussing the potential for sexual side effects before initiation of drug treatment and for continuing to reassess during follow-up visits. The TCAs have the potential for cardiotoxicity, which limits their use in older adults. Symptoms include QT prolongation that may worsen preexisting cardiac conduction problems (such as second-degree heart block). The newer antidepressants, such as the SSRIs and bupropion, are less cardiotoxic, and nefazodone at this time exhibit no evidence of cardiotoxicity.

Antidepressants that block the dopamine receptor, such as amoxapine, have the potential to produce symptoms of NMS. Mild forms of extrapyramidal symptoms and endocrine changes, including galactorrhea and amenorrhea, may develop. Amoxapine should be avoided in older adult patients because it may be associated with the development of tardive dyskinesia with this age group. Rare occurrences and only mild forms of extrapyramidal symptoms, such as tightness in the jaw and muscle spasms, may occur with any of the TCAs or SSRIs (Zullino, Delacrausaz, & Baumann, 2002).

The most common side effects of the SSRIs include headache, anxiety, insomnia, transient nausea, vomiting, and diarrhoea. Sedation may also occur, especially with fluvoxamine. Most often, these medications are given in the morning, but if daytime sedation occurs, they may be given in the evening. Venlafaxine (Effexor) has little effect on acetylcholine and histamine; thus, the risks for sedation and anticholinergic symptoms are low. However, higher doses are associated with sexual dysfunction, sedation, diastolic hypertension, increased perspiration, constipation, dry mouth, tremors, blurred vision, and asthenia or muscle weakness. Elevations in blood pressure and heart rate have been described, and nurses should monitor these vital sign parameters, especially in patients who have a preexisting history of coronary artery disease. Nurses need to be very familiar with nefazodone (Serzone) and the clinical issues related to its side effects. Nefazodone is a phenylpiperazine antidepressant that is structurally related to trazodone. Its most common side effects include sedation, dizziness, and orthostatic hypotension; less common is increased risk for seizures. Drug–drug interactions between nefazodone and triazolam and alprazolam have been reported, with increased plasma levels of these benzodiazepines, resulting in an enhancement of the psychomotor impairment caused by these agents. Bupropion (Wellbutrin) has a chemical structure unlike any of the other antidepressants. Some of its pharmacologic profile is due to effects on dopamine systems, in addition to effects on serotonin and norepinephrine.

Bupropion's activating effects may be experienced as agitation or anxiety by some patients. Others also experience insomnia and appetite suppression. Rarely, bupropion has produced psychosis, including hallucinations and delusions. Most likely, this is secondary to the stimulation of dopamine systems. Dopamine is also associated with reward and motivated behaviour, which accounts for the increasingly common use of bupropion, under the trade name of Zyban, as a smoking cessation agent. The slightly increased risk for experiencing seizures with bupropion use has received the most attention. It has been found that if the total daily dose of bupropion is no more than 450 mg and no individual dose is greater than 150 mg, the risk for seizures with bupropion is no greater than the risk with the other TCAs (Ferry & Johnston, 2003). Most important, bupropion has not been found to cause sexual dysfunction and often is used in individuals who are experiencing these side effects.

The MAOIs can produce anticholinergic side effects (dizziness, dry mouth, blurred vision, constipation, nausea, peripheral oedema, urinary hesitancy) but at a much reduced rate compared with the TCAs. Orthostatic hypotension and sexual dysfunction, including decreased libido, impotence, and anorgasmia, can occur with MAOIs. The most serious side effect of the MAOIs is their interaction with tyramine-containing foods and certain medications. The food interaction occurs because MAOIs block the breakdown of tyramine, a trace amine with vasoconstrictor properties. Increased levels of tyramine can cause severe headaches and hypertension, stroke, and, in rare instances, death. Patients who are taking MAOIs are placed on a low-tyramine diet. This diet has been difficult for some individuals to follow,

and concerns about the risk for severe hypertension have led many clinicians to rarely use the MAOIs (see Table 12.10).

MAOIs in use in Canada include phenelzine (Nardil) and tranylcypromine (Parnate). These are considered irreversible MAOIs because they form unbreakable covalent bonds with MAO. It takes at least 2 weeks to produce replacement enzyme molecules after discontinuation of use of the medication. Moclobemide is an example of a reversible MAOI that is available in Europe and Canada. Although it acts in the same way as the irreversible MAOIs, moclobemide forms weaker bonds that are short lasting. Therefore, a less restrictive diet may be used with moclobemide. In addition to food restrictions, many prescription and nonprescription medications that stimulate the sympathetic nervous system (sympathomimetics) produce the same risk for hypertensive crisis as do foods containing tyramine. The nonprescription medication interactions primarily involve diet pills and cold remedies. Patients should be advised to check the labels of any nonprescription drugs carefully for a warning against use with antidepressants, especially the MAOIs, and then consult their prescriber or pharmacist before consuming these medications. Patients should notify other health care providers, including dentists, that they are taking an MAOI before being prescribed or given any other medication.

Suicide is a major concern when working with individuals who are depressed. Systematic suicide risk

Table 12.10   Example of a Tyramine-Restricted Diet

Category of Food	Food to Avoid	Food Allowed
Cheese	All matured or aged cheeses All casseroles made with these cheeses, pizza, lasagna, etc. Note: All cheeses are considered matured or aged except those listed under the "Foods Allowed" column	Fresh cottage cheese, cream cheese, ricotta cheese, and processed cheese slices. All fresh milk products that have been stored properly (e.g., sour cream, yogurt, ice cream)
Meat, fish, and poultry	Fermented/dry sausage: pepperoni, salami, mortadella, summer sausage, etc. Improperly stored meat, fish, or poultry Improperly stored pickled herring	All fresh packaged or processed meat (e.g., chicken loaf, hot dogs), fish, or poultry Refrigerate immediately and eat as soon as possible
Fruits and vegetables	Fava or broad bean pods (not beans) Banana peel	Banana pulp All others except those listed in the "Food to Avoid" column
Alcoholic beverages	All tap beers	Alcohol: No more than two domestic bottled or canned beers or 4-fluid-oz glasses of red or white wine per day; this applies to nonalcoholic beer also; please note that red wine may produce a headache unrelated to a rise in blood pressure
Miscellaneous foods	Marmite concentrated yeast extract Sauerkraut Soy sauce and other soybean condiments	Other yeast extracts (e.g., brewer's yeast) Soy milk

Adapted from Gardener, D. M., Shulman, K. I., Walker, S. E., & Tailor, S. A. N. (1996). The making of a user-friendly MAOI diet. *Journal of Clinical Psychiatry, 57,* 99–104.

assessment should be done routinely before initiating antidepressant therapy, in the first 2 to 4 weeks of treatment and for longer if indicated. Some of these medications are more lethal than others. For example, the TCAs pose a significant risk for overdose and are more lethal in children. Symptoms of overdose and treatment are discussed more fully in Chapter 22, but for now, it is important to remember that this potential exists. Sometimes, the prescriber will provide the patient with only small amounts of the medication, requiring more frequent visits, and will closely monitor use. In general, newer antidepressant medications, such as the SSRIs, are associated with less risk for toxicity and lethality in overdose. Box 12.5 highlights some of the newest antidepressants being tested in clinical trials.

BOX 12.5 Novel Antidepressant Drug Development

Research into the neurobiology of depression has implicated other neurotransmitter and neuroendocrine systems in the aetiology of depression. This has led to the development of new antidepressants, many of which are in clinical trials at this time.

For example, the hypothalamic–pituitary–adrenal (HPA) axis, a major stress hormone system, shows evidence of overactivity and blunted feedback control in depression. The principal activator of the HPA axis is a hormone called *corticotropin-releasing hormone* (CRH). This hormone is produced in the hypothalamus and stimulates the pituitary to release adrenocorticotropic hormone, which stimulates the release of cortisol from the adrenal gland. In depression, excessive CRH leads to increased levels of cortisol. Increased levels of cortisol are associated with some of the symptoms in depression, such as difficulty concentrating, sleep disturbance, and lowered energy. This led to the CRH theory of depression (Holsboer & Ising, 2008) and prompted the development of CRH antagonists and glucocorticoid receptor antagonists as potential antidepressants. Despite strong evidence that they would have antidepressant properties, no effective CRH antagonists have yet to be developed.

Glutamate is the major excitatory neurotransmitter and has been implicated in many psychiatric and neuropsychiatric disorders, including depression. Ketamine, a specific glutamate receptor antagonist, was shown to attenuate acute suicidal ideation (DiazGranados et al., 2010). There are trials of IV ketamine infusions under way to determine its efficacy in reducing refractory depression.

PHASES OF MOOD STABILIZING AND ANTIDEPRESSANT THERAPY

Initiation Phase

Overcoming issues such as social stigma, viewing depression and mood disorders as a personal failing, fear about taking a medication, and the decreased energy and motivation associated with depression have made the decision to seek treatment a major hurdle. The nurse plays an important role in helping patient through the phases of drug therapy.

Stabilization Phase

The treatment goal for bipolar disorder is to prevent relapse of the current episode or cycling into the opposite pole. It lasts about 2 to 9 months after acute symptoms resolve. The usual pharmacologic procedure in this phase is to titrate the mood stabilizer while closely monitoring the patient for signs or symptoms of relapse. In depression, patients will experience a lag between starting drug therapy and complete drug effect. Nurses should warn patients about potential side effects, such as nausea and diarrhoea, associated with most antidepressant. Dose increases or the addition of other antidepressant agents occur in this phase.

Maintenance Phase

The goal of treating this phase is to sustain remission and to prevent new episodes or bipolar disorder or depression. The great weight of evidence favours long-term prophylaxis against recurrence after the effective treatment of acute episodes. It is recommended that long-term or lifetime prophylaxis with a mood stabilizer be prescribed after two manic episodes or one severe manic episode or if there is a family history of bipolar disorder. Careful monitoring and follow-up are essential during this phase to assess patient response to medications, adjust dosage if necessary, identify and address side effects, and provide patient support and education.

Discontinuation Phase

Both bipolar disorders are typically recurrent and progressive; long-term suppressive medication may be indicated. Unlike many psychiatric disorders, depressive disorders may be time limited; thus, medication therapy should be reviewed periodically. The decision to discontinue active treatment is generally based on factors that include the frequency and severity of past episodes, the persistence of dysthymic symptoms after recovery, the presence of comorbid disorders, and patient preference.

Patients may be reluctant to take prescribed antidepressant medications or may self-treat depression. The continuation of medication, as well as emphasizing potential drug–drug interactions, should be included in the teaching plan.

ANTIANXIETY AND SEDATIVE– HYPNOTIC MEDICATIONS

Sometimes called anxiolytics, antianxiety medications and sedative–hypnotic medications come from various pharmacologic classifications, including benzodiazepines, nonbenzodiazepines, and nonbarbiturate sedative–hypnotics, such as chloral hydrate. These drugs represent some of the most widely prescribed medications today for the short-term relief of anxiety or anxiety associated with depression.

Benzodiazepines

Commonly prescribed benzodiazepines include chlordiazepoxide (Librium), diazepam (Valium), lorazepam (Ativan), flurazepam (Dalmane), oxazepam (Serax), and clonazepam (Rivotril).

Indications and Mechanisms of Action

Benzodiazepines act as positive modulators at $GABA_A$ ion channels, increasing the ease of GABA binding to its binding site. This enhancement of GABA binding increases both the duration and frequency of channel opening and decreases the firing rate of the nerve cell. This inhibition of nerve cell firing allows this class of drugs to act as anticonvulsants, antianxiety medications, or hypnotic, depending on dose and pharmacokinetic properties. Other neurotransmitter systems are also involved in the effects of benzodiazepines. Of the various benzodiazepines in use to relieve anxiety (and treat insomnia), oxazepam (Serax) and lorazepam (Ativan) are often preferred for patients with liver disease and for older adult patients because of their short half-lives.

Pharmacokinetics

The variable rate of absorption of the benzodiazepines determines the speed of onset. Table 12.11 provides relative indications of the speed of onset, from very fast to slow, for some of the commonly prescribed benzodiazepines.

Chlordiazepoxide (Librium) and diazepam (Valium) are slow, erratic, and sometimes incompletely absorbed when given IM, whereas lorazepam (Ativan) is rapidly and completely absorbed when given IM. Lorazepam is also well absorbed by the sublingual route.

All the benzodiazepines are highly lipid soluble and highly protein bound. They are distributed throughout the body and enter the CNS quickly. Other drugs that compete for protein-binding sites may produce drug–drug interactions. The degree to which each of these drugs is lipid soluble affects its duration of action. Most of these drugs have active metabolites, but the degree of activity of each metabolite affects the duration of action and elimination half-life. Most of these drugs vary markedly in the length of half-life. Oxazepam, which is itself an active metabolite of diazepam, and lorazepam have no active metabolites and thus have shorter half-lives. Sustained presence of these drugs after discontinuation may be observed in older adult or obese patients.

Side Effects, Adverse Reactions, and Toxicity

The most commonly reported side effects result from the sedative and CNS depression effects of these medications. Drowsiness, intellectual impairment, anterograde memory impairment, ataxia, and reduced motor coordination are common adverse effects. If used for sleep, many of these medications, especially long-acting benzodiazepines, produce significant "hangover"

Table 12.11 Antianxiety and Sedative–Hypnotic Medications			
Generic (Trade) Drug Name	Usual Dosage Range (mg/day)	Half-Life (hours)	Speed of Onset After Single Dose
Benzodiazepines			
diazepam (Valium)	4–40	30–100	Very fast
chlordiazepoxide (Librium)	15–100	50–100	Intermediate
clorazepate (Tranxene)	15–60	30–200	Fast
prazepam (Centrax)	20–60	30–200	Very slow
flurazepam (Dalmane)	15–30	47–100	Fast
lorazepam (Ativan)	2–8	10–20	Slow–intermediate
oxazepam (Serax)	30–120	3–21	Slow–intermediate
temazepam (Restoril)	15–30	9.5–20	Moderately fast
triazolam (Halcion)	0.25–0.5	2–4	Fast
alprazolam (Xanax)	0.5–10	12–15	Intermediate
clonazepam (Rivotril)	1.5–20	18–50	Intermediate
Nonbenzodiazepines			
buspirone (BuSpar)	15–30	3–11	Very slow
zolpidem (Sublinox)*	5–10	2.6	Fast

*5 mg for women and people over 65

effects experienced on awakening. Flunitrazepam (Rohypnol), otherwise known as the "date rape" drug because of its ability to impair anterograde memory, is illegal in Canada. Older adults receiving repeated doses of medications, such as flurazepam (Dalmane), at bedtime may experience paradoxical confusion, agitation, and delirium, sometimes after the first dose. In addition, daytime fatigue, drowsiness, and cognitive impairments may continue while the person is awake. For the older adult, drowsiness mixed with mental confusion can lead to falls and hip fractures. Current clinical guidelines for drug treatments in older adults strongly recommend avoiding benzodiazepine use in this population (Maust et al., 2017). For most patients, the effects subside as tolerance develops; however, alcohol increases all these symptoms and potentiates CNS depression. Indeed, benzodiazepines have a wide therapeutic index but can be lethal when used with alcohol. Individuals using these medications should be warned to be cautious when driving or performing other tasks that require mental alertness. If these tasks are part of the person's work requirements, another medication may be chosen. Administered intravenously, benzodiazepines often cause phlebitis and thrombosis at the intravenous sites, which should be monitored closely and changed if redness or swelling develops.

Because **tolerance** develops to most of the CNS depressant effects, individuals who wish to experience the feeling of "intoxication" from these medications may be tempted to increase their own dosage. Psychological dependence is more likely to occur when using these medications for a longer period, which is the reason benzodiazepines are, for the most part, to be used as short-term therapies. Abrupt discontinuation of the use of benzodiazepines may result in a recurrence of the target symptoms, such as rebound insomnia or anxiety. Other withdrawal symptoms appear rapidly, including tremors, increased perspiration, palpitations, increased sensitivity to light, abdominal discomfort or pain, and elevations in systolic blood pressure. These symptoms may be more pronounced with the short-acting benzodiazepines, such as lorazepam. Gradual tapering is recommended for discontinuing the use of benzodiazepines after long-term treatment. When tapering short-acting medications, the prescriber may switch the patient to a long-acting benzodiazepine before discontinuing the use of the short-acting drug.

Individual reactions to the benzodiazepines appear to be associated with sensitivity to their effects. Some patients feel apathy, fatigue, tearfulness, emotional lability, irritability, and nervousness. Benzodiazepines do little for depression symptoms, except for sleep disturbance, and may even exacerbate anhedonia and difficulties concentrating. As such, their use in depression, even with significant comorbid anxiety, should be closely monitored. Gastrointestinal disturbances, including nausea, vomiting, anorexia, dry mouth, and constipation, may develop. These medications may be taken with food to ease the gastrointestinal distress.

Older adults are particularly susceptible to incontinence, memory disturbances, dizziness, and increased risk for falls when using benzodiazepines. Pregnant patients should be aware that these medications cross the placenta and are associated with an increased risk for birth defects, such as cleft palate, mental retardation, and pyloric stenosis. Infants born addicted to benzodiazepines often exhibit flaccid muscle tone, lethargy, and difficulties sucking. All the benzodiazepines are excreted in breast milk, and breast-feeding women should avoid using these medications. Infants and children metabolize these medications more slowly; therefore, more drug accumulates in their bodies.

Toxicity can develop with liver dysfunction or disease. Symptoms include worsening of the CNS depression, ataxia, confusion, delirium, agitation, hypotension, diminished reflexes, and lethargy. Rarely do the benzodiazepines cause respiratory depression or death. In overdose, these medications have a high therapeutic index and rarely result in death unless combined with another CNS depressant drug, such as alcohol.

Nonbenzodiazepines: Buspirone and Zolpidem

One of the nonbenzodiazepines, buspirone (BuSpar), was first synthesized in 1968 by Michael Eison, who was searching for an improved antipsychotic medication. Later, it was found that buspirone was effective in controlling the symptoms of anxiety but had no effect on panic disorders and little effect on obsessive–compulsive disorder. Another nonbenzodiazepine, zolpidem (Sublinox) is a medication for sleep that acts on the benzodiazepine–GABA receptor complex.

Indications and Mechanisms of Actions

These drugs are effective for treating anxiety disorders without the CNS depressant effects or the potential for abuse and withdrawal syndromes. Canadian treatment guidelines for generalized anxiety disorder caution against long-term use of benzodiazepines and, based on level I evidence, recommend either the SSRI, paroxetine, or the NSRI, venlafaxine (Katzman et al., 2014). Buspirone is also indicated for treating generalized anxiety disorder; therefore, its target symptoms include anxiety and related symptoms, such as difficulty in concentrating, tension, insomnia, restlessness, irritability, and fatigue. Because buspirone does not add to depression symptoms, it has been tried for treating anxiety that coexists with depression. In some instances, it is thought to potentiate the antidepressant actions of other medications.

Buspirone has no effect on the benzodiazepine–GABA complex but instead appears to control anxiety by blocking the serotonin subtype of receptor, 5-HT$_{1a}$, at both presynaptic reuptake and postsynaptic receptor sites. It has no sedative, muscle relaxant, or anticonvulsant effects. It also lacks potential for abuse.

Zolpidem (Sublinox), which is indicated for short-term insomnia treatment, appears to increase slow-wave (deep) sleep and to modulate GABA$_A$ receptors, but with less risk for tolerance or withdrawal issues compared with benzodiazepines.

Pharmacokinetics

Buspirone is rapidly absorbed but undergoes extensive first-pass metabolism. Food slows absorption but appears to reduce first-pass metabolism, increasing the bioavailability of the medication. Buspirone is given on a continual dosing schedule of three times a day because of its short half-life of 2 to 3 hours. Clinical action depends on reaching steady-state concentrations; taking this medication with food may facilitate this process.

Buspirone is highly protein bound but does not displace most other medications. However, it does displace digoxin and may increase digoxin levels to the point of toxicity. It is metabolized in the liver and excreted predominantly by the kidneys but also through the gastrointestinal tract. Patients with liver or kidney impairment should be given this medication with caution.

Buspirone cannot be used on a PRN basis; rather, it takes 2 to 4 weeks of continual use for symptom relief to occur. It is more effective in reducing anxiety in patients who have never taken a benzodiazepine.

Buspirone does not block the withdrawal of other benzodiazepines. Therefore, a switch to buspirone must be initiated gradually to avoid withdrawal symptoms. Nurses should closely monitor patients who are undergoing this change of medication for emergence of withdrawal symptoms from the benzodiazepines and report such symptoms to the prescriber.

Zolpidem is metabolized by the liver; it crosses the placenta and enters breast milk. It has a short half-life of 3 hours, which makes it an ideal hypnotic and is excreted in the urine.

Side Effects, Adverse Reactions, and Toxicity

Common side effects from higher-dose buspirone include dizziness, drowsiness, nausea, excitement, and headache. Most other side effects occur at an incidence of less than 1%. There have been no reports of death from an overdose of buspirone alone. Older adults, pregnant women, and children have not been adequately studied. For now, buspirone can be assumed to cross the placenta and is present in breast milk; therefore, its use should be avoided in pregnant women, and women who are taking this medication should not breastfeed.

Rebound effects, such as insomnia and anxiety, from zolpidem are minimal. There are minimal effects on respiratory function and little potential for abuse. Although very rare, there have been cases of sleepwalking, sleepdriving, and other complex behaviours while asleep attributed to zolpidem use (Dolder & Nelson, 2008).

■ STIMULANTS

Amphetamines were first synthesized in the late 1800s but were not used for psychiatric disorders until the 1930s. Initially, amphetamines were prescribed for a variety of symptoms and disorders, but their high abuse potential soon became obvious.

Methylphenidate, Pemoline, and Modafinil

Among the medications known as stimulants are methylphenidate (Ritalin), used for attention deficit hyperactivity disorder (ADHD); pemoline (Cylert), a CNS stimulant also used for hyperactivity and attention deficit disorders; and modafinil (Provigil), used for narcolepsy, a sleep disorder.

Indications and Mechanisms of Action

Medical use of these drugs is now restricted to a few disorders, including narcolepsy; ADHD, particularly in children; and obesity unresponsive to other treatments. However, stimulants are increasingly being used as an adjunctive treatment in depression and other mood disorders to address the anhedonia and low energy common to these conditions.

Dextroamphetamine (Dexedrine) indirectly stimulates the sympathetic nervous system, producing alertness, wakefulness, vasoconstriction, suppressed appetite, and hypothermia. Tolerance develops to some of these effects, such as suppression of appetite, but the CNS stimulation continues. Although the exact mechanism of action is not completely understood, stimulants cause a release of catecholamines, particularly norepinephrine and dopamine, into the synapse from the presynaptic nerve cell. They also block the reuptake of these catecholamines. Methylphenidate is structurally similar to the amphetamines but produces a milder CNS stimulation. Pemoline is structurally dissimilar from the amphetamines but produces the same pharmacologic actions. Pemoline predominantly affects the dopamine system and therefore has less effect on the sympathetic nervous system.

Although the stimulant effects of these medications may seem logically indicated for narcolepsy, a disorder in which the individual frequently and abruptly falls asleep, the indications for childhood ADHD seem less obvious. The aetiology and neurobiology of ADHD remain unclear, but psychostimulants produce a paradoxic calming of the increased motor activity characteristic of ADHD. Studies show that medication decreases disruptive activity during school hours, reduces noise and verbal activity, improves attention span and short-term memory, improves ability to follow directions, and decreases distractibility and impulsivity. Although these improvements have been well documented in the literature, the diagnosis of ADHD and subsequent use of psychostimulants with children remain a matter of controversy (see Chapter 30).

Off-Label Use

Psychostimulants have also been used for other psychiatric disorders, and nurses must be aware that these medications are outside of Health Canada–approved indications for the medications. Used alone, stimulants are not indicated for treating depression. However, research has found that these medications may be beneficial as adjunctive medications, especially in those with severe psychomotor retardation (Candy, Jones, Williams, Tookman, & King, 2008). In addition, these medications have relieved lethargy, boosted mood, and reduced cognitive deficits associated with chronic medically debilitating conditions, such as chronic fatigue syndrome, acquired immunodeficiency syndrome, and some types of cancer, but more research is needed. This use remains a matter of controversy, and psychostimulants should be used very cautiously in individuals who have a history of substance abuse.

Modafinil (Alertec) is a new wake-promoting agent used for treating excessive daytime sleepiness (EDS) associated with narcolepsy and other health states. Patients with EDS cannot stay awake in the daytime, even after getting enough nighttime sleep. Although modafinil is approved by Health Canada only for treating narcolepsy, it is being used for other mental health symptoms. For example, small studies support the use of modafinil as an augmentation to antidepressants in major depressive disorder to address fatigue.

Pharmacokinetics

Psychostimulants are rapidly absorbed from the gastrointestinal tract and reach peak plasma levels in 1 to 3 hours. Considerable individual variations occur between the drugs in terms of bioavailability, plasma levels, and half-life. Table 12.12 compares the primary psychostimulants used in psychiatry. Some of these differences are age dependent because children metabolize these medications more rapidly, producing shorter elimination half-lives. Methylphenidate (Ritalin) is available in a sustained release form and should not be chewed or crushed.

The psychostimulants appear to be unaffected by food in the stomach and should be given after meals to reduce the appetite-suppressant effects when indicated. However, changes in urine pH may affect the rates of excretion. Excessive sodium bicarbonate alkalizes the urine and reduces amphetamine secretion. An increased vitamin C or citric acid intake may acidify the urine and increase its excretion. Starvation from appetite suppression may have a similar effect. All these drugs are highly lipid soluble, crossing easily into the CNS and the placenta. Psychostimulants undergo metabolic changes in the liver, where they may affect, or be affected by, other drugs. They are primarily excreted through the kidneys; therefore, renal dysfunction may interfere with excretion.

The precise action of modafinil (Alertec) in promoting wakefulness is unknown. It does appear to have wake-promoting actions similar to sympathomimetic agents such as amphetamine and methylphenidate, although the pharmacologic profile is not identical.

Table 12.12 Psychostimulant Medications		
Generic (Trade) Name and Half-Life	Usual Dosage Drug Range (mg/day)	Side Effects
dextroamphetamine (Dexedrine); 6–7 hours	5–40	Overstimulation Restlessness Dry mouth Palpitations Cardiomyopathy (with prolonged use or high dosage) Possible growth retardation (greatest risk); risk reduced with drug holidays
methylphenidate (Ritalin); 2–4 hours	10–60	Nervousness Insomnia Anorexia Tachycardia Impaired cognition (with high doses) Moderate risk for growth suppression
pemoline (Cylert); 12 hours (mean)	37.5–112.5	Insomnia Anorexia with weight loss Elevated liver function tests (ALT, AST, LDH) Jaundice Least risk for growth suppression

ALT, alanine aminotransferase; AST, aspartate aminotransferase; LDH, lactic dehydrogenase.

It is absorbed rapidly and reaches peak plasma concentration in 2 to 4 hours. The absorption of modafinil may be delayed by 1 to 2 hours if taken with food. Modafinil is eliminated through liver metabolism, with subsequent excretion of metabolites through renal excretion. Modafinil may interact with drugs that inhibit, induce, or are metabolized by CYP2C19 isoenzymes, including phenytoin, diazepam, and propranolol. Concurrent use of modafinil and other drugs metabolized by CYP2C19 may lead to increased circulating blood levels of the other drugs.

Psychostimulants are usually begun at a low dose and increased weekly, depending on improvement of symptoms and occurrence of side effects. Initially, children with ADHD are given a morning dose so that their school performance may be compared from morning to afternoon. Rebound symptoms of excitability and talkativeness may occur when use of the medication is withdrawn or after dose reduction. These symptoms also begin about 5 hours after the last dose of medication, which may affect the dosing regimen for some individuals. The return of symptoms in the afternoon for children with ADHD may require that a second dose be given at school. Prescribers should work with parents to implement other interventions after school and on weekends when the psychostimulants are not used. Severity of symptoms may require that the medications be continued during these times, but this dosing schedule should be determined after careful evaluation on an individual basis. Use of these medications should not be stopped abruptly, especially with higher doses, because the rebound effects may last for several days.

Side Effects, Adverse Reactions, and Toxicity

Side effects associated with psychostimulants typically arise within 2 to 3 weeks after beginning the medication. From most to least common, these side effects include appetite suppression, insomnia, irritability, weight loss, nausea, headache, palpitations, blurred vision, dry mouth, constipation, and dizziness. Because of the effects on the sympathetic nervous system, some individuals experience blood pressure changes (both hypertension and hypotension), tachycardia, tremors, and irregular heart rates. Blood pressure and pulse should be monitored initially and after each dosage change. Pemoline is associated with elevated liver enzymes and produces hepatotoxicity in 1% to 3% of children taking the medication; therefore, liver function tests should be obtained at least every 6 months. Liver function returns to normal when use of the medication is discontinued.

Rarely, psychostimulants suppress growth and development in children. These effects are a matter of controversy, and research has produced conflicting results. Although the suppression of height seems unlikely to some researchers, others have indicated that psychostimulants may have an effect on cartilage. Height and weight should be monitored several times annually for children taking these medications and compared with prior history of growth. Weight should be monitored especially closely during the initial phases of treatment. These effects also may be minimized by drug "holidays," such as during school vacations.

Rarely, individuals may experience mild dysphoria, social withdrawal, or mild to moderate depression. These symptoms are more common at higher doses and may require discontinuing the medication. Abnormal movements and motor tics may also increase in individuals who have a history of Tourette's syndrome. Psychostimulants should be avoided by patients with Tourette's symptoms or a positive family history of the disorder. In addition, dextroamphetamine has been associated with an increased risk for congenital abnormalities. Because there is no compelling reason for a pregnant woman to continue to take these medications, patients should be informed and should advise their prescriber immediately if they plan to become pregnant or if pregnancy is a possibility.

Death is rare from overdose or toxicity of the psychostimulants, but a 10-day supply may be lethal, especially in children. Symptoms of overdose include agitation, chest pain, hallucinations, paranoia, confusion, and dysphoria. Seizures may develop, along with fever, tremor, hypertension or hypotension, aggression, headache, palpitations, rashes, difficulty breathing, leg pain, and abdominal pain. Maximum dosage for children is 40 mg per day, with potential death resulting from a 400-mg dose. Parents should be warned regarding the potential lethality of these medications and take preventive measures by keeping the medication in a safe place.

Side effects associated with modafinil include nausea, nervousness, headache, dizziness, and trouble sleeping. If the effects continue or are bothersome, patients should consult the prescriber. Modafinil is generally well tolerated, with few clinically significant side effects. It is potentially habit forming and must be used with great caution in individuals with a history of substance abuse or dependence.

■ NEW MEDICATIONS

Each country has its own approval process for new medications. In Canada, this process is controlled by Health Canada. Through various phases of drug testing, a new drug must be determined to have therapeutic benefit based on known physiologic processes, animal testing, and laboratory models of human disease and its potential toxicity predicted at doses likely to produce clinical improvement in humans (see Box 12.6 for more information). Then, the pharmaceutical company can begin research with human volunteers after filing an *investigational new drug* (IND) application.

BOX 12.6 Phases of New Drug Testing

- *Phase I*: Testing defines the range of dosages tolerated in healthy individuals.
- *Phase II*: Effects of the drug are studied in a limited number of individuals with the target disorder.
- *Phase III*: Extensive clinical trials are conducted at multiple sites throughout the country with larger numbers of patients. Efforts focus on corroborating the efficacy identified in phase II. Phase III concludes with a new drug application (NDA) being submitted to Health Canada.
- *Phase IV*: Postmarketing surveillance continues to detect new or rare adverse reactions and potentially new indications. During this period, adverse reactions from the new medication are required to be reported to Health Canada.

IMPLICATIONS FOR MENTAL HEALTH NURSES

Throughout the phases, side effects and adverse reactions are monitored closely. The studies are tightly controlled, and strict regulations are enforced at each step.

Clinical trials for new drugs usually involve patient populations that have no other health problems but the one under study. This is important to test the drug's effectiveness, but in clinical practice, many patients have other health problems, and postmarketing surveillance helps identify unforeseen benefits or adverse effects in most heterogeneous patient populations.

A newly approved drug is approved only for the indications for which it has been tested. However, there is often a widening of application for other health problems over time (called *off-label* uses).

In Canada, the pharmaceutical companies must follow strict guidelines in terms of product advertising and interaction with health professionals. For example, the companies are not permitted to advertise directly to the public, and there are stringent guidelines regarding any potential sales incentives offered to health professionals. This is to address potential ethical issues around influencing prescriber preferences.

Many new psychiatric medications, particularly the atypical antipsychotics and novel antidepressants, are in various phases of clinical testing and are expected to be released in the coming years. Keeping the phases of new drug development in mind will assist the nurse in understanding what to expect from drugs newly released to the market.

■ OTHER BIOLOGIC TREATMENTS

Biologic treatment is the term applied to treatments that work at a somatic, physical level but are nonpharmacologic in nature. There is a long history of using somatic therapies to treat neuropsychiatric illnesses. Throughout history, numerous treatments have been developed and used to change the biologic basis of what was thought, at the time, to cause psychiatric disorders. Insulin coma, atropine coma, hemodialysis, hyperbaric oxygen therapy, continuous sleep therapy, and ether and carbon dioxide inhalation therapies are examples of some of the historical treatments that seemed to relieve some symptoms, but results could not be replicated, or potential adverse effects proved too great a risk. Although the primary biologic interventions remain pharmacologic, some somatic treatments continue to show efficacy, whereas others have gained acceptance, remain under investigation, or show promise for the future. Common somatic treatments include the following: ECT, phototherapy, nutritional therapy, and, most recently, transcranial magnetic stimulation and vagus nerve stimulation (VNS).

Electroconvulsive Therapy

For hundreds of years, seizures have been known to produce improvement in some psychiatric symptoms. ECT was formally introduced in Italy in 1938. It is one of the oldest medical treatments available and remains safely in use today. Every year, over 1 million people in the world receive ECT for the treatment of severe depression (Payne & Prudic, 2009b). Although individuals with severe forms of depression, where delusions and/or paranoia are present, seem the best candidates for ECT, research has yet to determine accurate predictors of a person's response to ECT (Kellner et al., 2016). With ECT, a brief electrical current is passed through the brain to produce generalized seizures lasting 25 to 150 seconds. Short-acting anaesthetics and muscle relaxing agents are given before ECT, and the patient does not feel the stimulus or recall the procedure. A brief pulse stimulus, administered unilaterally on the nondominant side of the head, is associated with less confusion after ECT. However, some individuals require bilateral treatment for the effective resolution of depressive symptoms. Induction of a seizure is necessary to produce positive treatment outcomes. Because individual seizure thresholds vary and increase with age, the electrical impulse and treatment method also may vary. Older adults may experience longer postprocedure disorientation; however, it is unclear if changes in electric dose may improve this finding (Magne et al., 2016). Blood pressure and the ECG are monitored during the procedure. This procedure is repeated two or three times a week, usually for a total of 6 to 12 treatments. Because there is no particular difference in treatment efficacy and a twice-weekly regimen produces less accumulative memory loss, this treatment course is often chosen. After symptoms have improved, antidepressant medications are used to prevent relapse. Some patients who cannot take or do not experience response to antidepressant treatment may go on maintenance ECT treatments. Usually, once-weekly treatments are gradually decreased in frequency to once monthly. The number and frequency of treatments vary depending on the individual's response. Although coadministration of ketamine was thought to yield greater antidepressant effect, recent studies have shown no added benefit of this regime (Anderson et al., 2016).

Although ECT produces rapid improvement in depressive symptoms, its exact mechanism of antidepressant action remains unclear. From a neural perspective, ECT decreases the activity in the central nodes of the default mode network (Chau, Fogelman, Nordanskog, Drevets, & Hamilton, 2017). It is known to down-regulate β-adrenergic receptors in much the same way as antidepressant medications. However, unlike antidepressant therapy, ECT produces an up-regulation in serotonin, especially 5-HT$_2$. ECT also has several other actions on neurochemistry, including increased influx of calcium and effects on second messenger systems. People with higher levels of brain-derived neurotrophic factor (BDNF) experience higher levels of remission. This biologic marker may be used in the future as a test to predict ECT efficacy among individuals with major depression (Freire, de Almeida Fleck, & da Rocha, 2016).

Brief episodes of hypotension or hypertension, bradycardia or tachycardia, and minor arrhythmias are among the adverse effects that may occur during and immediately after the procedure but usually resolve quickly. Common aftereffects from ECT include headache, nausea, and muscle pain. Memory loss or disturbance is the most troublesome effect of ECT. Such cognitive side effects include *transient postictal* ("after seizure") *disorientation* that clears in minutes to hours and *anterograde amnesia* (amnesia for events occurring during and soon after a course of ECT). Nurses should document these symptoms and plan to interventions for subsequent ECT treatments. Other possible cognitive effects are *short-term retrograde amnesia* (gaps in memory about things occurring a few weeks or months before the ECT) that usually clears within weeks and *retrograde memory loss* (persistent, severe memory deficits) that occurs rarely (Payne & Prudic, 2009a). Many patients experience no amnesia at all. Memory loss occurring as part of the symptoms of untreated depression presents a confounding factor in determining the exact nature of the memory deficits from ECT. It is important to remember that patient surveys are positive, with most individuals reporting that they were helped by ECT and would have it again (Hirose, 2002).

ECT is contraindicated in patients with an increased intracranial pressure. Risk also increases in patients with recent myocardial infarction, recent cerebrovascular accident, retinal detachment, or pheochromocytoma (a tumour on the adrenal cortex) and in patients at high risk for complications from anaesthesia.

Light Therapy (Phototherapy)

Human circadian rhythms are set by time clues (zeitgebers) inside and outside the body. One of the most powerful regulators of these body patterns is the cycle of daylight and darkness. Research findings indicate that some individuals with depressive symptoms that worsen at specific times of the year (have a seasonal pattern) may experience disturbance in these normal body patterns or of circadian rhythms (Ekselius, Mårtensson, Pettersson, & Berglund, 2015; Kragh et al., 2017). For example, some individuals are more depressed during the winter months, when there is less light, and they improve spontaneously in the spring. (See Chapter 22 for a complete description of depression and mood disorders.) These individuals usually have symptoms that are somewhat different from classic depression, including fatigue, increased need to sleep, increased appetite and weight gain, irritability, and carbohydrate craving. Administering artificial light to these patients during winter months has reduced these depressive symptoms.

Light therapy, sometimes called phototherapy, involves exposing the patient to a specific type of artificial light source to relieve seasonal depression. Artificial light is believed to trigger a shift in the patient's circadian rhythm to an earlier time. Research remains ongoing. The light source must be very bright, full-spectrum light, usually 2,500 lux, which is about 200 times brighter than normal indoor lighting. Harmful ultraviolet light is filtered out.

Studies have shown that morning phototherapy produces a better response than either evening or morning and evening timing of the **phototherapy** session (Penders et al., 2016). Light banks with full-spectrum light may be put together by the individual or obtained from various companies now producing these light sources. Light visors, visors containing small, full-spectrum light bulbs that shine on the eyelids, have also been developed. The patient is instructed to sit in front of the lights at a distance of about 3 feet, engaging in a variety of other activities, but glancing directly into the light every few minutes. This should be done immediately upon waking and is most effective before 8 AM. The duration of administration may begin with as little as 30 minutes and increase to 2 to 5 hours. One to two hours is usually sufficient, and the antidepressant response begins in 1 to 4 days, with the full effect usually complete after 2 weeks. Full antidepressant effect is usually maintained with daily sessions of 30 minutes.

Side effects of phototherapy are rare, but eye strain, headache, and insomnia are possible. An ophthalmologist should be consulted if the patient has a preexisting eye disorder. In rare instances, phototherapy has been reported to produce mania. Irritability is a more common complaint. Follow-up visits with the prescriber or therapist are needed to help manage side effects and assess positive results.

Nutritional Therapies

The neurotransmitters necessary for normal healthy functioning are produced from amino acids taken in with the foods we eat. Many nutritional deficiencies may produce symptoms of psychiatric disorders. Fatigue, apathy, and depression are caused by deficiencies in iron, folic acid, pantothenic acid, magnesium, vitamin C, or biotin. Logically, treating these deficiencies with nutritional supplements should improve the psychiatric symptoms. The question becomes: Can nutritional supplements actually treat psychiatric disorders?

Older theories and related diets are based on the belief that food controls behaviour. High sugar intake was once thought to produce hyperactivity in children, and Benjamin Feingold developed a diet to eliminate food additives that he believed increased hyperactivity. More recently, advances in technology have led research to new investigations regarding dietary precursors for the bioamines. For example, tryptophan, the dietary precursor of serotonin, has been most extensively investigated as it relates to low serotonin levels and increased aggression. Individuals who have low tryptophan levels are prone to have lower levels of serotonin in the brain, resulting in depressed mood and aggressive behaviour (Young & Leyton, 2002). Some individuals with mild depression do respond to large amounts of tryptophan, and tryptophan has been used as an adjunct to antidepressant drugs. Many individuals are turning to dietary herbal preparations to address psychiatric symptoms, but the results are variable.

Despite increased use of St. John's wort for depression, ginkgo for cognitive impairment, and kava for anxiety, systematic reviews provide mixed evidence for their effectiveness. St John's wort is as effective for the treatment of mild depressive symptoms, but the drug–drug interactions are numerous and must be carefully evaluated. Birks and Grimley Evans (2009) found no evidence for the use of ginkgo for dementia, and kava was removed from the market for its high risk of toxicity. Nurses need to include an assessment of these agents into their overall patient assessment to understand the needs of the patient.

Though routine use of nutritional supplements cannot be routinely recommended, clear evidence exists to support the use of vitamin B1 (Thiamine) to prevent Wernicke's encephalopathy in people withdrawing from chronic alcohol use (Johnson, Wilson, & deBoisblanc, 2016). Other B vitamins, such as pyridoxine (B6) at high doses, can cause neurotoxic symptoms. More research is needed to identify the underlying mechanisms and relationships of dietary supplements and dietary precursors of the bioamines to mood and behaviour and psychopharmacologic medications. For now, it is important for the nurse to recognize that diet can have a significant impact on behaviour in sensitive individuals and that supplements can be a potential source of drug–drug interaction.

Newer Somatic Therapies

Repetitive transcranial magnetic stimulation (rTMS) and VNS are two emerging somatic treatments for psychiatric disorders. Both are ways to directly affect brain activity by stimulating nerve cell firing rates. While the interest in these therapeutic modalities originated between 15 and 20 years ago, more research is needed to better understand their utility in contemporary psychiatry.

Transcranial magnetic stimulation was introduced in 1985 as a noninvasive, painless method to stimulate the cerebral cortex. Underlying this procedure is the hypothesis that a time-varying magnetic field will induce an electrical field, which, in brain tissue, activates the inhibitory and excitatory neurons (Kanno, Matsumoto, Togashi, Yoshioka, & Mano, 2003), thereby modulating neuroplasticity in the brain. The low-frequency electrical stimulation from rTMS triggers lasting anticonvulsant effects in rats, and the therapeutic benefits of rTMS in humans are thought to be related to action similar to that produced by anticonvulsant medication. rTMS has been used for both clinical and research purposes. rTMS stimulation of the brain's prefrontal cortex may help some depressed patients in much the same way as ECT but without its side effects (Martin et al., 2003). In Alzheimer's disease, patient exposed to rTMS may improve in cognition, apathy, and dependence (Nguyen et al., 2017). The role of rTMS as a rehabilitative treatment in people with traumatic brain injury (TBI) is being explored (Neville et al., 2015).

VNS is the newest of the available somatic treatments (Pisapia & Baltuch, 2016). For years, scientists have been interested in identifying how autonomic functions modulate activity in the limbic system and higher cortex. The vagus nerve has traditionally been considered a parasympathetic efferent nerve that was responsible only for regulating autonomic functions, such as heart rate and gastric tone. However, the vagus nerve (cranial X) also carries sensory information to the brain from the head, neck, thorax, and abdomen, and research has identified that the vagus nerve has extensive projections of its sensory afferent connections to many brain areas (Armitage, Husain, Hoffmann, & Rush, 2003). VNS is primarily being used for the treatment of drug-resistant epilepsy (Morace et al., 2017).

PSYCHOSOCIAL ISSUES IN BIOLOGIC TREATMENTS

Many factors influence successful medication and other biologic therapies. Of particular importance are issues related to adherence. Adherence refers to following the therapeutic regimen, self-administering medications as prescribed, keeping appointments, and following other treatment suggestions. For instance, as adherence to oral antipsychotic medications is between 40% and 60%, a new tool, the *antipsychotic medication adherence scale*, is being developed to assist nurses and other clinicians to better detect potential nonadherence and plan interventions to increase rates of drug adherence (Martins et al., 2016). Box 12.7 lists some of the common reasons for nonadherence. It is also important to not conclude that the patient is nonadherent until a full assessment is completed.

The most often cited reasons for nonadherence are related to side effects of the medication. Improved functioning may be observed by health care professionals but not felt by the patient. Side effects may interfere with work performance or other important aspects of the individual's life. For example, a construction worker cannot afford to be drowsy and sedated while operating a crane at a construction site, or a woman in an intimate relationship may find anorgasmia intolerable. Nurses need to be sensitive to the patient's ability to tolerate side effects and to the impact that side effects have on the patient's life. Medication choice, dosing schedules, and prompt treatment of side effects may be crucial factors in helping patients to continue their treatment, even if the symptoms for which they initially sought help have improved.

Cognitive deficits associated with some psychiatric disorders may make it difficult for the individual to self-monitor, develop insight, make choices, remember to fill prescriptions, or keep appointments. Family members may have beliefs and attitudes that influence the individual not to take the medication. They may misunderstand or deny the illness; for example, "My wife's better, so she doesn't need that medicine anymore." Family members may be distressed when observable side effects occur. Akinesia, which has been linked to suicidal thoughts as a way to relieve the subjective discomfort, may be the most distressing side effect for family members of individuals who have schizophrenia (Meltzer, 2000; Niedermeyer, 2008). Patients may also be reluctant to disclose financial constraints, especially in relation to the cost of newer agents, and may try to stretch out the prescription or just not fill their prescription.

Adherence concerns must not be dismissed as the patient's or family's problem. Nurses should actively address this issue. A positive therapeutic relationship between the nurse and the patient and family must provide a strong sense of trust that side effects and other difficulties in treatment will be addressed and minimized. When individuals report distressing side effects, the nurse should immediately respond with assessment and interventions to reduce these effects or, at the very least, to validate the patient's concern. It is important to assess adherence often, asking questions in a nonthreatening, nonjudgmental manner.

Adherence can be improved by psychoeducation. This approach is most helpful if it addresses the individual's specific symptoms and concerns. For example, if the patient is having difficulty with understanding the purpose of the medication, it may be helpful to link taking it to a reduction of specific unwanted symptoms or improved functioning, such as continuing to work.

Other factors that interfere with adherence should also be assessed and plans developed to minimize their effect. For example, an individual who is being considered for clozapine therapy may have missed a number of appointments in the past. On assessment, the nurse may discover that it takes the individual 2 hours on three different busses each way to reach the clinic. The nurse can then assist with arranging for a home health nurse to visit the patient's apartment, draw blood samples for analysis, and assess side effects, thus decreasing the number of trips the patient must make to the clinic.

BOX 12.7 Common Reasons for Nonadherence With Medication Regimens

- Uncomfortable side effects and those that interfere with quality of life, such as work performance or intimate relationships
- Lack of awareness of or denial of illness
- Stigma
- Feeling better
- Limited psychoeducation and follow-up
- Difficulties in access to treatment and cost of newer drug therapies
- Substance abuse

SUMMARY OF KEY POINTS

- Psychopharmacology is the study of medications used to treat psychiatric disorders, including the drug categories of antipsychotics, mood stabilizers, antidepressants, antianxiety medications, and psychostimulants.
- PK refers to the how drugs move through the body. The phases are absorption, distribution, metabolism, and excretion.
- Pharmacodynamics refers to the actions of drugs on living tissue and the human body, with the focus primarily on drug actions at receptor sites, on transporters, and on enzyme activity.

- The importance of receptors is recognized in current psychopharmacology. Biologic action of many drugs depends on how their structure interacts with a specific receptor, functioning either as an agonist, reproducing the same biologic action as a neurotransmitter, or as an antagonist, blocking the response.
- A drug's ability to interact with a given receptor type may be judged on three qualities: selectivity—the ability to interact with specific types of receptors; affinity—the attraction the drug has for the binding site; and intrinsic activity—the ability to produce a certain biologic response.
- Many characteristics of specific drugs affect how well they act and how they affect patients. Nurses must be familiar with characteristics, adverse reactions, and toxicity of certain drugs to administer psychotropic medications safely, educate patients regarding their safe use, and encourage therapeutic adherence.
- Bioavailability describes the amount of the drug that actually reaches the systemic circulation.
- The wide variations in pharmacokinetic properties across individuals are related to physiologic differences caused by age, genetic makeup, other disease processes, and chemical interactions.
- Antipsychotic medications are drugs used in treating psychotic disorders, such as schizophrenia. They act primarily by blocking dopamine or serotonin postsynaptically. In addition, they have a number of actions on other neurotransmitters. Older typical antipsychotic drugs work on positive symptoms and are inexpensive, but they produce many side effects. Newer atypical antipsychotic drugs work on positive and negative symptoms; are much more expensive but have far fewer anticholinergic side effects; and are better tolerated by patients, but increase risk for metabolic disorders.
- Medication-related movement disorders are a particularly serious group of side effects that principally occur with the typical antipsychotic medications and that may be acute syndromes, such as dystonia, pseudoparkinsonism, and akathisia, or chronic syndromes, such as tardive dyskinesia.
- The mood stabilizers, or antimania medications, are drugs used to control wide variations in mood related to mania, but these agents may also be used to treat other disorders. Lithium and the anticonvulsants are chemically unrelated and act in different ways to stabilize mood.
- Antidepressant medications are drugs used primarily for treating symptoms of depression but are also used extensively for anxiety disorders and eating disorders. They act by blocking the reuptake of one or more of the monoamines, especially serotonin and norepinephrine. These medications vary considerably in their structure and action. Newer antidepressants, such as the SSRIs, have fewer side effects and are less lethal in overdose than the older TCAs.
- Antianxiety medications also include several subgroups of medications, but SSRIs, NSRIs, benzodiazepines, and nonbenzodiazepines are those principally used in psychiatry. Benzodiazepines act by enhancing the actions of GABA, whereas the nonbenzodiazepine buspirone acts on serotonin. Benzodiazepines can be used on a PRN basis, whereas buspirone must be taken regularly.
- Psychostimulants enhance neurotransmitter activity, acting at a number of different receptor sites. These medications are most often used for treating symptoms related to ADHD and narcolepsy.
- ECT uses the application of an electrical pulsation to induce seizures in the brain. These seizures produce a number of effects on neurotransmission that result in the fairly rapid relief of depressive symptoms.
- rTMS and VNS are two emerging somatic treatments for psychiatric disorders. They are both means to directly affect brain function through the stimulation of the nerves that are direct extensions of the brain.
- Phototherapy involves the application of full-spectrum light in the morning hours, which appears to reset circadian rhythm delays related to seasonal affective disorder and other forms of depression. Nutritional therapies are in various stages of investigation.
- Adherence refers to the ability of an individual to self-administer medications as prescribed and to follow other instructions related to medication treatment. Nonadherence is related to factors such as medication side effects, cost, stigma, and family influences. Nurses play a key role in educating patients and helping them to improve adherence.

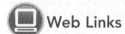 **Web Links**

www.ismp-canada.org This is the site for the Institute for Safe Medication Practices (ISMP), an independent, national, nonprofit organization focused on medication safety in health care settings. ISMP works with health care services, regulatory agencies, patient safety organizations, the pharmaceutical industry, and the public to promote safe practices by analyzing medication incidents, making recommendations for prevention of such incidents, and facilitating quality improvement.

References

Anderson, I. M., Blamire, A., Branton, T., Clark, R., Downey, D., Dunn, G., … Holland, F. (2016). Randomised-controlled trial of ketamine augmentation of ECT on neuropsychological and clinical outcomes in depression (ketamine-ECT study). *European Neuropsychopharmacology, 26,* S382.

Armitage, R., Husain, M., Hoffmann, R., & Rush, A. J. (2003). The effects of vagus nerve stimulation on sleep EEG in depression: A preliminary report. *Journal of Psychosomatic Research, 54*(5), 475–482.

Armstrong, S. C., Cozza, K. L., & Oesterheld, J. R. (2002). Med-psych drug-drug interactions update. *Psychosomatics, 43*(1), 77–81.

Baker, G. B., Urichuk, L. J., & Coutts, R. T. (1998). Drug metabolism and metabolic drug-drug interactions in psychiatry. *Journal of Child and Adolescent Pharmacology News Supplement, 1,* 1–8.

Bauer, M., & Gitlin, M. (2016). Treatment of mania with lithium. In *The essential guide to lithium treatment* (pp. 61–70). Cham, Switzerland: Springer International Publishing.

Bellivier, F., Belzeaux, R., Scott, J., Courtet, P., Golmard, J. L., & Azorin, J. M. (2017). Anticonvulsants and suicide attempts in bipolar I disorders. *Acta Psychiatrica Scandinavica, 135*(5), 470–478.

Bilici, M., Tekelioglu, Y., Efendioglu, S., Ovali, E., & Ulgen, M. (2003). The influence of olanzapine on immune cells in patients with schizophrenia. *Progress in Neuropsychopharmacology and Biological Psychiatry, 27*(3), 483–485.

Birks, J., & Grimley Evans, J. (2009) Ginkgo biloba for cognitive impairment and dementia. *Cochrane Database of Systematic Reviews,* (1). Art. No. CD003120. doi:10.1002/14651858.CD003120.pub3

Breit, S., & Hasler, G. (2016). Advantages and controversies of depot antipsychotics in the treatment of patients with schizophrenia. *Der Nervenarzt, 87*(7), 719–723.

Brunoni, A. R., Moffa, A. H., Sampaio-Júnior, B., Gálvez, V., & Loo, C. K. (2017). Treatment-emergent mania/hypomania during antidepressant treatment with transcranial direct current stimulation (tDCS): A systematic review and meta-analysis. *Brain Stimulation, 10*(2), 260–262.

Bschor, T., Baethge, C., Adli, M., Lewitzka, U., Eichmann, U., & Bauer, M. (2003). Hypothalamic-pituitary-thyroid system activity during lithium augmentation therapy in patients with unipolar major depression. *Journal of Psychiatry and Neuroscience, 28*(3), 210–216.

Candy, M., Jones, L., Williams, R., Tookman, A., & King, M. (2008). Psychostimulants for depression. *Cochrane Database of Systematic Reviews, 16*(2), CD006722.

Chau, D. T., Fogelman, P., Nordanskog, P., Drevets, W. C., & Hamilton, J. P. (2017). Distinct neural-functional effects of treatments with selective serotonin reuptake inhibitors, electroconvulsive therapy, and transcranial magnetic stimulation and their relations to regional brain function in major depression: A meta-analysis. *Biological Psychiatry: Cognitive Neuroscience and Neuroimaging, 2*(4), 318–326.

Chouinard, G., & Chouinard, V. A. (2008). Atypical antipsychotics: CATIE study, drug-induced movements disorder and resulting iatrogenic psychiatric-like symptoms, supersensitivity rebound psychosis and withdrawal syndromes. *Psychotherapy and Psychosomatics, 77*(2), 69–77.

Clarke, S. F., Karalliedde, L. D., Collignon, U., & Abeyratne, S. (2016). *Individual variability of adverse drug interactions.* In L. D. Karalliedde, S. J. Clarke, U. Gotel, & J. Karalliedde (Eds.), *Adverse drug interactions: A handbook for prescribers.* (pp. lxvii–lxxxi). Boca Raton, FL: CRC Press.

Corrado, A. C., & Walsh, J. P. (2016). Mechanisms underlying the benefits of anticonvulsants over lithium in the treatment of bipolar disorder. *NeuroReport, 27*(3), 131–135.

Cosci, F. (2016). Withdrawal symptoms after discontinuation of a noradrenergic and specific serotonergic antidepressant: A case report and review of the literature. *Personalized Medicine in Psychiatry, 1–2,* 81–84.

Crettol, S., De Leon, J., Hiemke, C., & Eap CB. (2014). Pharmacogenomics in psychiatry: From TDM to genomic medicine. *Clinical Pharmacology & Therapeutics, 95*(3), 254–257.

Dalfen, A. K. & Stewart, D. E. (2001). Who develops severe or fatal adverse drug reactions to selective serotonin reuptake inhibitors? *Canadian Journal of Psychiatry, 46*(3), 258–263.

DiazGranados, N., Ibrahim, L., Brutsche, N., Ameli, R., Henter, I. D., Luckenbaugh, D. A., ... Machado-Vieira, R. (2010). Rapid resolution of suicidal ideation after a single infusion of an NMDA antagonist in patients with treatment-resistant major depressive disorder. *Journal of Clinical Psychiatry, 71*(12), 1605–1611.

Dolder, C. R., & Nelson, M. H. (2008). Hypnosedative-induced complex behaviors: Incidence, mechanisms and management. *CNS Drugs, 22*(12), 1021–1036.

Dubovsky, S. L., Thomas, M., Hijazi, A., & Murphy, J. (1994). Intracellular calcium signalling in peripheral cells of patients with bipolar affective disorder. *European Archives of Psychiatry and Clinical Neuroscience, 243*(5), 229–234.

Eap, C. B. (2016). Personalized prescribing: A new medical model for clinical implementation of psychotropic drugs. *Dialogues in Clinical Neuroscience, 18*(3), 313.

Ekselius, L., Mårtensson, B., Pettersson, A., & Berglund, L. (2015). Bright white light therapy in depression: A critical review of the evidence. *Journal of Affective Disorders, 182,* 1–7

Ferry, L., & Johnston, J. A. (2003). Efficacy and safety of bupropion SR for smoking cessation: Data from clinical trials and five years of post-marketing experience. *International Journal of Clinical Practice, 57*(3), 224–230.

Freire, T. F. V., de Almeida Fleck, M. P., & da Rocha, N. S. (2016). Remission of depression following electroconvulsive therapy (ECT) is associated with higher levels of brain-derived neurotrophic factor (BDNF). *Brain Research Bulletin, 121,* 263–269.

Galeotti, N. (2017). Hypericum perforatum (St John's wort) beyond depression: A therapeutic perspective for pain conditions. *Journal of Ethnopharmacology, 200,* 136–146.

Gardener, D. M., Shulman, K. I., Walker, S. E., & Tailor, S. A. N. (1996). The making of a user-friendly MAOI diet. *Journal of Clinical Psychiatry, 57,* 99–104.

Goodwin, F. K., & Ghaemi, S. N. (2000). The impact of mood stabilizers on suicide in bipolar disorder: A comparative analysis. *CNS Spectrums, 5*(2), 12–19.

Granger, B. (1999). The discovery of haloperidol. *Encephale, 25*(1), 59–66.

Hale, G. M., Kane-Gill, S. L., Groetzinger, L., & Smithburger, P. L. (2016). An evaluation of adverse drug reactions associated with antipsychotic use for the treatment of delirium in the intensive care unit. *Journal of Pharmacy Practice, 29*(4), 355–360.

Hirose, S. (2002). ECT for depression with amnesia. *Journal of ECT, 18*(1), 60.

Holsboer, F., & Ising, M. (2008). Central CRH system in depression and anxiety—Evidence from clinical studies with CRH1 receptor agonists. *European Journal of Pharmacology, 583*(2–3), 350–357.

Izzo, A. A., Hoon-Kim, S., Radhakrishnan, R., & Williamson, E. M. (2016). A critical approach to evaluating clinical efficacy, adverse events and drug interactions of herbal remedies. *Phytotherapy Research, 30*(5), 691–700.

Johnson, P. J., Wilson, P. D., & deBoisblanc, M. B. (2016). Missed opportunities for health promotion intervention in the management of alcohol withdrawal syndrome. *The Journal of the Louisiana State Medical Society: Official Organ of the Louisiana State Medical Society, 168*(2), 35.

Kalapos, M. P. (2002). Carbamazepine-provoked hepatotoxicity and possible aetiological role of glutathione in the events. *Adverse Drug Reactions and Toxicological Reviews, 21*(3), 123–141.

Kanno, M., Matsumoto, M., Togashi, H., Yoshioka, M., & Mano, Y. (2003). Effects of repetitive transcranial magnetic stimulation on behavioural and neurochemical changes in rats during an elevated plus-maze test. *Journal of the Neurological Sciences, 211*(1–2), 5–14.

Katzman, M. A., Bleau, P., Blier, P., Chokka, P., Kjernisted, K., & Van Ameringen, M. (2014). Canadian clinical practice guidelines for the management of anxiety, posttraumatic stress and obsessive-compulsive disorders. *BMC Psychiatry, 14*(1), S1.

Kellner, C. H., Husain, M. M., Knapp, R. G., McCall, W. V., Petrides, G., Rudorfer, M. V., ... Prudic, J. (2016). A novel strategy for continuation ECT in geriatric depression: Phase 2 of the PRIDE study. *American Journal of Psychiatry, 173*(11), 1110–1118.

Kenicer, D., Ellahi, R., Davies, P., Walker, A., & Cheyne, A. (2016). Factors important to psychiatrists when prescribing depot antipsychotics. *Progress in Neurology and Psychiatry, 20*(3), 16–20.

Kennedy, S. H., Lam, R. W., McIntyre, R. S., Tourjman, S. V., Bhat, V., Blier, P., ... McInerney, S. J. (2016). Canadian network for mood and anxiety treatments (CANMAT) 2016 clinical guidelines for the management of adults with major depressive disorder: Section 3. Pharmacological treatments. *The Canadian Journal of Psychiatry, 61*(9), 540–560.

Kennedy, S. H., Segal, Z. V., Cohen, N. L., Levitan, R. D., Gemar, M., & Bagby, R. M. (2003). Lithium carbonate versus cognitive therapy as sequential combination treatment strategies in partial responders to antidepressant medication: An exploratory trial. *Journal of Clinical Psychiatry, 64*(4), 439–444.

Khan, A. Y., Salaria, S., Ovais, M., & Ide, G. D. (2016). Depot antipsychotics: Where do we stand? *Annals of Clinical Psychiatry, 28*(4), 289–298.

Klotz, U. (2007). The role of pharmacogenetics in the metabolism of antiepileptic drugs: Pharmacokinetic and therapeutic implications. *Clinical Pharmacokinetics, 46*(4), 271–279.

Kragh, M., Møller, D. N., Wihlborg, C. S., Martiny, K., Larsen, E. R., Videbech, P., & Lindhardt, T. (2017). Experiences of wake and light therapy in patients with depression: A qualitative study. *International Journal of Mental Health Nursing, 26*(2), 170–180.

Kulkarni, S. K., & Naidu, P. S. (2003). Pathophysiology and drug therapy of tardive dyskinesia: Current concepts and future perspectives. *Drugs of Today (Barcelona, Spain), 39*(1), 19–49.

Levy, G., Schupf, N., Tang, M. X., Cote, L. J., Louis, E. D., Mejia, H., ... Marder, K. (2002). Combined effect of age and severity on the risk of dementia in Parkinson's disease. *Annals of Neurology, 51*(6), 722–729.

Loscher, W. (2002). Basic pharmacology of valproate: A review after 35 years of clinical use for the treatment of epilepsy. *CNS Drugs, 16*(10), 669–694.

Magne, B. T., Engedal, K., Šaltytė, B. J., Bergsholm, P., Strømnes, D. G., Lødøen, G. T., & Tanum, L. (2016). Speed of recovery from disorientation may predict the treatment outcome of electroconvulsive therapy (ECT) in elderly patients with major depression. *Journal of Affective Disorders, 190*, 178–186.

Mahmood, I. (2016). Chapter 3: Developmental pharmacology: Impact on pharmacokinetics and pharmacodynamics of drugs. In I. Mahmood and G. Burckart (Eds.), *Fundamentals of Pediatric Drug Dosing.* (pp. 23–44). Cham, Switzerland: Springer International Publishing.

Marshall, J., Herzig, S. J., Howell, M. D., Le, S. H., Mathew, C., Kats, J. S., & Stevens, J. P. (2016). Antipsychotic utilization in the intensive care unit and in transitions of care. *Journal of Critical Care, 33*, 119–124.

Martin, J. L., Barbanoj, M. J., Schlaepfer, T. E., Thompson, E., Perez, V., & Kulisevsky, J. (2003). Repetitive transcranial magnetic stimulation for the treatment of depression: Systematic review and meta-analysis. *British Journal of Psychiatry, 182*, 480–491.

Martins, M. J., Pereira, A. T., Carvalho, C. B., Castilho, P., Lopes, A. C., Oliveira, A., … Madeira, N. (2016). Antipsychotic medication adherence scale (AMAS): Development and preliminary psychometric properties. *European Psychiatry, 33*, S305–S306.

Maust, D. T., Gerlach, L. B., Gibson, A., Kales, H. C., Blow, F. C., & Olfson, M. (2017). Trends in central nervous system–active polypharmacy among older adults seen in outpatient care in the United States. *JAMA Internal Medicine, 177*(4), 583–585.

Meltzer, H. Y. (2000). Side effects of antipsychotic medications: Physician's choice of medication and patient compliance. *Journal of Clinical Psychiatry, 61*(Suppl. 8), 3–4.

Melvin, C. L., Carey, T. S., Goodman, F., Oldham, J. M., & Ranney, L. M. (2008). Effectiveness of antiepileptic drugs for the treatment of bipolar disorder: Findings from a systematic review. *Journal of Psychiatric Practice, 14*(Suppl. 1), 9–14.

Meyer, J. M. (2007). Antipsychotic safety and efficacy concerns. *Journal of Clinical Psychiatry, 68*(Suppl. 14), 20–26.

Miller, C. H., & Fleischhacker, W. W. (2000). Managing antipsychotic-induced acute and chronic akathisia. *Drug Safety, 22*, 73–81.

Moisan, J., Gregoire, J., Gaudet, M., & Cooper, D. (2005). Exploring the risk of diabetes mellitus and dyslipidemia among ambulatory users of atypical antipsychotics: A population-based comparison of risperidone and olanzapine. *Pharmacoepidemiology and Drug Safety, 14*, 427–436.

Molina, J. D., Durán, M., López-Muñoz, F., Álamo, C., & Toledo-Romero, F. (2016). The role of antiepileptic drugs in bipolar depression. In F. López-Muñoz, V. Srinivasan, D. de Berardis, C. Álamo, T. A. Kato (Eds.), *Melatonin, neuroprotective agents and antidepressant therapy* (pp. 855–868). New Delhi: Springer India.

Morace, R., Di Gennaro, G., Quarato, P. P., D'Aniello, A., Mascia, A., Grammaldo, L., … Esposito, V. (2017). Vagal nerve stimulation for drug-resistant epilepsy: Adverse events and outcome in a series of patients with long-term follow-up. In M. Visocchi, H. M. Mehdorn, Y. Katayama, K. R. H. von Wild (Eds.), *Trends in reconstructive neurosurgery* (pp. 49–52). Cham, Switzerland: Springer.

Neville, I. S., Hayashi, C. Y., Hajj, S. A., Zaninotto, A. L. C., Sabino, J. P., Sousa, L. M., … Teixeira, M. J. (2015). Repetitive transcranial magnetic stimulation (rTMS) for the cognitive rehabilitation of traumatic brain injury (TBI) victims: Study protocol for a randomized controlled trial. *Trials, 16*(1), 440.

Nguyen, J. P., Suarez, A., Kemoun, G., Meignier, M., Le Saout, E., Damier, P., … Lefaucheur, J. P. (2017). Repetitive transcranial magnetic stimulation combined with cognitive training for the treatment of Alzheimer's disease. *Neurophysiologie Clinique/Clinical Neurophysiology, 47*(1), 47–53. doi:10.1016/j.neucli.2017.01.001

Nicolas, J. M., Bouzom, F., Chanteux, H., & Ungell, A. L. (2017). Oral drug absorption in pediatrics: The intestinal wall, its developmental changes and current tools for predictions. *Biopharmaceutics & Drug Disposition, 38*(3), 209–230.

Niedermeyer, E. (2008). Akinesia and the frontal lobe. *Clinical EEG and Neuroscience, 39*(1), 39–42.

Ott, M., Stegmayr, B., Salander Renberg, E., & Werneke, U. (2016). Lithium intoxication: Incidence, clinical course and renal function—A population-based retrospective cohort study. *Journal of Psychopharmacology, 30*(10), 1008–1019.

Painter, J. T., Owen, R., Henderson, K. L., Bauer, M. S., Mittal, D., & Hudson, T. J. (2017). Analysis of the appropriateness of off-label antipsychotic use for mental health indications in a veteran population. *Pharmacotherapy: The Journal of Human Pharmacology and Drug Therapy, 37*(4), 438–446.

Payne, N., & Prudic, J. (2009a). Electroconvulsive therapy Part 1. A perspective on the evolution and current practice of ECT. *Journal of Psychiatric Practice, 15*(5), 346–368.

Payne, N., & Prudic, J. (2009b). Electroconvulsive therapy Part II. A biopsychosocial perspective. *Journal of Psychiatric Practice, 15*(5), 369–390.

Penders, T. M., Stanciu, C. N., Schoemann, A. M., Ninan, P. T., Bloch, R., & Saeed, S. A. (2016). Bright light therapy as augmentation of pharmacotherapy for treatment of depression: A systematic review and meta-analysis. *The Primary Care Companion for CNS Disorders, 18*(5).

Pierre, J. M. (2005). Extrapyramidal symptoms with atypical antipsychotics: Incidence, prevention and management. *Drug Safety, 28*(3), 191–208.

Pisapia, J., & Baltuch, G. (2016). Vagus nerve stimulation. In C. Hamani, P. Holtzheimer, A. M. Lozano, & H. Mayberg (Eds.), *Neuromodulation in psychiatry* (325–334). West Sussex, UK: Wiley-Blackwell.

Post, R. M. (2016). Treatment of bipolar depression: Evolving recommendations. *Psychiatric Clinics of North America, 39*(1), 11–33.

Preston, S. T., & Hegadoren, K. (2004). Glass contamination in parenterally administered medication. *Journal of Advanced Nursing, 48*(3), 266–270.

Rezansoff, S. N., Moniruzzaman, A., Fazel, S., Procyshyn, R., & Somers, J. M. (2016). Adherence to antipsychotic medication among homeless adults in Vancouver, Canada: A 15-year retrospective cohort study. *Social Psychiatry and Psychiatric Epidemiology, 51*(12), 1623–1632.

Roerig, J. L., Steffen, K. J., & Mitchell, J. E. (2011). Atypical antipsychotic-induced weight gain: Insights into mechanisms of action. *CNS Drugs, 25*(12), 1035–1059.

Sabater, A., García-Blanco, A. C., Verdet, H. M., Sierra, P., Ribes, J., Villar, I., … Livianos, L. (2016). Comparative neurocognitive effects of lithium and anticonvulsants in long-term stable bipolar patients. *Journal of Affective Disorders, 190*, 34–40.

Schou, M. (1978). Lithium treatment. *Western Journal of Medicine, 128*(6), 535–536.

Simpson, G. M., & Angus, J. W. S. (1970). A rating scale for extrapyramidal side effects. *Acta Psychiatrica Scandinavica, 212*(Suppl.), 11–19.

Solomon, D. A., Keitner, G. I., & Ryan, C. E. (1998). Lithium plus valproate as maintenance polypharmacy for patients with bipolar I disorder: A review. *Journal of Clinical Psychopharmacology, 5*(2), 19–28.

Takeshima, M. (2017). Treating mixed mania/hypomania: A review and synthesis of the evidence. *CNS Spectrums, 22*(2), 177–185.

Tariot, P. N., Salzman, C., Yeung, P. P., Pultz, J., & Rak, I. W. (2000). Long-term use of quetiapine in elderly patients with psychotic disorders. *Clinical Therapeutics, 22*(9), 1068–1084.

Taylor, D. (2003). Ziprasidone in the management of schizophrenia: The QT interval issue in context. *CNS Drugs, 17*(6), 423–430.

Yatham, L. N., & Kesavan, M. (2017). The treatment of bipolar II disorder. In A. F. Carvalho, & E. Vieta (Eds.), *The treatment of bipolar disorder: Integrative clinical strategies and future directions* (pp. 108–122). Oxford, UK: Oxford University Press.

Young, S. N., & Leyton, M. (2002). The role of serotonin in human mood and social interaction: Insight from altered tryptophan levels. *Pharmacology, Biochemistry, and Behavior, 71*, 857–865.

Zhou, H. (2003). Pharmacokinetic strategies in deciphering atypical drug absorption profiles. *Journal of Clinical Pharmacology, 43*(3), 211–227.

Zintzaras, E. (2005). Statistical aspects of bioequivalence testing between two medicinal products. *European Journal of Drug Metabolism and Pharmacokinetics, 30*(1–2), 41–46.

Zullino, D., Delacrausaz, P., & Baumann, P. (2002). The place of SSRIs in the treatment of schizophrenia. *Encephale, 28*(5 Pt 1), 433–438.

13 Cognitive–Behavioural Interventions

Wendy Austin

Adapted from the chapter "Cognitive–Behavioural Therapy" by Tracey Tulley and Ruth Gallop

LEARNING OBJECTIVES

After studying this chapter, you will be able to:

- Explain the cognitive model.
- Describe the levels of cognition, including core beliefs, intermediate beliefs, automatic thoughts, and their interrelationship.
- Name and describe the 10 principles of cognitive–behavioural therapy.
- Identify cognitive treatment techniques.
- Identify behavioural treatment techniques.
- Define mindfulness.

KEY TERMS

- automatic thoughts • behavioural experiment
- cognitive schema • core beliefs • intermediate beliefs
- mindfulness

KEY CONCEPTS

- cognitive–behavioural therapy
- cognitive restructuring

One of the more significant achievements in modern psychotherapy is the knowledge gained of the central role of thought (cognition) in the development of core beliefs about self and the world. Cognitive–behavioural therapy (CBT) is a form of psychotherapy that uses that knowledge to identify, analyze, and ultimately change the habitually inflexible and negative cognitions about oneself, others, and the world at large that contribute to distressing emotional states and problematic behaviours (Beck, 2011). When thinking is modified, emotion and behaviour also change. The cognitive interventions in CBT are used to modify maladaptive thinking or beliefs; its behavioural interventions are aimed at decreasing maladaptive responses while increasing adaptive ones and at the learning of new behavioural practices (Craske, 2010).

Although special training is required to become a cognitive–behavioural (CB) therapist, its knowledge base is highly useful to nurses. Such knowledge can be used not only to help persons change unhealthy behaviours (e.g., poor eating habits), overcome avoidance behaviours, and deal with stress and anxiety but as an important approach to health promotion. Knowledge of CBT interventions also allows nurses to support persons undergoing CBT as a means of improving their lives.

CBT is the most widely researched form of psychotherapy, and given the robust findings from numerous controlled clinical trials, is recognized as an effective treatment for many mental health problems and disorders, including general anxiety disorder (GAD), social phobia, posttraumatic stress disorder (PTSD), bulimia nervosa, panic disorder, obsessive–compulsive symptoms,

depression, and pathologic gambling. There is evidence indicating that CBT is effective when delivered via teleconferencing (Marchand et al., 2011) and via the Internet (iCBT) (Carlbring, Degerman, Johnson, & Anderson, 2012; Paxling et al., 2011; Tilfors et al., 2008; Wootton, 2016) (see Box 13.1). As research shows that CBT for mental disorders is cost-effective, it is argued that greater access to publicly funded CBT in Canada may not only improve outcomes but result in cost savings (Myhr & Payne, 2006).

KEY CONCEPT

Cognitive–behavioural therapy is a psychotherapy focused on identifying, analyzing, and ultimately changing the habitually inflexible and negative cognitions about oneself, others, and the world that contribute to distress and problematic behaviours.

Although the assumptions underlying CBT can be traced back to ancient times and the Stoic philosopher Epictetus, psychiatrist Aaron Beck and psychologist Albert Ellis are acknowledged as having founded CBT as we know it today. From the mid-1950s to the early 1960s, when experimental and clinical psychology and psychiatry were ruled by behaviourism and psychoanalytic theory, Ellis and Beck, independently of each other, became increasingly dissatisfied with the ability of psychoanalysis to explain the struggles of their patients and its lack of scientific rigour. In treating their patients, they noted certain biases toward irrational and inflexible

BOX 13.1 Research for Best Practice

USING COGNITIVE–BEHAVIOUR THERAPY REMOTELY FOR OBSESSIVE–COMPULSIVE SYMPTOMS

Wootton, B. M. (2016). Remote cognitive-behavior therapy for obsessive-compulsive symptoms: A meta-analysis. Clinical Psychology Review, 43, 103–113.

The Aim: Remote cognitive–behaviour therapy (CBT) considered as "high intensity" involves the use of technology (via video link [vCBT] or telephone [tCBT]) to deliver treatment in real time, similar to face-to-face situations. "Low-intensity" remote CBT involves systematic acquisition of information and skills (via books [bCBT], computer resources [cCBT], Internet [iCBT]) rather than in face-to-face therapy. In this study, a meta-analytic approach was used to synthetize the results of existing, current research on remote CBT used for obsessive–compulsive disorder (OCD) symptoms to provide an evaluation of its efficacy.

Methods: Eighteen relevant research studies ($n = 823$) were identified through electronic databases (Scopus, Medline, PsycINFO) and previous reviews on the topic. To be included, the studies had to be a clinical trial or a case series targeting OCD symptoms, include a remote treatment, incorporate the CB technique of exposure and response prevention, and use the Yale-Brown O-C Scale as an outcome measure.

Findings: The meta-analysis found that both "high-" and "low-density" remote treatments for OCD produce a decrease in symptoms of a large magnitude. A meaningful difference between remote and face-to-face treatment outcomes was not found.

Implications: Individuals with OCD can have severe difficulty in accessing face-to-face treatment for their symptoms due to the restrictive nature of the symptoms. That remote CBT is efficacious for OCD symptoms is thus an important finding. It suggests that further development of remote CBT techniques is a worthwhile endeavour.

thought patterns that negatively influenced mood and behaviour. A radical idea at the time, they proposed that if these rigid and negative thought patterns could be changed, mood would improve and behaviour would become more functional. Although CBT is a mental health treatment, it is based on a cognitive model that is applicable to the experience of all humans in all situations. Life skills for coping with distress and problem solving can be learned using this model (see Box 13.2).

BOX 13.2 Preparing for the NCLEX: A Cognitive–Behavioural Approach

There is much at stake for nursing students taking credentialing examinations. Writing an examination like the NCLEX can create such anticipatory anxiety that examination performance is diminished. Distorted thinking translates into poor test-taking preparation and behaviour. Recognition of the way thinking impacts performance is an important first step to dealing with the issue. Self-assessment allows for the identification of specific knowledge deficits to be overcome, but negative thinking and problematic behaviours should also be identified. CB techniques such as cognitive restructuring, thought stopping, and visual imagery can then be used to help a student address test anxiety.

▣ THE COGNITIVE MODEL

The cognitive model forms the foundation of CBT, the essence of which is that humans respond primarily to cognitive representations of the environment, and that cognition mediates affect and behaviour (Beck, 2011). In simpler terms, the way we *think* about situations influences our emotions and our behaviour. Our emotions, behaviours, and thoughts all interact in complex and interconnected ways; however, the cognitive model places particular importance on thoughts as the "director" of our experiences (Fig. 13.1).

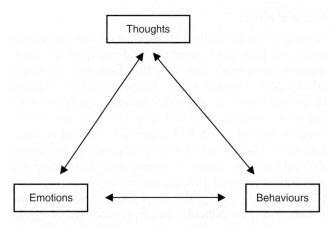

Figure 13.1. Interconnection between thoughts, emotions, and behaviours.

Cognitive theory suggests that one's perception of situations and events is particularly salient in guiding emotional and behavioural responses (Beck, 2011). Events in and of themselves do not cause us to feel and act in particular ways; rather, it is how we *understand* or think about what happens to us that affects how we feel about it and what we do about it. For example, think about what would go through your mind if you entered a party where the only other guest you knew had not yet arrived. Would you think, "This is a great opportunity to introduce myself to others. Maybe I'll meet some interesting people," or would you think, "Everyone is staring at me because I'm alone. If my friend does not show up in the next 15 minutes, I'm leaving"? The party itself is a relatively neutral event, but how you interpret the event will affect how you feel at the party and what you do or how you act. If your thought process tends toward the former, your emotions of excitement and enjoyment will propel you to stay and mingle with the other partygoers (your behaviour). If your thought process is more consistent with the latter, your anxiety and uncertainty will compel you to flee (your behaviour).

The different ways that individuals evaluate and respond to a particular situation or event are as varied as the individuals themselves. The particular reasons why individuals are so varied in their perceptions of situations and thereby their emotional and behavioural responses are in part accounted for by their core beliefs. See Box 13.3 for an example of students responding differently to the same situation. In summary, the cognitive model posits that when an emotion is felt, a thought is behind it, and when behaviour is enacted, a thought is behind it.

■ LEVELS OF COGNITION

Cognition is given primary importance in CBT. There are three levels of cognition that are considered: core beliefs, intermediate beliefs, and automatic thoughts.

Core Beliefs

Cognitive theory posits the existence of core knowledge structures that hold, organize, and interpret all information about one's view of self, others, and the world (Beck, 2011; Craske, 2010). These structures, referred to as core beliefs or **cognitive schema**, comprise basic beliefs so fundamental that they are often not articulated in explicit words but rather are accepted as absolute truths (Beck, 2011). **Core beliefs** assist in evaluating and assigning meaning to events and influencing the subsequent range of affective and behavioural responses (Beck & Emery, 1985). The deeply rooted nature of core beliefs and their difficulty in being accessed, or explicitly identified, mean that they are difficult to change. Examples of core beliefs are "I am inadequate"; "I am

---

> **BOX 13.3 Effect of Cognition on Feelings and Behaviour**
>
> In this example, four student nurses in the same clinical group respond to the same situation in four different ways, owing to different patterns of thinking, feeling, and acting.
>
> **The Situation:** A nursing instructor informs the clinical group that by the end of their shift each student is expected to seek out an opportunity to insert his or her first intravenous line. All students received the appropriate classroom teaching and lab practice with this skill.
>
> **Susanne** thinks, "I have been waiting so long to perform advanced clinical skills. I can hardly wait to give it a try." She feels excited and responds behaviourally by informing all staff in the morning report of her learning opportunity. She requests that any new intravenous starts be directed to her.
>
> **Dylan** thinks, "I understand the theory behind intravenous insertion, but I did not have much success in the lab. I know I need to fulfill this requirement, but I am not sure how I am going to do it without hurting someone and embarrassing myself." He feels anxious and uncertain and responds behaviourally by reluctantly informing his buddy nurse, midway through the shift, that he is required to meet this expectation.
>
> **Jasmine** thinks, "There is absolutely no way I am ready for this. I do not have the confidence or skill set to perform this task." She feels terrified and responds behaviourally by speaking to the clinical instructor privately informing her that she is feeling nauseous and must return home for the day.
>
> **Ella** thinks, "Once again I'm being told what to do without any regard for my own learning needs. No one can force me to comply." She feels outraged and angry and responds behaviourally by refusing to complete the skill as required.
>
> All the students were presented with the identical situation, and all received similar training to perform the required skill. The way in which each student *thought about* the situation, however, was very different and consequently led to emotions as varied as excitement and terror and behaviours as varied as approach and avoidance. It is not the situation itself that influenced how each of the students responded, but rather each individual's unique interpretation of the situation.
>
> Understanding the way thinking affects emotions and behaviours can be helpful in working with patients who are having difficulty adhering to treatment regimens.

unlovable"; "others are not trustworthy"; and "the world is an unsafe place."

Core beliefs hold both general and specific information about the self, others, and the world and influence the manner in which one negotiates one's way through life. If, for example, an individual holds the belief that she is a person worthy of love and that she will likely engage in mutually respectful and fulfilling relationships. Conversely, if the world is believed to be a hostile place in which people are not to be trusted, she may have an approach of hypervigilance and suspiciousness and may experience relationships as potentially dangerous. As one moves through life gathering and considering information, beliefs are processed in a way that is consistent with the view of self, others, and the world and become solidified. As such, core beliefs are self-confirming and self-perpetuating in nature, which contribute to their rigidity and global application (Beck, 2011).

Intermediate Beliefs

Existing at a more accessible level than core beliefs are cognitive products, which are often separated into two categories: **intermediate beliefs** and **automatic thoughts** (Beck, 2011). Intermediate beliefs consist of attitudes, rules or expectations, and assumptions that influence one's perceptions, affect, and behaviours. They often take the form of "if… then," "should," or "must" statements that are rigid and unrealistic. Assumptions, rules, and expectations may have arisen from the direct teaching or observation of important others early in life. One's cultural background also plays a role in one's understanding and tolerance of what is acceptable. Examples of intermediate beliefs include the following:

- If I'm not liked by everyone, it means I've failed.
- Assume the worst will happen because it usually does.
- If I show my vulnerability, I make myself open to attack.
- I must be the best in everything that I endeavour.
- Relationships make you open to rejection.

Automatic Thoughts

At an even more superficial level than intermediate beliefs are automatic thoughts. Automatic thoughts are the "knee-jerk," in-the-moment words and images generated in a particular situation (Beck, 2011). They may not be logical and are often difficult to "shut off." Automatic thoughts are the most superficial and accessible of the levels of cognition and thus are generally the first to be targeted in treatment. Although automatic thoughts are accessible, we are not always immediately conscious of their presence. Instead, we may be more aware of the accompanying emotion rather than the preceding spontaneous thought. In fact, the presence of a strong emotion is often a signal that an important thought is present. For example, when a car cuts you off on the freeway, you might be more likely to respond with anger than to be aware of the thought behind the emotion of anger ("Who do you think you are? You put the safety of my family at risk."). Part of the early therapeutic work of CBT is to bring automatic thoughts into our awareness and help us evaluate their impact (Beck, 2011).

Relationship Between Levels of Cognition

The relationship between automatic thoughts, intermediate beliefs, and core beliefs is demonstrated in the following two examples. There is a situation in which an individual is standing in a line and someone steps into the position in front of her. In the moment, the individual tells herself, "This person must not have realized I was already in line. I will tell him that I was first in line so that he can take his place behind me." These automatic thoughts occur spontaneously and reside at the most superficial level of cognition. The deeper intermediate beliefs, rules, and expectations that support these automatic thoughts may be "People do not intend to be malicious but can cause inconvenience," "It is necessary to follow social norms," and "The ability to assert oneself is important." Underlying these automatic thoughts and intermediate rules and expectations is a core belief, the deepest level of cognition, of "I am a valuable person who is worthy of respect." This example of the relationship between the three levels of cognition is illustrated in Figure 13.2. Another individual may process this same situation very differently. The same three levels of cognition still exist, although the content of each level is different. She may tell herself, "This person saw me standing here, and he intentionally stepped in front of me. He must think I am someone who can be easily exploited." The intermediate beliefs and rules that gave rise to these automatic thoughts are "I am not capable of speaking up for myself," "I expect that people will treat me with a lack of respect," and "I can't speak up for myself; therefore, I'll never get anywhere in life." In this example, the automatic thoughts and expectations are driven by core beliefs rooted in a sense of unworthiness, such as "I'm not deserving of respect."

Early experiences, past events, messages from others, and direct observations contribute to the formation of core beliefs and subsequent intermediate beliefs and automatic thoughts. In the individual whose early experiences were primarily nurturing, reliable, and positive, core beliefs are generally an accurate, realistic, and functional reflection of reality. However, the individual who experienced inconsistency, emotional unavailability, and cruelty may develop hypercritical beliefs about the self, others, and the world that are rigid, overgeneralized, and an inaccurate reflection of the current reality. These core beliefs contribute to emotions and behaviours that are intensely negative and harmful.

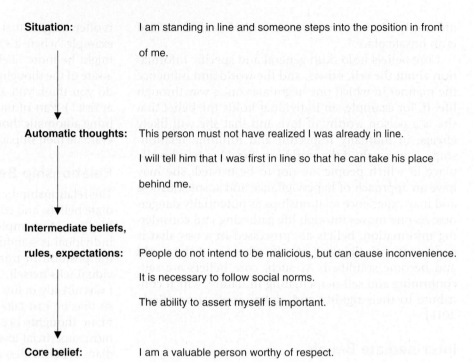

Situation: I am standing in line and someone steps into the position in front of me.

Automatic thoughts: This person must not have realized I was already in line.

I will tell him that I was first in line so that he can take his place behind me.

Intermediate beliefs, rules, expectations: People do not intend to be malicious, but can cause inconvenience.

It is necessary to follow social norms.

The ability to assert myself is important.

Core belief: I am a valuable person worthy of respect.

Figure 13.2. The relationship between levels of cognition.

PRINCIPLES OF COGNITIVE–BEHAVIOURAL THERAPY

CBT is grounded in a set of specific principles. Treatment strategies employed in CBT are specific to the disorder being treated; however, the basic principles remain common across disorders. The 10 principles that appear in Box 13.4 and are discussed below are based on the work of Beck (2011).

BOX 13.4 Ten Principles of CBT

1. CBT is based on an evolving CB formulation of the patient.
2. CBT requires a sound therapeutic alliance.
3. CBT emphasizes collaboration and active participation.
4. CBT is goal oriented and problem focused.
5. CBT initially emphasizes the present.
6. CBT is educative and emphasizes relapse prevention.
7. CBT aims to be time limited.
8. CBT sessions are structured.
9. CBT teaches how to identify, evaluate, and respond to dysfunctional thoughts and beliefs.
10. CBT uses a variety of techniques to change thinking, mood, and behaviour.

From Beck, J. (2011). *Cognitive therapy: Basics and beyond* (2nd ed.). New York, NY: Guilford Press.

Cognitive–Behavioural Formulation

A cognitive behavioural (CB) formulation begins during the patient's initial assessment and is reviewed and revised over the course of therapy. It outlines the typical thoughts and problematic behaviours that contribute to the current distress. The patient who presents with social anxiety may have the thoughts, "Showing my nervousness is a sign of weakness" and "I appear incompetent when I make presentations." Problematic behaviours that flow from these negative thoughts may include avoidance of any situation in which he or she might be the centre of attention (e.g., speaking up in meetings), overpreparing (e.g., memorizing a brief statement to be made during a meeting), and use of alcohol (e.g., reliance on several glasses of beer before attending a party where socializing is an expectation). The next component of the formulation involves collecting information on the factors that precipitated the onset of the current problem. The precipitating factor for the socially anxious patient may be starting a new job where there is an expectation to chair meetings, conduct staff training, and give presentations to outside agencies. A CB formulation also outlines the developmental issues that contributed to and continue to reinforce the current problem. For example, harsh criticism by parents for being less than perfect, being ridiculed and mocked by students while speaking in front of the class, and receiving below-average grades on oral presentations may all be predisposing factors for the socially anxious patient. Over his or her life, he or she may have systematically ignored his or her multiple successes and amplified his or her perceived social failures, which served to strengthen his or her beliefs about weakness and inadequacy.

The CB formulation is shared and modified with the patient as part of the collaborative relationship (see Box 13.4, principles 2 and 3). It is a framework that can be modified as new information becomes available. In addition to providing both a framework for guiding treatment and a means to enhancing therapeutic collaboration, it also demonstrates to the patient how part of one's experience can be broken down in order to gain a better understanding of the whole, and that one's "overwhelming" problems are composed of smaller, more manageable parts.

Strong Therapeutic Alliance

Therapeutic change would not be achievable without a strong therapeutic relationship consisting of trust, mutual respect, safety, empathy, warmth, and acceptance. Most patients enter therapy afraid, uncertain, and perhaps unsure if it will be helpful. Many have struggled for years on their own, perhaps too ashamed to seek help. Further, the personal histories of some patients render them highly mistrustful of those in positions of perceived power. It is the primary task of the therapist to create an environment in which patients feel free to disclose their anxieties and take risks, in which they feel attended to, listened to, and understood. The therapeutic relationship is discussed further in Chapter 6.

Time Limited and Brief

Many forms of psychotherapy are open-ended with respect to the length of treatment. Psychodynamic therapy, for instance, may continue for years. In contrast, CBT is a short-term treatment. An assumption of CBT is that the therapist will transfer knowledge and skills to the person in therapy and then further therapy becomes unnecessary (Butler, Fennell, & Hackmann, 2008). As example, the American Psychiatric Association recommends one CBT session per week for 10 to 15 weeks for persons with panic disorder (American Psychiatric Association, 2009). Maintenance CBT sessions lessen the likelihood of relapse for such patients (White et al., 2013). Severity and duration of the presenting problem, patient motivation, and the patient's ability to form and maintain a therapeutic relationship will determine the duration of CBT for a particular individual. The *Suitability for Short-term Cognitive Therapy Rating Scale* (SRS) developed at the Centre for Addiction and Mental Health in Toronto has predictive value regarding potential for CBT to be successful with a particular patient (Myhr, Talbot, Annable, & Pinard, 2007).

Goal Oriented, Problem Focused, and Change Oriented

Patients enter CBT with a clear idea of their struggles. With the therapist, they set realistic, measurable goals to be attained within the treatment period. Using cognitive and behavioural strategies (to be discussed), the patient works toward analyzing the current accuracy and logic of negative thinking patterns. Distortions in thinking are tested and are replaced with more accurate and flexible ways of evaluating self, others, and the world. Potential barriers to goal attainment are considered, and methods to overcome these obstacles are planned.

Structured and Directive

Although the content of each therapy session changes from week to week, sessions follow a similar structure throughout treatment. The structure of CBT provides clarity, reassurance, and a sense of control to the patient; it maintains focus and maximizes the ability to use the session effectively. It prepares the patient to be his or her own therapist upon therapy termination.

The therapist begins the session with a mood check, asks for a brief summary of the patient's week, collaboratively decides which problem areas will be discussed in the session (often referred to as agenda setting), requests feedback about the previous session, reviews and discusses the self-reflective exercise, addresses the agenda items, provides new self-reflective exercises, and elicits feedback about the session. Throughout the session, the therapist offers summaries of key areas. As the therapy progresses, the patient takes on the responsibility of providing these summaries and managing the structure in general.

Educative

The initial sessions of CBT are more therapist directed than later sessions and include education about the patient's presenting problem and the cognitive model of his or her particular disorder in addition to socializing the patient to CBT. Further on in CBT, therapists teach patients how to engage in cognitive restructuring, the process whereby habitually negative thought patterns are identified, evaluated, and modified. Providing patients information on the nature and course of their disorder not only helps them to understand their current struggles but also empowers them to engage in a collaborative approach to their care. An additional benefit of the educative nature of CBT is that it assists in preparing patients for the process of self-therapy; that is, it helps ensure that patients adopt the skills necessary to continue to change and prevent relapse after the specific therapy has ended.

Therapeutic Collaboration

CBT is a collaborative effort, with patient and therapist each bringing essential but different ingredients to the relationship and vital to achieving change. The patient assumes the role of equal partner in agenda setting, problem solving, and generating self-reflective exercises (see Box 13.4, principle 3). Because the content and the process of CBT are demystified and made transparent, it is possible for patients to truly take on a collaborative role. The therapist remains an active participant in the treatment; neither a neutral nor an authoritative stance would be appropriate in CBT.

Inductive Reasoning

Patients entering therapy often view their thoughts and feelings as facts and unshakeable truths: for example, "I know I am a stupid person. When I'm depressed, it means I'm weak." Patients of CBT are encouraged to view their thoughts and feelings as hypotheses; they are not rigid facts but are plausible explanations that will be put to test and revised as needed. The goal is to assist patients in attending to all the available facts and information in their hypothesis testing, not merely the "old ruts" of thinking in which they generally find themselves stuck. Patients are encouraged to "think like a scientist and search for objective facts" or "play detective to find all the evidence" when examining the validity and accuracy of their thoughts.

Socratic Questioning

CB therapists adopt a questioning stance, referred to as Socratic questioning, as a method to help patients to evaluate their thinking (e.g., negative thought patterns) and to aid in developing balanced thoughts. When a question is posed by the therapist, possible answers are generated. The patient is encouraged to view these answers as hypotheses capable of being examined and tested in the therapy. Socratic questioning is a reasoned dialogue; the intention is not for the patient to feel interrogated; rather, it is for the patient to come to his or her own broader perspective about the validity, accuracy, and functionality of his or her thought process (Beck, 2011).

Self-Reflective Exercises

One of the most effective ways of helping patients reflect on and practice newly developed skills and monitor progress is through the use of self-reflective exercises, sometimes referred to as homework exercises. Research indicates that homework compliance is a significant predictor of positive treatment outcome (Kazantzis, Whittington, & Dattilio, 2010). Self-reflective exercises are provided at the end of each session with the expectation that the patient will work on them throughout the week and be prepared to discuss them at the beginning of the following session. Providing the patient with materials that facilitate recollection of the assignment promotes homework completion. It is essential that therapists review the assigned exercise with the patient at the following session because this reinforces the therapist's commitment and investment in the process. Patients will be less likely to complete the exercises if they have little accountability and if they do not observe the therapist valuing the assignments. Review of the exercises also provides the therapist with clinically useful information. If patients state that they do not feel like completing the exercise, are too busy, or do not see the point, this provides the therapist with clinically relevant material that should be explored further in the therapy. For example, a patient may avoid attempting the exercises because he or she does not feel as though it will be done "right" or "good enough" or that he or she will appear "stupid, just like I always do," which would lead to humiliation. The therapist would then take the opportunity to explore these thoughts, as they may represent negative patterns of thinking that are generalized to situations beyond the completion of the exercises and warrant analyzing and modification. If the patient indicates an inability to complete the exercises because time is lacking, further exploration may reveal that either the exercises as assigned were in fact too detailed and labour intensive or that the patient has difficulty committing the personal time necessary to effect therapeutic change. It is important for the therapist to know whether the patient is experiencing new insights and a sense of accomplishment through completing the exercises: this assists in gauging where to direct therapy.

■ TREATMENT STRATEGIES

Both cognitive and behavioural techniques are used to effect change. Basic CBT strategies are outlined here. Advanced CBT strategies are beyond the scope of this text. Although treatment strategies are described here, advanced training and clinical supervision are essential to treatment delivery.

Cognitive Techniques

Cognitive techniques revolve primarily around cognitive restructuring, a process that follows a particular path of identifying, analyzing, and modifying the three levels of cognition, beginning with automatic thoughts and working through to core beliefs.

KEY CONCEPT

Cognitive restructuring is a process in which cognitions (automatic thoughts and intermediate and core beliefs) are identified, analyzed, and modified to effect positive change in mood and behaviour.

Identifying Automatic Thoughts

Awareness of one's thinking is the first step toward change. Early in treatment, patients are often unaware of their running internal negative dialogues about themselves, others, and the world. The accompanying emotion may be much more apparent to patients than the underlying negative, inflexible thoughts. When introducing patients to the skill of identifying automatic thoughts, a useful place to begin is to have them attend to shifts in or intensification of their emotions. When a strong emotion is felt or a new emotion is experienced, the question is asked, "What was going through your mind?" (Beck, 2011). This question often helps patients to attend to the thinking that drives their emotional experience. Another technique to elicit automatic thoughts is to ask the patient to recount a very recent problematic situation. The patient is encouraged to play back the situation in his or her mind using all the senses. As the patient visualizes the details of what happened, he or she is asked, "What does this situation say about you?" "What does it mean for how others will view you?" "What about this situation is bothering you the most?" "If the worst case scenario came from this situation, what do you think would happen?" (Greenberger & Padesky, 1995). Once automatic thoughts are identified, evaluation of their accuracy and usefulness is undertaken.

Evaluating Automatic Thoughts

The goal of evaluating automatic thoughts is to examine thoughts in detail to determine their accuracy. Patients consider both supporting and unsupporting evidence in relation to their automatic thoughts. They need to focus on objective facts rather than interpretations, assumptions, or opinions when generating evidence, although initially this may be difficult (Greenberger & Padesky, 1995). Finding evidence that is unsupportive of automatic thoughts can be aided by key questions such as, "What experiences have I had that show this thought is not always completely true?" "If someone I cared deeply about had this thought, what would I tell them?" "If someone who cared deeply about me knew I was thinking this, what would they say to me?" "What evidence is there that this thought is not 100% true?" (Greenberger & Padesky, 1995). When evaluating automatic thoughts, often patients conclude that the evidence for the automatic thought is weaker than the evidence against, and therefore that the thought is no longer as accurate and valid as it was once believed to be.

The following case example illustrates the process of evaluating automatic thoughts. A patient, Elizabeth, was reprimanded by her employer for not completing her monthly report, an essential part of her job. After exploring the emotions she experienced in this situation (fear and shame), she identified several negative automatic thoughts, including "My boss hates me," "I might lose my job," "He thinks I'm incompetent," "I'm not a responsible or trustworthy employee," and "I'm nothing but a screw-up." The therapist helped Elizabeth determine which automatic thought was most distressing to her ("I'm nothing but a screw-up"), and it was this

thought that became the one to be evaluated. Elizabeth was asked to find evidence to support the thought, "I'm nothing but a screw-up." Given that she was instructed to consider only objective information, and not her opinion, the following evidence was generated: "I failed two courses in one semester during my 1st year of university because I partied more than I studied," "I am sometimes late paying my credit card bill," and "I once had a boyfriend who told me I wouldn't get anywhere in life." Elizabeth's next task was to find evidence that does not support her thought, "I'm nothing but a screw-up." Reviewing key questions with her therapist, she was able to find nonsupporting evidence: "I generally receive above-average yearly performance appraisals from my boss," "In addition to working this job, I volunteer in my son's classroom two times a month, and I have been called invaluable," and "My best friend tells me that I'm a very organized mother."

Evaluating one's automatic thoughts also involves identifying cognitive distortions (thinking errors or problematic thinking styles). These are the characteristic and habitual ways people err in thinking about themselves or others (Burns, 1989). Thinking errors are problematic as they keep people locked into patterns of negative thinking and behaviour. Burns initially identified 10 types of thinking errors, a list that has been adapted and added to by others over time (Box 13.5). People tend to have a consistent pattern of thinking errors across a variety of situations. All people engage in distorted thinking; it is not a phenomenon limited to people with mental disorders. In CBT, the therapist works with the patient to first identify which thinking errors are being used. Patients are commonly given a handout listing all the cognitive errors with relevant examples of each. Such a handout guides patients through the process of identifying and labelling thinking errors. The next step is to examine the usefulness and validity of this style of thinking so that patients can respond to their thoughts in a more realistic, balanced manner. Through the process of correcting thinking errors, patients see that the negative automatic thoughts and beliefs they held about themselves, others, and the world at large are no longer valid. It is important to catch oneself when making the errors and inject a clearer way of looking at the situation. When we give ourselves more options for how to think, we give ourselves more options for how to feel and how to respond.

Returning to the case of Elizabeth, she identified that she routinely engages in distorted thinking by jumping to conclusions ("I might lose my job." "He thinks I'm incompetent.") and overgeneralization ("I'm not a responsible or trustworthy employee. I'm nothing but a screw-up"). Elizabeth worked with her therapist to increase her awareness of how frequently she engages in this style of thinking. Further, her therapist helped Elizabeth to realize the inaccuracy and destructiveness of this style of thinking.

BOX 13.5 Ten Thinking Errors

1. All-or-nothing thinking: The tendency to see things in black-and-white categories, with no shades of grey. Things are seen in extremes, either very good or very bad. "If I don't get a perfect evaluation, I'm a failure."

2. Overgeneralization: The assumption that one error/problem means a lifetime of the same error/problem. "If I lose this job, I will never succeed in making a living."

3. Mental filter: Filtering out the good things that happen and retaining only the negative. "When I received that award, I could see that Jane didn't think I deserved it."

4. Magnification/minimization: Overexaggeration of fears, imperfections, or errors. "There is absolutely no way I could have passed that exam. I've totally blown the course."

5. Jumping to conclusions: Concluding things that are not justified based on available evidence. "I saw Peter yawn during my presentation. Everyone was bored." It includes mind reading: "My coworker didn't say hello to me today because she's starting to dislike me" and fortune telling: "He didn't call me tonight. That's it. He'll never call again."

6. Labelling: Putting a negative label on yourself or others, a way to believe that no one can change. "My roommate is a slob. I have to keep everything tidy."

7. Personalization and blame: Making yourself feel responsible for things out of your control. "It is my fault our team lost the game. If only I hadn't dropped the ball in the first half."

8. Should/must statements: Thinking in terms of "should" and "must." "I must make no mistakes during the skill laboratory, no matter what."

9. Discounting the positives: Refusing to credit the positive aspects of situations. "John said that I looked great today. He must think that I look terrible most days."

10. Emotional reasoning: Believing something must be true because one "feels" it so strongly, ignoring any evidence to the contrary. "I know I've had people in my life who say I'm a good person, but it's hard to believe because I feel like I'm so bad."

From Burns, D. D. (1989). *The feeling good handbook: Using the new mood therapy in everyday life.* New York, NY: Morrow.

Modifying Automatic Thoughts

Modification of automatic thoughts is an essential component of CBT. The patient uses what he or she has learned about identifying and evaluating automatic thoughts to move toward modification. Modifying thoughts involves weighing evidence for and against an automatic thought in an effort to generate a new, more balanced way of thinking. This new way of thinking does not simply involve replacing negative thoughts with positive ones. Unquestioning acceptance of a positive stance can be as destructive as negative thinking because it does not take into account all available evidence (Greenberger & Padesky, 1995). The new way of thinking considers all aspects of one's experience so that one can arrive at a more broadened way of viewing oneself, others, or the world. In Elizabeth's case, she examined all her available evidence and recognized an alternative way of understanding her situation: "I have exceedingly high expectations of myself and find it very hard to give myself a break when I've done something I perceive as less than acceptable. I have screwed up in the past, but it's been relatively infrequently, and I do learn from my mistakes." A summary statement of the evidence regarding an automatic thought can be useful in the development of balanced thinking. For example, Elizabeth summarized her evidence by saying, "I've done things that are not responsible and have received negative messages from others of the same kind, but I also am currently successful in juggling many demanding roles and receive praise for my efforts." With this expanded view, patients generally report that they experience a positive shift in mood.

A useful, commonly used tool in CBT is the Thought Record (Greenberger & Padesky, 1995). It is a structured worksheet that records all the pertinent information about problematic and distressing situations and helps patients to make sense of why they feel and react in particular ways. Thought Records take all aspects of one's experience and organize them into information presented in seven columns: the situation, moods, automatic thoughts, evidence that supports the thoughts, evidence that does not support the thoughts, formation of balanced or alternative thoughts, and rerating of moods. At various points throughout the Thought Record, thoughts and emotions are rated and rerated on their degree of strength and believability (0% to 100%). Once the Thought Record is completed, the goal is for patients to experience a balanced or alternative thought that is rated as more believable than their original negative automatic thought accompanied by a decrease in the intensity of their originally identified emotions. Thought Records are completed during and between therapy sessions whenever problematic or distressing situations arise.

Students undergoing CB training routinely complete their own Thought Records to gain an increased awareness of their own thinking patterns and resulting emotions and behaviours, to encourage self-reflection and self-monitoring, and to become acquainted with the process of using the record. Thought Records may be shared with supervisors and discussed in supervision sessions.

Identifying and Modifying Intermediate Beliefs

The techniques of identifying and modifying automatic thoughts are used with intermediate beliefs or assumptions, as well as other techniques to get to the deeper level assumptions. Identifying assumptions can be aided by attending to the patterns of negative thoughts that emerge over the course of therapy, as these themes may suggest an underlying assumption or core belief. Identifying the rules that patients live by and expect of others may be useful. A commonly used method to uncover assumptions behind an automatic thought is the downward arrow technique (Burns, 1980), in which the therapist questions the meaning of the patient's thought until an assumption or a core belief about self, others, or the world is revealed. See Box 13.6 for an example. This technique can be used to reveal assumptions about others (What does x mean about other people?) or the world in general (What does x say about how the world works?). Once the assumption is revealed, the process of restructuring the assumption is initiated wherein the evidence for and against the assumption and alternative responses are considered. Behavioural experiments (to be discussed) are also an effective means to modify assumptions because they allow patients to use real-life situations to test the accuracy of beliefs.

Identifying and Modifying Core Beliefs

All the techniques discussed thus far, especially the downward arrow technique, are useful for identifying core beliefs. Deeply rooted core beliefs may require additional, advanced strategies beyond the scope of this chapter. Such strategies include discussing the early life experiences of the patient, as core beliefs may be better understood when the context in which they developed is considered. In-depth exploration wherein patients relive painful early experiences, however, is not appropriate in CBT.

Beck (2011) encourages the use of Core Belief Worksheets to identify core beliefs, to strengthen the believability of new core beliefs, and to weaken the influence of old core beliefs. The patient first identifies his or her old core belief and rates it out of 100 (e.g., "I'm undesirable," 70%), followed by his or her new core belief ("Once people get to know me, they can see that I'm a likeable person," 40%). Similar to the process of evaluating automatic thoughts, the patient gathers evidence that contradicts his or her old belief and supports his or her new belief ("Last week, someone in my running group gave me her number so we can arrange to go for a run together." "I have one friend who has stayed by my side despite all the things I've been through"). The final step is to gather evidence that supports the old belief with the addition of a cognitive reframe ("When my last girlfriend broke up with me, she said she could never love a person like me, but I was struggling with depression during our relationship; therefore, I couldn't bring much to the relationship," "People don't readily seek out my friendship, but I'm now realizing that I have given off signals to people to stay away. This was my way of protecting myself from the rejection I believed was inevitable"). Thus, a broader perspective is achieved that takes into account past and current experiences.

Behavioural Techniques

Behavioural strategies are primarily utilized in CBT as a way to test and challenge both old maladaptive thinking patterns and newly acquired rational thoughts. They may be used to modify symptoms when conducted in a manner that supports a change in cognition (Butler et al., 2008). Behavioural techniques must be considered and implemented within the larger scope of CBT. They are not employed in isolation, nor are they implemented without being linked back to the cognitive model of the particular disorder being treated.

Behavioural Strategies to Test Beliefs

Creating experiences to test and challenge core beliefs is an essential CBT treatment strategy called **behavioural experiments** (Beck, 2011). The validity and accuracy of old core beliefs are tested in real-life situations, thus increasing the believability of alternative thoughts. Without this behavioural component, the process of challenging the accuracy and validity of old thoughts and generating new thoughts may be little more than an intellectual exercise and may not lead to meaningful cognitive, emotional, or behavioural change. Behavioural

---

BOX 13.6 A Dialogue Using the Downward Arrow Technique

Patient: I didn't do the self-reflective exercise this week because it was too hard.

Therapist: What does that say about you that you found it too hard?

Patient: It says that I didn't pay enough attention in the session last week.

Therapist: And if that were true, that you didn't pay enough attention last week, what would that say about you?

Patient: It would say that I'm lazy.

Therapist: If it was true that you were lazy, what would that say about you?

Patient: It would say that I'm useless.

experiments can be challenging for patients because the prospect of putting new thoughts into action and testing old destructive ways of thinking can be anxiety producing.

Behavioural experiments can be presented to patients as an opportunity to "test-drive" their new thoughts to see what will really happen as a result. A typical behavioural experiment consists of the therapist and the patient collaboratively constructing an experiment to test a new belief. For example, the new belief, "I'm a likeable person," could be tested by constructing an experiment in which the patient plans to call an acquaintance from his running group and invite her to go for a run. The patient makes a prediction about what might happen in the course of the experiment ("She'll agree to go with me, but she'll find me a bit uninteresting"). Potential obstacles are considered ("I will become very nervous and talk very little; therefore, she'll think I'm boring"), as well as action that can be taken to manage the obstacles ("Remind myself that being nervous is okay when you are getting to know people for the first time. Remind myself that even if I don't talk much, I can't jump to the conclusion that she will think I'm boring"). The actual result of the experiment is reported ("We ran together for an hour and talked about our interests. I found out that we have many things in common, including that we both like classic films and we're both shy people. She told me that *Citizen Kane* is playing in 2 weeks and suggested that we see it together"). The patient then rates how much the result of the experiment supports his or her new belief (90%) and finally reflects on what was learned in the process of the experiment ("If I take more risks and show people who I really am, they can see that I'm a nice person and worth getting to know better"). Behavioural experiments are a powerful means of altering beliefs because they compel patients to take action on a thought. When patients are able to directly see the outcome of testing their beliefs, they are more likely to actually modify their beliefs.

Behavioural Strategies to Modify Symptoms

Numerous types of behavioural strategies for symptom reduction are available, including exposure techniques, relaxation training, and activity monitoring. Exposure therapy is utilized in panic disorder, panic disorder with agoraphobia, PTSD, social phobia, and obsessive–compulsive disorder. The common thread among all types of exposure is that they put the patient in contact with feared or avoided thoughts, emotions, behaviours, or situations (Craske, 2010). Through this process, three possible outcomes may occur: the patient's anticipated catastrophic outcome may be disconfirmed; the patient may become desensitized to the feared response; and the patient's ability to cope with the feared situation may be improved. Exposure-based techniques are very specific to the disorder being treated, and the protocols are extensive and comprehensive.

Relaxation strategies, such as controlled breathing and progressive muscle relaxation, may be employed with patients who have generalized anxiety disorder, panic disorder, and PTSD. Controlled breathing is the practice of learning how to breathe at an appropriate pace and depth so that this skill can be called on when faced with feared stimuli. The person learns to breathe from the diaphragm rather than the thorax (Craske, 2010). Patients are also educated about the effects of hyperventilation and breath holding, such as increased blood pressure and disturbance of the oxygen–carbon dioxide balance, and how these can worsen anxiety symptoms. Progressive muscle relaxation, or Jacobsonian relaxation (Jacobson, 1938), involves the practice of deliberately tensing and relaxing 12 groups of muscles, beginning with the feet and moving upward to the face. The technique teaches patients how to relax muscles and induce a sense of physical and mental calmness (see Chapter 23). Other relaxation techniques include mindfulness-based CBT (see below) and guided imagery (see Chapter 11).

Depressed individuals often benefit from activity scheduling, wherein daily activities and accompanying moods are recorded in a diary format (Beck, 2011). Many depressed patients become immobilized and believe that they must wait to feel better before engaging in activities. Activity monitoring encourages depressed individuals to instead engage in activity as a way to improve mood. Activity scheduling is useful for both pleasurable and avoided tasks and monitoring moods. It is beneficial for challenging beliefs ("There isn't anything that I enjoy doing," "I'm not good at doing anything") (Beck, Rush, Shaw, & Emery, 1979).

■ MINDFULNESS-BASED CBT

Mindfulness is a form of trained self-observation based on meditation practices (David, 2006). It involves learning to be present to what is happening to one in the immediate moment. Its core elements have been identified as attention (receptivity) and awareness (being deeply self-aware and self-monitoring), present-centredness (being in the moment), external events (the outer milieu's impact on the mind and body), and cultivation (the fostering of tranquility and insight); a fifth element, ethical-mindedness (social awareness) links mindfulness to its Buddhist origins as "sati" (Nilsson & Kazemi, 2016). Mindfulness can help people to disengage their "automatic pilot" in order to look more carefully at their convictions and thought patterns. The act of pushing away negative thoughts and emotions can actually increase distress. Mindfulness reduces that struggle and allows for calm. For those with long-standing problems, becoming mindful can be challenging. It takes time to experience mindful self-reflection with acceptance and an attitude of curiosity and compassion rather than self-judgement and distress (Butler et al., 2008). It takes practice to develop the skill of mindfulness, but being able to respond mindfully to a situation rather than with a habitually unhelpful response can make a significant positive difference (David, 2006).

■ CONCLUSION

The simple idea that emotion and behaviour are influenced by cognition has generated decades of empirical study, which indicates that CBT is a highly effective and cost-efficient treatment for individuals struggling with certain mental disorders. The active and collaborative nature of CBT, combined with its orientation toward change, makes it an easy fit with nursing, as is evidenced by the interest and broad appeal of CBT among nurses. Psychiatric and mental health nurses are strong advocates of self-reflection and awareness of how one's own experiences influence the therapeutic relationship. With appropriate training, nurses will find CBT to be useful to their therapeutic repertoire. CBT offers an empirically and theoretically sound means to improve the mental health of their patients.

SUMMARY OF KEY POINTS

- The cognitive model is based on the idea that the way we think about situations influences our emotion and behaviour.
- CBT is based on changing negative thought patterns as a means to improve mood and behaviour.
- CBT is the most widely researched form of psychotherapy used to treat many mental disorders, including PTSD, bulimia nervosa, panic disorder, and depression.
- There are 10 principles of CBT: CB formulation; strong therapeutic alliance; collaborative with active participation from the patient; goal oriented and problem focused; initially emphasizes the present; educative and looks to prevent relapse; time limited; structured; teaches identification, evaluation, and response to dysfunctional thoughts and beliefs; and uses a variety of techniques to change thinking, mood, and behaviour.
- Cognitive techniques involve cognitive restructuring, a process that follows the steps of identifying, analyzing, and modifying automatic thoughts through to core beliefs.
- Behavioural techniques are used within the cognitive model and are seen as opportunities to test new beliefs.
- Mindfulness is a form of self-awareness training based in meditation.

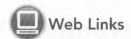 **Web Links**

www.anxietybc.com/cbt-home This website of the Anxiety Disorders Association of British Columbia (AnxietyBC) has information about CBT, including videos with real stories of individuals' use of CBT.

http://www.mindfulnessinstitute.ca/ The resources shared at the website of the *mindfulnessinstitute.ca* include information about the emerging research on mindfulness as well as program information.

References

American Psychiatric Association. (2009). Practice guideline for the treatment of patients with panic disorder. *American Journal of Psychiatry, 166*(5 Suppl), 1–68.

Beck, J. (2011). *Cognitive therapy: Basics and beyond* (2nd ed.). New York, NY: Guilford Press.

Beck, A. T., & Emery, G. (1985). *Anxiety disorders and phobias: A cognitive perspective.* New York, NY: Basic Books.

Beck, A. T., Rush, A. J., Shaw, B. F., & Emery, G. (1979). *Cognitive therapy of depression.* New York, NY: Guilford Press.

Burns, D. D. (1980). *Feeling good: The new mood therapy.* New York, NY: Morrow.

Burns, D. D. (1989). *The feeling good handbook: Using the new mood therapy in everyday life.* New York, NY: Morrow.

Butler, G., Fennell, M., & Hackmann, A. (2008). *Cognitive-behavioral therapy for anxiety disorders: Mastering clinical challenges.* New York, NY: The Guilford Press.

Carlbring, P., Degerman, N., Johnson, J., & Anderson, G. (2012). Internet-based treatment of pathological gambling with a three-year follow-up. *Cognitive Behavior Therapy, 4*(14), 321–334.

Craske, M. (2010). *Cognitive-behavioral therapy.* Washington, DC: American Psychological Association.

David, L. (2006). *Using CBT in general practice: The 10 minute consultation.* Bloxham, UK: Scion.

Greenberger, D., & Padesky, C. A. (1995). *Mind over mood.* New York, NY: Guilford Press.

Jacobson, E. (1938). *Progressive relaxation.* Chicago, IL: University of Chicago Press.

Kazantzis, N., Whittington, C., & Dattilio, F. (2010) Meta-analysis of homework effects in cognitive and behavioral therapy. *Clinical Psychology: Science & Practice, 17*(2), 144–156.

Marchand, A., Beaulieu-Prévost, D., Guay, S., Bouchard, S., Drouin, M. S., & Germain, V. (2011). Relative efficacy of cognitive-behavioral therapy administered by video conference for posttraumatic stress disorders: A six-month follow-up. *Journal of Aggression, Maltreatment & Trauma, 20*, 304–321.

Myhr, G., & Payne, K. (2006). Cost-effectiveness of cognitive-behavioural therapy for mental disorders: Implications for public health care funding policy in Canada. *Canadian Journal of Psychiatry, 51*(10), 662–669.

Myhr, G., Talbot, J., Annable, L., & Pinard, G. (2007). Suitability for short-term cognitive-behavioral therapy. *Journal of Cognitive Psychotherapy: An International Quarterly, 21*(4), 334–345.

Nilsson, H., & Kazemi, A. (2016). Reconciling and thematizing definitions of mindfulness: The big five of mindfulness. *Review of General Psychology, 20*(2), 183–193.

Paxling, B., Almlöv, J., Dahlin, M., Carlbring, P., Breitholtz, E., Eriksson, T., & Andersson, G. (2011). Guided Internet-delivered cognitive behavior therapy for generalized anxiety disorder: A randomized controlled trial. *Cognitive Behaviour Therapy, 40*(3), 159–173.

Tilfors, M., Carlbring, P., Furmark, T., Lewenhaupt, S., Spak, M., Eriksson, A., et al. (2008). Treating university students with social phobia and public speaking fears: Internet delivered self-help with or without live group exposure sessions. *Depression and Anxiety, 25*, 708–717.

White, K. S., Payne, L. A., Gorman, J. M., Shear, M. K., Woods, S. W., Saksa, J. R., & Barlow, D. H. (2013). Does maintenance CBT contribute to long-term treatment response of panic disorder with or without agoraphobia? A randomized controlled clinical trial. *Journal of Consulting and Clinical Psychology, 81*(1), 47–57.

Wootton, B. M. (2016). Remote cognitive-behavior therapy for obsessive-compulsive symptoms: A meta-analysis. *Clinical Psychology Review, 43*, 103–113.

14 Interventions With Groups

Carol Ewashen

Adapted from the chapter "Interventions with Groups" by Mary Ann Boyd

After studying this chapter, you will be able to:

- Discuss group concepts that are useful in understanding and leading groups.
- Compare the different roles and responsibilities of group members.
- Identify the important aspects of leading a group, such as member selection, leadership skills, seating arrangements, and ways of intervening with challenging group members.
- Differentiate types of groups: psychoeducational, cognitive–behavioural, supportive, psychotherapeutic, and self-help.
- Compare different nursing intervention groups.

- closed group • formal group roles • group cohesion • group dynamics • group leadership • groupthink • informal group roles • interactive groups • leadership styles • maintenance functions • open group • self-help groups • task functions • therapeutic factors

- group • group process

Participation in therapeutic groups has powerful treatment effects. Group treatment is effective and efficient for participants to further understand themselves in relation to others through interaction, gain new knowledge and social skills, conquer unwanted thoughts and feelings, and change behaviours. For effective interventions, the nurse must possess leadership skills that can shape, enhance, and monitor group interactions. The decisions regarding which interventions fit best are complex and dependent upon the purpose of the group. Competent group skill development requires the ability to critically select and modify techniques to best accommodate the particular practice conditions. This applies across diverse situations from providing patient and family education or conducting support groups to direct care provision, case management, and program leadership. Understanding group skills and dynamics is also increasingly relevant to contemporary health care education and service delivery with emphasis on effective interprofessional practice collaboration and teamwork (Canadian Interprofessional Health Collaborative, 2010); relationship communication for health care professionals (Pagano, 2015); racial and cultural diversity in groups (McRae & Short, 2010); and participatory and transformative pedagogies (Taylor & Cranston, 2012; Young & Paterson, 2007). A challenge in group intervention is the shift from a primarily individual focus to consideration of interpersonal and whole-group interactions. This chapter presents relevant group concepts for PMH nurses. Group leadership is explored with special emphasis on the groups relevant to PMH nursing practice.

■ GROUP: DEFINITIONS AND CONCEPTS

There are many different definitions of a group. Psychoanalytic tradition draws from the work of Sigmund Freud and considers group interaction as a recapitulation of the family of origin, interpreting unconscious conflicts and reexamining them. Contemporary psychodynamic theories consider groups a combination of group dynamics and interpersonal and intrapsychic transactions (Rutan & Stone, 2001). Yalom (1998) and Yalom and Leszcz (2005) suggest that a group is a social microcosm of interpersonal dynamics and advocate a here-and-now, self-reflective approach. The cognitive–behavioural approach considers a group a social arena for corrective change in maladaptive thinking and behaviour patterns, whereas, according to systems theory, a group consists of parts or components that exist to perform some activity or purpose. As group members interact, subsystems form, challenging leaders to understand boundary realignments and the effects of subcomponents on the system and to improve interpersonal communication. A more contemporary development, drawing from the rich history of group work and apparent across a wide range of settings, is the prevention group that utilizes a full range of group processes, constructive interactions, and positive group cohesion to reduce risk while promoting health and wellness (Harpine, 2013, 2015; Harpine, Nitza, & Conyne, 2010). A global, but rather simple, definition of a group is two or more people who are in an interdependent relationship with one another. The simplicity of the definition is misleading because interactions within groups, or group dynamics, are anything but simple. Group dynamics influence the group's development and process. In fact, it takes an astute observer to determine the real dynamics of a group and the effects. No matter the type of group, its theoretic orientation, or its purpose, group dynamics influence the effectiveness of a group intervention. Best practice requires that group facilitators understand and articulate the theoretical framework guiding their practice, including the rationale for use of specific techniques and interventions.

In this text, a group is defined as "two or more individuals who are connected to one another by social relationships" (Forsyth, 2006, p. 3). Groups are considered as social microcosms, dynamic living systems of interdependent relations, acquiring and expending energy, sustaining structure and functionalities, and responding to changing circumstances with capabilities for transformation (Forsyth & Diederich, 2014). As Susan Day states, "at the heart of group is a learning process in a social setting" (2014, p. 25). Groups can be further defined according to the number of people or the relationship of members. A dyad is a group of two people, such as a married couple, siblings, or parent and child. A triad is a group of three people. A family is a special type of group and is discussed in Chapter 15.

KEY CONCEPT

A **group** is "two or more individuals who are connected to one another by social relationships" (Forsyth, 2006, p. 3). "At the heart of group is a learning process in a social setting" (Day, 2014, p. 25)

Open Versus Closed Groups

A group can be viewed as either an open or a closed system. In an **open group**, new members are welcomed and provided time to learn group norms and expectations. For example, a newly admitted patient may join an anger management group that is part of an ongoing program in an inpatient unit. With new members, it is important to help them engage with the group by inviting member-to-member interaction. The advantage of an open group is that participants can join at any time. In addition, these groups can function on an ongoing basis and thus can be available to more people.

In a **closed group**, all members begin at the same time, and no new members are admitted. If a member of a closed group leaves, no replacement joins. Advantages of a closed group are that the participants get to know one another over time, the group becomes more cohesive, and members move concurrently through the group process. However, implementing closed-group interventions is often difficult, especially in tertiary settings where the length of stay is short and participant readiness for group work varies greatly.

Group Size

Group size is an important consideration in forming group programs. Many mental health professionals favour small groups, but large groups can also be effective. Whether to form a large or small group depends on the age of participants, the group's purpose, the leader's abilities, participant availability, and the resources available. Small groups (usually a minimum of 3 and no more than 10 members) become more cohesive, are less likely to form subgroups, and can provide a richer interpersonal experience than large groups. Small groups may function with one group leader, although many small groups are led by two people. An ideal small group is about seven to eight people in addition to the leader or leaders (Corey, 2013; Myers & Anderson, 2008).

Small groups often are used for people who are trying to deal with complex emotional issues such as depression, anxiety, eating disorders, substance use disorder, sexual abuse, or trauma. They are also ideal for individuals or families who require more specialized intervention such as families in recovery (Zimmerman & Winek, 2013). These groups work best if they are closed to new members or if new members are gradually introduced. One disadvantage of small groups relates to the loss of members. If places are unfilled, the group dynamics change, which may alter therapeutic effectiveness.

A large group (more than 10 members) can be therapeutic as well as cost-effective. Some research suggests that large intervention and prevention groups are effective for specific problems, such as smoking, or for settings such as schools and community (Harpine, 2013; McWhirter & McWhirter, 2010). A large group can be ongoing and open-ended. In large group intervention, a challenge for the nurse leader is to include all members in discussion, preventing a sense of alienation with the potential for member dropout.

Leading a group, whether large or small, is complex because of the number of potential interactions, relationships, and conflicts that can form. The leader needs both presentation and group leadership skills. Kottler and Englar-Carlson (2010) suggest that group work requires a different sort of mindset. It is insufficient to be purely a leader—a leader must practise in a therapeutic or facilitative manner while in the midst of a complex interactive event. Practitioners who take on *leadership* of groups require education and supervised training for competent, accountable, and ethical group practices. In large groups, the leader is often both a presenter of educative information and a facilitator of experiential learning among participants. In-depth reflection on participants' feelings and thoughts may not be the focus of group work. Depending on the theoretic orientation and the purpose of the group, leadership style and interventions must change to be effective in meeting the goals of small or large groups.

Group Development

In the same way that the development of the therapeutic relationship is a process (see Chapter 6), so too is the development of a group. Many researchers view group development as a sequence of phases, particularly in small groups (Table 14.1). Although models of group development differ, most follow a pattern of a beginning, middle, and ending stage (DeLucia-Waack, Kalodner, & Riva, 2014; Jacobs, Masson, & Harvill, 2009). These stages should be thought of not as a straight line with one preceding another, but as a dynamic and iterative process with continual revisiting and reexamining of group interactions, changes, and progress toward established goals.

KEY CONCEPT

Group process is the "what is happening" in the group and how members are interacting and relating with each other and as a whole group, involving nonverbal communications, group mood, and group atmosphere, including successes and tensions.

Beginning Stage

When a group begins, group members get to know one another and the group leader. The length of the beginning stage depends on, among other variables, the purpose of the group, the number of members, and the skill of the leader. It may last for only a few sessions or several. "Honeymoon" behaviours characterize the beginning of this stage, and "conflict" emerges at the end. During the initial sessions, members usually are polite and congenial, displaying behaviours typical of those in new social situations. They are "good" and often intellectualize problems; that is, by excessively using abstract thinking or generalizations, emotional conflict or stress is minimized. Members are usually anxious and sometimes act in ways that do not truly represent their feelings. In the first few sessions, members test whether they can trust one another. Sometime after the initial sessions, group members experience a period of conflict, either among themselves or with the leader. This conflict is a normal part of group development as members differentiate from each other, and many believe that negotiating conflict and differentiation satisfactorily is necessary to move into a productive working phase. Sometimes, one or more group members become the "scapegoat." While a scapegoat often performs a central function for the group, intervening to therapeutically process scapegoating is complex but necessary (Clark, 2002). Such situations challenge the leader to guide the group during this period by avoiding taking sides and treating all members respectfully.

Middle (Working) Stage

The middle, or working, stage of groups involves a real sharing of ideas and the development of closeness. A group-as-a-whole culture may emerge that is distinct from the individual personalities of its members. The group develops its own rules and rituals and has its own behavioural norms; for example, groups develop regular patterns of seating and interaction. Group norms are formed through the majority of members accepting or rejecting certain behaviour (Posthuma, 2001). During this stage, the group realizes its purpose. If the purpose

Table 14.1	Comparison of Models of Group Development	
Tuckman (1965)	**Garland, Jones, and Kolodny (1973)**	**Corey, Corey, and Corey (2013)**
Forming: Get to know one another and form a group	*Theme in all stages*: Closeness Pregroup *Forming*: Preparing for and deciding if this is the right group	*Preaffiliation*: Approach and avoidance; ambivalence around involvement
Storming: Tension and conflict occur; subgroups form and clash with each other	*Power and control*: Testing out and vying for status, authority, autonomy, influence and connection	*Initial stage*: Orienting; forming relations; establishing group structure and climate of trust
Norming: Develop norms for how to work with each other	*Intimacy*: More intense personal involvement and recognition of others; emergent growth	*Transition*: Emerging differences and potential for conflict
Performing: Reach consensus and develop cooperative relationships	*Differentiation*: Accept uniqueness of each with interdependence; cohesion	*Working*: Involved, interactive, and committed to engaging in productive group work
Adjourning: End of relationships and orientation to the future; sadness and appreciation	*Separation*: Moving apart; review and evaluation	*Final stage*: Consolidation of learning; sadness and anxiety with leaving

is education, the participants engage in learning new content or skills. If the aim of the group is to share feelings and experiences, these activities consume group meetings. During this stage, the group members take responsibility for starting on time, and the leader often needs to remind members when it is time to stop.

Ending (Termination) Stage

Ending, or termination, and saying goodbyes can be difficult for a group, especially a successful therapeutic one. During the final stages, members begin to separate and may grieve the loss of the group closeness while transitioning to reestablish themselves as individuals. Individuals terminate and say goodbyes from groups as they do from other relationships (see Chapter 6). One person may not show up at the last session, another person may bring up issues that the group has already addressed, and others may demonstrate anger or hostility. Most members of successful groups are sad as the group ends. During the last meetings, members may make arrangements for meeting after the group ends. Although these plans rarely materialize or continue, leaders should recognize these plans as part of the farewell process—saying goodbye to the group and to each other.

Roles of Group Members

There are two **formal group roles**, the leader and the members. In small groups, however, members often assume **informal group roles** or positions in the group with rights and duties that are directed toward one or more group members. Informal roles can be categorized as task, maintenance, or individual roles. One way to think of group roles is as the different hats members try on and learn from while involved in a group (Myers & Anderson, 2008; Posthuma, 2001). These roles can either facilitate or obstruct the group process and goals.

Task functions involve the business of the group or "keeping things focused." Individuals who assume this function keep the group focused on a main purpose. For any group to be successful, it must have members who assume some of these task roles, such as *information seeker* (asks for clarification), *coordinator* (spells out relationships between ideas), and *recorder* (keeper of the minutes). **Maintenance functions** facilitate the building of group-centred attitudes, behaviours, and processes. Members functioning in maintenance roles help by ensuring a consistent start time, assisting individuals to compromise, and encouraging everyone's participation. These members facilitate maintaining group cohesiveness and may have difficulty with group conflict and differentiation. The *harmonizer* (keeps the peace), *compromiser* (gives and takes), and *standard setter* (sets expectations) are examples of maintenance roles. In a successful group, members take on and learn from both group task and maintenance functions (Table 14.2). Leader and member responsibilities and functions shift depending upon the group stage and task.

Deviant roles are member roles that detract from group functioning (Myers & Anderson, 2008; Posthuma, 2001). These roles are considered dysfunctional to the group, often antagonistic to group building and group maintenance, and they may detract from the group purpose and cohesion; for example, someone who dominates the group conversation inhibits group interaction and work on task. When deviant roles dominate, the risk is that neither the group task nor group maintenance function is accomplished. Deviant role examples include the aggressor, blocker, recognition seeker, and dominator.

While acknowledged in scholarly and popular literature, member role classification and related functions in contemporary group work have become more controversial. Critiques include the dangers of decontextualizing, generalizing, and categorizing people as well as the potential "colonizing" effects when placing people in preexisting schemas that may negatively define people (Kottler & Englar-Carlson, 2010). While it is important for the leader to recognize that all groups function through a division of labour, the leader's primary responsibility is to facilitate all members in learning the functions of productive group work in relation to self, others, and group goals. This is especially challenging in contemporary practice where increasingly diverse and multicultural populations are served and where racial and cultural dynamics in group work and member roles cannot be underestimated or silenced (McRae & Short, 2010).

Group Communication

The main responsibilities of group leadership are to *actively listen* and to facilitate both verbal and nonverbal member-to-member communication to meet the treatment goals of the individual members and the entire group. Because of the number of people involved, developing trusting, working relationships within groups is more complicated than developing a single relationship with another person. The communication techniques used in establishing and maintaining individual relationships are similar for groups, but the leader also attends to the communication patterns among the members, the member-to-member communications.

Relational Communication

Group interaction can be viewed as relational communication that is dynamic and variable, with recognizable phases and interaction patterns oriented to growth and connection. Some patterns of interaction (e.g., sequences of speaking and acting) are more fixed while others are flexible (Clark, 2009). Relational communication posits that human beings yearn for connection, yet paradoxically, in developing increasingly complex relational

Table 14.2	Leader and Member Responsibilities and Functions	
Group Stage	**Leader**	**Member**
Pregroup: Formation of a group *Informed decision making*: How does this group fit with this member this purpose?	*Design and plan the group*: Purpose, structure, process, evaluation methods. Solicit group membership. Conduct pregroup screening interviews. Determine the group composition. Provide orientation to members.	To determine: Is the group right for me? Do I have enough knowledge to understand the group purpose and process? What do I want from the group experience? How do my expectations fit with the group expectations?
Initial Stage Orientation, exploration, and setting the structure of the group Creating a safe place Sharing information Engaging each other and as a whole group around purpose	Orient group members. Establish ground rules, norms, and expectations. Encourage all members to be involved and express expectations, reactions, and concerns. Clarify understandings. Be open with members' concerns and questions. Provide guidance yet encourage member interaction and initiative.	To work through: Will I be accepted? What will the leader think of me? What is expected of me? Establish trust. Form relations with others. Express thoughts, feelings, expectations, and reservations. Become involved. Set goals for self and self-in-relation to others. Be respectful of others. Learn well and share understandings.
Transition Increased anxiety and emergence of differences with potential for conflict Reluctance to voice concerns or frustrations	Teach members the value of recognizing conflict, naming the issue, and negotiating a win–win situation. Practise directness and tactfulness in naming issues in the here and now. Encourage members to share reactions while maintaining a safe environment. Intervene with sensitivity and prevent scapegoating of a particular member. Encourage participatory interaction. Reinforce learning of self in relation to others negotiating difference/conflict in group.	Recognize own defences and resistances. Recognize and express reactions to the group. Learn to constructively confront issues. Work through conflicts and differences rather than withdraw or form subgroups.
Working High trust High group cohesion High productivity Interactive with willingness to take risks Supportive hopeful climate	Exemplify caring confrontation, disclosure of issues, and support to others. Encourage member risk taking. Interpret meanings of behaviours and interpersonal patterns in group. Explore group themes. Encourage translating insight into action in daily living.	Practise openness with issues. Offer feedback to others. Practise new skills and behaviours in daily life. Initiate constructive challenge and support to others. Initiate active involvement with others.
Final Stage Saying goodbyes Reflection on learning, relations, changes made, and challenges ahead	Encourage saying of goodbyes to each other. Provide opportunity for members to provide feedback to each other. Reinforce changes made. Ensure members have the resources to enable further progress. Reemphasize the importance of confidentiality.	Acknowledge thoughts and feelings with leaving the group. Say goodbye to each member and to the leader. Review gains made and complete unfinished business. Evaluate the impact of the group. Plan for the future.

Adapted from Corey, M., Corey, G., & Corey, C. (2013). *Groups: Process and practice* (8th ed.). Belmont, CA: Brooks/Cole.

repertoires over time, patterns of disconnection also occur (Comstock, Duffey, & St. George, 2002; Fedele, 2004).

Interaction Patterns

Asking a colleague to observe and record content and interaction is a useful technique in determining the interaction patterns within a group; the leader may also use an audio or video recorder. In some groups, one person may always change the subject when another raises a sensitive topic. One person may always speak after another. People who sit next to each other tend to communicate among themselves. By analyzing the group event, content, process, and relational patterns, the leader can determine the existence of communication pathways and form interpretations—who is most liked in the group, who occupies a position of power, what subgroups have formed, where is connection growth-producing, and who is isolated and disconnecting from the group. Burtis and Turman's (2006) network analysis for group discussion provides a way to diagram connections among members, frequency of connections, and interactional patterns. Usually, those who are well liked or display leadership abilities tend to be chosen for interactions more often than do those who are less well liked (Fig. 14.1). In one study of communication networks, members who exhibited more dominant behaviours or whom the group perceived as being dominant emerged as more central to the group's communication networks and both sent and received more messages. The study also found that the task at hand affects the communication network. Groups that worked on low-complexity tasks had more centralized communication than when they worked on high-complexity tasks (Brown & Miller, 2000).

Group Themes

Group themes are the collective socioemotional and conceptual underpinnings of a group and express the members' underlying concerns or feelings, regardless of the group purpose. Themes that emerge in groups help members to understand group dynamics. Different groups have different themes. For example, three themes that emerged for a support group for grieving children included vulnerability, the importance of maintaining

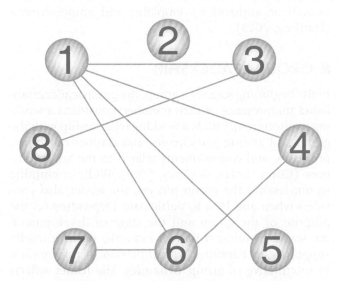

Figure 14.1. Network analysis of group discussion. In this analysis, response pattern was recorded during member interaction. Group members interacted with number *1* the most. Therefore, number *1* is the overchosen person. Numbers *5* and *7* are underchosen. Number *2* is never chosen and is determined to be the isolate.

memories, and the contribution of the group to the process of grieving. Although some predictable themes occur in groups, the obvious or assumed themes at the beginning may actually wind up differing as the process continues. In one hospice support group, the members seemed to be focusing on the memories of their loved ones. However, upon closer examination of the thematic content of group interactions, the discussion was revolving around financial planning for the future (Graham & Sontag, 2001).

Nonverbal Communication

Nonverbal communication is important to understanding group relations. All members, not just the group leader, observe the eye contact, posture, and body gestures of the participants. What is expressed is the result of individual and group, as well as internal and external, processes. For example, if one member is explaining a painful experience and another member looks away and tries to engage still another, the self-disclosing member may feel devalued and rejected because he or she interprets the behaviour as disruptive and disinterest. However, if the leader interprets the behaviour as anxiety over the topic, he or she may intervene and try to engage the other member in sharing reactions to the topic, the anxiety, and the impact on building relations with others.

The leader(s) should remain attuned to the nonverbal behaviour of group members during each session and the effect on group climate and process. Often, one or two people can set the overall mood of the group. Someone who comes to a session very sad or angry can set a tone of sadness or anger for the whole group. An astute group leader recognizes the effects of an individual's mood on the total group. If the purpose of the group is to process emotions, the group leader may invite member(s) to discuss emotional issues at the beginning of the session. The leader thus acknowledges the mood of the person(s) experiencing this and encourages discussion regarding the effect on other group members. If the group's purpose is inconsistent with self-disclosure of personal problems, the nurse should acknowledge the individual member's distress yet set limits while maintaining the group focus. In this instance, the nurse would limit repeated episodes of self-disclosure from the member(s) or others and redirect discussion to the group task.

Group Norms and Standards

Groups develop norms or rules and standards that establish acceptable group behaviours. Some norms are formalized, such as meeting as a group on time, but others are never really formalized. These standards encourage conformity of behaviour among group members. The group discourages deviations from these established norms. A group member has four options in relation to norms: conform, change the norm, be deviant, or leave the group (Posthuma, 2001). Open discussion that encourages healthy interaction while addressing unhelpful or problematic behaviours is one of the most successful ways of renegotiating group norms. *Leadership* is critical in establishing group norms consistent with the group goals to effect desired changes.

Group Cohesion

One of the goals of most group leaders is to foster **group cohesion**, a sense of "we-ness" as a group, with high levels of participation and involvement among members. Group cohesion is analogous to the therapeutic alliance in one-to-one relationships (MacKenzie, 1997). One of the first tasks of a good leader is to develop group cohesion through engaging all members in the group process. This involves close monitoring of the group atmosphere to develop a sense of belonging and commitment to the group goals. A particularly effective intervention for enhancing group cohesion is encouraging member-to-member interaction. In supportive and educational groups, leaders can promote social interaction with minimal supervision through organizing refreshment periods and team-building exercises. Cohesiveness is especially important in health education groups that focus on health maintenance behaviours such as exercise and weight control.

Dimock and Kass (2011) state that cohesion is like the glue that holds the group together and that if cohesion decreases, the group may begin to fall apart. Cohesion is a powerful force that motivates members and correlates with outcomes. In cohesive groups, members are committed to the existence of the group. In large heterogeneous groups, cohesiveness tends to be decreased, with subsequent decreased performance among group members in completing tasks. When members are strongly committed to completing a task and the leader encourages equal participation, cohesiveness promotes job satisfaction and higher performance (Steinhardt, Dolbier, Gottlieb, & McCalister, 2003). However, cohesiveness can be a double-edged sword. In very cohesive groups, members are more likely to transgress personal boundaries. Too much cohesiveness can exert powerful social pressure to conform to group standards with low tolerance for difference, while too little cohesiveness can result in mistrust, lack of engagement, and eventual disbanding of the group.

Groupthink and Decision Making

Groups that are strong and healthy encourage creativity, risk taking, differentiation, and change while remaining respectful of all members. Healthy groups encourage aligning with group norms and standards while remaining respectful of each member's unique contributions.

However, if feelings of unity become too intense and members are overly invested in maintaining the status quo, the phenomenon of **groupthink** can occur. Groupthink is the tendency of group members to isolate as a group, avoid conflict, maintain homogeneity, and adopt a closed-mindedness that is often congruent with a lack of impartial group leadership (Janis, 1982; Myers & Anderson, 2008). With groupthink, striving for uniformity overrides realistic, fair, and just appraisal of alternative courses of action. Members may not give honest feedback to each other for fear of censure. Empiric evidence of the effects of groupthink in organizations is lacking. Studies have shown that a closed *leadership* style and an external threat, particularly time pressure, appear to promote symptoms of groupthink and defective decision making (Neck & Moorhead, 1995).

Nurse leaders are responsible for mobilizing therapeutic and growth fostering factors to support healthy group development and prevent a stagnating groupthink consensus. What factors to mobilize and when depend on the type, purpose, and stage of the group. Supportive factors often emerge spontaneously and include universality, altruism, hope, and acceptance (MacKenzie, 1997). Other **therapeutic factors** proposed by Yalom and Leszcz (2005) are imparting information, corrective recapitulation of the primary family group, development of socializing techniques, imitative behaviours, catharsis, existential factors, cohesiveness, and interpersonal learning. Growth fostering relations are characterized by relational resilience and include the following dimensions: vitality and energy, capacity and desire for action, awareness of self in relation to others, self-worth, and desire for connection (Miller, 1986), as well as authenticity, empathy, and empowerment (Hartling, 2013).

■ GROUP LEADERSHIP

In the beginning stage of a group, the group leader establishes the presence of each member; constructs a working environment; builds a working relationship with the group and among participants; and clarifies outcomes, processes, and commitments related to the group purpose (Corey, Corey, & Corey, 2013). While attempting to understand the group process, the leader also considers when and how to participate. Depending on the purpose of the group and the stage of development, the leader position shifts, for example, from primarily supportive to educative with provision of information to interpretive of **group dynamics**. The leader reflects on, evaluates, and responds to promote effective group work. Leader intervention skills include attention to process while considering timing of interventions, when to clarify and when to interpret, when to intervene with individuals, and when to intervene with the group as a whole. Various techniques and strategies enhance the leader's ability to lead the group effectively and help the group attain its goals (Table 14.3).

One of the most important **group leadership** skills is active listening. A leader who practises active listening provides group members with someone who is responsive to what he or she says. A group leader who listens also models listening behaviour for others, helping them improve their skills. Listening enables the leader to process events and track interactions. The leader should be able to listen to the group members and formulate responses based on an understanding of the discussion. Members may need to learn to listen to one another,

track discussions without changing the subject, and learn to not speak while others are talking.

The leader tracks the verbal and nonverbal interactions throughout the group. Depending on the group purpose, the leader may keep this information private to understand the group process or may share the observations with the group. For example, if the purpose of the group is psychoeducational, the leader may use the information to facilitate the best learning environment. If the purpose of the group is to improve the self-awareness and interaction skills of members, the leader may point out patterns of interaction. The leader needs to be

Table 14.3	Techniques in Leading Groups	
Technique	**Purpose**	**Example**
Support: giving feedback that provides a climate of emotional support	Helps a person or group continue with ongoing activities Informs group about what the leader thinks is important Creates a climate for expressing unpopular ideas Helps the more quiet and fearful members speak up	"We really appreciate your sharing that experience with us. It sounds like it was quite painful."
Confrontation: challenging a participant (needs to be done in a supportive environment)	Helps individuals learn something about themselves Helps reduce some forms of disruptive behaviour Helps members deal more openly and directly with one another	"Tom, this is the third time that you have changed the subject when we have talked about spouse abuse. Is something going on?"
Information and suggestions: sharing expertise and knowledge that the members do not have	Provides information that members can use once they have examined and evaluated it Helps focus group's task and goals	"The medication that you are taking may be causing you to be sleepy."
Summarizing: statements at the end of the session that highlight the session's discussion, any problem resolution, and unresolved problems	Provides continuity from one session to the next Brings to focus still-unresolved issues Organizes past in ways that clarify Brings to focus themes and patterns of interaction	"This session we discussed Sharon's medication problems, and she will be following up with her physicians."
Clarification: restatement of an interaction	Checks on the meanings of the interaction and communication Avoids faulty communication Facilitates focus on substantive issues rather than allowing members to be sidetracked into misunderstandings	"What I heard you say was that you are feeling very sad right now. Is that correct?"
Probing and questioning: a technique for the experienced group leader that asks for more information	Helps members expand on what they were saying (when they are ready to) Gets at more extensive and wider range of information Invites members to explore their ideas in greater detail	"Could you tell us more about your relationship with your parents?"
Repeating, paraphrasing, highlighting: a simple act of repeating what was just said	Facilitates communication among group members Corrects inaccurate communication or emphasizes accurate communication	*Member*: "I forgot about my wife's birthday." *Leader*: "You forgot your wife's birthday."
Reflecting feelings: identifying feelings that are being expressed	Orients members to the feelings that may lie behind what is being said or done Helps members deal with issues they might otherwise avoid or miss	"You sound upset."
Reflecting behaviour: identifying behaviours that are occurring	Gives members an opportunity to see how their behaviour appears to others and to evaluate its consequences Helps members to understand others' perceptions and responses to them	"I notice that when the topic of sex is brought up, you look down and shift in your chair."

Adapted from Sampson, E., & Marthas, M. (1990). *Group process for the health professions* (pp. 222–224). Albany, NY: Delmar.

clear about the theoretical orientation and purpose of the group and tailor leadership strategies accordingly.

Understanding different group **leadership styles** can be useful in deciding which style fits which group situation. Leadership style is influenced by the group leader's personal characteristics and behaviours, theoretic background, and the group structure and purpose. Often leaders have a dominant style that fits more comfortably with who they are; however, developing a repertoire of different styles offers a wider range of interventions. Regardless of style, a leader remains fair and respectful, avoiding favouritism and encouraging participation and involvement of all members with each other. Other important skills include providing everyone with an opportunity to contribute and respecting everyone's ideas. A leader must also consider the degree of member disclosure warranted in each situation. In supportive and educative groups, leaders tend to be more expressive and interactive. A good rule of thumb in relation to leader self-disclosure is to consider whether the disclosure furthers the purposes of the group. A leader is responsible for understanding the intent and impact of leader self-disclosure on both individual members and the group as a whole. It is also assumed that a leader will engage in continuous learning through ongoing critical reflection with opportunity for regular supervision.

Some generally accepted guidelines in leading groups include establishing group structure and norms by setting start and stop times, arranging for the introduction of new members, and listening while other people talk. Leaders explain these group norms or rules at the first group meeting and continue structuring as an ongoing process. An important group rule is to always begin and end at the scheduled time. This sets a clear and reliable structure that helps reduce initial anxieties, educate members about group process, and encourage members to acquire skills that contribute to a successful group experience.

Typology of Leadership Styles

Whatever the leader's theoretic background, leadership styles can be viewed more traditionally as a continuum from direct to indirect, or, in keeping with contemporary literature, as transformational, authentic, and/or situational (Benson, 2010; Crowell, 2011). In the *direct leadership style*, the leader is actively authoritarian and controls the interaction by giving directions and information and allowing little discussion. The authoritarian leader literally tells the members what to do. On the other end of the continuum is *indirect leadership*, a form of laissez-faire, where the leader is primarily passive, reflects the group members' discussion, and offers little guidance or information to the group. Leadership is inadequate and lacking. Effective group leadership is flexible and considers the group task and when to intervene in situations that require attention. The challenge of providing leadership is to know what to do in specific situations so that the group and member goals can be met and group process furthered with enough freedom that members can make mistakes and recover in a supportive, caring learning environment. In transformational leadership, both leaders and members gain from one another, energized to perform beyond initial expectations (Grossman & Valiga, 2012), while authentic leadership promotes high ethical standards and relational transparency and instills powerful social processes that positively influence members and the group climate as a whole (Walumbwa, Luthans, Avey, & Oke, 2009). Nielsen (2013) examined the effect of leadership style on the occurrence of bullying in work groups. Laissez-faire leadership was associated with increased risk of exposure to bullying, while transformational and authentic leadership was associated with less risk.

Selecting the Members

Individuals can self-refer or be referred to groups. The leader is responsible for assessing the individual's suitability to the group. In instances where a new group is forming, the leader preplans, sets criteria for group membership, and invites members with the aim that the group can be well functioning and beneficial for each member. The leader should consider the following criteria when selecting members:

- Does the purpose of the group match the treatment goals of the potential member?
- Does the potential member have the social skills to function comfortably in the group?
- Can the potential member make a commitment to attending group meetings?

Arranging Seating

Spatial seating arrangements contribute to group comfort and interactive group communication. Over time, group members tend to sit in the same places. Where a person sits may offer different insights into group interaction. For example, those who consistently sit close to the group leader may desire power more so than those who sit far away, or those sitting closer to the leader may feel safer. Arranging a group in a circle with chairs comfortably close to one another without a table focuses group work on relations with each other and on communication. In therapeutic **interactive groups**, no one should sit outside the group, as this often indicates exclusion and/or resistance. If a table is necessary, a round table is preferable to a rectangular one that spatially identifies two distinct positions of power for those who sit at the ends.

Ideally, the session is held in a quiet, pleasant room with no distractions, adequate space, and the assurance of privacy and confidentiality. Holding a session in too large or too small a room may inhibit engaged communication and a sense of comfort.

Intervening With Challenging Group Behaviours

Behaviours problematic to the group task can occur in all groups. They can be challenging to the most experienced group leaders and frustrating to new leaders. When intervening with any problematic behaviour or situation, the leader must remember to support the integrity of the individual members and the group as a whole. It is important for the group leader to consider what might be escalating difficult behaviours and to remember that challenging or deviant members may serve a function for the group (American Group Psychotherapy Association, 2007). This could include releasing uncomfortable tension, speaking the unspeakable, or deflecting anger. One of the simpler therapeutic interventions with difficult member behaviour is to describe what is observed and let the member know how it is affecting others (Corey, 2013).

Monopolizing Group Time

Some people tend to monopolize a group by frequent talking or interrupting others. This behaviour is common in the beginning stages of group formation and usually represents anxiety that the member displaying such behaviour is experiencing. Within a few sessions, this person usually relaxes and spends less time monopolizing the group. However, for some people, monopolizing discussions is an established interpersonal style that will continue. Other group members usually find the behaviour mildly irritating in the beginning and extremely annoying as time passes. Members may drop out of the group to avoid that person. The leader needs to decide if, how, and when to intervene. The best case scenario is when savvy group members remind the monopolizer to let others speak. The leader can then support the group in reinforcing rules that allow everyone the opportunity to participate. However, the group often waits for the leader to act. There are a couple of ways to manage the situation. The leader can interrupt the monopolizer by acknowledging the member's contribution but redirecting the discussion to others, or the leader can become more directive and limit the discussion time per member.

"Yes, But..."

Some people have a patterned response to any suggestions from others. Initially, they agree with suggestions others offer them, but then they add "yes, but..." and give several reasons why the suggestions will not work for them. Leaders and members can easily identify this patterned response. In such situations, it is best to avoid problem solving for the member and encourage the person to develop his or her own solutions. The leader can role model problem-solving behaviour for the other members and encourage them to let the member develop a solution that would work specifically for him or her.

Disliked Member

In some groups, members clearly dislike one particular member. This situation can be challenging for the leader because it can result in considerable tension and conflict. This person could become the group scapegoat, a phenomenon that requires therapeutic intervention (Clark, 2002, 2009). Often, the group leader intervenes by showing respect for the disliked member and acknowledging his or her contribution. Depending on the group structure and purpose, one solution may be to move the person to a better-matched group. Whether the person stays or leaves, the group leader must be willing to accept anger, avoid displaying verbal and nonverbal behaviours that indicate that he or she too dislikes the group member or that he or she is displeased with the other members for their behaviour, and help the group members learn through processing what is happening in the group. In some instances, getting supervision from a more experienced group leader is useful. Defusing the situation may be possible by using conflict resolution strategies and discussing the underlying issues.

Group Conflict

Most groups experience periods of conflict. It is the avoidance of conflict that is problematic for a group. It is important that conflicts be acknowledged and the leader then decide how best to address the issues. Member-to-member conflict can be negotiated by using the conflict resolution process discussed in Chapter 11. Leader-to-member conflict is more complicated and often difficult for members to express because the leader has the hierarchical position of greater power. In this instance, the leader can use conflict resolution strategies, including encouraging members to directly express concerns, while remaining sensitive to the power differential. Group cohesion often increases as conflictual issues are effectively addressed.

■ TYPES OF GROUPS

Different types of groups are identified by the group goals and interactive processes or dynamics. The group leader assumes responsibility for ensuring group processes are in keeping with the group goals. Not every type of group is a therapy group. Over the past decade, the different types and specific uses of groups have grown, with increased research evidence of effectiveness. Type of group is increasingly responsive to emerging contemporary issues in research, education, and practice, for example, incarcerated women and addictions programs (Covington, 2013); group play interventions for children (Reddy, 2012); support group for fathers whose partners died from cancer (Yopp & Rosenstein, 2013); cardiovascular health promotion education for immigrant women (Fredericks & Guruge, 2015); effective group work in nurse education (Chapman, 2006); group prenatal care (Vonderheid, Klima, Norr, Grady, & Westdahl, 2013); and preventing health disparities (Stone & Kwan, 2016).

Structured Groups

Structured groups have an explicit structure predetermined by the group leader. These groups are often short term, oriented to education, and focus on a specific theme such as smoking prevention, substance abuse prevention, stress management, self-esteem for children, and parenting skills. Group goals focus primarily on education, psychosocial skill development, and task completion. In a mixed method research study, Kidd, Graor, and Murrock (2013) investigated the impact of a structured group "mindful eating intervention" on weight loss and depression in urban, underserved, obese women. The group mindfulness intervention was co-facilitated by an PMH clinical nurse specialist and a dietician. The study illustrated the benefits of social support, the significance of relationships, and the women's increased self-efficacy for weight loss.

Psychoeducational Groups

Psychoeducational groups are directed to specific concepts and teaching–learning aims. The process includes focused teaching with ample opportunity for questions, interactive discussions, and activities related to the topic.

The group leader primarily imparts information, promotes discussions, and facilitates experiential learning through structured activities. Psychoeducational groups include task groups that focus on completion of specific activities (e.g., planning a week's menu) and teaching groups that are used to enhance knowledge, improve skills, or solve problems. For example, van Santvoort, Hosman, van Doesum, and Janssens (2013) investigated the diverse needs of children of parents with mental illness or addiction participating in prevention support groups that offered social support, psychoeducation, and coping skills training. The authors concluded that given the heterogeneity in children's functioning and level of family risk, group interventions of different intensity and content should be considered as well as reaching children at an earlier age if prevention is a main aim. Other examples include medication groups, anger management groups, and stress management groups. Psychoeducational groups are formally planned, and members are purposefully selected. Members are asked to join specific groups because of the focus of the group. These groups are time limited and last for only a few sessions (Box 14.1).

BOX 14.1 **Research for Best Practice**

PSYCHOEDUCATIONAL GROUP NURSING INTERVENTION FOR RISK OF DEPRESSION WITH MOTHERS OF INTELLECTUALLY DISABLED CHILDREN

From Yıldırım, A., Aşilar, R. H., & Karakurt, P. (2013). Effects of a nursing intervention program on the depression and perception of family functioning of mothers with intellectually disabled children. Journal of Clinical Nursing, 22(1–2), 251–261.

Question: What are the effects of psychosocial education groups provided to mothers with intellectually disabled children on their risk of depression and their perception of family functioning?

Method: Mothers of intellectually disabled children (*n* = 75) attending a routine program at a private education and rehabilitation centre were randomly assigned to an intervention (*n* = 40) or a control (*n* = 35) group. Intervention group members attended four psychosocial educational sessions (120 minutes each) over 4 weeks, as well as the routine program. This group intervention involved topics such as care and education of a special needs child, family communication, problem-solving, and resources and use of strategies such as role play and homework. The control group attended only the routine program. Demographic data about the mother

and her child (e.g., ages, education, economic and work status, home helper) and answers to two open-ended questions re: child care challenges and need for support were gathered from all participants through one-to-one interviews. (These answers informed topics chosen in the educational intervention.) The Family Assessment Scale (FAS) and the Beck Depression Scale (BDS) were administered. The FAS and BDS were readministered to all participants one month after the completion of the programs.

Finding: No significant differences existed between the control and intervention group participants on the two pretest measure. Posttest results, however, indicated significant differences (*p* < 0001): the intervention group had a greater decrease in risk for depression as well as more positive perceptions of their family functioning.

Implications for Nursing: Psychosocial education groups conducted by nurses can be effective in the improvement of the mental health for mothers with intellectually disabled children. Group skills can be an important aspect of a nurse's skill set.

Cognitive–Behavioural Groups

The leader in cognitive groups identifies specific distorted thought patterns as the focus of change, whereas in behavioural groups, the leader targets specific behaviours to be modified. Cognitive and behavioural interventions may be combined to offer cognitive–behavioural group interventions. Cognitive interventions aim to modify distortions in attitudes and beliefs about self, the situation, and the future. Behavioural interventions modify behavioural excess, such as overly aggressive or sexual behaviour; behavioural deficits, such as social isolation or extreme passivity; and behaviours interfering with living, such as phobias and panic attacks (see Chapter 13). Cognitive–behavioural groups are often very structured with homework expectations for members.

Interactive Groups

Interactive groups include counselling and therapy groups. They may be focused and short-term or long-term experiential. Although some structure is predetermined by the group leader, group work primarily emphasizes dynamic, interactive group processes to allow for personal and interpersonal growth through experiential teaching and learning. With this focus, the group becomes, in a sense, a microcosm of society. Group goals focus on addressing personal and interpersonal problems in living as well as modifying and changing more long-standing maladaptive patterns of behaviour.

Supportive Therapy Groups

Supportive therapy groups are usually less intense than psychotherapy groups and focus on helping individuals cope with their illnesses and problems as well as build interpersonal connections. Implementing supportive therapy groups is one of the basic functions of the PMH nurse. In conducting this type of group, the nurse focuses on helping members cope with situations that are common for other group members. Counselling strategies are used. For example, a group of patients with bipolar illness, whose illness is stable, may discuss at a monthly meeting how to tell other people about the illness or how to cope with a family member who seems insensitive to the illness. Family caregivers of people with mental illnesses benefit from the support of the group as well as additional information about providing care for an ill family member. Innovations in this form of group work include a group quilting intervention with older African American women transitioning out of homelessness (Washington, Moxley, & Garriott, 2009).

Psychotherapy Groups

Groups that rely primarily on interpretive interventions are known as group psychotherapies. Psychotherapy groups differ depending on the theoretic perspective, including psychodynamic, interpersonal, and existential. These groups focus primarily on increasing cognitive and emotional insight as well as on improving interpersonal relations to help members face their life situations. In group psychotherapy, "therapeutic change is an enormously complex process" (Yalom, 1998, p. 7). At times, these groups can be extremely intense. Psychotherapy groups provide an opportunity for members to examine and resolve psychological and interpersonal issues within a safe environment. Mental health specialists who have a minimum of a master's degree and are trained in group psychotherapy lead such groups. When providing nursing care, communication with the group therapist is important for continuity and collaboration of care. Coulson and Morfett (2013) adeptly illustrate through qualitative data how group work inspired by Irvin Yalom's client-centred approach fosters healing and recovery for adult survivors of sexual abuse in childhood.

Self-Help Groups

Self-help groups are led by lay people, often a mental health consumer, who has experienced a specific problem or life crisis. These groups are generally structured, with supportive interaction among members. These groups do not explore psychodynamic issues in depth. Professionals usually do not attend these groups or serve as consultants. Alcoholics Anonymous, Overeaters Anonymous, and One Day at a Time (a grief group) are examples of self-help groups. A variation on lay-led self-help groups is the professional-led self-help group. Professional-led intervention can systematically strengthen group processes which in turn can contribute to social support and empowerment. This was shown by Stang and Mittelmark (2008) in a participatory action research study of three professionally led self-help groups for women recovering from breast cancer.

▍ COMMON NURSING INTERVENTION GROUPS

Common intervention groups led by nurses include medication, symptom management, anger management, self-care, and reminiscence groups. In addition, nurses lead many other groups, including stress management, relaxation groups, and women's groups. The key, as a nurse, to being a good group leader is to critically select and modify group interventions to best accommodate the primary focus of therapeutic change in relation to the unique conditions of the setting and the group membership (Garrick & Ewashen, 2001).

Medication Groups

Nurse-led medication groups are common in psychiatric nursing. Not all medication groups are alike, so the nurse must be clear regarding the purpose of each specific medication group (Box 14.2). A medication group can be used primarily to transmit information about

---

BOX 14.2 Medication Group Protocol

Purpose: Develop strategies that reinforce a self-medication routine.

Description: The medication group is an open, ongoing group that meets once a week to discuss topics germane to self-administration of medication. Members will not be asked to disclose the names of their medications.

Member Selection: The group is open to any person taking medication for a mental illness or emotional problem who would like more information about the medication, side effects, and staying on a regimen. Referrals from mental health providers are encouraged. Each person will meet with the group leader before attending the group to determine if the group will meet the individual's learning needs.

Structure: Format is a small group, with no more than eight members and one PMH nurse group leader facilitating a discussion about the issues. Topics are rotated.

Time and Location: 2 to 3 PM, every Wednesday at the Mental Health Centre.

Cost: No charge for attending.

Topics:

- How Do I Know if My Medications are Working?
- Side Effect Management: Is it Worth it?
- Hints for Taking Medications Without Missing Doses!
- Health Problems That Medication Affects
- (Other topics will be developed to meet the needs of group members.)

Evaluation: Short pretest and posttest for the instructor's use only.

---

medications, such as action, dosage, and side effects, or it can focus on issues related to medications, such as compliance, management of side effects, and lifestyle adjustments. Many nurses incorporate both perspectives.

To determine what an individual would like to learn, it is important to assess a potential member's medication knowledge before he or she joins the group. People with mental illness may have difficulty remembering new information so assessment of cognitive abilities is important. Assessing attention span, memory, and problem-solving skills gives valuable information that nurses can use in designing the group. The nurse should determine the members' reading and writing skills to select effective patient education materials.

Typically, the group members use various medications. The nurse should know which medications each member is taking, but to avoid violating patient confidentiality, the nurse needs to be careful not to divulge that information to other patients. If group members choose, they can share the names of their medications with one another. A small-group format works best, and the more interaction, the better. Using a lecture method of teaching is less effective than involving the members in the learning process. The nurse should expose the members to various audio and visual educational materials, including workbooks, videos, and handouts. The nurse should ask members to write down information to help them remember and learn through various modes. Evaluation of the learning outcomes begins with the first class. Nurses can develop and give pretests and posttests, which in combination can measure learning outcomes.

Symptom Management Groups

Nurses often lead groups that focus on helping patients with severe and persistent mental illnesses. Handling hallucinations, being socially appropriate, and staying motivated to complete activities of daily living are a few common topics. In symptom management groups, prevention of relapse is often a focus. Members learn when a symptom indicates that relapse is imminent and what to do to avoid relapse. Increasingly, the focus on treatment and relapse prevention extends to community settings and to diverse populations. Stacciarini's (2008) focus group study examined a community-based group intervention for treating depression in Puerto Rican women, identifying culturally relevant and appropriate, interactive interventions to increase participation and adherence to treatment, avoid cultural barriers, and empower participants.

Communication and Anger Management Groups

Communication and anger management are other common themes for nurse-led groups, often in inpatient settings. An inpatient communications group designed and implemented by Graham Paley, a nurse therapist, and colleagues incorporated supportive therapy, interpersonal learning, and a strengths-based focus. Evaluation, based on the Yalom model, identified the top four therapeutic factors as group cohesiveness, universality, catharsis, and member-to-member guidance (Paley, Danks, Edwards, Reid, & Rawse, 2013). The purposes of an anger management group are to discuss the concept of anger, identify antecedents to aggressive behaviour, and develop new strategies to deal with anger other than verbal and physical aggression (see Chapter 18). The treatment team refers individuals with a history of being verbally and physically abusive, usually to family members, to these groups to help them better understand their emotions and behavioural responses. Impulsiveness and emotional lability are problems for many of the group members. Anger management usually includes a discussion of associated stressful situations, events that trigger anger, feelings about the situation, and unmet personal needs.

■ SELF-CARE GROUPS

Another common nurse-led psychiatric group is a self-care group. People with psychiatric illnesses often have self-care difficulties and benefit from the structure that a group provides. These groups are challenging because members usually know how to perform these daily tasks (e.g., bathing, grooming, performing personal hygiene), but their illnesses cause a decrease in the motivation to complete them. The leader not only reinforces the basic self-care skills but also, more importantly, helps identify strategies that maintain motivation and provide structure to their daily lives. Contemporary self-care group interventions are increasingly complex and sophisticated in design. For example, Cespedes-Knadle and Munoz's (2011) *Teen Power*, a group mental health intervention for teens with Type I diabetes (who are at significant risk for depression) and a parallel support group for their caregivers involved a collaborative interdisciplinary team effort with the aim of improving diabetes management and adherence. An information–motivation–behavioural skills (IBM) model provided the theoretical underpinnings with a supportive-psycho-educational therapy format.

Reminiscence Groups

Reminiscence therapy has been shown to be a valuable intervention for older adults. In this type of group, members are encouraged to remember events from past years. Such a group is easily implemented. Usually, a simple question about an important family event will spark memories. Reminiscence groups are typically associated with people who have dementia and are having difficulty with recent memory. Recalling distant memories is comforting to older people and improves well-being. Reminiscence groups can also be used in caring for people with depression (Jones & Beck-Little, 2002) and in conjunction with cognitive therapy for affective symptoms in older adults (Puentes, 2004).

🍁 SUMMARY OF KEY POINTS

- The definition of group can vary according to theoretic orientation. A general definition of group is "two or more individuals who are connected to one another by social relationships" (Forsyth, 2006, p. 3) and "at the heart of group is a learning process in a social setting" (Day, 2014, p. 25). Group dynamics are the interactions within a group that constitute group development and process.

- Groups can be *open*, with every session available to new membership, or *closed*, with membership determined at the first session. Leading a group, whether small or large, is complex because dynamics change depending on different sizes of groups and clinical conditions.

- The group development process occurs in stages: beginning, middle (working), and ending (termination). These stages are not fixed but dynamic. Each stage challenges the leader to intervene in different ways. Success at the beginning stage prepares the group to take responsibility for addressing its purpose during the middle (working) stage.

- Although there are only two formal group roles—leader and member—there are many informal group roles. These roles are usually categorized according to purpose—task functions, maintenance functions, and individual-centred roles. Members who assume task functions encourage the group members to stay focused on the group's task. Those who assume maintenance functions concern themselves more with the group working together than the task itself. Deviant roles can detract from the work of the group as an individual member may increasingly become the focus of communication. Relational communication includes verbal and nonverbal communication, member-to-member connection and disconnection, and the communication network and group themes. Nonverbal communication is complex, open to misinterpretation, and involves eye contact, body posture, and mood of the group.

- Nurse leaders are responsible for mobilizing therapeutic factors to support healthy group development and prevent a stagnating groupthink. What factors to mobilize and when depend on the type, purpose, and developmental stage of the group.

- Seating arrangements affect group interaction. Fewer physical barriers, such as tables, improve potential for interactive communication. Everyone should be engaged as a member of the group and be invited to join in. Interactive groups should take place in a comfortable space with members facing one another in a circle arrangement.

- Leadership skills involve active listening, tracking verbal and nonverbal behaviours, remaining fair and respectful, avoiding favouritism, and encouraging participation and involvement of all members with each other.

- The leader should address challenges to the leadership, group process, or other members to determine whether to intervene and how. In some instances, the leader redirects a monopolizing member; at other times, the leader supports group members to provide feedback on the effects of the behaviour. Periods of group conflict occur in most groups during the transition from the beginning to the middle (working) phase.

- There are many different types of groups. PMH nurses lead psychoeducational and supportive therapy groups. Mental health specialists trained to provide intensive therapy lead psychotherapy groups and cognitive–behavioural groups. Self-help groups are led by participants themselves, and professionals assist only as requested.

- Medication, symptom management, anger management, self-care, and reminiscence groups are common nurse-led groups.

Web Links

agpa.org The American Group Psychotherapy Association (AGPA) is an interdisciplinary association for enhancing practice, theory, and research in group therapy. Extensive resources are available for members and nonmembers.

camh.net The Centre for Addiction and Mental Health (CAMH) offers valuable practical, educational, group, and research-based resources for health professionals in the field of addictions and mental health, including resources related to concurrent disorders, trauma, policy research, and health promotion.

cgpa.ca The Canadian Group Psychotherapy Association (CGPA) is a national organization dedicated to promoting group therapy practice and the enhancement of clinical knowledge and skills through training, continuing education, and research. CGPA is multidisciplinary, resulting in a rich and diverse membership. The association is responsible for setting national training standards and for accrediting regional training programs. CGPA has three levels of membership, reflecting a broad range of expertise and experience, from internationally acclaimed members to students of the mental health professions.

mentalhelp.net/selfhelp The American Self-Help Group Clearinghouse provides online self-help resources containing information on many different self-help groups.

References

American Group Psychotherapy Association. (2007). *Practice guidelines for group psychotherapy*. New York: Sage.

Benson, J. (2010). *Working more creatively with groups* (3rd ed.). New York, NY: Routledge.

Brown, T., & Miller, C. (2000). Communication networks in task-performing groups: Effects of task complexity, time, pressure, and interpersonal dominance. *Small Group Research, 31*(2), 131–157.

Burtis, J., & Turman, P. (2006). *Group communication pitfalls: Overcoming barriers to an effective group experience*. Thousand Oaks, CA: Sage.

Canadian Interprofessional Health Collaborative. (2010). *A national interprofessional competency framework*. Retrieved from http://www.cihc.ca/files/CIHC_IPCompetencies_Feb1210.pdf

Cespedes-Knadle, Y., & Munoz, C. (2011). Development of a group intervention for teens with Type 1 diabetes. *Journal of Specialists in Group Work, 36,* 278–295.

Chapman, H. (2006). Towards effective group-work in nurse education. *Nurse Education Today, 26*(4), 298–303.

Clark, A. (2002). Scapegoating: Dynamics and interventions in group counseling. *Journal of Counseling & Development, 80,* 271–276.

Clark, C. (2009). *Group leadership skills for nurses and health professionals* (5th ed.). New York: Springer.

Comstock, D., Duffey, T., & St. George, H. (2002). The relational-cultural model: A framework for group process. *Journal for Specialists in Group Work, 27*(3), 254–272.

Corey, G. (2013). *Theory and practice of group counseling* (8th ed.). Belmont, CA: Brooks/Cole.

Corey, M., Corey, G., & Corey, C. (2013). *Groups: Process and practice* (8th ed.). Belmont, CA: Brooks/Cole.

Coulson, L., & Morfett, H. (2013). Group work for adult survivors of sexual abuse in childhood. *Mental Health Practice, 17*(1), 14–21.

Covington, S. (2013). *Women and addiction: A gender responsive approach*. Retrieved from http://www.stephaniecovington.com/women-and-addiction.php

Crowell, D. (2011). *Complexity leadership: Nursing's role in health care delivery*. Philadelphia, PA: F.A. Davis.

Day, S. (2014). A unifying theory for group counselling and psychotherapy. In Delucia-Waack, J., Kalodner, C., & Riva, M. (Eds.). *The handbook of group counseling & psychotherapy* (2nd ed., pp. 24–33). Los Angeles, CA: Sage.

Delucia-Waack, J., Kalodner, C., & Riva, M. (2014). *The handbook of group counseling & psychotherapy* (2nd ed.). Los Angeles, CA: Sage.

Dimock, H. G., & Kass, R. (2011). *Making workgroups effective* (4th ed.). North York, ON: Captus Press.

Fedele, N. (2004). Relationships in groups: Connection, resonance, and paradox. In J. Jordon, M. Walker, & L. Hartling (Eds.), *The complexity of connection: Writings from the Stone Center's Jean Baker Miller Training Institute* (pp. 195–219). New York, NY: Guilford.

Forsyth, D. R. (2006). *Group dynamics*. Toronto, ON: Thomson Nelson.

Forsyth, D., & Diederich, T. (2014). Group dynamics and development. In J. Delucia-Waack, C. Kalodner, & M. Riva (Eds.). *The handbook of group counseling & psychotherapy* (2nd ed., pp. 34–45). Los Angeles, CA: Sage.

Fredericks, S., & Guruge, S. (2015). Promoting immigrant women's cardiovascular health redesigning patient education interventions. *Advances in Nursing Science, 38,* E13–E20.

Garland, J., Jones, H., & Kolodny, R. (1973). A model of stages of development in social work groups. In S. Bernstein (Ed.), *Explorations in group work: Essays in theory and practice* (pp. 17–71). Boston, MA: Milford House.

Garrick, D., & Ewashen, C. (2001). An integrated model for adolescent inpatient group therapy. *Journal of Psychiatric and Mental Health Nursing, 8,* 165–171.

Graham, M., & Sontag, M. (2001). Art as an evaluative tool: A pilot study. *Art Therapy, 18*(1), 37–43.

Grossman, S., & Valiga, T. (2012). *The new leadership challenge: Creating the future of nursing* (4th ed.). Philadelphia, PA: F.A. Davis.

Harpine, E. (2013). *Prevention groups*. Los Angeles, CA: Sage.

Harpine, E. (2015). *Group-centered prevention in mental health*. New York, NY: Springer.

Harpine, E., Nitza, A., & Conyne, R. (2010). Prevention groups: Today and tomorrow. *Group Dynamics: Theory, Research, and Practice, 14,* 268–280.

Hartling, L. M. (2013). Strengthening resilience in a risky world: It's all about relationships. In J. V. Jordon (Ed.). *The power of connection: Recent developments in relational-cultural theory* (pp. 49–68). New York, NY: Routledge.

Jacobs, E., Masson, R., & Harvill, R. (2009). *Group counseling strategies and skills*. Belmont, CA: Brooks/Cole.

Janis, I. (1982). *Groupthink* (2nd ed.). Boston, MA: Houghton-Mifflin.

Jones, E. D., & Beck-Little, R. (2002). The use of reminiscence therapy for the treatment of depression in rural-dwelling older adults. *Issues in Mental Health Nursing, 23,* 279–280.

Kidd, L., Graor, C., & Murrock, C. (2013). A mindful eating group intervention for obese women: a mixed methods feasibility study. *Archives of Psychiatric Nursing, 27,* 211–218.

Kottler, J., & Englar-Carlson, M. (2010). *Learning group leadership: An experiential approach*. Thousand Oaks, CA: Sage.

MacKenzie, R. K. (1997). *Time-managed group psychotherapy: Effective clinical applications*. Washington, DC: American Psychiatric Press.

McRae, M. B., & Short, E. L. (2010). *Racial and cultural dynamics in group and organizational life*. Los Angeles, CA: Sage.

McWhirter, P., & McWhirter, J. (2010). Community and school violence and risk reduction: Empirical supported prevention. *Group Dynamics: Theory, Research, and Practice, 14,* 242–256.

Miller, J. B. (1986). *What do we mean by relationships?* (Work in Progress, No. 22). Wellesley, MA: Stone Center Working Paper Series.

Myers, S., & Anderson, C. (2008). *The fundamentals of small group communication*. Thousand Oaks, CA: Sage.

Neck, C. P., & Moorhead, G. (1995). Groupthink remodeled: The importance of leadership, time pressure, and methodical decision-making procedures. *Human Relations, 48*(5), 537–557.

Nielsen, M. B. (2013). Bullying in work groups: The impact of leadership. *Scandinavian Journal of Psychology, 54,* 127–136.

Pagano, M. (2015). *Communication case studies for health care professionals: An applied approach*. New York, NY: Springer.

Paley, G., Danks, A., Edwards, K., Reid, C., & Rawse, H. (2013). Organizing an inpatient psychotherapy group. *Mental Health Practice, 16*(7), 10–15.

Posthuma, B. (2001). *Small groups in counseling and therapy: Process and leadership* (4th ed.). Boston, MA: Pearson Education.

Puentes, W. J. (2004). Cognitive therapy integrated with life review techniques: An eclectic treatment approach for affective symptoms in older adults. *Journal of Clinical Nursing, 13*, 84–89.

Reddy, L. A. (2012). *Group play interventions for children: Strategies for teaching prosocial skills.* Washington, DC: American Psychological Association.

Rutan, J. S., & Stone, W. N. (2001). *Psychodynamic group psychotherapy* (3rd ed.). New York: Guilford Press.

Sampson, E., & Marthas, M. (1990). *Group process for the health professions* (pp. 222–224). Albany, NY: Delmar.

Stacciarini, J. (2008). Focus groups: Examining a community-based group intervention for depressed Puerto Rican women. *Issues in Mental Health Nursing, 29*, 679–700.

Stang, I., & Mittelmark, M. (2008). Social support and interpersonal stress in professional-led breast cancer self-help groups. *International Journal of Mental Health Promotion, 10*(2), 15–25.

Steinhardt, M. A., Dolbier, C. L., Gottlieb, N. H., & McCalister, K. T. (2003). The relationship between hardiness, supervisor support, group cohesion, and job stress as predictors of job satisfaction. *American Journal of Health Promotion, 17*(6), 382–389.

Stone, J., & Kwan, V. (2016). How group processes influence, maintain, and overcome health disparities. *Group Process & Intergroup Relations, 19*, 411–414.

Taylor, E., & Cranston, P. (2012). *The handbook of transformative learning: theory, research, and practice.* San Francisco, CA: Jossey-Bass.

Tuckman, B. W. (1965). Development sequence in small groups. *Psychological Bulletin, 63*, 384–399.

Van Santvoort, F., Hosman, C., van Doesum, K., & Janssens, J. (2013). Children of mentally ill or addicted parents participating in preventive support groups. *International Journal of Mental Health Promotion, 14*, 198–213.

Vonderheid, S., Klima, C., Norr, K., Grady, M., & Westdahl, C. (2013). Using focus group and social marketing to strengthen promotion of group prenatal care. *Advances in Nursing Science, 4*, 320–355.

Walumbwa, F., Luthans, F., Avey, J., & Oke, A. (2009). Authentically leading groups: the mediating role of collective psychological capital and trust. *Journal of Organizational Behavior, 32*, 4–24.

Washington, O., Moxley, D., & Garriott, L. (2009). The telling my story: Quilting workshop. *Journal of Psychosocial Nursing, 47*(11), 42–52.

Yalom, I. D. (1998). *The Yalom reader: Selections from the work of a master therapist and storyteller.* New York, NY: Basic Books.

Yalom, I. D., & Leszcz, M. (2005). *The theory and practice of group psychotherapy* (5th ed.). New York, NY: Basic Books.

Yıldırım, A., Aşilar, R. H., & Karakurt, P. (2013). Effects of a nursing intervention program on the depression and perception of family functioning of mothers with intellectually disabled children. *Journal of Clinical Nursing, 22*(1–2), 251–261.

Yopp, J., & Rosenstein, L. (2013). A support group for fathers whose partners died from cancer. *Clinical Journal of Oncology Nursing, 17*, 169–173.

Young, L., & Paterson, B. (2007). *Teaching nursing: Developing a student-centered learning environment.* Philadelphia, PA: Lippincott, Williams & Wilkins.

Zimmerman, J., & Winek, J. (2013). *Group activities for families in recovery.* Thousand Oaks, CA: Sage.

CHAPTER

15 Family Assessment and Interventions

Cindy Peternelj-Taylor | Adapted from the chapter "Family Assessment and Interventions" by Peggy (Margaret) Simpson

LEARNING OBJECTIVES

After studying this chapter, you will be able to:

- Discuss the role families and caregivers provide in the support, advocacy, and recovery of people living with mental illness.
- Develop a genogram that depicts family history, relationships, and health patterns across three generations.
- Develop an ecomap to explore family networks of support that includes strengths and resources.
- Identify current family needs and concerns related to the mental illness.
- Develop a plan together with the family and health care team to address the identified family needs and concerns.

KEY TERMS

- ecomap • extended family • family development
- family life cycle • family structure • genogram
- immediate family • nuclear family • respite • transition times

KEY CONCEPTS

- comprehensive family assessment • family • 15-minute family interview

Mental illness affects families across the life span. Approximately 11 million Canadians, 15 years of age and older, have at least one family member with a mental illness or addiction (Pearson, 2015). Further, an estimated 1.2 million Canadian children and youth are affected by mental illness, and one in four Canadian seniors lives with a mental health issue or illness (MacCourt, 2013). The unique role that families play in promoting well-being, providing care, and facilitating recovery is finally being recognized. Families, however, are often poorly prepared for the inherent demands required of the primary caregiver role. Serious mental illness changes lives, and relationships of families, often with a "disturbing and destructive force" (Buckley & Scott, 2017, p. 55). Family engagement and involvement, however, is vital to successful management and well-being of members who experience mental health problems.

Evidence suggests that family-based interventions reduce relapse rates and improve recovery of patients while increasing family well-being. Family-based interventions are shown to be effective for patients with first-episode psychosis (Petrakis & Laxton, 2017); for bipolar disorder in adults and youth (Reinares et al., 2016); in families where parents have a mental illness (Reupert & Mayberry, 2016); and for diverse consumers experiencing mental illness and their families (Coker, Williams,

Hayes, Hamann, & Harvey, 2016). In outpatients with major depression, couples therapy is as effective as medication and often more acceptable to patients (Marshall & Harper-Jaques, 2008). Family-to-family interventions have also been shown to increase empowerment, knowledge, and coping and to reduce stress among family caregivers (Toohey, Muralidharan, Medoff, Lucksted, & Dixon, 2016). Well-supported family caregivers play an important role in the recovery journey of their ill relative.

In 2013, the Mental Health Commission of Canada (MHCC) published the *National Guidelines for a Comprehensive Service System to Support Family Caregivers of Adults with Mental Health Problems and Illnesses*. The *Guidelines*, a first for Canada, provide recommendations for mental health services that recognize and address the needs of family caregivers of adults with mental health problems and illnesses (MacCourt, 2013). The purpose of this chapter is to provide an overview of key concepts from the recommendations, as well as other sources, to enable nurses to effectively work with families as they navigate family life within the context of mental illness. This chapter includes ideas on how to assess family needs and concerns and how to enhance family strengths and resources to support persons experiencing illness and enhance their recovery journeys.

CHARACTERISTICS OF CANADIAN FAMILIES

The portrait of Canadian families continues to change. In 2011, Statistics Canada released *Fifty Years of Families in Canada: 1961 to 2011* highlighting the changing face of Canadian families. While marriage remains an important aspect of family life in Canada, there is now more diversity in the way families are configured. Married couples continue to form the predominant **family structure** in Canada, accounting for two thirds of all families. Since 2006, there are more common-law couples and lone-parent families. Between 2006 and 2011, common-law couples outnumbered lone-parent families. Same-sex married couples were counted in the 2006 census for the first time, and in 2011, the number of same-sex married couples nearly tripled, reflecting the first full 5-year period for which same-sex marriage had been legal across the country.

In Canada, the majority of children under the age of 14 live with married parents; however, an increasing number live with common-law parents. One in 10 children aged 14 and under lived in stepfamilies, while 0.5% of children in this age group were foster children in private households.

Over the past decade, more seniors aged 65 and over lived as part of a couple in a private household. During the same period, the proportion of senior women who lived alone declined; it remained relatively stable for senior men. About one in every 12 seniors lived in a collective dwelling, such as a nursing home or a residence for senior citizens. These characteristics are important when we begin to conceptualize family in the current Canadian context.

Definitions of family suggest that families are unique in that, unlike other organizations, they generally incorporate new members by birth, adoption, or marriage, and members leave only by divorce or death. Once considered a traditional family, the **nuclear family** is defined as two or more people living together and related by blood, marriage, or adoption. An **extended family** is defined as several nuclear families whose members may or may not live together but function as one group. McGoldrick, Garcia Preto, and Carter (2016) suggest that given the diversity of family forms, the term nuclear family is no longer appropriate due to its narrow association with a father and mother in intact first families. Instead, they recommend the use of the term **"immediate family,"** a more inclusive term that refers to "all household members and other family caretakers or siblings of children, whether in a heterosexual couple, single-parent, unmarried, remarried, gay, or lesbian household" (p. xxiv). It is the commitment to each other, rather than the biologic or legal status, that is the bond that defines family (McGoldrick et al., 2016). This definition of immediate family is consistent with Wright and Leahey's (2013) all-encompassing conceptualization of family, one that focuses on belonging, affection, and durability of the relationships in the context of a person's life; in essence,

"the family is who they say they are." Another way of conceptualizing family is a complex process where economics, emotion, context, and experiences are interwoven and multilayered (Doane & Varcoe, 2015). These latter conceptualizations seem to be an appropriate "fit" for the changing portrait of Canadian families.

Nurses interact with families in various ways. Because of the interpersonal and chronic nature of many mental illnesses, nurses may have frequent and long-term contact with families. Involvement may range from brief telephone contact, to meeting family members face to face once or twice, to treating the whole family as the unit of care. Families often share a unique history and investment in their relationships, caring for each other and promoting the welfare of family members. When one family member experiences the challenges associated with a serious mental health issue, the challenges are also experienced by other family members, often in complex ways. Family members are often thrust into the caregiving role, frequently ill prepared or equipped to deal with mental illness and all its ramifications (Grebeldinger & Buckley, 2016). The caregiving role can be challenging because of the unpredictable nature of many mental illnesses, the current barriers to family involvement in the mental health system, and the stigma associated with mental illness. In spite of such obstacles, family members fulfil an important role by providing support, advocating for the ill person, and contributing to the recovery process (MacCourt, 2013).

The provision of competent and holistic care to families includes ongoing access to information, guidance, and support so that families may effectively achieve their caregiving responsibilities, while enhancing their own health and well-being. However, nurses need to be mindful of issues of patient confidentiality as they respond to the family's need for information. The MHCC's *Guidelines* recognize that when families are well supported, they can enhance the recovery journey of their ill relatives and improve their quality of life and do so with less caregiving stress than when unsupported. The unpaid care provided by family caregivers makes a major contribution to Canada's health and social service systems (MacCourt, 2013).

KEY CONCEPT

Family is a group of people who are committed to each other and involved relationally in a complex process where economics, emotion, context, and experiences are interwoven and multilayered.

FAMILY CAREGIVERS

In 2012, a national survey was conducted on family caregivers, including those caring for people with mental illness. Characteristics of caregivers indicated that 54% were women, 60% were employed, 28% were sandwiched between caregiving and child-rearing, and 89% had been providing care for at least 1 year. Mental illness (e.g., depression, bipolar disorder, and schizophrenia) was the most common reason for parents caring for a sick child and accounted for 23% of family caregivers (Sinha, 2013). Additionally, over one million young carers in Canada (i.e., those under the age of 25), referred to as a "hidden army" by Stamatopoulos (2015), provide unpaid care to family members with chronic illness, disability, mental health issues, problems with substance abuse, and/or health challenges related to old age. Young carers are frequently from hidden and marginalized groups and are often both providers and recipients of care. It is critical that young carers are not only identified and supported but also provided with the necessary programming to prevent them from becoming secondary users of the health care system (Stamatopoulos, 2016).

Caregiving not only consumes time and energy but also impacts financial, emotional, and other resources. Families caring for adults living with mental illness frequently assist with shopping; banking; paying bills; preparing meals; housekeeping; childcare; monitoring symptoms; scheduling and coordinating appointments; managing behaviours, situations, and crises; and preventing relapses, while at the same time providing companionship and emotional and financial support. Many are also involved in providing housing and transportation, personal safety and hygiene, guidance, encouragement, and motivation. Family caregivers often assume an informal case management role; they advocate on their family member's behalf, navigate the health and social services systems, and contribute to continuity of care (MacCourt, 2013). Given the complex demands of caring for and supporting a family member experiencing mental illness, it is not surprising that families experience high levels of caregiver burden, which Wrosch, Amir, and Miller (2011) have equated with the burden reported by dementia caregivers.

Caregiver Burden

Caregiver burden is a common negative consequence experienced by family members who are involved in providing care for a family member with mental illness. Caregiver burden is simply defined as "a caregiver's subjective perception of hardship in providing necessary direct care to an ill individual which will change over time" (Mulud, 2016, p. 142). In a concept analysis of caregiver burden, Mulud (2016) concluded that caregiver burden represents a comingling of attributes (caregiver's subjective perception, hardship, changes over time), antecedents (unexpected events/illnesses, imbalance between demands and resources, negative coping), and consequences (psychological and physical morbidity, coping, and adaptation). Caregiver burden is further conceptualized as objective and subjective burden. Objective burden is associated with the practical objective aspects of care, including time and finances

(which may contribute to financial hardships and limitations on one's social life). Conversely, subjective burden is about how informal caregivers perceive the burden of care, often experienced as anxiety, depression, and relational problems related to the extent to which the ill person's presence, behaviour, and dependency are perceived as a source of worry, stress, and strain (Flyck, Fatouros-Bergman, & Koernig, 2015). In a study by Flyk et al. (2015), subjective burden in caregivers was found to be lower when patients had higher levels of functioning and when the health of the caregivers was good.

As noted, caring for a family member with a mental illness can exert both a physical and emotional toll on the caregiver. Analyzing data from the 2012 Canadian Community Health Survey–Mental Health, Pearson (2015) reported that about 10% of people who had one family member (defined as spouse or partner, children, parents, parents-in-law, grandparents, brothers and sisters, cousins, aunts, uncles, nieces, or nephews) with a mental illness reported having experienced symptoms themselves; the rate almost doubled for those with two or more family members with a mental illness. Of those with at least one family member with a mental illness, 35% reported that their time, energy, emotions, finances, or daily activities had been affected because of their family member's experiences with illness. Of those who perceived that their lives had been affected, 19% reported that they had experienced symptoms of a mental or substance use disorder themselves in the past 12 months, while two thirds (62%) reported that their family member's problems had caused them to become worried, anxious, or depressed. Interestingly, Ennis and Buntig (2013) found that people who perceived that their lives had been affected (as opposed to those who did not perceive an impact) were more likely to report that they had problems with their own mental health.

Clearly, caregiver burden is a distinct concept relevant to nursing practice. Nurses need to be cognizant of the burden and distress experienced by caregivers and prevent family caregivers from becoming "collateral casualties" of mental illness (MacCourt, 2013, p. 3). Through the identification of antecedents and consequences, nurses assess for the presence of burden in caregivers and implement specific interventions and programs for those at high risk for developing caregiver burden (Mulud, 2016). Flyck et al. (2015) concluded that interventions aimed at relieving burden in family caregivers should be congruent with the type of burden (objective vs. subjective) primarily experienced by the caregivers. Success in working with families is enhanced when clinicians are oriented to how mental illness impacts families.

Meeting the Needs of Families

Historically, the impact of mental illness on the family was mostly ignored, and any attention the family did receive focused on the role of the family in the aetiology of the illness. And while more recently, the family is finally beginning to be recognized as a partner in the ill person's recovery journey, family members are not consistently acknowledged or supported, and at times, they often feel blamed for the problems and issues associated with the mental illness. They are confronted with issues that can arise when health care professionals must balance the family need for information and support, with the individual family member's right to confidentiality. This can be particularly frustrating for family members who assume a primary caregiver role.

Family caregivers who participated in the development of the *National Guidelines for a Comprehensive Service System to Support Family Caregivers of Adults with Mental Health Problems and Illnesses* identified several ways health care providers can address their needs. Families need to:

- Know their relatives are receiving adequate care and services that facilitate their ability to maximize their quality of life
- Have their relationships and caregiving roles recognized by mental health service providers
- Be meaningfully involved in the assessment and treatment planning
- Receive information, skills, support and services from knowledgeable mental health care providers, so they can effectively provide care to their relative
- Receive family support and services to sustain their own health and emotional well-being (MacCourt, 2013).

Failure to address the needs of family caregivers increases their risk for developing mental health issues, compromises their physical health, reduces the effectiveness of their support of their ill relative, and increases costs to health and social service systems. On the other hand, enhancing caregiving capacity is clinically significant in terms of positive outcomes related to the relative's illness, family relationships with the ill person, improved medication adherence (El-Mallakh & Findlay, 2015; Farooq & Naeem, 2014; Miklowitz, George, Richards, Simoneau, & Suddath, 2003), fewer relapses and fewer hospitalizations (Falloon, 2005), and assisting with relapse prevention and promotion of recovery in their ill family member (Petrakis & Laxton, 2017).

CONTEXTUAL ISSUES TO CONSIDER WHEN WORKING WITH FAMILIES

Some important contextual issues to consider when working with families include stigma, access to services and respite, and diversity of families.

Stigma

Mental illness is highly stigmatized in society, and the stigma associated with mental health issues and diagnoses often extends to family members, a phenomenon known as stigma by association (Bos, Pryor, & Reeder, 2013). Thus, the stigma of mental illness harms not only persons with mental illness but also their family members (van der Sanden, Pryor, Studtterheim, Kok, & Bos, 2016). Families often experience difficulty coming to terms with mental illness in a family member, and may simply deny its existence and retreat in shame. Or worse yet, they may experience cognitive dissonance when faced with the realization that they too hold some of the negative stigmatizing beliefs commonly held by the general public. As a result, stigma may delay help seeking, which may in turn increase their isolation and decrease their ability to cope. Children of parents with mental illness are often wary of negative reactions of peers, and do not discuss their "family secret" (Gladstone, Boydell, Seeman, & McKeever, 2011, p. 283).

Access to Services and Respite

Families identify access to needed medical and social services as crucial to recovery. Social services include housing, income assistance, and legal and employment support. Information needs to be provided in an appropriate format and education level. It must be understandable to the family members (MacCourt, 2013).

Family members also need **respite** supports and services to provide relief from everyday caregiving responsibilities (Brighton et al., 2016). In 2005, the Schizophrenia Society of Canada conducted a national survey on the respite needs of people living with schizophrenia; 372 responses were received from individuals across the country who were identified as care providers. Of this group, 80% were female, with an average age of 63; the remaining 20% were male with an average age of 66. Of this group, 61% were not employed, while 41% were just beyond retirement. Conversely, the average age of care recipients was 49 years (Stuart, 2005). In essence, this data paints a picture of aging parents caring for aging adult children. In response to the questions "What does respite mean to you?" one respondent replied, "It means time to take care of my physical and mental needs so that I can be a better caregiver. Time to recharge and reconnect with my husband" (Stuart, 2005, p. 70). Although this study took place in 2005, it remains relevant today, as little has changed for family caregivers, who continue to have limited access to appropriate respite services.

In a study that explored the effect of respite services on carers of individuals with severe mental illness, three themes emerged (Brighton et al. 2016). In the first theme, respondents discussed the impact of caregiving on their health and well-being (experienced stress, depression and anxiety, and problems with their physical health). In the second theme, respondents discussed the impact of caregiving on their leisure activities, concluding that caregiving was too great a burden to engage in leisure activities. The final theme focused on the benefits of formal respite (i.e., a 5-day Recovery Camp) for care recipients. One participant remarked, "We went out for dinner, relaxed, put our feet up...didn't engage in other activities, just needed a rest, a break from looking after her" (Brighton et al., 2016, p. 37).

Nurses are ideally situated to assess, assist, and advocate for family members who are caregivers. Understanding caregiver burden and the importance of respite for family caregivers is imperative.

Diversity of Families

Canada is a multicultural and diverse society. Diversity is about difference and complexity. It includes such factors as age, ability, ethnicity, culture, faith, gender, education, income, language, and sexual orientation. Diversity is not a neutral concept; the social, political, and economic context of family life needs to be considered, and disparities and power imbalances addressed in the plan of care (Doane & Varcoe, 2015). Diversity is also apparent in the characteristics of individual family members, including the individual experiencing mental illness. Life cycle stage, gender, age, type and severity of illness, and type of treatments may influence needs.

Family configurations may include immediate, blended, or extended families. When "family" is defined as "who they say they are," then those in the circle of care, specifically those who protect the mentally ill individual and support his or her autonomy and recovery, may include unrelated individuals.

Determining the needs of families is a vital component of a comprehensive nursing assessment. When asked, families will let nurses know what has meaning, significance, and importance for them (Doane & Varcoe, 2015). Inquiring how the mental illness is influencing all members of the family will help the nurse understand the reciprocity between the illness and family functioning. In this way, nurses can gain understanding of the complex dynamics of familial context. They can learn about the way a particular family thinks about and organizes themselves around their member's mental illness, including the way the illness is interpreted, symptoms are managed, and mental health care resources are accessed and used.

■ FAMILY ASSESSMENT

The Canadian national *Guidelines* for services to support family caregivers of adults with mental problems and illness advocate a recovery-focused process (MacCourt, 2013). This means that caregivers as well as individuals with an illness are supported on their journey toward recovery and well-being. Principles in a recovery-focused approach include building relationships that foster hope, empowerment, self-determination, and responsibility. Five principles and values are outlined that are viewed as integral components of services. These include family engagement; respect and dignity; choice, determination, and independence; family caregiver needs; and family

caregiver sustainability (MHCC, 2009, 2015). These will be discussed in the context of a family nursing assessment recognizing the value of family, friends, and community.

The MHCC (2015), in its recovery guidelines, states "Recovery-oriented practice and service delivery recognizes the unique role of personal and family relationships in promoting well-being, providing care and fostering recovery across the lifespan; as well as recognizing the needs of families and caregivers themselves" (p. 44).

A comprehensive family assessment involves the collection of all relevant data related to family health, psychological and spiritual well-being, and social functioning. In this way, the nurse can identify problems, enhance family strengths, and generate solutions *with* the family to address their needs and concerns.

The assessment usually consists of a face-to-face interview with family members (although telephone- or videoconferencing may be an alternative) and may be conducted over several sessions. A comprehensive family assessment is appropriate when an individual is admitted to the hospital for psychiatric or mental health treatment. If the individual's admission status is voluntary, and he or she is deemed competent to make treatment decisions, permission to contact the family is in order (Box 15.1). Providing support to family caregivers does not require patient consent as long as confidentiality of patient information is maintained and respected.

Nurses also need to know to which social media (SM) sites families are referring. Knowing which sites families are using can assist in maximizing the use of appropriate and helpful information that is readily available while minimizing the effects of SM sites that may be potentially harmful. Assessing family members' use of SM provides opportunities for nurses to support families in making informed choices. Connecting families with reliable information, and communication channels, can be especially beneficial for those living in rural and remote areas, who are separated by distance, and have limited access to more traditional resources. Through SM, families can be provided with education regarding mental illness and information regarding specific family needs, peer support, and other useful family content (Risling, Risling, & Holstslander, 2017). Refer further to Web Links.

Engagement

In preparing for a family assessment, the nurse must take steps to promote a positive nurse–family relationship by enabling an atmosphere of trust, respect, dignity, and cooperation. This begins with the simple act of an introduction. The nurse provides an introduction by using his or her name and explaining his or her role for the meeting and the purpose of the meeting. During the meeting, the nurse calls the patient and family by name (Wright & Leahey, 2013). Many families do not know what to expect from the nurse, and this is the first step in decreasing their anxiety. Each family is unique, and

BOX 15.1 Family Mental Health Assessment

Family Name: _____

Family Members Present At Interview: _____

_____

_____

_____

Nurse Interviewer: _____

1. Referral route and presenting problem (include psychiatric diagnosis and current treatment): _____

_____

_____

2. Family composition (complete and attach a family genogram):

3. Family life cycle phase (include stage and any pertinent transitional issues):

_____

_____

4. Pertinent history of the problem:
   a. Explore what the family's most urgent concerns or needs are at this point in time
   b. Explore the effects of the mental health concern on all family members
   c. Developmental history (including family of origin, health or medical events)
   d. Communication patterns (for solving day-to-day issues or problems)
   e. Previous solutions
   f. Ethnicity/culture
   g. Ecomap showing social supports (internal and external), including financial, housing, educational, and legal resources

5. Strengths and problems (identify the family strengths, resources, and capabilities): _____

_____

_____

6. Summary (include urgent concerns and needs of family, strengths and resources, degree to which they wish to collaborate in care and discharge planning, any pertinent history, positive or negative relational patterns affecting illness symptoms, and preferred communication): _____

_____

7. Goals/plans (list interventions and family responses):

_____

_____

its needs, understanding of the situation, expectations for care, and previous experiences with the health care system are just some factors that should be explored at the beginning of a therapeutic relationship. More than the initial meeting may be necessary to build the relationship and complete the assessment.

KEY CONCEPT

A **comprehensive family assessment** is the collection of all relevant data related to family health, psychological well-being, and social functioning to identify problems for which the nurse can generate solutions with the family and enhance family strengths.

When working with families, the nurse must show understanding, competence, and caring. Listening to family members, valuing their contributions, acknowledging their knowledge and expertise, and addressing their immediate needs build confidence and trust with them. For example, a family that needs shelter or food is not ready to discuss a member's medication regimen until these basic needs are addressed. Families are encouraged to participate in the diagnosis, treatment, and recovery process of their ill family member; an approach that is balanced with the rights of that person that include privacy and confidentiality.

Genogram

The **genogram** is a structural assessment tool that may be used by the nurse to collect diverse information about family members, their relationships, and health and illness patterns over time. The genogram represents an engagement, assessment, and intervention tool. The tool is simple to use, requiring only a pencil and paper; alternatively, a computer program that has this feature can be used.

Genograms are schematic diagrams of families, listing family members and their relationships to one another. A genogram includes the age, dates of marriage/union and death, and geographic location of each member. Squares represent men and circles represent women; ages are listed inside the figures. Horizontal lines represent marriages/unions, with the date written on the line; vertical lines connect parents and children. Genograms can be particularly useful in understanding family history, composition, relationships, and illnesses (Fig. 15.1).

Genograms vary from simple to complex. The needs of the patient and family guide the level of assessment detail. In a small family with few concerns, the genogram can be simple. In a larger family with multiple concerns, the genogram can reflect these complexities.

Nurses can explore important events such as marriages, divorces, deaths, and geographic movements in relation to the presenting concern. Nurses should always include mental health issues and other significant health problems in the genogram. Questions are more meaningful to the family if they are designed to address the family's particular area of concern rather than a general exploration. The nurse can begin the interview by explaining to family members they will be having a conversation, so the nurse can better understand their situation, their needs and concerns, and their family or support network. The genogram as a tool should be explained and the offer made to provide family members with a copy should they desire one.

Ecomap

The purpose of the **ecomap** is to explore the context for family living. The ecomap is a diagram of the way the family is linked to the community, culture, and resources (Fig. 15.2). This is particularly useful to determine current and past access to mental health inpatient or outpatient/community services, support networks, cultural or religious affiliations, education, employment, and housing. The ecomap can be used as a starting point to identify family needs as well as family strengths and positive connections in terms of promoting family health. It can be most informative early in the assessment process and can be used to plan for discharge. Family members can actively participate in working on the ecomap during the assessment phase.

The family genogram is placed in a centre circle and labelled family or household. Outer circles represent significant people, organizations, and service providers

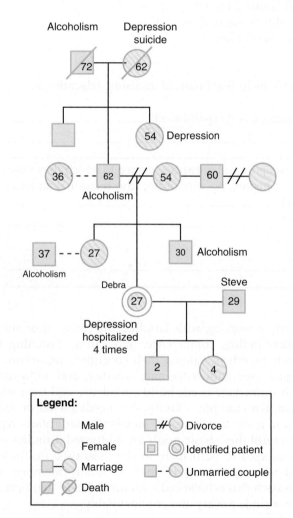

Figure 15.1. Analysis of genogram for Debra. Illness patterns are depression (maternal aunt and grandmother [suicide]) and alcoholism (brother, father, and grandfather). Relationship patterns show that parents are divorced and neither sibling is married.

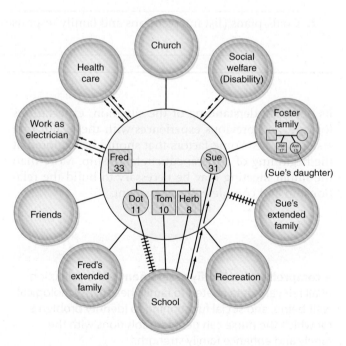

Figure 15.2. Ecomap.

in the context for living. Lines are drawn from the family to the outside circle and indicate the nature of the relationship. Straight lines indicate a strong connection, dotted lines indicate a tenuous relationship, and slashed or jagged lines indicate stressful or nonexistent relationships.

Analyzing Genogram and Ecomap Data

Genograms and ecomaps can be most useful in the assessment when the nurse analyzes the data for family composition, patterns of mental health in the family, individual family needs, and relationship strengths and problems (particularly related to the mental health concern).

Nurses can begin with family composition. Who is considered to be family? How large is the family? Where do family members live? In what way do the family members show support? A large family whose members live in the same city may have more support than a family in which distance separates members. Of course, this is not always the case. The nurse could also study the genogram for relationship and illness patterns. Who in the family are closer and further apart? How might marriage and divorce influence the relationships? What illness patterns might be observed across relationships or generations? For example, depression, gambling, or alcohol addiction might be evident in past generations and may be risk factors for present and future generations. Exploring the significance and meaning of these health issues with the family is important. This can lead to conversations with the family about family strengths and solution strategies that they have tried. It can improve their understanding of health promotion and illness prevention related to family health risks.

The ecomap may be constructed to further explore family connections. The nurse may ask questions like "What community agencies are you involved with now?" "Which are most and least helpful?" "How might you describe your work or school relationships?" "Which of your outside connections fosters your sense of well-being and gives you the most hope?" "What activities do you do, as a family, find rejuvenating?"

▌ FAMILY ASSESSMENT IN THE BIO/ PSYCHO/SOCIAL/SPIRITUAL DOMAINS

A comprehensive family assessment incorporates information related to the biologic, psychological, social, and spiritual domains.

Biologic Domain

Family assessment includes discussion of family members' physical and mental health status and how they affect family functioning. A family with multiple health problems, both physical and mental, will be trying to manage the symptoms and treatments, as well as obtain the financial and health care resources it needs.

Directly and matter of factly, the nurse should ask the family to identify any members who have had or have a physical or mental illness. The nurse can record family health status information on the genogram. This may include current and past physical or mental illness and disabilities. Stresses currently placed on the family and its resources may be indicated in the ecomap and in narrative form. It is important for the nurse to explore how the physical and mental health problems are affecting family functioning. For example, if a member requires frequent visits to a provider or hospitalizations, the whole family may feel the effects of focusing more time and financial resources on that member.

Exploring a family's history and experience with a mental disorder must be approached with respect and sensitivity. In most cultures, mental health problems are associated with stigma and shame (MHCC, 2012). How and with whom families share information about their ill member varies greatly, as illustrated in the following quote by a parent: "We went a long time without telling anyone what was going on partly because our son didn't want anyone to know and it would have freaked my family out" (MacCourt, 2013, p. 14).

If family members do not know if there is a family history of mental illness, the nurse could ask if anyone was treated for "nerves" or had a "nervous breakdown." Overall, a comprehensive family history of mental illness across multiple generations helps the nurse understand the significance of mental illness in the current generation. If one family member has a serious mental illness, the whole family can be affected. Exploring how this is unique to each family is important to planning care.

Psychological Domain

Assessment of the family's psychological domain focuses on the family's development and life cycle, communication patterns, stress and coping abilities, and problem-solving skills. One aim of the assessment is to understand how family members communicate with each other as they negotiate developmental and life transitions, including mental health problems and illnesses. It is important in terms of the recovery process for the nurse to explore coping styles and problem-solving abilities of family members relevant to the management of both crisis and long-term issues associated with their relative's mental illness. Identifying stressful events and assessing coping mechanisms, strengths, and resources should be a priority as a means to facilitate a family's recovery process.

Family Development

Family development is a broad term that refers to all the processes connected with the growth of a family, including changes associated with its economic situation, geographic location, migration, acculturation, and serious illness. In optimal family development, family members are relatively differentiated (capable of autonomous functioning) from one another, anxiety is low, and individuals have good emotional relationships with their own families of origin.

Family Life Cycles

There is a distinction between family life cycles and family development (McGoldrick et al., 2016). Family development refers to the unique path a family takes that is shaped by predictable and unpredictable events, such as illness or environmental disasters, and societal trends, such as an economic downturn. **Family life cycle** refers to a "typical" path most families go through related to the arrival and departure of family members through birth and death, couple unions and separations, and the raising and launching of children. It is important for nurses to model inclusivity and respect for the diversity of family forms or, as McGoldrick et al. (2016) state, to "widen our lens." Nurses will encounter a diversity of family forms in their clinical practice. Families may include parents who are unmarried, separated, or divorced and the children, biologic, adopted, or fostered. The family may be extended, including several generations in the same home. The nurse's focus regarding family development is not on categorizing the family but rather on understanding the relational processes that occur as the family evolves and responds to its member's mental illness.

The family life cycle is a process of expansion, contraction, and realignment of relationship systems to support the entry, exit, and development of family members in a functional way. There are many ways to go through life; while there is no single definitive list of stages of a family life cycle that is sufficiently inclusive (McGoldrick et al., 2016), a family's life cycle is conceptualized in terms of stages throughout the years. To move from one stage to the next, the family system undergoes changes (Table 15.1). Structural and potential structural changes within stages can usually be handled by rearranging the family system (first-order changes), whereas transition from one stage to the next requires changes in the system itself (second-order changes). In first-order changes, the family system is rearranged, such as when the youngest child enters schooling and the stay-at-home parent returns to work. The system is rearranged, but the structure remains the same. In second-order changes, the family structure does change, such as when a member moves away from the family home to live independently. Families may be transitioning through more than one stage depending on the family configuration. As suggested, the nurse may use this model to explore potential areas of stress related to the family transitions. Multiple transitions can trigger or exacerbate symptoms of mental illness.

Consider the following two situations:

A family transitioning through various life cycle stages experiences the emotional process and second-order changes occurring when one family member is experiencing an acute mental illness episode.

A family is affected when several life cycle changes are interrupted at the same time, such as the death of a grandparent, a job loss, and separation of the parents.

Transition times are any times of addition, subtraction, or change in status of family members. During transitions, family stresses are more likely to cause symptoms or difficulties. Significant family events, such as the death of a member or the introduction of a new member, also affect the family's ability to function. During these times, families may need help from the mental health system.

Cultural Diversity

Given Canada's multicultural climate, it is important for nurses to consciously attend to cultural diversity. One method for increasing sensitivity to culture has been by trying to identify distinctive characteristics or responses to life cycle transitions or disruptions such as mental illness within specific ethnic communities. Becoming conscious of the characteristics of particular ethnic groups is an important step toward developing an appreciation for cultural diversity, as long as these norms are remembered to be gross generalizations. Labelling and categorizing ethnic groups' behaviours according to general rules can help raise awareness of difference, but it can equally obscure the uniqueness of each family that nurses encounter. For the nurse, appreciating and validating ethnic differences, while at the same time acknowledging similarities, can feel like a delicate balancing act. Nurses must be mindful of the personal biases they bring to their practice. In the clinical example provided in Box 15.2, a particular generalization is at play in the description of Judy's rich familial connections and her location in a particular geographic region of Canada. This is an example of a cultural assumption.

Developing sensitivity to one's own beliefs about what constitutes normalcy and functionality in a family is a challenging and important endeavour. It is only in this process of self-reflection that the nurse will develop an awareness of the cultural norms and values that are guiding and creating the template against which the nurse is judging and assessing the family life cycle (Doane & Varcoe, 2015). Developing and maintaining sensitivity to ethnicity, culture, and power are important in helping the nurse to recognize issues of diversity (see Chapter 3).

Low-Income Families

Rates of psychological distress and mental disorders, including that of substance-related disorders and addiction, are much higher in the low-income population. These differences are statistically consistent across the Canadian sociodemographic strata: region/province, gender, age, marital status, immigration, first language,

Table 15.1   Phases of the Family Life Cycle

Family Life Cycle Phase	Emotional Process of Transition: Key Prerequisite Attitudes	Second Order Tasks/Changes of the System to Proceed Developmentally
1. Emerging young adults	Accepting emotional and financial responsibility for self	a. Differentiation of self in relation to family of origin b. Development of intimate peer relationships c. Establishment of self in respect to work and financial independence d. Establishment of self in community and larger society e. Establishment of one's worldview, spirituality, religion, and relationship to nature f. Parents shifting to consultative role in young adult's relationships
2. Couple formation: The joining of families	Commitment to new system	a. Formation of couple system b. Expansion of family boundaries to include new partner and extended family c. Realignment of relationships among couple, parents and siblings, extended family, friends, and larger community
3. Families with young children	Accepting new members into the system	a. Adjusting of couple system to make space for children b. Collaboration in child-rearing and financial and housekeeping tasks c. Realignment of relationships with extended family to include parenting and grandparenting roles d. Realignment of relationships with community and larger social system to include new family structure and relationships
4. Families with adolescents	Increasing flexibility of family boundaries to include children's independence and grandparents' frailties	a. Shift of parent–child relationships to permit adolescent to have more independent activities and relationships and to move more flexibly into and out of system b. Families helping emerging adolescents negotiate relationships with community c. Refocus on midlife couple and career issues d. Begin shift toward caring for older generation e. Realignment with community and larger social system to include shifting family of emerging adolescent and parents to new formation of relating
5. Launching children and moving on at midlife	Accepting multitude of exits from and entries into the system	a. Renegotiation of couple system as a dyad b. Development of adult-to-adult relationships between parents and grown-up children c. Realignment of relationships to include in-laws and grandchildren d. Realignment of relationships with community to include new constellation of family relationships e. Exploration of new interests/career, given the freedom from child care responsibilities f. Dealing with health needs, disabilities, and death of parents (grandparents)
6. Families in late middle age	Accepting shifting generational roles	a. Maintaining or modifying own and/or couple and social functioning and interests in face of physiologic decline: exploration of new familial and social role options b. Supporting more central role of middle generations c. Making room in the system for the wisdom and experience of the elders d. Supporting the older generation without over functioning for them
7. Families nearing the end of life	Accepting the realities of family members' limitations and death and the completion of one cycle of life	a. Dealing with loss of spouse, siblings, and other peers b. Making preparations for death and legacy c. Managing reversed roles in caretaking between middle and older generations d. Realignment of relationships with larger community and social system to acknowledge changing life cycle relationships

From McGoldrick, M., Garcia-Preto, N., & Carter, B. A. (Eds.) (2016). *Overview: The life cycle in its changing context: Individual, family, and social perspectives* (5th ed., pp. 1–44). Copyright 2016, reprinted by permission of Pearson Education Inc., Upper Saddle River, NJ.

and ethnic origin (Caron & Liu, 2010). People living in poverty struggle to make ends meet, and family members may face difficulties in meeting their own or other members' basic developmental needs. They may be homeless or living in unsafe conditions. To be poor does not mean that a family is dysfunctional, but poverty is

an important factor that can force even the healthiest families to crumble.

The life cycle may be condensed, such that family members leave their home, mate, have children, and become grandparents at much earlier ages than their working-class and middle-class counterparts do. Consequently, many

BOX 15.2 John and Judy Jones

John and Judy Jones were married 3 years ago, after their graduation from a small University in Eastern Canada. Judy's career choice required that she live on the East Coast, where she would be near her large family. John willingly moved with her and quickly found a satisfying position. After about 6 months of marriage, John became extremely irritable and depressed. He kept saying that his life was not his own. Judy was very concerned but could not understand his feelings of being overwhelmed. His job was going well,

and they had a very busy social life, mostly revolving around her family, whom John loved. They decided to seek counselling and completed the genogram below.

After looking at the genogram, both John and Judy began to realize that part of John's discomfort had to do with the number of family members who were involved in their lives. Judy and John began to redefine their social life, allowing more time with friends and each other.

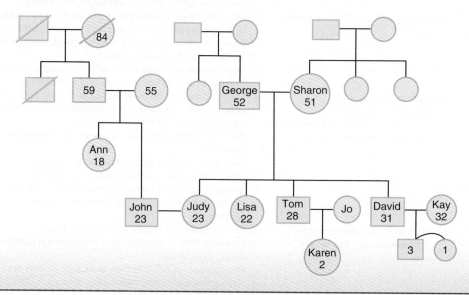

individuals in such families assume new roles and responsibilities before they are developmentally capable. The condensed life cycle creates adolescents whose educational opportunities are compromised (no time to complete school given the family demands), therefore limiting their employment skills. The cycle of poverty is thus reinforced.

Families living in poverty are subject to disruption via abrupt loss of members, loss of unemployment compensation, illness, death, imprisonment, or addiction. Men may die relatively young compared with their middle-class counterparts. Ordinary problems, such as transportation or a sick child, can become major crises because of a lack of resources.

Reliance on institutional supports is another distinguishing characteristic of families in poverty. Poor families are often forced to seek public assistance, which ultimately can result in additional stress in having to deal with a governmental agency.

Communication Patterns

Family communication patterns develop over a lifetime. Some family members communicate more openly and freely than others. In addition, family subgroups may

have unique communication patterns with one another. During the assessment, the nurse should observe the verbal and nonverbal communication of the family members. Who sits next to each other? Who talks to whom? Who answers most questions? Who volunteers information? Who changes the subject? Which subjects seem acceptable to discuss? Which topics are not discussed? How are partners intimate with each other? How are the family secrets or sensitive topics revealed? Does the nonverbal communication match the verbal communication? Nurses can use this information to help identify family problems, strengths, and communication issues.

Nurses should also assess the family for its daily communication patterns. Identifying which family members confide in one another is a place to start examining ongoing communication. Other areas include how often children talk with parents, which child talks to the parents most, and who is most likely to discipline the children. Another question considers how family members express positive and negative feelings. In determining how open or closed the family is, the nurse explores the type of information the family shares with nonfamily members. For example, one family may tell others about a member's mental illness, whereas another family may not discuss any illnesses with those outside the family.

Stress and Coping Abilities

One of the most important assessment tasks is to determine how family members deal with major and minor stressful events and their available coping skills. Some families seem able to cope with overwhelming stresses, such as the death of a member, major illness, or severe conflict, whereas other families seem to fall apart over relatively minor events. It is important for the nurse to listen to which situations a family appraises as stressful and help the family identify usual coping responses. The nurse can then evaluate these responses. Identifying what the family does well and acknowledging the family for these strengths are important. If the family's responses

are detrimental to health (e.g., substance abuse, physical abuse), the nurse may discuss the need to develop coping skills that lead to family well-being (see Chapter 17). The use of mindfulness within the context of a multifamily support holds promise for families coping with mental illness across the lifespan. See Box 15.3.

Problem-Solving Skills

Nurses assess family problem-solving skills by focusing on the more recent problems the family has experienced and determining the process that members used to solve them. For example, even with the most effective treatment, relapses are likely to occur; when a family member relapses, who is the one to ensure that he or she seeks treatment? Underlying the ability to solve problems is the decision-making process. Who makes and

---

BOX 15.3 Research for Best Practice

MINDFULNESS-BASED SUPPORT GROUP FOR FAMILIES

Whitehorn, D., Campbell, M. E., Cosgrove, P., Abidi, S., & Tibbo, P. G. (2017). A mindfulness-based support group for families in early psychosis: A pilot qualitative study. Journal of Mental Health and Addiction Nursing, 1(1), e30–e34.

Background: Support for family members of people with mental illness has long been considered an essential component of holistic and optimal care; unfortunately, it is all too often overlooked. A diagnosis of a psychotic disorder in one's child can be both disheartening and overwhelming for parents as they endeavour to support and care for their child, while struggling to manage their own responses to the impact of their child's illness on family life.

Purpose: This pilot study was implemented to explore both the feasibility and experiences of parents of young people in care for a first episode of psychosis with an Early Intervention Service (EIS) in Nova Scotia, who were engaged in a mindfulness-based support group.

Methods: Family members involved with the EIS were invited to participate in a 1-year research protocol during which time mindfulness, defined as "moment-to-moment, nonjudgmental awareness," practices were introduced. Ten self-selected parents (three fathers and seven mothers) volunteered to take part in the study, which included eight support group sessions. The first four sessions occurred weekly and introduced formal and informal mindfulness meditation in daily activities. The final four sessions took place over the remaining 11 months and focused on mindfulness practice and personal coping with life in general, and not specifically

in relation to having a child experiencing psychosis. Study participants were also asked to keep a diary of their mindfulness practices. During focus group discussions, participants were asked to reflect upon their experiences with mindfulness and mindfulness practice. Data analysis of the focus group interviews was guided by interpretive phenomenology.

Findings: All participants engaged in mindfulness activities in varying degrees and recognized some value in the experience of mindfulness, as cultivated in physical activities, and the nonjudgmental aspect of mindfulness. Mindfulness practice was associated with (1) a greater sense of ease, (2) increased awareness, (3) less emotional reactivity, and (4) improved interpersonal relationships. As one participant stated "when I don't react or I react differently from the way I would have habitually reacted…we can actually have a conversation…the relationship becomes different" (p. e32).

Implications for Practice: The family experience of mental illness is as varied as the families themselves. Including mindfulness, within the context of a multifamily support group, can contribute to a comprehensive program of support for families living with mental illness. Clinicians leading mindfulness activities need to be engaged in their own mindfulness practice and partake in ongoing professional development in order to support mindfulness practice in others. Further research is warranted, however, to explore the effectiveness of mindfulness interventions within the unique context of families coping with mental illness across the lifespan.

implements decisions? How does the family support each other? How does the family handle conflict? All these data provide information regarding the family's problem-solving abilities. Once these abilities are identified, the nurse can build on these strengths in helping families deal with additional problems.

Social Domain

An assessment of the family's social domain provides important data about the operation of the family as a system and its interaction within its environment. Areas of concern include the system itself, perspectives on understanding families, social and financial status, and formal and informal support networks.

Family Systems

Just as any group can be viewed as a system, a family can be understood as a system with interdependent members. Family system theories view the family as an open system whose members interact with their environment as well as among themselves. One family member's change in thoughts or behaviour can cause a ripple effect and change everyone else's (Wright & Leahey, 2013). For example, a father of a child with attention deficit hyperactivity disorder (ADHD) who decides to reinforce his child's positive efforts rather than focusing on negative actions may notice a change in the child's behaviour, which may in turn result in a reduction of the stress he feels when interacting with the child.

One common scenario in the mental health field is the effect of a patient's improvement on the family. With new medications and treatments, patients are more likely to be able to live independently, which subsequently changes the responsibilities and activities of family caregivers. Although family members may be relieved that their caregiving burden is lifted, they will be also adjusting to changes in the demands on their time and energies. This transition may not be easy because it is often less stressful to maintain familiar activities than to venture into uncharted territory. Families may seem as though they want to keep an ill member dependent, but, in reality, they are struggling with the change in their family system.

Wright and Leahey's (2013) Calgary Family Assessment Model (CFAM) and the Calgary Family Intervention Model (CFIM) are Canadian family nursing models that have been implemented successfully in mental health care settings (Leahey & Harper-Jaques, 2010; Marshall, Bell, & Moules, 2010). They are relational practice nursing models based on postmodernism, systems, cybernetics, communication and change theories, and the biology of cognition. These two models are multidimensional frameworks that conceptualize the family into structural, developmental, and functional categories. Each assessment category contains several subcategories. Structure is further categorized into internal (family, gender, sexual orientation, etc.), external (extended family

and larger systems), and contextual (ethnicity, race, social class, religion, spirituality, environment). Family developmental assessment is organized according to stages, tasks, and attachments. Functional assessment areas include instrumental (activities of daily living) and expressive (communication, problem-solving, roles, beliefs, influence, power, and alliances) (Wright & Leahey, 2013).

When the nurse uses CFAM/CFIM, relational practice develops and evolves during four stages: engagement, assessment, intervention, and termination. The nurse and the family are partners in care as each brings specialized expertise in managing health problems, as well as strengths and resources, to the relationship.

The *engagement* stage is the initial stage in which the family is greeted and made comfortable. In the *assessment* stage, needs are identified and relationships develop between family and health providers. During this stage, the nurse invites the family to tell its story. The nurse asks key questions and listens to the patient's and family members' expectations, hopes, questions, and ideas. The *intervention* stage is the core of the clinical work and involves providing a context in which recovery is facilitated (see Family Interventions section in this chapter). The nurse communicates regularly with the family to provide cognitive and emotional support. The *termination* phase refers to the process of evaluating the family interviews, recognizing the family efforts in their recovery journey, providing referrals if necessary, and, depending on the family's needs, extending an invitation for further interviews. The role of the family in promoting well-being and providing care to their loved one is to be recognized and their needs to be supported (MHCC, 2009, 2015).

Perspectives on Understanding Families

Nurses are looking to the ideas of postmodernism and social constructivism to enrich their understanding of families. These ideas support exploring how families make meaning in their lives and how they construct their reality in relation to their social environment. For instance, the constructivist influence invites nurses to understand that what they are seeing is a product of their own assumptions about people, families, and problems and their interactions with families. It is recognized that people are highly influenced by their current relationships and the environments in which they perceive their realities. Persons with mental illness and their families should therefore be encouraged to express their perspectives (their own "truth") on their situation. Nurses need to be respectful of family stories and viewpoints, within the parameters of values about human safety and rights, including self-determination and protection from interpersonal violence.

Nurses are also using a critical lens derived from feminist, poststructural, and postcolonial theories that support considerations of power, oppression, culture, economic conditions of life, social change, and emancipation. This critical perspective draws the nurse's attention to the sociopolitical, economic, and linguistic contexts within which families are situated and constituted. The focus can then be on exposing underlying sociopolitical structures that are advantaging some people/families and disadvantaging others. The goals are to explore social conditions and revise structures in ways that address inequities (Doane & Varcoe, 2015).

Social and Financial Status

Social status is often linked directly to financial status. The nurse should identify the occupations of the family members. Who works outside the home and inside the home? Who is primarily responsible for the family's financial support? Families of low social status are more likely to have limited financial resources, which can place additional stresses on the family. This information can be recorded on the ecomap and in narrative form. Nurses can use information on the family's financial status to determine whether to refer the family to social services.

Formal and Informal Support Networks

Networks both formal and informal are important in providing support to individuals and families. These networks are the links among the individual, family, and the community. Assessing the extent of formal support (e.g., hospitals, agencies) and informal support (e.g., extended family, friends, and neighbours) gives a clearer picture of the availability of support. In assessing formal support, the nurse could ask about the family's involvement with government institutions and self-help groups such as Alcoholics Anonymous or Strengthening Families Together (refer further to Web Links). Assessing the informal network is particularly important in cultural groups with extended family networks or close friends, because these individuals can be major sources of support to patients. This is important information to include in the ecomap. If the nurse does not ask about informal networks, these important people may be missed. Nurses can inquire whether family members volunteer at schools, local hospitals, or nursing homes. They can also ask whether the family attends religious services or activities.

Spiritual Domain

Families may find that their spiritual or religious beliefs and practices help promote their recovery by helping them to understand their experiences while strengthening their sense of meaning and purpose. For many families, their religious affiliations will play a key role in their everyday lives. These affiliations can influence the family's understanding of health and illness and of healing and treatment. Religious and spiritual practices can foster family and community support and may be a major resource to families. It is increasingly recognized that, in all faith groups, the help and guidance of religious leaders are frequently sought by families who have a mentally ill member (Aaron, 2008). Yet, research suggests that a majority of clergy (Christian clergy were studied) feel inadequate regarding their knowledge of mental illness (Farrell & Goebert, 2008). Unfortunately, mental health professionals do not tend to view religious leaders collaboratively (Leavey, Lowenthal, & King, 2007) even though they are frequently seen as conduits to the formal mental health system (Vermass, Greeen, Haley, & Haddock, 2017). Collaboration, however, could be of significant use to both groups, especially to individuals and families requiring assistance. Religious leaders can provide community-based support and assist health professionals, such as nurses, to understand patients' beliefs, which is important to informing treatment planning and to improving responses to crisis. Nurses and colleagues in turn can assist religious leaders to understand mental disorders and mental health issues and their treatment. Open communication can facilitate, for instance, appropriate use of complementary healing practices that can be a part of a group's religious beliefs, and more importantly, it may promote better trust in psychiatric treatment and care.

Collaborating with faith-based nurses (e.g., Christian parish nurses, Jewish congregational nurses, Muslim crescent nurses, etc.) can also be beneficial when working with family caregivers. In a study that explored the roles parish nurses employed in meeting the needs of family caregivers, four themes emerged in the data. Researchers found that parish nurses provided the gift of presence; they were the bearers of blessings, messengers of spiritual care; and they were involved in bridging challenges. In short, they were able to provide family caregivers with emotional, informational, and spiritual support (Grebeldinger & Buckley, 2016).

Finally, in addressing the spiritual domain of family nursing, it is important for the nurse to recognize that family members may differ widely in their religious beliefs and approach to spirituality. Such variation among members' perspectives, if it exists, should inform the family assessment. It may be a source of enrichment, distress, or both, for the family.

THE PYRAMID OF FAMILY CARE FRAMEWORK

The pyramid of the Family Care Framework, in the MHCC's national guidelines, identifies five levels of tasks for meeting the support needs of family caregivers (MacCourt, 2013). As one moves from the bottom to the top of the pyramid, the intensity of family intervention increases while the number of families who require the intervention decreases (Fig. 15.3). Nurses have the knowledge, skill, and competency to provide these services based on their level of education and advanced practice.

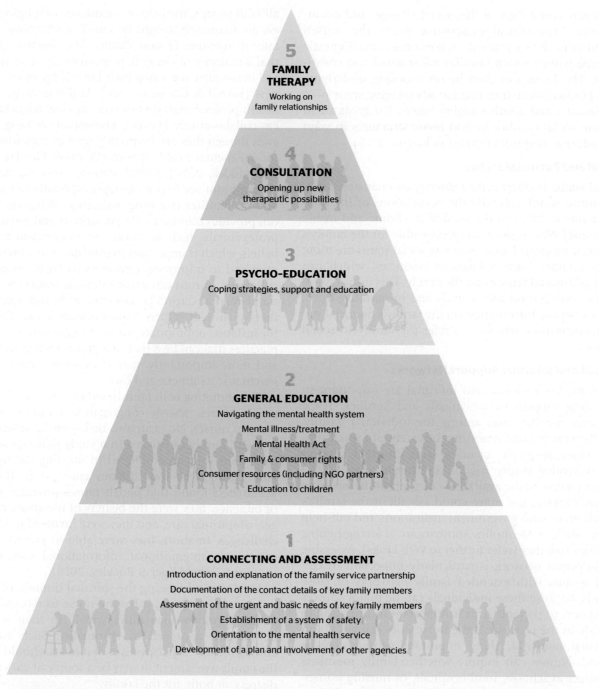

Figure 15.3. Pyramid of Family Care Framework. (Adapted from Mottaghipour, Y., & Bickerton, A. (2005). The pyramid of family care: A framework for family involvement with adult mental health services. *Australian e-Journal for the Advancement of Mental Health, 4*(3), 210–217. doi:10.5172/jamh.4.3.210)

Levels 1 (*connecting and assessment*) and 2 (*general education*) indicate the minimum level of service that should be available to all family caregivers. The need for level 1 and level 2 interventions should be assessed at each point of contact. One of the most important family interventions is education and health teaching related to the mental illness. As families have a central role in the treatment of mental illnesses, members need to learn about mental disorders, medications, actions, side effects, and overall treatment approaches and outcomes.

For example, families are often reluctant to have members take psychiatric medications because they believe the medications will "drug" the patient or become addictive. The family's beliefs about mental illnesses and treatment will often affect how patients manage their illness and recovery.

Level 3 (*psychoeducation*) refers to interventions in which recommendations are made to the family caregivers regarding coping strategies or specific ways to deal with the challenges of the mental illness. Level 4 (*consultation*) may be required by family caregivers with significant challenges in supporting an individual living with mental illness. Level 5 (*family therapy*) refers to interventions that work on family relationships and is designed to facilitate change in the family interactional system. Family therapy is useful for families who are having difficulty maintaining family integrity. Various theoretical perspectives are used in family therapy: more recently, therapies influenced by postmodernism, hermeneutics, and social constructionism have developed. These focus on collaborative, conversational approaches, and narrative and solution-based therapies. Family therapy can be short term or long term and is conducted by mental health specialists, including advanced practice psychiatric and mental health nurses. Few families require level 4 or 5.

■ FAMILY INTERVENTIONS

Each conversation the nurse has with a family member can be meaningful and healing, and it can effect change in the patient's and the family members' bio/psycho/social/spiritual integrity and functioning. Families with loved ones experiencing mental illness have reported that even a short meaningful conversation with a health care professional is significant. Therapeutic conversations, the heart of family nursing, are of central importance when working with family caregivers. Developing skill in therapeutic conversations that are sensitive to language, culture, setting, and time available allow nurses to "see" and "do" differently when working with family caregivers (Bell, 2016). In a study addressing a therapeutic conversation intervention with acute psychiatric patients and their families, Seveinbjarnardottir, Svararsdottir, and Wright (2013) found that family members receiving this type of intervention by nurses who were educated, trained, and supervised in this approach, built on the Calgary Family Assessment and Intervention models, perceived significantly higher cognitive and emotional support from nurses, compared to family members who received standard care. Therapeutic conversation in a brief family interview is purposeful and time limited. It is an opportunity to acknowledge and affirm the illness experience and patient and family expertise. Listening to the illness story is part of ethical nursing practice. Nurses have an opportunity to focus the conversations using language of recovery and strength while still addressing the needs and concerns of the family. Adopting therapeutic conversations as an intervention strategy, information sharing, emotional support, and patient and family involvement in decision-making can take place. Efforts should be made to enhance the family's choice, determination, and independence.

The "15-minute family interview" has been used effectively as a framework for family intervention. The following are some specific ideas for conducting a healing, productive, and efficient 15-minute family interview. They are condensed ideas from the CFAM and CFIM (Wright & Leahey, 2013) and consist of five key components: manners, therapeutic conversations, genogram and ecomap, therapeutic questions, and commending individual and family strengths:

- Begin the therapeutic conversation with a purpose in mind that can be accomplished in the time period you will be together with the family.
- Use manners to engage with the family by first introducing yourself with your name and your role.
- Provide a brief overview about the purpose of the interview.
- Assess, using a genogram and ecomap, the key areas of internal/external structure, function, and relationships.
- Identify family needs or concerns by asking key therapeutic questions.
- Commend the family on one or two strengths.
- Evaluate the usefulness of the meeting, and conclude the conversation.

KEY CONCEPT

The **15-minute family interview** is an assessment/intervention framework that consists of five key components: manners, therapeutic conversations, genogram and ecomap, therapeutic questions, and commending individual and family strengths.

Therapeutic Questions

Nurses can ask key questions to involve families in care. The questions need to fit with the context in which the nurse encounters the family. The purpose of the questions is to identify imminent needs of the family in supporting their caregiver sustainability. Questions should be built on the responses to the previous question.

Some useful questions include the following:

- What are your main concerns about this hospitalization or illness?
- What information would be most helpful for you at this time?
- How can we be most supportive to you now?
- Who in the family is most affected by the patient's illness?
- What is the most meaningful way to involve you in the care and treatment plan?

Commending Family and Individual Strengths

It is important to enhance the family's sense of worth. One way the nurse can accomplish this is to actively notice and distinguish the family's strengths, courage, resources, and capabilities in the form of a verbal *commendation*

(Limacher & Wright, 2003; Wright & Leahey, 2013). For a family that has been challenged, often for many years, with a serious mental health issue, to experience a direct, specific comment on their positive actions and solutions can be a powerful intervention. It can be as simple as a nurse telling them "I am impressed with your strength, your detailed knowledge about the medication regimen, and the way that you have stuck together to support one another by visiting the hospital and attending this family meeting." Families find participating in strength-based conversation enhances the recovery process.

Implementation

In implementing any family intervention, flexibility is essential, particularly when working with culturally diverse groups. To implement successful, competent family interventions, nurses need to be open to modifying the structure and format of the sessions. Longer sessions are often useful, especially when a translator or an interpreter is used. Nurses also need to respect and work with the changing composition of family and nonfamily participants (e.g., extended family members, intimate partners, friends and neighbours, community helpers) in sessions. Because of the stigma that some cultural groups associate with seeking help, nurses may need to hold intervention sessions in community settings (e.g., churches, schools) or at the family's home. Finally, ending face-to-face sessions with the family may need to be gradual. The family may need information for further support, consultation, or reengagement should the problems reoccur.

🍁 SUMMARY OF KEY POINTS

- Family is a group of people defined as "who they say they are" and involved relationally in a complex process where economics, emotion, context, and experiences are interwoven and multilayered. Families come in various compositions, including immediate, extended, multigenerational, single-parent, same-gender, and blended families. Cultural values and beliefs define family composition and roles.
- Families, whether they are relatives of individuals experiencing mental illness, or friends who make up a larger circle of support, have a unique role in promoting well-being, providing care, and facilitating recovery across the life span.
- Nurses complete a comprehensive family assessment when they care for families for extended periods or if a patient has complex mental health problems.
- In building relationships with families, nurses must establish credibility and competence with the family. Unless the nurse listens and addresses the family's immediate needs first, the family will have difficulty engaging in the challenges of caring for someone with a mental disorder.
- Families can be engaged and helped through education and programs like parenting and sibling support, financial assistance, peer support, and respite care. Wherever possible, families should be welcomed as partners in care and treatment of their loved ones and should be included in decision-making in a way that respects consent, confidentiality, and privacy.
- The genogram is an assessment and intervention tool that is useful in understanding health, relationships, and social functioning across several generations.
- In assessing the family biologic domain, the nurse determines physical and mental health status and its effects on family functioning.
- Family members are often reluctant to discuss the mental disorders of family members because of the stigma associated with mental illness. In many instances, family members do not know whether mental illnesses were present in other generations.
- The family psychological assessment focuses on family development, the family life cycle, communication patterns, stress and coping abilities, problem-solving skills, strengths, hope, and resourcefulness. Determining how these occur in relationships is key.
- The family life cycle is a process of expansion, contraction, and realignment of the relationship systems to support the entry, exit, and development of family members in a functional way. Families have unique patterns based on their context for living.
- The ecomap is a tool used to assess the family social domain, which includes relationships within formal and informal support networks. The ecomap is particularly useful in care planning and discharge.
- Religious leaders of all faiths may be a significant support to families with a mentally ill member in making meaning of their situation and in maintaining hope and spiritual strength.
- Family interventions focus on supporting the family's bio/psycho/social/spiritual integrity and functioning as defined by its members. Family nursing interventions include counselling, promotion of self-care activities, eliciting strengths and resources, purposefully commending the family, supportive therapy, education and health teaching, and the use of genograms and ecomaps. Mental health specialists, including advanced practice nurses, conduct family therapy.
- Education of the family is one of the most useful interventions. Teaching the family about mental disorders, life cycles, family systems, and family interactions can help the family develop a new understanding of family functioning and the effects of mental disorders on the family.

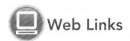

Web Links

http://www.cmha.ca/ Founded in 1918, the Canadian Mental Health Association (CMHA) champions mental health for all Canadians through advocacy, education, research and service. In doing so, CMHA helps people who experience mental illness and their families access the community-based resources they need to build resilience and support recovery in their own communities.

http://www.fameforfamilies.com Based in Toronto, the Family Association for Mental Health Everywhere (FAME) aims to facilitate "hope, acceptance, recovery and education," with an emphasis on self-care and individual responsibility.

http://www.heretohelp.bc.ca HeretoHelp represents a group of seven leading provincial mental health and addictions non-profit agencies, working collaboratively in the prevention and management of mental health and substance abuse problems. Here, readers will find excellent trustworthy resources regarding mental illness and addiction, specifically designed for family caregivers, including *Family Self-Care and Recovery from Mental Illness* and *A Toolkit for Families: A Resource for Families Supporting Children, Youth, and Adults with a Mental or Substance Use Disorder.*

https://www.mentalhealthcommission.ca Through this site, readers can access the *National Guidelines for a Comprehensive Service System to Support Family Caregivers of Adults with Mental Health Problems and Illnesses.* An evidence-informed comprehensive approach to meeting the needs of family caregivers is proposed and includes 41 recommendations intended to improve the capacity of caregivers to provide the best possible care to adults with mental illness while tending to their own well-being.

http://www.schizophrenia.ca The mission of the Schizophrenia Society of Canada is to improve the quality of life for those affected by schizophrenia and psychosis through education, support programs, public policy, and research. Through its provincial societies, individuals can take part in a variety of informative programs including *Strengthening Families Together,* a 10-week psychoeducational program for families and friends of individuals with schizophrenia and related disorders, and a *Partnership Program,* a public awareness campaign that features a person living with the illness, a family member, and a health care professional, who engage in educational presentations throughout local communities.

http://www.ourhealthyminds.com/family-handbook/ *Living with Mental Illness: A Guide for Family and Friends* was produced by Capital Health, Nova Scotia, to "make things a little easier" for family members, caregivers, or friends of someone living with an mental illness. This informative guide prepared by family members, caregivers, and mental health professionals includes information on understanding mental illness, managing mental illness, and supporting recovery.

References

Aaron, M. (2008). Spirituality, the heart of caring. *A Life in the Day, 12*(4), 23–26.

Bell, J. (2016). The central importance of therapeutic conversations in family nursing: Can talking be healing? *Journal of Family Nursing, 22*(4), 439–449.

Bos, A. E. R., Pryor, J. B., Reeder, G. D., & Stutterheim, S. E. (2013). Stigma: Advances in theory and research. *Basic Applied Social Psychology, 35*(1), 1–9.

Brighton, R. M., Patterson, C., Taylor, E., Moxham, L., Perlman, D., Sumskis, S., & Heffernan, T. (2016). The effect of respite services on carers of individuals with severe mental illness. *Journal of Psychosocial Nursing & Mental Health Services, 54*(12), 33–38.

Buckley, M. R., & Scott, S. K. (2017). Relational functioning: Understanding bipolar and related disorders. In J. A. Russo, J. K. Coker, & J. H. King (Eds.), *DSM-5® and family systems* (pp. 55–83). New York, NY: Springer Publishing Company, LLC.

Caron, J., & Liu, A. (2010). A descriptive study of the prevalence of psychological distress and mental disorders in the Canadian population: Comparison between low-income and non-low-income populations. *Chronic Diseases in Canada, 30*(3), 84–94.

Coker, F., Williams, A., Hayes, L., Hamann, J., & Harvey, C. (2016). Exploring the needs of diverse consumers experiencing mental illness and their families through family psychoeducation. *Journal of Mental Health, 25*(3), 197–203.

Doane, G. H., & Varcoe, C. (2015). *How to nurse: Relational inquiry with individuals and families in changing health care contexts.* Philadelphia, PA: Wolters Kluwer Health.

El-Mallakh, P., & Findlay, K. (2015). Strategies to improve medication adherence in patients with schizophrenia: The role of support services. *Neuropsychiatric Disease and Treatment, 11,* 1077–1090.

Ennis, E., & Bunting, B. P. (2013). Family burden, family health, and personal mental health. *BMC Public Health, 13,* 255. doi:10.1186/1471-2458-13-255

Falloon, I. (2005). Research on family interventions for mental disorders: Problems and perspectives. In N. Sartorius, J. Leff, J. J. López-Ibor, M. Maj, & A. Okasha (Eds.), *Families and mental disorders: From burden to empowerment* (pp. 235–257). Chichester, UK: Wiley.

Farooq, S., & Naeem, F. (2014). Tackling nonadherence in psychiatric disorders: Current opinion. *Neuropsychiatric Disease and Treatment, 10,* 1069–1077.

Farrell, J., & Goebert, D. (2008). Collaboration between psychiatrists and clergy in recognizing and treating serious mental illness. *Psychiatric Services, 59,* 437–40.

Flyck, L., Fatouros-Bergman, H., & Koernig, T. (2015). Determinants of subjective and objective burden of informal caregiving of patients with psychotic disorders. *International Journal of Social Psychiatry, 61*(7), 684–692.

Gladstone, B. M., Boydell, K. M., Seeman, M. V., & McKeever, P. D. (2011). Children's experiences of parental mental illness: A literature review. *Early Intervention in Psychiatry, 5,* 271–289.

Grebeldinger, T. A., & Buckley, K. M. (2016). You are not alone: Parish nurses bridge challenges for family caregivers. *Journal of Christian Nursing, 33*(1), 50–56.

Leahey, M., & Harper-Jaques, S. (2010). Integrating family nursing into a mental health urgent care practice framework: Ladders for learning. *Journal of Family Nursing, 16*(2) 196–212.

Leavey, G., Lowenthal, K., & King, M. (2007). Challenges to sanctuary. *Social Science and Medicine, 65*(3), 548–559.

Limacher, L. H., & Wright, L. M. (2003). Commendations: Listening to the silent side of a family intervention. *Journal of Family Nursing, 9*(2), 130–150.

MacCourt, P. (2013). *Family Caregivers Advisory Committee, Mental Health Commission of Canada. National guidelines for a comprehensive service system to support family caregivers of adults with mental health problems and illnesses.* Calgary, AB: Mental Health Commission of Canada. Retrieved from http://www.mentalhealthcommission.ca

Marshall, A., & Harper-Jaques, S. (2008). Depression and family relationships. *Journal of Family Nursing, 14*(1), 56–73.

Marshall, A., Bell, J., & Moules, N. (2010). Beliefs, suffering, and healing: A clinical practice model for families experiencing mental illness. *Perspectives in Psychiatric Care, 46*(3), 182–196.

McGoldrick, M., Garcia Preto, N., & Carter, B. A. (2016). *The expanding family life cycle: Individual, family and social perspectives* (5th ed.). New York, NY: Pearson.

Mental Health Commission of Canada. (2009). *Toward recovery and well-being: A framework for a mental health strategy for Canada.* Calgary, AB: Author.

Mental Health Commission of Canada. (2012). *Opening Minds program overview.* Retrieved from https://www.mentalhealthcommission.ca/English/initiatives/11874/opening-minds

Mental Health Commission of Canada. (2015). *Recovery guidelines.* Ottawa, ON: Author.

Miklowitz, D., George, E., Richards, J., Simoneau, T., & Suddath R. (2003). A randomized study of family-focused psycho-education and pharmacotherapy in the outpatient management of bipolar disorder. *Archives of General Psychiatry, 60,* 904–912.

Mottaghipour, Y., & Bickerton, A. (2005). The Pyramid of family care: A framework for family involvement with adult mental health services. *Australian e-Journal for the Advancement of Mental Health, 4*(3), 210–217. doi:10.5172/jamh.4.3.210

Mulud, Z. A. (2016). Caregiver burden in mental illness. In J. J. Fitzpatrick & G. M. McCarthy (Eds.), *Nursing concept analysis: Applications to research and practice* (pp. 141–150). New York, NY: Springer Publishing Company LLC.

Pearson, C. (2015, October). *The impact of mental health problems on family members.* Health at a Glance, Statistics Canada 82-624-X. Retrieved from http://www.statcan.gc.ca/pub/82-624-x/2015001/article/14214-eng.htm

Petraksis, M., & Laxton, S. (2017). Intervening early with family members during first-episode psychosis: An evaluation of mental health nursing psychoeducation within an inpatient unit. *Archives of Psychiatric Nursing, 31,* 48–54.

Reinares, M., Bonnin, C. M., Hidalgo-Mazzei, D, Sánchez-Moreno, J., Colm, R., & Vieta, E. (2016). The role of family interventions in bipolar disorder: A systematic review. *Clinical Psychology Review, 43,* 47–57.

Reupert, A., & Mayberry, D. (2016). What do we know about families where parents have a mental illness? A systematic review. *Child & Youth Services, 37*(2), 98–111.

Risling, T., Risling, D., & Holtslander, L. (2017). Creating a social media assessment tool for family nursing. *Journal of Family Nursing, 23*(1), 13–33.

Sinha, M. (2013). *Portrait of caregivers, 2012. Spotlight on Canadians: Results for the General Social Survey.* Statistics Canada. Catalogue no. 89-652-x-No. 001. Retrieved from http://www.statcan.gc.ca/pub/89-652-x/89-652-x2013001-eng.htm

Stamatopoulos, V. (2015). One million and counting: The hidden army of young carers in Canada. *Journal of Youth Studies, 18*(6), 809–822.

Stamatopoulos, V. (2016). Supporting young carers: A qualitative review of young carer services in Canada. *International Journal of Adolescence and Youth, 21*(2), 178–194.

Statistics Canada. (2011). *Fifty years of families in Canada: 1961 to 2011.* Retrieved from http://www12.statcan.gc.ca/census-recensement/2011/as-sa/98-312-x/98-312-x2011003_1-eng.cfm

Stuart, H. L. (2005). *Respite needs of people living with schizophrenia: A national survey of schizophrenia society members.* Toronto, ON: Schizophrenia Society of Canada. Retrieved from http://www.schizophrenia.ca/docs/SSCRespiteReportE.pdf

Sveinbjarnardottir, E., Svararsdottir, E., & Wright, L. (2013). What are the benefits of a short therapeutic conversation intervention with acute psychiatric patients and their families? A controlled before and after study. *International Journal of Nursing Studies, 50*(5), 593–602.

Toohey, M. J., Muralidharan, A., Medoff, D., Lucsted, A., & Dixon, L. (2016). Caregiver positive and negative appraisals. Effects of the National Alliance on Mental Illness Family-to-Family Intervention. *Journal of Nervous and Mental Disease, 204*(2), 156–159.

van der Sanden, R. L. M., Pryor, J. B., Stutterheim, S. E., Kok, G., & Bos, A. E. R. (2016). Stigma by association and family burden among family members of people with mental illness: The mediating role of coping. *Social Psychiatry & Psychiatric Epidemiology, 51,* 1233–1245.

Vermaas, J. D., Green, J., Haley, M., & Haddock, L. (2017) Predicting the mental health literacy of clergy: An informational resource for counselors. *Journal of Mental Health Counseling, 39*(3), 225–241.

Whitehorn, D., Campbell, M. E., Cosgrove, P., Abidi, S., & Tibbo, P. G. (2017). A mindfulness-based support group for families in early psychosis: A pilot qualitative study. *Journal of Mental Health and Addiction Nursing, 1*(1), e30–e34.

Wright, L. M., & Leahey, M. (2013). *Nurses and families: A guide to family assessment and intervention* (6th ed.). Philadelphia, PA: F.A. Davis.

Wrosch, C., Amir, E., & Miller, G. E. (2011). Goal adjustment capabilities, coping, and subjective well being: The sample case of caregiving for a family member with mental illness. *Journal of Personality and Social Psychology, 100*(5), 934–946.

Wendy Austin

LEARNING OBJECTIVES

KEY TERMS

After studying this chapter, you will be able to:

- Identify the relationship between work and mental health.
- Describe a psychologically healthy and safe workplace.
- Explain work–life balance.
- Discuss gender differences in paid work.
- Outline aspects of an inclusive work culture.
- Identify threats to workplace psychological health and safety.
- Define bullying and discuss workplace violence.
- Evaluate a health care environment for healthy workplace attributes.

- accommodation • bullying • burnout • compassion fatigue • hazards • incivility • job attitudes • job strain • risk • role overload • supported employment • underemployed • unemployed • work–life balance • work–life conflict

KEY CONCEPTS

- workplace health • work • workplace violence

The workplace has great potential as a setting in which the health of workers and their families can be protected and promoted. It offers a venue for health education, for workers to access preventive health services, and for links to primary health care (World Health Organization [WHO], 2009). This potential is being addressed globally through the WHO's (2013) *Global Plan of Action on Workers' Health (2008–2017)*, which is aimed at strengthening the links between workplace health, public health, and health systems and at improving working conditions everywhere. These aims, however, are far from being achieved.

Psychological health issues make up the greatest number of disability claims among Canadians; in a survey of human resources and health benefit managers, 83% and 85% of respondents cited mental health conditions as the reason for short- and long-term disability claims, respectively (Towers Watson, 2011). Almost 25% of Canadian workers are affected by mental health problems or disorders that will lead to absence from work, a significant drop in productivity ("presentism"), or job turnover. In Canada, the annual economic loss is estimated at $20 billion (Shain, Arnold, & GermAnn, 2013).

Of particular concern is the health and well-being of the health workforce: the health of everyone depends upon it (WHO, 2006). Nurses in particular are nearly twice as likely as other workers in Canada to be absent due to illness or injury (Berry & Curry, 2012). Nurses need to be able to address workplace health issues so

that better health promotion, prevention, and care are available to all Canadians, and they must recognize that their own health and that of their colleagues play a significant role in doing so. How can safe, compassionate, competent, ethical care be provided by individuals who are unhealthy, fatigued, and burned out? The rationale behind instructing airline passengers to put on their own oxygen masks before helping others can be applied here. Nurses must attend to their own well-being if they are to carry out their practice effectively.

Significant strides have been made in Canada toward improving workplace mental health. We are the first country to create national standards for psychological health and safety in the workplace (CSA Group, 2013). The standards, though voluntary, are a significant achievement, developed from legal and scientific research and through consultation with occupational health and safety experts, industry, unions, professional associations, and government agencies.

This chapter addresses psychological health and safety in the workplace. It considers the relation of work to health and well-being and the attributes of a healthy workplace. Outlined are some ways in which workplaces may support and accommodate individuals at **risk** for, or who have, mental health concerns. Workplace violence, including bullying, is discussed, and health care environments are considered as workplaces, particularly from the perspective of nurses.

■ WORK

Work is the term used to signify our paid employment, the job or task we perform to earn a living. In the lives of most people, however, work in its broadest sense is not restricted to places of employment. Some individuals work entirely within their homes, are not employees of any organization, and do not receive any monetary remuneration for their contribution to family, home, and community life.

Job attitudes, how people think and feel about their job, are important because one's job is important to his or her identity, health, and satisfaction with life (Judge & Kammeyer-Mueller, 2012). Facets of job satisfaction include satisfaction with work, supervision, coworkers, pay, and promotions. Of these, it is satisfaction with the work itself that is key to overall satisfaction (Herzberg, Mausner, & Snyderman, 2009; Judge & Kammeyer-Mueller, 2012). While the quality of workplace environments, particularly potential hazards (i.e., sources of physical and/or psychological harm), must be addressed, the quality of the work itself matters, too.

KEY CONCEPT

Work is "the job, occupation, or task one performs as a means of providing a livelihood" (Venes, 2009, p. 2502).

The Changing Nature of Work

Economic and technologic changes to the workplace, which are aimed at increasing short-term productivity and maximizing profits, continue to shape the nature of contemporary work. These changes include organizational restructuring and downsizing, decreased job stability, the frantic pace of work and life, and decreases in leisure time. The landscape of work continues to be transformed by factors such as the increasing turnover of work to machines and robotic devices, digital technology that allows production to occur anywhere on the globe while managed from a central location, and a decline in the need for middle management that contributes to downsizing (Blustein, 2008). This transformation of the nature of work has direct effects on the work life of Canadians.

One in three Canadians says he or she is a "workaholic" (Statistics Canada, 2007). Comparisons of available statistics, the 1991, 2001, and 2011–2012 National Work-Life Conflict Surveys, reveal that time in work seems to have increased across all job groups (Duxbury & Higgins, 2009, 2012). Whereas 1 in 10 respondents in the 1991 survey worked 50 or more hours per week, in 2001, the number had climbed to 1 in 4. In 2011–2012, the typical employee surveyed spent 50.2 hours per week in work-related activities. As well, it appears that employees find it increasingly difficult to complete their work during regular hours, as over half (54%) complete about 7 hours of supplemental work at home (Duxbury & Higgins, 2012). Unsurprisingly, the survey comparisons reveal that the perceived level of stress and depression among workers remains high while life satisfaction is seriously declining (Duxbury & Higgins, 2012). Nearly one in three Canadians indicates that issues such as financial concerns are distracting them while at work (Ipsos, 2016). Absenteeism increased from 2001 to 2011: 17% more individuals missed work due to ill health; an equivalent increase occurred due to child care challenges, and a 12% increase has been attributed to emotional and mental fatigue (Duxbury & Higgins, 2012). Although work has the potential to be a positive factor in sustaining health and well-being, work, or the lack of it, can have a negative effect on existing health problems and can contribute to the development of new ones.

Unemployment

Most governments identify an individual as **unemployed** when the person does not have paid employment, wants to be employed, and is actively seeking work. This definition, however, does not encompass individuals who are **underemployed**, those with insufficient work relative to hours, skills, income, or status, nor does it include "discouraged workers", those who want to work but have given up seeking it (Dooley, 2003; Dooley & Catalano, 2003). When considering a person's employment status, it may be more useful to consider employment along a continuum rather than as a dichotomous state of employed or unemployed.

Unemployment places individuals at risk for adverse health effects. A meta-analysis of the unemployment literature found that the unemployed had lower psychological and physical well-being than their employed counterparts (McKee-Ryan, Song, Wanberg, & Kinicki, 2005). When individuals have a strong attachment to the labour market or prior workplace, have high "breadwinning" responsibilities, or are disadvantaged in terms of occupational class, wage, or job quality, there is greater likelihood that unemployment will impair their mental health (Backhans & Hemmingsson, 2011). The WHO (2008) identifies the adverse effects of unemployment as including:

- Elevated blood pressure
- Increased depression and anxiety
- Increased visits to general medical practitioners
- Increased symptoms of coronary disease
- Greater stress
- Increased psychological morbidity
- An increase in the number of health problems
- An increase in family problems, particularly financial hardships

Social capital (i.e., social networks and social activities) does not seem to mediate the effect of unemployment on well-being (Winkelmann, 2009). Obtaining permanent employment after being in an unstable employment situation, however, can be health promoting as the probability of psychological symptoms decreases (Reine, Novo, & Hammarström, 2008). The adverse effects of job change go beyond those who have lost jobs. Family members of those who have lost their jobs can experience hardship and stigma (Dooley & Catalano, 2003). Insecurity regarding one's job contributes to a sense of insecurity regarding the future. Sharp and/or sustained rises in unemployment negatively impacts a community's well-being as people lose jobs, acquire debt, and become unable to maintain their lifestyle. When appropriate measures are not in place, such as adequate unemployment benefits, social services, and community support, the level of stress and mental health problems in a community rises (Gunnell, Platt, & Hawton, 2009).

Work and Gender

In industrialized nations, women make up nearly half of the paid workforce but remain underrepresented in decision-making positions (the "glass ceiling" continues to exist) and are paid less than men on the average (WHO, 2011). While gender stereotypes are less influential in determining job and career choices than they once were, males and females continue to be segregated into different types of work. Registered nurses in Canada, for instance, are overwhelmingly female, despite increases in males entering nursing programs ("Surge in numbers of male nursing students," 2012).

Gender segregation in types of work means that exposure to risk—the likelihood that harm may occur plus the severity of that harm (CSA Group, 2013)—differs between genders. For example, in a Statistics Canada survey, nearly one half of male nurses reported being physically assaulted by a patient the previous year, compared with one third of female nurses. It may be that the higher risk of abuse among male nurses involves greater exposure to violent patients and/or that male nurses tend to assume a primary role in responding to patient aggression and are protective of female staff (Shields & Wilkins, 2009). It is of note that work satisfaction for male nurses has been found to be associated with lower levels of experience with workplace aggression (Andrews, Stewart, Morgan, & D'Arcy, 2012).

Responses to workplace **hazards** may also have gender-based variation. Biologically, men and women may be affected differently by such hazards as toxins, due to hormonal differences; psychologically, women report work-related stress more frequently, perhaps due to less power and autonomy or vulnerability to harassment (WHO, 2011). Low control over work environment and conditions, however, has been found to correlate with hypertension in male workers but not in females (Smith, Mustard, Lu, & Glazier, 2013). Biology may shape response to job demands and control, as well.

Until rates of work-related injuries and disease are analyzed by gender, our understanding of its influence on workplace health will be insufficient. The dearth of research related to risks and health issues encountered in unpaid work (e.g., cooking, cleaning, care of family members, tending to the family business) contributed most often by women also leaves an important knowledge gap (WHO, 2011).

■ HEALTHY WORKPLACES

According to the WHO's framework, a healthy workplace exists when workers and managers continually collaborate to address health and safety concerns in the physical and psychosocial work environment, including the organization of work and workplace culture, and attend to health resources in the workplace and the community (Burton, 2010). The healthy workplace is an inclusive work culture: open, accessible, and accepting of workers with diverse backgrounds, demographics, and skills. Disparities between groups of workers or difficulties affecting specific workers (e.g., due to gender, ethnicity, or disability) are minimized or eliminated (Burton, 2010). A survey of over 4,000 Canadians found that 7 in 10 employed individuals considered their workplace to be healthy and their employer supportive of their personal needs (Ipsos Reid, 2007).

KEY CONCEPT

Workplace health is the promotion and maintenance of the health and well-being of workers through policies, programs, and practices that promote safety, minimize risk, and create a positive, responsive, equitable workplace culture and a supportive workplace climate.

The Psychologically Healthy and Safe Workplace

A psychologically healthy and safe workplace is one where workers understand their roles and believe that they can contribute to decisions about how their work is carried out. There is much evidence that both worker well-being and performance are improved when organizations understand the importance of flexible work design and give their employees as much choice and control as possible (Lowe, 2010). The Mental Health Commission of Canada's recognition of the key contribution that healthy workplaces can make toward the well-being of Canadians has informed the development of several resources for employers. The psychosocial factors for a healthy and safe workplace have been identified (see Table 16.1) and free resources to help employers assess and address these factors developed (Samra, Gilbert, Shain, & Bilsker, 2012). Box 16.1 describes research confirming the critical role that psychological health and safety plays across workplaces and occupations. The characteristics of psychologically

Table 16.1 Thirteen Psychosocial Factors in Workplace Health, Safety, and Well-Being

Factor	Objective for the Workplace	Benefits to Employees
1. Psychological support	Coworkers and supervisors provide support and appropriate responses to employees' psychological and mental health concerns.	Improved psychological health Increased productivity Reduced absenteeism and disability Successful and sustainable return to work
2. Organizational culture	An environment characterized by trust, honesty, and fairness	Higher job satisfaction and morale Improved teamwork and productivity Enhanced retention and recruitment Positive image in the community
3. Clear leadership and expectations	Effective leadership and support that help employees know what they need to do, how their work contributes, and whether there are impending changes	Clear expectations for job responsibilities and roles Positive morale and resiliency, particularly in times of stress and change Lessened frustration and conflict Greater trust in the employer
4. Civility and respect	An environment where employees and supervisors are respectful and considerate in their interactions with one another, as well as with clients and the public	Effective teamwork and positive morale Reduced conflict Fewer grievances and lessened legal risk Improved relationships with clients
5. Psychological competencies and requirements	There is a good fit between employees' interpersonal and emotional competencies and the requirements of the position they hold.	Enhanced performance and overall productivity Greater job satisfaction Increased retention of skilled staff Enhanced recruitment success
6. Growth and development	Employees receive encouragement and support in the development of their interpersonal, emotional, and job skills.	Increased employee competency Retention of skilled staff Effective succession planning/internal promotion Enhanced service quality
7. Recognition and reward	Appropriate, fair, and timely acknowledgement and appreciation of employees' efforts	Greater employee satisfaction, motivation, and loyalty Improved teamwork and positive employee morale Increased retention and enhanced recruitment of skilled staff Enhanced employee/labour relations
8. Involvement and influence	Employees are included in discussion about how their work is done and how important decisions are made.	Enhanced performance and productivity Greater employee motivation and job satisfaction Employees actively address challenges at work. Positive employee/labour relations
9. Workload management	Tasks and responsibilities can be accomplished successfully within the time available.	Enhanced performance and productivity Reduced stress and/or burnout Fewer job-related errors, incidents, accidents, and injuries Increased retention
10. Engagement	Employees feel connected to their work and motivated to do their job well.	Enhanced performance and productivity High morale and motivation Enhanced recruitment and increased retention of skilled staff Improved relationships with clients
11. Balance	An environment where there is recognition of the need for balance between the demands of work, family, and personal life	Greater job satisfaction and morale Reduced stress and burnout Enhanced performance and productivity Reduced absenteeism and disability
12. Psychological protection	An environment where employees' psychological safety is ensured	Reduced absenteeism and disability Reduced conflict Fewer job-related errors, incidents, accidents, and injuries Fewer grievances and lessened legal risk
13. Protection of physical safety	Management takes appropriate action to protect the physical safety of employees	Improved physical and psychological health and safety Fewer job-related errors, incidents, accidents, and injuries Reduced absenteeism and disability Improved labour–management relations Reduced legal and regulatory costs

© 2012 by Samra, J., Gilbert, M., Shain, M., & Bilsker, D (2012). Guarding Minds @ Work Organizational Review Worksheets. Vancouver, BC: Centre for Applied Research in Mental Health and Addiction, used with permission.

BOX 16.1 **Research for Best Practice**

EMPLOYERS' PERCEPTIONS AND ATTITUDES TOWARD THE CANADIAN NATIONAL STANDARD ON PSYCHOLOGICAL HEALTH AND SAFETY IN THE WORKPLACE: A QUALITATIVE STUDY

From Kunyk, D., Craig-Broadwith, M., Morris, H., Diaz, R., Reisdorfer, E., & Wang, J. (2016). Employers' perceptions and attitudes toward the Canadian national standard on psychological health and safety in the workplace: A qualitative study. International Journal of Law and Psychiatry, 44, 41–47. doi:10.1016/j.ijlp.2015.08.030

Background: Governments, employers, and other stakeholders are searching for policy solutions to the staggering societal and economic costs of mental illness and psychological injury in the workplace.

Purpose: The purpose of this study was to uncover organizational receptivity to a voluntary, comprehensive standard for dealing with psychological health and safety in the workplace.

Method: We conducted a series of five focus groups with participants from the fields of health care, construction/ utilities, manufacturing industries, business services, and finance. Their positions included management, consulting, human resources, health promotions, health and safety, mediation, and occupational health.

Findings: Our findings confirm and illustrate the critical role that psychological health and safety plays across workplaces and occupations. The standard resonated across the organizations and fit with their values but articulating its added value was challenging.

Implications: There appears to be a need for simplified engagement and implementation strategies of the standard that can be tailored to the nuanced differences between types and sizes of organizations. Those industries in the most need of improving psychological health and safety in the workplace were the least receptive to implementing the standard.

---

unsafe workplaces with increased risks to mental health have similarly been identified (Shain et al., 2013) (see Box 16.2).

The National Standard of Canada for Psychological Health and Safety in the Workplace outlines a systematic framework for employers to use in creating and sustaining healthy, safe workplaces. It includes ways to identify and eliminate environmental hazards and how to assess and control risks associated with hazards that cannot be removed (e.g., inherent job demands and stressors). The standard includes several application annexes with evidence-informed resources including sample implementation models, scenarios, and audit tools (CSA Group, 2013).

Work–Life Balance

A challenge for many people is to balance the demands of their paid employment with other aspects of their lives, such as family and community. Individuals have many roles beyond that of an employee. Nonwork roles, such as educational, cultural, recreational, and volunteer activities, are important to life satisfaction and contribute to the cohesion of a society (Lero, Richardson, & Korabik, 2009). **Work–life balance** is achieved when an individual finds a satisfactory interaction among all the domains of his or her life. This balance will not be the same for everyone but will differ based on personal values, family structure, life situations and expectations, and societal norms.

Work–life conflict occurs when work–life balance is upset, when the demands of work and nonwork roles directly interfere with an individual's ability to meet one or more of the roles. At the beginning of the 21st century, Health Canada funded the National Study on Balancing Work, Family, and Lifestyle from which six reports on work–life conflict in Canada were produced. It was noted that many workplaces operate as if the world of work is separate from the rest of an individual's life. For instance, about 40% of employee respondents stated that it was difficult to arrange their work schedules to meet personal or family commitments; about 75% noted that it was very difficult to be home from work when their children arrived after school; and about 25% either delayed or decided not to start a family or had fewer children because they did not believe that they could balance the demands of work and family (Duxbury & Higgins, 2009).

Heavy job demands (e.g., heavy workload, multiple and/or time-pressured tasks) are a primary antecedent of work–life conflict. In an attempt to meet job demands, workers may stay on the job after regular hours, take work home, or work on days off. These strategies interfere with successful fulfillment of other roles, such as those within the family. Working long hours can keep

---

BOX 16.2 The Psychologically Unsafe Workplace

RISKS TO MENTAL HEALTH IN THE WORKPLACE ARE MORE LIKELY TO OCCUR WHEN

- *Job demands and requirements of effort* consistently and chronically exceed worker skill levels or unreasonably exploit them or where work is distributed inequitably.
- *Job control or influence* is deliberately withheld from workers who lack discretion over the means, manner, and methods of their work (including "voice" or the perceived freedom to express views or feelings appropriate to the situation or context).
- *Reward*, such as praise, recognition, acknowledgement, and credit, is withheld from workers without good business reasons.
- *Fairness* is lacking in that there is consistent failure or refusal to recognize and accommodate the legitimate needs, rights, and claims of workers. Workers feel that decisions are made without attention to due process.
- *Support* with regard to advice, direction, planning, and provision of technical and practical resources and information (to the extent that they are available within the organization) is withheld from workers by choice rather than due to systematic organizational constraints.

Adapted from Shain, M., Arnold, I., & GermAnn, K. (2013). *The road to psychological health and safety: Legal, scientific and social foundations for a national standard for psychological safety in the workplace.* A working paper for the Mental Health Commission of Canada. Retrieved from www.mentalhealthcommission.ca

---

BOX 16.3 Work–Life Conflict Categories

- **Role overload**: The total demands on time and energy associated with the prescribed activities of multiple roles are too great to perform the roles adequately or comfortably.
- **Role interference**:
  - Work-to-family interference: role conflict when work demands and responsibilities hinder one from fulfilling family-role responsibilities
  - Family-to-work interference: role conflict when family demands and responsibilities make it more difficult to fulfill work role
  - Caregiver strain: strain related to the everyday responsibilities of providing necessary care or assistance to someone, such as a family member

Adapted from Higgins, C., Duxbury, L., & Lyons, S. (2008). *Reducing work-life conflict: What works? What doesn't?* Retrieved from Health Canada website: http://www.hc-sc.gc.ca/ewh-semt/pubs/occup-travail/balancing-equilibre/index-eng.php

---

one from attending family celebrations and children's school and sport events; preoccupation with or stress from work can strain family relationships. Family roles and responsibilities, in turn, can interfere with fulfilling one's role at work, as when caring for an ill family member means being absent from the job, or trouble at home impedes work functioning. A Canadian national survey of balancing work, child care, and eldercare among over 25,000 knowledge workers found that caregiver demands affected perceived energy levels, mental health, and productivity in the workplace (Duxbury & Higgins, 2013). Only 29% of males and 25% of females surveyed did not have child or eldercare responsibilities, while 17% and 20%, respectively, had both (Duxbury & Higgins, 2013). **Role overload** occurs when an individual is unable to satisfy role demands. See Box 16.3 for categories of work–life conflict.

Both the number of demands and the control individuals feel over such demands are factors in work–life conflict (Duxbury & Higgins, 2009; Lero et al., 2009). Such work and family conflicts are associated with health issues such as stress, anxiety, depression, sleep disturbances, suppressed immune functioning, poor dietary habits, lack of exercise, hypertension, and medication use, among others (Lero et al., 2009). Many individuals suffering role overload will cut back on sleep hours to try to complete more during the day; over 50% of full-time workers and 70% of evening-shift workers cut back on sleep (Williams, 2008).

The quality and availability of community supports, such as daycare or dependent care, can mitigate pressures on individuals and families, as can flexible working practices, such as varied hours of work, teleworking, opportunity for leave, and "family-friendly" workplaces (Lero et al., 2009; Lowe, 2010). In fact, flexible work design has been identified as the most effective solution for improving employee well-being, particularly when it is conceived in a holistic and systemic way (Lowe, 2010). This means that it encompasses elements related to supervisor and coworker support, job control (having some autonomy over how one's job is done and discretion to make job-related decisions), and job security, with employee assistance programs viewed as complementary (not separate) resources. More critical than formal policies of flexibility are employees' perceptions: if employees know that their supervisors will back them up when they make a decision, they will perceive they have flexibility; if they believe that taking advantage of work–family policies will have negative consequences for their career, they will not use them (Lowe, 2010). The perception of give and take in a workplace matters: workers need to feel they have some influence over their own work lives (Lowe, 2010).

THREATS TO WORKPLACE PSYCHOLOGICAL HEALTH AND SAFETY

Stress

Stress at work does not necessarily have a negative effect on employees; it depends upon the nature, intensity, and duration of the stress and upon the presence of protective factors (e.g., employees feel they have some control regarding their work situation) (Burton, 2010; WHO, 2005). Indications that an individual's stress is work related include awareness that he or she functions without any difficulty outside of the workplace and that stress is experienced when preparing for work or when thinking primarily about workplace issues (see Chapter 17 for a detailed discussion of stress).

When organizations commit to meeting Canada's voluntary national standard of psychological health and safety, they contribute to creating a less stressful workplace for their employees. There are many freely available resources for them to use, including the Comprehensive Workplace Health and Safety program of the Canadian Centre for Occupational Health and Safety, which addresses psychosocial work environment, workplace health promotion, and organizational community involvement (see Web Links). Proactive initiatives are to an organization's advantage: there are huge costs related to absenteeism, presentism, and voluntary employee turnover (Lowe, 2010; Shain et al., 2013).

Burnout

Burnout is a term used to indicate "exhaustion due to chronic job stress" (Venes, 2009, p. 332). It has been conceived further as "a psychological syndrome in response to chronic interpersonal stressors on the job with three dimensions: exhaustion, cynicism and detachment, and lack of a sense of accomplishment" (Maslach, Schaufeli, & Leiter, 2001, p. 399). The individual may initially experience physiologic arousal (e.g., anxiety, high blood pressure, insomnia) and then enter a phase of energy conservation (e.g., tiredness, apathy) leading to exhaustion (e.g., headaches, depression) (Pompili et al., 2006). Burnout has been associated with diseases of the circulatory, musculoskeletal,

and respiratory systems (Toppinen-Tanner, Ojajärvi, Väänänen, Kalimo, & Jäppinen, 2005).

Workplace Violence

Workplace violence encompasses far more than physical assault; it includes any type of intimidation, harassment, or abuse directed against a person in his or her place of employment. It is gaining attention as a serious global health, safety, and organizational problem rooted in broad cultural and socioeconomic factors (Chappell & Di Martino, 2006).

Some workers are at increased risk for violence due to factors related to their work situation. The Canadian Centre for Occupational Health and Safety (2012) has identified heightened workplace risk for employees who:

- Work with the public
- Handle money, valuables, or prescription drugs (e.g., cashiers, pharmacists)
- Carry out inspection or enforcement duties (e.g., government employees)
- Provide service, care, advice, or education (e.g., health care staff, teachers)
- Work in premises where alcohol is served (e.g., food and beverage staff)
- Work in community-based settings (e.g., nurses, social workers, and other home visitors)
- Have a mobile workplace (e.g., taxicab drivers)

KEY CONCEPT

Workplace violence is the intimidation, harassment, abuse, or assault of an individual in his or her place of employment.

Bullying

Bullying has three defining characteristics: it occurs repeatedly; there is intent to do emotional and/or physical harm; and a power difference exists between the victim and the aggressor (Canadian Council on Learning, 2008). Recognizing these is crucial to eliminating bullying. Labelling every conflict or criticism bullying diminishes the latter's seriousness, as does dismissing bullying behaviour as "joking" or "roughhousing." Forms of bullying are found in Table 16.2.

Under Canada's Criminal Code, physical bullying, which includes threats of physical aggression, can constitute assault; physical or cyberstalking can constitute criminal harassment. The police can be called to investigate such incidents by employees as well as employers.

Persons who are targets of bullying can experience a wide range of reactions, including anxiety, fatigue, chest and back pain, high blood pressure, headaches,

Table 16.2	Four Types of Bullying		
Physical	**Relational**	**Verbal**	**"Cyber"**
Threatening violence	Spreading gossip or rumours	Name-calling	Online verbal or relational
Pushing	Withholding job information	Verbal intimidation	bullying
Tripping	Overmonitoring of work	Insulting	Sending false e-mails under
Punching	Excessive or unjustified criticism	Mocking	victim's name
Kicking	Setting unrealistic goals	Attacking personal attributes	Forwarding private e-mails and
Stalking		Attacking private life	pictures
Forcibly confining			Online threats
			Cyberstalking

Adapted from Department of Criminal Justice Canada. (2003). *Stalking is a crime called criminal harassment*. Retrieved from http://canada.justice.gc.ca/eng/pi/fv-vf/pub/har/har.html, Canadian Council on Learning. (2008). *Bullying in Canada: How intimidation affects learning*. Retrieved from http://www.ccl-cca.ca/pdfs/LessonsInLearning/Mar-20-08-Bullying-in-Canad.pdf, and Public Services Health and Safety Association. (2010). *Bullying in the workplace: A handbook for the workplace*. Toronto, ON: Author.

sleep disturbance, recurrent nightmares, concentration difficulties, irritability, depression, and posttraumatic stress (Felblinger, 2008; Public Services Health and Safety Association, 2010). A wide range of psychosocial and professional support is therefore necessary to address bullying's many potentially traumatic effects. Such support needs to evolve. A Canadian qualitative study of men's experiences of surviving bullying at work found that a central concern of participants was a lack of workplace supports for addressing and resolving bullying; as well, some men felt that health care professionals were unwilling or unable to help manage emotional health problems (O'Donnell & MacIntosh, 2016).

Emergencies and Disasters

Traumatic events that constitute an emergency or disaster can affect those involved both physically and emotionally. A traumatic event can be an emergency such as a transportation accident, large chemical spill, nuclear incident, power outage, or terrorist threat, or it can involve a natural disaster such as a disease outbreak, fire, flood, earthquake, or tornado. The workplace can be affected directly by such events, but employees can also bring to the workplace the effect of such events on their personal lives. Health Canada has established a psychosocial emergency preparedness and response team to assist federal employees exposed to traumatic events such as emergencies and natural disasters (Health Canada, 2012). This group of professionals provides training in "resiliency building" for employees and managers, as well as consultation service to deal with the aftermath of a traumatic event.

The workplace may be a good and familiar place for employees to be following a traumatic event, as colleagues can comfort, console, and support one another. Responses to trauma can be planned and enacted together (e.g., holding memorial ceremonies, visiting the injured, attending funerals, setting up a relief fund for families). See Chapter 17 regarding response to trauma events.

▌ MENTAL HEALTH PROBLEMS AND DISORDERS IN THE WORKPLACE

Awareness of the potential for mental health issues among employees is an essential component of a psychologically healthy and safe workplace. It is important to recognize, for instance, that some employees may be more vulnerable than others, in the short or long term, to stress and other work-related threats to mental health. Such vulnerability may be associated with factors such as gender, age, health status, family situation, or life history.

Workplace strategies can be put in place to assist and support specific workers or groups of workers (Burton, 2010; WHO, 2005). Examples include workshops for employees nearing retirement, counselling for those exposed to traumatic events, interventions for those with substance-related problems, and support groups for single parents. Individuals with chronic health problems may require individually accommodated support, such as an adaption of work hours to include rest periods. Strategies can also include educating managers about particular topics (e.g., cross-cultural issues to enable them to assist recently immigrated employees).

While there is rarely a direct link between an individual's work situation and the onset of a mental disorder (except for severe trauma occurring on the job), workplace factors can affect the likelihood of mental health problems and disorders, increase the severity of an existing disorder, or impede treatment and rehabilitation (Samra et al., 2012). The workplace can also play a role in the prevention and early detection of disorders by improving knowledge of mental health problems and disorders within the organization. For instance, in regard to substance use problems, healthier attitudes and beliefs about the use of tobacco and psychoactive substances can be promoted and assistance made available to employees needing to deal with such a problem (Shain et al., 2002). Unfortunately, Canadian survey research ($n = 2,219$) indicates that one third of workers would not tell their managers if they were experiencing a mental health problem, predominately due to a fear of damaging their career. Decreasing this form of barrier to disclosure and the discrimination and stigma associated with it would better enable individuals to get the support they need (Dewa, 2014).

The Mental Health Commission of Canada (MHCC) offers Mental Health First Aid programs in which individuals learn how to recognize the signs and symptoms of a mental health problem or illness and how to find appropriate help (see Web Links). Using such a resource is not unlike employers' and employees' accessing training in first aid for physical injuries and illness. See Table 16.3 for work-related symptoms of common mental disorders.

Addressing mental health is economically worthwhile. It is estimated that the total annual economic cost from mental illness in Canada in 2018 will be nearly 60 billion dollars (Smetanin et al., 2011). Workplace mental health interventions can positively impact productivity, as well as absenteeism and financial outcomes (Wagner et al., 2016).

Accommodation

Employers in Canada are required to provide reasonable **accommodation** to special needs of current or potential employees. While an employer can show that a discriminatory policy or standard is necessary for a particular job (e.g., good vision for ambulance drivers), accommodation is otherwise a requirement under labour laws and human rights acts and prevents discriminatory employment practices. Accommodation involves primarily simple, oftentimes low-cost strategies. Examples of reasonable accommodation for people with mental health problems and disorders include the following (WHO, 2005):

- Changes in communication (e.g., requests put in writing for a clerk who becomes anxious with verbal instructions; positive feedback given, not just criticisms; opportunities for self-appraisal prior to evaluation; planning sessions with a coworker as needed)

- Modifications to the physical environment (e.g., quiet work space provided)
- Job modifications (e.g., opportunities to work at home; hiring an assistant, changing duties)
- Schedule modification (e.g., flexible working hours; rest periods or recuperation time; time allowed for medications or for treatment appointments; opportunity to start part-time work and move to full time)

There is strong research evidence that disability management programs are effective and that accommodating employee needs increases productivity and promotes greater trust between workers and employers (Burton, 2010).

Work and Persons Living With a Mental Disorder

Individuals living with mental disorders want, as others do, self-determination and life satisfaction through work. Work can help achieve relief from poverty, diminish reliance on social assistance, and promote social inclusion. Work can play an important role in recovery from mental illness and is a means to integrate persons with mental disorders back into their community. Nevertheless, finding appropriate employment remains difficult for persons with a mental disorder diagnosis: research has shown that a mental disorder may be a bigger barrier to employment than a physical disability (WISE Employment, 2012). "Unemployed" is the situation for up to 90% of Canadians with serious mental illness, many of whom aspire to be part of the workforce. This situation is sustained by barriers such as stigma and discrimination, income security policies that penalize earned income, and lack of support for getting and holding a job (Mental Health Commission of Canada [MHCC], 2013).

Supported employment (SE) is an approach to assisting people with disabilities, such as severe mental illness, in finding appropriate work and supporting them once employed through the services of trained professionals. The Aspiring Workforce research project, sponsored by

Table 16.3 Work-Related Symptoms of Common Mental Disorders		
Depression	**Anxiety Disorders**	**Burnout**
• Trouble concentrating	• Feeling apprehensive and tense	• Becoming cynical, sarcastic, and critical at work
• Trouble remembering	• Difficulty managing daily tasks	• Difficulty coming to work and getting started once at work
• Trouble making decisions	• Difficulty concentrating	• More irritable and less patient with coworkers, clients, customers
• Impairment of performance at work		
• Sleep problems		• Lack of energy to be consistently productive at work
• Loss of interest in work		
• Withdrawal: family, friends, and coworkers		• Tendency to self-medicate with alcohol or drugs
• Feeling pessimistic and hopeless		
• Feeling slowed down		
• Fatigue		

From Burton, J. (2010). *WHO healthy workplace framework and model: Background and supporting literature and practices*. Geneva, Switzerland: World Health Organization.

the MHCC and led by researchers from the Centre for Mental Health and Addiction, University of Toronto and Queen's University, identified existing and innovative practices in SE, which can help those with serious mental illness to achieve meaningful employment and income (MHCC, 2013). Through the means of literature reviews, client interviews, and service provider surveys, key insights and recommendations were evolved. These include that jobs should be matched to the client's interests and goals, that family and peer support must be part of the service, and that vocational, social skills, and cognitive training for clients should be provided as needed. Job accommodation needs to be addressed with clients and employers, and ongoing evaluation/support of their adaptation to one another should occur. Further, it is recommended that employment services be integrated with mental health services (MHCC). The reports of the Aspiring Workforce project are an important resource toward accessing the many capabilities of Canadians who live with a mental disorder and supporting their aspirations for employment.

NURSES AND WORKPLACE PSYCHOLOGICAL HEALTH AND SAFETY

The education, recruitment, and retention of workers in the health sector are a pressing global concern

(WHO, 2006). Nurses are the largest component of the health care workforce. They work across a wide range of settings, primarily on shift-work schedules, engaging with patients and families and all other members of the health care workforce (Kerr & Mustard, 2007). Nurses' health is a barometer of workplace health in the health sector. See Table 16.4 for recommendations for the workplace health, safety, and well-being of the nurse.

Nurses, Job Strain, and Burnout

The first Canadian National Survey of the Work and Health of Nurses revealed that psychosocial and interpersonal factors (e.g., work stress, low autonomy, and lack of respect) are more closely associated with health problems among nurses who work overtime (Statistics Canada, 2006). In this survey of approximately 19,000 regulated nurses, nearly one third had high **job strain**, defined as what happens when the psychological demands of a job exceed the worker's discretion of how to enact it. Many nurses (45% of female nurses and 51% of male nurses) believed they had only low support from coworkers. This percentage compared unfavourably with employed Canadians in general, of whom approximately 33% described low support. About 20% of nurses indicated that in the previous month, their mental health had made handling their workload difficult. Although **burnout** is usually considered as "long-term

Table 16.4	Recommendations for Workplace Health, Safety, and Well-Being of the Nurse
Organization practice recommendations	Organizations/nursing employers create and design environments and systems that promote safe and healthy workplaces, including strategies.
	Creating a culture, climate, and practices that support, promote, and maintain staff health, safety, and well-being
	Ensuring that the organization's annual budget includes adequate resources (human and fiscal) to implement and evaluate health and safety initiatives
	Establishing organizational practices that foster mutual responsibility and accountability by individual nurses and organizational leaders to ensure a safe work environment
	Being aware of the impact of organizational changes (such as restructuring and downsizing) on the health, safety, and well-being of nurses and be responsible and accountable for implementing appropriate supportive measures
	Implementing and maintaining education and training programs aimed at increasing awareness of health and safety issues for nurses (e.g., safe-lift initiative, employee rights, hazard awareness, etc.)
	Integrating health and safety best practices across all sectors of the health care system
Research recommendations	Researchers actively collaborate with health care partners to demonstrate the effectiveness of interventions aimed at improving nurse health, safety, and well-being using rigorous research and evaluation methodologies.
	Researchers make full use of existing databases on nurse health, including the National Survey on the Work and Health of Nurses, in order to improve understanding of the key factors contributing to healthy work environments for nurses and to develop and test best practice indicators.
Education recommendations	Nursing education institutions model the integration of health, safety, and well-being into their own workplace culture.
	Nursing education institutions incorporate information about the health, safety, and well-being of the nurse into the core curriculum of nursing education programs.
System recommendations	Governing/accreditation bodies incorporate the Organization Practice Recommendations from this Healthy Work Environments Best Practice Guideline in their quality health and safety standards for health care service and education organizations.

Source: Registered Nurses' Association of Ontario. (2008). *Workplace health, safety and well-being of the nurse.* Toronto, ON: Registered Nurses' Association of Ontario.

exposure to a work situation that is beyond the person's capacity to cope" (WHO, 2005, p. 18), newly graduated nurses in a Quebec study reported a high level of psychological distress (43%), and a majority (62%) stated that they planned to quit their current position and seek another job in nursing; some (13%) intended to quit nursing itself (Lavoie-Tremblay et al., 2008).

Another Canadian study found that nurses' burnout and mental health problems did not arise from empathic engagement with patients but rather from the way their work was organized, so that nurses found their sense of identity, self-esteem, and worth to be compromised (Alderson, 2008). The researcher pointed to problems with an organizational paradigm in which nurses' work is framed from an industrial perspective of productivity. Nurses find meaning in their work in their relationships with patients and families; these relationships "reinforce their identity and preserve their mental health" (p. 171).

Burnout is a serious threat to the quality of health care. Its effects reach far beyond the impact on an individual, harming the entire health care system as care standards are not met. For instance, researchers found that when burnout was reduced by 30%, there were 6,239 fewer nosocomial infections, with cost savings in the millions (Cimiotti, Aiken, Sloane, & Wu, 2012).

Nurses' Fatigue

In a survey study of 6,312 Canadian nurses, fatigue was identified as a major negative influence on safe practice. Organizational factors cited as preventing nurses from responding to their fatigue included workload, professional responsibility to be there for patients, feelings of not wanting to let down their colleagues, and the culture of doing more with less. Causes of fatigue reported by the nurses were workload, shift work, patient acuity, lack of time for professional development and mentoring, a decline in organizational leadership and decision-making processes, and inadequate time for "recovery" during and following work shifts (Canadian Nurses Association and Registered Nurses' Association of Ontario, 2010). That nurses' fatigue seriously affects safe practice is further evident in the finding that medication errors were positively associated with nurses working overtime on a regular basis, role overload, perceived staffing or resource inadequacy, as well as with low coworker support and low job security (Wilkins & Shields, 2008).

Compassion Fatigue

Compassion fatigue is the term used by caregiving professionals when they experience weariness, numbing of feelings like empathy, and relational disengagement from patients. Although it can appear as burnout, compassion fatigue seems to be rooted in prolonged exposure to others' suffering, coupled with one's own empathic responses. A review of the research literature suggests that the risk of compassion fatigue is increased by factors such as burnout and stress, heightened emotions of patients' families, the inability of the caregiver to maintain self-care, lack of social support, uncontrolled work stressors, lack of defined boundaries, degree of traumatic exposure, and lack of experience (Austin et al., 2013). In a qualitative study of registered nurses and registered psychiatric nurses with compassion fatigue, nurses described feelings of disconnection and disengagement from patients: "I couldn't give or open myself up to interact with the patients and their families ... You're going through the motions but there is some disconnection ... [you're] not really feeling their suffering." (Austin, Goble, Leier, & Byrne, 2009, p. 204). The nurses tried to overcome compassion fatigue by changing their practice area and schedule and by seeking out new knowledge, but they noted that changes to the health care system that improved support for compassionate caregiving were needed. The health care workplace has a role in preventing compassion fatigue. An overview of management strategies in a study by Lachman (2016) included recognition of the reality of compassion fatigue and its signs and symptoms, a workplace culture that supports dialogue and debriefing, stress-coping skills, and leaders supportive of a culture of caring.

Violence in the Health Care Workplace

Health care practitioners are at particularly high risk of workplace violence, and nurses are most at risk (Shields & Wilkins, 2009). Statistics Canada has reported that in the course of 1 year of providing direct care in hospitals or long-term care facilities, 34% of nurses were physically assaulted and 47% were emotionally abused by their patients (Shields & Wilkins, 2009). Factors identified by nurses who experienced abuse included being male, being relatively experienced, usually working noonday shifts, inadequate staffing and resources, poor nurse–physician relationships, and lack of support from coworkers and supervisors. Although many of these factors can be modified, nurses indicate that there is a culture of silence around incidents of violence, and many incidents go undocumented. The negative outcomes for nurses who experience abuse in the workplace include anger, fear, depression, anxiety, sleep disruption, increased sick leave, symptoms of posttraumatic stress disorder, and job dissatisfaction (Shields & Wilkins, 2009).

Standard IV of the Canadian Federation of Mental Health Nurses (CFMHN) practice standards—effectively manages rapidly changing situations—requires the psychiatric–mental health nurse to utilize safety measures to protect client, self, and colleagues from potentially abusive situations in the work environment (CFMHN, 2014) (see Chapter 5). The place to start is the identification of sources of violence, so discussion can begin and strategies be adopted for its prevention. Strategies may be as simple as providing timely information to patients and their friends and family, as this effectively lessens the risk of assault in health care settings, particularly in cases involving distress and long waiting periods (Chappell & Di Martino, 2006). Assigning tasks based on competencies and experience can also reduce contributing factors. Organizational pressures should be addressed. For example, appropriate staffing levels and shift lengths can reduce stress and avert aggression among staff and between workers and the public. Debriefing with those involved in the incident is helpful; counselling by qualified staff or outside specialists may be necessary in more serious cases.

Perhaps, the most essential approach to reducing violence in health care settings, however, is to ensure that everyday practice is grounded in courtesy, decency, and civility (Hesketh et al., 2003). Acceptable behaviours may require definition, systemic recognition, and support, while incivil behaviour should be confronted and addressed in a professional manner. **Incivility** is disrespectful speech or behaviour that involves such behaviour as making jokes at another persons' expense, interrupting or speaking over them, ignoring them or giving them the "silent treatment," or ignoring their input or opinions (Matthews & Ritter, 2016). In a survey study of approximately 1,000 new graduate nurses in Canada, it was found that civility norms (i.e., informal expectations of mutually respectful behaviour) were key to decreasing coworker incivility and to preventing early career burnout of the nurses (Laschinger & Read, 2016).

🍁 SUMMARY OF KEY POINTS

- Work influences self-identity, provides income, and plays a significant role in an individual's health and well-being. Unemployment and underemployment can cause psychological distress and negatively affect an individual's mental health. There are also adverse effects related to job change that go beyond those who have lost jobs.
- The nature of work has been changing across the globe due to economic and technologic developments; these changes are affecting the mental health of workers.
- Achieving work–life balance can be difficult. Work–life conflict occurs when one role interferes with meeting the demands of another.
- Gender differences continue to influence the situation of paid workers.
- Nurses need to understand the psychosocial factors that contribute to a healthy and inclusive workplace and the need for flexibility in sustaining a healthy workplace and for accommodating employees with mental health and/or other chronic health problems.

- The Mental Health First Aid and Working Mind programs of the MHCC are educational means of increasing literacy in mental health and decreasing stigma and discrimination.
- Work can help persons with mental disorders in their recovery and in the improvement of their well-being. The Supportive Employment approach facilitates acquiring and maintaining employment for persons with severe mental disorders.
- Bullying (physical, relational, verbal, and "cyber") involves repeated, intended harm to a person with less power than the aggressor.
- Nurses need to overcome a culture of silence related to workplace violence in health care settings.

 Web Links

www.cmha.ca The Canadian Mental Health Association provides information about their work in workplace mental health, including the employment of persons with mental health problems.

guardingmindsatwork.ca/info/index An excellent comprehensive and research-based resource for the promotion of psychological health and safety in the workplace, developed by the Centre for Applied Research in Mental Health and Addiction (CARMHA).

ccohs.ca The Canadian Centre for Occupational Health and Safety offers free resources including podcasts (also at iTunes) such as "Breaking the cycle of workplace bullying" and "Exploring psychosocial issues in the workplace."

www.hc-sc.gc.ca/ewh-semt/index-eng.php Health Canada provides many resources on workplace mental health, such as six reports on work–life conflict from the 2001 National Study on Balancing Work and Family.

mentalhealthfirstaid.ca Information about the mental health first aid programs can be found here.

www.mentalhealthcommission.ca/English/initiatives/11893/working-mind Details about the MHCC's educational program for managers and employees, The Working Mind, is at this site.

References

Alderson, M. (2008). Work structure in the chronic care setting: Possible consequences for nurses' mental health. *Canadian Journal of Nursing Research, 40*(3), 160–178.

Andrews, M. E., Stewart, N. J., Morgan, D. G., & D'Arcy, C. (2012). More alike than different: A comparison of male and female RNs in rural and remote Canada. *Journal of Nursing Management, 20*(4), 561–570.

Austin, W., Brintnell, S., Goble, E., Kagan, L., Kreitzer, L., Larsen, D., & Leier, B. (2013). *Lying down in the ever-falling snow: Canadian health professionals' experience of compassion fatigue.* Waterloo, ON: Wilfrid Laurier University Press.

Austin, W., Goble, E., Leier, B., & Byrne, P. (2009). Compassion fatigue: The experience of nurses. *Ethics and Social Welfare, 3*(2), 195–214.

Backhans, M., & Hemmingsson, T. (2011). Unemployment and mental health—Who is (not) affected? *European Journal of Public Health, 22*(3), 429–433.

Berry, L., & Curry, P. (2012). *Nursing workload and patient care.* Ottawa, ON: Canadian Federation of Nurses Unions.

Blustein, D. (2008). *The psychology of working: A new perspective for career development, counseling, and public policy.* Mahwah, NJ: Lawrence Erlbaum Associates Inc.

Burton, J. (2010). *WHO healthy workplace framework and model: Background and supporting literature and practices.* Geneva, Switzerland: World Health Organization.

Canadian Centre for Occupational Health and Safety. (2012). *Workplace violence*. Retrieved from http://www.ccohs.ca/oshanswers/psychosocial/violence.html

Canadian Council on Learning. (2008). *Bullying in Canada: How intimidation affects learning*. Retrieved from http://www.ccl-cca.ca/pdfs/LessonsInLearning/Mar-20-08-Bullying-in-Canad.pdf

Canadian Federation of Mental Health Nurses (CFMHN). (2014). *Canadian standards of psychiatric-mental health nursing* (4th ed.). Toronto, ON: Author.

Canadian Nurses Association and Registered Nurses' Association of Ontario. (2010). *Nurse fatigue and patient safety: Research report*. Retrieved from http://www2.cna-aiic.ca/cna/practice/safety/full_report_e/files/fatigue_safety_2010_report_e.pdf

Chappell, D., & Di Martino, V., (Eds.) (2006). *Violence at work* (3rd ed.). Geneva, Switzerland: International Labour Organization.

Cimiotti, J. P., Aiken, L. H., Sloane, D. M., & Wu, E. S. (2012). Nurse staffing, burnout, and health care-associated infection. *American Journal of Infection Control, 40*(6), 486–490.

CSA Group. (2013). *National Standard of Canada, CAN/CSA-Z1003-13/BNQ 9700-803/2013: Psychological health and safety in the workplace—Prevention, promotion, and guidance to staged implementation*. Retrieved from http://shop.csa.ca/en/canada/occupational-health-and-safety-management/cancsa-z1003-13bnq-9700-803201 3/invt/z10032013

Department of Criminal Justice Canada. (2003). *Stalking is a crime called criminal harassment*. Retrieved from http://canada.justice.gc.ca/eng/pi/fv-vf/pub/har/har.html

Dewa, C. S. (2014). Worker attitudes towards mental health problems and disclosure. *International Journal of Occupational and Environmental Medicine, 5*(15), 175–186.

Dooley, D. (2003). Unemployment, underemployment, and mental health: Conceptualizing employment status as a continuum. *American Journal of Community Psychology, 32*(1/2), 9–20.

Dooley, D., & Catalano, R. (2003). Introduction to underemployment and its social costs. *American Journal of Community Psychology, 32*(1/2), 1–7.

Duxbury, L., & Higgins, C. (2009). *Work-life conflict in Canada in the new millennium: Key findings and recommendations from the 2001 National Work-Life Conflict Study*. Ottawa, ON: Public Health Agency of Canada.

Duxbury, L., & Higgins, C. (2012). *Revisiting work-life issues in Canada: The 2012 National Study on Balancing Work and Caregiving in Canada*. Retrieved from http://newsroom.carleton.ca/wp-content/files/2012-National-Work-Long-Summary.pdf

Duxbury, L., & Higgins, C., in partnership with Desjardins Insurance. (2013). *Conclusions and implications: Balancing work, childcare and eldercare: A view from the trenches*. Retrieved from: https://sprott.carleton.ca/wp-content/files/Duxbury-BalancingWorkChildcareEldercare-ENG.pdf

Felblinger, D. M. (2008). Incivility and bullying in the workplace and nurses' shame responses. *Journal of Obstetric, Gynecologic, and Neonatal Nursing, 37*(2), 234–241.

Gunnell, D., Platt, S., & Hawton, K. (2009). Editorial: The economic crisis and suicide: Consequences may be serious and warrant early attention. *British Medical Journal, 338*, 1456–1457.

Health Canada. (2012). *Psychosocial emergency preparedness and response*. Retrieved from http://www.hc-sc.gc.ca/ewh-semt/occup-travail/empl/psychosoc-eng.php

Herzberg, F., Mausner, B., & Bloch Snyderman, B. (2009). *The motivation to work*. Piscataway, NJ: Transaction Publishers.

Hesketh, K. L., Duncan, S. M., Estabrooks, C. A., Reimer, M. A., Giovanetti, P., Hyndman, K., & Acorn, S. (2003). Workplace violence in Alberta and British Columbia hospitals. *Health Policy, 63*, 311–321.

Higgins, C., Duxbury, L., & Lyons, S. (2008). *Reducing work-life conflict: What works? What doesn't?* Retrieved from Health Canada website: http://www.hc-sc.gc.ca/ewh-semt/pubs/occup-travail/balancing-equilibre/index-eng.php

Ipsos. (2016). *Nearly one in three (29%) Canadians are distracted at work due issues related to financial concern*. Retrieved from http://ipsos-na.com/news-polls/pressrelease.aspx?id=7499

Ipsos Reid. (2007). *Mental health in the workplace: Largest study ever conducted of Canadian workplace mental health and depression. Public release*. Retrieved from http://www.mentalhealthroundtable.ca/dec_07/Ipsos%20Reid%20Nov%202007%20MentalHealthReport.pdf

Judge, T. A., & Kammeyer-Mueller, J. D. (2012). Job attitudes. *Annual Review of Psychology, 63*, 341–367.

Kerr, M., & Mustard, C. (2007). The challenge of effective workplace change in the health sector. *Healthcare Papers, 7*(Sp), 69–73.

Kunyk, D., Craig-Broadwith, M., Morris, H., Diaz, R., Reisdorfer, E., & Wang, J. (2016). Employers' perceptions and attitudes toward the Canadian national standard on psychological health and safety in the workplace: A qualitative study. *International Journal of Law and Psychiatry, 44*, 41–47. doi:10.1016/j.ijlp.2015.08.030

Lachman, V. D. (2016). Compassion fatigue as a threat to ethical practice: Identification, personal and workplace prevention/management strategies. *MedSurgNursing, 25*(4), 275–278.

Laschinger, H. K. S., & Read, E. A. (2016). The effect of authentic leadership, person-job fit, and civility norms on new graduate nurses: Experiences of coworker incivility and burnout. *Journal of Nursing Administration, 46*(11), 574–580.

Lavoie-Tremblay, M., Wright, D., Desforges, N., Gélinas, C., Marchionni, C., & Drevniok, U. (2008). Creating a healthy workplace for new-generation nurses. *Journal of Nursing Scholarship, 40*(3), 290–297.

Lero, D., Richardson, J., & Korabik, K. (2009). *Cost-benefit review of work-life balance practices—2009*. Gatineau, QC: Canadian Association of Administrators of Labour Legislation.

Lowe, G. (2010). *Creating sustainable organizations: How flexible work improves wellbeing and performance*. Retrieved from http://www.grahamlowe.ca/documents/258/

Maslach, C., Schaufeli, W. B., & Leiter, M. P. (2001). Job burnout. *Annual Review of Psychology, 52*, 397–422.

Matthews, R. A., & Ritter, K.-J. (2016). A concise, content valid, gender invariant measure of workplace incivility. *Journal of Occupational Health Psychology, 21*(3), 352–365.

McKee-Ryan, F. M., Song, Z., Wanberg, C. R., & Kinicki, A. J. (2005). Psychological and physical well-being during unemployment: A meta-analytic study. *Journal of Applied Psychology, 90*(1), 53–76.

Mental Health Commission of Canada. (2013). *The aspiring workforce: Employment and income for people with serious mental illness*. Retrieved from http://www.mentalhealthcommission.ca/sites/default/files/2016-06/Workplace_MHCC_Aspiring_Workforce_Report_ENG_0.pdf

O'Donnell, S. M., & MacIntosh, J. A. (2016). Gender and workplace bullying: Men's experience of surviving bullying at work. *Qualitative Health Research, 26*(3), 351–366.

Pompili, M., Rinaldi, G., Lester, D., Girardi, P., Ruberto, A., & Taterelli, R. (2006). Hopelessness and suicide risk emerge in psychiatric nurses suffering from burnout and using specific defence mechanisms. *Archives of Psychiatric Nursing, 20*(3), 135–143.

Public Services Health and Safety Association. (2010). *Bullying in the workplace: A handbook for the workplace*. Toronto, ON: Author.

Registered Nurses' Association of Ontario. (2008). *Workplace health, safety and well-being of the nurse*. Toronto, ON: Author.

Reine, I., Novo, M., & Hammarström, A. (2008). Does transition from an unstable labour market position to permanent employment protect mental health? Results from a 14-year follow-up of school-leavers. *BMC Public Health, 8*. Retrieved from http://www.biomedcentral.com/1471-2458/8/159

Samra, J., Gilbert, M., Shain, M., & Bilsker, D. (2012). *GuardingMinds@Work*. Vancouver, BC: Centre for Applied Research in Mental Health and Addiction (CARMHA). Retrieved from http://www.guardingmindsatwork.ca

Shain, M., Arnold, I., & GermAnn, K. (2013). *The road to psychological health and safety: Legal, scientific and social foundations for a national standard for psychological safety in the workplace*. A working paper for the Mental Health Commission of Canada. Retrieved from www.mentalhealthcommission.ca

Shain, M., Bender, A., Brenneman Gibson, J., Gnam, W., Siu, M., & Suuvali, H. (2002). *Mental health and substance use at work: Perspectives from research and implications for leaders*. A background paper prepared by the Scientific Advisory Committee to the Global Business and Economic Roundtable on Addiction and Mental Health. Retrieved from http://www.mentalhealthroundtable.ca/documents.html

Shields, M., & Wilkins, K. (2009). *Factors related to on-the-job abuse of nurses by patients*. Retrieved from Statistics Canada website: http://www.statcan.gc.ca/pub/82-003-x/2009002/article/10835-eng.htm

Smetanin, P., Stiff, D., Briante, C., Adair, C. E., Ahmad, S., & Khan, M. (2011). *The life and economic impact of major mental illnesses in Canada: 2011 to 2041*. RiskAnalytica, on behalf of the Mental Health Commission of Canada. Retrieved from www.mentalhealthcommission.ca

Smith, P., Mustard, C., Lu, H., & Glazier R. (2013). Comparing the risk associated with psychosocial work conditions and health behaviours on incident hypertension over a nine-year period in Ontario, Canada. *Canadian Journal of Public Health, 104*(1), e82–e86.

Statistics Canada. (2006). National survey of the work and health of nurses. *The Daily*. Retrieved from http://www23.statcan.gc.ca/imdb/p2SV.pl?Function=getSurvey&SDDS=5080&Item_Id=13648&lang=en

Statistics Canada. (2007). Workaholics and time perception. The Daily. Retrieved from http://www.statcan.gc.ca/daily-quotidien/070515/dq070515c-eng.htm

"Surge in numbers of male nursing students". (2012). *Canadian Nurse*. Retrieved from http://www.canadian-nurse.com/index.php?option=com_content&view=article&id=597%3Asurge-in-numbers-of-male-nursing-students&catid=4%3Aperspectives&Itemid=39&lang=en

Toppinen-Tanner, S., Ojajärvi, A., Väänänen, A., Kalimo, R., & Jäppinen, P. (2005). Burnout as a predictor of medically certified sick-leave absences and their diagnosed causes. *Behavioral Medicine, 31,* 18–27.

Towers Watson. (2011). Towers Watson study: Investing in workforce health generates higher productivity. Financial Post [Online]. Retrieved from www.financialpost.com

Venes, D. (Ed.) (2009). *Taber's cyclopedic medical dictionary* (21st ed.). Philadelphia, PA: F.A. Davis Company.

Wagner, S. L., Koehn, C., White, M. I., Harder, H. G., Schultz, I. Z., & Williams-Whitt, K. (2016). Mental health intervention in the workplace and work outcomes: A best-evidence synthesis of systematic reviews. *International Journal of Occupational and Environmental Medicine, 7*(1), 1–14.

Wilkins, K., & Shields, M. (2008). Correlates of medication error in hospitals. *Health Reports, 19*(2), Statistics Canada catalogue 82–003.

Williams, C. (2008). Work-life balance of shift workers. Retrieved from Statistics Canada website: http://www.statcan.gc.ca/pub/75-001-x/2008108/pdf/10677-eng.pdf

Winkelmann, R. (2009). Unemployment, social capital, and subjective well-being. *Journal of Happiness Studies, 10*(4), 421–430.

WISE Employment. (2012). SMEs attitudes to employing people who have a mental illness. Retrieved from http://www.wiseemployment.com.au/uploads/publications/Empowermental-McNair_Research.pdf

World Health Organization. (2005). *Mental health policies and programmes in the workplace.* Geneva, Switzerland: Author.

World Health Organization. (2006). *World Health Report 2006: Working together for health.* Geneva, Switzerland: Author.

World Health Organization. (2008). *World Health Report 2008: Primary health care: Now more than ever.* Geneva, Switzerland: Author.

World Health Organization. (2009). Occupational health. Retrieved from http://www.who.int/occupational_health/en/index.html

World Health Organization. (2011). Gender, work and health. Retrieved from http://whqlibdoc.who.int/publications/2011/9789241501729_eng.pdf

World Health Organization. (2013). WHO Global plan of action on worker's health (2008–2017): Baseline for implementation. Retrieved from http://www.who.int/occupational_health/who_workers_health_web.pdf

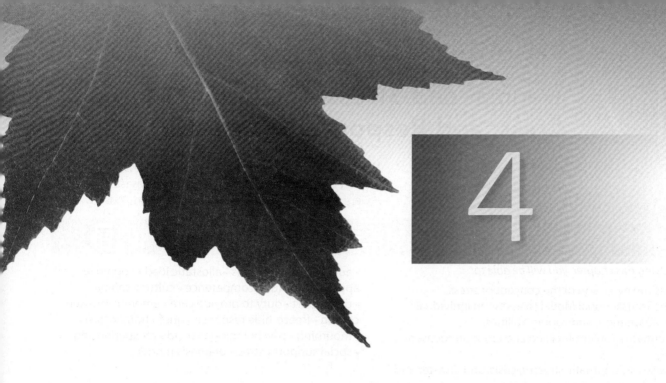

4

Challenges
to Mental
Health

17 Trauma- and Stressor-Related Disorders, Crisis, and Response to Disaster

Amy Bombay and
Wendy Austin

Adapted from the chapter "Trauma- and Stressor-Related Disorders, Crisis, and Response to Disaster" by Gerri Lasiuk, Kathleen Hegadoren, and Wendy Austin

LEARNING OBJECTIVES

After studying this chapter, you will be able to:

- Discuss the evolution of the concept of stress.
- Use the Transactional Model to assess an individual's stress, adaptation, and coping abilities.
- Differentiate problem-focused and emotion-focused coping.
- Define stress, traumatic stressor, crisis, and disaster and describe human responses to these.
- Define intergenerational trauma, collective trauma, and historical trauma and describe human responses to these.
- Understand the importance of trauma-informed care and differentiate between cultural competence, cultural humility, and cultural safety.
- Explain nursing assessment and interventions of trauma- and stressor-related disorders.
- Identify adaptive and maladaptive responses to disaster and indicators that a survivor may require psychiatric services.

KEY TERMS

- adaptation • allostasis • allostatic load • cognitive appraisal • cultural competence • cultural safety • dissupport • duty to provide care • emotion-focused coping • freeze-hide response • grief • homeostasis • mourning • psychological first aid • reexperiencing • social support • stress–diathesis model

KEY CONCEPTS

- collective trauma • coping • crisis • disaster • historical trauma • stress • trauma-informed care • traumatic stressor

Although stress has been the focus of considerable scientific, clinical, and general interest, most of us would be hard-pressed to explain what it is. As Selye (1980) quipped, "stress, like relativity, is a scientific concept which has suffered the mixed blessing of being too well known, and too little understood" (p. 127). Increasing acknowledgement of the pervasiveness of stressor and trauma experiences has resulted in increasing emphasis on the importance of providing clients with safe and supportive inpatient and care environments that can better serve people who are living with stress and/or who have had traumatic experiences (Harris & Fallot, 2001; Raja, Hasnain, Hoersch, Gove-Yin, & Rajagopalan, 2015). In this chapter, the concepts of stress, trauma, crisis, and disaster are described and the way that nurses can identify and address the needs of individuals experiencing these events are explained. The system level need for trauma-informed care is addressed.

■ STRESS

The Evolution of the Concept of Stress

The word stress comes from the Latin word *stringere*, meaning to draw tight (Cooper & Dewe, 2004), and the Middle English word *stresse*, which refers to hardship or distress (Harper, 2001). Throughout the 18th and 19th centuries, the word "stress" was used to denote *force*, *pressure*, or *strain*, which explains why the word "stress" was used almost exclusively by engineers before the beginning of the 20th century.

The early decades of the 20th century saw the rise of *psychosomatic medicine* and a shift away from the prevailing view of the body as a machine (Cooper & Dewe, 2004). Proponents of psychosomatic medicine believed that a mechanistic model was reductionistic and could not explain the role of the mind and spirit in health and illness. It was in this context that the concept of stress as hardship was taken up by biologic and social scientists as a possible explanation of disease and illness (Bartlett, 1998). Throughout the last century, our understanding of stress evolved through three distinct periods in which it was conceptualized as a physiologic response, as a stimulus, and, finally, as a transaction.

Stress as a Physiologic Response

Walter Cannon and Hans Selye, two pioneers in the study of stress, both conceptualized stress as a response to changing environmental conditions. Cannon (1939), a noted Harvard physiologist, is considered by many to be the father of modern stress research. In his book *The Wisdom of the Body*, he coined the term **homeostasis** to describe the body's ability to maintain a stable internal environment despite changing environmental conditions. Cannon's thesis was that environmental changes are perceived as threats to personal integrity or safety and signal a compensatory response mediated by the sympathetic branch of the autonomic nervous system (ANS). He also believed that strong emotions like fear and anger are fundamental to the stress response and have evolved because of their high survival value. "Fear," he wrote, "has become associated with the instinct to run, to escape; and anger or aggressive feeling, with the instinct to attack" (p. 227). This notion, later dubbed the *fight or flight* response, remains a key concept in discussions of stress.

Working at McGill University in Montreal, Selye (1956, 1974) developed his general **adaptation** syndrome theory. In this, Selye differentiated stress (a nonspecific response of the body to any demand placed on it) from stressors (events that initiate the response) and argued that stressors can be physical (e.g., infection, intense heat or cold, surgery, debilitating illnesses), psychological (e.g., psychological trauma, interpersonal problems), or social (e.g., lack of social support). Stressors can also be short term (acute) or long term (chronic).

According to Selye, the perception of a stressor triggers an automatic, total-body response. The first stage of this response is the *alarm reaction*, during which virtually all body systems (e.g., sense organs, brain, heart and blood vessels, lungs, digestive system, immune system) respond in a coordinated effort to mediate the stressor. If this effort is successful, the body returns to its normal state. If it is not successful and the stressor remains present for hours or days, the organism moves into the *stage of resistance*, and efforts to adapt continue. In circumstances in which the stressor becomes chronic or is extreme, the body moves into the *stage of exhaustion*, during which the individual's resources deplete, and exhaustion and death ensue.

Although Selye made significant contributions to our understanding of human stress, he was criticized for his notion that stress is a nonspecific response to diverse environmental stimuli. Selye's challengers (e.g., Mason, 1971; Mikhail, 1981) pointed out that many neuroendocrine responses are not general at all but very specific. Selye's critics argued that all stressors do not necessarily produce the same response in every individual, and what is a stressor for one person may not be a stressor for another (Lazarus & Folkman, 1984). The conceptualization of stress solely as a response was also challenged for its circular reasoning (i.e., an event is stressful because it elicits a stress response).

Stress as a Stimulus

Before the 1960s, the study of stress was a physiologic concept. By the middle of the last century, the disciplines of psychology and psychiatry were on the rise, and researchers and clinicians became interested in the psychological and emotional aspects of stress. With this came the notion that life changes or events were the stimuli (i.e., stressors) that evoked the stress response (e.g., Dohrenwend & Dohrenwend, 1974; Holmes & Rahe, 1967). Within this perspective, stress researchers explored associations between significant life events (e.g., marriage, birth, divorce, relocation, death) and stress. One of the most widely used tools in this type of research is the *Recent Life Changes Questionnaire* (RLCQ; Holmes & Rahe, 1967; see Table 17.1). A major problem with this conceptualization of stress is that stress-provoking stimuli can be identified only in retrospect, that is, only after a response occurs. Other criticisms are that it does not take into consideration the meaning the individual assigns to an item, the individual's coping abilities, or the implications of chronic or recurrent events (see Jones & Kinman, 2001).

Stress as a Person–Environment Transaction

The mid-1970s to the early 1990s was a critical period in stress research. During this period, a debate raged in the literature between two camps of stress researchers. One group favoured the view that critical life events (e.g., the presence of an objective event) mediate the experience of stress. Supporters "urged researchers to measure pure events, uncontaminated by perceptions, appraisals, or reactions" (Dohrenwend & Shrout, 1985, p. 782). On the other side, others maintained that it is the appraisal of an event (e.g., the subjective evaluation of an event or situation) that is critical to the stress experience (Lazarus, DeLongis, Folkman, & Gruen, 1985). Although the debate centred on measurement and other methodologic problems, Lazarus (1999) later wrote that what was at issue was the fundamental nature of stress and the person–environment relationship. In the end, the latter group prevailed, and the view of stress as a relationship between persons and their environment has become the dominant explanatory model.

In their seminal work *Appraisal and Coping*, Lazarus and Folkman (1984) conceptualized stress as resulting from a perceived imbalance between an individual's resources and the demands placed on them. Within their Transactional Model, stress depends on how a stressor

Table 17.1	Recent Life Changes Questionnaire	
Social Area	Life Changes	LCU Values*
Family	Death of spouse	105
	Marital separation	65
	Death of close family member	65
	Divorce	62
	Pregnancy	60
	Change in health of family member	52
	Marriage	50
	Gain of new family member	50
	Marital reconciliation	42
	Spouse begins or stops work	37
	Son or daughter leaving home	29
	In-law trouble	29
	Change in number of family get-togethers	26
Personal	Jail term	56
	Sex difficulties	49
	Death of a close friend	46
	Personal injury or illness	42
	Change in living conditions	39
	Outstanding personal achievement	33
	Change in residence	33
	Minor violations of the law	32
	Begin or end school	32
	Change in sleeping habits	31
	Revision of personal habits	31
	Change in eating habits	29
	Change in church activities	29
	Vacation	29
	Change in school	28
	Change in recreation	28
	Christmas	26
Work	Fired at work	64
	Retirement from work	49
	Trouble with boss	39
	Business readjustment	38
	Change to different line of work	38
	Change in work responsibilities	33
	Change in work hours or conditions	30
Financial	Foreclosure of mortgage or loan	57
	Change in financial state	43
	Mortgage (home, car, etc.)	39
	Mortgage or loan less than $10,000 (stereo, etc.)	26

Directions: Total the LCUs for your life change events during the past 12 months.
250 to 400 LCUs per year: Minor life crisis.
More than 400 LCUs per year: Major life crisis.
*LCU, Life change unit. The number of LCUs reflects the average degree or intensity of the life change.
From Rahe, R. H. (2000). Recent Life Changes Questionnaire (RLCQ) (1997). In T. H. Holmes & American Psychiatric Association (Eds.), *Task force for the handbook of psychiatric measures. Handbook of psychiatric measures* (pp. 235–237). Washington, DC: American Psychiatric Association.

is appraised in relation to the individual's resources for coping with it. The central premise is that stress is "neither an environmental stimulus, a characteristic of the person, nor a response, but a relationship between demands and the power to deal with them without unreasonable or destructive costs" (Coyne & Holroyd, 1982, p. 108).

Cognitive Appraisal

Lazarus and Folkman (1984) use the term **cognitive appraisal** to describe the process by which individuals examine the demands and constraints of a situation in relation to their own personal and network resources. Cognitive appraisal has two levels—primary and secondary. In primary appraisal, individuals evaluate the situation and determine whether they are in danger or under threat. If yes, they go on to secondary appraisal, during which the individual considers the options for dealing with the situation. According to Lazarus and Folkman, stress is the perception of threat or harm (primary appraisal) for which an individual has no effective response (secondary appraisal). Figure 17.1 depicts

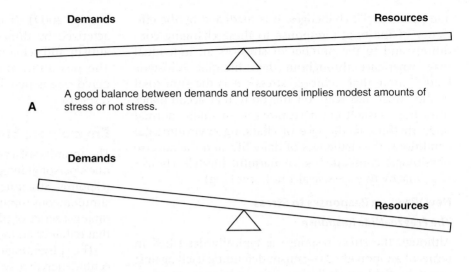

Demands   **Resources**

A A good balance between demands and resources implies modest amounts of stress or not stress.

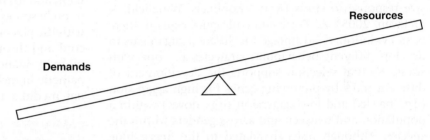

Demands

Resources

B High demands with few resources can result in a high stress balance.

Resources

Demands

C A low stress balance, which could imply boredom.

Figure 17.1. Lazarus's (1999) seesaw analogy of stress (with permission).

Lazarus's (1999, p. 59) seesaw analogy illustrating stress as a balance between environmental demands and personal resources.

KEY CONCEPT

According to the Transactional Model (Lazarus & Folkman, 1984), **stress** is the relationship between the person and the environment that is appraised as exceeding the person's resources and endangering his or her well-being.

New Understandings of the Stress and the Stress Response

In recent years, the concept of stress has been increasingly criticized for its lack of precision and specificity. Lazarus (1999) argued that while the concept of stress is a useful one, it is not a single, unitary phenomenon. This sentiment is echoed by Woolfolk, Lehrer, and Allen (2007) who contend that stress "is probably best thought of as a generic, nontechnical term, analogous to disease or to addiction" (p. 10). Until the term "stress" is replaced by a more precise label, it is a useful heuristic to aid communication among laypersons, health professionals, and researchers.

Allostasis

A recent refinement in our understanding of stress is the concept of **allostasis**. The word, which literally means *maintaining stability through change*, was coined by Sterling and Eyer (1988) to describe how the cardiovascular system adjusts to resting and active states of the body. Unlike the concept of homeostasis, which posits a single optimum state, allostasis reflects the notion that different environmental circumstances or conditions require different set points. For instance, individuals' ideal blood pressure when asleep is very different from their ideal blood pressure if they are bungee jumping (Sapolsky, 2004). Maintaining an allostatic balance in wide-ranging circumstances calls for continuous systemic adjustments throughout the whole body. For example, the hypothalamus regulates sleep and wakefulness and the production of adrenocortical hormones in response to the light–dark cycle that occurs as the earth rotates on its axis every day. When the light–dark cycle is altered (e.g., long flights across several time zones), the production of adrenocortical hormones is disrupted and alterations occur in the usual patterns of sleep, activity, appetite, and cognitive function (i.e., jet lag).

The term **allostatic load** (McEwen, 1998) refers to the cumulative negative effects on the body of continually having to adapt to changing environmental conditions and psychosocial challenges. It is mediated by the efficiency of the body's response to these changing conditions and to the number of stressors an individual may experience throughout their lifetime. Allostatic load is more than "chronic stress"; it is the sum total of the "wear and tear" on the body that accumulates from the constant effort required to maintain normal body rhythms in the face of changing environmental conditions, the challenges of daily life, and the adverse physiologic consequences of harmful lifestyle choices (e.g., inactivity, excessive alcohol, smoking).

New Views on Responses to Stress

The Freeze–Hide Response

Although the stress response is typically described in terms of an individual organism defending itself against threat by fighting or fleeing, other responses to stress have also been observed. One of these is the **freeze–hide response**, which is the tendency to produce a passive response to stress (Korte, Koolhaas, Wingfield, & McEwen, 2005). As Korte and colleagues explain, there is an evolutionary advantage for different organisms to develop different behavioural strategies to cope with stress. Natural selection supports the development of different traits by preserving genes for high aggression (e.g., hawks) and low aggression (e.g., doves) within a population and between and across genders within the species. Although research related to the freeze–hide response has been done with animals, it suggests that the stress response may actually be more differentiated than Canon predicted.

Tend and Befriend

Another line of research into the human stress response is one proposed by Taylor and colleagues (Taylor et al., 2000, 2002) who argue that males and females respond differently to stress. They theorize that women have the same physiologic response to stress but their resultant behaviours differ. They propose another alternative to fight-or-flight–type behavioural responses—which they call the *tend-and-befriend* behavioural response—characteristic of females of various species. According to these authors, the tend-and-befriend response also has evolutionary advantages and reflects the inclination of females towards affiliation, cooperation, and caretaking.

Tending involves nurturant activities designed to protect the self and offspring that promote safety and reduce distress; befriending is the creation and maintenance of social networks that may aid in this process (Taylor et al., 2000, p. 411).

As Taylor et al. (2000, 2002) explain, the biologic mediators of the tend-and-befriend response appear to involve oxytocin and female reproductive hormones. Oxytocin, dubbed the "love hormone," appears to have a role in a range of social behaviours including social memory, attachment, and bonding; sexual and maternal behaviour; trust; and aggression (Lee, Macbeth, Pagani, &

Young, 2009). It is also believed that disorders characterized by difficulties with social interactions (e.g., autism and schizophrenia) may also involve oxytocin. The possibility that the stress response may be gendered opens new horizons for exploring human stress responses.

Physiologic Stress Responses

The appraisal of a situation as dangerous or threatening to one's personal integrity triggers an automatic, total-body response. Structures in the brain receive and integrate simultaneous inputs from a number of sources and coordinate a series of physiologic and behavioural responses that enhance an individual's chances of survival.

The physiologic response to stress begins in the central nervous system (CNS) but quickly involves all body systems (refer to Table 17.2). The hypothalamus is responsible for maintaining the body's internal environment and for initiating the body's stress response, which it orchestrates through its dense neural connections with the posterior pituitary gland, brainstem, and spinal cord and through its endocrine links with the anterior pituitary gland. The hypothalamus activates the sympathetic branch of the ANS, which stimulates the adrenal medulla to secrete catecholamines and mediates

Table 17.2	Stress-Related Symptoms
System	**Symptom**
Physiologic	Headaches
	Fatigue
	Restlessness
	Sleep difficulties
	Indigestion
Emotional	Crying
	Feeling of pressure
	Easily upset
	Edginess
	Increased anger
	Feeling sick
	Nervousness
	Increased impatience
	Feeling of tension
	Overwhelmed
Cognitive	Memory loss
	Problems with decision-making
	Loss of humour
	Forgetfulness
	Feeling of tension
	Difficulty thinking clearly
Behavioural	Isolation
	Difficulty functioning
	Compulsive eating
	Lack of intimacy
	Intolerance
	Resentment
	Excessive smoking

Adapted with permission from Carpenito-Moyet, L. J. (2017). *Nursing diagnosis: Application to clinical practice* (15th ed.). Philadelphia, PA: Wolters-Kluwer.

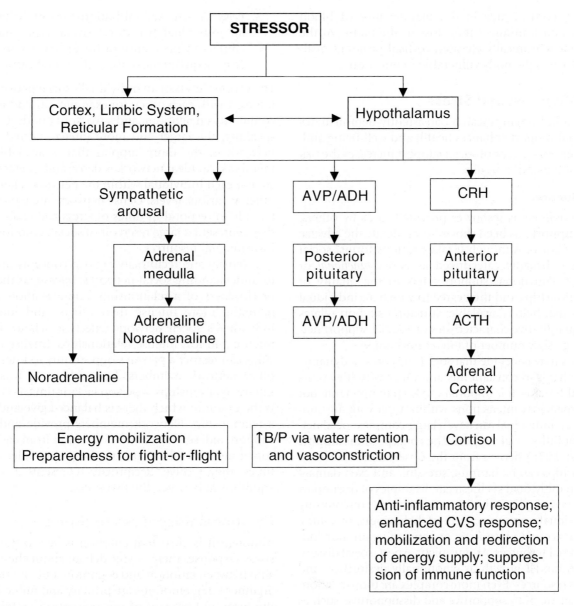

Figure 17.2. Physiologic responses to stress.

vigilance, arousal, activation, and mobilization (see Fig. 17.2). It also secretes corticotrophin-releasing hormone (CRH) to signal the anterior pituitary gland to release adrenocorticotropic hormone into the systemic circulation, which stimulates the adrenal cortex to secrete cortisol. Also through CRH, the hypothalamus excites firing of the locus coeruleus in the brainstem to increase norepinephrine in the CNS. The hypothalamus also synthesizes arginine vasopressin or antidiuretic hormone (AVP/ADH), which is released by the posterior pituitary gland and increases blood pressure by causing vasoconstriction and water retention.

The activities of the hypothalamic–pituitary–adrenocortical (HPA) axis and the sympathetic–adrenal medullary system operate within different time frames to provide the body with a wide range of defensive responses. Because the neural response of the ANS is instantaneous, it is the body's first line of defense against stressors. The release of AVP/ADH and corticosteroids is slightly slower and augments ANS effects. In the short term, these responses mobilize energy reserves (mainly in the form of glucose to skeletal muscles) and prepare the body to deal with the stressor by running away or fighting it off. If the stressor is prolonged, the body must make longer-term metabolic adjustments that ensure a sufficient supply of energy. Cortisol is essential to the body's sustained stress response because it mobilizes lipid stores and skeletal protein for energy, which allows the conservation of glucose energy for neural tissue. It also acts on the liver to elevate and stabilize blood glucose levels through gluconeogenesis and lipolysis. As well as having these metabolic effects, cortisol is an anti-inflammatory. By reducing the dilation and permeability of blood vessels, which is part of the inflammatory response, cortisol aids in the maintenance of blood pressure and minimizes fluid loss to the tissue. At the same time, chronically elevated cortisol prolongs healing and leaves the body vulnerable to infection.

Social Support and Stress

Animal and human research consistently demonstrates that social support enhances health and well-being and, conversely, that a lack of social support increases the risk of morbidity and mortality.

Social Support

Broadly defined as resources provided to us by others, **social support** has been shown to moderate the adverse effects of stress. Although it takes various forms, social support is broadly categorized as either *functional* or *structural*. Functional support refers to the quality of the relationships and the degree to which an individual believes that help is available; structural support relates to the quantitative characteristics of a social support network (e.g., size, number of interconnections).

Nurses may conclude that social support is a dynamic process that is in constant flux and varies with life events and health status. It is important to keep in mind that not all interpersonal interactions within a network are supportive; an individual can have a large, complex social network but little social support. The concept of **dissupport** (Malone, 1988) derives from the observation that some relationships can be harmful, stressful, and even damaging to an individual's self-esteem. Examples of dissupport include verbal, physical, or emotional abuse; discounting an individual's opinions, feelings, behaviours, or values; blocking access to resources; or consuming an individual's material resources. As one might expect, social dissupport can hinder growth, is emotionally destructive, and depletes resources. Even more complex are those relationships that are both supportive and dissupportive, such as those that provide tangible support (e.g., money) but are also emotionally destructive.

Social Network

We all live within networks of relationships among a defined set of people with whom we have regular face-to-face contact. It is through these relationships that we are socialized and acquire emotional support, material aid, services, and information. An individual's social network can be a resource, enhance the ability to cope with change, and influence the course of illness.

Contacts within a social network are categorized into three levels:

1. *Level I*—6 to 12 people with whom the person has intimate contact (e.g., one's closest family and friends)
2. *Level II*—30 to 40 people whom the person sees regularly (e.g., more distant family and friends, neighbours, coworkers)
3. *Level III*—the several hundred people with whom an individual has direct contact, but incidental contact in the course of his or her day-to-day life (e.g., acquaintances, the grocer, mail carrier)

The various levels of an individual's social network often intersect with each other; for example, a friend may be a confidant, a neighbour, and a workout buddy. Generally speaking, the larger and more interconnected a social network is, the more support that is available to its members. An ideal network is dense and interconnected so that each individual within the network relates to the other at various levels. Dense networks are typically better able to respond in times of stress and crisis because they represent a large reservoir of social, emotional, and instrumental resources.

Intensity and reciprocity are two concepts important to understanding social networks. *Intensity* is the degree or closeness of a relationship. Some relationships are naturally more intense than others, and ideally, an individual's social network reflects a balance between intense and less intense relationships. Intense relationships can restrict a person's opportunity to interact with other network members, but without at least a few intense relationships, a person lacks intimacy. *Reciprocity* is the extent to which there is balanced give-and-take in a relationship. Network members provide and receive support, aid, services, and information from each other; sometimes, members are on the giving side; at other times, they receive. Reciprocity represents a necessary equilibrium between the two states.

Emotional Responses to Stress

Although it is clear that emotion is key to the human stress response, there is still debate about the relationship between emotion and cognition. On one side is the argument that emotions are primary and influence both the form and content of our perceptions, while opponents believe that cognition is primary and gives rise to emotion. Consistent with his transactional view of stress, Lazarus (1991) takes a more integrative approach and contends that cognition and emotion are essentially simultaneous and interdependent. He and his colleagues define emotion as "complex, organized psychophysiologic reactions consisting of cognitive appraisals, action impulses, and patterned somatic reactions" (Folkman & Lazarus, 1991, p. 209).

Cognitive appraisal is fundamental to the experience of emotion because it colours the meaning of a situation or an event. Based on their research, Lazarus and colleagues believe that there are 15 basic emotions, each of which is elicited in response to a particular perception of what a situation or an event means to the individual (see Table 17.3). Anxiety, for example, is typically associated with the perception of a nonspecific threat or some uncertainty, whereas happiness reflects an appraisal of the person–environment condition that is beneficial.

Table 17.3 Fifteen Basic Emotions	
Emotion	**Relational Meaning**
Anger	A demeaning offense against me and mine
Anxiety	Facing an uncertain, existential threat
Fright	Facing an immediate, concrete, and overwhelming physical danger
Guilt	Having transgressed a moral imperative
Shame	Having failed to live up to an ego ideal
Sadness	Having experienced an irrevocable loss
Envy	Wanting what someone else has
Jealousy	Resenting a third party for the loss of or a threat to another's affection
Disgust	Taking in or being too close to an indigestible object or idea (metaphorically speaking)
Happiness	Making reasonable progress towards the realization of a goal
Pride	Enhancement of one's ego identity by taking credit for a valued object or achievement, either our own or that of someone or a group with whom we identify
Relief	A distressing goal-incongruent condition that has changed for the better or gone away
Hope	Fearing the worst but yearning for better
Love	Desiring or participating in affection, usually but not necessarily reciprocated
Compassion	Being moved by another's suffering and wanting to help

Adapted with permission from Lazarus, R. S. (1999). *Stress and emotion: A new synthesis*. New York, NY: Springer.

Patterned somatic reactions are the individual's own, unique experience of the physiologic changes associated with an emotion. For one person, a rush of energy is the salient feature of anger, whereas for another person, it is trembling and a feeling of weakness. These physical reactions motivate or inhibit action impulses. For example, the person who feels energized may attack an aggressor, whereas the person who experiences trembling and weakness is likely to withdraw.

Coping

According to Lazarus (1998), the following three principles are vital to an understanding of coping: (1) it continually changes over the course of an encounter; (2) it must be assessed independently of its outcomes; and (3) it consists of what an individual thinks and does in response to the perceived demands of a situation. With those principles in mind, coping is defined as "the efforts we take to manage situations we have appraised as being potentially harmful or stressful" (Kleinke, 2007, pp. 290–291). Coping reflects an individual's continual reappraisal of the person–environment relationship in light of changing conditions, as well as the success of his or her efforts to mitigate the situation. Those who evaluate their coping responses as effective are likely to feel competent and to repeat those responses in the future. Conversely, individuals who see their efforts as ineffective are likely to feel helpless and overwhelmed. Positive coping leads to adaptation, which is characterized by well-being and maximum social functioning. The inability to cope leads to maladaptation and contributes to ill health, a diminished self-concept, and deterioration in social functioning. These ideas are captured in the stress, coping, and adaptation models presented in Figures 17.3 and 17.4.

There are two general approaches to coping: problem focused and emotion focused. As Kleinke (2007) explains, problem-focused coping may be inner or outer directed. Outer-directed strategies attempt to eliminate or alter a situation or another's behaviour, while inner-directed strategies aim at altering one's own beliefs, attitudes, skills, responses, and so forth. In **emotion-focused coping**, individuals seek to manage their emotional distress (e.g., through exercise, prayer/meditation, expressing emotions, talking to friends). Table 17.4 contrasts problem-focused and emotion-focused coping.

Coping involves the continuous reevaluation or reappraisal of the changing person–environment relationship. Reappraisal incorporates feedback about the effects of coping and allows for continual processing of new information. No single coping strategy is effective in all situations. Throughout life, a repertoire of coping strategies is developed and adapted to suit different situations, and these strategies become ingrained into patterned responses. Well-adapted individuals are realistic in their appraisal of the demands upon them, are flexible in their use of coping resources, and remain open to learning new coping strategies. Poor reality testing, impaired judgement, inflexibility, limited coping strategies, and an unwillingness to acquire new resources can render individuals vulnerable to stress-related problems and illness.

KEY CONCEPT

Coping is an individual's constantly changing cognitive and behavioural efforts to manage specific external or internal demands that are appraised as taxing or exceeding the individual's resources.

Stress and Illness

For more than 50 years, accumulated research has demonstrated a relationship between stress and illness.

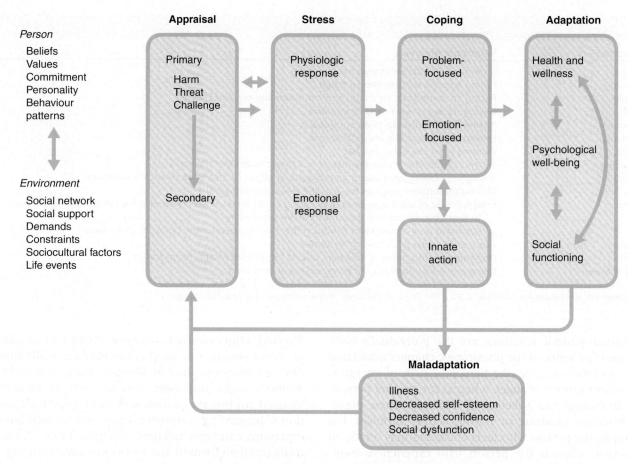

Figure 17.3. Stress, coping, and adaptation model.

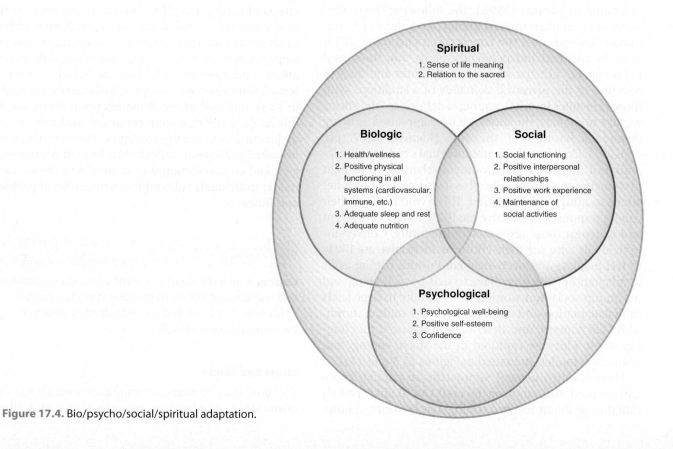

Figure 17.4. Bio/psycho/social/spiritual adaptation.

Table 17.4 Ways of Coping: Problem Focused Versus Emotion Focused	
Problem-Focused Coping	**Emotion-Focused Coping**
Outer directed When noise from the television in the apartment next door interrupts a student's studying, she experiences anxiety about being ready for an important exam the next day. She responds by asking her neighbour to turn the volume down.	A man dislikes visiting his wife's mother because she has two cats that roam her house freely, and the cat hair on all of the furniture irritates him. Rather than refusing to visit his mother-in-law, which causes conflict in his marriage, the man plans strategies that help him manage his distress during visits (e.g., long walks, a good book to distract him, thinking about how pleased his wife is).
Inner directed When an abused woman feels guilt about leaving her husband, she reminds herself that her children are much happier and doing well in school.	

Animal experiments in the 1950s and 1960s demonstrated that a number of stressors (e.g., isolation, crowding, exposure to predators, electrical shock) increased morbidity and mortality from tumours and infections (Sadock, Sadock, & Ruiz, 2015). In humans, acute academic exam stress is linked to a reduction in natural killer cells and increased activation of latent viruses (Glaser, Rice, Sherridan, & Fertel, 1987). Other studies demonstrate a correlation between exam stress and an increase in cytokines—proteins (produced by lymphocytes and other cells) that promote or inhibit an immune response (Lui et al., 2002). As well, Segerstrom and Miller's (2003) meta-analysis of 30 years of research on the effects of chronic stress associated with caring for a relative with dementia found a reduction in most measures of immune function.

The **stress–diathesis model** offers one explanation about the relationship between stress and mental health illness (Stanley & Burrows, 2005). This model proposes that preexisting genetic, biologic, and psychological vulnerabilities interact with negative or stressful life events to cause illness. Further, the model predicts an inverse relationship between vulnerability and stress such that the more vulnerable the individual, the smaller the stressor required to cause illness. Several lines of research conclude that the tendency to "nervousness, emotionality, "neuroticism," negative effect, anxiety, and being "high strung" runs in families and has a high genetic component, with 50% of these characteristics arising from genetic or biologic vulnerability" (Stanley & Burrows, 2005, p. 90).

Ineffective coping has other implications for health. For instance, if emotion-focused coping is used when a problem-focused approach is appropriate, stress is not relieved. In addition, if a coping strategy violates gender, ethnic, or cultural norms, stress is often exaggerated. Some coping strategies actually increase the risk for mortality and morbidity, such as the excessive use of alcohol, drugs, tobacco, or overeating. Although these strategies may provide some short-term stress relief, they often cause long-term secondary stress. The corollary is that healthy coping strategies such as exercising, adequate sleep, leisure activities, and good nutrition reduce the negative effects of stress and promote health and well-being.

Trauma- and Stressor-Related Disorders

Although historical and literary documents dating back to the third-century BCE describe human responses to extreme stress (e.g., natural disasters, combat, physical/sexual assault; Birmes, Hatton, Brunet, & Schmitt, 2003), modern psychiatry did not officially recognize them until 1980, when posttraumatic stress disorder (PTSD) appeared in the *Diagnostic and Statistical Manual of Mental Disorders (DSM)* (American Psychiatric Association [APA], 1980); 14 years later, acute stress disorder (ASD) was added as a diagnostic label (APA, 1994).

In the latest version of the *DSM* (APA, 2013), both PTSD and ASD were removed from the list of anxiety disorders and placed in a new category of disorders called *trauma- and stressor-related disorders*. All of the disorders in this category specify exposure to a traumatic or extremely stressful event as a diagnostic criterion. *Trauma* is from the Greek for *wound* and refers to an injury, physical and/or psychic (Oxford English Dictionary Online, 2013, December). A traumatic stressor is considered in the *DSM-5* to be "any event (or events) that may cause or threaten death, serious injury, or sexual violence to an individual, a close family member, or a close friend" (APA, 2013, p. 830). This change in criteria acknowledges that there are wide variations in individuals' responses to a traumatic experience.

KEY CONCEPT

A **traumatic stressor** is "any event (or events) that may cause or threaten death, serious injury, or sexual violence to an individual, a close family member, or a close friend" (APA, 2013, p. 830).

Acute Stress Disorder

A diagnosis of acute stress disorder (ASD) is made if an individual has experienced, personally or through witnessing others' experience(s), a severe threat in which life or injury is or appears to be at stake. This experience must then continue to affect the individual's mental health status in such areas as arousal, intrusive memories, and changes in behaviour and functioning. Refer to the *DSM-5* (2013) for APA's criteria for the traumatic event and for specific symptoms.

Posttraumatic Stress Disorder

A diagnosis of PTSD is made if an individual experiences or witnesses an authentic, severe threat of death or injury (including sexual injury) to self or others and this experience then affects the individual's mental health in specific ways. Reliving the traumatic experience through intrusive thoughts or images is a key symptom of PTSD. Avoidance of memories of the trauma (emotional avoidance) or external reminders of it (behavioural avoidance) may occur. Daily functioning can be affected by the inability to concentrate and by alterations in arousal level (e.g., hyperarousal and hypervigilance). PTSD may have negative effects on sleep and relationships, with some individuals experiencing a sense of being isolated and alone. Sareen (2014), in an overview of PTSD, notes that clinicians need to be aware that PTSD symptoms overlap with those of panic disorder, general anxiety disorder, and depression. The physical and mental effects of the trauma event on the individual need ongoing evaluation, as does risk for suicidal behaviour, which is increased with PTSD. Brief, self-report measures (e.g., the PTSD checklist and the Impact of Events Scale) can assist in this evaluation (Sareen, 2014). For symptom criteria for PTSD, please see the *DSM-5* (APA, 2013). Among the most common type of threats related to PTSD include witnessing the killing or injury of others and being in a life-threatening accident (Sareen, 2014). For children and adult refugees, precarious immigration status is associated with PTSD (Kronick, 2017).

Although more than half of individuals will experience a traumatic event at some time in their lives, most people will not develop PTSD (National Collaborating Centre for Mental Health, 2005). A survey study of adults in Ottawa regarding perceived personal threat in response to the terrorist attacks of September 11, 2001, found that the higher the appraisal of personal threat and distress experienced, the more likely it was that positive life changes (e.g., closer to family, refocused priorities) were made; these changes were reported to remain stable nearly a year later (Davis & Macdonald, 2004). For most people, adversity fosters resilience, not psychopathology. Preferred coping mechanisms tend to (1) focus on brief time intervals (e.g., think only about the next step), (2) maintain a view of oneself as competent and a view of others as willing and able to provide support, and (3) focus on the current implications

of the trauma and avoid regretting past decisions and actions.

Factors that predict the development of PTSD include being female, type and severity of the trauma, past trauma (including childhood physical, sexual, and emotional abuse), and availability of support at the time of the stressful event (Richardson, Naifeh, & Elhai, 2007). Since women are more likely to experience more high-impact trauma, they are also more likely than men to develop PTSD. It is the type of experience, such as interpersonal violence, that accounts for some of this difference (Amstadter, Aggen, Knudsen, Reichborn-Kjennerud, & Kendler, 2013; Kelly, Skelton, Patel, & Bradley, 2011; Maguen, Luxton, Skopp, & Madden, 2012; Rees et al., 2011). Women in the perinatal period have higher rates of PTSD compared with other times across the lifespan, likely due to exacerbation of preexisting PTSD symptoms (Seng et al., 2010). A study in which structured interviews of 8,441 members of the Canadian Armed Forces (CAF) regarding trauma exposure and PTSD found that PTSD rates were higher among female soldiers. Females had less exposure than males to warlike trauma but greater experience of sexual assault. Although members of the CAF have high exposure to trauma events (85.6% had such exposure), the rate of lifetime PTSD is moderate (6.6%) (Brunet, Monson, Lui, & Fikretoglu, 2015). Children (particularly those under the age of 10 years) are less likely to experience PTSD after trauma than are adults (National Collaborating Centre for Mental Health, 2005).

Treatments for PTSD include cognitive–behavioural therapy, psychotherapy, eye movement desensitization and reprocessing (EMDR), and medication. Treatment may need to be prolonged, and there are many who live with chronic persistent symptoms. Neurobiologic studies related to PTSD first began with Vietnam war veterans who still met criteria for PTSD 20 to 30 years after the war.

Intergenerational Transmission of Stress, Trauma, and Resilience

The processes by which the effects of stress and trauma experienced in one generation can be transmitted to the subsequent generations involve multiple factors and intersecting pathways (Bombay, Matheson, & Anisman, 2009, 2014a; Bowers & Yehuda, 2016; Dekel & Goldblatt, 2008). It is known that adverse experiences in childhood and adulthood may influence the risk for various health and social outcomes in offspring of those who encountered the stressor or trauma directly (Bombay et al., 2009, 2014b; Bowers & Yehuda, 2016; Dekel & Goldblatt, 2008). For example, the experiences of parents have been shown to be linked with the way their children appraise certain situations, including the way they appraise stressful experiences and their ability to contend with these stressors. These appraisals, in turn, can influence the coping strategies that are endorsed, which will also be influenced by the coping styles or predispositions that individuals bring with them. As a result, these individuals may be at increased risk of further stressor encounters, increased psychological and neurochemical reactivity to stressors, and the promotion of poor mental and physical health outcomes (Bowers & Yehuda, 2016).

This is not only one potential scenario demonstrating how trauma can be transmitted across generations, as other psychological, social, physiologic, cultural, and economic factors have also been shown to be involved in these intergenerational processes. The previous depiction of intergenerational transfer essentially portrays events within a family unit, but it is understood that stressful and traumatic events within this unit do not occur in isolation of other external and indirect factors that might contribute to, or protect against, the intergenerational transfer of stressor effects (e.g., sociocultural environment, physical environment, historical influences, and government policies). These factors, alone or in combination, may result in impaired abilities to provide an adequate early childhood environment for their children, which might result in the recapitulation of the events that occurred in the preceding generation. Of course, not all individuals whose parents face stress and trauma are destined to be at risk for negative outcomes throughout their lifetime, as the transmission of such risk across generations can be mitigated by various protective factors—including internal assets and external resources—that may buffer against the negative experiences faced by their parents (Bowers & Yehuda, 2016; Lee, Cheung, & Kwong, 2012).

Collective Trauma and Historical Trauma

It has been suggested that focusing solely on individual experiences of stress and trauma has resulted in the lack of appropriate consideration of the significant collective experiences and outcomes that can arise when a whole group of people encounter a traumatizing and/or adverse experience (Somasundaram, 2007). Collective trauma refers to instances in which a significant proportion of any given social group—based on political, racial, religious, cultural, or other factors—are collectively exposed to a traumatic event. Such experiences can be as random as a single natural disaster or purposely conducted by one group to another at one time or for an extended period (Bombay et al., 2009, 2014a). Increasing research has demonstrated the potential unique social and psychological outcomes at the collective or community level that can have significant long-term consequences (Somasundaram, 2007, 2014). In addition to the additive effects of individual trauma elicited by such collective experiences, effects at the family and community levels can modify social norms, dynamics, structures, and

functioning that are more than the sum of the individual-level effects. For example, community-level changes in the aftermath of mass trauma have included erosion of basic trust; collective silence; deterioration in social norms, morals, and values; and poor leadership (Bombay et al., 2014a, 2014b; Catani, Jacob, Schauer, Kohila, & Neuner, 2008; Saul, 2014; Somasundaram, 2007).

In addition to considering the collective nature of some traumatic events, it is also important to consider the traumatic events that the group had previously experienced. Similar to the allostatic overload associated with individual experiences of stress or trauma, the concept of historical trauma highlights the process by which the consequences of multiple collectively experienced adversities experienced by a group over time may be cumulative and be carried forward to subsequent generations if they outweigh contextual and group-level resilience factors (Evans-Campbell, 2008). For example, exposure to numerous collective traumas and stressors over generations that were intense, long lasting and affected a large proportion of the group, would be expected to be particularly at risk for individual- and group-level risk for negative outcomes associated with these experiences. This perspective allows events occurring across generations to be considered as part of a single traumatic trajectory, expanding the focus from isolated impacts of single events to also considering the interactions and synergies associated with numerous adversities over time (Bombay et al., 2014a, 2014b; Evans-Campbell, 2008).

Vulnerability, to a considerable extent, describes the current position of many indigenous people across the world, as the numerous collective traumas endured that were often intense, lasted from first contact until the present day, and impacted most members of this group. This was compounded by the suppression of spiritual and traditional practices during this time, which could have otherwise served as a resilience factor (Matheson, Bombay, Haslam, & Anisman, 2016). Indeed, historic trauma has been suggested and shown to be a contributing factor in relation to the high prevalence of certain psychosocial issues faced by First Nations and other Aboriginal groups (Braveheart-Jordan & DeBruyn, 1995; Duran, Duran, Brave Heart, & Yellow Horse-Davis, 1998; Robin, Chester, & Goldman, 1996).

Historical trauma can be considered a cumulative emotional and psychological wounding over the lifespan and across generations, emanating from massive group trauma experiences (Brave Heart, 2003). Increasing empirical research supports this concept, and intergenerational effects in relation to various mental health outcomes have been observed in the adult offspring of Indigenous adults in the United States and Canada who were affected by forced relocations (Walls & Whitbeck, 2012), or by the forced removal of Indigenous children to residential schools (Indian boarding schools in the United States), for the purposes of assimilation (Bombay et al., 2014a). For example, it was shown that Aboriginal adults in Canada who had a parent or grandparent who attended Indian residential schools were at greater risk for psychological distress and suicide attempts compared to those whose parents did not attend (Bombay et al., 2014a; McQuaid et al., 2017). Providing evidence for the cumulative nature of historical trauma events and experiences, it was also found that those with a parent and grandparent who attended—so with two previous familial generations who were directly affected—were at greater risk for these negative outcomes compared to those with only one previous generation who attended (i.e., parent or a grandparent) (McQuaid et al., 2017).

KEY CONCEPT

Collective trauma occurs when a traumatic event is experienced by a significant proportion of a given social group; it can have long-term consequences for the social group beyond its additive effect on individuals such that social norms, dynamics, functioning, and structure of the group may be modified.

KEY CONCEPT

Historical trauma is the process by which a social group is affected by the consequences of multiple, collectively experienced adversities across time that outweigh group resiliency factors, become cumulative, and are carried forward to subsequent generations such that the trauma may be considered as part of a single trajectory.

Responses to Collective and Historical Trauma

For collectivistic societies that place significant value on relationships, healing and recovery from collectively experienced trauma and stress must address the impacts on the collective and do so through integrated multi-level approaches (Somasundaram, 2007, 2014). Though both the DSM and World Health Organization (WHO) International Classification of Diseases (ICD) classification systems have traditionally been based on the individual, it has been argued that collective approaches will often have the most benefits from a public health perspective when resources are limited. For example, community-level mental health and psychosocial support interventions have been shown to help communities affected by disasters (Macy et al., 2004; Scholte & Ager, 2014; Somasundaram, 2007, 2014). Furthermore, community-based approaches enable interventions to reach a larger target population, as well as undertake preventive and promotional public mental health activities at the same time. Individuals and families can be expected to recover and cope when communities become functional, activating healing mechanisms

within the community itself (Somasundaram, 2007, 2014). It is important to recognize the manifestations of collective trauma, so that effective interventions at the community level can be used in these complex situations. Integrated holistic community approaches that were found useful in rebuilding communities include:

- creating public awareness;
- training of grass root workers;
- encouraging traditional practices and rituals;
- promoting positive family and community relationships and processes; and
- rehabilitation and networking with other organizations (Somasundaram, 2007, 2014).

In relation to the historical trauma of Indigenous peoples in Canada, indigenous researchers and scholars have expressed the need for multilevel assessment and intervention strategies to address factors related to health and wellness at individual, family, and community levels (Brave Heart, Chase, Elkins, & Altschul, 2011; Evans-Campbell, 2008). A long-term goal of historical trauma intervention research and practice is to reduce inequities faced by indigenous peoples by developing culturally responsive interventions driven by communities to improve quality of life and well-being. Through individual and community-based initiatives, as well as larger political and cultural processes, Aboriginal people in Canada are involved in healing their traditions, repairing the ruptures and discontinuities in the transmission of traditional knowledge and values, and asserting their collective identity and power.

Trauma-Informed Care

The term trauma-informed care has been used to describe ways in which health care providers collaborate to ensure that every part of health services for all clients is assessed and potentially modified in relation to considerations of how trauma can influence the life and experiences of someone seeking services (Raja et al., 2015). Such care is shaped by the principles of safety, choice, and control. Effective trauma-informed care is not simply designed to treat symptoms or disorders related to past adverse experiences, but it is also meant to ensure that staff are equipped with the knowledge to ensure that they do no further harm by traumatizing those already exposed to significant trauma (Elliott et al., 2005; Raja et al., 2015). Clients should find those providing their care to be compassionate and trustworthy.

KEY CONCEPT

Trauma-informed care is an approach to all clients that is based on knowledge of trauma and its effects with policies and practices incorporating principles of safety, choice, and control, as well as compassion, collaboration, and trustworthiness.

Health, social, and economic inequities continue to exist across certain racialized and marginalized groups in Canada and the United States, and interpersonal and systemic racism within the health care system contributes to these ongoing gaps (Allan & Smylie, 2015; Bombay, 2015; Braveman, Cubbin, Egerter, Williams, & Pamuk, 2010; Browne et al., 2012). In addition to systemic and more blatant forms of discrimination, implicit discrimination in the form of bias, attitudes, and beliefs, even without conscious intent or awareness, can influence provider behaviour in health care settings (Dovidio et al., 2008; Johnson, Saha, Arbelaez, Beach, & Cooper, 2004; Penner et al., 2010), clinical decision-making, and treatment recommendations, with potential detrimental consequences to the provision of effective and safe care (Green et al., 2007).

There is growing attention to the need for **cultural competence** in trauma-informed health care (Ardino, 2014; Huey, Tilley, Jones, & Smith, 2014; Imel et al., 2011). Culture, in this conception, is implied to be indistinguishable from ethnicity (Browne et al., 2009) rather than recognizing that we are all bearers of culture and espouse cultural values. Although it is clearly important to increase knowledge regarding differing culturally embedded world views, experiences and conceptualizations of health (Tervalon & Murray-Garcia, 1998), health care practitioners, community members, and researchers have advocated that cultural competence is not enough; we need *cultural safety* and *cultural humility* (Caron, 2017). *Cultural competence* implies a finite skill that can be acquired through training, whereas *cultural humility* is an active and continual engagement in a process of self-critique, reflection, acknowledgment, rectification of imbalances of power, and respectful community partnership in the provision of care (Kumagai & Lypson, 2009; Tervalon & Murray-Garcia, 1998). Approaching cultural competence as a sum of knowledge that can be acquired and implemented risks reductionism and may result in harm due to stereotyping and cultural assumptions when this information does not result in changes in practice or in the understanding for the need to adopt a particularly humble stance within cross-cultural interactions (Ben-Ari & Strier, 2010; Tervalon & Murray-Garcia, 1998). A concept compatible with cultural humility is **cultural safety**. Cultural safety was first conceived, developed, and advocated for within health care by Maori nurses in Aotearoa/New Zealand and was introduced as a requirement in nursing education in the early 1990s to redress Maori health and health care inequalities (Papps & Ramsden, 1996; Ramsden & Spoonley, 1993; Richardson, 2004). Central to cultural safety is an examination of colonial, interpersonal, and professional power relationships reflected through racism and discrimination (Allan & Smylie, 2015; Richardson & Carryer, 2005).

It is unlikely for a single paradigm to address the full complexity of intercultural interactions within health care settings, which must be understood in relation to historical contexts and power relations (Kirmayer, 2012). Adding to the complexity, patient's experiences and identities may include a variety of intersections, such as ethnicity, gender, immigrant experiences, sexuality, socioeconomic status, and ability, to name a few, which may interact to influence points of view and care needs (Quiros & Berger, 2015). However, health care provider perceptions and assumptions can and do interfere with care provision (Penner et al., 2010). The concept of cultural safety is potentially useful to improving intercultural care (Tervalon & Murray-Garcia, 1998) and is congruent with, and a core element of, trauma-informed care by creating a respectful and safe environment for all patients (Elliot et al., 2005) and working to reduce health inequities in primary care (Browne et al., 2012).

It is important to consider the impact of repetitive and/or chronic trauma experiences at not only an individual but also a collective or group level. There is growing awareness of repetitive and chronic trauma affecting generations and whole communities, as is the case with historical trauma (Bombay et al., 2014a, 2014b; Brave Heart et al., 2011). In addition to understanding the implications of colonization and other types of collective and historical trauma, it is equally important to adopt a strength-based perspective that respects individual and community resilience and empowerment within marginalized populations (Kirmayer, Sehdev, Whitley, Dandeneau & Isaac, 2009; Million, 2013). Within a Canadian context of colonization, it is imperative for health professionals within mainstream settings to recognize and work towards redressing the intergenerational impacts of the residential school system and other colonizing policies (TRC, 2015) as part of culturally safe trauma-informed care and to "create space for Indigenous healing strategies as part of treatment" (Linklater, 2014, p. 131).

Nursing Care of Individuals Affected by Stress

Nursing assessment of individuals experiencing stress attends to biologic, psychological, emotional, and environmental (physical and social), as well as coping resources. In particular, the nurse should explore recent changes (positive or negative) in the individual's life (e.g., trauma, loss, developmental milestones).

The overall goals of care for those individuals actively experiencing a stress response are to eliminate or moderate the stressor (if possible), to reduce untoward effects of the stress response, and to facilitate the maintenance or development of positive coping skills. The goals of care for individuals who are at high risk for stress (e.g., are experiencing significant life changes, have preexisting vulnerabilities, have limited coping mechanisms) are to recognize the potential for stress and to strengthen or develop positive coping skills. It is also important to educate clients about human stress responses as a way to help normalize bodily, emotional, and social responses, thereby helping the client to reappraise his or her own interpretation of these responses.

Biologic Domain

Biologic Assessment

Biologic data are essential for analyzing an individual's physical responses to stress, coping efforts, and adaptation. This information comes from the health history, physical examination, and diagnostic testing (as indicated; see Chapter 9). Nurses should pay particular attention to:

- Signs and responses indicating sympathetic and parasympathetic arousal (see Chapter 9)
- Alterations in vegetative functions (e.g., appetite and eating patterns, sleep, energy level, sexual activity)
- Chronic illness or conditions with a strong stress component (e.g., hypertension, migraine, chronic pain syndromes, irritable bowel syndrome)
- Evidence of immune system suppression (e.g., frequent infections)
- Physical appearance (e.g., deficits in grooming and hygiene; nonverbal indications of muscle tension, anxiety, or depression)
- Alterations in activity and exercise patterns

IN-A-LIFE

Maria Campbell (1940–)

Maria Campbell is a Métis woman and the eldest daughter of seven children. She was born in Park Valley, Saskatchewan, to parents of Scottish, aboriginal, and French descent. Her autobiography, *Halfbreed* (1973), recounts the first 33 years of her life and tells of how Maria lost her mother when she was only 12 years old, leaving her to care for her younger siblings. In an effort to keep her family together, young Maria married an abusive white man who reported her to child welfare authorities, and her siblings were placed in foster homes. Devastated, Maria moved to Vancouver, where her husband deserted her, and she turned to a life of drugs and prostitution. Alone and desperate, she attempted suicide twice and was hospitalized for psychiatric care. It was in the hospital that Maria joined Alcoholics Anonymous and began a journey of healing.

Campbell not only tells her own story but also speaks of the discrimination and racism that affects Métis people. In the book's introduction, she writes, "I write this for all of you, to tell you what it is like to be a half-breed woman in this country. I want to tell you about the joys and sorrows, the oppressing poverty, the frustrations and the dreams" (p. 8). Although Maria's story is one of stress and crises, it is also a story of courage and resilience. She is not a scared little girl but a strong, independent woman full of hope for herself and her people. She is a mother, grandmother, and great-grandmother.

Today, Maria is a Métis cultural leader and an officer of the Order of Canada (awarded in 2008). She continues to write; her translated work, *Stories of the Road Allowance People*, was republished in 2010. In 2012, she retired from the University of Saskatchewan, was awarded a Pierre Elliott Trudeau Fellowship, and joined the Métis Research Group, Institute of Canadian Studies, University of Ottawa. She is the recipient of many writing awards, including the Chalmers Award for best new play, and has four Honorary Doctorate degrees.

From Campbell, M. (1973). *Halfbreed*. Halifax, NS: Goodread Biographies.

As well, the biologic assessment of stress and coping considers the use of pharmacologic agents, including prescription and nonprescription medications, over-the-counter and herbal preparations, alcohol, tobacco, and illicit drugs. Some individuals begin or increase the frequency of using these agents as a way of coping with stress. At the same time, however, reliance on relaxants or mood-altering substances can become a secondary stressor and contribute to maladaptation. Understanding patterns of use (e.g., frequency, dose, circumstances, and effects) is important to assessing their role in stress management. The more important the substances are to a person's handling of stress, the greater the potential for abuse and addiction.

Interventions for the Biologic Domain

Individuals experiencing or at risk for untoward stress responses may benefit from a number of biologic interventions.

- The importance of (re)establishing regular routines for activities of daily living (e.g., eating, sleeping, self-care, leisure time) cannot be overstated. As well as ensuring adequate nutrition, sleep and rest, and hygiene, routines may help to structure an individual's time and give them a sense of personal control or mastery.

- Exercise can reduce the emotional and behavioural responses to stress. In addition to the physical benefits, regular exercise can provide structure to a person's life, enhance self-confidence, and increase feelings of well-being. Under stress, many individuals are not receptive to the idea of exercise, particularly if it has not been a part of their life. Exploration of usual activity patterns, as well as knowledge and beliefs about the value of exercise, will help to identify where the nurse may intervene.
- Activities such as yoga, meditation, deep breathing, and progressive muscle relaxation can help individuals mediate the physical stress response, improve sleep, and reduce pain. Nurses should also consider referring clients for hypnosis, biofeedback, or eye movement desensitization and reprocessing (EMDR) when indicated.
- Health teaching in such areas as nutrition, sleep hygiene, and medication management may also be a part of nursing interventions in this domain.

Psychological Domain

Psychological Assessment

Information about the psychological and emotional dimensions of stress may be forthcoming throughout the assessment process. In particular, the nurse should do the following:

- Observe for behavioural and affective indicators of stress response (e.g., energy level and general presentation; appearance, grooming, and hygiene; psychomotor agitation and retardation; facial expression; speech characteristics).
- Explore reports of recent changes in mood or current emotional distress (e.g., anxiety, fear, irritability, anger, tension, pressure, depression).
- Note alterations or impairment in mental status (e.g., suicidal ideation; self-deprecatory thoughts; impulsivity; ruminations; impaired concentration, problem-solving, or memory).
- Explore the individual's appraisal of significant life events (e.g., losses, physical or sexual abuse or assault, motor vehicle crashes, natural disasters, combat experience), the effect of those experiences, and the commitment to particular outcomes.
- Ask about alterations in day-to-day function or inability to fulfill responsibilities (e.g., family, work, school).
- Explore the individual's current resources and effectiveness of usual coping strategies.

Interventions for the Psychological Domain

Nursing interventions that support psychological functioning and facilitate lifestyle changes for persons coping with stress include cognitive–behavioural interventions (see Chapter 13), psychoeducational (individual or group) interventions (see Chapter 14), relaxation therapy, and assertiveness training.

Social Domain

Social Assessment

Information from a social assessment is invaluable to understanding an individual's coping resources. The ability to make healthy lifestyle changes is strongly influenced by one's social support system. Even the expression of stress is related to social factors, particularly ethnic and cultural expectations and values.

Social assessment also includes identification of the person's social network. The nurse should elicit the following information:

- Size and extent of the network, both relatives and nonrelatives, and the length and quality of the relationships
- Functions the network serves (e.g., intimacy, social integration, nurturance, reassurance of worth, guidance and advice, access to new contacts)
- Degree of reciprocity between the individual and others in the network (i.e., Whom provides support to the client? Whom does the client support?)
- Degree of interconnectedness among network members

Interventions for the Social Domain

Individuals who are coping with stressful situations often benefit from interventions that facilitate social functioning and promote the health and welfare of social network members. The education of the family regarding the client's disorder and their supportive involvement can be significant. The family and individual members may also require support, including respite. Referral to family therapy may be indicated.

Spiritual Domain

The challenges faced by individuals in times of stress and crisis can lead to an acute questioning about one's life choices and situation, about one's relationships, and about the meaning of one's very existence. Making sense of what is happening to you is fundamental to being human. If we want to believe in a "just world," one response may be to search for reasons that one deserves to be "punished" (Hafer & Bàgue, 2005). In his book *When Bad Things Happen to Good People*, Kushner (1981) describes how a personal tragedy compelled him to "rethink everything" he had been taught about God and God's ways (p. 1). He could not make sense of what was happening to his family and felt "a deep aching sense of unfairness" (p. 2). Ultimately, Kushner concluded that suffering happens in our natural world and that there are no exceptions for nice people; God gives humans strength to cope with their misfortunes and does not leave them to suffer alone. While his book reveals the search for meaning that a life crisis can inspire, his conclusions are his own. Others, even those in very similar circumstances, may choose a different resolution. For instance, lasting anger at the sacred power in which one believes may be the response if one feels totally abandoned or one may view the crisis situation as revealing direction for personal growth.

Nurses attending to the spiritual domain of their practice need to recognize the likely occurrence of such searching on the part of clients under duress or in crisis. Nurses need to refrain from providing their own answers to questions of meaning; rather, through listening, they need to provide support. Thoughtful questions may be helpful in understanding the client's perspective: Has your current stressful situation influenced the way you understand the world? Have your beliefs been affected? If so, in what way? What is sustaining you through this time? Are there spiritual acts, such as prayer or ritual, which you are finding helpful? What, if anything, can you take from this experience to help you in the future?

When a traumatic or crisis event is catastrophic in its scope, entire communities can struggle to understand the cause of what has happened and the meaning of the loss suffered. At one time in Western societies, disasters were understood as evidence of the wrath of the gods or God (Grandjean, Rendu, MacNamee, & Scherer, 2008). The Lisbon earthquake of 1755 is used to mark the beginnings of change in societal attitudes towards disaster: it is called the first modern disaster as it was attributed to "natural" rather than "supernatural" causes. The type of disaster influences this struggle, of course, and can affect the community's recovery (Furedi, 2007). Faith-based support in times of disaster may be absent from organized disaster response, but rituals and sacraments, group prayer, and action on beliefs regarding service and helping others can restore a sense of stability and comfort for those who feel a need to turn to their faith (Clements & Casani, 2016).

Spirituality can positively influence the response to disaster. In a study of psychiatric morbidity following a tsunami in a community with diverse religious beliefs, it was found that altruistic behaviour on the part of community leaders, religious faith, and spirituality (along with family systems and social support) were factors that positively affected the early coping of survivors (Math et al., 2008). In addition to their professional challenges, nurses responding to a disaster in their own community will have to address their personal reaction as members of the community with their own spiritual questions.

Evaluation and Treatment Outcomes

Evaluation is guided by treatment goals established in the plan of care. The goals of individual care relate to improved health, well-being, and social function. Depending on the level of intervention, there may also be goals for the family and other members of the client's social network. Family outcomes may relate to improved communication or social support (e.g., reduced caregiver stress). Social network outcomes focus on strengthening the social network and improving its function.

■ CRISIS

Our current understanding of the bio/psycho/social/spiritual implications of a crisis has its roots in Lindeman's (1944) study of bereavement among friends and relatives of the Coconut Grove nightclub fire in Boston in 1942. Four hundred and thirty-nine individuals died in that fire, which at the time was the worst single building fire in US history. In the course of his research, Lindeman learned that family and friends of those who died experienced somatic symptoms, feelings of anger and guilt, and preoccupation with the deceased. From this work, he developed a model that describes *grief as progressing through three stages*: shock and disbelief, acute mourning, and resolution. Lindeman concluded that grief is both a natural response to loss and necessary to survivors' mental health. He later extended his ideas about crisis to more common, yet significant, life events (e.g., the birth of a child, marriage, death) and hypothesized that the changes associated with these events cause emotional strain and require individuals to adapt to a new reality (Lindeman, 1956). These adaptive efforts lead to either mastery (psychological growth) or impaired functioning. Lindeman was convinced that by helping individuals through the bereavement process, mental health professionals could prevent later psychological and emotional problems. This thinking reflected two important trends that were germinating in psychiatry around the globe: the recognition of the potential for and the value of early intervention to prevent emotional and psychological problems and the movement from hospital-based to community-based psychiatric treatment.

Although Lindeman did much of the foundational work in the area of crisis, Gerald Caplan is widely acknowledged as the master architect of crisis intervention. A psychiatrist and close colleague of Lindeman's, Caplan (1961) equated mental health with a strong, mature ego, which he defined as (1) the capacity to withstand stress and maintain equilibrium, (2) an accurate perception of reality, and (3) a balanced repertoire of coping strategies based on sound reality testing. Caplan is believed to be the first to apply the term crisis in psychiatry, to relate the concept of homeostasis to crisis intervention, and to describe the stages of a crisis.

Caplan defined crisis as occurring "when a person faces an obstacle to important life goals, that is, for a time, insurmountable through the utilization of customary methods of problem solving" (1961, p. 18). More specifically, a crisis is a response in which psychological equilibrium is disrupted, usual coping methods are ineffective in restoring that equilibrium, and there is evidence of functional impairment (Caplan, 1961; Flannery & Everly, 2000). This disequilibrium causes a rise in inner tension and anxiety that, if it continues, engenders emotional upset and an inability to function (Caplan, 1961). Figure 17.5 summarizes the phases of crisis.

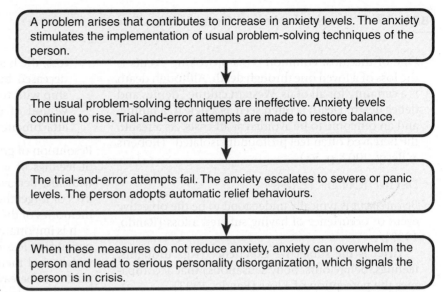

Figure 17.5. Phases of crisis response.

Although crises force individuals into uncharted territory, Caplan (1961) recognized that most individuals achieve resolution without professional help within 4 to 6 weeks. He viewed this time as a period of transition in which the individual, family, or group is more vulnerable to harm and, at the same time, more open to outside intervention. This prompted Caplan to advocate for community-based crisis services aimed at identifying maladaptive responses and intervening early to assist those involved to transform problems into opportunities for personal growth and new learning.

KEY CONCEPT

A **crisis** response occurs when an individual encounters an obstacle or problem that might affect his or her life goals and that cannot be solved by customary problem-solving methods. It is acute, is time limited, and may be developmental, situational, or interpersonal in nature.

Types of Crises

Situational Crisis

A situational crisis is any event that overwhelms an individual's coping resources and upsets his or her equilibrium. The precipitating event may be positive or negative, physiologic, psychological, or social in nature. Examples of situational crises include illness, the death of a loved one, separation or divorce, job loss, school problems, physical or sexual assault, or an unplanned pregnancy. Situational crises also result from less common occurrences such as accidents, natural or human-caused disasters, and acts of terrorism. Box 17.1 discusses the death of a loved one, a situational crisis that each of us will encounter in our lifetime.

Developmental Crisis

Theorists such as Erikson (1959) propose that human development proceeds sequentially through a series of stages, each with a new set of social roles and responsibilities. Stage theorists hold that demands from the social environment exert pressure on an individual to move on to the next developmental stage and that a failure to meet these new expectations precipitates a developmental crisis. Successful resolution of this crisis is necessary for movement into the next stage. Developmental crises are an expected part of maturation and are a time during which individuals acquire new skills and resources.

The concept of developmental crisis assumes that psychosocial development progresses in an orderly, easily identifiable process. Other developmental theories, such as those of Miller (1994) and Gilligan (1994), refute the notion that human development advances in stages (see Chapter 8). That being said, the concept of developmental crisis is useful for describing unfavourable person–environment relationships that relate to maturational events, such as leaving home for the first time, completing school, or the birth of one's first child.

Crisis or Not? The Effects of Balancing Factors

Aguilera (1998) believes that a stressful event developing into a crisis depends on three *balancing factors*: perception of the event, available situational supports, and coping mechanisms. As Figure 17.6 illustrates, the timely and successful resolution of a crisis is more likely if an individual has a realistic view of the situation, adequate supports available, and effective coping mechanisms.

BOX 17.1 Death of a Loved One: A Crisis Event

One of the most common crisis-provoking events is the loss of a loved one through death. Although death is a certainty for all of us, Western culture "denies and defies death. Death is often seen as a defeat, a failure, and an outcome to be avoided at all costs. As a result, the bereaved often feel profoundly isolated" (Roberts & Berry, 2002, p. 53).

DEFINITION OF TERMS

Bereavement is typically understood to be the objective event or occurrence of having suffered a loss (Rando, 1993).

Grief is the subjective experience (e.g., thoughts, feelings, behaviours, body sensations) that accompanies the perception of a loss (Rando, 1993).

Mourning is the external manifestation of grief, which is highly influenced by gender, ethnicity, culture, religion, and the cause of death (Wolfelt, 1999).

TASKS OF MOURNING

Worden (2003) describes the four tasks of mourning, which are necessary to the process of adapting to loss and reestablishing equilibrium. Unlike other theorists who conceptualize mourning in terms of *stages* or *phases*, which connote linearity, Worden emphasizes the issues that bereaved individuals must face and successfully negotiate as they come to terms with their new reality:

1. *Accepting the reality of the loss.* The first task of grieving is to accept the reality and full consequence of the loss. A part of this is recognizing the permanence of death and that life as it was is over forever.
2. *Working through the pain of grief.* It is important for the bereaved individual to experience and acknowledge the pain of grief. Denial or suppression of this pain prolongs grieving.
3. *Adapting to an environment in which the deceased is absent.* This adaptation requires the bereaved individual to adjust to a new reality, which involves developing a new self-identity (e.g., as a widow or single person) and taking on new social roles and responsibilities.
4. *Developing a new relationship with the deceased and reengaging with life.* In coming to terms with the

loss, the bereaved individual does not forget the deceased but rather establishes a new relationship with the deceased. This involves healing the wound of the severed attachment so that new attachments can be formed.

Resolution of grief is manifested by the gradual return of feelings of well-being and the ability to continue with life. Bereaved persons do not deny their former lives or forget their loved ones but find a way to weave memories of the past into the current reality.

It is important to keep in mind that although the experience of loss is universal, individual responses vary widely, and there is no one clearly defined course or process of bereavement or grieving. Grief is influenced by age, development, gender, history of loss and/or trauma, history of depression, the nature and quality of the relationship with the deceased, and the type of loss (e.g., anticipated, violent, traumatic). Research underscores that the experience and expressions of grief are influenced by such factors as familial relationships and expectations, social and cultural factors, and religion (Center for the Advancement of Health, 2004).

COMPLICATED GRIEF

Complicated grief is also termed abnormal, pathologic, chronic, or exaggerated grief. It refers to grief that does not seem to be advancing the bereaved individual towards acceptance and reorganization. Grief is complicated when an individual does not accomplish one or more of the tasks of mourning. Examples of this include denying the reality of one's loss, prolonged and intense emotions that do not seem to lessen over time, the apparent absence of mourning, and the inability to reinvest in life.

ROLE OF HEALTH CARE TEAMS IN SUPPORTING GRIEF

As members of the health care team, nurses participate in supporting bereaved individuals through the process of grieving. The goals of this care are to assist bereaved individuals with the tasks of mourning and to prevent complicated grief. Activities may include sitting in silence with the bereaved, active listening, assistance with practical needs, and referral for ongoing support.

Nursing Care of Individuals Experiencing Crisis

Crisis Intervention

Crisis intervention is the provision of emergency psychological care to assist victims in returning to an adaptive level of functioning and to prevent or moderate the

potentially negative effects of psychological trauma. Although there are several models of crisis intervention, virtually all of them incorporate the following principles:

1. **Early intervention.** By their nature, crises are acute and distressing events that overwhelm an

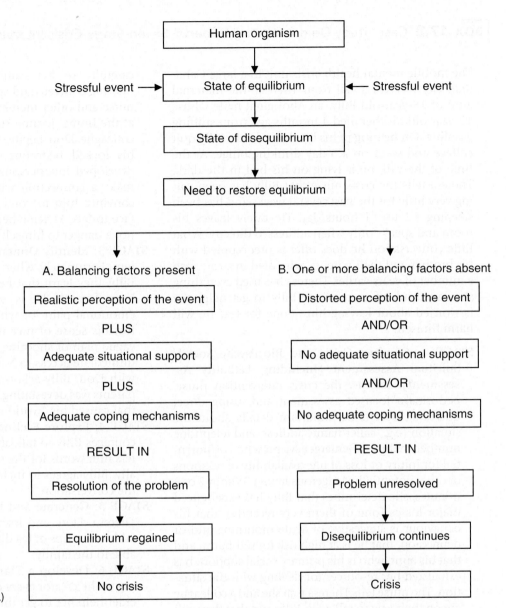

Figure 17.6. The effect of balancing factors in a stressful event. (From Aguilera, D. C. (1998). *Crisis intervention: Theory and methodology* (8th ed.). St. Louis, MO: Mosby.)

individual's coping resources. Inability to resolve a crisis in a timely manner renders those affected at higher risk for long-term health problems. Crisis intervention services are typically community based and operate 24 hours/day. Crisis teams provide telephone triage and counselling but may also travel to the scene of the crisis, where they work closely with other emergency service personnel (e.g., police officers, firefighters, and hospital emergency staff).

2. **Stabilization.** An immediate goal of all crisis intervention efforts is to prevent the situation from worsening. Stabilization involves mobilizing resources and support networks with the aim of minimizing harm and quickly restoring some semblance of order and routine.

3. **Facilitating understanding.** An important part of crisis intervention is helping individuals to develop an accurate understanding of the situation and its potential consequences. This usually involves listening to individuals' accounts of their experience and assisting them to identify and articulate their feelings about what is happening. Facilitating a clear understanding of a situation helps individuals to develop a realistic appraisal of the demands on them and aids the integration of the crisis into their cognitive schema.

4. **Focusing on problem-solving.** A primary task of crisis intervention is the identification and prioritization of immediate problems. Once achieved, interventions focus on assisting those involved to find short-term solutions.

5. **Encouraging self-reliance.** Encouraging and supporting individuals to participate in identifying and solving problems facilitate their return to independent function and the development of a sense of mastery (Flannery & Everly, 2000).

The case study in Box 17.2 uses Roberts' Seven-Stage Crisis Intervention Model (Fig. 17.7; Roberts, 1991) to illustrate the application of these principles to a clinical situation.

BOX 17.2 Case Study Demonstrating Roberts' Seven-Stage Crisis Intervention Model

The mobile mental health crisis unit in a large Canadian city receives a call from Theresa, the maternal aunt of 19-year-old Billy, an Aboriginal male whose 12-year-old brother died 4 months ago from sniffing gasoline. On hearing of his brother's death, Billy quit college and went on a 5-day drinking binge. At the time of the call, he is lying on his bed in the dark. Theresa tells the crisis nurse that Billy has been eating very little for the past several weeks and has been sleeping 12 to 14 hours/day. He rarely leaves his room and speaks only when addressed directly. What little conversation he does offer is preoccupied with his brother and their parents, who died in a car crash a number of years earlier. Theresa has tried everything she can think of to convince Billy to get help; she is worried about leaving him alone for fear he will harm himself.

STAGE 1: **Conduct Crisis and Bio/Psycho/Social/ Spiritual Assessment (Including Lethality Assessment).** Joanne, the crisis intervention nurse, performs a focused assessment and, using direct questions, ascertains important details about the situation (e.g., caller name, address, and telephone number; nature of emergency; presence of/potential for injury or loss of life; availability of weapons or other potentially dangerous items). Within 2 or 3 minutes, she determines that Billy has experienced major losses (one of them very recently), that his behaviour is suggestive of acute mourning and/or depression, that he is at high risk for self-harm, and that his aunt, who is his primary social support, has exhausted her resources for dealing with the situation. The nurse tells Theresa that she and a colleague are on their way to talk with Billy and that they will be bringing police assistance. The nurse decides to involve the police for two reasons. The first is that by their nature, crises are unpredictable situations and have some potential for violence; a police presence sometimes deters aggressive acting out, and if it does not, it ensures that there are trained personnel to effectively contain it. The second reason is that the police have authority, under provincial mental health legislation, to transport individuals for psychiatric assessment, even against their will. In order to do this, they must have evidence that the individual is in imminent danger to himself or herself or someone else.

STAGE 2: **Establish Rapport and a Working Therapeutic Relationship.** Joanne establishes rapport with Theresa on the telephone by listening carefully to her, validating her concerns, and offering concrete and specific assistance. When the nurse and other members of the crisis team arrive at the home, Joanne stays with Theresa while her colleague Don begins talking with Billy through his locked bedroom door. Don uses his well-developed interpersonal skills (see Chapter 6) to make a connection with the young man and to convince him to come out of his room and talk face-to-face. When it becomes apparent that Billy is not a danger to himself or others, the police leave.

STAGE 3: **Identify Dimensions of Presenting Problem.** Fortunately, when the crisis team speaks with Billy, they learn that he has not done anything to harm himself. He is experiencing a great deal of emotional pain for which he has few words, has lost his sense of meaning in life, and has only a vague plan of shooting himself. He does not have immediate access to a firearm. In his conversation with Don, Billy acknowledges that the loss of his parents was devastating, but it is his brother's death that caused his "world to crash apart."

STAGE 4: **Explore Feelings and Emotions.** Don encourages Billy to talk about his experience and offers him words for the things he is feeling. Eventually, Billy agrees to include his aunt and Joanne in the conversation.

STAGE 5: **Generate and Explore Alternatives.** Billy, Theresa, Don, and Joanne sit around the kitchen table with cups of tea discussing the supports available to the family.

STAGE 6: **Develop a Plan.** Theresa states that praying to the creator every day and speaking to a local elder help her to get through many difficult times. Billy says that he will pray with her every day, signs a written safety contract, and agrees to see an intake worker at the mental health centre for an assessment the next day. The safety contract specifies a number of things that Billy will do if he begins to feel overwhelmed again, including praying, talking to Theresa, and calling the crisis line.

STAGE 7: **Develop a Follow-Up Plan.** Joanne calls Theresa the next afternoon and learns that she and Billy had spent the evening talking and praying together. He had eaten breakfast and showered this morning before attending his appointment at the mental health centre. The intake worker referred Billy to a men's grief support group and was going to speak with the student counselling service at his college to arrange one-to-one counselling.

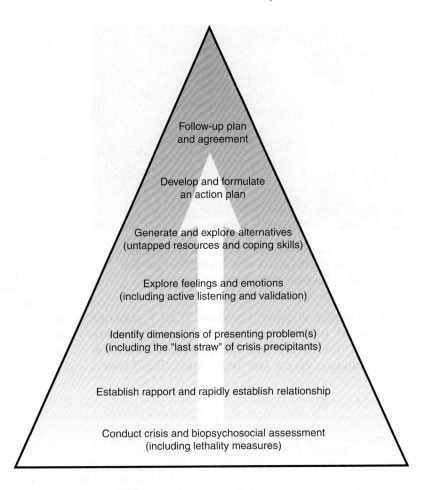

Follow-up plan
and agreement

Develop and formulate
an action plan

Generate and explore alternatives
(untapped resources and coping skills)

Explore feelings and emotions
(including active listening and validation)

Identify dimensions of presenting problem(s)
(including the "last straw" of crisis precipitants)

Establish rapport and rapidly establish relationship

Conduct crisis and biopsychosocial assessment
(including lethality measures)

Figure 17.7. Roberts' (1991) Seven-Stage Crisis Intervention Model.

Telephone Help Lines

Many health authorities now have telephone help lines, typically staffed by mental health professionals or trained volunteers, which offer support for problems such as child abuse, suicide, and family stress. These lines permit immediate access to a spectrum of support and intervention services for individuals who are experiencing a crisis or need help to manage life stressors.

Short-Stay Hospitalization and Community-Based Emergency Housing

Some health authorities also designate a few beds on their psychiatric units for short-stay crisis stabilization. Individuals are admitted to these beds for a brief period of inpatient care (typically 72 hours) when they have no supports in the community, need to have their medications assessed or stabilized, or require some other health service. Community-based emergency housings, such as shelters for children and youth who cannot remain at home, shelters for victims of domestic violence, and short- and long-term accommodations for individuals with serious and persistent mental illness, are also often available. These settings provide users with food, a place to stay, emotional support, and referrals to other community services.

■ RESPONSE TO DISASTER

Disasters are sudden, severe, and social phenomena. Defined, a disaster occurs when a hazard, originating in the geophysical or biologic environment or as the result of unintentional or malicious human action, exceeds a community's ability to cope (Ministers Responsible for Emergency Management, 2011). Disaster events have far-reaching effects. Malicious acts of terrorism have the greatest impact on mental health morbidity, while disasters caused by human and technologic error have a more moderate impact, and natural disasters have the least (Math, Kumar, Christine, & Cherian, 2013). Any disaster can cause extensive and sustained social and mental health problems, and challenge the resilience of all those affected. When the Fort McMurray wildfire occurred in May 2016, it necessitated the evacuation of all 88,000 residents and became Canada's most expensive natural disaster with recovery costs in billions of dollars (see Fig. 17.8). Although there was a vehicle collision in which two teenagers died on their journey away from the fire, amazingly, there were no deaths directly attributable to the fire. The psychological and social costs of this disaster, however, are incalculable and have the potential to affect the emergency responders and residents of Fort McMurray for years.

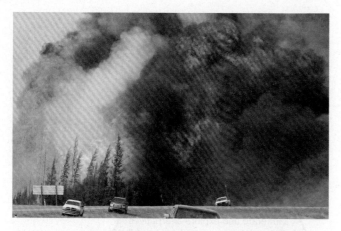

Figure 17.8. A giant fireball rips through the forest south of Fort McMurray, Alberta, May 7, 2016. (Photo: The Canadian Press/Jonathan Hayward, with permission.)

The Canada Disaster Database (CDC) contains information on disasters that have occurred since 1900 that directly affected Canadians and tracks significant disaster events (see Web Links). The disasters are categorized in the CDC as natural, conflict, or technology (see Table 17.5 for types of disasters). Disaster management needs to be intersectoral, be community based, and involve planning, mitigation, response, and recovery. Avoidance of disaster through prevention measures is critical, given the human and financial cost of these catastrophic events. The psychosocial and mental health aspects of disaster management and response must be integrated in a holistic way across the phases of disaster management rather than as an auxiliary endeavour.

KEY CONCEPT

A **disaster** is a social phenomenon that occurs when a hazard, originating in the geophysical or biologic environment or as the result of unintentional or malicious human action, exceeds a community's ability to cope (Ministers Responsible for Emergency Management, 2011).

Table 17.5	Types of Disasters With Selected Examples in Canada		
Natural			
	Biologic		
		Epidemic	March–August 2003
			SARS outbreak, 44 deaths, most in city of Toronto
		Infestation	October 2005
			Escherichia coli bacteria found in water supply of the Kashechewan reserve. 1,100 people evacuated, 74 people hospitalized
		Pandemic	
	Meteorologic–hydrologic		
		Avalanche	January–April 2003
			Rocky Mountains along the British Columbia–Alberta border experience deadliest avalanche season in over 30 years. Thirty people killed
		Cold Event	In 1947 in Snag, Yukon, temperatures dropped to −63°C, the lowest temperature recorded in North America. It is said that breath exhaled froze, making a hissing sound (The Canadian Encyclopedia, 2013).
		Drought	1990
			Parts of the Prairies stricken by cereal crop drought, estimated losses of half a billion dollars
		Flood	June 2013
			Worst flood in Alberta's history—4 people killed, 100,000 people displaced, damages estimated over $5 billion
		Hurricane	August 2011
			Tropical storm Irene hits Québec and the Maritime provinces. Power outages throughout the region, two people killed
		Tornado	June 2010
			An F2 tornado destroys 50 homes and causes $15 million worth of damage around the town of Midland, ON.
		Wildfire	May 2016 Wildfire at Fort McMurray, Alberta. Entire community of 88,000 evacuated with the fire causing billions of dollars in damages but, incredibly, no person died or was seriously injured.
		Winter storm	December 2010
			Canadian Forces assist Ontario Provincial Police in rescuing 237 motorists stranded on a highway in Lambton County. One man dies of exposure.
	Geologic		
		Earthquake	June 2010
			5.0-strength earthquake near Val-de-Bois, QC. A bridge collapses and a highway is closed. Three hundred houses lose power and a state of emergency is called.

Table 17.5   Types of Disasters With Selected Examples in Canada (*Continued*)

	Landslide	January 2005
		Landslide of mud, debris, and snow destroys two homes in North Vancouver. One person is killed and 100 homes are evacuated.
	Tsunami	
Conflict		
	Arson	January 1980
		Arsonists set fire to a social club in Chibougamau, QC, killing 45 people and injuring 55.
	Civil event	June 2011
		Hockey fans take to the streets of Vancouver, rioting, burning, and looting. Hundred and forty people taken to hospital with minor injuries, four serious injuries
	Hijacking	
	Terrorist	May 1984
		Shooting at the National Assembly of Québec kills 3 and injures 13.
Technologic		
	Fire	July 2007
		Hundreds of Edmonton residents affected by "wall of fire" that sweeps through neighbourhood, destroying 18 townhomes and damaging 76 more
	Hazardous chemicals	
	Infrastructure failure	August 2003
		Fifty million people throughout Ontario and the eastern United States affected by blackout (with power outages lasting over 48 h) caused by sagging transmission lines and untrimmed trees in Ohio
	Transportation	August 2011
		Flight en route from Yellowknife, NT, to Resolute Bay, NU, strikes a hill and crashes, killing four crewmembers and eight passengers.
	Explosion	July 2013
		Train carrying crude oil derails in the town of Lac-Mégantic, QC. Explosions kill 42 people, 5 missing and presumed dead. Half the town's centre is destroyed.
	Space event	January 1978
	Space launch	Space debris falls upon the Northwest Territories.

Adapted from the Canadian Disaster Database. (2017). *List of event types*. Retrieved from http://cdd.publicsafety.gc.ca/srchpg-eng.aspx; with information from The Canadian Encyclopedia. (2013). *Extreme-weather-in-Canada*. Retrieved from http://www.thecanadianencyclopedia.ca/en/article/extreme-weather-in-canada-feature/

Emergency Preparedness and Response

Role of the United Nations

The United Nations Office for Disaster Risk Reduction's (UNISDR) role is to work with nations to reduce natural hazards and their impact. This is a very important role given that among the top global risks in terms of likelihood are extreme weather events and major natural disaster events (World Economic Forum, 2017).

Disaster risk reduction involves analyzing and decreasing causal factors of disaster by decreasing exposure, reducing vulnerability, and increasing resiliency to hazards, improving preparation and early warning abilities regarding adverse events, and identifying wise approaches to sustaining the environment and usage of land and water (UNISDR, 2015a). The UNISDR publishes a global assessment report of disaster risk and management every 2 years. A global plan for disaster risk reduction is outlined in the Sendai Framework 2015–2030 using four priorities: understanding disaster risk; strengthening disaster risk governance; investing in resilience (economic, social, health, and cultural) of persons, communities, countries, and the environment;

and improving disaster preparedness in response, recovery, rehabilitation, and reconstruction (using a "build back better" approach) (UNISDR, 2015b). In Montréal in 2017, Canada hosted a meeting of countries and territories in the Americas where a regional disaster risk plan, aligned with the Sendai Framework, was endorsed (Public Safety Canada, 2017). Nurses across the Americas and the globe have a role in enhancing health infrastructure resilience and preparedness, as well as in the promotion of gender equitable and universally accessible (e.g., includes persons with disabilities) disaster preparedness, from response to reconstruction.

Role of Government

Canadians can expect their federal, provincial, and territorial governments to help them and their communities to mitigate and prepare for disaster and to assist them during such an event. When a disaster occurs here, our federal government mobilizes resources, coordinated through Public Safety and Preparedness Canada, when assistance is requested or when more than one province or territory is involved. Public Safety Canada is responsible for national policy, standards, and response systems related to disaster. The Public Health Agency of Canada's Centre for Emergency Preparedness and Response (CEPR) has information for the public concerning response to chemical, biologic, radiologic, and nuclear threats, as well as scenarios illustrating a natural and a possible bioterrorism threat and CEPR's role (see Web Links).

Health Canada is responsible for providing emergency health care to First Nations and Inuit communities, for working to decrease the adverse effects (health, economic) due to disaster, as well as for coordination of the response to a nuclear or radiologic emergency. Environmental and workplace health, including in emergencies and disasters, is also an area of activity (see Chapter 16 for information on emergencies in the workplace). Provincial and territorial governments' responsibilities, policies, and disaster plans can be found on their public Web sites. For example, British Columbia's disaster psychosocial response planning and delivery are addressed on their Web site (see Web Links).

Canada assists other nations in times of disaster and shares resources and information related to disaster mitigation, responsiveness, and recovery. For instance, Canada is a member of the International Initiative for Mental Health Leadership in which countries (e.g., Australia, New Zealand, England, United States) work together to improve mental health components of disaster planning and response.

Role of Nurses

Health care professionals play a key role across all phases of disaster: planning, mitigation, response, and recovery. Their society depends upon them to respond responsibly in times of disaster, with skill and expertise; they depend upon their society to reduce the risks they encounter in doing so (e.g., provision of antivirals, protective equipment, risk management protocols) and to plan for recovery and support in the aftermath (e.g., life and disability insurance; practical support). This reciprocal relationship must be evident in the planning phase onward, including the identification of threats to health care staff and their families and ways to mitigate them (e.g., child and elder care facilities for responders' family during a disaster).

The Canadian Nurses Association's (CNA, 2017) *Code of Ethics for Registered Nurses* identifies, as an obligation, nurses' **duty to provide care** (with appropriate precautions) during a disaster, communicable disease outbreak or pandemic. It is acknowledged that there may be circumstances when it is acceptable for a nurse to withdraw or refuse to provide care. The concept of unreasonable burden, such as ongoing threats to personal and family well-being, informs this decision. The Code provides examples of ethical decision-making models to assist the individual nurse and CNA's (2008) *Ethical*

Considerations for Nurses in a Natural or Human-Made Disaster, Communicable Disease Outbreak or Pandemic, part of the *Ethics in Practice for Registered Nurses* series, is a further resource.

The severe acute respiratory syndrome (SARS) global outbreak in 2003 is an example of the dangers nurses can face: 43% of the 251 confirmed cases in Canada were health care workers; three died and others were left with physical and psychosocial ailments, including respiratory problems and PTSD (O'Sullivan, 2009). A study of nurses' experiences during the SARS epidemic found that nurses did not feel prepared for a large-scale disaster and that they experienced role conflict as they put their families at risk (O'Sullivan et al., 2008). A relational ethics approach, with its focus on relationship, environmental context, ethical decisions as embodied actions, and the importance of dialogue, may be particularly useful to nurses in preparation for and response to disaster (Austin, 2008). CNA's (2012) position statement on emergency preparation and response supports the International Council of Nurses' (ICN) demand that nurses use strategies that respect human rights, social justice, and equity of access to health and social services for those affected by disaster (World Health Organization and the International Council of Nurses, 2009).

As the largest group in the health care workforce, it is highly problematic that nurses do not believe that they are sufficiently prepared to respond to disaster events; those who do feel prepared are those with previous participation in a disaster or disaster training (Labrague et al., 2017) (see Box 17.3). Optimally, nurses should have the basic knowledge and skills required in disaster response and public health emergencies, promote preparedness among their community and within the organization in which they practice, and be proactive at enhancing their professional competence in this area (e.g., participation in drills, disaster exercises) (Veenema et al., 2016). Nurses need to be involved across all aspects of disaster planning if they are to be fully cognizant of their roles and responsibilities when a disaster event occurs (Labrague et al., 2017).

Role of Individuals and Families

Public Safety Canada in collaboration with other government and nongovernment agencies has a *Get Prepared* initiative that assists Canadians and their families to prepare for the first 3 days following a disaster event. *Get Prepared* has three main components: know the risks and get prepared, make an emergency plan, and get an emergency kit. Guides to doing so, as well as a list of federal–provincial–territorial resources, are available for free (see Web Links); there is an emergency plan guide for persons with disabilities or special needs. A mobile "get prepared" site provides key steps to follow in particular types of emergencies such as floods, wildfires, and so on, as well as how to respond to an evacuation order (see Web Links).

BOX 17.3 Research for Best Practice

NURSE PREPAREDNESS FOR DISASTER

Labrague, L. J., Hammad, K., Gloe, D. S., McEnroe-Petitte, D. M., Fronda, D. C., Obeidat, A. A., ... Miranfurentes, E. C. (2017). Disaster preparedness among nurses: A systematic review of literature. International Nursing Review, *March 14. doi:10.1111/inr.12369 (Epub ahead of print).*

Question: Does research indicate that nurses are prepared for disaster response?

Method: A systematic review of the literature was conducted in which peer-reviewed publications from 2006 to 2016, which measured nurses' preparedness for disaster response, were explored. Primary databases used were SCOPUS, MEDLINE, PubMed, CINAHL, and PsycINFO. Seventeen articles were selected from 332 articles based on relevancy and methodologic soundness. All selected studies used a cross-sectional research design with a survey approach using questionnaires, with *n* ranging from 164 to 2647.

Findings: The research indicates that nurses are not sufficiently prepared for effective disaster response and do not feel confident in their ability to respond. The 2008 study of Canadian nurses, by O'Sullivan and colleagues and included in this review, indicated that most of the 685 nurse participants were uncertain whether or not their workplace had adequate institutional policies and programs for large-scale disasters. Increased confidence in response ability is associated with previous experience in a disaster event and with disaster-related training. Exercises that mimic actual events are viewed as particularly effective in training.

Implication for Practice: Nurses must be prepared for disaster if they are to ethically enact their role in mitigating the negative effects of disaster events on affected populations. Nursing education and health care organizations, as well as individual nurses, need to act if nurses are to overcome this deficit in their readiness to respond in times of public crisis and trauma.

As well as educating individuals and families in getting prepared for disaster, nurses have an obligation themselves to "anticipate, deliberate, and prepare" for disaster (CNA, 2008; WHO & ICN, 2009). They need to ensure that they and their family are prepared to cope on their own for 72 hours in the event of a disaster situation.

Phases of Disaster

Although the experience of disaster is unique to each individual and community, various phases of disaster can be delineated. It is important to recognize such phases (e.g., preparation, response, recovery, mitigation) as multilayered, complex, and influenced by the interaction of persons–community–environment rather than as discrete and constant categories. Phases of disaster focused on possible psychological and social responses from 1 to 3 days to 1 to 3 years are shown in Figure 17.9.

There are critical factors of disaster that can potentially shape aftermath reactions and postdisaster stress. These include causation (natural or human), degree of personal impact, size and scope, visible impact/low point, and the probability of recurrence (DeWolfe, 2000). When human intent causes a disaster (e.g., bombing), the stress reaction is greater than when the cause is "natural" (an "act of God"). Causes are not always clearly defined, such as when environmental degradation contributes to flooding. If an individual has high exposure to a disaster event or intimate personal loss, the disaster impact will usually be more intense; a disaster that destroys an entire community will have more negative and lasting impact than one of lesser scope. The recovery process is impeded when disasters are neither clearly visible nor defined (i.e., there is no "it's over and the rebuilding begins" moment), as in the case of toxic spills and nuclear accidents. With such disasters, the devastating consequences continue for years, resulting in chronic stress, fear, and anxiety. When there is a high probability that a disaster will reoccur in a community, the ongoing threat will affect recovery, particularly if disaster mitigation is not occurring (DeWolfe, 2000).

An international review of the effects of disaster on over 60,000 individuals in 102 different events indicates that effects are the greatest when two of the following are present:

- Extreme and widespread property damage.
- Serious and ongoing finance problems for the community.
- Human intent was the cause.
- High prevalence of trauma: injuries, loss of life (Norris, Friedman, & Watson, 2002, p. 246).

The spiritual impact that loss of home, possessions, community, and sense of belonging can have is difficult to quantify and to address (Hagen & Hagen, 2013).

Response to Mental Health and Illness in a Disaster

Natural recovery processes and community-based sources of help are foundational to disaster response. Research indicates that social cohesion in a community

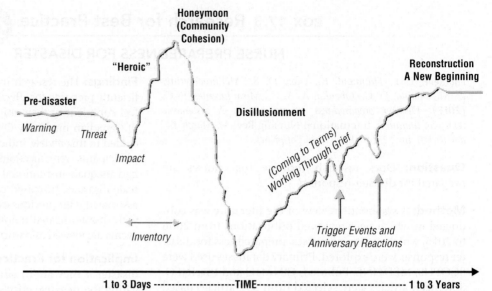

Figure 17.9. Sociopsychologic phases of disaster. (Reprinted from Zunin, L. M., & Meyers, D. (2000). *Phases of disaster: Training manual for human service workers in major disasters* (2nd ed., p. 5). Washington, DC: Department of Health and Human Services, Substance Abuse and Mental Health Services Administration, Center for Mental Health Services; DHHS Publication No. ADM 90-538.)

increases its resilience to disaster and is associated with a significant decrease in psychological distress (Greene, Paranjothy, & Palmer, 2015). Disaster events can increase social cohesion within a community (Cocking, 2013). The everyday cooperation of community members as survivors are comforted, fed, sheltered, and supported is as important as heroic acts and crucial to recovery. It is helpful to keep people in their normal groups if relocation is necessary and to facilitate their return to normal activities as soon as possible; disaster response should not undermine natural helping networks (Norris et al., 2002).

Key to community-level disaster response is the provision of accurate, timely information that allows informed action in meeting the rapidly changing circumstances inherent to disasters. In Canada, there is mandatory broadcaster participation in the public alerting system regarding disaster. Social networking (e.g., YouTube, Facebook, Twitter) has the potential to facilitate communication in times of disaster: it is broad in reach, user-friendly, and free. Nevertheless, there remain privacy, information accuracy, and trustworthiness concerns related to its use (Trainer & Goel, 2013). Information after disaster should be brief, basic, and focused on promoting coping among survivors. Three components to such information are recommended: reassurance and explanation about normal, to-be-expected reactions; advice to return to daily routines as soon as possible; and guidance regarding where to find help if needed (European Commission, 2008).

Psychological First Aid

The common model for mental health care delivery following a disaster is **psychological first aid** (PFA) (Rodriquez & Kohn, 2008; WHO, War Trauma Foundation, & World Vision International, 2011). As with medical first aid, PFA involves intervention with the purpose of immediate relief of distress and the

prevention of pathologic sequelae and can be performed by prepared nonprofessionals (Math et al., 2013). PFA competency domains have been identified as establishing rapport and stabilization at initial contact, performing screening and assessment, intervening in acute distress and fostering coping, triage for immediate or delayed care, referring/advocating for those requiring more intensive care, and being self-aware and self-caring (McCabe et al., 2014).

Much of the distress experienced by individuals at such times will be normative (i.e., grief, anger, and stress related to the trauma of a disaster event) and not require professional treatment (Prewitt Diaz, 2013). PFA involves promoting five key responses: sense of safety, calming, sense of self and community efficacy, connectedness, and hope (Hobfoll, Watson, & Bell, 2007; Prewitt Diaz, 2013). Hope for recovery can be supported through practical action: the provision of necessary services, housing and relocation, replacement of household goods, and employment help (Prewitt Diaz, 2013). See Table 17.6 for public health principles for disaster interventions.

The indications that an individual is not successfully coping with stress following a disaster event and may need assistance with stress management are listed in Box 17.4. Although it was once believed that PTSD, the mental disorder most often diagnosed in disaster-affected communities, could be prevented by psychological debriefing, the evidence now indicates otherwise. Single-session debriefing may even be harmful (European Commission, 2008). Professional help may be required for those experiencing persistent and complex grieving (Math et al., 2013).

Vulnerable Populations in Disaster

There are persons who are particularly "at risk" in a disaster situation. These include persons with communication difficulties (e.g., those who do not speak the area's

Table 17.6   Public Health Principles for Disaster Interventions (Early to Midterm)

Safety	Bring people to a safe place as much as possible.
	Provide accurate and organized information to help avoid threat.
	Advise media to enhance safety and resilience perceptions over threat.
	Monitor news exposure to children.
Calming	Help people directly solve concerns.
	Give information regarding safety of family and friends and if further danger is expected.
	Provide broad-scale outreach and psychoeducation using media, Web sites, and presentations.
	Giving false information to calm community is counterproductive and undermines credibility.
Self- and collective efficacy	Provide resources to restore dignity and losses and to rebuild.
	Involve those affected in decision-making policy and efforts to build self- and collective efficacy.
	Support activities conceived and implemented by the community.
	Support families who are often the main providers of mental health care after disasters.
Connectedness	Help individuals, particularly children, to reconnect with loved ones and neighbours.
	Conceive of temporary housing and assistance as "villages."
	Address negative social influences as much as possible.
Hope	Create advocacy programs to deal with "red tape" and the complex tasks that follow disaster.
	Support rebuilding of local economies.
	Involve community leaders in helping link the community with those who survived similar disasters, in memorializing and making meaning, and in helping people adapt to the change in their lives and environment, to build on their strengths.

Adapted from Hobfoll, S. E., Watson, P., & Bell, C. C. (2007). Five essential elements of immediate and mid-term mass trauma intervention: Empirical evidence. *Psychiatry, 70*, 283–315; Rodriquez, J. J., & Kohn, R. (2008). Use of mental health services among disaster survivors. *Current Opinion in Psychiatry, 21*, 370–378.

dominant language), those who are physically impaired (e.g., visually, hearing, mobility), those who are cognitively or psychologically impaired, those who are geographically or culturally isolated, and those who lack a

---

BOX 17.4   Indicators of Need for Assistance with Stress Management After a Traumatic Event

The following signs occurring for more than 2 to 4 weeks indicate that assistance with stress may be necessary:

Confusion; disorientation

Problems concentrating; short attention span

Changes in ability to see or hear

Becoming easily frustrated; continuous crying; frequent mood swings

Feelings of hopelessness

Overwhelming self-doubt and/or feelings of guilt

Reluctance to leave home

Fear of crowds, strangers, or being alone

Increased use of alcohol and/or other drugs, including prescription medication

Existing medical problems worsening

Adapted from Substance Abuse and Mental Health Services Administration. (2013). *Tips for survivors of a disaster or traumatic event: What to expect in your personal, family, work and financial life.* Rockville, MA: Author.

---

means of transportation when evacuation becomes necessary (Hagen & Hagen, 2013, p. 582). Issues for some at-risk populations are described below.

Aboriginal Peoples and Disaster

As Aboriginal communities in Canada are often geographically remote, as well as too often marginalized and dealing with poverty and lack of health and social services, they may be particularly vulnerable to disaster events. Problems that increase vulnerability have been lack of funding for on-reserve mitigation efforts and a complicated process for securing the necessary federal financial support after a disaster (Puxley, 2013). Getting the communities the necessary resources in a timely and culturally sensitive way seems key to good recovery, as the collective wisdom of many Aboriginal communities regarding survival in adverse conditions is already strong. Increasingly, experts are recognizing that lessons are to be learned from such traditional knowledge, lessons that can inform effective disaster management as a whole (Hagen & Hagen, 2013).

Notions of healing and tradition are central to contemporary efforts to confront the legacy of injustices and suffering brought on by colonization (Kirmayer, Brass, & Valaskakis, 2009). Any approach to health services with Aboriginal people must consider ongoing uses of tradition in the community and local efforts to assert cultural identity (Kirmayer et al., 2009). Indigenous researchers and scholars have expressed the need for multilevel assessment and intervention strategies to address factors related to health and wellness at individual, family, and community levels (Brave Heart et al., 2011; Evans-Campbell, 2008). A long-term goal of historical trauma intervention research and practice is to reduce inequities faced by indigenous people by developing culturally responsive interventions driven by communities to improve quality of life and well-being. Through individual and community-based initiatives, as well as larger political and cultural processes, aboriginal people in Canada are involved in healing their traditions, repairing the ruptures and discontinuities in the transmission of traditional knowledge and values, and asserting their collective identity and power.

Children and Adolescents

Children and adolescents will be strongly influenced in their response to disaster by the reactions of the adults around them. As with adults, assessment of children's and adolescents' reactions to a disaster event and their resulting mental health needs involves two components: screening and then clinical evaluation for those who are identified during screening as at risk for psychiatric disturbance, and for those who (or whose family/close associates) were directly exposed to the disaster (Pfefferbaum & North, 2013). PFA and related psychosocial interventions, such as use of play and art activities, can be effective in addressing normative psychological distress. Involving adolescents appropriately in disaster response tasks can help mitigate their distress. When clinical evaluation is required, it will involve a diagnostic assessment for psychopathology (such as PTSD) and the need for referral to professional care (Pfefferbaum & North, 2013).

Persons With an Existing Mental Disorder

As well as those individuals who develop mental health problems or symptoms of mental disorders (e.g., PTSD) as a result of experiencing a disaster event, persons with existing psychiatric disorders are at high risk for exacerbation of their symptoms, for poor emergency coping responses, and for difficulty achieving good recovery from their experience (Hagen & Hagen, 2013). During a disaster, mental health care infrastructures may be seriously damaged, displacing the resources normally accessed for ongoing care at a time when the need for services increases. The WHO (2013) projects that, during emergencies, rates of severe mental disorder among adult populations increase from preemergency rates of 2% to 3% to 4% to 5% and mild mental disorders from 10% to 15% to 20%. It is important that PTSD is not exclusively the focus in disaster management so that persons with other mental disorders, including addictions, will also receive assistance.

Disabled Persons

The disruption of infrastructure and support systems during a disaster disproportionally affects persons with disabilities: they are more likely to be left behind in evacuations, and disability can be a discriminating factor in allocation of scarce resources. The needs and perspectives of persons with disabilities must be included across all phases of disaster management if their vulnerability and risk are to be reduced. Article 11 in the United Nations Convention on the Rights of Persons with Disabilities (United Nations, 2006) identifies the obligation of nations to do so. Public Safety Canada's Emergency Preparedness Guide for People with Disabilities/Special Needs provides information about emergency packs, resources, and tips for helping persons with disabilities/special needs and addresses particular types of disability (e.g., mobility, hearing, vision, nonvisible disabilities like mental illness, heart disease) (see Web Links).

Ethnic Minorities

The symptoms of stress, anxiety disorders, and PTSD are identical across cultures (European Commission, 2008). Stress and distress can be reduced if disaster response information to ethnic minority communities is available in their mother tongue and if recovery efforts are culturally appropriate and involve key community figures. When possible, responders should adapt their approach to a person's culture. Things to consider include gender issues, touching, need for certain clothing items, and religious beliefs that will influence the meaning given to the disaster event (WHO et al., 2011).

Disaster Relief Workers

Volunteers are a major source of rescue and recovery assistance in times of disaster. The research on the postdisaster mental health of volunteer responders indicates that, compared with professional workers, volunteers have higher complaint levels, with the factors contributing to this being determined as "identification with victims as a friend, severity of exposure to gruesome events during disaster work, anxiety sensitivity, and lack of post-disaster social support" (Thormar et al., 2010, p. 529).

Summary

It is important that nurses understand the human experience of stress, crisis, and trauma so that they may respond appropriately to individuals, families, and communities in need. Such knowledge is important to nurses' professional self-development, as well, so that they can be confident and safe as they meet the challenges of health care practice. Being prepared to respond to disaster events is a responsibility that nurses share with other professionals; such preparation requires institutional support. Despite the adversity and challenges that disasters bring, there is also opportunity at such times to positively transform a community's approach to mental health care (WHO, 2013).

 SUMMARY OF KEY POINTS

- Many personal factors, such as personality patterns, beliefs, values, and commitment to an outcome, interact with environmental demands and constraints that produce a person–environment relationship.

- Stress occurs when a person–environment relationship is appraised as being unfavourable. Stress responses are simultaneously emotional and physiologic, leading to an innate tendency to act.
- Within the social network, social support can help a person cope with stress.
- Effective coping can be either problem focused or emotion focused. The outcome of successful coping is enhanced health, psychological well-being, and social functioning.
- A crisis is a severely stressful situation that causes exaggerated stress responses. The nursing process is similar for the person experiencing a stress response, except that increased attention is paid to safety issues.
- Nurses have an obligation to respond competently across all phases of disasters: planning, mitigation, response, and recovery. Nursing educators and administrators have a responsibility to assist nurses in achieving this competency.
- Natural recovery processes and community-based sources of help are foundational to successful disaster response and need to be supported. Timely information is key.
- Psychological first aid (PFA) is the common model for mental health delivery following a disaster.

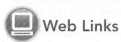 **Web Links**

www.getprepared.gc.ca The Government of Canada's public safety site, where "'72 Hours' Is your family prepared?" and other resources are freely available.

www.health.gov.on.ca/en/pro/programs/emb/pan_flu/pan_flu_plan.aspx An example of a governmental influenza pandemic plan (Ontario's) is available at this site.

www.health.gov.bc.ca/emergency/dstrs.html This is British Columbia's disaster psychosocial services Web site.

www.phac-aspc.gc.ca/cepr-cmiu/scenario-eng.php Two scenarios depicting disaster response by the Centre for Emergency Preparedness and Response (CEPR) can be found at this site.

www.publicsafety.gc.ca/cdd The Canada Disaster Database can be accessed here.

www.samhsa.gov/nctic/trauma-interventions This site describes six key principles of a trauma-informed approach.

www.http://trauma-informed.ca The Manitoba Trauma Information Centre is a resource for promoting trauma-informed relationships and practices.

ACKNOWLEDGEMENTS

The author thanks Flint Schwartz (MA) for his valuable contributions.

References

Aguilera, D. C. (1998). *Crisis intervention: Theory and methodology* (8th ed.). St. Louis, MO: Mosby.

Allan, B., & Smylie, J. (2015). *First Peoples, second class treatment: The role of racism in the health and well-being of Indigenous peoples in Canada*. Toronto, Canada: Wellesley Institute.

American Psychiatric Association (APA). (1980). *Diagnostic and statistical manual of mental disorders* (3rd ed). Washington, DC: Author.

American Psychiatric Association (APA). (1994). *Diagnostic and statistical manual of mental disorders* (4th ed.). Washington, DC: Author.

American Psychiatric Association (APA). (2013). *Diagnostic and statistical manual of mental disorders* (5th ed.). Washington, DC: Author.

Amstadter, A., Aggen, S., Knudsen, G. P., Reichborn-Kjennerud, T., & Kendler, F. (2013). Potentially traumatic event exposure, posttraumatic stress disorder, and Axis I and II comorbidity in a population-based study of Norwegian young adults. *Social Psychiatry and Psychiatric Epidemiology, 48*(2), 215–223.

Ardino, V. (2014). Trauma-informed care: Is cultural competence a viable solution for efficient policy strategies? *Clinical Neuropsychiatry, 11*(1), 45–51.

Austin, W. (2008). Relational ethics. In L. Given (Ed.), *The SAGE encyclopedia of qualitative research methods* (pp. 749–750). Thousand Oaks, CA: SAGE Publications, Inc.

Bartlett, D. (1998). *Stress: Perspectives and processes*. Philadelphia, PA: Open University Press.

Ben-Ari, A., & Strier, R. (2010). Rethinking cultural competence: What can we learn from Levinas? *British Journal of Social Work, 40*(7), 2155–2167. doi:10.1093/bjsw/bcp153

Birmes, P., Hatton, L., Brunet, A., & Schmitt, L. (2003). Early historical literature for post-traumatic symptomatology. *Stress and Health, 19*, 17–26.

Bombay, A., Matheson, K., & Anisman, H. (2009). Intergenerational trauma: Convergence of multiple processes among First Nations peoples in Canada. *Journal of Aboriginal Health, 5*(3), 6–47.

Bombay, A., Matheson, K., & Anisman, H. (2014a). The intergenerational effects of Indian Residential Schools: Implications for the concept of historical trauma. *Transcultural Psychiatry, 51*(3), 320–338.

Bombay, A., Matheson, K., & Anisman, H. (2014b). *Origins of lateral violence in aboriginal communities: A preliminary study of student-to-student abuse in Indian Residential Schools*. Ottawa, ON: Aboriginal Healing Foundation.

Bowers, M. E., & Yehuda, R. (2016). Intergenerational transmission of stress in humans. *Neuropsychopharmacology, 41*, 232–244.

Brave Heart, M. Y. H. (2003). The historical trauma response among natives and its relationship with substance abuse: A Lakota illustration. *Journal of Psychoactive Drugs, 35*, 7–13.

Brave Heart, M. Y., Chase, J., Elkins, J., & Altschul, D. B. (2011). Historical trauma among Indigenous Peoples of the Americas: concepts, research, and clinical considerations. *Journal of Psychoactive Drugs, 43*(4), 282–290.

Braveheart-Jordan, M., & DeBruyn, L. (1995). So she may walk in balance: Integrating the impact of historical trauma in the treatment of Native American Indian women. In J. Adleman & G. M. Enguidanos (Eds.), *Racism in the lives of women: Testimony, theory and guides to antiracist practice* (pp. 345–368). New York, NY: Haworth Press.

Braveman, P. A., Cubbin, C., Egerter, S., Williams, D. R., & Pamuk, E. (2010). Socioeconomic disparities in health in the United States: What the patterns tell us. *American Journal of Public Health, 100*(S1), S186–S196.

Browne, A. J., Varcoe, C., Smye, V., Reimer-Kirkham, S., Lynam, M. J., & Wong, S. (2009). Cultural safety and the challenges of translating critically oriented knowledge in practice. *Nursing Philosophy, 10*, 167–179. doi:10.1111/j.1466-769X.2009.00406.x

Browne, A. J., Varcoe, C. M., Wong, S. T., Smye, V. L., Lavoie, J., Littlejohn, D., … Fridkin, A. (2012). Closing the health equity gap: Evidence-based strategies for primary health care organizations. *International Journal for Equity in Health, 11*(1), 59.

Brunet, A., Monson, E., Lui, A., & Fikretoglu, D. (2015). Trauma exposure and posttraumatic stress disorder in the Canadian military. *The Canadian Journal of Psychiatry, 60*(11), 488–496. doi:10.1177/070674371506001104

Campbell, M. (1973). *Halfbreed*. Halifax, NS: Goodread Biographies.

Canadian Nurses Association. (2008). *Nurses' ethical considerations in a pandemic or other emergency*. Retrieved from http://www.cna-aiic.ca/~c/media/cna/page%20content/pdf%20en/2013/07/26/10/43/ethics_in_practice_august_2008_e.pdf

Canadian Nurses Association. (2012). *Position Statement (PS119): Emergency preparedness and response*. Toronto, ON: Authors.

Canadian Nurses Association. (2017). *Code of ethics for registered nurses*. Ottawa, ON: Author. https://www.cna-aiic.ca/en/on-the-issues/best-nursing/nursing-ethics#toc

Cannon, W. B. (1939). *The wisdom of the body*. New York, NY: WW Norton.

Caplan, G. (1961). *An approach to community mental health*. New York, NY: Grune & Stratton.

Caron, N. (2017, March). *Indigenous Health Interest Group*. Halifax, NS: Keynote address.

Carpenito-Moyet, L. J. (2017). *Nursing diagnosis: Application to clinical practice* (15th ed.). Philadelphia, PA: Wolters Kluwer.

Catani, C., Jacob, N., Schauer, E., Kohila, M., & Neuner, F. (2008). Family violence, war, and natural disasters: A study of the effect of extreme stress on children's mental health in Sri Lanka. *BMC Psychiatry, 8,* 33.

Center for the Advancement of Health. (2004). Report on bereavement and grief research. *Death Studies, 28,* 491–575.

Clements, B., & Casani, J. (2016). *Disasters and public health: Planning and response* (2nd ed.). Amsterdam, The Netherlands: Butterworth-Heineman/Elsevier.

Cocking, C. (2013). Collective resilience versus collective vulnerability after disasters: A social psychological perspective. In R. Arora & P. Arora (Eds.), *Disaster management: Medical preparedness, response and homeland security* (pp. 449–463). Wallingford, UK: CABI.

Cooper, G. L., & Dewe, P. (2004). *Stress: A brief history.* Malden, MA: Blackwell Publishing.

Coyne, J. C., & Holroyd, K. (1982). Stress, coping and illness: A transactional perspective. In T. Milton, C. Green, & R. Meagher (Eds.), *Handbook of clinical health psychology* (pp. 103–127). New York, NY: Plenum Press.

Davis, C. G., & Macdonald, S. L. (2004). Threat appraisals, distress and the development of positive life changes after September 11th in a Canadian sample. *Cognitive Behaviour Therapy, 33*(2), 68–78.

Dekel, R., & Goldblatt, H. (2008). Is there intergenerational transmission of trauma? The case of combat veterans' children. *American Journal of Orthopsychiatry, 78*(3), 281–289.

DeWolfe, D. J. (2000). *Training manual for mental health and human service workers in major disasters* (2nd ed.). Rockville, MD: Substance Abuse and Mental Health Services Administration (DHHS/PHS). Retrieved from http://www.samhsa.gov/dtac/FederalResource/Response/4-Training_Manual_MH_Workers.pdf

Dohrenwend, B. P., & Shrout, P. E. (1985). "Hassles" in the conceptualization and measurement of stress variables. *American Psychologist, 40*(7), 780–785.

Dohrenwend, B. S., & Dohrenwend, B. P. (1974). *Stressful life events: Their nature and their effects.* New York, NY: Wiley & Sons.

Dovidio, J. F., Penner, L. A., Albrecht, T. L., Norton, W. E., Gaertner, S. L., & Shelton, J. N. (2008). Disparities and distrust: The implications of psychological processes for understanding racial disparities in health and health care. *Social Science & Medicine, 67*(3), 478–486.

Duran, E., Duran, B., Brave Heart, M. Y. H., & Yellow Horse-Davis, S. (1998). Healing the American Indian Soul Wound. In Y. Danieli (Ed.), *International handbook of multigenerational legacies of trauma* (pp. 341–354). New York, NY: Plenum.

Elliott, D., Bjelajac, P., Fallot, R., Markoff, L., & Glover Reed, B. (2005). Trauma-informed or trauma-denied: Principles and implementation of trauma-informed services for women. *Journal of Community Psychology, 33*(4), 461–477.

Erikson, E. H. (1959). *Identity and the life cycle.* New York, NY: International Universities Press.

European Commission. (2008). *European multidisciplinary guideline: Early psychosocial interventions after disaster, terrorism and other shocking events.* Amsterdam, The Netherlands: Impact, the Dutch Knowledge & Advice Centre for Post-disaster Psychosocial Care.

Evans-Campbell, T. (2008). Historical trauma in American Indian/Native Alaska communities a multilevel framework for exploring impacts on individuals, families, and communities. *Journal of Interpersonal Violence, 23,* 316–338.

Flannery, R. B., & Everly, G. S. (2000). Crisis intervention: A review. *International Journal of Emergency Mental Health, 2*(2), 119–125.

Folkman, S., & Lazarus, R. S. (1991). The concept of coping. In A. Monat and & R. S. Lazarus (Eds.), *Stress and coping: An anthology* (3rd ed., pp. 209–227). New York, NY: Columbia University Press.

Furedi, F. (2007). The changing meaning of disaster. *Area, 39*(4), 482–489.

Gilligan, C. (1994). Joining the resistance: Psychology, politics, girls and women. In M. Berger (Ed.), *Women beyond Freud: New concept of feminine psychology* (pp. 99–145). New York, NY: Brunner Mazel.

Glaser, R., Rice, J., Sherridan, J., & Fertel, R. (1987). Stress-related immune suppression: Health implications. *Brain, Behavior, and Immunity, 1*(1), 7–20.

Grandjean, D., Rendu, A. -C., MacNamee, T., & Scherer, K. R. (2008). The wrath of the gods: Appraising the meaning of disaster. *Social Science Information, 47*(2), 187–204.

Green, A. R., Carney, D. R., Pallin, D. J., Ngo, L. H., Raymond, K. L., Iezzoni, L. I., & Banaji, M. R. (2007). Implicit bias among physicians and its prediction of thrombolysis decisions for Black and White patients. *Journal of General Internal Medicine, 22*(9), 1231–1238.

Greene, G., Paranjothy, S., & Palmer, S. R. (2015). Resilience and vulnerability to psychological harm from flooding: The role of social cohesion. *American Journal of Public Health, 105*(9), 1792–1796.

Hafer, C., & Bègue, L. (2005). Experimental research on just-world theory: Problems, developments, and future challenges. *Psychological Bulletin, 131*(1), 128–167.

Hagen, J., & Hagen, S. (2013). The immediate post-disaster reconstruction phase: Alternative care site settings and vulnerable populations. In R. Arora & P. Arora (Eds.), *Disaster management: Medical preparedness, response and homeland security* (pp. 575–590). Wallingford, UK: CABI.

Harper, D. (2001). *Online etymology dictionary.* Retrieved from http://www.etymonline.com

Harris, M., & Fallot, R. D. (2001). Envisioning a trauma-informed service system: A vital paradigm shift. *New Directions in Mental Health Services, 89,* 3–22.

Haskell, S., Gordon, K., Mattocks, K., Duggal, M., Erdos, J., Justice, A., & Brandt, C. (2010). Gender differences in rates of depression, PTSD, pain, obesity, and military sexual trauma among Connecticut war veterans of Iraq and Afghanistan. *Journal of Women's Health, 19*(2), 267–271.

Hobfoll, S. E., Watson, P., & Bell, C. C. (2007). Five essential elements of immediate and mid-term mass trauma intervention: Empirical evidence. *Psychiatry, 70,* 283–315.

Holmes, T., & Rahe, R. (1967). The social readjustment patient scale. *Journal of Psychosomatic Research, 11*(2), 213–218.

Huey Jr, S. J., Tilley, J. L., Jones, E. O., & Smith, C. A. (2014). The contribution of cultural competence to evidence-based care for ethnically diverse populations. *Annual Review of Clinical Psychology, 10,* 305–338.

Imel, Z. E., Baldwin, S., Atkins, D. C., Owen, J., Baardseth, T., & Wampold, B. E. (2011). Racial/ethnic disparities in therapist effectiveness: A conceptualization and initial study of cultural competence. *Journal of Counseling Psychology, 58*(3), 290.

Johnson, R. L., Saha, S., Arbelaez, J. J., Beach, M. C., & Cooper, L. A. (2004). Racial and ethnic differences in patient perceptions of bias and cultural competence in health care. *Journal of General Internal Medicine, 19*(2), 101–110.

Jones, F., & Kinman, G. (2001). Approaches to studying stress. In F. Jones, & J. Bright (Eds.), *Stress: Myth, theory & research* (pp. 17–44). London, UK: Prentice Hall.

Kelly, U. A., Skelton, K., Patel, M., & Bradley, B. (2011). More than military sexual trauma: Interpersonal violence, PTSD, and mental health in women veterans. *Research in Nursing and Health, 34*(6), 457–467.

Kirmayer, L., Brass, G., & Valaskakis, G. G. (2009). Conclusion: healing/intervention/tradition. In L. Kirmayer, & G. G. Valaskakis (Eds.), *Healing traditions: The mental health of Aboriginal Peoples in Canada* (pp. 440–472). Vancouver, BC: UBC Press.

Kirmayer, L. J., Shedev, M., Whitley, R., Dandeneau, S. F., & Isaac, C. (2009). Community resilience: Models, metaphors and measures. *Journal of Aboriginal Health, 5*(1), 62–117.

Kirmayer, L. J. (2012). Rethinking cultural competence. *Transcultural Psychiatry, 49,* 2, 149–164. doi:10.1177/1363461512444673

Kleinke, C. L. (2007). What does it mean to cope? In A. Monat, R. S. Lazarus, & G. Reevy (Eds.), *The Praeger handbook on stress and coping* (pp. 289–308). Westport, CT: Praeger.

Korte, S. M., Koolhaas, J. M., Wingfield, J. C., & McEwen, B. S. (2005). The Darwinian concept of stress: Benefits of allostasis and costs of allostatic load and the trade-offs in health and disease. *Neuroscience and Biobehavioral Reviews, 29*(1), 3–38.

Kronick, R. (2017). Mental health of refugees and asylum seekers: Assessment and intervention. *The Canadian Journal of Psychiatry,* e1–e7. doi:10.1177/0706743717746665

Kumagai, A. K., & Lypson, M. L. (2009). Beyond cultural competence: Critical consciousness, social justice, and multicultural education. *Academic Medicine, 84*(6), 782–787.

Kushner, H. (1981). *When bad things happen to good people.* New York, NY: Random House Inc.

Labrague, L. J., Hammad, K., Gloe, D. S., McEnroe-Petitte, D. M., Fronda, D. C., Obeidat, A. A., … Miranfurentes, E. C. (2017). Disaster preparedness among nurses: A systematic review of literature. *International Nursing Review,* March 14. doi:10.1111/inr.12369 (Epub ahead of print).

Lazarus, R. (1991). *Emotion and adaptation.* New York, NY: Oxford University Press.

Lazarus, R. S. (1998). *The life and work of an eminent psychologist: An autobiography of Richard S. Lazarus.* New York, NY: Springer.

Lazarus, R. S. (1999). *Stress and emotion: A new synthesis.* New York, NY: Springer.

Lazarus, R. S., DeLongis, A., Folkman, S., & Gruen, R. (1985). Stress and adaptation outcomes: The problem of confounded measures. *American Psychologist, 40*(7), 770–779.

Lazarus, R. S., & Folkman, S. (1984). *Stress, appraisal and coping.* New York, NY: Springer.

Lee, H. J., Macbeth, A. H., Pagani, J. H., & Young, W. S. (2009). Oxytocin: The great facilitator of life. *Progress in Neurobiology, 88*(2), 27–51.

Lee, T. Y., Cheung, C. K., & Kwong, W. M. (2012). Resilience as a positive youth development construct: A conceptual review. *Scientific World Journal, 2012*, 390450.

Lindeman, E. (1944). Symptomatology and management of acute grief. *American Journal of Psychiatry, 151*(6 Suppl.), 155–160.

Lindeman, E. (1956). The meaning of crisis in individual and family. *Teachers College Record, 57*, 310.

Linklater, R. (2014). *Decolonizing trauma work: Indigenous stories and strategies.* Blackpoint, NS & Winnipeg, Manitoba: Fernwood Publishing.

Lui, L. Y., Coe, C. L., Swenson, C. A., Kelly, E. A., Kita, H., & Busse, W. W. (2002). School examinations enhance airway inflammation to antigen challenge. *American Journal of Respiratory and Critical Care Medicine, 165*(8), 1062–1067.

Macy, R. D., Behar, L., Paulson, R., Delman, J., Schmid, L., & Smith, S. F. (2004). Community based, acute posttraumatic stress management: A description and evaluation of a psychosocial intervention continuum. *Harvard Review of Psychiatry, 12*, 217–228.

Maguen, S., Luxton, D., Skopp, N., & Madden, E. (2012). Gender differences in traumatic experiences and mental health in active duty soldiers redeployed from Iraq and Afghanistan. *Journal of Psychiatric Research, 46*, 311–316.

Malone, J. (1988). The social support and dissupport continuum. *Journal of Psychosocial Nursing and Mental Health Services, 26*(12), 18–22.

Mason, J. W. (1971). A re-evaluation of the concept of 'non-specificity' in stress theory. *Journal of Psychiatric Research, 8*(3), 323–333.

Math, S. B., John, J. P., Girimaji, S. C., Benegal, V., Sunny, B., Krishnakanth, K., ... Nagaraja, D. (2008). Comparative study of psychiatric morbidity among the displaced and non-displaced populations in the Andaman and Nicobar Islands following the tsunami. *Prehospital and Disaster Medicine, 23*(1), 29–34.

Math, S. B., Kumar, N. C., Christine, M. N., & Cherian, A. V. (2013). Disaster mental health: A paradigm shift from curative to preventative psychiatry. In R. Arora, & P. Arora (Eds.), *Disaster management: Medical preparedness, response and homeland security* (pp. 477–494). Wallingford, UK: CABI.

Matheson, K., Bombay, A., Haslam, A., & Anisman, H. (2016). Indigenous identity transformations: The pivotal role of student-to-student abuse in Indian residential schools. *Transcultural Psychiatry, 53*(5), 551–573.

McCabe, O. L., Everly Jr, G. S., Brown, L. M., Wendelboe, A. M., Hamid, N. H. A, Tallchief, V. L., & Links J. M. (2014). Psychological first aid: A consensus-derived, empirically supported, competency-based training model. *American Journal of Public Health, 104*(4), 621–628.

McEwen, B. S. (1998). Protective and damaging effects of stress mediators. *The New England Journal of Medicine, 338*(3), 171–179.

McQuaid, R. J., Bombay, A., McInnis, O. A., Humeny, C., Matheson, K., & Anisman, H. (2017). Suicide ideation and attempts among First Nations peoples living on-reserve in Canada: The intergenerational and cumulative effects of Indian Residential Schools. *Canadian Journal of Psychiatry, 62*(6), 422–430.

Mikhail, A. (1981). Stress: A psychophysiological conception. *Journal of Human Stress, 7*(2), 9–15.

Miller, J. (1994). Women's psychological development: Connections, disconnections, and violations. In M. Berger (Ed.), *Women beyond Freud: New concept of feminine psychology* (pp. 79–97). New York, NY: Brunner Mazel.

Million, D. (2013). Chapter 6: What will our nation be? In *Therapeutic nations: Healing in an age of Indigenous human rights* (pp. 123–145). Tucson, Arizona: The University of Arizona Press.

Ministers Responsible for Emergency Management. (2011, January). *An emergency management framework for Canada* (2nd ed.). Ottawa, ON: Emergency Management Policy Division, Public Safety Canada. Retrieved from http://www.publicsafety.gc.ca/cnt/rsrcs/pblctns/mrgnc-mngmnt-frmwrk/index-eng.aspx

National Collaborating Centre for Mental Health. (2005). *Post-traumatic stress disorder: The management of PTSD in adults and children in primary and secondary care.* NICE Clinical Guidelines, No. 26. Gaskell. Retrieved from http://publications.nice.org.uk/post-traumatic-stress-disorder-ptsd-cg26

Norris, F. H., Friedman, M. J., & Watson, P. J. (2002). 60,000 disaster victims speak: Part II. Summary and implications of the disaster mental health research. *Psychiatry, 65*(3), 240–260.

O'Sullivan, T. (2009, April). Spotlight on research: Caring about health workers project. *Health Policy Research Bulletin,* (15), 41–42.

O'Sullivan, T. L., Dow, D., Turner, M. C., Lemyre, L., Corneil, W., Krewski, D., ... Amaratunga C. A. (2008). Disaster and emergency management: Canadian nurses' perceptions of preparedness on hospital front lines. *Prehospital and Disaster Medicine, 23*(Suppl 1), 11–18.

Oxford English Dictionary Online. (2013, December). "trauma, n." Retrieved from http://www.oed.com.login.ezproxy.library.ualberta.ca/view/Entry/205242?redirectedFrom=trauma

Papps, E., & Ramsden, I. (1996). Cultural safety in nursing: The New Zealand experience. *International Journal for Quality in Health Care, 8*(5), 491–497.

Penner, L. A., Dovidio, J. F., West, T. V., Gaertner, S. L., Albrecht, T. L., Dailey, R. K., & Markova, T. (2010). Aversive racism and medical interactions with Black patients: A field study. *Journal of Experimental Social Psychology, 46*(2), 436–440.

Pfefferbaum, B., & North, C. (2013). Assessing children's disaster reactions and mental health needs: Screening and clinical evaluation. *Canadian Journal of Psychiatry, 58*(3), 135–142.

Prewitt Diaz, J. O. (2013). Community-based psychosocial support: an overview. In R. Arora & P. Arora (Eds.), *Disaster management: Medical preparedness, response and homeland security* (pp. 464–476). Wallingford, UK: CABI.

Public Safety Canada (2017, March 9). *Fifth regional platform for disaster risk reduction in the Americas endorses action plan demonstrating progress for Canada and Region.* Retrieved from http://www.newswire.ca/news-releases/fifth-regional-platform-for-disaster-risk-reduction-in-the-americas-endorses-action-plan-demonstrating-progress-for-canada-and-region-615822184.html

Puxley, C. (2013, November 19). First Nations to get disaster relief sooner, Ottawa says. *The Canadian Press.* Retrieved from theglobeandmail.com

Quiros, L., & Berger, R. (2015). Responding to the sociopolitical complexity of trauma: An integration of theory and practice, *Journal of Loss and Trauma, 20*(2), 149–159. doi:10.1080/15325024.2013.836353

Rahe, R. H. (2000). Recent Life Changes Questionnaire [RLCQ] [1997]. In T. H. Holmes & American Psychiatric Association (Eds.), *Task force for the handbook of psychiatric measures. Handbook of psychiatric measures* (pp. 235–237). Washington, DC: American Psychiatric Association.

Raja S, Hasnain M, Hoersch M, Gove-Yin S, Rajagopalan C. (2015). Trauma informed care in medicine: Current knowledge and future research directions. *Family & Community Health, 38*(3), 216–226.

Ramsden, I., & Spoonley, P. (1993). The cultural safety debate in nursing education in Aotearoa. *New Zealand Annual Review of Education, 3*, 161–174.

Rando, T. (1993). *Treatment of complicated mourning.* Champaign, IL: Research Press.

Rees, S., Silove, D., Chey, T., Ivancic, L., Steel, Z., Creamer, M., ... Forbes, D. (2011). Lifetime prevalence of gender-based violence in women and the relationship with mental disorders and psychosocial function. *Journal of the American Medical Association, 306*(5), 513–521.

Richardson, F., & Carryer, J. (2005). Teaching cultural safety in a New Zealand nursing education program. *Journal of Nursing Education, 44*(5), 201.

Richardson, J. D., Naifeh, J. A., & Elhai, J. D. (2007). Posttraumatic stress disorder and associated risk factors in Canadian peacekeeping veterans with health-related disabilities. *Canadian Journal of Psychiatry, 52*(8), 510–518.

Richardson, S. (2004). Aotearoa/New Zealand nursing: From eugenics to cultural safety. *Nursing Inquiry, 11*(1), 35–42.

Roberts, A. R. (1991). Conceptualizing crisis theory and the crisis model. In A. R. Roberts (Ed.), *Contemporary perspectives on crisis intervention and prevention* (pp. 3–17). Englewood Cliffs, NJ: Prentice-Hall.

Roberts, K. F., & Berry, P. H. (2002). Grief and bereavements. In K. K. Kuebler, P. H. Berry, & D. E. Heidrich (Eds.), *End of life care: Clinical practice guidelines* (pp. 53–63). Philadelphia, PA: WB Saunders.

Robin, R. W., Chester, B., & Goldman, D. (1996). Cumulative trauma and PTSD in American Indian communities. In A. J. Marsella, M. J. Friedman, E. T. Gerrity, & R. M. Scurfield (Eds.), *Ethnocultural aspects of posttraumatic stress disorder: Issues, research, and clinical applications* (pp. 239–253). http://dx.doi.org/10.1037/10555-009

Rodriquez, J. J., & Kohn, R. (2008). Use of mental health services among disaster survivors. *Current Opinion in Psychiatry, 21*, 370–378.

Sadock, B. J., Sadock, V. A., & Ruiz, P. (2015). *Kaplan and Saddock's synopsis of psychiatry* (11th ed.). Philadelphia, PA: Wolters Kluwer.

Sareen, J. (2014). Posttraumatic stress disorder in adults: Impact, comorbidity, risk factors, and treatment. *The Canadian Journal of Psychiatry, 59*(9), 460–467. doi:10.1177/070674371405900902

Sapolsky, R. M. (2004). *Why zebras don't get ulcers* (3rd ed.). New York, NY: Henry Holt.

Saul, J. (2014). *Collective trauma, collective healing: promoting community resilience in the aftermath of disaster.* New York, NY: Routledge.

Scholte, W. F., & Ager, A. (2014). Social capital and mental health: Connections and complexities in contexts of post conflict recovery. *Intervention, 12*(2), 210–218.

Segerstrom, S. C., & Miller, G. E. (2003). Psychological stress and the immune system in humans: A meta-analytic view of 30 years of inquiry. *Psychological Bulletin, 130*(4), 601–630.

Selye, H. (1956). *The stress of life.* New York, NY: McGraw-Hill.

Selye, H. (1974). *Stress without distress.* Philadelphia, PA: JB Lippincott.

Selye, H. (1980). The stress concept today. In I. L. Kutash, L. B. Schlesinger, & Associates (Eds.), *Handbook on stress and anxiety* (pp. 127–143). San Francisco, CA: Jossey-Bass.

Seng, J., Rauch, S., Resnick, H., Reed, C., King, A., Low, L., ... Liberzon, I. (2010). Exploring posttraumatic stress disorder symptom profile among pregnant women. *Journal of Psychosomatic Obstetrics and Gynecology, 31*(3), 176–187.

Somasundaram, D. (2007). Collective trauma in northern Sri Lanka: A qualitative psychosocialecological study. *International Journal of Mental Health Systems, 1*(5),1–27. doi:10.1186/1752-4458-1-5

Somasundaram, D. (2014). Addressing collective trauma: Conceptualisations and interventions. *Intervention, 12*(Suppl 1), 43–60.

Stanley, R. O., & Burrows, G. D. (2005). The role of stress in mental illness: The practice. In C. L. Cooper (Ed.), *Handbook of stress medicine and health* (2nd ed., pp. 87–100). Boca Raton, FL: CRC Press.

Sterling, P., & Eyer, J. (1988). Allostasis: A new paradigm to explain arousal pathology. In S. Fisher, & J. Reason (Eds.), *Handbook of life stress, cognition and health* (pp. 629–649). New York, NY: John Wiley & Sons.

Substance Abuse and Mental Health Services Administration (SAMHSA). (2013). *Tips for survivors of a disaster or traumatic event: What to expect in your personal, family, work and financial life*. Rockville, MA: Author.

Taylor, S. E., Klein, L. C., Lewis, B. P., Gruenewald, T. L., Gurung, R. A., & Updegraff, J. A. (2000). Biobehavioral responses to stress in females: Tend-and-befriend, not fight-or-flight. *Psychological Review, 107*(3), 411–429.

Taylor, S. E., Lewis, B. P., Gruenewald, T. L., Gurung, R. A. R., Updegraff, J. A., & Klein, L. C. (2002). Sex differences in biobehavioral responses to threat: Reply to Geary and Flinn. *Psychological Review, 109*(4), 751–753.

Tervalon, M., & Murray-Garcia, J. (1998). Cultural humility versus cultural competence: a critical distinction in defining physician training outcomes in multicultural education. *Journal of Health Care for the Poor and Underserved, 9*(2), 117–125.

The Canadian Encyclopedia. (2013). *Extreme-weather-in-Canada*. Retrieved from http://www.thecanadianencyclopedia.ca/en/article/extreme-weather-in-canada-feature/

Thormar, S. B., Gersons, B. P., Juen, B., Marschang, A., Djakababa, M. N., & Olff, M. (2010). The mental health impact of volunteering in a disaster setting: A review. *Journal of Nervous and Mental Disorders, 198*(8), 529–538.

Trainer, M., & Goel, A. (2013). The role of social networking in disaster management. In Arora, R., & Arora, P. (Eds.), *Disaster management: Medical preparedness, response and homeland security* (pp. 67–94). Wallingford, UK: CABI.

Truth and Reconciliation Commission of Canada (2015). *Calls to action*. Retrieved from http://www.trc.ca/websites/trcinstitution/File/2015/Findings/Calls_to_Action_English2.pdf

United Nations. (2006). *Convention on the rights of persons with disabilities*. Retrieved from http://www.un.org/disabilities/documents/convention/convoptprot-e.pdf

United Nations Office for Disaster Reduction (2015a). *Global assessment report*. Retrieved from https://www.unisdr.org/we/inform/gar

United Nations Office for Disaster Reduction (2015b). *The Sendai framework for disaster reduction 2015–2030*. Retrieved from http://www.unisdr.org/files/43291_sendaiframeworkfordrren.pdf

Veenema, T. G., Griffin, A., Gable, A. R., MacIntyre, L., Simons, R. N., Couig, M. P., et al (2016). Nurses as leaders in disaster preparedness and response—A call to action. *Journal of Nursing Scholarship, 48*(2), 187–200.

Walls, M. L., & Whitbeck, L. B. (2012). The intergenerational effects of relocation policies on indigenous families. *Journal of Family Issues, 33*, 1272–1293.

Washington, D., Davis, T., Martirosian, C., & Yano, E. (2013). PTSD risk and mental health care engagement in a multi-war era community sample of women veterans. *Journal of General Internal Medicine, 28*(7), 894–900.

Wolfelt, A. D. (1999). *Dispelling 5 common myths about grief*. Retrieved from http://www.griefwords.com/index.cgi?action=page&page=articles%2Fhelping7.html&site_id=2

Woolfolk, R. L., Lehrer, P. M., & Allen, L. M. (2007). Conceptual issues underlying stress management. In P. M. Lehrer, R. L. Woolfolk, & W. E. Sime (Eds.), *Principles and practice of stress management* (3rd ed., pp. 3–15). New York, NY: Guilford.

Worden, J. W. (2003). *Grief counseling and grief therapy: A handbook for the mental health practitioner*. New York, NY: Brunner-Routledge.

World Economic Forum. (2017).*The global risk report 2017*. Geneva: Author. Retrieved from reports.weforum.org/global-risks-2017/

World Health Organization (WHO). (2013). *Building back better: Sustainable mental health care after emergencies*. Geneva, Switzerland: Author.

World Health Organization and the International Council of Nurses. (2009). *ICN framework of disaster nursing competencies*. Retrieved from http://www.icn.ch/images/stories/documents/networks/DisasterPreparednessNetwork/Disaster_Nursing_Competencies_lite.pdf

World Health Organization, War Trauma Foundation and World Vision International. (2011). *Psychological first aid: Guide for field workers*. Geneva, Switzerland: WHO.

18 Anger, Aggression, and Violence

Phillip Woods

Adapted from the chapter "Anger, Aggression, and Violence" by Yvonne Savard

LEARNING OBJECTIVES

After studying this chapter, you will be able to:

- Explore feelings about the experience and expression of anger.
- Discuss the bio/psycho/social/spiritual factors that influence the expression of aggressive and violent behaviour.
- Discuss the theories used to explain anger, aggression, and violence.
- Identify the behaviour or actions that escalate and de-escalate violent behaviour.
- Recognize the risk for aggression towards nurses.
- Generate options for responding to the expression of anger and violent behaviour in clinical nursing practice.
- Apply the nursing process to the management of anger, aggression, and violence in clients.

KEY TERMS

- catharsis • emotional circuit • mindfulness • restraint • seclusion • violence

KEY CONCEPTS

- aggression • anger • assertiveness

Anger is considered a universal human emotion, identifiable across cultures, by theorists who believe that prototypical emotions exist (DiGiuseppe & Tafrate, 2007). We get our knowledge about emotion in several ways: personal knowledge, knowledge about others' emotions, social norms, and evolving conceptual knowledge (Faucher & Tappolet, 2008). Definitions of anger, aggression, and violence vary and are informed through such concepts as experience, beliefs, culture, and gender. Individuals and groups develop their own views of where the boundaries exist with these: verbally, nonverbally, and behaviourally. Theoretic distinctions can be made between anger, aggression, and violence, but clinically, their expression may be blurred. Each phenomenon may occur alone or in combination with one or both of the others.

Most societies develop norms for acceptable and unacceptable behaviour. Today, images and stories about aggressive and violent acts throughout the world appear daily in the media. Incidents such as mass killings are very rare but receive enormous coverage that strongly impacts public perception of the risk for violence, especially that posed by the mentally ill (Friedman & Michels, 2013). The societal debate remains ongoing over the significance of the effect of violence in movies, television, and video games on an individual's propensity for violence.

Like other places, health care settings are not immune to expressions of anger, aggression, and violence. In any setting, aggression and violence reflect the values of the individual, family, community, and society. Many people tend to minimize the frequency and severity of aggressive and violent acts; for example, couples who interact violently downplay the severity and effects of the episodes (Freeman, Schumacher, & Coffey, 2015). The expression of anger, aggression, and violence by clients and, sometimes, by their families is a tremendous challenge for nurses. This chapter discusses prominent theories about the nature of these phenomena and offers varying, sometimes controversial, models, theories, and evidence, with each discussion attempting to explain the phenomena of anger, aggression, and violence. Clinicians can choose a particular model as a basis for assessment, nursing diagnosis, planning, intervention, and evaluation. The chapter also explores how the nurse can apply the nursing process in managing angry, aggressive, or violent clients and in preventing or de-escalating situations that may lead to aggression or violence.

■ ANGER

Anger is "a normal human emotion, aroused by frequently occurring violations of our values, beliefs, or rights" (Thomas, 2005, p. 508). Anger is usually described as a temporary state of emotional arousal, in contrast to hostility, which is associated with a more enduring negative attitude (Thomas, 2001; see Chapter 34). Anger is part of the fight-or-flight response; although anger is portrayed as a bad emotion that always leads to aggression, this is often not the case. Thomas (2001) asserts that the expression of anger may prevent aggression and help to resolve a situation.

Language pertaining to anger is imprecise and confusing. The word *anger* is used to describe a wide range of feelings, from annoyance at having to wait at a red light when in a hurry to a severe emotional reaction to the news that a family member has been physically assaulted. Some of the words used interchangeably with anger include annoyance, frustration, temper, resentment, hostility, hatred, and rage. In addition, the word *angry* is used to describe both a transient emotional state and a personality trait. This imprecision is related to varying beliefs and theories, including the following (Novaco, 2007):

- Anger is a fixed quantity that either dams up or floods the system.
- Anger and aggression are linked. Anger is the feeling, and aggression is the behaviour; both result from an innate instinct.
- Anger is the instinctive response to a threat or to the inability to meet goals or desires.
- If outward expression of anger is blocked, then it turns inward and develops into depression.
- Anger arises out of feelings of hurt or anxiety.

Box 18.1 invites the reader to explore variations in responses to anger through the use of an experiential exercise.

BOX 18.1 Self-Awareness Exercise: Personal Experience of Anger

People's reactions differ when they experience anger. Some people report a sense of power, control, and calmness different from their usual experience; others report feeling shaky, tearful, and on the verge of collapse. Still others describe physical sensations of nausea and dizziness.

Think about the last time that you felt angry. List the body sensations and other emotions that you experienced. Now ask a friend, colleague, or family member to do the same. Compare lists. What are the similarities and differences between you? How will awareness of these differences help you in your clinical practice?

KEY CONCEPT

Anger is an affective state experienced as the motivation to act in ways that warn, intimidate, or attack those who are perceived as challenging or threatening. It occurs when there is a threat, delay, thwarting of a goal, or conflict between goals.

Experience of Anger

The experience of anger is an internal event that involves thoughts, images, and bodily sensations (Kassinove & Tafrate, 2006). The experience of anger can serve as a warning that demands are greater than available resources (Thomas, 2001). Yet, with the exception of anger that arises from specific neurologic damage or biochemical imbalances, angry episodes can be viewed also as social events (Thomas, 1998). The meaning of angry episodes develops from the beliefs held about anger and the interpretation given to the episode, and these are shaped by influences such as culture, language, and gender (Thomas, 2006). Anger is a normal human emotion; it is the dysfunctional expression of anger that may be threatening to the self or others.

Expression of Anger

Verbal (e.g., yelling) and motor behaviours (e.g., stomping one's foot) are involved in the expression of anger. Difficulties in expressing anger have often been associated with psychiatric health problems. Anger turned inwards has been implicated as a contributor to mood disorders, such as depression and somatoform disorder (Koh, Kim, Kim, & Park, 2005). Evidence from the Nova Scotia Health Survey (Davidson & Mostofsky, 2010) associated decreased constructive anger (discussing anger to resolve the situation) in men and increased destructive anger justification (blaming others for one's anger) in men and women with increased risk of coronary artery disease over a 10-year period.

Behavioural expressions of anger vary. In the 19th century, anger was viewed as sinful, dangerous, and destructive—an emotion to be contained, controlled, and denied. This negatively viewed emotion was to be dominated and conquered, and an ideal family life was free of anger. Husbands and wives were discouraged from expressing anger towards each other; parenting manuals promoted the suppression of anger in children (Thomas, 1993). This view contributed to the development of a powerful taboo against feeling and expressing anger. People who have accepted this persistent taboo may have difficulty even knowing when they are angry (Shannon, 2000).

During the early 20th century, Freud and Lorenz advocated the use of **catharsis**, the release of ideas through talking and expressing appropriate emotion, in the

Table 18.1	Examples of Behaviours on the Continuum of Aggression and Violence	
Term	**Description**	**Clinical Example**
Suspicious behaviour	Hypervigilance to external cues Attends more to cues that fit with current thinking patterns	A female client with a long history of delusional disorder (including the belief that her family wants to "lock her away") questions the motives of a community mental health nurse when she asks the client about her medication regimen. The client misperceives the nurse's inquiry as evidence of a conspiracy against her
Verbal hostility	Verbal comments that are sarcastic or blaming and often expressed with the intent to hurt others May be used as a means of getting attention or inviting others to take action	When administration of PRN medication is delayed, a client's mother comes to the nursing station and starts to yell. She states that the nurses do not care, are lazy, and should work harder. She also demands that someone give her daughter the analgesic. (Family members have been previously reported as using demanding behaviours to have needs met.)
Physical violence	Act of striking out, throwing an object, pushing, etc., that appears to be intended to cause harm to a person or object	A young man attending a mental health clinic has missed his appointment with the psychiatrist. When he finds out he cannot be scheduled to see her for another week, he yells at the receptionist, bangs his fist on the desk, and then picks up a chair and throws it at her

expression of anger. However, catharsis has been shown empirically to promote, not reduce, anger (Thomas, 1998). There is an old joke that expresses what research has shown: "How do you become a great performer?" Answer: "Practice, practice, practice." "How do you become a really angry person?" Answer: "Practice, practice, practice" (DiGiuseppe & Tafrate, 2007). Differences in expectations about how men and women should express anger also contribute to the confusion about anger. Varying beliefs about appropriate ways to express anger become apparent when a client and a nurse enter into a therapeutic relationship. Genetic predisposition, emotional development during infancy and childhood, and family environment influence the variations in expression for both the nurse and the client (Thomas, 2001, 2009). Previous experiences in expressing anger and reactions from others are also influential. Frequency, duration, intensity, and mode of expression are aspects of anger that can be explored and considered (Novaco, 2007). When the expression of anger has negative outcomes for the person in terms of personal distress (e.g., shame) and consequences (e.g., lost relationships), it may be considered dysfunctional (Kassinove & Tafrate, 2006).

■ AGGRESSION AND VIOLENCE

While anger is an emotion, aggression and violence are actions or behaviours. In this chapter, violence and aggression "refer to a range of behaviours or actions that can result in harm, hurt or injury to another person, regardless of whether violence or aggression is physically or verbally expressed, physical harm is sustained or the intention is clear" (National Institute for Health and Care Excellence, 2015, p. 5). Aggression and violent behaviour reflect a continuum from suspicious behaviour to extreme actions that threaten the safety of others or result in injury or death (see Table 18.1 for examples).

Research focused on inpatient psychiatric units has found that higher levels of aggression were associated with clients detained under mental health legislation (Bowers et al., 2011), high client turnover, unit doors being locked, and higher staffing ratios (Bowers et al., 2009). The imposition of restrictions on clients appeared to be associated with increased rather than reduced aggression. Reasons for aggression in these settings as identified by staff and patients included patient factors (e.g., psychotic symptoms), staff factors (e.g., lack of skill), and environmental factors (e.g., overcrowding, lack of access to outside space) (Bowers et al., 2011). Increasingly, the complexity of aggression and violence occurring in health care settings is being recognized. For instance, a systemic perspective of aggression and violence in mental health care has been proposed that identifies four related phenomena: environmental (e.g., layout of the unit, noise level), intrapersonal/client (e.g., age, gender, trauma, diagnosis), clinician (e.g., skills, stress level, attitude towards aggression), and mental health care system (e.g., policies, cultural factors, control orientation) (Cutcliffe & Riahi, 2013a, b).

Aggression does not occur in a vacuum. Therefore, a multidimensional framework (Fig. 18.1) is essential for understanding and responding to these behaviours.

KEY CONCEPT

Aggression is defined as verbal statements and/or physical actions that are intended to threaten.

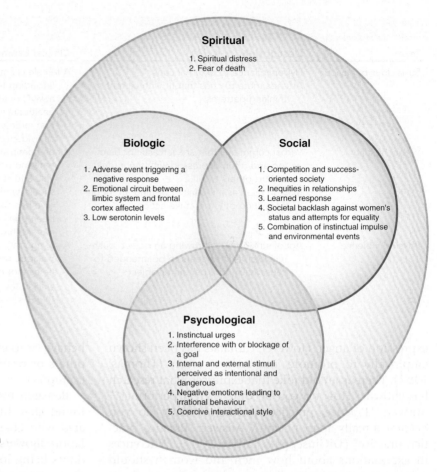

Figure 18.1. Aetiologies for clients with aggression.

MODELS OF ANGER, AGGRESSION, AND VIOLENCE

This section discusses some of the dominant theoretical explanations for anger, aggression, and violence. A single model or theory cannot yet fully explain anger, aggression, and violence; instead, the nurse must choose the most useful models for explaining a particular client's experience and for planning interventions.

Biologic Theories

From a biologic viewpoint, a tendency to have more frequent angry episodes may partially originate from developmental deficits, anoxia, malnutrition, toxins, tumours, or neurodegenerative diseases or trauma affecting the brain. Clients with a history of damage to the cerebral cortex are more likely to exhibit increased impulsivity, decreased inhibition, and decreased judgement than are those who have not experienced such damage. The interaction of neurocognitive impairment and social history of abuse or family violence increases the risk for violent behaviour (Scarpa & Raine, 1997). The odds of violent behaviour also increase when separate risk factors, such as untreated first-episode psychosis and substance use disorder, coexist in the same person (Latalova, 2014). Before reading additional research evidence, try the

---

BOX 18.2 Self-Awareness Exercise: Intensity of Anger

IMAGINE THIS SCENE

You are coming home late at night. You've been at the library studying for midterm examinations and are tired. As you come up the front walk, you trip over a skateboard, probably left by one of the neighbourhood children. Before you know it, you are sprawled across the front step.

What emotions threaten to overwhelm you at that moment? What contributes to the intensity of the anger that you feel?

- The pain where you scraped your leg across the cement?
- Your general state of tiredness?
- The fact that you skipped dinner?
- The five cups of coffee you had today?
- The careless children who left a toy in your way?

If the same thing had happened when you were well rested and feeling good, would the feeling and the intensity be the same?

anger exercise in Box 18.2. What does daily experience suggest about biologically based aspects of the experience and expression of anger?

Cognitive Neuroassociation Model

The cognitive neuroassociation model is one explanation for the interplay of biologic and other internal influences (Berkowitz, 1989; Miller, Pedersen, Earleywine, & Pollock, 2003). Initially, an adverse event (e.g., pain from tripping over a skateboard) triggers a primitive negative response. Peripheral receptors communicate this response to the spinal cord through the spinothalamic tract to the hypothalamus. The hypothalamus, which synthesizes input from throughout the nervous system, is part of the limbic system. The limbic system mediates primitive emotion and basic drives to produce behaviours for survival, such as the fight-or-flight response (Harper-Jaques & Reimer, 1992).

At first, cognitive appraisal is not involved in these rudimentary feelings of fear or anger, other than identifying the stimulus as aversive; however, higher-order cognitive processing quickly begins to take over. The brain associates the current experience of physiologic sensations with memories, ideas, and previously experienced expressive motor reactions. It then interprets and differentiates the experience. Depending on prior experience and associations, the response may be intensified or suppressed. It is this latter part of the process that is most amenable to modification through psychotherapy.

Neurostructural Model and the Emotional Circuit

The brain structures most frequently associated with aggressive behaviour are the limbic system and the cerebral cortex, particularly the frontal and temporal lobes. Harper-Jaques and Reimer (1992) propose the phrase **emotional circuit** to describe the interrelationship between the emotional processes of the limbic system and the neurocognitive processes of the frontal lobe and other parts of the cortex. They hypothesize that the functioning of this system determines the meaning a person gives to a particular situation. Thus, meaning is influenced by physiologic capability to perceive incoming messages, prioritize among competing stimuli, and interpret these messages in relation to stored ideas, beliefs, and memories.

Neurochemical Model and Low Serotonin Syndrome

In recent decades, knowledge has exploded about the complex role of neurotransmitters in human behaviour. Serotonin is a major neurotransmitter involved in mood, sleep, and appetite. Low serotonin levels are associated not only with depression but also with irritability, increased pain sensitivity, impulsiveness, aggression, vulnerability

to alcoholism, and obsessive–compulsive behaviour (Heinz, Mann, Weinberger, & Goldman, 2001).

Serotonin is sensitive to fluctuations in dietary intake of its precursor, tryptophan, which is found in high-carbohydrate foods. Once it crosses the blood–brain barrier, tryptophan is synthesized into serotonin within the 5-hydroxytryptophan neurons by interaction with the enzyme tryptophan hydroxylase. Normally, the amount of tryptophan available in the plasma is below saturation (i.e., below the amount that could be used if available). Tryptophan intake and the availability of binding sites on the plasma proteins affect the synthesis of serotonin. Thus, assessing overall dietary intake is relevant, particularly of good tryptophan sources, such as wheat, flour, corn, milk, and eggs. In one meta-analysis, a small inverse relationship between tryptophan level and aggression was found, highlighting that the literature continues to have contradictory findings and methodologic limitations (Duke, Begue, Bell, & Eisenlohr-Moul, 2013).

People with a history of aggressive behaviour have been found to have a lower-than-average level of serotonin. Studies of humans with known aggressive tendencies, such as violent offenders, have repeatedly shown lower-than-average concentrations of 5-hydroxyindoleacetic acid (5-HIAA), the major metabolite for serotonin (Soloff, Lynch, & Moss, 2000) and prefrontal cortex dysfunction (Best, Williams, & Coccaro, 2002). Similarly, the plasma concentration of tryptophan is lower in people with alcoholism who have a history of aggressive behaviour than in people with alcoholism and no such history. Criminals whose acts of violence were committed impulsively have lower levels of 5-HIAA than do criminals whose acts of violence were premeditated. Impulsivity and difficulty controlling anger are characteristic of borderline personality disorder, another condition associated with lower-than-normal serotonin levels (Paris, 2005). Hyperarousal, such as may occur through being constantly vigilant against possible risk to self, may contribute to aggressive behaviour.

This evidence for a biologic component to aggressive behaviour does not mean that only biologic means of treatment can be effective. Feedback between human behaviour and biochemistry is continuous; verbal suggestions and even early life stressors can affect biochemistry, just as biochemistry affects behaviour (Heinz et al., 2001). Environmental and learned behaviours influence the type and degree of aggression expressed, even by those for whom there is a biologic component (Soloff et al., 2000).

Psychological Theories

Several psychological explanations exist for aggressive and violent behaviours. This section discusses psychoanalytic, behavioural, and cognitive theories.

Psychoanalytic Theories

Psychoanalytic theorists view emotions as instinctual urges. They view suppression of these urges as unhealthy and as possible contributors to the development of psychosomatic or psychological disorders (Thomas, 1998). Freud struggled to understand the nature and expression of human aggressive behaviour. In his early works, he linked aggression with libidinal factors; however, this association did not explain destructive actions during wars and armed conflict. In his later writings, Freud identified aggression as a separate instinct, like the sexual instinct. He viewed aggression as an innate human quality that could be expressed when a person is provoked or abused. In doing so, he challenged the commonly held belief that human beings are essentially good.

Freud explained aggressive or violent behaviour as a combination of instinctual impulses and events in the environment that stimulated release of the instinctual urge. Freud's view fostered the use of catharsis. Therapeutic approaches, such as primal scream and nursing interventions that direct the client to "let it out" by pounding a pillow, find their origins in this theory (Tavris, 1989; Thomas, 1990). However, results of research studies have been mixed as to if catharsis is helpful in reducing anger (Verona & Sullivan, 2008). Venting can also have negative consequences when the action taken is hurtful to or blaming of others or damages property.

Erich Fromm (1900–1980), an American psychoanalyst best known for his application of psychoanalytic theory to social and cultural problems, believed that animals and humans share a form of aggression he called *benign*. This genetically programmed response was designed as a defence to protect oneself against a threat. The distinction between humans and animals is that human beings could reason. This capability provided them with options that are not available to animals. Thus, unlike animals, human beings are capable of behaving aggressively for reasons other than self-preservation. Fromm (1973) defined aggression in humans as any behaviour that causes or intends to cause damage to another person, animal, or object. Humans may foresee both real and perceived threats. Perceived threats that are based on distorted perceptions may lead to aggressive and violent behaviours; for example, the cognitive and information-processing deficits of clients with psychosis or schizophrenia (see Chapters 20 and 21) are frequently implicated in episodes of aggression and violence.

Behavioural Theories

The goal of behaviourists is to predict and control behaviour. Introspection has no role in these theories. One behavioural theory, drive theory, suggests that violent behaviour originates externally. A person experiences anger and acts violently in response to interference with or blocking of a goal. Laboratory experiments and the reality of everyday experience have proved the limitations of this theory (Thomas, 1990). Not all situations in which one's goal is blocked lead to anger or violence.

Another behavioural theory is social learning theory. In his research, Bandura (1973) drew attention to the role of learning and rewards in the expression of anger and violence. He studied interactions between mothers and children. The children learned that anger and aggressive behaviour helped them get what they wanted from their mothers. The children learned aggressive behaviour in a context that may have made them understand aggressive behaviour as appropriate. According to this view, people learn to be aggressive by participating in an aggressive environment. There is evidence, for instance, that playing violent video games is correlated with delinquency and violence even when other factors such as age, sex, race, and psychopathic personality traits are considered (DeLisi, Vaughn, Gentile, Anderson, & Shook, 2013).

Cognitive Theories

Cognitive theorists are interested in how people transform internal and external stimuli into useful information. They emphasize understanding how a person takes new information and fits it into an already developed schema. Beck (1976) proposed that cognitive schemas such as judgments, self-esteem, and expectations influence angry responses. In a situation perceived as intentional, dangerous, and unprovoked, the recipient's reaction will be intensified. The person's reaction will be further intensified if he or she views the offender as undesirable. In psychological disorders, cognitive processing may be compromised (Kornreich et al., 2016; Kurtz, Gagen, Rocha, Machado, & Penn, 2016).

Rational–emotive theory, a type of cognitive theory, considers cognition, affect, and behaviour to be interrelated psychological processes (Ellis, 1977). This theory regards anger as an inappropriate negative emotion because it stems from irrational beliefs. Change is directed at altering irrational beliefs by identifying and working to change them and their associated psychological processes. Cognitive theories inform us about how not to get angry in the first place not about what to do when we become angry (Novaco, 2007).

Sociocultural Theories

Sociocultural theories suggest violent behaviour has multiple determinants, including social experiences in family and peer settings and the social consequences (positive and negative) of physical aggression. These determinants can be influenced by the gender of the individual and the way that gender differences are conceived and enacted within a society (Snyder, Schrepferman, Brooker, & Stoolmiller, 2007).

Western society often is characterized by a competitive, success-oriented ideology that values the individual and individual accomplishments over collaboration and a sense of community. Self-esteem, particularly for men, may be based on social and economic status and influence over others and the environment (Thomas, 2003). The pursuit of status produces inequities in relationships, whereby one person is superior and the other is subordinate. A hazard inherent in the pursuit of status is the view that a person is entitled to have influence and control and that the "entitled person" has the right to use whatever means necessary to obtain status (Jenkins, 1990). These means may include force or disregarding the rights and needs of others. The entitled person may also begin to consider other people responsible for his or her thoughts, feelings, or actions. Such a belief in entitlement can be used to justify such actions as threatening, hurting, or murdering less powerful individuals.

Violence against women is a pressing global health issue. In 1993, the United Nations (UN) General Assembly adopted the UN Declaration on the Elimination of Violence against Women, asking countries to develop policies and take action. This resolution provides governments with a rationale to challenge men's position of entitlement and calls for societies to view women as equal partners with men. It has had an impact: women now have greater access to education, increased economic independence, and opportunities to control the frequency and number of pregnancies. Some believe, however, that these changes have led to a backlash against women's efforts to be equal, evident in continuing violence towards women (Tajaden & Thoennes, 2000).

A World Health Organization (WHO) study in 2005 revealed that the incidence of violence against women varies considerably across countries. For instance, the percentage of violence against a woman by a male partner ranged from 13% in Japan to 61% in Peru. Social factors related to violence against women included degree of economic inequality between males and females, level of women's mobility and autonomy, societal attitudes towards gender and towards violence, whether extended family or neighbours would intervene, and the level of crime and male-to-male violence (WHO, 2005).

Interactional Theory

Morrison (1998) challenges research and theories suggesting that aggression and violence are biologically or psychologically based. She asserts that these views lead to excusing the person's behaviour. She proposes that violence among people in psychiatric settings is the same as violence in other settings. Therefore, the client's behaviour should be considered a social problem and responded to on that basis. This challenge is grounded in several studies that examined the interactional style of the aggressive and violent individual. People with interactional styles that were argumentative or coercive were more likely to engage in aggressive or violent interchanges. Such people are often described as having a "chip on their shoulders." Morrison clearly states her view that the antecedent variables (e.g., history of violence, psychiatric diagnosis, length of hospitalization) and the mediating variable of interactional style are the primary reasons for the behaviour.

A lifespan approach to understanding aggressive behaviour can be taken, one that considers risks factors across the developmental spectrum (Liu, Lewis, & Evans, 2013). See Table 18.2 for characteristics and risk factors for aggressive behaviour across age groups.

Nursing Management: Human Response to Anger and Aggression

Aggression and violence often arise from an individuals' belief that their view of a situation is the only correct one. The first party considers other views wrong and in need of change. A second party's refusal to give in to the view of the first may lead to violence (Capra, 2002). Box 18.3 illustrates such a scenario in the clinical setting.

Contrary to popular belief, most clients who have mental health problems do not behave aggressively or violently. To develop a means of predicting aggressive and violent behaviours, researchers have examined the relationship between diagnosis and violence. They have also focused on the role of a person's history in predicting violence or examined demographics, client characteristics, and unit climate.

Although media attention highlights violence related to mental illness, research shows that "the mentally ill as a group pose little risk of violence" (Friedman & Michels, 2013, p. 455). Persons with severe mental illness, such as schizophrenia or bipolar depression, may be at a slightly higher risk for violent behaviour (Elbogen & Johnson, 2009; Swanson et al., 2006), but they are overwhelmingly more likely to be victims of violent crime (prevalence 6 to 23 times greater than others) (Teplin, McClelland, Abram, & Weiner, 2005). Research has also shown that factors additional to mental disorder increase the risk of violent behaviour such as historical, clinical, dispositional, and contextual factors (Elbogen & Johnson, 2009). Many possible causes have been identified for aggressive behaviours in individuals experiencing a psychiatric disorder, including the presence of comorbid substance abuse, dependence, and intoxication (Citrome, 2015; Elbogen & Johnson, 2009). As well, individuals experiencing symptom manifestation of hallucinations or delusions or those with neuropsychiatric deficits are identified as posing an increased risk for violence. Individuals with underlying antisocial personality traits may use violent acts as a means to achieve specific goals. Finally, environmental factors that are associated with aggressive behaviours are identified, including a chaotic or unstable home or hospital situation, which may further encourage maladaptive aggressive behaviours (Citrome, 2015; Elbogen & Johnson, 2009). An important consideration for the nurse is the course of violence related to changes in symptomatology (Bernstein & Saladino, 2007).

Table 18.2	Characteristics and Risk Factors for Aggressive Behaviour Across Age Groups	
Age Group	**Characteristics**	**Underlying and Contextual Risk Factors**
Toddlers	Crying, screaming, biting, kicking, throwing, and breaking objects	Genetic and biologic factors (e.g., birth complications, nutritional deficit)
School-age children	Aggressive behaviour peaks before age 2	Imitation of others' aggression (social learning theory)
	Teasing, irritability, bullying, fighting, cruelty to animals, and fire setting	After repeated exposure to specific social stimuli (social information-processing theory)
	Nonphysical aggressive behaviour (e.g., verbal, psychological) increases	Psychosocial and environmental factors (such as poor parenting)
	Symptoms of sexual or physical abuse to the child. It is important to assess for potential abuse in these clients.	
Adolescents	More serious aggressive behaviours and even violence appear	Aggressive behaviour that appears in only adolescence and disappears in later life (adolescence-limited antisocial behaviour)
	Gang activities including stealing, truancy, etc.	Learned aggressive behaviour in childhood that carried over into adolescence
	Cross-gendered aggressive behaviours, including dating violence, date rape, and sexual assault	Depression, family and other relationship difficulties, and a family history of suicide (or personal history of suicide attempts) may place an adolescent at greater risk for suicidal behaviour
	Suicide is the third leading cause of death for this group.	Substance abuse
Adults	Domestic violence, sexual abuse, child abuse, and homicide	Drug use
	Highest homicide rate among age groups	Traumatic brain injury to areas responsible for managing aggression and impulse control
Older adults	Older adults in nursing homes due to daily interactions with staff and other residents	The emergence of dementias such as Alzheimer's disease may result in misunderstanding of motives. Aggression may result from this confusion
	Aggressive behaviours aimed at caregivers centre on intimate care practices or those that cause pain.	The annual incidence of homicide–suicide is higher in adults 55 years and older and typically occurs more among couples
	Aggressive behaviour aimed at fellow residents in the context of excessive vocalization, territoriality, arguments with roommates, and general loneliness or frustration	Multifactorial aetiology

Adapted from Liu, J., Lewis, G., & Evans, L. (2013). Understanding aggressive behaviour across the lifespan. *Journal of Psychiatric and Mental Health Nursing, 20*(2), 156–168. Licensed © 2012 Blackwell Publishing.

BOX 18.3 CLINICAL VIGNETTE

PAUL'S ANGER

Paul, a new client on the unit, appears to be experiencing auditory hallucinations. The nurse approaches Paul, careful not to invade his personal space, and begins to walk with him. In an attempt to assess his current mental status, the nurse points out that he seems restless and asks if the voices have returned. Paul responds, "They are telling me this place isn't safe. The angel in the corner is signalling to me. She wants me to leave!" Paul starts to walk towards the door. In an attempt to offer an alternative point of view and orient him to the present, the nurse understands that what the client is seeing and hearing are hallucinations. The nurse attempts to increase Paul's feeling of safety by identifying his perceptions as hallucinations and reassuring him of his safety. "No I won't stay and you can't make me." Paul pushes the nurse aside and runs to the door.

What Do You Think?

If you were the nurse in this situation, what would be your next response? How would you acknowledge Paul's concerns and encourage him to stay?

Research, nevertheless, suggests that particular characteristics are predictive of violent behaviours. Low self-esteem that may be further eroded during hospitalization or treatment may influence a client to use force to meet his or her needs or to experience some sense of empowerment. Many people who have chronic mental health problems "fight" the experience and have difficulty accepting medical treatment. When admitted to the hospital, they may experience turmoil from both the illness and the anger at the additional loss of control that hospitalization mandates. Clients may resort to violence to force change or to regain or maintain control. Rewards from violence include attention from nursing staff and/or status and prestige among the client group (Harris & Morrison, 1995). For example, the client who behaves violently is observed more frequently and has more opportunities to discuss concerns with nurses. Impaired communication, disorientation, and depression have been found to be consistently associated with aggressive behaviour among nursing home residents with dementia (Talerico, Evans, & Strumpf, 2002).

Nurses bring their own perceptions and reactions to clinical settings. They respond to the behaviours of the clients and families for whom they care. Clients and families, in turn, react to nurses. Nurses' beliefs about themselves as individuals and professionals will influence their responses to aggressive behaviours. For example, the nurse who considers any expression of anger or aggression inappropriate will approach an agitated client in a manner different from that used by the nurse who considers agitated behaviour to be meaningful. In a phenomenologic study of client experiences of violent encounters (Carlsson, Dahlberg, Ekebergh, & Dahlberg, 2006), participants described wanting caregivers who were calm and confident and who did not respond to client anger by disconnecting (e.g., becoming cool and distant). They said that such reactions on the part of caregivers increased their despair and, with it, their aggression. When a caregiver genuinely related to the client as a person and seemed to recognize the suffering being experienced, the client's anger was diffused. The researchers found the clients to be "longing for authentic personal care" (p. 287). It is interesting to note that the Kings College London review of the literature found that reports of consequences of inpatient violence tended to focus on injuries of staff only (Bowers et al., 2011).

Duxbury and Whittington (2005) studied clients' and nurses' perspectives on inpatient aggression and violence. Clients believed poor communication on the part of staff played a significant role; nurses believed it was clients' mental illness that was most significant. Both noted that environmental conditions (e.g., restrictive and underresourced) play a role. Clients advocated for communication training for staff, while nurses looked for organizational deficits to be addressed. The nurse's ability to maintain personal control is challenged when faced with angry, provoking clients. Some clients who are experiencing emotional problems have an uncanny ability to verbally target a nurse's vulnerable characteristics. It is a usual response to become defensive when one feels vulnerable. However, when nurses lose control of their own responses, the potential for punitive interventions or the use of threats or sarcasm is greater.

Nurses in all areas of clinical practice need to understand angry emotions, know how to prevent aggression and violence, and respond proactively. To better prepare themselves to respond to different types of behaviour, many nurses take assertiveness training courses and workshops. Many nursing schools also teach assertiveness. Nurses should understand the phenomena of anger, aggression, and violence as meaningful behaviours that warrant attention rather than as disruptive behaviours to control.

KEY CONCEPT

Assertiveness is a set of behaviours and a communication style that is open, honest, direct, and confident. Assertiveness enables the expression of emotions, including anger, in a manner that assumes responsibility. It allows placement of boundaries and prevents acceptance of inappropriate aggression from others.

Predictors of Violence

When assessing a client, his or her history is probably the most important predictor of potential for violence. Important markers include previous episodes of rage and violent behaviour, escalating irritability, intruding angry thoughts, and fear of losing control. Extensive research has been undertaken to determine variables that are strongly associated with risk of violence. There is reasonable consensus in the literature that actuarial or statistical approaches are not the best way forward and the clinician should use a more structured professional judgement approach. One of the more prominent instruments to assist in prediction of violence risk is the HCR-20, now in its third version (Douglas, Hart, Webster, & Belfrage, 2013). The HCR-20 consists of 10 historical items (violence, other antisocial behaviour, relationships, employment, substance use, major mental disorder, personality disorder, traumatic experiences, violent attitudes, treatment or supervision response); 5 clinical items (insight, violent ideation or intent, symptoms of major mental disorder, instability, treatment or supervision response); and 5 risk items (professional service and plans, living situation, personal support, treatment or supervision response, stress and coping). Extensive research has been published on its predictive accuracy. Another prominent instrument utilized by nurses and other health care professionals to help with violence prediction in the short term is the Broset Violence Checklist (BVC) (Almvik, Woods, & Rasmussen,

Table 18.3 Physiologic and Behavioural Cues to Anger

Internal Signs	External Signs
• Increased pulse, respirations, and blood pressure • Chills and shudders • Prickly sensations • Numbness • Choking sensations • Nausea • Vertigo	• Increased muscle tone • Changes in body posture, clenched fists, set jaw • Changes to the eyes: eyebrows lower and draw together, eyelids tense, eyes assume a "hard" appearance • Lips pressed together to form a thin line, or in a square shape • Flushing or pallor • Goose bumps • Twitching • Sweating

2000). The BVC consists of six items predictive of violence: confusion, irritability, boisterousness, physical threats, verbal threats, and attacks on objects. Some physiologic and behavioural cues to anger are listed in Table 18.3.

Analysis and Outcome Identification

The nurse analyzes all assessment data across the biologic, psychological, and social domains to understand the dangers that the client's behaviour poses for self or others. The most common North American Nursing Diagnosis Association [NANDA] nursing diagnoses for clients experiencing intense anger and aggression are Risk for Self-Directed Violence and Risk for Other-Directed Violence (Herdman & Kamitsuru, 2014). NANDA also contains other diagnoses in Domain 11: Safety/Protection (class 3: violence) that may be relevant—Self-Mutilation, Risk for Self-Mutilation, and Risk for Suicide. Outcomes focus on aggression control.

Planning and Implementing Interventions

This section emphasizes the development of a partnership between the nurse and client, who work together to find solutions to prevent the recurrence of explosive episodes and to de-escalate volatile situations. However, sometimes the client's condition (e.g., advanced dementia) or the situation will prevent the development of a partnership. In such instances, the nurse must take the lead. The nurse who intervenes from within the context of the therapeutic relationship must be cognizant of the fit of a particular intervention. The nurse's action is based on his or her response to the client. The client's affective, behavioural, and cognitive response to the intervention provides information about its effects and guides the nurse's next response (Wright & Leahey, 2012; Fig. 18.2).

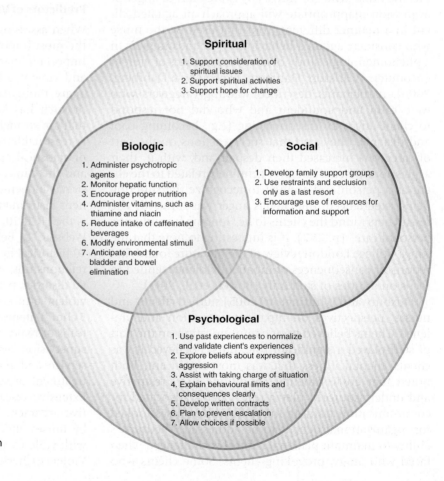

Figure 18.2. Interventions for clients with aggression.

The following assumptions are important to consider in planning interventions with this client population:

- The nurse and client collaborate to find solutions and alternatives to aggressive and violent outbursts.
- Anger is a normal emotion. All people have the right to express their anger. All people have a responsibility to express their anger in a way that does not, emotionally or physically, threaten or harm others.
- In most instances, the person who behaves aggressively or violently can assume responsibility for the behaviour.
- The nurse views the client from the perspective of acknowledging that the client has solved problems before and is only temporarily in need of help.
- The nurse understands that norms for behaviour are created within the context of a particular environment and are influenced by the client's history and culture.

Nurses who work collaboratively with potentially violent clients must also keep in mind that they can take certain actions to minimize personal risk:

- Using nonthreatening body language
- Respecting the client's personal space and boundaries
- Positioning themselves so that they have immediate access to the door of the room in case they need to leave the room
- Choosing to leave the door open to an office while talking to a client
- Knowing where colleagues are and making sure those colleagues know where they are
- Removing or not wearing clothing or accessories that could be used to harm them, such as scarves, necklaces, or dangling earrings

When a violent outburst appears imminent or occurs, immediate intervention is required and should be directed by a designated leader. Health care facilities will have protocols that outline leader designation and the crisis response process (see Box 18.4). It is each nurse's responsibility to be knowledgeable about the process in place so that an informed, coordinated team response can occur.

The nurse who works with potentially aggressive clients does so with respect and concern. The goal is to work with clients to find solutions. The nurse approaches these clients calmly, being mindful to use nonthreatening body language and to avoid violation of boundaries. In dealing with aggression, as in other aspects of nursing practice, the nurse will find that at times the best intervention is silence. It is easy to equate intervention with activity, the sense that "I must do something." But quiet calmness on the nurse's part may be enough to help a client regain control of his or her behaviour and perspective on the situation.

BOX 18.4 EMERGENCY

Guidelines for Crisis Response to Threatening or Violent Client Behaviour

1. Clear the immediate area of other persons.
2. Call for staff assistance as designated in unit policy. If possible to do so, safely, remove objects that may impede movement during a team response.
3. Brief responders and designated team leader regarding the status of the client, the situation preceding the threatening or violent behaviour, and any action that has been taken.
4. With team leader, plan intervention, including specific staff roles in the intervention. Responders should remove any items from their persons that may cause injury (e.g., watches, pens, pagers, jewellery).
5. The crisis response leader speaks clearly and calmly with the client and makes the response team's presence evident. The primary goal is to defuse the situation and prevent harm.
6. The options for intervention depend on the client's response. These include calming the client verbally and helping him/her to a safe area (e.g., client's room) or inviting the client to go with a staff member to "talk things over"; moving the client to a "time-out" space, sensory room, or seclusion area; or using chemical (i.e., medication) or physical restraints. The client may be offered a choice of these options by the team leader.
7. The team debriefs the crisis incident. Medical and/or supervisory staff are informed, as necessary. A report of the crisis incident is recorded.
8. There is postincident debriefing for the client, as appropriate.

Trying to clarify what has upset the client is important. The nurse can use therapeutic communication techniques to prevent a crisis or defuse a critical situation (see Box 18.5). During daily interactions with clients, nurses intervene in many creative and useful ways. The intervention alone does not serve as the solution; it is the process or art of offering the intervention within the context of the nurse–client relationship that is successful. These interventions will not be successful with all clients all the time. However, it is not the nurse or client's fault when an intervention is ineffective. The intervention simply did not fit the situation at that particular time.

Biologic Domain

Biologic Assessment

The nurse may encounter clients whose aggressive tendencies have been exacerbated by a biochemical imbalance. However, nurses must recognize that biologic

BOX 18.5

The Potentially Aggressive Client

Paul is a 23-year-old client in the high observation area of an inpatient unit. He is pacing back and forth. He is pounding one fist into his other hand. In the past 24 hours, Paul has been more cooperative and less agitated. The behaviour the nurse observes now is more like the behaviour that Paul displayed 2 days ago. Yesterday, the psychiatrist told Paul that he would be granted more freedom in the unit if his behaviour improved. The psychiatrist has just seen Paul and refused to change the restrictions on Paul's activities.

Ineffective Approach

Nurse: Paul, I can understand this is frustrating for you.

Paul: How can you understand? Have you ever been held like a prisoner?

Nurse: I do understand Paul. Now you must calm down or more privileges will be removed.

Paul: (voice gets louder) But I was told that calm behaviour would mean more privileges. Now you are telling me calm behaviour only gets me what I have got! Can't you talk to the doctor for me?

Nurse: No, Paul. I can't talk to the doctor. (Paul appears more frustrated and agitated as the conversation continues.)

Effective Approach

Nurse: Paul, you look upset (observation). What happened in your conversation with the psychiatrist? (seeking information)

Paul: Yesterday, he said calmer behaviour would mean

more freedom in the unit. I have tried to be calmer and not to swear. You said you noticed the difference. But today, he says "no" to more freedom.

Nurse: Some people might feel cheated if this happened to them (validation). Is that how you feel?

Paul: Yeah, I feel real cheated. Nothing I do makes a difference. That's the way it is here and that's the way it is when I am out of the hospital.

Nurse: Sounds like experiences like this leave you feeling pretty powerless (validation).

Paul: I don't have any power, anywhere. Sometimes when I have no power, I get mean. At least then people pay attention to me.

Nurse: In this situation with your doctor, what would help you feel that you had some power? (Inviting client partnership).

Paul: Well, if he would listen to me; if he would read my chart.

Nurse: I am a bit confused by the psychiatrist's decision. I won't make promises that your privileges will change but would it be okay with you if I talk with him?

Paul: That would make me feel like someone is on my side.

Critical Thinking Challenge

- In the first scenario, how did the nurse escalate the situation?
- Compare the first scenario with the second. How are they different?

---

alterations are neither necessary nor sufficient to account for most aggressive behaviours. In taking the client's history, the nurse listens for evidence of industrial exposure to toxic chemicals, missed doses of medications, alcohol intoxication, and withdrawal or premenstrual dysphoric disorder. Similarly, a history of even minor structural changes resulting in trauma, haemorrhage, or tumour may contribute to lowering a client's anger threshold and thus requires investigation.

Aggressive episodes that are mainly biologic in origin share certain characteristics (Corrigan, Yudofsky, & Silver, 1993):

- The client has a history or evidence of central nervous system lesion or dysfunction.
- Onset of the episode is sudden and relatively unprovoked.
- The outburst is less controlled than those associated with external influences.
- The episode has a clear beginning and ending.
- The client expresses remorse after the episode.

Sensory Impairment

The most common impairments are hearing loss and reduced visual acuity. A common component of nursing assessment documents is visual and hearing impairments. If a client cannot provide information about his or her hearing and vision, the nurse should ask a family member or friend. If there are impairments, the nurse should ensure that hearing aids are working for clients who use them and assess clients for access to glasses or contact lenses.

Interventions for the Biologic Domain

Administering and Monitoring Medications

Several classes of drugs are used in the management of aggressive behaviour. Important points for the nurse to consider in making decisions about client and family teaching, medication administration, and consultation with physicians and pharmacists are as follows:

- Evidence supports the use of *atypical antipsychotics*, such as clozapine (Clozaril), risperidone

(Risperdal), and olanzapine (Zyprexa), in reducing agitation (Caine, 2006). As with other psychotropic medications, the action of atypical antipsychotics is not fully understood. It is thought that they block dopamine and serotonin receptors. Extrapyramidal side effects are few, which makes these drugs easier to tolerate than the typical antipsychotics (see the drug profile on risperidone [Risperdal] in Chapter 12 for more information).

- *Selective serotonin reuptake inhibitors* (e.g., fluoxetine [Prozac], paroxetine [Paxil]) are increasingly being used for their antiaggressive effects, as well as for their antidepressant effects. Their effects on aggressive behaviour usually occur before their effects on depression.
- *β-Adrenergic receptor blockers*, such as propranolol (Inderal), has been reported in one systematic review to have some effect in reducing hostility and aggression (Victoroff, Coburn, Reeve, Sampson, & Shillcutt, 2014).
- *Lithium carbonate* has been effective in treating aggressive behaviour associated with brain injury (Burke, Loeber, & Birmaher, 2002).
- *Divalproex sodium* and *carbamazepine, oxcarbazepine, and phenytoin* have been shown to reduce aggressive behaviour in some studies (Huband, Ferriter, Nathan, & Jones, 2010).
- The liver metabolizes most psychotropic drugs (except lithium). The nurse should be alert to possible hepatic dysfunction in clients with a history of alcohol or drug abuse.

Managing Nutrition

The food clients eat can have a drastic effect on their mood and behaviour and those with long-standing poor dietary habits (e.g., clients with alcoholism) often have deficiencies of thiamine, niacin, and folic acid (Young, 2002). Prolonged use of alcohol can result in thiamine deficiency, which in turn can lead to increased irritability, disorientation, and paranoia, or even serious disorders (Horton, Duffy, Hollins Martin, & Martin, 2015). Encouraging clients to eat more whole grains, nuts, fruits, vegetables, organ meats, and milk, instead of "junk" foods, is important. The nurse may need to help clients with obtaining the resources needed to buy and prepare healthier food choices.

Caffeine is a potent stimulant (Lorist & Tops, 2003). Some inpatient psychiatric units have reduced clients' accessibility to coffee and other caffeinated beverages as a means of trying to reduce aggressive behaviour. Results have been mixed.

Psychological Domain

Psychological Assessment

The nurse interested in working with clients to prevent and manage aggressive and violent behaviours should observe them for disturbances in thought processing.

Clients may have disordered thoughts for various reasons, including associated psychiatric diagnoses. Some common diagnostic categories that the nurse needs to look for in the client's history are major depressive episode, bipolar disorder, delusional disorders, posttraumatic stress disorder, schizophrenia, and depersonalization. The nurse should also look for a current or past history of substance abuse because clients who abuse drugs, alcohol, or solvents may also exhibit disordered thought processing. Intoxication can trigger erratic thought processes and unpredicted violence. Some form of thought disorder may remain after a person is detoxified, becoming a permanent feature of the person's way of processing ideas. In addition, the nurse must look for acute and chronic medical conditions, such as brain tumour, encephalitis, electrolyte imbalance, and hepatic failure, which may also alter thought processing. The thought processes of greatest interest to the nurse in assessing a client's potential for aggression and violence are perception and delusion.

Perception

Perception is awareness of events and sensations and the ability to make distinctions between them. Clients with disordered perceptions may misinterpret objects or events. Such misperception is called an *illusion*. For example, a client may assume that a person walking towards him or her is going to strike out and thus take action to defend against this illusionary foe. The nurse can explore a client's perception by asking such questions as, "I noticed you were looking very cautious as I approached you. I wonder what you are thinking."

Delusions

Clients may maintain false or unreasonable beliefs, known as delusions, despite attempts to dissuade them from their point of view. The nurse may not notice any abnormalities in the client's behaviour or appearance until the client begins to discuss delusional ideas. Discussion of the delusions may precipitate aggressive or violent behaviour. To explore these false beliefs, the nurse could, with the client's consent, ask questions respectfully. The nurse should match the pacing of such questions to the client's responses. Attempts to dissuade the client from his or her beliefs are usually ineffective.

Interventions for the Psychological Domain

Psychological interventions help clients gain control over their expression of anger and aggressive behaviour. In some instances, these interventions eliminate the need for chemical (medications) or mechanical restraints. De-escalating potential aggression is always preferable to challenging or provoking a client.

Affective Interventions

Affective interventions are designed to reduce or increase intense emotions that may hinder the client from finding alternatives to the use of aggression or violence (Wright & Leahey, 2012). They include validating, listening to the client's illness experience, and exploring beliefs.

Validating. Clients who experience intense anger and rage can feel isolated. The nurse can reduce the client's feelings of isolation by acknowledging these intense feelings. By drawing on past experience with other clients, the nurse can also reassure the client that others have felt the same way.

Listening to the Client's Illness Experience. Often, clients and their family members are invited to provide details about past medical treatments, medications, hospitalizations, and therapies. What is overlooked is the experience of the health problem or the experience of interactions with professionals. Inviting clients and families to talk about their previous experience with the health care system may highlight both their concerns and resources. See Box 18.6 for an example of how a nurse uses this intervention to improve a client's care.

Exploring Beliefs. Exploring the client's beliefs about the expression of angry feelings can be useful. Discussion of beliefs that prevent clients from seeking alternate ways of handling distressing emotions and situations may help them to take charge of the situation.

Cognitive Interventions

Cognitive interventions are usually those that provide new ideas, opinions, information, or education about a particular problem. The nurse offers a cognitive intervention with the goal of inviting the client to consider other possibilities (Wright & Leahey, 2012). Examples include giving commendations, offering information, and providing education.

Giving Commendations. A commendation focuses on the client's behaviour pattern over time and highlights his or her strengths and resources (Limacher & Wright, 2003). For example, commending a client's decision to request medication or to remove herself from an overstimulating environment highlights the woman's ability to assume responsibility for thoughts and feelings that have previously invited aggressive behaviour.

Offering Information. Nurses can offer information or arrange opportunities for clients to receive information from other professionals. Clients may sometimes become agitated and threaten to harm the nurse because they do not know what is expected of them or they do not remember why they need to be in treatment. The nurse can tell them about unit expectations or the reasons for hospitalization. The nurse can also determine

---

BOX 18.6 CLINICAL VIGNETTE

MARY'S RAGE

Mary, a 22-year-old single woman, was a regular client at the crisis centre. During previous visits, she came alone or with her mother and demanded immediate attention. This time she comes with her mother. The receptionist groans and rolls her eyes as she describes this family to the new intake nurse. "They are obnoxious. It is best to handle them fast and get them out of here!"

Before the interview, the nurse reviews Mary's extensive file. She notes that on many occasions Mary was aggressive and violent while in the centre. The mother has complained to the local health authority about the centre on at least two occasions.

During the interview, the nurse asks the mother and daughter the following questions:

• What was the most useful thing that has happened during previous contacts at the centre?
• What was the least useful thing about previous contacts at the centre?

The family looks surprised to be asked these questions. They state that previous visits were useful only in providing them with written proof that Mary could not work. That information required by the social service agency ensured continuation of Mary's disability cheques. Furthermore, Mary and her mother state that they often left the centre feeling that the nurses were not interested in their concerns and believed that if Mary tried harder, her hallucinations would decrease. They add that they often waited 1 to 2 hours to be seen, whereas other clients were seen more quickly. Mary admits that she sometimes made a lot of noise in the waiting room to be seen sooner.

The nurse then asks, "What would need to happen during your visit today to make you feel that coming here was worthwhile?" The mother expresses interest in receiving information about hallucinations and how she could help Mary when she experiences them. Mary says she wants to know how to handle angry feelings.

the client's information needs by asking questions. One option in providing information, education, and support is to develop a family support group, which can provide a forum for responding to general concerns and questions at the same time.

In the mental health setting, the nurse must make behavioural limits and consequences clear. When possible, the nurse should match consequences to the client's interests and desires. For example, Jane was slamming doors and banging down dishes in the kitchen of the group home. The nurse approached her to discuss other means of expressing her anger. During the conversation, the nurse reminded Jane that further agitated behaviour would mean that Jane would not participate in a shopping trip planned that day. The trip was important to Jane, so she chose to discuss her concern with the nurse.

Providing Education. Nurses can offer education to clients and families about various topics, including anger management and strategies to control aggressive behaviours. Greater understanding about mental health problems and altered mental status may help to prevent aggression by clarifying misunderstandings. Effective use of debriefing techniques following a crisis situation can also provide nurses and clients insights to ineffective coping and further allow for client learning in the development of strategies for future behavioural change.

Behavioural Interventions

Behavioural interventions are designed to assist the client to behave differently (Wright & Leahey, 2012). Examples of such interventions include assigning behavioural tasks, using bibliotherapy, interrupting patterns, and providing choices.

Assigning Behavioural Tasks. Sometimes, the nurse may assign a behavioural task as a way to help the client maintain or regain control over aggressive behaviours. Behavioural tasks might include writing down a list of grievances that the client will discuss with the nurse or observing how other people take charge of anger and aggression. For example, the nurse may ask the client to observe clients or staff on the unit, people at a shopping mall, or particular movies or television shows to evaluate how other people in real or fictitious situations handle anger.

Using Bibliotherapy. In bibliotherapy, books, articles, and/or audiovisual materials are used as therapeutic tools. The nurse refers the client to a particular reference and then follow-ups with the client to discuss his or her impression of the ideas and information provided by it. A client might be referred to an article on anger management and then discuss with his nurse which, if any, ideas presented in it he might use to address his anger.

Interrupting Patterns. Although clients are not usually aware of it, escalation of feelings, thoughts, and behaviour from calmness to violence usually follows a particular pattern. Disruption of the pattern can sometimes be a useful means for preventing escalation and can help the client regain composure. Nurses can suggest several strategies to interrupt patterns:

- Counting to 10 or using a mantra (sacred name repetition)
- Removing oneself from interactions or stimuli that may contribute to increased distress
- Doing something different (e.g., reading, exercising, watching television)

Providing Choices. When possible, the nurse should provide the client with choices, particularly clients who have little control over their situation because of their condition. For example, the client who is experiencing a manic episode and is confined to her room may have few options in her daily schedule. However, she may be allowed to make choices about food, personal hygiene, and which pyjamas to wear.

Social Domain

Social Assessment

The nurse should evaluate factors related to the social domain that may be contributing to aggression or violence in a client. For example, are conditions in the client's home, family, or community leading to aggression or violent episodes? Are financial or legal troubles placing stress on the client that places him or her at risk?

Interventions for the Social Domain

Reducing Stimulation

Normally, people adjust their environments to suit their needs: some people like their music loud, whereas others want it soft; some people seek out the thrill of high-risk sports, whereas others prefer to be spectators. Within the context of a brain disorder or an unusually restrictive environment, such adjustments may not be within the client's control. A client with a brain injury, progressive dementia, or distorted vision may be experiencing intense and highly confusing stimulation, even though the environment, from the nurse or family's perspective, seems calm and orderly.

For people whose perceptions or thoughts are disordered from brain damage, degeneration, or other thought-processing difficulties, modification of the environment may be one of the main interventions. Likewise, introducing more structure into a chaotic environment can help decrease the risk for aggressive behaviour (Citrome, 2015). The nurse can make stimuli meaningful or can simplify and interpret the environment in many practical ways, such as by identifying people or equipment that may be unfamiliar, providing cues as to what is expected (e.g., posting signs with directions, putting toothbrush and toothpaste by the sink), and removing or silencing unnecessary stimuli (e.g., turning off paging systems). Considering the environment from the client's viewpoint is essential. Appropriate interventions include clarifying the meaning and purpose of people and objects in the environment, enhancing the client's sense of control and the predictability of the environment, and reducing other stimuli as much as possible (see Chapter 32).

Anticipating Needs

The nurse can anticipate many needs of clients. In assuming responsibility for clients with cognitive impairment, the nurse needs to know when the client last voided and the pattern of bowel movements. Regular toileting routines are not just interventions to prevent incontinence. Similarly, the anticipation of basic needs such as thirst and hunger is important, especially when working with adults or children who cannot readily express their needs. Other discomforts can arise from such conditions as ingrown toenails and adverse medication reactions.

The urge to void can be a powerful stimulus to agitated behaviour. It is not uncommon in a neurologic observation unit to see a young man with a recent head injury become violent just before spontaneously voiding. From a biologic perspective, such a client is probably normally sensitive or even hypersensitive to a full bladder. He probably also has sufficient cognitive function to recognize his need to void. Even some level of social inhibition may be operational in that he recognizes that voiding while lying on his back in bed, with strangers around, is inappropriate. But if he cannot speak or ask for help, he may become increasingly panic stricken. Thrashing around in bed, unable to communicate his need, he may strike out at staff.

The following scenario is the true account of how one nursing student dealt with another common situation. A 75-year-old woman was pacing around the nursing station of a psychogeriatric unit in an extended care facility, crying for her mother. Various people spoke kindly to her, trying to explain that her mother was not there. Donna, a nursing student, was studying the wandering behaviours of clients with Alzheimer's disease on the unit. Hypothesizing that there is purpose behind these actions, she walked alongside the woman. After talking a bit with her about the client's mother, Donna asked the client what she would like to do if her mother were there. Gradually, the client confided that she needed her mother to help her find the bathroom. Donna then offered to help the woman, walking her to the bathroom. After voiding copiously, the client seemed greatly relieved and settled down.

Using Seclusion and Restraint

Seclusion and **restraint** are controversial interventions to be used judiciously and only when other interventions have failed to control the client's behaviour. The availability of effective psychotropic medications since the 1950s has reduced the need for these interventions of last resort. Reasons usually cited for using them are to protect the client from injury to self or others, to help the client reestablish behavioural control, and to minimize disruption of unit treatment regimens. The controversy over these interventions and their potential to be applied punitively heightens the need for clear institutional standards for their use. The development and use of clear practice standards can reduce the likelihood that these interventions will be misused (College of Registered Psychiatric Nurses of British Columbia, 2015). Postseclusion debriefing for clients is being studied as a means of identifying and reducing traumatic effects of this intervention (Whitecross, Seeary, & Lee, 2013). A study of clients' experience before, during, and after seclusion and restraint found that client/carer communication was drastically affected and not viewed as therapeutic (Ling, Cleverley, & Perivolaris, 2015). The Registered Nurses' Association of Ontario (2012) have developed comprehensive clinical best practice guidelines on "Promoting Safety: Alternative Approaches to the Use of Restraints."

Lewis (2002) challenges the use of restraint as a primary intervention in forensic settings. Lewis presents nontouch interventions as an alternative to restraint. In contrast, Hibbs (2000) proposes the use of cognitive interventions with clients while they are restrained. These interventions are designed to challenge thought patterns that contribute to aggressive behaviours. PMH nurses choose to use restraint, as a necessary and last resort intervention, for safety, for maintaining control, and for its psychological impact; knowledge and perception of a client's behaviour and staffing composition can be influencing factors (Riahi, Thomson, & Duxbury, 2016) (see Box 18.7).

Evaluation is also important in tracking the use of seclusion and restraint. The Canadian Institute for Health Information (2011) reported that between 2006 and 2010 nearly one in four patients admitted to the Ontario mental health system had one or more forms of control intervention. Furthermore within this large group, 21% had physical/mechanical restraint and 20% seclusion intervention. On inpatient psychiatric units, the monitoring of restraints/seclusion as part of a primary prevention approach to restraint/seclusion reduction should also include such strategies as building staff skills and teamwork, promoting relationship-based care, using consultation for difficult cases, and making physical design safer (Johnson, 2010).

BOX 18.7 Research for Best Practice

EXPERIENCING SECLUSION IN A FORENSIC PSYCHIATRIC SETTING

Holmes, D., Murray, S. J., & Knack, N. (2015). Experiencing seclusion in a forensic psychiatric setting: A phenomenological study. Journal of Forensic Nursing, 11*(4), 200–213.*

Proposal: The use of restrictive measures (seclusion and restraint) is sometimes needed in mental health care. As little research has explored the lived experience, it is important to understand this from both patient and nurse perspectives.

Method: The researchers, through a modified Interpretative Phenomenological Analysis, wanted to understand how their participants viewed their surrounding world and understood their lived experiences. The sample consisted of 13 patients and 13 nurses who had experienced or used seclusion rooms in the past 6 months. Two different semistructured interview guides, with similar open-ended questions, were used for patients and nurses. Data were analyzed using content analysis.

Results: Similar themes emerged for both clients and nurses. For clients, these were experiencing seclusion, assessing quality of care, and space confinement. For the nurses, these were resorting to seclusion, observing and assessing patients, and experiencing seclusion.

Conclusions and Implications for Practice: For both patients and nurses, it was clear that maintaining a good therapeutic relationship was key to seclusion being other than "isolation." The structure of place in seclusion is not reducible to physical space but needs to be understood as lived (emotionally and through the senses) for seclusion to be a therapeutic, if last resort, measure.

Spiritual Domain

In addressing the spiritual domain of care for the client who is experiencing anger and aggression issues, contemplative practices, such as **mindfulness**, may be valuable to both the client and nurse (see Chapter 13). Mindfulness is being fully attentive in the "here and now" moment (Marlatt & Kristeller, 1999). The process of paying attention (without judgment) to what is happening can promote a connection to one's inner being and spirit. Acknowledging the present moment of reality is the beginning of transforming that reality (Kabat-Zinn, 1993). Mindfulness is similar to meditation: awareness of breathing and of the body is central to it. As well, it is about acting with attentiveness and concentration as one walks, eats, looks about, and carries out daily tasks of living. It is about being consciously aware of our body and mind, rather than thinking "about" experience (Sherman & Siporin, 2008). This meditative act can bring a sense of calmness within minutes.

Mindfulness can be found within most religious and spiritual traditions (Sherman & Siporin, 2008). It is a way to recognize one's connection with something beyond oneself, to realize that one is not separate nor alone, to experience serenity (Kreitzer, Gross, Waleekhachonloet, Reilly-Spong, & Byrd, 2009), and/or to search for meaning and purpose (Reed, 1992). Shapiro (2008, p. 3), who researches mindfulness, finds that individuals "often find their faith is deepened as a result of becoming more mindful."

Mindfulness in the health literature, however, is most often discussed as a cognitive behavioural technique. This practice tends to utilize a brief, structured format called mindfulness-based stress reduction (MBSR). MBSR programs, initially designed by Kabat-Zinn (1990, 1994), involve three basic techniques: meditation, body scan (involves directing one's attention through the entire body), and yoga. In addition to the resource of health care team members trained to teach mindfulness to clients, there are local community programs and educational tools, such as books and videos, which are available to learn about this contemplative practice. Aust and Bradshaw (2017) conclude that mindfulness as a therapy for psychosis is more beneficial than routine care.

Lown (2007) calls for mindfulness on clinicians' part when addressing anger in the clinician–client/family relationship. He notes that mindfulness in such an encounter allows one to be both a participant and an observer. In taking a moment to assess one's own response to the situation (e.g., anxiety; anger) and to focus on being present in a genuine way to the client/family member, one is better able to respond.

Interactional Processes

When nurses develop collaborative relationships with clients, they can assist the clients to not exhibit aggressive behaviour. Johnson, Martin, Guha, and Montgomery (1997) explored the experience of thought-disordered individuals before an aggressive incident. Three themes emerged from interviews with 12 clients who had a diagnosis of a thought disorder and a history of aggressive incidents:

- The strong influence of the external environment
- The use of aggressive behaviours to feel empowered briefly in a situation
- The occurrence of aggressive incidents, despite knowledge of strategies to control anger

A review of the research by Hamrin, Iennaco, and Olsen (2009) regarding factors affecting **violence** on psychiatric units showed that violence is influenced by complex interactions among clients, staff, and unit culture. For instance, a qualitative study of experienced mental health nurses found that participants identified workplace stressors (e.g., poor staffing skill mix, inadequate workplace design, and unsupported involuntary admissions) as contributing to increased pressure, fear, and uncertainty on units (Ward, 2013). A positive culture has appropriate levels of stimulation and meaningful client activities, as well as positive staff attitudes and values towards client care. Good assessment of client factors, including violence history, plays an important role. Therapeutic relationship strategies, including being available, being a client advocate, providing client education, and collaborating with the client in treatment planning, can decrease the potential for violence.

The skills the nurse uses in interactions with the client may invite escalation or de-escalation of a tense situation (Morrison, 1998). When the nurse uses communication skills to draw out the client's experience, together the nurse and client coevolve an alternative view of the problem. Some nursing writers (Leahey & Harper-Jaques, 1996; Wright & Leahey, 2012) have highlighted the importance of attending to notions of reciprocity and circularity when providing nursing care. For example, the nurse explores the meaning of the expression of aggressive behaviours with the client and the client's beliefs about the ability to control aggressive impulses. Or, the nurse and client could discuss the effects of the nurse's behaviours on the client and the effects of the client's behaviours on the nurse. Such an approach facilitates the development of an accepting and equal nurse–client relationship. The client is a partner invited to assume responsibility for inappropriate actions. This approach is in contrast to a hierarchical nurse–client relationship that emphasizes the nurse's role in controlling the client's behaviours and defining changes the client must make. In a collaborative approach, the nurse values the client's experience and acknowledges his or her strengths. The nurse asks the client to use those strengths to either maintain or resume control of behaviour.

In Western cultures, events are typically thought of in a linear fashion (Wright & Leahey, 2012). The nurse who uses a linear causality frame of reference to think about client aggression and violence will view the problem as follows:

PACING → leads to → THREATENING BEHAVIOURS
(Event A)   (Event B)

From this linear perspective, the nurse labels the client as the problem, and other factors assume secondary importance. The nurse might decide, first, to gain control over the client's behaviour. The nurse may base this decision on his or her affective response and previous experience (e.g., that threatening behaviours frighten other clients and disrupt the unit routine). The nurse's response to a client's behaviour could be to ask the client to stop yelling, to inform the client that the behaviour is inappropriate, or to suggest the use of medication if the client does not calm down. When one thinks based on linear causality, he or she assumes that event A (pacing) causes event B (threatening behaviour).

When one thinks using circular causality, he or she attempts to understand the link between behaviours and to determine how the threatening behaviour will influence a continuation or cessation of pacing. The nurse who engages in circular thinking will also know that his or her responses to the client will influence the situation. The nurse's responses will be in the domains of cognition (ideas, concepts, and beliefs), affect (emotional state), and behaviour. The nurse will be aware of the reciprocal influences of the nurse and client's behaviours (Wright & Leahey, 2012). In viewing the situation from a circular perspective, the nurse is interested in understanding how people are involved, rather than in discovering who is to blame. This perspective does not ignore individual responsibility for aggressive or violent actions, and it does not blame the victim. It does invite the nurse to consider the multiple influences on the expression of aggressive and violent behaviour.

Responding to Assault

In recent years, compelling scientific evidence that violence portrayed in the media is harmful to children has fostered debate about violence and its effects. As a result, television networks have taken both voluntary and legislated actions to limit violent programming during hours when children are generally watching programs. However, these gains in limiting access to violence have been countered by the growing availability of violent video games and websites.

Violence in health care settings threatens the safety of staff, clients, family members, and visitors yet remains an underreported problem. Close proximity to clients by health care staff presents a higher risk to experience acts of violence, with nurses the most frequent victims (Phillips, 2016).

In health care settings, nurses assume an active role in preventing and managing aggressive and violent behaviours. A review of the literature related to inpatient violence and aggression by the Mental Health Nursing Section of Kings College London's Institute of Psychiatry (Bowers et al., 2011) found that a majority of nurses reported experiencing violence at least once during their career, a rate much higher than that of psychiatrists. Categories of antecedents to violent and/ or aggressive incidents identified across studies were staff–client interaction, client behavioural cues (e.g., agitation, attention-seeking behaviour, increased motor activity, boisterousness, and confusion), client symptoms, mood cues, external/personal issues, and no clear cause (Bowers et al., 2011). Involuntary admission to a psychiatric facility or altered mental status in any setting may constrain the development of a trusting relationship between the nurse and client. Nurses are more likely than physicians to be involved with clients who are aggressive or potentially violent. It is nurses who play a major role in setting limits and defining boundaries (Bostrom, Boyd, & White, 2006).

Research shows that the incidence and severity of violence directed towards nurses are on the rise with the most common form of violence being verbal abuse followed by threatening behaviours (Luck, Jackson, & Usher, 2006). The Nova Scotia Department of Health (2006) indicated that 32% of nurses reported being physically assaulted by clients within the past year. Nurses commonly report emotional abuse, with 44% experiencing emotional abuse from a client (Canadian Institute for Health Information, 2005). Reported violence is higher in long-term care, general hospitals, and psychiatric facilities, but nurses who work in ambulatory care settings or community clinics are not immune to assault (Gerberich et al., 2004). Banerjee et al. (2012) report Canadian personal support workers in long-term care facilities to be six times more likely to experience violence directed towards them than their Nordic counterparts. The most common injury experienced by health care workers due to violence include strains to the body, such as the back (65%), and bruises/contusions (18%; WCB (Statistical Services, 2005)).

Variations in statistics can result from differences in definitions of violence, reporting practices, data collection and analysis, and underreporting. Rationale for underreporting is common and includes time constraints, staff attitudes, conflict between the traditional caring role and reporting the violence, belief that an individual will be blamed or perceived as inadequate, minimization of the event by the nurses involved or by their colleagues, and lack of understanding in the importance of data collection (Munro, 2002). Data, as identified by the WHO (2002), provide important information in the development of strategies to minimize violence. Lack of data limits health care facilities' ability to enact measures to protect their workers and others. The WHO (2014) reported on the status of violence prevention strategies in 133 countries and called for a scaling up of violence prevention programs, stronger legislation and enforcement of laws relevant for violence prevention, and enhanced services for victims of violence.

Reports of inpatient violence tend to be exclusively from the staff's perspective. Although data indicate one third of incidents are unprovoked, it may be that staff are not recognizing or not recording the antecedents of an incident. Clients' experiences need to be captured if the scope of antecedents is to be better understood (Bowers et al., 2011).

Assaults on nurses by clients can have immediate and long-term consequences (Henderson, 2003). Reported assaults range from verbal threats and minor altercations to severe injuries, rape, and murder. Any assault can produce severe consequences for the victim. Nonphysical violence towards nurses by clients or others can have long-lasting effects on nurses, such as posttraumatic stress disorder (Gerberich et al., 2005).

Lanza's research (Lanza, 1992) indicates that nurses experience a wide range of responses (Table 18.4) similar

Table 18.4 Nurses' Responses to Assault		
Response Type	**Personal**	**Professional**
Affective	• Irritability • Depression • Anger • Anxiety • Apathy	• Erosion of feelings of competence, leading to increased anxiety and fear • Feelings of guilt or self-blame • Fear of potentially violent clients
Cognitive	• Suppressed or intrusive thoughts of assault	• Reduced confidence in judgment • Consideration of job change
Behavioural	• Social withdrawal	• Possible hesitation in responding to other violent situations • Possible overcontrolling • Possible hesitation to report future assaults • Possible withdrawal from colleagues • Questioning of capabilities by coworkers
Physiologic	• Disturbed sleep • Headaches • Stomach aches • Tension	• Increased absenteeism from somatic complaints

to those of victims of any other type of trauma. However, because of their role as caregivers, nurses may suppress the normal range of feelings after an assault, believing that it is wrong to experience strong feelings of anger and fear in this situation. This belief may relate to the conflict nurses experience in having to care for clients who have hurt them.

Steps can be taken at a clinical and management level to reduce the risk for assaults on nurses by clients. A nursing-based framework that identifies three staff factors that are important to reduction of conflict in inpatient psychiatric units is the city model (Björkdahl, Hansebo, & Palmstierna, 2013; Bowers, 2009). These factors are positive appreciation of patients (i.e., psychological understanding of difficult behaviour promoted; humanistic values), self-regulation of emotional responses (i.e., awareness and control of feelings), and effective structure of rules and routine (i.e., teamwork, organizational support, clarity of rules, teamwork). This model, which aims to reduce conflict and containment, may not be fully applicable to forensic services, where the highest rates of violence are to be found and which can require high levels of containment (Bowers et al., 2011). Bowers (2014) introduced a Safewards model to address conflict and containment within mental health wards. This model has at its core: staff and patient modifiers, originating domains, flash points, conflict, and containment. The Safewards model is a popular approach globally, and evidence of its effectiveness continues to emerge including from a cluster randomized controlled trials (Bowers et al., 2015).

Clinically, nurses must be provided with training programs in the prevention and management of aggressive behaviour. These programs, like courses on cardiopulmonary resuscitation (CPR), impart both knowledge and skills. Like CPR training, the courses need to be made available to nurses and students regularly so that they have opportunities to reinforce and update what they have learned. It is assumed that nurses who have participated in preventive training programs as students or as professionals are more likely to effectively manage and reduce aggressive or violent situations. A systematic review concluded, however, that there is as yet insufficient evidence to determine if training for interventions such as de-escalation are effective and can improve safety (Price, Baker, Bee, & Lovell, 2015). Training programs need to address the complex interplay of factors related to violent client behaviour. Such training would inform staff about risk assessment, staff interactions, and unit milieu (primary); how to use de-escalation techniques (secondary); and how to control, manage, and perform a postassessment and documentation of an incident of violent patient behaviour (Björkdahl et al., 2013).

Evaluation and Treatment Outcomes

Treatment outcomes can be considered at both individual and aggregate levels. The desired outcome at the individual level is for the client to regain or maintain control over aggressive or potentially aggressive thoughts, feelings, and actions. The nurse may observe that the client shows decreased psychomotor activity (e.g., less pacing), has a more relaxed posture, speaks more directly about feelings of anger and personal needs, requires less sedating medication, shows increased tolerance for frustration and the ability to consider alternatives, and makes effective use of other coping strategies. Evidence of a reduction in risk factors may include decreased noise and confusion in the immediate environment, calmness on the part of nursing staff and others, and a climate of clear expectations and mutual acceptance and respect. In units, day hospitals, or group home settings, indicators of positive treatment outcomes might be a reduction in the number and severity of assaults on staff and other clients, fewer incident reports, and increased staff competency in de-escalating potentially violent situations.

Continuum of Care

Anger and aggression occur in all settings. During periods of extreme aggression, in which people are a risk to themselves or others because of a mental disorder, they are admitted to an acute psychiatric unit. Removing individuals from their environment and hospitalizing them in a locked psychiatric unit provide enough safety that the aggressive behaviour dissipates. Because uncontrolled anger and aggression interfere with their ability to function, people who have problems in these areas require referral to appropriate resources before these destructive behaviours erupt.

Additional understanding of the phenomena of anger, aggression, and violence as they occur in the clinical setting is needed. Research studies that have illuminated this problem from a nursing perspective need to be continued and expanded. Specific areas of study need to examine the links among biology, neurology, and psychology. In addition, further explorations of the reciprocal influence of client interactional style and treatment setting culture will assist in the development and management of humane treatment settings. Research suggests that the very language nurses use may be deemed oppressive and violent (Alex, Whitty-Rogers, & Panagopoulos, 2013). Finally, and perhaps most importantly, nurses must research the effectiveness of particular nursing interventions.

SUMMARY OF KEY POINTS

- Theories used to explain anger, aggression, and violence include the following types:
  - Neurobiologic, including the cognitive neuroassociation model, the neurostructural model (the emotional circuit), and the neurochemical model (low serotonin syndrome)
  - Psychological, including psychoanalytic theories, behavioural theories (e.g., drive theory,

social learning theory), and cognitive theories (e.g., rational–emotive theory)
- Sociocultural theories
- Interactional theory
- Biologic factors to assess in clients who display aggressive and violent behaviours include exposure to toxic chemicals, use of medications, substance abuse, premenstrual dysphoric disorder, trauma, haemorrhage, and tumour.
- Biologic intervention choices include administering medications and managing nutrition.
- Psychological factors to assess in clients who display aggressive and violent behaviours include thought processing (e.g., perception, delusion) and sensory impairment.
- Psychological intervention choices can be affective (e.g., validating, listening, exploring beliefs), cognitive (e.g., giving commendations, offering information, and providing education), or behavioural (e.g., assigning tasks, using bibliotherapy, interrupting patterns, providing choices).
- Social intervention choices include reducing stimulation, anticipating needs, and using seclusion or restraints.
- Mindfulness can be a component of addressing the spiritual domain of care. It is a contemplative practice that both clients and nurses may find useful in dealing with anger and situations involving aggression.
- Client aggression and violence are serious concerns for nurses in all areas of clinical practice. Training in and policies and procedures for the prevention and management of aggressive episodes should be available in all work settings.

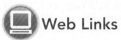 **Web Links**

http://www.cmha.ca/mental_health/feeling-angry/ Recommended short- and long-term solutions to dealing with one's anger can be found here.

http://cna-aiic.ca/~/media/cna/page-content/pdf-en/workplace-violence-and-bullying_joint-position-statement.pdf?la=en This is a link to the Canadian Nurses Association's Joint Position Statement on Workplace Violence and Bullying (May 2015).

http://www.crpnbc.ca/practice-support/topics-in-depth/restraint-and-seclusion/ This site provides links to the College of Registered Psychiatric Nurses of British Columbia's Restraint and Seclusion Information Decision Tree.

www.publichealth.gc.ca At this Public Health Agency of Canada site, information on violence prevention, and its impact on health can be found.

http://who.int/mediacentre/events/violence_health/en/ The World Health Organization's World Report on Violence and Health describes the magnitude and impact of violence throughout the world and includes national and regional data. The spectrum of violence is examined, with chapters devoted to child abuse, youth violence, violence by intimate partners, sexual violence, elder abuse, suicide, and collective violence.

http://www.rpnas.com/ The Registered Psychiatric Nurses Association of Saskatchewan site provides access to publications and position Statements. Of interest is a 2008 study: "Workplace Violence Isn't Always Physical: A One Year Experience of a Group of Registered Psychiatric Nurses."

http://www.rpnc.ca/sites/default/files/resources/pdfs/reportOnSafety.pdf At this College of Registered Psychiatric Nurses of Alberta site, there is a 2006 document submitted to the Office of Nursing Policy, Health Canada: "Report on Patient/Client Safety in Mental Health Settings: Issues, Professional Practice Concerns and Recommendations—A Call for Action."

References

Alex, M., Whitty-Rogers, J., & Panagopoulos, W. (2013). The language of violence in mental health: Shifting the paradigm to the language of peace. *Advances in Nursing Science, 36*(3), 229–242.

Almvik, R., Woods, P., & Rasmussen, K. (2000). The Brøset violence checklist (BVC): Sensitivity, specificity and inter-rater reliability. *Journal of Interpersonal Violence, 15*(12), 1284–1296. doi: 10.1177/08862600001501 2003

Aust, J., & Bradshaw, T. (2017). Mindfulness interventions for psychosis: A systematic review of the literature. *Journal of Psychiatric and Mental Health Nursing, 24*(1), 69–83. doi:10.1111/jpm.12357

Bandura, A. (1973). *Aggression: A social learning analysis.* New York, NY: Prentice-Hall.

Banerjee, A., Daly, T., Armstrong, P., Szebehely, M., Armstrong, H., & LaFrance, S. (2012). Structural violence in long-term, residential care for older people: Comparing Canada and Scandinavia. *Social Science and Medicine, 74*(3), 390–398. doi:10.1016/j.socscimed.2011.10.037.

Beck, A. T. (1976). *Cognitive therapy and emotional disorders.* New York, NY: International Universities Press.

Berkowitz, L. (1989). Frustration-aggression hypothesis: Examination and reformulation. *Psychological Bulletin, 106*(1), 59–73.

Bernstein, K. S., & Saladino, J. P. (2007). Clinical assessment and management of psychiatric patients' violent and aggressive behaviours in general hospital. *Medsurg Nursing, 16*(5), 301–331.

Best, M., Williams, J. M., & Coccaro, E. F. (2002). Evidence for a dysfunctional prefrontal circuit in clients with an impulsive aggressive disorder. *Proceedings of the National Academy of Sciences, 99*(12), 8448–8453.

Björkdahl, A., Hansebo, G., & Palmstierna, T. (2013). The influence of staff training on the violence prevention and management climate in psychiatric inpatient units. *Journal of Psychiatric and Mental Health Nursing, 20*, 396–404.

Bostrom, A. C., Boyd, M., & White, D. (2006). Coping with aggressive behavior in patients with schizophrenia. *Psychiatric Nurse: Counseling Points, 1*(2), 4–12.

Bowers, L. (2009). Association between staff factors and levels of conflict and containment on acute psychiatric wards in England. *Psychiatric Services, 60*(2), 231–239.

Bowers, L. (2014). Safewards: A new model of conflict and containment on psychiatric wards. *Journal of Psychiatric and Mental Health Nursing, 21*(6), 499–508. doi:10.1111/jpm.12129

Bowers, L., Allan, T., Simpson, A., Jones, J., Van Der Merwe, M., & Jeffery, D. (2009). Identifying key factors associated with aggression on acute inpatient psychiatric wards. *Issues in Mental Health Nursing, 30*, 260–271.

Bowers, L., James, K., Quirk, A., Simpson, A., Sugar, Stewart, D., & Hodsoll, J. (2015). Reducing conflict and containment rates on acute psychiatric wards: The Safewards cluster randomised controlled trial. *International Journal of Nursing Studies, 52*(9), 1412–1422.

Bowers, L., Stewart, D., Papadopoulos, C., Dack, C., Ross, J., Khanom, H., & Jeffery, D. (2011). *Inpatient violence and aggression: A literature review. Report from the Conflict and Containment Reeducation Research Programme.* London, UK: Institute of Psychiatry, King's College London.

Burke, J. D., Loeber, R., & Birmaher, B. (2002). Oppositional defiant disorder and conduct disorder: A review of the past 10 years, part II. *Journal of the American Academy of Child and Adolescent Psychiatry, 41*(11), 1275–1293.

Caine, E. D. (2006). Clinical perspectives on atypical antipsychotics for treatment of agitation. *Journal of Clinical Psychiatry, 67*(Suppl 10), 22–31.

Canadian Institute for Health Information. (2005). *A summary of highlights from the 2005 national survey of the work and health of nurses.* Ottawa, ON: Statistics Canada.

Canadian Institute for Health Information. (2011). *Restraint use and other control interventions for mental health inpatients in Ontario.* Ottawa, ON: Author.

Capra, F. (2002). *The hidden connections: Integrating the biological, cognitive and social dimensions of life into a science of sustainability.* New York, NY: Doubleday.

Carlsson, G., Dahlberg, K., Ekebergh, M., & Dahlberg, H. (2006). Patients longing for authentic personal care: A phenomenological study of violent encounters in psychiatric setting. *Issues in Mental Health Nursing, 27*(3), 287–305.

Citrome, L. (2015). *Aggression.* Retrieved from http://www.emedicine.com/Med/topic3005.htm

College of Registered Psychiatric Nurses of British Columbia. (2015). *Restraint & seclusion.* Port Moody, BC: Author. Retrieved from www.crpnbc.ca/practice-support/topics-in-depth/restraint-and-seclusion/

Corrigan, P. W., Yudofsky, S. C., & Silver, J. M. (1993). Pharmacological and behavioral treatment for aggressive psychiatric in-patients. *Hospital & Community Psychiatry, 44*(3), 125–133.

Cutcliffe, J., & Riahi, S. (2013a). Systematic perspective of violence and aggression in mental health care: Towards a more comprehensive understanding and conceptualization: Part 1. *International Journal of Mental Health Nursing, 22,* 558–567.

Cutcliffe, J., & Riahi, S. (2013b). Systematic perspective of violence and aggression in mental health care: Towards a more comprehensive understanding and conceptualization: Part 2. *International Journal of Mental Health Nursing, 22,* 568–578.

Davidson, K., & Mostofsky, E. (2010). Anger expression and risk of coronary heart disease: Evidence from the Nova Scotia Health Survey. *American Heart Journal, 159*(2), 199–206.

DeLisi, M., Vaughn, M., Gentile, D., Anderson, C., & Shook, J. (2013). Violent video games, delinquency and youth violence. *Youth Violence and Juvenile Justice, 11*(2), 132–142.

DiGiuseppe, R., & Tafrate, R. (2007). *Understanding anger disorders.* Oxford, UK: Oxford University Press.

Douglas, K. S., Hart, S. D., Webster, C. D., & Belfrage, H. (2013). *HCR-20V3: Assessing risk of violence—User guide.* Burnaby, BC: Mental Health, Law, and Policy Institute, Simon Fraser University.

Duke, A. A., Begue, L., Bell, R., & Eisenlohr-Moul, T. (2013). Revisiting the serotonin-aggression relation in humans: A meta-analysis. *Psychological Bulletin, 139*(5), 1148–1172.

Duxbury, J., & Whittington, R. (2005). Causes and management of patient aggression and violence: Staff and patient perspectives. *Journal of Advanced Nursing, 50*(5), 469–478.

Elbogen, E., & Johnson, S. (2009). The intricate link between violence and mental disorder: Results from the national epidemiologic survey on alcohol and related conditions. *Archives of General Psychiatry, 66*(2), 152–161.

Ellis, A. (1977). *Anger: How to live with and without it.* Secaucus, NJ: Citadel Press.

Faucher, L., & Tappolet, C. (2008). *The modularity of emotions.* Calgary, AB: University of Calgary Press.

Freeman, A. J., Schumacher, J. A., & Coffey, S. F. (2015). Social desirability and partner agreement of men's reporting of intimate partner violence in substance abuse treatment settings. *Journal of Interpersonal Violence, 30*(4), 565–579.

Friedman, R. A., & Michels, R. (2013). How should the psychiatric profession respond to the recent mass killings (editorial). *American Journal of Psychiatry, 170*(5), 455–458.

Fromm, E. (1973). *The anatomy of human destructiveness.* New York, NY: Holt, Rinehart and Winston.

Gerberich, S. G., Church, T. R., McGovern, P. M., Hansen, H., Nachreiner, N. M., Geisser, M. S., & Jurek, A. (2005). Risk factors for work-related assaults on nurses. *Epidemiology, 16,* 704–709.

Gerberich, S. G., Church, T. R., McGovern, P. M., Hansen, H. E., Nachreiner, N. M., Geisser, M. S., & Watt, G. (2004). An epidemiological study of the magnitude and consequences of work related violence: The Minnesota nurses' study. *Occupational and Environmental Medicine, 61,* 495–503.

Hamrin, V., Iennaco, J., & Olsen, D. (2009). A review of ecological factors affecting inpatient psychiatric unit violence: Implications for relational and unit culture improvements. *Issues in Mental Health Nursing, 30,* 214–226.

Harper-Jaques, S., & Reimer, M. (1992). Aggressive behavior and the brain: A different perspective for the mental health nurse. *Archives of Psychiatric Nursing, 6*(5), 312–320.

Harris, D., & Morrison, E. F. (1995). Managing violence without coercion. *Archives of Psychiatric Nursing, 9*(4), 203–210.

Heinz, A., Mann, K., Weinberger, D. R., & Goldman, D. (2001). Serotonergic dysfunction, negative mood states, and response to alcohol. *Alcoholism, Clinical and Experimental Research, 25*(4), 487–495.

Henderson, A. D. (2003). Nurses and workplace violence: Nurses' experiences of verbal and physical abuse at work. *Canadian Journal of Nursing Leadership, 16*(4), 82–98.

Herdman, T. H., & Kamitsuru, S. (Eds.). (2014). *NANDA International Nursing Diagnoses: Definitions and classification, 2015–2017.* Oxford, UK: Wiley Blackwell.

Hibbs, A. (2000). Cognitive therapy: A complementary strategy for expressed anger during the restraint of an aggressive individual. *The British Journal of Forensic Practice, 2*(2), 19–29.

Holmes, D., Murray, S. J., & Knack, N. (2015). Experiencing seclusion in a forensic psychiatric setting: A phenomenological study. *Journal of Forensic Nursing, 11*(4), 200–213.

Horton, L., Duffy, T., Hollins Martin, C., & Martin, C. R. (2015). Comprehensive assessment of alcohol-related brain damage (ARBD): Gap or chasm in the evidence? *Journal of Psychiatric & Mental Health Nursing, 22*(1), 3–14.

Huband, N., Ferriter, M., Nathan, R., & Jones, H. (2010). Antiepileptics for aggression and associated impulsivity. *Cochrane Database Systematic Reviews,* (2). Art. No.: CD003499. doi:10.1002/14651858.CD003499.pub3

Jenkins, A. (1990). *Invitations to responsibility.* Adelaide, Australia: Dulwich Centre Publications.

Johnson, M. E. (2010). Violence and restraint reduction efforts on inpatient psychiatric units. *Issues in Mental Health Nursing, 31,* 181–187.

Johnson, B., Martin, M. L., Guha, M., & Montgomery, P. (1997). The experience of thought disordered individuals preceding an aggressive incident. *Journal of Psychiatric and Mental Health Nursing, 4,* 213–220.

Kabat-Zinn, J. (1990). *Full catastrophe living: Using the wisdom of your body and mind to face stress, pain, and illness.* New York, NY: Dell.

Kabat-Zinn, J. (1993). Mindfulness meditation: Health benefits of an ancient Buddhist practice. In D. Goleman & J. Gurin (Eds.), *Mind/body medicine* (pp. 259–276). New York, NY: Consumer Reports Books.

Kabat-Zinn, J. (1994). *Wherever you go, there you are: Mindfulness meditation in everyday life.* New York, NY: Hyperion.

Kassinove, H., & Tafrate, R. C. (2006). Anger-related disorders: Basic issues, models, and diagnostic considerations. In E. L. Feindler (Ed.), *Anger-related disorders: A Practitioner's guide to comparative treatments* (pp. 1–28). New York, NY: Springer.

Koh, K. B., Kim, D. K., Kim, S. Y., & Park, J. K. (2005). The relation between anger expression, depression, and somatic symptoms in depressive disorders and somatoform disorders. *Journal of Clinical Psychiatry, 66*(4), 485–491.

Kornreich, C., Saeremans, M., Delwarte, J., Noel, X., Campanella, S., Verbanck, P., ... Brevers, D. (2016). Impaired non-verbal emotion processing in pathological gamblers. *Psychiatry Research, 236,* 125–129.

Kreitzer, M. J., Gross, C. R., Waleekhachonloet, O. A., Reilly-Spong, M., & Byrd, M. (2009). The brief serenity scale: A psychometric analysis of a measure of spirituality and well-being. *Journal of Holistic Nursing, 27*(1), 7–16.

Kurtz, M. M., Gagen, E., Rocha, N. B., Machado, S., & Penn, D. L. (2016). Comprehensive treatments for social cognitive deficits in schizophrenia: A critical review and effect-size analysis of controlled studies. *Clinical Psychology Review, 43,* 80–89.

Lanza, M. L. (1992). Nurses as client assault victims: An update, synthesis, and recommendations. *Archives of Psychiatric Nursing, 6*(3), 163–171.

Latalova, K. (2014). Violence and duration of untreated psychosis in first-episode patients. *International Journal of Clinical Practice, 68*(3), 330–335.

Leahey, M., & Harper-Jaques, S. (1996). Family–nurse relationship: Core assumptions and clinical implications. *Journal of Family Nursing, 2*(2), 133–151.

Lewis, D. M. (2002). Responding to a violent incident: Physical restraint or anger management as therapeutic interventions. *Journal of Psychiatric and Mental Health Nursing, 9*(1), 57–63.

Limacher, L. H., & Wright, L. M. (2003). Commendations: Listening to the silent side of a family intervention. *Journal of Family Nursing, 9*(2), 130–150.

Ling, S., Cleverley, K., & Perivolaris, A. (2015). Understanding mental health service user experiences of restraint through debriefing: A qualitative analysis. *Canadian Journal of Psychiatry, 60*(9), 386–92.

Liu, J., Lewis, G., & Evans, L. (2013). Understanding aggressive behaviour across the lifespan. *Journal of Psychiatric and Mental Health Nursing, 20*(2), 156–168.

Lorist, M. M., & Tops, M. (2003). Caffeine, fatigue, and cognition. *Brain and Cognition, 53*(1), 82–94.

Lown, B. (2007). Difficult conversations: Anger in the clinician-patient/family relationship. *Southern Medical Journal, 100*(1), 34–39.

Luck, L., Jackson, D., & Usher, K. (2006). Survival of the fittest, or socially constructed phenomena? Theoretical understandings of aggression & violence towards nurses. *Contemporary Nurse, 21*(2), 251–263.

Marlatt, G. A., & Kristeller, J. L. (1999). Mindfulness and meditation. In W. R. Miller, (Ed.), *Integrating spirituality into treatment*. Washington, DC: American Psychological Association.

Miller, N., Pedersen, W. C., Earleywine, M., & Pollock, V. E. (2003). Artificial theoretical model of triggered displaced aggression. *Personality and Social Psychology Review, 7*(1), 57–97.

Morrison, E. F. (1998). The culture of caregiving and aggression in psychiatric settings. *Archives of Psychiatric Nursing, 12*(1), 21–31.

Munro V. (2002). 'Why do nurses neglect to report violent incidents?' *Nursing Times, 98*(17), 38–40.

National Institute for Health and Clinical Excellence. (2015). *Violence and aggression: Short-term management of in mental health, health and community settings (NG 10)*. London, UK: Author. Retrieved from: www.nice.org.uk/guidance/ng10

The Nova Scotia Department of Health. (2006). The National Survey of the Work and Health of Nurses, 2005. Halifax, NS: Author.

Novaco, R. (2007). Anger dysregulation. In T. Cavell & K. Malcolm (Eds.), *Anger, aggression, and interventions for interpersonal violence* (pp. 3–54). London, UK: Lawrence Erlbaum Associates.

Paris, J. (2005). Borderline personality disorder. *Canadian Medical Association Journal, 172*(12), 1579–1583.

Phillips, J. P. (2016). Workplace violence against health care workers in the United States. *New England Journal of Medicine, 374*(17), 1661–1669. doi:10.1056/NEJMra1501998

Price, O., Baker, J., Bee, P., & Lovell, K. (2015). Learning and performance outcomes of mental health staff training in de-escalation techniques for the management of violence and aggression. *British Journal of Psychiatry, 206*(6), 447–455. doi:10.1192/bjp.bp.114.144576

Reed, P. G. (1992). An emerging paradigm for the investigation of spirituality in nursing. *Research in Nursing & Health, 15*, 349–357.

Registered Nurses' Association of Ontario. (2012). *Promoting safety: Alternative approaches to the use of restraints*. Toronto, ON: Author.

Riahi, S., Thomson, G., & Duxbury, J. (2016). An integrative review exploring decision-making factors influencing mental health nurses in the use of restraint. *Journal of Psychiatric and Mental Health Nursing, 23*(2), 116–128. doi:10.1111/jpm.12285

Scarpa, A., & Raine, A. (1997). Psychophysiology of anger and violent behavior. *Psychiatric Clinics of North America, 20*(2), 375–394.

Shannon, J. W. (2000). Understanding and managing anger: Diagnosis, treatment and prevention. Presentation by Mind Matters Seminar, April 2000, Calgary, Alberta.

Shapiro, S. L. (2008). Exploring the effects of mindfulness meditation on health, well-being, and spirituality. *Spirituality in Higher Education, 4*(2), 1–5.

Sherman, E., & Siporin, M. (2008). Contemplative theory and practice for social work. *Journal of Religion & Spirituality in Social Work, 27*(3), 259–274.

Snyder, K., Schrepferman, L., Brooker, M., & Stoolmiller, M. (2007). The roles of anger, conflict with parents and peers, and social reinforcement in the early development of physical aggression. In T. Cavell & K. Malcolm (Eds.), *Anger, aggression, and interventions for interpersonal violence* (pp. 187–214). London, UK: Lawrence Erlbaum Associates.

Soloff, P. H., Lynch, K. G., & Moss, H. B. (2000). Serotonin, impulsivity, and alcohol use disorders in the older adolescent: A psychobiological study. *Alcoholism, Clinical and Experimental Research, 24*(11), 1609–1619.

Swanson, J., Schwartz, M., Van Dorn, R., Elbogen, E., Wagner, H. R., Rosenheck, R., … Lieberman, J. (2006). A national study of violent behavior of persons with schizophrenia. *Archives of General Psychiatry, 63*(5), 490–499.

Tajaden, P., & Thoennes, N. (2000). *Findings from national violence against women survey*. Washington, DC: U.S. Department of Justice.

Talerico, K. A., Evans, L. K., & Strumpf, N. E. (2002). Mental health correlates of aggression in nursing home residents with dementia. *Gerontologist, 42*(2), 169–177.

Tavris, C. (1989). *Anger: The misunderstood emotion*. New York, NY: Simon & Schuster.

Teplin, L., McClelland, G., Abram, K., & Weiner, D. (2005). Crime victimization in adults with severe mental illness: Comparison with the National Crime Victimization Survey. *Archives of General Psychiatry, 62*(8), 911–921.

Thomas, S. P. (1990). Theoretical and empirical perspectives on anger. *Issues in Mental Health Nursing, 11*, 203–216.

Thomas, S. P. (1993). Women and anger. New York: Springer.

Thomas, S. P. (1998). Assessing and intervening with anger disorders. *Nursing Clinics of North America, 33*(1), 121–133.

Thomas, S. P. (2001). Teaching healthy anger management. *Perspectives in Psychiatric Care, 37*(2), 41–48.

Thomas, S. P. (2003). Men's anger: A phenomenological exploration of its meaning in a middle class sample of American men. *Psychology of Men & Masculinity, 4*(2), 163–175.

Thomas, S. P. (2005). Women's anger, aggression, and violence. *Health Care for Women International, 26*, 504–522.

Thomas, S. P. (2006). Culture and gender considerations in the assessment and treatment of anger-related disorders. In E. L. Feindler (Ed.), *Anger-related disorders: A practitioner's guide to comparative treatments* (pp. 71–96). New York, NY: Springer.

Thomas, S. P. (2009). *Transforming nurses' stress and anger: Steps toward healing* (3rd ed.). New York, NY: Springer.

Verona, E., & Sullivan, E. (2008). Emotional catharsis and aggression revisited: Heart rate reduction following aggressive responding. *Emotion, 8*(3), 331–340.

Victoroff, J., Coburn, K., Reeve, A., Sampson, S., & Shillcutt, S. (2014). Pharmacological management of persistent hostility and aggression in persons with schizophrenia spectrum disorders: A systematic review. *Journal of Neuropsychiatry & Clinical Neurosciences, 26*(4), 283–312.

Ward, L. (2013). Ready, aim fire! Mental health nurses under siege in acute inpatient facilities. *Issues in Mental Health Nursing, 34*, 281–287.

WCB Statistical Services. (2005). Fact sheet: Violence in health care and social assistance provincial overview. Vancouver, BC: Author.

Whitecross, F., Seeary, A., & Lee, S. (2013). Measuring the impacts of seclusion on psychiatry inpatients and the effectiveness of a pilot single-session post-seclusion counselling intervention. *International Journal of Mental Health Nursing, 22*, 512–521.

World Health Organization. (2002). *World report on violence and health*. Geneva, Switzerland: Author.

World Health Organization. (2005). *Multi-country study on women's health and domestic violence against women*. Geneva, Switzerland: WHO Press.

World Health Organisation. (2014). *Global status report on violence prevention 2014*. Geneva, Switzerland: WHO Press.

Wright, L. M., & Leahey, M. (2012). *Nurses and families: A guide to family assessment and intervention* (6th ed.). Philadelphia, PA: FA Davis.

Young, S. N. (2002). Clinical nutrition. 3. The fuzzy boundary between nutrition and psychopharmacology. *Canadian Medical Association Journal, 166*(2), 205–209.

19 Self-Harm Behaviour and Suicide

Elaine Santa Mina

Adapted from the chapter " Self-harm and Suicidal Behaviour" by B. Lee Murray and Wendy Austin

LEARNING OBJECTIVES

After studying this chapter, you will be able to:

- Define suicidal ideation, self-harm, parasuicide, suicidal behaviour, and suicide.
- Identify common myths about suicide.
- Describe population groups that have high rates of suicide.
- Discuss the rights of patients and other legal issues in the care of suicidal patients.
- Determine factors that affect the nurse's responsibility in assessment and intervention with suicidal individuals, including adolescents.
- List screening measures for depression, suicide intent, and psychiatric diagnostic measures.
- Discuss the process of a comprehensive suicide risk assessment.
- Identify suicide risk assessment factors, protective factors, and reasons for living.
- Describe factors that increase the risk for suicide completion.
- Describe the no self-harm contract (contracting for safety).
- Describe the nurse's responsibilities in promoting short- and long-term recovery in suicidal adult inpatients.
- Discuss the patient's and nurse's responsibilities in discharging the patient to the community.
- Identify potential impact on nurses and health care when a patient dies by suicide.
- Identify current issues in suicide.

KEY TERMS

- confidentiality • informed consent • involuntary hospitalization • least restrictive environment • no self-harm contract • parasuicide • self-harm • suicidal behaviour • suicidal ideation • suicide • suicide cluster • suicide contagion

KEY CONCEPTS

- helplessness • hopelessness • lethality • powerlessness • risk/rescue ratio

■ INTRODUCTION

The scope of human behaviours that are understood as self-harm and suicidal occur along a fluid and complex continuum of intent and self-destructiveness. The content of this chapter provides the information needed to understand self-harm and suicidality and to provide nurses with essential assessment skills and interventions to respond appropriately in care of patients, families, and communities who experience such distressful events. This chapter also explores the effect of this phenomenon on nurses and their requirements for self-care.

■ COMMON SUICIDE MYTHS

There are many myths about **suicide**, which, unfortunately if believed, may inhibit timely intervention and treatment. Some people think that people who talk about suicide will not actually "go through with it" and are just seeking attention. Others think that there are no warning signs and that they cannot "see it coming," and believe it is not preventable. It is also very common to think that suicidal people are weak or crazy. A most concerning myth about suicide is the false belief that taking to individuals about suicide will cause them to engage in suicide. If nurses hold

374

this myth, they may be hesitant to ask patients about their thoughts of suicidality and hence miss an opportunity for further assessment and intervention.

Definitions

Self-Harm

Self-harm is a broad classification of self-inflicted behaviours that cause destruction to body tissues (McKenzie & Gross, 2014). These self-inflicted actions may also be termed as self-injurious, self-destructive, parasuicidal, or nonsuicidal self-injury behaviours, and there is little consensus in terminology for this phenomenon. Intentions that motivate these behaviours may be multiple and complex (Butler & Malone, 2013). The behaviours may serve solely as a mechanism to relieve intense emotions and manage experiences of disassociation (Franklin & Nock, 2017), or be clouded with some sense of a wish to die. People who engage in self-harm behaviour are at risk to die by suicide. Trauma (including childhood physical or psychological abuse, sexual abuse, and neglect) has been linked to both **parasuicide** and suicidal ideation in adulthood (Long, Manktelow, & Tracey, 2012; McIntyre, Williams, Lavorato, & Patten, 2013; Molnar, Berkman, & Buka, 2001; Santa Mina, 2010).

Despite reasons alternative to dying, death may be the unanticipated outcome, as people can misjudge the lethality of their actions (Bergen et al., 2012). Our knowledge of motivations and risks for the spectrum of self-harm behaviours remains incomplete, as is our understanding of suicide, and its prevalence may be seriously underestimated. Self-harming individuals may not acknowledge that they engage in behaviour that tends to be socially unacceptable and frequently stigmatized. They may not seek out help, nor come to the attention of health or social services. People who engage in self-harm may do so impulsively or plan it in advance. Self-harm may be a single event or repetitive in nature. People may self-harm by one method only, for example cutting, or multiple methods, for example cutting and burning. Research is needed to more clearly define this phenomenon (Guo, Scott, & Bowker, 2003) and its association with suicide (Hawton & Harriss, 2008).

Suicidal Ideation

Suicidal ideation comprises the thoughts, ideas, and feelings that a person experiences that are about wanting to die and/or the wish to relieve oneself of severe emotional pain (Beck, Brown, & Steer, 1997). Suicidal ideation may be experienced in varying degrees of frequency (sporadic, intermittent, and continuous) and intensity (nonintrusive thoughts, intrusive thoughts, and triggers or associated risk factors; see section on Suicide Risk Factors). They may emanate within cogent thought processes and resultant actions may be assessed to be voluntary in nature. Or they may be a component of a psychotic thought process, from which the behavioural outcome may be assessed as involuntary. Suicidal thoughts may be expressed directly, verbally, or not spoken of at all. Sometimes, they may be expressed indirectly through changes in behaviours, such as suddenly taking care of one's affairs: financial, belongings, and dependents (Registered Nurses' Association of Ontario [RNAO], 2009).

Suicidal Plan

People who are in distress enough to consider suicide may act impulsively and not plan it out in advance (such as someone under the influence of alcohol or drugs or a sudden extreme emotional experience). Others may plan the suicide event in detail, possibly leaving a suicide note about the anticipated event, the method, location, circumstance, and time (RNAO, 2009).

Suicidal Behaviours

Suicidal behaviours are any self-inflicted behaviours for which the intent is to die. Intentions in suicidal behaviours may also include intentions associated with the spectrum of self-harm behaviours; however, the dominant motivation is the wish to die. Suicidal behaviours are described by type (e.g., overdose, gunshot, asphyxiation, hanging), lethality (low or nonlethal to fatal), and frequency (number of behaviours by type and how often or under what circumstances) (Beck, Schuyler, & Herman, 1974; RNAO, 2009).

Suicide Attempt

A suicide attempt is a self-destructive behaviour that did not result in death despite the expectation or intention that it would. Though the individual may receive support, help, and hospitalization and be grateful for such services, the intent to end one's life was present. Acts of suicide, despite the actual outcome, are defined as suicidal behaviour (Freedenthal, 2008).

Suicide: Completed Suicide

The definition of suicide is the self-termination of one's own life. The complex dimensions associated with suicide, however, are grounded in an individual's perceptions and experiences of life and specific factors that are known to put a person at risk to die by suicide (see risk factors). Suicide is associated with deep despair and distress; and death is perceived to be a solution to life's problems (Beck, Steer, Kovacs, & Garbin, 1985). Death by suicide has been highly stigmatized over recorded history and across societies, cultures, and faiths (Olson, 2013).

■ EFFECTS OF SUICIDE

Stigma and Suicide

Suicide, like mental illness, remains stigmatized in contemporary societies, as it has been for millennia. Until a few decades ago, suicide was considered a crime in Western nations and remains a crime today in some countries. The stigma of suicide can prevent people from voicing their suicidal thoughts or seeking help. When a person survives a suicidal act, the visibility of medical intervention can trigger stigmatization by others. Stigma may also be experienced by the survivors of persons who die by suicide, if blame for the loss is affixed to them. Those grieving the suicide may feel responsible for their loss and may not seek support. In this way, the stigma of suicide can significantly complicate bereavement (Olson, 2013). Nurses can do much to demystify suicide and prevent the stigmatization of those at risk through individual and public education.

Effect on Survivors

Worldwide, the rate of death by suicide is 10.7 per 100,000 population. In 2015, there were an estimated 788,000 suicide deaths worldwide (World Health Organization [WHO], 2017). If each suicide impacts only six or seven survivors, approximately 6 to 7 million people each year will lose someone close to them as a result of suicide. Suicide has devastating effects on everyone it touches, especially family and close friends. Prolonged suffering can be caused by the sudden shock, unanswered questions of "why," and potentially the discovery of the body (Knieper, 1999). Suicide bereavement is different than that experienced by families whose loved one's death is not self-inflicted. One's reaction to suicide death is very individual and depends on personal, sociocultural, and situational factors (Grad, 2011). Furthermore, those grieving the loss of someone from suicide are at an increased risk of developing suicidal ideation (Grad) and other mental health issues (Bolton et al., 2013). The grieving over the way the death occurred, the social processes that ensue, and the effect of the suicide on the family converge to establish a grieving process that is unique (Olson, 2013).

Family survivors of suicide report stigmatization, shame, and rejection. Insensitivity by others such as the media, police, medical examiners/coroners, and health care professionals may exacerbate grief. Nurses need to ensure that their response to survivors of suicide is compassionate and nonjudgmental. Simplistic explanations and clichés should be avoided. Survivors of suicide may need help in their search to understand what has happened. As their personal search for meaning regarding the death transpires, their coping abilities will mediate their grief response. It is an ongoing task, but recovery can be made easier by social support that helps address related psychological trauma (Mitchell, Gale, Garand, & Wesner, 2003).

Economic Effects

Estimating the economic cost of suicide is difficult. Nevertheless, in 2010, it was estimated that the total cost of suicide (direct and indirect costs) to Canadian society was approaching 3 billion dollars and is expected to increase substantively by 2035 if the current trajectory is not altered (Parachute, 2015).

Suicide remains a significant public health problem in Canada and places heavy demands on the health care system, despite efforts at both policy and clinical levels (e.g., to identify risk and protective factors, as well as to provide appropriate interventions). Suicide prevention is difficult because suicide is "the outcome of complex interactions among neurobiologic, genetic, psychobiologic, social, cultural, and environmental risk and protective factors" (Government of Canada, 2016; Guo et al., 2003). Nurses are in a unique position to contribute to preventive efforts. With knowledge of early risk assessment and interventions—understood within the context of a person's family, social world, and broader community—as well as with knowledge of how to engage with and respond to the actively suicidal person, nurses can make a difference by preventing the escalation or chronicity of the behaviour (Murray, 2003; RNAO, 2009).

Settings Where Nurses Work With Patients Who Are Suicidal and/or Families and Communities Affected by Suicide

Many nurses may be of the understanding that only those who work in mental health settings or emergency departments will work with people experiencing suicidality. However, human psychological and social distress may be found anywhere in society and hence anywhere in nursing practice. It is essential that all nurses, regardless of their area of practice and expertise, be knowledgeable of self-harm and suicide, the risk factors, and best practices for assessment and intervention for safety. Suicide affects all ages: children to elderly, all races and cultures, and socioeconomic groups. Individuals, families, friends, peers, communities, and cultural groups are all deeply affected by suicide. People struggle to know what to do when a patient, colleague, friend, loved one, or community experiences suicidality. The entire spectrum of self-harm and suicidal behaviours are very challenging for nurses and other health care professionals to address, to protect life, and to provide safety for all. This includes clinicians who care for those who are suicidal, as they may be vulnerable to vicarious trauma. Therefore, it is important that nurses are knowledgeable about self-harm and suicide, particularly because such behaviours can be a means of communicating to others one's despair (RNAO, 2009). Refer to Box 19.1 for information about suicide prevention internationally.

BOX 19.1 World Suicide Prevention Day

World Suicide Prevention Day is September 10th each year. It is significant that the **World Suicide Report (WSR)** is released on this day. The WSR presents the status of suicide prevention internationally. See www.iasp.info to learn of activities for this year.

EPIDEMIOLOGY OF SELF-HARM BEHAVIOUR AND SUICIDE

Rates of Suicidal Ideation

It is estimated that 36,560 (0.1%) people in Canada have unstated thoughts of suicide or suicidal ideation (Navaneelan, 2012). Suicidal acts tend to be seen as "cries for help" rather than overt expressions of a desire to die. A 17-country study found that, across all countries examined, 60% of people transitioned from suicidal ideation to their first suicide attempt within the first year of ideation onset. Prevalence estimates in low- and middle-income countries are similar to those in high-income countries for suicidal ideation (3.1% to 12.4% vs. 3.0% to 15.9%, respectively). Suicide plans are estimated to be at 0.9% to 4.1% in low-income countries versus 0.7% to 5.6% in high-income states (Nock et al., 2008).

Rates of Self-Harm and Suicidal Behaviour

Rates of self-harm and suicidal behaviours are likely generally underestimated. In Canada, the rates are highest among young women, whereas men are more likely to die from self-inflicted injuries (Canadian Institute of Health Information, 2011). Suicidal ideation and self-harm are more common among adolescents than other age groups. Self-harm behaviour in adolescents is often a way to communicate needs or wants, and often the need is for attention or care (Murray, 2003). As such, self-harm is an unacceptable means to acceptable ends and may communicate that the adolescent believes that something is wrong, life is tough, and things are becoming unbearable. Parasuicidal behaviour or self-injurious behaviour (e.g., cutting or self-mutilation) may also relieve or release certain emotions and feelings and may produce a tangible, physical pain to substitute for unfamiliar, unbearable psychological suffering (Franklin & Nock, 2017). Self-punishment is often identified with self-loathing, anger, guilt, and shame (Murray, 2003). Research assessing the risk of nonsuicidal self-injury using the Inventory of Statements about Self-Injury found, consistent with previous studies, that those who self-harm do so for a myriad of reasons, including self-punishment, sensation seeking, interpersonal influence, and marking distress (Klonsky & Glenn, 2009). Behaviour escalates if the purpose of the self-harm is not achieved, so feeling unheard or misunderstood can result in escalation of self-harm. Even if the purpose of self-harm behaviour is recognized, ignoring or minimizing the behaviour may escalate its intensity and frequency with increased attempts to get the message across (Murray, 2003).

In a Statistics Canada publication, Navaneelan (2012) reported that self-harm rates vary by gender and type as do rates of suicidal behaviour. Females are more likely to engage in self-harm by means of cutting and in suicide attempts by overdose. Males are more likely to engage in highly lethal suicide attempts such as gunshot and hanging. Suicide attempts also vary somewhat between low- and high-income countries (0.7% to 4.7% vs. 0.5% to 5.0%, respectively) (Nock et al., 2008). Although reliable data are lacking on the full impact of attempts at suicide that do not result in death, it is recognized that self-harm and suicide attempts can result in physical injury and emotional, psychological, and social trauma, acute and lengthy hospitalization, and community care.

Rates of Suicide

Suicide occurs in all age groups, social classes, and cultures. The WHO (2017) reports that nearly 1 million people suicide every year. Globally, suicide is a greater cause of death than war and homicide combined (Bertolote, Fleischmann, Butchart, & Besbelli, 2006; WHO, 2017).

Canadian Data

Canada ranks 41st in the world for reported suicides (WHO, 2012) and, within Canada, suicide is the ninth leading cause of death overall: seventh for men and thirteenth for women. Almost 4,000 Canadians die by suicide yearly (Navaneelan, 2012). The rate of suicide hovers between 10.7 and 11.3 per 100,000 between 2011 and 2014 (Statistics Canada, 2014). It is the leading cause of death for men aged 25 to 29 and 40 to 49 years and for women aged 30 to 34 years. It is also the leading cause of nonaccidental death for those aged 15 to 34 years. In the decade from 2000 to 2009, the most common means of death by suicide were by hanging, including strangulation and suffocation (44%), poisoning (25%), and firearms (16%). It is generally accepted that prevalence rates are underestimated. Death by suicide can be difficult to identify as it may be disguised as a motor vehicle collision or homicide, especially in young people, and there is time lag between the reporting of a death and identifying it as a suicide (Navaneelan, 2012).

Suicidality and Specific Populations

Suicide is more common among groups with specific risk factors and has been associated with loss, unemployment, transience, recent life events (e.g., financial problems, divorce, moving, problems with children), interpersonal distress, and earlier attempts. See Box 19.2 for a discussion of suicide and the Canadian military. Research indicates that, universally, suicide is strongly associated with chronic depression and most specifically with a pervasive sense of despair and hopelessness (Satyanarayana, Enns, Cox, & Sareen, 2009). The best predictor for suicide is a previous attempt.

Age

Children

Prepubertal Children

Self-harm is a growing concern among youth and adolescents. Adolescents at risk for body image concerns, peer pressure, and challenges of sexuality and those

BOX 19.2 Suicide and the Canadian Military

Understanding and preventing suicide is a priority within the Canadian Armed Forces (CAF). When eight suicides among our military personnel occurred in the first 3 months of 2014, this sudden spike prompted public concern (Brewster, 2014). Yet, suicides in the CAF are not significantly higher than in the Canadian population. A report on suicide mortality in the CAF from 1995 to 2015 confirms that fact, as well as indicates that there has been no overall statistically significant increase in suicide mortality in the CAF (Rolland-Harris, Cyr, & Zamorski, 2016). A trend over the past decade toward increased risk was found, however, for Regular Forces males with a history of deployment when compared with those without a deployment history, but this finding did not reach statistical significance. There was a significant increase in risk of suicide noted, from 2002 to 2015, for those who were part of army command compared with those in other commands. The report notes that the CAF mission in Afghanistan had a strong impact on some personnel deployed there and that there are links between trauma incurred during deployment, mental disorders, and suicide risk (Rolland-Harris et al., 2016). Examination of use of health care services (not necessarily direct access to mental health services) by personnel within the year prior to their suicide was high, approximately 93%, with over three quarters of these personnel accessing services within 30 days of their suicide. The report concludes that, while current trends in risks related to deployment and army command need to be recognized, suicide prevention in CAF requires consideration of many risk factors (Rolland-Harris et al., 2016).

A study that examined the association between suicidal ideation and self-reported symptoms of PTSD (see Chapter 17), major depressive disorder (see Chapter 22), and alcohol use disorder (see Chapter 26) in CAF combat and peace-keeping veterans seeking treatment at an Ontario operational stress injury clinic found that, although PTSD alone is associated with suicidal ideation, it was self-reported depressive symptom severity that was its most significant predictor (Richardson et al., 2012). About one quarter of Canadian military deaths are due to individual behaviours, particularly suicide, alcohol consumption, and tobacco use. The "healthy soldier effect" means that other risks seen in the general population due to lack of physical activity and poor diet are uncommon. Soldiers in combat, however, are more likely to smoke to deal with the stress of deployment and to abuse alcohol upon return home; combat veterans are more likely to have mental health problems. Targeting these behaviours seems important to a preventive mental health strategy (Tien et al., 2010).

---

with histories of childhood abuse are especially at risk for self-destructive behaviours.

Suicide is rare among children who are younger than 10 years of age. There were two reports of self-harm resulting in completed suicide in Canadian children this age in 2011 (Statistics Canada, 2014). However, suicides by children this age may be significantly underestimated, as many question whether children can fully understand the finality of death and intentionally kill themselves.

Adolescents/Youth

More teenagers die from suicide than from cancer, heart disease, birth defects, stroke, pneumonia, influenza, and chronic lung disease combined. In 2004, 156,000 adolescent deaths worldwide were the result of suicide (WHO, 2012). In 2011, 29 Canadian children aged 10 to 14 years (12.7% of all deaths within this age group) died due to intentional self-harm (Statistics Canada, 2014). Statistics Canada (2014) reports suicide to be the second leading cause of death for youth aged 15 to 24 years (499 deaths), making up 24.5% of all deaths in this age group. In 2011, 198 individuals aged 15 to 19 completed suicide. This represented one quarter (24.9%) of all deaths in this age group (Statistics Canada, 2014). Preadolescent and adolescent males are over three times more likely to complete suicide than are their female peers (17.9 vs. 5.3 per 100,000). Male and female Aboriginal youths in Canada, however, both die from suicide at rates higher than those in non-Aboriginal teens (Kirmayer, 2012), with Inuit males aged 15 to 19 committing suicide at 40 times the rate (500 per 100,000) of non-Inuit males the same age (Eggertson, 2013). Suffocation is the most common method used by Canadian adolescents, rather than firearms (Kirmayer, 2012).

Although the number of completed suicides is disturbingly high, the rate of attempted suicide is also alarming. The World Health Organization (2012) reports that, worldwide, suicidal behaviours of young people ages 15 to 25 have been increasing at an alarming rate and estimates this age group to be the most at risk in one third of countries. WHO, further estimates that for every suicide, there are 20 suicide attempts. Although exact suicide attempt rates in Canada are difficult to track, Langlois and Morrison (2002) report that 40.8, 152.2, and 117.9 per 100,000 Canadian youth aged 10 to 14, 15 to 19, and 20 to 29 years, respectively, attempted suicide.

Midlife

Worldwide trends indicate that the suicide rate increases with age (WHO, 2012). In Canada, however, suicide rates are at their highest at midlife (age 45 to 59) (Statistics Canada, 2014). Single people in this age group have double the suicide rates of other age groups. Divorced people aged 45 to 59 have a suicide rate 1.7 times higher than divorced people of other ages, while the suicide rate in persons widowed aged 40 to 59 years is 2.1 times higher than for the widowed 60 and older (Navaneelan, 2012). By age 55 to 60 years, however, suicide is the sixth leading cause of death falling to 17th by age 70 to 75 (Statistics Canada, 2014). As age increases, suicide rates as a cause of death within the age group decline, indicative of an increase in pathologic deaths occurring from cancers, heart attacks, and so on.

Elderly

Although other causes of death are more prominent, suicide risk is high among older adults (O'Connell, Chin, Cunningham, & Lawlor, 2004) and is an often-overlooked problem (Monette, 2012). Nationally, the ratio of suicide attempts to completions in older adults is 4 to 1. Older adults generally have a stronger intent to die, plan their suicide more carefully, and are more likely to use more lethal means of killing themselves than are younger people (Conwell & Duberstein, 2001). Of those aged 60 and older, 30% use hanging and 26% use firearms as a means to complete suicide (Navaneelan, 2012). The health challenges associated with aging may contribute to the rate of completed suicides, and because many older adults live alone, the chance of a suicide attempt being thwarted is often less than among younger people. Of all suicides in Canada in 2001, 19% were by people older than 60 years of age. Suicide is less stigmatized for this age group and may be viewed as more acceptable (Heisel & Duberstein, 2017).

For older adults, suicide is associated with less education, widowhood, previous attempts, depressive disorder, social isolation, financial difficulties, poor physical health and functioning, substance abuse, and loss of autonomy (Conwell, Duberstein, & Caine, 2002; Heisel & Duberstein, 2017). As in other age groups, major depressive disorder (MDD) is a significant factor in suicide. However, comorbid physical illnesses often make recognition of MDD difficult. In 2011, 71% to 95% of elderly people who completed suicide had a major psychiatric disorder at the time of death (Conwell, van Orden, & Caine, 2011; Heisel & Duberstein, 2017).

Regional Variations

Provincial statistics show varied rates of suicide across Canada (see Table 19.1). Eastern and central regions of the far north have some of the highest mortality rates from suicide in Canada (Navaneelan, 2012). In this table, the suicide rate per 100,000 people for Nunavut was 56.9,

Table 19.1   Canadian Suicide Statistics

Province/Territory	Suicide Rate*
Alberta	12.7
British Columbia	9.6
Manitoba	12.5
New Brunswick	13.2
Newfoundland and Labrador	8.8
Northwest Territories	21.9
Nunavut	56.9
Quebec	13.7
Saskatchewan	12.8
Yukon	5.7
National Average	10.4

*Per 100,000 people.

while for the Northwest Territories, it was 21.9 and for Québec, 13.7. These higher suicide rates may be due to a combination of factors. Many people in these regions live in rural or semirural environments where hunting (and ready access to firearms) is common; social isolation can occur due to low population per square kilometre; and the population is predominantly Indigenous, who experience rates of suicide higher than the national average. Within each province, rates of suicide are not consistent, because urban centres tend to have suicide rates lower than the national average, and demographic, social, cultural, and geographic factors affect rates of suicide.

Indigenous People

"I am here today because my ancestors, starving as they often were, fought to survive. Why did the old people strive to live ... and the young people now want to die?" (Nishnawbe Aski Nation Youth, 2004). The suicide rate among Indigenous populations in Canada is several times the national rate (Kumar, 2016; White & Jodoin, 2003). From 1999 to 2003, the Inuit suicide rate was more than 10 times the national rate (Government of Canada, 2006; Masecar, 2009), with Inuit males aged 15 to 19 years 40 times more likely to kill themselves than their non-Inuit peers (Eggertson, 2013; Inuit Tapiriit Kanatami, 2016). Suicide disproportionately affects Innu and Inuit populations in Canada (Pollack, Mulay, Valcour, & Jong, 2016). Unfortunately, many young Inuit see suicide as a viable option to cope with an untenable and hopeless living situation (Masecar, 2009). Among the Indigenous people of Canada, hanging is the most common method of committing suicide (49.2% for males, 45.8% for females), followed by firearms for men and drug overdoses for women (Kirmayer et al., 2007; Kumar, 2016).

Over a third of all deaths among Indigenous youth are attributable to suicide (Health Canada, First Nations and Inuit Health Branch, 2003). Conversely, the suicide rate for Indigenous people over the age of 70 drops below that for the general population. The risk factors for suicide among Indigenous people are the same as for non-Indigenous

---

BOX 19.3 Aboriginal Community Wellness Strategies

- Develop locally initiated, owned, and accountable programs.
- Suicide prevention should be the responsibility of the entire community.
- Focus on behavioural patterns of children and young people is crucial and requires the involvement of family and community.
- Suicide prevention must be addressed from the biologic, psychological, sociocultural, and spiritual perspectives.
- Long-term crisis and intervention programs must be developed.
- Suicide intervention strategies must be evaluated as needed.

From Health Canada, First Nations and Inuit Health Branch. (2003). *A statistical profile on the health of First Nations in Canada.* Ottawa, ON: Government of Canada.

(depression, abuse, poverty, isolation, etc.) (First Nations Information Governance Centre [FNIGC], 2012; Kirmayer et al., 2007) but are compounded by the effects of Indigenous-specific experiences such as colonization, the residential school system, and children being taken off reserves to be fostered or adopted by non-Indigenous families (Olson, 2013; Smye & Browne, 2002).

It is important to note that Indigenous suicide rates may be underreported. Data collected by Statistics Canada pertain only to status Aboriginals, thus excluding nonstatus First Nations, Métis, and Inuit people from the overall Indigenous suicide data. As well, the rate of accidental deaths among Indigenous people is four to five times higher than in the general population, and up to 25% of these deaths may be from suicide

(Inuit Tapiriit Kanatami, 2016; Royal Commission on Aboriginal Peoples, 1995; White & Jodoin, 2003).

Although the rate of suicide is higher for Indigenous people as compared with other Canadians, not every Indigenous community in Canada experiences high rates of suicide (Kirmayer et al., 2007; White & Jodoin, 2003). Marked differences can be noted between provinces and regions, and even between communities in the same geographic region. In studying suicide among British Columbia's Indigenous communities, Chandler and Lalonde (1998) discovered that some communities had suicide rates 800 times the national average, while in other communities, suicide was virtually unknown. They also identified six protective factors that may explain the differences in suicidal rates between communities (see Box 19.3). According to a Health Canada (2003) report, community wellness strategies may have the best chance of making a difference in suicide rates between Indigenous communities. Guidelines were suggested in developing such a strategy (see Box 19.4).

Despite widespread concern about the high rates of suicide in Indigenous populations, there are still no studies comparing rates across Indigenous groups, nor are there data showing the origins and effective interventions concerning suicide among Indigenous groups (Health Canada, 2003; Kirmayer et al., 2007). In Indigenous communities where there is autonomy and a strong sense of ownership, culture, and community, there are much lower rates of suicide (Kirmayer et al., 2007).

Gender

Worldwide, males complete suicide at a rate three times that of females, although women are four times more likely to attempt suicide than men (Health Canada, 2003; WHO, 2012). In Canada in 2011, a total of 2,781 males committed suicide (16.3 deaths per 100,000), compared to 947 females (5.4 deaths per 100,000) (Statistics Canada, 2014). The reasons for the difference

---

BOX 19.4 The Mental Health of Indigenous People in Canada: A Critical Review of the Research

Much of the available literature on suicidality in Indigenous people in Canada is in relation to colonialism and associated processes on the determinants of their health. The resultant themes of research into suicide and substance abuse have been questioned. To avoid continued patterns in colonial research, the following recommendations were raised as a result of this systematic review:

- Question whether health services and health data adequately address the specific mental health determinants or issues with respect to

the provision of health services with Indigenous populations.
- Consider that Métis peoples and urban or off-reserve populations are underrepresented in current research.
- Recognize that more research taking into account of the impacts of colonialism and the history of mental health research in Canada is required.

From Nelson, S. E., & Wilson, K. (2017). The mental health of Indigenous peoples in Canada: A critical review of research. *Social Science and Medicine, 176,* 9–112. doi:10.1016/j.socscimed.2017.01.021

are not entirely understood. Men are seven times more likely to use firearms than are women (20% vs. 3% of completed suicides), whereas women are twice as likely to die by poisoning (42%). Conversely, females are three to four times more likely to attempt suicide than are males, and hospitalization for attempts is 1.5 times greater in females than males (Navaneelan, 2012).

Factors that affect suicide risk differently by gender include experiences of violence, family upbringing, and economic deprivation. Exposure to violence, sexual assault, or both also increases women's risk for suicide (Koplin & Agathen, 2002; Nelson et al., 2002), while having a small child reduces it (Qin, Agerbo, Westergård-Nielson, Erikson, & Mortenson, 2000). Having a parent with a psychotic or affective disorder increases the risk for both sexes, but especially for women (von Borczyskowski, Lindlad, Vinnerlkjung, & Hjern, 2010). Being of low socioeconomic status increases the risk of suicide for men (but not women), while living in a highly urbanized environment increases the risk for women (von Borczyskowski et al., 2010). Economic deprivation is more likely to precipitate suicide in men but not necessarily in women (Piérard & Grootendorst, 2014). Although unemployment has long been associated with suicide in men, research has shown that for the long term, unemployed women also are at serious risk for suicide: unemployed women had a suicide rate three times that of employed women in a follow-up study of 9 years (Kposowa, 2001).

LGBTQ Sexual Orientation

In recent years, sexual orientation has been more openly addressed as a risk factor for suicide. "Coming out" can be a risk factor because of the possible negative reactions of others, particularly peers and family. Being unable to disclose sexual identity because it is unsafe to do so may contribute to a deep sense of isolation. During adolescence, when the major focus of a youth's life is on peers and sexuality, a gay, lesbian, bisexual, or transgender (GLBT) youth's search for self-identity may heighten depression and suicidal behaviour (Zhao, Montoro, Igartua, & Thombs, 2010). GLBT youth are also at a higher risk for suicide if they self-present with high levels of gender nonconformity (Liu & Mustanksi, 2012) or report being unsure as to their sexual identity (Zhao et al., 2010). As a predictor, GLBT victimization was the strongest—after suicide attempt history—for self-harm, associated with a 2.5-fold increased risk (Liu & Mustanksi, 2012). It is important to note that the risk factors associated with LGBTQ individuals are in addition to those common to all ages and sexual orientations. More recently, authors are offering alternative explanations to the traditional psychomedical reasons for self-harm and suicide in this cohort and suggest that these behaviours may be grounded in culturally embedded discourse that pathologizes nonnormative sexual orientation (McDermott & Roen, 2016).

KEY CONCEPT

Lethality refers to the probability that a person will complete suicide. Lethality is determined by the seriousness of the person's intent and the likelihood that the planned method will result in death. High lethality includes firearms, hanging, carbon monoxide poisoning, drowning, suffocation, or jumping from a great height.

KEY CONCEPT

Risk/rescue ratio refers to the lethality of means and the likelihood of rescue. Suicidal risk carries with it a progression of seriousness from suicidal ideation to completed suicide. Risk is lowest when intent is weak and the method used has low lethality. The likelihood of rescue is dependent on communication of intent and lower lethality of means.

■ RISK FACTORS

Major depressive disorders and physical, psychological, and social risk factors contribute to suicidal ideation. Physical factors include medical illness and alcohol and drug use; psychological factors include hopelessness, psychological distress, and low self-esteem; and external social risk factors include lack of social support, family problems, financial hardship, and legal problems. Childhood trauma (including physical abuse, sexual abuse, and childhood hunger) has been linked to both parasuicide and suicidal ideation in adulthood (McIntyre et al., 2013; Molnar et al., 2001).

Aetiology of Self-Harm Behaviour

Self-harm is more common among adolescents than other age groups. Research assessing the risk of nonsuicidal self-injury using the Inventory of Statements about Self-Injury found, consistent with previous studies, that those who self-harm do so for a myriad of reasons including self-punishment, sensation seeking, interpersonal influence, and marking distress (Klonsky & Glenn, 2009). Behaviour escalates if the purpose of the self-harm is not achieved, so feeling unheard or misunderstood can result in escalation of self-harm. Even if the purpose of self-harm behaviour is recognized, ignoring or minimizing the behaviour may escalate its intensity and frequency with increased attempts to get the message across (Murray, 2003).

Aetiology of Suicidality

The spectrum of suicidal thoughts, feelings, behaviours, and death by suicide occurs in the context of an individual's physiologic, psychological, and social situation and is usually triggered by stressors that are unmanageable and exceed typical coping efforts.

Vulnerabilities are enhanced by engagement in risky behaviours, often used in an effort to cope with stress. Risky behaviours related to suicide include fast, dangerous driving; tempting death; promiscuity; use of alcohol or drugs; and purchase of a handgun. Appropriate interventions guided by a comprehensive assessment of risk at this point can reduce the likelihood of suicidal behaviour. Most who attempt suicide have seen a health care professional at least 1 year prior to the attempt (Morrison & Laing, 2011). Edwin Shneidman (1985), a clinical psychologist and leading authority on suicide, has described common characteristics of suicide in his book *Definition of Suicide* (see Box 19.5).

A comprehensive assessment identifies the physical, psychological, and social factors that contribute to feelings of suicide (Fig. 19.1). These factors include changes in central nervous system neurotransmitters, engaging in negative thinking and risky behaviours, and deterioration of social relationships. The convergence of biologic, psychological, social, and spiritual factors can be directly linked to suicidal behaviour. Most will agree that suicide, like many other aspects of humanity, rarely lies within a single sphere of the bio/psycho/social/spiritual model. However, in order to facilitate learning, suicide will be discussed in relation to each of these spheres.

Biologic Theories

Biologic theories of suicide attempt to clarify the phenomenon of suicide by recognizing and interpreting physiologic, neurophysiologic, and hormonal changes. Psychopathologic changes are evident in most suicidal people. Major depressive disorders (MDD), sometimes

---

BOX 19.5 Shneidman's Common Characteristics of Suicide

1. **The common stimulus for suicide is unendurable psychological pain.**
   Faced with intolerable emotion and unacceptable anguish, people will sometimes opt for a cessation of consciousness. The core ambivalence in suicide reflects the conflict between survival and unbearable stress. The main clinical rule is reduce the suffering, often just a little bit, and the individual will choose to live.

2. **The common stressor in suicide is frustrated psychological needs.**
   Suicides are born, negatively, out of needs. Most suicides represent combinations of various needs. The clinical rule is address the frustrated needs and the suicide will not occur.

3. **The common purpose of suicide is to seek a solution.**
   Suicide is not a random act. It is a way out of a problem, dilemma, or crisis. It is the answer—seemingly the only available answer—to a real puzzler: How to get out of this? It is important to view each suicidal act as an urgently felt effort to answer a question, to resolve an issue, and to solve a problem.

4. **The common goal of suicide is "cessation of consciousness."**

5. **The common emotions in suicide are hopelessness and helplessness.**
   Often, people on the edge of committing suicide would be willing to live if things—life—were only a little bit better, a just noticeable difference. The common fear is that the inferno is endless and that one has to draw the line on one's suffering somewhere.

6. **The common internal attitude toward suicide is ambivalence.**

Something can be both "A" and "not A." We can both love and hate the same person. A prototypical suicidal state is one in which the individual feels that she or he has to do it and simultaneously yearns and even plans for rescue and intervention.

7. **The common cognitive state in suicide is "constriction" (tunnel vision).**
   Suicide cannot be understood as a psychosis, a neurosis, or a character disorder. It is a transient psychological constriction of affect and intellect. It is a narrowing of the range of options that leads to either/or thinking.

8. **The common interpersonal act in suicide is communication of intention.**
   The communication of suicidal intention is not always a cry for help. First, it is not always a cry; it can be a shout or a murmur or the nonverbal communication of something unspoken. The communication is not always for help; it can be for autonomy or any number of needs. Nonetheless, in most cases of suicide, there is some interpersonal communication related to that intended final act.

9. **The common action in suicide is regression or escape.**
   Suicide is a death in which the decedent removes him- or herself from intolerable pain and simultaneously from others in the world.

10. **Suicide is consistent with lifelong coping patterns.**
    "You can't fire me; I quit." "I'll leave her before she leaves me." Shneidman believes that suicide is not a random act and sometimes is reasonably predictable.

From Shneidman, E. (1985). *Definition of suicide.* New York, NY: John Wiley & Sons.

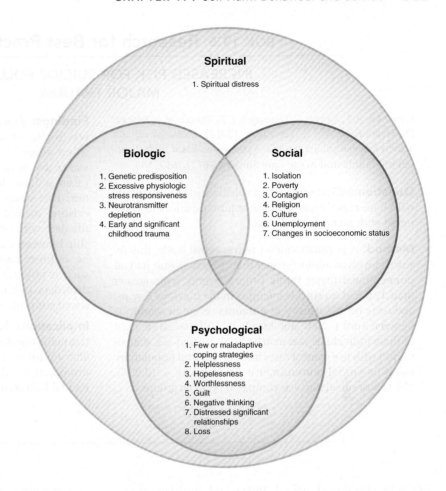

Figure 19.1. Bio/psycho/social/spiritual aetiologies of suicide.

comorbid with other psychiatric illnesses, are prevalent. Moreover, because suicide rates tend to be higher in families in which suicide has occurred, genetic and familial factors will be explored in this section. As well, a biologic explanation of increased suicide risk among those who experienced childhood sexual abuse and among those who have experienced a traumatic injury is considered (see Box 19.6 for the latter). Many adults who complete suicide have a psychiatric diagnosis, with depression being the most common condition (Mishara & Chagnon, 2011).

Considerable evidence exists showing a familial trend in suicide (McGuffin, Marusic, & Farmer, 2001; Qin, Agerbo, & Mortenson, 2003). First-degree relatives of individuals who have completed suicide have two to eight times the risk for suicide than do individuals in the general population (McGuffin et al., 2001). The genetic link to suicide is evident in studies of twins. Qin and colleagues (2003) showed that suicidal behaviour in one monozygotic twin increased the risk 11-fold for suicidal behaviour in the co-twin. Among adolescent female twins, genetic factors played a part in 35% of suicide attempts (Glowinski et al., 2001). Adoption studies have shown that among adults who experience mood disorders and were adopted as children, the suicide rate among the biologic relatives of the adoptees is much higher than the rate among the adoptive relatives.

Genetic abnormalities in the serotonergic neurotransmitter system may be responsible for the heightened familial risk for suicide (Mann, Brent, & Arango, 2001). Collectively, these studies demonstrate that the biologic risk for suicide appears to be independent of environmental factors.

MDD may develop when a person, vulnerable to depression because of genetic or other factors, is subjected to repeated or sustained stress. Stress responsiveness ultimately changes neurotransmitter and hormonal functioning to affect a depressed state (Hauenstein, 1996). Those who completed suicide had extremely low levels of the neurotransmitter serotonin, 5-hydroxytryptamine (5-HT; Mann, Oquendo, Underwood, & Arango, 1999), or lower levels of the neurotransmitter dopamine (Pitchot et al., 2001).

Other factors linked to suicide include childhood physical and sexual abuse, child hunger, and other psychosocial issues (Marshall, Galea, Wood, & Kerr, 2013; McIntyre et al., 2013). Child abuse has been described as a specific vulnerability for psychopathology and suicide (MacMillan et al., 2001). Enhanced vulnerability to MDD and suicide associated with child abuse are attributable to changes in the hypothalamic–pituitary–adrenal axis caused by intractable stress and altered serotonin and dopamine metabolism (Skodol et al., 2002). Evidence from twin studies suggests that the link

BOX 19.6 Research for Best Practice

INCREASED RISK FOR SUICIDE FOLLOWING MAJOR TRAUMA

From March, J., Sareen, J., Gawazjuk, J. P., Doupe, M., Chateau, D., Hoppensack, M., ... Logsetty, S. (2014). Increased suicidal activity following major trauma: A population-based study. Journal of Trauma and Acute Care Surgery, 76(1), 180–184.

Question: What is the risk of suicidality for individuals who have experienced a major traumatic injury as compared with a matched cohort?

Method: A population-level retrospective study, this research involved adults (greater than 18 years) who had an unintentional major injury (injury severity score greater than 12), had no suicide attempts in the previous 5 years, and were on the registry of a trauma centre in Manitoba between April 1, 2001, and March 31, 2011; *n* = 2,198. Each of these individuals was matched (i.e., on age, sex, date of injury) with five control cases from the general population, using provincial administrative databases (*n* = 10,990). The rate of suicidality was compared between groups.

Findings: Suicidality (suicides and suicide attempts) was higher in the trauma group. This persisted even when adjusted for anxiety, mood disorders, and substance use, as well as for residence (urban/rural), income (average household income), and physical comorbidities. This study is unique in that it controlled for preexisting mental illness and excluded individuals from the data with premorbid suicide attempts. The relationship between trauma and suicide may be direct or it may be indirect and mediated through postinjury factors such as physical immobility, mental health problems or disorders, or changes in social circumstances, including social support and marital status.

Implications for Practice: As individuals with major traumatic injuries are at a higher risk for suicidal behaviour after injury as compared to the general population, it is important to identify and assess those who may need mental health interventions and follow-up on discharge.

---

between childhood sexual abuse and biologic alterations contributing to psychopathology may be independent of other environmental influences. Several studies show that adult psychopathology is greater in abused twins when compared with nonabused co-twins (Bulik, Prescott, & Kendler, 2001; Kendler et al., 2000; Nelson et al., 2002). Additional specific features of the abuse, including severity, contributed to worse outcomes in the abused twins.

Psychological Theories

Coming to understand suicide as it is related to the human psyche is important. MDD, generalized anxiety disorder, personality disorders, bipolar disorder, schizophrenia, substance use disorders, and other psychiatric illnesses are frequently present in suicidal persons. The link between mental and substance use disorders and suicide is well documented and has been determined as responsible for approximately two thirds (22.5 million of the 36.2 million) disability adjusted life years (DALYs) allocated to suicide globally in 2010. The burden of mental and substance use disorder as a risk factor for suicide has elevated these disorders to the third leading disease category of global burden in 2010. Early prevention and detection and effective management of mental and substance use disorders—particularly major depressive disorders—have been determined as a key suicide prevention strategy (Ferrari et al., 2014).

A psychodynamic theoretical perspective conceptualizes suicidal behaviour as an intrapsychically determined phenomenon. From this conceptualization, a comprehensive understanding and formulation of intergenerational family dynamics, the individual's intrapsychic determinants, are important considerations for determining treatment modalities for suicidal individuals and their families (Morey, 2014). Suicide has been conceptualized psychologically as an excessive reaction arising from intense preoccupation with humiliation and disappointment (Leenaars, 1998) and driven by intolerable aloneness and isolation (Adler & Buie, 1996). Cognitive approaches also attribute suicide to learned helplessness and hopelessness as an automatic and pervasive pathologic scheme for organizing and interpreting experience. The widely used cognitive theory of depression espoused by Aaron Beck and his associates (Beck, 2011) accounts for how negative thoughts occur, how they tend to be repetitive and intrusive, and how they can lead to suicidal behaviour (see Chapter 13).

Attachment theory explains social isolation and disrupted interpersonal relationships as being a part of the spectrum of suicide (Lopez & Brennan, 2000). In this theory, adult behaviour is shaped by early interactions with the primary caregiver during infancy. Disturbed attachment results in the individual's inability to form meaningful relationships or in a constant concern about the viability of a lasting relationship. Suicide, in this conceptualization, is the result of conflicted or distant adult relationships and the social isolation that arises (Eng, Rimm, Fitzmaurice, & Kawacki, 2002). Muehlenkamp, Brausch, Quigley, and Whitlock (2013) suggest that treatments should focus on strengthening interpersonal bonds alongside emotion regulation.

Social Theories

Social factors are particularly important to the aetiology of suicide. As humans, we are inherently a part of the social fabric in which we exist. To be alive is to be in the world. Suicide, then, is the desire to estrange oneself from the world. Some suicidal people describe a desire to "feel nothing for a while," a temporary respite from life and the world.

Studying the social factors that contribute to rates of suicide, sociologist Emile Durkheim, at the end the 19th century, developed a theoretical framework outlining the social causes of suicide. Durkheim (1897, 2006) classified suicide under four headings: egoistic suicide, altruistic suicide, anomic suicide, and fatalistic suicide. These classifications of suicide are based on the degree of imbalance between social integration and moral regulation (Kendall, Lothian-Murray, & Linden, 2004).

Durkheim believed that the degree of social integration was a variable affecting rates of suicide. *Egoistic suicide* occurs among individuals who are not significantly bound to society. Some believe that the social isolation of single people is causally related to their higher rates of suicide when compared with their married counterparts. Conversely, *altruistic suicide* occurs when individuals become overly connected to society, for example, patriotic soldiers who kill themselves after a defeated battle because they are shamed.

Durkheim also acknowledged that extreme cases of social stability and social consensus contribute to rises in suicide rates. A society lacking a sense of purpose, social regulation, or community values experiences *anomic suicide*. This type of suicide occurs during times of financial depression. Contrastingly, in areas of overregulation and oppression, *fatalistic suicides* occur. Although Durkheim discussed little about fatalistic suicide, many use the suicide of slaves as an exemplar.

Contemporary sociologic investigations seek social structure models of influence on suicide. A theory explicated by Cohen and colleagues (2003) contends that socioeconomic status is a driving factor in what happens to an individual, affecting the physical and social structures available to him or her. For example, poverty represented by substandard housing affects other important neighbourhood social structures, such as schools, voluntary organizations, and jobs. People wishing to teach in these schools, help out, or conduct business in the neighbourhood are deterred by the neighbourhood deterioration. Poverty also reduces exposure to opportunities for individual advancement. Poverty

affects health outcomes directly, because of environmental hazards, or indirectly, through inadequate access to health care. Data exist to support this model of suicide. Ruiz-Perez and colleagues (2017) found that during times of economic deterioration, suicides increase. Socioeconomic deprivation and unemployment were found to be associated with suicide in several studies (Kposowa, 2001; Steenland, Halperin, Hu, & Walker, 2003). Unemployment may also pose an indirect risk for suicide through family tension arising from the loss of income and a normal social role. This loss may then lead to indignity, isolation, hopelessness, alcohol abuse, and violence. Wealth, too, brings with it a distinct set of worries and concerns. Importantly, suicide is at its greatest rates when a substantial change in social status occurs.

There is evidence to indicate that the social structure of marriage is a protective factor across all age groups, while divorce correlates to an increased risk of suicide. It is hypothesized that the social support and companionship provided by marriage help decrease the probability of suicide, while divorce increases a person's chance of developing depression (Navaneelan, 2012).

Suicide Contagion and Suicide Clusters

A social phenomenon, seen most frequently among adolescents, is **suicide contagion**. Several studies have shown that when one teenager takes his or her life, several more may follow (Olson, 2013; Poijula, Wahlberg, & Dyregrov, 2001; Zenere, 2009). The occurrence of suicide contagion can result in the development of a **suicide cluster**, which is defined as multiple suicidal behaviours or suicides that fall within a specific time frame and often specific geographical area (Olson, 2013). A *mass cluster* is often associated with media reports related to the suicide of celebrities (e.g., Marilyn Monroe and Kurt Cobain) or other cases of completed suicide with overwhelming attention generated by media saturation (e.g., Amanda Todd). Celebrity suicide is associated with increased completed suicides; considerable care must be taken when reporting suicides, particularly high-profile ones (Niederkrotenthaler et al., 2012). There is a direct relationship between media coverage of suicide and contagion (Scherr & Reinemann, 2011). This social phenomenon was originally termed the "Werther effect," after the young lover in Goethe (1774–1989) whose suicide inspired copycat suicides among young male readers. Some scholars, however, suggest that individuals who are influenced by such stories are already in a vulnerable state as a result of other precipitating factors and may not necessarily be influenced by media exposure of suicide (Westerlund, Schaller, & Schmidtke, 2009). Nevertheless, media guidelines have been developed to address the potential harm of suicide coverage, such as those of the Centers for Disease Control, the World Health Organization, and the Canadian Psychiatric Association. These guidelines emphasize collaboration between mental health professionals and the media to ensure that reporting is done in a way to reduce copycat suicidal behaviour. However, the realities of 21st-century technology—in which information about a person's suicide can readily be made available through YouTube, Twitter, and Facebook—can in part defeat the purpose of such guidelines.

In contrast to mass clusters, *point clusters* are suicides that occur close in time and space and often occur in settings such as hospitals, schools, prisons, and specific communities (Olson, 2013). Point clusters can be a major problem in Indigenous communities as individuals on reserves are closely related and share the same social predicaments: a single suicide affects the entire community (Kirmayer et al., 2007). This can also manifest as *echo clusters* that occur over an extended period of time after the original cluster (Masecar, 2009).

Bullying, Cyberbullying, and Suicide

Traditional bullying has been defined as aggressive intentional "harm doing" by one person or a group, generally carried out repeatedly over time, and which usually involves a power differential (Nansel et al., 2001). See Chapter 16, Table 16.2, for examples of the four types of bullying: physical, verbal, relational, and "cyber." People who are bullied tend to be at greater risk for suicide (Centers for Disease Control and Prevention [CDC], 2014; Ha, 2014). Cyberbullying has been defined as "willful and repeated harm inflicted through the use of computers, cell phones, and other electronic devices" (Hinduja & Patchin, 2010; p. 208). Across studies of the prevalence of cyberbullying among students, it seems that about 15% to 35% have been victims of cyber bullying while about 10% to 20% admit to cyberbullying others (Hinduja & Patchin, 2010; McLeod, 2011). A survey of nearly 2,000 randomly sampled adolescents revealed that those who had experienced cyberbullying, either as a victim or as an offender, were more likely to attempt suicide than those who had not experienced this form of peer aggression. Victimization had a stronger relationship to suicidal thoughts and behaviour than bullying (Hinduja & Patchin, 2010). Fisher and colleagues (2012) found that among 2,141 children aged 12 who had self-harmed, 56% were exposed to frequent bullying. This higher rate of self-harm existed even after children's premorbid emotional and behavioural problems, low IQ, and family environmental risks were taken into account. These researchers also found that the adolescents who did engage in self-harm were more likely to experience physical maltreatment by an adult, have a family history of suicidal behaviours, and suffer from mental illness such as conduct disorder and depression. Frequently, adolescents who completed suicide after experiencing bullying or cyberbullying had emotional and psychosocial issues in their lives such as low self-esteem and depression (CDC, 2014, 2016; Zetter, 2008), struggles with social and academic life (Flowers, 2006), and stressful life circumstances (Hinduja & Patchin, 2010). Clearly, the act of

suicide is a very complex phenomenon, and the relationship between cyberbullying and suicide requires further research. Many countries including Canada have initiated antibullying legislation and school policies.

IN-A-LIFE

Rehtaeh Parsons (1995–2013)

CYBERBULLYING, SUICIDE, AND PUBLIC RESPONSE

On April 4th, 2013, 17-year-old Rehtaeh Parsons attempted suicide and died 3 days later. Her suicide was preceded by 17 months of bullying following a gang rape of Rehtaeh that had been photographed and circulated online. Although Rehtaeh's rape had been reported to authorities at the time, RCMP and the prosecutor deemed there to be insufficient evidence to charge the perpetrators (Huffington Post, 2013). According to Rehtaeh's family, her suicide was prompted by depression brought on by the rape, the ongoing distribution of the photograph, bullying by her peers, and a continuous barrage of sexually explicit texts and Facebook posts. In the year prior to her death, Rehtaeh had been voluntarily hospitalized to treat her suicidality.

Rehtaeh's suicide was widely publicized and became a flash point online and across Canada about cyberbullying and victims' rights. Following the wishes of their daughter, who wanted to contact the media before her death, Rehtaeh's parents, Leah Parsons and Glenn Canning, have openly described what happened to her (Canadian Press, 2013). Leah Parsons also created a Facebook memorial page that went viral in popularity.

There was national outrage at what was perceived as a failure of the justice system (Huffington Post Canada, 2013). Online, the activist group Anonymous threatened to publicly identify Rehtaeh's rapists but stopped after Rehtaeh's mother requested the issue be settled in court (Huffington Post Canada, 2013; Ross, 2013). Initially, the Nova Scotia justice minister refused to open the case but, due to public pressure, it was later reopened (Huffington Post Canada, 2013). Not all publicity, however, was in support of Rehtaeh. Locally, a poster campaign was started in support of the accused, drawing concerns about vigilantism. Nationally, questions were raised about whether the sex was consensual (Blatchford, 2013), which drew the ire of many, including Rehtaeh's parents, as a case of victim blaming (Cross, 2013).

Since Rehtaeh's death, numerous changes have resulted. In August 2013, Nova Scotia passed a new

Cyber-Safety Act that would protect victims' identities during the investigative period, allow victims to sue aggressors, and, in the case of underage cyberbullies, hold their parents financially liable. Changes were also made to the province's Education Act, requiring principals to address known cases of bullying even if it happens off school property. A CyberSCAN Unit, the first in Canada, was also established in the province to investigate cases of cyberbullying (CBC News, 2013a). As well, both the school district where Rehtaeh was a student and the hospital that treated her a year earlier have investigated their handling of the situation and revised their practices. Following the renewed police investigation, two men were arrested and charged with the distribution of child pornography and one with the creation of child pornography (CBC News, 2013b). Supporters continue to hold sexual assault and cyberbullying awareness rallies (CTV News, 2014), while Glenn Canning and Leah Parsons continue to petition the government to improve national cyberbullying laws and mental health services for cyberbullying victims (Blatchford, 2015).

The problem of bullying, cyberbullying, and suicide remains. More recent publically reported incidents are Emilie Olson in 2014 (Alter, 2015); Alyssa Morgan, 2015 (Cruz, 2015); and 8-year-old Gabriel Taye, 2017 (Jorgensen & Chavez, 2017).

Spiritual Theories

Spirituality has reemerged as an important component of nursing care (Tinley & Kinney, 2007). Increasingly, it is recognized as a key component of holistic care. Spirituality, which can mean a search for meaning, connectedness (both intrapersonal and interpersonal), energy, and a person's worldview (Canadian Federation of Mental Health Nurses [CFMHN], 2014; Mandhouj & Huguelet, 2016; Pesut, 2003), is being recognized as a source of resilience and coping (Martin, 2002). Past studies have shown that people with spiritual involvement were at a decreased risk of substance abuse, addiction, and suicide (Benson, 1992; Koenig & Larson, 2001) and that, for some people with mental illness, spirituality was used as a coping resource and lowered the risk of substance abuse and suicide (Larson & Larson, 2003).

Suicide and Religion

Research regarding the impact of religion on suicide has not yielded consistent results (Leach, 2013; Rasic, Kisely, & Langille, 2011). It has been hypothesized that not only personal but also contextual differences in religious beliefs may determine an individual's willingness to consider suicide (Mandhouj & Huguelet, 2016). Greater moral objections to suicide in those with a religious affiliation may be protective against suicide attempts (Dervic et al., 2004). However, social scientists have not found that not believing in God or lack of religiosity is a causative factor leading to suicide. Rather, it is likely that an individual's belief that suicide is wrong is a strong deterrent to the act of suicide (Hilton, 2002; Leach, 2013).

Caring for People at Risk for, or Engaging in, Self-Harm and/or Suicidal Behaviours

Canadians have legal rights that health care providers must consider self-harm and/or suicide prevention and treatment. Patients always maintain their right to self-determination unless assessed to be incompetent. Patients have the right to be free from harm. Physically restraining or hospitalizing a patient against his or her will has the potential for both physical and emotional harm. Such action should be taken only when the patient is under the threat of imminent harm to self or others or when the patient's status is "not competent" under the relevant mental health act or is a risk to self and/or others. Nurses must be familiar with their provincial or territorial mental health legislation (see Chapter 7), understand patients' legal rights, and be able to explain them clearly.

Confidentiality

Disclosing information without the permission of patients violates their rights to privacy and anonymity and may damage the therapeutic relationship. Patients lose trust when the nurse shares their suicidal intent with others unless the nurse has specifically explained the limits of **confidentiality**. When informing the patient of existing limits of confidentiality, the nurse must be very clear and specific. The Canadian Nurses Association (CNA) has articulated the concept of confidentiality as safeguarding information acquired within a professional relationship, except when doing so, would cause significant harm (Canadian Nurses Association [CNA], 2017; CFMHN, 2014).

The CNA code of ethics is consistent with provincial legislation. Namely, patients have the right to confidentiality unless they are at risk for harming themselves or others or discloses any form of abuse of minors, including neglect and sexual, physical, psychological, and emotional abuses. In these situations, the nurse can enlist the help of others (e.g., outside of the health care team) to protect the patient's or others' safety.

Protecting the patient's right to confidentiality is a special concern when a minor child has suicidal intent. As with adult patients, the nurse is required to describe the right to confidentiality and its limits. The nurse must always consider informing parents or legal guardians of a child who has suicidal intent. The parents of a minor child retain the privilege to determine the right care for their child, and they need sufficient information to make good decisions. Before beginning any suicide risk assessment, nurses must let a child know that disclosure of self-harm may be shared with parents. Honesty about what the nurse can and cannot keep confidential ultimately increases a child's trust and often results in a more therapeutic relationship.

Informed Consent

Obtaining fully **informed consent** from patients protects their right to self-determination. However, nurses must inform suicidal patients about limits to their self-determination and work in collaboration with patients in their care. From the time that the nurse encounters a suicidal patient until a suitable placement is made in consultation with other members of the interprofessional team, the nurse must share with the patient his or her right to be placed in the least restrictive environment that will ensure safety. The **least restrictive environment** is the setting that puts the fewest constraints on patients' rights while still ensuring their safety. By informing patients about their choices, the nurse gains their trust and decreases the likelihood that **involuntary hospitalization** will be necessary.

The ethical requirement of beneficence, doing no harm, is critical when restraining patients against their will. Caring for patients who are suicidal and determined to get away is difficult without touching and actively restraining them. Still, nurses must do their best to disclose to patients the specifics of planned treatments, including restraints, and attempt to obtain their consent to proceed. Respect for the patient needs to be maintained throughout the process. (For further discussion of these issues, see Chapter 11.)

▌ NURSING ASSESSMENT AND INTERVENTIONS

The foundation of all nursing practice is the therapeutic relationship. Assessment and care for people who are experiencing any of the spectrum of self-harm and suicidal thoughts and behaviours must be grounded in the core principles of a therapeutic relationship. Persons experiencing suicidal ideation often experience hopelessness, helplessness, and powerlessness, which need to be assessed and integrated into their plan of care.

All patients who indicate verbally or nonverbally their intention to engage in any self-harm behaviour, or actually harm themselves, must be taken seriously and assessed for suicide risk. Self-harm and suicidal behaviours are seriously underreported and often not recognized by health care professionals. For example, a Statistics Canada study found that in Alberta, almost 60% of Albertans who committed suicide had recently visited an emergency room; nearly 90% had had a health visit (on average 17 visits) during the year before death (Morrison & Laing, 2011). Nurses play an essential role in suicide prevention because they practice in diverse health care settings and thus work with many different kinds of patients. Nurses are typically the first frontline health care providers to come in contact with a self-harming or suicidal patient and are pivotal in making a difference in the outcome and preventing death. A patient who is acutely suicidal is in a true psychiatric emergency. Nurses must act immediately and vigorously to prevent the patient's death (RNAO, 2009).

KEY CONCEPT

Hopelessness is a perception of having no hope that one's life situation or circumstance will change or improve. It is characterized by feelings of inadequacy and an inability to act on one's own behalf.

KEY CONCEPT

Helplessness is the perception of having limited ability or ambition to change one's current life situation. It is characterized by a sense of being unable to help oneself and a sense that there is a lack of support or protection.

KEY CONCEPT

Powerlessness is the perception of having no power or control over one's life circumstance, feeling that the world will never be fair, feeling helpless and totally ineffectual, or feeling one lacks legal or other authority.

Bio/Psycho/Social/Spiritual Domains

Nursing interventions based on a comprehensive assessment of risk provide a holistic approach to nursing care of the suicidal patient. The process of risk assessment will be discussed, followed by a discussion of nursing interventions in relation to the biologic, psychological, social, and spiritual aspects of the suicidal person.

Comprehensive Assessment of Risk

Comprehensive assessment provides a clear picture of self-harm and suicidal behaviour and guides possible interventions. (See Box 19.7 for Questions to Guide a Comprehensive Assessment of Risk; see Box 19.8 for Suicide Assessment Tools.)

Assessment includes collection of adequate data to provide a clear picture of the patient's life and relevant stressors from the patient's perspective. This includes a

---

BOX 19.7 Questions to Guide a Comprehensive Assessment of Risk

STRESSORS

What is troubling you most at the moment?

    Explore with curious questions in terms of all areas of the patient's life.

    Explore each area, asking the patient to tell you more.

    The idea is to get a clear picture of the patient's life situation and presenting stressors as the patient perceives them.

SYMPTOMS

Can you tell me about your sleep patterns?

    Explore using curious questions:

    Are you having difficulty sleeping?

    Do you want to stay in bed and sleep through the day?

Can you tell me about your eating habits?

    Explore using curious questions:

    Have you lost your appetite?

    Do you eat in an attempt to cope with difficulties?

What do you do for enjoyment?

    Explore with curious questions:

    Do you find you no longer enjoy activities you thought were enjoyable?

    How often do you use drugs or alcohol to cope?

PRIOR BEHAVIOUR

Have you ever thought of harming yourself?

    Explore with curious questions:

    Can you tell me about that (time, place, situation, feelings, meaning)?

    What was the self-harm about?

    What happened?

    What did you expect to happen?

    What did you want to happen?

CURRENT PLAN

Do you currently have a plan to harm yourself?

    Explore with curious questions:

    What would you do?

    Do you have access to the pills (other methods)?

    Have you picked a specific day or time?

RESOURCES AND SUPPORT

Do you have someone you recognize as supportive?

    Explore with curious questions:

    Who can you talk to about your concerns?

    Who can you confide in?

    Offer suggestions of a number of people the patient may not have thought of (e.g., parent's friend, colleague, clergy, coach).

---

good understanding of the patient's family, peers, and social relationships as well as workplace issues. Changes related to loss need to be explored to identify possible precipitating factors. Issues of abuse need to be discussed with thoughtfulness and sensitivity.

The broad spectrum of symptoms related to depression and hopelessness must be explored. (See Chapter 22 for assessment of depression.) Such symptoms include isolating or withdrawing from friends and family, sleep and eating disturbances, not enjoying or participating in

---

BOX 19.8 Suicide Assessment Tools

There are tools that can assist with risk assessment, such as the *Beck Scale for Suicide Ideation, Nurses' Global Assessment of Suicide Risk,* and the *Suicide Intent Scale* (see Perlman, Neufeld, Martin, Goy, and Hirdes, (2012)). Suicide risk assessment within the Tidal Model (Barker & Buchanan-Barker, 2005) includes a global assessment of risk (Cutcliffe & Barker, 2004) to determine the person's need for care and ongoing monitoring and reassessment. Its dimensions include initial screening, focused assessment; integration of the risk assessment; care planning, intervention, and implementation; and monitoring and reassessment.

Alternatively, the *Inventory of Motivation for Suicide Attempts* (IMSA), developed by May and Klonsky (2013), identifies two motivations. *Intrapersonal* motivations reveal the need to escape or relieve internal

emotions and thoughts and can be assessed using scales of hopelessness, psychache, escape burdensomeness, low belonging, and fearlessness. *Interpersonal* motivations reveal the desire to communicate with or influence another individual and can be assessed using scales of interpersonal influence and help seeking. To assess intent, the IMSA has 54 statements to be answered using a five-point Likert scale (e.g., "I attempted suicide because I...," "...was so lonely I couldn't handle it," "...hated myself so much," "...didn't fit in anywhere").

The *Suicide Risk Assessment Model* (Murray, 2003; Murray & Wright, 2006) can be used by nurses in any care setting and includes stressors, symptoms, prior behaviour, current plan, and available resources and support. It can be integrated as part of the focused suicide risk assessment in the Tidal Model.

activities that were enjoyed in the past, and having no sense of the future. Engaging in risky behaviours such as drug or alcohol use is commonly associated with suicide.

The patient should be assessed for other psychiatric disorders, especially those most commonly associated with suicidal behaviour (e.g., MDD, substance use disorder, panic disorder, anxiety disorder, schizophrenia). Severity of MDD is associated with a greater likelihood of suicide completion. For adolescents, a key question is whether any family member has attempted or completed suicide. The eight-item Suicide Intent Scale (Beck et al., 1997) is short and useful in determining whether a patient has a strong intent to die. Also of recommendation is the Beck Hopelessness Scale (Beck, Weissman, Lester, & Trexler, 1974), which assists in assessing the level of hopelessness. Although these references may seem dated, they are classics in the field, given Beck's pioneering work in this area. Assessment of hopelessness is important as it is highly associated with suicide.

Assessment of the context of both current and prior self-harm or suicidal behaviour begins to formulate an understanding of the complexities of behavioural motivations, unique to the individual. An exploration of prior behaviour also gives a message of interest and concern on the part of the health professional. A nonblaming, nonjudgmental approach allows further exploration and understanding of the patient's situation as the patient begins to trust the nurse within the context of the therapeutic relationship.

Assessment includes exploration of self-harm and suicidal behaviour from the perspective of the patient. Self-harm behaviour can be imitative, especially if it is interpreted as a way of coping with frustration and anger or a way of punishing self or others (Rew, Thomas, Horner, Resnick, & Beuhring, 2001). The exploration of the patient's motivations helps both the patient and the nurse to understand factors that put the patient at risk and work toward interventions that help the patient meet needs in healthier ways.

Having a Current Plan

Self-harm may be impulsive in nature, in response to overwhelming feelings of emotion and dissociation, and therefore may not be planned as such. People who engage in chronic self-harm behaviour may resort to their usual methods such as cutting and know when and under what triggers they will do this (refer further to self-harming behaviours in Chapter 27). Suicidal behaviour may also be impulsive. People who are under the influence of alcohol or other substances, or people with personality disorders who experience sudden emotionally negative feelings of abandonment and rage, may be at risk to impulsively end their lives. Patients with psychoses may respond impulsively to "voices" that direct them to kill themselves and are at considerable risk because of their inability to separate psychotic thinking from reality.

Suicide requires intent, a plan, knowledge of how to carry out the act, and few obstacles to completing it. Individuals who complete suicide have developed a method of ending their lives. They are less likely to have young children or other immediate responsibilities and may not be concerned with religious prohibitions concerning the act. The relationship between the availability of a method of suicide, the method's lethality, and suicide completion is strong. It is important for the nurse to ask whether the patient has a current plan for suicide and access to the means to end life. Further exploration of the plan gives the nurse a more accurate assessment of risks and guides appropriate interventions.

Protective Factors, Resources, and Support

There are many reasons that a person who may feel suicidal and have a plan may not carry it out. As much as someone may wish to die, that person may also have many reasons to stay alive. The state of ambiguity between wishing to live and wishing to die affords an opportunity to explore with the patient reasons for living, which are considered protective factors as they protect a person from acting on thoughts, feelings, and plans. It is important, therefore, to assess a patient's reasons for living. For some, it may be a child or parent to care for; for others, it may be against religious beliefs to take one's life; for others still, it may be a purpose in life as yet not fulfilled. Protective factors are not a guarantee that a person will not take his or her life, but they do offer a basis upon which a nurse can work with the patient to promote and sustain hope in living (Bongar, Sullivan, Kendrick, & Tomlins, 2017).

Resources and supports are also critical considerations for people at risk for self-harm and suicide. Lack of these may put patients at greatest risk. Suicidal people often feel socially isolated and struggle to identify and accept support from people in their immediate environment; therefore, it is important to explore supportive people in the patient's life. Interest in the patient's life and attention received during a thorough assessment are therapeutic and can also provide connectedness and engagement with the patient and family. Resources and supports not available through the patient's personal sphere of friends and family may need to be supplemented through any variety of community supports. Assessment of the patient's previous use of, access to, and benefits from community supports helps to plan the care post discharge from the hospital, crisis centre, or community agency. Assessment of financial resources, such as drug and benefit plans, is also important in considering the scope of available resources. See Web Links.

Method

Assessment of method and access to that method is important to ascertain potential lethality of any suicidal behaviour. Some researchers have provided evidence to indicate that the method of a suicide attempt holds meaning for the individual and understanding that meaning may also provide insight regarding motivation and lethality. Understanding access to method is also critical to creating a plan of care to ensure safety, for example removing pills to prevent overdoses, removing knives or sharp objects to prevent stabbings and other objects to prevent hangings. It is important to assess where all potential methods are kept or stored in relation to the patient to store away for safety. This includes knowing where firearms are stored safely.

Almost 60% of all firearm deaths are suicides, and firearms are used in nearly 20% of all suicide fatalities (Canada Safety Council, 2014). Gagné, Robitaille, Hamel, and St-Laurent (2010) report that when firearm restrictions were introduced in Canada, male firearm suicides declined. Although the accessibility of firearms is usually associated with rural areas, urban areas show the highest rates of completed suicides by firearms.

Assessment and Reassessment

Self-harm and suicide may be a single event in a person's life and with rapid interventions may resolve. However, as discussed, the thoughts and feelings underlying self-harm and suicide are complex, typically multifaceted and dynamic, which may make a very fluid situation for many people who suffer such despair. Hence, a suicidal state is often understood as existing along a continuum of wanting to live and wanting to die. A patient's thoughts and feelings may change rapidly with fluctuating personal and physical circumstances. That is why it is so important for nurses to be alert to subtle as well as overt changes in the patient's behaviours that may indicate a shift in suicidal thinking and reassess as often as required.

Documentation

The nurse must thoroughly document assessments and interactions with suicidal patients. This action is for both the patient's ongoing treatment and the nurse's protection. The nursing notes must reflect that the nurse took every reasonable action to provide for the patient's safety, inclusive of thorough assessments and reassessments. If a **no self-harm contract** has been instituted, the record must contain specific aspects of the contract.

Planning and Implementing Nursing Interventions

Thorough assessment becomes part of the intervention process. The health professional's genuine interest, concern, and exploration begin to establish a needed trusting relationship. Using this approach, health care professionals help patients identify what and who needs to change in their environment. This approach uncovers concrete areas of improvement or change. This empowerment addresses their feelings of hopelessness, helplessness, and powerlessness.

Understanding the purpose and meaning of the self-harm and suicidal behaviour guides the intervention strategies. It also gives the patient and family a sense of hope that things can change and that someone understands their situation and is willing to assist them in making changes.

If some or many of the risk factors for suicide are present in a member of a high-risk group, the nurse must determine what is necessary to ensure the patient's ongoing safety, which is the nurse's first priority. Until the nurse has identified a patient's safety needs and implemented a plan to ensure the patient's safety, the nurse must not leave the acutely suicidal person alone for any reason, not even briefly. Nursing care of acutely suicidal persons requires consultation within a team approach.

Contracting for Safety

Contracting for safety—having the patient agree and commit, in writing, to no self-harm or suicide attempt for an agreed upon period of time—is an intervention used extensively in some psychiatric settings (Knesper, 2011). Such contracts can only be negotiated after a thorough assessment of the patient has been completed. The nurse must consider patient competency in terms of being able to enter into a contract of this nature. The patient cannot be in a psychotic state or under the influence of alcohol or other drugs. Patients who have made a previous suicide attempt or who are extremely isolated are not good candidates for safety contracting. Legal and professional scholars disagree on the ability of children and adolescents to make decisions of this gravity on their own behalf. Involving parents in the decision about the appropriate environment for their suicidal child is important. Advantages and disadvantages of no self-harm contracts and several examples of contracts can be found in a review by Range and colleagues (2002). However, the use of safety contracts is underresearched; while their effectiveness depends upon the patient's ability to keep a commitment of this kind, the factors influencing this are not fully known or understood (Knesper, 2011).

Inpatient Care and Acute Treatment

Suicidal patients were once hospitalized for extended periods to ensure that the suicidal crisis had passed and to provide sufficient time to establish a solid base of treatment for the underlying psychiatric disorder. This is no longer the case. Hospitals are overly restrictive environments that may inhibit the patient's development of the self-reliance needed to return to the community. Objectives of hospitalization are to maintain the patient's safety, reduce or eliminate the suicidal crisis, decrease the level of suicidal ideation, initiate treatment for the underlying disorder, evaluate for substance abuse, reduce the patient's level of social isolation, and connect the patient and family with ongoing outpatient resources and therapy.

If the patient is assessed as acutely suicidal and is at considerable risk for completing suicide, the decision must be made whether to hospitalize the patient for the patient's safety. Safety in such cases is commonly determined by whether a patient may be a threat to self or others. Provincial law requires patients to be hospitalized only when they cannot make reasoned decisions to ensure their safety. The law also requires that the restriction of the patient occurs only when it provides a therapeutic effect. In considering the hospitalization of a patient, the nurse must consider how hospitalization will be useful in ensuring safety and relieving the patient's suicidal crisis.

Interventions for the Biologic Domain

Ensuring Safety

During the early part of the hospitalization, the most important way to reduce stress is to help the patient feel more secure and hopeful. Nurses can do so by ensuring the patient's safety with as little intrusion as possible on the person's exercise of free will. Achieving this goal can be difficult. The major deterrent to patients' completing suicide in psychiatric hospitals is their engagement in a therapeutic relationship and regular observation by nurses. Each hospital has its own specific protocol for maintaining patients' safety. In addition to nursing standards of care, hospital staffing and other policies that affect the degree to which a suicidal patient can be restrained may influence the procedures mandated for caring for patients.

Maintaining a safe environment includes observing the patient regularly for suicidal behaviour, removing dangerous objects, and providing counselling opportunities for the patient. Part of ensuring patient safety is helping patients to re-establish personal control by including them in decisions about their care and restricting their behaviour only as necessary. Ongoing and effective communication with the patient is key to allowing patients to disclose and discuss their life situation and the resulting emotions and behaviour. Patients often feel shaky in the first hours of psychiatric hospitalization, and it is comforting to know that a caring person is nearby. Observational periods can be used to help the patients express a broad range of feelings and strengthen their belief in their own abilities to keep themselves safe. The nurse can help the patient who is not skilled in self-expression or self-management skills to describe feelings more effectively and cite ways of managing safety needs. Then, at the next observation time, the nurse may have the opportunity to reinforce the patient's own safety behaviour. Thus, the observation period can be transformed from something negative (e.g., "The patient can't be trusted," "I am out of control") to something positive (e.g., "The patient is becoming safer," "Maybe I can keep myself safe after all"; Cardell & Pitula, 1999). As the patient becomes more confident in understanding and controlling self-harm behaviour, the frequency of observation periods can be reduced.

Seclusion and restraint are two modalities sometimes used in the inpatient settings to maintain patient safety. However, these restrictive interventions are extremely stressful for patients and may interfere with their recovery. Moreover, seclusion and restraint often are used to compensate for inadequate staffing numbers. Unduly restraining patients to prevent their suicide interferes with the development of trusting relationships between patients and health care providers. The stress associated with restraints contributes to the biochemical disarray of their underlying psychiatric disorders. Restraints prevent patients from managing their own dysphoric and anxiety symptoms and reinforce their sense of hopelessness and helplessness. Restraints also enhance patients' fears that they are "crazy" and incapable of controlling their impulses. These methods reinforce a patient's perception of being out of control and lessen his or her ability to form a partnership with mental health providers.

Assisting With Somatic Therapies

Suicidal patients with major depressive disorders will likely receive somatic therapies, and patients' response to them must be monitored. The major somatic therapies used in the treatment of suicidal behaviour are antidepressant medications and electroconvulsive therapy (ECT). ECT may be useful for selected patients with intractable suicidal ideation and severe depression. ECT may be used for people who do not experience response to medication or who do not tolerate antidepressant medications, such as older adults and those with comorbid medical disorders. Although the decision must be made carefully, ECT can be a lifesaving procedure for the acutely suicidal patient with MDD. Nurses need to be able to support patients in accepting and understanding this treatment (see Chapters 12 and 22).

The objective of medication for suicidal behaviour is to raise serotonin rapidly to a level that reduces suicide risk. To that end, third-generation and newer antidepressant medications should be used for those who are in imminent danger of harming themselves. These include fluoxetine (Prozac), sertraline (Zoloft), paroxetine (Serzone), bupropion (Wellbutrin), venlafaxine (Effexor), and citalopram (Celexa). These drugs generally are nontoxic and cause few side effects, especially after being taken for 1 to 2 weeks. They often are faster acting than the older drugs, but their onset of action varies. Especially useful are fluoxetine and paroxetine, which may be taken once a day. Sertraline also can be taken once a day, but achieving the proper dose can sometimes be difficult. Patients who take an overdose of these medications have much better outcomes than those who abuse first- and second-generation antidepressants.

The first- and second-generation antidepressants, including tricyclics and monoamine oxidase inhibitors, are equally effective for severe depression (Sutherland, Sutherland, & Hoehns, 2003). However, for those with suicidal behaviour, they may not be the best choice because these are highly toxic medications that people with suicidal intent can use to kill themselves. The resuscitation of a patient who has taken large amounts of one of these medications can be difficult because of cardiotoxicity; medical sequelae may be long term if the patient is saved. Also, the side effects of these early antidepressants may result in the patient stopping the use of prescribed medication while still having suicidal thoughts. The need for laboratory assessment for therapeutic drug levels is another disadvantage of these drugs. Blood monitoring requires the patient's cooperation when his or her motivation may be at its lowest.

Regardless of the medication that is prescribed, further ongoing assessment regarding the patient's suicidal ideation and behaviours is required. As a patient's depression is lifting, he or she may find that they may now have the energy to carry out their plan.

Assisting With Treatment for Substance Use

Suicidal behaviour is often associated with substance use disorders, especially among men. When substance use is an issue for the suicidal patient, the use must be addressed, or inpatient treatment of suicidal behaviour is only palliative, and the danger of the patient repeating a suicidal attempt is high. For men, substance use disorder may be the primary psychiatric disorder, with depression a side effect of it. For women, depression commonly is the primary psychiatric disorder, and substance use disorders result from attempts to medicate the underlying depressive condition. The nurse should help the patient understand the role that alcohol and other drugs play in his or her suicidal behaviour. Treatment for substance use disorders should be part of the treatment plan, as appropriate, including referral to specific inpatient or community-based programs. Refer further to Chapter 26.

Interventions for the Psychological Domain

It is important for nurses to use the hospitalization period to find out what may have precipitated or contributed to the suicidal crisis. Precipitating factors, and how the patient's coping process were ineffective, often become evident. After identifying extreme stressors experienced by the patient, the nurse and patient can help determine ways for the patient to avoid those stressors in the future or, if they cannot be avoided, to manage them more effectively.

During hospitalization, the nurse should evaluate the patient's ways of thinking about problems and generating solutions. Some patients, by virtue of their concurrent illness or social learning, have an unusually negative view of life. They may think such thoughts as, "I am no good," "Everything I do is useless," "I have no future," or "Nobody has ever liked me, and nobody ever will." Often patients are unable to recognize the connection between their stressors and their suicidal behaviour. Many patients have had very difficult and abusive experiences in their lives, and their ability to cope is threatened. It is important for the nurse to help the patient identify what needs to change in his or her life and how that change can come about most effectively. The prevention of further suicidal behaviour is dependent on the patient's belief that he or she can make changes with the necessary support and resources and that there is hope for the future. (See Box 19.9 for examples of effective and ineffective dialogue with a patient.)

Interventions for the Social Domain

Improving Communication

Some suicidal patients can identify family and friends who are willing to help, but in many cases, patients are concerned about burdening these people or do not feel comfortable sharing their concerns with others. Helping the suicidal patient express these concerns and arrive at ways of reducing them is important. In other cases, because of trauma and abuse, patients may have difficulty identifying anyone in their lives as supportive. These patients are usually at a high risk for suicide because of their perception of aloneness and lack of connection with any significant other. The nurse needs to assist the patient in identifying people in the patient's life who may be supportive and make appropriate referrals to professionals with expertise in the area. Within the confines of therapeutic boundaries, the nurse can also be one of the supportive people in the patient's life if the nurse is successful in establishing a professional relationship with the patient.

Networking and Discharge Planning

Another concern may be patients' embarrassment about the hospitalization and their emotional state. Through education, the nurse can do much to destigmatize the situation for both the patient and significant others. Before discharge, it is ideal for the patient to be able to name people who can act as a support. When supportive people are present, with the patient's permission, the nurse can work with them to begin to develop a network for the patient to rely on to remain safe. It is important for the patient and supportive family and friends to have a plan to contact another person, either a confidante or a mental health care provider, when they have questions or distressing thoughts or feel unable to manage or control suicide thoughts and behaviours.

Educating the Patient and Family

The objectives of patient and family education are to increase the patient's understanding of the origins of his or her suicidal behaviour, establish effective treatment for depression, provide for ongoing and seamless outpatient treatment, devise a plan for managing future suicidal ideation, identify supportive others in the community, establish a plan to make contact with these people and community resources, and continue with drug and alcohol treatment. These objectives are demanding for both the nurse and patient during a brief hospitalization.

BOX 19.9

THERAPEUTIC DIALOGUE

Suicide

When Caroline sought medical care from her nurse practitioner for a cold, the nurse observed more than a cough and runny nose. Caroline appeared downcast and unusually sad. As the nurse and patient talked, the subject of family life came up, and Caroline began to cry softly. As the words tumbled out, she said that she had been unhappy for a long time. When she was very young, she recalled being happy, but things changed when her brother was born, 4 years after her. When she was 5 years old, her father began to abuse her sexually, continuing to do so until he moved out when she was 12. Caroline suspects her mother knew of the abuse, but did nothing about it. Two years ago, Caroline's father completed suicide. She feels relieved about his death but frustrated that she never got a chance to tell him how angry she was with him. Caroline's relationship with her mother has not improved. She says that her mother favours her brother and is always telling her she won't amount to anything. Caroline begins to cry harder.

Ineffective Approach

Nurse: Clearly, many things are troubling you. Don't you think that things seem worse now because you have a cold?

Caroline: Well, that could be. What are you going to do to make me feel better?

Nurse: Give you some medicine to help you sleep and clear your nose. I think you should see a psychiatrist, too.

Caroline: I don't need a psychiatrist. I came here for my cold.

Nurse: I know you did, but you seem to be depressed.

Caroline: What are you, some kind of social worker? I am just tired.

Nurse: I am a nurse, and you seem down to me. Are you thinking about suicide?

Caroline: I don't think you know what you're talking about. I want to go now. Could you give me my medicine?

Effective Approach

Nonjudgmental, curious questions; painting a picture helps the nurse and the patient.

Nurse: It seems as though many things have been piling up on you. Does it seem that way to you, too?

Caroline: It sure does. I've just been trying to get through one day at a time, but now with this cold and no sleep, I feel like I can't go on.

Nurse: When you say you can't go on, what do you mean by that?

Caroline: Lately, I have been thinking about running away to some place where I can't be found and maybe starting over. But then I think, where would I go? Where would I stay? Who would take care of me?

Nurse: When you think that your plan for escape won't work, what happens?

Caroline: (Starting to cry again.) Then, I think that maybe it would be better if I just did what my father did. I really don't think anyone would miss me.

Nurse: So you think you might take your life, like your Dad did?

Caroline: Yeah, and what really scares me is lately I have been thinking about that a lot. I keep saying to myself, "You're just tired," but I am so exhausted now that I can't chase the thoughts away.

Nurse: So do you think about suicide every day?

Caroline: It seems like I never stop thinking about it.

Nurse: Is there anything you can do to make the thoughts go away?

Caroline: Nothing. (Silence.)

Nurse: What would you do?

Caroline: I think I would get as many pills as I could find, drink a lot of alcohol, and maybe smoke some pot and just go to sleep.

Nurse: Do you have enough pills at home to kill yourself?

Caroline: (wan smile): I was hoping that sleeping medicine from you might do the job.

Nurse: It seems like you might need help getting through this time in your life. Would you like some help?

Caroline: I honestly don't know—I just want to sleep for a long time.

Critical Thinking Challenge

- In the first interaction, the nurse made two key blunders. What were they? What effect did they have on the patient? How did they interfere with the patient's care?
- What did Caroline do that might have contributed to the nurse's behaviours in the first interaction?
- In the second interaction, the nurse did several things that ensured reporting of Caroline's suicidal ideation. What were they? What differences in attitude might differentiate the nurse in the first interaction from the nurse in the second?

In addition to trying to reduce the stigma that the patient and family may associate with suicide, the nurse must provide education about depression, substance use, suicidal behaviour, and treatments. When possible, the nurse should schedule educational sessions to include significant others so that they will better understand the patient's illness and also learn what is necessary in providing outpatient care.

Interventions for the Spiritual Domain

There can be a gap between how a patient defines his or her spirituality and the ability of health care professionals to understand and participate in their patient's spirituality in a therapeutic way (Tacey, 2003; Webb, 2005). Nurses not only must understand the influences within the bio/psycho/social/spiritual domains on their patients' experiences but also must understand how their spirituality, meaning and purpose in life, encompasses the other three domains. In order to understand suicide from patients' perspectives, it is important to be open to patients' concepts of spirituality, their thoughts and feelings around the meaning of suicide, and what it is like to contemplate killing oneself (Tacey, 2003). The lived experience of suicide contemplation needs to be heard in a caring way. Nurses, by providing a patient with the time and space to explore their meaning of life, their spirituality, and their concept of death and dying, may gain insight into the factors that precipitate the patient's suicidal thoughts and behaviours.

Evaluation and Treatment Outcomes

The most desirable treatment outcome is the patient's return to the community. Because most hospitalizations for suicidal behaviour are brief, discharge planning must begin immediately after the patient is admitted. The nurse needs to explain to the patient that hospitalization is likely to be short term and should immediately begin to form a partnership with the patient and family to ensure a smooth transition to the community. Partnering means empowering patients to engage in self-care as soon as possible by helping to provide the tools they need to manage.

Identifying Continuing Sources of Social Support

Appropriate referrals to professionals in the community and available resources and support are important. The community nurse or therapist requires adequate information to continue with effective interventions after discharge. In addition, engaging family and friends in the patient's ongoing care and finding sources of help in the community, such as church groups, clubhouses, drop-in centres, or other social groups, is a necessary task. A patient's inability to name any significant others or social groups often means a poor outpatient course.

Establishing an Outpatient Care Plan

At the time of discharge, the patient is still considered very ill. Most suicides occur during the first week after discharge, and many happen within the first 24 hours. Before the patient's release, a specific, concrete plan for outpatient care must be in place. The care plan includes scheduling an appointment for outpatient care, providing for continuing medication until the first outpatient treatment visit, ensuring postrelease contact between the patient and significant others, providing for access to emergency psychiatric care, and arranging the patient's environment so that it provides both structure and safety.

At discharge, the patient should have enough medication on hand to last until the first community nurse visit or follow-up appointment. At that time, the community nurse can assess the patient's level of stability and determine whether a full prescription can be given safely to the patient. At that visit, the patient and community nurse can establish a plan of care that specifies the intensity of outpatient care. Very unstable patients may need two to three outpatient visits per week in the early days after hospitalization to maintain their safety in the community.

Patients and significant others must have a plan for their ongoing supervision. This plan must be established in such a way that the patient does not feel undermined in their ability to manage self-care but is reassured that help will be available when needed. The family members or friends involved must feel that they are resources for the patient but not responsible for the patient's life or death. In the end, it is the patients, not their supporters, who must bear responsibility for their safety. Patients who feel connected to, but not dependent on significant others, will be most likely to maintain safety in the community.

The patient's outpatient environment should be made as safe as possible before discharge. The nurse must share the care plan with family members so that they can remove any objects in the patient's environment that could be of assistance in completing suicide. The nurse must explain this measure to patients to reinforce their sense of self-control. It is important to be reasonable in deciding what to remove from the environment. Patients who are truly determined to kill themselves after discharge may ultimately complete suicide.

Finally, there should be some continuity between inpatient and outpatient care. Nurses must tell their patients specifically how to obtain emergency psychiatric care, and provide patients with written instructions, and ensure that emergency contact numbers are placed in their phones. It is helpful for community nurses, in addition to visits, to call periodically during the few first weeks after discharge to assess how the patient is doing. This contact will help the patient to feel valued and connected to others. Lack of continuity is thought to contribute to significant suicide mortality after hospital discharge (Hulten & Wasserman, 1998).

Short-Term Outcomes

Short-term outcomes for the suicidal patient include maintaining the patient's safety, averting suicide, and mobilizing the patient's resources. Whether patients are hospitalized or cared for in the community, their emotional distress must be reduced. This often is accomplished in an environment that restricts suicidal behaviour and provides sustained emotional support. The treatment during the suicidal crisis should also set the stage for meeting long-term objectives.

Long-Term Outcomes

Long-term outcomes must focus on maintaining the patient in psychiatric treatment, enabling the patient and family to identify and manage suicidal crises effectively, and widening the patient's support network.

Impact on Nurses

Avoiding Compassion Fatigue

Professional work centred on relief of emotional suffering involves empathy as a key tool. Over time, being empathetic can become exhausting, even when the caregiver is diligently maintaining self-care skills. Compassion fatigue is a genuine concern and one that may result in diminished capacity to function at work, at home, and within personal and professional relationships. The symptoms of compassion fatigue include intrusive thoughts or images of patients' situations or trauma, difficulty separating work from personal life, lower frustration tolerance, hypervigilance, decreased feelings of confidence, diminished sense of purpose or enjoyment of career, and sleep disturbances or nightmares. The nurse may begin to avoid the stress through absenteeism or presentism (i.e., being physically present but not truly engaged in one's role). These signal that a nurse's health is at risk (Mathieu, 2012). Caring for suicidal patients who are close to one's own age or who have a history of being abused or neglected in childhood enhances the risks.

To care successfully for suicidal patients or others in crisis, nurses must attend to their own well-being. Self-care with attention to nutrition, rest, and exercise facilitates managing stress physiologically. Self-awareness is integral to good nursing practice, particularly in terms of one's feelings of anxiety and vulnerability. Debriefing (i.e., sharing experiences and feelings) about stressful situations and one's response to them with a colleague and developing supports within the team so that members do not feel isolated but that care burdens are shared are helpful strategies. Compassion fatigue may not be recognized as such by the fatigued health care professional; it is often caring others who realize their colleague is in trouble (Austin et al., 2013). Many health regions in Canada are ensuring that their staff are knowledgeable regarding compassion fatigue, as well as self-care, stress management strategies, and critical stress debriefing.

Prevention

As suicide is a global concern, the World Health Organization adopted suicide prevention as an integral component of its mental health action plan (WHO, 2013). Canada's mental health strategy, *Changing Directions, Changing Lives*, also contains a comprehensive suicide prevention strategy that cuts across the six identified strategic directions (Mental Health Commission of Canada, 2012). It includes improving frontline practitioner suicide prevention training, supporting suicide awareness and prevention programs in schools and workplaces, decreasing the stigma associated with suicide, supporting the families of persons who are suicidal, improving screening for suicidality, supporting research into suicide and its causes, and addressing social factors like poverty that increase suicide risk for specific groups. For the strategic directions of Canada's mental health strategy, see Chapter 1, Box 1.3.

 ## SUMMARY OF KEY POINTS

- Self-harm and suicidal behaviour are a means of communicating that something is wrong in one's life—that life is difficult or intolerable.
- Self-harm and suicide are common and major public health problems that accompanies disturbance in emotion regulation, dissociation, depression, and hopelessness.
- People who engage in self-harm are likely to do so repeatedly.
- People who engage in self-harm are at greater risk to die by suicide.
- Parasuicide is more common among women than among men.
- Men have a higher rate of completed suicide because of the use of more lethal means (e.g., guns, hanging).
- Suicidal behaviour may be associated with genetic and biologic origins, as well as psychological, social, and spiritual factors.
- People who threaten suicide have rights that must be preserved.
- The "no self-harm" contract (i.e., contracting for safety) is a potential means of increasing the suicidal patient's safety in the community.
- The major objectives of brief hospital care are to maintain the patient's safety, reestablish the patient's biologic equilibrium, strengthen the patient's cognitive coping skills, and develop an outpatient support system.
- The nurse who cares for suicidal patients is vulnerable to compassion fatigue and must take steps to sustain personal mental health.

 ## Web Links

iasp.info The International Association for Suicide Prevention is dedicated to preventing suicidal behaviour, alleviating its effects, and providing a forum for discussion. It is the largest international organization dedicated to suicide prevention and to the alleviation of the effects of suicide.

suicideinfo.ca/ The Centre for Suicide Prevention was founded in 1981, as a branch of the Canadian Mental Health Association. The mission of the Centre is "to educate people with the information, knowledge and skills necessary to respond to people at risk of suicide."

suicideinfo.ca/wp-content/uploads/2016/09/Aboriginal-Cyberbullying.pdf The Centre for Suicide Prevention published this fact sheet in 2011 regarding the extent and effect of cyberbullying in the Aboriginal youth community. It provides stay safe rules for Internet use.

suicideprevention.ca/ The purpose of the Canadian Association for Suicide Prevention is "to reduce the suicide rate in Canada and to minimize the consequences of suicidal behaviour." It achieves its purpose through the provision of educational material and resources. It is not a crisis line.

who.int/mediacentre/factsheets/fs398/en The World Health Organization published this online media fact sheet about suicide on March 2011. It has links to its key publications and the work the WHO does regarding mental health, substance abuse, and suicide. It provides data on worldwide suicide rates per 100,000.00 and the global imperative to prevent suicide.

who.int/mental_health/suicide-prevention/world_report_2014/en This link is to the World Health Organization report, *Preventing suicide: A global imperative*. It is available in several different languages free of charge.

ACKNOWLEDGMENT

The author thanks Ms. Bukama Muntu for support with the literature, presentation, and organization of content.

References

Adler, G., & Buie, D. H., Jr. (1996). Aloneness and borderline psychopathology: Possible relevance of child development issues. In J. T. Maltsberger & M. J. Goldblatt (Eds.), *Essential papers on suicide* (pp. 356–378). New York, NY: New York University Press.

Alter, M. (2015). Uncovered evidence shows bullying was a factor in Emilie Olsen's suicide. *WCPO Cincinnati*. Retrieved from http://www.wcpo.com/longform/emilie-olsen-uncovered-evidence-shows-bullying-was-factor-in-13-year-old-suicide

Austin, W., Brintnell, E. S., Goble, E., Kagan, L., Kreitzer, L., Larsen, D. J., & Leier, B. (2013). *Lying down in the ever-falling snow: Canadian health professionals' experience of compassion fatigue*. Ottawa, ON: Wilfrid Laurier Press.

Barker, P., & Buchanan-Barker, P. (2005). *The Tidal model: A guide for mental health professionals*. New York, NY: Brunner-Routledge.

Beck, A. T. (2011). *Cognitive behavior therapy: Basics and beyond* (2nd ed.). New York, NY: Guilford.

Beck, A. T., Brown, G. K., & Steer, R. A. (1997). Psychometric characteristics of the scale for suicide ideation with psychiatric outpatients. *Behaviour Research and Therapy, 35*, 1039–1046.

Beck, A. T., Schuyler, D., & Herman I. (1974). Development of suicidal intent scales. In A. T. Beck II, L. P. Resnik, & D. J. Lettieri (Eds.), *The prediction of suicide*. Bowie, MD: Charles Press.

Beck, A. T., Steer, R. A., Kovacs, M., & Garbin, M. G. (1985). Hopelessness and eventual suicide: A 10 year prospective study of patients hospitalized with suicidal ideation. *American Journal of Psychiatry, 142*(5), 559–563.

Beck, A. T., Weissman, A., Lester, D., & Trexler, L. (1974). The measurement of pessimism: The Hopelessness Scale. *Journal of Consulting and Clinical Psychology, 42*(6), 861–865.

Benson, P. (1992). Religion and substance use. In J. E. Schumaker (Ed.), *Religion and mental health* (pp. 211–220). New York, NY: Oxford University Press.

Bergen, H., Hawton, K., Ness, J., Cooper, J., Steeg, S., & Kupur, N. (2012). Premature death after self-harm: A multicenter cohort study. *Lancet, 380*, 1568–1574.

Bertolote, M., Fleischmann, A., Butchart, A., & Besbelli, N. (2006). Suicide, suicide attempts and pesticides: A major hidden public health problem. *Bulletin of the World Health Organization, 84*(4). Retrieved from http://www.who.int/bulletin/volumes/84/4/editorial30406html/en/

Blatchford, C. (2013). Why there may never be a case against the alleged Rehtaeh Parsons rapists. *The National Post*. Retrieved from http://fullcomment.nationalpost.com/2013/04/26/christie-blatchford-why-there-will-never-be-a-case-against-the-rehtaeh-parsons/

Blatchford, C. (2015, January). Boy in notorious Rehtaeh Parson photo talks for the first time about what happened. Retrieved from http://nationalpost.com/opinion/christie-blatchford-boy-in-notorious-rehtaeh-parsons-photo-talks-for-first-time-about-what-happened

Bolton, J. M., Au, W., Leslie, W. D., Martens, P. J., Enns, M. W., Roos, L. L., ... Sareen, J. (2013). Parents bereaved by offspring suicide: A population-based longitudinal case–control study. *JAMA Psychiatry, 70*(2), 158–167.

Bongar, B., Sullivan, G., Kendrick, V., & Tomlins, J. (2017). Evaluating and managing suicide risk with the adult patient. In P. M. Kleespies (Ed.), *The Oxford handbook of behavioral emergencies and crises* (pp. 115–125). New York, NY: Oxford University Press. doi:10.1093/oxfordhb/9780199352722.013.10

Brewster, M. (2014). Military top doc confirms 8 suicides in 2014. Retrieved from *National Newswatch* website, http://www.nationalnewswatch.com/2014/04/08/military-top-doc-confirms-8-suicides-in-2014/#.U44XoSjyK_I

Bulik, C. M., Prescott, C. A., & Kendler, K. S. (2001). Features of childhood sexual abuse and the development of psychiatric and substance use disorders. *British Journal of Psychiatry, 179*, 444–449.

Butler, A. M., & Malone, K. (2013). Attempted suicide v. non-suicidal self-injury: Behaviour, syndrome or diagnosis? *British Journal of Psychiatry, 202*, 324–325. doi:10.1192/bjp.bp.112.113506

Canada Safety Council. (2014). *Proper handling and storage of firearms*. Retrieved from https://canadasafetycouncil.org/safety-canada-online/article/proper-handling-and-storage-firearms

Canadian Federation of Mental Health Nurses. (2014). *Canadian standards for psychiatric-mental health nursing* (4th ed.). Toronto, ON: Author.

Canadian Institute for Health Information. (2011). *Health indicators: 2011*. Ottawa, ON: Author. Retrieved from https://secure.cihi.ca/free_products/health_indicators_2011_en.pdf

Canadian Nurses Association. (2017). *Code of ethics for registered nurses*. Ottawa, ON: Author.

Canadian Press. (2013). Rehtaeh Parsons wanted to go public before her death. *CBC News*. Retrieved from http://www.cbc.ca/news/canada/nova-scotia/rehtaeh-parsons-wanted-to-go-public-before-her-death-1.1895085

Cardell, R., & Pitula, C. R. (1999). Suicidal inpatients' perceptions of therapeutic and non-therapeutic aspects of constant observation. *Psychiatric Services, 50*(8), 1066–1070.

CBC News. (2013a). Child porn charges against 2 teens in Rehtaeh Parsons case. *CBC News*. Retrieved from http://www.cbc.ca/news/canada/nova-scotia/child-porn-charges-against-2-teens-in-rehtaeh-parsons-case-1.1320438

CBC News. (2013b). N.S. cyberbullying legislation allows victims to sue. *CBC News*. Retrieved from http://www.cbc.ca/news/canada/nova-scotia/n-s-cyberbullying-legislation-allows-victims-to-sue-1.1307338

Centers for Disease Control and Prevention. (2014). *The relationship between bullying and suicide: What we know and what it means for schools*. Chamblee, GA: Centers for Disease Control and Prevention, National Centre for Injury and Control. Retrieved from https://www.cdc.gov/violenceprevention/pdf/bullying-suicide-translation-final-a.pdf

Centers for Disease Control and Prevention (2016). *Understanding Bullying Factsheet 2016*. Chamblee, GA: Centers for Disease Control and Prevention, National Center for Injury Prevention and Control. Retrieved from https://www.cdc.gov/violenceprevention/pdf/bullying_factsheet.pdf

Chandler, M. J., & Lalonde, C. (1998). Cultural continuity as a hedge against suicide in Canada's First Nations. *Transcultural Psychiatry, 35*(2), 191–219.

Cohen, D. A., Mason, K., Bedimo, A., Sckibner, R., Basolo, V., & Farley, T. A. (2003). Neighborhood physical conditions and health. *American Journal of Public Health, 93*(3), 467–471.

Conwell, Y., & Duberstein, P. R. (2001). Suicide in elders. *Annals of the New York Academy of Sciences, 932*, 132–150.

Conwell, Y., Duberstein, P. R., & Caine, E. D. (2002). Risk factors for suicide in later life. *Biological Psychiatry, 52*, 193–204.

Conwell, Y., van Orden, K., & Caine, E. D. (2011). Suicide in older adults. *Psychiatric Clinics of North America, 34*(2), 451–468.

Cross, A. (2013). 'It's always about the victim': Rehtaeh Parsons' parents respond to Christie Blatchford's column. *The National Post*. Retrieved from http://news.nationalpost.com/2013/04/26/its-always-about-the-victim-rehtaeh-parsons-father-responds-to-christie-blatchfords-column/

Cruz, E. (2015). Bullied teen dies by suicide; Mom says school's attitude was 'Toughin Up'. *Advocate*. Retrieved from http://www.advocate.com/bisexuality/2015/05/09/bullied-teen-dies-suicide-mom-says-school-told-daughter-toughen?pg=full

CTV News. (2014). Rehtaeh Parsons' supporters march for awareness. *CTV News*. Retrieved from http://www.ctvnews.ca/canada/rehtaeh-parsons-supporters-march-for-awareness-1.1762455

Cutcliffe, J., & Barker, P. (2004). The Nurses' Global Assessment of Suicide Risk (NGASR): Developing a tool for clinical practice. *Journal of Psychiatric and Mental Health Nursing, 11*(4), 393–400. Retrieved from http://works.bepress.com/john_cutcliffe/164/

Dervic, K., Oquendo, M. A., Grunebaum, M. F., Ellis, S., Burke, A. K., & Mann, J. J. (2004). Religious affiliation and suicide attempt. *American Journal of Psychiatry, 161*, 2303–2308.

Durkheim, E. (1897, 2006). *On suicide.* London, UK: Penguin.

Eggertson, L. (2013). Risk of suicide 40 times higher for Inuit boys. *Canadian Medical Association Journal, 185*(15), E701–E702.

Eng, P. M., Rimm, E. B., Fitzmaurice, G., & Kawachi, I. (2002). Social ties and change in social ties in relation to subsequent total and cause-specific mortality and coronary heart disease incidence in men. *American Journal of Epidemiology, 155*(8), 700–709.

Ferrari, A. J., Norman, R. E., Freedman, G., Baxter, A. J., Pirkis, J. E., Harris, M. G., … Whiteford, H. A. (2014). The burden attributable to mental and substance use disorders as risk factors for suicide: Finding from the Global Burden of Disease Study 2010. *PLoS One, 9*(4), 1–11.

First Nations Information Governance Centre. (2012). *First Nations Regional Health Survey (RHS) 2008/10: National report on adults, youth and children living in First Nations communities.* Ottawa, ON: Author.

Fisher, H. L., Moffitt, T. E., Houts, R. M., Belsky, D. W., Arseneault, L., & Caspi, A. (2012). Bullying victimization and risk of self harm in early adolescence: Longitudinal cohort study. *British Medical Journal, 344*, e2683. doi:10.1136/bmj.e2683

Flowers, J. (2006). Cyber-bullying hits community. *Addison County Independent.* Retrieved from http://www.addisonindependent.com/node/280

Franklin, J. C., & Nock, M. K. (2017). Nonsuicidal self-injury and its relation to suicidal behavior. In P. M. Kleespies (Ed.), *The Oxford Handbook of Behavioral Emergencies and Crises* (pp. 401–416). New York, NY: Oxford University Press. doi:10.1093/oxfordhb/9780199352722.013.29

Freedenthal, S. (2008). Assessing the wish to die: A 30-year review of the Suicide Intent Scale. *Archives of Suicide Research, 12*(4), 277–298.

Gagné, M., Robitaille, Y., Hamel, D., & St-Laurent, D. (2010). Firearms regulation and declining rates of male suicide in Quebec. *Injury Prevention, 16*(4), 247–253.

Glowinski, A. L., Bucholz, K. K., Nelson, E. C., Fu, Q., Madden, P., Reich, W., & Heath, A. C. (2001). Suicide attempts in an adolescent female twin sample. *Journal of the American Academy of Child and Adolescent Psychiatry, 40*(11), 1300–1307.

Goethe, J. W. (1774/1989). *The sorrows of young Werther* (Trans. M. W. Hulse). Harmondsworth, UK: Penguin.

Government of Canada. (2006). *The human face of mental health and mental illness in Canada 2006.* Ottawa, ON: Minister of Public Works and Government Services of Canada.

Government of Canada. (2016). *Working together to prevent suicide in Canada: The Federal Framework for Suicide Prevention.* Retrieved from https://www.canada.ca/en/public-health/services/publications/healthy-living/suicide-prevention-framework.html

Grad, O. (2011). The sequelae of suicide: Survivors. In R. C. O'Connor, S. Platt, & J. Gordon (Eds.), *International handbook of suicide prevention; Research, policy and practice* (pp. 561–576). New York, NY: John Wiley and Sons.

Guo, B., Scott, A., & Bowker, S. (2003). *Suicide prevention strategies: Evidence from systematic reviews. HTA 28.* Edmonton, AB: Heritage Foundation for Medical Research.

Ha, L. (2014). A snapshot of bullying. *Victims of Crime Research Digest, 7*, 2–9. Retrieved from http://www.justice.gc.ca/eng/rp-pr/cj-jp/victim/rd7-rr7/rd7-rr7.pdf

Hauenstein, E. (1996). A nursing practice paradigm for depressed rural women: Theoretical basis. *Archives of Psychiatric Nursing, 10*(5), 283–292.

Hawton, K., & Harriss, L. (2008). How often does deliberate self-harm occur relative to each suicide? A study of variations by gender and age. *Suicide and Life-Threatening Behavior, 38*(6), 650–660.

Health Canada. (2003). *Acting on what we know: Preventing youth suicide in First Nations.* Retrieved from http://www.hc-sc.gc.ca/fniah-spnia/pubs/promotion/_suicide/prev_youth-jeunes/index-eng.php

Health Canada, First Nations and Inuit Health Branch. (2003). *A statistical profile on the health of First Nations in Canada.* Ottawa, ON: Author.

Heisel, M., & Duberstein, P. (2017). Working sensitively and effectively to reduce suicide risk among older adults: A humanistic approach. In P. M. Kleespies (Ed.), *The Oxford Handbook of Behavioral Emergencies and Crises* (pp. 115–125). New York, NY: Oxford University Press. doi:10.1093/oxfordhb/9780199352722.013.25

Hilton, S. C. (2002). Active Latter-day Saints seven times less likely to commit suicide. *American Journal of Epidemiology, 155*, 413–419.

Hinduja, S., & Patchin, J. W. (2010). Bullying, cyberbullying, and suicide. *Archives of Suicide Research, 14*, 206–221.

Huffington Post. (2013). Rehtaeh Parsons, Canadian girl, dies after suicide attempt; parents allege she was raped. *The Huffington Post.* Retrieved from http://www.huffingtonpost.com/2013/04/09/rehtaeh-parsons-girl-dies-suicide-rape-canada_n_3045033.html

Huffington Post Canada. (2013). Rehtaeh Parsons suicide: Web calls on Anonymous to act after Nova Scotia Teen's death (Update: Anonymous Responds). *The Huffington Post Canada.* Retrieved from http://www.huffingtonpost.ca/2013/04/10/rehtaeh-parsons-suicide-anonymous_n_3052495.html

Hulten, A., & Wasserman, D. (1998). Lack of continuity: A problem in the care of young suicides. *Acta Psychiatrica Scandinavica, 97*(5), 326–333.

Inuit Tapiriit Kanatami. (2016). *National Inuit suicide prevention strategy.* Ottawa, ON: Author. Retrieved from www.itk.ca

Jorgensen, S., & Chavez, N. (2017). Video shows 'bullying' incident days before 8-year-old took his life. *CNN.* Retrieved from http://www.cnn.com/2017/05/13/health/ohio-boy-suicide-bullying/index.html

Kendall, D., Lothian-Murray, J., & Linden, R. (2004). *Sociology: In our time* (3rd ed.). Scarborough, ON: Thompson Canada Inc.

Kendler, K. S., Bulik, C. M., Silberg, J., Hettema, J. M., Myers, J., & Prescott, C. A. (2000). Childhood sexual abuse and adult psychiatric and substance use disorders in women: An epidemiological and co-twin control analysis. *Archives of General Psychiatry, 57*(10), 953–959.

Kirmayer, L. (2012). Changing patterns in suicide among young people [Commentary]. *Canadian Medical Association Journal, 184*(9), 1015–1016.

Kirmayer, L. J., Brass, G. M., Holton, T., Paul, K., Simpson, C., & Tait, C. (2007). *Suicide among Aboriginal people in Canada.* Ottawa, ON: Aboriginal Healing Foundation.

Klonsky, E. D., & Glenn, C. R. (2009). Assessing the functions of non-suicidal self-injury: Psychometric properties of the Inventory of Statements about Self-injury (ISAS). *Journal of Psychopathology and Behavioral Assessment, 31*, 215–219.

Knesper, D. J. (2011). *Suicide prevention and research: Suicide attempts and suicide details subsequent to discharge from emergency rooms and psychiatric units. American Association of Suicidology, and Suicide Prevention Research Center.* Newton, MA: Education Development Centre.

Knieper, A. J. (1999). The suicide survivor's grief and recovery. *Suicide and Life-Threatening Behavior, 29*(4), 353–364.

Koenig, H. G., & Larson, D. B. (2001). Religion and mental health: Evidence for an association. *International Review of Psychiatry, 13*, 67–78.

Koplin, B., & Agathen, J. (2002). Suicidality in children and adolescents: A review. *Current Opinion in Pediatrics, 14*, 713–717.

Kposowa, A. J. (2001). Unemployment and suicide: A cohort analysis of social factors predicting suicide in the U.S. National longitudinal mortality study. *Psychological Medicine, 31*(1), 127–138.

Kumar, N. (2016). *Aboriginal Peoples' Survey, 2012: Lifetime suicidal thoughts among First Nations living off reserve, Métis and Inuit aged 26 to 59: Prevalence and associated characteristics.* Statistics Canada Catalogue no. 89-653-X2016008. Retrieved from http://www.statcan.gc.ca/pub/89-653-x/89-653-x2016008-eng.pdf

Langlois, S., & Morrison, P. (2002). Suicide deaths and suicide attempts. *Health Reports, 13*(2), 9–22.

Larson, D., & Larson, S. B. (2003). Spirituality's potential relevance to physical and emotional health: A brief review of quantitative research. *Journal of Psychology and Theology, 31*, 37–51.

Leach, M. (2013). *Cultural diversity and suicide ethnic, religious, gender, and sexual orientation perspectives.* New York, NY: Routledge.

Leenaars, A. A. (1998). *Suicide notes: Predictive clues and patterns.* New York, NY: Human Sciences Press.

Liu, R. T., & Mustanksi, B. (2012). Suicidal ideation and self-harm in lesbian, gay, bisexual and transgender youth. *American Journal of Preventive Medicine, 42*(3), 221–228.

Long, M., Manktelow, R., & Tracey, A. (2012). We are all in this together: Working towards a holistic understanding of self-harm. *Journal of Psychiatric and Mental Health Nursing, 20*, 105–113.

Lopez, F. G., & Brennan, K. A. (2000). Dynamic processes underlying adult attachment organization: Toward an attachment theoretical perspective on the health and effective self. *Journal of Counseling Psychology, 47*(3), 283–300.

MacMillan, H. L., Fleming, J. E., Streiner, D. L., Lin, E., Boyle, M. H., Jamieson, E., … Beardslee, W. R. (2001). Childhood abuse and lifetime psychopathology in a community sample. *American Journal of Psychiatry, 158*(11), 1878–1883.

Mann, J. J., Brent, D. A., & Arango, V. (2001). The neurobiology and genetics of suicide and attempted suicide: A focus on the serotonergic system. *Neuropsychopharmacology, 24*(5), 467–477.

Mann, J. J., Oquendo, M., Underwood, M. D., & Arango, V. (1999). The neurobiology of suicide risk: A review for the clinician. *Journal of Clinical Psychiatry, 60*(Suppl 2), 7–11.

Mandhouj, O., & Huguelet, P. (2016). Why it is important to talk about religion. In P. Courtet (Ed.), *Understanding suicide: From diagnosis to personalized treatment.* Cham, Switzerland: Springer International Publishing.

Marshall, B. D. L., Galea, S., Wood, E., & Kerr, T. (2013). Longitudinal associations between types of childhood trauma and suicidal behavior among substance users: A cohort study. *American Journal of Public Health, 103*(9), e69–e75.

Martin, G. (2002). Spirituality and suicide prevention. *Auseinetter, 15*(2), 3–4.

Masecar, D. (2009). *Suicide clusters: A discussion.* Ottawa, ON: First Nations Inuit Health Branch, Health Canada.

Mathieu, F. (2012). *The compassion fatigue handbook.* New York, NY: Taylor & Francis Group, LLC.

May, A. M., & Klonsky, E. D. (2013). Assessing motivations for suicide attempts: Development and psychometric properties of the Inventory of Motivations for Suicide Attempts. *Suicide and Life-Threatening Behavior, 43*(5), 532–546.

McDermott, E., & Roen, K. (2016). *Queer youth, suicide and self-harm: Troubled subjects, troubling norms.* London, UK: Palgrave Macmillan. doi: 10.1057/9781137003454

McGuffin, P., Marusic, A., & Farmer, A. (2001). What can psychiatric genetics offer suicidology. *Journal of Crisis Intervention and Suicide, 22*(2), 62–65.

McIntyre, L., Williams, J. V. A., Lavorato, D. H., & Patten, S. (2013). Depression and suicide ideation in late adolescence and early adulthood are an outcome of child hunger. *Journal of Affective Disorders, 150,* 123–129.

McKenzie, K. C., & Gross, J. J. (2014). Nonsuicidal self-injury: An emotion regulation perspective. *Psychopathology, 47,* 207–219. doi:10.1159/000358097

McLeod, S. (2011). *Cyberbullying. Centre for Suicide Prevention's Straight Talk: Youth Suicide Prevention Workbook.* Retrieved from http://csp.cloud8.ion-linehosting.net/LinkClick.aspx?fileticket=U9Oo1Hz3LCs=&tabid=516

Mental Health Commission of Canada. (2012). *Changing directions, changing lives: The mental health strategy for Canada.* Calgary, AB: Author.

Mishara, B. L., & Chagnon, F. (2011). Understanding the relationship between mental illness and suicide and the implications for suicide prevention. In R. C. O'Connor, S. Platt, & J. Gordon (Eds.), *International handbook of suicide prevention: Research, policy and practice* (pp. 609–623). New York, NY: John Wiley & Sons.

Mitchell, A. M., Gale, D. D., Garand, L., & Wesner, S. (2003). The use of narrative data to inform the psychotherapeutic process with suicide survivors. *Issues in Mental Health Nursing, 24,* 91–106.

Molnar, B., Berkman, L. F., & Buka, S. L. (2001). Psychopathology, childhood sexual abuse and other childhood adversities: Relative links to subsequent suicidal behaviour in the U.S. *Psychological Medicine, 31*(6), 965–977.

Monette, M. (2012). Senior suicide: An overlooked problem. *CMAJ, 184*(17), E855–E856.

Morey, C. M. (2014). The influence of intergenerational family dynamics of suicidal behavior: Conceptualization, assessment, and intervention. *Smith College Studies in Social Work, 84*(1), 5-22.

Morrison, K. L., & Laing, L. (2011). Adults' use of health services in the year before death by suicide. *Health Reports, 22*(3), 1–8.

Muehlenkamp, J. J., Brausch, A. M., Quigley, K., & Whitlock, J. L. (2013). Interpersonal features and functions of non-suicidal self-injury. *Suicide and Life-Threatening Behavior, 43,* 67–80.

Murray, B. L. (2003). Self-harm among adolescents with developmental disabilities: What are they trying to tell us? *Journal of Psychosocial Nursing, 41*(11), 37–45.

Murray, B. L., & Wright, K. (2006). Integration of a suicide risk assessment and intervention approach: The perspective of youth. *Journal of Psychiatric and Mental Health Nursing, 13*(2), 157–161.

Nansel, T. R., Overpeck, M., Pilla, R. S., June Ruan, W., Simons-Morton, B., & Scheidt, P. (2001). Bullying behaviors among U.S. youth: Prevalence and association with psychosocial adjustment. *Journal of the American Medical Association, 285*(16), 2094–2100.

Navaneelan, T. (2012). *Suicide rates: An overview.* Statistics Canada. Retrieved from http://www.statcan.gc.ca/pub/82-624-x/2012001/article/11696-eng.htm

Nelson, E. C., Heath, A. C., Madden, P. A. F., Cooper, M. L., Dinwiddie, S. H., Bucholz, K. K., & Martin, N. G. (2002). Association between self-reported childhood sexual abuse and adverse psychosocial outcomes: Results from a twin study. *Archives of General Psychiatry, 59,* 139–145.

Nelson, S. E., & Wilson, K. (2017). The mental health of Indigenous peoples in Canada: A critical review of research. *Social Science and Medicine, 176,* 9–112. doi:10.1016/j.socscimed.2017.01.021

Niederkrotenthaler, T., Fu, K., Yip, P. S., Fong, D. Y. T., Stack, S., Cheng, Q., & Pirkis, J. (2012). Changes in suicide rates following media reports on celebrity suicide: A meta-analysis. *Journal of Epidemiology and Community Health, 66*(11), 1037–1042. Published online April 21, 2012. doi:10.1136/jech-2011-200707

Nishnawbe Aski Nation. (2004). *What's wrong? Depression, suicide and Aboriginal teenagers.* Retrieved from https://sites.google.com/site/northernontarioaboriginalyouth/

Nock, M. K., Borges, G., Bromet, E. J., Alonso, J., Angermeyer, M., Beautrais, A., & Williams, D. (2008). Cross-national prevalence and risk factors for suicidal ideation, plans and attempts. *British Journal of Psychiatry, 192,* 98–105.

O'Connell, H., Chin, A., Cunningham, C., & Lawlor, B. A. (2004). Recent developments: Suicide in older people. *British Medical Journal, 329,* 895–899.

Olson, R. (2013). *InfoExchange 10: Suicide contagion and suicide clusters.* Calgary, AB: Centre for Suicide Prevention.

Parachute. (2015). *The cost of injury in Canada.* Toronto, ON: Author.

Perlman, C. M., Neufeld, E., Martin, L., Goy, M., & Hirdes, J. P. (2012). *Suicide risk assessment guide: A resource for health care organizations.* Toronto, ON: Ontario Hospital Association and Canadian Patient Safety Institute.

Pesut, B. (2003). Developing spirituality in the curriculum: Intrapersonal connectedness, interpersonal connectedness. *Nursing Education Perspectives, 24,* 290–294.

Piérard, E., & Grootendorst, P. (2014). Do downturns cause desperation? The effects of economic conditions on suicide rates in Canada. *Applied Economics, 46*(10), 1081–1092.

Pitchot, W., Hansenne, M., Gonzalez Moreno, A., Pinto, E., Reggers, J., Fuchs, S., … Ansseau, M. (2001). Reduced dopamine function in depressed patients is related to suicidal behaviour but not its lethality. *Psychoneuroendocrinology, 26,* 689–696.

Poijula, S., Walberg, K. E., & Dyregrov, A. (2001). Adolescent suicide and suicide contagion in three secondary schools. *International Journal of Emergency Mental Health, 3*(3), 163–168.

Pollack, N. J., Mulay, S., Valcour, J., & Jong, M. (2016). Suicide rates in Aboriginal communities in Labrador, Canada. *American Journal of Public Health, 106*(7), 1309–1315.

Qin, P., Agerbo, E., & Mortensen, P. B. (2003). Suicide risk in relationship to socioeconomic, demographic, psychiatric, and familial factors: A national register-based study of all suicides in Denmark, 1981–1997. *American Journal of Psychiatry, 160*(4), 765–772.

Qin, P., Agerbo, E., Westergård-Nielson, N., Erikson, T., & Mortenson, P. B. (2000). Gender differences in risk factors for suicide in Denmark. *British Journal of Psychiatry, 177,* 546–550.

Range, L. M., Campbell, C., Kovac, S. H., Marion-Jones, M., Aldridge, H., Kogos, S., & Crump, Y. (2002). No-suicide contracts: An overview and recommendations. *Death Studies, 26,* 51–74.

Rasic, D., Kisely, S., & Langille, D. B. (2011). Protective associations of important of religion and frequency of service attendance with depression risk, suicidal behavior, and substance use in adolescents in Nova Scotia, Canada. *Journal of Affective Disorders, 132,* 389–395.

Registered Nurses' Association of Ontario. (2009). *Assessment and care of adults at risk for suicidal ideation and behaviour.* Toronto, ON. Author.

Rew, L., Thomas, N., Horner, S. D., Resnick, M. D., & Beuhring, T. (2001). Correlates of recent suicide attempts in a triethnic group of adolescents. *Journal of Nursing Scholarship, 33*(4), 361–367.

Richardson, J. D., St Cyr, K. C. M., McIntyre-Smith, A. M., Haslam, D., Elhai, J. D., & Sareen, J. (2012). Examining the association between psychiatric illness and suicidal ideation in a sample of treatment-seeking Canadian peacekeeping and combat veterans with posttraumatic stress disorder. *Canadian Journal of Psychiatry, 57*(8), 496–504.

Rolland-Harris, E., Cyr, E., & Zamorski, M. A. (2016). *2016 Report on suicide mortality in the Canadian Armed Forces (1995–2015). SGR-2016-005.* Ottawa, ON: Minister of National Defense.

Ross, S. (2013). Who failed Rehtaeh Parsons?. *Herald News.* Retrieved from http://www.thechronicleherald.ca/metro/1122345-who-failed-rehtaeh-parsons

Royal Commission on Aboriginal Peoples. (1995). *Choosing life: Special report on suicide among Aboriginal people.* Ottawa, ON: Communication Group.

Ruiz-Perez, I., Rodriquez-Barranco, M., Rohas-Garcia, A., & Mendoza-Garcia, O. (2017). Economic crisis and suicide in Spain: Socio-demographic and regional variability. *European Journal of Health Economics, 18*(3), 313–320.

Santa Mina, E. E. (2010) Self-Harm Intentions: Can they be distinguished based upon a childhood physical and sexual abuse history? *Canadian Journal of Nursing Research, 42*(4), 122–143.

Satyanarayana, S., Enns, M. W., Cox, B. J., & Sareen, J. (2009). Prevalence and correlates of chronic depression in the Canadian Community Health Survey: Mental health and well-being. *Canadian Journal of Psychiatry, 54,* 389–398.

Scherr, S., & Reinemann, C. (2011). Belief in a Werther effect: Third-person effects in the perceptions of suicide risk for others and the moderating role of depression. *Suicide and Life-Threatening Behavior, 41*(6), 624–634.

Shneidman, E. (1985). *Definition of suicide.* New York, NY: John Wiley & Sons.

Skodol, A. E., Gunderson, J. G., Pfohl, B., Widiger, T. A., Livesley, J. W., & Siever, L. J. (2002). The borderline diagnosis I: Psychopathology, comorbidity, and personality structure. *Biological Psychiatry, 51,* 936–995.

Smye, V., & Browne, A. (2002). 'Cultural Safety' and the analysis of health policy affecting aboriginal people. *Nurse Researcher, 9*(3) 42–56.

Statistics Canada. (2014). Deaths and mortality rate (age standardization using 1991 population, by selected grouped causes and sex, Canada provinces and territories age group and sex, Canada. In *CANSIM Table 102-0561*. Ottawa, ON: Author. Retrieved from www5.statcan.gc.ca/cansim/a26?lang=eng&id=1020561

Steenland, K., Halperin, W., Hu, S., & Walker, J. T. (2003). Deaths due to injuries among employed adults: The effects of socioeconomic class. *Epidemiology, 14*(1), 74–79.

Sutherland, J. E., Sutherland, S. J., & Hoehns, J. D. (2003). Achieving the best outcome in treatment of depression. *Journal of Family Practice, 53*(3), 118–126.

Tacey, D. (2003). *The spirituality revolution*. Sydney, Australia: Harper Collins.

Tien, H. C. N., Acharya, S., & Redelmeier, D. A. (2010). Preventing deaths in the Canadian military. *American Journal of Preventive Medicine, 38*(3), 331–339.

Tinley, S. T., & Kinney, A. Y. (2007). Three philosophical approaches to the study of spirituality. *Advances in Nursing Science, 30*, 71–80.

von Borczyskowski, A., Lindlad, F., Vinnerlkjung, B., & Hjern, A. (2010). Gender differences in risk factors for suicide: Findings from a Swedish national cohort study. *Canadian Journal of Psychiatry, 55*(2), 108–111.

Webb, D. (2005). Bridging the spirituality gap. *Australian e-Journal for the Advancement of Mental Health, 4*(1), 1–9.

Westerlund, M., Schaller, S., & Schmidtke, A. (2009). The role of mass-media in suicide prevention. In D. Wasserman, & C. Wasserman (Eds.), *Oxford textbook of suicidology and suicide prevention: A global perspective* (pp. 515–525). Oxford, UK: Oxford University Press.

White, J., & Jodoin, N. (2003). *Aboriginal youth: A manual of promising suicide prevention strategies*. Retrieved from http://www.suicideinfo.ca/csp/go.aspx?tabid=144

World Health Organization. (2012). *Suicide prevention programme*. Retrieved from http://www.who.int/mental_health/prevention/suicide/suicideprevent/en/

World Health Organization (2013). *Mental Health Action Plan 2013–2020*. Geneva, Switzerland: World Health Organization. Retrieved from http://apps.who.int/iris/bitstream/10665/89966/1/9789241506021_eng.pdf?ua=1

World Health Organization. (2017). *Suicide*. Retrieved from http://www.who.int/mediacentre/factsheets/fs398/en/

Zenere, F. (2009). Suicide clusters and contagion. *Principal Leadership, 10*(2), 12–16.

Zetter, K. (2008). *Dead teen's mother testifies about daughter's vulnerability in MySpace suicide case—Update. Wired*. Retrieved from https://www.wired.com/2008/11/lori-drew-pla-1/

Zhao, Y., Montoro, R., Igartua, K., & Thombs, B. D. (2010). Suicidal ideation and attempt among adolescents reporting "unsure" sexual identity or heterosexual identity plus same-sex attraction or behavior: Forgotten groups? *Journal of the American Academy of Child and Adolescent Psychiatry, 49*(2), 104–113.

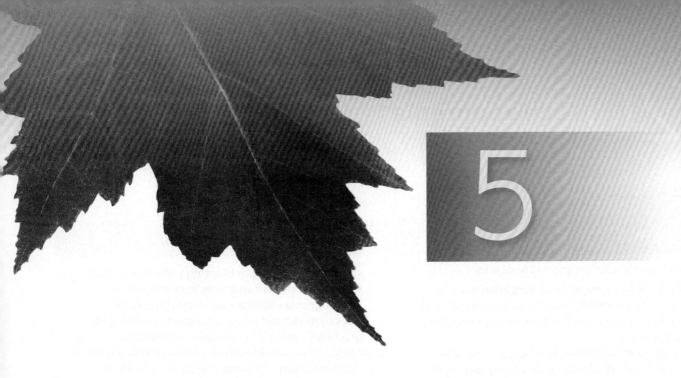

Care and Recovery

for Persons With a Psychiatric Disorder

CHAPTER

20 Schizophrenia

Tanya Park

Adapted from the chapter "Schizophrenia" by Jane Hamilton Wilson

LEARNING OBJECTIVES

After studying this chapter, you will be able to:

- Distinguish key symptoms of schizophrenia.
- Analyze the prevailing biologic, psychological, and social theories that are the basis for understanding schizophrenia.
- Analyze human response to schizophrenia with emphasis on hallucinations, delusions, and social isolation.
- Formulate nursing diagnoses based on a bio/psycho/social/spiritual assessment of persons with schizophrenia.
- Formulate nursing interventions that address specific diagnoses based on a continuum of care.
- Analyze special concerns within the nurse–patient relationship common to treating those with schizophrenia.
- Identify the expected outcomes and their evaluation.

KEY TERMS

- affective flattening or blunting • affective lability
- akathisia • alogia • ambivalence • anhedonia
- anosognosia • apathy • avolition • delusions
- disorganized behaviour • duration of untreated psychosis • dystonic • echolalia • echopraxia
- extrapyramidal side effects • first-episode psychosis
- hallucinations • illusions • negative symptoms
- neurocognition • positive symptoms • stereotypy
- tangentiality • tardive dyskinesia • waxy flexibility
- word salad

KEY CONCEPTS

- disorganized symptoms • negative symptoms
- neurocognitive impairment • positive symptoms

Schizophrenia has fascinated and confounded healers, scientists, and philosophers for centuries. It is one of the most severe complex mental illnesses and is present in all cultures, races, and socioeconomic groups. Its symptoms have historically been attributed to possession by demons, considered punishment by gods for evils done, or accepted as evidence of the inhumanity of its sufferers. These explanations have resulted in enduring stigma for people with a diagnosis of this disorder. Today, such stigma persists despite numerous national efforts to educate the Canadian public. All nurses need to understand this disorder and advocate to correct stereotyping and misperceptions. The Mental Health Commission of Canada (MHCC) has identified combating the stigma of mental illness and preventing discrimination as important priorities in improving the mental health of Canadians (MHCC, 2007). Educating the public and the media about mental illness is a priority. In fact, in 2012, the Mental Health Commission published a strategy document entitled *Changing Directions: Changing Lives* (MHCC, 2012). This document is the first national mental health strategy, which focuses upon better mental health care for all. Canadians with serious mental illnesses such as schizophrenia are likely to be the beneficiaries of the enactment of the evidence-based approaches to enhance mental health, reduce stigmatization of those with serious mental illness, and reduce barriers to meaningful employment.

◼ CLINICAL COURSE

In the late 1800s, Emil Kraepelin first described the course of the disorder he called *dementia praecox*. In the early 1900s, Eugene Bleuler renamed the disorder *schizophrenia*, meaning *split minds*, and began to determine that there was not just one type of schizophrenia but rather a group of schizophrenias. These pioneering physicians had a great influence on the current diagnostic conceptualizations of schizophrenia that emphasize the heterogeneity of the disorder in terms of the course of illness and positive and negative symptoms. In contemporary times, researchers at the University of Alberta, collaborating with IBM scientists, have developed neuroimaging-based means of objectively assessing individuals for schizophrenia and for predicting the severity of specific symptoms (Dhariwal, 2017; Gheiratmand et al., 2017).

Overview of Schizophrenia

The clinical picture of schizophrenia is highly variable and complex. Individual symptoms differ from one another, and the experience for a single individual may be different from episode to episode. For some individuals, the illness onset is slow and insidious; for others, it is sudden, seemingly coming from out of the blue. Similarly, the course of schizophrenia is also unique and unpredictable. About 25% to 30% of people with schizophrenia experience a complete remission after one or several psychotic episodes (Barak & Aizenberg, 2012). However, early intervention, including pharmacologic and phase-specific psychosocial interventions, shows promise for increasing the rate of recovery in people with first-onset schizophrenia (Amminger et al., 2011).

Although schizophrenia is treatable, it remains a serious and potentially disabling illness. As is the case with most chronic illnesses, the emphasis must be upon maximizing wellness while minimizing the disability. It is important to note that recovery does not mean cure. There is not one predictable outcome for an individual with schizophrenia. There may be a variety of outcomes depending on how the illness affects the person, his or her family, and the kind and type of treatment received. Nurses in both inpatient and community settings have an opportunity to help patients live well with schizophrenia (Box 20.1).

Acute Illness Period

Initially, the illness behaviours may be both confusing and frightening to the patient and the family. At first, the changes (often called prodromal symptoms) may be subtle and, as they often begin in late adolescence, can even be confused with the anxiety and moodiness of teenage years. However, at some point, the changes in thought and behaviour become so disruptive or bizarre that they can no longer be overlooked. These changes herald the beginning of psychosis. Typically, family and friends become aware that something is not right. Changes might include episodes of staying up all night for several nights, withdrawal from social activities, incoherent conversations, and irritability or aggressive acts against self or others. For example, one patient's parents reported their son sneaking around their home for several days peeking out from behind the curtains and complaining that their home was under surveillance. Another father described his son's first delusional–hallucination episode as so convincing that it was frightening. His son began visiting cemeteries and making "mind contact" with the deceased. He saw his deceased grandmother walking around in the home and was certain that there were pipe bombs in objects in his home. Another patient believed that he had been visited by space aliens who wanted to unite their world with Earth and assured him that he would become the leader of his country.

These experiences are collectively referred to as indicators of **first-episode psychosis**, or the initial episode of psychosis, which most often occurs in adolescence or early adult life (see Box 20.2). This early stage of illness, defined as the first 3 to 5 years following the onset of symptoms, is considered a critical period for intervention (Melau et al., 2011). Excellent early intervention has been found to lead to more favourable recovery outcomes, leading to many early intervention programs being developed in Canada and around the world. In general, the threefold aim of these programs has been to reduce the **duration of untreated psychosis** (DUP), intervene appropriately at this early stage of illness, and prevent subsequent relapse and minimize the disability (Amminger et al., 2011; Malla, Norman, & Joober, 2005).

BOX 20.1 Quality of Life: The Importance of Understanding Individual Meanings

In May 2008, the Schizophrenia Society of Canada commissioned a Canada-wide survey to learn how it can support people living with schizophrenia and their families to recover the best quality of life possible. The survey results also provide an insight into the meaning of quality of life. The participants who responded to survey included people with schizophrenia and their families or caregivers. There were 433 consumers and 570 family members or caregivers that responded to the survey, and they shared what quality of life meant to them in this survey.

The survey results demonstrated that hope, optimism, and a belief in recovery are critical. There is an overwhelming belief by people living with schizophrenia that recovery is possible. Family and caregivers are also critical components of the recovery journey and people living with schizophrenia need their family, friends, and professionals to remain optimistic and to nurture the belief that recovery is possible—particularly when they are unwell and not feeling hopeful. Health care professionals are challenged to move beyond their focus of symptom management to a model that includes supporting recovery from a body, mind, and spirit perspective.

Source: Schizophrenia Society of Canada. (2009). *QUALITY OF LIFE: As defined by people living with schizophrenia & their families.* Schizophrenia Society of Canada. Retrieved from www.schizophrenia.ca/docs/FINALSSCQOLReport.pdf

BOX 20.2 First-Episode Psychosis

First-episode psychosis simply refers to the first time someone experiences psychotic symptoms or a psychotic episode. A psychotic episode occurs in three phases. The length of each phase varies from person to person.

Phase 1. *Prodrome*: The early signs may be vague and hardly noticeable. There may be changes in the way some people describe their feelings, thoughts, and perceptions, which may become more difficult over time.

Phase 2. *Acute*: Clear psychotic symptoms are experienced, such as hallucinations, delusions, or confused thinking.

Phase 3. *Recovery*: Psychosis is treatable: Most people recover. The pattern of recovery varies from person to person. Despite common misperceptions, recovery from a first episode of psychosis is more probable than not. With help, many never have another psychotic episode.

Adapted from the Early Psychosis Prevention and Intervention Centre. Retrieved from http://www.eppic.org.au

These efforts have led to new hope for individuals who develop schizophrenia.

As the DUP increases, patients are less and less able to care for their basic needs, such as eating, sleeping, and bathing. Substance use is common. Functioning at school or work deteriorates. Dependence on family and friends increases, and those persons recognize the individual's need for treatment. In the acute phase, individuals with schizophrenia are at high risk for suicide and may require hospitalization to protect themselves or others.

Initial treatment for schizophrenia focuses upon thorough assessment and the alleviation of symptoms through the initiation of medications, decreasing the risk for suicide through safety measures, normalizing sleep, and reducing substance misuse. Functional deficits may persist during this period, and the patient and family must begin to learn to cope with these. Emotional blunting diminishes the ability and desire to engage in hobbies, vocational activities, and relationships. Limited participation in social activities may spiral into numerous skill deficits, such as difficulty engaging others interpersonally. Similarly, cognitive deficits may lead to problems recognizing patterns in situations and transferring learning and behaviours from one circumstance to another similar one.

Stabilization Period

After the initial diagnosis of psychosis and the initiation of treatment, stabilization of schizophrenia symptoms becomes the focus. Symptoms become less acute but may still be present. Treatment is intense during this period as medication regimens are established and patients adapt to various medication side effects. With appropriate assistance and support, patients and their families begin to adjust to the idea of a family member having a serious mental illness. Ideally, the misuse of substances is eliminated. Socialization with others begins to increase, and rehabilitation begins.

Maintenance and Recovery Period

After the patient's condition is stabilized, his or her focus is upon recovery efforts to regain a previous level of functioning and improve quality of life. Medication treatment of schizophrenia has generally contributed to an improvement in the symptom remission of people with this disorder; however, no medication has cured it. Faithful medication management tends to make the impairments in functioning less severe when they do occur, and to diminish the extremes individuals might experience. As with any chronic illness, stresses of life and major crises can contribute to exacerbations of acute symptoms.

Clearly, family support and involvement are extremely important at this time. Once the initial diagnosis is made, patients and families can be educated to watch for early signs of potential relapse and know how to cope with it. This is one of the important themes throughout the nursing process for people with schizophrenia. One of the key goals in the treatment of schizophrenia is to avoid subsequent relapses after the remission of the first episode. This can be challenging. The long-term prognosis with regard to relapse is most certainly influenced by a patient's willingness to remain on maintenance antipsychotic treatment and by accessing and engaging in other therapies and supports.

Relapses

Relapses can occur at any time during treatment and recovery. Relapse is not inevitable; however, it occurs with sufficient regularity to be a major concern in the treatment of schizophrenia. Relapses can occur and are detrimental to the successful management of this disorder. With each subsequent relapse, rehabilitation is prolonged, and there is a longer period of time required to recover. Combining medications and psychosocial treatment greatly diminishes the severity and frequency of recurrent relapses (Emsley, Chiliza, Asmal, & Harvey, 2013).

One of the major reasons for relapse is nonadherence to the medication regimen. Even with newer medications, nonadherence leading to relapse continues to be a problem. Discontinuing the use of medications almost certainly leads to a relapse and may actually be a stressor that causes a severe and rapid relapse (Freudenreich & Cather, 2012). Lower relapse rates are, for the most part, among groups who were following an effective continuing treatment regimen.

Table 20.1 Fostering Recovery From Schizophrenia	
Factors That Encourage Recovery	**Factors That Hinder Recovery**
• Early detection • Short duration of untreated psychosis • Optimal treatment including medication, education, individual counselling, and family education and support • Supportive social network • Stable and safe living environment • Access to meaningful activity • Companionship • Attention to physical health • Quick resolution of psychotic symptoms • Hope for the future	• Late detection • Long duration of untreated psychosis • Fragmented, inadequate, or inaccessible care • Little support from the social environment • Excess stress, tension, and conflict in the personal environment • Idleness, boredom • Isolation, loneliness • Neglect of physical health and abuse of street drugs or other substances • Persistent, unremitting psychotic symptoms • Hopelessness and despair

Adapted from Onken, S. J., Dumont, J. M., Ridgway, P., Dornan, D. H., & Ralph, R. O. (2002). Mental health recovery: What helps and what hinders? In *A national research project for the development of recovery facilitating system performance indicators.* Retrieved from https://www.nasmhpd.org/sites/default/files//MHSIPReport%281%29.pdf

Several factors contribute to relapse reduction and to optimal prognostic outcomes and recovery (see Table 20.1). Patients, their families, and members of the treatment team need to be familiar with ways to enhance recovery. It is also important to provide a realistically hopeful attitude for the future.

Many other factors can trigger a relapse: the degree of impairment in cognition and coping that leaves patients vulnerable to stressors; the accessibility of community resources, such as public transportation, housing, entry-level and low-stress employment, and social services; income supports that buffer the day-to-day stressors of living; the degree of stigmatization that the community holds for mental illness, which undermines the self-concept of patients; and the responsiveness of family members, friends, and supportive others (e.g., peers and professionals) when patients need help.

Diagnostic Criteria

Schizophrenia has been described as a mixture of positive and negative symptoms since the 19th century (Young, Halari, & Gray, 2013). **Positive symptoms**, or "first rank," symptoms reflect an excess or distortion of normal functions, including delusions, hallucinations, and thought disturbances. **Negative symptoms**, or "second rank" symptoms, reflect a lessening or loss of normal functions, such as restriction or flattening in the range and intensity of emotion (affective flattening or blunting), reduced fluency and productivity of thought and speech (alogia), withdrawal and inability to initiate and persist in goal-directed activity (avolition), and inability to experience pleasure (anhedonia).

The *DSM-5* criteria for diagnosing schizophrenia include necessary symptomatology, duration of symptoms, evaluation of functional impairment, and elimination of alternate hypotheses that might account for the symptoms (APA, 2013). In the past, several schizophrenia subtypes were recognized: paranoid, disorganized, catatonic, undifferentiated, and residual. However, there was growing belief that this subtyping was not useful

for predicting the course and response to treatment. The diagnostic criteria are listed in Box 20.3.

KEY CONCEPT

Positive (first rank) symptoms reflect an excess or distortion of normal functions, including delusions and hallucinations.

KEY CONCEPT

Negative (second rank) symptoms reflect a lessening or loss of normal functions, such as restriction or flattening in the range and intensity of emotion (**affective flattening or blunting**), reduced fluency and productivity of thought and speech (**alogia**), withdrawal and inability to initiate and persist in goal-directed activity (**avolition**), and inability to experience pleasure (**anhedonia**).

Positive Symptoms of Schizophrenia

Delusions are fixed false beliefs that usually involve a misinterpretation of experience. For example, patients believe someone is reading their thoughts or plotting against them. Types of delusions include the following:

- *Grandiose*: the belief that one has exceptional powers, wealth, skill, influence, or destiny
- *Nihilistic*: the belief that one is dead or a calamity is impending
- *Persecutory*: the belief that one is being watched, ridiculed, harmed, or plotted against
- *Somatic*: beliefs about abnormalities in bodily functions or structures

Hallucinations are perceptual experiences that occur without actual external sensory stimuli. They can involve any of the five senses, auditory, visual, olfactory (smell), gustatory (taste), tactile, and somatic, but *visual*

BOX 20.3 DSM-5 Diagnostic Criteria: Schizophrenia

A. Two (or more) of the following, each present for a significant portion of time during a 1-month period (or less if successfully treated). At least one of the must be (1), (2), or (3):
   1. Delusions
   2. Hallucinations
   3. Disorganized speech (e.g., frequent derailment or incoherence)
   4. Grossly disorganized or catatonic behaviour
   5. Negative symptoms (i.e., diminished emotional expression or avolition)
B. For a significant portion of the time since the onset of the disturbance, level of functioning in one or more major areas, such as work, interpersonal relations, or self-care, is markedly below the level achieved prior to the onset (or when the onset is in childhood or adolescence, there is failure to achieve expected level of interpersonal, academic, or occupational functioning).
C. Continuous signs of the disturbance persist for at least 6 months. This 6-month period must include at least 1 month of symptoms (or less if successfully treated) that meet Criterion A (i.e., active-phase symptoms) and may include periods of prodromal or residual symptoms. During these prodromal or residual periods, the signs

of the disturbance may be manifested by only negative symptoms or by two or more symptoms listed in Criterion A present in an attenuated form (e.g., odd beliefs, unusual perceptual experiences).
D. Schizoaffective disorder and depressive or bipolar disorder with psychotic features have been ruled out because either (1) no major depressive or manic episodes have occurred concurrently with the active-phase symptoms or (2) if mood episodes have occurred during active-phase symptoms, they have been present for a minority of the total duration of the active and residual periods of the illness.
E. The disturbance is not attributable to the physiologic effects of a substance (e.g., a drug of abuse, a medication) or another medical condition.
F. If there is a history of autism spectrum disorder or a communication disorder of childhood onset, the additional diagnosis of schizophrenia is made only if prominent delusions or hallucinations, in addition to the other required symptoms of schizophrenia, are also present for at least 1 month (or less if successfully treated).

Reprinted with permission from the *Diagnostic and Statistical Manual of Mental Disorders*, Fifth Edition, (Copyright 2013). American Psychiatric Association.

---

and *auditory* are more common. Auditory hallucinations are more common than are visual ones. For example, the patient hears voices carrying on a discussion about his or her own thoughts or behaviours.

Negative Symptoms of Schizophrenia

Negative symptoms are not as dramatic as positive symptoms, but they can interfere greatly with the patient's ability to function day to day. Because expressing emotion is difficult for them, people with schizophrenia laugh, cry, and get angry less often. Their affect is flat, and they show little or no emotion when personal loss occurs. They also suffer from **ambivalence**, which is the concurrent experience of equally strong opposing feelings so that it is impossible to make a decision. The **avolition** may be so profound that simple activities of daily living, such as dressing or combing hair, may not get done. **Anhedonia** prevents the person with schizophrenia from enjoying activities. People with schizophrenia may have limited speech and difficulty saying anything new or carrying on a conversation. These negative symptoms cause the person with schizophrenia to withdraw and experience feelings of severe isolation.

Neurocognitive Impairment

Neurocognitive impairment exists in schizophrenia and may be independent of positive and negative symptoms.

Neurocognition includes short- and long-term memory, vigilance or sustained attention, verbal fluency or the ability to generate new words, and executive functioning, which includes volition, planning, purposive action, and self-monitoring behaviour. Working memory is a concept that includes short-term memory and the ability to store and process information.

This impairment is independent of the positive symptoms. That is, cognitive dysfunction can exist even if the positive symptoms are in remission. Not all areas of cognitive functioning are impaired. Long-term memory and intellectual functioning are not necessarily affected. However, for many people with this disorder, symptoms may have interfered with completing educational opportunities. Neurocognitive dysfunction often is manifested in disorganized symptoms.

KEY CONCEPT

Neurocognitive impairment in memory, vigilance, and executive functioning is related to poor functional outcome in schizophrenia (Addington & Addington, 2006; Mesholam-Gately, Giuliano, Faraone, Goff, & Seidman, 2009).

Disorganized symptoms of schizophrenia are those things that make it difficult for the person to understand and respond to the ordinary sights and sounds of daily living. These include disorganized speech and thinking and **disorganized behaviour**.

Disorganized Thinking

Examples of disturbed speech and thinking patterns can be found in Chapter 10, specifically in Boxes 10.4 and 10.5.

Disorganized perceptions often create oversensitivity to colours, shapes, and background activities. **Illusions** occur when the person misperceives or exaggerates stimuli that actually exist in the external environment. This is in contrast to hallucinations, which are perceptions in the absence of environmental stimuli. Ancillary symptoms that may accompany schizophrenia include anxiety, depression, irritability, and hostility.

Disorganized Behaviour

Disorganized behaviour (which may manifest as a very slow, rhythmic, or ritualistic movement), coupled with disorganized speech, makes it difficult for someone with schizophrenia to partake in daily activities. Examples of disorganized behaviour include the following:

- Aggression—behaviours or attitudes that reflect rage, hostility, and the potential for physical or verbal destructiveness (usually comes about if the person believes that someone is going to do him or her harm)
- Agitation—inability to sit still or attend to others, accompanied by heightened emotions and tension
- Catatonic excitement—a hyperactivity characterized by purposeless activities and abnormal movements such as grimacing and posturing
- Echopraxia—involuntary imitation of another person's movements and gestures
- Regressed behaviour—behaving in a manner of a less mature life stage; childlike and immature
- Stereotypy—repetitive, purposeless movements that are idiosyncratic to the individual and to some degree outside of the individual's control
- Hypervigilance—sustained attention to external stimuli as if expecting something important or frightening to happen
- Waxy flexibility—posture held in odd or unusual fixed position for extended periods of time

Schizophrenia in Special Populations

Children

The diagnosis of schizophrenia is rare in children prior to adolescence. When it does occur in children aged 5 or 6 years, the symptoms are essentially the same as in adults. In this age group, hallucinations tend to be visual and delusions less developed. Because disorganized speech and behaviour may be explained better by other disorders that are more common in childhood, those disorders should be considered before applying the diagnosis of schizophrenia to a child (APA, 2013).

However, some studies suggest that the likelihood of children later experiencing schizophrenia can be predicted. Developmental abnormalities in childhood, including delays in the attainment of speech and motor development, problems in social adjustment, and poorer academic and cognitive performance, have been found to be present in individuals who experience schizophrenia in adulthood. Specific factors that appear to predict schizophrenia in adulthood include problems in motor and neurologic development, deficits in attention and verbal short-term memory, poor social competence, positive formal thought disorder–like symptoms, and severe instability of early rearing environment (Niemi, Suvisaari, Tuulio-Henriksson, & Lonnqvist, 2003).

Older Adults

As with other members of society, people with schizophrenia do grow old. For older persons who have had schizophrenia since young adulthood, this may be a time in which they experience some improvement in symptoms or relapse fluctuations. Their lifestyle probably is dependent on the effectiveness of earlier treatment, the support systems that are in place (including relationships with family members and professionals), and the interaction between environmental stressors and the patient's functional impairments.

In late-onset schizophrenia (when the diagnostic criteria are met after the age of 45 years), women are affected more than are men. The presentation of late-onset schizophrenia is most likely to include positive symptoms, particularly paranoid or persecutory delusions. Cognitive deterioration and affective blunting occur less frequently. Social functioning is more intact. Many individuals with diagnoses of late-onset schizophrenia have disturbances in sensory functions, primarily hearing and vision losses (APA, 2013). The cost of caring for older persons with schizophrenia remains high because many are no longer cared for in an institution, and community-based treatment has developed more slowly for this age group than for younger adults.

■ EPIDEMIOLOGY

Schizophrenia occurs in approximately 1% of the population in all cultures and countries. Variations in the incidence and prevalence rates across studies can be explained by the definition of schizophrenia and the sampling method used. Its economic costs are enormous. Direct costs include treatment expenses, and indirect costs include lost wages, premature death, and incarceration. In addition, employment among people with schizophrenia is one of the lowest of any group with disabilities (Crowther, Marshall, Bond, & Huxley, 2001; MHCC, 2013a). The costs of schizophrenia in terms of individual and family suffering are inestimable.

People with schizophrenia tend to cluster in the lowest social classes in industrialized countries and urban communities. For some, the symptoms of the illness are so pervasive that it is difficult for these individuals to maintain any type of gainful employment. Homelessness is a problem for those with severe and persistent symptoms of schizophrenia. Somewhere between 30% and 40% of people who are homeless are estimated to be suffering from mental illness, and of those, 20% to 25% are living with concurrent disorders, that is, with addiction and other health problems (Standing Senate Committee on Social Affairs, Science and Technology, 2006). A Canadian study, conducted by the MHCC (2013b), entitled *At Home/Chez Soi* reinforces the need for secure and safe housing for individuals suffering from serious mental illness.

Risk Factors

Risk factors for schizophrenia include stresses in the perinatal period (e.g., starvation, poor nutrition, infections), obstetrical complications, and genetic and family susceptibilities (Picchioni & Murray, 2007). Canadian researchers have discovered rare genetic changes that may be responsible for the onset of schizophrenia. This discovery gives new support to the notion that multiple rare genetic changes may contribute to schizophrenia and other brain disorders (Centre for Addiction and Mental Health, 2013). There has been some evidence that parental age may also be a risk factor (Byrne, Agerbo, Ewald, Eaton, & Mortensen, 2003). Early birth cohort studies suggest that the incidence of schizophrenia may be higher among individuals born in urban settings than those born in rural ones and may be somewhat lower in later-born birth cohorts (Harrison et al., 2003). Infants affected by maternal stressors may have conditions that create their own risk, such as low birth weight, short gestation, and early developmental difficulties. In childhood, stressors may include central nervous system (CNS) infections.

Age of Onset

Most people with schizophrenia have the disorder diagnosed in late adolescence or early adulthood. When schizophrenia begins prior to age 25, symptoms seem to develop more gradually, and negative symptoms predominate throughout the course of the disease. People with early-onset schizophrenia experience a greater number of neuropsychological problems. Disruptions occur in the achievement of milestone events of early adulthood, such as achieving in education, work, and long-term relationships (Csernansky, 2003).

Gender Differences

Men are typically diagnosed with schizophrenia earlier than are women. The median age of onset for men is in the middle 20s, whereas the median age of onset for women is in the late 20s. These gender differences have received attention because of hypotheses about sex-linked genetic aetiologies. For instance, estrogen may play a protective role against the development of schizophrenia that disappears as estrogen levels drop during menopause (Kulkarni, Hayes, & Gavrilidis, 2012). This may account for the higher median age of onset and a more favourable treatment outcome in women.

Ethnic and Cultural Differences

Increasingly, efforts are being made to consider culture and ethnic origin when diagnosing the disorder and treating individuals with symptoms of schizophrenia (APA, 2013). Although symptoms of schizophrenia appear to be clearly defined, it is possible to find cultures in which what appears to be a hallucination may be considered a vision or a religious experience. In addition, behaviours such as averting eyes during a conversation or minimizing emotional expression may be culturally bound, yet easily misinterpreted by clinicians of a different cultural or ethnic background.

Individuals of various racial groups may have varying diagnosis rates of schizophrenia. However, it is important to note that these findings may reflect a misdiagnosis of the disorder based on a cultural bias of the clinician. Prevalence studies indicate a lower incidence of schizophrenia in Asian versus non-Asian countries. It is not known if this difference is due to methodologic, genetic, environmental, or sociologic variables such as stigma and underreporting (Goldner, Hsu, Waraich, & Somers, 2002).

Familial Differences

First-degree biologic relatives (children, siblings, parents) of an individual with schizophrenia have a 10 times greater risk for schizophrenia than does the general population (APA, 2013). Other relatives may have an increased risk for disorders within the "schizophrenia spectrum" (a group of disorders with some similarities of behaviour, such as schizoaffective disorder and schizotypal personality disorder) (APA, 2013). Refer further to Chapter 21. It is still not clear whether genetic vulnerability is present in all cases of schizophrenia. It is possible that those genetic vulnerabilities are in terms of psychosis in general and that the expression of these vulnerabilities can take various forms (Costain & Bassett, 2014).

Comorbidity

Several somatic and psychological disorders coexist with schizophrenia. It is estimated that nearly 50% of patients with schizophrenia have a comorbid medical condition, but many of these illnesses are misdiagnosed or underdiagnosed (Isane, Nitkin, & Gastaldo, 2010). More attention is being paid to the causes of mortality among people with schizophrenia. Several physical disorders have been identified, including vision and dental problems, heart disease, hypertension, diabetes, and sexually transmitted diseases (Laursen, Munk-Olsen, & Vestergaard, 2012; Manu, Dima, Shulman, Vancampfort, De Hert, & Correll, 2015).

Depression

Depression may also be observed in patients with schizophrenia. This is an important symptom for several reasons. First, depression may be the evidence that the diagnosis of a mood disorder is more appropriate (see Chapter 22). Second, depression is not unusual in all stages of schizophrenia and deserves attention. Third, the suicide rate (10%) among individuals with schizophrenia is higher than that of the general population. Risk factors for suicide are male gender, chronic illness with frequent relapses, frequent short hospitalizations, a negative attitude toward treatment, impulsive behaviour, parasuicide (nonfatal self-harm or gesture), psychosis, and depression (De Hert, McKenzie, & Peuskens, 2001). Periods of untreated psychosis exceeding 1 year and treatment with older typical antipsychotic drugs also have been associated with a higher risk for suicide attempts (Harkavy-Friedman, 2007).

Diabetes Mellitus

There is increasing interest in the relationship between diabetes mellitus and schizophrenia. An association between glucose regulation and psychiatric disorders has been established. Research indicates that diabetes can exacerbate cognitive deficits in persons with schizophrenia, mainly in immediate memory and attention (Han et al., 2013). Also of growing concern is the possibility that people with schizophrenia may be more prone to type II diabetes, with two to three times greater prevalence than the general public (Cohn, 2012). Some suggest that this may be attributable to inherent characteristics (Leucht, Burkard, Henderson, Maj, & Sartorius, 2007). Evidence that supports this view includes a higher rate of type II diabetes in first-degree relatives of people with schizophrenia and higher rates of impaired glucose tolerance and insulin resistance among people with schizophrenia. However, obesity, which is associated with type II diabetes, is a growing problem, in general, and is complicated in schizophrenia treatment by the tendency of individuals to gain weight once their disease is managed with medications. Weight gain in some individuals may be attributed to a return to a healthier living situation in which regular meals are available and symptoms that interfere with obtaining food regularly (e.g., delusions) are decreased. For other individuals, weight gain may result from the antipsychotic drug (either typical or atypical) selected for their treatment. Not surprisingly,

weight gain is often cited as a reason for nonadherence to antipsychotic medications.

Substance Use

Substance use and abuse are common among Canadian society. Estimates suggest that up to 10% of the Canadian population use substances like cannabis, with up to 25% of people with schizophrenia using cannabis (Imtiaz et al., 2015). Cannabis use has been associated with an increased risk of psychosis onset (Carlson, 2013). There is debate in the literature on the effect of cannabis on mental health and in particular psychotic illnesses like schizophrenia, with Hill (2015) stating that if cannabis is related to the development of schizophrenia, then incidence of the disease would have increased. Hill goes on to outline, however, that there is evidence of increased cannabis use by people with schizophrenia, particularly in the prodromal period, likely in an attempt to manage psychotic symptoms (Hill, 2015). With the imminent introduction of decriminalization laws in Canada, it is important to acknowledge what is known and unknown about the risks of using cannabis. Hill (2015) suggests highlighting the association of cannabis use with schizophrenia, while acknowledging that health professionals should not confuse correlation with causation. Another commonly used substance is tobacco. The prevalence of tobacco smoking in people experiencing their first episode of psychosis has been reported as more than 50% (Grossman et al., 2017). Given that smoking has been "casually linked to diseases of nearly all organs of the body, to diminished health status, and to harm the fetus" (United States Department of Health and Human Services, 2014, p. 5), it is important that nurses provide support and alternatives to reduce tobacco use (see Chapter 26).

■ AETIOLOGY

Since the 1970s, hypothetical causes of schizophrenia have changed dramatically (Gur & Gur, 2005; Murray & Bramon, 2005; Walker, Kestler, Bollini, & Hochman, 2004). Purely psychological theories have been replaced by a neurobiologic model that says that patients with schizophrenia have a biologic predisposition or vulnerability that is exacerbated by environmental stressors. Individuals with schizophrenia are thought to have a genetically or biologically determined sensitivity that leaves them vulnerable to an overwhelming onslaught of stimuli from without and within. These inherent vulnerabilities include cognitive, psychophysiologic, social competence, and coping deficits that alter the individual's ability, both cognitively and emotionally, to manage life events and interpersonal situations (Box 20.4 and Fig. 20.1). This section describes the various observations and current theories about the cause of schizophrenia. However, it is important to note that the exact cause of schizophrenia remains elusive.

BOX 20.4 Vulnerabilities Experienced by People With Schizophrenia

COGNITIVE DEFICITS

- Deficits in processing complex information
- Deficits in maintaining a steady focus of attention
- Inability to distinguish between relevant and irrelevant stimuli
- Difficulty forming consistent abstractions
- Impaired memory

PSYCHOPHYSIOLOGIC DEFICITS

- Deficits in sensory inhibition
- Poor control of autonomic responsiveness

SOCIAL SKILLS DEFICITS

- Impairments in processing interpersonal stimuli, such as eye contact or assertiveness

- Deficits in conversational capacity
- Deficits in initiating activities
- Deficits in experiencing pleasure

COPING SKILLS DEFICITS

- Overassessment of threat
- Underassessment of personal resources
- Overuse of denial

Adapted from McGlashan, T. H. (1994). Psychosocial treatments of schizophrenia: The potential relationships. In N. C. Andreasen (Ed.), *Schizophrenia: From mind to molecule* (pp. 189–215). Washington, DC: American Psychiatric Press.

Biologic Theories

Theories and research about the biologic vulnerability for schizophrenia focus on incorporating multiple observations into a coherent explanation. These observations include the course of the illness already described, possible brain structure changes identified by postmortem and neuroimaging techniques, familial patterns, and pharmacologic effects on behaviour and neurotransmitter functions in the brain. One theory about the cause of schizophrenia focuses on neurodevelopment of the brain from the prenatal period through adolescence. Research efforts are making progress in

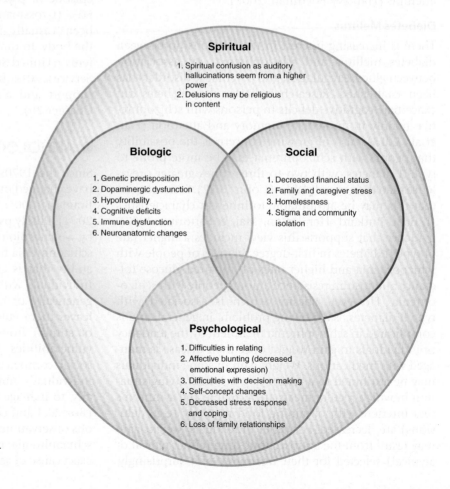

Figure 20.1. Bio/psycho/social/spiritual aetiologies for patients with schizophrenia.

depicting the neurobiologic substrate of schizophrenia (Kaneko & Keshavan, 2012; Keshavan, Tandon, Boutros, & Nasrallah, 2008).

Neuroanatomic Findings

Postmortem and neuroimaging brain studies of patients with schizophrenia show four consistent changes in brain anatomy:

- Decreased blood flow to the left globus pallidus early in the disease
- Absence of normal blood flow increase in frontal lobes during tests of frontal lobe functioning, such as working memory tasks
- Thinner cortex of the medial temporal lobe and a smaller anterior portion of the hippocampus
- Decreases in gray matter and enlarged lateral and third ventricles and widened sulci (Chance, Esiri, & Crow, 2003)

These findings are being used as a basis for exploring the influence of genetic loading, obstetric complications, and differences in familial and nonfamilial patients with schizophrenia (Falkai et al., 2003).

Familial Patterns

Evidence supports a familial or genetic base for schizophrenia. First-degree relatives (including siblings and children) are 10 times more likely to experience schizophrenia than are individuals in the general population (APA, 2013). Concordance for schizophrenia is higher among monozygotic (identical) twins than among dizygotic (fraternal) twins, although the rate is not perfectly concordant.

Genetic researchers have sought to identify specific genes responsible for schizophrenia, but replicated results are emerging very slowly (Tsuang, Stone, & Faraone, 2001). The infrequency of reproducible results is likely attributable to the heterogeneity of the disorder, which may not be consistent with a single gene theory. A model that includes several genes is more likely to explain the development of schizophrenia. Two possible locations are on the long arm of chromosome 22 and on chromosome 6 (Kandel, Schwartz, & Jessell, 2000).

Neurodevelopment

Theory and research attempt to explain how genes or events early in life (especially perinatal events such as infections or obstetric irregularities) would cause schizophrenia yet manifest symptoms only after years—in adolescence or young adulthood. The neurodevelopmental theory explains and reconciles the inconsistent neuroanatomic brain changes that have been found and links them to early development. Neurodevelopmental models of aetiology remain dominant and are fueling advances in epidemiology, imaging, and genetics. It is likely that future whole-genome association studies will

further tease out the gene–gene and gene–environment interactions (Rapoport, Addington, & Frangou, 2005).

Brain development from prenatal periods through adolescence requires several coordinated molecular activities, including cell proliferation, cell migration, axonal outgrowth, pruning of neuronal connections, programmed cell death, and myelination. All these activities require coordinated development, usually through the activation and inactivation of proteins by genes. Any of these processes could be disrupted by (1) inherited genes that place the individual at risk for schizophrenia, (2) a wild-type allele of this gene that is activated in adolescence or early adulthood, or (3) genetic sensitizing that leaves the individual susceptible to environmental causes or lesioning during some adverse perinatal event. In addition, several maturational events normally occur during puberty that may affect brain development: (1) changes in dopaminergic, serotonergic, adrenergic, glutamatergic, gamma-aminobutyric acid (GABA)ergic, and cholinergic neurotransmitter systems and substrates; (2) a complex combination of synaptic pruning along with substantial brain growth in some areas of the cortex; and (3) changes in the steroid hormonal environment (Chou, Halldin, & Farde, 2003).

Neurotransmitters, Pathways, and Receptors

Theories about the cause and pathophysiology of schizophrenia have been generated from decades of pharmacologic research and management of the disorder. For years, the leading hypothesis about the neurobiology of schizophrenia has been based on observations of drug actions. The *dopamine hypothesis* of schizophrenia arose from observations that antipsychotic drugs (Table 20.2), which so successfully ameliorate or reduce the positive symptoms of schizophrenia, act primarily by blocking postsynaptic dopamine receptors in the brain. In addition, other drugs that enhance dopamine function, such as amphetamines or cocaine, cause behavioural symptoms similar to those of schizophrenia and paranoid subtype in humans and bizarre stereotyped behaviour in monkeys. Antipsychotic drugs stop these drug-induced behaviours. Based on these observations, researchers concluded that schizophrenia was a syndrome of hyperdopaminergic action in the brain.

This older, straightforward hypothesis of dopamine hyperactivity is clearly complicated by more recent findings. Positron emission tomography (PET) scan findings suggest that in schizophrenia, there is a general reduction in brain metabolism, with a relative hypermetabolism in the left side of the brain and in the left temporal lobe. Abnormalities exist in specific areas of the brain, such as in the left globus pallidus (Anticevic & Lisman, 2017). These findings support further exploration of differential brain hemisphere function in schizophrenia (Fig. 20.2).

Other PET studies show *hypofrontality* or a reduced cerebral blood flow and glucose metabolism in the prefrontal cortex of people with schizophrenia and hyperactivity in the limbic area (Buchsbaum, 1990; Figs. 20.3 and 20.4).

Table 20.2 Selected Antipsychotic Drugs Currently Available in Canada		
First Generation or Typical		
Generic Name	Chemical Class	Route
Chlorpromazine hydrochloride	Phenothiazines	Oral, intramuscular, intravenous
Fluphenazine	Phenothiazines	Oral, intramuscular, subcutaneous
Perphenazine	Phenothiazines	Oral
Prochlorperazine	Phenothiazines	Oral, intramuscular, intravenous, per rectum
Trifluoperazine hydrochloride	Phenothiazines	Oral
Thiothixene	Thioxanthene	Oral
Haloperidol	Phenylbutylpiperidines	Oral, intramuscular
Pimozide	Phenylbutylpiperidines	Oral
Second Generation or Atypical		
Generic Name	Chemical Class	Route
Clozapine	Dibenzodiazepines	Oral
Loxapine succinate	Dibenzodiazepines	Oral
Loxapine hydrochloride	Dibenzodiazepines	Intramuscular
Asenapine maleate	Dibenzodiazepines	Sublingual
Olanzapine	Dibenzodiazepines	Oral, intramuscular
Quetiapine fumarate	Dibenzodiazepines	Oral
Risperidone	Benzisoxazoles	Oral, intramuscular
Ziprasidone hydrochloride monohydrate	Benzisoxazoles	Oral, intramuscular
Lurasidone hydrochloride	Benzisoxazoles	Oral
Paliperidone	Benzisoxazoles	Oral, intramuscular
Aripiprazole	Quinolinone	Oral, intramuscular

Adapted from Lilley, L. L., Collins, S. R., Synder, J., & Swart, B. (2017). *Pharmacology for Canadian health care practice* (3rd ed.). Toronto, ON: Elsevier Canada.

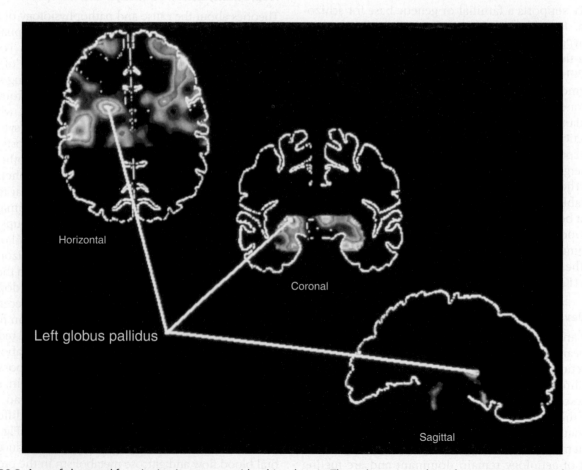

Figure 20.2. Area of abnormal functioning in a person with schizophrenia. These three views show the excessive neuronal activity in the left globus pallidus (portion of the basal ganglia next to the putamen). (Courtesy of John W. Haller, PhD, Departments of Psychiatry and Radiology, Washington University, St. Louis, MO.)

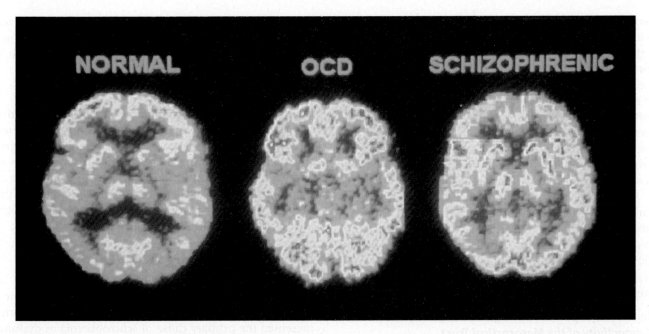

Figure 20.3. Metabolic activity in a control subject (*left*), a subject with obsessive–compulsive disorder (OCD) (*centre*), and a subject with schizophrenia (*right*). (Courtesy of Monte S. Buchsbaum, MD, The Mount Sinai Medical Center and School of Medicine, New York, NY.)

In addition, several types of dopamine receptors (labelled D_1, D_2, D_3, D_4, and D_5) and dopamine are found in five pathways that innervate different parts of the brain (Kandel et al., 2000) (see Chapter 9). Based on the current understanding of schizophrenia, the following discussion relates the neurobiologic changes to the clinical symptoms.

Positive Symptoms: Hyperactivity of Mesolimbic Tract

Positive symptoms of schizophrenia (e.g., hallucinations and delusions) are thought to be caused by dopamine *hyperactivity* in the mesolimbic tract, which regulates memory and emotion. It is hypothesized that this hyperactivity could result from an overactive modulation of

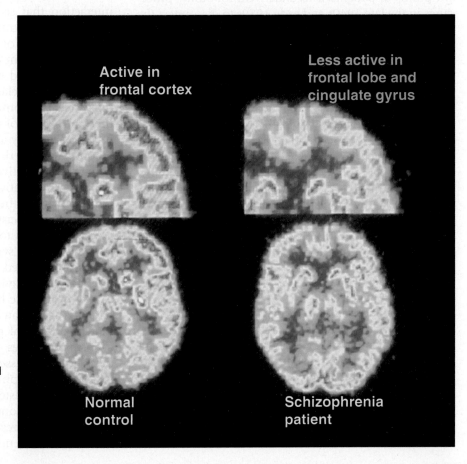

Figure 20.4. PET scan with ^{18}F-deoxyglucose shows metabolic activity in a horizontal section of the brain in a control subject (*left*) and in an unmedicated patient with schizophrenia (*right*). *Red* and *yellow* indicate areas of high metabolic activity in the cortex; *green* and *blue* indicate lower activity in the white matter areas of the brain. The frontal lobe is magnified to show reduced frontal activity in the prefrontal cortex of the patient with schizophrenia. (Courtesy of Monte S. Buchsbaum, MD, The Mount Sinai Medical Center and School of Medicine, New York, NY.)

neurotransmission from the nucleus accumbens (Kandel et al., 2000). Another explanation for dopaminergic hyperactivity in the mesolimbic tract is hypoactivity of the mesocortical tract, which normally inhibits dopamine activity in the mesolimbic tract by some type of feedback mechanism. In schizophrenia, the primary defect may be in the mesocortical tract, where dopaminergic function is diminished, thereby decreasing the inhibitory effects on the mesolimbic tract. This disinhibition may be responsible for the overactivity of dopamine in the mesolimbic tract, resulting in the positive symptom cluster (Kandel et al., 2000).

Support for this interconnection between the mesocortical and the mesolimbic tracts has been found in laboratory animals. Destruction of the mesocortical tract of animals resulted in increased activity in the mesolimbic tract, especially in the nucleus accumbens. A compensatory increase in mesolimbic neurons is a suggested mechanism by which this overactivity occurs.

Negative Symptoms and Cognitive Impairment: Hypoactivity of the Mesocortical Tract

Negative symptoms and cognitive impairment are thought to be related to hypoactivity of the mesocortical dopaminergic tract, which by its association with the prefrontal and neocortex contributes to motivation, planning, sequencing of behaviours in time, attention, and social behaviour (Jibson & Tandon, 2000; Kandel et al., 2000). Negative symptoms, such as poor motivation and planning and flat affect, are remarkably similar to the symptoms of patients who underwent lobotomy procedures in the late 1940s and early 1950s to disconnect the frontal cortex from the rest of the brain. Monkeys who have had dopamine in the prefrontal cortex depleted have difficulty with cognitive tasks. Finally, PET scans of energy metabolism suggest a reduced metabolism in frontal and prefrontal areas (Davidson & Heinrichs, 2003).

Role of Other Dopamine Pathways

The tuberoinfundibular dopaminergic tract is active in prolactin regulation and may be the source of neuroendocrine changes observed in schizophrenia. The nigrostriatal dopaminergic tract modulates motor activity and is believed to be the site of the **extrapyramidal side effects** of antipsychotic drugs, such as pseudoparkinsonism and **tardive dyskinesia** (abnormal involuntary movements). This may also be the site of some motor symptoms of schizophrenia, such as stereotypic behaviour.

Role of Other Receptors

Other receptors are also involved in dopamine neurotransmission, especially serotonergic receptors. It is becoming clear that schizophrenia does not result from the dysregulation of a single neurotransmitter or biogenic amine (e.g., norepinephrine, dopamine, serotonin). Investigators are also hypothesizing a role for glutamate and GABA (Ghose et al., 2003) because of the complex interconnections of neuronal transmission and the complexity and heterogeneity of schizophrenia symptoms. The N-methyl-D-aspartate

class of glutamate receptor is being studied because of the actions of phencyclidine (PCP) at these sites and the similarity of the psychotic behaviours that are produced when someone takes PCP (see Figs. 20.2 to 20.4).

Neural Connectivity

Manifestations of poor mental coordination include difficulty in a variety of functions, such as measuring time or space; making inferences about relationships; and coordinating the processing, priority setting, retrieval, and expression of information. It is being hypothesized that there may be a basic developmental disorder of the neural connectivity involving multiple molecular mechanisms (Benes, 2000; Penn, 2001; Sallet et al., 2003).

Psychological Theories

Several psychological frameworks have been used to explain the aetiology of schizophrenia. Before biologic and neurochemical discoveries, these psychological theories presented the primary cause of schizophrenia as dysfunctional parenting in early childhood development. Families often were blamed (e.g., the "schizophrenogenic mother" was suggested as a cause) and alienated by mental health professionals. These theories are no longer held valid, and neurochemical–biologic theories have replaced them.

Social Theories

There are no social theories believed to explain schizophrenia, but some theories focus on patterns of family interaction that seem to affect the eventual outcome and social adjustment of individuals with schizophrenia. The theory of expressed emotion (EE) correlates certain family communication patterns with an increase in symptoms and relapse in patients with schizophrenia. Families are classified as high EE families when they make negative comments about family members; when there are aspects of speech that connote criticism, hostility, and negativity about the patient; and when they are emotionally "overly involved" with the patient, such as being overprotective or self-sacrificing. Low EE families make fewer negative comments and show less overinvolvement with the patient. Families that rate high in the areas of criticism, hostility, and battles for control are hypothesized to be associated with increases in the patient's positive symptoms and relapse.

Research related to emotional expressiveness is contradictory and divisive. Although families categorized as low in EE have been shown to accept the patient as having a legitimate illness and have an understanding that interpersonal problems can exacerbate the illness (Weisman, Gomes, & Lopez, 2003), families high in EE have not been associated with either a greater family history of schizophrenia or the chronicity of the illness (Subotnik, Goldstein, Nuechterlein, Woo, & Mintz, 2002; Wuerker, Long, Haas, & Bellack, 2002).

Although this research might contribute to the understanding of how negative family interaction affects the patient, there are negative consequences to categorizing families in this dualistic manner. Professionals and society may tend to erroneously blame families for causing relapse or limit the patient's contact with the family, thus further alienating families who are so vital to the care and support of the patient.

There are numerous social barriers that prevent people with mental illness from getting the care they need. One of the major ones is the social stigma that surrounds mental illnesses (see Chapter 3). Box 20.5 describes the impact of living with a stigmatized illness. Another barrier is difficulty accessing recovery-oriented mental health services that provide comprehensive interventions, resources, and continuity of care. A Canadian study found that individuals experiencing symptoms of psychosis for the first time tried an average of 2.3 times to obtain help. The average length of time the psychosis remained untreated was almost 2 years (Addington, van Mastrigt, Jutchinson, & Addington, 2002; Standing Senate Committee on Social Affairs, Science and Technology, 2006). Mental health service delivery systems are often fragmented, with the quality and types of services varying between communities. Canada's remote rural regions present particular challenges to the provision of timely, comprehensive mental health care. Stigma is an ongoing issue, which prevents individuals from seeking timely mental health assistance.

■ INTERDISCIPLINARY TREATMENT

The most effective treatment approach for individuals with schizophrenia involves a variety of disciplines, including nursing (and nurse practitioners), psychiatry, psychology, social work, occupational and recreational therapies, pastoral counselling, peer support workers, and others. Pharmacologic management is the responsibility of the physicians, nurses, and pharmacists; the members of the mental health team can implement various psychosocial interventions. Various health professionals are necessary because of the complex nature of schizophrenia symptoms and the continuum of interventions required to enhance best outcomes. Inpatient teams are often the starting point, but the spectrum of interventions must include outpatient teams and community-based, recovery-oriented programs.

A considerable amount of overlap exists among these professionals and the therapeutic interventions and services they perform. Individual, group, and family education or counselling may be provided by nurses, psychiatrists, psychologists, certified social workers, and pastoral counsellors. Nurses, along with occupational and recreational therapists, can help patients with schizophrenia cope with the disruptions in their day-to-day functioning caused by cognitive and social deficits associated with negative symptoms. Teams of professionals working in partnership with self-help and peer support programs can shape a favourable recovery environment for stabilizing and enhancing the lives of people who have schizophrenia. However, barriers to this type of treatment abound and include access; inadequate funding; limitations on physician fee reimbursements; staff shortages (in particular, skilled mental health nurses); large caseloads; insufficient inpatient opportunities; and insufficient community

---

BOX 20.5 CLINICAL VIGNETTE

GRADUATE STUDENT EXPERIENCE

BGW, born in 1985, spent most of his teenage years using drugs and alcohol, behaviour that started when he was 11. He and his small group of friends spent their teenage years outside of school running around on bicycles. He failed 8th grade, repeated it, and made it to 10th grade. He was removed permanently from school at the age of 16. His dress included a dirty denim jacket or Army fatigues, torn tee shirts with rock band logos, and tight-fitting jeans. At age 16, he was hospitalized for a psychotic episode initiated by LSD; it was the scariest moment of his life. His mind had been getting fuzzier every day; he had dabbled with black magic and Satanism. Later, he admitted that for years, he had been trapped in a fantasy land, only partially explained by his drug use.

Years of treatment followed, and even with abstinence from drugs, his mental status fluctuated. Once antipsychotic agents were prescribed, he began to feel like himself. He was motivated to complete his high school diploma and entered college. He kept his mental illness a secret. While in graduate school, his thoughts, feelings, and behaviours began to change. His thinking became delusional, his moods unpredictable, and his behaviours illogical. Finally, he was hospitalized once again, and his condition was stabilized with medications. Currently, he is reapplying to graduate school and this time vowing to keep people close to him aware of his mental status.

Adapted from Oxford University Press and the Maryland Psychiatric Research Center. (2002). Graduate student in peril: A first person account of schizophrenia. *Schizophrenia Bulletin, 28*(4), 745–755.

supports, facilities, and social services. Despite these barriers, nurses can contribute significantly to interdisciplinary care given nursing's emphasis on patients' responses to their illness; their functional adaptation; their holistic needs, including physical and psychosocial requirements; and their attention to family support.

■ PRIORITY CARE ISSUES

Several special concerns exist when working with people with schizophrenia. About 20% to 50% of people with the diagnosis of schizophrenia attempt suicide, and 10% commit suicide either as a result of psychosis in acute stages or in response to depression in the chronic phase (Canadian Psychiatric Association, 2005; Hettige, Bani-Fatemi, Kennedy & De Luca, 2017). A systematic review of the literature found consensus for a 5% lifetime risk for suicide for persons with schizophrenia (Hor & Taylor, 2010). Suicide assessment should always be done with a person who is experiencing a psychotic episode. In an inpatient unit, patient safety concerns extend to potential aggressive actions toward self, staff, and other patients during episodes of psychoses. A priority of care during times of acute illness is treatment with antipsychotic medications.

During the recovery phase of schizophrenia, patients need help in accepting their illness and developing hopeful expectations for their future. They also need help to avoid social isolation through improved social and vocational skills and living arrangements that ensure contact with others (Frese, Knight, & Saks, 2009). Interventions that focus on psychosocial goals can address the hopelessness that may lead to suicide.

■ FAMILY RESPONSE TO DISORDER

Few families have had experience with mental illness to help them deal with the manifestations of schizophrenia. The first episode of psychosis is often accompanied by mixed emotions of disbelief, shock, fear, and care and concern for the family member. Hope that this is an isolated or transient episode may also be present. Families initially may seek reasons for the psychotic episode, attributing it to taking illicit drugs or to extraordinary stress or fatigue. Others, particularly parents, may blame themselves. They often do not know how to comfort their ill family member and may find themselves fearful of his or her behaviours. If the patient is hostile and aggressive toward family members, the family may respond with anger and hostility along with fear, confusion, and anxiety. During these episodes, some families may have to seek help from police or a crisis response team to control the situation. Coming to terms with the mental illness of a loved one is often described as an experience of catastrophic proportions (Addington, McCleery, & Addington, 2005; Wilson, 2012).

The initial period of illness for a patient and family that receive a diagnosis of schizophrenia is extraordinarily challenging. Often, during the initial phase of treatment, families are the primary caregivers for an ill relative. This necessitates that families have opportunities for explanation, education about the illness, and access to timely support. As families acknowledge the meaning of the diagnosis and the potential long-term rehabilitation required, they often feel overwhelmed, angry, and depressed (Wilson, 2012). More than 50 years have passed since the original theories of the schizophrenogenic family were popularized, but the notion of parents as potential causal factors in serious mental illness remains. Diagnostic labels are imbued with history and still resonate with fear and apprehension. During the early moments, when families receive the diagnostic proclamation, they generally hold the same unenlightened notions of schizophrenia as others within our culture. It is imperative then, for nurses and other health care providers, to provide families with useable explanations that assist them in thinking about themselves in a way that reduces any notions of blame or self-reproach. Families are often fearful that the future they once anticipated will not be realized or will take a very different form. Nurses can help families hold the hope for their ill relative.

The issue of family caregiving for a relative with serious mental illness has received attention from the MHCC. A working group from the commission developed a comprehensive guide for caregivers that contains many useful recommendations. Nurses should familiarize themselves with the recommendations contained in this document entitled, *National Guidelines for a Comprehensive Service System to Support Family Caregivers of Adults with Mental Health Problems and Illnesses* (MHCC, 2013c).

Nursing Management: Human Response to Disorder

The nursing management of the patient with schizophrenia usually lasts many years. Different phases of the illness require various nursing interventions at varying intensity. During exacerbation of symptoms, many patients are hospitalized for stabilization. During periods of relative stability, the nurse helps patients maintain a therapeutic regimen, develop positive mental health strategies, devise strategies to prepare for and cope with the stress, and reclaim their lives as much as possible.

Because of the complexity of this major psychiatric disorder, the nursing management for each domain is discussed separately. In reality, the nursing process steps overlap in all domains. For example, medication management is a direct biologic intervention; however, the effects of medications also are seen in psychological functioning. In the clinical area, effective nursing management requires an integration of the assessment data from all domains into meaningful interventions. Nursing interventions should cover all domains, including biologic, psychological, social (including family functioning), and spiritual. See Nursing Care Plan 20.1 and Interdisciplinary Treatment Plan 20.1.

NURSING CARE PLAN 20.1

PATIENT WITH FIRST-EPISODE PSYCHOSIS: PROBABLE SCHIZOPHRENIA

JT is a 19-year-old man who was brought to the hospital following his return from college, where he had locked himself in his room for 3 days. He was talking to non-existent people in a strange language. His room was covered with small pieces of notepaper with single words on them. His parents were summoned and immediately made arrangements for him to be assessed and, if necessary, subsequently hospitalized.

Setting: Psychiatric Intensive Care Unit

Baseline Assessment: JT is a 6'1", 145-pound young man whose appearance is dishevelled. He has not slept for 4 days and appears frightened. He is hypervigilant, pacing, and mumbling to himself. He is vague about past drug use, but his parents do not believe that he has used drugs. He appears to be hallucinating, conversing as if someone is in the room. He is confused and unable to write, speak, or think coherently. He is disoriented to time and place. Lab values are within normal limits except Hgb, 10.2, and Hct, 32. He has not eaten for several days.

Associated Psychiatric Diagnosis	Medications
Schizophrenia	Risperidone (Risperdal), 2 mg bid, then titrate to 3 mg if needed Lorazepam (Ativan), 2 mg PO or IM for agitation PRN
Psychosocial and contextual issues: educational problems (failing), social problems (withdrawn from peers)	

Nursing Diagnosis 1: Disturbed Thought Processes

Defining Characteristics	Related Factors
Inaccurate interpretation of stimuli (people thinking his thoughts) Cognitive impairment—attention, memory, and executive function impairment Suspiciousness Hallucinations	Uncompensated alterations in brain activity

Outcomes

Initial	Long Term
Decrease or eliminate hallucinations	Use coping strategies to deal with hallucinations or delusions if they reappear
Accurate interpretation of the environment (stop thinking that people are thinking his thoughts)	Communicate clearly with others
Improvement in cognitive functioning (improved attention, memory, and executive functioning)	Maintain cognitive functioning

(Continued)

NURSING CARE PLAN 20.1 *(Continued)*

Interventions	Rationale	Ongoing Assessment
Initiate a nurse–patient relationship by using an accepting, nonjudgmental approach. Be patient.	A therapeutic relationship will provide patient support as he begins to deal with the realization that he has experienced a first-episode psychosis and that diagnosis, although uncertain at this stage, could be the onset of schizophrenia. Be patient and offer information in small, gradual ways. Information processing is likely to be slow at this time.	Determine the extent to which JT is willing to trust and engage in a relationship.
Administer risperidone as prescribed. Observe for effects, side effects, and adverse effects. Begin teaching about the medication and its importance, once symptoms subside.	Risperidone is a D_2 and 5-HT2A antagonist and is indicated for the management of psychotic disorders.	Make sure JT swallows the pills. Monitor for relief of positive symptoms and assess side effects, especially extrapyramidal. Monitor BP for orthostatic hypotension and body temperature increase (neuroleptic malignant syndrome [NMS]).
During hallucinations and delusional thinking, assess significance (is it frightening, voices telling him to hurt himself or others?). Reassure JT that you will keep him safe. (Do not try to convince JT that his hallucinations are not real.) Redirect to the here and now.	It is important to understand the context of the hallucinations and delusions to be able to provide the appropriate interventions. By avoiding arguments about the content, the nurse will enhance communication.	Assess the meaning of the hallucination or delusion to the patient. Determine whether he is a danger to himself or others. Determine whether the patient can be redirected.
Assess the ability for self-care activities.	Disturbed thinking may interfere with JT's ability to carry out activities of daily living (ADLs).	Continue to assess: determine whether the patient can manage self-care.

Evaluation

Outcomes	Revised Outcomes	Interventions
Hallucinations and delusions began to decrease within 5 days.	Participate in unit activities according to interdisciplinary treatment plan.	Encourage attendance at treatment activities.
He is oriented to time, place, and person. Attention and memory are improving.	Agree to continue to take antipsychotic medications as prescribed.	Teach JT about medications. Teach JT about first-episode psychosis initially and schizophrenia when diagnosis is confirmed.

Nursing Diagnosis 2: Risk for Violence

Defining Characteristics	Related Factors
Assaultive toward others, self, and environment	Frightened, secondary to auditory hallucinations and delusional thinking
Presence of pathophysiologic risk factors: delusional thinking	Poor impulse control Dysfunctional communication patterns

NURSING CARE PLAN 20.1 *(Continued)*

Outcomes

Initial	Long Term
Avoid hurting self or assaulting other patients or staff. Decrease agitation and aggression.	Control behaviour with assistance from staff and parents.

Interventions

Interventions	Rationale	Ongoing Assessment
Acknowledge the patient's fears, hallucinations, and delusions.	Hallucinations and delusions change an individual's perception of environmental stimuli. A patient who is frightened will respond because of his need to stay safe.	Determine whether the patient is able to hear you. Assess his response to your comments and his ability to concentrate on what is being said.
Offer the patient choices of maintaining safety: keeping distance from others, medication for relaxation, etc.	By having choices, he will begin to develop a sense of control over his behaviour.	Observe the patient's nonverbal communication for evidence of increased agitation.
Administer lorazepam, 2 mg, for agitation. Oral route is preferable over injection.	Exact mechanisms of action are not understood, but this medication is believed to potentiate the inhibitory neurotransmitter GABA, relieving anxiety and producing sedation.	Observe for a decrease in agitated behaviour.
JT gradually decreased agitated behaviour. Lorazepam was given regularly for the first 2 days.	Demonstrate control of behaviour by resisting hallucinations and delusions.	Teach JT about the effects of hallucinations and delusions. Problem solve ways of controlling hallucinations if they occur. Emphasize the importance of taking medications.

Many nursing diagnoses apply to a person with schizophrenia. This is particularly true given that schizophrenia affects so many aspects of an individual's functioning and that symptoms can be observed in cognitive, emotional, family, social, and physical functioning. The applicable diagnoses can be categorized into the phases in which they are most likely to appear. However, it is important to note that even though they have been sorted into these categories, they may still represent recovery challenges in other phases. It is also important to note that the periods between exacerbations of symptoms are actually very important phases for pursuing recovery goals.

Biologic Domain
Biologic Assessment

The following sections highlight the important assessment areas for people with schizophrenia.

Current and Past Health Status and Physical Examination

It is important to conduct a thorough history and physical examination to rule out medical illness or substance abuse that could cause the psychiatric symptoms. It is also important to screen for comorbid medical illnesses that need to be treated, such as diabetes mellitus, hypertension, and cardiac disease, or a family history of such disorders. People with schizophrenia have a higher mortality rate from physical illness and often have smoking-related illnesses, such as emphysema, and other pulmonary, cardiac, and cancer problems. The nurse should determine whether the patient smokes tobacco, which not only affects the patient's health but also can affect the clearance of medications.

Physical Functioning

The negative symptoms of schizophrenia are often manifested in terms of impairment in physical functioning. Self-care often deteriorates, and sleep may be

Interdisciplinary Treatment Plan 20.1

Patient With First-Episode Psychosis: Probable Schizophrenia

Admission Date	Date of This Plan	Type of Plan: Check Appropriate Box					
05/03/14		☐ Initial	☐ Master	☐ 30	☐ 60	☐ 90	☐ Other

Treatment Team Present:
A. Barton, MD; J. Jones, RN; C. Anderson, RPN; B. Thomas, PhD; T. Toon, SW; J. Barker, Rec T; F. Huffern, OT; H. Kitchen, Peer Support Worker (PeerSW)

DIAGNOSIS (DSM-5)

Schizophreniform disorder, possible schizophrenia
Context: Educational problems (failing)
Social problems (withdrawn from peers)

ASSETS (MEDICAL, PSYCHOLOGICAL, SOCIAL, EDUCATIONAL, VOCATIONAL, RECREATIONAL)

1. First episode of psychosis. No evidence of drug use.
2. Premorbid functional level appears to be normal.
3. Maintained good grades in high school.
4. Has supportive family members.

Prob. No.	Date	Problem/Need	Code	Code	Date	
1	3/5/14	Is hallucinating and had delusional thoughts. Unable to communicate with parents or staff.	T			
2	3/5/14	Is aggressive and is striking out at staff and unfamiliar people.	T			
3	3/5/14	Dropped out of college because of thoughts and behaviours.	X			
4	3/5/14	Family members are very upset about their son's psychiatric symptoms.	T			

CODE	T = Problem must be addressed in treatment.
	N = Problem noted and will be monitored.
	X = Problem noted, but deferred/inactive/no action necessary.
	O = Problem to be addressed in aftercare/continuing care.
	I = Problem incorporated into another problem.
	R = Resolved.

No. 1 Problem/Need	Date Identified	Problem Resolved Discontinuation Date	
Is hallucinating and has delusional thoughts. Unable to communicate with parents or staff.	3/5/14		

Objective(s)/Short-Term Goals	Target Date	Achievement Date	
1. Reduce report and observations of hallucinations and delusions.	3/15/14		

Treatment Interventions	Frequency	Person Responsible	
1. Antipsychotic therapy for hallucinations and delusions. Administer and monitor for adherence, effect, and side effects.	As prescribed	MD/RN	
2. Monitor the frequency of hallucinations and delusions.	Close observation for 24–48 hours and then according to RN judgment	RN/RPN/LPN	
3. Attend symptom management group as symptoms subside.	Daily	PhD, RN, RPN	

Interdisciplinary Treatment Plan 20.1 (Continued)

ASSETS (MEDICAL, PSYCHOLOGICAL, SOCIAL, EDUCATIONAL, VOCATIONAL, RECREATIONAL)

No. 2 Problem/Need	Date Identified	Problem Resolved/Discontinuation Date	
Is aggressive and is striking out at staff and unfamiliar people.	3/5/14		

Objective(s)/Short-Term Goals	Target Date	Achievement Date	
1. De-escalate aggressive behaviour.	3/15/14		

Treatment Interventions	Frequency	Person Responsible	
1. Keep the patient in a quiet, nonstimulating environment. Assign a private room.	Ongoing	RN/RPN/LPN	
2. Administer antianxiety medication as needed.	PRN	MD/RN/RPN	
3. Use de-escalation techniques when approaching the patient.	Ongoing	Everyone	
4. Assign to anger management group, if needed when psychotic symptoms decrease.	In 1 week	RN/RPN/LPN	

No. 4 Problem/Need	Date Identified	Problem Resolved/Discontinuation Date	
Family members are very upset about their son's psychiatric symptoms.	3/5/14		

Objective(s)/Short-Term Goals	Target Date	Achievement Date	
Increase the family's comfort levels with mental illness.	3/15/14		

Treatment Interventions	Frequency	Person Responsible	
1. Meet with the family members each time they visit. Provide support, counselling and education to the family.	Ongoing	RPN/RN/MD	
2. Encourage the family to attend family support group.	Weekly	RN/SW/PeerSW	
3. Provide community resources for the treatment of mental illness.	When visiting	RN/RPN/PeerSW	

Responsible QMHP		**Client or Guardian**		**Staff Physician**	
Signature	Date	Signature	Date	Signature	Date

nonexistent during acute phases. Information regarding physical functioning may best be collected from family members.

Nutritional Assessment

A nutritional history should be completed to determine baseline eating habits and preferences. Medications can alter normal nutrition, and the patient may need to limit calories or fat consumption.

Fluid Imbalance Assessment

Although quite rare, the nurse should remain alert for signs of polydipsia and polyuria to identify disordered water balance (Goldman, 2009). Patients suspected of having disordered water balance should be assessed for signs and symptoms of hyponatraemia, water intoxication, excessive urination, incontinence, or periodically elevated blood pressure. Signs and symptoms of hypervolaemia that may be evident include puffiness of the face or eyes, abdominal distention, and hypothermia. These patients should be weighed daily, and their urine specific gravity and serum sodium levels should be monitored (Goldman, 2009).

Pharmacologic Assessment

Baseline information about the initial psychological and physical functioning should be obtained before the initiation of medication (or as early as possible). Side effects of medications should be assessed. Patients are often physically awkward and have poor coordination, motor abnormalities, and abnormal eye tracking. Before medication begins, standardized assessment of abnormal motor movements should be conducted using one of several assessment tools designed for that purpose, such as the Abnormal Involuntary Movement Scale (AIMS) (Guy, 1976) (see Appendix C), the Dyskinesia Identification System: Condensed User Scale (DISCUS) (Sprague & Kalachnik, 1991) (Fig. 20.5), or the Simpson-Angus Rating Scale (Simpson & Angus, 1970) (see Appendix B), which is designed for Parkinson-like symptoms.

Nursing Diagnoses for Biologic Domain

Typical nursing diagnoses focusing on the biologic domain for the person during all phases of schizophrenia include self-care deficit and disturbed sleep pattern. During a relapse, ineffective therapeutic regimen management, imbalanced nutrition, excess fluid volume, and sexual dysfunction are possible diagnoses. Constipation may occur if the patient takes anticholinergic medications.

Interventions for Biologic Domain

Nursing interventions during the initial acute phase of schizophrenia include prompt, safe, and informed administration of antipsychotic medications. During any stage, attention to self-care needs and the patient's ability to maintain hygiene and adequate nutrition are important.

Promotion of Self-Care Activities

For many individuals with schizophrenia, the plan of care will include specific interventions to enhance self-care, nutrition, and overall health knowledge. Negative symptoms commonly leave patients unable to initiate these seemingly simple activities. Developing a daily schedule of routine activities (e.g., showering and shaving) can help the patient structure the day. Most patients actually know how to perform self-care activities (e.g., hygiene, grooming) but are not motivated (avolition) to carry them out consistently. Interventions include developing a schedule with the patient for various hygiene activities and emphasizing the importance of maintaining appropriate self-care activities.

Activity, Exercise, and Nutritional Interventions

Encouraging activity and exercise is necessary, not only to maintain a healthy lifestyle but also to counteract the side effects of psychiatric medications that cause weight gain. Because the diagnosis of schizophrenia is usually made in late adolescence or early adulthood, it is possible to establish solid exercise patterns early.

During episodes of acute psychosis, patients are unable to focus on eating. Often when patients begin atypical antipsychotic medications, normal satiety and hunger responses change, and overeating or weight gain can become a problem. Promoting healthy nutrition is a key intervention. Maintaining healthy nutrition and monitoring calorie intake also become important because of the effect many medications have on eating habits. Patients report that appetite increases and cravings for food develop when some neuroleptic medications are initiated.

Weight gain is one of the reasons some patients become resistant to taking medication. It also may be a contributing factor to the development of type II diabetes mellitus. As such, this places patients at greater risk for several health complications and early death.

Monitoring for diabetes and managing weight are important activities for all care providers to perform (Gough, 2005; Stahl, 2013). Patients should be screened for risk factors of diabetes, such as family history, obesity as indicated by a body mass index (BMI) exceeding or equal to 27, and age older than 45 years. Patients' weight should be measured at regular intervals and their BMI calculated. Blood pressure readings should be taken regularly. Laboratory findings for triglycerides, HDL cholesterol, and glucose level should be monitored and reviewed regularly as well. All providers should be alert to the development of diabetic ketoacidosis, particularly in patients known to have diabetes who begin taking new antipsychotic agents. A program to address weight gain should be initiated at the earliest sign of weight gain (probably between 5 and 10 pounds over desired body weight). Reduced caloric intake may be accomplished by increasing the patient's access to affordable, healthful, and easy-to-prepare foods. Behavioural management of weight gain includes keeping a food diary, diet teaching, and exercise and weight management support groups.

Thermoregulation Interventions

Patients with schizophrenia may have disturbed body temperature regulation. In winter, they may seem to be oblivious to cold weather. In the heat of summer, they may dress for winter. Observing patients' responses to temperatures helps identify problems in this area. In patients who are taking psychotropic medications, body temperature needs to be monitored, and the patient needs to be protected from extremes in temperature. Sun safety is also important, and regular use of a sunscreen product to avoid skin damage from sunburn should be recommended.

Pharmacologic Interventions

Early in the 20th century, somatic treatment of schizophrenia included hydrotherapy (baths), wet-pack

| | NAME | I.D. |

(HEALTH CARE FACILITY)
Dyskinesia Identification System:
Condensed User Scale (DISCUS)

CURRENT PSYCHOTROPICS/ANTI-
CHOLINERGIC AND TOTAL MG/DAY

_____ ____ mg
_____ ____ mg
_____ ____ mg
_____ ____ mg

See Instructions on the Other Side

EXAM TYPE (check one)
- ☐ 1. Baseline
- ☐ 2. Annual
- ☐ 3. Semi annual
- ☐ 4. D/C—1 month
- ☐ 5. D/C—2 months
- ☐ 6. D/C—3 months
- ☐ 7. Admission
- ☐ 8. Other

COOPERATION (check one)
- ☐ 1. None
- ☐ 2. Partial
- ☐ 3. Full

SCORING

0—**Not present** (movements not observed or some movements observed but not considered abnormal)

1—**Minimal** (abnormal movements are difficult to detect or movements are easy to detect but occur only once or twice in a short nonrepetitive manner)

2—**Mild** (abnormal movements occur infrequently and are easy to detect)

3—**Moderate** (abnormal movements occur frequently and are easy to detect)

4—**Severe** (abnormal movements occur almost continuously **and** are easy to detect)

NA—**Not assessed** (an assessment for an item is not able to be made)

ASSESSMENT
DISCUS Item and Score (circle one score for each item)

FACE
1. Tics.. 0 1 2 3 4 NA
2. Grimaces............................... 0 1 2 3 4 NA

EYES
3. Blinking................................. 0 1 2 3 4 NA

ORAL
4. Chewing/Lip Smacking.......... 0 1 2 3 4 NA
5. Puckering/Sucking/Thrusting Lower Lip........ 0 1 2 3 4 NA

LINGUAL
6. Tongue Thrusting/Tongue in Cheek........ 0 1 2 3 4 NA
7. Tonic Tongue........................ 0 1 2 3 4 NA
8. Tongue Tremor...................... 0 1 2 3 4 NA
9. Athetoid/Myokymic/Lateral Tongue........ 0 1 2 3 4 NA

HEAD/NECK/TRUNK
10. Retrocollis/Torticollis........... 0 1 2 3 4 NA
11. Shoulder/Hip Torsion........... 0 1 2 3 4 NA

UPPER LIMB
12. Athetoid/Myokymic Finger–Wrist–Arm........ 0 1 2 3 4 NA
13. Pill Rolling........................... 0 1 2 3 4 NA

LOWER LIMB
14. Ankle Flexion/Foot Tapping........ 0 1 2 3 4 NA
15. Toe Movement..................... 0 1 2 3 4 NA

EVALUATION

1. Greater than 90 d neuroleptic exposure? : YES NO
2. Scoring/intensity level met? : YES NO
3. Other diagnostic conditions? : YES NO
(if yes, specify)
_____
_____
_____

4. Last exam date: _____
Last total score: _____
Last conclusion: _____

Preparer signature and title for items 1–4 (if different from the physician):

5. Conclusion (circle one):

A. No TD (if scoring prerequisite met, list other diagnostic conditions or explain in comments)
B. Probable TD
C. Masked TD
D. Withdrawal TD
E. Persistent TD
F. Remitted TD
G. Other (specify in comments)

6. Comments:
_____
_____
_____
_____
_____
_____

COMMENTS/OTHER
_____
_____
_____
_____

TOTAL SCORE (items 1–15 only)

EXAM DATE

RATER SIGNATURE AND TITLE | NEXT EXAM DATE | CLINICIAN SIGNATURE | DATE

From Sprague, R. L., & Kalachnik, J. E. (1991). Reliability, validity, and a total score cutoff for the Dyskinesia Identification Scale System: Condensed User Scale (DISCUS) with mentally ill and mentally retarded populations. *Psychopharmacology Bulletin, 27,* 51–58.

Figure 20.5. The dyskinesia identification system. (From Sprague, R. L., & Kalachnik, J. E. (1991). Reliability, validity, and a total score cutoff for the dyskinesia identification scale system: Condensed user scale (DISCUS) with mentally ill and mentally retarded populations. *Psychopharmacology Bulletin, 27,* 51–58.)

sheets, insulin shock therapy, electroconvulsive therapy, psychosurgery, and occupational and physical therapies. But in the early 1950s, treatment of schizophrenia drastically changed with the accidental discovery that a drug, chlorpromazine, used to induce anaesthesia also calmed patients with schizophrenia. Optimism persists as older medications continue to be used effectively while offering clues into the workings of the brain and as new discoveries about the brain lead to more precise medications for treating schizophrenia.

Antipsychotic drugs have the general effect of blocking dopamine transmission in the brain by blocking D_2 receptors to some degree (see Chapter 12). Some also block other dopamine receptors and receptors of other neurotransmitters to varying degrees. For the most part, the antidopamine effects are not specific to the mesolimbic and mesocortical tracts associated with schizophrenia, but instead travel to all the dopamine receptor sites throughout the brain. This results in desirable antipsychotic effects but also creates some unpleasant and undesirable side effects. The effects of antipsychotic drugs on other neurotransmitter systems may account for additional side effects.

The newer antipsychotic drugs, often referred to as second generation or atypical antipsychotics, such as risperidone (Risperdal; Box 20.6), olanzapine (Zyprexa), quetiapine (Seroquel), paliperidone (Invega), ziprasidone (Zeldox), and aripiprazole (Abilify) appear to be more efficacious and safer than conventional antipsychotics. They are available in a variety of formulations. Risperidone (Consta) and paliperidone (Invega Sustenna) are both available in a long-acting injectable form. They are effective in treating negative and positive symptoms. These newer drugs also affect several other neurotransmitter systems, including serotonin. This is believed to contribute to their overall antipsychotic effectiveness.

Monitoring and Administering Medications

Antipsychotic medications are the treatment of choice for patients with psychosis. The use of conventional or typical antipsychotics (e.g., haloperidol, Thorazine) decreased dramatically with the introduction of the second generation of antipsychotics. Generally, it takes 1 to 2 weeks for antipsychotic drugs to effect a change in symptoms. During the stabilization period, the type of drug selected should be given an adequate trial, generally 6 to 12 weeks, before considering a change in the drug prescription. If treatment effects are not seen, another antipsychotic agent may be tried. Clozapine (Clozaril) use may be initiated when no other atypical antipsychotic is effective (see Box 20.7 for more information about clozapine). Clozapine is exceptional in that it often works even when other medications have failed; however, because it requires monitoring of white blood cell counts, it is not the first choice for treatment.

BOX 20.6 **DRUG PROFILE**

Drug Profile Risperidone (Risperdal; Consta, Long-Acting Injectable)

Drug Class: Atypical antipsychotic.

Receptor Affinity: Antagonist with high affinity for D_2 and 5-HT_2, also histamine (H_1) and α_1- and α_2-adrenergic receptors, weak affinity for D_1 and other serotonin receptor subtypes; no affinity for acetylcholine or beta-adrenergic receptors.

Indications: Psychotic disorders such as schizophrenia, schizoaffective illness, bipolar affective disorder, and major depression with psychotic features.

Routes and Dosage: 1-, 2-, 3-, and 4-mg tablets and liquid concentrate (1 mg/mL). 25, 50, and 75 mg long-acting IM.

Adult Dosage: Initial dose typically 1 mg bid. Maximal effect at 6 mg/day. Safety not established above 16 mg/day. Use lowest possible dose to alleviate symptoms.

Geriatric: Initial dose, 0.5 mg/day, increase slowly as tolerated.

Children: Safety and efficacy with this age group have not been established.

Injection: Initiate 25 or 50 mg with oral supplementation for 2 to 3 weeks. Then, injections only, every 2 to 3 weeks. Given IM in gluteal area.

Half-Life (Peak Effect): mean, 20 hours (1 hour, peak active metabolite = 3 to 17 hours).

Select Adverse Reactions: Insomnia, agitation, anxiety, extrapyramidal symptoms, headache, rhinitis, somnolence, dizziness, headache, constipation, nausea, dyspepsia, vomiting, abdominal pain, hypersalivation, tachycardia, orthostatic hypotension, fever, chest pain, coughing, photosensitivity, and weight gain.

Warning: Rare development of NMS. Observe frequently for early signs of tardive dyskinesia. Use caution with individuals who have cardiovascular disease; risperidone can cause ECG changes. Avoid its use during pregnancy or while breast-feeding. Hepatic or renal impairments increase plasma concentration.

Specific Patient/Family Education

- Notify the prescriber if tremor, motor restlessness, abnormal movements, chest pain, or other unusual symptoms develop.
- Avoid alcohol and other CNS depressant drugs.
- Notify the prescriber if pregnancy is possible or planning to become pregnant. Do not breastfeed while taking this medication.
- Notify the prescriber before taking any other prescription or over-the-counter (OTC) medication.
- It may impair judgment, thinking, or motor skills; avoid driving or other hazardous tasks.
- During titration, the individual may experience orthostatic hypotension and should change positions slowly.
- Do not abruptly discontinue.

BOX 20.7 DRUG PROFILE ℞

Drug Profile Clozapine (Clozaril)

Drug Class: Atypical antipsychotic

Receptor Affinity: D_1 and D_2 blockade, antagonist for 5-HT_2, H_1, α-adrenergic, and acetylcholine. These additional antagonist effects may contribute to some of its therapeutic effects. It produces fewer extrapyramidal effects than standard antipsychotics with lower risk for tardive dyskinesia.

Indications: Severely ill individuals who have schizophrenia and have not responded to standard antipsychotic treatment. Unlabelled use for other psychotic disorders, such as schizoaffective disorder and bipolar affective disorder.

Routes and Dosage: Available only in tablet form, 25- and 100-mg doses.

Adult Dosage: Initial dose of 25 mg PO bid or qid may gradually increase in 25 to 50 mg/day increments, if tolerated, to a dose of 300 to 450 mg/day by the end of the 2nd week. Additional increases should occur no more than once or twice weekly. Do not exceed 900 mg/day. For maintenance, reduce the dosage to the lowest effective level.

Children: Safety and efficacy with children younger than 16 years have not been established.

Half-Life (Peak Effect): 12 hours (1 to 6 hours).

Select Adverse Reactions: Drowsiness, dizziness, headache, hypersalivation, tachycardia, hypo-/hypertension, constipation, dry mouth, heartburn, nausea/vomiting, blurred vision, diaphoresis, fever, weight gain, hematologic changes, seizures, tremor, and akathisia.

Warning: Agranulocytosis, defined as a granulocyte count of less than 500 mm^3, occurs at about a cumulative 1-year incidence of 1.3%, most often within 4 to 10 weeks of exposure, but it may occur at any time. Required registration with the clozapine. *Patient management system,* a WBC count before initiation, and weekly WBC counts while taking the drug and for 4 weeks after its discontinuation. Rare development of NMS. No confirmed cases of tardive dyskinesia, but it remains a possibility. Increased seizure risk at higher doses. Use caution with individuals who have cardiovascular disease; clozapine can cause ECG changes. Cases of sudden, unexplained death have been reported. Avoid its use during pregnancy or while breastfeeding.

Specific Patient/Family Education

- Need informed consent regarding the risk for agranulocytosis. Weekly blood draws are required. Notify the prescriber immediately if lethargy, weakness, sore throat, malaise, or other flu-like symptoms develop.
- Notify the prescriber if pregnancy is possible or planning to become pregnant. Do not breastfeed while taking this medication.
- Notify the prescriber before taking any other prescription or OTC medication. Avoid alcohol or other CNS depressant drugs.
- It may cause drowsiness and seizures; avoid driving or other hazardous tasks.
- During titration, the individual may experience orthostatic hypotension and should change positions slowly.
- Do not abruptly discontinue.

Adherence to a prescribed medication regimen is the best approach to preventing relapse. In these days of spending constraints and funding shortfalls, inpatient facilities are discharging patients before a judgment can be made about the efficacy of a given drug treatment. Nurses and other mental health professionals are charged with ensuring the continuation of these stabilization protocols and to also ensure that outpatient caregivers assume the responsibility for maintaining this stabilization phase of treatment and continue to monitor and manage the patient's symptoms. Outpatient systems should avoid the immediate manipulation of dosages and medications during the stabilization phase unless a medical emergency ensues.

Given the nature of a chronic illness like schizophrenia, patients generally face a lifetime of taking antipsychotic medications. Rarely is discontinuation of medications prescribed; however, many patients stop taking medications on their own. Some situations that require the cessation of medication use are neuroleptic malignant syndrome (NMS) (see *Emergency!* later in this chapter) and agranulocytosis (dangerously low level of circulating neutrophils). Agranulocytosis is most commonly experienced with clozapine (Clozaril) therapy. Discontinuation is an option when tardive dyskinesia develops. Discontinuation of medications, other than in circumstances of a medical emergency, should be achieved by gradually lowering the dose over time. This diminishes the likelihood of withdrawal symptoms, which include withdrawal dyskinesia and withdrawal psychosis.

Monitoring Extrapyramidal Side Effects

Parkinsonism that is caused by antipsychotic drugs is identical in appearance to Parkinson's disease and tends to occur in older patients. The symptoms are believed to be caused by the blockade of D_2 receptors in the basal ganglia, which throws off the normal balance between acetylcholine and dopamine in this area of the brain and effectively increases acetylcholine. The symptoms are managed by re-establishing the balance between acetylcholine and dopamine by reducing the dosage of the antipsychotic (increasing dopamine activity) or adding an anticholinergic drug (decreasing acetylcholine

Table 20.3 Nursing Interventions for Anticholinergic Side Effects

Effect	Intervention
Dry mouth	Sips of water; hard candies and chewing gum (preferably sugar-free)
Blurred vision	Avoid dangerous tasks; teach the patient that this side effect will diminish in a few weeks
Decreased lacrimation	Artificial tears if necessary
Mydriasis	May aggravate glaucoma; teach the patient to report eye pain
Photophobia	Sunglasses
Constipation	High-fibre diet; increased fluid intake; laxatives as prescribed
Urinary hesitancy	Privacy; run water in sink; warm water over perineum
Urinary retention	Regular voiding (at least every 2–3 h) and whenever urge is present; catheterize for residual; record intake and output; evaluate benign prostatic hypertrophy
Tachycardia	Evaluate for pre-existing cardiovascular disease; sudden death has occurred with thioridazine (Mellaril)

activity), such as benztropine (Cogentin) or trihexyphenidyl (Artane). Discontinuation of the use of anticholinergic drugs should never be abrupt, which can cause a cholinergic rebound and result in withdrawal symptoms, such as vomiting, excessive sweating, and altered dreams and nightmares. Thus, the anticholinergic drug dosage should be reduced gradually (tapered) over several days. If a patient experiences **akathisia** (physical restlessness), an anticholinergic medication may not be particularly helpful. Table 20.3 lists the anticholinergic side effects of antiparkinson drugs and several antipsychotic medications and interventions to manage them.

Dystonic reactions are also believed to result from the imbalance of dopamine and acetylcholine, with the latter being dominant. Young men seem to be more vulnerable to this particular extrapyramidal side effect. This side effect, which develops rapidly and dramatically, can be very frightening for patients as their muscles tense and their body contorts. The experience often starts with stiffness experienced in the muscles and can rapidly escalate to oculogyric crisis, in which the muscles that control eye movements tense and pull the eyeball so that the patient is looking toward the ceiling. This may be followed rapidly by torticollis, in which the neck muscles pull the head to the side, or retrocollis, in which the head is pulled back, or orolaryngeal–pharyngeal hypertonus, in which the patient has extreme difficulty swallowing. The patient may also experience contorted extremities. These symptoms occur early in antipsychotic drug treatment, when the patient may still be experiencing psychotic symptoms. Experiencing these side effects may compound the patient's fear and anxiety and requires a quick response. The immediate treatment is to administer benztropine (Cogentin), 1 to 2 mg, or diphenhydramine (Benadryl), 25 to 50 mg, intramuscularly or intravenously. This is followed by daily administration of oral anticholinergic drugs and, possibly, by a decrease in antipsychotic medication (see Box 20.8 for more information about benztropine).

Akathisia appears to be caused by the same biologic mechanism as other extrapyramidal side effects. Patients are restless and report that they feel driven to keep moving. They are very uncomfortable. Frequently, this response is misinterpreted as anxiety or increased psychotic symptoms, and the patient may be inappropriately given increased dosages of the antipsychotic drug, which only perpetuates the side effect. If possible, the dose of the antipsychotic drug should be reduced. A beta-adrenergic blocker such as propranolol (Inderal), 20 to 120 mg, may be required. Failure to manage this side effect is a leading cause of patients ceasing to take antipsychotic medications.

Tardive dyskinesia (impaired voluntary movement, resulting in fragmented or incomplete movements), **tardive dystonia**, and **tardive akathisia** are less likely to appear in individuals taking atypical, rather than conventional, antipsychotics. Table 20.4 describes these and associated motor abnormalities. Tardive dyskinesia is late-appearing abnormal involuntary movements (dyskinesia). It can be viewed as the opposite of parkinsonism both in observable movements and in aetiology. Whereas muscle rigidity and the absence of movement characterize parkinsonism, constant movement characterizes tardive dyskinesia. Typical movements involve the mouth, tongue, and jaw and include lip smacking, sucking, puckering, tongue protrusion, the bon-bon sign (where the tongue rolls around in the mouth and protrudes into the cheek as if the patient were sucking on a piece of hard candy), athetoid (wormlike) movements in the tongue, and chewing. Other facial movements, such as grimacing and eye blinking, also may be present.

Movements in the trunk and limbs are frequently observable. These include rocking from the hips, athetoid movements of the fingers and toes, jerking movements of the fingers and toes, guitar strumming movements of the fingers, and foot tapping. The long-term health problems for people with tardive dyskinesia are choking associated with loss of control of muscles used for swallowing and compromised respiratory function leading to infections and, possibly, respiratory alkalosis.

Because the movements resemble the dyskinetic movements of some patients who have idiopathic Parkinson's disease and who have received long-term treatment with L-dopa (a direct-acting dopamine

BOX 20.8 DRUG PROFILE Rx

Benztropine Mesylate (Cogentin)

Drug Class: Antiparkinson agent

Receptor Affinity: Blocks cholinergic (acetylcholine) activity, which is believed to restore the acetylcholine/dopamine balance in the basal ganglia.

Indications: Used in psychiatry to reduce extrapyramidal symptoms (acute medication-related movement disorders), including pseudoparkinsonism, dystonia, and akathisia (not tardive syndromes), due to neuroleptic drugs such as haloperidol. Most effective with acute dystonia.

Routes and Dosage: Available in tablet form, 0.5-, 1-, and 2-mg doses, also injectable 1 mg/mL.

Adult Dosage: For acute dystonia, 1 to 2 mg IM or IV usually provides rapid relief. No significant difference in the onset of action after IM or IV injection. Treatment of emergent symptoms may be relieved in 1 or 2 days, with 1 to 2 mg orally two to three times per day. Maximum daily dose is 6 mg/day. After 1 to 2 weeks, withdraw the drug to see if continued treatment is needed. Medication-related movement disorders that develop slowly may not respond to this treatment.

Geriatric: Older adults and very thin patients cannot tolerate large doses.

Children: Do not use in children younger than 3 years. Use with caution in older children.

Half-Life: 12 to 24 hours, very little pharmacokinetic information is available.

Select Adverse Reactions: Dry mouth, blurred vision, tachycardia, nausea, constipation, flushing or elevated temperature, decreased sweating, muscular weakness or cramping, urinary retention, urinary hesitancy, dizziness, headache, disorientation, confusion, memory loss, hallucinations, psychoses, and agitation in toxic reactions,

which are more pronounced in elderly people and occur at smaller doses.

Warning: Avoid its use during pregnancy or while breast-feeding. Give with caution in hot weather due to a possible heatstroke. Contraindicated with angle-closure glaucoma, pyloric or duodenal obstruction, stenosing peptic ulcers, prostatic hypertrophy or bladder neck obstructions, myasthenia gravis, megacolon, or megaesophagus. It may aggravate the symptoms of tardive dyskinesia or other chronic forms of medication-related movement disorder. Concomitant use of other anticholinergic drugs may increase the side effects and risk for toxicity. Coadministration of haloperidol or phenothiazines may reduce serum levels of these drugs.

Specific Patient/Family Education

- Take with meals to reduce dry mouth and gastric irritation.
- Dry mouth may be alleviated by sucking sugarless candies, adequate fluid intake, or good oral hygiene; increase the intake of fibre and fluids in diet to avoid constipation; stool softeners may be required. Notify the prescriber if urinary hesitancy or constipation persists.
- Notify the prescriber if rapid or pounding heartbeat, confusion, eye pain, rash, or other adverse symptoms develop.
- It may cause drowsiness, dizziness, or blurred vision; use caution while driving or performing other hazardous tasks requiring alertness. Avoid alcohol and other CNS depressants.
- Do not abruptly stop this medication because a flu-like syndrome may develop.
- Use caution in hot weather. Ensure adequate hydration. It may increase the susceptibility to heatstroke.

---

agonist that crosses the blood–brain barrier), the suggested hypothesis for tardive dyskinesia includes the supersensitivity of the dopamine receptor in the basal ganglia.

There is no consistently effective treatment; however, antipsychotic drugs mask the movements of tardive dyskinesia and have periodically been suggested as a treatment. This is counterintuitive because these are the drugs

Table 20.4 Extrapyramidal Side Effects of Antipsychotic Drugs

Side Effect	Symptoms
Parkinsonism or pseudoparkinsonism	Resting tremor, rigidity, bradykinesia/akinesia, masklike face, shuffling gait, and decreased arm swing
Acute dystonia	Intermittent or fixed abnormal postures of the eyes, face, tongue, neck, trunk, and extremities
Akathisia	Obvious motor restlessness evidenced by pacing, rocking, and shifting from foot to foot; subjective sense of not being able to sit or be still; these symptoms may occur together or separately
Tardive dyskinesia	Abnormal dyskinetic movements of the face, mouth, and jaw; choreoathetoid movements of the legs, arms, and trunk
Tardive dystonia	Persistent sustained abnormal postures in the face, eyes, tongue, neck, trunk, and limbs
Tardive akathisia	Persisting, unabating sense of subjective and objective restlessness

Adapted from Lilley, L. L., Collins, S. R., Synder, J., & Swart, B. (2017). *Pharmacology for Canadian health care practice* (3rd ed.). Toronto, ON: Elsevier Canada.

that cause the disorder. Newer antipsychotic drugs, such as clozapine, may be less likely to cause the disorder. The best management remains prevention through prescription of the lowest possible dose of antipsychotic drug over time that minimizes the symptoms of schizophrenia, prescription of these drugs for psychotic symptoms only, and early case finding by regular systematic AIMS screening of everyone receiving these drugs (see Table 20.4).

Orthostatic hypotension is another side effect of antipsychotic drugs. The primary antiadrenergic effect is decreased blood pressure, which may be general or orthostatic. Patients may be protected from falls by teaching them to rise slowly and by monitoring blood pressure before doses of the drug. The nurse should monitor and document lying, sitting, and standing blood pressures when any antipsychotic drug therapy begins.

Hyperprolactinaemia can occur and is associated with the use of haloperidol and risperidone. When dopamine is blocked in the tuberoinfundibular tract, it can no longer repress prolactin, the neurohormone that regulates lactation and mammary function. The prolactin level increases and, in some individuals, side effects appear. **Gynaecomastia** (enlarged breasts) can occur among both sexes and is understandably distressing to individuals who may be experiencing delusional or hallucinatory body image disturbances. **Galactorrhoea** (lactation) also may occur. Menstrual irregularities and sexual dysfunction are also possible. If these symptoms appear, the medication should be reduced or changed to another antipsychotic agent. Evidence for long-term consequences of hyperprolactinaemia is still lacking.

Weight gain is related to antipsychotic agents, especially olanzapine and clozapine, which have major antihistaminic properties. Patients may gain as much as 20 or 30 pounds within 1 year. Increased appetite and weight gain are often distressing to patients. Diet teaching and monitoring may have some effect on this side effect. Another solution is to increase the accessibility of healthful, easy-to-prepare food. Although nausea and vomiting can occur with the use of these drugs, they most often mask nausea.

Sedation is another possible side effect of antipsychotic medication. Patients should be monitored for the sedating effects of antipsychotic agents that are antihistaminic. In elderly patients, sedation can be associated with falls.

Screening for new-onset diabetes in patients taking antipsychotic drugs should be conducted regularly. An association has been made between new-onset diabetes mellitus and the administration of atypical antipsychotic agents, especially olanzapine and clozapine (Gough, 2005). Patients should be assessed and monitored for clinical symptoms of diabetes. Fasting blood glucose tests are commonly ordered for these individuals.

Cardiac arrhythmias may also occur. Prolongation of the QT interval is associated with torsade de pointes (polymorphic ventricular tachycardia) or ventricular fibrillation. The potential for drug-induced prolonged QT interval is associated with many drugs, for example, the antipsychotic agent ziprasidone (Zeldox) may be more likely than other drugs to prolong the QT interval and change the heart rhythm. For these patients, baseline electrocardiograms may be ordered. Nurses should observe these patients for cardiac arrhythmias.

Agranulocytosis is a reduction in the number of circulating granulocytes and decreased production of granulocytes in the bone marrow that limits one's ability to fight infection. Agranulocytosis can develop with the use of all antipsychotic drugs, but it is most likely to develop with clozapine use. Although laboratory values below 500 cells/mm^3 are indicative of agranulocytosis, often, granulocyte counts drop to below 200 cells/mm^3 with this syndrome.

Patients taking clozapine must have regular blood tests. White blood cell and granulocyte counts should be measured before the treatment is initiated and at least weekly or twice weekly after the treatment begins. Initial white blood cell counts should be above 3,500 cells/mm^3 before treatment initiation; in patients with counts of 3,500 to 5,000 cells/mm^3, cell counts should be monitored three times a week if clozapine is prescribed. Any time the white blood cell count drops below 3,500 cells/mm^3 or granulocytes drop below 1,500 cells/mm^3, the use of clozapine should be stopped, and the patient should be monitored for fever and infections.

A faithfully implemented program of blood monitoring, however, should not replace careful observation of the patient. It is not unusual for blood cell counts to drop precipitously in a period of 2 to 3 days. This may not be discovered when the patient is on a strict weekly blood monitoring schedule. Any reported symptoms that are reminiscent of a bacterial infection (e.g., fever, pharyngitis, weakness) should be a cause for concern, and immediate evaluation of blood count status should be undertaken. Because patients are frequently discharged before the critical period of risk for agranulocytosis, patient and family education about these symptoms is also essential so that they will report these symptoms and obtain blood monitoring if necessary. In general, granulocytes return to normal within 2 to 4 weeks after discontinuing use of the medication.

Drug–Drug Interactions

Several potential drug–drug interactions are possible when administering antipsychotic medications. One of the cytochrome P450 enzymes responsible for the metabolism of olanzapine and clozapine is 1A2. If either olanzapine or clozapine is given with another medication that inhibits this enzyme, such as fluvoxamine (Luvox), the antipsychotic blood level would increase and possibly become toxic. On the other hand, cigarette smoking can also induce 1A2 and lower concentration of drugs metabolized by this enzyme, such as olanzapine and clozapine. Individuals that smoke may require a higher dose of these medications than do non-smokers (Levin & Rezvani, 2007). Similarly, individuals that are unable to smoke (due to smoke-free policies) or have quit smoking are at risk of increased antipsychotic blood levels and possible toxicity. This effect may be of high relevance when an individual is discharged from a nonsmoking institution to a community setting.

Several atypical antipsychotic agents, including clozapine, quetiapine, and ziprasidone, are metabolized by the 3A4 enzyme. Weak inhibitors of this enzyme include the antidepressants fluvoxamine, nefazodone, and norfluoxetine (an active metabolite of fluoxetine). Potent inhibitors of 3A4 enzyme include ketoconazole (antifungal drug), protease inhibitors, and erythromycin. If these drugs are given with clozapine, quetiapine, or ziprasidone, the antipsychotic level will rise. In addition, the mood stabilizer carbamazepine (Tegretol) is a 3A4 inducer. When this drug is given with clozapine, quetiapine, or ziprasidone, the antipsychotic dose should be increased to compensate for the 3A4 induction. If the use of carbamazepine is discontinued, the dosage of the antipsychotic agent needs to be adjusted (Stahl, 2008).

Risperidone, clozapine, and olanzapine are substrates for the enzyme 2D6. Theoretically, antidepressants (fluoxetine and paroxetine) that inhibit this enzyme could increase these antipsychotics' levels. However, this is not usually clinically significant (Stahl, 2008).

TEACHING POINTS

Nonadherence to the medication regimen is an important factor in relapse. Patients and their families must be made aware of the importance of consistently taking medications. Medication education should cover the association between medications and the amelioration of symptoms (in general as well as individualized for the patient), side effects and their management, and coaching as to when to report medication effects.

EMERGENCY

Neuroleptic Malignant Syndrome

In NMS, severe muscle rigidity develops with elevated temperature and a rapidly accelerating cascade of symptoms (occurring during the next 48 to 72 hours), which can include two or more of the following: hypertension, tachycardia, tachypnea, prominent diaphoresis, incontinence, mutism, leukocytosis, changes in the level of consciousness ranging from confusion to coma, and laboratory evidence of muscle injury (e.g., elevated creatinine phosphokinase). NMS occurs in about 1% of those who receive antipsychotic drugs, especially the

conventional antipsychotics such as haloperidol and other drugs that block dopamine, such as metoclopramide (Montoya, Ocampo, & Torres-Ruiz, 2003). Up to one third of patients experiencing NMS die as a result of the syndrome. NMS is probably underreported and may account for unexplained emergency room deaths of patients taking these drugs who do not have diagnoses because their symptoms do not seem serious. The presenting symptom is a temperature greater than 37.5°C (usually between 38.3°C and 39.4°C) with no apparent cause.

The most important aspects of nursing care for patients with NMS relate to recognizing symptoms early, stopping the administration of any neuroleptic medications, and initiating supportive nursing care. In any patient with fever, fluctuating vital signs, abrupt changes in levels of consciousness, or any of the symptoms presented in Box 20.9, NMS should be suspected. The nurse should be especially alert for early signs and symptoms of NMS in high-risk patients, such as those who are agitated, physically exhausted, or dehydrated, or those who have an existing medical or neurologic illness. Patients receiving parenteral or higher doses of oral neuroleptic drugs or lithium concurrently must also be

> **BOX 20.9** Diagnostic Criteria for Neuroleptic Malignant Syndrome (NMS)*
>
> 1. Treatment with neuroleptics within 7 days of onset (2 to 4 weeks for depot neuroleptic medications)
> 2. Hyperthermia
> 3. Muscle rigidity
> 4. Five of the following:
>   - Change in mental status
>   - Tachycardia
>   - Hypertension or hypotension
>   - Tachypnea or hypoxia
>   - Diaphoresis or sialorrhoea
>   - Tremor
>   - Incontinence
>   - Creatinine phosphokinase elevation or myoglobinuria
>   - Leukocytosis
>   - Metabolic acidosis
> 5. Exclusion of other drug-induced, systemic, or neuropsychiatric illnesses
>
> *All five items are required concurrently.
> Adapted from Lilley, L. L., Collins, S. R., Synder, J., & Swart, B. (2017). *Pharmacology for Canadian health care practice* (3rd ed.). Toronto, ON: Elsevier Canada.

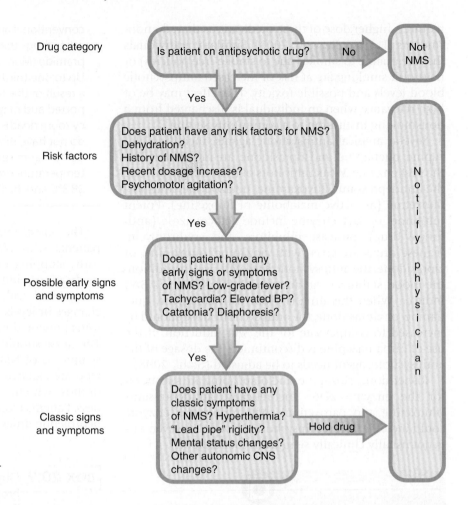

Figure 20.6. Action tree for "holding" a neuroleptic drug because of suspected NMS.

carefully assessed. The nurse should carefully monitor fluid intake and fluid and electrolyte status.

To prevent NMS from developing in a patient with signs or symptoms of the disorder, the nurse should immediately discontinue the administration of any neuroleptic drugs and notify the physician. In addition, the nurse should hold any anticholinergic drugs that the patient may be taking. A common error made by nurses who fail to analyze the patient's total clinical picture (including vital signs, mental status changes, and laboratory values) is to continue the use of neuroleptic drugs. Figure 20.6 shows how to decide whether to withhold an antipsychotic medication. Medical treatment includes administering several medications. Dopamine agonist drugs, such as bromocriptine (modest success), and muscle relaxants, such as dantrolene or benzodiazepine, have been used. Antiparkinsonism drugs are not particularly useful. Some patients experience improvement with electroconvulsive therapy.

The vital signs of the patient with symptoms of NMS must be monitored frequently. In addition, it is important to check the results of the patient's laboratory tests for increased creatine phosphokinase, elevated white blood cell count, elevated liver enzymes, or myoglobinuria. The nurse must be prepared to initiate supportive measures or anticipate emergency transfer of the patient to a medical–surgical or an intensive care unit.

Treating high temperature (which frequently exceeds 39°C) is an important priority for these patients. High body temperature may be reduced with a cooling blanket and acetaminophen. Because many of these patients experience diaphoresis, temperature elevation, or dysphagia, it is important to monitor fluid hydration. Another important aspect of care for patients with NMS is safety. Joints and extremities that are rigid or spastic must be protected from injury. The treatment of these patients depends on the facility and availability of medical support services.

EMERGENCY

Anticholinergic Crisis

There is also a potential for abuse of anticholinergic drugs. Some patients may find the anticholinergic effects of these drugs on mood, memory, and perception pleasurable. Although at toxic dosages, patients may experience disorientation and hallucinations, lesser doses may cause patients to experience greater sociability and euphoria. Anticholinergic crisis is a potentially life-threatening medical emergency caused by an overdose of or sensitivity to drugs with anticholinergic properties. This syndrome (also called anticholinergic delirium)

(Continued)

may result from an accidental or intentional overdose of antimuscarinic drugs, including atropine, scopolamine, or belladonna alkaloids, which are present in numerous prescription drugs and over-the-counter (OTC) medicines. The syndrome may also occur in psychiatric patients who are receiving therapeutic doses of anticholinergic drugs, especially when such agents are combined with other psychotropic drugs that produce anticholinergic side effects. Numerous drugs commonly prescribed in psychiatric settings produce anticholinergic side effects, including tricyclic antidepressants and some antipsychotics. As a result of either drug overdose or drug sensitivity, these anticholinergic substances may produce an acute delirium or a psychotic reaction resembling schizophrenia. More severe anticholinergic effects may occur in older patients, even at therapeutic levels (Ramnarine & Ahmad, 2016; Stahl, 2008).

The signs and symptoms of anticholinergic crisis are dramatic and physically uncomfortable (Box 20.10). This disorder is characterized by elevated temperature; parched mouth; burning thirst; hot, dry skin; decreased salivation; decreased bronchial and nasal secretions; widely dilated eyes (bright light is painful); decreased ability to accommodate visually; increased heart rate; constipation; difficulty urinating; and hypertension or hypotension. The face, neck, and upper arms may become flushed because of reflex blood vessel dilation. In addition to peripheral symptoms, patients with anticholinergic psychosis may experience neuropsychiatric symptoms of anxiety, agitation, delirium, hyperactivity, confusion, hallucinations (especially visual), speech difficulties, psychotic symptoms, or seizures. The acute psychotic reaction that is produced resembles schizophrenia. The classic description of anticholinergic crisis is summarized in the following mnemonic: "Hot as a hare, blind as a bat, mad as a hatter, dry as a bone."

In general, episodes of anticholinergic crisis are self-limiting, usually subsiding in 3 days. However, if untreated, the associated fever and delirium may progress to coma or cardiac and respiratory depression. Although rare, death is generally due to hyperpyrexia and brainstem depression. Once the use of the offending drug is discontinued, improvement usually occurs within 24 to 36 hours.

A specific and effective antidote, physostigmine (an inhibitor of anticholinesterase) is frequently used for treating and diagnosing anticholinergic crisis. Administration of this drug rapidly reduces both the behavioural and the physiologic symptoms. However, the usual adult dose of physostigmine is 1 to 2 mg intravenously, given slowly during a period of 5 minutes because rapid injection of physostigmine may cause seizures, profound bradycardia, or heart block. Physostigmine is relatively short acting, so it may need to be given several times during the course of treatment. This drug provides relief from symptoms for a period of 2 to 3 hours. In addition to receiving physostigmine, patients who intentionally overdose on large amounts of anticholinergic drugs are treated by gastric lavage, administration of charcoal, and catharsis. The dose may be repeated after 20 or 30 minutes.

It is important for the nurse to be alert for signs and symptoms of anticholinergic crisis, especially in elderly people and children, who are much more sensitive to the anticholinergic effects of drugs, and in patients who are receiving multiple medications with anticholinergic effects. If signs and symptoms of the syndrome occur, the nurse should discontinue the use of the offending drug and notify the physician immediately.

Other Somatic Interventions

Electroconvulsive therapy is suggested as a possible alternative when the patient's schizophrenia is not being successfully treated by medication alone. Research supports using electroconvulsive therapy as an augmentation to antipsychotic therapy (Tharyan & Adams, 2005). For the most part, this is not indicated unless the patient is experiencing catatonia or has a depression that is not treatable by other means.

BOX **20.10** **EMERGENCY**

Signs and Symptoms of Anticholinergic Crisis

Neuropsychiatric signs: confusion, recent memory loss, agitation, dysarthria, incoherent speech, pressured speech, delusions, ataxia, and periods of hyperactivity alternating with somnolence, paranoia, anxiety, or coma

Hallucinations: accompanied by "picking," plucking, or grasping motions, delusions, or disorientation

Physical signs: unreactive dilated pupils; blurred vision; hot, dry, flushed skin; facial flushing; dry mucous membranes; difficulty swallowing; fever; tachycardia; hypertension; decreased bowel sounds; urinary retention; nausea; vomiting; seizures; or coma

---

BOX 20.11 Standardized Scales Used in Assessing Symptoms of People With Schizophrenia

SCALE FOR THE ASSESSMENT OF NEGATIVE SYMPTOMS (SANS)

Available from Nancy C. Andreasen, MD, PhD, Department of Psychiatry, College of Medicine, The University of Iowa, Iowa City, IA 52242. Copyright 1984 (see Box 20.14).

SCALE FOR THE ASSESSMENT OF POSITIVE SYMPTOMS (SAPS)

Available from Nancy C. Andreasen (see above) (see Box 20.13).

ABNORMAL INVOLUNTARY MOVEMENT SCALE (AIMS)

Guy, W. (1976). *ECDEU: Assessment manual for psychopharmacology (DHEW Publication No. 76-338)*. Washington, DC: Department of Health Education and Welfare, Psychopharmacology Branch.

BRIEF PSYCHIATRIC RATING SCALE (BPRS)

Overall, J. E., & Gorham, D. R. (1988). The brief psychiatric rating scale (BPRS): Recent developments in ascertainment and scaling. *Psychopharmacology Bulletin, 24*, 97–99.

DYSKINESIA IDENTIFICATION SYSTEM: CONDENSED USER SCALE (DISCUS)

Sprague, R. L., & Kalachnik, J. E. (1991). Reliability, validity, and a total score cutoff for the dyskinesia identification scale system: Condensed user scale (DISCUS) with mentally ill and mentally retarded populations. *Psychopharmacology Bulletin, 27*(1), 51–58 (see Table 20.4).

SIMPSON-ANGUS RATING SCALE

Simpson, G. M., & Angus, J. W. (1970). A rating scale for extrapyramidal side effects. *Acta Psychiatrica Scandinavica, 212*, 11–19. Copyright 1970, Munksgaard International Publishers, Ltd.

Psychological Domain

Although schizophrenia is a brain disorder, the psychological manifestations are the most difficult to assess and treat. Many of these psychological manifestations improve with the use of medications, but they are not necessarily eliminated.

Psychological Assessment

Several assessment scales have been developed and received considerable reliability and validity testing to help evaluate positive and negative symptom clusters in schizophrenia. Box 20.11 lists the standardized instruments used in assessing symptoms of people with schizophrenia. These include the Scale for the Assessment of Positive Symptoms (SAPS) (Box 20.12), the Scale for the Assessment of Negative Symptoms (SANS) (Box 20.13), and the Positive and Negative Syndrome Scale (PANSS) (Kay, Fiszbein, & Opler, 1987), which assesses both symptom clusters in the same instrument. Tools that list symptoms, such as the Brief Psychiatric Rating Scale (BPRS) (Overall & Gorham, 1988) (see Appendix A), SANS, or SAPS, can also be used to help patients self-monitor their symptoms.

Information about prediagnosis experiences usually requires retrospective reporting by the patient or the family. This reporting is generally reliable for the frankly psychotic symptoms of delusions and hallucinations; however, negative symptoms are more difficult to date. In fact, negative symptoms vary from an imperceptive deviation from normal to a clear impairment. Negative symptoms probably occur earlier than do positive symptoms and are less easily noted by the patient and significant others.

Responses to Mental Health Problems

Schizophrenia robs people of mental health and imposes social stigma. People with schizophrenia struggle to maintain control of their symptoms, which affects every aspect of their life. The person with schizophrenia displays a variety of interrelated symptoms and experiences deficits in several areas. More than half of patients report the following prodromal symptoms (in order of frequency): tension and nervousness, lack of interest in eating, difficulty concentrating, disturbed sleep, decreased enjoyment and loss of interest, restlessness, forgetfulness, depression, social withdrawal from friends, feeling laughed at, more religious thinking, feeling bad for no reason, feeling too excited, and hearing voices or seeing things.

Because schizophrenia is a disorder of thoughts, perceptions, and behaviour, it is sometimes not recognized as an illness by the person experiencing the symptoms. Many people with thought disorders do not believe that they have a mental illness. Their denial of mental illness and the need for treatment poses problems for the family and clinicians. This lack of insight or **anosognosia** in schizophrenia has previously been interpreted as a primary symptom of the illness, namely, a defensive mechanism rather than a neurologically based condition. However, research suggests a neuropsychologic interpretation of the lack of insight in schizophrenia (Pia & Tamleto, 2006). Ideally, in lucid moments, patients recognize that their thoughts are really delusions, that their perceptions are hallucinations, and that their behaviour is disorganized. In reality, many patients do not believe that they have a mental illness but agree to treatment to please their family and clinicians.

BOX 20.12 Scale for the Assessment of Positive Symptoms

0 = None; 1 = Questionable; 2 = Mild; 3 = Moderate; 4 = Marked; 5 = Severe

Hallucinations

1. *Auditory Hallucinations* 0 1 2 3 4 5
   The patient reports voices, noises, or other sources that no one else hears.
2. *Voices Commenting* 0 1 2 3 4 5
   The patient reports a voice that makes a running commentary on his behaviour or thoughts.
3. *Voices Conversing* 0 1 2 3 4 5
   The patient reports hearing two or more voices conversing.
4. *Somatic or Tactile Hallucinations* 0 1 2 3 4 5
   The patient reports experiencing peculiar physical sensations in the body.
5. *Olfactory Hallucinations* 0 1 2 3 4 5
   The patient reports experiencing unusual smells that no one else notices.
6. *Visual Hallucinations* 0 1 2 3 4 5
   The patient sees shapes or people that are not actually present.
7. *Global Rating of Hallucinations* 0 1 2 3 4 5
   This rating should be based on the duration and severity of the hallucinations and their effect on the patient's life.

Delusions

8. *Persecutory Delusions* 0 1 2 3 4 5
   The patient believes that he or she is being conspired against or in some way persecuted.
9. *Delusions of Jealousy* 0 1 2 3 4 5
   The patient believes that his spouse is having an affair with someone.
10. *Delusions of Guilt or Sin* 0 1 2 3 4 5
    The patient believes that he has committed some terrible sin or done something unforgivable.
11. *Grandiose Delusions* 0 1 2 3 4 5
    The patient believes that he has special powers or abilities.
12. *Religious Delusions* 0 1 2 3 4 5
    The patient is preoccupied with false beliefs of a religious nature.
13. *Somatic Delusions* 0 1 2 3 4 5
    The patient believes that somehow his body is diseased, abnormal, or changed.
14. *Delusions of Reference* 0 1 2 3 4 5
    The patient believes that insignificant remarks or events refer to him or have some special meaning.

15. *Delusions of Being Controlled* 0 1 2 3 4 5
    The patient feels that his feelings or actions are controlled by some outside force.
16. *Delusions of Mind Reading* 0 1 2 3 4 5
    The patient feels that people can read his mind or know his thoughts.
17. *Thought Broadcasting* 0 1 2 3 4 5
    The patient believes that his thoughts are broadcast so that he or others can hear them.
18. *Thought Insertion* 0 1 2 3 4 5
    The patient believes that thoughts that are not his own have been inserted into his mind.
19. *Thought Withdrawal* 0 1 2 3 4 5
    The patient believes that thoughts have been taken away from his mind.
20. *Global Rating of Delusions* 0 1 2 3 4 5
    This rating should be based on the duration and persistence of the delusions and their effects on the patient's life.

Bizarre Behaviour

21. *Clothing and Appearance* 0 1 2 3 4 5
    The patient dresses in an unusual manner or does other strange things to alter his appearance.
22. *Social and Sexual Behaviours* 0 1 2 3 4 5
    The patient may do things considered inappropriate according to usual social norms (e.g., masturbating in public).
23. *Aggressive and Agitated Behaviour* 0 1 2 3 4 5
    The patient may behave in an aggressive, agitated manner, often unpredictably.
24. *Repetitive or Stereotyped Behaviour* 0 1 2 3 4 5
    The patient develops a set of repetitive actions or rituals that he must perform over and over.
25. *Global Rating of Bizarre Behaviour* 0 1 2 3 4 5
    This rating should reflect the type of behaviour and the extent to which it deviates from social norms.

Positive Formal Thought Disorder

26. *Derailment* 0 1 2 3 4 5
    A pattern of speech in which ideas slip off track onto ideas obliquely related or unrelated.
27. *Tangentiality* 0 1 2 3 4 5
    Replying to a question in an oblique or irrelevant manner.
28. *Incoherence* 0 1 2 3 4 5
    A pattern of speech that is essentially incomprehensible at times.

(Continued)

BOX 20.12 Scale for the Assessment of Positive Symptoms (Continued)

29. *Illogicality*   0 1 2 3 4 5
A pattern of speech in which conclusions are reached that do not follow logically.
30. *Circumstantiality*   0 1 2 3 4 5
A pattern of speech that is very indirect and delayed in reaching its goal idea.
31. *Pressure of Speech*   0 1 2 3 4 5
The patient is distracted by nearby stimuli that interrupt his or her flow of speech.
32. *Distractible Speech*   0 1 2 3 4 5
The patient's speech is rapid and difficult to interrupt; the amount of speech produced is greater than that considered normal.
33. *Clanging*   0 1 2 3 4 5
A pattern of speech in which sounds, rather than meaningful relationships, govern word choice.

34. *Global Rating of Positive Formal*   0 1 2 3 4 5
Thought Disorder
This rating should reflect the frequency of abnormality and the degree to which it affects the patient's ability to communicate.

Inappropriate Affect
35. *Inappropriate Affect*   0 1 2 3 4 5
The patient's affect is inappropriate or incongruous, not simply flat or blunted.

From Nancy C. Andreasen, MD, PhD, Department of Psychiatry, College of Medicine. The University of Iowa, Iowa City, IA 52242. Copyright 1984 Nancy C. Andreasen. Reprinted with permission.

BOX 20.13 Scale for the Assessment of Negative Symptoms

0 = None; 1 = Questionable; 2 = Mild; 3 = Moderate; 4 = Marked; 5 = Severe

Affective Flattening or Blunting
1. *Unchanging Facial Expression*   0 1 2 3 4 5
The patient's face appears wooden; it changes less than expected as the emotional content of discourse changes.
2. *Decreased Spontaneous Movements*   0 1 2 3 4 5
The patient shows few or no spontaneous movements and does not shift position, move extremities, etc.
3. *Paucity of Expressive Gestures*   0 1 2 3 4 5
The patient does not use hand gestures, body position, etc., as an aid to expressing ideas.
4. *Poor Eye Contact*   0 1 2 3 4 5
The patient avoids eye contact or "stares through" interviewer even when speaking.
5. *Affective Nonresponsivity*   0 1 2 3 4 5
The patient fails to smile or laugh when prompted.
6. *Lack of Vocal Inflections*   0 1 2 3 4 5
The patient fails to show normal vocal emphasis patterns; is often monotonic.
7. *Global Rating of Affective Flattening*   0 1 2 3 4 5
This rating should focus on the overall severity of symptoms, especially unresponsiveness, eye contact, facial expression, and vocal inflections.

Alogia
8. *Poverty of Speech*   0 1 2 3 4 5
The patient's replies to questions are restricted in amount and tend to be brief, concrete, and unelaborated.

9. *Poverty of Content of Speech*   0 1 2 3 4 5
The patient's replies are adequate in amount but tend to be vague, overconcrete, or overgeneralized, and they convey little information.
10. *Blocking*   0 1 2 3 4 5
The patient indicates, either spontaneously or with prompting, that his train of thought was interrupted.
11. *Increased Latency of Response*   0 1 2 3 4 5
The patient takes a long time to reply to questions; prompting indicates that the patient is aware of the question.
12. *Global Rating of Alogia*   0 1 2 3 4 5
The core features of alogia are poverty of speech and poverty of content.
13. *Grooming and Hygiene*   0 1 2 3 4 5
The patient's clothes may be sloppy or soiled, and the patient may have greasy hair, body odour, etc.
14. *Impersistence at Work or School*   0 1 2 3 4 5
The patient has difficulty seeking or maintaining employment, completing schoolwork, keeping house, etc. If an inpatient, he or she cannot persist at ward activities, such as OT, playing cards, etc.
15. *Physical Anergia*   0 1 2 3 4 5
The patient tends to be physically inert. He or she may sit for hours and does not initiate spontaneous activity.

BOX 20.13 Scale for the Assessment of Negative Symptoms *(Continued)*

16. *Global Rating of Avolition–Apathy*   0 1 2 3 4 5
Strong weight may be given to one or two prominent symptoms if particularly striking.

Anhedonia–Asociality

17. *Recreational Interests and Activities*   0 1 2 3 4 5
The patient may have few or no interests. Both the quality and the quantity of interests should be taken into account.

18. *Sexual Activity*   0 1 2 3 4 5
The patient may show a decrease in sexual interest and activity or in enjoyment when active.

19. *Ability to Feel Intimacy and Closeness*   0 1 2 3 4 5
The patient may display an inability to form close or intimate relationships, especially with the opposite sex and family.

20. *Relationships With Friends and Peers*   0 1 2 3 4 5
The patient may have few or no friends and may prefer to spend all of his or her time isolated.

21. *Global Rating of Anhedonia–Asociality*   0 1 2 3 4 5
This rating should reflect the overall severity, taking into account the patient's age, family status, etc.

Attention

22. *Social Inattentiveness*   0 1 2 3 4 5
The patient appears uninvolved or unengaged. He or she may seem "spacey."

23. *Inattentiveness During Mental Status Testing*   0 1 2 3 4 5
Tests of "serial 7s" (at least five subtractions) and spelling "world" backward: Score: 2 = 1 error; 3 = 2 errors; 4 = 3 errors.

24. *Global Rating of Attention*   0 1 2 3 4 5
This rating should assess the patient's overall concentration, clinically and on tests.

From Nancy C. Andreasen, MD, PhD, Department of Psychiatry, College of Medicine, The University of Iowa, Iowa City, IA 52242. Copyright 1984 Nancy C. Andreasen. Reprinted with permission.

Mental Status and Appearance

The patient with schizophrenia may look eccentric or dishevelled or have poor hygiene and bizarre dress. The patient's posture may suggest lethargy or stupor.

Mood and Affect

Patients with schizophrenia often display altered mood states. In some cases, they may show heightened emotional activity; others may display severely limited emotional responses. Affect, the outward expression of mood, is categorized on a continuum: flat (emotional expression entirely absent), blunted (expression of emotions present but greatly diminished), and full range. Inappropriate affect is marked by incongruence between the emotional expression and the thoughts expressed. Other common emotional symptoms include the following:

- **Affective lability**—abrupt, dramatic, unprovoked changes in the type of emotions expressed
- **Ambivalence**—the presence and expression of two opposing feelings, leading to inaction
- **Apathy**—reactions to stimuli are decreased; diminished interest and desire

Speech

Speech patterns may reflect obsessions, delusions, pressured thinking, loose associations, or flight of ideas and neologisms. Speech is an indicator of thought content and other mental processes and is usually altered. An assessment of speech should note any difficulty articulating words (dysarthria) and difficulty swallowing (dysphagia) as indicators of medication side effects. In many instances, what an individual says is as important as how it is said. Both content and speech patterns should be noted.

Thought Processes and Delusions

Delusions can be distinguished from strongly held ideas by the degree of conviction with which the belief is held despite clear contradictory evidence (APA, 2013). Culture must be considered when evaluating delusions. Delusional beliefs are those not sanctioned or held by a cultural or religious subgroup.

Bizarre delusions alone are sufficient to diagnose schizophrenia. It can often be difficult to distinguish between bizarre and nonbizarre delusions. Nonbizarre delusions generally have themes of jealousy and persecution and are derived from ordinary life experiences. For example, a woman believes that her husband, from whom she has recently separated, is trying to poison her, or a man believes that members of the Mafia are trying to kill him because, when he was in high school, he reported to the principal that several of his classmates were selling drugs at school.

Bizarre delusions are those that are implausible, not understandable, and not derived from ordinary life experiences. Bizarre delusions often include delusions of control (that some outside force controls thoughts and actions), thought broadcasting (that others can read or hear one's thoughts), thought insertion (that someone has placed thoughts into one's mind), and thought withdrawal (that someone is removing thoughts from one's mind) (APA, 2013). For example, a patient who has been with a hypnotist for 2 months reports that the hypnotist continued to read his mind and was "picking his brain away piece by piece." Another patient was convinced that

BOX 20.14

THERAPEUTIC DIALOGUE

The Patient With Delusions

John joined the nurse in a game of pool. The following conversation occurred as they played.

Ineffective Approach

John: The RCMP put a transmitter in my molar, here (points to his right cheek).

Nurse: No one would put a transmitter in your tooth; come on, the RCMP isn't looking for you.

John: You get the striped balls. Yeah, they want to monitor me while I'm here. I know that they have the real Governor General here in the hospital. They are trying to get the Prime Minister to intervene with the Ontario Police. Mark from Ottawa told me that.

Nurse: The Governor General can't possibly be here; I saw him on television this morning.

John: Maybe—he does have lighter hair and has different-coloured contacts to disguise his eyes, but they're just trying to keep people from knowing what they're doing.

Nurse: John, he isn't in the hospital; if he were, I would know it because I work here.

John: (With anger) You don't know anything! You are probably from the RCMP also. I have nothing else to say to you.

Effective Approach

John: The RCMP put a transmitter in my molar, here (points to his right cheek).

Nurse: Oh. Which balls are mine?

John: You get the striped ones. Yeah, they want to monitor me while I'm here. I know that they have the real

Governor General here in the hospital. They are trying to get the Prime Minister to intervene with the Ontario Provincial Police. Mark from Ottawa told me that.

Nurse: Do you suppose that you saw someone who looks like the Governor General?

John: Maybe—he does have lighter hair and has different-coloured contacts to disguise his eyes. But they're just trying to keep people from knowing what they're doing.

Nurse: You sound a little overwhelmed with all the information you have.

John: No, no. I can handle it. The RCMP can't do anything to me, I'll never talk. They are trying to confuse me so that I stay away from the Governor General. They all think they can keep me from my mission.

Nurse: Who is it that worries you, John?

John: Everyone in the government. The RCMP, CSIS, CRA—all those alphabets.

Nurse: It must be rather frightening to feel all these people are looking for you. You must be scared a lot of the time.

John: It's scary but I can handle it. I've handled it all my life.

Nurse: You've been in scary situations all your life?

John: Yeah. I don't know. Maybe not scary, just hard. I never seemed to be able to do as well as my parents wanted—or as I wanted.

Critical Thinking Challenge

- How did the nurse's argumentative responses cause the patient to react in the first scenario?
- What effective communication techniques did the nurse use in the second scenario?

---

a computer chip was placed in her vagina during a gynaecologic examination and that this somehow directly influenced her physical movements and her thoughts.

Assessing and judging the content of the delusion and exploring other aspects of the delusional experience are helpful in understanding the significance of these false beliefs. The underlying feeling that accompanies the delusion should be identified. Other aspects to consider include the conviction with which the delusion is held; the extent to which other aspects of the individual's life are incorporated into or affected by the delusion; the degree of internal consistency, organization, and logic evident in the delusion; and the amount of pressure (in terms of preoccupation and concern) individuals feel in their lives as a result of the delusion (see Box 20.14).

Hallucinations

Hallucinations are the most common example of disturbed sensory perception observed in patients with schizophrenia. Hallucinations can be experienced in all

sensory modalities; however, auditory hallucinations are the most common in schizophrenia. Some specific hallucinations may be sufficient to diagnose schizophrenia, such as hearing voices conversing with each other or carrying on a discussion with someone who is not there. Because most individuals will not spontaneously share their hallucinatory experiences with an interviewer, the nurse may need to rely on indirect evidence in the patient's behaviour, such as (1) pauses during conversations in which the individual seems preoccupied or appears to be listening to someone other than the interviewer, (2) looking toward the perceived source of a voice, or (3) responding to the voices in some manner. Although patients may not spontaneously share their hallucinations, many validate observations of the examiner or admit to a history of hallucinations when asked (see Box 20.15).

Disorganized Communication

The other aspect of thought content and processes that may be altered in schizophrenia is the organization of

BOX **20.15**

THERAPEUTIC DIALOGUE

The Patient With Hallucinations

The following conversation took place in a dayroom with several staff members present. The patient was potentially very violent. Although it is a good example of dealing with someone who is hallucinating, it is not a situation that should be taken lightly. Always make certain that you have a means to leave a situation (i.e., you are not in the corner of a room) and that you have sufficient staff members close by to ensure safety. Take careful note of whether the patient has a potential weapon near at hand.

Jason approached the nurse and asked to play pool. The nurse debated about playing but chose to play because Jason appeared distracted and the game might give him something to focus on.

Ineffective Approach

Nurse: Shall I break?

Jason: (Had been looking off to his right, but turns and looks directly at the nurse.) Yeah, go ahead. (Looks at the table briefly and then turns to look out the door and down the hallway.)

Nurse: (Breaking the pool balls without putting any in a pocket.) It's your turn. You can hit any ball that you'd like.

Jason: (Turning back to the table.) Huh? (Shaking his head as he stared at the table.) What?

Nurse: You know, Jason, you really should pay attention.

Jason: (Hits a ball in and moves to the other side of the table. Stops in line with the next shot but doesn't bend down to take aim. Stands very still and then shakes his head slightly and quickly. Leans down to take aim and then stands up again.)

Nurse: Jason. (Looks at the nurse.) Jason! Are you going to play or not? I don't have all day.

Jason: Oh yeah. (Leans down, takes aim, and misses.)

Nurse: (Moves to where the next shot is. Position is near where Jason is standing. The nurse watches him carefully, moving closer to him.) Please move over, Jason.

Jason: No. (Doesn't move. In peripheral vision, the nurse sees Jason's lips move and he again looks to his right and shakes his head in a staccato motion, as if trying to shake something out of his head.)

Effective Approach

Nurse: Shall I break?

Jason: (Had been looking off to his right, but turns and looks directly at the nurse.) Yeah, go ahead. (Looks at the table briefly and then turns to look out the door and down the hallway.)

Nurse: (Breaking the pool balls without putting any in a pocket.) Your turn; you can hit any ball that you'd like.

Jason: (Turning back to the table.) Huh? (Shakes his head as he stares at the table.) What?

Nurse: You can hit any ball you like. I didn't get any.

Jason: (Hits a ball in and moves to the other side of the table. Stops in line with the next shot but doesn't bend down to take aim. Stands very still and then shakes his head slightly and quickly. Leans down to take aim and then stands up again.)

Nurse: Jason. (He looks at nurse.) Are you aiming at the 10 ball?

Jason: Oh yeah. (Leans down, takes aim, and misses.)

Nurse: (Moving to where her next shot is. The position is very close to where Jason is standing. The nurse watches him carefully while moving closer to him.) Here, let me take this shot.

Jason: Oh. (Moves back. In peripheral vision, the nurse sees Jason's lips move and again he looks to his right and shakes his head in a staccato motion, as if trying to shake something out of his head.)

Nurse: I missed again. (Moves away from the table and turns to Jason, who moves up to the table. He leans down and then stands up again. His lips move again as he turns his head to the right and then looks over his back toward the doorway.) Jason. Jason. (He looks at the nurse.) You have the striped ones.

Jason: (Nods and leans down to take a shot, which he makes. He then misses the next shot. He stands up and moves back from the table, again looking back toward the doorway. He shakes his head.)

Nurse: (Watches him closely and moves to the opposite side of the table, making the next shot. Lining up the next shot, Jason leans the pool cue against the table, looks past the nurse, and turns and walks away toward the door. Looks down the hallway, takes a few steps, stops for a minute or so, turns back into the room, and again looks past the nurse. Sits down and shakes his head again. Holds his head in his hands, with his hands covering his ears. The nurse picks up his pool cue and places both against the wall, out of the way. The nurse, recognizing that Jason is likely experiencing auditory hallucinations, remains where she can observe him, noting, as well, that another staff member is near at hand.)

Critical Thinking Challenge

- How did the nurse's impatience translate into Jason's behaviour in the first scenario?
- What effective communicating techniques did the nurse use in the second scenario?

expressed thoughts. Impaired verbal fluency (ability to produce spontaneous speech) is commonly present. Abrupt shifts in the focus of conversation are a typical symptom of disorganized thinking. The most severe shifts in focus may occur after only one or two words (**word salad**), after one or two phrases or sentences (flight of ideas or loose associations), or somewhat less severely as a shift that occurs when a new topic is repeatedly suggested and pursued from the current topic (**tangentiality**). In some individuals, speech may be a simple repetition of words or phrases spoken by others (**echolalia**).

Cognitive Impairments

Although cognitive impairments in schizophrenia vary widely from patient to patient, several primary problems have been identified:

- Attention may be increased and sustained on external stimuli over a period of time (hypervigilance).
- The ability to distinguish and focus on relevant stimuli may be diminished.
- Familiar cues may go unrecognized or be improperly encoded.
- Information processing may be diminished, leading to inappropriate or illogical conclusions from available observations and information (Sheffield et al., 2014).

Cognitive impairments are not easy to recognize. By relying only on clinical assessment, the nurse can miss the extent of the impairment. Using a standardized instrument such as the Mini-Mental Status Examination (MMSE), the Cognitive Assessment Screening Instrument (CASI), or the 7-Minute Screen can provide a screening measurement of cognitive function (see Chapter 10). If impairment is suspected, neuropsychologic testing by a qualified psychologist may be necessary.

Memory and Orientation

Impairments in orientation, memory, and abstract thinking may be observed. Orientation to time, place, and person may remain relatively intact unless the patient is particularly preoccupied with delusions and hallucinations. Although all aspects of memory may be affected in schizophrenia, registration or the recall within seconds of newly learned information may be particularly diminished. This affects the individual's short- and long-term memories. The ability to engage in abstract thinking may be impaired.

Insight and Judgment

Individuals display insight when they display evidence of knowing their own thoughts, the reality of external objects, and their relationship to these. Judgment is the ability to decide or act on a situation. Insight and judgment are closely related to each other and depend on cognitive functions that are frequently impaired in people with schizophrenia (Pia & Tamleto, 2006).

Behavioural Responses

During periods of psychosis, unusual or bizarre behaviour often occurs. These behaviours can usually be understood within the context of the patient's disturbed thinking. The nurse needs to understand the significance of the behaviour to the individual. One patient moved the family furniture into the yard because he thought that evil spirits were hiding in the furniture. His bizarre behaviour was an attempt to protect his family. Another patient painted a sequence of numbers on his bedroom walls. He said that the numbers were the language of the angels. His bizarre thoughts were at the basis of his behaviour.

Because of the negative symptoms, specifically avolition, patients may not seem interested or organized to complete their normal daily activities. They may stay in bed most of the day or refuse to take a shower. Many times, they will agree to get up in the morning and go to school or work, but they never get around to it. Several specific behaviours are associated with schizophrenia, including **stereotypy** (idiosyncratic repetitive, purposeless movements), **echopraxia** (involuntary imitation of others' movements), and **waxy flexibility** (posture held in odd or unusual fixed position for extended periods). In some cases, certain behaviours need to be evaluated carefully to distinguish them from movements that are associated with medication side effects, such as grimacing, stereotypic behaviour, or agitation.

Self-Concept

Self-concept is usually poor, for people with schizophrenia. Patients often are aware that they are hearing voices others do not hear. They recognize that they are different from others and are often afraid of "going crazy." Many are aware of the loss of expectations for their future achievements. The pervasive stigma associated with having a mental illness contributes to poor self-concept. Body image can be disturbed, especially during periods of hallucinations or delusions. One patient believed that her body was infected with germs and she could feel them eating away her insides.

Stress and Coping Patterns

Stressful events are often linked to psychiatric symptoms. It is important to determine stresses from the patient's perspective because a stressful event for one may not be stressful for another (see Chapter 17). It is also important to determine typical coping patterns, especially negative coping strategies, such as the use of substances or aggressive behaviour.

Risk Assessment

Because of high suicide and attempted suicide rates among patients with schizophrenia, the nurse needs to assess patients risk for self-injury: Do patients speak of suicide, have delusional thinking that could lead to dangerous behaviour, and have command hallucinations telling them to harm themselves or others? Do patients have homicidal ideations? Do patients have access to weapons? Do patients lack social support and the skills to be meaningfully engaged with other people or a vocation? Substance-related disorders are also common among patients with schizophrenia, and nurses should assess for substance misuse or abuse.

Nursing Diagnoses for Psychological Domain

Many nursing diagnoses can be generated from data collected assessing the psychological domain. Disturbed thought processes can be used for delusions, confusion, and disorganized thinking. Disturbed sensory perception is appropriate for hallucinations or illusions. Other examples of diagnoses include disturbed body image, low self-esteem, disturbed personal identity, risk for violence, ineffective coping, and knowledge deficit.

Interventions for Psychological Domain

All the psychological interventions, such as counselling, conflict resolution, behaviour therapy, and cognitive interventions, are appropriate for patients with schizophrenia. The following discussion focuses on applying these interventions.

Special Issues in the Nurse–Patient Relationship

The development of the nurse–patient relationship with patients with schizophrenia centres on developing trust and accepting the person as a worthy human being. People with schizophrenia are often reluctant to engage in any relationship because of previous rejection and, in some instances, an underlying suspicion that is a part of the illness. If they are having hallucinations, their images of other people may be distorted and frightening. They struggle to trust their own thoughts and perceptions, and engaging in an interaction with another human being may prove too overwhelming.

The nurse should approach the patient in a calm and caring manner. Engaging the patient in a relationship may take time. Brief interactions are best for a patient who is experiencing psychosis. Being consistent in interactions and following through on promises will help establish trust within the relationship.

Establishing a therapeutic relationship is crucial, especially with patients who deny that they are ill. Patients are more likely to agree to treatment if these recommendations are made within the context of a safe, trusting relationship. Even if some patients deny having mental illness, they may take medication and attend treatment activities because they trust the nurse.

Management of Disturbed Thoughts and Sensory Perceptions

Although antipsychotic medications may relieve positive symptoms, they do not always eliminate hallucinations and delusions. The nurse must continue helping the patient develop creative strategies for dealing with these sensory and thought disturbances. Information about the content of the hallucinations and delusions is needed, not only to determine whether the medications are effective but also to assess safety and the meaning of these thoughts and perceptions to the patient. In caring for a patient who is experiencing hallucinations or delusions, nursing actions should be guided by three general patient outcomes:

- Decrease the frequency and intensity of hallucinations and delusions.
- Recognize that hallucinations and delusions are symptoms of a brain disorder.
- Develop strategies to manage the recurrence of hallucinations or delusions.

When interacting with a patient who is experiencing hallucinations or delusions, the nurse must remember that these experiences are real to the patient. The nurse should never tell a patient that these experiences are not real. Discounting the experiences blocks communication. It also is dishonest to tell the patient that you are having the same hallucinatory experience. It is best to validate the patient's experiences and identify the meaning of these thoughts and feelings to the patient. For example, a patient who believes that he or she is under surveillance by the police probably feels frightened and suspicious of everyone. By acknowledging how frightening it must be to always feel like you are being watched, the nurse focuses on the feelings that are generated by the delusion, not the delusion itself. The nurse can then offer to help the patient feel safe within this environment. The patient, in turn, begins to feel that someone understands him or her.

TEACHING POINTS 🍎

Teaching patients that hallucinations and delusions are part of the disorder becomes easier after the medication begins working and a therapeutic relationship is established. Once patients believe and acknowledge that they have a mental illness and that some of their thoughts are delusions and some of their perceptions are hallucinations, they can develop strategies to manage their symptoms.

Self-Monitoring and Relapse Prevention

Patients benefit greatly by learning techniques of self-regulation, symptom monitoring, and relapse prevention. By monitoring events, time, place, and stimuli surrounding the appearance of symptoms, the patient can begin to predict high-risk times for symptom recurrence. Cognitive behavioural therapy is often used in helping patients monitor and identify their emerging symptoms in order to prevent relapse (see Chapter 13).

Another important nursing intervention is to help the patient identify who and where to talk about delusional or hallucinatory material. Unfortunately, because self-disclosure of these symptoms immediately labels someone as having a mental illness, patients should be encouraged to evaluate the environment for negative consequences of disclosing these symptoms. It may be fine to talk about it at home but not at the grocery store.

Enhancement of Cognitive Functioning

After identifying deficits in cognitive functioning, the nurse and the patient can develop interventions that target specific deficits. The most effective interventions usually involve the whole treatment team. If the ability to focus or attend is an issue, patients can be encouraged to select activities that improve attention, such as computer games. For memory problems, patients can be encouraged to make lists and to write down important information.

Executive functioning problems are the most challenging for these patients. Patients who cannot manage daily problems may have planning and problem-solving impairments. For these patients, developing interventions that closely simulate real-world problems may help. Through coaching, the nurse can teach and support the development of problem-solving skills. For example, during hospitalizations, patients are given medications and reminded to take them on time. They are often instructed in a classroom setting but rarely have an opportunity to practice self-medication and figure out what to do if their prescription expires, the medications are lost, or they forget their medications. Yet, when discharged, patients are expected to take medication at the prescribed dose at the prescribed time. Interventions are needed that are designed to have patients actively engage in problem-solving behaviour with real problems. Cognitive remediation strategies are being developed to assist with these difficulties. Computerized remediation strategies appear promising, but more research is required (Subramaniam et al., 2012).

Another approach to helping patients solve problems and learn new strategies for dealing with problems is solution-focused therapy, which focuses on the strengths and positive attributes that exist within each person. For example, patients can be asked to identify the most important problem from their perspective. This focuses the patient on the issue that he or she deems important.

Behavioural Interventions

Behavioural interventions can be very effective in helping patients improve motivation and organize routines and daily activities, such as maintaining a regular schedule and completing activities. Reinforcement of positive behaviours (e.g., getting up on time, completing hygiene, going to treatment activities) can easily be included in a treatment plan. In the hospital, patients gain ward privileges by following an agreed-upon treatment plan.

Stress and Coping Skills

Developing skills to cope with personal, social, and environmental stresses are important to everyone, but particularly to those with a severe mental illness. Stresses can easily trigger symptoms that patients are trying to avoid. Establishing regular counselling sessions to support the development of positive coping skills is helpful for both the hospitalized patient and those in the community. Another interesting innovation is the development of digital applications, which are purported to assist with coping with delusions and hallucinations. One such application is *CopingTutor* (Gottlieb, 2012), which includes presentations, games, and self-help worksheets. The download is available for a small cost.

Patient Education

Cognitive deficits (difficulty in processing complex information, maintaining steady focus of attention, distinguishing between relevant and irrelevant stimuli, and forming abstractions) may challenge the nurse planning educational activities. Evidence indicates that people with schizophrenia may learn best in an errorless learning environment; that is, they are directly given correct information and then encouraged to write it down. Asking questions that encourage guessing is not as effective in helping them retain information. Trial-and-error learning is avoided. In one study, a group of people with schizophrenia who were taught using an errorless learning approach improved work skill in two entry-level job tasks (index card filing and toilet tank assembly) and performed better than the group that was instructed with conventional trial-and-error instructions (Kern, Green, Mintz, & Liberman, 2003; Kern, Liberman, Kopelowicz, Mintz, & Green, 2002).

Education sessions should occur in an environment with minimal distractions. Terminology should be clear and unambiguous. Visual aids can supplement verbal information, but these materials should have simple information stated in simple language. The nurse takes care not to overcrowd the visual material or incorporate images that draw attention away from the important content. Teaching should occur in small segments with frequent reinforcement. Most important of all, teaching should occur when the patient is ready. Regular assessments of cognitive abilities with standardized instruments can help determine this readiness. These suggestions can be adapted for teaching during any phase of the illness.

Skill-training interventions should be designed to compensate for cognitive deficits. To help patients learn to process complex activities, such as catching a bus, preparing a meal, or shopping for food or clothing, nurses should break the activity into small parts or steps and list them for the patient's reference. For example:

- Make sure you have the correct bus fare in your pocket
- Leave your apartment with keys in the hand
- Close the door
- Walk to the corner
- Turn right and walk three blocks to the bus stop

Family Education

Because having a family member with schizophrenia is a life-changing event for the family and friends who provide care and support, educating patients and their families or significant others is crucial. It is a primary concern for the mental health nurse. Family support and education are crucial to help patients maintain their treatment. Education should include information about the disease course, treatment regimens, support systems, and life management skills (see Box 20.16). The most important factor to reinforce during patient and family education is the consistent taking of medication (Wilson, 2012).

Social Domain

Social Assessment

Several difficulties with social functioning occur in schizophrenia. As the disorder progresses, individuals can become increasingly socially isolated. On a one-to-one basis, this occurs because the individual seems unable to connect with people in his or her environment. Several aspects of the symptoms already discussed can contribute to this, for example, emotional blunting and anhedonia (the inability to form emotional attachment and experience pleasure). Cognitive deficits that contribute to difficult social functioning include problems with the face and affect recognition, deficiencies in recall of past interactions, problems with decision-making and judgment in conflictual interactions, and poverty of speech and language. Poor functioning and the inability to complete activities of daily living are manifested in poor hygiene, malnutrition, and social isolation.

Social Systems

In schizophrenia, support systems become very important in maintaining the patient in the community. The individual may become socially isolated if the treatment and management occur in long-term care facilities and group homes away from family and friends. One challenge in treating schizophrenia is to identify and maintain the patient's links with family and significant others. Assessment of the patient's formal support (e.g., family caregivers, health care providers) and informal support (e.g., neighbours, friends) should be conducted.

Quality of Life

People with schizophrenia often have a poor quality of life, especially older people who may have spent many years in a long-term hospital. The nurse should assess the patient's quality of life and how it could be improved. Simple changes, such as arranging for a different roommate or improving access to social activities by meeting transportation needs, can greatly improve a patient's quality of life. Stable housing is key to making any improvements to the patient's quality of life (MHCC, 2013b).

Family Assessment

The assessment of the family can take many forms, and the family assessment guide presented in Chapter 15 can be used. In many instances, the patient will be young and living with his or her parents. This is most often the case when a young person experiences the first episode of psychosis. Often, the nurse's first contact with the patient and family is in the initial phases of the disorder. The family is dealing with the shock and disbelief of seeing a child with a mental illness that may have lifelong consequences. Ideally, in this instance, the assessment process may be extended over several sessions to provide the family with support and education about the disorder. Certainly, the emergence of psychotic illness is a distressing and confusing time, not only for young persons experiencing these perplexing changes but also for their parents.

The family, and in particular the parents, play a critical role in early intervention for psychosis, both as a vehicle for early identification and treatment, and as a supportive context for recovery. Understanding of this caregiving experience was gleaned from a qualitative study that employed a phenomenologic approach to uncover four distinct stories: *a story of Protection, a story of Loss, a story of Stigma,* and a final story of *Enduring Love* (Wilson, 2012). The experiences of parent caregivers suggest that health care providers, and nurses in particular, can have more discretion, insight, and discernment in clinical approaches and might also serve to shape future policies, which will recognize and affirm the strengths and resilient capacities of families. Nursing assessment and approaches, which focus upon family resilience and strengths, is most effective.

Because women with schizophrenia generally have better treatment outcomes than do men, many will marry and have children. These women experience the same life stresses as other women and may find themselves single parents, raising children in poverty-stricken conditions. Managing a psychiatric illness and trying to

---

BOX 20.16

Psychoeducation Checklist: Schizophrenia

When working with the person with schizophrenia and their family or caregiver, be sure to include the following topic areas in the education plans:

- ✓ Psychopharmacologic agents, including drug action, dosage, frequency, and possible adverse effects. Stress the importance of adherence to the prescribed regimen
- ✓ Management of hallucinations
- ✓ Coping strategies such as self-talk, getting busy
- ✓ Management of the environment
- ✓ Use of contracts that detail the expected behaviours, with goals and consequences
- ✓ Community resources
- ✓ Community educational opportunities for families
- ✓ Family peer supports/family navigator contacts in the community

be an effective parent in a socially stigmatizing society are exceedingly challenging because of the lack of financial resources and social support. This family will need an extensive assessment of financial need and social support. The family life cycle model presented in Chapter 15 can also be used as a framework for the assessment.

Nursing Diagnoses for Social Domain

The nursing diagnoses generated from the assessment of the social domain are typically impaired social interaction, ineffective role performance, disabled family coping, and interrupted family processes. Outcomes will depend on the specific diagnostic area.

Interventions for Social Domain

Promoting Patient Safety

Although violence is not a consistent behaviour of people with schizophrenia, it is always a concern during the initial phase when hallucinations or delusions may put patients at risk for harming themselves or others. Nonviolent patients who are experiencing hallucinations and delusions can also be at risk for victimization by more aggressive patients. The patient who is hallucinating needs to be protected. This protection may include increased staff monitoring and, if necessary, a safer environment in a secluded area.

The nurse's best approach to avoiding violence or aggression is to demonstrate respect for the patient and the patient's personal space, assess and monitor for signs of fear and agitation, and use preventive interventions before the patient loses control. Medications should be administered as ordered. Because most antipsychotic and antidepressant medications take 1 to 2 weeks to begin moderating the patient's behaviour, the nurse must be vigilant during the acute illness.

Reducing environmental stimulation is particularly important for individuals who are experiencing hallucinations but can be helpful for all patients when signs of fear and agitation are observed. Allowing patients to use private rooms or seclusion for brief periods can be an important preventive method.

Other techniques of managing the environment (milieu management) have been found to be helpful in inpatient settings. One researcher who examined aggression and violence in psychiatric hospitals found violent behaviour to be associated with the following predictors: a history of violence, a coercive interaction style of using violence to obtain what is desired, and an environment in which violence is inadvertently rewarded, for example, by gaining staff attention (Morrison & Love, 2003). Morrison (1992) proposed the following methods to help avoid acts of violence or aggression:

- Take a thorough history that includes information about the patient's past use of violence.
- Help the patient to talk directly and constructively with those with whom he or she is angry, rather than venting anger to staff about a third person.
- Set limits with consistent and justly applied consequences.
- Involve the patient in formulating a contract that outlines patient and staff behaviours, goals, and consequences.
- Schedule brief but regular time-outs to allow the patient some privacy without the attention of staff either before or after the time-out (these time-outs may be patient activated).

Staff members need to have planned sessions after all incidents of violence or physical management in which the event is analyzed. These sessions allow staff members to learn how to better manage these situations and evaluate patients' cues. With sensitive leadership, these sessions can help staff to learn more about the interaction of patient and staff characteristics that can contribute to these incidents (Box 20.17).

Convening Support Groups

People with mental illness benefit from support groups that focus on daily problems and the stress of dealing with a mental illness. These groups are useful throughout the continuum of care and help reduce the risk for suicide. In the hospital setting, the focus of the group can be simply sharing the experience of living with a mental illness. In the community, a regular support group can provide interaction with people with similar problems and issues and the opportunity to share stories of recovery. Friendships often develop from these groups.

Implementing Milieu Therapy

Individuals with schizophrenia can be hospitalized or live in group homes for a long period of time. It is unrealistic to expect people who have an illness that interferes with their ability to live with family members to live in peace and harmony with complete strangers. Arranging the treatment environment to maximize recovery is crucial to the rehabilitation of the patient.

Developing Psychiatric Rehabilitation Strategies

Rehabilitation strategies are used to support the individual's recovery and integration into the community. Community-based psychosocial rehabilitation programs usually offer long-term intensive case management services to adults with schizophrenia. Programs provide a continuum of services to meet the changing needs of people with psychiatric disabilities. Patients set rehabilitation goals, and services are then provided to help "clients" (most programs do not use the term "patients") reach their goals. Services range from daily home visits to providing transportation, occupational training, and group support. Social skills training shows much promise for patients with schizophrenia, both individually and in groups. This is a method for teaching patients specific behaviours needed for social interactions. The skills are taught by lecture, demonstration, role-playing, and homework assignments (see Chapters 11 and 14).

BOX 20.17 **Research for Best Practice**

CIGARETTE SMOKING, CANNABIS, AND FIRST-EPISODE PSYCHOSIS

Grossman, M., Bowie, C. R., Lepage, M., Malla, A. K., Joober, R., & Iyer, S. N. (2017). Smoking status and its relationship to demographic and clinical characteristics in first episode psychosis. Journal of Psychiatric Research, 85, 83–90.

Question: Past research has not controlled for cannabis use in cigarette smokers with people who are experiencing a first-episode psychosis. This study aimed to determine the prevalence and patterns of cigarette smoking and its co-use with cannabis in first-episode psychosis and to examine the demographic, clinical, cognitive, and functional characteristics associated with cigarette smoking status.

Methods: All participants ($n = 140$) of the study were from a First-Episode Psychosis Program specializing in early intervention. This study used various tools to collect information. To determine diagnosis, the Structured Clinical Interview for DSM-IV was used; to determine smoking status the Chemical Use, Abuse, and Dependence Scale was used along with a brief interview. Neurocognitive assessment data was also collected and a functional assessment using the Strauss Carpenter Level of Functioning Scale.

Findings: The prevalence of smoking in this study was more than half (53%) of participants. 34% were categorized as light/moderate (1 to 19 cigarettes/day) and 19% as heavy smokers (>20 cigarettes/day). 34% of participants reported smoking cannabis daily. There was a high association between cigarette smoking and cannabis use. Nonsmokers had more education, better neurocognitive performance, and higher levels of functioning than did smokers.

Implications for Practice: This study demonstrated that people experiencing a first-episode psychosis used tobacco and cannabis at high rates, and neurocognitive and functional impairments were more pronounced in light/moderate smokers. It is essential that all health care professionals provide every opportunity to support people with decreasing and ceasing tobacco and cannabis use, as it is apparent that decreased use will lead to a better neurocognitive and functional outcome.

Nurses may be team members and involved in case management or provision of services. These and other psychological treatment approaches, combined with breakthroughs in biologic therapy, continue to help improve the functioning and quality of life for patients with schizophrenia.

Family Interventions

When schizophrenia first becomes apparent, the patient and family must negotiate the mental health system for the first time (in most cases)—a challenge that almost equals that of confronting the family member's illness. In most provincial jurisdictions, the mental health system is complex and is usually ignored unless a family member becomes seriously mentally ill. The system includes inpatient and outpatient clinics supported by provincial health insurance and publicly funded community mental health clinics and hospitals.

Family members should be encouraged to participate in educational and support groups that help family members deal with the realities of living with a loved one with a mental illness. Family members should be given information about local community and provincial resources and organizations such as mental health associations and those that can help families negotiate the complex system. See Nursing Care Plan 20.2 for care of a patient with a more persistent form of schizophrenia.

Spiritual Domain

Many people living with schizophrenia find comfort in their spirituality, as well as the strength to deal with life events that interfere with their recovery journeys. Religious or spiritual beliefs can be a resource for both patients and their families. Such beliefs may help, for instance, to reappraise difficult events into a positive light (e.g., God gives us only difficulties that we are able to handle). A relationship with the sacred through ritual, prayer, worship, meditation, or other spiritual activities may offer solace, peace, and serenity. These activities may also help to structure the daily lives of individuals with schizophrenia, an important rehabilitation goal. The experience of living with a serious and chronic illness, however, can also cause a crisis of faith or lead one to question the purpose and meaning of one's life. This may be especially true if one's illness brings stigma and rejection by the members of one's community. The sense of connection and hope that supports spiritual growth may be diminished if one is labelled "crazy" by others.

Spiritual nursing care actively supports patients in their efforts to sustain and enhance their spirituality. This support can take many forms, from safeguarding the dignity

NURSING CARE PLAN 20.2

PATIENT WITH SCHIZOPHRENIA

MP is a 53-year-old woman who was brought to the crisis support clinic by her community nurse case manager. MP had made a number of telephone calls to her case manager and to the police in rapid succession in the previous 24 hours to report that her next-door neighbour was spying on her. When the nurse case manager arrived, MP was very agitated and distrusting. The case manager also received a call from MP's landlord to report that MP has been making threatening hand gestures to neighbours from her apartment window. MP disclosed to her nurse case manager that her neighbours had tampered with her medications and that she had not been taking them for several days. MP was acutely paranoid and agreed to a hospitalization to keep her safe. She had been attending the Community Clubhouse Program but had not been there for 2 weeks.

She failed to attend her follow-up appointment at the mental health clinic to pick up her biweekly dosette of pills.

Setting: Crisis Support Team: Psychosocial Rehabilitation Unit

Baseline Assessment: MP is a 5'4", 155-pound woman whose appearance is dishevelled. She has not slept for 2 days and appears frightened. She is hypervigilant, suspicious, irritable, and wringing her hands. She is vague about when she last took her treatment medications. She is oriented to time and place and person. Lab values are within normal limits. She has a history of at least 12 former admissions to the psychiatric ward for self-discontinuation of treatment medications.

Associated Psychiatric Diagnosis	Medications
Schizophrenia	Olanzapine, 5 mg bid Lorazepam (Ativan), 2 mg PO or IM for agitation PRN
Social problems/context: Landlord threatening to evict MP from her apartment. Estranged from her two adult sons. Support system limited to a few acquaintances at the clubhouse.	

Nursing Diagnosis 1: Ineffective Health Maintenance

Defining Characteristics	Related Factors
MP does not remember when she last took her medications. Two weeks of pills are still in the dosette box. MP has not taken the pills for at least 2 weeks, possibly more. MP has not attended the Clubhouse program for 2 weeks. MP did not attend her appointment at the clinic to get a refill of pills in her dosette. MP has been calling the police and the case manager several times in the past 24 hours.	Paranoid delusions are contributing to her thought disturbance. Suspiciousness is contributing to her reluctance to leave her apartment. Inability to make thoughtful judgments. Ineffective individual coping.

Outcomes

Initial	Long Term
Restarts medications in the hospital. Agreement from MP to a referral to the ACT team. Increased ability to self-administer medications. Demonstrates willingness to take her medications independently while in hospital using a blister pack dosette.	MP will communicate her understanding of and demonstrate follow-through with the mutually agreed on health maintenance plan. MP will show the ability to perform health maintenance activities needed to function in her apartment independently with ACT team assistance.

NURSING CARE PLAN 20.2 *(Continued)*

Interventions

Interventions	Rationale	Ongoing Assessment
Take initial steps to help MP feel safe in the hospital setting.	When a person feels safe, trust is more likely to develop.	Determine when MP's suspiciousness is diminishing. Assess when she is ready to discuss plans for discharge.
Listen carefully, making eye contact. Make efforts to clarify what MP is thinking and feeling.	Listening attentively will help MP to feel safe and cared for.	
Contact all community care providers and convene an interdisciplinary meeting to discuss possible changes to the current community care plan.	A meeting of all care providers will provide a forum to explore alternative support/treatment solutions to improve MP's health maintenance once discharged.	Assess MP's readiness for discharge and transition to the ACT team in addition to returning to the community clubhouse.
	ACT team will be able to increase visitation to MP's home at more frequent intervals. ACT team will provide a more intense level of support.	

Evaluation

Outcomes	Revised Outcomes	Interventions
MP's delusions begin to decrease.	MP meets with the ACT team and agrees to include this team in her follow-up health maintenance plan.	Problem solve ways for MP to respond to ongoing worries and suspicions.
MP uses some distraction techniques to draw her away from focusing upon the neighbours.		Develop a written, mutually agreed-upon relapse prevention and crisis action plan and send to all community care partners.

Nursing Diagnosis 2: Disturbed Thought Processes

Defining Characteristics	Related Factors
Inaccurate interpretation of stimuli (neighbours tampering with her medications) Cognitive impairment—attention, memory, and executive function impairment Suspiciousness Hallucinations (hears voices telling her that her sons are in danger)	Uncompensated alterations in brain activity

Outcomes

Initial	Long Term
Decrease or eliminate hallucinations.	Use coping strategies to deal with hallucinations or delusions if they reappear.
Have accurate interpretation of the environment. Exhibits some reality-based thinking. Demonstrates improvement in cognitive functioning (improved attention, memory, and executive functioning). Interacts appropriately with others.	Communicate clearly with others. Maintain cognitive functioning.

(Continued)

NURSING CARE PLAN 20.2 *(Continued)*

Interventions

Interventions	Rationale	Ongoing Assessment
Initiate a nurse–patient relationship by using an accepting, nonjudgmental approach. Be patient.	A therapeutic relationship will provide patient support as she begins to deal with the realization that she is in hospital once again. Be patient and offer reassurance as required until MP feels safe. Do not argue with the false beliefs.	Determine the extent to which MP is willing to trust and engage in a relationship. Make every effort to help MP attend to real rather than internal stimuli, orient her to the real situation, and encourage MP to focus upon distracting concrete activities. Make determined efforts to steer thinking in alternate directions.
Administer olanzapine as prescribed. Observe for effects, side effects, and adverse effects. Begin teaching about the potential switch to an injectable form of antipsychotic medication.	Olanzapine is a D_2 and $5\text{-}HT_{2A}$ antagonist and is indicated for the management of psychotic disorders.	Make sure MP swallows the pills. Monitor for relief of positive symptoms and assess side effects, especially extrapyramidal. Monitor BP for orthostatic hypotension and body temperature increase (NMS).
Assess the ability for self-care activities.	Disturbed thinking may interfere with MP's ability to carry out ADLs.	Continue to assess: determine whether the patient can manage self-care.

Evaluation

Outcomes	Revised Outcomes	Interventions
Delusions began to decrease within 6 days.	Participate in Community Clubhouse activities as soon as possible to bridge the transition from hospital back to the community.	Encourage attendance at the Clubhouse while in hospital to reconnect with the activity/recreational group, which MP enjoys.

Nursing Diagnosis 3: Anxiety Related to Fears About Neighbours

Defining Characteristics	Related Factors
Constantly asking nurses for reassurance that her neighbours are not on the unit. Presence of pathophysiologic risk factors: delusional thinking.	Frightened, secondary to **paranoia** (feelings of being unsafe), and delusional thinking.

Outcomes

Initial	Long Term
MP is able to describe a reduction in anxiety.	MP will demonstrate decreased anxiety while at home.
Decreased agitation, gesturing, and pacing.	MP will refrain from gesturing at neighbours.

NURSING CARE PLAN 20.2 *(Continued)*

Interventions

Interventions	Rationale	Ongoing Assessment
Acknowledge MP's fear and paranoid delusions. Be genuine and empathetic.	Anxiety and delusions change an individual's perception of environmental stimuli. A patient who is frightened will respond because of her need to stay safe.	Assess her response to your comments and her ability to concentrate on what is being said.
Reassure MP verbally at frequent intervals. Make frequent brief supportive contacts. Acknowledge MP's distress.	It is helpful to validate the anxious feelings MP is experiencing.	Observe MP's nonverbal communication for evidence of increased anxiety and agitation.
Administer lorazepam, 2 mg, for agitation. Oral route is preferable over injection.	Exact mechanisms of action are not understood, but this medication is believed to potentiate the inhibitory neurotransmitter GABA, relieving anxiety and producing sedation.	Observe for a decrease in anxiety.

Evaluation

Outcomes	Revised Outcomes	Interventions
MP gradually decreased anxious behaviour. Lorazepam was given regularly for the first 4 days.	Demonstrate control of behaviour by resisting delusions.	Teach MP about the effects of delusions. Problem solve ways of controlling hallucinations if they occur. Emphasize the importance of taking medications.

of the patient to understanding the potential impact of hallucinations on spiritual needs to ensuring spiritual activities can occur. In psychiatric and mental health settings, there may be reluctance on the part of staff to consider the spirituality of a patient who is experiencing the psychotic symptoms of delusions and hallucinations, especially if there are religious overtones to the "voices" and/or fixed beliefs. Knowledge of the patient and of the disease, along with a broad, rich understanding of spirituality, should nevertheless enable the nurse and other staff to address the spiritual domain of care. Employing a relational ethics approach can move the nurse to consider the context and environment of the patient's situation to safeguard dignity (Wilson, 2009) (see Chapter 7).

Evaluation and Treatment Outcomes

Outcome research related to schizophrenia has redefined previous ways of thinking about the course of the disorder. Schizophrenia was once considered to have a progressively long-term and downward course, but it is now known that schizophrenia can be successfully treated and managed. In one older but significant study, the researchers interviewed patients 20 to 25 years after diagnosis and found that 50% to 66% experienced significant improvement or recovery (Harding, Zubin, & Strauss, 1987). This study is important because it occurred before the development of atypical antipsychotic agents. Today, we can be hopeful that even more people can experience improvement or recover from schizophrenia.

Continuum of Care

Continuity of care has been identified as a major goal of community mental health systems for patients with schizophrenia, because they are at risk for becoming "lost" to services if left alone after discharge. Careful attention to discharge planning encourages follow-up care in the community. In fact, many mental health systems require an outpatient appointment before discharge to better facilitate this transition. Treatment of schizophrenia occurs across a variety of settings. Not only inpatient hospitalization but also partial hospitalization, day treatment, and crisis stabilization and continuing community care can be used effectively.

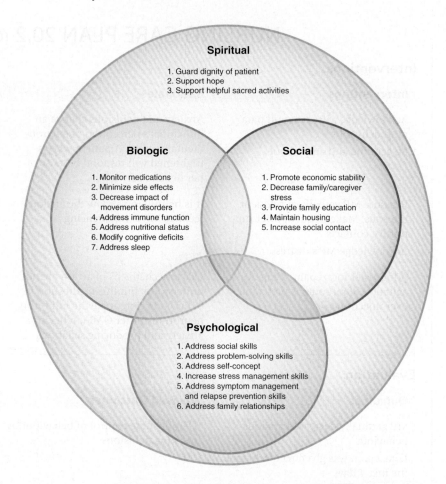

Spiritual
1. Guard dignity of patient
2. Support hope
3. Support helpful sacred activities

Biologic
1. Monitor medications
2. Minimize side effects
3. Decrease impact of movement disorders
4. Address immune function
5. Address nutritional status
6. Modify cognitive deficits
7. Address sleep

Social
1. Promote economic stability
2. Decrease family/caregiver stress
3. Provide family education
4. Maintain housing
5. Increase social contact

Psychological
1. Address social skills
2. Address problem-solving skills
3. Address self-concept
4. Increase stress management skills
5. Address symptom management and relapse prevention skills
6. Address family relationships

Figure 20.7. Bio/psycho/social/spiritual interventions for patients with schizophrenia.

Inpatient-Focused Care

Much of the previous discussion concerns care in the inpatient setting. Today, inpatient hospitalizations are brief and focus on patient stabilization. Many times, patients are involuntarily admitted for a short period. During the stabilization period, the status is changed to voluntary admission, whereby the patient agrees to treatment.

EMERGENCY CARE

Emergency care ideally takes place in a hospital emergency room, but the crisis often occurs in the home. Patients are usually relapsing and do not recognize their bizarre or aggressive behaviours as symptoms. In many urban communities, a specially trained crisis team is sent to assess the emergency and recommend further treatment. Patients are brought to the emergency room not only because of relapse but also because of medication side effects. Nurses should refer to the previous discussion for nursing management.

Community Care

Most of the care of patients with schizophrenia will be in the community through publicly supported mental health delivery systems. Community services include assertive community treatment, outpatient therapy, case

management, and psychosocial rehabilitation, including clubhouse programs. For a very small number of patients with a community treatment order in effect that delineates the conditions required to live in the community, services must be congruent with those conditions (see Chapter 7). For all patients in the community, health care should be integrated in a holistic manner with physical health care. Nurses should be especially vigilant that patients with mental illnesses receive proper primary and medical health care.

Mental Health Promotion

In some cases, it is less the disorder itself threatening the mental health of the person with schizophrenia than the stresses of seeking care and services. Health care systems are complex and are often at the mercy of a system rule that is outdated. Development of assertiveness and conflict resolution skills can help the person in negotiating access to systems that will provide services. Developing a positive support system for stressful periods will help promote a positive outcome (Fig. 20.7).

SUMMARY OF KEY POINTS

- The person with schizophrenia displays a complex myriad of symptoms typically categorized as positive symptoms (those that exist but should not), such as delusions or hallucinations and disorganized thinking and behaviour, and negative symptoms (characteristics that should be there but are lacking), such as alogia, avolition, anhedonia, and affective blunting.

- In the past, the diagnosis and treatment of schizophrenia focused on the more observable and dramatic positive symptoms (i.e., delusions and hallucinations), but scientists have shifted their focus to the disorganizing symptoms of cognition.

- The clinical presentation of schizophrenia occurs in three phases: phase 1, first-episode psychosis, entails the initial diagnosis and first treatment; phase 2 includes periods of stabilization between episodes of overt signs and symptoms but during which the patient needs sustained treatment; and phase 3 includes periods of exacerbation or relapse that require hospitalization or more frequent contacts with mental health professionals and increased use of resources.

- Biologic theories of what causes schizophrenia include genetic, infectious–autoimmune, neuroanatomic, and dopamine hypotheses. The last is supported by the advanced technology of PET scan findings and the understanding of the mechanisms of antipsychotic medications.

- Biologic assessment of the patient with schizophrenia must include a thorough history and physical examination to rule out any medical illness or substance abuse problem that might be the cause of the patient's symptoms, assessment of risk for self-injury or injury to others, and documentation of baseline health information before medications are administered. Several standardized assessment tools are available to help assess characteristic abnormal motor movements.

- Several nursing interventions address the biologic domain: promotion of self-care activities (activity, exercise, and nutritional), thermoregulation, and fluid balance interventions. In general, the antipsychotic drugs used to treat schizophrenia block dopamine transmission in the brain but also cause some troublesome and sometimes serious side effects, primarily anticholinergic side effects and extrapyramidal side effects (motor abnormalities). Newer antipsychotic agents block serotonin as well as dopamine. The nurse should be familiar with these drugs, their possible side effects, and the interventions required to manage side effects.

- The extrapyramidal side effects of antipsychotic drugs can appear early in drug treatment and include acute parkinsonism or pseudoparkinsonism, acute dystonia, and akathisia, or they can appear late in treatment after months or years. The primary example of late-appearing extrapyramidal side effects is tardive dyskinesia, which is a severe syndrome of abnormal motor movements of the mouth, tongue, and jaw.

- Psychological assessment must include equal attention to manifestations of both positive and negative symptoms and a concentrated focus on the cognitive impairments that make it so difficult for patients to manage their disorder. Several standardized assessment tools assess for positive and negative symptoms. Developing the nurse–patient relationship is essential in helping patients manage disturbed thoughts and sensory perceptions. Interventions should be designed to enhance cognitive functioning. Patient and family education are critical interventions for the person with schizophrenia.

- Because schizophrenia is a lifetime disorder and patients require the continued support and care of mental health professionals and family or friends, one of the primary nursing interventions is ensuring that patients and families are properly educated about the course of the disorder, the importance of medication adherence, and the need for consistent care and support. Research is demonstrating that interaction between patients and their families is key to the success of long-term treatments and outcomes.

 Web Links

cmha.ca This is the site of the Canadian Mental Health Association, a charitable organization that promotes mental health and supports the resilience and recovery of those with mental illness.

eppic.org.au This is the site of the Early Psychosis Prevention and Intervention Centre, Melbourne, Australia. It has excellent downloadable and printable fact sheets in multiple language formats for patient/family education.

mentalhealth.com Internet Mental Health provides extensive information on schizophrenia.

mentalhealthcommission.ca The Mental Health Commission of Canada (MHCC) website contains all the reports of the commission and the National Strategy for Mental Health. It also offers access to Collaborative Spaces, an electronic repository of recovery-oriented mental health resources and discussions.

nami.org This is the site of the National Alliance on Mental Illness, which is the largest grassroots organization for people with mental illness and their families in the United States.

narsad.org This is the site of the U.S. National Alliance for Research on Schizophrenia and Depression, which is a national organization that raises and distributes money for research.

psychcentral.com/blog/archives/2013/09/20/top-10-free-mental-health-apps/ Top 10 free mental health apps are available for download here.

psychosissucks.ca This is a British Columbia early psychosis intervention site with links to other excellent resources.

www.schizophrenia.ca This is the site of the Schizophrenia Society of Canada, an organization committed to alleviating suffering caused by schizophrenia.

unsuicide.wikispaces.com/Mental+Health+Apps#.UmR4dRaKYp8 A collection of apps for mental health, some of which are available for download free of charge.

References

Addington, J., & Addington, D. (2006). The impact of cognitive functioning on outcome. *Schizophrenia Research, 86*(S1), 27.

Addington, J., McCleery, A., & Addington, D. (2005). Three-year outcome of family work in an early psychosis program. *Schizophrenia Research, 79*(1), 107–116.

Addington, J., van Mastrigt, S., Jutchinson, J., & Addington, D. (2002). Pathways to care: Help seeking behaviour in first episode psychosis. *Acta Psychiatrica Scandinavica, 106*(5), 358–364.

American Psychiatric Association. (2013). *Diagnostic and statistical manual of mental disorders* (5th ed.). Arlington, VA: Author.

Amminger, G. P., Henry, L. P., Harrigan, S. M., Harris, M. G., Alvarez-Jimenez, M., Herrman, H., ... McGorry, P. D. (2011). Outcome in early-onset schizophrenia revisited: Findings from the Early Psychosis Prevention and Intervention Centre long-term follow-up study. *Schizophrenia Research, 131*(1–3), 112–119.

Anticevic, A., & Lisman, J. (2017). How can global alteration of excitation/inhibition balance lead to the local dysfunctions that underlie schizophrenia? *Biological Psychiatry, 81*(10), 818–820. doi:http://dx.doi.org/10.1016/j.biopsych.2016.12.006

Barak, Y., & Aizenberg, D. (2012). Clinical and psychosocial remission in schizophrenia: Correlations with antipsychotic treatment. *BioMedCentral Psychiatry, 12*, 108, 1–5.

Benes, F. M. (2000). Emerging principles of altered neural circuitry in schizophrenia. *Brain Research. Developmental Brain Research, 31*(2–3), 251–269.

Buchsbaum, M. (1990). The frontal lobes, basal ganglia, and temporal lobes as a site for schizophrenia. *Schizophrenia Bulletin, 16*(3), 377–387.

Byrne, M., Agerbo, E., Ewald, H., Eaton, W. W., & Mortensen, P. B. (2003). Parental age and risk of schizophrenia: A case–control study. *Archives of General Psychiatry, 60*(7), 673–678.

Canadian Psychiatric Association. (2005). Clinical practice guidelines: Treatment of schizophrenia. *Canadian Journal of Psychiatry, 50*(S1), 1–48.

Carlson, N. R. (2013). *Physiology of behavior* (11th ed.). New York, NY: Pearson.

Centre for Addiction and Mental Health. (2013). *CAMH scientists discover genetic changes that may contribute to the onset of schizophrenia.* Retrieved from http://www.camh.ca/en/hospital/about_camh/newsroom/news_releases_media_advisories_and_backgrounders/current_year/Pages/CAMH-scientists-discover-genetic-changes-that-may-contribute-to-the-onset-of-schizophrenia-.aspx

Chance, S. A., Esiri, M. M., & Crow, T. J. (2003). Ventricular enlargement in schizophrenia: A primary change in the temporal lobe? *Schizophrenia Research, 62*(1–2), 123–131.

Chou, Y. H., Halldin, C., & Farde, L. (2003). Occupancy of 5HT(1A) receptors in clozapine in the primate brain: A PET study. *Psychopharmacology, 166*(3), 234–240.

Cohn, T. (2012). The link between schizophrenia and diabetes. *Current Psychiatry, 11*(10), 29–34, 46.

Costain, G., & Bassett, A. S. (2014). Individualizing recurrence risks for severe mental illness: Epidemiologic and molecular genetic approaches. *Schizophrenia Bulletin, 40*(1), 21–23. doi:10.1093/schbul/sbt133

Crowther, R., Marshall, M., Bond, G., & Huxley, P. (2001). Vocational rehabilitation for people with severe mental illness. *Cochrane Database of Systematic Reviews,* (2): CD003080. doi:10.1002/14651858.CD003080.

Csernansky, J. G. (2003). Treatment of schizophrenia: Preventing the progression of disease. *Psychiatric Clinics of North America, 26*(2), 367–379.

Davidson, L. L., & Heinrichs, R. W. (2003). Quantification of frontal and temporal lobe brain-imaging findings in schizophrenia: A meta-analysis. *Psychiatry Research, 122*(2), 69–87.

De Hert, M., McKenzie, K., & Peuskens, J. (2001). Risk factors for suicide in young people suffering from schizophrenia: A long-term follow-up study. *Schizophrenia Research, 47*(2–3), 127–134.

Dhariwal, M. (July 21, 2017). U of A research shows faster, more accurate schizophrenia diagnosis possible with artificial intelligence. *CBC News,* 1–2. Retrieved from cbc.ca/news/Canada/Edmonton/university-alberta-schizophrenia-research-machine-intelligence-institute-1.4216437

Emsley, R., Chiliza, B., Asmal, L., & Harvey, B. (2013). The nature of relapse in schizophrenia. *BioMedCentral Psychiatry, 13*, 50. Retrieved from http://www.biomedcentral.com/1471-244X/13/50

Falkai, P., Schneider-Axmann, T., Honer, W. G., Vogeley, K., Schonell, H., Pfeiffer, U., ... Tepest, R. (2003). Influence on genetic loading, obstetric complications, and premorbid adjustment on brain morphology in schizophrenia: A MRI study. *European Archives of Psychiatry and Clinical Neuroscience, 253*(2), 92–99.

Frese, F. III, Knight, E., & Saks, E. (2009). Recovery from schizophrenia: With views of psychiatrists, psychologists, and others diagnosed with this disorder. *Schizophrenia Bulletin, 35*(2), 370–380.

Freudenreich, O., & Cather, C. (2012). Antipsychotic medication nonadherence: Risk factors and remedies. *Focus, 10*(2), 124–129.

Gheiratmand, M., Rish, I., Cecchi, G. A., Brown, M. R. G., Greiner, R., Polosecki, P., ... Dursun, S. M. (2017). Learning stable and predictive network-based patterns of schizophrenia and its clinical symptoms. *NPJ Schizophrenia, 3*, 22, doi:10.1038/s41537-017-0022-8

Ghose, S., Weickert, C. S., Colvin, S. M., Coyle, J. T., Herman, M. M., Hyde, T. M., & Kleinman, J. E. (2003). Glutamate carboxypeptidase II gene expression in the human frontal and temporal lobe in schizophrenia. *Neuropsychopharmacology, 29*(1), 117–125.

Goldman, M. B. (2009). The mechanism of life-threatening water imbalance in schizophrenia and its relationship to the underlying psychiatric illness. *Brain Research Review, 61*(2), 210–220.

Goldner, E. M., Hsu, L., Waraich, P., & Somers, J. M. (2002). Prevalence and incidence studies of schizophrenia disorders: A systematic review of the literature. *Canadian Journal of Psychiatry, 47*(9), 833–843.

Gottlieb, J. (2012). *CopingTutor App.* Cognitive Health Innovations Inc. Retrieved from https://www.copingtutor.com/.

Grossman, M., Bowie, C. R., Lepage, M., Malla, A. K., Joober, R., & Iyer, S. N. (2017). Smoking status and its relationship to demographic and clinical characteristics in first episode psychosis. *Journal of Psychiatric Research, 85*, 83–90.

Gough, E. (2005). Diabetes and schizophrenia. *Practical Diabetes, 22*(1), 23–26.

Gur, R. E., & Gur, R. C. (2005). Neuroimaging in schizophrenia: Linking neuropsychiatric manifestations to neurobiology. In B. J. Sadock & V. A. Sadock (Eds.), *Comprehensive textbook of psychiatry* (pp. 1396–1408). Philadelphia, PA: Lippincott Williams & Wilkins.

Guy, W. (1976). *ECDEU: Assessment manual for psychopharmacology* (DHEW Publication No. 76-338). Washington, DC: Department of Health Education and Welfare, Psychopharmacology Branch.

Han, M., Huang, X. F., Chen, D. C., Xiu, M., Kosten, T. R., & Zhang, X. Y. (2013). Diabetes and cognitive deficits in chronic schizophrenia: A case–control study. *PLoS ONE, 8*(6), e66299. doi:10.1371/journal.pone.0066299

Harding, C., Zubin, J., & Strauss, J. (1987). Chronicity in schizophrenia: Fact, partial fact or artifact? *Hospital and Community Psychiatry, 38*(5), 477–486.

Harkavy-Friedman, J. M. (2007). Risk factors for suicide in patients with schizophrenia. *Psychiatric Times, 25*(2). Retrieved from http://www.psychiatrictimes.com/articles/risk-factors-suicide-patients-schizophrenia

Harrison, G., Fouskakis, D., Rasmussen, F., Tynelius, P., Sipos, A., & Gunnell, D. (2003). Association between psychotic disorder and urban place of birth is not mediated by obstetric complications or childhood socioeconomic position: A cohort study. *Psychological Medicine, 33*(4), 723–731.

Hettige, N. C., Bani-Fatemi, A., Kennedy, J. J., & De Luca, V. (2017). Assessing the risk for suicide in schizophrenia according to migration, ethnicity and geographical ancestry. *BMC Psychiatry, 17*, 63.

Hill, M. (2015). Be clear about the real risks. *Nature, 525*, S14.

Hor, K., & Taylor, M. (2010). Suicide and schizophrenia: A systematic review of rates and risk factors. *Journal of Psychopharmacology, 24*(Suppl. 4), 81–90.

Imtiaz, S., Shield, K. D., Roerecke, M., Cheng, J., Popova, S., Kurdyak, P., Fischer, B., & Rehm, J. (2015). The burden of disease attributable to cannabis use in Canada in 2012. *Addiction, 111*, 653–662.

Isane, D., Nitkin, K., & Gastaldo, D. (2010). Addressing physical health problems experienced by people with schizophrenia in Canada: A critical literature review/Les problèmes de santé physique chez les personnes atteintes de schizophrénie au Canada: une recension critique de la littérature. *Canadian Journal of Nursing Research, 42*(3), 124–140.

Jibson, M. D. & Tandon, R. (2000). Treatment of schizophrenia. In D. L. Dunner, & J. E. Rosenbaum (Eds.), *The psychiatric clinics of North America annual of drug therapy* (Vol. 7, pp. 83–113). Philadelphia, PA: WB Saunders.

Kandel, E. R., Schwartz, J. H., & Jessell, T. M. (2000). *Principles of neural science* (4th ed.). New York, NY: McGraw-Hill.

Kaneko, Y., & Keshavan, M. (2012) Cognitive remediation in schizophrenia. *Clinical Psychopharmacology and Neuroscience, 10*(3), 125–135.

Kay, S. R., Fiszbein, A., & Opler, L. A. (1987). The Positive and Negative Syndrome Scale (PANSS) for schizophrenia. *Schizophrenia Bulletin, 13*, 261–276.

Kern, R. S., Green, M. V., Mintz, J., & Liberman, R. P. (2003). Does 'errorless learning' compensate for neurocognitive impairments in the work rehabilitation of persons with schizophrenia? *Psychological Medicine, 33*(3), 433–442.

Kern, R. S., Liberman, R. P., Kopelowicz, A., Mintz, J., & Green, M. F. (2002). Applications of errorless learning for improving work performance in persons with schizophrenia. *American Journal of Psychiatry, 159*(11), 1921–1926.

Keshavan, M., Tandon, R., Boutros, N., & Nasrallah, H. (2008). Schizophrenia, "just the facts": What we know in 2008. Part 3: Neurobiology. *Schizophrenia Research, 106*(2–3), 89–107.

Kulkarni, J., Hayes, E., & Gavrilidis, E. (2012). Hormones and schizophrenia. *Current Opinions in Psychiatry, 25*(2), 89–95.

Laursen, T. M., Munk-Olsen, T., & Vestergaard, M. (2012). Life expectancy and cardiovascular mortality in persons with schizophrenia. *Current Opinions in Psychiatry, 25*, 83–88.

Leucht, S., Burkard, T., Henderson, J., Maj, M., & Sartorius, N. (2007). Physical illness and schizophrenia: A review of the literature. *Acta Psychiatrica Scandinavica, 116*(5), 317–333.

Levin, E., & Rezvani, A. (2007). Nicotinic interactions with antipsychotic drugs, models of schizophrenia and impacts on cognitive function. *Biochemical Pharmacology, 74*(8), 1182–1191.

Lilley, L. L., Collins, S. R., Synder, J. S., & Swart, B. (2017). *Pharmacology for Canadian health care practice* (3rd ed.). Toronto, ON: Elsevier Canada.

Malla, A., Norman, R., & Joober, R. (2005). First episode psychosis, early intervention and outcome: What have we learned? *Canadian Journal of Psychiatry, 50*(14), 881–891.

Manu, P., Dima, L., Shulman, M., Vancampfort, D., De Hert, M., & Correll, C. U. (2015). Weight gain and obesity in schizophrenia: Epidemiology, pathobiology, and management. *Acta Psychiatrica Scandinavica, 132*(2), 97–108.

Melau, M., Jeppesen, P., Thorup, A., Bertelsen, M., Peterson, L., Krarup, G., & Nordentoft, M. (2011). The effect of five years versus two years of specialised assertive intervention for first episode psychosis—OPUS II: Study protocol for a randomized controlled trial. *Trials, 12*, 72.

Mental Health Commission of Canada (MHCC). (2007). *A time for action: Tackling stigma and discrimination.* Retrieved from http://www.mentalhealthcommission.ca/English/Pages/AntiStigmaCampaign.aspx

Mental Health Commission of Canada (MHCC). (2012). *Changing directions: Changing lives. The mental health strategy for Canada.* Retrieved from http://www.mentalhealthcommission.ca/English/node/721

Mental Health Commission of Canada (MHCC). (2013a). *Aspiring workforce: Employment and income for people with serious mental illness.* Retrieved from http://www.mentalhealthcommission.ca/English/node/7606

Mental Health Commission of Canada (MHCC). (2013b). *At home/Chez soi.* Retrieved from http://www.mentalhealthcommission.ca/English/initiatives-and-projects/home?routetoken=ff8ead4644148979334f1198d0bb826f&terminitial=38

Mental Health Commission of Canada (MHCC). (2013c). *National guidelines for a comprehensive service system to support family caregivers of adults with mental health problems and illnesses.* Retrieved from http://www.mentalhealthcommission.ca/English/node/8601/#sthash.FZdfsot1.dpuf

Mesholam-Gately, R., Giuliano, A., Faraone, S., Goff, K., & Seidman, L. (2009). Neurocognition in first-episode schizophrenia: A meta-analytic review. *Neuropsychology, 23*(3), 315–336.

Montoya, A., Ocampo, M., & Torres-Ruiz, A. (2003). Neuroleptic malignant syndrome in Mexico. *Canadian Journal of Clinical Pharmacology, 10*(3), 111–113.

Morrison, E. F. (1992). A coercive interactional style as an antecedent to aggression in psychiatric patients. *Research in Nursing and Health, 15*, 421–431.

Morrison, E. F., & Love, C. C. (2003). An evaluation of four programs for the management of aggression in psychiatric settings. *Archives in Psychiatric Nursing, 17*(4), 146–155.

Murray, R. M., & Bramon, E. (2005). Developmental model of schizophrenia. In B. J. Sadock & V. A. Sadock (Eds.), *Comprehensive textbook of psychiatry* (pp. 1381–1396). Philadelphia, PA: Lippincott Williams & Wilkins.

Niemi, L. T., Suvisaari, J. M., Tuulio-Henriksson, A., & Lonnqvist, J. K. (2003). Childhood developmental abnormalities in schizophrenia: Evidence from high-risk studies. *Schizophrenia Research, 60*(2–3), 239–258.

Onken, S. J., Dumont, J. M., Ridgway, P., Dornan, D. H., & Ralph, R. O. (2007). Mental health recovery: What helps and what hinders? In *A national research project for the development of recovery facilitating system performance indicators.* Retrieved from https://www.nasmhpd.org/sites/default/files/MHSIPReport%281%29.pdf; http://www.mhsret.org/documents/ROSIPilotMeasuresV7.pdf

Overall, J. E., & Gorham, D. R. (1988). The Brief Psychiatric Rating Scale (BPRS): Recent developments in ascertainment and scaling. *Psychopharmacology Bulletin, 24*, 97–99.

Oxford University Press and the Maryland Psychiatric Research Center. (2002). Graduate student in peril: A first person account of schizophrenia. *Schizophrenia Bulletin, 28*(4), 745–755.

Penn, A. A. (2001). Early brain wiring: Activity-dependent processes. *Schizophrenia Bulletin, 27*(3), 336–347.

Pia, L., & Tamleto, M. (2006). Unawareness in schizophrenia: Neuropsychological and neuroanatomical findings. *Psychiatry and Clinical Neurosciences, 60*(5), 531–537.

Picchioni, M. M., & Murray, R. M. (2007). Schizophrenia. *British Medical Journal, 335*(7610), 91–95.

Ramnarine, M., & Ahmad, D. A. (2016, July 28). *Anticholinergic toxicity clinical presentation.* Medscape. Retrieved from http://emedicine.medscape.com/article/812644-clinical

Rapoport, J., Addington, A., & Frangou, S. (2005). The neurodevelopmental model of schizophrenia: Update 2005. *Molecular Psychiatry, 10*, 434–449.

Sallet, P. C., Elkis, H., Alves, T. M., Oliveira, J. R., Sassi, E., Campi de Castro, C., … Gattaz, W. F. (2003). Reduced cortical folding in schizophrenia: An MRI morphometric study. *American Journal of Psychiatry, 160*(9), 1606–1613.

Sheffield, J. M., Gold, J. M., Strauss, M. E., Carter, C. S., Macdonald, A. W. III, Ragland, J. D., … Barch, D. M. (2014). Common and specific cognitive deficits in schizophrenia: Relationships to function. *Cognitive, Affective, & Behavioral Neuroscience, 14*(1), 161–174.

Simpson, G. M., & Angus, J. W. S. L. (1970). A rating scale for extrapyramidal side effects. *Acta Psychiatrica Scandinavica, 212*, 11–19.

Sprague, R. L., & Kalachnik, J. E. (1991). Reliability, validity, and a total score cutoff for the Dyskinesia Identification Scale System: Condensed User Scale (DISCUS) with mentally ill and mentally retarded populations. *Psychopharmacology Bulletin, 27*, 51–58.

Stahl, S. (2013). *Stahl's essential psychopharmacology: Neuroscientific basis and practical application* (4th ed.). Cambridge, UK: Cambridge University Press.

Standing Senate Committee on Social Affairs, Science and Technology. (2006). *Out of the shadows at last: Transforming mental health, mental illness and addiction services in Canada.* Retrieved from http://www.parl.gc.ca/39/1/parlbus/commbus/senate/Com-e/SOCI-E/rep-e/rep02may06-e.htm

Subotnik, K. L., Goldstein, M. J., Nuechterlein, K. H., Woo, S. M., & Mintz, J. (2002). Are communication deviance and expressed emotion related to family history of psychiatric disorders in schizophrenia? *Schizophrenia Bulletin, 28*(4), 719–729.

Subramaniam, K., Luks, T., Fisher, M., Simpson, G., Nagarajan, S., & Vinogradov, S. (2012). Computerized cognitive training restores neural activity within the reality monitoring network in schizophrenia. *Neuron, 73*(4), 842–853.

Tharyan, P., & Adams, C. E. (2005). Electroconvulsive therapy for schizophrenia. *Cochrane Database of Systematic Reviews, 18*(2), CD000076.

Tsuang, M. T., Stone, W. S., & Faraone, S. V. (2001). Genes, environment and schizophrenia. *British Journal of Psychiatry, 178*(Suppl. 40), S18–S24.

United States Department of Health and Human Services. (2014). *The health consequences of smoking: A report of the surgeon general.* Atlanta, GA: U.S. Department of Health Services, Centers for Disease Control and Prevention, National Center for Chronic Disease Prevention and Promotion, Office on Smoking and Health.

Walker, E., Kestler, L., Bollini, A., & Hochman, K. M. (2004). Schizophrenia: Etiology and course. *Annual Review of Psychology, 55*, 401–430.

Weisman, A. G., Gomes, L. G., & Lopez, S. R. (2003). Shifting blame away from ill relatives: Latino families' reactions to schizophrenia. *Journal of Nervous and Mental Disease, 191*(9), 574–581.

Wilson, J. H. (2009). Moving beyond policy rhetoric: Building a moral community for early psychosis intervention. *Journal of Psychiatric and Mental Health Nursing, 16*(7), 621–628.

Wilson, J. H. (2012). *First episode psychosis: The experience of parent caregivers.* Doctoral dissertation, University of Alberta, Edmonton, AB.

Wuerker, A. K., Long, J. D., Haas, G. L., & Bellack, A. S. (2002). Interpersonal control, expressed emotion, and change in symptoms in families of persons with schizophrenia. *Schizophrenia Research, 58*(2–3), 281–292.

Young, A., Halari, R., & Gray, R. (2013). Negative symptoms in schizophrenia: Meeting the challenge. *Progress in Neurology and Psychiatry, 17*(5), 33–36.

CHAPTER

21 Schizoaffective, Delusional, and Other Psychotic Disorders

Diana Clarke and
Shelley Marchinko

LEARNING OBJECTIVES

After studying this chapter, you will be able to:

- Define schizoaffective disorder and distinguish the major differences and similarities among schizophrenia, schizoaffective, and mood disorders.
- Discuss the important epidemiologic findings related to schizoaffective disorder.
- Explain the primary elements involved in assessment, nursing diagnoses, nursing interventions, and evaluation of patients with schizoaffective disorder.
- Define delusional disorder and name the subtypes of this disorder.
- Discuss the theories related to the aetiology of delusional disorder.
- Explain the nursing care of patients with delusional disorder.
- Identify the essential features of schizophreniform disorder, brief psychotic disorder, substance-/medication-induced psychotic disorder, and psychotic disorder due to another medical condition.

KEY TERMS

- bizarre delusions • delusional disorder • erotomanic delusion • grandiose delusion • jealous delusion • misidentification • persecutory delusion • schizoaffective disorder • somatic delusion

KEY CONCEPTS

- delusions

Psychiatric and mental health nurses care for patients who have psychiatric disorders involving underlying psychoses other than schizophrenia, depressive disorders, and bipolar and related disorders. These disorders include schizoaffective, delusional, brief psychotic, and schizophreniform disorders and are classified as per DSM-5 under schizophrenia spectrum and other psychotic disorders. Psychotic disorders also may be induced by medications or other substances or be a symptom of another medical disorder. This chapter introduces these disorders and describes the associated nursing care. Their common element is the state of psychosis in which an individual can experience hallucinations, delusions, or disorganized thoughts, speech, or behaviour (positive symptoms) and/or diminished emotional expression, anhedonia, and avolition (negative symptoms) (see Chapter 20 for further delineation of positive and negative symptoms).

■ SCHIZOAFFECTIVE DISORDER

Clinical Course

Schizoaffective disorder is a complex and persistent psychiatric illness. This disorder was recognized in 1933 by Kasanin, who described varying degrees of symptoms of both schizophrenia and mood disorders (depressive disorders and/or bipolar and related disorders) beginning in youth. All his patients were well adjusted before the sudden onset of symptoms that erupted after the occurrence of a specific environmental stressor. Since Kasanin's time, debate and controversy about the status of this disorder have been extensive, resulting in many different definitions and classifications that remain under consideration (van Os, Linscott, Myin-Germeys, Delespaul, & Krabbendam, 2009). Schizoaffective disorder was not recognized as a separate disorder in the *Diagnostic and Statistical Manual* (*DSM*) of the American

Psychiatric Association (APA) until the *DSM-III-R* in 1987; its definition included symptom duration. Debate about the status of this disorder continues (Malaspina et al., 2013). A systematic review of clinical trial studies comparing schizoaffective disorder with schizophrenia and mood disorders suggests that schizoaffective disorder occupies an intermediate position between the latter disorders, but no clear-cut distinctions between schizoaffective disorder and schizophrenia or schizoaffective disorder and a mood disorder could be established (Cheniaux et al., 2008). A survey of psychiatrists' attitudes toward schizoaffective disorder found that while almost all had used the diagnosis in clinical practice and most considered the diagnosis to be clinically useful, there was little agreement about its nature, its relationship to other mental disorders, or its aetiology (Rowe & Clark, 2008). Schizoaffective disorder remains a separate disorder in the *Diagnostic and Statistical Manual of Mental Disorders, 5th ed. (DSM-5)* (APA, 2013).

Schizoaffective disorder is characterized by intervals of intense symptoms alternating with quiescent periods, during which psychosocial functioning is adequate. The episodic nature of this disorder is characteristic. It is at times marked by symptoms of schizophrenia; at other times, it appears to be a depressive disorder, or bipolar disorder. In other cases, both psychosis and pervasive mood changes occur concurrently. Patients feel that they are on a "chronic roller-coaster ride" of symptoms that are often more difficult to cope with than the individual problem of schizophrenia, a depressive disorder, or bipolar disorder. The long-term outcome of schizoaffective disorder is generally better than that of schizophrenia but worse than that for depressive disorders or bipolar disorder. This group of patients resembles the mood disorders group in work function and the schizophrenia group in social function (Bottender, Strauss, & Moller, 2010).

Clinical Features

Mental health providers find schizoaffective disorder difficult to conceptualize, diagnose, and treat because the clinical picture is often very complex and varies from episode to episode over time, and its validity as a diagnosis remains controversial (Malaspina et al., 2013). Patients often have misdiagnoses of schizophrenia or conversely of depression with psychotic features or bipolar disorder. The difficulty in conceptualizing schizoaffective disorder is reflected in the controversy regarding the diagnostic criteria. Although it has been argued that this disorder should be named either *schizophrenia with mood symptoms* or *mood disorder with schizophrenia symptoms*, the fifth edition of the *DSM* (APA, 2013) has left it as a separate diagnosis midway along the schizophrenia spectrum between schizophrenia and schizophreniform disorder.

To receive a diagnosis of schizoaffective disorder, a patient must have an uninterrupted period of illness when there is a major depressive, manic, or mixed episode along with some symptoms of schizophrenia, such as delusions, hallucinations, or other indicative symptoms. (See Chapter 20 for the DSM-5 criteria for schizophrenia.) As well, although the person's problems with mood are present much of the time, the positive symptoms of schizophrenia must be experienced without the mood symptoms at some time. To clarify this disorder further, two related subtypes of schizoaffective disorder have been identified (APA, 2013). For the American Psychological Association diagnostic criteria for schizoaffective disorder and its subtypes, please see the DSM-5.

Epidemiology and Risk Factors

The lifetime prevalence of schizoaffective disorder is estimated to be around 0.3% (APA, 2013) but is very difficult to track. This disorder occurs less commonly than does schizophrenia. The incidence of schizoaffective disorder is relatively constant across populations in varied geographic, climatic, industrial, and social environments. Environmental contributions are minimal.

IN-A-LIFE

Louis Riel (1844–1885)

MÉTIS LEADER

Public Persona

Louis Riel, leader of the Métis in Manitoba and Saskatchewan, has been remembered as the man who negotiated for the establishment of Manitoba as a province and who led the fight for the protection of Métis and Aboriginal land and rights in Western Canada. Arrested for treason in 1884, he showed symptoms of grandiosity and paranoid delusions. He was declared "sane" by the superintendent of the Asylum for the Insane in Toronto, stood trial, and was hanged in 1885.

Personal Realities

Riel had numerous episodes of profound depression, apparent psychosis, and delusional thinking throughout his life. At times, he believed he had been substituted for the real Louis Riel who had died. At other times, he talked about his "mission" to form a new religion and replace the Pope. He was hospitalized and committed to insane asylums on numerous occasions. In retrospect, he has been "diagnosed" variably in the literature with paranoid schizophrenia, schizoaffective disorder, and bipolar disorder.

From Perr, I. N. (1992). Religion, political leadership, charisma and mental illness: The strange story of Louis Riel. *Journal of Forensic Science, 37*(2), 574–584; Waite, P. (1987). Between three oceans: Challenges of a continental destiny. In C. Brown (Ed.), *The illustrated history of Canada* (pp. 279–373). Toronto, ON: Lester & Orpen Dennys.

Age of Onset

Schizoaffective disorder can affect individuals across the life span, although in children, the disorder is rare and is often indistinguishable from early-onset schizophrenia. In the older adult, this disorder becomes complicated because of frequent comorbid medical conditions. The typical age of onset for this disorder is early adulthood, and the most common type presented is bipolar. Cases of later onset of schizoaffective disorder are typically found to be of the depressive type (APA, 2013). Earlier age of onset is associated with longer illness, more severe illness, and worse outcomes (APA, 2013).

Gender

Schizoaffective disorder is more likely to occur in women than in men, which may be accounted for by a greater incidence of the depressive type in women (APA, 2013). It is not yet clear if this is related to biologic differences or to a diagnostic bias. Because women, on average, have more supportive social networks than do men and tend to be behaviourally less violent when ill, they can more readily be cared for by family at home and may not come to the attention of mental health services in the same manner as do men (MacDougall, Luckett, & Jones, 2007). While women are reported to have better outcomes than men in terms of symptom control and sometimes employment (those typically examined in research), there are other outcomes particularly relevant to women (friendships, romantic relationships, family relationships, reproductive decisions, parenting, custody loss of children, psychological and socioeconomic independence, physical attractiveness, victimization, generativity, reproductive and metabolic side effects of medications) that may contribute to mood symptoms and that have not been adequately explored (Chernomas, Clarke, & Chisholm, 2000; Chernomas, Reiger, Karpa, Clarke, Marchinko, & Demczuk, 2017; Judd, Armstrong, & Kulkarni, 2009; MacDougall et al., 2007).

Ethnicity and Culture

While patterns of mental health services use may differ among ethnic and racial groups (Delphin-Rittman, Flanagan, Andres-Hyman, Ortiz, Amer, & Davidson, 2015), no specific associations with race, geographic area, or class have been demonstrated (Siris & Lavin, 1995). Culturally sensitive assessment is crucial especially if the patient's and the clinician's cultural backgrounds differ. Some beliefs and cultural practices may appear delusional to one culture but be acceptable in another.

Family

Some authorities support a familial association in schizoaffective disorder, but a clear familial pattern has not been established. Relatives of patients with diagnoses of schizoaffective disorder appear to be at increased risk for this disorder, schizophrenia, or both (APA, 2013). Whether this familial clustering is related to genetic risk factors, nongenetic environmental and cultural factors, or a combination of both is not yet clear (van Os et al., 2009).

Comorbidity

Schizoaffective disorder may be associated with substance abuse. Men may be more likely to engage in antisocial behaviour. Twenty-five percent of patients with diagnoses of schizoaffective disorder experience postpsychotic depression and panic attacks. The incidence of general medical disorders for those with schizoaffective disorder is also found to be above the base rate for the general population (APA, 2013).

Patients with schizoaffective disorder are at high risk for suicide. The risk for suicide in patients with psychosis is increased by the presence of depression. Risk for suicide is increased with the use of alcohol or substances, cigarette smoking, previous attempts at suicide, and previous hospitalizations (Potkin et al., 2003; Seguin et al., 2006).

Aetiology

Biologic Theories

Although the aetiologies of schizophrenia, depressive disorders, and bipolar disorder have been investigated extensively, the aetiology of schizoaffective disorder remains unresolved.

Neuropathologic

Magnetic resonance imaging (MRI) and computed tomography (CT or CAT) scans have been used in the study of schizoaffective disorder for more than 20 years (Crow & Harrington, 1994; Lewine, Hudgins, Brown, Caudle, & Risch, 1995). A 2016 systematic review of the neuropsychological and neuroimaging underpinnings of schizoaffective disorder (Madre et al., 2016) concluded that the abnormalities associated with it resemble schizophrenia more than bipolar disorder suggesting that schizoaffective disorder may be closer to schizophrenia than bipolar disorder on the psychosis spectrum.

Genetic

As noted above, familial clustering may be related to genetics or environmental risk factors or both (van Os et al., 2009). Results from family, twin, and adoption studies vary but suggest that schizoaffective disorder shows significant familial overlap with both schizophrenia and bipolar disorder, the latter particularly when mania is seen in the patient presentation (Cardno & Owen, 2014).

Biochemical

Before 1999, the prevailing neurochemical hypothesis, overactivity of dopamine pathways, was based on observations of the effects of psychoactive drugs on psychotic symptoms (Jacobson & Tarraza, 2013). More recently, other neurochemicals under investigation are serotonin and glutamate (Andreasen & Black, 2006; Nasrallah, 2011).

Psychological and Social Theories

No current psychodynamic, behavioural, cognitive, or developmental theories of causation explain schizoaffective disorder. It is clear, however, that the psychological and social sequelae of a diagnosis of schizoaffective disorder can be overwhelming for the patient and family. The experience of psychosis is much more than simply the symptoms and can result in issues of loss, a need to learn how to seek help, and a desire to learn how to rebuild one's life within the context of the illness (McCarthy-Jones, Marriott, Knowles, Rowse, & Thompson, 2013). While historical hypotheses related to overprotective, rigid families have been disproven, family dynamics nevertheless play an important role in influencing the clinical course of the disorder (Jacobson & Tarraza, 2013).

Interprofessional Treatment

Because this disorder is persistent, these individuals are constantly trying to manage complex symptoms. Patients with schizoaffective disorder benefit from a comprehensive treatment plan and a cohesive interprofessional treatment team. Integral to this team is the patient (and often his or her family) who needs to be an active participant in treatment planning. Ideally, most of the treatment occurs within the patient's natural environment, and hospitalizations are limited to times of symptom exacerbation, when symptoms are so severe or persistent that extended care in a protected environment is necessary.

Pharmacologic intervention is needed to stabilize the symptoms, and it presents specific challenges. Long-term atypical antipsychotic agents are as effective as the traditional combination of a standard antipsychotic agent and an antidepressant drug. Mood stabilizers, such as lithium or valproic acid, may also be used. A combination of antipsychotic and antidepressant agents is sometimes used (see Chapter 12).

After the patient's condition has stabilized (i.e., the patient exhibits a decrease in positive and negative symptoms), the treatment that led to remission of symptoms should be continued. Titrating antipsychotic agents to the lowest dose that provides suitable protection may enable optimal psychosocial functioning while slowing recurrence of new episodes. Patients with schizoaffective disorder will likely need to remain on medication for the disorder. Electroconvulsive therapy (see Chapter 12) is considered when symptoms are refractory to other interventions or when the patient's life is at risk and a rapid improvement is required (Pompili et al., 2012).

The treatment plan is revised regularly, and symptoms are monitored to guide medication management. Psychiatric mental health nursing interventions in hospital and in community care are guided by the nursing diagnoses. Psychotherapy may help manage interpersonal relationships and mood changes. Social services are often needed to obtain disability benefits or services. Use of advanced practice clinicians helps to provide continuity of care (Jacobson & Tarraza, 2013).

Priority Care Issues

Patients with schizoaffective disorder may be at least as susceptible to suicide (see Chapter 19) as those with depressive disorder (Potkin et al., 2003). Living with a persistent psychotic disorder that has a mood component makes suicide a real risk. A review of completed suicides in New Brunswick has further suggested that comorbidity with substance abuse may increase the risk (Seguin et al., 2006).

Nursing Management: Human Response to Schizoaffective Disorder

Biologic Domain

Assessment

Assessment of patients with schizoaffective disorder is similar to assessment of those with schizophrenia, depressive disorder, or bipolar disorder. A careful history from the patient and family is crucial. The history should contain a description of the full range and duration of symptoms the patient has experienced and those observed by the family; this information is important for predicting outcomes. A patient who has had symptoms for a relatively long period of time may have greater difficulty in overcoming effects of the psychosis resulting in deterioration in functioning.

A thorough system assessment is important to discover any physiologic problems the patient is experiencing, such as sleep pattern disturbances, difficulties with self-care, or poor nutritional habits.

Nursing Diagnoses for Biologic Domain

Common nursing diagnoses for the biologic domain are *disturbed thought process, disturbed sensory perception,* and *disturbed sleep patterns.* Because of the variety of problems in patients with schizoaffective disorder, almost any nursing diagnosis could be generated. The persistent nature of this disorder lends itself to numerous and varied problems that must all be addressed (see Nursing Care Plan 21.1).

NURSING CARE PLAN 21.1

PATIENT WITH SCHIZOAFFECTIVE DISORDER

Ms. B is a 28-year-old divorced woman with a 4-year-old daughter. They reside with Ms. B's parents. Ms. B is a hairdresser and tries to work, but she becomes stressed in the workplace, which results in her being fired. She has never applied for disability. Her parents are stressed because of the exacerbations of her illness and caring for her child.

Ms. B has had numerous hospitalizations for aggressive behaviour, nonadherence with medications, and receiving medications from various physicians, which result in inappropriate psychiatric management. She is medication seeking and is often prescribed benzodiazepines and diet pills by her primary care physician.

The patient has an ingrained delusional system that makes it hard to introduce reality orientation and feedback. She believes that her ex-husband has sexually abused their child. She has gone to numerous attorneys to try to prosecute her ex-husband to no avail because of the lack of evidence to prove any abuse.

For the last 2 years, Ms. B has believed that a bank guard is in love with her. She is adamant about him protecting her and her child. She states that he watches over them. They

have no contact other than speaking to each other when she enters the bank. She has been seeing a man the past 9 months but states that she really does not care much for him and that it is hard for her to move forward in the relationship because she loves the bank guard.

Medications have included antidepressants, neuroleptics (typical and atypical), mood stabilizers, benzodiazepines, sleep medications, and anticonvulsants. She often complains of being depressed and yet does not take the antidepressant medications when they are prescribed.

Setting: Intensive Care Psychiatric Unit in a General Hospital

Baseline Assessment: Ms. B is admitted to the hospital through the emergency department. She was hearing voices and was delusional. She has not been taking medications for several months. She is oriented in all spheres and well-nourished but unkempt. She is verbalizing delusions about a man at the bank. She cannot sleep well and reportedly goes outdoors at night and yells at a bank guard. Reality feedback increases her agitation. She denies any problems.

Associated Psychiatric Diagnosis and Other Conditions That May Be a Focus of Clinical Attention	Medications
Schizoaffective disorder Relational problems Economic problem (no income) Occupational problem (unemployed) Nonadherence to medical treatment	None

Nursing Diagnosis 1: Ineffective Individual Coping

Defining Characteristics	Related Factors
Inability to meet role expectations	Chronicity of the condition
Anxiety	Inadequate psychological resources secondary to delusions
Delusions	Inadequate coping skills
Inability to problem solve	Inadequate psychological resources to adapt to residential setting

Outcomes

Initial	Discharge
1. Identify coping patterns	5. Manage own behaviour
2. Identify stressors	6. Adherence to medication regimen
3. Identify personal strengths	7. Reduction of delusions
4. Accept support through the nursing relationship	

NURSING CARE PLAN 21.1 *(Continued)*

Interventions

Interventions	Rationale	Ongoing Assessment
Initiate a nurse–patient relationship to develop trust.	Through the use of the nurse–patient relationship, the patient will be able to maintain adherence to the treatment plan.	Determine whether the patient is able to relate to the nurse.
Facilitate the identification of stressors in the patient's environment.	To be able to cope with stressors, they need to be identified by the patient.	Assess whether the patient is able to identify and verbalize stressors.
Develop a wellness plan in collaboration with the patient	The patient needs to develop healthy and realistic strategies to handle environmental stressors.	Determine whether patient-identified strategies are realistic.
Help the patient to identify personal strengths.	By identifying personal strengths, the patient will increase confidence in using coping strategies.	Assess the patient's ability to incorporate coping strategies into her daily routine.
Assist the patient to understand the disorder and its management.	By understanding the disorder, the patient can develop ways to manage her disorder.	Assess the patient's level of understanding of the disease.
Facilitate emotional support for the family.	Supported family is better equipped to support the patient.	Assess the family's ability to seek emotional support from the staff.
Identify coping skills that have been effective in the past and teach new coping skills.	By developing positive coping skills, anxiety and agitation will decrease.	Assess the patient's ability to learn the skills to manage stressors.

Evaluation

Outcomes	Revised Outcomes	Interventions
Within the nursing relationship, Ms. B. was able to understand how coping skills can reduce stressors.	Support the patient's ability to recognize stressors and apply coping skills.	Discuss stressors and means of applying coping skills.
Increased insight into what behaviour is appropriate has helped the patient to decrease verbalization of delusions.	Provide ongoing support to maintain the present level of functioning.	Discuss behaviour and provide reality feedback.

Nursing Diagnosis 2: Disturbed Thought Processes

Defining Characteristics	Related Factors
Delusions	Ingrained delusions
Impulsivity	Decreased ability to process secondary to delusions
Medication noncompliance	

(Continued)

NURSING CARE PLAN 21.1 *(Continued)*

Outcomes

Initial	Discharge
1. Maintain reality orientation	4. Identify situations that contribute to delusions
2. Communicate clearly with others	5. Identify how delusions affect life situations
3. Express delusional material less frequently	6. Use coping strategies to deal with delusions
	7. Recognize changes in behaviour

Interventions

Interventions	Rationale	Ongoing Assessment
Promote adherence to medication regimen.	Medication will reduce delusions.	Assess for side effects: heat intolerance, neuroleptic malignant syndrome (NMS), renal failure, constipation, dry mouth, increased appetite, salivation, nausea, vomiting, tardive dyskinesia, seizures, somnolence, agitation, insomnia, dizziness, metabolic syndrome, and weight gain.
Discuss actions, effects, and side effects of planned medications and assess patient's level of tolerance for the relative side effect profiles.	The more knowledgeable patients are about medication, the more likely they will agree to take the medications.	Assess ability to understand information.
Support reality testing through helping the patient to differentiate thoughts and feelings in relation to situations.	When comparing thoughts with the situations, patients can develop skills to refute delusions.	Assess for medication compliance.
Monitor verbalization of delusional material.	To determine whether medication is reducing delusional thoughts	Assess verbalization of delusional material.
Identify stressors that promote delusions.	If the patient is able to identify stressors that promote delusions, she can manage the stressors to effectively decrease delusions.	Assess the patient's ability to recognize stressors when they occur. Encourage use of crisis planning or wellness planning tools.
Assist the patient in developing skills to deal with delusions (recognizing delusional themes can help the patient in distinguishing between reality-based and non–reality-based patterns).	Even though medication can reduce the occurrence of delusions, they may continue in some people with decreased intensity. Cognitive–behavioural skills are important in dealing with these altered thoughts.	Monitor the patient's ability to handle delusions.

NURSING CARE PLAN 21.1 (Continued)

Evaluation

Outcomes	Revised Outcomes	Interventions
Delusions will be less ingrained.	Continue to practice skills in reality orientation and communication.	Support verbalization of reality-based thoughts.
The patient verbalized action, effect, dosage, and side effects of medications.	Take prescribed medication regularly.	Give positive feedback for understanding of medication.
Medication adherence		Encourage patient to be forthright about her adherence to the medication regimen.

Summary: Ms. B was discharged from the hospital. Verbalization of delusions had not decreased. She was less anxious. She is presently on Risperdal 2 mg AM and hs, Effexor XR 75 mg AM, Xanax 0.5 mg AM, and Seroquel 50 mg hs. Her mother is helping by filling a weekly medication box. At times, Ms. B is questioning her delusions.

Interventions for Biologic Domain

Patient Education

Interventions are based on the needs identified in the bio/psycho/social/spiritual assessment (Fig. 21.1). Helping the patient to establish a regular sleep pattern by using a routine can promote or reestablish normal rest patterns. Focusing with the patient on the principles of good nutrition and identifying any barriers to healthy eating can improve nutritional status. Working with the patient can help identify self-care deficits, especially those caused by lack of motivation. For deficits created

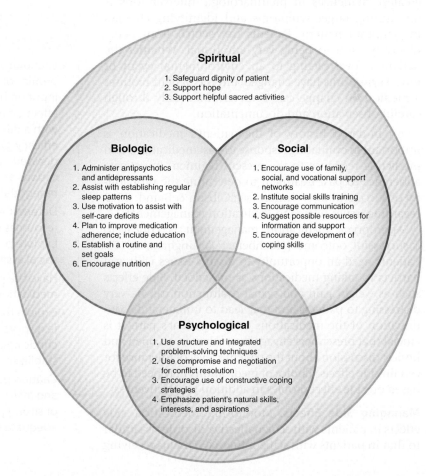

Figure 21.1. Bio/psycho/social/spiritual interventions for patients with schizoaffective disorder.

by severe mood symptoms, establishing a routine and setting goals can be useful.

Pharmacologic Interventions

An in-depth history of the patient's medication is important in evaluating response to past medications and predicting response to the present regimen. Mood and psychotic symptoms are equally important and should be evaluated throughout treatment. Atypical antipsychotic agents are generally prescribed because of their efficacy (see Chapter 20). Clozapine, reported effective for schizoaffective disorder by several authorities, can reduce hospitalizations and risk for suicide in treatment-refractory patients although it carries with it significant side effect risk. Atypical antipsychotic agents may have thymoleptic (mood stabilizing), as well as antipsychotic, effects. Quetiapine has been found effective in this respect. Dosage is the same as that used for treating schizophrenia, but lower dosage ranges may also be effective.

In many cases, symptoms of depression disappear when psychotic symptoms decrease. If depressive symptoms persist, adjunctive use of an antidepressant agent may be helpful (see Chapter 22). Mood stabilizers, which can decrease the frequency and intensity of episodes, may be an alternative adjunctive medication for mood states associated with the bipolar type.

Administering and Monitoring Medications. One of the greatest challenges in pharmacologic interventions is monitoring target symptoms and identifying changes in symptom pattern. Patients can switch from being relatively calm to being very emotional. Whether the patient is overreacting to an environmental event or mood symptoms have changed and the patient requires a medication change can be determined only through careful observation and documentation.

An in-depth history of the patient's medication is important in evaluating response to past medications and predicting response to the present regimen. Investigate adherence to past treatment to determine the probability of successful intervention (see Gibson & Brand, 2013 regarding issues related to medication management).

Appropriate medication management is critical to a successful outcome (Hochberger & Lingham, 2017). Patients need an opportunity to discuss issues with and barriers to taking medications as prescribed. Side effects such as weight gain and sexual dysfunction can be very distressing to patients and may lead to unilateral discontinuation of the medications on the patient's part. It is crucial that prescribers engage the patient in an open and honest discussion about the patient's level of tolerance for certain side effects. Choice of medications may need to be based on side effect profiles in addition to effectiveness.

Managing Side Effects. Monitoring medication side effects in patients with schizoaffective disorder is similar to that in patients with schizophrenia. Patients receiving antipsychotic medications need to be aware of extrapyramidal symptoms and the possibility of developing metabolic syndrome—a triad of diabetes, dyslipidemia, and hypertension with associated obesity (DeHert, Schreurs, Vancampfort, & Winkel, 2009; Shirzadi & Ghaemi, 2006). Regular monitoring of abdominal obesity and fasting blood glucose has been shown to be a cost-effective screening test to detect patients at high risk for cardiovascular morbidity (Straker et al., 2005). Counselling regarding nutrition and healthy lifestyle choices (e.g., smoking cessation, physical exercise) is paramount with these patients.

Monitoring for Drug Interactions. Although using lithium alongside antipsychotic medications is common practice, particularly in cases of acute mania or hypomania (Stovall, 2016), caution must be used. A few patients taking haloperidol and lithium have experienced an encephalopathic syndrome, followed by irreversible brain damage (Boora, Xu, & Hyatt, 2008). Lithium may interact similarly with other antipsychotic agents. It may also prolong the effects of neuromuscular blocking agents. Use of nonsteroidal anti-inflammatory drugs may increase plasma lithium levels. Diuretics and angiotensin-converting enzyme inhibitors should be prescribed cautiously with lithium, which is excreted through the kidney.

TEACHING POINTS

- Encourage the patient to discuss the side effect profiles of the medications planned. Seek patient's input on his/her level of tolerance for the side effects. If necessary, negotiate for a medication with a different side effect profile but comparable efficacy. Once a medication regimen has been decided upon, advise the patient to take medications as prescribed. Reevaluate regularly and renegotiate as needed.

- Determine whether the patient has sufficient resources to purchase and obtain medications. Explore provincial medication plans for those on social assistance.

- Have the patient write down the prescribed medication and time of administration.

- Explain the target symptom for each medication (e.g., psychosis and mood for atypical antipsychotic agents, mood for antidepressant and mood stabilizer drugs).

- Caution patients about orthostatic hypotension and instruct them to get up slowly from a lying or sitting position. Also advise them to maintain adequate fluid intake.

(Continued)

- Advise patients to contact their case coordinators or health care providers immediately if they experience dramatic changes in body temperature (neuroleptic malignant syndrome), inability to control motor movement (dystonia), or dizziness.
- Advise patients to maintain a relationship with a primary health care provider for regular monitoring of general health and wellness.
- Advise patients to avoid over-the-counter medications unless their primary health care provider is consulted.
- Advise patients taking olanzapine and clozapine to monitor body weight and report any rapid weight gain.
- Advise patients to report symptoms of diabetes mellitus (frequent urination, excessive thirst, etc.).

Psychological Domain

Assessment

The level of insight experienced by patients into their illnesses may play a role in the course and treatment of schizoaffective disorder. Patients with schizoaffective disorder tend to have better insight than those with schizophrenia (Pini, Cassano, Dell'Osso, & Amador, 2001). Stressors should be evaluated because they may trigger symptoms. Uncovering or exploratory techniques that may reveal, for example, past episodes of abuse should generally be avoided. During periods of psychosis or profound depression, mental status and reality contact may be compromised. Assessment of anxiety level or reactions to stressful situations is important because the combination of these symptoms with psychosis increases the patient's risk for suicide. Discussing the experience of the illness in the patient's life is also crucial. Understanding the symptoms and their sequelae from the patient's point of view will greatly facilitate the satisfactory engagement in planning for wellness and recovery.

Nursing Diagnoses for Psychological Domain

In schizoaffective disorder, individuals vacillate between mood dysregulation and disturbed thinking. Typical nursing diagnoses for this domain include hopelessness, powerlessness, *ineffective coping,* and *low self-esteem.*

Interventions for Psychological Domain

Using appropriate interpersonal modalities is important to help the patient, family, and social and vocational support networks cope with the onslaught of acute episodes and recuperative periods. Patients with schizoaffective disorder have fewer awareness deficits than do patients with schizophrenia. Structured, integrated, and problem-solving psychotherapeutic interventions should be used to develop or increase the patient's insight.

BOX 21.1 Psychoeducation Checklist

SCHIZOAFFECTIVE DISORDER

When caring for the patient with schizoaffective disorder, be sure to include the caregiver as appropriate and address the following topic areas in the teaching plan:

- Psychopharmacologic agents (antipsychotic or antidepressants), if used, including drug action, dosage, frequency, and possible adverse effects
- Methods to enhance adherence
- Sleep measures
- Consistent routines
- Goal setting
- Nutrition
- Support networks
- Problem-solving
- Positive coping strategies
- Social and vocational skills training

Psychoeducational interventions can help to decrease symptoms, enhance recognition of early regression, and hone psychosocial skills (see Boxes 21.1 and 21.2).

The collaborative development of a crisis plan or a "wellness" plan when individuals are able to do so can help patients identify triggers and prodromal symptoms of decompensation and allow them to preplan coping mechanisms and ways to engage supports to mitigate the effects of illness (Copeland, 2005). Such plans have been well researched in the United Kingdom and have been shown to decrease the need for involuntary hospitalization (Papageorigiou, King, Jonhohamed, Davison, & Dawson, 2002; Sutherby et al., 1999). Evidence from a Manitoba study suggests that facilitating patients in planning their community care through the use of a Wellness Planner (including crisis planning and personal goal setting) can increase their sense of empowerment and improve their quality of life (Marchinko & Clarke, 2011).

Social Domain

Assessment

Social dysfunction is common in patients with a diagnosis of schizoaffective disorder. Premorbid adjustment, such as marital status and adolescent social adjustment, may influence both patients' level of functioning at the time of diagnosis and their prognoses. Assessment of social skill deficits and problems with interpersonal conflicts should be made. Assessment of an adult patient's childhood may provide clues to the patient's current level of social functioning. Assess the patient's use of fantasy and fighting as a means of coping. Patients who report the most severe peer rejection present with the angriest dispositions and display antisocial behaviours.

BOX 21.2

THERAPEUTIC DIALOGUE

Ms. B's "Delusions"

Ineffective Communication

Nurse: Hello, Ms. B. What has been happening?
Patient: The guy from the bank keeps me up all night.
Nurse: That's not possible.
Patient: He's there all the time to look after me.
Nurse: No, he's not. You just think that.
Patient: No, he really is. He is helping me.
Nurse: He does not even know who you are.

Effective Communication

Nurse: Hello, Ms. B. How have you been?
Patient: That guy from the bank is really bothering me.
Nurse: What is happening?
Patient: He keeps me up all night. I go out in the street to yell at him.
Nurse: Have you actually seen him at night?
Patient: No, but I know he is there.
Nurse: Can he be there when you cannot see him?
Patient: I guess he can't.
Nurse: Does it seem that the thoughts about him come from your mind?
Patient: This might be.
Nurse: Your illness often causes thoughts that are not based in reality.
Patient: It seems real but yet so unreal. Those are sort of stupid thoughts.

Critical Thinking Challenge

- How could the nurse's approach in the first scenario have prevented development of a therapeutic relationship?
- How can the second scenario benefit the patient in developing insight into her delusions?
- Discuss the differences between the two approaches.

Nursing Diagnoses for Social Domain

Because of their mood and thought disturbances, these individuals will have significant problems in the social domain. Typical nursing diagnoses include *compromised family coping*, *impaired home maintenance*, and *social isolation*.

Interventions for Social Domain

Social skills training is useful for remediating social deficits and may result in positive social adjustment. Support for independent maintenance of daily activities is crucial (Milbourn, McNamara, & Buchanan,

2015). Positive results include improved interpersonal competence, decreased symptom severity, and personal empowerment leading to recovery (Kurtz & Maeser, 2008). Help in identifying feelings and developing realistic goals, along with supportive therapy, can integrate insight into the disease process. Engaged and collaborative crisis planning between the patient and the mental health care provider can help the patient and family recognize oncoming decompensation and take appropriate steps to improve coping. Education focusing on conflict–resolution skills, promoting compromise, negotiation, and expression of negative feelings can help the patient achieve positive social adjustment. Social skills can be improved through role-playing and assertiveness training. Supportive, nurturing, and nonconfrontational interventions help to minimize anxiety and improve understanding (see Box 21.2).

Helping the patient to develop coping skills is essential. Teach communication skills to decrease conflicts and environmental negativity. Memory is linked with development of social skills; psychotic symptoms may interfere with retention of these skills, resulting in slower learning. These patients require long-term, intensive social training. Cognitive–behavioural therapy (CBT) has been demonstrated to be useful for individuals living with psychotic illness and a trial of CBT is recommended in the UK-based National Institute for Health and Care Excellence (NICE) guidelines for management of psychosis and schizophrenia in adults (Bird et al., 2010; Dickerson & Lehman, 2011; Kuipers, Yesufu-Udechuku, Taylor, & Kendall, 2014).

Families are at risk for ineffective coping. Family members face many of the same issues faced by families of patients with schizophrenia and are often puzzled by the patient's emotional overreaction to normal daily stresses. Frequent arguments may lead to verbal and physical abuse.

Spiritual Domain

As with persons living with schizophrenia, the spiritual domain of care is very significant for persons living with schizoaffective disorder (see Chapter 20). With schizoaffective disorder more than with schizophrenia, the person is likely to experience emotional turmoil that is seriously disruptive to a sense of serenity the person may have achieved. Spiritual nursing care can support patients particularly in times of despair. Finding meaningful ways to cope with such a serious illness, one that often brings social rejection and isolation, becomes a life challenge. Religious or spiritual beliefs may be a comfort, and a relationship with the sacred through ritual, prayer, or other activities may offer daily comfort. Mindfulness-based strategies may also be of significant benefit (Guadiano, 2005).

Spiritual support should be understood as an ongoing need. The nurse also needs to strive to understand the potential impact of other symptoms, such as hallucinations and delusions, on spiritual needs and to assist persons with schizoaffective disorder to engage in spiritual activities that are satisfying to them.

Evaluation and Treatment Outcomes

Teaching skills to patients with schizoaffective disorder often takes longer than teaching other patients. The nurse evaluating progress related to interventions must be patient if outcomes are not completely met. Psychoeducation results in increased knowledge of the illness and treatment, increased medication compliance, fewer relapses and hospitalizations, briefer inpatient stays, increased social function, decreased family tension, and lighter family burdens (Bartholomeusz & Allot, 2012). Maintain realistic outcomes and praise small successes to promote positive outcomes (Fig. 21.2).

Continuum of Care

Inpatient Focus Care

Hospitalization may be required during acute psychotic episodes or when suicidal ideations are present. This structured environment protects the patient from self-harm (i.e., suicidal, assaultive, financial, legal, vocational, or social) (Jensen & Clough, 2016). During periods of acute psychosis, offering reassurance in a soft, nonthreatening voice and avoiding confrontational stances within a context of trauma-informed care (Corbin, Rich, Bloom, Delgado, Rich, Wilson, 2011) will help the patient begin to trust the staff and nursing care (see Chapter 6). Avoid seclusion and restraint and keep environmental stimulation to a minimum. Use the patient's coping capabilities to reinforce constructive aspects of functioning and enable a return to autonomy. If the patient has advance directives, adhere to the patient's wishes as much as possible.

Family Intervention

Helping families support the patient at home or in a community placement is an integral part of nursing care. With the patient's permission, key family members can be included in home visits to learn about symptoms, medications, and side effects. By collaborating with family members, the nurse can strengthen the patient's willingness to follow treatment, monitor symptoms, and continue with rehabilitation and recovery. Families should be encouraged to seek out self-help support groups in the community- and/or family-directed psychoeducation programming. Early interventions focused on family members and other individuals in a caregiving role can improve quality of life and reduce distress (Yesufu-Udechuku et al., 2015).

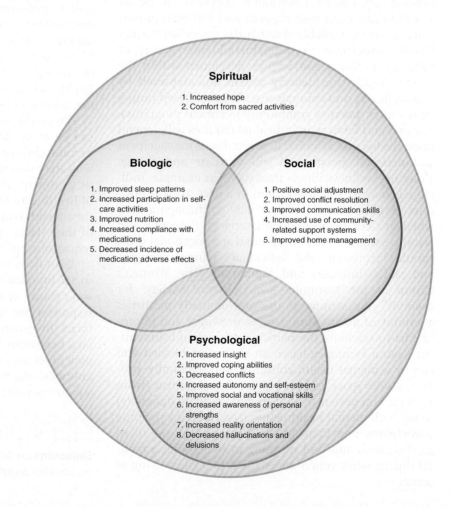

Figure 21.2. Bio/psycho/social/spiritual outcomes for patients with schizoaffective disorder.

EMERGENCY CARE

Emergency care may be needed during symptom exacerbation. Psychosis, mood disturbance, and medication-related adverse effects account for most emergency situations. During an exacerbation of psychosis, patients may become agitated or aggressive. Assaultive behaviour can be managed by using therapeutic techniques (see Chapter 18) and pharmacologic management. If medications are used, benzodiazepines such as lorazepam are usually given. Patients are then evaluated for antipsychotic therapy. Possible medication-related adverse effects include NMS as a reaction to dopamine antagonists or serotonin intoxication, especially if the patient is taking an atypical antipsychotic agent and a selective serotonin reuptake inhibitor (see Chapter 12). Suicidality (ideation and intent) must always be assessed (Clarke, Brown, & Giles-Smith, 2008) (see Chapter 19).

Community Care Within a Recovery Framework

Although this illness is episodic and chronic, within the framework of recovery, patients must be supported along their journey to becoming the best, most fulfilled persons they can be. Community supports can be on a continuum from peer support and self-help groups (such as those available through the Canadian Mental Health Association or the Schizophrenia Society of Canada) to clinics and services developed within the mental health care delivery system and delivered by mental health professionals (e.g., hospital-based outpatient clinics, assertive community treatment programs). The care and services an individual requires will depend upon the balance achieved between illness management and personal growth and will fluctuate and change along the wellness/illness trajectory. For example, individuals may be able to function in a peer support position, helping others, but then may go through a time when in need of peer support services. Programs and resources that foster building social and vocational skills should incorporate the individual's natural strengths and skills, interests, and aspirations. The Women's Group at the Manitoba Schizophrenia Society, for example, runs writing groups and annually publishes a volume of poetry, short stories, drawings, and photographs to celebrate the participants' accomplishments. Art Beat, a Winnipeg-based art studio established and run by a mental health consumer and his family, provides studio space and support for aspiring artists (from painters and potters to weavers and jewellery designers) living with mental health issues (see Web Links). Some participants find their artistic expression allows them to cope with and find meaning in living with a mental illness, while others are enabled to make a living as artists.

■ DELUSIONAL DISORDER

Delusional disorders rarely bring an individual to the attention of mental health care providers. As such, they are not well studied in a systematic manner (Ibanez-Casa & Cervilla, 2012). The person with a **delusional disorder** is more likely to be encountered in a medical–surgical rather than a psychiatric setting. As this disorder often remains undiagnosed, nurses practising in nonpsychiatric settings need to be able to recognize and understand it in order for meaningful care to be provided.

Clinical Course

Delusional disorder is a psychotic disorder characterized by nonbizarre, logical, stable, and well-systemized delusions that occur in the absence of other psychiatric symptoms. Delusions are false, fixed beliefs (not in keeping with one's culture) and unchanged by reasonable arguments. Although delusions are a symptom of many psychotic disorders, in delusional disorder, the delusions typically are nonbizarre delusions; that is, they are characterized by adherence to possible situations that could occur in real life and are plausible in the context of the person's ethnic and cultural background. More rare are **bizarre delusions** that are clearly implausible and are not derived from ordinary life experiences (APA, 2013).

Examples of real-life situations include being followed, poisoned, infected, loved at a distance, or deceived by a spouse or lover. A diagnosis of delusional disorder is based on the presence of one or more nonbizarre delusions for at least 1 month, nor attributed to other psychiatric disorders (Sadock, Sadock, & Ruiz, 2015). Delusions are the primary symptom of this disorder, and other psychotic features are not typically seen.

The course of delusional disorder is variable. Onset can be acute, or the disorder can occur gradually and become chronic. Patients with this disorder usually live with their delusions for years, rarely receiving psychiatric treatment. They are seldom brought to the attention of health care providers unless their delusion relates to their health (somatic delusion), or they act on the basis of their delusion and violate legal or social rules. Full remissions can be followed by relapses.

Apart from the direct impact of the delusion, psychosocial functioning is not markedly impaired. The person's clarity of thinking and behaviour and emotional responses are usually consistent with the delusional focus. In general, behaviour is not odd or bizarre. In fact, behaviour is remarkably normal, except when the patient focuses on the delusion. At that time, thinking, attitudes, and mood may change abruptly and the person focuses on the delusional concern (APA, 2013).

KEY CONCEPT

Delusions are false, fixed beliefs unchanged by reasonable arguments.

Clinical Features

Delusional disorder is characterized by the presence of nonbizarre delusions, which can be of various forms such as a belief that one is being persecuted, or loved by a celebrity, or that one's partner is unfaithful, or that one has a serious disease despite proof otherwise. (See below for subtypes.) A patient who has met criterion A for schizophrenia does not receive a diagnosis of delusional disorder (see Chapter 20 for criterion A). See the DSM-5 for the APA diagnostic criteria for delusional disorder and the various forms of delusions.

If mood episodes occur with this disorder, the total duration of the mood episode is relatively brief compared with the total duration of the delusional period. The delusion is not caused by the direct physiologic effects of substances (i.e., cocaine, amphetamines, marijuana) nor by a general medical condition (i.e., Alzheimer's disease, systemic lupus erythematosus). Because delusional disorder is uncommon and possesses features that are characteristic of other illnesses, the differential diagnosis has a clear-cut logic. It is a diagnosis of exclusion requiring careful evaluation. Distinguishing this disorder from schizophrenia and depressive disorders with psychotic features or bipolar disorder is difficult (APA, 2013).

The prevalence of delusional disorder is estimated to be about 0.2% to 0.3% within the general population with the most common subtype being persecutory (Sadock et al., 2015). It is a rare disease even in psychiatric samples. Research data are limited because numbers of recorded case studies and participants are small, and the studies lack systematic description, assessment, and diagnosis.

Subtypes

Erotomanic Delusions

The **erotomanic delusion**, also known as de Clérambault syndrome, is characterized by the belief that the patient is loved intensely by the "loved object," who is usually married, of a higher socioeconomic status, or otherwise unattainable. Patients believe that the loved object's position in life would be in jeopardy if their true feelings were known. In addition, they are convinced that they are in amorous communication with the loved object. The loved object is often a public figure (e.g., movie star, politician) but may also be a common stranger. The patient may have minimal or no contact with the loved object and often keeps the delusion secret, but efforts to contact the loved object through letters, telephone calls, gifts, visits, surveillance, and stalking are also common. The patient may in many cases transfer his or her delusion to another loved object. Clinical patients are mostly women who do not usually act out their delusions. Men may more often come into contact with the law in their pursuit of the loved object or in a misguided effort to rescue the loved object from some imagined danger. This disorder is difficult to control, contain, or treat. Orders of protection are generally ineffective, and criminal charges of stalking or harassment that lead to incarceration are ineffective as a long-term solution to the problem (Petherick, 2013). The result is repeated arrests and psychiatric examinations, followed by ineffective treatment. Patients are rarely motivated to seek psychiatric treatment.

Grandiose Delusions

Patients presenting with a **grandiose delusion** are convinced they have a great, unrecognized talent or have made an important discovery. A less common presentation is the delusion of a special relationship with a prominent person (i.e., an adviser to the Prime Minister) or of actually being a prominent person (i.e., the Prime Minister). In the latter case, the person with the delusion may regard the actual prominent person as an impostor. Other grandiose delusions may be religious in nature, such as a delusional belief that he or she has a special message from a deity (APA, 2013).

Jealous Delusions

The **jealous delusion** is focused on the unfaithfulness or infidelity of a spouse or lover. The belief arises from "evidence" that cannot stand up to scrutiny, such as a smile at a stranger or spots on sheets. The delusional individual may try to gather further proof by following the loved one or by investigating the imagined lover, prior to a confrontation regarding the infidelity (APA, 2013).

Delusions of jealousy are difficult to treat and may diminish only with separation, divorce, or the death of the spouse or lover. Except in the elderly, such patients generally are male. Jealousy is a powerful, potentially dangerous emotion. Aggression, even violent behaviour, may result. Litigious behaviour is common, and symptoms with forensic aspects are often seen. Care is essential in determining how to work with these patients (Sadock et al., 2015).

Persecutory Delusions

Persons with a **persecutory delusion** believe that they are the focus of some treachery, whether it be a scheme to cheat, trick, or obstruct them or one to malign or physically injure them. They may attempt to seek justice through the police, the courts, or government and/or take action on their own and behave violently to those whom they believe are persecuting them. The course may be chronic, although the patient's preoccupation with the delusional belief often waxes and wanes.

Somatic Delusions

Somatic delusions involve bodily sensations. These patients believe they have physical ailments or bodily deformities. The delusion occurs in the absence of other medical or psychiatric conditions. Somatic delusions are manifested in the following beliefs (Munro, 1999):

- A foul odour is coming from the skin, mouth (delusions of halitosis), rectum, or vagina.
- Insects have infested the skin (delusional parasitosis).

- Internal parasites have infested the digestive system.
- A certain body part is misshapen or ugly (contrary to visible evidence).
- Parts of the body are not functioning (e.g., large intestine, bowels).

The delusion of infestation by insects cannot occur without sensory perceptions, which constitute tactile hallucinations. The patient vividly describes crawling, itching, burning, swarming, and jumping on the skin surface or below the skin. The patient maintains the conviction that he or she is infested with parasites in the absence of objective evidence to the contrary.

Patients with somatic delusions present a dilemma for health care systems because of their excessive use of health care resources. They seek repeated medical consultations with dermatologists, entomologists, infectious disease specialists, and general practitioners, but they refuse psychiatric referral. Studies of somatic delusions have been marred by methodologic uncertainties, and factors limiting investigation include rarity of the disease, lack of contact with psychiatrists, and noncompliance with the medication regimen. A differential diagnosis of delirium or a major neurocognitive disorder must be ruled out (APA, 2013). A variant of the somatic subtype is body dysmorphic disorder, which is classified under Obsessive–Compulsive and Related Disorders in the *Diagnostic and Statistical Manual of Mental Disorders*, 5th ed. (*DSM-5*).

Unspecified Delusions

In the mixed subtype, no one delusional theme predominates, and the patient presents with two or more types of delusions. In the unspecified subtype, the delusional beliefs cannot be clearly determined, or the predominant delusion is not described as a specific type. There may be feelings of depersonalization and derealization or negative-associated paranoid features. The delusions can be short-lived, recurrent, or persistent. This subtype also includes delusions of **misidentification** (i.e., illusions of doubles), also known as Capgras syndrome, wherein a familiar person is replaced by an impostor. For example, the patient may believe that close family members have assumed the persona of strangers or that people they know can change into other people at will. This type of delusion occurs rarely and has been found to be associated with acute psychosis with rapid onset (Salvatore et al., 2014).

Shared Delusional Disorder

Shared delusional disorder (or folie à deux) is an occasionally seen phenomenon where the delusional ideas of one individual (the primary) are transferred to another individual (the secondary) living in close proximity. Most common associations are between adult siblings (typically female) living together, for example, parent/offspring, or sibling/sibling, followed closely by husband/wife pairings (Arnone, Patel, & Tan, 2006; Jolfaei, Isfahani, & Bidaki, 2011). Social isolation can be a contributing factor. This diagnosis does not appear in the *DSM-5*; rather, *delusional symptoms in partner of individual with delusional disorder* is noted in the "other specified" category (APA, 2013).

Epidemiology and Risk Factors

Delusional disorder is relatively uncommon in clinical settings (APA, 2013). The best estimate of its prevalence in the population is about 0.03%, but precise information is lacking (APA, 2013). Lifetime morbidity is between 0.05% and 0.1% because of the late age of onset. Few risk factors are associated with delusional disorder. Patients can live with their delusions without psychiatric intervention because their behaviour is normal, although if delusions are somatic, patients risk unnecessary medical interventions. Acting on delusions carries a risk for intervention by law enforcement agencies or the legal system. Suicide attempts are neither more nor less common than in the general population (Grunebaum et al., 2001).

Age of Onset

Delusional disorder can begin in adolescence and occurs in middle to later adulthood. Onset occurs at a later age than among patients with schizophrenia. A prevalence of 2% to 4% has been reported in the elderly (APA, 2013).

Gender

Gender does not appear to affect the overall frequency of most delusional disorders, although men present with more severe symptoms and worse functionality (Portugal et al., 2010). Patients with erotomanic delusions are generally women; in forensic settings, most people with this disorder are men. Men also tend to experience more jealous delusions, except in the elderly population, in which women outnumber men (APA, 2013).

Ethnicity and Culture

A person's ethnic, cultural, and religious background must be considered in evaluating the presence of delusional disorder. The content of delusions varies between cultures and subcultures, as culture provides a framework for people's "bizarre and extraordinary experiences" (Jacobson & Tarraza, 2013, p. 199).

Family

No increased risk due to familial and genetic factors is known.

Aetiology

The cause of delusional disorder is unknown. The only major feature of this condition is the formation and persistence of the delusions. Possible neurophysiologic and neuropsychological causes of delusional disorder have not been extensively researched, and theories of causation are contradictory. Delusional beliefs have been considered as dysfunctional extremes of cognitive and emotional mechanisms with adaptive significance but lacking in flexibility. This hypothesis places delusions on a continuum with "normalcy" and as a possible function of high vigilance toward threat and a search for safety (Abdel-Hamid & Brüne, 2008). No social theories of causation are addressed in the literature.

Possible medical reasons for delusions, especially in cases of sudden onset, need to be carefully ruled out. Disorders of the basal ganglia, toxic–metabolic conditions, dementias, and substance-related disorders can produce delusions in some persons (Sadock et al., 2015).

Biologic Theories

Neuropathologic

In patients with delusional disorder, MRIs show a degree of temporal lobe asymmetry. However, these differences are subtle and delusional disorder may involve a neurodegenerative component (Ota et al., 2003), most likely located in the right hemisphere (Colheart, 2010). The tactile hallucinations of somatic delusions may arise from sensory alterations in the nervous system (Abdel-Hamid & Brüne, 2008) or from sensory input that has been misinterpreted because of subtle cortical changes associated with aging.

Genetic and Biochemical

Delusional disorder is probably biologically distinct from other psychotic disorders, yet little or no attention has been paid to genetic factors. Delusions may involve faulty processing of essentially intact perceptions, whereby perceptions become linked with an interpretation that has deep emotional significance but no verifiable basis (Conway et al., 2002; McGuire, Junginger, Adams, Burright, & Donovick, 2001). Alternately, a complex, malfunctioning dopaminergic system may lead to delusions (Morimoto et al., 2002). This explanation could lead to the argument that a particular delusion depends on the "circuit" that is malfunctioning. Denial of reality has been linked to right posterior cortical dysfunction. Some authors have proposed a combination of biologic and early life experiences as aetiologic components (Bentall, Corcoran, Howard, Blackwood, & Kinderman, 2001).

Interprofessional Treatment

Few, if any, interdisciplinary treatments are associated with delusional disorder because patients rarely receive attention from health care providers. Pharmacologic intervention is often based on symptoms. For example, patients with somatic delusions are treated for the specific complaints with which they present. Use of benzodiazepines may be common with this disorder because complaints are vague.

Priority Care Issues

By the time a patient with a diagnosis of delusional disorder is seen in a psychiatric setting, he or she generally has had the delusion for a long time. It is deeply ingrained and many times unshakable, even with psychopharmacologic intervention. These patients rarely comply with medication regimens.

Male patients who have the erotomanic subtype are likely to require special care because they are more likely than other patients to act on their delusions (e.g., by continued attempts to contact the loved object or by stalking). This group is generally seen in forensic settings.

Nursing Management: Human Response to Delusional Disorder

Biologic Domain

Assessment

Body systems are assessed to evaluate any physical problems. In people with somatic delusional disorder, assessment may be difficult because of the number and variety of presenting symptoms. Complaints are explored to develop a complete symptom history and to determine whether symptoms have a physical basis or are delusional. Past history of each symptom should be determined because this information may affect outcome. The more recent the onset is, the more favourable the prognosis.

Most patients who receive diagnoses of delusional disorder do not experience functional difficulties or impairments. Self-care patterns may be disrupted in patients with the somatic subtype by the elaborate processes used to treat perceived illness (e.g., bathing rituals, creams). Sleep may be disrupted because of the central and overpowering nature of the delusions.

A complete medication history, past and present, is also important to determine the patient's past response and what agents the individual perceives as effective. Examining the patient's records for tests and procedures may help to substantiate the individual's symptoms.

Nursing Diagnoses for the Biologic Domain

The nursing diagnoses for the biologic domain depend on the type of delusions that are manifested and the response to these symptoms. For example, for a woman with the somatic delusion that insects are crawling on her, *disturbed sensory perception (tactile)* would be appropriate. For others who are fearful of poisoning, *imbalanced nutrition, less than body requirements*, may be a useful diagnosis. Refusal of all medication may support a nursing diagnosis of *ineffective therapeutic regimen management*.

Interventions for Biologic Domain

Interventions are based on the problems identified during assessment (Fig. 21.3) and addressed individually. The nurse helps the patient to establish routines that can resolve problems and promote healthy functioning. A mechanism for managing the patient's medication regimen is developed.

Somatic Interventions

Treating somatic disorder is difficult because of the patient's insistence that the problem is not psychiatrically related. Realistic and modest goals are most

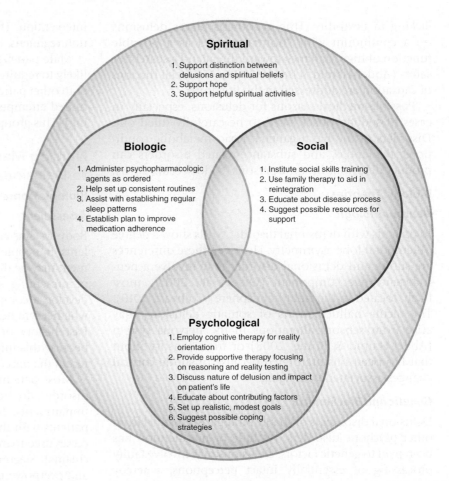

Spiritual
1. Support distinction between delusions and spiritual beliefs
2. Support hope
3. Support helpful spiritual activities

Biologic
1. Administer psychopharmacologic agents as ordered
2. Help set up consistent routines
3. Assist with establishing regular sleep patterns
4. Establish plan to improve medication adherence

Social
1. Institute social skills training
2. Use family therapy to aid in reintegration
3. Educate about disease process
4. Suggest possible resources for support

Psychological
1. Employ cognitive therapy for reality orientation
2. Provide supportive therapy focusing on reasoning and reality testing
3. Discuss nature of delusion and impact on patient's life
4. Educate about contributing factors
5. Set up realistic, modest goals
6. Suggest possible coping strategies

Figure 21.3. Bio/psycho/social/spiritual interventions for patients with delusional disorder.

sensible. Establishing a therapeutic relationship is a goal for which to strive.

Pharmacologic Interventions

The literature available about using psychiatric medications in delusional disorder is sparse, and the available reports conflict. Antipsychotic agents are useful in improving acute symptoms by decreasing agitation and the intensity of the delusion. They may also be effective in the long term, but little formal information exists to support this theory.

Administering and Monitoring Medications

Patients often do not adhere to medication regimens and require monitoring of target symptoms. Look for an opportunity to discuss medications and to identify issues the patient may have with them.

Managing Side Effects

Management of side effects is similar to that in other disorders that have a delusional component. The nurse assesses for neuroleptic malignant syndrome, extrapyramidal side effects, weight gain, and sedation.

Monitoring for Drug Interactions

Interactions are similar to those seen with medications for other disorders. A detailed list of prior and current medications must be elicited from patients, especially those with somatic delusions, because they may be receiving medications from several practitioners.

Psychological Domain

Assessment

Patients with delusional disorder show few, if any, psychological deficits, and those that do occur are generally related directly to the delusion. Use of the Minnesota Multiphasic Personality Inventory, a clinical scale that identifies paranoid symptom deviation, may be useful in substantiating the diagnosis.

Mental status is not generally affected. Thinking, orientation, affect, attention, memory, perception, and personality are generally intact. Presenting reality-based evidence in an attempt to change the person's delusion can be helpful in determining whether the belief can be altered with sufficient evidence. If mental status is altered, this fact is generally brought to the health professional's attention by a third party, such as a family member, neighbour, physician, the police, or attorney. In these cases, the person usually has acted in some manner that draws attention to himself or herself. Talk with the person to grasp the nature of the delusional thinking: its theme, impact on the person's life, complexity, systematization, and related features.

Nursing Diagnosis for Psychological Domain

Numerous nursing diagnoses could be generated based on the assessment of the psychological domain. *Ineffective denial, impaired verbal communication, deficient knowledge,* and *risk for loneliness* are some examples. Nursing diagnoses of *disturbed self-concept, disturbed self-esteem,* anxiety, *fear,* and powerlessness may also be generated.

TEACHING POINTS

Patients may need help and information in order to take the medication as prescribed. Determine whether the patient has sufficient resources to purchase and obtain medications and explain target symptoms for each medication. Caution patients not to take over-the-counter medications without consulting their provider.

Interventions for Psychological Domain

Patients with delusional disorder are treated most effectively in outpatient settings with supportive therapy that allays the person's anxiety. Initiating discussion of the troubling experiences and consequences of the delusion and suggesting a means for coping may be successful. Assisting the person toward a more satisfying general adjustment is desirable (see Box 21.3).

Insight-oriented therapy is not useful because there is no benefit in trying to prove the delusion is not true, arguing the person out of the delusion, or telling the individual that the delusion is imaginary. Cognitive therapy with supportive therapy that focuses on

---

BOX 21.3 Psychoeducation Checklist

DELUSIONAL DISORDER

When caring for the patient with delusional disorder, be sure to include the caregiver, as appropriate, and address the following topic areas in the teaching plan:

- Psychopharmacologic agents (antipsychotic or antidepressants), if used, including drug action, dosage, frequency, and possible adverse effects
- Identification of troubling experiences
- Consequences of delusions
- Realistic goal setting
- Positive coping strategies
- Safety measures
- Social training skills
- Family participation in therapy

reasoning or reality testing to decrease delusional thinking, or modifying the delusion itself, may be helpful (see Chapter 13). Educational interventions can aid the patient in understanding how factors such as sensory impairment, social and physical isolation, and stress contribute to the intensity of this disorder.

In certain instances, hospitalization is needed in response to dangerous behaviour that could include aggressiveness, poor impulse control, excessive psychological tension, unremitting anger, and threats. If hospitalization is required, the person needs to be approached tactfully. Legal assistance may be necessary (Reid, 2005).

Suicide can be a concern, but most patients are not at risk. A British interview study with nurses identified as having expertise in working with acutely psychotic patients found that the nurses emphasized the importance of being respectfully attentive and supportive to these patients, including determining how their psychotic symptoms were affecting their emotions, functioning, and experiences. The nurses described the need to be empathetic, engage the patient in ordinary conversation when possible, and help them focus on the here and now. When necessary, it should be gently acknowledged that the patient's delusional ideas are not shared by the care team (Bowers, Brennan, Winship, & Theodoridou, 2009).

Social Domain

Assessment

A common characteristic of individuals with delusional disorder is normal behaviour and appearance unless their delusional ideas are being discussed or acted on. The cultural background of the person with delusional disorder has to be evaluated. Ethnic and cultural systems have different beliefs that are accepted within their individual context but not outside their group. Problems can occur in social, occupational, or interpersonal areas. In general, the person's social and marital functioning is more likely to be impaired than his or her intellectual or occupational functioning. Most are employed, although generally they hold low-paying jobs. Supportive family members and friends can mean a more positive outcome for the person living with a delusional disorder.

Life difficulties are often related to the delusion; it is important to assess the person's capacity to act in response to it. What is his or her level of impulsiveness (i.e., related to behaviours of suicide, homicide, aggression, or violence)? Uncertainty in assessment can be mitigated by establishing as complete a picture of the person as possible, including his or her subjective experiences and concrete psychopathologic symptoms.

Nursing Diagnoses for the Social Domain

Several nursing diagnoses can be generated from the assessment data for the social domain. Examples are *ineffective coping, interrupted family processes,* and *ineffective role performance.*

Interventions for Social Domain

People with diagnoses of delusional disorder often become socially isolated. The secretiveness of their delusions and the importance the delusions have in their lives are central to this phenomenon. Social skills training tailored to the patient's specific deficits can help to improve social adaptation. Family therapy can help the person reintegrate into the family; family education and patient education will enhance understanding of the patient and the disease process. However, group therapy is usually not beneficial because the patient lacks insight into the origin of the delusion. Families face many of the same issues as families of patients with other disorders involving delusions and are at risk for ineffective coping.

Spiritual Domain

Nurses may hesitate to address the spiritual domain of a person who is experiencing delusional thinking, especially if there are religious overtones to fixed beliefs. This hesitancy may lie in an awareness that another's religious beliefs may seem so different to one's own that they may seem "fixed" and "false." Trying to understand the way a person's religious or spiritual beliefs are being shaped by his or her delusional disorder may seem a daunting task. If the nurse's response, however, is to be as sensitive and receptive as possible to the person's values (as revealed in his or her general behaviour and expression of pleasure and fears as well as by pre-illness choices and goals), then spiritual care may begin. Attending to the person's ultimate need to find meaning in life is what is required. This is grounded in thoughtful caring and attention to "the little things" that matter to the person, as well as through a hopeful, encouraging attitude that may foster hope in the patient (Carr, 2008).

Evaluation and Treatment Outcomes

For patients with delusional disorders, the greater the lack of insight and the poorer the adherence to treatment regimens, the more difficult it is to teach the individual. The patient rarely, if ever, develops full insight, and the symptoms related to the original diagnosis are not likely to disappear completely. In evaluating progress, the nurse must remember that outcomes are often not met completely. The nurse should maintain realistic outcomes and praise small successes to promote positive outcomes (Fig. 21.4).

Continuum of Care

Inpatient Focus Care

Hospitalization rarely occurs and is usually precipitated by legal or social violations. It is important to avoid confrontational situations; use the patient's coping abilities

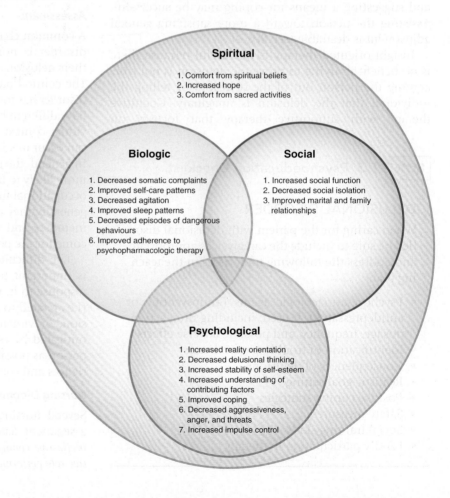

Figure 21.4. Bio/psycho/social/spiritual outcomes for patients with delusional disorder.

to reinforce constructive aspects of functioning to enable a return to autonomy.

Family Intervention

Family therapy may be helpful. By helping the family to develop mechanisms to cope with the patient's delusions, nurses help the family to be more supportive and understanding of the patient.

Community Treatment

Patients with diagnosis of delusional disorder are treated most effectively in an outpatient setting. They should be encouraged to seek psychiatric treatment. Medications are not often used with delusional disorder, but antipsychotic agents or benzodiazepines are helpful during exacerbations. Other treatments include supportive therapy, development of coping skills, cognitive therapy, and social skills training. Family therapy may be helpful.

EMERGENCY CARE

Emergency care is seldom required, unless the patient has had an incident with the law or legal system. The patient may be agitated or aggressive because the delusion, which is perceived as real, has been interrupted.

■ OTHER PSYCHOTIC DISORDERS

Other disorders have psychoses as their defining features. The nursing care for patients with these disorders is not discussed specifically, but care used with other disorders can be applied to the disorders presented here.

Schizophreniform Disorder

The essential features of schizophreniform disorder are identical to those of criteria A for schizophrenia, with the exception of the duration of the illness, which is less than that for schizophrenia (see Chapter 20). Some research has suggested that this disorder may be an early manifestation of schizophrenia (van Os et al., 2009). Altered social or occupational functioning may occur but is not necessary. Most patients experience interruption in one or more areas of daily functioning (APA, 2013).

Brief Psychotic Disorder

In brief psychotic disorder, the episode is brief (at least 1 day) but may last up to 1 month. The onset is sudden and includes at least one of the positive symptoms of schizophrenia (see Chapter 20). Although episodes are brief, impairment can be severe, and supervision may be required to protect the person. Suicide is a risk, especially in younger patients. A predisposition to develop a brief psychotic disorder may include pre-existing personality disorders (APA, 2013). The person's ethnic and cultural background should also be considered in relation to the social or religious context of the symptoms presented. This disorder is uncommon but usually appears in early adulthood (Sadock et al., 2015).

Substance-/Medication-Induced Psychotic Disorder

This psychotic disorder involves prominent hallucinations or delusions that are the direct physiologic effects of medication or a substance. This effect is indicated as the symptoms develop during or after intoxication or withdrawal of a substance or after exposure to medication capable of producing the symptoms. The symptoms do not occur exclusively during the course of a delirium and cause clinically significant distress or impairment of functioning (APA, 2013).

Psychotic Disorder Due to Another Medical Condition

Evidence shows that the hallucinations and/or delusions causing clinically significant distress or impairment in functioning are the direct pathophysiologic consequence of another medical condition and are not better explained by another mental disorder or delirium (APA, 2013).

Other Specified Presentations

In the APA diagnostic system, when symptoms characteristic of psychotic disorders cause clinically significant distress or impairment of functioning but do not meet the full criteria of a diagnostic class, they can be designated using *DSM-5* notation as "other specified" (APA, 2013). An example is *persistent auditory hallucinations* that occur without other features.

❖ SUMMARY OF KEY POINTS

- Schizoaffective disorder has symptoms typical of both schizophrenia and depressive disorders and/or bipolar disorders but is a separate disorder. Although these patients experience mood problems most of the time, the diagnosis of schizoaffective disorder depends on the presence of positive symptoms (i.e., delusions or hallucinations) without mood symptoms at some time during the uninterrupted period of illness.

- Although controversy and discussion continue about whether schizoaffective disorder is truly a separate disorder, the *DSM-5* identifies it as separate.

- Patients with schizoaffective disorder have fewer awareness deficits and appear to have more insight than do patients with schizophrenia, a fact that can be used in teaching patients to control symptoms, recognize early regression, and develop psychosocial skills.

- Nursing care for patients with schizoaffective disorder is focused on minimizing psychiatric symptoms through promoting medication maintenance and on helping patients maintain optimal levels of functioning and self-care. Interventions centre on developing social and coping skills through supportive, nurturing, and nonconfrontational approaches. The nurse must be constantly attuned to the mood state of the patient and help the patient learn to solve problems, resolve conflict, and cope with social situations that trigger anxiety.

- Delusional disorder is characterized by stable, well-systematized, and logical nonbizarre delusions that could occur in reality and are plausible in the context of the patient's ethnic and cultural background. These delusions may or may not interfere with an individual's ability to function socially. Patients typically deny any psychiatric basis for their problem and refuse to seek psychiatric care. Patients whose delusions relate to somatic complaints are often seen on medical–surgical units of hospitals. Diagnosis otherwise is often made only when patients act on the basis of their delusions and violate the law or social rules.

- Delusional disorder is further classified as a particular subtype, depending on the nature and content of the patient's delusions, including erotomanic, grandiose, jealous, somatic, mixed, and unspecified.

- Patients with delusional disorder usually do not experience functional difficulties or mental status impairments. Their thinking, orientation, affect, attention, memory, perception, and personality generally remain intact.

- Other psychotic disorders, distinguished particularly by duration of symptoms or specifically identified cause, include schizophreniform disorder, brief psychotic disorder, substance-/medication-induced disorder, and psychotic disorder due to another medical condition.

- The therapeutic relationship is crucial to the successful treatment of the patient with any psychotic disorder. Nurses must be aware of the patient's fragile self-esteem and unusual vulnerabilities and try to establish a trusting relationship through a flexible, nonjudgemental approach that promotes empathy, trust, and support.

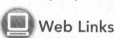 **Web Links**

www.artbeatstudio.ca Art Beat is a Winnipeg-based art studio established by a mental health consumer and his family. The Web site provides examples of the studio's stated vision to "enable consumers of mental health services to engage in artistic expression that promotes recovery, empowerment, and community."

www.mentalhealthcommission.ca/sites/default/files/KEC MHFAPsychosisGuidelines ENG 0 1.pdf Here, readers will find the *Mental Health First Aid Canada Psychosis First Aid Guidelines*. These were developed to help members of the Canadian public assist someone who may be experiencing a psychotic episode until professional help becomes available.

www.mentalhealth.com Internet mental health Web site that provides the American and European description of schizoaffective disorder and its treatment.

www.mentalhealthcommission.ca/sites/default/files/ MHCC RecoveryGuidelines ENG 0.pdf Guidelines for recovery oriented care from the Mental Health Commission of Canada.

cnia.ca/cna-learning-module-de-stigmatizing-practices-and-mental-illness A national training program for nurses and other health care professionals that specifically confront mental health stigma and discrimination in the health care environment: the module is made available from the Canadian Nurses Association in partnership with the Mental Health Commission of Canada and the Mood Disorders Association of Canada.

References

Abdel-Hamid, M., & Brüne, M. (2008). Neuropsychological aspects of delusional disorder. *Current Psychiatry Reports, 10,* 229–234.

American Psychiatric Association. (2013). *Diagnostic and statistical manual of mental disorders* (5th ed.). Washington, DC: Author.

Andreasen, N. C., & Black, W. (2006). *Introductory textbook of psychiatry* (4th ed.). Arlington, VA: American Psychiatric Publishing.

Arnone, D., Patel, A., & Tan, G. M. -Y. (2006). The nosological significance of Folie à Deux: A review of the literature. *Annals of General Psychiatry, 5,* 11. doi:10.1186/1744-859x-5-11

Bartholomeusz, C. F., & Allott, K. (2012). Neurocognitive and social cognitive approaches for improving functional outcome in early psychosis: Theoretical considerations and current state of evidence. *Schizophrenia Research and Treatment, 2012,* 815315. doi:10.1155/2012/815315

Bentall, R. P., Corcoran, R., Howard, R., Blackwood, N., & Kinderman, P. (2001). Persecutory delusions: A review and theoretical integration. *Clinical Psychology Review, 21*(8), 1143–1192.

Bird, V., Premkumar, P., Kendall, T., Whittington, C., Mitchell, J., & Kuipers, E. (2010). Early intervention services, cognitive-behavioural therapy and family intervention in early psychosis: Systematic review. *British Journal of Psychiatry, 197,* 350–356. doi:10.1192/bjp.bp.109.074526

Boora, K., Xu, J., & Hyatt, J. (2008). Encephalopathy with combined lithium-risperidone administration. *Acta Psychiatrica Scandinavia, 117,* 394–395.

Bottender, R., Strauss, A., & Moller, H. J. (2010). Social disability in schizophrenic, schizoaffective, and affective disorder 15 years post first admission. *Schizophrenia Research, 116,* 9–15.

Bowers, L., Brennan, G., Winship, G., & Theodoridou, C. (2009). *Talking with acutely psychotic people: Communication skills for nurses and others spending time with people who are very mentally ill.* London, UK: City University.

Cardno, A. G., & Owen, M. J. (2014). Genetic relationships between schizophrenia, bipolar disorder, and schizoaffective disorder. *Schizophrenia Bulletin, 40*(3), 504–515. doi:10.1093/schbul/sbu016

Carr, T. (2008). Mapping the processes and qualities of spiritual nursing care. *Qualitative Health Research, 18*(5), 686–700.

Cheniaux, E., Landeira-Fernandez, J., Telles, L., Lessa, J., Dias, A., Duncan, T., & Versiani, M. (2008). Does schizoaffective disorder really exist? A systematic review of the studies that compared schizoaffective disorder with schizophrenia or mood disorders. *Journal of Affective Disorders, 106,* 209–217.

Chernomas, W. M., Clarke, D. E., & Chisholm, F. A. (2000). Perspectives of women living with schizophrenia. *Psychiatric Services, 51*(12), 1517–1521.

Chernomas, W., Reiger, K., Karpa, J., Clarke, D., Marchinko, S., & Demczuk, L. (2017). Young women's experiences of psychotic illness. *JBI Database of Systematic Reviews and Implementation Reports, 15*(3), 694–737. doi:10.11124/JBISRIR-2016-002942

Clarke, D., Brown, A. M., & Giles-Smith, L. (2008). Triaging suicidal patients: Sifting through the evidence. *International Emergency Nursing, 16,* 165–174.

Colheart, M. (2010). The neuropsychology of delusions. *Annals of the New York Academy of Medicine, 1189*(Suppl. 1), E1–E15. doi:10.1111/j.1749-6632.2010.05495.x

Conway, C. R., Bollini, A. M., Graham, B. G., Keefe, R. S., Schiffman, S. S., & McEvoy, J. P. (2002). Sensory acuity and reasoning in delusional disorder. *Comprehensive Psychiatry, 43*(3), 175–178.

Copeland, M. (2005). *Community links: Pathways to reconnection and recovery program implementation manual.* Waterbury, VT: Vermont State Department of Mental Health.

Corbin, T. J., Rich, J. A., Bloom, S. L., Delgado, D., Rich, L. J., & Wilson, A. S. (2011). Developing a trauma-informed emergency department-based intervention for victims of urban violence. *Journal of Trauma and Dissociation, 12,* 510–525. doi:10.1080/15299732.2011.593260

Crow, T. J., & Harrington, C. A. (1994). Etiopathogenesis and treatment of psychosis. *Annual Review of Medicine, 45,* 219–234.

DeHert, M., Schreurs, V., Vancampfort, D., & VanWinkel, R. (2009). Metabolic syndrome in people with schizophrenia: A review. *World Psychiatry, 8,* 15–22.

Delphin-Rittman, M. E., Flanagan, E. H., Andres-Hyman, R., Ortiz, J., Amer, M. M., & Davidson, L. (2015). Racial-ethnic differences in access, diagnosis, and outcome in public sector inpatient mental health treatment. *Psychological Services, 12*(2), 158–166.

Dickerson, F. B., & Lehman, A. F. (2011). Evidence-based psychotherapy for schizophrenia. *Journal of Nervous and Mental Disease, 199*(8), 520–526.

Gibson, S., & Brand, S. (2013). Understanding treatment non-adherence in schizophrenia and bipolar mood disorder: A survey of what services users do and why. *BMC Psychiatry, 13,* 153.

Grunebaum, M. F., Oquendo, M. A., Harkavy-Friedman, J. M., Ellis, S. P., Li, S., Haas, G. L., … Mann, J. J. (2001). Delusions and suicidality. *American Journal of Psychiatry, 158*(5), 742–747.

Guadiano, B. A. (2005). Cognitive behavior therapies for psychotic disorders: Current empirical status and future directions. *Clinical Psychology: Science and Practice, 12*(1), 33–50.

Hochberger, J. M., & Lingham, B. (2017). Utilizing Peplau's interpersonal approach to facilitate medication self-management for psychiatric patients. *Archives of Psychiatric Nursing, 31,* 122–124.

Ibanez-Casas, I., & Cervilla, J. A. (2012). Neuropsychological research in delusional disorder: A comprehensive review. *Psychopathology, 45,* 84–101. doi:10.1159/000327899

Jacobson, L., & Tarraza, M. (2013). Integrative management of psychotic symptoms. In K. R. Tusaie & J. J. Fitzpatrick (Eds.), *Advanced practice psychiatric nursing* (pp. 182–229). New York: Springer.

Jensen, L., & Clough, R. (2016). Assessing and treating the patient with acute psychotic disorders. *Nursing Clinics of North America, 51,* 185–197.

Jolfaei, A. G., Isfahani, M. N., & Bidaki, R. (2011). Folie à deux and delusional disorder by proxy in a family. *Journal of Research in Medical Sciences, 16*(Suppl. 1), S453–S455.

Judd, F., Armstrong, S., & Kulkarni, J. (2009). Gender sensitive mental healthcare. *Australasian Psychiatry, 17,* 105–111.

Kasanin, J. (1933). The acute schizo-affective psychoses. *American Journal of Psychiatry, 13,* 97–126.

Kuipers, E., Yesufu-Udechuku, A., Taylor, C., & Kendall, T. (2014). Management of psychosis and schizophrenia in adults: Summary of updated NICE guidelines. *British Medical Journal, 348,* g1173. doi:10.1136/bmj.g1173

Kurtz, M. M., & Maeser, K. T. (2008). A meta-analysis of controlled research on social skills training for schizophrenia. *Journal of Consulting and Clinical Psychology, 76,* 491–504.

Lewine, R. R., Hudgins, P., Brown, F., Caudle, J., & Risch, S. C. (1995). Differences in qualitative brain morphology findings in schizophrenia, major depression, bipolar disorder, and normal volunteers. *Schizophrenia Research, 15*(3), 253–259.

MacDougall, V., Luckett, K., & Jones, M. (2007). Women's experiences of psychosis: Recognition of gendered differences. In R. Velleman, E. Davis, G. Smith, & M. Drage (Eds.), *Changing outcomes in psychosis: Collaborative cases from practitioners, users, and carers* (pp. 117–134). Leicester, UK: Blackwell.

Madre, M., Canales-Rodriguez, E. J., Ortiz-Gil, J., Murru, A., Torrent, C., Bramon, E., … Amann, B. L. (2016). Neuropsychological and neuroimaging underpinnings of schizoaffective disorder: A systematic review. *Acta Psychiatrica Scandinavica, 134*(1), 16–30. doi:10.1111/acps.12564

Malaspina, D., Owen, M. J., Heckers, S., Tandon, R., Bustillo, J., Schultz, S, … Carpenter, W. (2013). Schizoaffective disorder in the DSM-5. *Schizophrenia Research, 150,* 21–25. doi:10.1016/j.schres.2013.04

Marchinko, S., & Clarke, D. (2011). The wellness planner: Empowering consumers in self-care. *Archives of Psychiatric Nursing, 25,* 284–293.

McCarthy-Jones, S., Marriott, M., Knowles, R., Rowse, G., & Thompson, A. R. (2013). What is psychosis? A meta-synthesis of inductive qualitative studies exploring the experience of psychosis. *Psychosis: Psychological, Social and Integrative Approaches, 5,* 1–16.

McGuire, L., Junginger, J., Adams, S. G. Jr., Burright, R., & Donovick, P. (2001). Delusions and delusional reasoning. *Journal of Abnormal Psychology, 110*(2), 259–266.

Milbourn, B., McNamara, B., & Buchanan, A. (2015). The lived experience of everyday activity for individuals with severe mental illness.

Health Sociology Review, 24(3), 270–282. doi:10.1080/14.2015.103474746124

Morimoto, K., Miyatake, R., Nakamura, M., Watanabe, T., Hirao, T., & Suwaki, H. (2002). Delusional disorder: Molecular genetic evidence for dopamine psychosis. *Neuropsychopharmacology, 26*(6), 794–801.

Munro, A. (1999). *Delusional disorder.* Cambridge, MA: Cambridge University Press.

Nasrallah, H. A. (2011). The primary and secondary symptoms of schizophrenia: Current and future management. A bridge to the future; redefining the scientific paradigm in the treatment of schizophrenia. *Current Psychiatry, 10*(Suppl. 9), S4–S9.

Ota, M., Mizukami, K., Katano, T., Sato, S., Takeda, T., & Asada, T. (2003). A case of delusional disorder, somatic type with remarkable improvement of clinical symptoms and single photon emission computed tomography findings following modified electroconvulsive therapy. *Progress in Neuro-Psychopharmacology & Biological Psychiatry, 27*(5), 881–884.

Papageorigiou, A., King, M., Jonhohamed, A., Davison, D., & Dawson, J. (2002). Advanced directives for patients compulsorily admitted to hospital with serious mental illness. *British Journal of Psychiatry, 181,* 513–519.

Perr, I. N. (1992). Religion, political leadership, charisma, and mental illness: The strange story of Louis Riel. *Journal of Forensic Sciences, 37*(2), 574–884.

Petherick, W. (2013). *Profiling and serial crime* (3rd ed.). Philadelphia, PA: Elsevier Inc.

Pini, S., Cassano, G. B., Dell'Osso, L., & Amador, X. F. (2001). Insight into illness in schizophrenia, schizoaffective disorder, and mood disorders with psychotic features. *American Journal of Psychiatry, 158*(1), 122–125.

Pompili, M., Lester, D., Dominici, G., Longo, L., Marconi, G., Forte, A., … Girardi, P. (2013). Indications for electroconvulsive treatment in schizophrenia: A systematic review. *Schizophrenia Research, 146*(1–3), 1–9. http://dx.doi.org/10.1016/j.schres.2013.02.005

Portugal, E., Gonzalez, N., Vilaplana, M., Haro, J. M., Usall, J., & Cervilla, J. A. (2010). Gender differences in delusional disorder: Evidence from an outpatient sample. *Psychiatric Research, 177,* 235–239.

Potkin, S. G., Alphs, L., Hsu, C., Krishnan, K., Anand, R., Young, F. K., et al. (2003). Predicting suicidal risk in schizophrenic and schizoaffective patients in a prospective two-year trial. *Biological Psychiatry, 54*(4), 444–452.

Reid, W. (2005). Delusional disorder and the law. *Journal of Psychiatric Practice, 11*(2), 126–130.

Rowe, R., & Clark, T. (2008). A survey of psychiatrists' attitudes to schizoaffective disorder. *International Journal of Psychiatry in Clinical Practice, 12*(1), 25–30.

Sadock, B. J., Sadock, V. A., & Ruiz, P. (2015). *Kaplan and Sadock's synopsis of psychiatry* (11th ed.). Philadelphia, PA: Wolters Kluwer Health/Lippincott Williams & Wilkins.

Salvatore, P., Bhuvaneswar, C., Tohen, M., Khalsa, H. M., Maggini, C., & Baldessarini, R. J. (2014). Capgras' Syndrome in first episode psychotic disorders. *Psychopathology, 47*(4), 261–269. doi:10.1159/000357813

Seguin, J., Lesage, A., Chawky, N., Guy, A., Daigle, F., Girard, G., & Turecki, G. (2006). Suicide cases in New Brunswick from April, 2002 to May 2003: The importance of better recognizing substance and mood disorder comorbidity. *Canadian Journal of Psychiatry, 51,* 581–586.

Shirzadi, A. A., & Ghaemi, S. N. (2006). Side effects of atypical antipsychotics: Extrapyramidal symptoms and the metabolic syndrome. *Harvard Review of Psychiatry, 14,* 152–164.

Siris, S. G., & Lavin, M. R. (1995). Other psychotic disorders. In H. Kaplan & B. Sadock (Eds.), *Comprehensive textbook of psychiatry* (6th ed.). Baltimore, MD: Williams & Wilkins.

Stovall, J. (2016, December). *Bipolar disorder in adults: Pharmacotherapy for acute mania and hypomania.* UptoDate.

Straker, D., Correll, L. U., Kramer-Ginsberg, E., Abdulhamid, N., Koshy, F., Rubens, E., … Manu, P. (2005). Cost-effective screening for metabolic syndrome in patients treated with second-generation antipsychotic medications. *American Journal of Psychiatry, 162,* 1217–1221.

Sutherby, K., Szmukler, G. I., Halpern, A., Alexander, M., Thornicroft, G., Johnson, C., & Wright, S. (1999). A study of 'crisis cards' in a community psychiatric service. *Acta Psychiatrica Scandinavica, 100,* 56–61.

Van Os, J., Linscott, R. J., Myin-Germeys, I., Delespaul, P., & Krabbendam, L. (2009). A systematic review and meta-analysis of the psychosis continuum: Evidence for a psychosis proneness-persistence-impairment model of psychotic disorder. *Psychological Medicine, 39,* 179–195.

Waite, P. (1987). Between three oceans: Challenges of a continental destiny. In C. Brown (Ed.), *The illustrated history of Canada* (pp. 279–373). Toronto, ON: Lester & Orpen Dennys.

Yesufu-Udechuku, A., Harrison, B., Mayo-Wilson, E., Young, N., Woodhams, P., Shiers, D., … Kendall, T. (2015). Interventions to improve the experience of caring for people with severe mental illness: Systematic review and meta-analysis. *British Journal of Psychiatry, 206,* 2268–2274. doi:10.1192/bjp.bp.114.147561

22 Depressive, Bipolar, and Related Disorders

Carol Rupcich

Adapted from the chapter "Mood Disorders" by Yvonne M. Hayne

LEARNING OBJECTIVES

After studying this chapter, you will be able to:

- Describe the impact of underdiagnosed and untreated mood disorders as a major public health problem.
- Differentiate the clinical characteristics and describe the course of various mood disorders.
- Analyze human responses to mood disorders, distinguishing the experience of symptoms as distinct from the subjective experience of bearing a clinical diagnosis of such a disorder.
- Analyze prevailing biologic, psychological, and social theories, while taking into account spiritual considerations as a basis in caring for patients with mood disorders.
- Identify needs based on the holistic assessment of patients with mood disorders.
- Formulate nursing interventions on a continuum of care for individuals experiencing specific diagnoses of mood disorder.
- Identify expected outcomes and evaluate the response to implementations of care.
- Analyze special concerns within the nurse–patient relationship common to treating people with mood disorders.

KEY TERMS

- affect • bipolar • cyclothymic disorder• depressive episode • dysthymic disorder • euphoria • hypomanic episode • mixed features • rapid cycling • unipolar

KEY CONCEPTS

- mania • mood

The World Health Organization (WHO) (2009) identifies major depression as a serious public health concern and estimates that by the year 2030, it will be the main cause of disease burden globally. Depression not only directly affects a person's quality of life but also impacts the family and society (Lepine & Briley, 2011). A study using mental health data from the 2012 Canadian Community Health Survey indicated that during a 12-month period prior to the survey, 5.4% of Canadians age 15 years and older met the criteria for mood disorder symptoms. In those surveyed, 4.7% indicated major depression and 1.5% reported bipolar disorder. The lifetime rate for a mood disorder in Canadians was estimated at 12.6% (approximately 3.5 million people) with symptoms of depression in 11.3% of the population and bipolar disorder profiles in 2.6% of Canadians. The prevalence of mood disorders was greatest in the group 15 to 24 years of age with females reflecting

significantly higher levels of depression than males (Pearson, Janz, & Ali, 2013). Indeed, studies show that the lifetime rate of major depression is 1.7 to 2.7 times greater in females than in males, with risk increasing especially between adolescence and mid-50s, perhaps triggered by fluctuations in female hormones (Albert, 2015; Bryson, 2012). Reflecting this higher prevalence rate of depression in women, in Canada between 2007 and 2011, women were prescribed antidepressants twice as often as were men (Rotermann, Sanmartin, Hennessy, & Arthur, 2014).

Studies show the connection of depressive disorders with the incidence of chronic conditions such as hypertension, arthritis, back problems, and diabetes (Canadian Mental Health Association, 2008, 2013). Further, "the risk of death by all causes is increased in depressed patients who are twice as likely to die prematurely compared with the general population" (Lepine

& Briley, 2011, p. 5). A major concern is the extent that untreated mood disorders are concurrent with elevated suicide rates. These "premature and preventable" deaths prompted the WHO to declare the necessity of building awareness and improving treatments to stop such dire consequences (WHO, 2006). Caring, connecting, and a holistic perspective, primary tenets of nursing, foster a unique therapeutic context that places the nurse in a key position to prevent suicide through the identification, treatment, and referral of individuals experiencing a mood disorder.

Common features of depressive disorders, and bipolar and related disorders, as described in the fifth edition of the American Psychiatric Association's *Diagnostic and Statistical Manual of Mental Disorders* (*DSM-5*) (APA, 2013), "include the presence of sad, empty, or irritable mood, accompanied by somatic and cognitive changes that significantly affect the individual's capacity to function" (p. 155). In depressive and bipolar-related disorders, mood is the primary alteration rather than thought or perceptual disturbances. Several terms describe **affect**, or the observable expression of mood (APA, 2013), such as the following:

- *Blunted*: Significantly reduced intensity of emotional expression
- *Flat*: Absent or nearly absent affective expression
- *Inappropriate*: Discordant affective expression accompanying speech content or ideation
- *Labile*: Varied, rapid, and abrupt shifts in affective expression
- *Restricted or constricted*: Mildly reduced in range and intensity of emotional expression

Primary mood disorders include depressive (**unipolar**) and **bipolar** (manic–depressive) disorders. Although the *DSM-5* has separated its discussion of Depressive Disorders from Bipolar and Related Disorders, what endure related to both groupings are the common features noted above. Specific criteria differentiating the diagnostic classification of these disorders are detailed according to "issues of duration, timing, or presumed aetiology" (APA, 2013, p. 155). While several *mood categories* are described in the *DSM-5*, this chapter focuses primarily on the following disorders:

- *Depressive disorders*: Major depressive disorder, single or recurrent; and dysthymic disorder
- *Bipolar disorders*: Bipolar I disorder, bipolar II disorder, and cyclothymic disorder
- *Mood disorder* caused by a general medical condition
- *Substance-induced mood disorder*

Two additional identifiers within the category of mood disorders warrant mention. First, *postpartum-onset specifier* is distinguished by the onset of an episode within 3 to 4 weeks postpartum (Sadock, Sadock, & Ruiz, 2015). Second, *seasonal depression* is a recognized,

recurrent, annual pattern of depressive symptoms with a specific onset related to seasonal light deprivation, typically occurring during the fall and winter months, followed by symptom cessation in the spring and summer. Seasonal variations in mood occur most commonly in northern latitudes. Therefore, this disorder may be especially relevant to Canadians. Somatic treatment with phototherapy is shown to benefit some people suffering with depressive symptoms in such environmental situations (Melrose, 2015).

The advantages of diagnosing a mood disorder early (e.g., early intervention, community nursing support) can be constrained by the adverse effect of a psychiatric diagnosis as a negative social label. Accessing effective care can be sabotaged by the need to keep the diagnosis hidden, even from oneself (Davis, 2014). Increased awareness is a principal "weapon against stigma" and fundamental to combating misperceptions. Awareness would lead to clarity in detection, to acceptance by patients and their families, and ultimately to the required support and treatment (Kuhl, Kupfer, & Regier, 2011).

KEY CONCEPT

Mood is the predominant, pervasive, and sustained emotion colouring the patient's perception of the world and ability to function in it. Normal variations in mood, such as sadness, euphoria, and anxiety, occur as responses to specific life experiences and are time limited, not associated with significant functional impairment.

■ DEPRESSIVE DISORDERS

Clinical Course

The criteria in the *DSM-5* indicate that a major depressive disorder can occur as a single episode, although episodes often recur. To constitute a **major depressive episode** (MDE), either a depressed mood or a loss of interest or pleasure in nearly all activities must be present for at least 2 weeks. Additionally, four of the following seven symptoms are usually present: disruption in sleep, appetite (or weight), concentration, or energy; psychomotor agitation or retardation; excessive guilt or feelings of worthlessness; and suicidal ideation (see Box 22.1 for the APA's DSM-5 criteria). Patients often report feeling depressed, hopeless, or discouraged. If a person complains of feeling sad and empty, a depressed mood may be inferred from their facial expression and demeanour. Depression may also be demonstrated by other behaviours such as withdrawal and excessive ruminations typically with the theme of guilt (Barnhill, 2014)

The course of major depression is variable, but increasingly, this illness is considered persistent and recurrent. Over time, episodes can increase in frequency, severity,

BOX 22.1 DSM-5 Diagnostic Criteria: Major Depressive Disorder

A. Five (or more) of the following symptoms have been present during the same 2-week period and represent a change from previous functioning; at least one of the symptoms is either (1) depressed mood or (2) loss of interest or pleasure.

1. Depressed mood most of the day, nearly every day, as indicated by either subjective report (e.g., feels sad, empty, hopeless) or observation made by others (e.g., appears tearful). (**Note:** In children and adolescents, can be irritable mood.)

2. Markedly diminished interest or pleasure in all, or almost all, activities most of the day, nearly every day (as indicated by either subjective account or observation).

3. Significant weight loss when not dieting or weight gain (e.g., a change of more than 5% of body weight in a month) or decrease or increase in appetite nearly every day. (**Note:** In children, consider failure to make expected weight gain.)

4. Insomnia or hypersomnia nearly every day.

5. Psychomotor agitation or retardation nearly every day (observable by others, not merely subjective feelings of restlessness or being slowed down).

6. Fatigue or loss of energy nearly every day.

7. Feelings of worthlessness or excessive or inappropriate guilt (which may be delusional) nearly every day (not merely self-reproach or guilt about being sick).

8. Diminished ability to think or concentrate, or indecisiveness, nearly every day (either by subjective account or as observed by others).

9. Recurrent thoughts of death (not just fear of dying), recurrent suicidal ideation without a specific path, or a suicide attempt or a specific plan for committing suicide.

B. The symptoms cause clinically significant distress or impairment in social, occupational, or other important areas of functioning.

C. The episode is not attributable to the physiologic effects of a substance or to another medical condition.

D. The occurrence of the major depressive disorder is not better explained by schizoaffective disorder, schizophrenia, schizophreniform disorder, delusional disorder, or other specified and unspecified schizophrenia spectrum and other psychotic disorders.

E. There has never been a manic episode or a hypomanic episode.

Reprinted with permission from the *Diagnostic and Statistical Manual of Mental Disorders,* Fifth Edition, (Copyright 2013). American Psychiatric Association.

and duration (Yatham et al., 2013). The number of episodes and the amount of time major depression is left untreated influence the prognosis (Palazidou, 2012). Complicating the course of major depression may be the frequently occurring bidirectional link between alcohol dependence and this disorder. Research suggests that alcohol dependence is related to an increased risk for a MDE (Bulloch, Lavorato, Williams, & Patten, 2012). Further, suicide as a result of major depression underscores the serious and lethal progression this disorder can take. Yet, despite the potentially problematic course of major depression, it is important to note that a large number of people experiencing a depressive episode are likely to recover fully from it (Klein & Allmann, 2014).

Dysthymic disorder is a milder, chronic form of major depressive disorder. Eating and sleeping behaviours are affected (too little or too much); the individual has low energy, difficulty concentrating and making decisions, low self-esteem, and feelings of hopelessness. When an MDE overlaps dysthymia, it is often referred to as "double depression" (McInnis, Reba, & Greden, 2014, p. 375).

Depressive Disorders in Special Populations

Children and Adolescents

Depressive disorders in children have manifestations similar to those seen in adults, with some exceptions in presentation and developmental expression. In major depressive disorder, children are less likely to present with psychosis, but when they do, auditory hallucinations are more common than are delusions. They are also less likely to express subjectively, hopelessness and dysphoria, and tend to have anxiety symptoms characterized as internalizing disorders, which are often expressed somatically in the form of stomachaches and headaches. Externalizing behavioural abnormalities, such as fear of separation, are often demonstrated in young children (Hammen, Ruolph, & Abaied, 2014; Statistics Canada, 2012). In adolescence, major depressive disorder is twice as common in female as in male populations, while prepubertal boys and girls are noted to be equally affected. Insomnia, hypersomnia, and an irritable instead of sad mood may predominate in a depressed adolescent. The risk for suicide is real in children and adolescents and peaks during the midadolescence in girls and late adolescence in boys (Hammen et al., 2014). See Chapter 19 regarding suicidal behaviour.

Older Adults

The aging demographic in Canada necessitates that nurses take a leadership role in ensuring that the health care needs of the older adult are met (Canadian Nurses Association, 2012a, 2012b), especially depression in this population. Older patients experiencing depressive symptoms do not always meet the full criteria for major depression, and this disorder can manifest comorbidly with dementia, complicating the presentation of both conditions. It is estimated that 8% to 20% of older adults in the community, and as many as 37% in primary care settings, experience depressive symptoms. Treatment is successful in 60% to 80%, but response to treatment is slower than in younger adults. Depression in older adults often is associated with chronic illnesses, such as heart disease, stroke, and cancer; symptoms may be somatically focused. Suicide is a very serious risk for older adults, especially males. In Canada, significant mortality rates due to suicide are reported in people older than 80 years of age. Statistics also reflect more deaths by suicide in older adults between the years 2005–2009, from 110 to 146 suicides, respectively. Rates were substantially higher among males than among females (Statistics Canada, 2012).

Canada's Indigenous Populations

Very limited and variable data exist regarding the prevalence rates of major depression in Canada's indigenous population. When compared to the general population, however, there are significantly elevated rates of suicide in indigenous peoples, which may reflect a high incidence of depression (Bellamy & Hardy, 2015; Davis, 2014). Colonization, the multigenerational effects of trauma experiences from residential schools, the transgenerational transfer of depression, marginalization (Kielland & Simeone, 2014), and banning of spiritual practices are factors implicated in MDEs in Canada's indigenous people (Firestone et al., 2015). Pertinent is that depressive symptoms evidenced among Canada's indigenous peoples may be quite distinct with respect to their own unique cultural practices (Firestone et al., 2015). The spiritual beliefs of this population play a vital part in their mental health, and the use of a term such as "spirit" to connote mood does not fit with Western descriptions of depression (Bellamy & Hardy, 2015). Thus, it is critical that nurses possess a clear understanding of how each indigenous person conceptualizes his or her depression to ensure accurate assessment and intervention.

Epidemiology

An analysis by Bromet et al. (2011), of 18 epidemiologic surveys conducted to determine the prevalence, course,

IN-A-LIFE

James Eugene Carrey (1962–)

CANADIAN-BORN ACTOR AND COMEDIAN

Public Persona

Jim Carrey grew up in Toronto. His fame as a comedian began on *The Carol Burnett Show* at the age of ten. His stage talents ripened through the comedy routines he performed for classmates throughout his school years. Carrey, a high school dropout, began his acting career in comedy clubs and with bit-part television and movie performances. His unique on-screen characteristics were recognized quickly, and he became a box-office success. Jim Carrey is well known for his performances in such films as *The Mask, Eternal Sunshine of the Spotless Mind,* and *A Christmas Carol.* He was inducted into Canada's Walk of Fame in 2004.

Personal Reality

Carrey publicly discussed his struggle with depression on *60 Minutes* (November 2004), exposing a serious, complicated side of himself as a person who was continually questioning himself and the world. Carrey was candid about periods of desperation in his life: the poverty, deprivation, and anger that marked some of his early childhood and adolescence; the struggles through two failed marriages; the highs and the lows bordering on despair; and the extended use of Prozac that helped him "out of a jam." Through it all, Jim, using the mask of *comedy* as a shield, maintains "life is beautiful" and that he is committed to giving full expression to the "realness" of his being.

Source: Leung, R. (2004, November). Carrey: Life is too beautiful. *60 Minutes, CBS NEWS.* Retrieved from http://www.cbsnews.com/stories/2004/11/18/60minutes/main656547.shtml

and sociodemographic correlates of major depression in low- to middle-income countries throughout the world, suggests a widely variable but meaningful prevalence of this illness. In the 10 high-income countries surveyed, a greater occurrence of major depression at 14.6% and 5.5% (on average) was noted as compared to 11.1% and 5.9% in the eight low- to middle-income countries. In another epidemiologic review of depression across cultures, Kessler and Bromet (2013) noted that 20% of adults and up to 50% of children and adolescents reported depressive symptoms during recall periods from 1 to 6 weeks. However, in the surveys where a structured diagnostic interview was used, the point prevalence (i.e., the number of people with this illness during a specific time period divided by the number of people in the population), for a DSM MDE, was much lower than the number of depressive symptoms reported. This difference indicates that a large number of people experienced subclinical depression, which is highly important to identify as a substantial number of MDEs emerge from this context (Kessler et al., 2014).

In Canada, to evaluate national trends in the prevalence of major depression during the past two decades, data were examined from a series of representative Canadian surveys, conducted from 1994 to 2012. No increase in the yearly prevalence of major depression over time was noted and stability was evident in a 4.7% annual prevalence rate in 2012 and a 4.8% annual prevalence rate in 2002 (Patten et al., 2015, p. 34). Specific factors associated with this stability are unclear, but it may be that heightened public recognition of depression, increased mental health literacy, improved diagnosis, and treatment as well as increased antidepressant use have exerted an effect (Patten et al., 2015; Simpson, Meadows, Francis, & Patten, 2012).

Despite some evidence that major depression in Canada may be stabilizing, it remains a serious public health concern as it occurs so commonly and has a chronic–recurrent trajectory. Moreover, this illness presents comorbidly with other medical disorders, and particularly endocrine disorders, cardiovascular disease, neurologic disorders, autoimmune conditions, infectious diseases, and cancer (Freedland & Carney, 2014), as well as nutritional deficiencies, and as a direct physiologic effect of a substance such as corticosteroid treatment (McInnis, Riba, & Greden, 2014). Further, major depression usually coexists with other mental illnesses, particularly anxiety and substance-use disorders. Importantly, major depression predicts serious role performance impairments, which have significant personal and social economic ramifications (Kessler & Bromet, 2013). Thus, the magnitude of major depression as a significant public health problem occurring throughout the life span must register with nurses practicing in all health care contexts.

Ethnic and Cultural Differences

While prevalence rates in Canada are said to be unrelated to race, culture can influence the experience and communication of depressive symptoms. Canada is a country of vast regional differences and numerous "microidentities" populated by indigenous and non-indigenous peoples. Many groups of inhabitants, such as those of Ukrainian and Asian cultures, maintain "homeland" beliefs and ideologies that may influence how individual patients experience and express emotional disturbances. Culture may dictate an iron resolve to keep feelings in check or unexpressed. In some cultures, somatic symptoms, rather than sadness or guilt, may predominate. Complaints of "nerves" and headaches (in Ukrainian cultures); weakness, tiredness, or

"imbalance" (in Chinese and other Asian cultures); or problems of the "heart" (in Middle Eastern cultures) may be ways of expressing experience of depression. Although culturally distinctive experiences must be distinguished from symptoms, it is imperative that a symptom not be dismissed merely because it may be viewed as a culture-specific norm. It is important for the nurse to be cognizant of emergent Canadian immigration trends; Syrian, Latin American, south Asian, Indian, and African populations may have their own ways of characterizing a depressive disorder. Nurses must be equipped to care for an increasingly diverse population. To achieve this aim, culturally competent mental health nursing care must value different beliefs and multiple ways of knowing, engaging, and expressing so that proper assessments may be conducted in a culturally and linguistically sensitive manner (International Council of Nurses, 2013).

Risk Factors

Depression is so common that it is sometimes difficult to identify risk factors. The Adverse Childhood Experiences study indicates devastating risk links between childhood emotional, physical, and sexual abuses and subsequent life experiences of depression (Felitti, 2007). Other generally acknowledged risk factors include the following:

- Prior episode of depression
- Family history of depressive disorder
- Lack of social support
- Stressful life events
- Current substance use
- Medical comorbidity
- Economic difficulties

Aetiology

The aetiology of major depression is undoubtedly understood as biopsychosocial with the spiritual component increasingly recognized. In the biologic domain, a proliferation of research over the past 50 years has led to a clear understanding that multifactorial biologic disturbances are involved in the aetiology of major depression. Box 22.2 explores research into differences in the level of depressive symptoms of men and women.

Genetics

Family, twin, and adoption studies conducted to determine a heritable aetiology for major depression suggest a genetic liability for this disorder. Twin studies offer compelling data that major depressive disorder is demonstrated more commonly among first-degree biologic relatives of people with this illness than among the general population (Sadock et al., 2015). New understandings about genetics and major depression continue to emerge through research in linkage studies examining coinheritance of genetic markers for major depression. However, the extent to which shared gene–environment factors influence familiality remains unclear. Advances

BOX 22.2 Research for Best Practice

GENDERED DEPRESSION: VULNERABILITY OR EXPOSURE TO WORK AND FAMILY STRESSORS?

Marchand, A., Bilodeau, J., Demers, A., Beauregard, N., Durand, P., & Haines, V. (2016). Gendered depression: Vulnerability or exposure to work and family stressors? Social Science and Medicine, 166, 160–168. Retrieved from http://dx.doi.org/10.1016/j.socscimed.2016.08.021

Question: Are differences in the level of depressive symptoms of men and women explained by differentials in their vulnerability and exposure to work and family circumstances, as well as the mediating effects of work-to-family conflict (WFC) and family-to-work conflict (FWC)? Two hypotheses were advanced: the vulnerability hypothesis (women react more intensely than do men to stressful conditions) and the exposure hypothesis (the distribution of psychosocial risks and resources in the workplace and in the family are gendered).

Method: Data in this study were derived from the Salveo Study, which occurred from 2009 to 2012. It included a random sample of 1,935 employees (women constituted 48.9% of the sample) working in Quebec, Canada. Multilevel path analysis models were used to test the differential exposure hypothesis; gender stratification of the data was used to test for a differential vulnerability hypothesis.

Results: Both hypotheses were supported. Differences in vulnerability and exposure risks did impact depressive symptoms in men and women, with exposure risks having the most empirical support. Overall, it was the WFC that had a mediating effect between work–family stressors and depression (i.e., increased depression levels in women). In terms of the vulnerability hypothesis, results indicated only one gendered pathway, and it pertains to the relationship between WFC and depression. For men, lower skill utilization and higher job security were associated with higher depressive symptoms;

psychological demands and abusive supervisors were the only work factors associated with women's higher symptoms. Couple-related problems and WFC were associated with higher depressive symptoms in both genders, with child-related problems associated with increased symptoms for women. The importance of the relationship between family income and WFC was greatest in women. When work, family, and WFC factors were accounted for, differences in symptoms of depression between women and men were not significant because variables such as working hours, irregular work schedules, and skill acted as mediators for both genders. Increased working hours and irregular work schedules were also associated with WFC. More women than men reported higher WFC, but fewer working hours, a more regular work schedule, and lower skill use.

Nursing Implications: Nurses must be cognizant that the higher rate of depression in women compared with men may be related to differential social experiences that are formed by gendered social structures and gendered organizations. Despite increased gender equity in home life, women typically take on and juggle more family responsibilities while simultaneously working in occupational environments that do not afford them the same possibilities as men. Gendered role meanings for women are fundamentally linked to work–family conflict, and significant role strain may occur in women in the domains of work and family. Nurses need to integrate into their assessments how work and family domains are influencing depressive symptoms in men and women so more effective nursing interventions can be implemented. As well, assessing women for gendered role strain, promoting individual self-care, and offering family support in the context of gendered work–family conflict may decrease a vulnerability to depression.

---

in epigenetics are enhancing the understanding of how early life experiences can trigger changes in the association between gene and environment expression, which results in mood disorders (Lau, Lester, Hodgson, & Eley, 2014).

Neurobiologic Hypotheses

The evolution of early neurobiologic theories has resulted in new paradigms regarding the cause of depression in which it is attributed to a wide range of complex and intertwining neurobiologic abnormalities. Advances in the neurobiology of depression are seen in the areas of increased phasic rapid eye movement sleep, poor sleep

maintenance, elevated cortisol levels, impaired cellular immunity, and decreased activity in the dorsolateral prefrontal cortex, low levels of the serotonin metabolite 5-hydroxy-indoleacetic acid (5-HIAA), and increases in limbic responses. Depression is also linked to abnormalities in either the excretion of the neurotransmitters norepinephrine (NE), dopamine (DA), and serotonin (5-HT) or their receptor functions. The homeostasis of these neurotransmitters, and their cellular responses to stress, can be disrupted so that an increase or decrease results depending on how stressful events are cognitively processed and encoded. Other notable developments in the neurobiology of clinical depression are related to newer neuroimaging capabilities that have identified brain regions and structures integral to the expression of depressive symptoms such as decreased hippocampal volume (Thase, Hahn, & Berton, 2014).

Neuroendocrine and Neuropeptide Hypotheses

Major depressive disorder is associated with multiple endocrine alterations, specifically of the hypothalamic–pituitary–adrenal axis, the hypothalamic–pituitary–thyroid axis, the hypothalamic–growth hormone axis, and the hypothalamic–pituitary–gonadal axis. Increased hypothalamic–pituitary–adrenal axis (HPA) activity is considered the trademark of the human stress response. Sustained hypercortisolism damages the integrity of HPA axis regulation and in doing so plays an important role in the pathophysiology of depression. Hyperactivity of the HPA and increased levels of glucocorticoid hormones, features seen in depressed people, are attributed to a disrupted feedback regulation possibly due to altered glucocorticoid receptor functioning. Glucocorticoid receptor involvement in depression is evident in recent research evidence concerning the role of the amygdala in the aetiology of major depression. Results obtained from studying postmortem brain tissue of people diagnosed with major depression showed increased expression of glucocorticoid protein levels in amygdala tissue (Wang et al., 2014). There is also mounting evidence that components of neuroendocrine axes (e.g., neuromodulatory peptides such as corticotropin-releasing factor) may themselves contribute to depressive symptoms. Evidence also suggests that the secretion of these hypothalamic and growth hormones is controlled by many of the neurotransmitters implicated in the pathophysiology of depression (Sadock et al., 2015).

Psychoneuroimmunology

Psychoneuroimmunology is a recent area of research into a diverse group of proteins known as *chemical messengers* between immune cells. These messengers, called cytokines, signal the brain and serve as mediators between immune and nerve cells. The connection between brain–immune interactions and susceptibility to major depression is a complex and ongoing study (Thase et al., 2014).

Psychological Theories

Psychodynamic Factors

Most psychodynamic theorists acknowledge some debt to Freud's drive theory, which ascribes the aetiology of depression to an early lack of love, care, warmth, and protection, with resultant anger, guilt, and helplessness turned inward (McWilliams, 2011). A more current hypothesis about the onset of depression implicates uncorrected negatively biased associative processing leading to a "cognitive vulnerability" or specific predisposition that interacts with life stressors (Hammen et al., 2014).

Behavioural Factors

Behaviourists hold that depression occurs primarily as the result of a severe reduction in rewarding activities or an increase in unpleasant events in one's life. The resultant depression then leads to further restriction of activity, thereby decreasing the likelihood of experiencing pleasurable activities, which in turn intensifies the mood disturbance.

Developmental Factors

Developmental theorists pose that depression results from early adverse life events that become formed and progressively evolve into core dysfunctional attitudinal patterns, activated in later life by stressful events that lead to depression. Early experiences such as child maltreatment, parental loss possibly through death or emotionally inadequate parenting, as well as other factors such as a disrupted attachment system, and negative familial interactional influences can lead to a vulnerability for major depression (Hammen et al., 2014).

Social Theories

Family Factors

Family theorists Wright and Leahey (2013) contend that the family is who they say they are (p. 55). Wright and Leahey ascribe maladaptive "circular" patterns in family interactions as contributing to the onset of depression in family members. Disruption to family dynamics deriving from multiple causes can manifest as depression experienced by an individual's single family member. Nurses should be vigilant in identifying if the individual's depressive experience is symptomatic of family distress. In such cases, a "family unit" assessment and assistance may be warranted and, indeed, possibly the best predictor of a positive outcome for the individual (see Chapter 15).

Social Factors

Social isolation, deprivation, and financial distress are risk factors for ensuing depression. Depression may also follow loss and adverse or traumatic life events, especially those that involving the loss of an important human relationship or role in life. Grieving after the loss of a loved one has been regarded as a normal process unless it endures for inordinate and extensive time periods and ultimately results in the symptoms equated with major depression. The dawn of the *DSM-5* has generated debate related to *grief* and whether or not it warrants labelling as a diagnostic mental disorder. For many, this topic became a contentious issue instigating debate about what "should" be considered normal, and/or normal variations of grieving, and why that should earn entry and be labelled within the rubric of mental disorder. Grief is said to be "an inescapable part" of the human condition and medicalizing what is regarded as normal bereavement "could run the risk of pathologizing the cultural norms established for individuals who grieve the death of a loved one" (Fox & Jones, 2013, p. 113). However, both grief and depression may follow a major loss and possess overlapping features, introducing a complexity to each experience. Thus, the *grief diagnosis* may be thought of as a way to identify any harmful extremes of a grief response in order to facilitate treatment of an associated depression (Ogden & Simmonds, 2014). Helping patients process their feelings about a loss gives them the opportunity to understand this experience in a meaningful way and could prevent progression into a depressive episode.

Interdisciplinary Treatment

Although depressive disorders are the most commonly occurring mental disorders, they are usually treated within the primary care setting, not the psychiatric setting. Patients with depression enter mental health settings when their symptoms become so severe that hospitalization is needed, usually for suicide attempts or if they self-refer because of incapacitation. Interprofessional treatment of these disorders, which are often lifelong, needs to include a wide array of health professionals in all areas. The specific goals of treatment are to

- Reduce/control symptoms and, if possible, eliminate signs and symptoms of the depressive syndrome
- Improve occupational and psychosocial functioning as much as possible
- Reduce the likelihood of relapse and recurrence

Priority Care Issues

The overriding concern for people with mood disorders is safety. In depressive disorders, suicide risk must be evaluated and suicide assessments should be done frequently to protect the patient (see Chapter 19).

Family Response to Disorder

Depression in one member affects the whole family. Spouses, children, parents, siblings, and friends experience frustration, guilt, anger, and even mental health issues when the functional ability of the family member is compromised by depression. It is often hard for others to understand the depth of the mood and how disabling it can be. Financial hardship can occur when the family member cannot work and spends days in bed. The lack of understanding and difficulty of living with a person with depression can lead to family estrangement. Moreover, a mood disorder such as bipolar disorder, characterized by unpredictability, can have profound effects on family members. Qualitative nursing research, concerned with close family members who have a relative with a bipolar mood disorder, highlights that nurses need to provide holistic support to both the individual affected by this illness and his or her family

in order to affect the unpredictability it causes in their life and to make life more liveable for them. Nurses can be facilitators in three key areas for families: recognizing and ensuring appropriate distance keeping among family members so adequate reflection about the illness can occur, encouraging daily stability and structure, and fostering transparent communication among family members (Rusner, Carlsson, Brunt, & Nystrom, 2013).

Nursing Management: Human Response to Depressive Disorder

The diagnosis of major depressive disorder is made when *DSM-5* criteria are met. An awareness of the risk factors for depression, a comprehensive bio/psycho/social/spiritual assessment, and a history of the patient's illness and any past treatment are key to formulating a treatment plan and to evaluating outcomes. Interviewing a family member or close friend about the patient's day-to-day functioning and specific symptoms may be helpful in determining the course of the illness, current symptoms, and level of functioning.

Depression during pregnancy and the postpartum period warrants special consideration. A mood disorder in these contexts is particularly important to identify and treat as it has the potential to disrupt the maternal–foetal bond as well as the postpartum maternal–infant bond. Such outcomes also have negative ramifications for infant attachment, which in turn can affect the infant's mental health and developmental trajectory (BC Reproductive Mental Health Program & Perinatal Services, 2014). In their first year of life, approximately 1 in 11 infants will experience their mother's MDE (Center on the Developing Child at Harvard University, 2009). Infants need an environment that supports and nurtures their capabilities for emotional regulation, one that is protective and fosters a positive developmental trajectory. Symptoms of depression can inhibit the mother's ability to respond sensitively to her infant (Tronick & Reck, 2009). However, the treatment of pregnant and postpartum women with antidepressant medications presents a unique challenge due to the potential effects of these medications on the foetus and breast-feeding infants. When decisional conflict arises about this topic, a risk and benefit discussion about both the impact of the medications and untreated maternal depression is always necessary (BC Reproductive Mental Health Program & Perinatal Services, 2014). Nurses must always examine if they are playing a role in fostering stigmatization toward women choosing to take antidepressants during pregnancy (Stepanuk, Fisher, Wittmann-Price, Posmontier, & Bhattacharya, 2013).

Biologic Domain

Assessment

Symptoms of depression can be similar to some medical problems or side effects of medication therapies;

therefore, a biologic assessment must include a physical systems review and thorough history of medical problems, with special attention to CNS function, endocrine function, anaemia, chronic pain, autoimmune illness, diabetes, or menopause. Additional medical history includes surgeries, medical hospitalizations, head injuries, episodes of loss of consciousness, and pregnancies, childbirths, miscarriages, and abortions. Also, a complete list of prescribed, over-the-counter (OTC) medications and herbal supplements should be compiled, including the reason for taking them. Information about the frequency and dosage of prescribed OTC medications and supplements should be obtained, and any abrupt discontinuation of medications warrants further assessment. With depressive disorders, the nurse must always assess the lethality of the medication being taken. For example, if a patient has sleep medications at home, the patient should be questioned about the number of pills in the bottle. The use of alcohol, marijuana, other mood-altering medications, as well as herbal substances must be assessed as they can cause drug–drug interactions (see Chapter 12).

Physical examination is recommended with baseline vital signs and laboratory tests, which include a comprehensive blood chemistry panel, complete blood count, liver function tests, thyroid function tests, urinalysis, and electrocardiogram. Biologic assessment also includes evaluating the patient for the characteristic neurovegetative symptoms listed below.

- *Appetite and weight changes* are a set criterion in major depression (APA, 2013): Changes from baseline can include decrease or increase in appetite with or without significant weight loss or gain (i.e., a change of more than 5% of body weight in 1 month). Weight loss occurs when not dieting, and weight gain presents more as an atypical feature of depression. Older adults with moderate to severe depression need to be assessed for dehydration as well as weight changes.
- *Sleep disturbance*: The most common sleep disturbance associated with major depression is insomnia. DSM-5 (APA, 2013) addresses varied forms of insomnia, such as initial insomnia (difficulty falling asleep), middle insomnia (waking up during the night and having difficulty returning to sleep), or terminal insomnia (waking too early and being unable to return to sleep). Less frequently, the sleep disturbance is hypersomnia (prolonged sleep episodes at night or increased daytime sleep). The patient with either insomnia or hypersomnia complains of not feeling rested upon awakening (see Chapter 28).
- *Decreased energy, tiredness, and fatigue*: Fatigue associated with depression is a subjective experience of feeling tired regardless of how much sleep or physical activity a person has had. Even the smallest tasks require substantial effort (APA, 2013).

- *Loss of interest or pleasure* is to some degree always present (APA, 2013): Activities that brought pleasure in the past (e.g., hobbies, golfing, etc.) hold no interest in periods of depression.

Physical assessment should also include current weight with any changes noted and assessment of loss of appetite, sleep habits and related disturbances, fatigue factors, and loss of interest.

Nursing Diagnoses for Biologic Domain

Several nursing diagnoses could be formulated based on assessment data, including Disturbed Sleep Pattern, Imbalanced Nutrition, Fatigue, Ineffective Coping, and Nausea. Other diagnoses that should be considered are Ineffective Activity Planning and Sexual Dysfunction.

Interventions for Biologic Domain

Weeks or months of disturbed sleep patterns and nutritional imbalances worsen the progression of depressive disorders. Counselling and education should be aimed at establishing normal sleep patterns and healthy nutrition to help patients move toward remission or recovery. Health teaching about physical care should focus on encouraging patients to practise positive sleep hygiene measures such as avoiding any caffeine intake prior to sleep and avoiding the use of electronics in bed (see Chapter 28 on Sleep–Wake Disorders). Patients should be encouraged to eat well-balanced meals regularly. Activity and exercise are also very important for improving depressed mood state. Most people find that regular exercise is hard to maintain, and people who are depressed may find it impossible. When teaching about exercise, it is important to start with the patient's current activity level and increase it slowly. For example, if the patient is spending most of the time in bed, encouraging the patient to get dressed every day and walk for 5 or 10 minutes may be all that the patient can tolerate. Gradually, patients should be encouraged to have a regular exercise programme.

Pharmacologic Interventions

A cornerstone of treatment for mood disorders is pharmacologic intervention with antidepressants and mood stabilizers. Patients may be reluctant to take prescribed medications or may self-treat. Continuing medication and emphasizing any potential drug–drug interactions should always be included in the patient teaching plan. A complete discussion of antidepressants and mood stabilizers as well as the nurse's role related to them is found in Chapter 12. Lithium, a mood stabilizer typically situation specific to bipolar disorder, warrants special inclusion in this chapter.

Other Biologic Interventions

Biologic treatments, the term applied to treatments working at a somatic or physical level, are nonpharmacologic in nature. Historically, somatic therapies were developed and used as treatments to change the physiologic mechanisms thought to be the prevailing cause of psychiatric disorders. Early somatic treatments believed to relieve mania, psychosis, and depressive symptoms included insulin or atropine coma, hemodialysis, hyperbaric oxygen therapy, continuous sleep therapy, lobotomies, as well as ether and carbon dioxide inhalation therapies. Seizures were also noted to improve some psychiatric symptoms, and this effect led to seizure induction as a treatment modality. Camphor-induced seizures, prevalent in the 16th century, were used to reduce psychosis and mania symptoms. Other chemicals administered as inhalants were also used to induce a seizure, but difficulty controlling their adverse reactions and sometimes-fatal results rendered them prohibitive. The advent of pharmacologic therapies replaced these somatic treatments with the exception of electroconvulsive therapy (ECT), which has remained an efficacious and safely used treatment for depression. ECT is one of several neuromodulatory approaches (i.e., modulates the activity of neural networks implicated in the pathophysiology of depression) to treat depression. In the past 10 years, new neuromodulatory modalities have emerged such as transcranial magnetic stimulation and vagus nerve stimulation (VNS). These modalities developed in conjunction with advances in engineering and neuroimaging, and they show some promise as research continues to investigate their efficacy as future treatments for depression (Rosa & Lisanby, 2012). Other biologic interventions such as phototherapy and nutritional therapy are gaining some acceptance too but remain under inquiry.

Electroconvulsive Therapy

ECT was formally introduced in Italy in 1938 to treat mental illness. Each year, over one million people in the world receive ECT as treatment (Payne & Prudic, 2009). ECT, however, is not a first-line treatment for depression but rather used to treat patients whose disorder is refractory, patients who are intolerant to initial drug treatments, and patients who are so severely ill that rapid treatment is required (e.g., patients with malnutrition, catatonia, or suicidality). ECT is also used in other disorders, such as mania and schizophrenia, when other treatments have failed. Although patients with a severe form of depression, with psychosis present, are considered the best candidates for ECT, reliable predictors of a person's response to this modality remain unclear.

The ECT procedure involves the administration of a muscle relaxant followed by an anaesthetic. An electrical current is then passed through the brain to produce generalized seizures lasting 25 to 150 seconds. A brief pulse stimulus, administered unilaterally on the nondominant side of the head, is associated with less confusion post ECT. However, some individual patients require bilateral treatment for effective resolution of depressive symptoms. Bilateral lead placement, with increased voltage, is associated with more negative cognitive outcomes (George, Taylor, Short, Snipes, & Pelic, 2014; Gitlin, 2014). Seizure induction appears to be necessary to produce positive treatment outcomes. Individual seizure thresholds vary and increase with age; therefore, the electrical impulse and treatment method also may differ. Typically, the lowest possible electrical stimulus necessary to produce seizure activity is used. Blood pressure and ECG monitoring occur during the procedure. The ECT procedure is repeated two or three times weekly, usually for 6 to 12 treatments in total. Twice-weekly regimes are favoured because they produce less accumulative memory loss. After symptoms have improved, an aggressive trial of antidepressant medications is used for relapse prevention. Some patients who cannot tolerate or do not respond to antidepressant treatment may go on maintenance ECT treatments where once-weekly treatments are gradually decreased to once monthly. ECT can be administered to inpatients and outpatients.

The exact antidepressant action of ECT is unclear. Positron emission tomography (PET) scans show an increase in glucose and blood flow followed by a marked decrease, particularly in the frontal lobes. This decreased blood flow is a mechanism thought to have antidepressant effects. ECT also affects all neurotransmitters, but it particularly down-regulates β-adrenergic receptors in much the same way as do antidepressant medications. However, unlike antidepressant therapy, ECT produces an up-regulation in serotonin, especially 5-HT$_2$. Additionally, ECT also exerts other effects on neurochemistry, including increased influx of calcium and effects on second messenger systems (Gitlin, 2014).

Brief, usually transient episodes of hypotension or hypertension, bradycardia or tachycardia, and minor arrhythmias are among the adverse effects that may occur during and immediately after the procedure. Cognitive side effects include *transient postictal* ("after seizure") *disorientation* that clears in minutes to hours (Cusin & Dougherty, 2012; Sadock et al., 2015). Common aftereffects from ECT include headache, nausea, and muscle pain. Memory loss or disturbance is the most troublesome effect of ECT with *anterograde amnesia* (amnesia for events occurring during and soon after a course of ECT) that varies in severity. In this context, a patient might find a diary helpful. Other possible cognitive effects are *short-term retrograde amnesia* (gaps in memory about things occurring a few weeks or months before the ECT) that usually clears within weeks and *retrograde memory loss* (persistent, severe memory deficits) that rarely occurs (Sadock et al., 2015). Many patients experience no amnesia at all. Since memory loss is a symptom of untreated depression, it can present as a confounding factor in determining the extent of memory deficits related to ECT.

ECT is contraindicated in patients with an increased intracranial pressure. Risk also increases in patients with recent myocardial infarction, recent cerebrovascular accident, retinal detachment, or pheochromocytoma (an adrenal cortex tumour) and in patients at high risk for complications from anaesthesia. The nursing care for patients undergoing ECT is to provide educational and emotional support for the patient and family, assess baseline or pretreatment levels of functioning, prepare the patient for the ECT process, and monitor and evaluate the patient's response to the treatment and communicate it to the ECT team so treatment modifications can occur if necessary.

New Somatic (Neuromodulatory) Therapies

Repetitive transcranial magnetic stimulation (rTMS) and VNS are two recognized somatic treatments for depression. Both directly affect brain activity by stimulating nerve cell firing rates. Transcranial magnetic stimulation was introduced in 1985 as a noninvasive, painless method to stimulate the cerebral cortex. Rapidly alternating magnetic fields are applied to the scalp at subconvulsive levels. Underlying this procedure is the hypothesis that a time-varying magnetic field will induce an electrical field, which, in brain tissue, activates the inhibitory and excitatory neurons thereby modulating neuroplasticity in the brain (Cusin & Dougherty, 2012). The low-frequency electrical stimulation from rTMS triggers lasting anticonvulsant effects in rats, and the therapeutic benefits of rTMS in humans are considered related to action similar to that produced by anticonvulsant medication. rTMS relies on the cumulative effects of intermittent application that may occur four to five times a week for 40 minutes while the patient is awake (Sabella, 2014). rTMS stimulation of the brain's prefrontal cortex may help some depressed patients in much the same way as ECT but without the cognitive side effects. Thus, it has been proposed as an alternative to ECT in managing symptoms of depression. Research is mixed about the efficacy of this procedure, and more investigation about it as a treatment modality is necessary. Side effects of rTMS include mild headaches (Rosa & Lisanby, 2012; Sabella, 2014).

VNS is a new somatic treatment that requires the surgical implantation of a pulse generator that delivers chronic intermittent electrical signals at low frequency to the vagus nerve (Shah, Regina, & Frazer, 2014). VNS was initially used for treatment refractory epilepsy, and mood improvement was noted in patients with epilepsy that received this treatment (Cusin & Dougherty, 2012). For years, scientists have been interested in identifying how autonomic functions modulate activity in the limbic system and higher cortex. The vagus nerve has traditionally been considered a parasympathetic efferent nerve responsible only for regulating autonomic functions, such as heart rate and gastric tone. However, the vagus nerve (cranial X) also carries sensory information to the brain from the head, neck, thorax, and abdomen. Research identified that the vagus nerve has extensive projections of its sensory afferent connections to many brain areas. Although the basic mechanism of action of VNS is unknown, incoming sensory, or afferent, connections of the left vagus nerve directly project into many of the very same brain regions implicated in depressive disorders. It is also thought that VNS changes levels of several neurotransmitters implicated in the development of major depression, including serotonin, norepinephrine, GABA, and glutamate. Chronic VNS may cause side effects such as cough, pharyngitis, throat discomfort, dyspnea, headache, nausea, and vomiting (Shah et al., 2014). Presently, it is used as an adjunct to pharmacologic treatment and can be combined with ECT if the patient's depression is particularly treatment resistant (Cusin & Dougherty, 2012).

Other Somatic Treatments

Light Therapy (Phototherapy)

Another somatic therapy is phototherapy, used in seasonal affective disorder. Human circadian rhythms are set by time clues (zeitgebers) inside and outside the body (Sadock et al., 2015). One of the most powerful regulators of these body patterns is the cycle of daylight and darkness. Individuals vulnerable to seasonal depression may experience disturbances either in these normal body patterns or in circadian rhythms. They usually have symptoms that are somewhat different from classic depression, such as irritability, fatigue, and increased need to sleep, increased appetite and weight gain, and carbohydrate craving. Administering artificial light to such patients during winter months has reduced these depressive symptoms (Melrose, 2015). Phototherapy involves exposing the patient to a specific type of artificial light source to relieve seasonal depression. Artificial light is believed to trigger a shift in the patient's circadian rhythm to an earlier time. The light source must be very bright, full-spectrum light, usually 2,500 lux, which is about 200 times brighter than normal indoor lighting. Harmful ultraviolet light is filtered out. Exposure to this light source has produced improvement and relief of depressive symptoms for significant numbers of seasonally depressed individuals. It does not produce change for individuals who are not seasonally depressed. Morning phototherapy is thought to produce a better response than either evening or morning and evening timing of the phototherapy session (Lewy et al., 2010). Light banks with full-spectrum light are readily available. Light visors, visors containing small, full-spectrum light bulbs that shine on the eyelids, have also been developed. The patient is instructed to sit in front of light banks at a distance of about 3 feet, engaging in a variety of other activities, but glancing directly into the light every few minutes. This action should be done immediately on rising and is most effective before 8 AM. The duration of administration may begin with as little as 30 minutes and increase to 2 to 5 hours. One to two hours is usually sufficient, and the antidepressant response begins in 1 to 4 days, with the full effect usually complete after 2 weeks. Full antidepressant effect is usually maintained with daily sessions of 30 minutes. Side effects of phototherapy are rare, but eyestrain, headache, and insomnia are possible. An ophthalmologist should be consulted if the patient has a preexisting eye disorder. In rare instances, phototherapy has been reported to produce mania. Melatonin may also be used in conjunction with phototherapy to treat seasonal affective disorder (Lewy et al., 2010). Follow-up visits with the phototherapy prescriber are necessary to help manage side effects and assess positive results.

Nutritional Therapies

The neurotransmitters necessary for normal healthy functioning are produced from amino acids absorbed with the foods we eat. Nutritional deficiencies, such as deficits in iron, folic acid, pantothenic acid, magnesium, vitamin C, or biotin, may produce symptoms of psychiatric disorders such as fatigue, apathy, and depression. Logically, treating these deficiencies with nutritional supplements should improve the psychiatric symptoms. In 1967, Linus Pauling espoused this idea as a theory and posited psychiatric disorders were caused by an ascorbic acid deficiency. He implemented *megavitamin therapy* or *orthomolecular therapy* as a treatment for schizophrenia that included administering large doses of ascorbic acid and other vitamins. Initial interest in Pauling's hypothesis resulted in scepticism when his research and claims could not be proven. Research about the role of vitamins as a treatment for depression continues. Some moderate, short-term improvement in depressive symptoms and quality of life noted when methylated vitamin B complex was administered to patients diagnosed with an MDE or a related depressive disorder (Lewis et al., 2013). Others have speculated that depression may be caused by oxidative stress, and they suggest that treatment to reduce this process with antioxidants, such as vitamin E and curcumin, may be effective in mitigating depression (Scapagnini, Davinelli, Drago, Lorenzo, & Oriani, 2012).

Previous theories purported that diets and specific foods control behaviour. High sugar intake was thought to produce hyperactivity in children, and Benjamin Feingold developed a diet to eliminate food additives he believed increased hyperactivity. Recent advances in technology led researchers to identify dietary precursors for the bioamines. As an example, tryptophan (5-HTP), a dietary precursor of serotonin, has been extensively investigated in relation to low serotonin levels. Some patients with mild depression and insomnia respond to tryptophan (100 mg to 2 g daily), which has been used as an adjunct to antidepressant drugs (Sadock et al., 2015).

Many patients are turning to dietary herbal preparations to address psychiatric symptoms. More than 17% of the adult population has used herbal preparations to address their mood or emotions. Dietary herbal preparations such as St. John's wort are used to treat depression. Cui and Zheng (2016) conducted a meta-analysis the effectiveness and safety of St John's wort extract and found this herbal remedy was effective in mild to moderate depression. However, more research in this area is needed. It is important to note that unlike pharmaceutical supplements, herbal preparations are often unregulated; therefore, the contents available may vary significantly.

Systematic reviews provide mixed evidence for the effectiveness of ginkgo for cognitive impairment and kava for anxiety. Birks and Grimley Evans (2009) found no evidence for the use of ginkgo for dementia, and kava was removed from the market for its high risk of liver toxicity (Sadock et al., 2015). Nurses, using a nonjudgmental approach, must assess phytomedicinal use by the patient during the initial assessment to determine any drug interactions and to understand the patient's treatment preferences.

Medications may also influence the development of nutritional deficiencies that may worsen psychiatric symptoms. For example, drugs with strong anticholinergic actions often produce impaired or enhanced gastric motility, which may lead to the generalized malabsorption of vitamins and minerals. Additionally, many nutritional supplements have toxicities of their own when given in excess. For example, daily ingestion of more than 100 mg pyridoxine (vitamin B_6) can produce neurotoxic symptoms, photosensitivity, and ataxia. Robust research is needed to identify how the underlying mechanisms of supplements and dietary precursors of the bioamines are related to mood, behaviour, and psychopharmacologic medications. It is important for nurses to recognize that diet can affect mood and behaviour, and dietary supplements have the potential to cause drug–drug interaction.

Psychosocial Issues in All Biologic Treatments

Many factors influence the success of medication and other biologic therapies and notably adherence. Adherence refers to following the therapeutic regimen, self-administering medications as prescribed, keeping appointments, and following other treatment suggestions. It exists on a continuum and can be conceived of as full, partial, or absent.

Psychological Domain

Assessment

The mental status examination is an effective clinical tool to evaluate the psychological aspects of major depression, which causes disturbances in mood, affect, thought processes and content, cognition, memory, and attention. The comprehensive mental status examination is described in detail in Chapter 10.

Mood

The person with depression has a sustained period of feeling depressed, sad, or hopeless and may experience anhedonia (loss of interest or pleasure). The patient may report "not caring anymore" or not feeling any enjoyment in activities that were previously considered pleasurable. In some individuals, this may include a decrease in or loss of libido and sexual function. Depressed mood may be severe enough to provoke thoughts of suicide.

Numerous assessment scales are available for assessing depression. Easily administered self-report questionnaires can be valuable detection tools. These questionnaires cannot be the sole basis for making a diagnosis of MDE, but they are sensitive to depressive symptoms. A commonly used self-report scale questionnaire is the Beck Depression Inventory (BDI). The Hamilton Rating Scale for Depression (HAM-D; see Appendix E) is a clinician-completed rating scale often used and may be somewhat more precise than self-report questionnaires in detecting depression.

Thought Content

Individuals with depression often have an unrealistic, negative evaluation of their worth or have guilty preoccupations or ruminations about minor past failings. Neutral or trivial day-to-day events are interpreted as evidence of personal defects and contain an exaggerated sense of responsibility for untoward events. As a result, feelings of helpless, hopeless, worthless, and powerless may ensue. Thus, an exploration of the patient's perspective on self, the world, and the future should be included in the overall assessment, as should the possible occurrence of disorganized thought processes (e.g., tangential or circumstantial thinking) and perceptual disturbances (e.g., hallucinations, delusions).

Suicidal Behaviour

Patients with major depressive disorder are high risk for suicide. Suicide risk is dynamic and should be assessed initially and throughout the course of treatment. Suicidal ideation can be passive in nature with thoughts that range from a belief that others would be better off if the person were dead, to active thoughts of death with an organized plan for committing suicide. The frequency, intensity, and lethality of these thoughts may vary and can help determine the seriousness of intent. The more specific the plan and the more accessible the means, the more serious is the intent. Risk factors that must be carefully considered are the availability and adequacy of social supports, past history of suicidal ideation or behaviour, presence of psychosis or substance abuse, and decreased ability to control suicidal impulses. Importantly, behavioural indicators toward suicide, such as hoarding medications to overdose, need to be determined and immediately addressed. Questioning to verify behavioural indicators determines if the person has a plan and is actually acting on it. Such questions should be interfaced with a deliberate Suicide Risk Assessment (see Chapter 19).

Cognition and Memory

Many individuals with depression report an impaired ability to think, concentrate, or make decisions. They may appear easily distracted or complain of memory difficulties. In older adults with major depressive disorder, memory difficulties may be the chief complaint and may be mistaken for early signs of a dementia. When the depression is fully treated, the memory problem often improves or fully resolves.

Nursing Diagnoses for Psychological Domain

Nursing diagnoses focusing on the psychological domain of the patient with a depressive disorder are numerous. If patient data lead to the diagnosis of Risk for Suicide, a formal assessment of suicidality must occur. Other nursing diagnoses include Hopelessness, Risk for Situational Low Self-Esteem, Ineffective Coping, Decisional Conflict, Spiritual Distress, and Complicated Grieving.

Interventions for Psychological Domain

Often pharmacotherapy is used in conjunction with psychosocial and psychoeducational treatments. The most effective therapies for patients with severe or recurrent major depressive disorder are combinations of psychotherapy (including interpersonal therapy [IPT], cognitive–behavioural therapy [CBT], behaviour therapy) and pharmacotherapy. Adding a course of CBT may be an adjunct strategy for preventing relapse in patients who have had only a partial response to pharmacotherapy alone (see Chapter 12). Moreover, a combination of medication and psychotherapy may be particularly useful in more complex situations (e.g., depression in the context of concurrent, chronic general medical or other psychiatric disorders or in patients who fail to respond completely to either treatment alone). Further, depressive symptomatology can be complicated by stressful lifestyle circumstances, perhaps presenting as work-related or located in social aspects of an individual's life. CBT and other psychotherapies (individual, marital, or group) can be helpful in addressing such situational life complexities. Mindfulness-based cognitive therapy is increasingly valued as a supportive intervention modality that can be implemented in community health programmes by nurse therapists (Cowen, Harrison, & Burns, 2012, p. 250).

Therapeutic Relationship

One of the most effective therapeutic tools for treating any psychiatric disorder is the therapeutic alliance, a helpful and trusting relationship between clinician and patient. The alliance is built from a number of activities, including the following:

- Establishment and maintenance of a supportive relationship
- Availability in times of crisis
- Vigilance regarding dangerousness to self and/or others
- Education about the illness and treatment goals
- Encouragement and feedback concerning progress
- Guidance regarding the patient's interactions with the personal and work environment
- Realistic goal setting and monitoring

Interacting with patients with depression can be challenging because they tend to be withdrawn and have difficulty expressing feelings and engaging in interpersonal interactions. The therapeutic alliance partly depends on winning the patient's trust through a warm and empathic stance within the context of professional boundaries (see Chapter 6). Understanding the individual's personal experience of receiving a psychiatric diagnosis enables the nurse to respond more effectively.

Cognitive Therapy

Cognitive therapy is successful in reducing depressive symptoms during the acute phase of major depression (APA, 2013). Techniques such as monitoring thoughts, emotions, and actions are used to identify irrational, distorted thinking and beliefs. The use of cognitive therapy in the acute phase of treatment, combined with medication, has grown in the past few years. Cognitive therapy is also considered first-line treatment for outpatients with mild to moderate depression outpatients. Varied modalities for implementing cognitive therapy have been made convenient through computer-assisted technology, with some early promise in this area and more research needed. For example, a meta-analysis of the research in computerized CBT demonstrated short-term reduction in depression but no significant long-term clinical and functional outcomes for patients with depression (So et al., 2013).

Behaviour Therapy

Behaviour therapy for depression encompasses behavioural activation techniques, which are effective in the treatment of patients with depression and particularly when they are combined with pharmacotherapy. Therapeutic techniques include activity scheduling, self-control therapy, social skills training, and problem-solving.

See Chapter 13 for cognitive–behavioural interventions.

Interpersonal Therapy

IPT is a form of brief therapy that is used to recognize, explore, and resolve any current interpersonal losses, role confusion and transitions, social isolation, and deficits in social skills that may precipitate depressive states (Stuart & Robertson, 2012). It is based on a biopsychosocial stress-diathesis model. In IPT losses must be mourned and related affects appreciated, role confusion and transitions must be recognized and resolved, and social skills deficits must be overcome to acquire social supports.

Family and Marital Therapy

Patients who experience high family stress are at risk for greater future severity of illness, higher use of health services, and higher health care expenses. Family and marital problems may be an outcome of major depressive disorders but can also increase susceptibility to the disorder and, in some instances, inhibit recovery. Assisting the adjustment of the partner, and of all family members, may be invaluable in averting a relapse of depression for the recovering patient. Since marital and family problems are common among patients with mood disorders; comprehensive treatment requires that these problems be assessed and interventions suggested to ensure the family is part of the therapeutic system. Many family-nursing interventions (see Chapter 15) may be used by the nurse in providing targeted family-centred care. These include

- Monitoring patient and family for indicators of stress
- Teaching stress management techniques
- Counselling family members on coping skills for their own use
- Providing necessary knowledge of options and support services
- Facilitating family routines and rituals
- Assisting family to resolve feelings of guilt
- Assisting family with conflict resolution
- Identifying family strengths and resources with family members
- Facilitating communication among family members

Group Therapy

The role of group therapy in treating depression is based on clinical experience rather than on systematic, controlled studies. It may be particularly useful for depression associated with bereavement or chronic medical illness. Patients may benefit from the example of others who have dealt successfully with similar losses or challenges. Survivors can gain self-esteem as successful role models for new group members. Medication support groups can provide information to the patient and to family members regarding prognosis and medication issues, thereby providing a psychoeducational forum (see Chapter 14).

Teaching Patients and Families

Patients with depression and their close family members often incorrectly believe that their illness is their own fault and that they should be able to "pull themselves up by their bootstraps" or "snap out of it." It is vital to educate patients and their families about the nature, prognosis, and treatment of depression to dispel these false beliefs and unnecessary associated guilt.

Patients need to know the full range of suitable treatment options before consenting to participate in treatment. Nurses can provide opportunities for patients to question, discuss, and explore their feelings about past, current, and planned use of medications and other treatments. Developing strategies to enhance adherence and to raise awareness of early signs of relapse can be important aids to making treatment more effective.

Social Domain

Assessment

Social assessment focuses on the patient's developmental history, family psychiatric history, patterns of relationship, education and work history, the quality of their support system, and the impact of physical or sexual abuse on their interpersonal functioning (see Chapter 10). Depression can colour a patient's perception of the quality of their relationships therefore including a family member or close friend in the assessment process can be helpful. Changes in patterns of relating (especially social withdrawal) and changes in occupational functioning are commonly reported and may represent a significant deterioration from baseline behaviour. Increased use of "sick days" may occur. The family's level of support and understanding of the disorder also need to be assessed.

Nursing Diagnoses for Social Domain

Nursing diagnoses common for the social domain include Compromised Family Coping, Ineffective Role Performance, Interrupted Family Processes, and Caregiver Role Strain (if the patient is also a caregiver).

Interventions for Social Domain

Patients experiencing depression often withdraw from daily activities such as engaging in family routines, attending work, and participating in community events. During hospitalization, patients often withdraw to their rooms and refuse to participate in unit activities. Nurses are challenged to help the patient balance the need for privacy with the need to return to normal social functioning. Patients with depression should never be approached in an overly enthusiastic manner; this approach may be irritating and block communication. On the other hand, patients should be encouraged to set realistic goals to reconnect with family and community. Explaining to patients the importance of attending social activities, however much they may not feel like doing so, will promote the recovery process.

Milieu Therapy

While hospitalized, milieu therapy (see Chapter 11) helps patients with depression maintain socialization

skills and continue to interact with others. When depressed, people are often unaware of their environment and withdraw into themselves. On a psychiatric unit, patients with depression should be encouraged to attend and participate in unit activities. These individuals have a decreased energy level and thus may be moving more slowly than others; however, their efforts should be acknowledged.

Safety

In many cases, patients are admitted to the psychiatric hospital because of a suicide attempt. Suicide risk is dynamic and should continually be evaluated, especially at transition points in the patient's care such as when there is a change in the care level, prior to anticipated leaves from hospital, and at discharge. During the depths of depression, patients may not have the energy to complete a suicide, but as they begin to feel better, and their energy increases, they may be at a greater risk. If a previously depressed patient appears to have become energized overnight, he or she may have decided to commit suicide and thus may be relieved the decision is finally made. The nurse may misinterpret the mood improvement as a positive move toward recovery; however, this patient may be very intent on suicide. Emphasis is always on protecting the patient and ensuring the development of a strong therapeutic alliance, which fosters a hopeful milieu. Ongoing, careful monitoring must take place to maintain safety. It is imperative to collaborate with the patient in the development of a written suicide safety plan to help the patient to stay safe in the hospital and community (see Chapter 19).

Consumer-Oriented Interventions

Nurses are exceptionally well positioned to engage patients and their families in the active process of improving daily functioning, increasing knowledge and skill acquisition, and increasing independent living. Consumer-oriented support groups can help to enhance the self-esteem and the support network of participating patients and their families. Advice, encouragement, and the sense of group camaraderie may make an important contribution to recovery. Organizations providing support and information about depression (and bipolar disorder) include the Canadian Mental Health Association (CMHA), Canadian Alliance on Mental Illness and Mental Health, the Mood Disorders Society of Canada (MDSC), the Native Mental Health Association of Canada (NMHAC), and the Organization for Bipolar Affective Disorders (OBAD). Many other Internet resources are available that can provide patients and families with education and support for mood disorders (see website section below).

Interventions for Family Members

The family needs education and support during and after the treatment of a family member with depression.

Nurses should be attentive to family distress and caregiver burden and provide appropriate support and education. Because major depressive disorder can recur, the family needs information about specific antecedents to a family member's depression and what steps to take. For example, one patient may routinely become depressed during the fall of each year, with the initial symptom manifesting as excessive sleepiness. For another patient, a major loss, such as a child going to college or the death of a pet, may precipitate a depressive episode. Families of older patients need to be aware of the possibility of depression and related symptoms, which may occur after the deaths of friends and relatives. Families of children who are depressed often misinterpret depression as behaviour problems.

Spiritual Domain

Understanding the relevance of spirituality in today's varied arenas of "pluralistic" health care can be daunting and even problematic, particularly given the varied interpretations of spirituality as a concept. Koenig (2012) recognizes that aspects of spirituality and religion overlap and identifies "the transcendent" (or divine) as an important commonality in both. Religious or spiritual involvement is considered a positive correlate to less stress, decreased depression, decreased suicide, as well as better coping. Moreover, constructs associated with spirituality such as forgiveness, flourishing, and resilience may serve as protective factors in mental health recovery (Tuck & Anderson, 2014). However, religion can also increase guilt and despair in some populations that view themselves as failures when they are unable to live up to the high standards of their faith. Therefore, health care providers must take into account the religious and spiritual activities of their patients and recognize the potential of spirituality as both an important mental health resource and possible stressor (Bonelli et al., 2012).

Assessment

Spirituality involves thoughts and feelings that contribute meaning, purpose, connectedness, and hope about one's existence (Rogers & Wattis, 2015). When a person experiences depression, he or she may have despairing thoughts and express a lack of spiritual well-being. Conducting a spiritual assessment not only facilitates the implementation of holistic care (Rogers & Wattis, 2015) but also facilitates exploration of how this integral component is related to the patient's mental health recovery (Bonelli et al., 2012; Gomi, Starnino, & Canda, 2014). The intensely personal and intimate nature of this domain justifies a cautionary and tentative approach. Patients with mood disorders may feel especially guarded in discussing their spirituality, fearing that clinicians may belittle or "pathologize" their experience. In attending to the spiritual domain, Hodge (2015) endorses an initial basic spiritual screening, and then if deemed advisable, this screening should be followed by an in-depth spiritual assessment.

Spiritual Screening and In-depth Assessment

An initial spiritual screening can determine the persons' basic needs related to their religious affiliation and if they desire additional attention in this domain. Queries posed tentatively and with sensitivity are more likely to have the desired effect of eliciting concerns, should they exist. This initial assessment gives an indication of whether or not spirituality is an organizing principle in the depressed person's life and if further assessment is appropriate (Gomi et al., 2014). Spiritual screening questions may include those developed from the collective feedback of a focus group composed of mental health providers and consumers tasked to delineate spiritual assessment questions: "Is spirituality, (religion or faith) important to you? Has it been in your past, or is it something that you would like to explore as part of your recovery?" (Gomi et al., 2014, p. 452). The predominant focus in a spiritual assessment is directly on the patient's understanding of spirituality and its importance in their lives. The intent of the assessment is an exploration of the person's religious history and/or spiritual practice and how they might wish to have spiritual concerns included in their recovery work (Gomi et al., 2014). Within an interprofessional context, this exploration may also default to (or be done in consultation with) pastoral counsellors or clinicians deemed most proficient in addressing the spiritual dimension of a patient's experience. The spiritual assessment can also help to determine if more support for the patient is necessary, such as ensuring contact with a religious representative (e.g., minister, priest, chaplain, elder, imam, rabbi). If indicated, a spiritual assessment can be followed by an in-depth spiritual history using a tool that identifies themes in the patient's spiritual concerns and recognizes the impact of those concerns on the patient's condition (Borneman, Ferrell, & Puchalski, 2010). A broadly used and researched model of spiritual history taking, implemented to help establish relevant care, is based on the acronym FICA: "F—faith, presence of faith and specific beliefs that give the person's life meaning. I—importance; what is the importance and influence of faith and beliefs on the person's life? C—community, is there any spiritual or religious community involvement? A—address in care, how can health care providers use the information about spirituality in the person's care? (Borneman et al., 2010, p. 166).

Nursing Diagnoses for Spiritual Domain

Nursing diagnoses pertaining to the spiritual domain focus on distress of the spirit. Very often these are situation specific. Within the realm of mood disorders, these are often expressed as disturbances in one's belief system related to loss of hope, uncertainty about the meaning of life, suffering, discouragement, and despair.

Interventions for Spiritual Domain

Spiritual interventions can have positive outcomes for patients suffering depression and other mood disorders. Where need presents, appropriate people can intervene with patients by way of guided conversations, personal life storytelling, and ritual experiences. Spiritual activities can be encouraged, including prayer, the reading of religious texts, and attendance at devotional services or ceremonies. Such care modalities may serve to relieve distress, make meaning of suffering, nurture hope, promote spiritual resolution, and foster wellness.

Evaluation and Treatment Outcomes

The major goals of treatment are to help the patient to be as independent as possible and to achieve stability, remission, and recovery from major depression. It is often a lifelong struggle for the individual. An ongoing evaluation of the patient's symptoms, functioning, and quality of life should be carefully documented in the patient's record in order to monitor treatment outcomes.

Continuum of Care

If the prevalence of major depressive disorders in Western countries escalates, it is not unrealistic to speculate that demands for services will increasingly threaten the capacity for service delivery (Carta et al., 2012). Nurses can expect to encounter individuals with depressive disorders in all areas of practice. Initially, they may present in inpatient and outpatient medical and primary care settings, emergency departments (EDs), and inpatient and outpatient mental health settings (see Chapter 4). Thus nurses must be able to recognize depression in their patients and make appropriate interventions or

referrals. The continuum of care, however, goes beyond these settings and may include partial hospitalization or day treatment programmes; individual, family, or group psychotherapy; home visits; and psychopharmacotherapy. Although most patients with major depression are treated in outpatient settings, brief hospitalization may be required if the patient is suicidal or psychotic.

Nurses working on inpatient units provide a wide range of direct services, including administering and monitoring medications and monitoring target symptoms, conducting psychoeducational groups, and, more generally, structuring and maintaining a therapeutic environment. Community nurses are well situated to detect undiagnosed depressive disorders and make appropriate referrals. Nurses providing home care, by virtue of their in-home role, can be particularly helpful in helping both patients living with a mood disorder and their families to address the everyday challenges this illness brings.

Nursing practice requires a coordinated, ongoing interaction among patients, families, and providers to deliver comprehensive services. This includes using the complementary skills of other disciplines for forming overall goals, plans, and decisions and for providing continuity of care as needed. Integrated multidisciplinary care aimed at holistic interventions is key to achieving the remission of symptoms and physical well-being, restoring baseline occupational and psychosocial functioning, and reducing the likelihood of relapse or recurrence (Fig. 22.1).

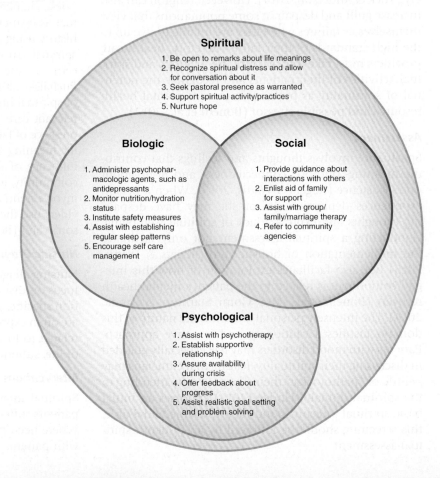

Figure 22.1. Holistic interventions for patients with major depressive disorder.

BIPOLAR DISORDERS (MANIC–DEPRESSIVE DISORDERS)

Diagnostic Criteria

Bipolar disorders are distinguished from depressive disorders by the occurrence of manic or hypomanic (i.e., mildly manic) episodes in addition to depressive episodes. The *DSM-5* divides bipolar disorders into bipolar I (characterized by one or more manic episodes generally with a major depressive occurrence), bipolar II (periods of major depression accompanied by at least one incidence of hypomania), and **cyclothymic disorder** (periods of hypomanic episodes and depressive episodes that do not meet full criteria for an MDE) (see Box 22.3 for the APA's DSM-5 criteria) (Fig. 22.2).

A manic episode is characterized by **euphoria**, a state of elation experienced as a heightened sense of well-being. During a manic episode, the patient often mani-

---

BOX 22.3 DSM-5 Diagnostic Criteria: Bipolar I Disorder

For a diagnosis of bipolar I disorder, it is necessary to meet the following criteria for a manic episode. The manic episode may have been preceded by and may be followed by hypomanic or MDEs. (Refer to Box 22.1 for the DSM-5 Diagnostic Criteria for Major Depressive Episodes.)

MANIC EPISODE

A. A distinct period of abnormally and persistently elevated, expansive, or irritable mood and abnormally and persistently increased goal-directed activity or energy, lasting at least 1 week and present most of the day, nearly every day (or any duration if hospitalization is necessary).

B. During the period of mood disturbance and increased energy or activity, three (or more) of the following symptoms (four if the mood is only irritable) are present to a significant degree and represent a noticeable change from usual behaviour:
1. Inflated self-esteem or grandiosity
2. Decreased need for sleep (e.g., feels rested after only 3 hours of sleep)
3. More talkative than usual or pressure to keep talking
4. Flight of ideas or subjective experience that thoughts are racing
5. Distractibility (i.e., attention too easily drawn to unimportant or irrelevant external stimuli), as reported or observed
6. Increase in goal-directed activity (either socially, at work or school, or sexually) or psychomotor agitation (i.e., purposeless non–goal-directed activity)
7. Excessive involvement in activities that have a high potential for painful consequences (e.g., engaging in unrestrained buying sprees, sexual indiscretions, or foolish business investments)

C. The mood disturbance is sufficiently severe to cause marked impairment in social or occupational functioning or to necessitate hospitalization to prevent harm to self or others, or there are psychotic features.

D. The episode is not attributable to the physiologic effects of a substance (e.g., a drug of abuse, a medication, or other treatment) or to another medical condition.

HYPOMANIC EPISODE

A. A distinct period of abnormally and persistently elevated, expansive, or irritable mood and abnormally and persistently increased activity or energy, lasting at least 4 consecutive days and present most of the day, nearly every day.

B. During the period of mood disturbance and increased energy or activity, three (or more) of the following symptoms (four if the mood is only irritable) have persisted, represent a noticeable change from usual behaviour, and have been present to a significant degree:
1. Inflated self-esteem or grandiosity
2. Decreased need for sleep (e.g., feels rested after only 3 hours of sleep)
3. More talkative than usual or pressure to keep talking
4. Flight of ideas or subjective experience that thoughts are racing
5. Distractibility (i.e., attention too easily drawn to unimportant or irrelevant external stimuli), as reported or observed
6. Increase in goal-directed activity (either socially, at work or school, or sexually) or psychomotor agitation (i.e., purposeless non-goal-directed activity)
7. Excessive involvement in activities that have a high potential for painful consequences (e.g., engaging in unrestrained buying sprees, sexual indiscretions, or foolish business investments)

C. The episode is associated with an unequivocal change in functioning that is uncharacteristic of the individual when not symptomatic.

D. The disturbance in mood and the change in functioning are observable by others.

E. The episode is not severe enough to cause marked impairment in social or occupational functioning or to necessitate hospitalization. If there are psychotic features, the episode is, by definition, manic.

F. The episode is not attributable to the physiologic effects of a substance (e.g., a drug of abuse, a medication, or other treatment).

Reprinted with permission from the *Diagnostic and Statistical Manual of Mental Disorders*, Fifth Edition, (Copyright 2013). American Psychiatric Association.

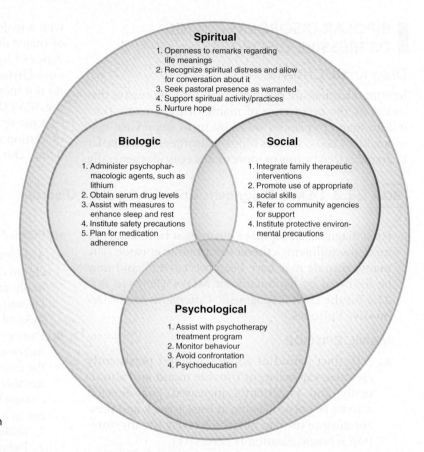

Spiritual
1. Openness to remarks regarding life meanings
2. Recognize spiritual distress and allow for conversation about it
3. Seek pastoral presence as warranted
4. Support spiritual activity/practices
5. Nurture hope

Biologic
1. Administer psychopharmacologic agents, such as lithium
2. Obtain serum drug levels
3. Assist with measures to enhance sleep and rest
4. Institute safety precautions
5. Plan for medication adherence

Social
1. Integrate family therapeutic interventions
2. Promote use of appropriate social skills
3. Refer to community agencies for support
4. Institute protective environmental precautions

Psychological
1. Assist with psychotherapy treatment program
2. Monitor behaviour
3. Avoid confrontation
4. Psychoeducation

Figure 22.2. Holistic interventions for patients with bipolar I disorder.

fests an expansive mood, in which he or she shows an inappropriate lack of restraint in expressing feelings and frequently overvalues his or her own importance. Expansive qualities include an unceasing and indiscriminate enthusiasm for interpersonal, sexual, or occupational interactions and involve behaviours the patient later regrets and that have a high potential for painful consequences. It is important to note that an irritable rather than euphoric mood is often the first sign of mania. This irritability manifests as easy annoyance and anger, particularly when the patient's wishes are challenged or thwarted. Additionally, in manic episodes the mood can be labile, altering between euphoria, depression, and irritability within minutes or hours. Other symptoms include inflated self-esteem or grandiosity, which may range from unusual self-confidence to delusions about possessing special powers or abilities. Delusions occur in 75% of patients experiencing mania, and they can be either congruent or incongruent with the mood state (Sadock et al., 2015). As well in a manic episode, there is frequently a decreased need for sleep, pressured speech (excessive talkativeness), racing thoughts, distractibility, and a decrease in goal-directed activity or psychomotor agitation. As the mania increases, the patient feels more pressured to speak and at times is difficult to interrupt. Speech can become incoherent and associations in thought become quite loose and even disorganized. When thoughts skip rapidly among seemingly unrelated topics with a decreased

logical connection between them, it is termed flight of ideas. Further, decreased inhibition, impulsivity, and distractibility in bipolar disorder can negatively affect cognition in diffuse areas such as *attention* and *concentration* (Conus, Macneil, & McGorry, 2014; Sadock et al., 2015). During a manic episode, patients experience an increase in energy that manifests as pressure of activity, often with less sleep to feel rested. The patient often remains awake for long periods at night or wakes up several times a night, full of energy. Increased motor activity and agitation, which may be purposeful at first (e.g., cleaning the house), may deteriorate into inappropriate or disorganized actions. The patient may get involved unrealistically in several new endeavours, such as overspending sprees, or in reckless sexual encounters, drug or alcohol use, or other high-risk activities such as driving too fast or taking up dangerous sports. Frequently hospitalization may be required to prevent self-harm.

Other psychiatric disorders have symptoms resembling a manic episode. Borderline personality disorder, attention deficit disorder, and substance abuse involving stimulants should be ruled out when assessing for mania. When considering any symptoms of bipolar disorder, it must be noted that the *DSM-5* criteria indicate that the presenting disturbances must be severe enough to cause marked impairment in social activities, occupational functioning, and interpersonal relationships (APA, 2013).

The criteria describing a **hypomanic episode** are the same as those detailed in a manic episode, with the exception of a longer duration of time noted in the expression of symptoms during the latter. An important feature, in hypomania, is that generally no marked impairment in social or occupational functioning occurs. Moreover, should there be fluctuations in the way the patient presents throughout the duration of an acute illness episode, for example, demonstrating high anxiety, agitation, and irritability alternating with the occurrence of depressive symptoms, the patient may be described as having **mixed features**. Such presentations can occur when the criteria for a manic or hypomanic episode are present. Mixed symptoms can also be associated with an MDE. If a patient presents with symptoms that meet full episode criteria for both mania and depression simultaneously, the diagnosis would rightfully be "manic episode, with mixed features" (*DSM-5*), (APA, 2013, p. 150). Hypomanic episodes can be considered less intense manic episodes.

KEY CONCEPT

Central features of **mania** include overactivity, elevated or irritable mood, and grandiose ideas of self-importance (Cowen et al., 2012).

Secondary Mania

Underlying medical disorders such as certain metabolic abnormalities, neurologic disorders, CNS tumours, and particular medications can cause mania. Further, mania can be precipitated by some medical treatments, steroid therapy of particular note. As well, certain substances of abuse such as stimulants and cocaine induce mania (Ketter & Chang, 2014). This range of precipitants requires the nurse to consider them as distinct possibilities for mania onset if there is no previous history of bipolar disorder.

Clinical Course

Bipolar disorder is a chronic, cyclic disorder (Yatham et al., 2013). With mixed states of mania, extreme turmoil can occur with possible suicidal ideation presenting especially high risk. Bipolar disorders can lead to severe functional impairments, resulting in job losses and financial duress and culminating in alienation from family, friends, and coworkers.

Epidemiology

Distribution and Onset

Bipolar disorder affects approximately 1% of the world's population globally irrespective of ethnicity and socioeconomic status and it is a leading cause of disability in the younger population (Alonso et al., 2011; Grande, Berk, Birmaher, & Vieta, 2016). The results of a Canadian epidemiologic study conducted by McDonald et al. (2015) estimated the prevalence of bipolar I and bipolar II disorders at 0.87% and 0.57%, respectively.

The mode of onset for bipolar disorder can be variable, manifesting as a mild retarded depression, hypersomnia, or as an episode of overt psychosis. Onset may also be characterized by several depressive episodes preceding the first manic occurrence (Sadock et al., 2015). Bipolar onset often occurs in adolescence; paediatric bipolar disorder (PBD) is rare, has a much earlier onset, and must be distinguished from attention deficit hyperactivity disorder (ADHD), which has a much earlier onset (Brus, Solanto, & Goldberg, 2014). Depression may be the initial presentation in children, though the hallmark of PBD is demonstrations of intense rage. Children may display seemingly unprovoked rage episodes for as long as 2 to 3 hours. The symptoms of bipolar disorder reflect the developmental level of the child. Whereas children younger than 9 years exhibit more irritability and emotional lability, older children exhibit more classic symptoms, such as euphoria and grandiosity. The first contact with the mental health system often occurs when the behaviour becomes disruptive and these children may have comorbid psychiatric disorders such as ADHD and conduct disorder (Youngstrom & Algorta, 2014). Noteworthy is that, on average, the delay between onset of bipolar disorder and diagnosis can range from 5 to 10 years (Berk et al., 2007).

Recognizing bipolar disorder in the older adult can be challenging as it occurs less frequently than in younger populations and the symptoms are often atypical. Mood changes are likely to manifest as irritability rather than euphoria and anger instead of excessive spending may dominate the clinical presentation. Moreover, geriatric patients with mania often demonstrate more neurophysiologic abnormalities and cognitive disturbances such as confusion and disorientation, which can be confused with dementia or delirium (Blazer & Hybels, 2014). Therefore, a careful history must be obtained where mood symptoms duration and presentation and a previous history are identified. The use of new medications must also be identified. When possible, collaborative sources should be included in the assessment of bipolar problems in an older adult patient.

Gender, Ethnic, and Cultural Differences

Although no significant gender differences have been found in the lifetime prevalence of bipolar I disorder, the incidence of bipolar II disorder is reportedly greater in females than males (Ketter & Chang, 2014)). In addition, some data indicate that female patients with bipolar disorder are at greater risk for depression whereas male patients are prone to manic episodes (Corcoran & Walsh, 2009).

While prevalence rates in Canada are said to be unrelated to race and ethnicity, data from research studies suggest immigration is a risk factor for mood disorders, including bipolar disorder, particularly if migration occurs during early childhood. Specifically, those from infancy to 5 years of age had the highest prevalence rates and risk for mood disorders when compared to their migration generation cohorts and especially adults (Islam, 2015). These data invite speculation about how those subject to mood-related disorders are affected by the process of transitioning and what situational circumstances dispose new migrants to affective reactivity. Factors that could give the young this vulnerability include the sense of being remote from one's homeland, feeling situationally isolated in a land where language and local customs are experienced as "strange," and living where they experience transgenerational distress related to their parents' social status loss and precarious employment prospects. The need exists for studies to identify contextual circumstances that may dispose to possible "immigration risk." At this time, no significant differences in prevalence have been found based on race or ethnicity.

Comorbidity

Medical comorbidity in patients with bipolar disorder is a significant issue as it complicates diagnosis and management of the illness and may have a negative impact on patient outcomes (APA, 2013). Sylvia et al. (2015) analyzed data from a clinical research study regarding medical burden in bipolar patients and found high rates of cardiovascular, metabolic, and alcohol disorders. Cardiovascular comorbidities, and associated problems, such as low HDL and high triglycerides, were suggested to be related to weight gain during depression as well as the medications prescribed. Noteworthy in this data analysis is that mania was negatively related to cardiac and metabolic problems but positively correlated to alcohol problems (Sylvia et al., 2015). Substantial evidence exists suggesting that bipolar disorder in and of itself is an independent risk factor for weight gain, diabetes mellitus, hypertension, dyslipidaemia, cardiovascular disease, and metabolic syndrome (Chennattucherry & Mok, 2010). How these medical problems, specifically rates of obesity, in bipolar disorder interact is difficult to determine due the confounding variables of medication side effects and unhealthy lifestyle choices. Preventing and treating obesity in patients with bipolar disorder could decrease the morbidity and mortality related to physical illness, enhance psychological well-being, and possibly improve the course of the disorder (Chennattucherry & Mok, 2010).

Other comorbid psychiatric conditions are anxiety disorders (most prevalent: panic disorder and social phobia) and substance use, notably alcohol and marijuana. Individuals with a comorbid anxiety disorder are more likely to experience a more severe course. In a report for the Canadian Centre for Substance Abuse, Schutz and Young (2009) suggested that a history of substance use complicates the course of bipolar illness by decreasing treatment adherence and chances for remission.

Aetiology

Current theories of the aetiology of bipolar disorders are associated with chronic abnormalities of neurotransmission, which are thought to result in compensatory but maladaptive changes in brain regulation. In addition, the use of controlled structural and functional imaging studies of patients with mood disorders have generated hypotheses that CNS dysfunction is associated with specific structural brain abnormalities and functional CNS alterations (Johnson, Cuellar, & Peckham, 2014).

Chronobiologic Theories

Sleep and schedule disturbances are important aspects of depression and can predict mania. Sleep patterns appear to be regulated by an internal biologic clock centred in the hypothalamus (see Chapter 9). Events that cause sleep deprivation such as time zone changes and childbirth may trigger symptoms. A number of neurotransmitter and hormone levels follow circadian patterns; therefore, sleep disruption may lead to biochemical abnormalities that affect mood. Preliminary research evidence suggests that bipolar disorder can be characterized by biologic and behavioural disturbances in the individual's circadian rhythm and sleep deprivation as well as life events that disrupt schedules can trigger manic symptoms (Johnson et al., 2014).

Sensitization and Kindling Theory

Sensitization (increase in response to a drug with repetition of the same dosage) and the related phenomenon of kindling (subthreshold stimulation of a neuron generates an action potential; see Chapter 12) refer to animal models. Repeated chemical or electrical stimulation of certain regions of the brain produces stereotypical behavioural responses or seizures. The amount of the chemical or electricity required to evoke the response or seizure decreases with each experience. These phenomena have been used as models to explain why, over time, affective episodes, particularly those seen in patients with bipolar disorder, recur in shorter and shorter cycles and with less relation to environmental precipitants. It is hypothesized that repeated affective episodes might be accompanied by the progressive alteration of brain synapses that lower the threshold for future episodes and increase the likelihood of illness. The kindling theory also helps explain the value of using antiseizure medication, such as carbamazepine and valproic acid, for mood stabilization.

Genetic Factors

A risk factor for bipolar disorder is having a first-degree relative, and particularly a parent, with this illness. The genetic basis for the development of bipolar disorder is increasingly seen in results from family, adoption, and twin studies that indicate in bipolar disorder familial pattern can be seen (Sadock et al., 2015). Such results show a 1% incidence rate in the general population, compared with a 7% incidence rate for first-degree relatives of a patient with bipolar disorder, and 60% for a monozygotic twin of a bipolar patient (Payne, Potash, & DePaulo, 2005). Modes of genetic transmission and the cumulative effects of multiple genes interacting with environmental influences have yet to be definitively identified. Compelling longitudinal study (Duffy, 2012; Duffy et al., 2010) is being done in the area of genetic associations between parents with bipolar disorder and the risks this might pose to their offspring. As evidence mounts, an increase in our understanding as to the nature of possible neurodevelopmental correlates may occur. Likely a vulnerability to bipolar disorder is related to many genetic risk factors interacting with family and environment specific influences. Genomic studies support this model and research continues to identify candidate genes, structural genomic variations, and protein damaging mutations in individual genes possibly implicated in transmitting bipolar disorder (Kerner, 2014).

Psychological and Social Theories

Bipolar disorder encompasses two extremes of a continuum; depression locates at one end and mania at the other. In regard to depression, most psychological and social theories of mood disorders focus on loss as its cause in genetically vulnerable individuals. Mania is considered to be a biologically rooted condition, but when viewed from a psychological perspective, it is usually regarded as a state that arises from an attempt to overcompensate for depressed feelings rather than a disorder in its own right.

Interdisciplinary Treatment of Disorder

Patients with bipolar disorder struggle with the complexity of their illness and must be treated by an interdisciplinary team. Nurses, physicians, social workers, psychologists, occupational, and recreation therapists all have valuable expertise for bipolar patients. For children with bipolar disorder, schoolteachers and counsellors are included in the team. In older adults, the primary care physician is an integral part of the team. An important treatment goal is to minimize and prevent either manic or depressive episodes as the fewer the episodes, the more likely the person can live a normal, productive life. Another important goal is to provide psychoeducation and support for the client and family about the disorder so to assist them in managing it.

Priority Care Issues

During a manic episode, protecting the patient is a priority. During a manic episode poor judgement and impulsivity result in risk-taking behaviours that can have dire consequences for the patient and family. For example, the person suddenly begins excessively spending money and partying. As well, during a manic episode, the patient may believe that he or she has supernatural powers, such as the ability to fly, and then may act on them. During a manic phase suicidality as result of poor judgement and poor impulse control may increase. When the patient recovers from a manic episode, he or she may be devastated by the consequences of poor judgement and impulsivity so that suicide is considered as a way to deal with shame. Nurses play an important role in promoting improved self-esteem after patients experience a manic episode.

Family Response to Disorder

Bipolar disorder can devastate families, who often feel that they are on an emotional roller coaster if they have difficulty understanding the mood shifts. They can be burdened by their family member's problematic behaviours (e.g., impulsive behaviour during manic episodes, such as excessive debt, assault charges, and sexual infidelities) and the disruption of household routine. Family members can also experience emotional distress and become significant users of mental health resources themselves. It is important to understand, however, that families do report developing coping strategies that make life more liveable for them such as finding respite from caring for ill relatives and ensuring appropriate boundaries (Rusner et al., 2013). Nurses must recognize that families can feel strained to the limit when a family member has bipolar disorder and that they too need support, education, and assistance navigating the mental health system.

Nursing Management: Human Response to Bipolar Disorder

The nursing care of patients with bipolar disorder can be one of the greatest challenges in psychiatric nursing. In general, the behaviour of patients with bipolar disorder is often symptom free between episodes. Nursing care of a patient experiencing bipolar disorder should be approached in a multifaceted and compassionate manner during periods of acute illness and during states of remission.

Biologic Domain

Assessment

In the biologic domain, the assessment emphasis is on evaluating symptoms of mania and, most particularly, changes in sleep patterns. In the manic phase of bipolar disorder, the patient often experiences sleeplessness, resulting in irritability and physical exhaustion. Eating habits usually change during a manic or depressive episode, and the nurse should therefore assess changes in diet and body weight. Patients with mania may experience malnutrition and fluid imbalance. The nurse must monitor laboratory studies, such as electrolytes and thyroid functioning. Abnormal thyroid function can be responsible for the mood and behavioural disturbances. Excessive use of alcohol and other substances may also occur, and therefore, the individual must also be assessed for these behaviours. Special attention should focus on the use of alcohol and other substances. Usually, a drug screen is ordered to determine current use of substances. A further concern during a manic phase is that patients often become hypersexual and engage in risky sexual practices. Changes in sexual practices should be explored.

Pharmacologic Assessment

When a patient is in a manic state, previous use of antidepressants should be assessed as they can precipitate such an episode. In such cases, antidepressant use should be discontinued. Often, manic or depressive episodes occur after patients stop taking their mood stabilizer, at which time the reason for stopping the medication should be explored. Patients may stop taking their medications because of side effects or because they no longer believe they have a mental disorder. As well, patients with known bipolar disorder who take antidepressants without attendant mood stabilizers could be at risk for a manic episode.

Nursing Diagnoses for Biologic Domain

Among nursing diagnoses in this domain are Disturbed Sleep Pattern, Sleep Deprivation, Imbalanced Nutrition, Hypothermia, Risk for Deficient Fluid Volume, and Noncompliance (related to treatment measures). If patients are in the depressive phase of illness, the previously discussed diagnoses for depression should be considered.

Interventions for Biologic Domain

Physical Care

In a state of mania, the patient's primary physical needs are rest, adequate hydration and nutrition, and reestablishment of physical well-being. Self-care has usually deteriorated. For a patient who is unable to sit long enough to eat, snacks and high-energy and finger foods that can be eaten while moving should be provided. Alcohol should be avoided. Sleep hygiene is a priority but may not be realistic until medications take effect. Limiting stimuli is important in decreasing agitation and promoting sleep.

Teaching Points

Once the patient's mood stabilizes, the nurse should focus on monitoring changes in physical functioning in sleep or eating behaviour and teaching patients to identify antecedents to mood episodes. A regular sleep routine should be maintained if possible. High-risk times for manic episodes, such as changes in work schedule (day to night), should be avoided if possible. The postpartum period is a particularly high-risk period for exacerbation of bipolar illness as women are very sleep deprived. They should be encouraged to sleep when the baby sleeps and advised to obtain childcare respite if possible. Patients with a bipolar disorder should be taught to monitor the amount of their sleep each night and report a pattern of decreased sleep and sleeplessness as this may indicate a shift toward a manic episode.

Lithium Carbonate and Related Nursing Interventions

Pharmacotherapy is essential in treating bipolar disorder to achieve two goals: the rapid control of symptoms and the prevention of future episodes—or, at least, reduction in their severity and frequency. Pharmacotherapy continues through the various phases of bipolar disorder; see Chapter 12.

The mainstay of therapy for bipolar disorder is mood-stabilizing drugs and notably lithium carbonate (Lithium), which has an impressive efficacy profile in the treatment of this disorder. Lithium is the most widely used mood stabilizer in bipolar disorder (see Box 22.4). It is a very effective treatment for euphoric mania but less so in mania with mixed features, **rapid cycling** bipolar disorder, and secondary manias and in the presence of comorbid substance abuse. The supplemental use of antipsychotics is often a beneficial adjunct to treatment with Lithium. Due to its significant side-effect burden (Table 22.1), Lithium can be poorly tolerated, and small differences in dose or blood levels can cause adverse and even life-threatening outcomes because of its narrow therapeutic index (McKnight et al., 2012).

Lithium is a salt, and the interaction between lithium levels and sodium levels in the body and the relationship between lithium levels and fluid volume in the body remain crucial issues in its safe, effective use. High sodium levels in the body lower the lithium level and vice versa. Thus, changes in dietary sodium intake can affect lithium blood levels that, in turn, may affect therapeutic results or increase the incidence of side effects. The same applies to fluid volume. If body fluid decreases significantly because of a hot climate, strenuous exercise, vomiting, diarrhoea, fever, a drastic reduction in fluid intake, or diuretic use then lithium levels can rise sharply, causing an increase in side effects, progressing to lethal lithium toxicity (Ketter & Chang, 2014). Prior to lithium administration, a physical assessment that includes laboratory tests to determine electrolytes, thyroid and renal functioning, an electrocardiogram, a baseline pregnancy test, weight status and concomitant medications are necessary. The nurse must also be cognizant that lithium has serious

BOX 22.4 DRUG PROFILE

Lithium (Eskalith)

Drug Class: Mood stabilizer

Generic Name: Lithium carbonate

(Trade) Name: (Eskalith, Lithane)

Receptor Affinity: Alters sodium transport in nerve and muscle cells, increases norepinephrine uptake and serotonin receptor sensitivity, slightly increases intraneuronal stores of catecholamines, and delays some second messenger systems. Exact mechanism of action is unknown.

Indications: Treatment and prevention of manic episodes in bipolar affective disorder. Used successfully in a number of off-label uses such as prophylaxis of cluster headaches, bulimia, etc.

Routes and Dosage: Dosing is done according to clinical response, side effects, and serum levels. Targeted dosages are between 900 and 1,800 mg/daily by mouth. 150-, 300-, and 600-mg capsules. Lithobid, 300-mg slow-release tablets; Eskalith CR, 450-mg controlled-release tablets. Lithium citrate, 300 mg/5 mL liquid form.

Adult: In acute mania, optimal response is usually 600 mg tid or 900 mg bid. Obtain serum levels twice weekly in acute phase. Maintenance: Use lowest possible dose to alleviate symptoms and maintain serum level of 0.6 to 1.2 mEq/L. In uncomplicated maintenance, obtain serum levels every 2 to 3 months. Do not rely on serum levels alone. Monitor patient side effects.

Geriatric: An increased risk for toxic effects; use lower doses, and monitor frequently.

Children: Safety and efficacy in children younger than 12 years has not been established.

Half-Life (Peak Effect): Mean, 24 hours (peak serum levels in 1 to 4 hours). Steady state reached in 5 to 7 days.

Select Adverse Reactions: Weight gain. A common side effect of lithium is hand tremors and dosage needs to be monitored.

Warning: Avoid use during pregnancy or while breastfeeding. Hepatic or renal impairments increase plasma concentration.

There is a fine line between therapeutic levels and toxicity levels. Mindfulness is required in use of lithium as a treatment agent.

Specific Patient/Family Education:

- Avoid alcohol or other CNS depressant drugs.
- Notify the prescriber if pregnancy is possible or planned. Do not breast-feed while taking this medication.
- Notify the prescriber before taking any other prescription, OTC medication, or herbal supplements.
- May impair judgement, thinking, or motor skills; avoid driving or other hazardous tasks.
- Do not abruptly discontinue use.

Table 22.1 Lithium Blood Levels and Associated Side Effects

Plasma Level	Side Effects or Symptoms of Toxicity
<1.5 mEq/L Mild side effects	Metallic taste in the mouth
	Fine hand tremor (resting)
	Nausea
	Polyuria
	Polydipsia
	Diarrhoea or loose stools
	Muscular weakness or fatigue
	Weight gain
	Oedema
	Memory impairments
1.5–2.5 mEq/L Moderate toxicity	Severe diarrhoea
	Dry mouth
	Nausea and vomiting
	Mild to moderate ataxia
	Incoordination
	Dizziness, sluggishness, giddiness, vertigo, cognitive slowing
	Slurred speech
	Tinnitus
	Blurred vision
	Fine motor tremor
	Muscle irritability or twitching
	Asymmetric deep tendon reflexes
	Increased muscle tone
>2.5 mEq/L Severe toxicity	Cardiac arrhythmias
	Blackouts
	Nystagmus
	Coarse tremor, clonic limb movements
	Fasciculations, seizures
	Visual or tactile hallucinations, delirium
	Oliguria, renal failure
	Peripheral vascular collapse, death
	Confusion
	Seizures
	Coma and death

Source: Data from Ferrando, S., Owen, J., & Levenson, J. (2014). Psychopharmacology. In R. Hales, S. Yudofsky, & L. Roberts (Eds.), *The American psychiatric publishing textbook of psychiatry* (6th ed., pp. 929–1003). Washington, DC: American Psychiatric Publishing.

interactions with medications and other substances as seen in Table 22.2. Table 22.3 describes nursing interventions for lithium side effects.

Psychological Domain

Assessment

The assessment of the psychological domain should follow the process explained in Chapter 10. Individuals with bipolar disorder can usually participate in many parts of the assessment.

Mood

By definition, bipolar disorder is a disturbance of mood. If the patient is depressed, using an assessment tool for depression may help determine the severity of depression. If mania predominates, evaluating the

Table 22.2 Lithium Interactions With Medications and Other Substances

Substance	Effect of Interaction
Angiotensin-converting enzyme inhibitors, such as: • Captopril • Lisinopril • Quinapril	Increases serum lithium; may cause toxicity and impaired kidney function
Acetazolamide	Increases the renal excretion of lithium, decreases lithium levels
Alcohol	May increase serum lithium level
Caffeine	Increases lithium excretion, increases lithium tremor
Carbamazepine	Increases neurotoxicity, despite normal serum levels and dosage
Fluoxetine	Increases serum lithium levels
Haloperidol	Increases neurotoxicity, despite normal serum levels and dosage
Loop diuretics, such as furosemide	Increases lithium serum levels but may be safer than thiazide diuretics; potassium-sparing diuretics (amiloride, spironolactone) are safest
Methyldopa	Increases neurotoxicity without increasing serum lithium levels
Nonsteroidal anti-inflammatory drugs, such as: • Diclofenac • Ibuprofen • Indomethacin • Piroxicam	Decreases renal clearance of lithium Increases serum lithium levels by 30%–60% in 3–10 days Aspirin and sulindac do not appear to have the same effect
Osmotic diuretics, such as: • Urea • Mannitol • Isosorbide	Increases renal excretion of lithium and decreases lithium levels
Sodium chloride	High sodium intake decreases lithium levels; low-sodium diets may increase lithium levels and lead to toxicity. Caution warranted regarding salt intake
Thiazide diuretics, such as: • Chlorothiazide • Hydrochlorothiazide	Promotes sodium and potassium excretion; increases lithium serum levels; may produce cardiotoxicity and neurotoxicity
TCAs	Increases tremor; potentiates pharmacologic effects of TCAs

Table 22.3 Interventions for Lithium Side Effects

Side Effect	Intervention
Oedema of the feet or hands	Monitor intake and output; check for possible decreased urinary output. Monitor sodium intake. The patient should elevate the legs when sitting or lying. Monitor weight.
Fine hand tremor	Provide support and reassurance if it does not interfere with daily activities. Tremor worsens with anxiety and intentional movements; minimize stressors. Notify the prescriber if it interferes with the patient's work and compliance will be an issue. More frequent smaller doses of lithium may also help.
Mild diarrhoea	Take lithium with meals. Provide for fluid replacement. Notify the prescriber if becomes severe; may need a change in medication preparation or may be early sign of toxicity.
Muscle weakness, fatigue, or memory and concentration difficulties	Provide support and reassurance; this side effect will usually pass after a few weeks of treatment. Short-term memory aids such as lists or reminder calls may be helpful. Notify the prescriber if becomes severe or interferes with the patient's desire to continue treatment.
Metallic taste	Suggest sugarless candies or throat lozenges. Encourage frequent oral hygiene.
Nausea or abdominal discomfort	Consider dividing the medication into smaller doses or give it at more frequent intervals. Give medication with meals.
Polydipsia	Reassure the patient that this is a normal mechanism to cope with polyuria.
Polyuria	Monitor intake and output. Provide reassurance and explain nature of side effect. Also explain that this causes no physical damage to the kidneys. Withhold medication.
Toxicity	Notify the prescriber. Use symptomatic treatments.

quality of the mood (elated, grandiose, irritated, or agitated) becomes important. Usually, mania is determined by clinical observation.

Cognition

In a **depressive episode**, the patient may not be able to concentrate enough to complete cognitive tasks, such as those called for in the Mini-Mental State Exam. During the acute phase of a manic or depressive episode, mental status may be abnormal, and in a **manic episode**, insight and judgement is impaired by extremely rapid, disjointed, and distorted thinking. Moreover, feelings such as grandiosity can interfere with normal executive functioning.

Thought Disturbances

Psychosis commonly occurs in patients with bipolar disorder, especially during acute mania episodes. Auditory hallucinations and delusional thinking may constitute the clinical picture. In children and adolescents, psychosis may not be easily detected, due to possible differential disorders such as ADHD.

Stress and Coping Factors

Stress and coping are critical assessment areas for a patient with bipolar disorder. A stressful event often triggers a manic or depressive episode. In some instances, there may be no apparent stress precipitating the episode, but it is important to discuss the possibility of a specific trigger. Determining the patient's usual coping skills for stresses lays the groundwork for developing interventional strategies. Negative coping skills, such as substance use or aggression, should be identified because these skills need to be replaced with more appropriate and functional coping.

Risk Assessment

Patients with bipolar disorder are at high risk for suicide. A complex interplay between the illness, environment, and person is considered the likely cause of suicide (Schaffer, Sinyor, Reis, Goldstein, & Levitt, 2014). Violent behaviours may occur during severe manic episodes, particularly when irritability, poor insight, limited judgement, as well substance abuse and personality disorder problems, are present; thus, patients should be assessed promptly for suicidal or homicidal risk. Behavioural control of violence is often achieved through medicating the patient to prevent harm (Volavka, 2013).

Nursing Diagnoses for Psychological Domain

Nursing diagnoses associated with the psychological domain of bipolar disorder include Disturbed Sensory Perception, Disturbed Thought Processes, Defensive Coping, Risk for Suicide, Risk for Other-Directed Violence, Risk for Self-Directed Violence, and Ineffective Coping.

Interventions for Psychological Domain

Pharmacotherapy is the primary treatment for bipolar disorder, but structured psychotherapies and adjunctive therapies for bipolar disorder have notable benefits. Research about psychotherapy for bipolar disorder has focused predominantly on patients with a chronic illness course. However, researchers are exploring the feasibility of implementing a new therapy for patient. Family-focused therapy has also been shown to have primary benefit in preventing relapse. Other modalities such as psychoeducation, IPT, and social rhythm therapy are adjunct therapies for reducing relapses (Parikh et al., 2013; Parikh & Velyvis, 2010). Integration of these therapies is fundamental to reducing depression and preventing possible relapses. Through early intervention, these therapies can be effective in promoting appropriate lifestyle management, improving medication adherence, and ultimately preempting intense symptom reoccurrence (Garland & Duffy, 2010).

Other risk factors for illness reoccurrence include obesity, high rates of nonadherence to medication therapy, marital conflict, separation, divorce, unemployment, and underemployment. The goals of psychosocial interventions aim to address these risk factors and associated features, which are difficult to address with pharmacotherapy alone. Of particular importance to the intents of interventions in this domain are improving medication adherence, decreasing the number and length of hospitalizations and relapses, enhancing social and occupational functioning, improving quality of life, increasing the patient's and family's acceptance of the disorder, and reducing the suicide risk (Davis, 2014).

Psychoeducation

Psychoeducation is designed to provide information on bipolar disorder, treatment, and recovery, and it usually focuses on medication adherence. Research suggests that psychoeducation, particularly in a group context, that specifically includes information about the importance of adherence to medications in addition to relapse prevention is effective in averting relapses and decreasing mania (Bond & Anderson, 2015). Nurses can provide psychoeducational information and identify any obstacles to recovery. Other important psychoeducational interventions nurses can implement include teaching patients to recognize warning signs and symptoms of relapse and offering strategies to help cope with residual symptoms and functional impairments. As well, resistance to accepting the illness and to taking medication, the symbolic meaning of taking medication, and worries about the future should be discussed openly. In the interest of improved medication adherence, it is helpful to listen carefully to patients' concerns about the medication, the dosing schedules, any changes in dosage, and side effects. Health teaching and weight management should be a component of any psychoeducation programme. In addition to individual variations in body weight, many of the antipsychotic and mood stabilizing medications are associated with weight gain. Monitoring weight and developing individual weight management plans that include exercise can reduce the relapse risk that is related to medication cessation, which is related to these concerns. Nurses must also be cognizant of the fact that poverty can negatively impact the patient's ability to maintain a healthy diet. Overall, the plan to support adherence should be made to fit the attitude, knowledge, and skills of the individual patient.

Psychotherapy

Psychotherapy is an integral aspect of bipolar disorder treatment. Often treatment of the depression is overlooked due to a focus on medication adherence. In addition to addressing the depression, psychotherapy can temper the stressors that trigger episodes and increase the patient's acceptance of the need for medication. Patients should be encouraged to keep their appointments with the therapist, communicate their needs, and provide feedback on the efficacy of their treatment. Kay Redfield Jamison offers important qualitative support for the benefits of psychotherapy and medications in treating bipolar disorder in her book *An Unquiet Mind* (1995).

Social Domain

Assessment

One of the tragedies of bipolar disorder is its effect on social and occupational functioning. Cultural views of mental illness profoundly influence the patient's acceptance of the disorder (Davis, 2014). During illness episodes, patients often behave in ways that jeopardize their social relationships. Losing a job or going through a divorce are common events. When performing an assessment of social function, the nurse should identify changes resulting from a manic or depressive episode.

Nursing Diagnoses for Social Domain

Nursing diagnoses for adults can include Ineffective Role Performance, Interrupted Family Processes, Impaired Social Interaction, Impaired Parenting, Compromised Family Coping, and Caregiver Role Strain. Another relevant diagnosis specific to children and adolescents in a family coping with a member with bipolar disorder is Delayed Growth and Development.

Interventions for Social Domain

Interventions focusing on the social domain are integral to nursing care for all ages. During mania, patients usually violate others' boundaries. Roommate selection for patients requiring hospital admittance needs to be carefully considered. If possible, a private room is ideal

because patients with bipolar disorder tend to irritate others, who quickly tire of the intrusiveness. These patients may miss the cues indicating anger and aggression from others. The nurse should protect the patient experiencing mania from self-harm, as well as harm from other patients.

Support groups are helpful for people with this disorder. Participating in groups allows the person to meet others with the disorder and learn management and preventive strategies. Support groups also are helpful in dealing with the stigma associated with mental illnesses (see Box 22.5).

Family Interventions

Marital and family interventions are often needed at different periods in the life of a person with bipolar disorder. For the family with a child with this disorder, additional parenting support and skills may be needed to manage the child's behaviours. The goals of family interventions are to help the family understand and cope with the disorder. Interventions may range from occasional counselling sessions to intensive family therapy. Research indicates family psychoeducation, as an adjunct treatment to pharmacotherapy, is effective in assisting families to cope, in decreasing the risk for relapse and hospitalization, and in improving outcomes at 6 months postintervention (Kolostoumpis et al., 2015) (see Box 22.6).

Spiritual Domain

The nursing approach to the spiritual domain in the care of the person with a bipolar disorder is the same as for the person with a major depressive disorder.

Evaluation and Treatment Outcomes

Desired treatment outcomes are mood stabilization and enhanced quality of life. Primary tools for evaluating outcomes are nursing observation and patient self-report (see Nursing Care Plan 22.1).

Continuum of Care

Inpatient Management

Inpatient admission is the treatment setting necessary when patients are severely psychotic or are an immediate threat to themselves or others. In acute mania, nursing interventions focus on patient safety, because patients in this state are prone to injury due to hyperactivity and are often unaware of injuries they sustain. Patients are often impulsive, disinhibited, and interpersonally inappropriate during acute mania. Redirecting conversation as well as behaviour and implementing boundaries is required when a patient is talking or acting inappropriately. Removal to a quieter environment may be necessary if other interventions have not been successful, but

BOX 22.5 Stigma

Receiving a diagnosis of bipolar disorder can be a stigmatizing experience that affects the lives and self-esteem of individuals with this disorder (Thome et al., 2012). In a phenomenological study, Hayne (2001) examined the response to receiving a psychiatric diagnosis, as differentiated from experiencing the illness itself. Emphasized in the lived description of psychiatric diagnosis was the notion that the diagnosis places the individual in a context of reflective self-knowledge. Below are excerpts of the experiences of two participants, Matt and Jeff, as well as before and after drawings that exemplify their perceptions of a "legitimized/delegitimized self." Matt desperately wanted to avoid being "abnormal." A diagnosis spelled "insanity" and he shuddered at the prospect of it. Why not "bizarre experience" or something less caustic? The diagnosis threatened to reveal "a secret he held to himself about himself," confronting him with, "I am flawed! Not, I have a flaw, but, I am flawed!" He sketches "diagnosis" in "Before" and "After" self-profiles. Prediagnosis self has a halo to arc dark (blue) hair (he interprets this as ominous). With diagnosis, there is no evading the ill-fated knowledge and Matt accommodates the diagnosis, colouring his hair bright (green) to represent hope

and "self-acceptance." Jeff views embracing the diagnosis as central in to his mental illness experience in that it supplied him "a battleground for living." Prior to diagnosis, he felt empty, forlorn, immobilized ("a scarecrow, suspended in a field"). Diagnosis resulted in "knowledge made knowledgeable" to him. With that he was able to reformulate (pictured as a snowman). Someone "cared" enough to assist this reconstituting (the therapeutic encounter). Therefore, he is not cold as a snowman (scarf); he wears a smile. Rediscovery of his personal significance (top hat) equips him to take up his future (hands outstretched). The nursing implications from this research are that it fosters a greater understanding of the significance of receiving a psychiatric diagnosis and this knowledge may better prepare nurses to help patients sustain hope and self-acceptance. As well, it encourages nurses to implement early intervention strategies that address shame and stigma. It is also knowledge that may be transferred to understanding the potential life-changing ramifications of any medical diagnosis.

Diagnosis: Matt Before and After.
Diagnosis: Jeff Before and After.

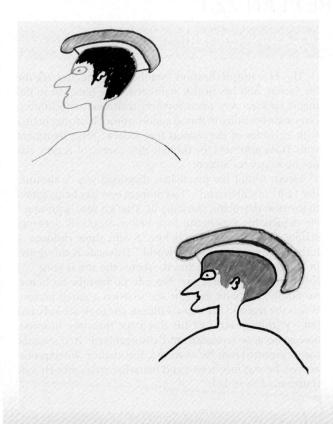

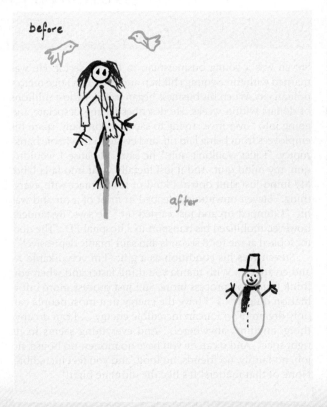

| BOX **22.6** Psychoeducation Checklist: |
| Bipolar I Disorder |

When caring for the family and their family member who has a bipolar I disorder, be sure to include the following topic areas in the teaching plan:
- Psychopharmacologic agents, including drug action, dosage, frequency, and possible adverse effects
- Medication regimen adherence
- Strategies to decrease agitation and restlessness
- Safety measures
- Self-care management
- Follow-up laboratory testing
- Support services

---

the patient should be carefully monitored. The nurse should avoid a confrontational approach and instead, respectfully implement limits.

Medication management including control of side effects is a major nursing responsibility during inpatient hospitalization. Nurses should be familiar with drug–drug interactions (Chapter 12) and with interventions to help control side effects.

Intensive Outpatient Programmes

When hospitalization is not necessary, or in order to prevent or shorten hospitalization, intensive outpatient programs for several weeks of acute-phase care during a manic or depressive episode are used. These programs are usually called *partial hospitalization* or *day hospitalization*. Close medication monitoring and milieu therapies that foster the restoration of a patient's previous adaptive abilities are the major nursing responsibilities in these settings. Setting up frequent office visits and crisis telephone calls are additional nursing interventions that can help to shorten or prevent hospitalization. Psychoeducation that includes the patient and significant others are alternatives. Severely and persistently ill patients may need ongoing intensive treatment, but the frequency of visits can be decreased for patients whose conditions stabilize and who enter the continuation or the maintenance phase of treatment.

NURSING CARE PLAN 22.1

THE PATIENT WITH BIPOLAR DISORDER

Steven was a young businessman in the oil sector. He was married with three young children and lived in a large metropolitan city. When his business began to fail, he lost millions of dollars within weeks. He describes feeling desperate and going into "overdrive" trying to save the company, spare his employees from being laid off, and evade an inevitable bankruptcy. "I just wouldn't quit," he says. "Because I wouldn't quit, my mind quit. And it just literally went into la-la-land. My mind just shut down. I kind of lost contact with everything." Steven unwittingly stepped in front of a car and was hit. "I jumped up and just carried on," he says. Bystanders, however, mobilized his transport to a hospital ED. "The doctor looked at me for 8 seconds and said 'manic depressive!'"

Steven sees his condition as a gift: "I'm very likable … and creative…. With mania you think faster and when you think faster you process more. So I just process more information quicker…. "I have the energy that most people can only dream of … I mean incredible energy … I can do anything, anytime, anywhere…. And everything seems in its right space. And it can be you have no money, no house, no job, no family, no friends, no food, and you feel incredible. None of that matters! It's like the ultimate high!"

The first hospitalization established a medical regime for Steven, and his health stabilized for a time. An initial manic episode very often involves treatment with lithium carbonate resulting in mood stabilization. Recurring mania with episodes of depression may benefit from treatment with TCAs and MAOIs, though this course of action was not necessary for Steven.

Steven found his psychiatric diagnosis was "a destructive (gift) of difference!" "I went from one day being gifted to the next day being mentally ill. That's a very large step." He depicts his experience in a before-diagnosis drawing, stating, "I had everything before: a wife, three children, a home! The sun shone in my world." This state is contrasted in an after-diagnosis portrayal, where "the sun is gone." "I lost it all. There is just me! No job, no friends, no home, no family! My wife thought she married a gifted person. When she realized the mental illness, she took the kids and left." Within months of his discharge from the hospital, Steven became confused and disorganized. A restaurant owner reported him for causing a disturbance. When police arrived, he was incoherent and behaving erratically. He was transported to an ED.

NURSING CARE PLAN 22.1 *(Continued)*

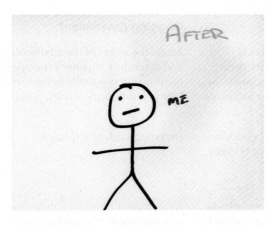

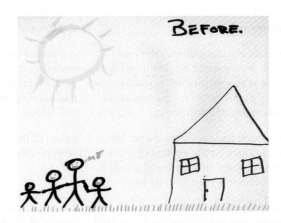

Setting: Acute Care Psychiatric Unit in a General Hospital

Baseline Assessment: From the ED, Steven is admitted to acute care inpatient services where he presents with symptoms of mixed bipolar mood disorder. His mood is quite labile and he is easily irritated. His speech is pressured.

He is unable to account for his behaviour and is exhibiting flight of ideas. Historical records indicate his prior admission and discharge on lithium, which he admits he did not take. When asked why he stopped his medication he states, "I completely disagreed with it. I didn't think that my gift needed treatment."

Diagnostic Features	Medications
Bipolar I disorder	L-Thyroxine 0.1 mg q AM × 1 day
Hypothyroidism	Clonazepam 0.5 mg bid for sleep and agitation
Social problems (Divorce finalized 18 months ago. Ex-wife has full custody of three children. Patient has supervised visitations.)	Carbamazepine added on transfer to be titrated up to 400 mg tid

Setting: Acute Care Psychiatric Unit in a General Hospital

Associated Features	Related Factors
Potential for life-threatening injury	Elation and expansive feelings
Poor judgement and impulse control	Excitement vacillating with desolation
Lack of support system	Loss secondary to finances/job, divorce

Goals of Care

Initial	Discharge
1. Will seek out appropriate support	5. Will discuss the complexity of his illness
2. Will comply with unit regulations	6. Will express antecedents of treatment related to mania and depression
3. Will participate in programme activities	7. Will discuss need for adherence to meds
4. Will achieve balance in activities of daily living (e.g., rest, hydration, nutrition)	8. Will identify antecedents and indicators of impending illness exacerbation

(Continued)

NURSING CARE PLAN 22.1 *(Continued)*

Interventions	Rationale	Ongoing Assessment
Initiate a nurse–patient relationship; demonstrate acceptance of the patient as a worthwhile human being through the use of nonjudgemental statements and behaviour.	A sense of worthlessness often underlies despair. A positive therapeutic relationship can maintain the patient's dignity and foster improved self-esteem.	Assess the stages of the relationship and determine whether a therapeutic relationship is actually being formed. Identify indicators of trust.
Initiate suicide precautions per hospital policy. Apply vigilant observation routines. Implement individual suicide safety plan with patient.	Safety of the individual is a priority with people who have poor impulse control.	Determine risk of self-harm.
Help the client to develop a relapse prevention plan that includes seeking professional mental health support when she or he feels suicidal.	A relapse prevention plan can help the patient maintain wellness and safety by encouraging the resistance of impulses and providing a stepwise plan to address any exacerbation of symptoms.	Determine the patient's ability to commit to the relapse plan.
	A relapse prevention plan requires an understanding of *denial* as an expected coping mechanism. This coping mechanism should be connected with the client's underlying emotional struggle with his or her illness.	

Evaluation

Outcomes	Revised Outcomes	Interventions
Has not harmed self; denies self-harm thoughts/intent. Identifies people and resources to assist when suicidality heightens	Absence of risk or self-harm intent will continue.	Discontinue precautions incrementally; maintain ongoing assessment for safety.
Made a suicide safety plan with nurse, agrees to keep it after discharge	Maintains suicide safety plan and reviews it regularly with outpatient mental health provider	Support and reinforce this suicide safety plan, updating it regularly.

Associated Impaired Sense of Self and Self-Esteem

Defining Characteristics	Related Factors
Expressions of grandiosity vacillating with expressions of shame and guilt Lack of success in business endeavours and relationships	Labile mood (elation and despair noted) Feelings of abandonment secondary to separation from significant others Feelings of failure secondary to bankruptcy and relationship problems Unrealistic expectations of self

Goals of Care

Initial	Discharge
1. Realistic self-appraisal	3. Verbalize acceptance of personal limitations
2. Modify excessive and unrealistic self-expectations	4. Report freedom from untoward symptoms
	5. Avoid behavioural risks

NURSING CARE PLAN 22.1 *(Continued)*

Interventions	Rationale	Ongoing Assessment
Enhance the patient's sense of self by being attentive; validate interpretation of what is being said or experienced; help to make consistent, realistic verbalizations.	By showing respect and helping the patient frame happenings realistically, the nurse can support and help build the patient's sense of self.	Determine whether the patient confirms realistic interpretation of situations and verbalizes with moderation in rate and volume.
Assist to reframe and redefine negative statements ("not a failure, but a setback").	Reframing an event positively can help the patient view the situation in an alternative way and it directs dialogue toward enhancing change.	Assess whether the patient can actually view the world in a different way.
Problem-solve with the patient about how to approach finding satisfying employment.	Work is very important to adults. Bankruptcy can decrease self-esteem. Focusing on the possibility of a future job can provide hope.	Assess the patient's problem-solving ability. Note indicators of realistic plans.
Encourage positive physical habits (healthy eating patterns, exercise, adequate sleep).	A healthy lifestyle promotes well-being, increasing self-esteem.	Determine willingness to consider making lifestyle changes.
Teach the patient to validate consensually with others.	Low self-esteem is generated by negative interpretations of the world. Through consensual validation, the patient can determine whether others view situations in the same way.	Assess the patient's ability to participate in this process.
Teach constructive self-appraisal. Helpful exercises might include self-affirmations, imagery, use of humour, meditation/prayer, and relaxation.	There are many different approaches that can be practiced to increase self-esteem.	Assess the patient's energy level and ability to focus on learning new skills.
Assist in establishing appropriate personal boundaries.	In an attempt to meet their own needs, people with a compromised sense of self often violate other people's boundaries and/or allow others to take advantage of them. Helping patients establish their own boundaries will improve the likelihood of needs being met in an appropriate manner.	Assess the patient's ability to understand the concept of boundary violation and its significance.
Provide an opportunity within the therapeutic relationship to express thoughts and feelings. Use open-ended statements and questions. Encourage expression of both positive and negative statements.	The individual with compromised self-esteem may have difficulty expressing thoughts and feelings. Varied outlets for expression may help improve how thoughts and feelings are expressed.	Monitor thoughts and feelings that are expressed in order to help the patient examine them.
Explore opportunities for positive socialization.	Individuals with insecurity issues may be in social situations that reinforce artificial self-evaluation. Helping the patient identify new positive situations will present other options.	Assess whether the new situations are potentially positive or are a re-creation of other negative (self-aggrandizing) situations.
Steven began to modify excessive and unrealistic expectations of self.	Strengthen ability to affirm realistic aspects and examine expectations related to work and relationships.	Refer to mental health clinic for cognitive behavioural psychotherapy.
Verbalized defeatist thinking related to finding worthwhile employment	Identify important aspects of tentative employment so that he can begin looking for a job that has those characteristics.	Attend a support group that focuses on job interviewing skills.
As Steven's mood stabilized, he was able to sleep through the night, and he began eating again. He also expressed positive thoughts about his future.	Maintain a stable mood to promote a positive and realistic self-concept.	Monitor mood and identify antecedents to mood escalation and/or depression.

(Continued)

NURSING CARE PLAN 22.1 *(Continued)*

Associated Ineffective Individual Coping

Defining Characteristics	Related Factors
Verbalization in inability to cope or ask for help Reported difficulty with life stressors Compromised ability to problem-solve Alteration in social participation Disinhibited behaviour resulting in self-risk Distorted thought and self-control Substance abuse	Altered mood (alternating mania and depression) caused by changes secondary to body chemistry (bipolar disorder) Altered mood caused by changes secondary to intake of mood-altering substance (alcohol) Unsatisfactory support system Sensory overload secondary to excessive activity Unreliable psychological resources for consistency of employment

Goals of Care

Initial	Discharge
1. Accept support through the nurse–patient relationship.	6. Practise new coping skills.
2. Identify areas of ineffective coping.	7. Focus on realistic strengths.
3. Examine current efforts at coping.	
4. Identify realistic areas of strength.	
5. Learn new coping skills.	

Interventions	Rationale	Ongoing Assessment
Identify current stresses in Steven's life, including the acceptance of bipolar disorder.	When the patient verbalizes areas of concern, he will be able to focus on one issue at a time. If he identifies the mental disorder as a stressor, he will more likely be able to develop strategies to deal with it.	Determine whether Steven is able to identify problem areas realistically. Continue to assess for self-risk behaviours.
Identify Steven's strengths in dealing with past stressors.	By focusing on past successes, he can identify strengths and build on them in the future.	Assess if Steven can identify any previous successes in his life.
Assist Steven in discussing, selecting, and practicing positive coping skills (jogging, yoga, volunteer work).	New coping skills take a conscious effort to learn and will at first seem strange and unnatural. Practising these skills will help build a repertoire of coping strategies.	Assess whether Steven follows through on learning new skills.
Educate the patient on the use of alcohol and its relationship to bipolar disorder.	Alcohol is an ineffective coping strategy that can exacerbate the symptoms of bipolar disorder.	Assess for the patient's willingness to control drinking.
Assist the patient in coping with bipolar disorder, beginning with education about it.	A mood disorder is a major stressor in a patient's life. To manage the stress, the patient needs a knowledge base.	Determine Steven's knowledge about bipolar disorder.
Administer lithium as ordered (give with food or milk). Reinforce the action, dosage, and side effects. Review laboratory results to determine whether lithium is within therapeutic limits. Assess for toxicity. Recommend a normal diet with normal salt intake; maintenance of adequate fluid intake.	Lithium carbonate is effective in the treatment of bipolar disorder, but it must be managed. The patient should have a thorough knowledge of the medication and side effects.	Assess for target action, side effects, and toxicity.

NURSING CARE PLAN 22.1 *(Continued)*

Goals of Care

Hypothyroidism Interventions	Rationale	Ongoing Assessment
Administer thyroid supplement as ordered. Review thyroid functioning laboratory results. Discuss the symptoms of hypothyroidism and how they are similar to depression. Emphasize the importance of taking lithium and L-thyroxine. Explain about the long-term effects of lithium on thyroid functioning.	Hypothyroidism can be a side effect of lithium carbonate and also mimics symptoms of depression.	Determine whether the patient understands the relationship between thyroid dysfunction and lithium carbonate.

Evaluation

Outcomes	Revised Outcomes	Interventions
Clonazepam 0.5 mg bid for sleep and agitation		
Steven is easily engaged in a therapeutic relationship. He examined the areas in his life where he coped ineffectively.	Establish a therapeutic relationship with a therapist at the mental health clinic.	Refer to mental health clinic.
He identified his strengths and how he coped with stressors, especially his illness, in the past.	Continue to view illness as a potential stressor that can disrupt life.	Seek advice immediately if there are any problems with medications.
He learned new problem-solving skills and reported that he learned a lot about his medication. He plans to adhere to medication regimen.	Continue to practise new coping skills as stressful situations arise.	Discuss with the therapist the outcomes of using new coping skills.

Spectrum of Care

In today's health care climate, with efforts to reduce hospitalization, most patients with bipolar disorder are treated as outpatients. Hospitalizations are usually brief, and treatment focuses on restabilization. Patients with mood disorders are likely to need long-term medication regimens and supportive psychotherapy to function in the community. Therefore, medication regimens and additional treatment planning need to be tailored to individual needs. Patients need extended and continued follow-up to monitor medication trials and side effects, reinforce self-care management, and provide continued psychosocial support (see Chapter 4).

Mental Health Promotion

Mental health promotion activities should be the focus during remissions. During this period, patients have an opportunity to learn new coping skills that promote positive mental health. Stress management and relaxation techniques can be practised for use when needed. A plan for managing emerging symptoms can also be developed during this period.

SUMMARY OF KEY POINTS

- Mood disorders are characterized by persistent or recurring disturbances in mood that cause significant psychological distress and functional impairment. Mood disturbances can be broadly categorized as manic or dysphoric (typified by exaggerated feelings of elation or irritability) or depressive or dysthymic (typified by feelings of sadness, hopelessness, loss of interest, and fatigue).
- Primary mood disorders include both depressive disorders (unipolar depression) and manic–depressive disorders (bipolar disorders).

- Genetics undoubtedly play a role in the aetiology of mood disorders. Risk factors include family history of mood disorders; prior mood episodes; lack of social support; stressful life events; substance abuse; and medical problems, particularly chronic or terminal illnesses.

- The recommended depression treatment guidelines include antidepressant medication, alone or with psychotherapeutic management or psychotherapy; ECT for severe depression; or phototherapy for patients with seasonal depressive symptoms.

- Nurses must be knowledgeable about antidepressant medications: their therapeutic effects and associated side effects, toxicity, dosage ranges, and contraindications. Nurses must also be familiar with ECT protocols and associated interventions. Patient education and the provision of emotional support during and after the course of treatment are also nursing responsibilities.

- Many symptoms of depression, such as weight and appetite changes, sleep disturbance, decreased energy, and fatigue, are similar to those of medical illnesses. Assessment includes a thorough medical history and physical examination to detect or rule out medical or psychiatric comorbidity.

- Bio/psycho/social/spiritual assessment includes assessing medical and health status; mood; speech patterns; thought content and processes; suicidal, filicidal, or homicidal thoughts; cognition and memory; social factors such as patterns of relationship, quality of support systems, and changes in occupational functioning; and spiritual beliefs and practices. Several self-report scales, such as the BDI and the Hamilton Rating Scale, are helpful in evaluating depressive symptoms.

- Establishing and maintaining a therapeutic nurse–patient relationship is key to successful outcomes. Nursing interventions that foster the therapeutic relationship include being available in times of crisis, providing understanding and education to patients and their families regarding goals of treatment, providing encouragement and feedback concerning the patient's progress, providing guidance in the patient's interpersonal interactions (within the work environment, the community), and helping to set and monitor realistic goals.

- Psychosocial interventions for mood disorders include self-care management, cognitive therapy, behaviour therapy, IPT, patient and family psychoeducation regarding the nature of the disorder and treatment goals, marital and family therapy, and group therapy that includes medication maintenance support groups and other consumer-oriented support groups.

- Bipolar disorders are characterized by one or more manic episodes or mixed mania (co-occurrence of manic and depressive states) that cause marked impairment in social activities, occupational functioning, and interpersonal relationships and may require hospitalization to prevent self-harm.

- Manic episodes are periods in which the patient experiences abnormally and persistently elevated, expansive, or irritable mood characterized by inflated self-esteem, decreased need to sleep, excessive energy or hyperactivity, racing thoughts, easy distractibility, and inability to stay focused. Other symptoms can include hypersexuality and impulsivity.

- Similar to treatment of major depressive disorder, pharmacotherapy is the cornerstone of treatment of bipolar illness, but adjunctive psychosocial interventions are also needed. Pharmacologic therapy includes treatment with mood stabilizers alone or in combination with antipsychotics or benzodiazepines if psychosis, agitation, or insomnia is present and antidepressants for unremitted depression.

- ECT is a valuable alternative for patients with severe mania that do not respond to other treatment.

- Recent major advances in bipolar disorder treatment research validate the efficacy of integrated psychosocial and pharmacologic treatment involving family or couples therapies, psychoeducational programmes, and individual cognitive–behavioural or interpersonal therapies.

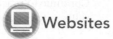 **Websites**

ccsa.ca Canadian Centre on Substance Abuse website where information exists issues related to alcohol and mood disorders.

canmat.org The site of the Canadian Network for Mood and Anxiety Treatment has information for health professionals and the public, including guidelines for management and treatment of mood disorders.

camimh.ca The Canadian Alliance on Mental Illness and Mental Health (CAMIMH) offers information on services of member mental health organizations for health care practitioners, consumers, and their families. The organization is committed to raising mental health awareness and making accessibility to care and support for the mentally ill and their families a priority for government and communities.

cmha.ca This is the site of the Canadian Mental Health Association, which uses a wellness model to approach such topics as mental fitness and how it is defined, acquired, and maintained across the life span.

cpa.ca The Canadian Psychological Association takes an advisory role for people wanting to know about issues and care alternatives. Areas of focus include mental health problems related to mood disorders and the psychological factors necessary to maintain wellness in the context of such mood-related disorders.

cdrin.org Canadian Depression Research and Intervention website. It discusses the coalitions participating in an endeavour to promote research by collaborating with provincial and national organizations about depression and PTSD.

internationalbipolarfoundation.org International bipolar foundation (IBPF) organization (nonprofit) that offers information in 60 languages about bipolar disorder and its treatment. There are videos and webinars available as well as resources for families and caregivers.

isbd.org International Society for Bipolar Disorder Professional international organization publishing the journal Bipolar Disorder. It supports research about bipolar treatment and has sections for patients and families.

mdsc.ca The Mood Disorders Society of Canada (MDSC) is a volunteer organization with a commitment to optimizing the quality of life for people with mood disorders. The MDSC gives a voice to consumers by establishing a national research agenda and developing strategies of care.

nccah-ccnsa.ca National Collaborating Centre for Aboriginal Health website containing information, webinars, and publications about the health and mental health of indigenous populations.

nimh.nih.gov The site of the National Institute of Mental Health (NIMH) provides a forum for worldwide research into mental illness. In addition to offering a wealth of information on the latest research, the site offers education information pamphlets on depression, bipolar disorder, and other mental illnesses that can be ordered or printed free of charge. These publications are in the public domain and can be reproduced without copyright infringement, as long as authorship is acknowledged.

nmhac.ca This site is the Native Mental Health Association of Canada which developed from the Canadian Psychiatric Association of Mental Health. NMHAC offers educational information and understanding to promote culturally relevant mental health care for Indigenous peoples.

nnmh.ca This is the site of the National Network for Mental Health, which functions as an advocate and educational resource for Canadian mental health consumers and their families and friends. The organization's goal is to unite and empower individuals.

obad.ca This is the site of the Organization for Bipolar Affective Disorders (OBAD). This organization offers peer support for anyone affected by mood disorders, aiming to assist them to be active in their recovery and gain a sense of resolution in their lives.

obad.ca/bpkids.org This is the site of the Child & Adolescent Bipolar Foundation (CABF), a parent-led, not-for-profit membership organization that maintains an extensive website of information and support for families and youth who have bipolar disorder. The organization has a large professional advisory board of experts in the field, including Kay Redfield Jamison, author of *An Unquiet Mind* (1995), a book about her own struggles with bipolar disorder. While much of the information is available to anyone visiting the website, for a donation families and professionals can obtain membership access to chat rooms and other resources.

suicideprevention.ca This is the site of the Canadian Association for Suicide Prevention, which provides information on suicide and resources related to its prevention—the location of crisis centres, survivor support groups, and related library materials. Guidelines to minimize the suicide risk of loved ones are available here.

statcan.gc.ca Statistics Canada website contains statistical information about depression and bipolar disorder

psychguides.com/bipolar A copy of *Treatment of Bipolar Disorder: A Guide for Patients and Families* can be downloaded from this site.

mobilemoodkit.com This application assists the user to create helpful, intuitive, and scientifically sound tools to improve the lives of people who suffer from depression.

who.int/mental_health/management/depression/who_paper_depression_wfmh_2012.pdf The World Health Organization (2012) report titled *Depression: A Global Crisis* is available here.

References

Albert, R. (2015). Why is depression more prevalent in women? *Journal of Psychiatry and Neuroscience, 40*(4), 219–221. doi:10.1503/jpn.150205

Alonso, J., Petukhova, M., Vilagut, G., Chatterji, S., Heeringa, S., Ustun, T., … Kessler, R. (2011). Days out of role due to common physical and mental conditions: Results from the WHO World Mental Health Surveys. *Molecular Psychiatry, 16*, 1234–1246. doi:10.1038/mp.2010.101

American Psychiatric Association. (2013). *Diagnostic and statistical manual of mental disorders* (5th ed.). Arlington, VA: Author.

Barnhill, J. W. (2014). The psychiatric interview and mental status examination. In R. Hales, S. Yudofsky, & L. Roberts (Eds.), *The American psychiatric publishing textbook of psychiatry* (6th ed., pp. 3–29). Washington, DC: American Psychiatric Publishing.

BC Reproductive Mental Health Program & Perinatal Services BC. (2014). *Best practice guidelines for mental health disorders in the perinatal period.* British Columbia, Canada: Author. Retrieved from http://www.perinatalservicesbc.ca/Documents/Guidelines-Standards/Maternal/MentalHealthDisordersGuideline.pdf

Bellamy, S., & Hardy, C. (2015). Understanding depression in Aboriginal communities and families. *National Collaborating Centre for Aboriginal Health.* Retrieved from http://www.nccah-ccnsa.ca/Publications/Lists/Publications/Attachments/150/2015-10-07-RPT-MentalHealth03-Depression-BellamyHardy-EN-Web.pdf

Berk, M., Dodd, S., Callaly, P., Berk, L., Fitzgerald, P., de Castella, A. R., … Kulkarni, J. (2007). History of illness prior to a diagnosis of bipolar disorder or schizoaffective disorder. *Journal of Affective Disorders, 103*, 181–186. doi:10.1016/j.jad.2007.01.027

Birks, J., & Grimley Evans, J. (2009). Gingko biloba for cognitive impairment and dementia. *Cochrane Database of Systematic Reviews, 1*, CD003120. doi:10.1002/14651858.CD003120.pub3

Blazer, D., & Hybels, C. (2014). Depression in later life: Epidemiology, assessment, impact, and treatment. In I. Gotlib & C. Hammen (Eds.), *Handbook of depression* (3rd ed., pp. 429–447). New York, NY: The Guilford Press.

Bond, K., & Anderson, I. M. (2015). Psychoeducation for relapse prevention in bipolar disorder: A systematic review of efficacy in randomized controlled studies. *Bipolar Disorder, 17*, 349–362. doi:10.1111/bdi.12287

Bonelli, R., Dew, R., Koenig, H., Rosmarin, D., & Vasegh, S. (2012). Religious and spiritual factors in depression: Review and integration of the research. *Depression Research and Treatment, 2012:962860*, 1–8. doi:10.1155/2012/962860

Borneman, T., Ferrell, B., & Puchalski, C. (2010). Evaluation of the FICA tool for spiritual assessment. *Journal of Pain and Symptom Management, 40*(2), 163–173. doi:10.1016/j.jpainsymman.2009.12.019

Bromet, E., Andrade, L., Hwang, I., Sampson, N., Alonso, J., Girolamo, G., … Kessler, R. (2011). Cross-national epidemiology of DSM-IV major depressive episode. *BMC Medicine, 9*(90), 1–16. doi:10.1186/1741-7015-9-90

Brus, M., Solanto, M., & Godlberg, J. (2014). Adult ADHD vs. bipolar disorder in the DSM-5 era: A challenging differentiation for clinicians. *Journal of Psychiatric Practice, 29*(6), 428–437. doi:10.1097/01.pra.0000456591.20622.9e

Bryson, C. (2012). Women's health. In *Research News. Alberta innovates—Health solutions.* Edmonton, AB: McCallum Printing Group Inc.

Bulloch, A., Lavorato, D., Williams, J., & Patten, S. (2012). Alcohol consumption and major depression in the general population: The critical importance of dependence. *Depression and Anxiety, 29*(12), 1058–1064. doi:10.1002/da.22001

Canadian Mental Health Association. (2008). *The relationship between mental health, mental illness and chronic physical conditions.* Retrieved from ontario.cmha.ca/public_policy/the-relationship-between-mental-health-mental-illness-and-chronic-physical-conditions/#

Canadian Mental Health Association. (2013). *Connection between mental and physical health.* Retrieved from http://ontario.cmha.ca/mental-health/connection-between-mental-and-physical-health/

Canadian Nurses Association. (2012a). *A nursing call to action: The health of our nation, the future of our health system.* National Expert Commission. Retrieved from https://www.cna-aiic.ca/~/media/cna/files/en/nec_report_e.pdf

Canadian Nurses Association. (2012b). *Position statement: Mental Health Services.* Retrieved from https://www.cna-aiic.ca/~/media/cna/page-content/pdf-en/ps85_mental_health_e.pdf?la=en

Carta, M. G., Mura, G., Lecca, M. E., Moro, M. F., Bhat, K. M., Angermeyer, M. C., ... Akiskal, H. S. (2012). Decreases in depression over 20 years in a mining area of Sardinia: Due to selective migration? *Journal of Affective Disorders, 141,* 255–260. doi:10.1016/j.jad.2012.03.038

Center on the Developing Child at Harvard University. (2009). *Maternal depression can undermine the development of young children: Working paper no. 8.* Retrieved from http://www.developingchild.harvard.edu

Chennattucherry, J. J., & Mok, Y. M. (2010). Physical health issues. In A. H. Young, I. N. Ferrier, & E. E. Michalak (Eds.), *Practical management of bipolar disorder* (pp. 106–119). New York, NY: Cambridge University Press.

Conus, P., Macneil, C., & McGorry, P. (2014). Public health significance of bipolar disorder: Implications for early intervention and prevention. *Bipolar Disorders, 16*(5), 548–556. doi:10.1111/bdi.12137

Corcoran, J., & Walsh, J. (2009). Bipolar disorder. In J. Corcoran & J. Walsh (Eds.), *Mental health in social work* (pp. 216–241). Boston, MA: Pearson Education.

Cowen, P., Harrison, P., & Burns, T. (2012). Mood disorders. In P. Cowen, P. Harrison, & T. Burns (Eds.), *Shorter oxford textbook of psychiatry* (pp. 205–253). Oxford, UK: Oxford University Press.

Cui, Y., & Zheng, Y. (2016). A meta-analysis on the efficacy and safety of St John's wort extract in depression therapy in comparison with selective serotonin uptake inhibitors in adults. *Neuropsychiatric Disease and Treatment, 12,* 1715–1723. doi:10.2147/NDT.S106752

Cusin, C., & Dougherty, D. (2012). Somatic therapies for treatment-resistant depression: ECT, TMS, VNS, DBS. *Biology of Mood and Anxiety Disorders, 2*(14), 1–9. doi:10.1186/2045-5380-2-14

Davis, S. (2014). *Community mental health in Canada: Theory, policy, and practice.* Vancouver, BC: UBC Press.

Duffy, A. (2012). The nature of the association between childhood ADHD and the development of bipolar disorder: A review of prospective high-risk studies. *American Journal of Psychiatry, 169*(12), 1247–1255. doi.org/10.1176/appi.ajp.2012.11111725

Duffy, A., Alda, M., Hajek, T., Sherry, S. B., & Grof, P. (2010). Early stages in the development of bipolar disorder. *Journal of Affective Disorders, 121*(1–2), 127–135. doi:10.1016/j.jad.2009.05.022

Felitti, V. (2007). The tragic imprint of childhood adversity. In *Alberta Mental Health Board (AMHB), Mending Minds: Information Supplement.* Proceedings of the Mental Health Research Showcase, Alberta, Canada.

Ferrando, S., Owen, J., & Levenson, J. (2014). Psychopharmacology. In R. Hales, S. Yudofsky, & L. Roberts (Eds.), *The American psychiatric publishing textbook of psychiatry* (6th ed., pp. 929–1003). Washington, DC: American Psychiatric Publishing.

Firestone, M., Smylie, J., Maracle, S., McKnight, C., Spiller, M., & O'Campo, P. (2015). Mental health and substance abuse in an urban First Nations population in Hamilton Ontario. *Canadian Journal of Public Health, 106*(6), 375–371. doi:10.17269/CJPH.106.4923

Fox, J., & Jones, D. (2013). DSM-5 and bereavement: The loss of normal grief. *Journal of Counseling & Development, 91,* 113–119. doi:10.1002/j.1556-6676.2013.00079.x

Freedland, K., & Carney, R. (2014). Depression and medical illness. In I. Gotlib & C. Hammen (Eds.), *Handbook of depression* (3rd ed., pp.122–141). New York, NY: The Guilford Press.

Garland, E. J., & Duffy, A. (2010). Treating bipolar disorder in the early stages of illness. In A. H. Young, I. N. Ferrier, & E. E. Michalak (Eds.), *Practical management of bipolar disorder* (pp. 73–83). New York, NY: Cambridge University Press.

George, M., Taylor, J., Short, E., Snipes, J., & Pelic, C. (2014). Brain stimulation therapies. In R. Hales, S. Yudofsky, & L. Roberts (Eds.), *The American psychiatric publishing textbook of psychiatry* (6th ed., pp. 1005–1036). Washington, DC: American Psychiatric Publishing.

Gitlin, M., (2014). Phamacotherapy and other somatic treatments. In I. Gotlib & C. Hammen (Eds.), *Handbook of depression* (3rd ed., pp. 492–512). New York, NY: The Guilford Press.

Gomi, S., Starnino, V., & Canda, E. (2014). Spiritual assessment in mental health recovery. *Community Mental Health, 50,* 447–453. doi:10.1007/s10597-013-9653-z

Grande, I., Berk, M., Birmaher, B., & Vieta, E., (2016). Bipolar disorder. *The Lancet, 387*(10027), 1561–1572. doi:10.1016/S0140-6736(15)00241-X

Hammen, C., Rudolf, K., & Abaied, J. (2014). Child and adolescent depression. In E. Mash & R. Barkley (Eds.), *Child psychopathology* (3rd ed., pp. 225–263). New York, NY: Guilford Press.

Hayne, Y. (2001). *To be diagnosed—The experience of persons with chronic mental illness (Unpublished Dissertation).* Edmonton, AB: University of Alberta.

Hodge, D. R. (2015). Administering a two-stage spiritual assessment in healthcare settings: A necessary component of ethical and effective care. *Journal of Nursing Management, 23,* 27–38. doi:10.1111/jonm.12078

International Council of Nurses. (2013). *ICN code of ethics for nurses. Cultural and linguistic competence.* Retrieved from http://www.icn.ch/images/stories/documents/publications/position_statements/B03_Cultural_Linguistic_Competence.pdf

Islam, F. (2015). Immigrating to Canada during early childhood associated with increased risk for mood disorders. *Community Mental Health, 51,* 723–732. doi:10:1007/s10597-015-9851-y

Jamison, K. R. (1995). *An unquiet mind.* Toronto, ON: Random House.

Johnson, S., Cuellar, A., & Peckham, A. (2014). Risk factors for bipolar disorder. In I. Gotlib & C. Hammen (Eds.). *Handbook of depression* (3rd ed., pp. 315–333). New York, NY: The Guilford Press.

Kerner, B. (2014). Genetics of bipolar disorder. *The Application of Clinical Genetics, 7,* 33–42. doi:10.2147/TACG.S39297

Kessler, R., & Bromet, E. (2013). The epidemiology of depression across cultures. *Annual Review of Public Health, 34,* 119–138. doi:10.1146/annurev-publhealth-031912-114409

Kessler, R., De Jonge, P., Shahly, V., van Loo, P., Wang, P., & Wilcox, M. (2014). Epidemiology of depression. In I. Gotlib & C. Hammen (Eds.), *Handbook of depression* (3rd ed., pp. 7–24). New York, NY: The Guilford Press.

Ketter, T., & Chang, K. (2014). Bipolar and related disorders. In R. Hales, S. Yudofsky, & L. Roberts (Eds.), *The American psychiatric publishing textbook of psychiatry* (6th ed., pp. 311–352). Washington, DC: American Psychiatric Publishing.

Kielland, N., & Simeone, T. (2014). *Current issues in mental health in Canada: The mental health of First Nations and Inuit communities.* No. 2014-02-E. Ottawa, ON: Library of Publications. Retrieved from http://www.lop.parl.gc.ca/content/lop/ResearchPublications/2014-02-e.pdf

Klein, D., & Allmann, A. (2014). Course of depression: Persistence and recurrence. In I. Gotlib & C. Hammen (Eds.), *Handbook of depression* (3rd ed., pp. 64–83). New York, NY: The Guilford Press.

Koenig, H. G. (2012). Religion, spirituality, and health: The research and clinical implications. *International Scholarly Research Network Psychiatry, 2012,* 1–31. doi:10.5402/2012/278730

Kolostoumpis, D., Bergiannaki, J., Peppou, L., Louki, E., Fousketaki, S., Patelakis, A., & Economou, M. (2015). Effectiveness of relatives' psychoeducation on family outcomes in bipolar disorder. *International Journal of Mental Health, 44*(4), 290–302. doi:10.1080/00207411.2015.1076292

Kuhl, E. A., Kupfer, D. J., & Regier, D. A. (2011). Patient-centered revisions to the DSM-5. *Virtual Mentor, 13*(12), 873–879. doi:10.1001/virtualmentor.2011.13.12.stas1-1112

Lau, J., Lester, K., Hodgson, K., & Eley, T. (2014). The genetics of mood disorders. In I. Gotlib & C. Hammen (Eds.), *Handbook of depression* (3rd ed., pp. 165–181). New York, NY: The Guilford Press.

Lepine, J. P., & Briley, M. (2011). The increasing burden of depression. *Neuropsychiatric Disease and Treatment, 7*(Suppl 1), 3–7. doi:10.2147/NDT.S19617

Leung, R. (2004, November). Carrey: Life is too beautiful. *60 Minutes, CBS NEWS.* Retrieved from http://www.cbsnews.com/stories/2004/11/18/60minutes/main656547.shtml

Lewis, J., Tiozzo, E., Melillo, A., Leonard, S., Chen, L., Mendez, A., ... Konefal, J. (2013). The effect of methylated vitamin B complex on depressive and anxiety symptoms and quality of life in adults with depression. *International Scholarly Research Notices Psychiatry, 621453,* 1–7. doi:10.1155/2013/621453

Lewy, A., Emens, J., Songer, J., Sims, N., Laurie, A., Fiala, S., & Buti, A. (2010). Winter depression: Integrating mood, circadian rhythms, and the sleep/wake and light/dark cycles into a bio-psycho-social-environmental model. *Sleep Medicine Clinics, 4,* 285–299. doi:10.1016/j.jsmc.2009.02.003

Marchand, A., Bilodeau, J., Demers, A., Beauregard, N., Durand, P., & Haines, V. (2016). Gendered depression: Vulnerability or exposure to work and family stressors? *Social Science and Medicine, 166,* 160–168. Retrieved from http://dx.org/10.1016/jsocscimed.2016.08.021

McDonald, K., Bulloch, A., Duffy, A., Bresee, L., Williams, J., Lavorato, D., & Patten, S. (2015). Prevalence of bipolar I and II disorder in Canada. *Canadian Journal of Psychiatry, 60*(3), 151–156. Retrieved from https://www.ncbi.nlm.nih.gov/pubmed/25886691

McInnis, M., Riba, M., & Greden, J. (2014). Depressive disorders. In R. Hales, S. Yudofsky, & L. Roberts (Eds.), *The American psychiatric publishing textbook of psychiatry* (3rd ed., pp. 3–29). Washington, DC: American Psychiatric Publishing.

McKnight, R., Adida, M., Budge, K., Stockton, S., Goodwin, G., & Geddes, J. (2012). Lithium toxicity profile: A systematic review and meta-analysis. *The Lancet, 379*(9817), 721–728. doi:10.1016/S0140-6736(11)61516-X

McWilliams, N. (2011). *Psychoanalytic diagnosis: Understanding personality structure and clinical process* (2nd ed.). New York, NY: The Guilford Press.

Melrose, S. (2015). Seasonal affective disorder: An overview of assessment and treatment approaches. *Depression Research and Treatment, 2015,* 178564, 1–6. doi.org/10.1155/2015/178564

Ogden, S., & Simmonds, J. (2014). Psychologists' and counsellors' perspectives on prolonged grief disorder and its inclusion in diagnostic manuals. *Grief Counselling and Psychotherapy Research, 14*(3), 212–219. doi:10.1080/14733145.2013.790456

Palazidou, E. (2012). The neurobiology of depression. *British Medical Bulletin, 101,* 127–145. doi:10.1093/bmb/lds004

Parikh, S. V., & Velyvis, V. (2010). Psychosocial interventions in bipolar disorder: Theories, mechanisms and key clinical trials. In A. H. Young, I. N. Ferrier, & E. E. Michalak (Eds.), *Practical management of bipolar disorder* (pp. 44–62). New York, NY: Cambridge University Press.

Parikh, S., Hawke, L., Zaretsky, A., Beaulieu, S., Patelis-Siotis, I., MacQueen, G., … Cervantes, P. (2013). Psychosocial interventions for bipolar disorder and coping style modification: Similar clinical outcomes, similar mechanisms? *Canadian Journal of Psychiatry, 58*(8), 482–486. Retrieved from https://www.researchgate.net/profile/Sagar_Parikh/publication/256098502_Psychosocial_Interventions_for_Bipolar_Disorder_and_Coping_Style_Modification_Similar_Clinical_Outcomes_Similar_Mechanisms/links/00b7d52714b597f3d7000000.pdf?origin=publication_list

Patten, S., Williams, J., Lavorato, D., Fiest, K., Bulloch, K., & Wang, J. (2015). The prevalence of major depression is not changing. *Canadian Journal of Psychiatry, 60*(1), 31–43. Retrieved from https://www.ncbi.nlm.nih.gov/pubmed/25886547

Payne, N., & Prudic, J. (2009). Electroconvulsive therapy part II: A biopsychosocial perspective. *Journal of Psychiatric Practice, 15*(5), 369–390. doi:10.1097/01.pra.0000361278.73092.85

Payne, J. L., Potash, J. B., & DePaulo, J. R. (2005). Recent findings on the genetic basis of bipolar disorder. *Psychiatric Clinics of North America, 28*(2), 481–498. doi:10.1016/j.psc.2005.01.003

Pearson, C., Janz, T., & Ali, J. (2013). *Mental and substance use disorders in Canada. Health at a Glance.* No. 82-624-X. Statistics Canada. Retrieved from http://www.statcan.gc.ca/pub/82-624-x/2013001/article/11855-eng.pdf

Rogers, M., & Wattis, R. (2015). Spirituality in nursing practice. *Nursing Standard, 29,* 51–57. Retrieved from https://www.researchgate.net/publication/277412258_Spirituality_in_nursing_practice

Rosa, M., & Lisanby, S. (2012). Somatic treatments for mood disorders. *Neuropsychopharmacology Reviews, 37,* 102–116. doi:10.1038/npp.2011.225

Rotermann, M., Sanmartin, C., Hennessy, D., & Arthur, M. (2014). Prescription medication use by Canadians aged 6 to 79. *Health Reports.* No. 82-003-x, 1–9. Retrieved from http://www.statcan.gc.ca/pub/82-003-x/2014006/article/14032-eng.pdf

Rusner, M., Carlsson, G., Brunt, D., & Nystrom, M. (2013). Towards a more liveable life for close relatives of individuals diagnosed with bipolar disorder. *International Journal of Mental Health Nursing, 22,* 162–169. doi:10.1111/j.1447-0349.2012.00852.x

Sabella, D. (2014). Treating depression with transcranial direct current stimulation. *American Journal of Nursing, 114*(6), 66–70. doi:10.1097/01.NAJ.0000450438.73619.27

Sadock, J., Sadock, V., & Ruiz, P. (2015). *Kaplan & Sadock's synopsis of psychiatry: Behavioral science/clinical psychiatry* (11th ed.). Philadelphia, PA: Wolters Kluwer.

Scapagnini, G., Davinelli, S., Drago, F., Lorenzo, A., & Oriani, G. (2012). Antioxidants as antidepressants. *CNS Drugs, 26*(6), 477–490. doi:10.2165/11633190-000000000-00000

Schaffer, A., Sinyor, M., Reis, C., Goldstein, B. I., & Levitt, A. J. (2014). Suicide in bipolar disorder: Characteristics and subgroups. *Bipolar Disorders, 16,* 732–740. doi:10.1111/bdi.12219

Schutz, C., & Young, A. (2009). *Mood disorders and substance use disorders. Concurrent disorders.* Canadian Centre on Substance Abuse, 38–47. Retrieved from http://www.ccsa.ca/Resource%20Library/ccsa-011811-2010.p

Shah, A., Carreno, F., & Frazer, A. (2014). Therapeutic modalities for treatment resistant depression: Focus on vagal nerve stimulation and ketamine. *Clinical Psychopharmacology and Neuroscience, 12*(2), 83–89. doi:10.9758/cpn.2014.12.2.83

Simpson, K., Meadows, G., Frances, A., & Patten, S. (2012). Is mental health in the Canadian population changing over time? *Canadian Journal of Psychiatry, 57*(5), 324–331. Retrieved from http://www.ncbi.nlm.nih.gov/pubmed/22546065

So, M., Yagamuchi, S., Hashimoto, S., Mitsuhiro, S., Furukawa, T., McCrone, P. (2013). Is Computerized CBT really helpful for adult depression? A meta-analytic re-evaluation of CCBT for adult depression in terms of clinical implementation and methodological validity. *BMC Psychiatry, 13*(113), 1–14. doi:10.1186/1471-244X-13-113

Statistics Canada. (2012). *Suicides and suicide rate, by sex and by age group.* Ottawa, ON: Author. Retrieved from http://www.statcan.gc.ca/tables-tableaux/sum-som/l01/cst01/hlth66a-eng.htm

Stepanuk, K., Fisher, K., Wittmann-Price, R., Posmontier, B., & Bhattacharya, A. (2013). Women's decision-making regarding medication use in pregnancy for anxiety and/or depression. *Journal of Advanced Nursing, 69*(11), 2470–2480. doi:10.1111/jan.12122

Stuart, S., & Robertson, M. (2012). *Interpersonal psychotherapy: A clinician's guide.* Boca Raton, FL: CRC Press.

Sylvia, L., Shelton, R., Kemp, D., Bernstein, E., Friedman, E., Benjamin, D.B., … Calabrese, J. (2015). Medical burden in bipolar disorder: Findings from the Clinical and Health Outcomes Initiative in Comparative Effectiveness for Bipolar Disorder Study (CHOICE). *Bipolar Disorders, 17,* 212–223. doi:10.1111/bdi.12243

Thase, M. E., Hahn, C., & Berton, O. (2014). Neurobiological aspects of depression. In I. Gotlib & C. Hammen (Eds.), *Handbook of depression* (3rd ed., pp. 182–199). New York, NY: The Guilford Press.

Thome, E., Dargel, A., Migliavacca, F., Potter, W., Jappur, D., Kapczinski, F., & Cereser, K. (2012). Stigma experiences in bipolar patients: The impact upon functioning. *Journal of Psychiatric and Mental Health Nursing, 19,* 665–671. doi:10.1111/j.1365-2850.2011.01849.x

Tronick, E., & Reck, C. (2009). Infants of depressed mothers. *Harvard Review of Psychiatry, 17*(2), 147–156. doi:10.1080/10673220902899714

Tuck, I., & Anderson, L. (2014). Forgiveness, flourishing, and resilience: The influences of expressions of spirituality on mental health recovery. *Issues in Mental Health Nursing, 35*(4), 277–282. doi:10.3109/01612840.2014.885623

Volavka, J. (2013). Violence in schizophrenia and bipolar disorder. *Psychiatrica Danubina, 25*(1), 24–33. Retrieved from http://www.hdbp.org/psychiatria_danubina/pdf/dnb_vol25_no1/dnb_vol25_no1_24.pdf

Wang, Q., Verweij, E., Krugers, H., Joels, M., Swaab, D., & Lucassen, P., (2014). Distribution of the glucocorticoid receptor in the human amygdala: Changes in mood disorder patients. *Brain Structure and Function, 219,* 1615–1626. doi:10.1007/s00429-013-0589-4

World Health Organization. (2006). *Building awareness—Reducing risks: Suicide and mental illness.* Retrieved from http://www.who.int/mediacentre/news/releases/2006/pr53/en/

World Health Organization. (2009). *The global burden of disease: 2004 update.* Geneva, Switzerland: Author. Retrieved from http://www.who.int/healthinfo/global_burden_disease/2004_report_update/en/

Wright, L. M., & Leahey, M. (2013). *Nurses and families: A guide to family assessment and intervention* (6th ed.). Philadelphia, PA: FA Davis.

Yatham, L., Kennedy, S., Parikh, A., Schaffer, A., Beaulieu, S., Alda, M., … Berk, M. (2013). Canadian Network for Mood and Anxiety Treatments (CANMAT) and International Society for Bipolar Disorders (ISBD) collaborative update of CANMAT guidelines for the management of patients with bipolar disorder: Update 2013. *Bipolar Disorders, 15*(1), 1–44. doi:10.1111/bdi.12025

Youngstrom, E., & Algorta, G. (2014). Pediatric bipolar disorder. In E. Mash & R. Barkley (Eds.), *Child psychopathology* (3rd ed., pp. 264–316). New York, NY: Guilford Press.

23 Anxiety, Obsessive–Compulsive, and Related Disorders

Emily Jenkins and Lynn Musto

Adapted from the chapter "Anxiety and Obsessive-Compulsive Disorders" by Kathleen Hegadoren and Gerri Lasiuk

LEARNING OBJECTIVES

After studying this chapter, you will be able to:

- Discuss anxiety as an adaptive human response to a perceived threat.
- Identify the physical, cognitive, and social manifestations of anxiety.
- Describe the neurobiologic correlates of anxiety.
- Differentiate "normal" anxiety, worry, and anxiety disorder.
- Identify the shared and unique features of specific anxiety disorders.
- Describe the treatments available for anxiety.

KEY TERMS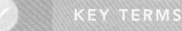

- allostasis • cognitive–behavioural therapy
- depersonalization • derealization • distraction
- existential anxiety • exposure therapy • fear • fear conditioning • generalized anxiety disorder • hoarding disorder • obsessive–compulsive disorder • panic disorder (PD) • paresthesia • phobias • positive self-talk
- systematic desensitization • worry

KEY CONCEPTS

- anxiety • compulsion • obsession • panic

In recent decades, we have gained considerable insight into the mechanisms and processes that influence the experience of anxiety. Importantly, researchers have started to clarify the physiologic mechanisms that underpin the mind–body–brain connection. Clearer understanding of the integrated nature of physiologic and mental processes has highlighted the bidirectional relationship between mind and body. While physiologic responses can shape behaviour, the opposite is also true; thoughts can change behaviour and influence physiologic processes (Geller & Porges, 2014; Mallorqui-Bague et al., 2016). This knowledge has been used to inform treatment of anxiety disorders to the extent that a range of modalities is being used to intervene with people diagnosed with anxiety disorders, such as mind–body techniques, cognitive–behavioural therapies, or a combination of mindfulness and cognitive therapies and pharmaceutical interventions.

Although fear and anxiety are common human experiences, they are complex ones that involve both physiologic and psychological processes (LeDoux, 2015). Most of us would be challenged to define them precisely or explain how they are similar and different. In the literature, a few authors do argue that fear and anxiety are indistinguishable; however, most experts claim that they are distinct phenomena (Perusini & Fanselow, 2015) with different aetiologies, response patterns, intensity, and time courses (see Sylvers, Lilienfeld, & LaPrairie,

2011 for a full discussion). In this chapter, we endorse the position that fear and anxiety are distinct but related emotions that function "to signal danger, threat, or motivational conflict and to trigger appropriate adaptive responses" (Steimer, 2002, p. 233). We define **fear** as an emotional response to a specific and proximal threat to an organism's life or integrity—for example, being held at gunpoint or encountering a snarling dog (Nebel-Schwalm & Davis, 2013). Anxiety, on the other hand, is an emotion characterized by the apprehension or dread of a potentially threatening or uncertain outcome (Sylvers et al., 2011). Stated differently, fear is a "primitive alarm in response to present danger" (Barlow, 2002, p. 104), whereas anxiety is a "future-oriented" state (Barlow, 2002, p. 64) that helps one prepare for *potentially aversive* situations. Based on these definitions, the key differences between anxiety and fear relate to characteristics of the trigger (stimulus). Characteristics of the trigger include its immediacy or temporal orientation (i.e., whether it exists in the present or future) and its ambiguity or specificity (Nebel-Schwalm & Davis, 2013). A related concept is **worry**, which has been defined as thoughts and images centering on adverse outcomes that engender negative affect and are relatively uncontrollable (Borkovec, Robinson, Pruzinsky, & DePree, 1983). Fear and anxiety are emotions, and worry involves negative thoughts and images; worry is considered a symptom of fear and anxiety.

The anxiety disorders are a family of disorders that all share excessive fear or anxiety as their core symptom; specific anxiety disorders differ from one another based on their key feature(s) (e.g., panic attacks, phobias) (American Psychiatric Association [APA], 2013). The anxiety disorders discussed in this chapter include **generalized anxiety disorder** (GAD), social anxiety disorder (social phobia), **panic disorder** (PD), and specific phobias (grouped as anxiety disorders in the *Diagnostic and Statistical Manual of Mental Disorders*, 5th edition (*DSM-5*) (APA, 2013)). In earlier versions of the *DSM*, **obsessive–compulsive disorder (OCD)** was categorized as an anxiety disorder and while it will be discussed in this chapter, in the *DSM-5*, it is grouped under obsessive–compulsive and related disorders (which includes body dysmorphic disorder, **hoarding disorder**, trichotillomania, and excoriation disorder). Acute stress disorder (ASD) and posttraumatic stress disorder were also previously considered to be anxiety disorders but now appear in the newly created category Trauma- and Stressor-Related Disorders (discussed in Chapter 17).

Significant anxiety and anxiety disorders are not restricted to mental health practice; they are seen across all practice settings and continua of care. Indeed, inpatient psychiatric care is rare in instances where an anxiety disorder is the primary diagnosis. More common to inpatient settings are anxiety disorders that are comorbid with disorders such as severe depression or schizophrenia. Outpatient psychiatric clinics, primary care services, general practice settings, chronic disease management clinics, and private practitioners all provide various types of treatment for individuals experiencing an anxiety disorder. Anxiety disorders are often difficult to treat and symptoms often persist over many years. These disorders are thus frequently chronic in their longitudinal course, with acute episodes occurring in response to stressors or other health problems (Antai-Otong, 2016).

NORMAL VERSUS ABNORMAL ANXIETY RESPONSE

From an evolutionary perspective, an emotion is a transient response to a specific stimulus that produces an arousal reaction characterized by changes in subjective feelings and behaviour (Critchley, 2003). At low to moderate intensities, acute anxiety is an adaptive response to a perceived threat and can motivate one to act. On the other hand, when anxiety is extreme or chronic, it can produce paralysis and inaction. An anxiety disorder differs from adaptive ("normal") anxiety in that it is greater than expected in intensity and/or duration for one's age and the situation, and it interferes with one's quality of life and ability to function (APA, 2013).

McEwen (2005) conceptualizes normal responses to stress as **allostasis**, the adaptive processes that maintain homeostasis through the production of various brain and peripheral stress-related chemicals. These mediators of the stress responses promote adaptation to perceived threat or stress. However, they also contribute to allostatic load, the cumulative wear and tear on biologic systems that over time that can increase the risk for stress-related disorders and physical health problems like cardiovascular and metabolic disorders.

The perception of a threat triggers physical and emotional changes in all individuals. A normal emotional response to anxiety consists of three parts: physiologic arousal, cognitive processes, and coping strategies. Physiologic arousal is the signal that an individual is facing a threat. During this part of the anxiety process, sensory input is increasing. Next, cognitive processes in the brain decipher the various inputs and yield judgements about the extent of danger and whether the perceived threat should be approached or avoided. Behaviours include "fight" or "flight" (i.e., escape) as described by Selye (1956) and later updated to include "freeze" (i.e., immobilization) (Porges, 2007). Finally, coping strategies can be used to resolve the threat. Table 23.1 summarizes many physical, affective, cognitive, and behavioural symptoms associated with anxiety.

KEY CONCEPT

Anxiety is an emotion characterized by apprehension or dread of a potentially threatening or uncertain outcome. It is triggered by the perception of a threat and is manifested in physical, emotional, cognitive, and/or behavioural ways.

■ OVERVIEW OF ANXIETY DISORDERS

As a group, anxiety disorders represent the most common of all mental illnesses in Canada and around the globe. Research informing Canadian clinical practice guidelines for the management of anxiety disorders and OCD reports the lifetime prevalence of anxiety disorders to be "as high as 31% higher than the lifetime prevalence of mood disorders and substance use disorders" (Katzman et al., 2014, p. 1). They are the most treated psychiatric disorders in childhood and adolescence (Merikangas et al., 2010), and evidence suggests a relationship between childhood separation, anxiety disorders, and atopic disorders (asthma, hives, hay fever, and eczema) and adult-onset PD (Copeland, Angold, Shanahan, & Costello, 2014). In fact, symptoms of anxiety disorder often begin in adolescence (Meyer, Hajcak, Torpey-Newman, Kujawa, & Klein, 2015; Kessler, Petukhova, Sampson, Zaslavsky, & Wittchen, 2012). Multiple factors contribute to the development of anxiety disorders in childhood, including genetic inheritance, as well as parental behaviours and modelling and stressful life events at key developmental stages (Compton, 2014).

Table 23.1	Symptoms of Anxiety	

Physical		
Cardiovascular	**Neuromuscular**	**Gastrointestinal**
Sympathetic	Increased reflexes	Loss of appetite
Palpitations	Startle reaction	Revulsion towards food
Heart racing	Eyelid twitching	Abdominal discomfort
Increased blood pressure	Insomnia	Diarrhoea and vomiting
	Unsteadiness	
Respiratory		**Eyes**
Rapid breathing	**Skin**	Dilated pupils
Difficulty getting air	Face flushed or pale	
Shortness of breath	Sweating	**Urinary Tract**
Pressure of chest	Feeling hot or cold	Pressure to urinate
Shallow breathing		
Lump in throat		
Choking sensations		
Gasping		

Affective	Cognitive	Behavioural
Edgy	**Sensory–Perceptual**	Inhibited
Impatient	Feeling dazed	Tonic immobility
Uneasy	Objects seem blurred/distant	Flight
Nervous	Environment seems different/unreal, feelings of	Avoidance
Wound up	depersonalization	Impaired coordination
Anxious	Self-consciousness	Restlessness
Fearful	Hypervigilance	Postural collapse
Apprehensive		Hyperventilation
Scared	**Thinking Difficulties**	Jumpy
Frightened	Cannot recall important things	Jittery
Alarmed	Confused	
Terrified	Difficulty focusing attention	
	Difficulty concentrating	
	Fear of losing control or not being able to cope	
	Fear of physical injury or death	
	Fear of going crazy	
	Fear of negative evaluation	
	Frightening visual images	
	Repetitive fearful ideation	

Adapted from Beck, A. T., Emery, C., & Greenberg, R. L. (1985). *Anxiety disorders and phobias: A cognitive perspective* (pp. 23–27). New York, NY: Basic Books.

Children and adolescents with anxiety disorders are more likely to demonstrate of suicidal behaviour, drug and alcohol dependence, and educational underachievement later in life (Essau, Lewinsohn, Olaya, & Seely, 2015).

Anxiety disorders remain common in adulthood. Statistics Canada's (2013) *Community Health Survey of Mental Health* found that 2.6% of Canadians 15 years and older reported symptoms meeting the diagnostic criteria for GAD in the previous 12 months. Like many mental disorders, there appear to be differences in prevalence across gender, with girls and women more likely than boys and men to be diagnosed with any anxiety disorder during their lifetime (Katzman et al., 2014). For example, lifetime prevalence of social anxiety was found to be 4.2% in men and 5.6% in women in an American-based community sample (Xu et al., 2012). In terms of aetiology, specific anxiety disorders show more evidence of genetic vulnerability, particularly PD, OCD, and

phobias, while environmental factors have also been identified as contributing to the development of anxiety disorders (Goes, McCusker, Bienvenu, & MacKinnon, 2012).

Anxiety may exist as a primary disorder, but as noted earlier, it often cooccurs with other psychiatric and/or physical conditions (Hofmeijer-Sevink et al., 2013). In fact, this comorbidity can contribute to challenges in distinguishing between symptoms of anxiety and symptoms of physical conditions that share similar features (e.g., shortness of breath, racing heart). Evidence from community-based samples indicates that persons diagnosed with an anxiety disorder will likely have at least one comorbid psychiatric disorder, either concomitantly or in their lifetime (for a full discussion, see Merikangas & Swanson, 2010). Individuals who live with chronic anxiety report more functional impairment, increased use of both psychiatric and nonpsychiatric health care services, and decreased productivity than those in the general population (Kessler, Chiu, Demler, Merikangas, & Walters, 2005). After adjusting for sociodemographic factors and other mental disorders, the presence of any anxiety disorder is significantly associated with suicidal ideation and suicide attempts (Anderberg, Bogren, Mattisson, & Brådvik, 2016).

Generalized Anxiety Disorder

GAD is characterized by unwarranted, enduring anxiety across life situations, especially those in which the individual feels a lack of control. These anxiety symptoms significantly impact the person's functioning and bring with it associated physical symptoms. Thus, the amount of time spent worrying; the degree of control one has over one's worrying; and the impact on personal, social, and occupational functioning are key components of the assessment of GAD. GAD can be a debilitating disorder with serious impact on quality of life (Antai-Otong, 2016; Barrera & Norton, 2009). (For the APA criteria for GAD, please see the DSM-5.)

GAD is a common anxiety disorder. Most community-based population studies report lifetime prevalence rates of GAD ranging between 2% and 9%, depending on the country and the definitional and measurement criteria employed (Haller, Cramer, Lauche, Gass, & Dobos, 2014; Kessler et al., 2012; Moffitt et al., 2010). In a Canadian sample, the prevalence estimates of GAD were reported at 2.6% (Public Health Agency of Canada, 2016). Onset of GAD is often early in life and often follows a chronic course with more severe symptoms being triggered by acute stressors. Persons living with GAD often feel powerless to change, frustrated with life, demoralized, and hopeless, and comorbid depression is very common (Almeida, Draper, Pirkis, & Snowdon, 2012; Antai-Otong, 2016; Lamers et al., 2011). In fact, less than one third of those with GAD are without a comorbid disorder (Lamers et al., 2011). Rovira and colleagues (2012) reported that 7.9% of those attending a primary care setting had GAD, highlighting the importance of comprehensive mental and physical health assessment in these settings. Assessment of persons with GAD must include the assessment of mood, somatic symptoms, specific worries, and worry management strategies employed. A standardized questionnaire, such as the Generalized Anxiety Disorder Scale (GAD-7), may help assess the severity of the symptoms and health impacts (Spitzer et al., 2006).

Social Anxiety Disorder

Social anxiety disorder (social phobia) involves a marked or intense fear of social situations in which the individual feels scrutinized and negatively evaluated by others. People with social anxiety disorder appear to be highly sensitive to disapproval or criticism, tend to evaluate themselves negatively, and have poor self-esteem and a distorted view of personal strengths and weaknesses. These individuals magnify personal flaws and underrate any talents, and the resulting fear or anxiety is out of proportion to the actual risk of being negatively evaluated. Generalized social anxiety disorder brings with it reduced quality of life (Wong, Gordon, & Heimberg, 2012) and in children is associated with significant decreases in school performance (Nail et al., 2015). Despite substantial functional impairment, treatment seeking usually results from a comorbid mental disorder (Ertekin et al., 2015). (For the American Psychological Association [APA] criteria of social anxiety disorder, please see the DSM-5.)

The onset of social anxiety disorder usually occurs in early adolescence. There are two subtypes of this disorder: generalized social phobia and specific social phobia. Generalized social phobia is diagnosed when an individual experiences fears related to most social situations, including public performances and social interactions. These individuals are likely to demonstrate deficiencies in social skills, and their phobias interfere with their ability to function. Individuals with specific social phobias fear and avoid only one or two specific social situations. Classic examples of the latter are eating, writing, or speaking in public or using public bathrooms.

Social phobia has a lifetime prevalence of 8% to 13% in the general population (Kessler et al., 2012). In a Canadian community sample, 12-month prevalence estimates of social phobia were 2.6% for men and 3.4% for women (Xiangfei & D'Arcy, 2012). In certain subpopulations, rates are even higher. For example, one systematic review of individuals with chronic obstructive pulmonary disorder reported prevalence of social phobia to be between 5% and 11% (Willgoss & Yohannes, 2013), and in the Canadian military, the estimates were as high as 8.2% (Mather, Stein, & Sareen, 2010). Further, research has shown that people who experience both social phobia and depression have more severe symptoms and greater functional impairment than those with social phobia alone. It has also been found that individuals who experience these two disorders in tandem tend to be younger and have an earlier diagnosis of major depression (Adams et al., 2016).

Panic Disorder

PD is characterized by repeated episodes of panic. These panic "attacks" are abrupt surges of intense fear or discomfort that peak within minutes and are associated with multiple key physical and cognitive symptoms (see Boxes 23.1 and 23.2). Panic attacks can occur in response to a serious threat but can also occur "out of the blue" with no apparent triggering environmental stimulus or stressor. PD is characterized by recurrent unexpected panic attacks and fear of prompting another attack, which limits the individual's ability to function socially, occupationally, and interpersonally.

BOX 23.1 CLINICAL VIGNETTE

PANIC DISORDER (PD)

M, a 22-year-old man, has experienced several life changes, including a recent engagement, loss of his father to cancer and heart disease, graduation from college, and entrance to the workforce as a computer engineer in a large inner-city company. Because of his active lifestyle, his sleep habits have been poor. He frequently uses sleeping aids at night and now drinks a full pot of coffee to start each day. He has started smoking to "relieve the stress." While sitting in heavy traffic on the way to work, he suddenly experienced chest tightness, sweating, shortness of breath, feelings of being "trapped," and foreboding that he was going to die. Fearing a heart attack, he went to an emergency room, where his discomfort subsided within a half hour. After several hours of testing, the doctor informed him that his heart was healthy. During the next few weeks, he experienced several episodes of feeling trapped and slight chest discomfort on his drive to work. He fears future "attacks" while sitting in traffic and while in his crowded office cubicle.

What Do You Think?

- What risk factors does M have that might contribute to the development of panic attacks?
- What lifestyle changes do you think would help M reduce stress?

PD is a chronic condition with exacerbations and remissions. Lifetime prevalence estimates vary widely (1.4% to 20.5%), depending on the age of the sampled population and the methodologic approaches used to study it. In Canada, the lifetime prevalence of PD is estimated at 3.7% (Government of Canada, 2006). Recent longitudinal data suggest that having panic attacks increases the risk of developing a mood and/or anxiety

BOX 23.2 DSM-5 Diagnostic Criteria: Panic Disorder

A. Recurrent unexpected panic attacks. A panic attack is an abrupt surge of intense fear or intense discomfort that reaches a peak within minutes, and during with time four (or more) of the following symptoms occur:
Note: The abrupt surge can occur from a calm state or an anxious state.
  1. Palpitations, pounding heart, or accelerated heart rate
  2. Sweating
  3. Trembling or shaking
  4. Sensations of shortness of breath or smothering
  5. Feelings of choking
  6. Chest pain or discomfort
  7. Nausea or abdominal distress
  8. Feeling dizzy, unsteady, light-headed, or faint
  9. Chills or heat sensations
  10. **Paresthesias** (numbness or tingling sensations)
  11. **Derealization** (feelings of unreality) or **depersonalization** (being detached from oneself)
  12. Fear of losing control or "going crazy"
  13. Fear of dying
Note: Culture-specific symptoms (e.g., tinnitus, neck soreness, headaches, uncontrollable screaming or crying) may be seen. Such symptoms should not count as one of the four required symptoms.

B. At least one of the attacks has been followed by 1 month (or more) of one or both of the following:
  1. Persistent concern or worry about additional panic attacks or their consequences (e.g., losing control, having a heart attack, "going crazy").
  2. A significant maladaptive change in behaviour related to the attacks (e.g., behaviours designed to avoid having panic attacks, such as avoidance of exercise or unfamiliar situations).
C. The disturbances is not attributable to the physiologic effects of a substance (e.g., a drug of abuse, a medication) or another medical conditions (e.g., hyperthyroidism, cardiopulmonary disorders).
D. The disturbance is not better explained by another mental disorder (e.g., the panic attacks do not occur only in response to feared social situations, as in social anxiety disorder; in response to circumscribed phobic objects or situations, as in specific phobia; in response to obsessions, as in obsessive–compulsive disorder; in response to reminders of traumatic events, as in posttraumatic stress disorder; or in response to separate from attachment figures, as in separation anxiety disorder).

Reprinted with permission from the *Diagnostic and Statistical Manual of Mental Disorders*, Fifth Edition, (Copyright 2013). American Psychiatric Association.

disorder in the future (Asselmann, Wittchen, Lieb, Höfler, & Beesdo-Baum, 2014). Higher rates of PD occur in women and among those 30 to 59 years, with a mean age of onset at 23 years (Kessler et al., 2006, 2012). Several risk factors have been implicated in the development of PD, including previous triggered panic attacks, a family history of psychological difficulties, childhood trauma, being female, and history of mood disorder (Kinley, Walker, Enns, & Sareen, 2011; Tibi et al., 2013). Adolescents with PD may be at higher risk for suicidal thoughts or attempt suicide more often than their peers (Kanwar et al., 2013).

In addition to comorbid psychiatric disorders, certain physical health problems are also common among individuals with PD, including vertigo, cardiac disease, gastrointestinal disorders, and asthma. One might ponder whether these medical conditions produce similar somatic sensations to anxiety and over time increase the risk of development of PD. The population with both physical health problems and panic symptoms reports poorer quality of life than do those without such comorbidity.

PD can occur with and without agoraphobia. Those who experience PD with agoraphobia tend to have more coexisting anxiety disorders, anxiety attacks, and anticipatory anxiety than do patients who have PD without agoraphobia. Women appear more likely to experience PD with agoraphobia (Inoue, Kaiya, Hara, & Okazaki, 2016) and to have poorer outcomes manifesting as missed work time and more frequent visits to health care providers (e.g., family doctor, emergency department visits) (McLean, Asnaani, Litz, & Hofmann, 2011).

Panic attacks are typically accompanied by fear of death because their symptoms often mimic those of a heart attack, which are both physically taxing and psychologically frightening to patients. Affected individuals often seek emergency medical care because they feel as if they are dying, but most will have normal results upon cardiac workup. People experiencing panic attacks may also believe that the attacks stem from an underlying major medical illness. Even with sound medical testing and assurance of no underlying disease, it can be difficult for individuals with PD to feel reassured. Recognition of the seriousness of the panic attacks should be communicated to the patient. However, individuals with PD continue to experience panic attacks with or without predisposing conditions (Box 23.1).

KEY CONCEPT

Panic can be a normal but extreme, overwhelming form of anxiety often initiated when an individual is placed in a real or perceived life-threatening situation.

IN-A-LIFE

Charles Darwin (1809–1882)

THEORY OF EVOLUTION

Public Persona

Charles Darwin, credited as the first scientist to gain wide acceptance of the theory of natural selection, might never have published his 1859 seminal work, *Origin of the Species by Means of Natural Selection*, had it not been for his psychiatric illness. Born in England, Charles Darwin, the grandson of a famous poet, inventor, and physician, was expected to accomplish great things. However, his childhood years were troublesome. When he was sent to Cambridge to study medicine, card playing and drinking became his main activities. After meeting a botanist, however, his life changed and he embarked on a 5-year expedition to the Pacific Coast of South America.

Personal Realities

Darwin described his sensation of fear, accompanied by troubled beating of the heart, sweat, and trembling of muscles. Thought to have PD, he constantly worried about what he thought he knew until he finally published his ideas on paper. He died in 1882 and was buried in Westminster Abbey.

Source: Darwin, C. (1887). *The life and letters of Charles Darwin.* New York, NY: Appleton & Co.

Agoraphobia and Other Specific Phobias

Panic attacks can lead to the development of **phobias** or persistent, unrealistic fears of situations, objects, or activities. People with phobias will go to great lengths to avoid the feared objects or situations to deter panic attacks. Box 23.3 presents examples of common phobias. Agoraphobia, fear of certain environments such as open spaces (including shopping malls), travelling on public transportation (buses, subways), or being in closed and crowded spaces (elevators, theatres) often cooccurs with PD and often leads to avoidance behaviours. Fear arising in places with limited opportunity to escape or when outside alone are also characteristic of agoraphobia (APA, 2013). The process often begins with an intense, irrational fear of being in an open space, being alone, or being in a public place where escape might be difficult or embarrassing. The person fears that if a panic attack occurred, help would not be available, so he or she begins to avoid such situations. Such avoidance interferes with routine functioning and eventually renders the person afraid to leave the safety of home. Some affected individuals continue to face feared

---

BOX 23.3 Common Phobias

Acrophobia (fear of heights)
Agoraphobia (fear of open spaces)
Ailurophobia (fear of cats)
Algophobia (fear of pain)
Arachnophobia (fear of spiders)
Brontophobia (fear of thunder)
Claustrophobia (fear of closed spaces)
Cynophobia (fear of dogs)
Entomophobia (fear of insects)
Haematophobia (fear of blood)
Microphobia (fear of germs)
Nyctophobia (fear of night or dark places)
Ophidiophobia (fear of snakes)
Phonophobia (fear of loud noises)
Photophobia (fear of light)
Pyrophobia (fear of fire)
Topophobia (stage fright)
Xenophobia (fear of strangers)
Zoophobia (fear of animal or animals)

---

situations but with significant trepidation (i.e., going in public only to pay bills or to take children to school).

Specific phobia (i.e., simple phobia) is a disorder marked by an irrational fear of a specific object or situation that the person realizes is unreasonable. The lifetime prevalence varies by subtype, with highest occurrence among those with natural environment phobias (8.9% to 11.6%), followed by situational phobias (5.2% to 8.4%), animal phobias (3.3% to 7%), and blood injection injury phobias (3.2% to 4.5%) (LeBeau et al., 2010).

Exposure to the stimulus object or situation engenders anxiety; the intensity of anxiety is usually related to both the proximity of the object and the degree to which escape is possible. For example, anxiety heightens as a cat approaches a person who fears cats and lessens when the cat moves away. At times, the level of anxiety can escalate to a full panic attack, particularly when the person must remain in a situation from which escape is deemed impossible. Fear of specific objects is fairly common, and the diagnosis of specific phobia is not made unless the fear significantly interferes with functioning or causes marked distress.

Careful assessment differentiates simple phobia from other diagnoses with overlapping symptoms. Blood injection injury–type phobia merits special consideration here because the phobia is fairly common across all health care settings. Before beginning a procedure, nurses should routinely ask whether the person has had any prior difficulty and should continue to monitor the person closely during and afterwards. The physiologic processes exhibited during phobic exposure to

a procedure or treatment (e.g., needle poke, suturing) includes a strong vasovagal response, which significantly increases blood pressure and pulse, followed by the deceleration of the pulse and lowering of blood pressure resulting in fainting. Factors that predispose individuals to specific phobias include prior traumatic events; unexpected panic attacks in the presence of the phobic object or situation; observation of others experiencing a trauma; or repeated exposure to information warning of dangers, such as parents' repeatedly warning young children that dogs bite.

Obsessive–Compulsive and Related Disorders

This cluster of disorders includes OCD, body dysmorphic disorder, hoarding disorder, trichotillomania (also known as hair pulling disorder), and excoriation disorder (skin picking disorder) (APA, 2013). OCD and hoarding disorder will be discussed in this chapter.

OCD is a psychiatric disorder characterized by severe obsessions (repetitive, intrusive thoughts), compulsions (repetitive, ritualistic behaviours), or both. A key feature of OCD is the relationship between obsessions and compulsions; the obsessions cause anxiety, and the compulsions are an attempt to reduce or eliminate it. Obsessive thinking and/or compulsive behaviours are not necessarily signs of a psychiatric disorder if they are not persistent and do not significantly interfere with the person's ability to function. However, when they are severe and persistent, obsessions can interfere with a person's reality testing and judgment to the degree that most of their day is spent performing actions in an attempt to minimize severe anxiety. Affected individuals feel chronically anxious and powerless to control the obsessions and compulsions.

Commons patterns seen in OCD are that of fear of contamination (e.g., from dirt, germs), pathologic doubt (e.g., requiring repeated checking that an action was carried out, such as windows closed), and need of symmetry (e.g., table settings, desktop) (Sadock, Sadock, & Ruiz, 2015). Common compulsions include handwashing, checking and arranging things, and counting. Individuals who perform checking rituals repeatedly check locks, stoves, and/or switches; check for errors; or check that they have not harmed someone or themselves. For example, after hitting a bump in the road, an individual may obsess for hours over whether they hit someone. Some individuals with OCD have somatic fears and frequently seek medical treatment for physical symptoms, often just to get reassurance. Other compulsions include arranging things in perfect symmetry, counting rituals, or doing-and-undoing rituals (e.g., repeatedly turning on and off the alarm clock).

Persons with religious obsessions ruminate over the meaning of sins and whether they have followed the letter of the law. In the case of religious obsessions and compulsions, a diagnosis of OCD is not made unless the thoughts or rituals clearly exceed cultural or religious norms, occur at inappropriate times as described by members of the same religion or culture, or interfere with social obligations. (For the APA criteria for Obsessive–Compulsive Disorder, please see the DSM-5.)

The prevalence of OCD is similar across community samples drawn from different countries. For example, lifetime prevalence estimates of OCD in a mixed Asian population were reported as 3.0% (Subramaniam, Abdin, Vaingankar, & Chong, 2012), 2.3% in an American sample (Ruscio, Stein, Chiu, & Kessler, 2010), and 3.5% in a Swiss population (Fineberg et al., 2013). Each of these studies reported men as having a younger age of onset than women. The typical age of onset of OCD is in the early 20s to mid-30s, although symptoms of OCD can begin in childhood. Despite this early onset, it takes an average of 8 years following the onset of symptoms before individuals access professional help (Stengler et al., 2013).

The most common reasons that individuals with OCD seek professional help include higher symptom severity, poor quality of life, and concurrent mental disorder (García-Soriano, Rufer, Delsignore, & Weidt, 2014). For instance, researchers have estimated that 78% of individuals with OCD will experience a comorbid mental disorder, with depression, GAD, social anxiety disorder, and PD commonly co-occurring (Hofmeijer-Sevink et al., 2013; Lochner et al., 2014). Because children subscribe to myths, superstition, and magical thinking and obsessive and ritualistic behaviours, OCD may go unnoticed in younger persons. However, it is increasing concerns about social, academic, and personal impairments that differentiate common childhood behaviours from OCD. Predictors of poorer treatment outcomes for adults include earlier age of onset; longer duration of symptoms; high symptom severity; comorbidity with other mental disorders, especially depression; a family history of OCD or other anxiety disorders; personality disorders; and sexual obsessions, as well as hoarding and compulsions (Jakubovski et al., 2013; Skapinakis et al., 2016). In children, the predictors of poorer outcomes also include severity and family history of OCD, but family accommodation of OCD behaviours has also been demonstrated to predict poorer outcomes (Strauss, Hale, & Stobie, 2015).

KEY CONCEPT

Obsessions are unwanted, intrusive, and persistent thoughts, impulses, or images that are incongruent with the person's usual thought patterns and cause significant anxiety and distress. The person tries to ignore, suppress, or neutralize the thoughts by some other thought or action but is unable to do so.

KEY CONCEPT

Compulsions are behaviours performed repeatedly, in a ritualistic fashion, with the goal of preventing or relieving anxiety and distress caused by obsessions.

Hoarding Disorder

Sometimes, individuals with OCD may exhibit hoarding behaviours; in fact, hoarding was originally considered as a symptom or subtype of OCD. As per the DSM-5, hoarding is now recognized as a discreet diagnostic syndrome (APA, 2013). Hoarding disorder is characterized by the excessive acquisition of and inability or unwillingness to discard material possessions. Accumulated possessions clutter active living areas and become barriers to their use for daily living. There is impairment in social, occupational, and family functioning. Individuals who hoard may feel compelled to check their belongings repeatedly to see that all is accounted for and they may check the garbage to ensure that nothing of value has been discarded. Hoarding is a "debilitating psychiatric disorder that can lead to considerable health risks, functional impairment, family conflict, and substantial financial burden for sufferers, family members, and the community" (Stekettee et al., 2015, p. 728).

Individuals who hoard may collect items that appear to have no apparent value. Some hoarders collect newspapers, decorations, and other collectables; others hoard animals. Excessive accumulation of objects creates fire hazards, insect and rodent infestations, food contamination, unsanitary living conditions, and associated health hazards (Elsenhauer, 2017; Kress, Stargell, Zoldan, & Paylo, 2016). The clutter can be so severe that individuals with hoarding disorder have been found dead in their homes after being trapped in a "clutter avalanche" (Brakoulias & Milicevic, 2015). (For APA criteria for Hoarding Disorder, please see the DSM-5.)

Hoarding disorder is a chronic progressive disorder affecting approximately 2% to 6% or the population. Similar to anxiety disorders, females tend to be overrepresented in clinical samples. Symptoms often are present during adolescence and become increasingly severe as individuals age. The disorder is most prevalent in older adults, with 50 being the average age of those seeking treatment. Hoarding behaviours can be seen in approximately 20% of persons with dementia and 14% of those with brain injury (Sadock et al., 2015). Individuals with hoarding disorder frequently present with a co-occurring mood or anxiety disorder, with high rates of comorbid OCD or Attention Deficit Hyperactivity Disorder (ADHD). Individuals with hoarding disorder rarely voluntarily seek treatment, as greater than 50% of those with the disorder experience poor insight (Kress et al., 2016). Instead, they may be pressured to seek treatment by family members, public health officials, and/or mental health professionals. It is not uncommon for a number of community services to be involved including the fire department, public health, animal control, law enforcement, mental health services, and public works (Brakoulias & Milicevic, 2015; Elsenhauer, 2017; Kress et al., 2016). Cognitive–behavioural therapy that includes a focus on decision-making skills can be an effective treatment approach, with aspects of the therapy occurring in home (Sadock et al., 2015).

AETIOLOGIC THEORIES OF ANXIETY DISORDERS

There are many similarities and overlaps among aetiologic theories of the various anxiety disorders, and the various theories are not mutually exclusive.

Genetic Theories

Genetic theories of the aetiology of anxiety disorders focus on genetic vulnerabilities that increase anxiety sensitivity, childhood maltreatment, environmental stressors, and dysregulations of neurotransmitter systems or the neural circuits that underpin fear and **fear conditioning** (Hovens, Giltay, Spinhoven, van Hemert, & Penninx, 2015; Nuss, 2015; Trzaskowski, Zavos, Haworth, Plomin, & Eley, 2012). One meta-analysis of genetic studies of anxiety disorders found that genes account for 30% to 50% of the risk for PD and that the risk for first-degree relatives was five times that of the general population (Shimada-Sugimoto, Otowa, & Hettema, 2015). "Groundbreaking" research findings have linked a variation in the promoter region of the serotonin transporter gene to stress sensitivity and anxiety symptoms (Ming et al., 2015; Schiele et al., 2016), which has become a model for genetic susceptibility to mood and anxiety disorders. However, some researchers question whether the significance of this theory has been overestimated as a result of publication bias (de Vries et al., 2016). This area of research remains very active. For example, links have been shown between the serotonin transporter and specific brain enzyme polymorphisms and anxiety/rejection sensitivity in women (Gressier, Calati, & Serretti, 2016). However, social conditioning may play a role in anxiety sensitivity or in overestimating the degree of threat, both of which may increase the risk to develop anxiety disorders. Mundo, Richter, Sam, Macciardi, and Kennedy (2000) discovered a link between the pathogenesis of OCD and the 5-HT$_{1D\beta}$ receptor gene. This discovery may lead to breakthroughs in pharmacologic treatments for OCD (Corregiari, Bernik, Cordeiro, & Vallada, 2012).

Neurobiology of Anxiety

The concept of learned associations provides a useful framework to understand the nature of emotional responsiveness and how anxiety can be manifested in our emotions, thoughts, and behaviour. Advances in research methods and neuroimaging techniques have also increased our understanding of the roles of different neurotransmitters and the regions of the brain involved in anxiety and specific anxiety disorders.

Fear conditioning is a type of learning during which an organism is conditioned to associate a neutral stimulus with an aversive one. Over time, the neutral stimulus elicits an automatic emotional response previously associated with the aversive one, and the individual is conditioned to respond with fear to what was once a neutral stimulus. The anxiety and fear response can further generalize to similar stimuli and become a pattern of response to stimuli that are tangentially similar to the original (e.g., a fear of dogs can generalize to all furry animals). This has led to the belief that anxiety disorders reflect an exaggeration of the normal fear response. Extinction (the gradual decrease in a conditioned fear response) can occur when repeated exposure to the conditioned stimulus does not elicit an anxiety or fear response, although the memory is still there and can be reestablished to produce the fear response in the face of a similar threat. These dynamics partially explain the chronicity of anxiety disorders and have also shaped many of the current interventions and treatments for anxiety and anxiety disorders.

The major structures of the brain involved in fear conditioning are the hippocampus and the amygdala. The hippocampus is involved with memory acquisition and storage. Short-term memory is thought to be related to enhancement of glutamate neurotransmission, while longer-term memory is considered to be the result of long-term synaptic potentiation, a process whereby synaptic activity is enhanced by increased gene expression and protein synthesis. The amygdala is a crucial area for encoding and storing fearful memories. Studies using functional magnetic resonance imaging (fMRI) have shown increased amygdalar activity during associative learning (i.e., pairing stimuli with previously experienced stimuli and the prior emotional responses).

The Role of Neurotransmitters and Neuropeptides

Serotonin (5-hydroxytryptamine [5-HT]) is indirectly implicated in the aetiology of anxiety disorders in that drugs that facilitate serotonergic neurotransmission are effective in treating anxiety and panic symptoms. Indeed, selective serotonin reuptake inhibitors (SSRIs) are considered first-line pharmacotherapy for patients with anxiety. Norepinephrine is implicated in anxiety disorders because of its effects on the systems associated with the physical sensations of anxiety—the cardiovascular, respiratory, and gastrointestinal systems via stimulation of the sympathetic arm of the autonomic nervous system. Cell bodies of norepinephrine neurons in the brain are located in the locus coeruleus, which is one of the internal regulators of sleep and alertness. Electrical stimulation of the locus coeruleus in monkeys increases fear and anxiety, and studies indicate that norepinephrine-based medications (i.e., serotonin–norepinephrine reuptake inhibitors—SNRIs) are effective in the treatment of anxiety, in some cases more so than SSRIs, particularly in addressing the somatic symptoms that so often accompany these disorders (Dell'Osso et al., 2010).

Gamma-aminobutyric acid (GABA) is the most abundant inhibitory neurotransmitter in the brain. Very small GABAergic neurons (interneurons) affect the firing rates of neurons distributed throughout the brain, which explains why GABA has such pervasive effects within the brain. Although a direct role of GABA in fear conditioning or anxiety disorders has yet to be clearly demonstrated, drugs that enhance GABA neurotransmission are commonly used to treat anxiety symptoms during the day and to help with sleep disturbance that often accompanies significant anxiety.

Corticotropin-releasing hormone (CRH) is a neuropeptide and hormone found in many areas of the brain; it is the initial hormone released from the hypothalamus that activates one of the major stress response systems, the hypothalamic–pituitary–adrenal (HPA) axis. CRH receptors are widely distributed in the hypothalamus, as well as brain regions associated with fear and fear conditioning. Activation of the HPA axis results from many stimuli, including perception of threat, and increases arousal, attention to environmental cues, and glucose availability to skeletal muscles to promote survival responses like "fight or flight." Cortisol, the final output of the HPA axis in humans, is significantly elevated during panic attacks (Bandelow et al., 2000) and appears to decrease or become blunted among those experiencing persistent stress or panic states, such as PD (Wintermann, Kirschbaum, & Petrowski, 2016). Increasing levels of cortisol act as negative feedback to decrease further release of CRH; however, many other neurotransmitters and neuropeptides help regulate the HPA axis. CRH receptor antagonists were suggested as a mechanism to treat anxiety, but no drugs based on this mechanism are currently on the market.

Cholecystokinin (CCK) became a neuropeptide of interest when administered in challenge tests; CCK induces panic attacks in patients with PD and, to a much lesser degree, in people without PD (Ruland et al., 2015). High concentrations of CCK are found in the cerebral cortex, amygdala, and hippocampus—areas implicated in fear and stress responses. Although specific CCK_B receptor antagonists would be a potential treatment mechanism, these compounds did not show sufficient efficacy to be marketed. Other neurochemicals have been associated with anxiety, including growth hormone (GH), female sex hormones, arginine vasopressin (AVP), and oxytocin (OT). In healthy subjects, stimulating α-adrenergic receptors elevates GH. This process is blunted in individuals with PD (Sallee, Sethuraman, Sine, & Liu, 2000).

Neuroactive steroids, including the various metabolites of progesterone, have been implicated in the development of panic attacks, which may help to explain why women show an increased susceptibility to PD (Lovick, 2014). AVP and OT help regulate the activity of the HPA axis in a gender-specific fashion, with AVP being able to stimulate the axis independent of CRH and OT decreasing further release of CRH, thus dampening down HPA axis activity. Indeed, OT has been central to two gender-specific theories of stress responses in women (Kumsta & Heinrichs, 2013; Munro et al., 2013).

Neuroimaging Data Related to Specific Anxiety Disorders

The increasing sophistication of neuroimaging techniques has enabled researchers to better understand the physiology of anxiety and the involved neural network or circuits. Most neuroimaging work related to anxiety disorders has focused on PD, with recent magnetic resonance imaging (MRI) studies demonstrating significant volumetric reductions in gray matter in the fronto-limbic regions, thalamus, brainstem, and cerebellum and decreased white matter volume in the fronto-limbic, thalamocortical, and cerebellar pathways (Konishi et al., 2014). Studies have also demonstrated consistent increases in blood supply or glucose uptake (indicators of increased neuronal activity) in the amygdala of those with PD, GAD, or social anxiety disorder (Demenescu et al., 2013; Makovac et al., 2016; Sladky et al., 2015). Functional MRI studies also identify abnormal activation patterns in response to provocation paradigms. Consistent findings across neuroimaging studies have led to a consensus that there is a close relationship between the prefrontal cortex and amygdala. The amygdala is activated when an individual is confronted with a novel or fearful situation. Learning from experience that a stressor can be coped with, is under control, or no longer requires attention is termed "emotional processing" and is associated with specific regions of the prefrontal cortex (Sánchez-Navarro et al., 2014). However, cumulative data suggest a distinction between two classes of anxiety disorders. Those disorders involving intense fear and panic (i.e., PD and specific phobias) seem to be characterized by hypoactivity of distinct prefrontal cortex areas, thus disinhibiting the amygdala. Disorders that involve worry and rumination, such as GAD or cognitions of negative consequences in social anxiety disorder, seem to be more associated with hyperactivity of the prefrontal cortex (Greenberg, Carlson, Cha, Hajcak, & Mujica-Parodi, 2012; Kawashima et al., 2016).

Psychodynamic Theories

Psychodynamic theories focus on the psychological influences on human behaviour, feelings, and emotions, and explore how these relate to early life experience. As noted at the beginning of the chapter, research from developmental neuroscience supports our understanding of how early life experiences lay a template in the brain and body that shapes the response to stressors across the lifespan (Schore, 2001, 2014). A particular contribution of psychodynamic theories to the understanding of anxiety disorders is their emphasis on the important role of separation and loss on the development of anxiety. Patients with anxiety disorders report greater numbers and severity of recent personal losses at symptom onset than do healthy controls. Childhood risk factors for the development of GAD or major depression in adulthood include "maternal internalizing symptoms, low SES (socioeconomic status), maltreatment, inhibited temperament, internalizing problems and conduct problems, and high scores on negative emotionality" (Moffitt et al., 2007, p. 448). Further, research in the area of childhood trauma and neglect demonstrates the potential consequences of neglect and abuse including long-lasting alterations in the neural networks of the brain, whereby adaptive traits become maladaptive. For example, being in a constant state of fear arousal "can become, over time, the persisting state of anxiety" (Perry, 2008, p. 108). Having said this, these risk factors or environmental and social conditions are part of a complex constellation of elements that contribute to experiences of anxiety and other mental disorders. Protective factors, such as supportive school-based relationships, may mitigate the negative impact of these and other risk factors.

Nursing Management of Significant Anxiety Symptoms and Specific Anxiety Disorders

Primary anxiety disorders are usually treated in primary care settings, in outpatient clinics, or by private practitioners. Hospitalization is limited to acute exacerbation of anxiety or panic symptoms or comorbid mental disorders such as depressive disorder or schizophrenia. Given the comorbidity of significant anxiety and GAD among individuals with chronic physical health conditions such as cardiovascular problems, assessment of anxiety should be part of the overall approach to chronic disease management.

Assessment within a bio/psycho/social/spiritual framework is the foundation of holistic care. Physiologic symptoms tend to be the impetus for patients to seek health care. Often, persons with PD are initially seen in emergency rooms, as they seek treatment for their panic attack. Biologic, psychological, social, and spiritual assessments unveil potential contributing factors and identify sources of strength that can guide the nurse to develop an individual action plan.

Biologic Domain

Assessment

Once it is determined that anxiety symptoms have led to significant impairment in occupational, social, and interpersonal functioning, the nurse should assess for any potential environmental triggers and obtain a detailed history of any previous similar experiences. Questions to ask the patient might include the following:

- What did you experience preceding and during times of increased anxiety or a panic attack, including physical symptoms, feelings, and thoughts? Have you ever experienced some of these symptoms before? If so, under what circumstances?
- Has anyone in your family ever had similar experiences?
- What do you do when you have these experiences that help you to feel less anxious?
- What has helped you in the past to manage your symptoms?

Substance Use

Assessment for panicogenic substance use, such as sources of caffeine intake, pseudoephedrine, amphetamine, cocaine, or other stimulant use, may rule out contributory issues either related or unrelated to PD. Patients with anxiety disorders may use alcohol to self-treat their symptoms. Details of typical alcohol and other substance use are an important part of the assessment.

Sleep Patterns

Sleep is often disturbed in patients with anxiety disorders. Panic attacks can occur during sleep, and the patient may fear sleep for this reason. Nurses should closely assess the impact of sleep disturbance as it can increase the risk of further panic attacks and the development of major depressive disorder.

Interventions for Biologic Domain

These interventions can assist individuals with either severe anxiety or panic symptoms.

Physical Activity

Interventions that focus on the physical aspects of anxiety and panic are particularly helpful in reducing the number and severity of the attacks, giving patients an increasing sense of accomplishment and control. Routine leisure walking can create time for reappraisal and reflection of triggering stimuli. Active participation in an exercise program may help individuals reassess automatic thinking that relates increased heart rate and shortness of breath with a physical crisis. Physical activity can also improve sleep.

Breathing Control

Hyperventilation is common for people with anxiety disorders. Often, people are unaware that they take rapid, shallow breaths when they become anxious. Other common sensations are choking and pressure on the chest, restricting normal breathing. Teaching breathing control is a simple intervention that has immediate results. Begin by encouraging the person to simply observe the rate, pattern, and depth of their breathing. Next, invite the person to perform the following abdominal or diaphragmatic breathing exercise:

- Sit in an upright position, feet flat on the floor, and arms supported on the side-arms of a chair or on your lap. (Rationale: This position increases the capacity of the lungs to fill with air and for the limbs to be comfortably supported.)
- Place your hand on your abdomen, slightly above your umbilicus (bellybutton).
- Inhale slowly through the nose to the count of four and feel your abdomen rise.
- Exhale slowly through the mouth to the count of six and feel your abdomen fall.
- As you exhale, feel all of your muscles relax and let go.
- Repeat a series of 10 slow abdominal breaths, followed by normal breathing.

Abdominal breathing may also be used to interrupt an episode of panic as it begins. Once individuals have learned to identify their own early signs of panic, they can use abdominal breathing to divert or decrease the severity of the attack.

Nutrition Planning

Patients need to work towards reducing and eventually eliminating stimulants such as caffeine from their diet. Many over-the-counter (OTC) remedies, especially "energy drinks" used to boost energy or increase mental performance, have high levels of caffeine. The nurse should also assess for other potential sources of stimulants, which are found in some cold remedies and herbal products, and provide information about substitutes.

Relaxation Techniques

Teaching the patient relaxation techniques is another way to help with anxiety and anxiety disorders. Many individuals are unaware of the tension they carry in their bodies and first need to learn to monitor their own tension. Isometric exercises and progressive muscle relaxation are helpful methods to learn to differentiate muscle tension from muscle relaxation. This method of relaxation is also helpful when individuals have difficulty clearing the mind, focusing, or visualizing a scene, which are often required in other forms of relaxation such as meditation. Box 23.4 provides one method of progressive muscle relaxation.

Pharmacotherapy for Anxiety and Anxiety Disorders

As mentioned previously, there are known neurotransmitter systems associated with anxiety and anxiety disorders, but not all of these associations have led to specific drug therapies. For example, drugs such as propranolol act primarily on β-adrenergic receptors and reduce the

---

BOX 23.4 Progressive Muscle Relaxation

Choose a quiet, comfortable location where you will not be disturbed for 20 to 30 minutes. Your position may be lying or sitting, but all parts of your body should be supported, including your head. Wear loose clothing and remove restrictive items such as glasses and shoes.

Begin by closing your eyes and clearing your mind. Moving from head to toe, focus on each part of your body and assess the level of tension. Visualize each group of muscles as heavy and relaxed.

Take two or three slow abdominal breaths, pausing briefly between each breath. Imagine the tension flowing from your body.

Each muscle group listed below should be tightened (or tensed isometrically) for 5 to 10 seconds and then abruptly released; visualize this group of muscles as heavy, limp, and relaxed for 15 to 20 seconds before tightening the next group of muscles. There are several methods to tighten each muscle group, and suggestions are provided below. Each muscle group may be tightened two to three times until relaxed. Do not over tighten or strain. You should not experience pain.

- Hands (tighten by making fists)

- Biceps (tighten by drawing forearms up and "making a muscle")
- Triceps (extend forearms straight, locking elbows)
- Face (grimace, tightly shutting mouth and eyes; open mouth wide and raise eyebrows)
- Neck (pull head forward to chest and tighten neck muscles)
- Shoulders (raise shoulders towards ears; push shoulders back as if touching them together)
- Chest (take a deep breath and hold for 10 seconds)
- Stomach (suck in your abdominal muscles)
- Buttocks (pull buttocks together)
- Thighs (straighten your legs and squeeze the muscles in thighs and hips)
- Leg calves (pull toes carefully towards you, avoid cramps)
- Feet (curl toes downwards and point toes away from your body)

Finally, repeat several deep abdominal breaths and mentally check your body for tension. Rest comfortably for several minutes, breathing normally, and visualize your body as warm and relaxed. Get up slowly when you are finished.

peripheral symptoms of anxiety, but they have limited effectiveness against panic symptoms.

Selective Serotonin and Serotonin–Norepinephrine Reuptake Inhibitors (SSRIs and SNRIs)

The SSRIs and SNRIs are generally considered the first-line pharmacotherapy long-term treatment for most anxiety disorders (Bandelow et al., 2015; Bereza, Machado, Ravindran, & Einarson, 2012; Fineberg, Brown, Reghunandan, & Pampaloni, 2012). Overall, SSRIs and SNRIs produce fewer side effects than do other drugs used to treat anxiety, are safer to use, and are not lethal in the event of overdose. Details regarding these two classes of antidepressants can be found in Chapter 12.

Tricyclic Antidepressant Therapy

Like the SSRIs and the SNRIs, the TCAs imipramine (Tofranil), nortriptyline (Pamelor), and clomipramine (Anafranil) reduce anxiety and panic symptoms, through their inhibition of serotonin and norepinephrine reuptake. However, this class of drugs also interacts with many more neurotransmitter systems, and these drugs carry with them significant side effects. Thus, they are usually only considered in the event that SSRIs or SNRIs have failed to produce remission of symptoms. Details regarding this class of antidepressants can be found in Chapter 12.

Benzodiazepine Therapy

All benzodiazepines produce anxiolytic action, and their therapeutic onset is much faster (hours, not weeks) than that of antidepressants. Therefore, benzodiazepines are tremendously useful in treating intensely distressed patients. However, evidence to support their use in long-term treatment of anxiety disorder is limited and should only be used for short periods of time for acute anxiety and sleep disturbance (Offidani, Guidi, Tomba, & Fava, 2013). Alprazolam (Xanax), lorazepam (Ativan), and clonazepam (Rivotril) are widely used for anxiety disorders. They are well tolerated but carry the risk for withdrawal symptoms like rebound anxiety and sleep disturbance upon discontinuation of use.

Administering and Monitoring Benzodiazepines

Treatment may include administering benzodiazepines concurrently with antidepressants for the first 4 weeks and then tapering the benzodiazepine. This strategy provides rapid symptom relief but avoids the complications of long-term benzodiazepine use. Details regarding this class of drugs can be found in Chapter 12. Short-acting benzodiazepines, such as alprazolam and lorazepam, are associated with rebound anxiety or anxiety that increases after the peak effects of the medication have decreased. Medications with short half-lives should be given in three or four small doses spaced throughout the day, with a higher dose at bedtime to allay anxiety-related insomnia. Clonazepam, a longer-acting benzodiazepine, requires less frequent dosing and has a lower risk for rebound anxiety. Rebound anxiety and insomnia are also common with higher dosing regimens and the abrupt cessation of benzodiazepine treatment. Benzodiazepines should be used with extreme caution to treat anxiety in the elderly due to significantly increasing the risk of falls and anterograde memory difficulties, which can be misinterpreted as signs of dementia (van Strien, Koek, van Marum, & Emmelot-Vonk, 2013).

Psychological Domain

Assessment

A complete psychological assessment is necessary to determine patterns of anxiety, characteristic symptoms, and the person's emotional, cognitive, and behavioural responses (see Chapter 10). A comprehensive assessment includes overall mental status, suicidal tendencies and thoughts, cognitive thought patterns, avoidance behaviour patterns, and any comorbid depression symptoms. Patients' perceptions regarding their symptoms are discussed, as well as present and past coping strategies.

Self-Report Scales

Self-evaluation can be difficult in anxiety disorders. Specific triggers are often no longer present or have generalized so that it is difficult to be aware of subtle associations that increase symptoms. Several tools are available to characterize and rate the patient's state of anxiety and to differentiate between different anxiety disorders. Examples of these symptom and behavioural rating scales are provided in Box 23.5. The majority of these tools are self-report measures and, as such, are limited by the individual's self-awareness and openness. However, the Hamilton Rating Scale for Anxiety (HAM-A), provided in Table 23.2, is an example of a scale rated by the clinician (Hamilton, 1959). This 14-item scale reflects both psychological and somatic aspects of anxiety.

Assessment of Thought Patterns

Catastrophic misinterpretations of trivial physical symptoms can trigger intense anxiety and panic symptoms. Once identified, these sensations and associated thoughts should serve as a basis for individualizing patient education to address the resulting fear. Table 23.3 presents an example of a scale to assess catastrophic misinterpretations of the symptoms of panic. Several studies have found that individuals who have strategies for coping with uncomfortable sensations and feel a sense of control have fewer severe panic attacks. Individuals who fear loss of control during a panic attack often make the following types of statements:

- "I feel trapped."
- "I think I might die."
- "I'm afraid others will know, or I'll hurt someone."
- "I feel alone. I can't help myself."
- "I'm losing control."

BOX 23.5 Rating Scales for Assessment of Panic Disorder and Anxiety Disorder

PANIC SYMPTOMS

Panic-Associated Symptom Scale (PASS; Argyle et al., 1991)

Acute Panic Inventory (Dillon, Gorman, Liebowitz, Fyer, & Klein, 1987)

National Institute of Mental Health Panic Questionnaire (NIMH PQ; Scupi, Maser, & Uhde, 1992)

COGNITIONS

Anxiety Sensitivity Index (Reiss, Peterson, & Gursky, 1986)

Agoraphobia Cognitions Questionnaire (Chambless, Caputo, Bright, & Gallagher, 1984)

Body Sensations Questionnaire (Chambless et al., 1984)

PHOBIAS

Mobility Inventory for Agoraphobia (Chambless, Caputo, Jasin, Gracely, & Williams, 1985)

Fear Questionnaire (Marks & Matthews, 1979)

ANXIETY

State-Trait Anxiety Inventory (STAI; Spielberger, Gorsuch, & Luchene, 1976)

Penn State Worry Questionnaire (PSWQ; Meyer, Miller, Metzger, & Borkovec, 1990)

Beck Anxiety Inventory (Beck, Epstein, Brown, & Steer, 1988)

Table 23.2 Hamilton Rating Scale for Anxiety

Hamilton (1959) designed this scale to help clinicians gather information about states of anxiety. The symptom inventory provides scaled information that classifies anxiety behaviour and assists the clinician in targeting behaviours and achieving outcome measures. Provide a rating for each indicator based on the following scale:

0 = None   1 = Mild   2 = Moderate

3 = Severe   4 = Severe, grossly disabling

Item	Symptoms	Rating
Anxious mood	Worries, anticipation of the worst, fearful anticipation, irritability	
Tension	Feelings of tension, fatigability, startle response, moved to tears easily, trembling, feelings of restlessness, inability to relax	
Fear	Fear of dark, strangers, being left alone, animals, traffic, crowds	
Insomnia	Difficulty falling asleep, broken sleep, unsatisfying sleep and fatigue on waking, dreams, nightmares, night terrors	
Intellectual (cognitive)	Difficulty concentrating, poor memory	
Depressed mood	Loss of interest, lack of pleasure in hobbies, depression, early waking, diurnal swings	
Somatic (sensory)	Tinnitus, blurred vision, hot and cold flushes, feelings of weakness, picking sensation	
Somatic (muscular)	Aches and pains, twitching, stiffness, myoclonic jerks, grinding of teeth, unsteady voice, increased muscular tone	
Cardiovascular symptoms	Tachycardia, palpitations, chest pain, throbbing of vessels, fainting feelings, heart missing beat	
Respiratory symptoms	Pressure or constriction in chest, choking feelings, sighing, dyspnea	
Gastrointestinal symptoms	Difficulty swallowing, wind, abdominal pain, burning sensation, abdominal fullness, nausea, vomiting, borborygmi (stomach rumbling), looseness of bowels, loss of weight, constipation	
Genitourinary symptoms	Frequent micturition, urgent micturition, amenorrhea, menorrhagic, development of frigidity, premature ejaculation, loss of libido, impotence	
Autonomic symptoms	Dry mouth, flushing, pallor, tendency to sweat, giddiness, tension headache, raising of hair	
Behaviour at interview	Fidgeting, restlessness or pacing, tremor of hands, furrowed brow, strained face, sighing or rapid respiration, facial pallor, swallowing, belching, brisk tendon jerks, dilated pupils, exophthalmos	

From Hamilton, M. (1959). The assessment of anxiety states by rating. *British Journal of Medical Psychology, 32,* 54.

Table 23.3	Panic Attack Cognition Questionnaire

Rate each of the following thoughts according to the degree to which you believe each thought contributes to your panic attack.

1 = Not at all   2 = Somewhat
3 = Quite a lot   4 = Very much

Thought	Rating
I'm going to die.	
I'm going insane.	
I'm losing control.	
This will never end.	
I'm really scared.	
I'm having a heart attack.	
I'm going to pass out.	
I don't know what people will think.	
I won't be able to get out of here.	
I don't understand what is happening to me.	
People will think I'm crazy.	
I'll always be this way.	
I am going to throw up.	
I must have a brain tumour.	
I'll choke to death.	
I'm going to act foolish.	
I'm going blind.	
I'll hurt someone.	
I'm going to have a stroke.	
I'm going to scream.	
I'm going to babble or talk funny.	
I'll be paralyzed by fear.	
Something is physically wrong with me.	
I won't be able to breathe.	
Something terrible will happen.	
I'm going to make a scene.	

Adapted from Panic attack cognitions questionnaire in Clum, G. A. (1990). *Coping with panic: A drug-free approach to dealing with anxiety attacks.* Pacific Grove, CA: Brooks/Cole.

Such individuals also tend to show low self-esteem, feelings of helplessness, demoralization, and overwhelming fears of experiencing panic attacks. They may have difficulty with assertiveness or expressing feelings.

Interventions and Therapies Within the Psychological Domain

Current clinical guidelines for the treatment of anxiety disorders suggest that either pharmacotherapy or specific psychotherapies can be efficacious and, in the short term, a combination of both modes of therapy can be superior to using only one or the other in isolation (Cuijpers et al., 2014; Huhn et al., 2014). Nurses can assist individuals to identify triggers and eventually learn to manage their responses.

Peplau (1989) was one of the first to develop guidelines for nursing interventions for treating individuals experiencing problems with anxiety. These interventions help the person attend to and react to input other than the subjective experience of anxiety. Although Peplau's work is almost 30 years old, many of the interventions she described are still relevant today (see Table 23.4). Box 23.6 offers a comparison of effective and ineffective dialogue with a person with an anxiety disorder.

Distraction

Once individuals can identify the early symptoms of panic, they can learn to use **distraction** behaviours to shift their attention away from the uncomfortable physical sensations. Distraction activities include initiating a conversation with a nearby person or engaging in a physical activity (e.g., walking, gardening, house cleaning). Performing simple, repetitive activities such as snapping a rubber band against the wrist, counting backwards from 100 by threes, and counting objects along the roadway are other strategies for deterring an attack.

Table 23.4	Nursing Interventions Based on Degrees of Anxiety

Degree of Anxiety	Nursing Interventions
Mild	Learning is possible. The nurse assists the patient to use the energy that anxiety provides to encourage learning.
Moderate	The nurse needs to check his or her own anxiety so that the patient does not empathize with it. Encourage the patient to talk: to focus on one experience, to describe it fully, then to formulate the patient's generalizations about that experience.
Severe	Learning is less possible. Allow relief behaviours to be used but do not ask about them. Encourage the patient to talk: ventilation of random ideas is likely to reduce anxiety to a moderate level. When this is observed by the nurse, proceed as above.
Panic	Learning is impossible. The nurse needs to stay with the patient. Allow pacing and walk with the patient. No content inputs to the patient's thinking should be made by the nurse. (They burden the patient, who will distort them.) Pick up on what the patient says, for example, Pt: "What's happening to me—how did I get here?" N: "Say what you notice." Short phrases by the nurse—direct, to the point of the patient's comment, and investigative—match the current attention span of the patient in panic and therefore are more likely to be heard, grasped, and acted on, with the patient's responses gradually reducing the anxiety in a helpful way. Do not touch the patient; patients experiencing panic are very concerned about survival, are experiencing grave threat to self, and usually distort intentions of all invasions of their personal space.

Adapted from Peplau, H. (1989). Theoretical constructs: Anxiety, self, and hallucinations. In A. O'Toole & S. Welt (Eds.), *Interpersonal theory in nursing practice: Selected works of Hildegard E. Peplau.* New York, NY: Springer.

BOX 23.6

THERAPEUTIC DIALOGUE

Panic Disorder With Agoraphobia

Mark, a 55-year-old Caucasian man, was admitted 4 days ago to the psychiatric unit with exacerbation of anxiety symptoms and panic attacks during the last 3 weeks. He has a 30-year history of uncontrolled anxiety that is refractory to medications and psychotherapies. On admission, he stated that he feels suicidal at times because he thinks that his life is not within his control. He feels embarrassed, angry, and "trapped" by his disorder. During the past 24 hours, Mark is seen crying at times; he also isolates himself in his room. Michelle, Mark's nurse, enters his room to make a supportive contact and to assess his current mental status.

Ineffective Approach

Nurse: Oh…. Why are you crying?

Patient: (Looks up, gives a nervous chuckle) Obviously, because I'm upset. I am tired of living this way. I just want to be normal again. I can't even remember what that feels like.

Nurse: You look normal to me. Everyone has bad days. It'll pass.

Patient: I've felt this way longer than you've been alive. I've tried everything and nothing works.

Nurse: You're not the first depressed person that I've taken care of. You just need to go to groups and stay out of your room more. You'll start feeling better.

Patient: (Angrily) Oh, it's just that easy. You have no idea what I'm going through! You don't know me! You're just a kid.

Nurse: I can help you if you help yourself. A group starts in 5 minutes, and I'd like to see you there.

Patient: I'm not going to no damn group! I want to be alone so I can think!

Nurse: (Looks about anxiously) Maybe I should come back after you've calmed down a little.

Effective Approach

Nurse: Mark, I noticed that you are staying in your room more today. What's troubling you?

Patient: (Looks up) I feel like I've lost complete control of my life. I'm so anxious and nothing helps. I'm tired of it.

Nurse: I see. That must be difficult. Can you tell me more about what you are feeling right now?

Patient: I feel like I'm going crazy. I worry all the time about having panic attacks. They make me scared I'm going to die. Sometimes I think I'd be better off dead.

Nurse: (Remains silent, continues to give eye contact)

Patient: Do you know what it's like to be a prisoner to your emotions? I can't even go out of the house sometimes, and when I do, it's terrifying. I don't know what to think anymore.

Nurse: Mark, you have lived with this disorder for a long time. You say that the medications do not work to your liking, but what has helped you in the past?

Patient: Well, I learned in relaxation group that panic symptoms are probably caused by chemicals in my brain that are not working correctly. I learned that medications can help, but they don't work well for me. I tried an exposure plan and relaxation techniques to deal with my fears of leaving the house and my chronic anxiety. That did help some, but it's scary to do.

Nurse: It sounds like you have learned much about your illness, one that can be treated, so that you don't always have to feel this way.

Patient: This is easier to say right now when I'm here and can get help if I need it. It's hard to remember this when I'm in the middle of a panic attack and think I'm dying.

Nurse: It's harder when you're alone?

Patient: Much harder! And I'm alone so much of the time.

Nurse: Let's talk about some ways you can manage your panics when you're alone. Tell me some of the techniques you've learned.

Critical Thinking Challenge

- What tone is established by the nurse's opening question in the first scenario?
- Which therapeutic communication techniques did the nurse use in the second scenario to avoid the pitfalls encountered in the first scenario?
- What information was uncovered in the second scenario that was not touched on in the first?
- What predictions can you make about the interpersonal relationship likely to develop between the nurse and the patient in each scenario?

Positive Self-Talk

During states of increased anxiety and panic, individuals can learn to counter frightening or negative thoughts with positive coping statements, also called **positive self-talk**. Examples of positive self-talk include "This is only anxiety and it will pass"; "I can handle these symptoms"; and "I'll get through this." These positive statements are most effective when they are grounded in truth, because they offer the individual a focal point and challenge fear-provoking thoughts (e.g., "I am going to die," or "I can't handle this"). Some individuals carry positive statements written on a small card in their purse or wallet or on a handheld device. These messages can quickly be retrieved and read at the onset of panic symptoms.

Cognitive–Behavioural Therapy

Cognitive–behavioural therapy (CBT) is a model of psychotherapy developed in the late 1950s and is highly effective first-line psychotherapy for the treatment of anxiety disorders. Self-help manuals based on CBT principles and online structured modules have also been shown to be effective. It is also an effective treatment for depression, sleep problems, chronic pain, and eating disorders and tends to have fewer side effects and better treatment retention as compared to pharmacotherapy (Hunsley, Elliot, & Therrien, 2013). CBT is often recommended as the first line of treatment for anxiety disorders, depending on accessibility and acceptability to the patient (Hunsley et al., 2013). There is evidence that individuals prefer psychological interventions such as CBT to medication, and psychosocial interventions are first-line treatment for children, adolescents, and pregnant and breast-feeding women (Khouzam, 2009; McHugh, Whitton, Peckham, Welge, & Otto, 2013). Although CBT principles are applied in many different situations, the basic principles are simple and remain constant (Burns, 1999): (1) Thoughts, feelings, behaviours (actions, choices), and body sensations affect each other. (2) Because thoughts, feelings, behaviours (actions, choices), and body sensations are connected, even small changes in one area can affect the others. (3) CBT focuses on events and situations in the "here and now" and does not try to understand how or where they began. (4) CBT encourages self-awareness. And (5) CBT emphasizes learning and practicing new skills (homework).

CBT is a highly effective approach for treating severe anxiety, GAD, PD, and social anxiety disorder. The goal of CBT is to help individuals manage their anxiety by challenging anxiety-provoking thoughts. CBT strategies include psychoeducation, self-monitoring, cognitive restructuring, and somatic exercises. CBT is offered to individuals and groups and over a 12- to 20-week period, although longer treatment may be necessary to maintain an initial response. (See Chapter 13, *Cognitive–Behavioural Interventions*.)

Clinicians have started to combine the principles of CBT with other treatment modalities, such as mindfulness, to achieve better outcomes with patients who have challenging anxiety disorders and/or OCD (Fairfax & Barfield, 2010; Kumar, Sharma, Narayanaswamy, Kandavel, & Reddy, 2016). Jeffrey Schwartz (1996/2016), a research psychiatrist at the University of California, developed a four-step self-treatment method for patients struggling with OCD, which combines aspects of mindful awareness with the principles of CBT identified previously. The four steps are listed in Box 23.7. Components of mindfulness that seem to be effective in helping people shift their thoughts are mindful awareness, or dispositional mindfulness, being aware of one's present-moment experiences, thoughts, and sensations, in a nonjudgmental way, and the selective focusing of attention (Hoge et al., 2015; Kumar et al., 2016).

BOX 23.7 **A four-step self-treatment method, from Schwartz, J. M. (2016). *Brain lock*. New York, NY: Harper Collins.**

The four steps are:

1. Relabel—whereby the patient learns to recognize the thought for what it is, an obsessive thought or a compulsive urge.
2. Reattribute—when the person recognizes that the messages they are receiving are false and a result of a medical condition.
3. Refocus—is when the person intentionally engages in a different activity, thereby focusing their attention on different, more pleasurable, activity.
4. Revalue—as the person becomes more adept at recognizing OCD symptoms, they recognize the symptoms as distractions and devalue the thoughts and compulsions. At the same time, the person can begin to revalue their lives.

Importantly, built into each of the steps is a *fifteen-minute rule* whereby the intent is for the person to delay their response to the obsessive thought or compulsion by 15 minutes. During this time, the patient is reminded to be mindfully aware that they are relabelling, reattributing, or refocusing their attention. You can see how these four steps integrate mindful awareness in aid of cognitive restructuring.

Exposure therapy is the treatment of choice for agoraphobia, specific phobias, and OCD. Patients are repeatedly exposed to increasingly complex and real or simulated anxiety-provoking situations until they become desensitized and anxiety subsides. **Systematic desensitization**, another exposure method used to desensitize patients, exposes the patient to a hierarchy of feared situations that the patient has rated from least to most feared. The patient is taught to use muscle relaxation as levels of anxiety increase through multisituational exposure. Planning and implementing exposure therapy requires special training. Because of the multitude of outpatients in treatment for agoraphobia, exposure therapy would be a useful tool for home health psychiatric nurses. Outcomes of home-based exposure treatment are similar to clinic-based treatment outcomes.

Psychoeducation programs help to educate patients and families about the symptoms of anxiety and panic. Individuals with PD legitimately fear "going crazy," losing control, or dying because of their physical symptoms. Attempting to convince a patient that such fears are groundless only heightens anxiety and impedes communication. Information and physical evidence, such as electrocardiogram results and laboratory test results, should be presented in a caring and open manner that demonstrates acceptance and understanding of the patient's situation.

Box 23.8 suggests topics for individual or small group discussion. It is especially important to cover such topics as the differences between panic attacks and heart attacks, the difference between PD and other psychiatric disorders, and the effectiveness of various treatment methods.

Social and Occupational Domains

Individuals with anxiety disorders often deteriorate socially as the disorder takes its toll on relationships with family and friends. Occupational success and work satisfaction are often compromised. If the disorder becomes severe enough, the person may experience extreme isolation. Therefore, it is an important area for assessment and active intervention if necessary.

Assessment

During the assessment, the nurse needs to assess the patient's understanding of how anxiety or panic symptoms and associated avoidance behaviours have affected their social and work life along with that of the family. Pertinent questions include the following:

- How has the disorder affected your family's social life?
- How has the disorder affected your work and work–life balance?

BOX 23.8 Psychoeducation Checklist

When caring for the patient with anxiety disorders, be sure to include the following topic areas in the teaching plan:

- Psychopharmacologic agents (anxiolytics or antidepressants) if ordered, including drug action, dosage, frequency, and possible adverse effects
- Breathing control measures
- Potential dietary triggers
- Exercise
- Progressive muscle relaxation
- Distraction behaviours
- Relevant psychotherapies and where they are available
- Time and specific stress management strategies
- Positive coping strategies

- What limitations related to travel has the disorder placed on you or your family?
- What coping strategies have you used to manage the symptoms?
- How has the disorder affected your family members or others? (Fig. 23.1)

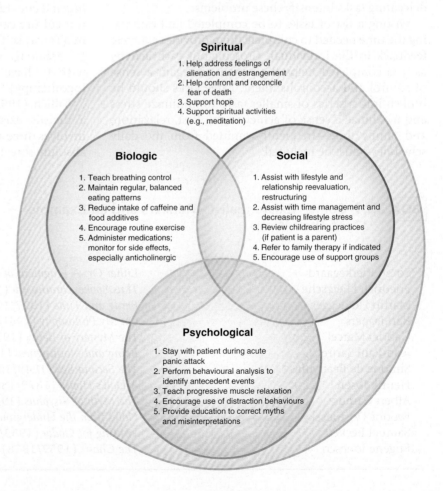

Spiritual
1. Help address feelings of alienation and estrangement
2. Help confront and reconcile fear of death
3. Support hope
4. Support spiritual activities (e.g., meditation)

Biologic
1. Teach breathing control
2. Maintain regular, balanced eating patterns
3. Reduce intake of caffeine and food additives
4. Encourage routine exercise
5. Administer medications; monitor for side effects, especially anticholinergic

Social
1. Assist with lifestyle and relationship reevaluation, restructuring
2. Assist with time management and decreasing lifestyle stress
3. Review childrearing practices (if patient is a parent)
4. Refer to family therapy if indicated
5. Encourage use of support groups

Psychological
1. Stay with patient during acute panic attack
2. Perform behavioural analysis to identify antecedent events
3. Teach progressive muscle relaxation
4. Encourage use of distraction behaviours
5. Provide education to correct myths and misinterpretations

Figure 23.1. Bio/psycho/social/spiritual interventions for patients with panic disorder.

Cultural Factors

Cultural competence calls for the understanding of cultural knowledge, cultural awareness, cultural assessment skills, and cultural practice. Therefore, cultural differences must be considered in the assessment of anxiety disorders. Different cultures interpret anxiety-related sensations, feelings, or understandings differently. "Nervousness" may be more accepted by some cultural groups, and several cultures do not have a word to describe "anxiety" or to denote "anxiousness" but instead may use words or meanings to suggest somatic complaints. In addition, showing anxiety may be a sign of weakness in some cultures (Hofmann, Asnaani, & Hinton, 2010).

Interventions for Social and Occupational Domains

Individuals with anxiety disorders, especially those with significant anxiety sensitivity, may need assistance in reevaluating their lifestyles. Casual comments by friends or coworkers can be misinterpreted or overinterpreted and be triggers for intense anxiety or panic symptoms. Time management can be a useful tool. In the workplace or at home, underestimating the time needed to complete a chore or being overly involved in several activities at once increases stress and anxiety. Procrastination, lack of assertiveness, and difficulties with prioritizing or delegating tasks intensify these problems.

Writing a list of tasks to be completed and estimating the time needed to complete them provides concrete feedback to the individual. Crossing-out each activity as it is completed helps the patient to regain a sense of control and accomplishment. Large tasks should be broken into a series of smaller tasks to minimize stress and maximize a sense of achievement. Rest, relaxation, and family time—frequently omitted from the daily schedule—must be included.

Family Response to Anxiety Disorders

Affected families often have difficulty with overall communication. Parents with agoraphobia may become discouraged and self-critical regarding their child-rearing abilities, which may cause their children to be overly dependent. Parents with PD may inadvertently cause excessive fears, phobias, or excessive worry in their children. Family members may get frustrated with the chronic nature of anxiety disorders and show irritation when anxiety symptoms are exacerbated by acute stressors.

Pregnancy can increase anxiety symptoms for women who have preexisting anxiety disorders. Assessment of mood and anxiety symptoms both in the antepartum and the postpartum period, as well as available resources to manage such symptoms, should be part of routine maternity care.

Spiritual Domain

Anxiety can be understood as basic to the human condition. Existentialist thinkers (see Box 23.9) argue that, because we humans are aware of our own mortality, the apprehension that death will end our existence fills us with foreboding. This **existential anxiety** must be accepted and faced, or it can subvert our everyday life. We can feel alienated and estranged (not at home) in the world. We look to find meaning in our lives, a *raison d'étre*. Existentialists note that, as neither nature nor culture can do this for us, individual humans are, in a sense, self-making. Frankl (1992), in *Man's Search for Meaning*, wrote about how it is every human's wish to have a meaningful life (see Chapter 8 for logotherapy).

Tillich (1952), the author of *The Courage to Be* and a theistic existentialist, finds that existential anxiety involves three areas of apprehension: fate and death (the absolute threat to self), emptiness and meaninglessness

---

BOX 23.9 Some "Existentialist" Thinkers and an Example of Their Work

Søren Kierkegaard	*Either Or: A Fragment of a Life* (1843/1944)
Friedrich Nietzsche	*Thus Spoke Zarathustra* (1883/1985)
Martin Heidegger	*Being and Time* (1927/1962)
Karl Jaspers	*On My Philosophy* (1941/1955)
Gabriel Marcel	*The Mystery of Being* (1951)
Jean-Paul Sartre	*Being and Nothingness* (1943/1956)
Simone de Beauvoir	*The Second Sex* (1949/1953)
Henrik Ibsen	*A Doll's House* (1879/1889)
Albert Camus	*The Myth of Sisyphus* (1942/1955)
Fyodor Dostoevsky	*Notes from the Underground* (1864/1918)
Samuel Beckett	*Waiting for Godot* (1953/1955)
Eugène Ionesco	*The Chairs* (1952/1958)

(worry that there is no ultimate meaning), and guilt and condemnation (perceived threats to one's identity). Being human involves confronting and reconciling such anxiety.

Researchers are exploring the importance of understanding the relation between existential anxiety and clinical anxiety. The existential anxiety scale (EAS) has been developed, for instance, based on Tillich's theory. Early results suggest that existential anxiety, as measured by the EAS, is common and associated with symptoms of anxiety and depression (Weems, Costa, Dehon, & Berman, 2004). In a critical review of the literature, Koslander, Barbosa da Silva, and Roxberg (2009) concluded that "it is evident that addressing patients' existential and spiritual needs helps them improve mentally" (p. 40). They argue that an existential perspective should be an element of mental health care.

EVALUATION AND TREATMENT OUTCOMES

Patients can be assisted to keep a daily log of the severity of anxiety and the frequency, duration, and severity of anxiety symptoms and panic episodes. This log will be a basic tool for monitoring progress as symptoms decrease. A number of self-help books can provide a rich source of reinforcement of simple interventions that can attenuate the intensity and frequency of panic symptoms. Rating scales may also be helpful to monitor changes in misinterpretations or other symptoms related to panic. Figure 23.2 illustrates a number of examples of bio/psycho/social/spiritual treatment outcomes for individuals with PD.

CONTINUUM OF CARE

As with any disorder, the continuum of patient care across multiple settings is crucial. Individuals are treated in the least restrictive environment that will meet their safety needs.

Inpatient Care

Inpatient settings provide care and treatment for individuals experiencing severe anxiety with comorbid depression, increased risk of suicide, or poor treatment response to typical treatment strategies.

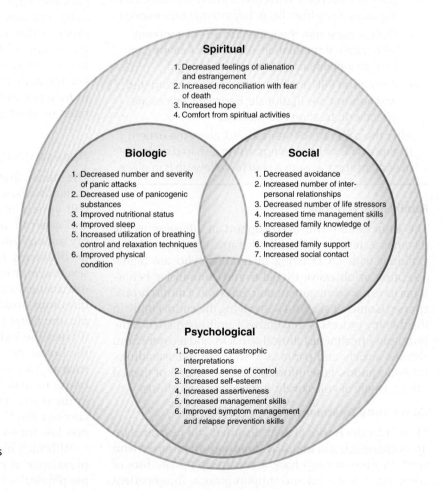

Figure 23.2. Bio/psycho/social/spiritual outcomes for patients with PD.

EMERGENCY CARE

Because individuals with PD are likely to first present for treatment in an emergency room or primary care setting, nurses and nurse practitioners working in these settings should be involved in early recognition and referral. Consultation with a psychiatrist or mental health professional by the primary care provider can decrease both anxiety symptoms and costs to the health care system (Archer et al., 2012; Goorden et al., 2014). Several interventions may be useful in reducing the number of emergency room visits related to panic symptoms. Psychiatric consultation and patient teaching can be provided in the emergency department, including the following:

- Stay with the person and maintain a calm demeanour. (Rationale: Anxiety often produces more anxiety, and a calm presence will help calm the patient.)
- Reassure the patient that you will not leave, that this episode will pass, and that he or she is in a safe place. (Rationale: A person experiencing a panic episode often fears dying and cannot see beyond the panic attack.)
- Give clear, concise directions, using short sentences. Do not use medical jargon. (Rationale: A person in the throes of panic is in crisis and has difficulty shifting focus away from his or her internal experience.)
- Walk or pace with the patient to an environment with minimal stimulation. (Rationale: Activity can help an individual focus excessive energy.)
- Administer PRN anxiolytic medications as ordered and appropriate. (Rationale: Benzodiazepines are effective in treating acute panic.)

After the panic attack has resolved, allow the patient to express his or her feelings. Using a shared decision-making process, ensure a plan for follow-up is in place.

Family Interventions

The entire family will need support in adjusting to the disorder. A referral for family therapy may be indicated. Children with OCD living in families who are highly accepting of obsessive thoughts and compulsive behaviours have poorer treatment outcomes and a more chronic course (Gomes et al., 2014). Involving the entire family in the therapy process is imperative. Families experience the symptoms, treatments, clinical setbacks, and recovery from chronic anxiety and panic as a unit. Misunderstandings, misconceptions, false information, and stigma of mental illness, singly or collectively, impede recovery efforts.

Community Treatment

Most individuals with anxiety disorders will be treated on an outpatient basis, and it is important that nurses who work in these settings have access to up-to-date lists of community resources and support groups. In outpatient or primary care settings, nurses are directly involved in treatment, collaborative care management (Muntingh

et al., 2016), conducting psychoeducation groups on relaxation and breathing techniques, and teaching symptom management. Advanced practice nurses conduct CBT and individual and family psychotherapies.

Recovery from anxiety disorders involves the engagement of individuals in self-management of their anxiety disorder. Self-management of anxiety disorders is explored by Coulombe and colleagues in Box 23.10.

ASSESSMENT AND TREATMENT ISSUES SPECIFIC TO OBSESSIVE–COMPULSIVE DISORDER

Symptoms of OCD can be difficult to treat because of the pathology of the disorder, and individuals diagnosed with OCD are treated in specific outpatient programs. Short-term hospitalization may be necessary for treatment of comorbid depression and for treatment refractory symptoms. When this occurs, it is important to have a clear plan of care and to ensure that all staff members follow it consistently (Box 23.11).

Individuals with OCD do not consider their compulsions pleasurable. Often, they recognize them as odd and may initially try to resist them. Resistance eventually fails, and patients incorporate repetitive behaviours into daily routines, performing activities in a specific, ritual order. If this sequence is disturbed, the person experiences extreme anxiety until the process can be repeated in the correct sequence. Interpersonal relationships suffer, and patients may actively isolate themselves. Indeed, individuals with OCD are more likely to be young, separated or divorced, and unemployed.

Assessment

The nurse should assess the type and severity of the patient's obsessions and compulsions. Most individuals will appear neatly dressed and groomed, cooperative, and eager to answer questions. Orientation and memory are not usually impaired, but these individuals may be distracted by obsessive thoughts. Individuals with severe symptoms may be preoccupied with fears or with discussing their obsessions, but in most instances, direct questions must be asked to reveal symptoms. For example, the nurse may begin indirectly by asking how long it takes the individual to dress in the morning or leave the house, but usually follow-up questions are needed, such as "Do you find yourself frequently returning to the house to make sure that you have turned off the lights or the stove, even when you know that you have already checked this?" "Does this happen every day?" "Are you ever late for work or for important appointments?"

Although individuals with OCD do not have a higher prevalence of physical disease, some may report multiple physical symptoms. In patients with late-onset OCD (after 35 years of age) or in children who develop symptoms after a febrile illness, cerebral pathology should be

BOX 23.10 **Research for Best Practice**

PROFILES OF RECOVERY FROM MOOD AND ANXIETY DISORDERS

Coulombe, S., Radziszewski, S., Meunier, S., Provencher, H., Hudon, C., Roberge, P., Provencher, M. D., & Houle, J. (2016). Profiles of recovery from mood and anxiety disorders: A person-centred exploration of people's engagement in self-management. Frontiers in Psychology, 7, 584. doi:10.3389/fpsyg.2016.00584

Purpose: The purpose of this study was to identify profiles underlying mental health recovery including participant characteristics and associations with specific criterion variables.

Methods: One hundred and forty-nine participants with diagnoses of anxiety disorder depression or bipolar disorder were recruited from community organizations located in Quebec and France. In this quantitative study, participants completed a number of questionnaires addressing self-management, clinical recovery, personal recovery, as well as specific criterion variables (including personal goal appraisal, social participation, self-care, and coping strategies).

Findings: Utilizing a latent profile analysis, three profiles emerged: the *Floundering* profile, the *Flourishing* profile, and the *Struggling* profile. Those in the *Floundering* profile rarely engaged in self-management strategies,

experienced moderately severe symptoms, and reported the lowest positive mental health. Individuals in this group were more likely to be male, single, and with a low income. Those in the *Flourishing* profile frequently used self-empowerment strategies, experienced the least severe symptoms, and reported the highest mental health. Participants in this group had the most favourable scores on personal goal appraisal, social participation, self-care, and coping. Participants in the *Struggling* profile actively engaged in self-management strategies focused on symptom reduction and a healthy lifestyle, despite the fact that they reported high symptom severity and moderately high positive mental health.

Implications for Nursing: Recovery is a multifaceted process and individuals in this study used a variety of approaches to promote their mental health and recovery (and not solely focused on symptom reduction strategies). The importance of individualized person-centred care is critical. Nurses should work *with* their patients by exploring recovery-oriented strategies being utilized, utilizing teachable moments to encourage diversity in self-care management and recovery strategies, and to offer patients positive feedback to assist them with building confidence.

---

excluded. Patients whose compulsions involve washing should be checked for dermatologic lesions caused by repetitive handwashing, excessive cleaning with caustic agents, or bathing. Osteoarthritis joint damage secondary to cleaning rituals may also be observed.

Identifying the degree to which the OCD symptoms interfere with the patient's daily functioning is important. Several rating scales can be used to identify symptoms and monitor improvement. Examples of these scales are provided in Box 23.12. The Yale-Brown

BOX 23.11 CLINICAL VIGNETTE

OBSESSIVE–COMPULSIVE DISORDER

Robert, a 32-year-old man, is a new patient at a local psychiatric unit. He admitted himself to have his medicines evaluated because his obsessive thoughts and depression have worsened since his recent divorce. While in the hospital, he has quickly become viewed as a "problem patient" because he hoards linens and demands a new bar of soap for each of his five daily showers. He is compelled to open and close his door five times when he leaves or enters his room but does not know why. This behaviour has led to arguments with his roommate. In an effort to "help him," the staff locked his bathroom door to prevent him from showering so frequently. He tried to enter his bathroom to shower and panicked when the staff refused to allow him to shower, telling him "You can live without it." After receiving PRN medication for extreme anxiety, Robert signed out of the hospital against medical advice because of embarrassment and anger towards the nursing staff.

What Do You Think?

- How could the staff have handled the situation differently in order not to disrupt Robert's or the unit's clinical care?
- What nursing interventions might be appropriate in providing Robert's care?

BOX 23.12 Rating Scales for Assessing Obsessive–Compulsive Symptoms

Yale-Brown Obsessive–Compulsive Scale (Y-BOCS; Goodman et al., 1989)

The Maudsley Obsessional–Compulsive Inventory (MOC; Rachman & Hodgson, 1980)

The Leyton Obsessional Inventory (Cooper, 1970)

Obsessive–Compulsive Scale (Y-BOCS) is a popular, clinician-rated 16-item scale that obtains separate subtotals for the severity of obsessions and compulsions. The Maudsley Obsessive–Compulsive Inventory is a 30-item, true–false, self-assessment tool that may help the individual to recognize individual symptoms.

Nurses must consider sociocultural factors when evaluating OCD. At times, cultural or religious beliefs may be misunderstood and mistaken for obsessions or compulsions. Shame and embarrassment over the irrational thoughts and behaviours often lead to social isolation and relational difficulties. The time demands related to the compulsions often lead to decreased occupational success. Assessment of current level of functioning in social, occupational, and personal spheres is therefore important.

Family Response to Disorder

Individuals whose OCD symptoms are severe are more likely to demonstrate social skill deficits and have more difficulties with intimacy; consequently, they are less likely to marry. Some studies have also shown higher divorce rates for individuals with OCD, particularly when comorbid with other mental disorders (Fineberg et al., 2013). They also have higher rates of celibacy, possibly because they fear becoming contaminated.

OCD often diminishes the quality of family relationships. Individuals with this disorder may ask family members to become involved in their rituals of checking or providing repeated reassurance (Strauss et al., 2015). Those with OCD can become very angry and frustrated with family members for failing to comply with their requests for help with rituals. This can result in verbal and even physical altercations. Many family members find themselves modifying routines to suit a patient's symptoms and report this to be at least moderately distressing for them (Futh, Simonds, & Micali, 2012). The most troublesome symptoms of OCD for families to cope with include the patients' ruminations, long-standing unemployment, rituals, noncompliance with medication, depression, withdrawal from social and family contact, lack of motivation, and excessive arguing (Cooper, 1996; Peris et al., 2012). Spouses report a variety of issues such as sexual difficulties, overwhelming feelings of frustration, anger, guilt, and fatigue, and disrupted family and social life. Other relatives report moderate to severe burden in coping with an individual with OCD. They state that they have poor social relationships and neglect their hobbies due to their relative's illness (Cicek, Cicek, Kayhan, Uguz, & Kaya, 2013).

Treatment

Specific clinical pharmacotherapy reviews for OCD support that long-term SSRIs are the first-line treatment of choice (Fineberg et al., 2012; Poppe et al., 2016). Although extremely rare, psychosurgery has been used to treat extremely severe OCD that has not responded to prolonged and intensive drug treatment, behavioural therapy, or a combination of the two. Modern stereotactic surgical techniques that produce lesions of the cingulum (a bundle of connective pathways between the two hemispheres) or the anterior limb of the internal capsule (a region near the thalamus and part of the circuit connecting to the cortex) may bring about substantial clinical benefit in some patients without causing significant morbidity (Brown et al., 2016; Kim et al., 2003). Other treatment options include radiotherapy and deep brain stimulation in which electrical current is applied through an electrode inserted into the brain (Blomstedt, Sjöberg, Hansson, Bodlund, & Hariz, 2013).

For the patient with cleaning or handwashing compulsions, attention to skin condition is necessary. Encourage the patient to use tepid water when washing and hand cream after washing. Remove harsh, abrasive soaps and replace with moisturizing soaps. The treatment team should work with the patient to decrease the frequency of washing by structuring time schedules and time-limited washing.

Specific Psychotherapeutic Interventions for OCD

The front-line psychotherapeutic treatments for OCD are exposure with response prevention (ERP) and CBT. During ERP, the person is exposed to situations or objects that are known to induce anxiety but is asked to refrain from performing the ritualistic behaviours. One goal of this procedure is to help the patient understand that resisting the rituals while exposed to the object of anxiety is less stressful and time consuming than performing the rituals. Another goal is to confound the expectation of distressing outcomes and eventually extinguish the compulsive behaviours. Cognitive restructuring is another intervention to teach the patient to restructure dysfunctional thought processes by defining and testing them (Beck, Emery, & Greenberg, 1985). Its goal is to alter the patient's immediate, dysfunctional appraisal of a situation and perception of long-term consequences.

Community Treatment

Partial hospitalization programs and day treatment programs care for most patients with OCD. They allow patients to maintain significant independence while beginning medications and behavioural therapies. Specific day treatment psychotherapy programs for OCD are available in some larger urban centres. Specific outpatient clinics may also be available. Self-help groups and self-help books can also help patients keep their symptoms under control.

ASSESSMENT AND TREATMENT ISSUES SPECIFIC TO HOARDING DISORDER

Assessment

Individuals experiencing hoarding disorder often also experience physical health conditions such as fibromyalgia, chronic fatigue syndrome, and obesity; thus, a compressive physical and mental status assessment should be completed. When assessing patients, multiple sources of information are included in the overall assessment including police reports, public health reports, and reports from family members (with the patient's consent). Objective measures such as the Saving Inventory—Revised (Frost, Steketee, & Grisham, 2004) or the Hoarding Rating Scale—Interview (Tolin, Frost, & Steketee, 2010) are also useful formal measures for assessment.

Family Response

Hoarding disorder can have a negative impact on the health and well-being of family members and significant others. Those who live with a person with hoarding disorder frequently experience embarrassment because of the cluttered living environment and frustration with the individual's unwillingness or inability to change. Family members may not be aware of the individuals hoarding and as a result experience shock and disbelief, while others may be aware, but fear judgement and shame, for not being able to assist the person (Kress et al., 2016).

Treatment

Treatment for hoarding disorder is complex and consists of a combination of treatment approaches including cognitive behaviour therapy, psychopharmacological treatment, family assistance, and multidisciplinary community based care. Traumatic life events have been associated with the onset of hoarding; thus, trauma-informed approach to working with individuals is warranted. CBT, however, is the gold standard treatment for hoarding disorder, focusing specifically on three areas of hoarding: disorganization, difficulty discarding items, and excessive acquisition. Antidepressants such as paroxetine (Paxil) and extended release venlafaxine (Effexor XR) have been effective in improving symptoms of hoarding disorder and comorbid symptoms of depression and anxiety (Brakoulias & Milicevic, 2015; Kress et al., 2016). The importance of the nurse–patient relationship

cannot be overemphasized. Patents with hoarding disorder need to be treated with respect. Nurses need to exercise self-awareness, be careful not to judge patients (or their families), and mitigate their treatment expectations. Community-based approaches that include mental health services and the inclusion of professional organizations that can assist with home clean out can be very helpful (Bratiotis et al., 2013).

 SUMMARY OF KEY POINTS

- Anxiety-related disorders are the most common of all psychiatric disorders and significantly impair individuals' social and occupational functioning.
- The anxiety disorders are a family of disorders that share excessive fear or anxiety as their core symptom; specific anxiety disorders differ from one another according their key feature(s).
- Significant anxiety and anxiety disorders are seen across all practice settings and along the continuum of care.
- Although anxiety can be a primary diagnosis, it is more often comorbid with other psychiatric disorders (e.g., depression, schizophrenia) and/or physical illnesses (e.g., coronary artery disease, irritable bowel disease).
- Those experiencing anxiety disorders have high levels of physical and emotional symptoms and often experience comorbid or concurrent diagnoses with other anxiety disorders, substance use disorder, or depression. These disorders often significantly impair individuals' abilities to function socially, occupationally, and personally.
- Treatment approaches for all anxiety-related disorders include pharmacotherapies, psychological treatments, or often a combination of both.
- Current research points to a combination of biologic, psychological, social, and spiritual factors that cause persistent anxiety. Other research demonstrates that there are also personality traits that predispose individuals to anxiety disorders, including low self-esteem, external locus of control, some negative family influences, and some traumatic or stressful precipitating event. These components combine to yield a true bio/psycho/social/spiritual theory of causation.
- Nurses employ interventions from each of the dimensions—biologic, psychological, social, and spiritual—in the care of persons experiencing anxiety. Approaching these individuals with knowledge of the disorders, understanding, and with a calm demeanour is key. Nurses can be instrumental in crisis intervention, medication management, and psychoeducation. Psychoeducation is crucial in the management of anxiety disorders and includes methods to help patients understand and manage

anxiety symptoms (e.g., diaphragmatic breathing, stress reduction, relaxation techniques), education regarding medication side effects and management, and education of family members to understand these disorders.

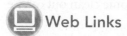

Web Links

Anxiety BC is a nonprofit established in 1999, whose mission is to "promote awareness of anxiety disorders and support access to evidence based resources and treatment." Anxiety BC is a member of the BC Partners for Mental Health and Addictions and is a leader in developing online, self-help, and evidence-based resources.

Anxiety Disorders Association of Canada is dedicated to the awareness, prevention, and treatment of anxiety disorders in Canada and to improve the lives of Canadians who experience anxiety disorders.

The Canadian Network for Mood and Anxiety Treatments (CANMAT) is a federally incorporated, academically based, not-for-profit research organization linking health care professionals from across Canada who have a special interest in mood and anxiety disorders.

References

Adams, G. C., Balbuena, L., Meng, X., & Asmudson, G. J. G. (2016). When social anxiety and depression go together: A population study of comorbidity and associated consequences. *Journal of Affective Disorders, 206*, 48–54.

Almeida, O. P., Draper, B., Pirkis, J., & Snowdon, J. (2012). Anxiety, depression, and comorbid anxiety and depression: Risk factors and outcome over two years. *International Psychogeriatrics, 24*(1), 1622–1632.

American Psychiatric Association (APA). (2013). *Diagnostic and statistical manual of mental disorders* (5th ed.). Washington, DC: Author.

Anderberg, J., Bogren, M., Mattisson, C., & Brådvik, L. (2016). Long-term suicide risk in anxiety—The Lundby study 1947–2011. *Archives of Suicidal Research, 20*, 463–475.

Antai-Otong, D. (2016). Caring for the patient with an anxiety disorder. *Nursing Clinics of North America, 51*, 173–183.

Archer, J., Bower, P., Gilbody, S., Lovell, K., Richards, D., Gask, L., … Coventry, P. (2012). Collaborative care for depression and anxiety problems. *Cochrane Database of Systematic Reviews, 10*, CD006525.

Argyle, N., Deltito, J., Allerup, P., Maier, W., Albus, M., Nutzinger, D., … Rasmussen, S. (1991). The panic-associated symptom scale: Measuring the severity of panic disorder. *Acta Psychiatrica Scandinavica, 83*, 20–26.

Asselmann, E., Wittchen, H.-U., Lieb, R., Höfler, M., & Beesdo-Baum, K. (2014). Associations of fearful spells and panic attacks with incident anxiety, depressive, and substance use disorders: A 10-year prospective-longitudinal community study of adolescents and young adults. *Journal of Psychiatric Research, 55*, 8–14.

Bandelow, B., Reitt, M., Röver, C., Michaelis, S., Görlich, Y., & Wedekind, D. (2015). Efficacy of treatments for anxiety disorders: A meta-analysis. *International Clinical Psychopharmacology, 30*(4), 183–192.

Bandelow, B., Wedekind, D., Pauls, J., Brooks, A., Hajak, G., & Ruther, E. (2000). Salivary cortisol in panic attacks. *American Journal of Psychiatry, 157*, 454–456.

Barlow, D. H. (2002). *Anxiety and its disorders: The nature and treatment of anxiety and panic*. New York, NY: Guilford Press.

Barrera, T. L., & Norton, P. J. (2009). Quality of life impairment in generalized anxiety disorder, social phobia, and panic disorder. *Journal of Anxiety Disorders, 23*(8), 1086–1090.

Beck, A. T., Emery, C., & Greenberg, R. L. (1985). *Anxiety disorders and phobias: A cognitive perspective*. New York, NY: Basic Books.

Beck, A. T., Epstein, N., Brown, G., & Steer, R. (1988). An inventory for measuring clinical anxiety: The Beck Anxiety Inventory. *Journal of Consulting and Clinical Psychology, 56*, 893–897.

Bereza, B. G., Machado, M., Ravindran, A. V., & Einarson, T. R. (2012). Evidence-based review of clinical outcomes of guideline-recommended pharmacotherapies for generalized anxiety disorder. *Canadian Journal of Psychiatry, 57*(8), 470–478.

Blomstedt, P., Sjöberg, R. L., Hansson, M., Bodlund, O., & Hariz, M. I. (2013). Deep brain stimulation in the treatment of obsessive-compulsive disorder. *World Neurosurgery, 80*(6), 245–253.

Borkovec, T. D., Robinson, E., Pruzinsky, T., & DePree, J. A. (1983). Preliminary exploration of worry: Some characteristics and processes. *Behaviour Research and Therapy, 21*(1), 9–16.

Brakoulias, V., & Milicevic, D. (2015). Assessment and treatment of hoarding disorder. *Australian Psychiatry, 23*(4), 358–360.

Bratiotis, C., Steketee, G., Davidwo, J., Samuels, J., Tolin, D., & Frost, R. (2013). Use of services by people who hoard objects. *Best Practices in Mental Health, 9*, 39–51.

Brown, L. T., Mikell, C. B., Youngerman, B. E., Zhang, Y., McKahnn, G. II, & Sheth, S. A. (2016). Dorsal anterior cingulotomy and anterior capsulotomy for severe, refractory obsessive-compulsive disorder: A systematic review of observational studies. *Journal of Neurosurgery, 124*(1), 77–89.

Burns, D. (1999). *Feeling good: The new mood therapy*. New York, NY: Plume.

Chambless, D. L., Caputo, G. C., Bright, P., & Gallagher, R. (1984). Assessment of fear in agoraphobics: The Body Sensations Questionnaire and the Agoraphobic Cognitions Questionnaire. *Journal of Consulting and Clinical Psychology, 52*, 1090–1097.

Chambless, D. L., Caputo, G. C., Jasin, S. E., Gracely, E. J., & Williams, C. (1985). The mobility inventory for agoraphobia. *Behaviour Research and Therapy, 23*, 35–44.

Cicek, E., Cicek, I. E., Kayhan, F., Uguz, F., & Kaya, N. (2013). Quality of life, family burden and associated factors in relatives with obsessive-compulsive disorder. *General Hospital Psychiatry, 35*(3), 253–258.

Clum, G. A. (1990). *Coping with panic: A drug-free approach to dealing with anxiety attacks*. Pacific Grove, CA: Brooks/Cole.

Compton, S. N. (2014). Predictors and moderators of treatment response in childhood anxiety disorders: Results from the CAMS trial. *Journal of Consulting and Clinical Psychology, 82*(2), 212–224.

Cooper, J. (1970). The Leyton Obsessional Inventory. *Psychiatric Medicine, 1*, 48.

Cooper, M. (1996). Obsessive-compulsive disorder: Effects on family members. *American Journal of Orthopsychiatry, 66*, 296–304.

Copeland, W. E., Angold, A., Shanahan, L., & Costello, E. J. (2014). Longitudinal patterns of anxiety from childhood to adulthood: The Great Smoky Mountains study. *Journal of the American Academy of Child & Adolescent Psychiatry, 53*(1), 21–33.

Corregiari, F. M., Bernik, M., Cordeiro, Q., & Vallada, H. (2012). Endophenotypes and serotonergic polymorphisms associated with treatment response in obsessive-compulsive disorder. *Clinics, 67*(4), 335–340.

Coulombe, S., Radziszewski, S., Meunier, S., Provencher, H., Hudon, C., Roberge, P., Provencher, M. D., & Houle, J. (2016). Profiles of recovery from mood and anxiety disorders: A person-centered exploration of people's engagement in self-management. *Frontiers in Psychology, 7*, 584. doi:10.3389/fpsyg.2016.00584

Critchley, H. (2003). Emotion and its disorders. *British Medical Bulletin, 65*, 35–47.

Cuijpers, P., Sijbrandij, M., Koole, S. L., Andersson, G., Beekman, A. T., & Reynolds, C. F. III. (2014). Adding psychotherapy to antidepressant medication in depression and anxiety disorders: A meta-analysis. *World Psychiatry, 13*(1), 56–67.

Darwin, C. (1887). *The life and letters of Charles Darwin*. New York, NY: Appleton & Co.

de Vries, Y. A., Roest, A. M., Franzen, M., Munafò, M. R., & Bastiaansen, J. A. (2016). Citation bias and selective focus on positive findings in the literature on the serotonin transporter gene (5-HTTLPR), life stress and depression. *Psychological Medicine, 46*(14), 2971–2979.

Dell'Osso, B., Buoli, M., Baldwin, D. S., & Carlo Altamura, A. (2010). Serotonin norepinephrine reuptake inhibitors (SNRIs) in anxiety disorders: A comprehensive review of their clinical efficacy. *Human Psychopharmacology: Clinical and Experimental, 25*, 17–29.

Demenescu, L. R., Kortekass, R., Cremers, H. R., Renken, R. J., van Tol, R. M. J., van der Wee, N. J. A., … Aleman, A. (2013). Amygdala activation and its functional connectivity during perception of emotional faces in social phobia and panic disorder. *Journal of Psychiatric Research, 47*(8), 1024–1031.

Dillon, D. J., Gorman, J. M., Liebowitz, M. R., Fyer, A. J., & Klein, D. F. (1987). Measurement of lactate-induced panic and anxiety. *Psychiatry Research, 20*, 97–105.

Elsenhauer, A. (2017, February). Preparing for patients with hording disorder. *EMSWorld*, pp. 45–47.

Ertekin, E., Çelebi, F., Koyuncu, A., Uysal, Ö, Demir, E. Y., & Tükel, R. (2015). Predictors of early or late treatment seeking in patients with social anxiety disorder. *Annals of Clinical Psychiatry, 27*(4), 236–241.

Essau, C. A., Lewinsohn, P. M., Olaya, B., & Seely, J. R. (2015). Anxiety disorders in adolescents and psychosocial outcomes at age 30. *Journal of Affective Disorders, 163*, 125–132.

Fairfax, H., & Barfield, J. (2010). A group-based treatment for clients with Obsessive Compulsive Disorder (OCD) in a secondary care mental health setting: Integrating new developments within cognitive behavioural interventions—An exploratory study. *Counselling and Psychotherapy Research, 10*(3), 214–221.

Fineberg, N. A., Brown, A., Reghunandan, S., & Pampaloni, I. (2012). Evidence-based pharmacotherapy of obsessive-compulsive disorder. *International Journal of Neuropsychopharmacology, 9*, 1–19.

Fineberg, N. A., Hengartner, M. P., Bergbaum, C., Gale, T., Rössler, W., & Angst, J. (2013). Lifetime comorbidity of obsessive-compulsive disorder and sub-threshold obsessive-compulsive symptomatology in the community: Impact, prevalence, socio-demographic and clinical characteristics. *International Journal of Psychiatry in Clinical Practice, 17*(3), 188–196.

Frankl, V. (1992). *Man's search for meaning: An introduction to logotherapy* (4th ed.). Boston, MA: Beacon Press.

Frost, R. O., Steketee, G., & Grisham, J. (2004). Measurement of compulsive hoarding: Saving Inventory-Revised. *Behaviour Research and Therapy, 42*, 1163–1182.

Futh, A., Simonds, L. M., & Micali, N. (2012). Obsessive-compulsive disorder in children and adolescents: Parental understanding, accommodation, coping and distress. *Journal of Anxiety Disorders, 26*(5), 624–632.

García-Soriano, G., Rufer, M., Delsignore, A., & Weidt, S. (2014). Factors associated with non-treatment of delayed treatment seeking in OCD sufferers: A review of the literature. *Psychiatry Research, 220*, 1–10.

Geller, S. M., & Porges S. W. (2014). Therapeutic presence: Neurophysiological mechanisms mediating feeling safe in therapeutic relationships. *Journal of Psychotherapy Integration, 24*(3), 178–192.

Goes, F. S., McCusker, M. G., Bienvenu, O. J., & MacKinnon, D. F. (2012). Co-morbid anxiety disorders in bipolar disorder and major depression: Familial aggregation and clinical characteristics of co-morbid panic disorder, social phobia, specific phobia and obsessive-compulsive disorder. *Psychological Medicine, 42*(7), 1449–1459.

Gomes, J. B., Van Noppen, B., Pato, M., Braga, D. T., Meyer, E., Bortoncello, C. F., & Cordioli, A. V. (2014). Patient and family factors associated with family accommodation in obsessive-compulsive disorder. *Psychiatry and Clinical Neurosciences, 68*(8), 621–630.

Goodman, W., Price, L., Rasmussen, S., Mazure, C., Fleischmann, R. L., & Hill, C. L. (1989). The Yale-Brown Obsessive Compulsive Scale (Y-BOCS): Part 1. Development, use and reliability. *Archives of General Psychiatry, 46*, 1006–1011.

Goorden, M., Muntingh, A., van Marwijk, H., Spinhoven, P., Adèr, H., van Balkom, A., … Hakkaart-van Roijen, L. (2014). Cost utility analysis of a collaborative stepped care intervention and generalized anxiety disorders in primary care. *Journal of Psychosomatic Research, 77*(1), 57–63.

Government of Canada. (2006). *The Human Face of Mental Health and Mental Illness in Canada, 2006.* Minister of Public Works and Government Services Canada. Catalogue no.: HP5-19/2006E.

Greenberg, T., Carlson, J. M., Cha, J., Hajcak, G., & Mujica-Parodi, L. (2012). Ventromedial prefrontal cortex reactivity is altered in generalized anxiety disorder during fear generalization. *Depression and Anxiety, 30*(3), 242–250.

Gressier, F., Calati, R., & Serretti, A. (2016). 5-HTTLPR and gender differences in affective disorders: A systematic review. *Journal of Affective Disorders, 190*, 193–207.

Haller, H., Cramer, H., Lauche, R., Gass, F., & Dobos, G.J. (2014). The prevalence and burden of subthreshold generalized anxiety disorder: A systematic review. *BMC Psychiatry, 14*, 128.

Hamilton, M. (1959). The assessment of anxiety states by rating. *British Journal of Medical Psychology, 32*, 54.

Hofmann, S. G., Asnaani, M. A. A., & Hinton, D. E. (2010). Cultural aspects in social anxiety and social anxiety disorder. *Depression and Anxiety, 27*(12), 1117–1127.

Hofmeijer-Sevink, M., van Oppen, P., van Megen, H. J., Batelaan, N. M., Cath, D. C., … van Balkom, A. J. (2013). Clinical relevance of comorbidity in obsessive compulsive disorder: The Netherlands OCD Association study. *Journal of Affective Disorders, 150*(3), 847–854.

Hoge, E. A., Bui, E., Goetter, E., Robinaugh, D. J., Ojserkis, R. A., Fresco, D. M., & Simon, N. M. (2015). Change in decentering mediates improvement in anxiety in mindfulness-based stress reduction for Generalized Anxiety Disorder. *Cognitive Therapy and Research, 39*, 228–235.

Hovens, J. G. F. M., Giltay, E. J., Spinhoven, P., van Hemert, A. M., & Penninx, B. W. J. H. (2015). Impact of childhood life events and childhood trauma on the onset and recurrence of depressive and anxiety disorders. *Journal of Clinical Psychiatry, 76*(7), 931–938.

Huhn, M., Tardy, M., Spineli, L. M., Kissling, W., Förstl, H., Pitschel-Walz, G., … Leucht, S. (2014). Efficacy of pharmacotherapy and psychotherapy for adult psychiatric disorders: A systematic overview of meta-analyses. *JAMA Psychiatry, 71*(6), 706–715.

Hunsley, J., Elliott, K., & Therrien, Z. (2013). *The efficacy and effectiveness of psychological treatments.* Retrieved from the Canadian Psychologist Association website: http://cpa.ca/thecpastore/purchasecpapublications TheEfficacyAndEffectivenessofPsychologicalTreatments_web.pdf

Inoue, K., Kaiya, H., Hara, N., & Okazaki, Y. (2016). A discussion of various aspects of panic disorder depending on presence or absence of agoraphobia. *Comprehensive Psychiatry, 69*, 132–135.

Jakubovski, E., Diniz, J. B., Valerio, C., Fossaluza, V., Belotto-Silva, C., Gorenstein, C., … Miguel, E. (2013). Clinical predictors of long-term outcome in obsessive-compulsive disorder. *Depression and Anxiety, 30*(8), 763–772.

Kanwar, A., Malik, S., Prokop, L. J., Sim, L. A., Feldstein, D., Wang, Z., & Murad, M. H. (2013). The association between anxiety disorders and suicidal behaviors: A systematic review and meta-analysis. *Depression and Anxiety, 30*, 917–929.

Katzman, M. A., Bleau, P., Blier, P., Chokka, P., Kjernisted, K., & Van Ameringen, M. (2014). Canadian clinical practice guidelines for the management of anxiety, posttraumatic stress and obsessive-compulsive disorders. *BMC Psychiatry, 14*(Suppl. 1), S1.

Kawashima, C., Tanaka, Y., Inoue, A., Nakanishi, M., Okamoto, K., Maruyama, Y., … Akiyoshi, J. (2016). Hyperfunction of left lateral prefrontal cortex and automatic thoughts in social anxiety disorder: A near-infrared spectroscopy study. *Journal of Affective Disorders, 206*, 256–260.

Kessler, R. C., Chiu, W. T., Demler, O., Merikangas, K. R., & Walters, E. E. (2005). Prevalence, severity, and comorbidity of 12-month DSM-IV disorders in the National Comorbidity Survey Replication. *Archives of General Psychiatry, 62*(6), 617–627.

Kessler, R. C., Chiu, W. T., Jin, R., Ruscio, A. M., Shear, K., & Walters, E. E. (2006). The epidemiology of panic attacks, panic disorder, and agoraphobia in the National Comorbidity Survey Replication. *Archives of General Psychiatry, 63*(4), 415–424.

Kessler, R. C., Petukhova, M., Sampson, N. A., Zaslavsky, A. M., & Wittchen, H. U. (2012). Twelve-month and lifetime prevalence and lifetime morbid risk of anxiety and mood disorders in the United States. *International Journal of Methods in Psychiatric Research, 21*(3), 169–184.

Khouzam, H. R. (2009). Anxiety disorders: Guidelines for effective primary care, part 2, treatment. *Consultant, 49*(4), 1–2.

Kim, C. H., Chang, J. W., Koo, M. S., Kim, J. W., Suh, H. S., Park, I. H., & Lee, H. S. (2003). Anterior cingulotomy for refractory obsessive-compulsive disorder. *Acta Psychiatrica Scandinavica, 107*(4), 241–243.

Kinley, D. J., Walker, J. R., Enns, M. W., & Sareen, J. (2011). Panic attacks as a risk for later psychopathology: Results from a nationally representative survey. *Depression and Anxiety, 28*(5), 412–419.

Konishi, J., Asami, T., Hayano, F., Yoshimi, A., Hayasaka, S., Fukushima, H., … Hirayasu, Y. (2014). Multiple white matter volume reductions in patients with panic disorder: Relationships between orbitofrontal gyrus volume and symptom severity and social dysfunction. *PLoS One, 9*(3), e92862. doi:10.1371/journal.pone.0092862

Koslander, T., Barbosa da Silva, A., & Roxberg, A. (2009). Existential and spiritual needs in mental health care: An ethical and holistic perspective. *Journal of Holistic Nursing, 27*(1), 34–42.

Kress, V. E., Stargell, N. A., Zoldan, C. A., & Paylo, M. J. (2016). Hoarding disorder: Diagnosis, assessment and treatment. *Journal of Counseling & Development, 94*, 83–90.

Kumar, A., Sharma, M. P., Narayanaswamy, J. C., Kandavel, T., & Reddy, Y. C. J. (2016). Efficacy of mindfulness-integrated cognitive behavior therapy in patients with predominant obsessions. *Indian Journal of Psychiatry, 58*, 366–371.

Kumsta, R., & Heinrichs, M. (2013). Oxytocin, stress and social behavior: Neurogenetics of the human oxytocin system. *Current Opinion in Neurobiology, 23*(1), 11–16.

Lamers, F., van Oppen, P., Comijs, H. C., Smit, J. H., Spinhoven, P., Anton, J. L. M., … Penninx, B. W. J. H. (2011). Comorbidity patterns of anxiety and depressive disorders in a large cohort study: The Netherlands Study of Depression and Anxiety (NESDA). *Journal of Clinical Psychiatry, 72*(3), 341–348.

LeBeau, R. T., Glenn, D., Liao, B., Wittchen, H. U., Beesdo-Baum, K., Ollendick, T., & Craske, M. G. (2010). Specific phobia: A review of DSM-IV specific phobia and preliminary recommendations for DSM-V. *Depression and Anxiety, 27*(2), 148–167.

LeDoux, J. (2015). *Anxious: Using the brain to understand and treat fear and anxiety.* London, UK: Penguin Books.

Lochner, C., Fineberg, N. A., Zohar, J., Van Ameringen, M., Juven-Wetzler, A., Alfredo Carlo Altamura, A. C., … Stein, D. J. (2014). Comorbidity in obsessive–compulsive disorder (OCD): A report from the International College of Obsessive–Compulsive Spectrum Disorders (ICOCS). *Comprehensive psychiatry, 55*(7), 1513–1519.

Lovick, T. A. (2014). Sex determinants of experimental panic attacks. *Neuroscience & Biobehavioural Reviews, 46*(3), 465–471.

Makovac, E., Meeten, F., Watson, D. R., Herman, A., Garfinkel, S. N., Critchley, H. D., & Ottaviana, C. (2016). Alterations in amygdala-prefrontal functional connectivity account for excessive worry and autonomic dysregulation in generalized anxiety disorder. *Biological Psychiatry*, 80(10), 786–795.

Mallorquí-Bagué, N., Bulbena, A., Pailhez, G., Garfinkel, S. N., & Critchley, H. D. (2016). Mind-body interactions in anxiety and somatic symptoms. *Harvard Review of Psychiatry*, 24(1), 53–60.

Marks, I. M., & Matthews, A. M. (1979). Brief standard self-rating for phobic patients. *Behaviour Research and Therapy*, 17, 263–267.

Mather, A. A., Stein, M. B., & Sareen, J. (2010). Social anxiety disorder and social fears in the Canadian military: Prevalence, comorbidity, impairment, and treatment-seeking. *Journal of Psychiatric Research*, 44(14), 887–893.

McEwen, B. (2005). Stressed or stressed out: What is the difference? *Journal of Psychiatry and Neuroscience*, 30, 315–318.

McHugh, R. K., Whitton, S. W., Peckham, A. D., Welge, J. A., & Otto, M. W. (2013). Patient preference for psychological vs pharmacologic treatment of psychiatric disorders: A meta-analytic review. *Journal of Clinical Psychiatry*, 74(6), 595–602.

McLean, C. P., Asnaani, A., Litz, B. T., & Hofmann, S. G. (2011). Gender differences in anxiety disorders: Prevalence, course of illness, comorbidity and burden of illness. *Journal of Psychiatric Research*, 48(8), 1027–1035.

Merikangas, K. R., He, J. P., Burstein, M., Swanson, S. A., Avenevoli, S., Cui, L., … Swendsen, J. (2010). Lifetime prevalence of mental disorders in U.S. adolescents: Results from the National Comorbidity Survey Replication—Adolescent Supplement (NCS-A). *Journal of the American Academy of Child and Adolescent Psychiatry*, 49(10), 980–989.

Merikangas, K. R., & Swanson, S. A. (2010). Comorbidity in anxiety disorders. In M. B. Stein & T. Steckler (Eds.), *Behavioral neurobiology of anxiety and its treatment* (Vol. 2, pp. 37–59). New York, NY: Springer.

Meyer, A., Hajcak, G., Torpey-Newman, D. C., Kujawa, A., & Klein, D. N. (2015). Enhanced error-related brain activity in children predicts the onset of anxiety disorders between the ages of 6 and 9. *Journal of Abnormal Psychology*, 124(2), 266–274.

Meyer, T., Miller, M., Metzger, R., & Borkovec, T. (1990). Development and validation of the Penn State Worry Questionnaire. *Behaviour Research and Therapy*, 28(6), 487–495.

Ming, Q. M., Zhang, Y., Yi, J., Wang, X., Zhu, X., & Yao, S. (2015). Serotonin transporter gene polymorphism (5-HTTLPR) L allele interacts with stress to increase anxiety symptoms in Chinese adolescents: A multi-wave longitudinal study. *BMC Psychiatry*, 15, 248.

Moffitt, T. E., Caspi, A., Harrington, H., Milne, B. J., Melchior, M., Goldberg, D., & Poulton, R. (2007). Generalized anxiety disorder and depression: Childhood risk factors in a birth cohort followed to age 32. *Psychological Medicine*, 37, 441–452.

Moffitt, T. E., Caspi, A., Taylor, A., Kokaua, J., Milne, B. J., Polanczyk, G., & Poulton, R. (2010). How common are common mental disorders? Evidence that lifetime prevalence rates are doubled by prospective versus retrospective ascertainment. *Psychological Medicine*, 40, 899–909.

Mundo, E., Richter, M., Sam, F., Macciardi, F., & Kennedy, J. (2000). Is the 5-HT (1D beta) receptor gene implicated in the pathogenesis of obsessive-compulsive disorder? *American Journal of Psychiatry*, 157(7), 1160–1161.

Munro, M. L., Brown, S. L., Pournajafi-Nazarloo, H., Carter, C. S., Lopez, W. D., & Seng, J. S. (2013). In search of an adult attachment stress provocation to measure effect on the oxytocin system: A pilot validation study. *Journal of the American Psychiatric Nurses Association*, 19(4), 180–191.

Muntingh, A. D. T., van der Feltz-Cornelis, M., van Marwijk, H. W. J., Spinhoven, P., & van Balkom, A. J. L. M. (2016). Collaborative care for anxiety disorders in primary care: A systematic review. *BMC Family Practice*, 17, 62. doi:10.1186/s12875-016-0466-3

Nail, J. E., Christofferson, J., Ginsburg, G. S., Drake, D., Kendall, P. C., McCracken, J. T., … Sakolsky, D. (2015). Academic impairment and impact of treatments among youth with anxiety disorders. *Child & Youth Care Forum*, 44, 327–342.

Nebel-Schwalm, M., & Davis, T. E. (2013). Nature and etiological models of anxiety disorders. In E. Storch & D. McKay (Eds.), *Handbook of treating variants and complications in anxiety disorders* (pp. 3–21). New York, NY: Springer.

Nuss, P. (2015). Anxiety disorders and GABA neurotransmission: A disturbance of modulation. *Neuropsychiatric Disease and Treatment*, 11, 165–175.

Offidani, E., Guidi, J., Tomba, E., & Fava, G. A. (2013). Efficacy and tolerability of benzodiazepines versus antidepressants in anxiety disorders: A systematic review and meta-analysis. *Psychotherapy and Psychosomatics*, 82(6), 355–362.

Offord, D. R., Boyle, M. H., Campbell, D., Goering, P., Lin, E., Wong, M., & Racine, Y. A. (1996). One-year prevalence of psychiatric disorder in Ontarians 15 to 64 years of age. *Canadian Journal of Psychiatry*, 41(9), 559–563.

Peplau, H. (1989). Theoretic constructs: Anxiety, self, and hallucinations. In A. O'Toole & S. Welt (Eds.), *Interpersonal theory in nursing practice: Selected works of Hildegard E. Peplau*. New York, NY: Springer.

Peris, T. S., Sugar, C. A., Bergman, R. L., Chang, S., Langley, A., & Piacentini, J. (2012). Family factors predict treatment outcome for pediatric obsessive-compulsive disorder. *Journal of Consulting and Clinical Psychology*, 80(2), 255–263.

Perry, B. D. (2008). Child maltreatment: A neurodevelopmental perspective on the role of trauma and neglect in psychopathology. In T. P. Beauchaine & S. P. Hinshaw (Eds.), *Child and adolescent psychopathology* (pp. 93–128). Hoboken, NJ: John Wiley & Sons.

Perusini, J. N., & Fanselow, M. S. (2015). Neurobehavioural perspectives on the distinction between fear and anxiety. *Learning & Memory*, 22, 417–425.

Poppe, C., Müller, S. T., Greil, W., Walder, A., Grohmann, R., & Stübner, S. (2016). Pharmacotherapy for obsessive compulsive disorder in clinical practice—Data of 842 inpatients from the International AMSP Project between 1994 and 2012. *Journal of Affective Disorders*, 200, 89–96.

Porges, S. W. (2007). The Polyvagal perspective. *Biological Psychology*, 74(2), 116–143. doi.org/10.1016/j.biopsycho.2006.06.009

Public Health Agency of Canada. (2016). Report from the Canadian chronic disease surveillance system: Mood and anxiety disorders in Canada, 2016. Retrieved from http://healthycanadians.gc.ca/publications/diseases-conditions-maladies-affections/mood-anxiety-disorders-2016-troubles-anxieux-humeur/alt/mood-anxiety-disorders-2016-troubles-anxieux-humeur-eng.pdf

Rachman, S., & Hodgson, R. (1980). *Obsessions and compulsions*. New York, NY: Prentice-Hall.

Reiss, S., Peterson, R. A., & Gursky, D. M. (1986). Anxiety sensitivity, anxiety frequency, and the prediction of fearfulness. *Behaviour Research and Therapy*, 24, 1–8.

Rovira, J., Albarracin, G., Salvador, L., Rejas, J., Sánchez-Iriso, E., & Cabasés, J. M. (2012). The cost of generalized anxiety disorder in primary care settings: Results of the ANCORA study. *Community Mental Health Journal*, 48(3), 372–383.

Ruland, T., Domschke, K., Schütte, V., Zavorotnyy, M., Kugel, H., Notzon, S., … Zwanzger, P. (2015). Neuropeptide S receptor gene variation modulates glutamatergic anterior cingulate cortex activity during CCK-4 induced panic. *Pharmacopsychiatry*, 25(10), 1677–1682.

Ruscio, A. M., Stein, D. J., Chiu, W. T., & Kessler, R. C. (2010). The epidemiology of obsessive-compulsive disorder in the National Comorbidity Survey Replication. *Molecular Psychiatry*, 15(1), 53–63.

Sadock, B. J., Sadock, V. A., & Ruiz, P. (2015). *Kaplan & Sadock's synopsis of psychiatry: Behavioral sciences/clinical psychiatry* (11th ed.). Philadelphia, PA: Wolters Kluwer.

Sallee, F., Sethuraman, G., Sine, L., & Liu, H. (2000). Yohimbine challenge in children with anxiety disorders. *American Journal of Psychiatry*, 157, 1236–1242.

Sánchez-Navarro, J. P., Driscoll, D., Anderson, S. W., Tranel, D., Bechara, A., & Buchanan, T. W. (2014). Alterations of attention and emotional processing following childhood-onset damage to the prefrontal cortex. *Behavioral Neuroscience*, 128(1), 1–11.

Schiele, M. A., Ziegler, C., Schartner, C., Romanos, M., Pauli, P., Zwanzger, P., … Domschke, K. (2016). Interaction of serotonin transporter gene (5-HTT) variation, childhood maltreatment and general self-efficacy on anxiety traits—Adding a dimension? *European Neuropsychopharmacology*, 26, (Suppl. 2), S164.

Schore, A. N. (2001). Minds in the making: Attachment, the self-organizing brain, and developmentally-oriented psychoanalytic psychotherapy. *British Journal of Psychotherapy*, 17(3), 299–328.

Schore, A. N. (2014). The right brain is dominant in psychotherapy. *Psychotherapy*, 51(3), 388–397. doi.org/10.1037/a0037083

Schwartz, J. M. (1996/2016). *Brain lock*. New York, NY: Harper Collins.

Scupi, B. S., Maser, J. D., & Uhde, T. W. (1992). The National Institute of Mental Health Panic Questionnaire: An instrument for assessing clinical characteristics of panic disorder. *Journal of Nervous and Mental Disease*, 180, 566–572.

Selye, H. (1956). *The stress of life*. New York, NY: McGraw-Hill.

Shimada-Sugimoto, M., Otowa, T., & Hettema, J. M. (2015). Genetics of anxiety disorders: Genetic epidemiological and molecular studies in humans. *Psychiatry and Clinical Neurosciences*, 69(7), 388–401.

Skapinakis, P., Caldwell, D., Hollingworth, W., Bryden, P., Fineberg, N., Salkovskis, P., … Lewis, G. (2016). A systematic review of the clinical effectiveness and cost-effectiveness of pharmacological and psychological interventions for the management of obsessive-compulsive disorder in children/adolescents and adults. *Health Technology Assessment Monograph*, 20(43), 1–392.

Sladky, R., Höflich, A., Küblböck, M., Kraus, C., Baldinger, P., Moser, E., ... Windischberger, C. (2015). Disrupted effective connectivity between the amygdala and orbitofrontal cortex in social anxiety disorder during emotion discrimination revealed by dynamic causal modeling for fMRI. *Cerebral Cortex, 25*(4), 895–903.

Spielberger, C. D., Gorsuch, R. L., & Luchene, R. E. (1976). *Manual for the State-Trait Anxiety Inventory.* Palo Alto, CA: Consulting Psychologists Press.

Spitzer, R. L., Kroenke, K., Williams, J. B. W., & Löwe, B. (2006). A brief measure for assessing generalized anxiety disorder: The GAD-7. *Archives of Internal Medicine, 166,* 1092–1097.

Statistics Canada. (2013). Canadian community health survey: Mental health, 2012. Retrieved from http://www.statcan.gc.ca/daily-quotidien/130918/dq130918a-eng.pdf

Steimer, T. (2002). The biology of fear- and anxiety-related behaviors. *Dialogues in Clinical Neuroscience, 4*(3), 231–249.

Steketee, G., Kelley, A. A., Wernick, J. A., Muroff, J., Frost, R. O., & Tolin, D. F. (2015). Family patterns of hording symptoms. *Depression and Anxiety, 32,* 728–736.

Stengler, K., Olbrich, S., Heider, D., Dietrich, S., Riedel-Heller, S., & Jahn, I. (2013). Mental health treatment seeking among patients with OCD: Impact of age of onset. *Social Psychiatry and Psychiatric Epidemiology, 48*(5), 813–819.

Strauss, C., Hale, L., & Stobie, B. (2015). A meta-analytic review of the relationship between family accommodation and OCD symptom severity. *Journal of Anxiety Disorders, 33,* 95–102.

Subramaniam, M., Abdin, E., Vaingankar, J. A., & Chong, S. A. (2012). Obsessive-compulsive disorder: Prevalence, correlates, help-seeking and quality of life in a multiracial Asian population. *Social Psychiatry and Psychiatric Epidemiology, 47*(12), 2035–2043.

Sylvers, P., Lilienfeld, S. O., & LaPrairie, J. L. (2011). Differences between trait fear and trait anxiety: Implications for psychopathology. *Clinical Psychology Review, 31,* 122–137.

Tibi, L., van Oppen, P., Aderka, I. M., van Balkom, A. J. L. M., Batelaan, N. M., Spinhoven, P., ... Anholt, G. E. (2013). Examining determinants of early and late age at onset in panic disorder: An admixture analysis. *Journal of Psychiatric Research, 47*(12), 1870–1875.

Tillich, P. (1952). *The courage to be.* New Haven, CT: Yale University Press.

Tolin, D. F., Frost, R., & Steketee, G. (2010). A brief interview for assessing compulsive hoarding: The Hoarding Rating Scale—Interview. *Psychiatric Research, 178,* 147–152.

Trzaskowski, M., Zavos, H. M. S., Haworth, C. M. A., Plomin, R., & Eley, T. C. (2012). Stable genetic influence on anxiety-related behaviours across middle childhood. *Journal of Abnormal Child Psychology, 40*(1), 85–94.

van Strien, A. M., Koek, H. L., van Marum, R. J., & Emmelot-Vonk, M. H. (2013). Psychotropic medications, including short acting benzodiazepines, strongly increase the frequency of falls in elderly. *Maturitas, 74*(4), 357–362.

Weems, C., Costa, N., Dehon, C., & Berman, S. (2004). Paul Tillich's theory of existential anxiety: A preliminary conceptual and empirical examination. *Anxiety, Stress, and Coping, 17*(4), 383–399.

Willgoss, T. G., & Yohannes, A. M. (2013). Anxiety disorders in patients with COPD: A systematic review. *Respiratory Care, 58*(5), 858–866.

Wintermann, G.-B., Kirschbaum, C., & Petrowski, K. (2016). Predisposition or side effect of the duration: The reactivity of the HPA-axis under psychosocial stress in panic disorder. *International Journal of Psychophysiology, 107,* 9–15.

Wong, J., Gordon, E. A., & Heimberg, R. G. (2012). Social anxiety disorder. In P. Sturmey & M. Hersen (Eds.), *Handbook of evidence-based practice in clinical psychology (part II).* Hoboken, NJ: John Wiley & Sons.

Xiangfei, M., & D'Arcy, C. (2012). Common and unique risk factors and comorbidity for 12-month mood and anxiety disorders among Canadians. *Canadian Journal of Psychiatry, 57*(8), 479–487.

Xu, Y., Schneier, F., Heimberg, R. G., Princisvalle, K., Liebowitz, M. R., Wang, S., & Blanco, C. (2012). Gender differences in social anxiety disorder: Results from the national epidemiological sample on alcohol and related conditions. *Journal of Anxiety Disorders, 26*(1), 12–19.

24 Somatic Symptom and Related Disorders

Duncan Stewart MacLennan

LEARNING OBJECTIVES

After studying this chapter, you will be able to:

- Explain the concept of somatization and its presentation in people with mental health problems.
- Discuss epidemiologic factors related to somatic symptoms.
- Compare the etiologic theories of somatic symptom and related disorders from a bio/psycho/social/spiritual perspective.
- Contrast the major differences between somatic symptoms and factitious disorders.
- Discuss human responses to somatic symptom and related disorders.
- Apply the elements of nursing management to a patient with somatic symptom and related disorders.

KEY TERMS

- factitious disorder • malingering • pseudoneurologic symptoms • somatic symptom and related disorder

KEY CONCEPT

- somatization

The connection between the mind and the body has been described for centuries. **Somatic symptom and related disorders** describes conditions in which a psychological state contributes to the development of physical symptoms or illness. For example, "broken heart syndrome" or Takotsubo cardiomyopathy causes the heart to enlarge and pump poorly in response to very stressful situations (such as the death of a loved one). In contrast, the term somatization is used when unexplained physical symptoms occur in the presence of psychological distress or psychiatric illness. This chapter explores the concept of somatization and explains the care of patients experiencing somatic symptom disorders.

Although somatization occurs commonly in many psychiatric disorders, including depression, anxiety, and psychosis, it is the *primary* symptom of somatic symptom disorders. Somatic symptom and related disorders occur when a person experiences physical symptoms causing psychological distress or abnormal patterns of thought (American Psychiatric Association [APA], 2013). The prevalence of somatic symptoms and related disorders in general practice ranges from 10% to 23%, often occurring comorbidly with anxiety or depressive disorders (Hilderink, Collard, Rosmalen, & Oude Voshaar, 2013; Steinbrecher, Koerber, Frieser, & Hiller, 2011). A **factitious disorder** is one in which the patient simulates or inflicts injury on himself or herself or others in order

to receive medical treatment or for another secondary purpose. Unlike other somatic symptom disorders, the physical symptoms in a factitious disorder are deliberately produced by the patient.

Historically, people with "medically unexplained symptoms" were said to have a somatic symptom disorder. This diagnostic approach relied on the assumption that all other likely or possible diagnoses were fully explored *and* excluded. Practitioners were reluctant to diagnose somatic symptom or related disorders, in part, due to the impossible task of excluding other alternative diagnoses. This reluctance contributed to treatment delays.

In 2013, the American Psychiatric Association responded to the complexity contributing to the seemingly under-diagnoses of somatic symptom and related disorders by significantly revising earlier diagnostic criteria in the fifth edition of the Diagnostic and Statistical Manual of Mental Disorders (DSM-5). These newer criteria have been criticized primarily due to the shifted focus on treating patients' distress to a symptom (whether arising from a physical cause or not). These criteria are feared to inappropriately cause the mislabelling of many people with mental illness (Frances, 2013) by failing to clearly distinguish mental illness from normal variants in human expression (Wakefield, 2016; Wygant, Arbisi, Bianchini, & Umlauf, 2017). A case report, for instance, describes anterior cutaneous nerve entrapment syndrome (ACNES) being misdiagnosed as a somatic symptom disorder. The patient subsequently endured many months of chronic pain and developed depressive symptoms. After months of inappropriate psychotherapy for a misdiagnosed somatic symptom disorder, the patient underwent surgery to remove the source of the painful stimuli. The symptoms (including depression) subsequently disappeared (Arts, Buis, & de Jonge, 2016; Longstreth, 2016).

This chapter presents the nursing care of patients experiencing somatic symptoms and related disorders. Somatization is explained in detail because it is the core symptom of all somatic symptom and related disorders.

KEY CONCEPT

Somatization is the term used when unexplained physical symptoms are present that are related to psychological distress or psychiatric illness.

SOMATIZATION

Anyone who feels the pain of a sore throat or the ache of influenza has a somatic symptom (from *soma*, meaning body). Somatization, however, occurs when a person has disturbed ways of feeling, thinking, and behaving when experiencing a distressing somatic symptom. With the current understanding of somatization, the focus is on how an individual reacts to a somatic symptom rather than the previous focus on the lack of explanatory medical diagnosis. This change has the following impact: (1) fewer inappropriate mental illness diagnoses in people coping well with unexplained somatic symptoms, (2) increased diagnosis and treatment of somatic symptom and related disorders among those responding abnormally to a medically explained somatic symptom, and (3) a potential underdiagnosis of medically explained causes for a symptom. Clinicians must be cognizant that, at present, no perfect diagnostic tool exists to accurately diagnose somatic symptom or related disorders infallibly. Rather, clinicians must remain open to the possibility of a misdiagnosis and revise treatment options accordingly.

With somatization, individuals typically develop a preoccupation, amplify, and seek medical care for the somatic symptoms. People with somatization disorders often view their personal problems in physical rather than psychosocial terms. For example, a person quits her job due to being chronically tired instead of recognizing that she is emotionally distressed from a coworker's constant harassment.

SOMATIC SYMPTOM DISORDER

Somatic symptom disorder is a condition characterized by emotional distress and a disruption of daily living caused by one or more physical symptoms. Somatic

symptom disorders, especially those occurring over a long period of time expressed by many symptoms and co-occurring with depression or anxiety, contribute to significant disability (Kushwaha, Sinha, Chadda, & Mehta, 2014). Therefore, there remains an urgent need to properly identify and treat individuals with this disorder.

Clinical Course

In somatic symptom disorder, patients have one or more clinically significant somatic concerns that may involve several body systems. Physical symptoms in somatic symptom disorder occur in all body systems, such as gastrointestinal (nausea, vomiting, diarrhoea), neurologic (headache, backache), or musculoskeletal (aching legs). The physical symptom, which may be present all the time or may come and go, will typically last 6 months or longer. These individuals perceive themselves as being "sicker than sick" and report all aspects of their health as poor. They often cannot work or take part in routine activities of daily living. Since no medical explanation of the symptom can be identified, these individuals often become frustrated with primary health care providers. Consequently, they seek opinions from many health care providers until they find one who will give them new medication, hospitalize them, or perform surgery. People with somatic symptom disorder sometimes cause frustration among health care providers. Nurses need to recognize their feelings and deal with them in a constructive way. This may include discussing their feelings with the colleague who is their mentor or clinical supervisor.

Because a psychiatric diagnosis of somatic symptom disorder is made only after numerous unexplained physical problems, psychiatric and mental health nurses do not usually care for these individuals early in the disorder; rather, these patients are more likely to have been encountered initially by nurses in primary care and medical–surgical settings.

Diagnostic Criteria

The diagnosis is made when there is an *abnormal* response to a somatic symptom. It is important to remember that not all people experiencing an "unexplained symptom" have a somatic symptom disorder. Like many other disorders, a diagnosis may only be considered if the symptom is found to be interfering with the patient's quality of life, social interactions, or other areas of functioning (APA, 2013; Fava, Cosci, & Sonino, 2017). For the diagnostic criteria for somatic symptom disorders, see the DSM-5. Alternatively, the Diagnostic Criteria for Psychosomatic Research, initially published in 1995, are also commonly used in both research and practice (Cosci & Fava, 2016).

The Somatic Symptom Disorder—B Criteria Scale (SSD-12) is a newly developed tool, based on the diagnostic criteria outlined in the DSM-5 (Toussaint et al., 2016). The SSD-12 is one of the first tools being developed and validated using the newer "B criterion" of the DSM-5. The B criterion of the DSM 5 is used to diagnose severity of illness and may prove to be a useful tool for diagnosing and monitoring somatic symptom disorder (Barsky, 2016).

Somatic Symptom Disorder in Special Populations

Evidence suggests that this disorder occurs in all populations and cultures. However, the type and frequency of somatic symptoms may differ across cultures.

Children

Although many children experience unexplained symptoms, somatic symptom disorder is not usually diagnosed until adolescence. While some degree of somatization may be a normal element of childhood development and coping, early detection and treatment may impact longer-term outcomes by decreasing functional disability and health care utilization later in life (Tierney & Walker-Harding, 2017). Children at increased risk for somatic symptom disorder use fewer and less effective coping strategies. Further, children who are insecure, internalize their emotions, or tend toward perfectionism experience somatic symptom disorder more frequently (Malas, Ortiz-Aguayo, Giles, & Ibeziako, 2017). Peer relationships seem to influence the development of somatic complaints among youth. Increased somatization occurs among youth who received greater punitive responses to emotional disclosures by peers (Parr, Zeman, Braunstein, & Price, 2016). Therefore, decreasing bullying behaviour among youth may decrease present and future somatic symptom disorder impairments.

Older Adults

Somatic symptom disorder occurs in the older adult but less prevalently than in other age groups (Hilderink et al., 2013). New onset of somatic symptoms in later life warrants a thorough investigation for hidden medical or psychiatric disorders. Subjective lack of well-being (never feeling good), rather than objective health measures, may be an indicator of somatization (Schneider et al., 2003). In the older adult, somatic symptoms can represent many things, such as depression or bereavement.

Epidemiology

Somatic symptom disorder occurs more prevalently among individuals less than 65 years (10% to 21%) when compared to older adults (1.5% to 13%) (Hilderink et al., 2013). This difference may reflect a biased approach to attribute somatic complaints by older patients to mere aging.

Gender, Ethnic, and Cultural Differences

It was initially thought that females experienced somatic symptom disorder more frequently than did males; however, Karkhanis and Winsler (2016) demonstrated no significant gender differences. Validating and responding to emotional expressions (e.g., anger, sadness), especially among children, provide for a better understanding of the emotional reaction and seemingly provide a space to help the individual develop more effective coping mechanisms to overcome emotional distress.

Norms, values, perceptions, and expectations about illness and wellness are culturally based. In cultures in which great stigma toward mental illness exists, the expression of psychological distress can occur through physical symptoms. In Iranian culture, for instance, somatization (primarily pain) is a central feature of clinical depression (Firoozabadi, Bahredar, & Seifsafari, 2013). Cultural differences also influence how nurses recognize and manage somatization. Despite cultural and ethnic differences, the comorbidity of depression and somatic symptoms is consistent around the world (APA, 2013). In many areas, however, sets of somatic symptoms hold cultural meaning to describe feelings of distress. For instance, "burning in the head" can be an idiom for "burnout" (Kirmayer & Sartorius, 2007). Refugees, however, do exhibit more somatic symptoms than the general population (Rohlof, Knipscheer, & Kleber, 2014). Given the current rise in refugees fleeing war and terrorism around the world, identifying and addressing somatic symptoms among the refugee population is increasingly relevant.

Comorbidity

Somatic symptom disorder frequently coexists with other psychiatric disorders, most commonly depression and anxiety. Somatic symptom disorder may also become more pronounced when coupled with existing impairment from other medical conditions (Kohlmann, Gierk, Hilbert, Brähler, & Löwe, 2016). A disproportionately high number of people who eventually receive diagnoses of somatic symptom disorder have been treated for irritable bowel syndrome, polycystic ovary disease, fibromyalgia, and other functional somatic syndromes (Warren, Langenberg, & Clauw, 2013). Many of these patients have had prior investigations or treatments associated with a functional somatic syndrome. For instance, women with chronic pelvic pain have undergone hysterectomies, while those with irritable bowel syndrome have experienced many invasive diagnostic tests such as endoscopy/colonoscopy.

Aetiology

The cause of somatic symptom disorder is unknown. The following are theories regarding the development of the disorder.

Biologic Theories

Neuropathologic Theory

The neuropathology of somatic symptom disorder is unknown. Evidence suggests decreased activity in certain brain areas, such as the caudate nuclei, left putamen, and right precentral gyrus (Garcia-Campayo, Sanz-Carrillo,

Baringo, & Ceballos, 2001; Hakala et al., 2002). These findings indicate that hypometabolism may be associated with somatization.

Genetic

Although somatization disorder has been shown to run in families, the exact transmission mechanism is unclear. Because many women with somatization disorder live in chaotic families, environmental influence could explain the high prevalence in first-degree relatives.

There is research that suggests that genetic variability within the serotoninergic and hypothalamic–pituitary–adrenal axis (HPA) may contribute to somatization (Holliday et al., 2010). This has led to early drug trials using serotonergic agents to evaluate for clinical effect in treating somatic symptom disorders. While these agents may improve symptoms of depressive and anxiety disorders, they have not demonstrated significant efficacy in reducing somatic disorder symptoms (Holster, Hawks, & Ostermeyer, 2017).

Biochemical Changes

Research thus far is insufficient to identify specific biochemical changes that would lead to somatization disorder. However, because these patients experience other psychiatric symptoms, such as depression or panic, clearly many neurobiologic changes occur. The HPA axis is currently being studied for potential links between proinflammatory cytokines and somatization (Rief, Hennings, Riemer, & Euteneuer, 2010). As an update, suppression of the HPA axis has been found to increase gastrointestinal symptoms in major depression (Karling, Wikgren, Adolfsson, & Norrback, 2016). A clearer link between HPA axis and expression of somatic symptoms seems to be emerging.

Psychological Theories

Somatization has been explained as a form of social or emotional communication, meaning the bodily symptoms express an emotion that cannot be verbalized. The adolescent who experiences severe abdominal pain after her parents' argument or the wife who receives nurturing from her husband only when she has back pain are two examples of how the body expresses emotions. From this perspective, somatization may be a way of maintaining relationships. With time, physical symptoms develop automatically in response to perceived threats. Finally, somatic symptom disorder develops when somatizing begins to interfere with daily life or pervades thought. Research is indicating that lack of social support, perceived violence within the community, and external stressors can contribute to somatization (Hart, Hodgkinson, Belcher, Hyman, & Cooley-Strickland, 2013; Karkhanis & Winsler, 2016).

Social Theories

While somatic symptom disorder occurs everywhere, the symptoms may vary between cultures. The

BOX 24.1 Somatization in Chinese Culture

In Chinese tradition, the health of the individual reflects a balance between positive and negative forces within the body: five elements at work in nature and in the body control conditions (fire, water, wood, earth, metal); five viscera (liver, heart, spleen, kidneys, lungs); five emotions (anger, joy, worry, sorrow, fear); and five climatic conditions (wind, heat, humidity, dryness, cold). All illness is explained by imbalances among these elements. Because emotion is related to the circulation of vital air within the body, anger is believed to result from an adverse current of vital air to the liver. Emotional outbursts are seen as results of imbalances among the natural elements, rather than results of the person's behaviour.

The stigma of mental illness in the Chinese culture is so great that it can have an adverse effect on a family for many generations. If problems can be attributed to natural causes, the individual and family are less responsible, and stigma is minimized. Rather, a more culturally acceptable term for symptoms of mental distress—the closest translation of which would be *neuraesthenia*—comprises somatic complaints of headaches, insomnia, dizziness, aches and pains, poor memory, anxiety, weakness, and loss of energy.

conceptualization of somatic symptom disorder is primarily a product of Western culture. In non-Western societies, where the mind–body distinction is not made and symptoms have different meanings and explanations, these physical manifestations are not labelled as a psychiatric disorder (Box 24.1). For example, within Chinese culture as well as in some Latin American countries, depression is more likely described with somatic symptoms, such as headaches, gastrointestinal disturbances, or complaints of "nerves," rather than with the sadness or guilt associated with major depression (Jorge, 2003; Yick, Shibusawa, & Agbayani-Siewert, 2003).

Risk Factors

Somatic symptom disorder tends to "run in families," and children of mothers with multiple unexplained somatic complaints are themselves more likely to have somatic problems. Substance use and depressive and anxiety disorders seem to be risk factors, and women with somatic symptom disorder appear more likely to have been sexually abused as children than do those with other psychiatric conditions, such as mood disorders (Steine et al., 2017). Individuals with depression are especially likely to experience somatization (Silverstein et al., 2013).

Interdisciplinary Treatment

The care of patients with somatic symptom disorder involves three approaches:

- Providing long-term general management of the chronic condition
- Conservatively treating symptoms of comorbid psychiatric and physical problems
- Providing care in special settings, including group treatment

The cornerstone of management is trust. Ideally, the patient sees only one health care provider at regularly scheduled visits. During each primary care visit, the provider should conduct a partial physical examination of the organ system in which the patient has complaints. Physical symptoms are to be treated conservatively using the least intrusive approach. In the mental health setting, the use of cognitive–behaviour therapy (CBT; see Chapter 13) has produced significant clinical benefits beyond other current treatment methods such as antidepressants or supportive psychotherapy (Williams & Gorfinkle, 2016). In a review of 31 clinical trials, patients treated with CBT showed more improvement than control subjects did in 71% of the studies. Benefits were observed irrespective of the amelioration of psychological distress (Kroenke & Swindle, 2000). Increasingly, exposure-based CBT via the Internet has demonstrated

effect in treating somatic symptom disorders (Hedman, Axelsson, Andersson, Lekander, & Ljótsson, 2016).

Nursing Management: Human Response to Disorder

Somatization is the primary response to this disorder. The defining characteristics, depicted in the bio/psycho/social/spiritual model (Fig. 24.1), are so well integrated that separating the psychological and social dimensions is difficult. The most common characteristics include the following:

- Reporting the same symptoms repeatedly
- Receiving support from the environment that otherwise might not be forthcoming (e.g., gaining a spouse's attention because of severe back pain)
- Expressing concern about the physical problems inconsistent with the severity of the illness

Biologic Domain

During the assessment interview, allow enough time for the patient to explain all medical problems; a hurried assessment interview blocks communication.

Assessment

Past medical treatment may have been ineffective because it did not address the underlying psychiatric disorder. However, nurses typically see these patients for coexistent

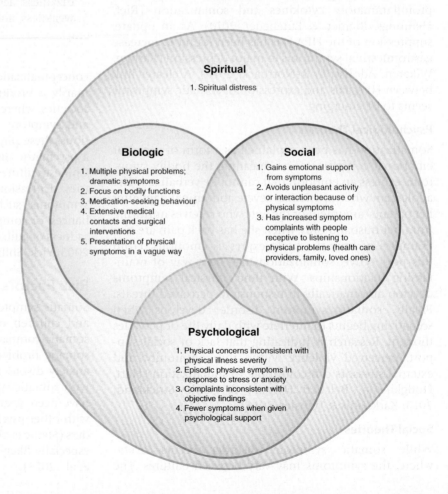

Figure 24.1. Bio/psycho/social/spiritual characteristics of patients with somatic symptom disorder.

problems related to the psychiatric disorder, such as depression, rather than for the somatic symptom disorder itself. While taking the patient's history, the nurse will discover that the individual has had medical problems or multiple surgeries and realize that somatic symptom disorder is a strong possibility. If the patient has not already received a diagnosis of somatic symptom disorder, the nurse should screen for it by determining the presence of the most commonly reported problems associated with this disorder, which include dysmenorrhoea, lump in throat, vomiting, shortness of breath, burning in sex organs, painful extremities, and amnesia. If the patient has these symptoms, he or she should be seen by a mental health provider qualified to make the diagnosis.

Review of Systems

Although these patients' symptoms have usually received considerable attention from the medical community, a careful review of systems is important to ensure that nothing is overlooked. Even as the nurse continues to see the patient for mental health reasons, an ongoing awareness of biologic symptoms is important, particularly because these symptoms are de-emphasized in the overall management.

Pain is the most common problem in people with this disorder. Because it is usually related to symptoms of all the major body systems, it is unlikely that a somatic intervention such as an analgesic will be effective on a long-term basis. The nurse must remember that although there is potentially no medical explanation for the pain, the patient's pain is real and has serious psychosocial implications. A careful assessment should include the following questions:

- What is the pain like?
- What is the extent of the pain?
- When is the pain at its best? Worst?
- What has worked in the past to relieve the pain?

Physical Functioning

The actual physical functioning of these individuals is often limited. They usually have problems with sleep, fatigue, activity, and sexual functioning. Assessment of these areas will generate data to be used in establishing nursing diagnoses. The amount and quality of sleep are important, as are the times when the individual sleeps. For example, an individual may sleep a total of 6 hours each diurnal cycle, but only from 2 to 6 AM, plus a 2-hour afternoon nap.

Fatigue is a constant problem, and a variety of physical problems, such as pain, interferes with normal activity. These patients report overwhelming lack of energy, which makes maintaining usual routines or accomplishing daily tasks difficult. Fatigue is accompanied by the inability to concentrate on simple functions, leading to decreased performance and disinterest in social activities. Patients tend to be apathetic and often have little energy (see Clinical Vignette, Box 24.2).

 BOX 24.2 CLINICAL VIGNETTE

SOMATIC SYMPTOM DISORDER AND STRESS

Ms. J, age 42 years, has been coming to the mental health clinic for 2 years for her "nerves." She has only seen her primary health care provider for prescription medication. She has been referred to the nurse's new "Stress Management Group" because she is experiencing side effects of all the medications that have been tried. The psychiatrist has diagnosed somatic symptom disorder and wants her to learn to manage her "nerves" without medication.

At the first meeting with the nurse, Ms. J was preoccupied with chest pain and bloating that had been ongoing for the past 6 months. Her chest pain is constant and sharp at times. The pain does not prevent her from going to her job as a waitress but does interfere with meal preparation at night for her family and her ability to have sexual intercourse. She has numerous other physical problems, including allergies to certain perfumes, dysmenorrhoea, ovarian polycystic disease (ovarian cysts), chronic urinary tract infections, and rashes. She is constantly fatigued and has frequent leg cramps. She states that she is too tired to prepare dinner for her family. On days off from work, she takes a nap in the afternoon, sleeping until evening. She is unable to fall asleep at night.

She believes that she will soon have to have her gallbladder removed because of occasional referred pain to her back and nausea that occurs a couple hours after eating. She is not enthusiastic about a stress management group and does not believe that it will help her problems; however, she has agreed to consider it, while insisting that the psychiatrist continue prescribing diazepam (Valium).

What Do You Think?

- How would you prioritize Ms. J's physical symptoms?
- What strategies would you use in the group to help Ms. J explore the roots of her stress and fatigue?

Female patients with this disorder usually have had multiple gynaecologic problems. The reason is not known, but symptoms of dysmenorrhoea, painful intercourse, and pain in the sex organs suggest involvement of the hypothalamic–pituitary–gonadal axis. Physiologic indicators, such as those produced by laboratory tests, are not available. However, a careful assessment of the patient's menstrual history, gynaecologic problems, and sexual functioning is important. The physical manifestations of somatic symptom disorder often lead to altered sexual behaviour.

Pharmacologic Assessment

A psychopharmacologic assessment of these patients is challenging. Patients with somatic symptom disorder frequently see many different health care providers, perhaps seeing seven or eight different providers within a year. Because they often receive medications from each provider, they are usually taking a large number of drugs. They tend to protect their sources and may not truthfully identify the actual number of medications they are ingesting. A thorough pharmacologic best possible medication history (BPMH) and assessment of all current home medications, herbal supplements, over-the-counter vitamins, and medications is needed not only because of the number of medications but also because these individuals frequently may have multiple drug–drug interactions and unusual side effects. Moreover, because of their somatic sensitivity, they often report side effects to many medications.

Patients with somatic symptom disorder spend much of their life trying to find out what is wrong with them. When one provider after another finds little or no explanation for their symptoms, they may become anxious. To alleviate their anxiety, they either self-medicate with over-the-counter medications and substances of abuse (e.g., alcohol, marijuana) or find a provider who prescribes an anxiolytic. Because the anxiety of their disorder cannot be treated within a few weeks with an anxiolytic agent, they may become dependent on medication that should not have been prescribed in the first place.

Although anxiolytics have a place in therapeutics, some are addictive and therefore not recommended for long-term use. They also tend to complicate the treatment of somatic symptom disorders. Unfortunately, by the time a patient with a somatic symptom disorder sees a mental health provider, he or she has often already begun taking one or more benzodiazepine agents. Often, the reason a patient agrees to see a mental health provider is that the primary health provider has refused to continue prescribing an anxiolytic until the patient has undergone psychiatric evaluation.

Nursing Diagnoses for the Biologic Domain

Because somatic symptom disorder is a chronic illness, a patient could receive almost any one of the nursing diagnoses at some point in life. At least one nursing diagnosis likely will be related to the individual's physical state. Fatigue, pain, and disturbed sleep patterns are usually supported by the assessment data. The challenge in devising outcomes for these problems is to avoid focusing on the biologic aspects and instead help the patient overcome the fatigue, pain, or sleep problem through bio/psycho/social/spiritual approaches.

Interventions for the Biologic Domain

Nursing interventions that focus on the biologic dimension become especially important because medical treatment must be conservative, and aggressive pharmacologic treatment must be avoided. Each time a nurse sees the patient, time spent on the physical complaints should be limited. The goal is to help the person better understand the meaning behind the physical manifestations of the somatic symptom disorder. Several biologic interventions, including pain management, activity enhancement, nutrition regulation, relaxation, and pharmacologic interventions, may also be useful in caring for patients with somatic symptom disorder.

Pain Management

Pain is a primary issue, but a single approach to its management rarely works. After a careful pain assessment, the nurse should encourage nonpharmacologic management strategies (see Caudill-Slosberg, 2002). If gastrointestinal pain is frequent, for example, eating and bowel habits should be explored and modified where possible. For back pain, exercises and consultation from a physical therapist may be useful. And while headaches are particularly challenging, self-monitoring and tracking them engage the patient in the therapeutic process and help to identify psychosocial triggers.

Activity Enhancement

Helping the patient establish a daily activity routine, especially during times when the patient does not work, may alleviate some of the difficulty with sleeping. Encouraging good sleep hygiene with established patterns and times for sleeping and waking is especially helpful. Although patients typically use various reasons to avoid activity, regular exercise is important to improve the overall physical state. The nurse needs to work with the patient to foster adequate movement for healthier living.

Nutrition Regulation

Patients with somatic symptom disorder often have gastrointestinal problems including special nutritional needs. The nurse should discuss with the patient the nutritional value of foods. Because these individuals often take medications that lead to weight gain, weight control strategies may be discussed (see Chapter 11). Overweight individuals should be given suggestions for healthy, low-calorie foods. Patients should be taught about balancing dietary intake with activity levels to increase their awareness of food choices.

Relaxation

Patients taking anxiolytic medication for stress reduction can also be taught relaxation techniques. The challenge is to help a patient develop strategies for routine practice and evaluation of effect. The nurse may consider a variety of techniques, including simple relaxation techniques, distraction, and guided imagery (see Chapter 11).

Psychopharmacologic Interventions

No particular medication is recommended for somatic symptom disorder. However, psychiatric symptoms of comorbid disorders, such as depression and anxiety, may be treated pharmacologically as appropriate. Patients with this disorder often suffer from depression and anxiety. While depressed mood itself is not an indication to initiate antidepressant treatment, when a depressive disorder is present, aggressive psychopharmacologic management is indicated. A wide variety of drugs are available, including the selective serotonin reuptake inhibitors (SSRIs), tricyclic antidepressants (TCAs), and monoamine oxidase inhibitors (MAOIs; see Chapters 12 and 22). Patients with somatic symptom disorder usually take several different antidepressants throughout the course of the disorder. Evidence should be sought that the depressive symptoms are cleared before discontinuing use of the medication.

Amitriptyline is one of the TCAs found effective in treating not just depression (see Chapters 12 and 22) but also the chronic pain and headaches common in people with somatic symptom disorder. Increasingly, drugs such as tramadol (an analgesic agent) are being used to treat comorbid pain syndromes. Both drugs have an effect on the serotonin, and caution is required to prevent the development of serotonin syndrome.

Anxiety associated with a somatic symptom disorder is more difficult than is depression to treat pharmacologically. Nonpharmacologic approaches such as biofeedback or relaxation are preferred. Benzodiazepines should be avoided because of the high potential for abuse and physiologic dependence associated with these medications. Buspirone (BuSpar), a nonbenzodiazepine, does not lead to tolerance or withdrawal and, although not as potent as benzodiazepines, may be useful for relief of anxiety. Other agents, such as the SSRIs, are effective in the management of generalized anxiety and panic disorders and may be effective in the management of anxiety associated with somatic symptom disorder.

Monitoring Medications, Interactions, and Side Effects

In somatic symptom disorder, patients are usually treated in the community, where they often use multiple over-the-counter and prescription medications. Once the nurse completes a BPMH of all current home medicinal substances, including self-prescribed and over-the-counter remedies, vitamins and herbal supplements, etc., the information should be documented and reported to the rest of the interdisciplinary team. The nurse questions and listens carefully to determine the full scope of medications, how they are used, and effects that the patient attributes to each substance. Using the BPMH, an evaluation of possible drug–drug interactions needs to be completed by the prescriber through a medication reconciliation process. The nurse needs to work with the patient, pharmacist, nurse practitioner, and physician to support the patient in maintaining a safe and effective pharmacotherapeutic regime. Individuals with somatic symptom disorder often have idiosyncratic reactions to their medications. Side effects should be assessed, but the patient should be encouraged to compare the benefits of the medication with any problems related to side effects.

In working with patients with somatization disorder, the nurse must always monitor for drug–drug interactions. Medications patients are taking for physical problems could interact with psychiatric medications. Patients may be taking alternative medicines, such as herbal supplements (e.g., Valarian for management of anxiety), and these also need to be evaluated for possible adverse interactions. The patient should be encouraged to use the same pharmacy to fill all prescriptions so that possible reactions can be checked.

Psychological Domain

The cognitive functioning of individuals with somatic symptom disorder is usually within normal limits. However, these individuals seem preoccupied with personal illnesses and often keep a record of symptoms and illnesses. They constantly focus on bodily functions, and "living with diseases" truly becomes a way of life.

Individuals with somatic symptom disorder usually have intense emotional reactions to life stressors. They often have a series of personal crises beginning at an early age. Typically, a new symptom or medical problem develops during times of emotional stress. It is critical that the physical assessment data be linked to psychological and social events. A history of major psychological events should be compared with the chronology of physical problems. Special attention should be paid to any history of sexual abuse or trauma in the patient's younger years. Early sexual abuse also may interfere with self-esteem, belonging, and sexual fulfilment in adulthood.

Response to physical symptoms is often exaggerated, such as interpreting a simple cold as pneumonia or a brief chest pain as a heart attack. Family members may not believe the physical symptoms are real, instead viewing them as attention-seeking behaviour, since the symptoms often do improve when the patient receives attention. For example, a woman who has been in bed for 3 weeks with severe back pain may suddenly feel much better once her children visit her.

Assessment

While gathering information from the biologic domain, the nurse concurrently assesses mental status in the psychological domain. Components include appearance, psychomotor behaviour, mood, affect, perception, thought content and process, sensorium, insight, and judgment (see Chapter 10).

Nursing Diagnoses for the Psychological Domain

Nursing diagnoses related to the psychological domain and typical of people with somatic symptom disorder include anxiety, ineffective sexuality patterns, impaired social interactions, ineffective coping, and ineffective therapeutic regimen management.

Interventions for the Psychological Domain

The choice of psychological intervention depends on the specific problem the patient is experiencing. Cognitive–behavioural therapy, which helps the patient identify, connect, and change feelings, thoughts, and behaviour, is the most effective treatment for somatic symptom disorder (Williams & Gorfinkle, 2016). Supportive psychotherapy, counselling, and patient education are also useful strategies. The most important and ongoing intervention is the development and maintenance of a therapeutic relationship.

Development of a Therapeutic Relationship

The most difficult yet crucial aspect of nursing care is developing a sound, person-centred, positive, and helping nurse–patient relationship. Without it, the nurse is just one more provider who fails to meet the patient's needs and expectations. Developing this relationship requires time and patience. Therapeutic communication techniques are used to help the patient explore underlying psychosocial and spiritual problems related to the physical manifestations of the disorder (Box 24.3).

During periods when symptoms of other psychiatric disorders surface, additional therapeutic interventions may be needed (see Chapter 6). For example, the occurrence of depression requires additional supportive or cognitive approaches.

Counselling

Counselling, with a focus on problem-solving, is needed from time to time. These patients may have chaotic

---

BOX 24.3

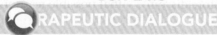
THERAPEUTIC DIALOGUE

Establishing a Relationship

Ineffective Approach

Nurse: Good morning, Ms. C.

Patient: I'm in so much pain. Take that breakfast away.

Nurse: You don't want your breakfast?

Patient: Can't you see? I hurt! When I hurt, I can't eat!

Nurse: If you don't eat now, you probably won't be able to have anything until lunch.

Patient: Who cares. I have no intention of being here at lunchtime. I don't belong here.

Nurse: Ms. C, I don't think that your doctor would have admitted you unless there is a problem. I would like to talk to you about why you are here.

Patient: Nurse, I'm just here. It's none of your business.

Nurse: Oh.

Patient: Please leave me alone.

Nurse: Sure, I will see you later.

Effective Approach

Nurse: Good morning, Ms. C.

Patient: I'm in so much pain. Take that breakfast away.

Nurse: (Silently removes the tray, pulls up a chair, and sits down.)

Patient: My back hurts.

Nurse: Oh, when did the back pain start?

Patient: Last night. It's this bed. I couldn't get comfortable.

Nurse: These beds can be pretty uncomfortable.

Patient: My back pain is shooting down my leg.

Nurse: Does anything help it?

Patient: Sometimes if I straighten out my leg it helps.

Nurse: Can I help you straighten out your leg?

Patient: Oh, it's OK. The pain is going away. What did you say your name is?

Nurse: I'm Susan Miller, your nurse while you are here.

Patient: I won't be here long. I don't belong in a psychiatric unit.

Nurse: While you are here, I would like to spend time with you.

Patient: OK, but you understand I do not have any psychiatric problems.

Nurse: We can talk about whatever you want. But, since you want to get out of here, we might want to focus on what it will take to get you ready for discharge.

Critical Thinking Challenge

- What communication mistakes did the nurse in the first scenario make?
- What communication strategies helped the patient feel comfortable with the nurse in the second scenario? How is the second scenario different from the first?

lives and need support through a multitude of crises. Although they sometimes appear flamboyant and self-assured, their constant complaints may irritate others. The consequences of their impaired social interactions must be examined within a counselling framework. The nurse helps the patient identify stressors, explore related thoughts and feelings, and develop positive coping responses.

Patient Education: Health Teaching

Health teaching is useful throughout the nurse–patient relationship. These patients have many questions about illnesses, symptoms, and treatments. Emphasis should be upon positive health care practices rather than the effects of serious illness. Because of problems in managing medications and treatment, the therapeutic regimen needs constant monitoring; this provides ample opportunity for teaching. One area that might require special health teaching is impaired sexuality. Because of their history of physical problems related to the reproductive tract, patients may have difficulty carrying out normal sexual activity, such as masturbation, intercourse, reaching orgasm, and so forth. Basic teaching about sexual function is often needed (see Box 24.4).

Social Domain

People with somatic symptom disorder spend excessive time seeking medical care and attending to their multiple illnesses. Because they believe themselves to be very sick, they also often believe that they are disabled and cannot work; their unemployment rate is therefore high. While these individuals are rarely satisfied with health care providers who can find no basis for a medical diagnosis, their social network may consist more of these providers than of their peers. Identifying a support network requires sorting out health care providers from their family and friends.

Assessment

It is important to identify both beneficial and harmful relationships within the patient's family. Family members may become weary of the patient's constant physical complaints. In assessing relations, however, it is important that other members with social problems and psychiatric disorders be identified, as the individual suffering from somatic symptom disorder may live in a chaotic family with multiple challenges.

Symptoms of somatic symptom disorder may disrupt the family's social life. A change in routine or a major life event often precipitates a symptom's appearance. For example, a patient planning a vacation with the family may decide at the last minute that she cannot go because her back pain has returned and she will be unable to sit in the car. Such family disruptions are common.

Nursing Diagnoses for the Social Domain

Some of the nursing diagnoses related to the social domain that are typical of people with somatic symptom disorder include risk for caregiver role strain, ineffective community coping, disabled family coping, and social isolation.

Interventions for the Social Domain

Patients with somatic symptom disorders may be isolated from family and community. Strengthening relationships and encouraging social activity often become the focus of nursing care. The nurse should help the patient identify individuals with whom contact is desired, encourage him or her to reinitiate a relationship, and ask for a commitment to contact them. The nurse should counsel the patient about talking too much about his or her symptoms with these individuals and emphasize that medical information should be shared with the nurse.

Group Interventions

Although these patients may not be good candidates for insight group psychotherapy, they do benefit from cognitive–behavioural groups that focus on developing coping skills for everyday life (Hedman et al., 2016). For female patients, participation in groups that address feminist issues should be encouraged; this may help to strengthen their assertiveness skills and improve self-esteem (Fig. 24.2).

When leading a group that has members with somatic symptom disorder, redirection can keep the group from giving too much attention to a person's illness. However, these individuals need reassurance and support while in a group. The patient may report feeling as though he or she does not fit in with or belong in the group; in reality, he or she is likely feeling insecure and threatened in the situation. The group leader needs to show patience and understanding in order to engage the individual effectively in meaningful group interaction.

BOX 24.4 Psychoeducation Checklist: Somatic Symptom Disorder

When caring for the patient with somatic symptom disorder, be sure to include the following topic areas in the teaching plan:

- Psychopharmacologic agents if ordered, including drug, action, dosage, frequency, and possible adverse effects
- Nonpharmacologic approaches to pain relief
- Exercise
- Nutrition
- Social interaction
- Appropriate health maintenance practices
- Problem-solving
- Relaxation and anxiety-reduction techniques
- Sexual functioning

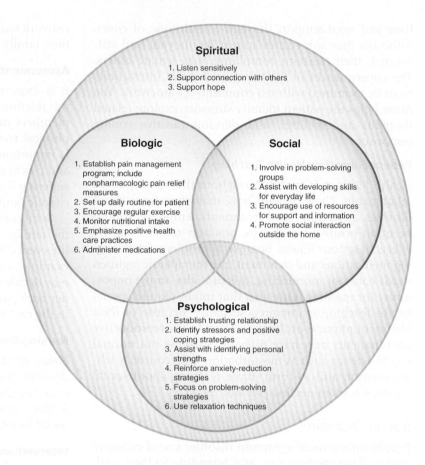

Figure 24.2. Bio/psycho/social/spiritual interventions for patients with somatic symptom disorder.

Family Interventions

The results of a family assessment often reveal a need for education about the disorder, helpful strategies for dealing with the patient's symptoms, and, usually, help in developing more effective communication and problem-solving strategies. Many people with somatic symptom disorder have experienced a chaotic family life and, potentially, physical and/or sexual abuse. The nurse must assess and offer interventions such as those identified through a thorough family assessment (see Chapter 15).

Spiritual Domain

The spiritual domain assesses how people with a somatic symptom disorder connect experiences, make meaning of their disorder, and find purpose in life. Somatic symptom disorder produces a continuous physical awareness of the body's pain or distress. Over time, patients may begin to resent their bodies, become bitter by living in a world of ongoing challenges, and experience conflict with their religious beliefs. A spiritual assessment provides important information needed to help patients regain spiritual health.

Assessment

To assess spiritual health, nurses enquire about topics such as meaning, ambiguity, and hope using questions such as: What is "being ill" like for you? What

does "being ill" mean in your life? Personal strengths are assessed with questions such as: What brings joy and peace to you? How has your illness changed the way you understand the world? Do you have spiritual beliefs that have been affected by your illness experience? Questions to elicit information about connections with self, others, and a higher power include: How are you right now? What sustains or heals your spirit? Who is significant to you? How do you feel connected to the world and events around you? Are there spiritual acts, such as prayer, that you find helpful (Burkhardt & Nagai-Jacobson, 2008)?

Nursing Diagnoses for the Spiritual Domain

Nursing diagnoses related to the spiritual domain and typical of people with somatic symptom disorder include hopelessness, spiritual distress, and potential for enhanced spiritual well-being.

Interventions for the Spiritual Domain

Individuals with somatic symptom disorders sometimes feel estranged from others. For individuals who belong to a religious group, this can include estrangement from their faith communities. Nurses intervene by creating a safe and caring environment to help the person explore deep questions related to connection, meaning, and purpose. Trust, rapport, and a mutual plan for care are developed with the use of presence, empathy,

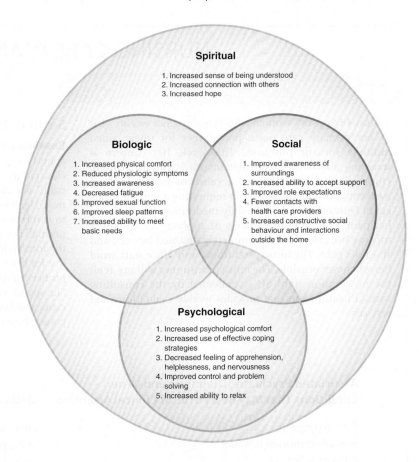

Figure 24.3. Bio/psycho/social/spiritual outcomes for patients with somatic symptom disorder.

and sensitivity. Based on the person's assessed needs, nurses may also facilitate religious practices, assist with life review or reminiscence therapy, or make a referral to a spiritual care expert (Chida, Schrempft, & Steptoe, 2016).

Evaluation and Treatment Outcomes

The outcomes for patients with somatic symptom disorder must be realistic and formulated with the patient. Because this is a lifelong disorder, small successes should be expected. Specific outcomes should be identified. Over time, there should be a gradual reduction in the number of health care providers the individual contacts and gradual improvement in the ability to cope with stresses (Fig. 24.3).

Continuum of Care

For individuals experiencing somatic symptom disorder, mental health services ranging from inpatient care to health promotion may occur in various health care settings over the course of life.

Inpatient Care

Ideally, individuals with somatic symptom disorder will spend minimal time in the hospital. Inpatient stays occur when their comorbid psychiatric disorders become

symptomatic. In order to provide consistency of care during inpatient care, the patient should be the responsibility of one primary nurse who provides or oversees all the nursing care. The inpatient nurse must establish a relationship with the patient (and family) and consult other nursing staff members about this disorder.

EMERGENCY CARE

The emergencies these individuals experience may be physical (e.g., chest pain, back pain, gastrointestinal symptoms) or stress responses related to a psychosocial crisis. Careful assessment must be used so as not to overlook the symptoms of acute and/or potentially fatal illness.

Community Treatment

Individuals with somatic symptom disorder can spend a lifetime in the health care system and still have little continuity of care. Switching from provider to provider is detrimental to their long-term care. Most are outpatients. When they are hospitalized, it is usually for evaluation of physical problems. When their comorbid psychiatric disorders, such as depression, become symptomatic, these patients may also be hospitalized for a short time (see Nursing Care Plan 24.1).

NURSING CARE PLAN 24.1

THE PATIENT WITH SOMATIZATION DISORDER

SC is a 48-year-old woman who is making her weekly visit to her primary care nurse practitioner for unexplained multiple somatic problems. This week, her concern is recurring abdominal pain that fits no symptom pattern. Upon physical examination, a cause of her abdominal pain could not be found. She is requesting a refill of lorazepam (Ativan), which is the only medication that "relieves her pain." She is in the process of applying for disability income because of being completely disabled by neck and shoulder pain. The nurse practitioner and office staff avoid her whenever possible. The nurse practitioner will not refill the prescription until SC is evaluated by the consulting mental health team that provides weekly evaluations and services.

Setting: Primary Care Office

Baseline Assessment: SC is a 48-year-old obese woman who appears very angry. She resents being forced to see a psychiatric clinician for "the only medication that works to alleviate her pain." She denies any psychiatric problems or emotional distress. Her hair is in disarray; she says that it is too much trouble to comb her hair. Cognitive aspects of mental status appear normal, but she admits to being slightly depressed and takes the lorazepam for her "nerves." She says she has nothing to live for but denies any thoughts of suicide. She is dependent on her children for everything and feels very guilty about it. She spends most of her waking hours going to various clinicians and taking combinations of medications to relieve her pains. She has no friends or nonfamily social contacts.

Associated Psychiatric Diagnosis and Other Conditions That May Be a Focus of Clinical Attention	Medications
R/O depression	Premarin, 1.2 mg daily
Somatic symptom disorder	lorazepam (Ativan), 1 mg tid
S/P gastric bypass	ranitidine HCL (Zantac), 150 mg bid
S/P carpel tunnel release	simethicone 125 mg qid with meals
Chronic shoulder, neck pain, vertigo	Calcium carbonate, 1,000 mg daily
Social problems (father died 6 months ago, divorced 9 months)	Multiple vitamin, daily
	zopiclone (Imovane), 7.5 mg at hs PRN
Economic problems (small pension)	ibuprofen, 600 mg q6h PRN pain
Occupational problems (potential disability)	

Nursing Diagnosis 1: Chronic Low Self-Esteem

Defining Characteristics	Related Factors
Self-negating verbalizations (long standing)	Feeling unimportant to family
Hesitant to try new things	Feeling rejected by ex-husband
Expresses feelings of guilt	Constant physical problems interfering with normal social activities
Evaluates self as being unable to cope with events	

Outcomes

Initial	Long-term
Identify need to increase self-esteem.	Participate in individual or group therapy for self-esteem building.

NURSING CARE PLAN 24.1 *(Continued)*

Interventions

Interventions	Rationale	Ongoing Assessment
Establish rapport with the patient.	Individuals with low self-esteem feel vulnerable and may be reluctant to discuss true feelings.	Ask the patient for her perceptions of care and the helping relationship.
Encourage the patient to spend time dressing and grooming appropriately.	Confidence and self-esteem improve when a person looks well groomed.	Monitor responses.
Encourage the patient to discuss various somatic problems, as well as psychological and interpersonal issues.	Patients with somatic symptom disorder need time to express their physical problems. It helps them feel valued. The best way to build a relationship is to acknowledge physical symptoms.	Monitor time that the patient spends explaining physical symptoms.
Explore opportunities for SC to meet other people with similar, nonmedical interests.	Focusing SC on meeting others will improve the possibilities of increasing contacts.	Observe willingness to identify other interests besides physical problems.

Evaluation

Outcomes	Revised Outcomes	Interventions
SC admitted to having low self-esteem but was very reluctant to consider meeting new people.	Focus on building self-esteem.	Identify activities that will enhance self-esteem.

Nursing Diagnosis 2: Ineffective Therapeutic Regimen Management

Defining Characteristics	Related Factors
Choices of daily living ineffective for meeting health care goal Verbalizes difficulty with prescribed regimens	Inappropriate use of benzodiazepine agents

Outcomes

Initial	Long-term
Openly discuss the use of medications.	Use nonpharmacologic means for stress reduction.

(Continued)

NURSING CARE PLAN 24.1 *(Continued)*

Interventions

Interventions	Rationale	Ongoing Assessment
Clarify the frequency and purpose of taking lorazepam.	Unsupervised polypharmacy is common.	Carefully track self-report of medication use; assess drug adherence and safety.
Educate the patient about the effects of combining medications.	Education about combining medication is the beginning of helping the patient become independent in medication management.	Observe the patient's ability and willingness to consider potential adverse effects.
Explore ways to gradually reduce the number of medications, including other means of managing physical symptoms.	Help the patient to identify appropriate ways and means to manage health care regimens.	Evaluate the patient's ability to problem solve.

Evaluation

Outcomes	Revised Outcomes	Interventions
Patient disclosed the use of medications but was unwilling to consider changing ineffective use of medication.	Identify next step if the nurse practitioner or physician does not refill prescription.	Discuss the possibility of not being able to obtain lorazepam. Refer the patient to mental health clinic for further evaluation.

Mental Health Promotion

Patients with somatic symptom disorder are encouraged to focus on staying healthy rather than on the symptoms of their illness. For these individuals, approaching the topic of health promotion usually has to be within the context of preventing further problems. Setting aside time for themselves and identifying activities that meet their psychological and spiritual needs, such as connecting with their faith group, are important in maintaining a healthy balance.

▌ OTHER SOMATIC SYMPTOM AND RELATED DISORDERS

The following discussion summarizes other somatic symptom and related disorders and highlights the primary focus of nursing management.

Illness and Anxiety Disorder

The exclusion of hypochondriasis from the *DSM-5* has brought about the emergence of illness anxiety as a new *DSM* disorder. The majority of individuals previously diagnosed with hypochondriasis seemingly fit well into the criteria for somatic symptom disorder. With *illness anxiety disorder*, patients experience excessive anxiety and

preoccupation with having or acquiring a serious illness. Physical symptoms, if present, are a minor aspect of this diagnosis. Persistent worry regarding illness invades multiple aspects of an individual's life. For instance, illness becomes a frequent topic of discussion as they repeatedly discuss illness within their social circle and seek reassurance from family and friends. They will spend hours researching suspected illnesses and continuously examine their body for signs of illness. This impacts their quality of life, potentially limiting activities of daily living (looking after family, going to work) and, in extreme cases, results in the inability to go to work or school.

The prevalence rate between men and women is similar, and although the aetiology is unknown, it is proposed that a serious childhood illness or abuse may be a precursor (Hovens, Giltay, Hemert, & Penninx, 2016). Careful evaluation of illness anxiety disorder must be carried out and other psychiatric illnesses, such as obsessive–compulsive disorder, delusional disorder, and generalized anxiety, excluded.

Several interventions have been effective in reducing patients' fears of experiencing serious illnesses. Cognitive–behavioural therapy, stress management, and group interventions lead to a decrease in intensity and increase in control of symptoms (Tyrer, Eilenberg,

Fink, Hedman, & Tyrer, 2016). It is unknown whether the positive outcomes result from the intervention itself or from the symptom validation and increased attention given to the patient. Nursing management should include listening to the patient's report of symptoms and fears, validating it by acknowledging that the fears may be real, asking the patient to monitor symptoms in a journal, and encouraging the patient to bring the journal to clinical visits. By seeing the symptom pattern, the nurse can continue assessment and help the patient better understand the significance and implications of symptoms. The outcome of this approach should be to decrease fear and achieve better symptom control.

Conversion Disorder

Conversion disorder, also known as functional neurologic symptom disorder, is the somatization of neurologic conditions such as paralysis. Symptoms associated with conversion disorder are called **pseudoneurologic symptoms**. Patients with conversion disorder present with symptoms of impaired coordination or balance, paralysis, aphonia (inability to produce sound), difficulty swallowing or a sensation of a lump in the throat, and urinary retention. They also may have loss of sensation, vision problems, blindness, deafness, seizures, and hallucinations (Levenson & Sharpe, 2017). Females experience conversion disorder two to three times more frequently than do males (APA, 2013). These symptoms do not follow neurologic pathways but rather the individual's conceptualization of the problem. The nurse must understand that the physical sensation is real for the patient. There is evidence of a relationship between childhood trauma (e.g., sexual abuse) or stressful life events and conversion disorder (Roelofs & Pasman, 2017). In approaching this patient, the nurse treats the conversion symptom as a real symptom that may have distressing psychological aspects. The nurse intervenes by acknowledging the pain and helps the patient deal with it. As trust develops within the nurse–patient relationship, the nurse can help the patient develop approaches to solving everyday problems.

IN-A-LIFE

Emily Carr (1871–1945)

CANADIAN PAINTER AND WRITER

Public Persona

Emily Carr was an accomplished artist and writer best known for her vivid depictions of Indigenous culture and Canadian West Coast nature. Influenced by early educational sojourns in San Francisco, England, and France and later encouraged by the important artists known as the Group of Seven, Carr developed her unique impressionistic style in both painting and writing. Embellished with dramatizations and idealism, works like *Growing Pains* autobiographically depict the struggle of her life. Raised in a strict Victorian home, Carr has been described as rebellious, overweight, irritable, and socially insecure.

Personal Realities

Carr's career was interrupted many times with bouts of poor health. Just more than 100 years ago, Carr was treated in an English sanatorium. Many of the symptoms she described were representatives of what today is called illness anxiety disorder, clinical depression, and/or conversion disorder.

PSYCHOLOGICAL FACTORS AFFECTING OTHER MEDICAL CONDITIONS

Within this category, patients engage in behaviours that negatively impact the outcome of an existing medical condition. In mild cases, patients may, for instance, not take their antidiabetic medication appropriately and intentionally increase their risk for diabetic complications. In more severe cases, the patient's behaviour may lead to life-threatening complications and risk of death. For example, a patient may ignore a life-threatening infection rather than seek help. This diagnosis can only be established in the absence of other diagnoses that may better characterize or explain such risky behaviour, such as major depressive disorder, delusion disorder, or posttraumatic stress disorder (APA, 2013).

FACTITIOUS DISORDERS

The other type of psychiatric disorder characterized by somatization is **factitious disorder**. Patients with this disorder intentionally cause an illness or injury to receive the attention of health care workers. These individuals are motivated solely by the desire to become a patient and develop a dependent relationship with a health care provider. There are two classes of factitious disorders: factitious disorder imposed on self and factitious disorder imposed on another. See the DSM-5 for more specific details on their diagnostic criteria.

Factitious Disorder, Imposed on Self

Although feigned illnesses have been described for centuries, it was not until 1951 that the term *Munchausen's syndrome* was used to describe the most severe form of this disorder, which was characterized by fabricating a physical illness, having recurrent hospitalizations, and going from one provider to another (Asher, 1951). Today, this disorder is called factitious disorder and is differentiated from **malingering**, in which the individual who intentionally produces illness symptoms is motivated by another specific self-serving goal, such as being classified as disabled or avoiding work.

Patients with factitious disorder injure themselves covertly. The illnesses are produced in such a manner that the health care provider is tricked into believing that a true physical or psychiatric disorder is present. The self-produced physical symptoms appear as medical illnesses such as seizure disorders, wound-healing disorders, the abscess processes (introduction of infectious material below the skin surface), and feigned fever (rubbing the thermometer).

Epidemiology

The estimated prevalence of factitious disorders is between 0.5% and 2% (Fischer, Beckson, & Dietz, 2017). The prevalence of factitious disorder is difficult to determine because its secretive nature interferes with traditional epidemiologic research methods. Recovery from this condition is seldom addressed in academic literature and effective treatment approaches are not well known.

Nursing Management: Human Response to Disorder

The overall goal of treatment is for the patient to replace the dysfunctional, attention-seeking behaviours with positive behaviours. To begin treatment, the patient must acknowledge the deception, but confrontation does not appear to lead to acknowledgment. Nonetheless, a supportive, nonpunitive approach may be beneficial in order to establish a therapeutic relationship and encourage psychotherapy (Fischer et al., 2017). The mental health team has to accept and value the patient as a human being who needs help. As the pattern of self-injury is well established, giving up the behaviours is difficult.

Assessment

Early childhood experiences, particularly instances of abuse, neglect, or abandonment, should be identified in order to understand the underlying psychological dynamics of the individual and the role of self-injury. Family assessment is important; relationships become strained as family members become aware of this disorder's self-inflicted nature.

Nursing Interventions

The fabrications and deceits may provoke anger and a sense of betrayal in the nurse. To be effective with these patients, the nurse must be aware of these feelings and resolve them by developing a better understanding of the underlying psychodynamic issues. Therapeutic confrontation in the context of a helping relationship can be effective if the patient feels supported and accepted and

if there is clear communication between the patient, the mental health care team, and family members. All care should be centralized within one facility, and the patient should see providers regularly, even when not in active crisis. The treatment goal is recovery not confession.

Factitious Disorder, Imposed on Another

Within the category of factitious disorder, the *DSM-5* includes a rare but dramatic disorder, factitious disorder imposed on another, once called *Munchausen's by proxy.* It involves a person's inflicting injury on another—often a mother on her own child—hoping thereby to gain the attention of a health care provider. These actions include inducing seizures, poisoning, or smothering. This most severe form of child abuse is usually identified in the emergency room or by critical care nurses. The mother rarely admits to injuring the child and thus is not amenable to treatment; if this is the case, the child is removed from the mother's care. This form of child abuse is distinguished from other forms by the routine, unwitting involvement of health care workers, who subject the child to physical risk and emotional distress through tests, procedures, and medication trials.

 ## SUMMARY OF KEY POINTS

- Somatic symptom and related disorders are manifested as psychological distress and abnormal thought patterns in relation to physical symptoms, independent of whether the symptom may be medically explained or not.
- Factitious disorders are manifested by individuals intentionally inflicting or feigning injury or illness on themselves or others in order to gain medical attention.
- Somatization is affected by sociocultural and traumatic childhood experiences. It occurs more frequently in those with lower levels of education or socioeconomic class, and less frequently in older adults.
- Illness anxiety disorder occurs when an individual's preoccupation with having or acquiring an illness causes excessive distress.
- Conversion disorder manifests as one or more somatic symptoms involving altered voluntary motor or sensory function. This disorder is two to three times more prevalent in females.
- Patients with somatic symptom disorder are often seen on the medical–surgical units of hospitals and can go years without receiving a correct diagnosis. In most cases, they eventually receive mental health treatment because of comorbid conditions such as depression and panic.
- The development of the nurse–patient relationship is crucial to assessing these patients and identifying appropriate nursing diagnoses and interventions. Because these patients deny any psychiatric

basis for their problem and continue to focus on their symptoms having a medical basis, the nurse must take a nonjudgmental, open approach that acknowledges the symptoms while helping the patient explore and understand his or her behaviour and focus on new ways of coping with stress.

- Health teaching is important in helping the individual develop positive lifestyle changes in place of somatization responses. Identifying personal strengths and supporting the development of positive skills improve self-esteem and personal confidence. Teaching the use of biofeedback and relaxation provides the patient with positive coping skills.

 Web Links

dsm.psychiatryonline.org This Web site holds the "DSM Library." You can search the Web site for information regarding somatic symptom and other disorders.

intelihealth.com InteliHEALTH provides health information. Somatic symptom disorder can be found through a search on this Aetna Web site.

mental-health-matters.com/disorders This is the site of Mental Health Matters, a Web site for consumers and professionals, which describes several psychiatric disorders, including somatic symptom disorder.

References

American Psychiatric Association (APA). (2013). *Diagnostic and statistical manual of mental disorders* (5th ed.). Washington, DC: Author.

Arts, M., Buis, J., & de Jonge, L. (2016). Misdiagnosis of anterior cutaneous nerve entrapment syndrome as a somatization disorder. *European Psychiatry, 33*, S478. doi:10.1016/j.eurpsy.2016.01.1392

Asher, R. (1951). Münchredsen's syndrome. *Lancet, 1*, 339–341.

Barsky, A. J. (2016). Assessing the new DSM-5 diagnosis of somatic symptom disorder. *Psychosomatic Medicine, 78*(1), 2–4. doi:10.1097/PSY.0000000000000287

Burkhardt, M. A., & Nagai-Jacobson, M. G. (2008). Spirituality and health. In B. M. Dossey & L. Keegan (Eds.), *Holistic nursing: A handbook for practice* (5th ed., pp. 617–645). Toronto, ON: Jones and Bartlett Publishers.

Caudill-Slosberg, M. A. (2002). *Managing pain before it manages you* (rev. ed.). New York, NY: Guilford Press.

Chida, Y., Schrempft, S., & Steptoe, A. (2016). A novel religious/spiritual group psychotherapy reduces depressive symptoms in a randomized clinical trial. *Journal of Religion and Health, 55*(5), 1495–1506. doi:10.1007/s10943-015-0113-7

Cosci, F., & Fava, G. A. (2016). The clinical inadequacy of the DSM-5 classification of somatic symptom and related disorders: An alternative trans-diagnostic model. *CNS Spectrums, 21*(04), 310–317. doi:10.1017/S1092852915000760

Fava, G. A., Cosci, F., & Sonino, N. (2017). Current psychosomatic practice. *Psychotherapy and Psychosomatics, 86*(1), 13–30. doi:10.1159/000448856

Firoozabadi, A., Bahredar, M. J., & Seifsafari, S. (2013). Somatization as central manifestation of depression in Iranian culture. *European Psychiatry, 28*(1), 1.

Fischer, C. A., Beckson, M., & Dietz, P. (2017). Factitious disorder in a patient claiming to be a sexually sadistic serial killer. *Journal of Forensic Sciences, 62*(3), 822–826. doi:10.1111/1556-4029.13340

Frances, A. (2013). The new somatic symptom disorder in DSM-5 risks mislabeling many people as mentally ill. *BMJ, 346*. doi:10.1136/bmj.f1580

Garcia-Campayo, J., Sanz-Carrillo, C., Baringo, T., & Ceballos, C. (2001). A SPECT scan in somatization disorder patients: An exploratory study of eleven cases. *The Australian and New Zealand Journal of Psychiatry, 35*(3), 359–363.

Hakala, M., Karlsson, H., Ruotsalainen, U., Koponen, S., Bergman, J., Stenman, H., … Niemi, P. (2002). Severe somatization in women is associated with altered cerebral glucose metabolism. *Psychological Medicine, 32*(8), 1379–1385.

Hart, S. L., Hodgkinson, S. C., Belcher, H. M. E., Hyman, C., & Cooley-Strickland, M. (2013). Somatic symptoms, peer, and school stress, and family and community violence exposure among urban elementary school children. *Journal of Behavioral Medicine, 36*, 454–465. doi:10.1007/s10865-012-9440-2

Hedman, E., Axelsson, E., Andersson, E., Lekander, M., & Ljótsson, B. (2016). Exposure-based cognitive–behavioural therapy via the internet and as bibliotherapy for somatic symptom disorder and illness anxiety disorder: Randomised controlled trial. *The British Journal of Psychiatry, 209*(5), 407–413.

Hilderink, P. H., Collard, R., Rosmalen, J. G. M., & Oude Voshaar, R. C. (2013). Prevalence of somatoform disorders and medically unexplained symptoms in old age populations in comparison with younger age groups: A systematic review. *Ageing Research Reviews, 12*(1), 151–156.

Holliday, K. L., MacFarlane, G. J., Nicholl, B. I., Creed, F., Thomson, W., & McBeth, J. (2010). Genetic variations in neuroendocrine gene associated with somatic symptoms in the general population: Results from the EPIFUND study. *Journal of Psychosomatic Research, 68*(5), 469–474. doi:10.1016/j.jpsychores.2010.01.024

Holster, J., Hawks, E. M., & Ostermeyer, B. (2017). Somatic symptom and related disorders. *Psychiatric Annals, 47*(4), 184–191.

Hovens, J. G., Giltay, E. J., Hemert, A. M., & Penninx, B. W. (2016). Childhood maltreatment and the course of depressive and anxiety disorders: The contribution of personality characteristics. *Depression and Anxiety, 33*(1), 27–34. doi:10.1002/da.22429

Jorge, J. R. (2003). Depression in Brazil and other Latin American countries. *Seishin Shinkeigaku Zasshi, 105*(1), 9–16.

Karkhanis, D. G., & Winsler, A. (2016). Temperament, gender, and cultural differences in maternal emotion socialization of anxiety, somatization, and anger. *Psychological Studies, 61*(3), 137–158. doi:10.1007/s12646-016-0360-z

Karling, P., Wikgren, M., Adolfsson, R., & Norrback, K. F. (2016). Hypothalamus-pituitary-adrenal axis hypersuppression is associated with gastrointestinal symptoms in major depression. *Journal of Neurogastroenterology and Motility, 22*(2), 292. doi:10.5056/jnm15064

Kirmayer, L. J., & Sartorius, N. (2007). Cultural models and somatic syndromes. *Psychosomatic Medicine, 69*(9), 832–840.

Kohlmann, S., Gierk, B., Hilbert, A., Brähler, E., & Löwe, B. (2016). The overlap of somatic symptoms, anxiety and depression: A population based analysis. *Journal of Psychosomatic Research, 85*, 68. doi:10.1016/j.jpsychores.2016.03.167

Kroenke, K., & Swindle, R. (2000). Cognitive-behavioral therapy for somatization and symptom syndromes: A critical review of controlled clinical trials. *Psychotherapy and Psychosomatics, 69*(4), 205–215.

Kushwaha, V., Sinha, D. K., Chadda, R. K., & Mehta, M. (2014). A study of disability and its correlates in somatization disorder. *Asian Journal of Psychiatry 8*, 56–58. doi:10.1016/j.ajp.2013.10.016

Levenson, J. L., & Sharpe, M. (2017). The classification of conversion disorder (functional neurologic symptom disorder) in ICD and DSM. *Handbook of Clinical Neurology, 139*, 189. doi:10.1016/B978-0-12-801772-2.00016-3

Longstreth, G. F. (2016). Carnett's legacy: Raising legs and raising awareness of an often misdiagnosed syndrome. *Digestive Diseases and Sciences, 61*(2), 337–339. doi:10.1007/s10620-015-3885-4

Malas, N., Ortiz-Aguayo, R., Giles, L., & Ibeziako, P. (2017). Pediatric somatic symptom disorders. *Current Psychiatry Reports, 19*(2), 11. doi:10.1007/s11920-017-0760-3

Parr, N. J., Zeman, J., Braunstein, K., & Price, N. (2016). Peer emotion socialization and somatic complaints in adolescents. *Journal of Adolescence, 50*, 22–30. doi:10.1016/j.adolescence.2016.04.004

Rief, W., Hennings, A., Riemer, S., & Euteneuer, F. (2010). Psychobiological differences between depression and somatization. *Journal of Psychosomatic Research, 68*(5), 495–502. doi:10.1016/j.jpsychores.2010.02.001

Roelofs, K., & Pasman, J. (2017). Stress, childhood trauma, and cognitive functions in functional neurologic disorders. *Handbook of Clinical Neurology, 139*. doi:10.1016/B978-0-12-801772-2.00013-8

Rohlof, H. G., Knipscheer, J. W., & Kleber, R. J. (2014). Somatization in refugees: A review. *Social Psychiatry and Psychiatric Epidemiology, 49*(11), 1793–1804.

Schneider, G., Wachter, M., Driesch, G., Kruse, A., Nehen, H. G., & Heuft, G. (2003). Subjective body complaint as an indicator of somatization in elderly patients. *Psychosomatics, 44*(2), 91–99.

Silverstein, B., Edwards, T., Gamma, A., Ajdaric-Gross, V., Rossier, W., & Angst, J. (2013). The role played by depression associated with somatic symptomatology in accounting for gender differences in the prevalence of depression. *Social Psychiatry and Psychiatric Epidemiology, 48*, 257–263.

Steinbrecher, N., Koerber, S., Frieser, D., & Hiller, W. (2011). The prevalence of medically unexplained symptoms in primary care. *Psychosomatics, 52*(3), 263–271. doi:10.1016/j.psym.2011.01.007

Steine, I. M., Winje, D., Krystal, J. H., Bjorvatn, B., Milde, A. M., Grønli, J., ... Pallesen, S. (2017). Cumulative childhood maltreatment and its dose–response relation with adult symptomatology: Findings in a sample of adult survivors of sexual abuse. *Child Abuse & Neglect, 65,* 99–111. doi:10.1016/j.chiabu.2017.01.008

Tierney, C. D., & Walker-Harding, L. R. (2017). Early intervention for functional somatic symptoms using psychological interventions highlights the need for a medical home care model for pediatric patients. *The Journal of Pediatrics, 187*:15–17. doi:10.1016/j.jpeds.2017.04.028

Toussaint, A., Murray, A. M., Voigt, K., Herzog, A., Gierk, B., Kroenke, K., ... Löwe, B. (2016). Development and validation of the somatic symptom disorder–B criteria scale (SSD-12). *Psychosomatic Medicine, 78*(1), 5–12.

Tyrer, P., Eilenberg, T., Fink, P., Hedman, E., & Tyrer, H. (2016). Health anxiety: The silent, disabling epidemic. *BMJ, 25*(353), i2250. doi:10.1136/bmj.i2250

Wakefield, J. C. (2016). Diagnostic issues and controversies in DSM-5: Return of the false positives problem. *Annual Review of Clinical Psychology, 12,* 105–132. doi:10.1146/annurev-clinpsy-032814-112800

Warren, J. W., Langenberg, P., & Clauw, D. J. (2013). The number of existing functional somatic syndromes (FSSs) is an important factor for new, different FSSs. *Journal of Psychosomatic Research, 74*(1), 12–17. doi:10.1016/j.jpsychores.2012.09.002

Williams, D. T., & Gorfinkle, K. (2016). Somatic symptom disorders: Update on diagnosis and treatment. *Journal of the American Academy of Child & Adolescent Psychiatry, 55*(10), S356. doi:10.1016/j.jaac.2016.07.111

Wygant, D. B., Arbisi, P. A., Bianchini, K. J., & Umlauf, R. L. (2017) Waddell non-organic signs: New evidence suggests somatic amplification among outpatient chronic pain patients. *The Spine Journal, 17*(4), 505–510. doi:10.1016/j.spinee.2016.10.018

Yick, A. G., Shibusawa, T., & Agbayani-Siewert, P. (2003). Partner violence, depression, and practice implications with families of Chinese descent. *Journal of Cultural Diversity, 10*(3), 96–104.

CHAPTER

25 Eating Disorders

Kathryn Weaver

LEARNING OBJECTIVES

After studying this chapter, you will be able to:

- Distinguish the characteristics of eating disorders.
- Describe biologic, psychological, and social aetiologic theories of anorexia nervosa, bulimia nervosa, and binge-eating disorder within the broader spiritual dimension.
- Explain the importance of body image, body dissatisfaction, and gender identity in developmental theories that explain aetiology of anorexia nervosa, bulimia nervosa, and binge-eating disorder.
- Appreciate the role obesity plays in the development of anorexia nervosa and bulimia nervosa and as a consequence of binge-eating disorder.
- Describe the neurobiology, neurochemistry, and physiologic consequences associated with anorexia nervosa, bulimia nervosa, and binge-eating disorder.
- Explain the impact of sociocultural norms on the development of eating disorders.
- Describe the risk factors and protective factors associated with the development of eating disorders.
- Formulate nursing diagnoses for individuals with eating disorders.
- Develop nursing interventions for individuals with anorexia nervosa, bulimia nervosa, and binge-eating disorder.
- Analyze special concerns within the nurse–client relationship for the nursing care of individuals with eating disorders.
- Identify strategies for the prevention and early detection of eating disorders.

KEY TERMS

- anorexia nervosa • binge-eating disorder
- body image • body mass index • bulimia nervosa
- cue elimination • self-monitoring

KEY CONCEPTS

- body dissatisfaction • body image distortion • dietary restraint • drive for thinness • enmeshment
- interoceptive awareness • maturity fears • social comparison

---

Eating disorders are commonly believed to date from the time of ancient Rome with rich people gorging themselves and vomiting in designated places called vomitoriums. However, this belief is most likely mistaken because the written account by Stoic Seneca (4 BC to AD 65) of people vomiting so they might eat and eating so they may vomit was metaphorically referring to the excesses of Rome (Pappas, 2016). In actual fact, the term *vomitorium* referred to the stadium exits from which crowds rapidly disgorged, and not to special rooms for the purpose of purging. Parallels between religious practices and eating disorders have also been drawn. To illustrate, the story of Saint Catherine of Siena (1347–1380) provides a medieval example of self-starvation honoured by the Catholic Church. Fasting in response to the death of her sister and opposing her parents' demand that she be married, Catherine starved herself and tirelessly cared for the sick and the poor, denying her own needs until she died from malnutrition at 33 (Forcen, 2013). Although Saint Catherine became a model of virtue through starvation, reconceptualizing her fasting practice as a present-day eating disorder may minimize basic differences in the symbolic meaning and the sociocultural contexts. Later on during the Enlightenment, English physician Richard Morton, in the midst of the tuberculosis epidemics in 1694, described the case of a woman who suffered a "nervous consumption" as the cause of her wasting (Forcen, 2015). "Anorexia nervosa" was coined around 1873 by Sir William Withey Gull and "hysterical anorexia" by Ernest Charles Lasègue the same year (Valente, 2016). Both anorexic disorders refer to a set of phenomena that resemble the construct of "anorexia" used today: loss of weight, food refusal, amenorrhoea, and hyperactivity. The first Canadian publication on anorexia nervosa was by New Brunswick physician Peter Inches (1895) who described a 17-year-old with low weight, loss of menses, and "almost complete refusal of food of any kind" (p. 74).

This chapter focuses on **anorexia nervosa** (AN), **bulimia nervosa** (BN), and **binge-eating disorder** (BED) with other eating issues that do not fully meet clinical criteria for AN, BN, or BED discussed. The role of obesity in the development of eating disorders and as a specific consequence of BED is considered. A transdiagnostic approach to eating disorders is based on the idea that all eating disorders have comparable characteristics and underlying core psychopathology that is reflected in similar attitudes and behaviours and evidenced by the high number and frequency of persons moving from one diagnosed eating disorder to another (Dudek, Ostaszewski, & Malicki, 2014). Drawing on the pioneering transdiagnostic model of Fairburn (e.g., Fairburn & Cooper, 2014), eating disorders are understood as sharing the same set of dysfunctional self-worth beliefs. For persons living with eating disorders, their sense of self-esteem is primarily determined by their ability to control weight and shape. Consequently, they attempt to follow various dieting regimes, often extremely restrictive or irrational, such as complete avoidance of carbohydrates or eating 400 kcal a day. Breaking any of these rules, virtually unavoidable due to their restrictiveness, usually prompts a binge-eating episode, which leads to even stricter dietary restrictions and is often accompanied by a sense of guilt. For some people, a binge-eating episode is followed by compensatory behaviour (e.g., induced vomiting, strenuous physical exercise, or intake of laxatives), which, in turn, increases the risk of another binge through a dysfunctional belief that compensatory behaviour helps control weight. Some persons who do not use compensation use binge eating to cope with stressful life events and negative emotions or as a diversion or mood regulator. Over time, these persons may experience overweight and obesity. In individuals who rarely or never engage in binge eating, dietary restrictions cause gradual loss of body mass, leaving them underweight.

To recap, manifestations of eating disorders (e.g., dieting, binge eating, weight fluctuations, and preoccupation with weight and shape) overlap significantly and thus may be viewed holistically within a continuum of eating experiences (Fig. 25.1). On one end is *unrestricted eating*, whereupon eating and appearance are not at issue for the individual. For most, this is a time of healthy eating, exercise, weight, and **body image**; however, unrestricted eating can include binge eating. *Watchful eating* includes paying attention to food composition and calories, tracking calories, and physical activity for the purpose of modifying daily energy balance. At this stage, the individual is becoming dissatisfied with body appearance, engages in watchful eating, and may weigh self more than usual, relating weight changes to calories ingested or expended. The individual's identity is shifting to one of a dieter and/or

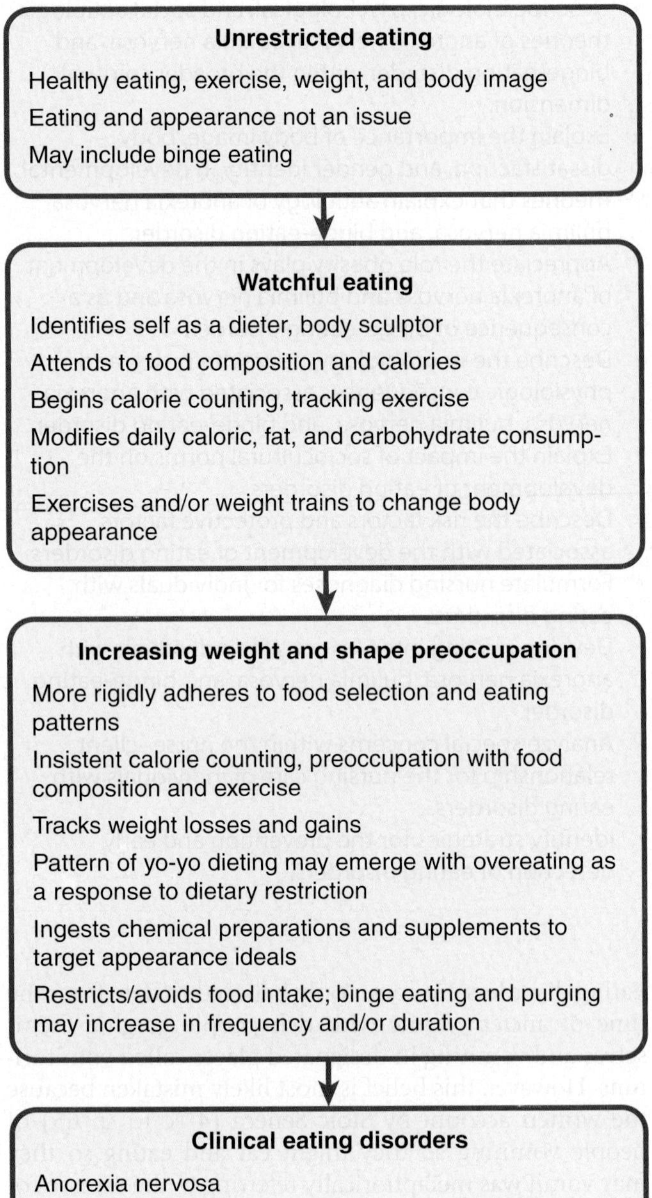

Unrestricted eating

Healthy eating, exercise, weight, and body image

Eating and appearance not an issue

May include binge eating

↓

Watchful eating

Identifies self as a dieter, body sculptor

Attends to food composition and calories

Begins calorie counting, tracking exercise

Modifies daily caloric, fat, and carbohydrate consumption

Exercises and/or weight trains to change body appearance

↓

Increasing weight and shape preoccupation

More rigidly adheres to food selection and eating patterns

Insistent calorie counting, preoccupation with food composition and exercise

Tracks weight losses and gains

Pattern of yo-yo dieting may emerge with overeating as a response to dietary restriction

Ingests chemical preparations and supplements to target appearance ideals

Restricts/avoids food intake; binge eating and purging may increase in frequency and/or duration

↓

Clinical eating disorders

Anorexia nervosa

Binge-eating disorder

Bulimia nervosa

Other specified feeding or eating disorder (*DSM-5*)

Figure 25.1. Continuum of eating experiences.

body sculptor. Watchful eating is not the same as mindful eating, an emerging healthy weight regulation approach for maintaining a nonjudgmental awareness of physical feelings, thoughts, and perceptions in the present moment and for recognizing one's own cues of physical hunger and satiety in order to make decisions about what and how much to eat, choose foods that are nutritious and pleasurable, and not participate in other activities while eating (Lofgren, 2015). Next on the continuum of eating experiences, *increasing weight and shape preoccupation* entails the individual more rigidly adhering to food selection and eating patterns, insistently comparing energy expended to energy ingested and tracking weight losses and gains. A pattern of dietary restriction in response to weight gain may follow. *Orthorexia* is a term that describes a dietary pattern in which an individual restricts intake to include only "healthy" foods such as vegetables or organic foods, but in doing so develops significant problems, such as an obsession with food and severe weight loss (American Psychiatry Association [APA], 2017). Chemical preparations and supplements may also be obtained and used to target appearance ideals. Episodes of restricting or avoiding food intake, binge eating, and purging may develop. At the far end of the continuum, as the disturbed eating increases in frequency and/or duration, *clinical eating disorders* emerge as full clinical eating disorders of AN, BN, BED, and other partial clinical disorders. Individuals may cycle back and forth among these disorders. Definition, clinical course, aetiologies, and interventions for the different eating disorders are considered separately in this chapter. Yet, because their risk factors and prevention strategies are similar, these are discussed under one heading.

IN-A-LIFE

Sarah Morin: Successful Student Advocate

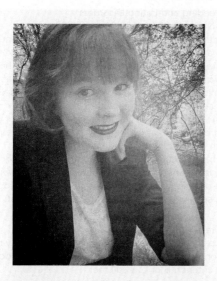

FIGHTING MORE THAN FOOD

Sarah Morin (2016) began feeling particularly self-conscious about her looks when she was about 11 years old. When she turned 12, she started skipping meals. By the time she reached 13, she "looked like a corpse" with her sallow skin stretched across knobbly bones. She was roughly 165 cm tall and her weight hovered around 27 kg (about half of what it should have been). Her heart rate was usually below 40 beats per minute, while an average heart rate for a 13-year-old is between 60 and 100. Size double-zero jeans were baggy on her and extra-small shirts intended to be tight drooped off her body. Her long hair fell out in clumps. Her eyes appeared desperate and vacant. Perpetually cold, she wore several layers to keep warm and hide her malnourished body from others.

Sarah was hospitalized with anorexia nervosa when she was 13. "Lying on one of those hospital beds with the fake plastic mattress that you would stick to in the heat of summer … with five heavy heated blankets stacked on top of [her], but … still shivering" (Morin, 2017), she recalls looking at her mother's tearful face and at the beeping monitor while her heart rate fell further and further down to 20—18—14—10—9.

Now 19, "fully recovered," and a 2nd year journalism student at St. Thomas University, Fredericton, NB, Sarah believes her experience with an eating disorder will always be a part of her, although no longer an impediment or a hindrance on the life she lives or on her hopes and goals for the future. Sarah is an exceptionally strong advocate for increased awareness and local resources. "New Brunswick is the only province without a treatment facility. Had I lived here when I was 13, I likely would not be alive to write this commentary" (Morin, 2017). Sarah was instrumental in working to get St. Thomas University to proclaim Feb. 1–7, 2017, as Eating Disorder Awareness Week. She hopes this recognition would help those struggling with an eating disorder at the university feel a bit more comfortable and supported in their community. She believes no one should ever have to watch their heart rate drop as low as hers.

Sources: Morin, S. (2017, February 6). Eating disorders need more attention, funding. *The Aquinian*. Retrieved from http://theaquinian.net/eating-disorder-awareness-commentary/
Morin, S. (2016, January 27). Fighting more than just food. *The Aquinian*. Retrieved from http://theaquinian.net/fighting-just-food/

■ ANOREXIA NERVOSA

The term "anorexia nervosa" is deceptive as its literal meaning is lack or absence of appetite of nervous origin. Persons with AN suffer, rather, from a deep fear of becoming fat that is accompanied by a disturbance in the way in which they perceive and experience their body. This fear, not lack of appetite, is what motivates their refusal to maintain an even minimally normal weight (Vandereycken & van Deth, 1994).

Clinical Course

Although the risk of eating disorders occurs across the lifespan, the onset of AN is usually in adolescence or early adulthood (Statistics Canada, 2015). This onset is often associated with a stressful transition (e.g., leaving home) and can be slow with serious dieting present long before an emaciated body is noticed. Eating disorders in later life are frequently unrecognized or masked behind medical conditions, depression, or the natural changes of aging. Roy, Shatenstein, Gaudreau, Morais, and Payette (2015) found approximately 50% of 67- to 84-year-old Quebec men and women dissatisfied with their bodies and misperceived their current body sizes. Among those dissatisfied with their body weight, 90.7% perceived themselves as being too fat, and only 9.3% perceived themselves as being too thin; the prevalence of body weight dissatisfaction was higher among women as compared with men. Although the importance given to body image as it relates to physical appearance was lower in comparison with younger populations, tensions regarding the aging body (e.g., appearance versus health) as well as a double standard of aging were reported. Further, results of an Internet survey of older women (n = 245; aged 60 to 90) indicate that factors associated with eating pathology—perfectionism, depression, and sociocultural pressure to be thin—match those reported for younger women (Midlarsky, Marotta, Pirutinsky, Morin, & McGowan, 2017).

The long-term outcome of AN has improved during the past 20 years because awareness has increased early detection. Still, prognosis is variable, and less than 50% recover (Errichiello, Iodice, Bruzzese, Gherghi, & Senatore, 2016; Steiger, 2017). Currently, AN is regarded as a chronic condition, with relapses characterized by significant weight loss. Poor outcome is predicted by lifetime presence of vomiting and a higher level of trait anxiety (Zerwas et al., 2013). In a large Finnish population-based study, unrecovered women were more likely to suffer from depressive symptoms prior to eating disorder onset, remain unemployed, describe dissatisfaction with their current partner/spouse, and report high perfectionism than recovered women (Keski-Rahkonen et al., 2014). Accounting for duration of illness in this analysis, premorbid depression was solely and significantly associated with decreased likelihood of recovery. Positive prognostic factors include impulsivity at onset (Zerwas et al., 2013), shorter duration of illness, shorter duration of first

inpatient treatment, and insight (Errichiello et al., 2016). Available evidence suggests that autonomously motivated individuals (those who experience participation in therapy as a choice made with personally meaningful reasons and freely chosen goals) have better outcomes in treatment for AN than do those whose motivations are externally controlled (Thaler et al., 2016).

AN has a higher all-cause mortality than do all other psychiatric disorders with the exception of substance abuse and postpartum admission (Chesney, Goodwin, & Fazel, 2014). Low self-reported vitality, high scores in eating control, and poor reported health status have been associated with poor health-related quality of life in AN (Pohjolainen et al., 2014).

Diagnostic Criteria

The diagnostic criteria for full clinical AN have been refined in the *DSM-5* (see Table 25.1). Changes include

Table 25.1 Diagnostic Characteristics for Anorexia Nervosa

DSM-5: Feeding and Eating Disorders
Anorexia Nervosa: 307.1 (F50.01 or F50.02)
A. Restriction of energy intake relative to requirements leading to a significantly low body weight in the context of age, sex, developmental trajectory, and physical health. *Significantly low weight* is defined as a weight that is less than minimally normal or, for children and adolescents, less than that minimally expected.
B. Intense fear of gaining weight or becoming fat, or persistent behavior that interferes with weight gain, even though at a significantly low weight.
C. Disturbance in the way in which one's body weight or shape is experienced, undue influence of body weight or shape on self-evaluation, or persistent lack of recognition of the seriousness of the current low body weight.

Specify if:
In partial remission:
After full criteria for anorexia nervosa were previously met, criterion A has not been met for a sustained period, but either criterion B or C is still met.

In full remission:
After full criteria for anorexia nervosa were previously met, none of the criteria have been met for a sustained period of time.

Specify current severity:
The minimum level of severity is based, for adults, on current BMI (see below) or for children and adolescents, on BMI percentile. The ranges below are derived from World Health Organization categories for thinness in adults; for children and adolescents, corresponding BMI percentiles should be used. The level of severity may be increased to reflect clinical symptoms, the degree of functional disability, and the need for supervision.

Mild: BMI > 17 kg/m²
Moderate: BMI = 16–16.99 kg/m²
Severe: BMI = 15–15.99 kg/m²
Extreme: BMI < 15 kg/m

Reprinted with permission from the *Diagnostic and Statistical Manual of Mental Disorders*, Fifth Edition, (Copyright 2013). American Psychiatric Association.

revision of the weight-loss criterion, clarification that fear of weight gain does not need to be verbalized if behaviours interfering with weight gain can be observed, and elimination of the criterion of amenorrhoea. These revised criteria increased the population prevalence of AN by 60% among community-based young adult women (Mustelin et al., 2016). The *DSM-5* uses **body mass index** (BMI) cutoffs to denote severity. BMI, calculated as weight in kilograms/height in metres squared, defines limits of body weight as agreed upon by the Centers for Disease Control and Prevention and the World Health Organization. For example, a BMI below 16.5 kg/m^2 for an adult is considered to indicate severe underweight.

AN is categorized as (1) restricting or (2) binge–purge type. The purging associated with the binge–purge type may occur through self-induced vomiting or misuse of laxatives, diuretics, or enemas even after eating a normal or small-sized meal or snack. Many of the clinical features associated with AN result from malnutrition or semistarvation. Classic research with volunteers who semistarved, and observations of prisoners of war and conscientious objectors, have demonstrated that these states of starvation are characterized by food preoccupation, binge eating, depression, obsession, and apathy.

A central feature of AN is a distortion in body image, the mental picture of one's own body (Mitchison et al., 2017). Body image constructs include dissatisfaction, overvaluation, and preoccupation with weight and/or shape. Overvaluation is the assignment of excessive importance to body weight and/or shape in evaluating one's self-worth, whereas dissatisfaction with weight/shape is the negative evaluation of one's body weight and/or shape. Preoccupation is excessive thinking about weight and/or shape. Mustelin et al. (2017) found preoccupation with weight and shape a potent predictor of distress and eating disorder behaviours in girls and dietary restraint in boys, whereas the preoccupation, overvaluation, and dissatisfaction with weight and shape contributed equally to distress and binge eating in boys. Given that young men may also hold stigmatizing views of body image disorders and thinness-oriented concerns and behaviours as being less masculine, Mitchison et al. suggested that boys in their study who were aware of their weight/shape dissatisfaction may have been more prone to self-criticism and, in turn, higher levels of distress. Regarding eating disorder behaviours, preoccupation had the strongest direct and indirect effects on binge eating in girls, whereas overvaluation had the strongest effects on binge eating in boys.

KEY CONCEPT

Body image distortion occurs when the individual perceives his or her body disparately from how the world or society views it.

Neurobiology, Neurochemistry, and Physiologic Consequences of Anorexia Nervosa

Essential to the diagnosis of AN are semistarvation behaviours, relentless drive for thinness or a morbid fear of becoming fat, and signs and symptoms resulting from the starvation. Individuals living with AN ignore body signals or cues, such as hunger and weakness, and concentrate all efforts on controlling food intake. Their entire mental focus narrows to one goal: weight loss. Typical thought patterns are "If I gain half of a kilo, I'll keep gaining. I'll never stop until I am the same size as the fat woman in the circus." Such all-or-nothing thinking keeps these individuals on rigid regimens for weight loss. Their behaviours become organized around food-related activities, such as preparing food, counting calories, and reading cookbooks. Much behaviour concerning what, when, and how they eat is ritualistic; for example, they may cut food into tiny pieces, refuse to eat in the presence of others, or fix elaborate meals for others that they themselves do not eat. Box 25.1 lists common psychological characteristics.

BOX 25.1 Psychological Characteristics Related to Eating Disorders

Anorexia Nervosa
  Decreased interoceptive awareness
  Sexuality conflict/fears
  Maturity fears
  Ritualistic behaviours
  Perfectionism
  Dietary restraint

Bulimia Nervosa
  Impulsivity
  Boundary problems
  Limit-setting difficulties
  Dietary restraint

Binge-Eating Disorder
  Negative mood
  Self-deprecation
  Social insecurity

Anorexia, Bulimia Nervosa, and Binge-Eating Disorder
  Difficulty expressing anger
  Low self-esteem
  Body dissatisfaction
  Powerlessness
  Ineffectiveness
  Obsessiveness
  Compulsiveness
  Nonassertiveness
  Cognitive distortions

Because individuals with AN feel inadequate, many fear emotional maturation and the unknown challenges the next developmental stages will bring. For some, remaining physically small symbolizes remaining childlike; weight loss becomes a way to experience control and combat feelings of inadequacy and ineffectiveness. Every lost kilogram is viewed as a success, and weight loss often confers a feeling of virtuousness. Perfectionism is an important characteristic found in adults (Petersson, Johnsson, & Perseius, 2017; Wade & Tiggemann, 2013) and adolescents (Wade, Wilksch, Paxton, Byrne, & Austin, 2015) with AN.

Individuals living with AN may avoid conflict; have difficulty expressing negative emotions, especially anger (Oldershaw, Lavender, Sallis, Stahl, & Schmidt, 2015); and have an overwhelming sense of shame and guilt. In addition, they may have difficulty defining feelings because they are confused about or unsure of emotions and visceral cues, such as hunger; therefore, their responses to cues are inaccurate and inappropriate. Often, they cannot name the feelings they are experiencing. This uncertainty and confusion in interpreting signals from the body is called a lack of interoceptive awareness, and it is thought to be partially responsible for developing and maintaining the eating disorder (Khalsa et al., 2015).

Because of the ritualistic behaviours, all-encompassing focus on food and weight, and feelings of inadequacy that accompany AN, social contacts are gradually reduced and the person becomes isolated. With more severe weight loss come other symptoms, such as apathy, depression, and even mistrust of others.

The nutritional compromise associated with AN may affect most organs and can produce physiologic disturbances that include cardiac arrhythmias, loss of bone density, neuronal deficits, and hormonal changes (e.g., amenorrhoea, decreased libido). When extremely underweight, individuals with AN may exhibit major depressive disorder (APA, 2013). Table 25.2 presents the medical complications, signs, and symptoms of AN and the other eating disorders that result from starving or binge eating and purging. For instance, purging behaviours may cause electrolyte disturbances. It has been identified that individuals with AN who have diabetes mellitus

Table 25.2 Complications of Eating Disorders	
Body System	**Symptoms**
From Starvation to Weight Loss	
Musculoskeletal	Loss of muscle mass and loss of fat (emaciation)
	Osteopenia (*bone mineral* deficiency) and less frequently, osteoporosis
Metabolic	Hypothyroidism (symptoms include lack of energy, weakness, intolerance to cold, and bradycardia)
Cardiac	Hypoglycaemia and decreased insulin sensitivity
Gastrointestinal	Bradycardia, hypotension, loss of cardiac muscle, small heart, cardiac arrhythmias including atrial and ventricular premature contractions, prolonged QT interval, ventricular tachycardia, and sudden death
	Delayed gastric emptying, bloating, constipation, abdominal pain, gas, and diarrhoea
Reproductive	Amenorrhoea, low levels of luteinizing hormone and follicle-stimulating hormone, and irregular periods
Dermatologic	Dry, cracking skin and brittle nails due to dehydration, lanugo (fine baby-like hair over body), oedema, and acrocyanosis (bluish hands and feet); hair thinning
Hematologic	Leucopenia, anaemia, thrombocytopaenia, hypercholesterolaemia, and hypercarotenaemia
	Abnormal taste sensation (possible zinc deficiency)
Neuropsychiatric	Neurologic deficits in cognitive processing of new information; decreased total brain volume; increased brain ventricular size
	Apathetic depression, mild organic mental symptoms, sleep disturbances, and fatigue
Related to Purging (Vomiting and Laxative Abuse)	
Metabolic	Electrolyte abnormalities, particularly hypokalaemia and hypochloremic alkalosis; hypomagnesaemia; increased blood urea nitrogen
Gastrointestinal	Salivary gland and pancreatic inflammation and enlargement with increase in serum amylase; oesophageal and gastric erosion (oesophagitis); dysfunctional bowel with haustral dilation; superior mesenteric artery syndrome
Dental	Erosion of dental enamel (perimyolysis), particularly frontal teeth with decreased decay
Neuropsychiatric	Seizures (related to large fluid shifts and electrolyte disturbances), mild neuropathies, fatigue, weakness, and mild organic mental symptoms
Cardiac	Ipecac cardiomyopathy arrhythmias
Binge Eating to Weight Gain	
Gastrointestinal	Heartburn; abdominal discomfort; bloating; gastric rupture; symptoms of fullness may interrupt sleep
Metabolic	Gall bladder disease; type 2 diabetes
Cardiac	Hypertension and hypercholesterolaemia
Musculoskeletal	Arthritis
Respiratory	Shortness of breath; asthma; sleep apnoea; snoring

may "purge" through decreasing insulin doses to subsequently decrease carbohydrate metabolism (McCavill & Weaver, 2014).

Drive for thinness is an intense physical and emotional process that overrides all physiologic body cues.

Interoceptive awareness is a term used to describe the sensory response to emotional and visceral cues, such as hunger.

Epidemiology

The prevalence of AN in Canada is 0.3% to 1% (Statistics Canada, 2015), similar to that of most Western countries. AN appears to be more prevalent within ethnic minorities and in other countries than previously recognized or reported. Cultural change may be associated with increased vulnerability to eating disorders, especially when values about physical aesthetics are involved (Kimber, Georgiades, Jack, Couturier, & Wahoush, 2015; Mustafa, Zaidi, & Weaver, 2017).

Age of Onset

The age of onset is typically between 14 and 16 years, with the highest incidence rates for females aged 15 to 19 years. Adolescents are vulnerable because of stressors associated with their development, especially concerns about body image, autonomy, and peer pressure, and their susceptibility to such influences as the media, which extols an ideal body type and discusses dieting and exercise as ways to achieve success, popularity, and power. In a large representative population-based sample of Quebec youths aged 13 and 16 years, body dissatisfaction was found to increase the likelihood of using healthy and unhealthy behaviours among adolescent girls and was associated with more frequent use of unhealthy behaviours among boys. Healthy behaviours included practicing physical activity; consuming daily breakfast; eating more vegetables (other than potatoes), fruits, whole wheat bread, and milk (as a beverage); and limiting fat and sugar intake. Unhealthy behaviours included following a hypocaloric diet (less than 1,000 cal per day), doing intensive workouts for weight loss or gain, smoking, skipping meals, fasting for 1 day, and taking dietary supplements (for increasing muscle mass such as creatine and amino acid steroids) (Roy & Gauvin, 2013). As well, 3.8% of this study's girls and 1.5% of boys reported using disordered health behaviours that included taking laxatives, diet pills (for appetite suppression), and ergogenic products such as steroids. Nationally, a significant proportion of Canadian students with overweight (21%) and obesity (27%) reported they were "doing something" to lose weight, although it is unknown if they were using healthy and productive weight-loss practices (Public Health Agency of Canada, 2015). At the international level, adolescents report that the prevalence of binge eating and purging has almost doubled from age 14 to age 16 (Bartholdy et al., 2017). According to Moore, McKone, and Mendle (2016), recollections of disliking the physical changes of puberty and feeling underprepared relate to disordered eating symptoms, feelings of ineffectiveness, and difficulties with interpersonal relationships in the postpubertal period.

Gender Differences

Anorexia nervosa occurs predominantly in females (90% of cases or more) and is one of the most common psychiatric conditions in young women (Statistics Canada, 2015). This disparity may be attributed to society's influence on females to achieve an ideal body type and to men's reluctance to seek help for what is widely perceived as a female issue. Box 25.2 highlights findings about eating disorders in males, while Box 25.3 summarizes current research regarding the perspectives of Canadian women about the meaning of activity to AN.

Ethnic and Cultural Differences

Contextual variables that may influence eating disorders include level of acculturation, socioeconomic status, peer socialization, family structure, and immigration. In Canada, approximately 30% of children and adolescents under the age of 18 live in an immigrant family (Statistics Canada, 2013). Greater exposure to fast-food outlets and less exposure to supermarkets selling familiar nutritious foods and opportunities for physical activity such as walking or cycling contribute to Canadian immigrants' adoption of unhealthy eating and exercise habits, which may increase the likelihood of developing higher BMI (Boisvert & Harrell, 2013). Results from a scoping review focusing on body image dissatisfaction among ethnic minority children and adolescents within Canada and the United States suggest these individuals experience higher levels of body image dissatisfaction compared to their white counterparts (Kimber, Couturier, Georgiades, Wahoush, & Jack, 2015). In other research, a 19-year-old woman who immigrated to Ontario reported actively changing her eating habits after seeing her cousin in a bathing suit and feeling like she could not wear the same swimwear.

> I was bigger and I didn't think that it would be nice looking. I was like okay, I can't wear that and I want to. So then I started just not eating, I think I was worse than her even, she would actually eat kind of normally, but I just went overboard. (Kimber et al., 2015, p. 126)

BOX 25.2 Boys and Men With Eating Disorders

Eating disorders have been present in males for as long as in females. Indeed, the first case of loss of appetite in the absence of medical disease was described by Morton (1694, as cited in Robinson, Mountford, and Sperlinger, 2013) in a 16-year-old boy. Males get eating disorders with increasing prevalence now than in years past. Reports in the Canadian Medical Association Journal (Collier, 2013) convey a ratio of male-to-female Canadian cases of approximately 1:4.

Boys and men involved in an occupation or a sport with a greater emphasis on weight classes and aesthetic ideals such as wrestling, weight lifting, dancing, jockeying, and body building exhibit high rates of weight and shape preoccupation, intensive body modification practices, binge eating, and BN (National Eating Disorders Collaboration, 2017). The presence of excessive exercise that may have been used as a compensatory behaviour to offset intake has been documented by two publications. The first describes stress fractures presenting in 8.7% of males hospitalized in a British Columbia tertiary inpatient treatment centre for eating disorders (Coelho, Kumar, Kilvert, Kunkel, & Lam, 2015). The second reports a severely malnourished Ontario male adolescent with AN who developed primary spontaneous pneumothorax presumably from the sudden increase in intrathoracic pressure during vigorous exercise (Loung, Cooney, Fallon, Langer, & Katzman, 2016).

There are indications that men and boys who are hospitalized for AN exhibit severe medical complications, with high levels of osteopenia and osteoporosis (Coelho et al., 2015; Sabel, Rosen, & Mehler, 2014).

Commonly, males only seek treatment or receive a correct medical diagnosis when symptoms become severe. The stigma associated with having a "female disease" may contribute to a delay in seeking help.

Most of the risk factors for eating disorders apply to males and females (e.g., perfectionism, bullying, dieting, trauma, childhood obesity). For men, the social construct of masculinity or "masculine shape" is more commonly manifested as the pursuit of a muscular, lean physique rather than a lower body weight. Anabolic steroid use may indicate body preoccupation. The images of perfect male bodies coming from pop culture, sports figures, and the media can lead to feelings of low self-esteem in young men, which contribute to the body image disturbance associated with AN. The unique cultural messages males are exposed to can increase their vulnerability toward developing an eating disorder. These messages extol the ideal physical body shape for men as lean and muscular to the exclusion of other male body types, as well as the notion that males need to be in control. Thus, when coping with particular issues beyond their control, males can sometimes displace these anxieties onto their bodies to manifest control through excessive exercise and dieting.

Preventive methods must include maintaining a healthy body image and healthy self-esteem. The masculine body shape portrayed in society is often not realistic. Teaching young men that there is not one "right way" to be/look like a man is essential in preventing eating disorders (Cottrell & Williams, 2016).

Familial Predisposition

There is increased risk among first-degree biologic relatives of individuals with AN (Statistics Canada, 2015). Female relatives also have high rates of depression, leading researchers to hypothesize that a shared genetic factor may influence the development of both disorders.

Comorbidity

Data from the Canadian Community Health Survey of Mental Health and Well-Being indicate that the lifetime prevalence of eating problems is 1.7% among Canadians; almost half of those with eating problems also had mood or anxiety disorders and reported more unmet needs (Meng & D'Arcy, 2015). Comorbid major depression is common in AN (Zerwas et al., 2013), as are obsessive–compulsive disorder (OCD) (Reas, Rø, Karterud, Hummelen, & Pedersen, 2013; Zerwas et al., 2013), and anxiety disorders such as posttraumatic stress, avoidant personality disorder (Zerwas et al.,

2013), and alcohol abuse/dependence (Baker et al., 2013; Zerwas et al., 2013). Baker et al. (2013) found that women with combined AN and alcohol use disorder had higher impulsivity scores and higher prevalence of depression and borderline personality disorder than did women with AN only. Increased severity from combined psychological disturbance could interfere with treatment and decrease the likelihood of recovery. Comorbid conditions may resolve when AN has been treated successfully. At other times, symptoms of a premorbid condition, such as OCD, remain even though an individual has recovered, leading many to believe that anxiety may actually influence the development of the disorder.

Aetiology

Some risk factors and aetiologic factors for eating disorders overlap. For example, dieting is a risk factor for the development of AN, but it is also a biologic aetiologic factor, and in its most serious form—starving—it is also

BOX 25.3 Research for Best Practice

ACTIVITY EXPERIENCES OF CANADIAN WOMEN LIVING WITH ANOREXIA NERVOSA

Moola, F. J., Gairdner, S., & Amara, C. (2015). Speaking on behalf of the body and activity: Investigating the activity experiences of Canadian women living with anorexia nervosa. Mental Health and Physical Activity, 8, 44–55. doi:10.1016/j.mhpa.2015.02.002

Background: Historically, exercise was regarded as a symptom of AN, and persons with AN were prescribed bed rest. Given the advantages activity offers, the tenet that women with AN be restricted from activity has been questioned. Research is needed to distinguish healthy and unhealthy activity and to bring forward clients' perspectives on the clinical management of activity during treatment.

Purpose: To investigate how Canadian women with AN experience the moving body and their emic perspectives on the management of activity during treatment.

Methods: A thematic analysis informed by feminist embodiment theory was used to explore the perspectives of eleven women between the ages of 18 and 40 who recounted experiences of hospitalization in mental health facilities, eating disorders units, or general hospitals. The interviews were examined for recurring patterns of meaning. These were refined through a constant comparing, contrasting, and sorting process to distil the central, conceptual meaning captured within each theme.

Findings: From "becoming anorexic" to "life after discharge from hospital," complex experiences characterized women's relationship to activity, which included pleasure, pain, punishment, and the pursuit of thinness. During the events leading to hospitalization, women's relationship to activity became a "pathologic" process of becoming entrenched in the eating disorder. They exercised in solitary environments despite physical weakness and bodily pain. At the height of AN, the women reached critical crisis points in which their "broken bodies" could no longer withstand the combined stress of intense activity and reduced nutrition. Medical interventions were characterized by the cessation of all activity and marked a prolonged period of sedentariness. Women experienced refeeding as distressing and causing extreme anxiety; engaging in secretive activity reduced anxiety. "Getting kicked out of treatment" was the consequence of being caught exercising. The culture of secrecy permeated the broader treatment milieu as clients would routinely "help each other cheat" by concealing activity from the staff who were perceived as regarding all activities as "symptoms." The activity restrictions were "like trying to get through life without moving!" To the women hospitalized for AN, the activity restrictions exacerbated bodily image distress and anxiety, reduced autonomy, and resulted in their confusion about what is and is not a symptom. Post hospitalization, some participants were able to healthily engage in activity without incurring health deteriorations by incorporating rest days and varied routines, "listening to the body," and "staying connected." The women expressed that treatment programs should prepare them for posthospitalization activity challenges through incorporating therapeutic activity education and counselling. The findings draw attention to how the "physical activity and mental health conversation" should perhaps be extended to people living with eating disorders.

Implications for Nursing: Although the activity restrictions were designed by staff to protect the women from what was considered a dangerous symptom, it is evident from the findings that the extreme restrictions placed on young women who are already excessively self-restrictive might further damage their fragile sense of autonomy and set up conditions of secrecy and deceit. Women's accounts that are attentive to their bodies can help inform ethical treatment. Such accounts need to penetrate the culture of paternalism that surrounds the care of AN.

---

a symptom. Most experts agree that eating disorders are multidimensional and multidetermined. Figure 25.2 depicts the aetiologic factors for AN within their larger spiritual dimension.

Biologic Theories

The many comorbid conditions, such as depression and OCD, associated with the diagnosis of AN may have a shared aetiology. Although the relationship between these clinical manifestations and the biologic changes caused by starvation is not well understood, many of the biologic changes noted in AN are determined to be the result of starvation and thus are state, rather than trait or causative, factors. Little evidence exists to substantiate that dysregulations in appetite–satiety systems cause AN. Appetite dysregulation is best viewed as the end product or result of an interaction between the environment and physiology. The bio/psycho/social/spiritual model of this interaction best explains the aetiology (see Fig. 25.2).

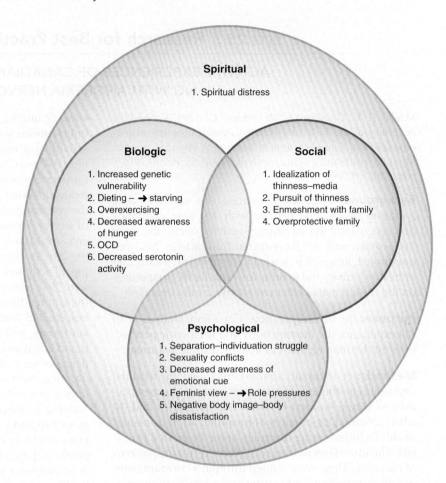

Spiritual

1. Spiritual distress

Biologic

1. Increased genetic vulnerability
2. Dieting – → starving
3. Overexercising
4. Decreased awareness of hunger
5. OCD
6. Decreased serotonin activity

Social

1. Idealization of thinness–media
2. Pursuit of thinness
3. Enmeshment with family
4. Overprotective family

Psychological

1. Separation–individuation struggle
2. Sexuality conflicts
3. Decreased awareness of emotional cue
4. Feminist view – → Role pressures
5. Negative body image–body dissatisfaction

Figure 25.2. Bio/psycho/social/spiritual aetiologies for clients with AN.

Neuropathologic Theories

Magnetic resonance imaging and computed tomography disclose changes in the brain (e.g., smaller brain volumes, cerebral ventricular enlargement, and decreased grey matter volume) of individuals with AN who have significant weight loss. In the largest study sample to date of neuroimaging and persons with AN, Fonville, Giampietro, Williams, Simmons, and Tchanturia (2014) found a correlation between grey matter volume loss and duration of illness. The correlation with duration of illness supports the implication of cerebellar atrophy in the maintenance of low weight and disrupted eating behaviour and illustrates its role in the chronic phase of anorexia nervosa. The grey matter changes may not fully return to normal after months of weight restoration.

Genetic Theories

The field of genetics in AN and other eating disorders is still in an early stage. Twin and family studies provide clear evidence of genetic contribution to AN risk (Brandys, de Kovel, Kas, van Elburg, & Adan, 2015). Shih and Woodside (2016) call for a focused effort to understand gene–diet interactions in AN as this will lead to a more personalized treatment approach and promote discovery of novel nutritional and pharmacologic interventions.

Biochemical Theories

Undernutrition and weight regulatory behaviours such as vomiting and laxative abuse can lead to a range of biochemical problems in AN, most commonly hypokalaemia and hypophosphatemia in persons who engage in vomiting, laxative abuse, or diuretic use. Hypochloremic metabolic alkalosis may develop in clients who vomit, and hyperchloremic metabolic acidosis may develop in those who abuse laxatives (Campbell & Peebles, 2014). Hyponatraemia may result from excessive water ingestion and chronic energy deprivation or diuretic misuse; low urea and creatinine concentrations may mask dehydration or renal dysfunction (Stheneur, Bergeron, & Lapeyraque, 2014). Hypoglycaemia is common (Rosen et al., 2016). Most persons admitted with AN have altered regulation of the hypothalamic–pituitary–thyroid axis during starvation with low T3 and low-normal free T4 and thyroid-stimulating hormone (Dickstein, Franco, Rome, & Auron, 2014). It is uncertain whether these neurobiologic factors contribute to the development of the eating disorder or result from the physiologic alterations caused by the eating disorder (Kaye, Wierenga, Bailer, Simmons, & Bischoff-Grethe, 2013).

Neurotransmitter and neuroendocrine abnormalities, such as blunted serotonergic function in low-weight clients, must be viewed with caution as causative factors because these disturbances are considered state related and tend to normalize after symptom remission and weight gain. To illustrate, Gauthier et al. (2014) found anxiety and depressive symptoms decreased in the course of refeeding in AN and concluded that bioavailability or tryptophan (TRP; an essential amino acid that is a precursor for synthesis of the neurotransmitter serotonin) could be a factor contributing to the decrease in anxiety and depressive symptoms. As well, O'Hara et al. (2016) noted emaciation and physical activity were, in part, mediated by dopaminergic reward processes as the symptoms observed in the acute stage were not present when dopamine was depleted.

Psychological Theories

The most widely accepted theory of AN is psychodynamic. In this theory, key tasks of separation–individuation and autonomy are interrupted. Struggles around identity and role, body image formation, sexuality, and maturity fears predominate (Treasure & Cardi, 2017). During early adolescence, when individuals begin to establish their independence and autonomy, some may feel inadequate or ineffective. Dieting and weight control may be viewed as a means to defend against these feelings. In later adolescence, when separation–individuation is a developmental task, similar conflicts arise when an adolescent is ill prepared for this stage and feels inadequate and ineffective in going forward emotionally. Because AN is usually diagnosed between 14 and 18 years of age, developmental struggles of adolescence are one acceptable theory of causation (Le Grange et al., 2014; Rohde, Stice, & Marti, 2015).

Studies have shown that girls and boys begin to differ dramatically in self-esteem just before adolescence. At the time self-doubt increases in girls, pubertal weight gain can also occur, resulting in a more rounded, mature female shape. These normal developmental occurrences can add to confusion about identity. Such confusion and self-doubt are further promoted by conflicting messages that girls receive from society about their roles in life. Girls may interpret expectations about how they should look, what roles they should perform, and what they should achieve in society as pressures to achieve "all." They often try to please others to avoid conflicts around perceived expectations. Similarly, Burns and Kehler (2014) found the intersection of masculinity, health, and physical education in school spaces produced a normative discourse that has reduced health to the singular measure of adolescent boy's BMI. This discourse has defined masculinity through a muscular body unattainable by most young men and not required for a healthy life. One youth expressed his discomfort with the surveillance and competition of physical education and his embarrassment over the inability to perform as "not my best moment," adding:

> I felt really uncomfortable because, like, there would also be girls in the class, so obviously it [felt] really embarrassing to not be one of the kids who could actually do pull-ups. And for girls it didn't really matter that much

cuz they would literally go up there, um, give it their best shot, and pretty much none of them got a pull-up. But then there were the guys, and that's when everyone really paid attention cuz, like, as a guy you were supposed to be, I guess stronger than a woman, so, I don't know. I guess it was pretty embarrassing when I couldn't do a pull-up. (Burns & Kehler, 2014, p. 14)

Boys who feel overwhelmed by such experiences may react by engaging in disordered eating/unhealthy weight behaviours. Feminists have focused on role pressure to partly explain the increase in eating disorders and the greater prevalence in females. Box 25.4 outlines some feminist assumptions regarding role, feminism, eating disorder development, and applicability to both women and men.

KEY CONCEPT

Maturity fears or feeling overwhelmed by adult responsibilities are often underlying issues for individuals with AN. Starvation is viewed as a response to these fears.

Social Theories

The media, the fashion industry, and peer pressure are significant social influences in the development of eating disorders. Magazines and television shows depict young girls and adolescents with thin and often emaciated bodies as glamorous to young women. In a study with 179 youth aged 10 to 17 years, media influence to lose weight was found a significant predictor of engagement in unhealthy weight control behaviours for girls with average to low self-esteem, while media influence to lose weight was related to frequency of engaging in unhealthy weight control behaviours for boys with higher BMIs (Mayer-Brown, Lawless, Fedele, Dumont-Driscoll, & Janicke, 2016). Among a sample of 110 five-year-old girls, 34% reported at least a moderate level of dietary restraint that was correlated with weight bias favouring thinner bodies and greater internalization of the thin ideal, media exposure, and appearance conversations (talking about clothes, looks, and hairstyles) with peers. Media exposure and appearance conversations were the strongest predictors of the girls' dietary restraint (Damiano, Paxton, Wertheim, McLean, & Gregg, 2015).

Body dissatisfaction resulting from perceiving one's own body as falling short of an ideal may include dissatisfaction about one's weight, shape, size, or even a certain body part. In a study that investigated relationships between actual body weight, body weight perception, and weight control practices among Mauritius male and female teenagers using a questionnaire-based survey, weight-loss behaviours were more prevalent among girls (Bhurtun & Jeewon, 2013). The most commonly reported methods to lose weight included reducing fat intake (84.6%), exercising (80.8%), increasing intake

---

BOX 25.4 Feminist Ideology and Eating Disorders

Feminist scholars claim that women are socialized to avoid self-expression in the face of conflict, seek attachment through putting others first, judge self by external standards, and present an outward compliant self. These societal factors and gender beliefs specific to Western cultures foster a view of one's self as the way an outside observer would see one; this may fuel constant body monitoring and comparison to societal standards, shame, and disordered eating (Borowsky, Eisenberg, Bucchianeri, Piran, & Neumark-Sztainer, 2016; Carr, Green, & Ponce, 2015).

Body size and weight are aspects of identity upon which difference is identified. Social and health discourses have co-constructed a body hierarchy that positions slender people as the norm and fat people as the "other." In doing so, the ideal slender body type is conferred with implicit and explicit advantages and privileges that include greater likelihood for employment, romantic relationships, popularity, and protection from peer victimization. In contrast, fat or overweight people are marginalized as individuals to be laughed at, presumed as lazy and ugly, and in need of health advice. Understanding the extent to which ideals and discourses about body weight and shape act to delimit social and class status can help address the influence of the internalization of such ideals (van Amsterdam, 2013).

Feminists take issue with the biomedical explanation of eating disorders, seeing it as limiting and patriarchal. In a culture that rewards thinness and toned bodies but simultaneously peddles consumer products encouraging excess, it can be difficult for anyone to decipher how to attain a body identified as healthy and ideal (LaMarre & Rice, 2016). The everyday sexism and historically lower social status experienced by women as well as sexual abuse and violence are seen as pathways that expose women to risk for body disturbances (Borowsky et al., 2015). The recovery of society must take place if the prevalence of eating disorders is to decrease. For this to occur, women must be emancipated, have a voice, and be socialized differently so their stories and perspectives may be known (Penny, 2013). Feminism, by promoting critical evaluation of social imperatives and encouraging questioning of physical appearance norms, may buffer persons from self-destructive body image concerns and disordered eating. Feminist beliefs are associated with more positive body image, lower drive for thinness, and better ability to cope with societal pressures to look and act a certain way (Kinsaul, Curtin, Bazzini, & Martz, 2014). Penny (2013) asserts that "maybe women who are plain, or large, or old, or differently abled, or who simply don't give a damn what they look like because they're too busy saving the world or rearranging their sock drawer, have as much right to take up space as anyone else" (p. 38).

Principles of the feminist relational model apply to males with eating disorders. A feminist relational approach proposes that, in growing up, boys may long for connection but are pushed to become autonomous before they have developed the ability to identify their feelings and needs. The increase in eating disorders among males reveals a need to explore their gender roles and expectations, globalized exposure to media images of idealized male bodies, and the possibility that men express distress through their bodies. This approach focuses less on individual pathology and more on individuals' responses to pressures, expectations, roles, or environment (Webb, 2014). Contextualizing men's body-related responses within sociopolitical realities may enable greater understanding.

---

of fruits and vegetables (73.1%), and decreasing intake of sugar (66.7%). Among the weight-loss teens, body weight perception was poorly associated with actual weight status in that 88.5% perceived themselves as overweight even though only 19.2% were overweight. The perception of self as overweight when at an acceptable weight for height is not exclusive to Mauritius adolescents. Blackburn et al. (2016) compared anthropometric data from 428 Quebec men and women aged 18 to 35 years with their actual 3D image to evaluate the relationship between women and men's perception of their "real" body, ideal body image, and levels of self-esteem. In both women and men, the most important factor explaining higher level of self-esteem was higher satisfaction with aspects of one's body. In men, a distorted body image, either by seeing themselves as thinner than the reality or by not having a good perception of their body shape, improved self-esteem. Media pressure was not significant in men. However, women who had a higher level of internalization of media ideals as personal standards of attractiveness were found to have a lower level of self-esteem. Women who claimed to never expect a change in their silhouette before buying new clothes, as well as those who attempted to control their weight in the last year, showed better self-esteem.

Social comparison theory helps explain how sociocultural pressure may influence the development of eating disorders. The central premise of social comparison theory is that people have an innate drive to evaluate their own standing on a wide range of characteristics, and in the absence of objective standards, people compare themselves with others in the social environment to obtain information about their own qualities or performance (Homan & Lemmon, 2016). Appearance comparisons with those considered more attractive are referred to as upward appearance comparisons, whereas comparisons made with those considered less attractive are called downward appearance comparisons. Lin and Soby (2016), in surveying online responses of 325 female college students aged 18 to 25, found that women who engaged in upward or downward appearance comparisons were more likely to exhibit higher levels of drive for thinness and dietary restraint. There was a positive relationship between upward comparisons and body dissatisfaction or negative body talk. Lin and Soby concluded that women who do not engage in upward and downward appearance comparisons at all may be at the lowest risk for negative body image. Arcelus et al. (2013) suggest that social comparisons are related to uncertainties about the self and self-esteem and that women who compare themselves with inappropriate targets such as idealized images are more vulnerable toward developing eating disorders. In other studies, the process of social comparison, based upon physical and/or personality features, was found to increase the likelihood of negative self-evaluation, body dissatisfaction, and disturbed eating behaviours due to feelings of insecurity (Chrisler, Fung, Lopez, & Gorman, 2013; Sharpe, Damazer, Treasure, & Schmidt, 2013; Ty & Francis, 2013).

KEY CONCEPT

Body dissatisfaction is the belief that one's current body size differs from a highly valued ideal body size and that this difference deserves negative appraisal and may be expressed through comments including "I feel too fat/too gross." Body dissatisfaction has been related to low self-esteem, depression, dieting, binge eating, and purging.

KEY CONCEPT

Social comparison—evaluating oneself against idealized others, such as models or attractive peers—is a major factor in body dissatisfaction, weight anxiety, and disturbed eating.

Family Responses

Early family theories and observations classically labelled the family of the individual with AN as *enmeshed*, overprotective, rigid, and unable to resolve conflicts. In an enmeshed family, boundaries that define individual autonomy are weak: One member may relay communication from another to a third; excessive togetherness may intrude on privacy. An enmeshed, overprotective, and rigid family engenders and maintains the eating disorder, whereas a highly cohesive and flexible family style is considered more favourable for the son or daughter's well-being and move into maturation and independence. In studying factors related to dysfunctional family functioning, Anastasiadou et al. (2016) found both fathers' and mothers' anxiety and depressive symptom scores, accommodation and enabling behaviours, and the perception of their family as rigid, related to the symptom severity of their children. In the case of the mothers, negative caregiving experience and emotional overinvolvement related to higher levels of eating disorder attitudes and behaviours. In the case of fathers, criticism levels were associated with eating disorder symptom severity. These results support a multidetermined and contextual view of eating disorders, which takes into consideration, both theoretically and methodologically, whether family functioning precedes, maintains, or comes as a consequence of the eating disorder. Research conceptualizations support the idea that no particular pattern of functioning exists in families of clients with eating disorders.

Overprotectiveness is defined as acting on a high degree of concern for another. Parental overprotectiveness may hinder the child's development of autonomy and competence. Family *rigidity* refers to maintaining the status quo and avoiding change and conflict often through being heavily committed to a strong moral code or religious orientation. Laghi et al. (2017) researched whether 36 adolescents with AN and their parents differ from healthy controls in perceptions of family functioning. The findings highlighted a general agreement among family members, except that mothers and daughters had a different view of the dimension of rigidity; in particular, daughters with AN rated their families as characterized by less rigidity compared to mothers. When compared to controls, findings confirmed that girls with AN had a worse perception of family functioning and were less satisfied about their families. These adolescents with AN rated family environment as poorly communicative, characterized by a low level of emotional bonding between family members and by a low ability to change when circumstances require. Laghi et al. suggest these dimensions could represent the aspects on which treatment should be focused, to enable family members to improve their abilities and learn how to act with a better use of functional patterns. In addition, the discrepancy found between daughters and mothers stresses the importance of taking into consideration the different views of family members, as such information may represent an essential resource in health care settings.

KEY CONCEPT

Enmeshment refers to an extreme form of intensity in family interactions.

Spiritual Theories

Core struggles in eating disorders are spiritual in nature. One woman framed her AN symptoms as having a beneficial spiritual meaning, "Like maybe [God] wanted me to go through that, and He let me choose that so I could get through difficult situations in my life" (Buser, Parkins, & Buser, 2014, p. 104). Spirituality involves developing a personal quest for understanding answers to ultimate questions about life, meaning, and a relationship with the transcendent (Akrawi, Bartrop, Potter, & Touyz, 2015) and having a sense of purpose or meaning in life (Cottingham, Davis, Craycraft, Keiper, & Abernethy, 2014). Young women's struggles in the formation of their body image, sense of self, relationship building, and connection with the world often reflect an underlying personal journey to achieve a stable positive self-identity, a larger purpose in life, and a sustained connectedness with others—all necessary conditions for spiritual development (Zhang, 2013). As well, women may turn to the pursuit of thinness as a method of acquiring meaning when religion has failed to meet their deep-seated needs for meaning, purpose, and value (Rider et al., 2014).

Historically, the example of Catherine of Sienna (1347–1380), who fasted as part of extreme asceticism, demonstrated profound preoccupation with eating.

Few systematic studies have examined an aetiologic connection between religiosity (devotion to the rituals and traditions of a religion) and AN. Sipilä et al. (2017) found no evidence that either higher personal or parental religiosity is significantly associated with lifetime AN in their population-based Finnish twin cohort. However, they could not exclude the possibility that religiosity might have a positive effect on body image. Weinberger-Litman et al. (2016) suggest that individuals who are intrinsically motivated toward religion are more internally motivated in general and are less likely to make decisions based on appearance or externalities. Intrinsic religious orientation may serve as a buffer to the development of disordered eating and body dissatisfaction via lower levels of thin-ideal internalization (Weinberger-Litman et al., 2016).

Risk Factors

Similar risk factors may put individuals at risk for AN, BN, and BED. The risk factors are classified in the same way as are the aetiologic categories: biologic, psychological, social, and spiritual (Fig. 25.3).

Biologic

Biologic risk factors include dieting, altered metabolic rate, and a history of overweight or obesity. Dieting

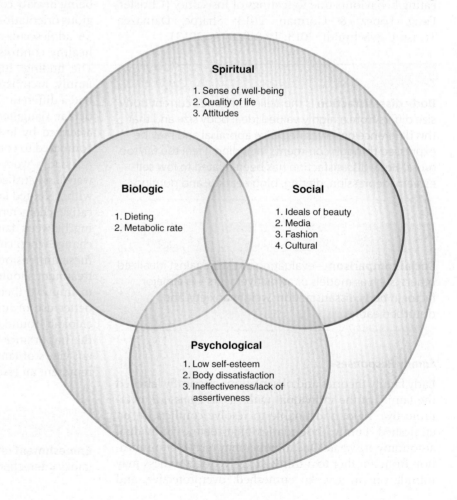

Figure 25.3. Bio/psycho/social/spiritual risk factors for eating disorders.

despite weight loss and an increase in basal metabolic rate are the most studied biologic risk factors. Individuals diet because of body dissatisfaction, a need for control, an actual weight gain, and the fear of weight gain. Girls at risk for developing AN may begin to diet in response to a prepubertal weight increase. The starvation of AN may lead to binge eating followed by purging as a compensatory behaviour when restricting food intake is no longer effective or not possible to maintain (Fairburn & Cooper, 2014). For individuals at risk for BN, purging ensues because of fear of becoming fat, and further dieting occurs in response to the binge eating and its associated negative effect. Those who develop obesity as a consequence of BED may have a history of "yo-yo" dieting also known as weight cycling, which has impaired their metabolic response (amount of calories burned daily) so that over time their dieting efforts become ineffective as the cycle of gaining weight back and attempting to lose the weight recurs (Ellis, 2016).

High-level exercise and compulsive physical activity have been associated with eating disorder symptoms of dietary restraint, weight and shape concerns, obsession with food, poor concentration, drive for thinness, body dissatisfaction, and binge eating (Rizk et al., 2015). Adolescents with a history of overweight or obesity represent a substantial portion of treatment-seeking adolescents with restrictive eating disorders (Lebow, Sim, & Kransdorf, 2015) and individuals with BED (Hilbert et al., 2014). Further, adolescent eating, weight, and shape concerns mediate the relationship between parent-perceived childhood overweight at age 10 and later risk for a binge-eating or purging eating disorder (Allen, Byrne, & Crosby, 2015). Eating disorder symptoms at 12 years of age are greater body dissatisfaction for both sexes and, for girls only, higher depressive symptoms (Evans et al., 2017). For both males and females, higher eating disorder symptoms at 9 years of age significantly predict higher eating disorder symptoms at age 12 years. Dietary restraint at 7 years of age predicts boys' but not girls' eating disorder symptoms at age 12. Adolescent girls around the age of 13 years are more likely to use disordered eating behaviours to relieve depressive symptoms, and reciprocally, disordered eating gives rise to negative self-evaluations and depressed affect (Evans et al., 2017). Early-appearing hyperactivity/inattention is a risk factor for adolescent binge eating (Sonneville et al., 2015).

Pubertal growth puts girls at increased risk relative to boys given that the pubertal physical changes (e.g., increased adiposity) move them away from society's ideal body shape for women, while physical changes in boys (i.e., increased muscle mass and shoulder width) move them closer to the sociocultural valued changes for men's body shape and size, such as athletic ability. The timing of puberty rather than puberty itself may play a role in body satisfaction for boys (de Guzman & Nishina, 2014). Late-maturing boys are more likely to

have higher levels of body dissatisfaction, be less popular with their peers, have more conflict with parents, and show more depressive symptoms. Girls who mature early have been found to be at the greatest risk of body dissatisfaction (Klump, 2013) and also tend to be less popular, have poorer self-esteem, and have higher levels of depression than do later-maturing girls.

Psychological

Depressive symptoms and low self-esteem are two psychological risk factors associated with restrictive eating (Haynos, Watts, Loth, Pearson, & Neumark-Stzainer, 2016). In writing of their experiences with AN, women expressed constant performance anxiety, low self-esteem, depressed state of mind, and self-destructive behaviours, and engaged in self-harm practices of cutting, vomiting, or extreme physical training stating "Nothing cures pain as effectively as pain" (Dahlborg Lyckhage, Gardvik, Karlsson, Törner, & Berndtsson, 2015, p. 4). Adolescent girls who are dissatisfied with their body experience body shame, which may lead to development of disturbed eating behaviours (Mustapic, Marcinko, & Vargek, 2015). Body shame encompasses negative feelings about the self in general. Those girls and women whose eating behaviours are disordered feel bad about themselves in relation to their bodies and eating difficulties, more so than they do about their behaviours. Instead of seeing their eating problems as a problematic set of behaviours and cognitions that are separate from the self, they view them as reflections of their self-worth. Women with restricting AN report higher scores on perceived physical appearance and global self-worth than do those with the binge-eating–purging subtype or BN (Obeid, Buchholz, Boerner, Henderson, & Norris, 2013). This may be because those with restrictive behaviours achieve the "thin ideal" and the goals they set out to accomplish.

Comparing Canadian female populations of both undergraduate students ($n = 155$) and clients beginning treatment for eating disorders ($n = 97$), Kelly, Vimalakanthan, and Carter (2014) found client self-esteem a negative predictor, client BMI a positive predictor, and client fear of self-compassion the strongest predictor of eating disorder symptoms. For the study's student population, low self-compassion was the strongest predictor of eating disorder symptoms. Self-compassion is the tendency to respond to one's own suffering by adopting an attitude of caring and kindness rather than judgment and by viewing personal pain as common within humanity rather than as isolating. As such, self-compassion is positively correlated with self-esteem and also with acknowledging one's role in setbacks, learning from, and improving upon one's mistakes (Schoenefeld & Webb, 2013). Self-compassion is thus a frightening experience for individuals who feel undeserving of compassion and worry about lowered personal standards. Research has demonstrated that resilience or protective factors, such as satisfaction with life and having an engaged life, can mediate psychological risk factors of low self-esteem and body dissatisfaction among 13- to 18-year-old male and female adolescents and can help prevent eating disorder development (Góngora, 2014). Understandably, developing resilience (turning away from deep dissatisfaction with life toward acting on one's determination to change) preceded the experience of recovery in women with AN and BN (Las Hayas et al., 2016).

Childhood sexual abuse is associated with all eating disorders with binge-eating behaviours (AN binge–purge [AN-BP]), BN, BED, and subclinical forms of BN and BED (Micali et al., 2017). Sexual abuse perpetrated by a nonstranger was twice as prevalent among women with AN-BP, but as prevalent as sexual abuse by a stranger for BN and BED. Childhood unhappiness was associated with higher odds of developing restricting AN, BN, BED, and subclinical purging. Childhood life events of parental separation or divorce were positively associated with all but subclinical eating disorders. Reporting low maternal warmth was also associated with increased odds for BN, BED, and subclinical binge-eating and purging disorders. Women who reported a more oppressive relationship with parents had higher odds of AN-BP, BED, subclinical BN, AN, and purging.

An external locus of control was associated with BED and interpersonal sensitivity with all eating disorders (Micali et al., 2017). Better maternal care was protective for BN, while perceived criticism and parental expectations of perfectionism were associated with bulimic behaviours (La Mela et al., 2015). In addition to perfectionism, the trait of impulsivity is a risk factor for BN that may largely be genetically determined (Slof-Op't Landt et al., 2013). In a sample of college women, those with eating issues were clustered into groups (dysregulated, rigid, and adaptive) associated with adjustment difficulties and specific family disturbances (Perkins, Slane, & Klump, 2013). Women in the dysregulated group reported the least parental empathy, warmth, and affection and the most parental hostility, intrusion, and maternal overprotection

LGBT students report a significantly higher prevalence of disordered eating than heterosexual students. Although the prevalence of disordered eating behaviours for most sexual orientation groups decreased between 1999/2001 and 2011/2013, the odds of fasting, using diet pills, and purging to control weight remain mostly unchanged for bisexual females and increased (at least twice the odds for each variable) among lesbians (Watson, Adjei, Saewyc, Homma, & Goodenow, 2017).

Researchers have found a relationship between stress, anxiety, depression, and binge eating (Rosenbaum &

White, 2015). Women report higher levels of binge-eating symptoms, anxiety, and stress than men; women have higher rates of BED. Rosenbaum and White (2015) recommended further study of the idea that binge eating may serve to decrease one domain (i.e., anxiety) but increase another (i.e., depression). Comparing 107 clients with BED and 107 clients with bulimia nervosa (BN), matched for duration of illness, clients with BED reported a greater number of traumatic events in the 6 months preceding onset, with bereavement, separation from a family member and accident events more often (Degortes et al., 2014). In a study with older men, Rosenberger and Dorflinger (2013) found that depressive symptoms, lower self-efficacy in sticking with healthier eating habits (e.g., eating smaller portions), higher self-classified weight, and perceived barriers to physical activity (e.g., lack of time, social support, energy level, and willpower) significantly predicted binge eating.

Social

In families, weight teasing and parental underinvolvement are correlates of childhood BED (Saltzman & Liechty, 2016). Although family meals protect against dieting for girls whose families engaged in no or low-level weight-related teasing, exposure to family meals became a risk factor for engaging in dieting when weight teasing was present (Loth et al., 2015). Appearance-related teasing by mothers, fathers, siblings, and peers was associated with higher body dissatisfaction among girls and appearance-related teasing by fathers was associated with a greater drive for muscularity among boys (Schaefer & Salafia, 2014). Sibling teasing was reported more frequently than teasing from mothers or fathers, and the odds of being teased by siblings increased dramatically if adolescents were teased by either parent. Beyond adolescence, men who receive negative commentary (compared to positive commentary) are more likely to experience eating pathology and body dissatisfaction and report more dieting behaviours (Schuster, Negy, & Tantleff-Dunn, 2013).

Media, the fashion industry, and society's focus on the ideal body type are social risk factors for eating disorders. In addition, peer pressure and attitudes reinforce societal messages regarding the importance of thinness or popularity. Some adolescents reported that dieting, binge eating, and purging were learned behaviours, resulting from peer pressure and a perceived need to conform. As demonstrated by their scores on eating behaviour scales, young women who experienced weight-related teasing by peers during childhood and adolescence were more likely to develop disturbed eating behaviours and eating disorders than were their non–weight-teased peers. Those who recalled their weight at ages 6, 12, or 16 years as being heavier than average reported having endured weight teasing more frequently and greater distress than their lighter counterparts (Quick, McWilliams, &

Byrd-Bredbenner, 2013). In addition to girls, boys who reported more teasing about their weight and appearance by friends or peers showed greater concurrent body dissatisfaction (Webb & Zimmer-Gembeck, 2014). School-level weight-related teasing is also associated with greater depressive symptoms in boys (Lampard, MacLehose, Eisenberg, Neumark-Sztainer, & Davison, 2014). Bullying predicts eating disorder symptoms for both bullies and victims, with victims displaying increases in anorexic, bulimic, and binge-eating symptoms and bullies having high prevalence of both binge eating and vomiting. The experience of criticizing/teasing others may sensitize bullies to their own physical attributes and shortcomings; bullies may experience regret or guilt following bullying incidents, and this contributes to impulsive eating behaviours (Copeland et al., 2015).

Although peers increase in importance throughout adolescence, romantic partners become primary sources of personal feedback and satisfaction during adulthood. In a community-based study that represented a range of eating disorders, women reported the onset of symptoms as triggered by abusive intimate relationships, weight-related teasing from a partner, and coping with neglect or overcontrolling by a partner through binge eating or restriction (Mitchison, Dawson, Hand, Mond, & Hay, 2016).

The ways in which individuals cope with weight stigma from the public can be seen as risk factors for promoting or prolonging adverse eating behaviours. For example, exposure to weight-stigmatizing stimuli in individuals with obesity and BED leads to increased calorie consumption and reinforces binge-eating intentions and behaviour. Negative stereotypes toward individuals with BN and AN promote social rejection and limit help seeking (Puhl & Suh, 2015). People were found more resistant to having social contact with a person experiencing AN compared to a person with obesity or cancer (Zwickert & Rieger, 2013).

Athletes are at greater risk for developing eating disorders. The actual performance demands of a sport and the sports environment itself can intensify body- and weight-related concerns because of such factors as pressure from coaches and parents, social comparisons with teammates, team weigh-ins, physique-revealing uniforms, and judging criteria. Elite athletes are particularly at risk (Martinsen & Sundgot-Borgen, 2013). Ballet dancers are at high risk because of the need to maintain a particular appearance and performance; both male and female athletes are at risk for developing eating disorders. In particular, boys and men involved in weight-classed sports that necessitate weight restrictions, such as wrestling, bodybuilding, rowing, ski jumping, and swimming, are more likely to engage in pathogenic eating and weight control behaviours than are endurance athletes (Chatterton & Petrie, 2013).

Spiritual

Research into the relationship of spirituality and eating pathology is emerging and findings conflictive. Some research suggests that specific aspects of religious involvement are protective against the development of body dissatisfaction and dysfunctional eating. For example, seeing one's body as having sacred qualities is associated with more body satisfaction and less body objectification (Henderson & Ellison, 2015; Jacobson, Hall, & Anderson, 2013). Daily spiritual experiences and having a stronger commitment to one's religion, praying more, and using positive religious coping have been associated with more body satisfaction and fewer unhealthy eating habits (Homan & Cavanaugh, 2013; Piko & Brassai, 2016). Spirituality's general emphasis on greater purpose and connectedness may encourage individuals to define themselves more by their contributions to society or relationships than by their appearance, perhaps promoting self-acceptance regardless of their discrepancy or similarity to a cultural ideal. In other research, the importance of religion in one's life has been recently correlated with greater eating pathology. Goulet, Henrie, and Szymanski (2017) suggest that women who place greater importance on religion may be more attentive to religious teachings about fasting for religious purposes or reconciliation for sins (e.g., gluttony). As well, worrying about being deserted by God/Higher Power (Buser & Bernard, 2013) or seeking to avoid attachment to God/Higher Power (Strenger, Schnitker, & Felke, 2016) are each associated with increased levels of bulimic symptoms. Attendance and prayer were found to buffer the relationship between binge eating and self-esteem in a large national sample of young women (Henderson & Ellison, 2015).

Interdisciplinary Treatment

Treatment of the client with AN focuses on initiating nutritional rehabilitation, resolving conflicts around body image disturbance, increasing effective coping, addressing the underlying conflicts related to maturity fears and role conflict, and assisting the family with healthy functioning and communication. The preferred method of treatment is outpatient care that includes family-based interventions if the client is a child or adolescent (Findlay, Pinzon, Taddeo, Katzman, & Canadian Paediatric Society Adolescent Health Committee, 2013). The acuity of the eating disorder is carefully monitored. Inpatient hospital admission is warranted if health deteriorates and the client meets the criteria outlined in Table 25.3. Clients are often ambivalent about being admitted for weight restoration. Considering the difficulty clients experience in consenting to relinquish the AN, Woodside et al. (2016) describe an approach to admission for severe and enduring AN as the adult client and clinician mutually negotiating a set of goals

Table 25.3 Criteria for Hospitalization of Children, Adolescents, and Adults With Eating Disorders

Presence of one or more of the following:	
Medical	**Psychiatric**

• Weight loss that is:
  ≤75% below median BMI for age, sex, and height
  Rapid, e.g., greater than 15% in 1 month
  Associated with physiologic instability unexplained by another
    medical condition
  Rapidly approaching weight at which physiologic instability occurred
    in the past
• BMI < 16 for adults
• Heart rate for children, adolescents, and adults (resting daytime)
  <40 bpm
• ECG abnormalities (e.g., bradycardia, other cardiac arrhythmias,
  prolonged QT)
• Cardiac oedema
• Hemodynamic compromise (bradycardia, hypotension, hypothermia)
• Orthostasis
• Hypoglycaemia
• Electrolyte disturbance (hypokalaemia, hyponatraemia,
  hypophosphataemia, and/or metabolic acidosis or alkalosis)
• Acute medical complications due to starvation (e.g., syncope,
  seizures, cardiac failure, pancreatitis)
• Comorbid medical or psychiatric condition that hinders appropriate
  ate outpatient treatment (e.g., severe depression, suicide ideation,
  obsessive–compulsive disorder, type 1 diabetes)
• Uncertainty of the diagnosis of an eating disorder
	• Acute food refusal
	• Suicidal thoughts or actions
	• Significant comorbid diagnosis that interferes with the
	  treatment of an eating disorder (e.g., severe depression,
	  OCD, anxiety)
	• Failure of outpatient treatment
	• Uncontrollable binge eating and/or purging
	• Inadequate social support and/or follow-up medical or
	  psychiatric care

Source: Academy for Eating Disorders' Medical Care Standards Committee. (2016). *Eating disorders: A guide to medical care: Critical points for early recognition & medical risk management in the care of individuals with eating disorders.*
AED REPORT (3rd ed.). Retrieved from http://www.aedweb.org/images/updatedmedicalcareguidelines/AED-Medical-Care-Guidelines_English_02.28.17_NEW.pdf

and plan with no preconceived notions, aside from the goals being realistic for the setting and consistent with the maintenance or improvement of health.

Treatment goals are developed around medical stabilization, nutritional rehabilitation to achieve weight restoration, management of refeeding and its potential complications, and interruption of purging/compensatory behaviours. For full recovery from an eating disorder, weight restoration alone is not a sufficient end goal. It is important that distorted body image and other disordered thoughts/behaviours, psychological comorbidities, and social or functional impairments be addressed (Academy of Eating Disorders [AED], 2016). Treatment requires an interdisciplinary approach of professionals who together strive to meet the multidisciplinary needs of the client (Lock et al., 2015). Dieticians plan a weight-increasing program; physicians, nurses, psychologists, and social workers monitor the refeeding process and its effects and establish the intensive therapies that must be instituted after the refeeding phase. Team members may include a consulting psychiatrist, occupational therapist, and dentist. Family must be considered members of the team.

Individuals with AN are often intelligent, engaging, and (with the exception of their emaciated state)

appear nonimpaired. Because of this, they may be erroneously perceived as less sick (Parry, 2014). It is therefore important to remember the high rates of mortality and medical complications among individuals with eating disorders. If they are severely malnourished and their somatic systems are seriously compromised, a medical unit might be the choice for the initial intensive refeeding phase that requires close monitoring (see Table 25.2).

The intensive therapies needed to help clients with their underlying issues (e.g., body dissatisfaction and low self-esteem) and families with communication typically begin after refeeding because concentration is usually impaired in the severely undernourished individual with anorexia. During this phase of treatment, a privilege-earning program is often implemented in which positive reinforcers, such as having visitors and receiving passes to go outside the hospital, are earned based on weight gain. After an acceptable weight (at least 85% of ideal) is established, the client may be discharged to a partial hospitalization program or an intensive outpatient program. Art therapy and psychodrama may be more effective than traditional group therapy for adolescents with eating disorders during the acute phases, when the concentration required for verbal therapy may be impaired. Art therapy can provide access to feelings and emotions that have long been repressed or suppressed, and this increases bodily awareness, helping to clarify problems central to the position of the anorexia such as identity (Kramer, 2015). Family therapy typically begins while the individual is still hospitalized.

Pharmacologic Interventions

Many experts claim that the symptoms of AN, such as body distortion and hyperactivity, are primarily the result of starvation, which causes changes in brain chemistry. Therefore, restoring weight influences symptom remission more than psychopharmacology. It is generally held that the core symptoms of AN are unresponsive to psychotropic medications; however, these medications may be useful in treating comorbid psychiatric conditions and preventing relapses (Garner, Anderson, Keiper, Whynott, & Parker, 2016; Milano et al., 2013). The use of tricyclic antidepressants is discouraged, as they generally failed to accelerate weight regain in clinical trials (Mitchell, Roerig, & Steffen, 2013) and may increase susceptibility to hypotension and cardiac arrhythmias (Milano et al., 2013). Research has demonstrated that selective serotonin reuptake inhibitors (SSRIs) are not efficacious for the early treatment of AN (Mitchell et al., 2013), possibly because low body weights cause low protein stores, and protein is needed for SSRI metabolism. However, some clinical experts have found that the SSRIs can be effective later, during outpatient treatment and after weight restoration to address symptoms such as obsessiveness, ritualistic behaviours, and perfectionism. SSRIs must be used with caution, and the client's weight must be constantly monitored because, during the initiation phase, some of the SSRIs may cause weight loss. Bupropion is contraindicated because of increased risk of seizures (American Society of Health-System Pharmacists, 2017). Lebow, Sim, Erwin, and Murad (2013) found no evidence that atypical antipsychotics are useful in the treatment of either the cognitive or weight-loss symptoms of AN and, despite having a positive effect on depression, can increase anxiety in an AN population. Lebow et al. suggested that atypical antipsychotics, which have been shown to increase hunger and thus promote weight gain in other samples, are not enough to overcome the eating disorder drive for thinness. Marzola et al. (2015) found promising results on the effectiveness of aripiprazole augmentation in reducing eating-related obsessions and compulsions, although caution is needed when interpreting these findings as those clients who were started with an augmentation agent were characterized by greater clinical severity upon admission than those who received SSRIs as monotherapy.

There is no evidence to support the efficacy of mood stabilizers (e.g., lithium) for treating AN. These medications should be used if comorbid bipolar disorders are identified (Tseng, Chang, Liao, & Chen, 2017) and with extreme caution in clients with dehydration and compromised renal function (Williams, 2014). Investigation of prokinetic agents to alleviate gastrointestinal (GI) complaints associated with refeeding (e.g., bloating, early satiety) resulted in removal of cisapride (Prepulsid) from the market because of potentially fatal cardiac effects (Kerr, 2016). Oestrogen replacement therapy in the form of oral contraceptive pills has not been found effective in preventing osteopenia/osteoporosis in AN (Bergström et al., 2013). A practical reason to refrain from using hormonal therapy is that it may cause resumption of menses, which in turn may give a false sense of being cured and reinforce denial in women who are still at a low weight. The use of bisphosphonates to improve bone density has shown to increase bone mass density in women with AN; however, no improvement was found in adolescents with AN (Misra & Klibanski, 2014). These differing results in adults versus adolescents with AN may reflect differences in bone turnover in the two age groups. Also, bisphosphonates have an extremely long half-life and can persist in the body for many years after the discontinuation of treatment. Because of this possible effect on foetal bone development, their use is cautioned in adolescents and young women of reproductive age.

Body weight is the most important determinant of bone density; optimal intervention promotes weight restoration. Therefore, standard treatment for anorexia nervosa consists of nutritional rehabilitation and psychotherapy. There is little evidence supporting the use of medications. Although a few randomized trials suggest that adjunctive antipsychotics may possibly enhance weight gain, other psychotropic drugs have demonstrated little or no benefit in accelerating weight gain or relieving psychological symptoms (Walsh, 2017).

Priority Care Issues

In a 20-year study of 246 treatment-seeking female clients with AN or BN, risk of premature death among those with lifetime AN peaked within the first 10 years, resulting in a standardized mortality ratio of 7.7% (Franko et al., 2013). Predictors of mortality in AN included long duration of illness, alcohol abuse, low BMI, and poor social adjustment. The *Government of Canada's Report of the Standing Committee on the Status of Women* (2014) estimates the overall mortality rate for AN at between 10% and 15%. Together, AN and BN kill approximately 1,000 to 1,500 Canadians per year. The true lethality of eating disorders is hidden when death certificates do not record eating disorders as the cause of death, but instead record the medical complication that killed the person or, if applicable, suicide, as the cause of death.

Stigma is an issue that may impede seeking treatment. Because eating disorders are perceived as trivial and self-inflicted, affected individuals believe they are personally responsible for their condition (Griffiths, Mond, Murray, & Touyz, 2015). Studies within university settings have found individuals with AN more stigmatized than obesity and perceived as having significantly more psychological problems and impairment than individuals with obesity (Murakami, Essayli, & Latner, 2016; Zwickert & Rieger, 2013). However, Bannatyne and Abel (2015) found lower levels of reported blame-based stigma among university students when the aetiology of AN was conceptualized as biologic rather than sociocultural.

Nursing Management: Human Response to Anorexia Nervosa Disorder

Establishing therapeutic alliance with individuals with AN may be difficult initially because they may be suspicious and mistrustful. They often express fear of adults, especially health care professionals, whom they believe want to "make them fat." Because of their low body weight and starvation, they are often impatient and irritable. A matter of fact, accepting approach is important. Providing a rationale for all interventions helps build trust. Power struggles over eating are common; remaining nonreactive is a challenge. In avoiding such power struggles, the nurse monitors and reduces personal feelings of frustration and need for control (see Box 25.5).

Nursing management involves bio/psycho/social/ spiritual assessment and interventions (see Nursing Care Plan 25.1).

Biologic Domain

Assessment

A thorough evaluation of the client's body systems is important because many systems can be compromised by starvation. A detailed history from both the individual with AN and the family, including the length and duration of symptoms, such as avoiding meals and over exercising, is necessary to assess altered nutrition. The longer the duration of these behaviours typically means more difficult and prolonged recovery.

Nursing Diagnoses for Biologic Domain

A primary nursing diagnosis is Imbalanced Nutrition: Less Than Body Requirements.

BOX 25.5

THERAPEUTIC DIALOGUE

The Client With an Eating Disorder

Ineffective Approach

Nurse: You haven't eaten your lunch yet.
Client: I can't. I'm already fat.
Nurse: Look at you, you're skin and bones.
Client: I'll eat when I go out this afternoon on pass.
Nurse: You can't go on pass. You have to start realizing that you are sick. Because you can't take care of yourself, we are in charge.
Client: You're trying to control me.
Nurse: We are trying to be responsible.
Client: I won't eat!
Nurse: Then you will also lose the next pass.
Client: Well I won't go out! At least I won't get fatter.

Effective Approach

Nurse: You haven't eaten your lunch.
Client: I can't. I'm already fat.
Nurse: You're uncomfortable with how you see yourself and with eating?
Client: I'll eat when I go out on pass.

Nurse: You and I and the other members of your treatment team wrote your behavioural plan together. You know then that you will not be able to go out because your pass is dependent on you eating both breakfast and lunch.
Client: You're trying to control me.
Nurse: The plan is to help you learn to take control over the eating disorder. It sure does mean a lot of hard work for you. How can I help you right now with this meal?
Client: What if I eat half?
Nurse: You are to eat all of it. Why don't I sit here while you eat? Eating is scary for you. We can talk about other choices you have on the unit; tonight, you can choose the movie or board games.
Client: Okay, at least I have some choices.

Critical Thinking Challenge

- What effect did the first interaction have on the client's behaviour? Why?
- In the second interaction, what theories and interventions regarding eating disorders did the nurse use in her approach to the client?

NURSING CARE PLAN 25.1

Maddison is a 19-year-old university student from Nova Scotia who is 163 cm (5'4") tall and weighs 44.4 kg (98 pounds). A 2nd year Arts student, she initially sought treatment at the Student Health Centre for diarrhoea, cramps, gas, and bloating, saying "I think I have a nervous stomach." She tells the nurse that she is having difficulty sleeping, is stressed out to the point of wanting to stay in bed all day, and states "I feel like such a waste of a university education. I have been trying so hard to be my best and do well. But I can't seem to function. It might be best if I took enough sleeping pills to never wake up!"

Maddison believes that her eating is out of control. Unwanted eating binges as often as once or twice a day have provoked her to try to avoid the feared weight gain through taking laxatives in addition to self-inducing vomiting after eating what she perceives as too much. "I force myself to vomit when I eat regular salad dressing instead of fat-free. I shouldn't be eating so much and it takes so long to get it all back out of my stomach! But I can't let myself get fat again like I was in high school. I felt sad all the time then, as I do now. But never again will I let others call me 'Fatty Maddy' or take advantage of me." She added "I'm so on my own. I can't go out with my friends because they always want to go and eat or drink with them. I don't want them to find me puking in the restaurant or bar toilet. They say I am lucky to have such a fast metabolism. Little do they know that inside I am falling apart! Right now I can't handle the 25-minute bus ride home from the university without binging and purging. I even developed the insane habit of bingeing on chips in the back of the bus and throwing up into my empty Red Bull can. I pray to God that nobody ever saw it!"

Maddison was hospitalized for suicidality and assessment of anorexia nervosa, binge–purge type.

Setting: Inpatient Psychiatric Unit

Baseline Assessment: Maddison appears dishevelled and tearful. She discloses she has been watching her diet since high school and began using laxatives to help prevent her from gaining as she sometimes binges on potato chips and energy drinks. Her symptoms of binge eating and purging worsened over the past month as a result of realizing past sexual abuse by an older relative. She is depressed and angry and has not told anyone about the abuse.

History: Maddison lives alone in an apartment just outside city limits. She weighs herself before and after every meal or snack. She lost 12 kg since graduating from high school 2 years ago, by skipping meals and restricting the quantity of food consumed. She had tried using diet tea and slimming pills on a few occasions. Despite being underweight, she perceives herself as being too fat. She acknowledges the frequency of self-induced vomiting as 7 to 10 times per week; she takes 6 Ex-Lax tablets daily "to hurry the food out of my system." Maddison has occasionally experienced heart palpations, weakness, dizziness, and fatigue. She feels ashamed and guilty about binge eating, self-induced vomiting, and laxative use. She perceives her weight to be much higher than she wishes and desires a slimmer face and thinner legs. She feels that she deserves punishment for her eating behaviour and is contemplating suicide.

Physical findings include dehydration and swollen parotid glands. BMI = 16.7. Laboratory results are all within normal range except for slightly elevated amylase level (116 µ/L suggesting she has been vomiting) and slight metabolic alkalosis (elevated serum bicarbonate level = 33 mmol/L). The only slightly elevated serum bicarbonate level despite vomiting may relate to her misuse of laxatives, which decreases serum bicarbonate levels due to loss of alkaline fluid from the bowel. Her electrocardiogram shows sinus bradycardia. Her menstruation is irregular, 3 to 4 days duration every 30 to 45 days. Her scores on the drive for thinness, bulimia, interoceptive awareness, and perfectionism subscales of the Eating Disorder Inventory (EDI) are significantly increased when compared with the scores of normal female undergraduates in North America.

Upon admission, Maddison's fluoxetine hydrochloride dose was increased from 20 mg to 40 mg. She is encouraged to participate in the psychiatric unit milieu by normalizing her mealtime frequency to three times daily with an evening snack to reduce the binge-eating and purging episodes. She is also expected to start interpersonal therapy (IPT) and attend the unit's stress management group that aims to improve coping strategies.

Associated Psychiatric Diagnosis	**Medications**
Anorexia nervosa Binge-eating/purging type	

(Continued)

NURSING CARE PLAN 25.1 (Continued)

Nursing Diagnosis 1: Risk for Suicide

Defining Characteristics	Related Factors
Feelings of worthlessness	History of sexual trauma
Difficulty sleeping, wanting to stay in bed all day	History of obesity and weight discrimination
Feels hurt, sad, deserving of punishment, angry	She wants to never again be victimized
"I feel like such a waste of a university education … It might be best if I took enough sleeping pills to never wake up!"	

Outcomes

Initial	Long Term
Agrees to seek out nurse if feeling suicidal	Develops self-compassion, self-acceptance
Remains safe from self-harm	Develops alternative and positive ways of coping

Interventions

Interventions	Rationale	Ongoing Assessment
Initiate a nurse–client relationship, convey acceptance of Maddison as a deserving, worthwhile person.	The nurse–client relationship builds trust and acceptance.	Assess the development of trust.
Initiate suicide precautions as per institution policy. Frequent regular round-the-clock observations.	Maddison's safety is the priority of care.	Determine risk of self-harm.
Support Maddison to contact sexual assault centre for information, self-care skills training, therapeutic/social support, and assistance with reconciliation measures as wanted.	Coping strategies and support can facilitate moving past the trauma, rebuilding sense of control and self-worth, and developing resilience.	Evaluate self-care capacity.
Help promote sleep hygiene.	Attention to environment, limiting consumption of caffeine, and establishing a regular bedtime routine improves sleep.	Assess quality of sleep by asking if Maddison feels rested upon awakening.

Outcomes

Entered a no-harm contract with the nurse. Agrees to continue the contract with outpatient clinic nurse after discharge. Has not harmed self; denies self-harm ideas/intentions.

Connects with others via participation in the unit milieu and community supports.

Nursing Diagnosis 2: Imbalanced Nutrition: Less Than Body Requirements

Defining Characteristics	Related Factors
Underweight; BMI below healthy range	Purging (self-induced vomiting and laxative misuse)
Electrolyte and metabolic disturbances	Decreased potassium level from vomiting and laxative use
Weakness, dizziness, and fatigue	Dehydrated

NURSING CARE PLAN 25.1 *(Continued)*

Outcomes

Initial	Long Term
Adhere to meal and snack schedule of hospital. This decreases the incidence of binge eating, which is often precipitated by starvation and fasting.	Eats three nondieting meals and at least one snack per day. Maintains healthy BMI
Ceases purging for 1 week	Develops positive ways of managing emotions and stress rather than binging and purging

Interventions

Interventions	Rationale	Ongoing Assessment
Continue to develop a therapeutic relationship with Maddison. Encourage her to verbalize feelings such as anxiety related to food, weight, and situations associated with or that trigger binge eating.	Through relationship with the nurse and examining her feelings, Maddison may be more likely to cooperate with the nutritional regimen.	Determine anxiety level when discussing food, body image, and weight. Support Maddison in following her nutritional regimen.
Monitor meals and snacks; record the amount eaten.	Skipping meals triggers hunger, which may precipitate an episode of binge eating. Binge eating triggers the compulsion to purge.	Assess Maddison's ability to complete regularly scheduled meals.
Teach to incorporate adequate daily fibre intake.	To restore normal peristalsis without laxatives.	Monitor BM pattern.
Encourage making a journal of incidents and feelings before, during, and after binge episode.	To increase understanding and responsibility taking.	Assist Maddison in identifying triggers to binge eating.
Monitor Maddison's behaviour after meals and snacks for purging. Monitor vital signs daily, electrolytes regularly.	Physical signs of impending complications include evidence of purging, hypotension, and hypokalaemia. Reduce potential for cardiac arrhythmia associated with hypokalaemia from purging.	Monitor vital signs, weight, and electrolytes, especially potassium.
Assist Maddison to identify activities to try if she feels compelled to purge. Contract with Maddison to approach the nurse when she feels the urge to binge or purge so that feelings and alternative ways of coping can be explored.	Positive coping skills will enable her to build capacity to hold and mitigate distress.	Monitor restless behaviour. Evaluate her practice of activities to delay a binge or purge.
Provide psychoeducational intervention. Teach risks of laxative dependency, foods to meet potassium needs, dangers of caffeine-laced energy drinks and slimming pills, importance of adequate water intake, ineffectiveness and risks of purging to prevent weight gain, and role of potassium in heart and muscle function.	Increase awareness of health needs and risks.	Observe comprehension of material.

(Continued)

NURSING CARE PLAN 25.1 (Continued)

Evaluation

Outcomes	Revised Outcomes	Interventions
Maddison cooperates with meal regimen.	Ceases purging episodes for 1 week. Approaches nurse if she feels driven to binge or purge.	Regular blood work. Praise her successes. Arrange for discharge to outpatient or community clinic.
She has begun to acknowledge the seriousness of her illness and the life-threatening aspects of dieting and purging.	Establish and maintain regular, adequate nutritional eating habits.	Participation in relapse prevention classes.

Nursing Diagnosis 3: Disturbed Body Image/Body Experience

Defining Characteristics	Related Factors
Verbalizes that she is too fat	Inaccurate perceptions of physical appearance secondary to anorexia nervosa Desires a slimmer face and thinner legs
"I have been trying so hard to be my best and do well" but not able to function at this level.	Believes that she is failing to measure up to an internalized desired ideal
Hides body in baggy, loose fitting clothing	History of depression, sexual trauma, weight loss, and dieting.

Outcomes

Initial	Long Term
Verbalizes feelings related to changing body shape and weight	Acknowledges negative consequences of too little fat on body
Identifies beliefs about controlling body size	Identifies positive aspects of her body and its ability to function

Interventions

Interventions	Rationale	Ongoing Assessment
Explore Maddison's beliefs and feelings about body. Maintain a nonjudgmental approach. Provide opportunities to talk about her experiences of being teased about body changes or sexual abuse.	The past experiences of sexual trauma and weight-related teasing may lead to negativity toward her body. To help Maddison gain a more positive body image, an understanding of her own views is important.	Monitor for statements that identify perceptions of her body. Is her view *distorted* or *dissatisfied*? Monitor for PTSD symptom and need for trauma-oriented psychotherapy.
Assist Maddison in identifying positive and realistic physical characteristics.	In AN, the body is viewed negatively. By focusing on parts of the body that are positive, such as the eyes or hands, or that enhance function, such as strong legs for running, Maddison can begin to experience a positive image of her body.	Observe for her reaction to her body. Which areas are viewed positively? Observe for negative statements related to body size and self-esteem.
Clarify Maddison's views about an ideal body.	Many societal cues idealize an unrealistically thin female body.	Monitor for statements indicating external pressures to lose weight.
Provide education related to normal growth of women's bodies and the protective role of fat.	Providing education will help in reinforcing a broader view of the importance of a healthy body.	Assess willingness to learn information.

NURSING CARE PLAN 25.1 *(Continued)*

Evaluation

Outcomes	Revised Outcomes	Interventions
Maddison revealed her belief that she is too fat. She has difficulty identifying aspects of her self and body she likes. She believes that those who are overweight have lost control of their lives.	Maddison accepts alternative beliefs related to her own abilities and body.	Gradually, focus on other positive aspects of Maddison's whole self and body. Challenge her beliefs about loss of personal control and overweight.
Willing to read information about normal body functioning.	Maddison accepts a new view of body functioning as a complex phenomenon.	Discuss the biologic aspect of the development of body weight. Emphasize multiple factors that determine body weight.

Nursing Diagnosis 4: Spiritual Distress Related to Loss of Relationship With Self and Others

Defining Characteristics	Related Factors
Questions or expresses inner conflict about her self, the meaning or purpose of her life	"I'm so on my own. I can't go out with my friends."
Evinces guilt, hopelessness, despair, and/or abandonment	Tearful, depressed, and angry
Withdrawal from, or absence of, relationships	Believes others would treat her negatively if they knew she binges and purges
Guilt and shame about disordered eating behaviours and abuse	Secretive vomiting. Has not disclosed past sexual abuse to anyone

Outcomes

Initial	Long Term
Begins to expresses inner distress in acceptable ways (e.g., talking, journalling, art work)	Spiritual health as evidenced by: Using a type of spiritual experience/expression that provides her comfort Connecting with others to share thoughts, feelings, and beliefs

(Continued)

NURSING CARE PLAN 25.1 *(Continued)*

Interventions

Interventions	Rationale	Ongoing Assessment
Model self-awareness and acceptance without harsh self-judgment.	Maddison will not trust a nurse who does not demonstrate self-comfort.	Ask: How do you feel about the changes in your life that have come about because of the eating disorder? The abuse?
Create an accepting, nonjudgmental atmosphere.	Providing ongoing, unconditional support establishes rapport and therapeutic relationship, which promotes communication, open expression, and opportunity to explore inner world of meaning and experience.	Assess her ability to see and affirm her self-worth and identity. What does she see as her strengths? Does she define herself as *the eating disorder*? The younger victim *(Fatty Maddy)*?
Spend nontask time with Maddison.	Being with the person who is suffering gives meaning to his or her experience. It confirms to Maddison that she is important and of value. The nurse's presence helps alleviate the client's sense of isolation, anxiety, and abandonment.	Is she feeling distant and disconnected from others? What are her relations with family? Does she know what she does and does not have control over? Does she accept her human limitations within the context of her traumatic experiences?
Encourage Maddison to experience and verbalize feelings, perceptions, and fears	Helps her access potential healing resources to well-being. Releasing emotions can provide energy and freedom.	Assess her ability to name and identify her feelings.
Encourage her to identify values that guide her everyday behaviour and her actions in times of crisis, loss, and tragedy.	Helps her clarify values and beliefs by reflecting on past behaviours. Experience is a major source for values development.	Assess her ability to challenge counterproductive beliefs.
Observe and listen empathetically to her communication, offering patience, repetition, and reassurance over an extended period of time.	Listening to the "unacceptable" helps the process of finding meaning, healing, growth, and reentering life with a renewed sense of purpose and connection to others and self.	Assess her growth beyond the prior traumatic experiences. Does she accept herself and her past? What, if anything, would she change now?
Help Maddison tell her story about the eating disorder and any painful traumatic experiences in descriptive rather than evaluative terms.	Storytelling minimizes self-judgment and allows emergence of patterns that aid understanding.	Monitor her capacity for informed understanding.
Help Maddison develop a healthy, positive outlook through such things as letter writing, meditation, and/or imagery.	Helps her access potential healing resources to enhance well-being and reduce negative affectivity.	Assess her ability to care for self.

Evaluation

Outcomes	Revised Outcomes	Interventions
She has begun to acknowledge the meaning of the eating disorder in her life but has not developed a non–self-blaming understanding of the abuse.	Establish and maintain appropriate self-care strategies that include adequate nutrition and eating practices and self-development.	Participation in comprehensive and individualized treatment program.

Interventions for Biologic Domain

Weight restoration is the chief intervention during the hospital or initial stage of treatment for AN (Fig. 25.4). The nurse will encounter resistance to eating and weight gain and carefully monitors and records all intake as part of the weight gain protocol. For instance, an adult with an eating disorder who is significantly malnourished, and has had very low intake prior to hospitalization, might be safely started at approximately 1,600 kcal per day and increased by 300 kcal per day every 2 to 3 days until consistent weight gain of at least 1 to 2 kg (2 to 4 pounds) per week is achieved. Children and adolescents are in a state of growth and development. Their treatment goal weights and nutritional needs will change as they continue to grow and develop. Supplemental enteral feeds may be indicated when rates of weight gain are low less than 1 kg (2 pounds) per week (AED, 2016).

Methods of refeeding that "start low and go slow" have been replaced by more rapid refeeding with close medical monitoring during inpatient treatment. According to AED (2016), the risk of refeeding syndrome is related to the degree of malnutrition at presentation (i.e., less than 70% median BMI in adolescents, BMI less than 15 in adults). Refeeding syndrome is a rare but potentially fatal condition that can occur during refeeding of severely malnourished individuals. After prolonged starvation, the body begins to use fat and protein to produce energy because there are not enough carbohydrates.

Upon refeeding, there is a surge of insulin (because of the ingested carbohydrates) and a sudden shift from fat to carbohydrate metabolism. One of the key features of refeeding syndrome is hypophosphatemia (abnormally low levels of phosphate in the blood), which occurs primarily because the insulin surge during food ingestion leads to a cellular uptake of phosphate. Phosphate dysregulation affects almost every system in the body and can lead to leucocyte dysfunction, respiratory failure, cardiac failure, hypotension, arrhythmias, seizures, coma, and sudden death (Tetyana, 2013, p. 2).

Weight-increasing protocols usually take the form of a behavioural plan, using positive reinforcements (e.g., outings or passes) and negative reinforcements (e.g., returning to bed rest). The reinforcements are incremental, informed by client preferences, and based on progress. For example, phone calls, walks around the unit, and walks outside the hospital occur before the day passes and then weekend passes. These protocols provide consistent responses to food avoidance behaviours and are carried out in a caring and supportive context. However, activity restrictions may be perceived negatively by clients (see Box 25.3). During the implementation of negative reinforcements, the client is helped to see that these actions are not punitive. On rare occasions when the client is unable to recognize or accept the eating disorder as harmful, nasogastric tube feedings may be necessary to enable weight restoration.

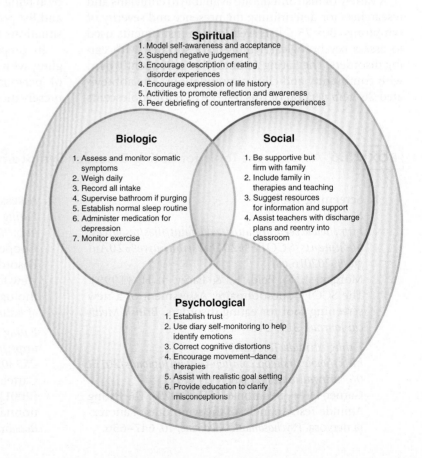

Figure 25.4. Bio/psycho/social/spiritual interventions for individuals with AN.

Menses history also is assessed. Most young women with AN have reached menarche but may have experienced amenorrhoea for some months because of starvation. A return to regular menses signifies substantial body fat restoration. Sleep disturbance is also common, and these individuals may sleep little but usually awaken in an energized state. A structured, healthy sleep routine is established to conserve energy and calorie expenditure. To further conserve energy, clients are often relegated to bed rest until a certain amount of weight is regained. Exercise is generally not permitted during refeeding and only with caution after this phase. Inpatient clients are closely supervised because they are often found exercising in their rooms (or while on bed rest).

Psychological Domain

Assessment

The psychological symptoms that individuals with AN experience are listed in Box 25.1. The classic symptoms — low weight, unrealistic expectations and thinking, and ritualistic behaviours—may be noted during a clinical interview. Conflicts that underlie this disorder, such as maturity or independence fears and feelings of ineffectiveness, may not be apparent during the interview. Assessing individuals with low self-esteem and high social anxiety may be particularly difficult, as clients may believe the clinician is negatively evaluating them, whereas their low self-worth may make them feel that they are not worth the effort of referral or therapy.

A variety of instruments are available to clinicians and researchers for determining the presence and severity of symptoms. Box 25.6 lists well-known instruments used to assess psychological symptoms associated with eating disorders. The Eating Attitude Test is frequently used with community and clinical populations. The abbreviated 26-item version of this test, EAT-26 for adolescents and adults, is readily available online (http://www.eat-26.com/) and is particularly useful in screening for eating disorder risk in high school students, in university students, and in other groups such as athletes. The results can help identify the most significant symptoms and indicate if an individual should be referred for evaluation of an eating disorder.

Nursing Diagnosis for Psychological Domain

Two common nursing diagnoses in AN are Anxiety and Disturbed Body Image.

Interventions for Psychological Domain

Most individuals with AN experience interoceptive awareness problems (inability to experience visceral cues and emotions) and use a somatic complaint such as "I feel bloated" or "I'm fat" to replace a negative emotion such as guilt or anger. Although these complaints may be related to refeeding, they often are part of body dissatisfaction. Research into the experiences of women with eating disorders has demonstrated body shame as a major theme influencing self-criticism (Kelly & Carter, 2013), nondisclosure (Dimitropoulos, Freeman, Muskat, Domingo, & McCallum, 2016), and social rank perceptions (Matos, Ferreira, Duarte, & Pinto-Gouveia, 2015). To make it possible for women to speak about such feelings, the nurse can normalize the shame experience in conversation with the client and can encourage clients to keep a journal, help them to identify feelings by having them write a description of the "fat feeling" and list possible underlying emotions and troublesome situations next to this description.

In preparing to interact with an individual struggling with AN, the clinician must first make meaning of personal experiences with eating issues and self-preservation strategies. Self-awareness and acceptance

---

BOX 25.6 Assessment Tools for Eating Disorder Symptoms

1. Screening Tools

SCOFF
http://www.ceed.org.au/sites/default/files/resources/documents/SCOFF%20Questionnaire%20August%202016.pdf
Morgan, J. F., Reid, F., & Lacey, J. H. (1999). The SCOFF questionnaire: Assessment of a new screening tool for eating disorders. *British Medical Journal, 319*, 1467–1468.

Eating Attitude Test (EAT)
http://www.drshepp.com/wp-content/uploads/2015/06/eatingattitudestest.pdf
Garner, D. M., & Garfinkel, P. E. (1979). The Eating Attitude Test: An index of the symptoms of anorexia nervosa. *Psychosomatic Medicine, 10*, 647–656.

2. Assessment/Diagnostic Measures

Eating Disorder Examination
http://rcpsych.ac.uk/pdf/EDE_16.0.pdf
Cooper, Z., & Fairburn, C. G. (1987). The Eating Disorder Examination: A semi-structured interview for the assessment of the specific psychopathology of eating disorders. *International Journal of Eating Disorders, 6*, 1–8.

Eating Disorder Examination Questionnaire (EDE-Q)
https://www.phenxtoolkit.org/toolkit_content/PDF/PX230104.pdf
Carter, J. C., Stewart, D. A., & Fairburn, C. G. (2001). Eating Disorder Examination Questionnaire: Norms for adolescent girls. *Behaviour Research and Therapy, 39*, 625–632.

BOX 25.6 Assessment Tools for Eating Disorder Symptoms (*Continued*)

Eating Disorder Inventory-3 (EDI-3) and EDI-3 Symptom Checklist (EDI-3-SC)
http://river-centre.org/wp-content/uploads/2015/10/EDI-3-Scale.pdf
Garner, D. M. (2011). *Eating Disorder Inventory-3: Professional manual.* Odessa, FL: Psychological Assessment Resources.

Yale-Brown-Cornell Eating Disorder Scale (YBC-EDS)
https://www.phenxtoolkit.org/toolkit_content/PDF/PX650501.pdf
Mazure, C. M., Halmi, K. A., Sunday, S. R., Romano, S. J., & Einhorn, A. M. (1994). Yale-Brown-Cornell Eating Disorder Scale: Development, use, reliability, and validity. *Journal of Psychiatric Research, 28,* 425–445.

Three-Factor Eating Questionnaire-R18
http://www.med.umich.edu/pdf/weight-management/TFEQ-r18.pdf
de Lauzon, B., Romon, M., Deschamps, V., Lafay, L., Borys, J-M., Karlsson, J., ... Fleurbaix Laventie Ville Sante Study Group. (2004). The Three-Factor Eating Questionnaire-R18 is able to distinguish among different eating patterns in a general population. *Journal of Nutrition, 134*(9), 2372–2380.

3. **Tests of Body Dissatisfaction/Body Image**
Body Shape Questionnaire (BSQ)
http://www.psyctc.org/tools/bsq/
Cooper, P., Taylor, M., Cooper, Z., & Fairburn, C. (1987). The development and validation of the BSQ. *International Journal of Eating Disorders, 6,* 485–494.

Colour-a-Person Test
Wooley, S. C., & Kearney-Cooke, A. (1986). Intensive treatment of bulimia and body image disturbance. In K. D. Brownell & J. P. Foreyt (Eds.), *Handbook of eating disorders: Physiology, psychology and treatment of obesity, anorexia, and bulimia* (pp. 476–502). New York, NY: Basic Books.

Body Parts Dissatisfaction Scale
http://www.midss.org/sites/default/files/body_parts_dissatisfaction_scale.pdf
Corning, A. F., Gondoli, D. M., Bucchianeri, M. M., & Blodgett-Salafia, E. H. (2010). Preventing the development of body issues in adolescent girls through intervention with their mothers. *Body Image, 7,* 289–295.

Body Dissatisfaction Scale
http://www.nspb.net/index.php/nspb/article/view/249
Mutale, G. T., Dunn, A., Stiller, J., & Larkin, R. (1996). Development of a body dissatisfaction scale assessment tool. *The New School Psychology Bulletin, 13*(2), 47–57.

4. **Tests of Emotional and Cognitive Components**
Cognitive Behavioural Dieting Scale
Martz, D. M., Sturgis, E. T., & Gustafson, S. B. (1996). Development and preliminary validation of the Cognitive Behavioral Dieting Scale. *International Journal of Eating Disorders, 19,* 297–309.

Emotional Eating Scale
Arrow, B., Kenardy, J., & Agras, W. S. (1995). The Emotional Eating Scale: The development of a measure to assess coping with negative affect by eating. *International Journal of Eating Disorders, 18,* 79–90.

Compulsive Eating Scale
www.moray.gov.uk/downloads/file93345.doc
Kagan, D. M., & Squires, R. L. (1984). Compulsive eating, dieting, stress, and hostility among college students. *Journal of College Student Personnel, 25*(3), 213–220.

The Restraint Scale (RS)
Herman, C. P., & Polivy, J. (1975). Anxiety, restraint, and eating behavior. *Journal of Abnormal Psychology, 84,* 66–72.

Three-Factor Eating Questionnaire Cognitive Restraint Scale (TFEQ-R)
http://www.med.umich.edu/pdf/weight-anagement/TFEQ-r18.pdf
Stunkard, A. J., & Messick, S. (1985). The Three-Factor Eating Questionnaire to measure dietary restraint, disinhibition, and hunger. *Journal of Psychosomatic Research, 29,* 71–83.

5. **Behavioural Tests**
Test Meals
Andersen, A. E. (1995). A standard test meal to assess treatment response in anorexia nervosa patients. *Eating Disorders, 3,* 47–55.

6. **Risk Factors Identification**
The McKnight Risk Factor Survey
http://bml.stanford.edu/resources/documents/MRFS_6-12_WEB.pdf
Shisslak, C. M., Renger, R., Sharpe, T., Crago, M., McKnight, K. M., Gray, N., ... Taylor, C. B. (1999). Development and evaluation of the McKnight Risk Factor Survey for assessing potential risk and protective factors for disordered eating in preadolescent and adolescent girls. *International Journal of Eating Disorders, 25*(2), 195–214. (Versions available for younger and older children.)

cannot be effectively modelled without having engaged in this critical self-development. In Box 25.7, an upper-level psychology student poetically reflected on her concern with appearance that influenced the development of an eating disorder. This student was receptive to exploring underlying factors and points of interest with her peers in a campus peer-led education and support group for students with eating issues.

Box 25.8 outlines the "It's Not about Food" intervention project at the University of New Brunswick.

Understanding Feelings

Identifying feelings, such as anxiety and fear, and especially negative emotions, such as anger, helps individuals decrease conflict avoidance and develop effective strategies for managing these feelings. It is unhelpful to attempt to change distorted body image by pointing out that the individual is actually too thin. This characteristic is often the last to resolve itself, and it may take years for individuals to see their bodies realistically. Imaginal exposure may help individuals face the fear of hypothetical fatness in breaking the avoidance–anxiety cycle (Levinson, Rapp, & Riley, 2014). Individuals may continue to fear becoming fat but no longer be driven to act on the distortion by starving. The fear of becoming fat eventually lessens with time.

Relying on positive and well-timed interactions, nurses may contribute to productive physical outcomes and a positive client experience. Clients have indicated that their motivation to adhere to care was derived from having strong relationships with their nurses (Zugai, Stein-Parbury, & Roche, 2013). The nurse can help individuals restructure the way they view the world, especially relative to food, eating, weight, and shape. Faulty ways of viewing these situations result in ineffective coping. Table 25.4 lists some cognitive distortions commonly experienced by individuals with eating disorders and some typical restructuring responses that challenge the distortion, which the nurse can present as more realistic ways of perceiving situations. Other therapies, such as movement and dance therapy, can help individuals experience pleasure from their bodies, although dance should be used cautiously during refeeding because of energy-expenditure concerns. Women with eating disorders who participated in equine-assisted therapy described noticing new sensations and feelings that they had previously not been able to feel at a corporeal level or that they actively avoided feeling; they experienced a sort of "reattunement" to themselves and the world through their horses that interrupted some of their habitual ways of attuning and helped to quiet eating disorder thoughts and ways of being (Sharpe, 2014). Imagery and relaxation are often used to overcome distortions and decrease anxiety.

Psychotherapy

IPT is a type of treatment that focuses on uncovering and resolving developmental and psychological issues

---

BOX 25.7 Spirituality of the Clinician: Beginning the Journey

SELF-EXAMINATION

Mirror, Mirror

Mirror, mirror on the wall, who's the cutest girl of all?

For all I know it can't be me, I am much too fat you see.

The girl you show has great big thighs, a flabby stomach, a large waist size.

She's not at all what I want to be, but she's not the only girl I see

Because behind her, peeking out, is another girl, without a doubt.

I like this girl. This girl is thin. She beckons me. She draws me in.

All the promises of beauty and grace. She is very thin and has a pretty face.

She tells me what I have to do, in order to look just like her too.

If I listen, follow one rule, I'll be the thinnest girl at school.

The rule is that I cannot eat. I must be good. I must mustn't cheat.

I listen to what she has to say. I eat nothing, I obey.

She becomes my truest friend, and she'll stay with me until the end.

And when the pounds start coming off, I think it's good, I'm pulling it off.

But then I find she's not so nice. Her words, they cut me deep like ice.

She tells me I am worthless, fat. Something she cannot look at.

I try harder so she will stay. But there has to be another way.

She says that she has got me beat. I will not tell, I cannot eat.

That's when I find I cannot stop. The mirror, well it was just a prop.

To get me into in this place, so she could thrive, could have a face.

Now I'm something that she owns, condemned to die, just skin and bones.

Because every time the mirror lied, it was Ana's voice, deep inside.

By Leslie Marie
University of New Brunswick

BOX 25.8 Research for Best Practice

"IT'S NOT ABOUT FOOD!"

Weaver, K. (2015). Peer-led teaching and support to reduce eating disorders on campus. Proceedings of the 2014 AAU Teaching Showcase, XVIII, 78–92. https://ojs.library.dal.ca/auts/article/view/6721/5906

Purpose: To describe the advanced nursing practice-research program, "It's Not about Food" (INAF), designed to identify and address knowledge and social support needs of university women with self-identified eating issues, and the specific support rendered by upper-level nursing students who served as peer facilitators.

Methods: A short film depicting the peer learning process was produced to orient students to the INAF program. At the end of the 6 weeks of INAF groups, quantitative questionnaires were distributed and collected. INAF participants and also peer facilitators were invited to participate in interviews to explore their experiences within INAF. Mixed-method evaluation of the project involved descriptive statistics and thematic analysis of interview data.

Findings: The majority of participants found INAF helpful, especially in terms of information, support, and peer facilitation. Although their eating habits did not significantly change over the course of the six weekly groups, attending INAF facilitated professional help seeking. For INAF participants, the group served as a "safe zone" for enabling understanding and contemplation of personal and health changes including self-care. From the perspectives of the peer facilitators, the most salient finding was learning to preserve rapport, a strategy that helped them develop greater relational competency, professional satisfaction, and leadership capacity. Interrelated aspects of preserving rapport were keeping conversations flowing, reaching common understanding, nurturing "breakthrough" (aha moments) among participants, and knowing the person beyond the eating issue.

Implications for Nursing: The establishment of the INAF program in NB (a province without a publicly funded eating disorder treatment facility), and on the campus of the largest university in the province, was an opportunity to support those affected in meaningful ways. The key finding that attending INAF facilitated professional help seeking is significant because persons experiencing eating issues often minimize or hide symptoms from health professionals. Willingness to seek professional help conveys the power of INAF in assisting participants to break away from the secrecy and containment of their eating issues. The nursing duty to help clients from a highly stigmatized group make positive behaviour changes requires opportunities to build knowledge of the client issues and available resources; to participate in interdisciplinary training, briefing, and postsession debriefing with cofacilitators; and, above all, to learn to preserve rapport.

Table 25.4 Cognitive Distortions Typical of Patients with Eating Disorders, With Restructuring Statements	
Distortion	**Clarification or Restructuring**
Dichotomous or all-or-nothing thinking "I've gained 1 kilo (2 pounds), so I'll be up by 50 kilos (100 pounds) soon."	"You have not ever gained 50 kilos (100 pounds), but I understand that gaining 1 kilo (2 pounds) is scary."
Magnification "I binged last night, so I can't go out with anyone."	"Feeling bad and guilty about a binge are difficult feelings, but you are in treatment and you have been monitoring and changing your eating."
Selective abstraction "I can only be happy 5 kilos (10 pounds) lighter." or "People will only love me if I am thin."	"When you were 5 kilos (10 pounds) lighter, you were hospitalized. You can choose to be happy about many things in your life." "People love you for being you—your kindness, sense of humour, and so on. Let's talk about qualities that make you a good friend/sister."
Overgeneralization "I didn't eat anything yesterday and did okay, so I don't think *not* eating for a week or two will harm me."	"Any starvation harms the body, whether or not outward signs are apparent to you. The more you starve, the more problems your body will encounter."
Catastrophizing "I purged last night for the first time in 4 months—I'll never recover." or "I am so evil—if I have whipped cream on my latte, my stomach will be over my jeans like a muffin in the tin."	"Recovery includes ups and downs, and it is expected you will still have some mild but infrequent symptoms." "No, that's not true. You are working hard to ensure you take in enough to meet your body's needs, such as the extra energy it takes you to walk all the way to the coffee shop."

underlying the disorder. Role transitions, conflicts, and interpersonal deficits leading to social isolation or chronically unsatisfactory relationships typically are the focus (Melville, 2016). Cognitive behavioural therapy (CBT) may also be incorporated to continue to address faulty beliefs about food and social interactions; CBT has been shown to be effective in treating many of the problems which are often a feature of AN such as depression, anxiety, low self-esteem, and obsessions/compulsions (Galsworthy-Francis & Allan, 2014). Refer further to Chapter 13. A third treatment option, specialist supportive clinical management (SSCM), includes education, care, support, and therapeutic alliance that promotes adherence to treatment through use of praise, reassurance, and advice. Supportive clinical management emphasizes the resumption of normal eating and the restoration of weight; verbal and written information are provided on weight maintenance strategies, energy requirements, and relearning to eat normally (McIntosh et al., 2016). Family-based therapy is currently the only treatment for adolescents with anorexia that is supported by scientific evidence. In particular, behaviourally based family therapy (FBT or "Maudsley family therapy") for adolescents with eating disorders is superior to individual therapy (Couturier, Kimber, & Szatmari, 2013). No one specialist treatment has been shown to be best for treatment of adults with AN (Kass, Kolko, & Wilfley, 2013). However, a significant therapy effect was found using each—CBT, IPT, and SSCM (McIntosh et al., 2016).

Client Education

As weight is restored and concentration improved, individuals with AN can maximally benefit from psychoeducation. Although these individuals have much knowledge about food and calories, they also have misinformation that needs clarifying. For example, they are often unclear about the role of "fats" in a healthy diet and try to be as "fat free" as possible. A thorough assessment of their knowledge is important because they may need information on the importance of including all nutrients in a healthy diet. Furthermore, individuals with AN are often perfectionistic; they may set unrealistic goals and end up frustrated. Teaching them to set smaller, progressive, attainable eating goals is one of the most helpful interventions. To help these clients learn to develop appropriate goals around food and other activities, the nurse can help them consider essential topic areas pertinent to their recovery (see Box 25.9) and patiently support them to gain skill in formulating realistic, attainable goals.

Social Domain

Nursing Diagnosis for Social Domain

Ineffective Coping is a predominant nursing diagnosis regarding the social domain.

BOX 25.9 Psychoeducation Checklist: Anorexia Nervosa

When caring for the client with AN, be sure to include the following topic areas in the teaching plan:

- Psychopharmacologic agents, if used (rarely), including drug, action, dosage, frequency, and possible adverse effects
- Nutrition and eating patterns
- Effect of restrictive eating or dieting
- Weight monitoring
- Safety and comfort measures
- Avoidance of triggers
- Self-monitoring techniques
- Trust
- Realistic goal setting
- Resources

Interventions for Social Domain

Younger individuals with AN who may have lost some school time because of hospitalization may find integrating back into a school and classroom setting difficult. Shame and guilt about having an eating disorder and being hospitalized need to be addressed. Because these clients typically have isolated themselves before hospitalization and treatment, renewing friendships and relationships with peers may provoke anxiety. Involving school nurses and teachers in the reentry process may help.

When parents are informed that their child has a diagnosis of anorexia nervosa, tension begins:

> The atmosphere in the house was horrendous, you know because it takes over, actually the whole house really, because you trying to get her to eat and she's sitting there in tears and its horrendous and it's the worst thing ever and its happening under your nose and you know it's dreadful. (McCormack & McCann, 2015, p. 144)

In learning to help manage the eating disorder, parents may experience social isolation, financial difficulties, worry for siblings, strained spouse relationships, powerlessness, hardship, shame, and especially self-blame (Svensson, Nilsson, Levi, & Suarez, 2013). Further, parents may feel lost alongside their child with the eating disorder and in need of information, support, and inclusion in treatment decisions (Weaver, Martin-McDonald, & Spiers, 2016). Box 25.10 provides a list of general strategies that may assist families and friends.

Nurses are able to help family members manage feelings, increase effective communication and capacity to provide helpful nonintrusive support, decrease protectiveness, and resolve guilt. Successful family treatment addresses underlying issues such as negative body image, intergenerational coalitions between parents and children, fear of separation, and undeveloped marital

BOX 25.10 What Family and Friends Can Do to Help Those With Eating Disorders

- Tell the person you are concerned, you care, and you would like to help. Suggest that the person seek professional help from a physician or therapist.
- If the person refuses to seek professional help, encourage reaching out to an adult, such as a teacher, school nurse, or counsellor.
- Do not discuss weight, the number of calories being consumed, or particular eating habits. Do try to talk about things other than food, weight, counting calories, and exercise.
- Avoid making comments about a person's appearance. Concern about weight loss may be interpreted as a compliment; comments regarding weight gain may be felt as criticism.
- It will not help to become involved in a power struggle. You cannot force the person to eat.
- You can offer support. Ultimately, however, the responsibility and the decision to accept help and to change rest with the person.
- Read and educate yourself regarding these disorders.
- Care for yourself (e.g., have periods of rest as a way to regain energy).

relationships. Goals in the therapy include helping the parents work together, strengthening silenced voices, bringing out repressed emotions, and keeping conversations going between family members (Gerstein & Pollack, 2016). Family are helped to focus on such issues as separation–individuation, autonomy, ineffective communication, symptom interruption, and practical issues, such as how to effectively monitor food intake. A major focus is to help family members see each other's strengths and begin to work together to address the eating issue.

Parents worry about the siblings (Svensson et al., 2013). Often, siblings become resentful of the attention the individual with an eating disorder gets from the parents. It is helpful to have siblings attend family sessions to discuss these feelings and the effect the illness has had on them. Further research is needed to explore social support to individuals with eating disorders and to identify best approaches that enable nurses and other care providers reduce the occurrence of unhelpful interactions.

Spiritual Domain

Overcoming eating disorders requires attention to the individual in his/her physical, psychological, social, and spiritual fullness. Core components of recovery

can be having input into one's own recovery and sense of empowerment (Fogarty & Ramjan, 2016). Empowerment was experienced through regaining some control through learning new coping strategies and skills such as increasing self-worth and respect to help combat the disorder. Spiritual interventions entail establishing trust, rapport, consistency, and support while enabling clients to voice and make meaning of their eating disorder experience. The nurse helps clients recognize patterns, identify, and clarify values. Encouraging activities that promote reflection and self-awareness helps clients access potential solutions to well-being and reduce depression, anxiety, relationship distress, social role conflict, and eating disorder symptoms. Some important skills during treatment are learning to resist comparing self with others and to impart self-kindness; one participant attributed her recovery to having developed a deeper sense of her own identity, a connection to what she loves, and an ability to be present in a relationship despite having imperfections (Lea, Richards, Sanders, McBride, & Allen, 2015). The quality of alternate relationships, such as with a pet or a "higher (spiritual) being," may be as important as those with family and friends (Hay, 2013, p. 734).

The need for ongoing self-awareness on the part of the nurse is critical when interacting with an individual whose body has served as a container for pain, suffering, and disgust and has subsequently been starved, stuffed, or purged. The nurse may encounter body countertransference or the phenomenon of experiencing a similar type of discomfort in the nurse's own body (Jirak Monetti, 2014). The nurse must be attuned to these body sensations and anticipate this phenomenon throughout the working relationship. It is necessary to understand and process countertransference issues concerning nurses'/therapists' relationships with their own weight, eating patterns, and body image; clients' tendencies to scrutinize and comment about nurses'/therapists' bodies; and the degree of self-disclosure in the therapeutic relationship (Seah, Tham, Kamaruzaman, & Yobas, 2017). Clients having therapy for eating disorders report wanting the service provider to be genuinely curious, elicit trust, have eating disorder expertise to inform the therapy, engage in therapy by listening and sharing in conversations, and work in environments that reflect the therapists' care and creation of a place participants consider "safe" and "comfortable." Participants described genuine curiosity as therapists being interested in their clients' experiences, in tentative and nonjudgmental ways (Lefebvre, 2016). Nurses have to be able to express interest in clients when they say they binged, threw up, or ate without hunger. Nurses need to investigate, in great detail, their instances of hating their bodies or of shaming themselves because of their bodies (Gutwill, 2017). Without awareness and self-monitoring, the nurse may communicate any personal body discomfort to the client. Individual or group peer debriefing sessions are helpful to manage such countertransference.

Evaluation and Treatment Outcomes

Among the varied factors influencing the outcome of treatment for AN, discharge BMI was found the singularly best predictor of full recovery from AN (Lock et al., 2013; Vall & Wade, 2015). This finding emphasizes the crucial need for full weight restoration during treatment. Intensive ongoing outpatient treatment, including nutritional counselling and support, can prevent relapse and facilitate full recovery. Many of the instruments used to assess eating disorder symptoms (see Box 25.6) can be used throughout the individual's treatment to evaluate attitudes and thinking processes. Nurses are ideally positioned within hospital and community health treatment settings to help individuals with AN recover.

Continuum of Care

Hospitalization

AN in its acute stage requires hospitalization.

EMERGENCY CARE

Death may result from cardiac problems associated with starvation and suicide. However, emergency care is not usually needed for individuals with AN. Family members and peers usually notice the weight loss and emaciation before the individual's systems are compromised to the degree that they require emergency treatment. The individual is admitted immediately for inpatient care if systems are compromised or if the individual is suicidal. In hospital, individuals are evaluated for discharge to day hospitalization or outpatient therapy, depending on the resources available, the extent of family support, and comorbidity. In both instances, the individual and family participate in a combination of individual and family therapy. Family therapy, initiated in the hospital, is continued more intensively after discharge (see Chapter 15).

Outpatient Treatment

After weight restoration, treatment of AN may take place on an outpatient basis and involve continued individual and family therapy, nutrition counselling to reinforce healthy eating patterns and attitudes, and physician visits to monitor weight and evaluate somatic recovery. Support groups that pay respect to the views and needs of each participant and provide a continuous feedback cycle can help participants develop a sense of empowerment, allow their voices to be heard, and foster a belief they could begin new relationships and friendships (Nicholls, Fogarty, Hay, & Ramjan, 2016). However, support groups are not a substitute for therapy. This is because some self-directed support groups that

lack professional leadership can actually delay or prevent needed professional treatment. In particular, online communities may validate the proanorexic identity in the cycle of disclosure–response exchanges (Chang & Bazarova, 2016). The role of support groups to maintain recovery requires further study.

■ BULIMIA NERVOSA

Until about 35 years ago, BN was thought to be a subtype of AN. However, findings from extensive investigations identified BN as a separate entity. Individuals with BN are usually older at onset than are those with AN. The usual treatment is outpatient therapy. Outcomes are better for BN than for AN, and mortality rates are lower.

Clinical Course

There are few outward signs associated with BN. Individuals binge and purge in secret and are typically of normal weight; therefore, BN does not come to the attention of parents and peers as quickly as AN. Consequently, treatment can be delayed for years as individuals attempt on their own to get their eating under control. Once treatment is undertaken and completed, they are capable of full recovery, except when personality disorders and comorbid serious depression are also present.

Individuals with BN may present as overwhelmed and overly committed and have difficulty with setting limits and establishing appropriate boundaries. They have many rules regarding food and food restriction, and they feel ashamed, guilty, and disgusted about binge eating and purging. They may also be impulsive in other areas of their lives, such as spending.

BN Symptomatology

According to Mayo Clinic Staff (2016), persons struggling with BN may purge through self-induced vomiting; misusing laxatives, diuretics, or enemas; or fasting, strict dieting, or excessive exercise after eating only a small snack or a normal-size meal. BN can be hard to overcome when individuals are preoccupied with their weight and body shape and severely judge self-perceived flaws.

Dietary restriction serves to regulate painful feelings. It may also alter one's perceptual reactivation to food cues, making them more irresistible. Restriction may make persons who diet more prone to feel distress over their dietary "failures," especially if dieting has become a way to overcome body dissatisfaction and to compensate for distress through binge eating. Pearson, Riley, Davis, and Smith (2014) identified both state-based and trait-based ways in which girls increase their risk to begin engaging in the impulsive behaviour of binge eating and purging. With state-based ways, the experience of negative mood in girls attempting to restrain eating leads to the depletion of self-control and thus increased risk for loss of control over eating. With trait-based ways, increased negative urgency, or the tendency to act rashly when distressed, increases risk for loss of control. These behaviours, when reinforced, put girls at further risk for developing BN. Consequently, whether the eating is influenced by hunger, the attraction of forbidden foods, or internal needs to assuage perceived failure, restraining one's intake may instigate a drive toward repletion and subsequent overeating.

As shown in Figure 25.5, dietary restraint leads to hunger. Hunger may occur in response to inadequate intake or as hedonic hunger, the drive to eat to obtain pleasure in the absence of an energy deficit. Persons living with BN scored higher for measures of hedonic hunger compared to persons with AN, and there was a trend for those with AN-BP type to score higher than those with AN restrictive type (AN-R) (Witt & Lowe, 2014). Rapid ingestion of food during a short period of time (binge eating) is followed by feelings of guilt, remorse, and often self-contempt, leading to purging. To assuage the out-of-control feeling, severe dieting referred to as dietary restraint is instituted. Restrictions are viewed as "rules," such as no sweets or fats. Each binge seems to influence stricter rules about what cannot be consumed, leading to more frequent binge eating, subsequent guilt, and self-loathing. Purging or dietary restraint may follow (Fig. 25.5). Accurso, Lebow, Murray, Kass, and Le Grange (2016) found adolescents over 16 who practiced weight suppression while having a higher BMI engaged in more frequent binge eating, while those with a low current

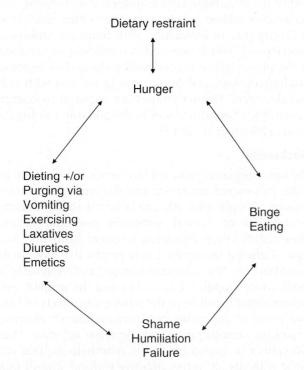

Figure 25.5. Binge–purge cycle.

BMI engaged in less frequent binge eating. The binge–purge cycle prompts clinicians to focus the treatment on interventions related to weight suppression and dietary restraint as well as purging behaviours.

KEY CONCEPT

Dietary restraint, a cognitive effort to restrict food intake for the purpose of weight loss or the prevention of weight gain, was originally described to explain the differences between the eating patterns of obese individuals and those of normal-weight people. Restraint is often initiated as a response to weight gain, and the sustained effort to monitor and control food intake characterizes successful long-term weight maintenance.

Epidemiology

Approximately 1% to 3% of young women develop BN in their lifetime (Statistics Canada, 2015). Using symptom frequency of once a week criteria, the lifetime prevalence (proportion of a population who, at some point in life up to the time of assessment, ever had the characteristic) of BN was reported as 2.15% in a large UK sample of midlife women (Micali et al., 2017), while the period prevalences (proportion of a population who has the characteristic at any point during a given time period) of AN and BED were reported as 3.64% and 1.96%, respectively.

Age of Onset

Typically, the onset of BN begins in adolescence or early adulthood (Statistics Canada, 2015) and may coincide with a developmental transition (e.g., leaving home to attend university) or psychosocial stress such as from unexpected loss of a close relative (Su et al., 2016).

Gender Differences

In the community setting, one case in four of BN is a male (Dr. Blake Woodside, Director of the Program for Eating Disorders at Toronto General Hospital, as cited by Kirkey (2013)).

Ethnic and Cultural Differences

BN is related to culture in the same way as AN. In Western cultures and those becoming westernized in their norms, the focus on achieving an idealized thin body underlies the dieting and dietary restraint that set up the trajectory toward an eating disorder. Hispanic and White women have higher reported rates than do Asian and African Americans. There is a paucity of research exploring ethnic and culture differences among Canadian women.

Familial Differences

First-degree relatives of women with BN are more likely to have eating disorders than control group members and women with other psychiatric disorders (Woodside,

2013). Families of clients with BN also have higher rates of substance abuse, particularly alcoholism, mood disorders, and obesity. Underlying traits such as impulsivity and perfectionism may largely be genetically determined (Slof-Op't Landt et al., 2013).

Comorbidity

Common comorbid conditions are substance misuse (Mann et al., 2014), depression (Keski-Rahkonen et al., 2013), and anxiety disorders (Hocaoglu, 2017). For both men and women, anxiety disorders are the most common comorbidity. Anxiety disorders may start in the childhood period before the diagnosis of the eating disorder, leading to the question: Are anxiety disorders also risk factors for the development of BN? PTSD was found to be approximately three times more frequent in individuals with BN and AN-BP as opposed to those with AN-R (Hocaoglu, 2017). Males with BN had the highest levels of general anxiety syndrome comorbidity (Ulfvebrand, Birgegård, Norring, Högdahl, & von Hausswolff-Juhlin, 2015). BN has been significantly associated with suicidality above and beyond risk predicted by comorbid mood, anxiety, or substance use disorders (Bodell, Joiner, & Keel, 2013). There is a higher occurrence of BN in clients with attention deficit hyperactivity disorder (ADHD) compared to controls; Keshen and Ivanova (2013) described the responses to a course of psychostimulants for five clients with comorbid BN and ADHD as decreased binge/purging and improved ADHD symptoms. Cluster B disorders, such as borderline personality disorder (BPD), are also identified frequently with BN. The presence of a comorbid diagnosis of BN among women with BPD is significantly and uniquely associated with recent suicidal ideation and with self-harm behaviour and suicide attempts during treatment (Reas, Pedersen, Karterud, & Rø, 2015). Women with premenstrual syndrome and premenstrual dysphoric disorder have higher odds of having BN, independent of comorbid mental health conditions (Nobles et al., 2016).

Aetiology

Some of the predisposing or risk factors for BN overlap with theories of causality (see Fig. 25.2). For example, dieting may put an individual at risk for developing BN. The dieting can turn into dietary restraint, which can lead to binge eating and purging in vulnerable individuals. The interplay of other risk factors (e.g., body dissatisfaction and separation–individuation issues) also helps explain the development of this disorder.

Biologic Theories

Dieting may occur in girls as young as 9 years of age. At 12 years, girls had significantly higher depressive symptom scores than boys and they had significantly higher body dissatisfaction than boys at 7, 9, and 12 years of age. Predictors of early dieting for males and females include personal factors of weight concern, weight importance, and depressive symptoms (Loth, MacLehose, Bucchianeri, Crow, & Neumark-Stainer, 2014). Higher eating disorder symptoms at 9 years have significantly predicted higher eating disorder symptoms at 12 years for both boys and girls, while greater dietary restraint at 7 years was a significant predictor for boys (Evans et al., 2017). Dieting is believed to affect the neurotransmitters, including serotonin, which are involved in appetite, satiety, and eating patterns of BN. Levels of cholecystokinin (CCK), a hormone associated with satiation, previously found to be low in some individuals with BN, were found to be similar in comparison to controls; however, a positive correlation was found between the BN groups' CCK response and urge to vomit following ingestion of a test meal (Hannon-Engel, Filin, & Wolfe, 2013). This suggests that persons experiencing BN may become sensitive to or uncomfortable with the sensations associated with the release of the satiety hormone, which triggers an episode of vomiting and subsequent feeling of relief. As in AN, overexercising has also contributed to some of the symptoms of BN.

Neuropathologic

The changes in the brain are the result rather than the cause of eating dysregulation. As with AN, these changes resolve when symptoms such as dietary restraint, binge eating, and purging remit.

Genetic

A specific gene responsible for BN has not been identified. However, research suggests that genes acting within the dopamine system influence both eating- and personality-related psychopathology either directly or indirectly (i.e., in interaction with traumatic childhood experiences). This is believed to contribute to variations in the presentation of comorbid traits and to increased psychopathology and body mass in women with bulimia disorders. Further studies are required to confirm heritability of abnormalities in BN and other eating disorders (Rikani et al., 2013).

Biochemical

The most frequently studied biochemical theories in BN relate to lowered serotonin and dopamine neurotransmission. People with BN are believed to have altered modulation of central serotonin neuronal systems (Sree, 2013). Even following recovery from BN, findings of altered serotonin levels persist that potentially contribute to BN symptomatology and responses to medication. Dopamine is considered the primary neurotransmitter involved in the reinforcing effects of food. Low levels of dopamine can increase hunger; increased dopamine concentration can decrease appetite. These differences in dopamine levels may help explain why those with BN are more attentive to food stimuli (Sue, Wing Sue, Sue, & Sue, 2016).

Psychological and Social Theories

Psychological factors in the aetiology of BN have been studied extensively, and most experts believe that these factors converge with environmental or sociocultural factors within individuals who have a biologic predisposition, causing symptoms to develop. Stress precedes the occurrence of bulimic behaviours, and increases in negative affect following stressful events may function as maintenance factors for bulimic behaviours (Goldschmidt et al., 2014). As with AN, psychoanalytic developmental theories that explain separation–individuation are important in causality. Because the age of onset for BN is late adolescence/early adulthood, leaving home (e.g., for employment or educational opportunities) may represent the first physical separation for adolescents unprepared for the emotional separation. Analysis of interviews conducted with women receiving online therapy to help with BN revealed the life–historical development of BN as stemming from low self-esteem, poor self-concept, a negative view of the future, and concerns about the impact of the disorder on their family. The women spoke of isolation and shame associated with BN and expressed a sense that their eating problems were a significant burden in their lives, for example, "I thought I was just a horrible, horrible person and all I deserved was to be who I am" (McClay, Waters, McHale, Schmidt, & Williams, 2013, p. 5).

The same sociocultural factors regarding societal focus on the ideal body type that underlie AN play a significant role in the development of BN.

Cognitive Theory

Within the view of BN as a disorder of thinking, distortions are the basis of behaviours such as binge eating and purging. Core low self-esteem is exacerbated by dependence on perfectionist standards toward weight, shape, and eating control. Interpersonal problems maintain the binge-eating and purging symptoms of BN through heightened sensitivity to perceiving interpersonal problems and repeated experience of these problems that further exacerbates and contributes to the core low self-esteem (Lampard & Sharbanee, 2015). For instance, cues such as stress related to interpersonal difficulties (e.g., an argument with a loved one), negative emotions, physiologic state (e.g., hunger, fullness), and environment (e.g., the presence of attractive food, a remark about the person's weight or how much one is eating, catching sight of self in a mirror) may activate personal negative self-beliefs (e.g., "I'm unlikeable," or "I'm a failure"). This activation typically generates considerable emotional distress. Eating provides a distraction from negative thoughts and emotions and is commonly associated with a decrease in intensity of emotional states. Thus, eating is initially interpreted positively and linked to positive beliefs (e.g., "Eating will take away my painful feelings"). However, eating can also be closely linked

with negative beliefs about the potential consequences (e.g., "I'll gain weight"). The person with BN is caught in a state of conflict in which both positive and negative beliefs about eating coexist. The binge provides only temporary relief from the original distress and is subject to negative interpretation (e.g., as a sign of failure) that, in turn, reinforces the negative self-beliefs in the first place. In contrast, purging may result when negative beliefs about eating dominate positive beliefs and the person switches from eating to vomiting or other compensatory behaviour. Once the compensatory behaviour has ceased, any initial sense of relief at having gotten rid of the food starts to dissipate and the negative consequences of yet another episode of binge eating and purging, negative mood, and arousal start to increase again. These cognitive and triggering theories are viewed as an explanation for maintaining the binge eating once it has been established, rather than an explanation of causality (Ristea & Drăgoi, 2014).

Family

As with AN, the convergence of many factors at a vulnerable stage of individual development contribute to the development of BN. Originating with work at the Maudsley Hospital in London in the late 1970s, a paradigm shift directed attention away from presuming an aetiologic role for family dynamics and toward regarding the family as a resource in therapy, easing parents' guilt, and promoting an attitude of inclusion (Reel, 2013).

Spirituality and Attachment Theory

BN is symbolic of a difficulty in finding other more satiating ways to deal with important needs and emotional issues, some of which may not be accessible to awareness. BN may thus be connected to one's identity and purpose in life, covering a true hunger for meaning about where one belongs. It can be frightening for individuals to accept and acknowledge their spirituality, because it means confronting greater issues about death, life, and one's place in the world.

Attachment theory describes one's relationship with a main early caregiver and the subsequent development of internal working models, which may guide one's view of self and the nature of relationships with others. Attachment can be conceptualized as being either secure or insecure. Investigating the link between attachment to God/Higher Power and BN with college students, Buser and Gibson (2016) found significant links between insecure attachments to God/Higher Power and bulimic symptoms. It may be that an individual who fears being abandoned by God/Higher Power and questions God's/Higher Power's love is more vulnerable to accepting sociocultural messages and pressures about body image. Also, an individual who places little value on having a relationship with God/Higher Power may feel upset about this lack of a personal spiritual connection, experience unpleasant emotions, and then use bulimic behaviours to alleviate the negative emotions (Buser & Gibson, 2016).

Risk Factors

The risk or predisposing factors for BN are included in Figure 25.3.

Interdisciplinary Treatment

Individuals with BN benefit from a comprehensive multifaceted treatment approach that usually takes place in an outpatient setting, except when the client is suicidal or when past outpatient treatment has failed (see Table 25.3). Therapy for BN focuses on psychological issues, including boundary setting and separation–individuation conflicts and on changing problematic behaviours and dysfunctional thought patterns and attitudes, especially about eating, weight, and shape. Intensive psychotherapy and pharmacologic interventions are necessary. Nutrition counselling helps stabilize and normalize eating, which means stopping the binge–purge cycle. Support groups may also be involved. Family therapy is not usually a part of the treatment, because many people with BN live on college campuses away from home or are older and on their own. Usually, the treatment becomes less intensive as symptoms remit. In short, therapeutic relationships, nutrition counselling, and cognitive interventions are priorities in the nursing care of individuals with eating disorders.

Priority Care Issues

Given the comorbid conditions of depression, anxiety, substance misuse, and BPD, some individuals with BN may become suicidal. They are also often at risk for self-mutilation. Because they display high levels of impulsivity (e.g., shoplifting, overspending), financial and legal difficulties have been associated with BN.

Nursing Management: Human Response to Bulimia Nervosa Disorder

The primary nursing diagnoses for clients with BN are Imbalanced Nutrition: Less Than or More Than Body Requirements, Powerlessness, Anxiety, and Ineffective Coping.

Therapeutic Relationship

Individuals with BN experience shame and guilt and have an intense need to please and be liked. They are too ashamed to discuss their symptoms but do not want to disappoint others, so they may discuss more superficial social or unrelated issues in an attempt to engage the nurse. A nonjudgmental approach stressing the importance of the relationship and outlining its purpose is important from the outset. Explaining the nature of the

relationship and the goals of therapy will help clarify the boundaries (see Chapter 6).

Biologic Domain

Most individuals with BN maintain normal weights. Those who purge risk fluid and electrolyte abnormalities, particularly hypokalaemia that contributes to muscle weakness and fatigability, cardiac arrhythmias, palpitations, and cardiac conduction defects. Neuropsychiatric disturbances, such as poor concentration and attention, and sleep disturbances are common.

Assessment

The nurse assesses current eating patterns, determines the number of times a day the individual binges and purges, and notes dietary restraint practices. Sleep patterns, oral health, and exercise habits are also important.

Nursing Diagnoses for Biologic Domain

Imbalanced Nutrition: Less Than/More Than Body Requirements and Disturbed Sleep Pattern are typical nursing diagnoses for the biologic domain.

Interventions for Biologic Domain

If the client is admitted to the hospital, all food intake is strictly monitored to normalize eating. Bathroom visits are also supervised to prevent purging. Outpatients are asked to record their intake, binges, and purges to establish a foundation for changing behaviours with psychotherapy. Because individuals with BN have chaotic lifestyles and are often overcommitted, sleep may be a low priority. Sleep-deprived individuals may assume that food would be helpful, and they begin to eat, triggering a binge. To encourage regular sleep patterns, individuals are encouraged to go to bed and rise at about the same time every day. Clients who purge by inducing vomiting are instructed in proper oral care practices to mitigate enamel erosion and caries.

Pharmacologic Interventions

Pharmacotherapy is effective for symptom remission in BN. Antidepressant treatment may additionally benefit comorbid affective symptoms (Milano et al., 2013; Mitchell et al., 2013). Fluoxetine (Prozac) has been the most studied medication for BN in clinical trials (see Box 25.11) and is U. S. Food and Drug Administration approved for treatment of an eating disorder (Dalkilic, 2013). Effective doses are usually 60 mg per day, a higher dosage than that used to treat depression. Weight is monitored as decreased appetite and weight loss are common during the first few weeks of administration. It is also important to monitor the intake of medication for possible purging after administration. The effect of the medication depends on the time taken for its absorption. Bupropion (Wellbutrin) is contraindicated for the treatment of BN due to its seizure risk (Mitchell et al., 2013).

BOX 25.11 DRUG PROFILE

Fluoxetine Hydrochloride (Prozac)

Drug Class: Selective serotonin reuptake inhibitor

Receptor Affinity: Inhibits central nervous system neuronal uptake of serotonin with little effect on norepinephrine; thought to antagonize muscarinic, histaminergic, and α-adrenergic receptors.

Indications: Treatment of depressive disorders, most effective in major depression, obesity, bulimia, and OCD

Routes and Dosage: Available in 10- and 20-mg pulvules and 20 mg per 5 mL oral solution

Adults: 20 mg per day in the morning, not to exceed 80 mg per day. Full antidepressant effect may not be seen for up to 4 weeks. If no improvement, dosage is increased after several weeks. Dosages above 20 mg per day may be administered on a once-a-day (morning) or BID schedule (i.e., morning and noon). For eating disorders, typically, 60 mg per day, administered in the morning, is recommended for reducing the frequency of binge eating and vomiting.

Geriatric: Administer at lower or less frequent doses; monitor responses to guide dosage.

Children: Safety and efficacy have not been established.

Half-Life (Peak Effect): 2 to 3 days (6 to 8 hours)

Selected Adverse Reactions: Headache, nervousness, insomnia, drowsiness, anxiety, tremors, dizziness, light-headedness, nausea, vomiting, diarrhoea, dry mouth, anorexia, dyspepsia, constipation, taste changes, upper respiratory infections, pharyngitis, painful menstruation, sexual dysfunction, urinary frequency, sweating, rash, pruritus, weight loss, asthenia, and fever.

Warnings: Avoid use in pregnancy and while breast-feeding. Use with caution in clients with impaired hepatic or renal function and diabetes mellitus. Possible risk for toxicity if taken with tricyclic antidepressants.

Special Client and Family Education:

- Be aware that the drug may take up to 4 weeks to get full antidepressant effect.
- Take the drug in the morning or in divided doses, if necessary.
- Report any adverse reactions.
- Avoid driving a car or performing hazardous activities because the drug may cause drowsiness or dizziness.
- Eat small, frequent meals to help with complaints of nausea and vomiting.

TEACHING POINTS

Individuals should be instructed to take medication as prescribed. SSRIs should be taken in the morning because they can cause insomnia. Individuals should be informed that any weight loss they initially experience is temporary and is usually regained after a few weeks, when the medication dosage has stabilized. Treatment dropout is high (Schnicker, Hiller, & Legenbauer, 2013); monitoring adverse effects and eliciting the client's understanding of the reasons why the clinician recommended the pharmacotherapy may help direct interventions.

Psychosocial Domain

Assessment

Psychological assessment focuses on cognitive distortions—cues or stimuli that lead to dysfunctional behaviour affecting symptom development—and knowledge deficits. The psychological characteristics typical of individuals with BN are presented in Box 25.1. Examples of cognitive distortions present in BN are given in Table 25.4. These thought patterns form the basis for "rules" and lead the way to destructive eating patterns. During routine history taking, individuals may relate many of these distortions. Situations that produce feelings of

being overwhelmed and powerless need to be explored, as does the individual's ability to set boundaries, control impulsivity, and maintain quality relationships. These underlying issues may precipitate binge eating. Several assessment tools are available to gauge such characteristics as body dissatisfaction and impulsivity (see Box 25.6). Body dissatisfaction should be openly explored. Mood is evaluated because many people with BN also have depression.

Nursing Diagnoses for Psychosocial Domain

Deficient Knowledge and Disturbed Thought Processes are among the common diagnoses for the psychosocial domain.

Interventions for Psychosocial Domain

CBT is the most empirically supported treatment for BN. In a recent clinical trial, the majority (95.7%) of persons participating in CBT exhibited fewer binge and/or vomit and/or laxative use behaviours compared to persons treated using a different treatment (71.4%) (MacDonald, McFarlane, Dionne, David, & Olmsted, 2017). CBT is usually conducted in a group, with one or two sessions a week. CBT has also been effectively delivered in guided self-help format (Naeem et al., 2017). IPT has had positive outcomes but may take longer to change binge-eating and purging symptoms. Behavioural therapy alone has not been as effective as CBT. While binge eating may persist, little work can be done on underlying interpersonal issues, such as boundary setting, because the client feels out of control with eating. Therefore, cognitive therapy is begun first, to address the distorted thinking processes influencing dietary restraint, binge eating, and purging. Decreasing these symptoms will help eliminate the out-of-control feelings.

Behavioural Techniques

The behavioural techniques, such as **cue elimination** and response prevention, require self-monitoring to individualize the therapy. **Self-monitoring** is accomplished using a diary, in which the individual records binges, purges, precipitating emotions, and environmental cues including physiologic/nutritional and psychological pressures to eat, as well as individuals and situations that may be associated with negative feelings such as depression, anger, or anxiety. Self-monitoring enables further understanding of the eating problem, identifies progress, and helps clients develop awareness of what is happening *in the moment* so that they can begin to change behaviours that may have seemed automatic or beyond their control (Herrin & Larkin, 2013). The client's records are jointly reviewed at each session, and any difficulties are addressed in the session. Emotional and environmental cues are identified, and alternative responses are formulated, tried, and reinforced. When

a cue or stimulus leads to a dysfunctional or unhealthy response, the response can be eliminated, or an alternate, healthier response to the cue can be substituted, tried, and then reinforced. The client is encouraged to focus on longer-term consequences (e.g., social isolation) rather than shorter-term relief of uncomfortable feelings. The proliferation of health-related apps with self-monitoring of eating habits as a major feature may be helpful for people with eating disorders and for eating disorder professionals. There is a need to evaluate the clinical utility of such apps (Fairburn & Rothwell, 2015). Figure 25.6 gives two examples of behavioural interventions. In example 1, for the individual with AN, the response is modified or altered to a healthier one; in example 2, for the individual with BN, the cue is changed to produce a different, healthier response. Other techniques, such as postponing binges and purges through distraction, a technique to interrupt the cycle, are also effective.

Psychoeducation

The nurse can assist clients to understand the binge–purge cycle and the role of rigid rules in contributing to this cycle. The value of eating meals regularly to ward off hunger and reduce the possibility of a binge is important. Individuals who misuse laxatives are taught that although these drugs produce water weight loss, they are ineffective for true, lasting weight loss. Moreover, individuals also need information about potassium depletion, electrolyte imbalances, dehydration, and the medical consequences of binge eating and purging. Other topics for psychoeducation are included in Box 25.12. Psychoeducation is effective for clients with BN while

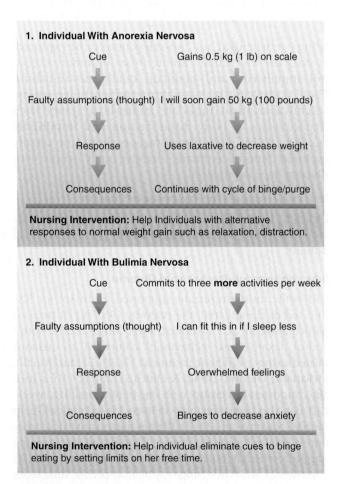

Figure 25.6. Examples of the relationship of cues, thoughts, and responses: behavioural interventions.

BOX 25.12 Psychoeducation Checklist: Bulimia Nervosa

When caring for the individual with BN, be sure to include the following topic areas in the teaching plan:

- Psychopharmacologic agents, if used, including drug, action, dosage, frequency, and possible adverse effects
- Binge–purge cycle and effects on body
- Nutrition and eating patterns
- Hydration
- Avoidance of cues
- Cognitive distortions
- Limit-setting
- Appropriate boundary setting
- Assertiveness
- Resources
- Self-monitoring and behavioural interventions
- Realistic goal setting

on a treatment waiting list (Tatham, Athanasia, Dodd, & Waller, 2016) and subsequently promotes higher rates of engagement and completion of therapy (Brewin et al., 2016). Yet, psychoeducation was not found to significantly increase readiness to change and confidence in ability to control binge eating (Vella-Zarb, Mills, Westra, Carter, & Keating, 2015).

TEACHING POINTS

Psychoeducation for individuals with BN focuses on setting boundaries and healthy limits, developing assertiveness, learning nutritional concepts related to healthy eating, discussing societal definitions of beauty, and clarifying misconceptions about food. Research findings related to semistarvation, weight regulation, dieting, obesity, and the sociocultural milieu that influences the development and perpetuation of eating disorders are discussed. Cognitive distortions are addressed because of their role in dietary restraint and resultant binge eating. Measures such as Garner's abbreviated Eating Attitudes Test (EAT-26; see Box 25.6) can be used to assess clients' eating concerns before, during, and after psychoeducation.

Family Assessment and Intervention

For parents, their child's purging behaviour elicits stronger emotional reactions than binge eating (Hoste, Lebow, & Le Grange, 2015). Parents express similar dissatisfaction with their families as do clients (Fisher & Bushlow, 2015). National eating disorder associations recommend that families engage in self-care activities such as speaking about their experiences to help lessen the shame and obtaining support (National Eating Disorders Association [NEDA], 2013; National Eating Disorders Information Centre [EDIC], 2014).

Group Therapy

Group therapy is cost-effective and effectively increases learning because individuals learn from each other as well as from the nurse or other therapist. Some experts have recommended 12-step programs for treating BN. However, many clinicians who work in this specialty have noted that these programs, with their strict rules, can be counterproductive for individuals with BN, who already have stringent rules (e.g., dietary restraint) and are "abstinent" in many ways that lead to binge eating. Broad parameters regarding food choices (e.g., allowing all foods in moderation), together with knowledge about healthy eating, are encouraged instead. As symptoms subside, individuals can concentrate on underlying

interpersonal issues in therapy, such as feelings of inadequacy and low self-esteem, and can work with other group members to develop assertiveness.

Spiritual Domain

Assessment

The role of spirituality in the lives of individuals with BN can be assessed through their expressions of loss and powerlessness, self-care capacity, quality of relationships, history of conflicts and painful traumatic experiences, attitudes about food and overeating, harm avoidance strategies, self-directedness, and self-judgments. The nurse must strive to see the person beyond the dieting, binge-eating, and purging behaviours. Women with a diagnosis of BN who are depressed have displayed identity problems associated with lifetime suicide attempt (Pisetsky et al. 2015). This finding suggests the need to monitor depression severity as the most important target of treatment and suicide prevention.

Nursing Diagnoses for Spiritual Domain

Loss and Powerlessness are among the common diagnoses for the spiritual domain.

Interventions for Spiritual Domain

Research has demonstrated an association between therapeutic alliance (the bond between the client and nurse or therapist) and overall BN symptoms; a negative association was found between the therapeutic alliance and posttreatment purge frequency and a positive association between therapist and client ratings of the tasks carried out in therapy and improvements in binge eating and vomiting (Zaitsoff, Pullmer, Cyr, & Aime, 2015). Given the importance of therapeutic alliance, the nurse encourages clients to express feelings of loss and powerlessness without negative self-judgment. Clients will benefit from exploring what they do and do not have control over and to accept their human limitations. Those who binge eat and purge can learn to delay these behaviours through engaging in activities such as journal writing, affirming positive self-worth, meditation, and imagery. These strategies may help clients with BN to build support from self and to help deal with comorbid depression and anxiety. Nurses can further help create the context for clients with BN to enlist support from others.

Evaluation and Treatment Outcomes

Individuals with BN may have better recovery outcomes than do those with AN. Outcomes have improved since the early 1990s, partially because of earlier detection, research on treatments that are most effective, and neuropharmacologic research and advances. Recovery from BN has been described by women as a process of beginning with renewed self-esteem. There is progress from feeling stuck in BN, getting ready to change, breaking free of bulimia symptomatology, and grasping a new reality of self-acceptance. The process is back and forth between progress and relapse, and women express strong ambivalence about leaving the illness behind. Essential for their recovery is developing a unique explanation of the cause of their illness. These findings indicate a need for care that bolsters women's self-efficacy through strengthening beliefs in their own abilities and instilling hope for recovery (Lindgren, Enmark, Bohman, & Lundström, 2015).

In another study that defined recovery as abstinence from binge eating and purging and BMI greater than 18.5, recovery rates of 15.6% at the end of treatment and 19.8% at 62-week follow-up were reported for a sample of 96 adults with BN (Yu, Agras, & Bryson, 2013). Relapse was reported as 60% when recovery was defined as abstinence from binge eating and purging. The researchers recommended using the term "remission" for individuals who no longer binge eat and purge at the end of treatment and "recovered" for those maintaining abstinence for a prolonged period of follow-up (Yu et al., 2013). Decreased likelihood of recovery was associated with a history of lifetime major depressive disorder and high drive for thinness at the time of assessment (Keski-Rahkonen et al., 2013). In a meta-analysis of treatment outcome, more frequent binge–purge behaviours at baseline predicted worse outcome at end of treatment and follow-up; a lower level of drive to exercise was predictive of good outcomes across end of treatment and 6-month follow-up (Vall & Wade, 2015). Midlife adults (greater than 40 years) were found to have higher rates of poor outcome or death compared to youth (12 to 18 years) and young adults (18 to 39 years); good outcome was achieved by only 5.9% of midlife adult clients compared to 14% of young adult and 27.5% of youth clients. Such factors as alcohol and/or drug misuse and endocrine concerns predicted poor outcome or death for midlife adults seeking treatment. Specialized treatment focusing on quality of life, comorbid medical concerns, interpersonal connection, and emotion regulation is encouraged.

Continuum of Care

Individuals with BN are less likely than those with AN to require hospitalization. However, those with extreme dehydration and electrolyte imbalance, depression and suicidality, or symptoms that have not remitted with outpatient treatment need hospitalization. After treatment, referrals to recovery groups and support groups are important to prevent relapse.

■ BINGE-EATING DISORDER

BED was introduced into the *DSM-IV* as a provisional diagnosis in 2004 (APA, 2000) and included in the *DSM-5* (APA, 2013) as its own category of eating disorders (Refer to DSM-5 for full diagnostic criteria). BED is more prevalent than either AN or BN and is not uncommon in men.

Lifetime prevalence for BED in Canada is 3.5% (Canadian Psychology Association, 2014). It is associated with overweight and high comorbidity comparable to that of BN. When diagnosed, the usual treatment is outpatient therapy.

Clinical Course

Investigators have shown that individuals with BED, when compared to those with BN, have lower dietary restraint and are higher in weight, even though many are not obese. It has been estimated that 10% to 30% of obese individuals have BED. In a community study that completed annual diagnostic interviews during the entire adolescent period, the peak age for onset of BED was between 18 and 20 years. The findings revealed that about a quarter of the women reported shifting from binge–purge symptoms into BED, while an equal number reported moving from binge-eating symptoms into BN (Stice, Marti, & Rohde, 2013). In a separate study, a man with BED expressed:

> There is still something really shameful about binge eating ... because that's like admitting that's all there is: you massively overeat food; you lose all control around food. I think that compounds the isolation ... you feel as if you're an oddity, as if you are completely alone. (Spyrou, 2014, p. 54)

In another account, BED was personified as a powerful "instinct that takes over, that compels me to ... eat the bad things" (Spyrou, 2014, p. 50). Attributing the binge eating to this external powerful compulsion provides the means to deny personal responsibility for the binge eating until "after the binge I am in so much pain, all I can focus on is how disgusted I feel ... and how I am going to add to my stretch marks" (Spyrou, 2014, p. 49).

Outward signs associated with BED may include overweight, obesity, and associated consequences such as gallbladder disease and arthritis. Through these manifestations, BED may come to the attention of family and peers. Treatment can be delayed for years as individuals attempt on their own or with commercial weight-loss programs to control their eating. Outcomes have not been extensively studied; poor prognosis is expected given the difficulty of attempting to achieve and maintain weight loss and in cases in which mood and anxiety disorders are also present.

Individuals with BED may miss work, school, or social activities to binge eat. Those who become obese often are extremely distressed by their binge eating, feel bad about themselves, and are preoccupied with their appearance. Most feel ashamed, may avoid social gatherings, and try to hide their problem. Often, they are so successful that close family members and friends do not know that they binge eat.

Diagnostic Criteria

BED shares with the other major eating disorders of AN and BN a high body dissatisfaction (Schmitz, Schnicker,

& Legenbauer, 2016). BED differs from AN and BN in terms of dietary restraint and drive for thinness. In AN, for example, an excessively strong drive for thinness and fear of weight gain may trigger restriction, refusal of normal food amounts, and subsequently lead to underweight. In contrast, in BN and BED, excessive food intake related to loss of control while eating may trigger fear of weight gain, but in the case of BN, inappropriate compensatory behaviours (e.g., self-induced vomiting or misuse of laxatives). Women who have been diagnosed with BED neither compensate for binge eating directly nor counterregulate its effect indirectly by restrictive eating between the episodes of binge eating. As a consequence, weight differs between the diagnostic groups, from underweight in AN to possible overweight in BED (Schmitz et al., 2016). Persons with BED are typically ashamed of their eating and try to conceal symptoms from others.

Binge-Eating Disorder in Special Populations

BED is more prevalent among those seeking weight-loss treatment (Faulconbridge & Bechtel, 2014). BED is more prevalent in certain clinical populations, including persons with diabetes (Raevuori et al., 2015) and obese older men (Reas & Stedal, 2015).

Epidemiology

BED is understudied in children and adolescents but appears to be rarer in younger clients than adults (Lock et al., 2015). BED in individuals with type 2 diabetes is more common than AN or BN. A community survey conducted by the World Health Organization in 12 nations (including the United States, New Zealand, and countries in Latin America and Europe) reported country-specific lifetime prevalence estimates for BED as consistently higher than for BN (Kessler et al., 2013).

Age of Onset

Onset of binge eating typically begins in late adolescence or early adulthood, often after a period of significant dieting or weight loss (Lock et al., 2015). Data from the 2004 Canadian Community Health Survey (CCHS) identified that overweight and obese adult Canadians underreported their weight. Approximately 25% reported being overweight or obese, while approximately 59% were overweight or obese based on measured weight and height from the CCHS (Schermel et al., 2014). Canadians are also dissatisfied with their appearance. Only 11% are completely satisfied with their looks, according to a global survey based on interviews conducted across 22 countries (Kozicka, 2015). The survey findings were gendered with 13% of Canadian males completely satisfied with their looks, compared to 9% of females. The survey also found that 9% of Canadian teens are not at all satisfied with their looks, which is much higher than the global average of 3%. These results begin to inform an understanding of body dissatisfaction among Canadians that requires further study to determine if persons affected are initiating dietary restraint or engaging in unhealthy weight practices to modify shape, weight, and appearance.

Gender Differences

A ratio of 1.5 to 2 adult females to 1 male experiences BED.

Ethnic and Cultural Differences

BED prevalence does not differ across Asian American ethnic subgroups or between Asian Americans as a group compared with non-Latino Whites; however, Asian Americans as a group are less likely than Whites to endorse BED symptoms (Lee-Winn, Mendelson, & Mojtabai, 2014). This suggests that Asian Americans would be diagnosed with BED less frequently than non-Latino Whites and that the lower prevalence of BED diagnosis may lead to under recognition of problematic binge eating and underutilization of clinical care.

Familial Differences

BED may run in families, reflecting a genetic influence. First-degree relatives report significantly higher lifetime rates of anxiety disorders, mood disorders (in particular, bipolar I or II disorder and any depressive disorder), and eating disorders than the first-degree relatives of those without BED (Bulik & Trace, 2013).

Comorbidity

BED is associated with medical conditions related to obesity, including diabetes, hypertension, dyslipidaemias, sleep problems/disorders, and pain conditions; BED may be related to these conditions independent of obesity and co-occurring psychiatric disorders (Olguin et al., 2017). Prospective data suggest that BED may be associated with type 2 diabetes and with metabolic syndrome in adults and children (Mitchell, 2016). In a prospective multicenter observational study of 242 adolescents with severe obesity, the most common comorbid conditions were dyslipidaemia (74.4%), chronic back or joint pain (58.3%), obstructive sleep apnea (56.6%), and hypertension (45.0%) (Zeller et al., 2015). BED or binge-eating behaviour is also associated with asthma and GI symptoms and disorders and, among women, with menstrual dysfunction, pregnancy complications, intracranial hypertension, and polycystic ovary syndrome (Olguin et al., 2017).

Mood and substance use disorders co-occur frequently among clients with BED. Grilo, White, Barnes, and Masheb (2013) found that 67% of persons seeking treatment for obesity and binge eating in primary care had at least one additional lifetime psychiatric disorder with mood (49%), anxiety (41%), and substance use (22%) disorders most common and 37% had at least one current psychiatric disorder with anxiety (27%) and mood (17%) most common. In persons diagnosed with BED, depression scores were significantly high (Çelik et al., 2015). Further to this, BED was associated with elevated odds of suicide ideation, plan, and attempt among adults and adolescents; adolescents experience suicidality onset following BED onset and adults experience suicidality onset prior to BED onset (Forrest, Zuromski, Dodd, & Smith, 2017). Thus, the presence of BED in adolescence may serve as a marker for more severe symptomatology that precedes the occurrence of suicidality. Psychiatric comorbidity was associated with the severity.

Complications

Medical complications of BED include above comorbidities of obesity, diabetes, hypertension, high cholesterol, gallbladder disease, kidney disease and/or failure, heart disease, arthritis, certain types of cancer, bone deterioration, menstrual irregularities, ovarian abnormalities, complications of pregnancy, depression, anxiety, and suicidal thoughts. BED is also associated with impaired quality of life and increased health care utilization. Obese individuals with BED may also experience the consequences of stigma such as increased risk of depression, economic hardship, isolation, and social withdrawal. These stigmatized individuals have negative body image, poorer psychosocial functioning, and higher incidence of binge eating. They have reported feelings of discouragement and social inadequacy, which in turn have generated insecurity, social escape, and relationship difficulties. Persons with BED have been deemed more responsible for their condition than persons with AN and BN. When BED has led to obesity, these persons are blamed more for their condition than any other target, even though obese individuals with BED are held less personally responsible for their condition than obese individuals without BED (Ebneter & Latner, 2013). Perceived weight discrimination increases the health risks of obesity and can contribute to health decline (Sutin & Terracciano, 2013).

As a stigmatized condition, obesity negatively affects the relationship between clients and health care providers. Obese clients have reported feeling that health care professionals' ambivalence toward their health needs amplified the extent to which the obese persons felt personally responsible for their condition. This contributed to their ambivalence in relation to accessing and using services. For example, they cancelled medical appointments if they believed they would be weighed (Phelan et al., 2015) and were less probable to undergo clinical breast examination (Atkins et al., 2013) and gynaecologic examination or Papanicolaou smear testing (Qaseem, Humphrey, Harris, Starkey, & Denberg, 2014).

Aetiology

It is postulated that binge eating functions to modulate negative emotional states. When individuals with BED experience negative affect, they may lack effective strategies for managing these emotions or else their typically functional strategies for coping with negative emotions do not work. These individuals are inclined to behave in an impulsive fashion to a negative affective state (Danner et al., 2013). They may be able to anticipate long-term negative consequences but do not chose more advantageous behaviour given their impulsive nature. Along with this, they may lack motional clarity or ability to determine what emotion is being felt (Gianini, White, & Masheb, 2013). Examining the association between coping strategies and emotion regulation in individuals who report binge-eating symptoms, Mac Vie (2016) found a positive association between self-reported binge-eating behaviour and self-reported difficulties regulating emotions and a negative association between self-reported binge-eating behaviour and self-reported positive coping strategies. Moreover, Coffino, Orloff, and Hormes (2016) found that the relationships between impulsivity, dietary restraint, and binge-eating severity were moderated by body weight. In their under- and normal-weight sample, dietary restraint mediated the relationship between impulsivity and binge-eating severity. In the overweight and obese sample, impulsivity had a direct effect on binge-eating severity, but because this relationship was not mediated by dietary restraint, impulsivity may be a more proximal antecedent to binge episodes in overweight and obese individuals, who do not engage in dietary restraint.

Biologic Theories

While AN and BN tend to be characterized by high levels of most forms of dietary restraint, including extreme restrictive behaviours, BED tends to be associated with low levels of dietary restraint The peculiar food choice (e.g., fats, sweets, and snacks) that clients make during binge-eating episodes has been related to the hypothesis of a "hedonic deprivation," where eating impulsiveness can be triggered by restrictions on palatable foods during everyday life (Amianto, Ottone, Daga, & Fassino, 2015).

Genetic

Significantly increased rates of BED were reported in first-degree family members of individuals with BED, a finding corroborated by twin studies (Trace, Baker, Peñas-Lledó, & Bulik, 2013). Candidate gene association studies of binge eating have examined neurotransmitter systems or genetic variants implicated in appetite and obesity, including the serotonin and dopamine systems. Research on the dopamine and the µ-opioid receptor genes suggests that a predisposing risk factor for BED may be a heightened sensitivity to reward, which could manifest as a strong dopamine signal in the brain's striatal region (Davis, 2015). However, candidate gene studies have not clearly confirmed the involvement of any one gene or genetic pathway. In other research, individuals with a specific mutation in the location of the FTO gene were found to have higher circulating levels of the "hunger hormone," ghrelin, in their blood, which means they start to feel hungry again soon after eating a meal. Individuals with the FTO gene variation were 20 percent more likely to binge eat; girls specifically were 30 percent more likely to binge eat (Micali, Field, Treasure, & Evans, 2015).

Using gene mapping and gene validation, Kirkpatrick et al. (2016) identified cytoplasmic FMR1-interacting protein 2 (CYFIP2)—a protein complex active in the outer layers of the cortex, hippocampus, and striatum and in Purkinje cells of the cerebellum—as a major genetic risk factor for binge eating. In addition, they observed that decreased myelination could be a neuropathologic consequence of binge eating. Because changes in the brain as a consequence of binge eating were predictive of decreased myelination, therapeutically promoting remyelination may represent a novel treatment avenue for promoting recovery in BED.

Psychological and Social Theories

Binge eating is significantly positively related to BMI and depression, negative mood, feelings of ineffectiveness, negative self-esteem and significantly negatively related to somatic complaints and all aspects of health-related qualities of life (Pasold, McCracken, & Ward-Begnoche, 2014).

Individuals with BED show higher harm avoidance scores than obese individuals who do not binge eat. Harm avoidance manifests as pessimistic worry in anticipation of problems, fear of uncertainty, social inhibition, shyness with strangers, passivity, and rapid fatigability (Grave, Calugi, El Ghoch, & Marchesini, 2014). Among 192 female clients with eating disorders in an outpatient eating disorders unit of a European hospital, those with BED reported moderate/severe childhood emotional abuse (30.77%), childhood sexual abuse (19.23%), and moderate/severe childhood emotional neglect (34.62%) (Guillaume et al., 2016). Some individuals with past abuse describe experiences of dissociation and emotional numbing while binge eating (Rosenbaum & White, 2013). Beyond childhood abuse, women have attributed the development of their eating disorder to their relationship with an abusive partner. The abuse was most commonly reported as weight-related teasing, overcontrol, or neglect. One women described the daily experience of this abuse and the impact on her self-esteem and behaviour as:

> a vicious cycle—the more I ate, the more I became overweight. The more overweight I became, the more cruel he became... It sort of started with the fat jokes, like 'oh you're getting podgy'... He'd go: 'You just worked out for an hour, so you can't eat such and such'... And then he'd go and do something and I'd quickly go to the fridge and just shove whatever I could in my mouth 'cause I'd be starving. And then quickly finish before he got back because heaven forbid he see that I was eating something... And I think I would be like halfway through and feel 'oh well I might as well keep eating

> because what's the point? And I'm doing this exercise and I'm not losing weight and he still calls me fat and I'm still fat.' (Mitchison et al., 2016, p. 7–8 of 13)

Obese individuals with BED are more likely to request professional psychological help than obese non–binge-eating individuals. Their greater sense of social insecurity and the impairment in interpersonal relationships associated with being overweight may contribute to this issue, and the intrinsic feeling of ineffectiveness and self-deprecation maintained by social stigmatization promotes the vicious circle leading to binge eating through negative feedback on self-esteem.

Cognitive Theory

The concept of overvaluation of shape and weight is central in interpreting BED through cognitive theory because overvaluation contributes to many of the symptoms related to BED, including preoccupation with thoughts about food and eating, weight, and shape; repeated body checking or avoidance (an individual avoiding looking at their body or reflections in mirrors); and attempts at dietary restraint (Edwards, 2013). Through a cognitive lens, overvaluation could be interpreted as a cognitive distortion deriving from (a) how individuals filter, process, organize, and assign meanings to internal and environmental stimuli and (b) the schemas, or core beliefs, that individuals hold about themselves. For example, an individual may have a negative self schema related to being overweight ("I am ugly") or many negative self schemas that are interrelated ("I am worthless because I am ugly") and thus easily activated by many events or stimuli. Also, an individual who is overweight would likely regularly encounter events or stimuli that could be interpreted as demeaning, embarrassing, or discriminating. With a negative core schema of ugliness activated, individuals would interpret and filter the information they receive to confirm their ugliness and their worthlessness because they connect their body/appearance with their worth.

The cognitive profile of BED clients is characterized by a poorer performance in decision-making, poorer cognitive flexibility, lower accuracy, a lack of attention, and difficulty adapting to changes in a new situation compared to clients with AN and healthy controls. BED clients' longer average time in providing answers could be explained by slowed thinking as a characteristic symptom of clients with depression (Aloi et al., 2015).

Disinhibition occurs once the "diet" is broken: The individual will no longer maintain control and will compensate through overeating (Vázquez & Rodríguez, 2013). Because of the inflexibility of these eating schemes, any minor transgression can lead to an all-or-nothing reaction whereby attempts to control eating are abandoned and result in a binge. The tendency to evaluate self-worth in terms of weight and shape and the dichotomous (black-and-white) thinking style, together with having unrealistic weight goals, low self-efficacy, and poor coping or problem-solving skills, have been identified as significant psychological predictors of higher frequency of binge eating at 12-month follow-up after completing treatments for BED (Grilo, White, Gueorguieva, Wilson, & Masheb, 2013).

Spiritual Theories

Underlying reasons for eating without being hungry include subjective experiences of distress and disconnection that do not encourage trust in others and prior relationships characterized by insecurity. Individuals who come to regard food as a kind of substitute attachment object may use it to fill the emptiness, often hiding their food and eating from others and thus increasing their sense of disconnection from self and others. Research by Homan and Lemmon (2014) indicates that a secure sense of attachment to God is associated with a lower risk of developing an eating disorder as well as a more positive body image. This is described in other research as "I realize that my 'interior' is more important than what I look like" (Zhang, 2013, p. 1246). Examining the relationship between religion and obesity using data from a large nationally representative sample, Krause and Hayward (2016) found the odds of being obese higher for study participants who received the least amount of spiritual support from religious others. Participants with higher spiritual support and/or emotional support scores had the lowest odds of being obese. Krause and Hayward indicate that some people experience significant personal growth when confronted by a stressful life event and that having a sympathetic and understanding religious other available to work through ambiguous feelings about God may go a long way toward alleviating the psychological distress. Krause and Neal suggest that having an anxious attachment to God is a stressor, and people who are exposed to acute stress tend to eat more even when they are not hungry. Higher rate of exposure to stress has been associated with a greater risk of becoming obese (Kiecolt-Glaser et al., 2015). Having a secure relationship with God may provide benefits are not unlike the benefits that arise from close relationships with human beings.

Risk Factors

The risk or predisposing factors for BED are included in Figure 25.3.

Interdisciplinary Treatment

Women with BED have self-identified their most common treatment priorities as mood concerns (72.2%), weight loss (66.7%), and body image/food issues (50%). Among those with obesity, a greater proportion of these women indicated body image/food issues were their top treatment priorities, suggesting that these persons may be more apt to seek treatment beyond weight management for their problematic eating patterns (Rosenbaum et al., 2016). The treatment methods for BED in current use include CBT, interpersonal psychotherapy, medications, self-help support groups, and commercial weight-loss and exercise programs. Surgical interventions are recommended for morbidly obese (BMI > 40) adult clients for whom other weight-loss attempts have failed (Neff, Olbers, & Le Roux, 2013). Clients receiving bariatric surgery for obesity were found to have lower scores for quality of life compared with non-BED obese individuals (Costa & Pinto, 2015). This finding makes it more critical that treatment provides opportunities for improving self-esteem, body experience, and problem-solving skills as suggested by Amianto et al. (2015). As with the treatment of AN and BN, a comprehensive interdisciplinary approach is needed. The treatment goals focus on reducing binge eating, effecting and maintaining weight loss if overweight or obese, restructuring dysfunctional thinking about food and appearance, alleviating comorbid depression and anxiety, and addressing harassment. Treatment occurs in an outpatient setting, except for when the client is hospitalized for bariatric surgery.

Nutrition counselling is an important treatment component focusing on portion size and control, the role of emotions on eating behaviours, healthy food and nutrient choices, self-monitoring, and strategies to delay binge eating. A pilot trial with chromium supplementation resulted in greater reductions in binge frequency, weight, fasting glucose, and symptoms of depression for those treated with chromium versus placebo (Brownley, Von Holle, Hamer, La Via, & Bulik, 2013). These findings require replication and are not considered within treatment guidelines. Clients may also access commercial weight-loss and fitness programs. Alternative therapies monitored by holistic health professionals may also be helpful, such as relaxation and yoga.

Priority Care Issues

Comorbid obesity, overweight, depression, and anxiety can contribute to cardiac and other health crises. The risk of type 2 diabetes is significant in the presence of obesity.

Nursing Management: Human Response to Binge-Eating Disorder

The primary nursing diagnoses for clients with BED may include Imbalanced Nutrition: More Than Body Requirements, Impaired Physical Mobility, Activity Intolerance, Anxiety, Ineffective Coping, and Ineffective Health Maintenance. The nurse establishes a therapeutic relationship and through this connection helps the client monitor self-care abilities including dietary intake and activity, teaches and models effective problem-solving, and suggests nutritional recommendations, taking into account the client's individual needs.

Therapeutic Relationship

Individuals with BED may experience a great deal of shame and guilt in response to negative judgements of their obesity and eating behaviours. They often are reluctant to participate in formal fitness programs for fear of being ridiculed. They may opt out of such programs when they believe they have nothing in common with other group members. Often, those who have BED suffer with the disorder for years, feeling very lonely. The nurse builds a relationship of trust through modelling a self-accepting, nonjudgmental approach, and discussing the role of the nurse–client relationship with respect to the goals of therapy (see Chapter 6). As discussed previously, the hallmarks of BED are low self-esteem experiences, weak therapeutic alliance, and low mastery and clarification experiences which, in turn, predict treatment dissatisfaction with and early discontinuation of care (Amianto et al., 2015). In examining the alliance–outcome relationship across 20 sessions of group therapy for BED, previous session alliance was significantly associated with lower subsequent session binge eating (Tasca, Compare, Zarbo, & Brugnera, 2016). This finding suggests that nurses, by attending to the quality of the therapeutic relationship, may help clients reduce binge eating.

Biologic Domain

Most individuals with BED become overweight or obese. The medical consequences of cardiovascular disease, diabetes, and arthritis as well as other health threats are considered in all aspects of the nursing process.

Assessment

The nurse assesses current binge-eating patterns and associated symptoms of gastric distress (e.g., acid regurgitation, heartburn, dysphagia, bloating, upper abdominal pain, diarrhoea, urgency, and constipation). Physical mobility, activity, and sleep patterns are also evaluated.

Nursing Diagnoses for Biologic Domain

Imbalanced Nutrition: More Than Body Requirements, Impaired Physical Mobility, and Activity Intolerance are examples of nursing diagnoses for the biologic domain.

Interventions for Biologic Domain

Clients are asked to record their intake, binges, and feelings associated with food and eating to form a foundation for changing behaviours. Clients should be monitored for complications such as diabetes, cardiovascular disease, and arthritis.

Pharmacologic Interventions

Lisdexamfetamine dimesylate (Vyvanse), a prescription medicine used for the treatment of attention deficit hyperactivity disorder (ADHD) in clients 6 years and above, is the first medication with an approved indication for the treatment of moderate to severe BED in adults in Canada (Shire, 2015). It is not known if Vyvanse is safe and effective for weight loss in the treatment of obesity. Topiramate and orlistat are currently used in the long-term treatment of obesity. Investigations have shown that topiramate (an antiepileptic agent) has been effective in decreasing binge eating and appetite. Topiramate has demonstrated efficacy in the treatment of BED-related obesity (Mitchell et al., 2013). Orlistat inhibits GI lipase, an enzyme that breaks down triglycerides in the intestine so that triglycerides from the diet are prevented from being hydrolyzed into absorbable free fatty acids and are excreted undigested, thus preventing approximately 30% of dietary fat from being absorbed. In a double-blind trial comparing Orlistat with polyglucosamine (a low molecular weight substance that binds fats to make them nonbioavailable yet partially eliminated or used by colonic bacteria as a fuel), both medications yielded weight loss; however, BMI and waist circumference reduction were more consistent with polyglucosamine than with orlistat (Stoll, Bitterlich, & Cornelli, 2017). Polyglucosamine side effects of stomach ache, bloating, nausea, vomiting, constipation, palpitations, and mood swings were reasons cited by participants for withdrawing from the study. The side effects resulting from orlistat's mode of action, which include oily spotting, liquid stools, faecal urgency or incontinence, flatulence, and abdominal cramping, were not cited by participants. Further research will confirm the feasibility of polyglucosamine in the treatment of obesity associated with BED. Other medications, usually SSRIs, may treat anxiety and depression symptomatology. Fluoxetine (Prozac) is often used to reduce binge eating (see Box 25.11).

TEACHING POINTS

Individuals taking the above weight-loss agents should be informed that weight will be regained if the medication is stopped unless lifestyle interventions that include physical activity and stress management are incorporated. Those taking antiobesity drugs should be instructed in what side effects to expect. The instructions for SSRI use are contained in Chapter 12.

Psychosocial Domain

Assessment

Psychological assessment for the individual with BED is similar to that for the individual with BN, requiring identification of cognitive distortions and knowledge deficits. Dissociation is evaluated given that binge eating may be a means to escape negative emotion (Vanderlinden, Claes, De Cuyper, & Vrieze, 2015). Symptoms of mood and anxiety disorders are explored in-depth in Chapters 22 and 23, respectively.

Nursing Diagnoses for Psychosocial Domain

Common diagnoses for the psychosocial domain include Anxiety, Ineffective Coping, Deficient Knowledge, and Social Isolation.

Interventions for Psychosocial Domain

Psychotherapy and structured self-help, both based on cognitive–behavioural interventions, are recommended as the first-line treatments for BED (Amianto et al., 2015). A longer course of treatment (i.e., 20 sessions or more) is associated with better BED remission than is a briefer course (Thompson-Brenner et al., 2013). When BED is an aspect of complex trauma-related disorders, it must be treated in sequenced stages commonly consisting of three different phases: (a) establishing safety, stabilization, and symptom reduction; (b) confronting, working through and integrating traumatic memories; and (c) identity integration and rehabilitation (Vanderlinden et al., 2015). Special attention must be paid to the development of a trustful therapeutic alliance, which can be very challenging in the beginning and throughout treatment. Treatment must also educate clients (and families) about dissociation and related impulsive behaviours. Compared to eating disorder clients without complex trauma and dissociation, the nurse must be aware that both the weight-loss and/or binge-eating behaviours may function to avoid confrontation with painful emotions and memories rather than to avoid confrontation with body weight. In any event, the nurse must try to motivate and help clients normalize eating habits and weight through teaching techniques to monitor and change eating habits, as well as to change the way they respond to difficult and stressful situations. CBT is superior to fluoxetine for BED (Reas & Grilo, 2014). Therapist-led individual treatment has been associated with better outcomes of remission and treatment completion than self-help individual treatment. Compared with therapist-led group therapy, self-help group participants who received self-help in a group format were three times more likely to drop out and 3.58 times more likely to continue binge eating at termination (Thompson-Brenner et al., 2013).

Family

There is little research into family needs; families of individuals with BED may need support themselves.

Psychoeducation

The nurse can assist the individual with BED to eat appropriately portioned meals at regular intervals to reduce hunger and binge eating. Individuals also need information about the medical consequences of binge eating. Other topics for psychoeducation are included in Box 25.13.

BOX 25.13 Psychoeducation Checklist: Binge-Eating Disorder

When caring for the individual with BED, consider the following topics:

- Health and lifestyle
- How weight reduction can be attained
- Applied knowledge about food and healthy eating
- Principles of dieting
- The importance of being present of one's body and choices
- Relaxation techniques
- Stress management
- The importance of physical activity
- Strength training: instruction and practical exercises
- Accessing resources: computers as an aid in eating well and achieving nutritional goals
- Planning for holidays

Spiritual Domain

Assessment

The nurse assesses the client's reported satisfaction with relationships and lifestyle choices, is watchful of client expressions of self-judgment and self-acceptance, and enables the client to describe any painful traumatic experiences with harassment and discrimination. The nurse listens to client stories of social exclusion, developmental interruption, and denied extracurricular opportunities such as shopping for clothing, attending parties, and participating in recreational/sporting events.

Nursing Diagnoses for Spiritual Domain

Potential diagnoses for the spiritual domain include Ineffective Protection: Reduced Quality of Life and Impaired Self-Identity. Individuals with BED who binge eat in response to various biopsychosocial experiences, environmental cues, trauma, and nonevents may struggle to protect themselves from such underlying issues as isolation and discrimination, filling themselves with food without awareness of deeper unmet needs.

Interventions for Spiritual Domain

Provide clients with BED opportunities to discuss any experiences of stress, relationship conflict, and trauma. Support them to narrate themes of disappointment and pain in response to stigma. Through the safety of the nurse–client relationship, they can develop their capacity to reconnect with self, others, and, when appropriate, the larger universal life force. The nurse may offer anticipatory guidance to individuals who need to catch up with developmental milestones such as dating and intimacy that were missed due to the overarching presence of eating disorder symptoms of social withdrawal and low self-esteem.

Evaluation and Treatment Outcomes

In a random trial to test brief and long-term clinical efficacy of enhanced and standard CBT in obese clients with BED, control participants regained on average most of the weight they had lost during the inpatient treatment program, while participants receiving enhanced CBT had improved weight loss at 1-year follow-up (Cesa et al., 2013). In a trial comparing effectiveness of CBT with IPT, longer duration of the eating disorder (equal to or greater than 8 years) and higher levels of the importance of shape were associated with the severity of eating disorder features at 60-week follow-up (Cooper et al., 2016). Those with low self-esteem at baseline who received CBT had lower scores on the severity of eating disorder features than those who received IPT. For those whose baseline self-esteem scores were higher, there was no relative advantage for either treatment. These findings point to the need for early intervention and treatment and for addressing overevaluation of the importance of shape.

TEACHING POINTS

Keeping in mind that many BED clients are overweight or obese and may have experienced harassment, psychoeducation focuses on principles of dieting, lifestyle changes to maintain weight loss, the importance of being self-aware, relaxation techniques, strength training, and stress management. High attrition rate is reported for psychoeducational programs (Amianto et al., 2015). Therefore, attend to client emotional comfort, briefing, and debriefing.

Long-term outcome studies indicate that BED may have a more favourable remission rate than other eating disorders. The severity, persistence, and duration, as well as suicide risk, for BED are comparable (Bernstein, 2017). The majority of RCTs for CBT have reported remission rates greater than 50%. CBT has generally not produced meaningful weight loss, but has demonstrated improvements in eating disordered psychopathology, depression, social adjustment, and self-esteem that are generally well maintained at 1-year to 4-year follow-up. Individual and group treatments appear to produce similar results. Poor treatment outcomes have been associated with a history of weight problems during childhood, high levels of emotional eating at baseline, overvaluation of weight and shape, interpersonal dysfunction, and low group cohesion during group CBT. The presence of a cluster B personality disorder (e.g., borderline, histrionic, antisocial, and narcissistic personality disorders) predicts higher levels of binge eating at 1-year follow-up (Saules, Carey, Carr, & Sienko, 2015). Positive

treatment outcomes have been associated with low levels of emotional eating at baseline, older age of onset, weight-loss history that is negative for amphetamine use, and decreases in depressive symptoms during treatment; early response to treatment (defined as a 65% to 70% reduction in binge eating within 4 weeks of starting treatment) tends to be associated with greater long-term (i.e., 1 to 2 year) remission from BED and lower eating disorder psychopathology, across the varied psychological treatment approaches (Saules et al., 2015).

Continuum of Care

Although individuals do not require hospitalization for BED, the consequence of obesity may involve hospitalization for surgical intervention such as gastric bypass or gastric banding surgery (Neff, Olbers, & Le Roux, 2013).

■ PREVENTION OF EATING DISORDERS

Eating disorders are among the most preventable mental disorders. National eating disorder awareness and advocacy groups work toward educating the general public, those at risk, and those who work with groups at risk, such as teachers, coaches, and college student health centre staff. They promote greater awareness of early signs of eating disorders and available resources to those at risk for developing eating disorders. They also monitor the media, striving to remove unhealthy advertisements and articles in magazines appealing to vulnerable individuals. A list of online resources is found in the Web Links.

Prevention and early detection strategies for parents and schoolteachers are often the focus of school nurses and community mental health nurses. Specific strategies to promote positive body image in children have included the Body Project, based on the principal of cognitive dissonance and designed to encourage high school and college students to explore the costs of pursuing the thin ideal. The Body Project has been found to reduce risk for onset of eating disorders (including BED) through 3-year follow-up compared with assessment only controls (Field & Sonneville, 2013). The Body Project Canada is currently offered in Newfoundland and Labrador (http://edfnl.ca/body-project-canada/). A related project, Healthy Weight Intervention, involves teaching participants how to make small gradual changes in their diets and exercise to effectively reduce future onsets of BED and obesity after 1-year follow-up (Field & Sonneville, 2013). A school-based program called Weigh to Eat targets unhealthy dieting and binge eating via 10 weekly hour-long session conducted within classes during the school day. The goals are to change knowledge, attitudes, and behaviours related to nutrition and weight control; improve body and self image; and promote greater self-efficacy in dealing with social pressures regarding excessive eating and dieting. Weigh to Eat produced marked improvement in knowledge, healthy weight control behaviours, dieting, and binge eating at 6-month follow-up, and the effects for binge eating remained significant after 2-year follow-up (Field & Sonneville, 2013). Other prevention programs include British Columbia's Web-based resources designed for elementary school teachers (http://keltymentalhealth.ca/sites/default/files/eating_disorders_-_resources_for_educators.pdf), a children's picture book called *Shapesville* that has increased the appearance satisfaction and awareness of healthy eating in 5- to 9-year-old girls (https://www.edcatalogue.com/small-book-fills-big-need-for-children/), and Healthy Buddies (healthybuddies.ca/index.htm), a program designed for elementary school children encouraging positive attitudes toward physical activity, nutrition, and mental health. National and provincial eating disorder associations also contain information about available prevention programs (e.g., http://www.mirror-mirror.org/eating-disorder-prevention-programs.htm). Successful overweight and obesity prevention programs are delivered in school settings with program leaders having access to specialist support (Carcieri, 2015).

Other strategies for parents and children appear in Table 25.5 and are based on research of risk factors and protective factors. These protective factors mainly concerned the quality of family relationships. They included family composition (living in a two parent household and, for girls, having a greater number of full siblings to "dilute" parental expectations and pressure as opposed to having half-siblings that reflect the fact that these families were more likely to have experienced adverse events such as loss of a parent or divorce), satisfaction with family life (greater family connectedness, positive family communication and clear family boundaries), social support (feeling loved/supported by family and loved by friends), healthy family environment around eating and weight (positive atmosphere at family meals, frequent family meals, and avoiding comments about weight) (Langdon-Daly & Serpell, 2017). Dieting, low self-esteem, and body dissatisfaction are examples of risk factors underlying the development of eating disorders that can be reversed with early identification and intervention.

FUTURE DIRECTIONS IN EATING DISORDER KNOWLEDGE

The classification of eating disorders underwent significant revision in 2013 with the *DSM-5*. Refer to the DSM-5 (2013) for comprehensive detailing of AN, BN, and BED as well as other feeding and eating disorders that require ongoing research and development.

Society has begun to engage in an effort to help young individuals resist developing eating disorders. Many of the Web Links have online help and resources for young individuals, families, teachers, and health care professionals.

 SUMMARY OF KEY POINTS

- AN, BN, and BED have some common symptoms, risk factors, and aetiologic factors, and individuals may migrate between the different diagnostic entities, which are discrete disorders.
- Eating disorders are best viewed along a continuum that includes normal unrestricted eating, mild disturbed eating, increasing weight and shape preoccupation, and clinical eating disorders. Because these symptomologic patterns occur more frequently than full eating disorders, they may be overlooked; however, once identified, they can be prevented from worsening.
- Similar factors predispose individuals to the development of AN, BN, and BED, and these factors represent a bio/psycho/social/spiritual model of risk that threatens health and well-being. Identifying risk factors assists with prevention strategies.
- Aetiologic factors contribute in combination to the development of eating disorders; no one factor provides a complete explanation.
- Mood and anxiety disorders are significantly more frequent in individuals with eating disorders than the general community.
- All of the eating disorders have physical, emotional, social, and spiritual consequences that influence health, well-being, and even life.
- Treatment of AN almost always includes hospitalization for refeeding; BN and BED are treated primarily on an outpatient basis.
- For individuals with BN, CBT improves symptoms sooner than does IPT. For individuals with AN,

Table 25.5 Prevention Strategies for Parents and Children	
Education for Parents	**Education for Children**
Real vs. ideal weight	Peer pressure regarding eating and weight
Influence of attitudes, behaviours, and teasing	Menses, puberty, and normal weight gain
Ways to increase self-esteem	Strategies for obesity
Role of media: TV and magazines	Ways to develop or improve self-esteem
Signs and symptoms	Body image traps: media and retail clothing
Interventions for obesity	Adapting and coping with problems
Boys at risk also	Reporting friends with signs of eating disorders
Observe for rituals	**Screening:** for risk factors
Supervision of eating and exercise	**Assessment:** for treatment
	Follow-up: monitor for relapse

family therapy plus individual IPT are the most effective. Research on best practice for BED is in its infancy; CBT and weight reduction behavioural therapy may foster remission.

- Pharmacotherapy can be effective for BN and BED but less so for AN, especially during acute malnourishment.
- Individuals with eating disorders require responsive treatment addressing both specific (e.g., eating behaviour) and nonspecific (e.g., underlying) vulnerabilities.
- The outcomes for BN are better than those for AN and BED. The type and severity of comorbid conditions and the length of the illness influence outcomes.

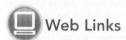 Web Links

bana.ca This site of the Bulimia Anorexia Nervosa Association (BANA) at the University of Windsor has information on specialized treatment education, support services for individuals affected directly and indirectly by eating disorders, and prevention of eating disorders, negative body image, and low self-esteem.

daniellesplace.org Danielle's Place, Burlington, ON, became a part of ROCK (Reach Out Centre for Kids) in April 2015. Programming includes groups for children and youth up to age 17—body image and self-esteem group for girls through grades 4 to 8, *Boy Zone* for boy's body issues, an eating disorder workshop series, anxiety management group, yoga, meditation, and an active parenting group.

edac-atac.ca Eating Disorders Association of Canada–Association des Troubles Alimentaires du Canada (EDAC/ARAC) is a Canadian organization of professionals in the field of eating disorders and related areas. The mandate is to promote a reflective, responsive approach in the provision of services among providers.

edfofcanada.com The Eating Disorder Foundation of Canada supports local community awareness campaigns, education in the schools, and fundraising toward establishing treatment programs, transition housing, and ongoing research.

edoyr.com Eating Disorders of York Region (EDOYR), a grassroots, community-based, registered nonprofit organization provides eating disorder and substance addiction help/support through an expressive, therapeutic art program funded by the Ontario Trillium Foundation.

feast-ed.org Families Empowered and Supporting Treatment of Eating Disorders (F.E.A.S.T) is an international organization providing information on evidence-based treatment and mutual support to caregivers of eating disorder clients with over 6,000 members on four continents.

hopesgarden.org Hope's Garden Eating Disorder Support and Resource Centre provides services free of charge for individuals 18 years and older who struggle with disordered eating. The programs include art therapy and help participants increase confidence, self-esteem, self-sufficiency, and peer support networks.

kidshelp.sympatico.ca This Kids Help Phone site offers a toll-free (1-800-668-6868) national telephone counselling service for Canadian children and youth experiencing violence, alcohol or drug abuse, or issues related to suicide or who are suffering from an eating disorder. It features tips for parents and others.

lookingglassbc.com Residential care, Summer Camp, online peer support group, educational scholarships, and family support to those affected by eating disorders.

nedic.ca The National Eating Disorder Information Centre (NEDIC) provides information and resources for individuals, families, friends, and teachers on eating disorders and weight preoccupation.

nied.ca The National Initiative for Eating Disorders aims to increase awareness and education of the chronic situation facing persons living with eating disorders and their families in Canada and to ensure eating disorders are included in mental health discussions, policies, mental health organizations, programs, decisions, campaigns, and agendas.

sheenasplace.org This site describes Sheena's Place, Canada's first community-based centre to offer services at no cost to people affected by severe eating and body image issues. The site provides information and support to parents, siblings, friends, spouses, partners, teachers, and other care providers.

something-fishy.org A website (available in English and French) about eating disorders that is dedicated to raising awareness. It emphasizes that eating disorders are *not* about food and weight but are symptoms of something deeper going on, inside.

References

Academy of Eating Disorders' Medical Care Standards Committee. (2016). *Eating disorders: A guide to medical care: Critical points for early recognition and medical risk management in the care of individuals with eating disorders* (3rd ed.). Retrieved from http://www.aedweb.org/images/updatedmedicalcareguidelines/AED-Medical-Care-Guidelines_English_02.28.17_NEW.pdf

Accurso, E. C., Lebow, J., Murray, S. B., Kass, A. E., & Le Grange, D. (2016). The relation of weight suppression and BMIz to bulimic symptoms in youth with bulimia nervosa. *Journal of Eating Disorders, 4*, 1–6. doi:10.1186/s40337-016-0111-5

Akrawi, D., Bartrop, R., Potter, U., & Touyz, S. (2015). Religiosity, spirituality in relation to disordered eating and body image concerns: A systematic review. *Journal of Eating Disorders, 3*(1), 1–24. doi:10.1186/s40337-015-0064-0

Allen, K., Byrne, S., & Crosby, R. (2015). Distinguishing between risk factors for Bulimia Nervosa, Binge Eating Disorder, and Purging Disorder. *Journal of Youth and Adolescence, 44*(8), 1580–1591. doi:10.1007/s10964-014-0186-8

Aloi, M., Rania, M., Caroleo, M., Bruni, A., Palmieri, A., Cauteruccio, M. A., … Segura-García, C. (2015). Decision making, central coherence and set-shifting: A comparison between Binge Eating Disorder, Anorexia Nervosa and Healthy Controls. *BMC Psychiatry, 15.* doi:10.1186/s12888-015-0395-z

American Psychiatric Association. (2000). *Diagnostic and statistical manual of mental disorders* (4th ed., Text revision). Washington, DC: Author.

American Psychiatric Association. (2013). *Diagnostic and statistical manual of mental disorders* (5th ed.). Washington, DC: Author.

American Psychiatric Association. (2017). *Orthorexia: Can healthy eating become unhealthy?* Retrieved from https://www.psychiatry.org/news-room/apa-blogs/apa-blog/2016/06/orthorexia-can-healthy-eating-become-unhealthy

American Society of Health-System Pharmacists, Inc. (2017). *Bupropion.* MedlinePlus U.S. National Library of Medicine. Retrieved from https://medlineplus.gov/druginfo/meds/a695033.html

Amianto, F., Ottone, L., Daga, G. A., & Fassino, S. (2015). Binge-eating disorder diagnosis and treatment: A recap in front of DSM-5. *BMC Psychiatry, 15*, 70. doi:10.1186/s12888-015-0445-6

Anastasiadou, D. Sepulveda, A. R., Parks, M., Cuellar-Flores, I., & Graell, M. (2016). The relationship between dysfunctional family patterns and symptom severity among adolescent patients with eating disorders: A gender-specific approach. *Women and Health, 56*(6), 695–712. http://dx.doi.org.proxy.hil.unb.ca/10.1080/03630242.2015.1118728

Arcelus, J., Haslam, M., Farrow, C., & Meyer, C. (2013). The role of interpersonal functioning in the maintenance of eating psychopathology: A systematic review and testable model. *Clinical Psychology Review, 33*(1), 156–167. https://doi.org/10.1016/j.cpr.2012.10.009

Arrow, B., Kenardy, J., & Agras, W. S. (1995). The Emotional Eating Scale: The development of a measure to assess coping with negative affect by eating. *International Journal of Eating Disorders, 18,* 79–90.

Atkins, E., Madhavan, S., LeMasters, T., Vyas, A., Gainor, S. J., & Remick, S. (2013). Are obese women more likely to participate in a mobile mammography program? *Journal of Community Health, 38*(2), 338–348. http://doi.org/10.1007/s10900-012-9619-z

Baker, J. H., Thornton, L. M., Strober, M., Brandt, H., Crawford, S., Fichter, M. M., … Bulik, C. M. (2013). Temporal sequence of comorbid alcohol use disorder and anorexia nervosa. *Addictive Behaviors, 38*(3), 1704–1709. https://doi.org/10.1016/j.addbeh.2012.10.005

Bannatyne, A. J., & Abel, L. M. (2015). Can we fight stigma with science? The effect of aetiological framing on attitudes towards anorexia nervosa and the impact on volitional stigma. *Australian Journal of Psychology, 67*(1), 38–46. doi:10.1111/ajpy.12062

Bartholdy, S., Allen, K., Hodsoll, J., O'Daly, O. G., Campbell, I. C., Banaschewski, T., … Gallinat, J. (2017). Identifying disordered eating behaviours in adolescents: How do parent and adolescent reports differ by sex and age? *European Child and Adolescent Psychiatry, 26*(6), 691–701. doi:10.1007/s00787-016-0935-1

Bergström, I., Crisby, M., Engström, A. M., Hölcke, M., Fored, M., Jakobsson Kruse, P., & Of Sandberg, A. M. (2013). Women with anorexia nervosa should not be treated with estrogen or birth control pills in a bone-sparing effect. *Acta Obstetricia et Gynecologica Scandinavica, 92*(8), 877–80. doi: 10.1111/aogs.12178.

Bernstein, B. E. (2017). Prognosis: Binge-Eating Disorder (BED). *Medscape,* April 10, 2017. Retrieved from http://emedicine.medscape.com/article/2221362-overview#a7

Bhurtun, D. D., & Jeewon, R. (2013). Body weight perception and weight control practices among teenagers. *ISRN Nutrition,* 2013, 395125. doi:10.5402/2013/395125

Blackburn, M.-E., Auclair, J., Dion, J., Lessard, I., Bellemare, J., & Lapalme, L. (2016). Body dissatisfaction and self-esteem: Perception vs reality. *Appearance Matters 7,* London. http://ecobes.cegepjonquiere.ca/media/tinymce/Publication-Sante/AfficheMEBlack_30Juin16_3.pdf

Bodell, L. P., Joiner, T. E., & Keel, P. K. (2013). Comorbidity-independent risk for suicidality increases with bulimia nervosa but not with anorexia nervosa. *Journal of Psychiatric Research, 47*(5), 617–621. doi:10.1016/j.jpsychires.2013.01.005

Boisvert, J. A., & Harrell, W. A. (2013). Sociocultural and psychological considerations of pediatric obesity and eating disorder symptomatology in Canadian immigrants. *Journal of Pediatric Biochemistry, 3,* 23–33. doi:10.3233/JPB-120073

Borowsky, H. M., Eisenberg, M. E., Bucchianeri, M. M., Piran, N., & Neumark-Sztainer, D. (2016) Feminist identity, body image, and disordered eating. *Eating Disorders, 24*(4), 297–311. doi:10.1080/10640266.2015.1123986

Brandys, M. K., de Kovel, C. G., Kas, M. J., van Elburg, A. A., & Adan, R. A. (2015). Overview of genetic research in anorexia nervosa: The past, present and the future. *International Journal of Eating Disorders, 48*(7), 814–825. doi:10.1002/eat.22400

Brewin, N., Wales, J., Cashmore, R., Plateau, C. R., Dean, B., Cousins, T., & Arcelus, J. (2016). Evaluation of a motivation and psycho-educational guided self-help intervention for people with eating disorders (MOPED). *European Eating Disorders Review, 24*(3), 241–246. doi:10.1002/erv.2431

Brownley, K. A., Von Holle, A., Hamer, R. M., La Via, M., & Bulik, C. M. (2013). A double-blind, randomized pilot trial of chromium picolinate for binge eating disorder: Results of the Binge Eating and Chromium (BEACh) study. *Journal of Psychosomatic Research, 75*(1), 36–42.

Bulik, C. M., & Trace, S. E. (2013). The genetics of binge-eating disorder. In J. Alexander, A. Goldschmidt, & D. Le Grange (Eds), *A clinician's guide to binge eating disorder* (pp. 26–41). New York, NY: Routledge.

Burns, J., & Kehler, M. (2014). Boys, bodies and negotiated school spaces: When boys fail the litmus test. *Culture, Society and Masculinities, 6*(1), 3–18. doi:10.3149/CSM.0601.3

Buser, J. K., & Bernard, J. M. (2013). Religious coping, body dissatisfaction, and bulimic symptomatology. *Counseling and Values, 58*(2), 158–176. doi:10.1002/j.2161-007X.2013.00031.x.

Buser, J. K., & Gibson, S. (2016). Attachment to god/higher power and bulimic symptoms among college women. *Journal of College Counseling, 19,* 124–137. doi:10.1002/jocc.12036

Buser, J. K., Parkins, R. A., & Buser, T. J. (2014). Thematic analysis of the intersection of spirituality and eating disorder symptoms. *Journal of Addictions and Offender Counseling, 35*(2), 97–113. doi:10.1002/j.2161-1874.2014.00029.x

Campbell, K., & Peebles, R. (2014). Eating Disorders in Children and Adolescents: State of the art review. *Pediatrics, 134*(3), 582–592. doi: 10.1542/peds.2014-0194

Canadian Psychological Association (CPA). (2014). *Expanded brief to the house of commons standing committee on the status of women: Eating disorders amongst girls and women.* Retrieved from http://www.cpa.ca/docs/File/News/2014/eating_disorders_brief_final_2014-05-29.pdf

Carcieri, E. (2015). *Should schools have eating disorder prevention programs?* Mirror Mirror. http://www.mirror-mirror.org/eating-disorder-prevention-programs.htm

Carr, E. R., Green, B., & Ponce, A. P. (2015). Women and the experience of serious mental illness and sexual objectification: Multicultural feminist theoretical frameworks and therapy recommendations. *Women and Therapy, 38*(1–2), 53–76. doi:10.1080/02703149.2014.978216

Çelik, S., Kayar, Y., Akçakaya, R. Ö., Uyar, E. T., Kalkan, K., Yazısız, V., … Yücel, B. (2015). Correlation of binge eating disorder with level of depression and glycemic control in type 2 diabetes mellitus patients. *General Hospital Psychiatry, 37*(2), 116–119. doi:10.1016/j.genhosppsych.2014.11.012

Cesa, G. L., Manzoni, G. M., Bacchetta, M., Castelnuovo, G., Conti, S., Gaggioli, A., … Riva, G. (2013). Virtual reality for enhancing the cognitive behavioral treatment of obesity with binge eating disorder: Randomized controlled study with one-year follow-up. *Journal of Medical Internet Research, 15*(6), e113.

Chang, P. F., & Bazarova, N. N. (2016). Managing stigma: Disclosure-response communication patterns in pro-anorexic websites. *Health Communication, 31*(2), 217–229. doi:10.1080/10410236.2014.946218

Chatterton, J. M., & Petrie, T. A. (2013). Prevalence of disordered eating and pathogenic weight control behaviors among male collegiate athletes. *Eating Disorders, 21*(4), 328–341.

Chesney, E., Goodwin, G. M., & Fazel, S. (2014). Risks of all-cause and suicide mortality in mental disorders: A meta-review. *World Psychiatry, 13*(2), 153–160

Chrisler, J. C., Fung, K. T., Lopez, A. M., & Gorman, J. A. (2013). Suffering by comparison: Twitter users' reactions to the Victoria's Secret fashion show. *Body Image, 10*(4), 648–652.

Coelho, J. S., Kumar, A., Kilvert, M., Kunkel, L., & Lam, P. (2015). Male youth with eating disorders: Clinical and medical characteristics of a sample of inpatients. *Eating Disorders, 23*(5), 455–461. doi:10.1080/10640266.2015.1027119

Coffino, J. A., Orloff, N. C., & Hormes, J. M. (2016). Dietary restraint partially mediates the relationship between impulsivity and binge eating only in lean individuals: The importance of accounting for body mass in studies of restraint. *Frontiers in Psychology, 7,* 1499. doi:10.3389/fpsyg.2016.0149

Collier, R. (2013). Treatment challenges for men with eating disorders. *Canadian Medical Association Journal, 185*(3), E137–E138.

Cooper, Z., Allen, E., Bailey-Straebler, S., Basden, S., Murphy, R., O'Connor, M. E., & Fairburn, C. G. (2016). Predictors and moderators of response to enhanced cognitive behaviour therapy and interpersonal psychotherapy for the treatment of eating disorders. *Behaviour Research and Therapy, 84,* 9–13. doi:10.1016/j.brat.2016.07.002

Copeland, W. E., Bulik, C. M., Zucker, N., Wolke, D., Lereya, S. T., & Costello, E. J. (2015). Does childhood bullying predict eating disorder symptoms? A prospective, longitudinal analysis. *International Journal of Eating Disorders, 48*(8), 1141–1149. doi:10.1002/eat.22459

Costa, A. J. R. B., & Pinto, S. L. (2015). Binge eating disorder and quality of life of candidates to bariatric surgery. *Arquivos Brasileiros de Cirurgia Digestiva (São Paulo), 28*(Suppl. 1), 52–55. https://dx.doi.org/10.1590/S0102-6720201500S100015

Cottingham, M. E., Davis, L., Craycraft, A., Keiper, C. D., & Abernethy, A. D. (2014). Disordered eating and self-objectification in college women: Clarifying the roles of spirituality and purpose in life. *Mental Health, Religion and Culture, 17*(9), 898–909. doi:10.1080/13674676.2014.950558

Cottrell, D. B., & Williams, J. (2016). Eating disorders in men. *Nurse Practitioner, 41*(9), 49–55.

Couturier, J., Kimber, M., & Szatmari, P. (2013). Efficacy of family-based treatment for adolescents with eating disorders: A systematic review and meta-analysis. *International Journal of Eating Disorders, 46*(1), 3–11.

Dahlborg Lyckhage, E., Gardvik, A., Karlsson, H., Törner, J. M., & Berndtsson, I. (2015). Young women with anorexia nervosa. *SAGE Open, 5*(1), 1–8. doi:10.1177/2158244015577654

Dalkilic, A. (2013). Psychopharmacological treatments in eating disorders and comorbid conditions. *Klinik Psikofarmakoloji Bulteni, 23,* S26.

Damiano, S. R., Paxton, S. J., Wertheim, E. H., McLean, S. A., & Gregg, K. J. (2015). Dietary restraint of 5-year-old girls: Associations with internalization of the thin ideal and maternal, media, and peer influences. *International Journal of Eating Disorders, 48*(8), 1166–1169. doi:10.1002/eat.22432

Danner, U. N., Evers, C., Sternheim, L., van Meer, F., van Elburg, A. A., Geerets, T. A. M., … de Ridder, D. T. D. (2013). Influence of negative affect on choice behavior in individuals with binge eating pathology. *Psychiatry Research, 207*, 100–106. http://dx.doi.org/10.1016/j.psychres.2012.10.016

Davis, C. (2015). The epidemiology and genetics of binge eating disorder (BED). *CNS Spectrums, 20*(6), 522–529. doi:https://doi.org/10.1017/S1092852915000462

de Guzman, N. S., & Nishina, A. (2014). A longitudinal study of body dissatisfaction and pubertal timing in an ethnically diverse adolescent sample. *Body Image, 11*(1), 68–71. http://dx.doi.org/10.1016/j.bodyim.2013.11.001

Degortes, D., Santonastaso, P., Zanetti, T., Tenconi, E., Veronese, A., & Favaro, A. (2014). Stressful life events and binge eating disorder. *European Eating Disorders Review, 22*(5), 378–382. doi:10.1002/erv.2308

Dickstein, L. P., Franco, K. N., Rome, E. S., & Auron, M. (2014). Recognizing, managing medical consequences of eating disorders in primary care. *Cleveland Clinic Journal of Medicine, 81*, 255–263.

Dimitropoulos, G., Freeman, V. E., Muskat, S., Domingo, A., & McCallum, L. (2016). "You don't have anorexia, you just want to look like a celebrity": Perceived stigma in individuals with anorexia nervosa. *Journal of Mental Health, 25*(1), 47–54. http://dx.doi.org.proxy.hil.unb.ca/10.3109/09638237.2015.1101422

Dudek, J., Ostaszewski, P., & Malicki, S. (2014). Transdiagnostic models of eating disorders and therapeutic methods: The example of fairburn's cognitive behavior therapy and acceptance and commitment therapy. *Roczniki Psychologiczne/Annals of Psychology, XVII, 1*, 25–39. Retrieved from https://www.kul.pl/files/1024/Roczniki_Psychologiczne/2014/1/RPsych2014nr1pp025-039_Dudek_Ostaszewski_MalickiEN.pdf

Ebneter, D. S., & Latner, J. D. (2013). Stigmatizing attitudes differ across mental health disorders: A comparison of stigma across eating disorders, obesity, and major depressive disorder. *Journal of Nervous and Mental Disease, 201*(4), 281–285. doi:10.1097/NMD.0b013e318288e23f

Edwards, L. M. (2013). Theoretical analysis of binge eating disorder through the perspectives of self psychology and cognitive theory/cognitive behavioral therapy, and an explanation of blending these perspectives. Theses, Dissertations, and Projects. Paper 578. Smith College School for Social Work. Retrieved from http://scholarworks.smith.edu/cgi/viewcontent.cgi?article=1655&context=theses

Ellis, M. (2016, December 5). "Brain thinks yo-yo dieting is a famine, causing weight gain." *Medical News Today*. Retrieved from http://www.medicalnewstoday.com/articles/314527.php.

Errichiello, L., Iodice, D., Bruzzese, D., Gherghi, M., & Senatore, I. (2016). Prognostic factors and outcome in anorexia nervosa: A follow-up study. *Eating and Weight Disorders, 21*, 73–82. doi:10.1007/s40519-015-0211-2

Evans, E. H., Adamson, A. J., Basterfield, L., Le Couteur, A., Reilly, J., Reilly, J., & Parkinson, K. N. (2017). Risk factors for eating disorder symptoms at 12 years of age: A 6-year longitudinal cohort study. *Appetite, 108*, 12–20. https://doi.org/10.1016/j.appet.2016.09.005

Fairburn, C. G., & Cooper, Z. (2014). Eating disorders: A transdiagnostic protocol. In D. H. Barlow (Ed.), *Clinical handbook of psychological disorders: A step-by-step treatment manual* (5th ed., pp. 670–702). New York, NY: Guilford.

Fairburn, C. G., & Rothwell, E. R. (2015). Apps and eating disorders: A systematic clinical appraisal. *International Journal of Eating Disorders, 48*(7), 1038–1046. doi:10.1002/eat.22398

Faulconbridge, L. F., & Bechtel, C. F. (2014). Depression and disordered eating in the obese person. *Current Obesity Reports, 3*(1), 127–136. http://doi.org/10.1007/s13679-013-0080-9

Field, K. D., & Sonneville, K. R. (2013). Prevention. In J. Alexander, A. B. Goldschmidt, & D. Le Grange (Eds.), *A clinician's guide to binge eating disorder* (pp. 218–228). New York, NY: Routledge.

Findlay, S., Pinzon, J., Taddeo, D., Katzman, D. K., & Canadian Paediatric Society, Adolescent Health Committee. (2013). Family-based treatment of children and adolescents with anorexia nervosa: Guidelines for the community physician. *Paediatrics and Child Health, 15*(1), 31–35.

Fisher, M., & Bushlow, M. (2015). Perceptions of family styles by adolescents with eating disorders and their parents. *International Journal of Adolescent Medicine end Health, 27*(4), 443–449. doi:10.1515/ijamh-2014-0058

Fogarty, S., & Ramjan, L. M. (2016). Factors impacting treatment and recovery in Anorexia Nervosa: Qualitative findings from an online questionnaire. *Journal of Eating Disorders, 64*, 1–9. doi:10.1186/s40337-016-0107-1

Fonville, L., Giampietro, V., Williams, S. C. R., Simmons, A., & Tchanturia, K. (2014). Alterations in brain structure in adults with anorexia nervosa and the impact of illness duration. *Psychological Medicine, 44*(9), 1965–1975. https://doi.org/10.1017/S0033291713002389

Forcen, F. E. (2013). Anorexia mirabilis: The practice of fasting by Saint Catherine of Siena in the late middle ages. *American Journal of Psychiatry, 170*(4), 370–371. Retrieved from https://login.proxy.hil.unb.ca/login?url=http://search.proquest.com.proxy.hil.unb.ca/docview/1368604407?accountid=14611

Forcen, F. E. (2015). The practice of holy fasting in the late middle ages: A psychiatric approach. *Journal of Nervous and Mental Disease, 203*(8), 650–653.

Forrest, L. N., Zuromski, K. L., Dodd, D. R., & Smith, A. R. (2017). Suicidality in adolescents and adults with binge-eating disorder: Results from the national comorbidity survey replication and adolescent supplement. *International Journal of Eating Disorders, 50*(1), 40–49. doi:10.1002/eat.22582

Franko, D. L., Keshaviah, A., Eddy, K. T., Krishna, M., Davis, M. C., Keel, P. K., & Herzog, D. B. (2013). A longitudinal investigation of mortality in anorexia nervosa and bulimia nervosa. *American Journal of Psychiatry, 170*, 917–925.

Galsworthy-Francis, L., & Allan, S. (2014). Cognitive behavioural therapy for anorexia nervosa: A systematic review. *Clinical Psychology Review, 34*(1), 54–72. https://doi.org/10.1016/j.cpr.2013.11.001

Garner, D. M. (2011). *Eating disorder inventory-3: Professional manual.* Odessa, FL: Psychological Assessment Resources.

Garner, D. M., Anderson, M. L., Keiper, C. D. Whynott, R., & Parker, L. (2016). Psychotropic medications in adult and adolescent eating disorders: Clinical practice versus evidence-based recommendations. *Eating and Weight Disorders, 21*, 395–402. doi:10.1007/s40519-016-0253-0

Garner, D. M., & Garfinkel, P. E. (1979). The Eating Attitude Test: An index of the symptoms of anorexia nervosa. *Psychosomatic Medicine, 10*, 647–656.

Gauthier, C., Hassler, C., Mattar, L., Launay, J-M., Callebert, J., Steiger, H., … Godart, N. (2014). Symptoms of depression and anxiety in anorexia nervosa: Links with plasma tryptophan and serotonin metabolism. *Psychoneuroendocrinology, 39*, 170–178. https://doi.org/10.1016/j.psyneuen.2013.09.009

Gerstein, F., & Pollack, F. (2016). Two case studies on family work with eating disorders and body image issues. *Clinical Social Work Journal, 44*(1), 69–77. doi:10.1007/s10615-015-0566-x

Gianini, L. M., White, M. A., & Masheb, R. M. (2013). Eating pathology, emotion regulation, and emotional overeating in obese adults with binge eating disorder. *Eating Behaviors, 14*(3), 309–313. http://doi.org/10.1016/j.eatbeh.2013.05.008

Goldschmidt, A. B., Lavender, J. M., Li, C., Wonderlich, S. A., Crosby, R. D., Engel, S. G., … Mitchell, J. E. (2014). Ecological momentary assessment of stressful events and negative affect in bulimia nervosa. *Journal of Consulting and Clinical Psychology, 82*(1), 30–39. doi:10.1037/a0034974

Góngora, V. C. (2014). Satisfaction with life, well-being, and meaning in life as protective factors of eating disorder symptoms and body dissatisfaction in adolescents. *Eating Disorders, 22*(5), 435–449. doi:10.1080/10640266.2014.931765

Goulet, C., Henrie, J., & Szymanski, L. (2017). An exploration of the associations among multiple aspects of religiousness, body image, eating pathology, and appearance investment. *Journal of Religion and Health, 56*, 493–506. doi:10.1007/s10943-016-0229-4

Government of Canada. Report of the Standing Committee on the Status of Women. (2014). *Eating disorders among girls and women in Canada.* Retrieved from http://www.parl.gc.ca/HousePublications/Publication.aspx?DocId=6772133

Grave, D. R., Calugi, S., El Ghoch, M., Marzocchi, R., & Marchesini, G. (2014). Personality traits in obesity associated with binge eating and/or night eating. *Current Obesity Reports, 3*(1), 120–126. doi:10.1007/s13679-013-0076-5

Griffiths, S., Mond, J. M., Murray, S. B., & Touyz, S. (2015). The prevalence and adverse associations of stigmatization in people with eating disorders. *International Journal of Eating Disorders, 48*(6), 767–774. doi:10.1002/eat.22353

Grilo, C. M., White, M. A., Barnes, R. D., & Masheb, R. M. (2013). Psychiatric disorder comorbidity and correlates in an ethnically diverse sample of obese patients with binge eating disorder in primary care settings. *Comprehensive Psychiatry, 54*(3), 209–216.

Grilo, C. M., White, M. A., Gueorguieva, R., Wilson, G. T., & Masheb, R. M. (2013). Predictive significance of the overvaluation of shape/weight in obese patients with binge eating disorder: Findings from a randomized controlled trial with 12-month follow-up. *Psychological Medicine, 43*(6), 1335–1344.

Guillaume, S., Jaussent, I., Maimoun, L., Ryst, A., Seneque, M., Villain, L., … Courtet, Ph. (2016). Associations between adverse childhood experiences and clinical characteristics of eating disorders. *Science Reports, 6*, 35761. doi:10.1038/srep35761

Gutwill, S. (2017). *Transference and countertransference in working with eating problems—Part 1*. Retrieved from https://www.edcatalogue.com/transference-countertransference-working-eating-problems/

Hannon-Engel, S. L., Filin, E. E., & Wolfe, B. E. (2013). CCK response in bulimia nervosa and following remission. *Physiology and Behavior, 122*, 56–61. http://doi.org/10.1016/j.physbeh.2013.08.014

Hay, P. H. (2013) A qualitative exploration of influences on the process of recovery from personal written accounts of people with anorexia nervosa. *Women and Health, 53*(7), 730–740. doi:10.1080/03630242.2013.821694

Haynos, A. F., Watts, A. W., Loth, K. A., Pearson, C. M., & Neumark-Stzainer, D. (2016). Factors predicting an escalation of restrictive eating during adolescence. *Journal of Adolescent Health, 59*(4), 391–396. http://dx.doi.org/10.1016/j.jadohealth.2016.03.011

Henderson, A., & Ellison, C. (2015). My body is a temple: Eating disturbances, religious involvement, and mental health among young adult women. *Journal of Religion and Health, 54*(3), 954–976. doi:10.1007/s10943-014-9838-y

Herrin, M., & Larkin, M. (2013). Self monitoring. In *Nutrition counseling in the treatment of eating disorders* (2nd ed., pp. 140–149). New York, NY: Routledge.

Hilbert, A., Pike, K. M., Goldschmidt, A. B., Wilfley, D. E., Fairburn, C., Dohm, F.-A., … Striegel Weissman, R. (2014). Risk factors across the eating disorders. *Psychiatry Research, 220*(1–2), 500–506. https://doi.org/10.1016/j.psychres.2014.05.054

Hocaoglu, C. (2017). Eating disorders with comorbid anxiety disorders. In *Eating disorders—A paradigm of the biopsychosocial model of illness* (pp. 99–122). Retrieved from http://www.intechopen.com/books/eating-disorders-a-paradigm-of-the-biopsychosocial-model-of-illness

Homan, K. J., & Cavanaugh, B. N. (2013). Perceived relationship with god fosters positive body image in college women. *Journal of Health Psychology, 18*(12), 1529–1539. doi: 10.1177/1359105312465911.

Homan, K. J., & Lemmon, V. A. (2014). Attachment to God and eating disorder tendencies: The mediating role of social comparison. *Psychology of Religion and Spirituality, 6*(4), 349–357. http://dx.doi.org/10.1037/a0036776

Homan, K. J., & Lemmon, V. A. (2016). Perceived relationship with God moderates the relationship between social comparison and body appreciation. *Mental Health, Religion and Culture, 19*(1), 37–51, doi: 10.1080/13674676.2016.1140372

Hoste, R. R., Lebow, J., & Le Grange, D. (2015). A bidirectional examination of expressed emotion among families of adolescents with bulimia nervosa. *The International Journal of Eating Disorders, 48*(2), 249–252. http://doi.org/10.1002/eat.22306

Inches, P. R. (1895). Anorexia nervosa. *Maritime Medical News, 7*, 73–75.

Jacobson, H. L., Hall, M. L., & Anderson, T. L. (2013). Theology and the body: Sanctification and bodily experiences. *Psychology of Religion and Spirituality, 5*(1), 41–50. doi:10.1037/a0028042

Jirak Monetti, C. (2014). *Somatic countertransference experiences of nurse therapeutic touch practitioners: A content analysis.* Dissertation submitted to the Graduate School–Newark Rutgers, The State University of New Jersey. https://rucore.libraries.rutgers.edu/rutgers-lib/43818/PDF/1/

Kass, A. E., Kolko, R. P., & Wilfley, D. E. (2013). Psychological treatments for eating disorders. *Current Opinion in Psychiatry, 26*(6), 549–555. http://doi.org/10.1097/YCO.0b013e328365a30e

Kaye W. H., Wierenga, C. E., Bailer, U. F., Simmons, A. N., & Bischoff-Grethe, A. (2013). Nothing tastes as good as skinny feels: The neurobiology of anorexia nervosa. *Trends in Neuroscience, 36*(2), 110–120.

Kelly, A. C., & Carter, J. C. (2013). Why self-critical patients present with more severe eating disorder pathology: The mediating role of shame. *British Journal of Clinical Psychology, 52*(2), 148–161. doi:10.1111/bjc.12006

Kelly, A. C., Vimalakanthan, K., & Carter, J. C. (2014). Understanding the roles of self-esteem, self-compassion, and fear of self-compassion in eating disorder pathology: An examination of female students and eating disorder patients. *Eating Behaviors, 15*(3), 388–391. doi:10.1016/j.eatbeh.2014.04.008

Kerr, M. (2016). Prokinetic agents: Cisapride. *Healthline.* Retrieved from http://www.healthline.com/health/gerd/prokinetics#1

Keshen, A., & Ivanova, I. (2013). Reduction of bulimia nervosa symptoms after psychostimulant initiation in patients with comorbid ADHD: Five case reports. *Eating Disorders: The Journal of Treatment and Prevention, 21*(4), 360–369. doi:10.1080/10640266.2013.797828

Keski-Rahkonen, A., Raevuori, A., Bulik, C. M., Hoek, H. W., Rissanen, A., & Kaprio, J. (2014). Factors associated with recovery from anorexia nervosa: A population-based study. *International Journal of Eating Disorders, 47*(2), 117–123. doi:10.1002/eat.22168

Keski-Rahkonen, A., Raevuori, A., Bulik, C. M., Hoek, H. W., Sihvola, E., Kaprio, J., … Rissanen, A. (2013). Depression and drive for thinness are associated with persistent bulimia nervosa in the community. *European Eating Disorders Review, 21*(2), 121–129.

Kessler, R. C., Berglund, P. A., Chiu, W. T., Deitz, A. C., Hudson, J. I., Shahly, V., … Xavier, M. (2013). The prevalence and correlates of binge eating disorder in the World Health Organization World Mental Health Surveys. *Biological Psychiatry, 73*(9), 904–914.

Khalsa, S. S., Craske, M. G., Li, W., Vangala, S., Strober, M., & Feusner, J. D. (2015). Altered interoceptive awareness in anorexia nervosa: Effects of meal anticipation, consumption and bodily arousal. *International Journal of Eating Disorders, 48*(7), 889–897. http://doi.org/10.1002/eat.22387

Kiecolt-Glaser, J. K., Habash, D. L., Fagundes, C. P., Andridge, R., Peng, J., Malarkey, W. B., & Belury, M. A. (2015). Daily stressors, past depression, and metabolic responses to high-fat meals: A novel path to obesity. *Biological Psychiatry, 77*(7), 653–60.

Kimber, M., Couturier, J., Georgiades, K., Wahoush, O., & Jack, S. M. (2015). Ethnic minority status and body image dissatisfaction: A scoping review of the child and adolescent literature. *Journal of Immigrant and Minority Health, 17*(5), 1567–1579. doi:http://dx.doi.org.proxy.hil.unb.ca/10.1007/s10903-014-0082-z

Kimber, M., Georgiades, K., Jack, S. M., Couturier, J., & Wahoush, O. (2015). Body image and appearance perceptions from immigrant adolescents in Canada: An interpretive description. *Body Image, 15*, 120–131. https://doi.org/10.1016/j.bodyim.2015.08.002

Kinsaul, J. A. E., Curtin, L., Bazzini, D., & Martz, D. (2014). Empowerment, feminism, and self-efficacy: Relationships to body image and disordered eating. *Body Image, 11*(1), 63–67. https://doi.org/10.1016/j.bodyim.2013.08.001

Kirkey, S. (2013). Anorexia hitting men increasingly hard: One in three cases in new study is male. *National Post.* Retrieved from http://life.nationalpost.com/2013/01/21/anorexia-hitting-men-increasingly-hard-one-in-three-cases-in-new-study-is-male/

Kirkpatrick, S. L., Goldberg, L. R., Yazdani, N., Babbs, R. K., Wu, J., Reed, E. R., … Bryant, C. D. (2017). Cytoplasmic FMR1-interacting protein 2 is a major genetic factor underlying binge eating. *Biological Psychiatry, 81*(9), 757–769. doi:10.1016/j.biopsych.2016.10.021

Klump, K. L. (2013). Puberty as a critical risk period for eating disorders: A review of human and animal studies. *Hormones and Behavior, 64*(2), 399–410. https://doi.org/10.1016/j.yhbeh.2013.02.019

Kozicka, P. (2015). 1 in 5 Canadian women not satisfied with their appearance: Survey. *Global News, May 29, 2015.* http://globalnews.ca/news/2025789/1-in-5-canadian-women-not-satisfied-with-their-appearance-survey/

Kramer, J. L. (2015). Art therapy in the treatment of eating disorders. *Salucore.* Retrieved from https://www.edcatalogue.com/art-therapy-in-the-treatment-of-eating-disorders/

Krause, N., & Hayward, R. D. (2016), Anxious attachment to God, spiritual support, and obesity: Findings from a recent nationwide survey. *Journal for the Scientific Study of Religion, 55*, 485–497. doi:10.1111/jssr.12284

La Mela, C., Maglietta, M., Caini, S., Casu, G. P., Lucarelli, S., Mori, S., & Ruggiero, G. M. (2015). Perfectionism, weight and shape concerns, and low self-esteem: Testing a model to predict bulimic symptoms. *Eating Behaviors, 19*, 155–158. doi:10.1016/j.eatbeh.2015.09.002.

Laghi, F., Pompili, S., Zanna, V., Castiglioni, M. C., Criscuolo, M., Chianello, I., … Baiocco, R. (2017). How adolescents with anorexia nervosa and their parents perceive family functioning? *Journal of Health Psychology, 22*(2), 197–207. doi:10.1177/1359105315597055

LaMarre, A., & Rice, C. (2016). Normal eating is counter-cultural: Embodied experiences of eating disorder recovery. *Journal of Community and Applied Social Psychology, 26*(2), 136–149. doi:10.1002/casp.2240

Lampard, A. M., & Sharbanee, J. M. (2015). The cognitive-behavioural theory and treatment of bulimia nervosa: An examination of treatment mechanisms and future directions. *Australian Psychologist, 50*, 6–13. doi:10.1111/ap.12078

Lampard, A., MacLehose, R., Eisenberg, M., Neumark-Sztainer, D., & Davison, K. (2014). Weight-related teasing in the school environment: Associations with psychosocial health and weight control practices among adolescent boys and girls. *Journal of Youth and Adolescence, 43*(10), 1770–1780. doi:10.1007/s10964-013-0086-3

Langdon-Daly, J., & Serpell, L. (2017). Protective factors against disordered eating in family systems: A systematic review of research. *Journal of Eating Disorders, 5*, 1–15. doi:10.1186/s40337-017-0141-7

Las Hayas, C., Padierna, J. A., Muñoz, P., Aguirre, M., del Barrio, A. G., Beato-Fernández, L., & Calvete, E. (2016) Resilience in eating disorders: A qualitative study. *Women and Health, 56*(5), 576–594. doi:10.1080/03630242.2015.1101744

Le Grange, D., O'Connor, M., Hughes, E. K., Macdonald, J., Little, K., & Olsson, C. A. (2014). Developmental antecedents of abnormal eating attitudes and behaviors in adolescence. *International Journal of Eating Disorders, 47*(7), 813–824. doi:10.1002/eat.22331

Lea, T., Richards, P. S., Sanders, P. W., McBride, J. A., & Allen, G. K. (2015). Spiritual pathways to healing and recovery: An intensive single-N study of an eating disorder patient. *Spirituality in Clinical Practice, 2*(3), 191–201. doi:10.1037/scp0000085

Lebow, J. Sim, L. A., Erwin, P. J., & Murad, H. (2013). The effect of atypical antipsychotic medications in individuals with anorexia nervosa: A systematic review and meta-analysis. *International Journal of Eating Disorders*, 13(4), 332-33

Lebow, J., Sim, L. A., & Kransdorf, L. N. (2015). Prevalence of a history of overweight and obesity in adolescents with restrictive eating disorders. *Journal of Adolescent Health*, 56(1), 19-24. doi:10.1016/j.jadohealth.2014.06.005.

Lee-Winn, A., Mendelson, T., & Mojtabai, R. (2014). Racial/Ethnic disparities in binge eating: Disorder prevalence, symptom presentation, and help-seeking among Asian Americans and Non-Latino Whites. *American Journal of Public Health*, 104(7), 1263-1265. http://doi.org/10.2105/AJPH.2014.301932

Lefebvre, D. B. (2016). Client perspectives of psychotherapy for eating disorders in community practice settings. Published PhD Thesis. University of Ottawa. http://hdl.handle.net/10393/34130

Levinson, C. A., Rapp, J., & Riley, E. N. (2014). Addressing the fear of fat: Extending imaginal exposure therapy for anxiety disorders to anorexia nervosa. *Eating and Weight Disorders*, 19, 521-524. doi:10.1007/s40519-014-0115-6

Lin, L., & Soby, M. (2016). Appearance comparisons styles and eating disordered symptoms in women. *Eating Behaviors*, 23, 7-12. https://doi.org/10.1016/j.eatbeh.2016.06.006

Lindgren, B., Enmark, A., Bohman, A., & Lundström, M. (2015). A qualitative study of young women's experiences of recovery from bulimia nervosa. *Journal of Advanced Nursing*, 71(4), 860-869. doi:10.1111/jan.12554

Lock, J., Agras, W. S., Grange, D., Couturier, J., Safer, D., & Bryson, S. W. (2013). Do end of treatment assessments predict outcome at follow-up in eating disorders? *International Journal of Eating Disorders*, 46(8), 771-778. doi:10.1002/eat.22175

Lock, J., LaVia, M., & American Academy of Child and American Academy of Child and Adolescent Psychiatry Committee on Quality Issues. (2015). Practice parameter for the assessment and treatment of children and adolescents with eating disorders. *Journal of American Academy of Child and Adolescent Psychiatry*, 54(5), 412-425.

Lofgren, I. E. (2015). Mindful eating. *American Journal of Lifestyle Medicine*, 9(3), 212-216. doi:10.1177/1559827615569684; http://journals.sagepub.com.proxy.hil.unb.ca/doi/abs/10.1177/1559827615569684

Loth, K., MacLehose, R., Bucchianeri, M., Crow, S., & Neumark-Stainer, D. (2014). Personal and socio-environmental predictors of dieting and disordered eating behaviors from adolescence to young adulthood: 10-Year longitudinal findings. *Journal of Adolescent Health: Official Publication of the Society for Adolescent Medicine*, 55(5), 705-712. http://doi.org/10.1016/j.jadohealth.2014.04.016

Loth, K., Wall, M., Choi, C., Bucchianeri, M., Quick, V., Larson, N., & Neumark-Sztainer, D. (2015). Family meals and disordered eating in adolescents: Are the benefits the same for everyone? *International Journal of Eating Disorders*, 48(1), 100-110. doi:10.1002/eat.22339

Loung, R. P. Y., Cooney, M., Fallon, E. M., Langer, J. C., & Katzman, D. K. (2016). Pneumothorax in a young man with anorexia nervosa. *International Journal of Eating Disorders*, 49, 895-898. doi:10.1002/eat.22558

Mac Vie, J. D. (2016). The association between emotion regulation strategies and symptoms of binge eating disorder (Order No. 10146447). Available from ProQuest Dissertations & Theses A&I; ProQuest Dissertations & Theses Global (1829545297). Retrieved from ttps://login.proxy.hil.unb.ca/login?url=http://search.proquest.com.proxy.hil.unb.ca/docview/1829545297?accountid=14611

MacDonald, D. E., McFarlane, T. L., Dionne, M. M., David, L., & Olmsted, M. P. (2017). Rapid response to intensive treatment for bulimia nervosa and purging disorder: A randomized controlled trial of a CBT intervention to facilitate early behavior change. *Journal of Consulting and Clinical Psychology*, 85(9), 896-908. doi: 10.1037/ccp0000221

Mann, A. P., Accurso, E. C., Stiles-Shields, C., Capra, L., Labuschagne, Z., Karnik, N. S., & Le Grange, D. (2014). Factors associated with substance use in adolescents with eating disorders. *Journal of Adolescent Health*, 55(2), 182-187. doi: 10.1016/j.jadohealth.2014.01.015

Martinsen, M., & Sundgot-Borgen, J. (2013). Higher prevalence of rating disorders among adolescent elite athletes than controls. *Medicine and Science in Sports and Exercise*, 45(6), 1188-1197.

Marzola, E., Desedime, N., Giovannone, C., Amianto, F., Fassino, S., & Abbate-Daga, G. (2015). Atypical antipsychotics as augmentation therapy in anorexia nervosa. *PLoS ONE*, 10(4), e0125569. http://doi.org/10.1371/journal.pone.0125569

Matos, M., Ferreira, C., Duarte, C., & Pinto-Gouveia, J. (2015). Eating disorders: When social rank perceptions are shaped by early shame experiences. *Psychology and Psychotherapy: Theory, Research and Practice*, 88(1), 38-53. doi:10.1111/papt.12027

Mayer-Brown, S., Lawless, C., Fedele, D., Dumont-Driscoll, M., & Janicke, D. M. (2016). The effects of media, self-esteem, and BMI on youth's unhealthy weight control behaviors. *Eating Behaviors*, 21, 59-65. https://doi.org/10.1016/j.eatbeh.2015.11.010

Mayo Clinic Staff. (2016). *Bulimia nervosa*. http://www.mayoclinic.org/diseases-conditions/bulimia/home/ovc-20179821

McCarvill, R., & Weaver, K. (2014). Primary care of female adolescents with type 1 diabetes mellitus and disordered eating behavior. *Journal of Advanced Nursing*, 70(9), 2005-2018. doi:10.1111/jan.12384 PMID: 24628439

McClay, C. A., Waters, L., McHale, C., Schmidt, U., & Williams, C. (2013). Online cognitive behavioral therapy for bulimic type disorders, delivered in the community by a nonclinician: Qualitative study. *Journal of Medical Internet Research*, 15(3), e46. doi:10.2196/jmir.2083

McCormack, C., & McCann, E. (2015). Caring for an adolescent with anorexia nervosa: Parent's views and experiences. *Archives of Psychiatric Nursing*, 29(3), 143-147. https://doi.org/10.1016/j.apnu.2015.01.003

McIntosh, V. V. W., Jordan, J., Carter, J. D., Luty, S. E., Carter, F. A., McKenzie, J. M., … Joyce, P. R. (2016). Assessing the distinctiveness of psychotherapies and examining change over treatment for anorexia nervosa with cognitive-behavior therapy, interpersonal psychotherapy, and specialist supportive clinical management. *International Journal of Eating Disorders*, 49, 958-962. doi:10.1002/eat.22555

Melville, N. A. (2016). IPT effective for depression, anxiety, eating disorders. *Medscape*. Retrieved from http://www.medscape.com/viewarticle/861812#vp_2

Meng, X., & D'Arcy, C. (2015). Comorbidity between lifetime eating problems and mood and anxiety disorders: Results from the Canadian Community Health Survey of Mental Health and Well-being. *European Eating Disorders Review*, 23(2), 156-162. doi:10.1002/erv.2347

Micali, N., Field, A. E., Treasure, J. L., & Evans, D. M. (2015). Are obesity risk genes associated with binge eating in adolescence? *Obesity*, 23(8), 1729-1736. doi:10.1002/oby.21147

Micali, N., Martini, M. G., Thomas, J. J., Eddy, K. T., Kothari, R., Russell, E., … Treasure, J. (2017). Lifetime and 12-month prevalence of eating disorders amongst women in mid-life: A population-based study of diagnoses and risk factors. *BMC Medicine*, 15, 1-10. doi:10.1186/s12916-016-0766-4

Midlarsky, E., Marotta, A. K., Pirutinsky, S., Morin, R. T., & McGowan, J. C. (2017). Psychological predictors of eating pathology in older adult women. *Journal of Women and Aging*, 3, 1-15. doi:10.1080/08952841.2017.1295665

Milano, W., De Rosa, M., Milano, L., Riccio, A., Sanseverino, B., & Capasso, A. (2013). The pharmacological options in the treatment of eating disorders. *ISRN Pharmacology*, 2013, 352865. http://doi.org/10.1155/2013/352865

Misra, M., & Klibanski, A. (2014). Anorexia nervosa and bone. *The Journal of Endocrinology*, 221(3), R163-R176. http://doi.org/10.1530/JOE-14-0039

Mitchell, J. E. (2016). Medical comorbidity and medical complications associated with binge-eating disorder. *International Journal of Eating Disorders*, 49(3), 319-323. doi:10.1002/eat.22452

Mitchell, J. E., Roerig, J., & Steffen, K. (2013). Biological therapies for eating disorders. *International Journal of Eating Disorders*, 46(5), 470-477.

Mitchison, D., Dawson, L., Hand, L. Mond, J., & Hay, P. (2016). Quality of life as a vulnerability and recovery factor in eating disorders: A community-based study. *BMC Psychiatry*, 16, 328. doi:10.1186/s12888-016-1033-0

Mitchison, D., Mond, J., Hay, P., Griffiths, S., Murray, S. B., Bentley, C., … Harrison, C. (2017). Disentangling body image: The relative associations of overvaluation, dissatisfaction, and preoccupation with psychological distress and eating disorder behaviors in male and female adolescents. *International Journal of Eating Disorders*, 50(2), 118-126. doi:10.1002/eat.22592

Moore, S. R., McKone, K. M. P., & Mendle, J. (2016). Recollections of puberty and disordered eating in young women. *Journal of Adolescence*, 53, 180-188. https://doi.org/10.1016/j.adolescence.2016.10.011

Morin, S. (2016, January 27). Fighting more than just food. *The Aquinian*. http://theaquinian.net/fighting-just-food/

Morin, S. (2017, February 6). Eating disorders need more attention, funding. *The Aquinian*. http://theaquinian.net/eating-disorder-awareness-commentary/

Murakami, J. M., Essayli, J. H., & Latner, J. D. (2016). The relative stigmatization of eating disorders and obesity in males and females. *Appetite*, 10, 77-82. https://doi.org/10.1016/j.appet.2016.02.027

Mustafa, N., Zaidi, A. U., & Weaver, R. R. (2017). Conspiracy of silence: Cultural conflict as a risk factor for the development of eating disorders among second-generation Canadian South Asian women. *South Asian Diaspora*, 9(1), 33-49. Retrieved from http://works.bepress.com/robert-weaver/1/

Mustapic, J., Marcinko, D., & Vargek, P. (2015). Eating behaviours in adolescent girls: The role of body shame and body dissatisfaction. *Eating and Weight Disorders*, 20(3), 329-335. doi:10.1007/s40519-015-0183-2

Mustelin, L., Silen, Y., Raevuori, A., Hoek, H. W., Kaprio, J., & Keski-Rahkonen, A. (2016). The DSM-5 diagnostic criteria for anorexia nervosa may change its population prevalence and prognostic value. *Journal of Psychiatric Research, 77*, 85–91. https://doi.org/10.1016/j.jpsychires.2016.03.003

Naeem, F., Johal, R. K., Mckenna, C., Calancie, O., Munshi, T., Hassan, T., ... Ayub, M. (2017). Preliminary evaluation of a 'formulation-driven cognitive behavioral guided self-help (fCBT-GSH)' for crisis and transitional case management clients. *Neuropsychiatric Disease and Treatment, 13*, 769–774.

National Eating Disorder Association. (2013). Eating disorders affect families for the bad and the good. Retrieved from www.nationaleatingdisorders.org/eating-disorders-affect-families-bad-and-good

National Eating Disorder Information Centre. (2014). Ideas for families. Retrieved from http://nedic.ca/give-get-help/prevention-health-promotion

National Eating Disorders Collaboration. (2017). NEDC fact sheet—Eating disorders in males. http://www.nedc.com.au/eating-disorders-in-males

Neff, K. J., Olbers, T. T., & Le Roux, C. W. (2013). Bariatric surgery: The challenges with candidate selection, individualizing treatment and clinical outcomes. *BMC Medicine, 11*(1), 1–17.

Nicholls, D., Fogarty, S., Hay, P., & Ramjan, L. M. (2016). Participatory action research for women with anorexia nervosa. *Nurse Researcher, 23*(5), 26–30.

Nobles, C. J., Thomas, J. J., Valentine, S. E., Gerber, M. W., Vaewsorn, A. S., & Marques, L. (2016). Association of premenstrual syndrome and premenstrual dysphoric disorder with bulimia nervosa and binge-eating disorder in a nationally representative epidemiological sample. *International Journal of Eating Disorders, 49*(7), 641–650. doi:10.1002/eat.22539

Obeid, N., Buchholz, A., Boerner, K. E., Henderson, K. A., & Norris, M. (2013). Self-esteem and social anxiety in an adolescent female eating disorder population: Age and diagnostic effects. *Eating Disorders, 21*(2), 140–153.

O'Hara, C. B., Keyes, A., Renwick, B., Giel, K. E., Campbell, I. C., & Schmidt, U. (2016). Evidence that illness-compatible cues are rewarding in women recovered from anorexia nervosa: A study of the effects of dopamine depletion on eye-blink startle responses. *PLoS ONE, 11*(10), 1–16. doi:10.1371/journal.pone.0165104

Oldershaw, A., Lavender, T., Sallis, H., Stahl, D., & Schmidt, U. (2015). Emotion generation and regulation in anorexia nervosa: A systematic review and meta-analysis of self-report data. *Clinical Psychology Review, 39*, 83–95. https://doi.org/10.1016/j.cpr.2015.04.005

Olguin, P., Fuentes, M., Gabler, G., Guerdjikova, A. I., Keck, P. E., & McElroy, S. L. (2017). Medical comorbidity of binge eating disorder. *Eating and Weight Disorders, 22*(1), 13–26. doi:10.1007/s40519-016-0313-5

Pappas, S. (2016, August 28). Purging the myth of the vomitorium. *Scientific American*. Retrieved from https://www.scientificamerican.com/article/purging-the-myth-of-the-vomitorium/

Parry, L. (2014, August 27). You don't have to be stick thin to be anorexic, warn experts: Fivefold increase in 'normal weight' teens being admitted to hospital with the eating disorder. *Mail Online*. Retrieved from http://www.dailymail.co.uk/health/article-2735559/You-dont-stick-anorexic-warn-experts-Fivefold-increase-normal-weight-teens-admitted-hospital-eating-disorder.html

Pasold, T. L., McCracken, A., & Ward-Begnoche, W. L. (2014). Binge eating in obese adolescents: Emotional and behavioral characteristics and impact on health-related quality of life. *Clinical Child Psychology and Psychiatry, 19*(2), 299–312. doi:10.1177/1359104513488605

Pearson, C. M., Riley, E. N., Davis, H. A., & Smith, G. T. (2014). Research review: Two pathways toward impulsive action: An integrative risk model for bulimic behavior in youth. *Journal of Child Psychology and Psychiatry, 55*(8), 852–864. doi:10.1111/jcpp.12214

Penny, L. (2013). I don't want to be told I'm pretty as I am. I want to live in a world where that's irrelevant. *New Statesman, 142*(5156), 38.

Perkins, P. S., Slane, J. D., & Klump, K. L. (2013). Personality clusters and family relationships in women with disordered eating symptoms. *Eating Behaviors, 14*(3), 299–308.

Petersson, S., Johnsson, P., & Perseius, K. (2017). A Sisyphean task: Experiences of perfectionism in patients with eating disorders. *Journal of Eating Disorders, 5*, 1–11. doi:10.1186/s40337-017-0136-4

Phelan, S., Burgess, D., Yeazel, M., Hellerstedt, W., Griffin, J., & van Ryn, M. (2015). Impact of weight bias and stigma on quality of care 2266 and outcomes for patients with obesity. *Obesity Reviews, 16*(4), 319–326. http://doi.org/10.1111/obr.1

Piko, B. F., & Brassai, L. A. (2016). A reason to eat healthy: The role of meaning in life in maintaining homeostasis in modern society. *Health Psychology Open, 3*(1), 1–4. doi:10.1177/2055102916634360

Pisetsky, E. M., Wonderlich, S. A., Crosby, R. D., Peterson, C. B., Mitchell, J. E., Engel, S. G., ... Crow, S. J. (2015). Depression and personality traits associated with emotion dysregulation: Correlates of suicide attempts in women with bulimia nervosa. *European Eating Disorders Review, 23*(6), 537–544. doi:10.1002/erv.2401

Pohjolainen, V., Ryynänen, O. P., Räsänen, P., Roine, R. P., Koponen, S., & Karlsson, H. (2014). Bayesian prediction of treatment outcome in anorexia nervosa: A preliminary study. *Nordic Journal of Psychiatry, 7*, 1–6. doi:10.1002/eat.20676

Public Health Agency of Canada. (2015, February 24). *Health behaviour in school-aged children in Canada: Focus on relationships*. Retrieved from http://healthycanadians.gc.ca/publications/science-research-sciences-recherches/health-behaviour-children-canada-2015-comportements-sante-jeunes/index-eng.php#c9a6

Puhl, R., & Suh, Y. (2015). Stigma and eating and weight disorders. *Current Psychiatry Reports, 17*, 10. doi:10.1007/s11920-015-0552-6

Qaseem, A., Humphrey, L. L., Harris, R., Starkey, M., Denberg, T. D., & for the Clinical Guidelines Committee of the American College of Physicians. (2014). Screening pelvic examination in adult women: A clinical practice guideline from the American College of Physicians. *Annals of Internal Medicine, 161*, 67–72. doi:10.7326/M14-0701

Quick, V. M., McWilliams, R., & Byrd-Bredbenner, C. (2013). Fatty, fatty, two-by-four: Weight-teasing history and disturbed eating in young adult women. *American Journal of Public Health, 103*(3), 508–515.

Raevuori, A., Suokas, J., Haukka, J., Gissler, M., Linna, M., Grainger, M., & Suvisaari, J. (2015). Highly increased risk of type 2 diabetes in patients with binge eating disorder and bulimia nervosa. *International Journal of Eating Disorders, 48*(6), 555–562. doi:10.1002/eat.22334

Reas, D. L., & Grilo, C. M. (2014). Current and emerging drug treatments for binge eating disorder. *Expert Opinion on Emerging Drugs, 19*(1), 99–142. http://doi.org/10.1517/14728214.2014.879291

Reas, D. L., Pedersen, G., Karterud, S., & Rø, Ø. (2015). Self-harm and suicidal behavior in borderline personality disorder with and without bulimia nervosa. *Journal of Consulting and Clinical Psychology, 83*(3), 643–648. doi:10.1037/ccp0000014

Reas, D. L., Rø, O., Karterud, S., Hummelen, B., & Pedersen, G. (2013). Eating disorders in a large clinical sample of men and women with personality disorders. *International Journal of Eating Disorders, 46*, 801–809.

Reas, D. L., & Stedal, K. (2015). Eating disorders in men aged midlife and beyond. *Maturitas, 81*(2), 248–255. https://doi.org/10.1016/j.maturitas.2015.03.004

Reel, J. R. (Ed.) (2013). *Eating disorders: An encyclopedia of causes, treatment, and prevention*. Santa Barbara, CA: Greenwood.

Rider, K. A., Terrell, D. J., Sisemore, T. A., & Hecht, J. E. (2014). Religious coping style as a predictor of the severity of anorectic symptomology. *Eating Disorders, 22*(2), 163–179. doi:10.1080/10640266.2013.864890

Rikani, A. A., Choudhry, Z., Choudhry, A. M., Ikram, H., Asghar, M. W., Kajal, D., ... Mobassarah, N. J. (2013). A critique of the literature on etiology of eating disorders. *Annals of Neurosciences, 20*(4), 157–161. doi:10.5214/ans.0972.7531.200409

Ristea, S., & Drăgoi, A. I. (2014). Bulimia nervosa: A short theoretical review of the cognitive-behavioral conceptualization and approach. *Romanian Journal of Cognitive Behavioral Therapy and Hypnosis, 1*(2), 1–11. Retrieved from http://www.rjcbth.ro/articles/V1I2_Silvia%20Ristea_RJCBTH.pdf

Rizk, M., Lalanne, C., Berthoz, S., Kern, L., EVHAN Group, & Godart, N. (2015). Problematic exercise in anorexia nervosa: Testing potential risk factors against different definitions. *PLoS One, 10*(11), e0143352. http://doi.org/10.1371/journal.pone.0143352

Robinson, K. J., Mountford, V. A., & Sperlinger, D. J. (2013). Being men with eating disorders: Perspectives of male eating disorder service users. *Journal of Health Psychology, 18*, 176–186.

Rohde, P., Stice, E., & Marti, C. N. (2015). Development and predictive effects of eating disorder risk factors during adolescence: Implications for prevention efforts. *International Journal of Eating Disorders, 48*(2), 187–198. doi:10.1002/eat.22270

Rosen, E., Sabel, A. L., Brinton, J. T., Catanach, B., Gaudiani, J. L., & Mehler, P. S. (2016). Liver dysfunction in patients with severe anorexia nervosa. *International Journal of Eating Disorders, 49*(2), 153–160. doi:10.1002/eat.22436

Rosenbaum, D. L., & White, K. S. (2013). The role of anxiety in binge eating behavior: A critical examination of theory and empirical literature. *Health Psychology Research, 1*(2). doi:10.4081/hpr.2013.e19

Rosenbaum, D. L., & White, K. S. (2015). The relation of anxiety, depression, and stress to binge eating behavior. *Journal of Health Psychology, 20*(6), 887–898. doi:10.1177/1359105315580212

Rosenbaum, D. L., Kimerling, R., Pomernacki, A., Goldstein, K. M., Yano, E. M., Sadler, A. G., ... Frayne, S. M. (2016). Binge eating among women veterans in primary care: Comorbidities and treatment priorities. *Women's Health Issues, 26*(4), 420–428. doi:10.1016/j.whi.2016.02.004

Rosenberger, P. H., & Dorflinger, L. (2013). Psychosocial factors associated with binge eating among overweight and obese male veterans. *Eating Behaviors, 14*(3), 401–404.

Roy, M., & Gauvin, L. (2013). Associations between different forms of body dissatisfaction and the use of weight-related behaviors among a representative population-based sample of adolescents. *Eating and Weight Disorders, 18*(1), 61–73. doi:10.1007/s40519-013-0007-1

Roy, M., Shatenstein, B., Gaudreau, P., Morais, J. A., & Payette, H. (2015). Seniors' body weight dissatisfaction and longitudinal associations with weight changes, anorexia of aging, and obesity. *Journal of Aging and Health, 27*(2), 220–238. doi:10.1177/0898264314546715

Sabel, A. L., Rosen E., & Mehler, P. S. (2014) Severe anorexia nervosa in males: Clinical presentations and medical treatment. *Eating Disorders, 22*, 209–220.

Saltzman, J. A., & Liechty, J. M. (2016). Family correlates of childhood binge eating: A systematic review. *Eating Behaviors, 22*, 62–71. https://doi.org/10.1016/j.eatbeh.2016.03.027

Saules, K. S., Carey, J., Carr, M. M., & Sienko, R. M. (2015). Binge-eating disorder: Prevalence, predictors, and management in the primary care setting. *Journal of Clinical Outcomes Management, 22*(11), 512–528. Retrieved from http://www.turner-white.com/pdf/jcom_nov15_binge.pdf

Schaefer, M. K., & Salafia, E. H. B. (2014). The connection of teasing by parents, siblings, and peers with girls' body dissatisfaction and boys' drive for muscularity: The role of social comparison as a mediator. *Eating Behaviors, 15*(4), 599–608. https://doi.org/10.1016/j.eatbeh.2014.08.018

Schermel, A., Mendoza, J., Henson, S., Dukeshire, S., Pasut, L., Emrich, T. E., … L'Abbé, M. R. (2014). Canadians' perceptions of food, diet, and health—A national survey. *PLoS ONE, 9*(1), e86000. https://doi.org/10.1371/journal.pone.0086000

Schmitz, C., Schnicker, K., & Legenbauer, T. (2016). Influence of weight on shared core symptoms in eating disorders. *Behavior Modification, 40*(5), 777–796. doi:10.1177/0145445516643487

Schnicker, K., Hiller, W., & Legenbauer, T. (2013). Drop-out and treatment outcome of outpatient cognitive-behavioral therapy for anorexia nervosa and bulimia nervosa. *Comprehensive Psychiatry, 54*(7), 812–823. doi:10.1016/j.comppsych.2013.02.007

Schoenefeld, S. J., & Webb, J. B. (2013). Self-compassion and intuitive eating in college women: Examining the contributions of distress tolerance and body image acceptance and action. *Eating Behaviors, 14*(4), 493–496. doi:10.1016/j.eatbeh.2013.09.001

Schuster, E., Negy, C., & Tantleff-Dunn, S. (2013). The effects of appearance-related commentary on body dissatisfaction, eating pathology, and body change behaviors in men. *Psychology of Men and Masculinity, 14*(1), 76–87. doi:10.1037/a0025625

Seah, X. Y., Tham, X. C., Kamaruzaman, N. R., & Yobas, P. (K). (2017). Knowledge, attitudes and challenges of healthcare professionals managing people with eating disorders: A literature review. *Archives of Psychiatric Nursing, 31*(1), 125–136. https://doi.org/10.1016/j.apnu.2016.09.002

Sharpe, H. (2014). Equine-facilitated counselling and women with eating disorders: Articulating bodily experience. *Canadian Journal of Counselling and Psychotherapy/Revue canadienne de counseling et de psychothérapie, 48*(2), 127–152.

Sharpe, H., Damazer, K., Treasure, J., & Schmidt, U. (2013). What are adolescents' experiences of body dissatisfaction and dieting, and what do they recommend for prevention? A qualitative study. *Eating and Weight Disorders, 18*(2), 133–141.

Shih, P. B., & Woodside, D. B. (2016). Contemporary views on the genetics of anorexia nervosa. *European Neuropsychopharmacology, 26*(4), 663–673. https://doi.org/10.1016/j.euroneuro.2016.02.008

Shire US Inc. (2015). *Vyvanse® for adults with moderate to severe binge eating disorder.* Retrieved from http://www.vyvanse.com/binge-eating-disorder-treatment

Sipilä, P., Harrasova, G., Mustelin, L., Rose, R., Kaprio, J., & Keski-Rahkonen, A. (2017). 'Holy anorexia'-relevant or relic? Religiosity and anorexia nervosa among Finnish women. *International Journal of Eating Disorders, 50*(4), 406–414. https://doi.org/10.1002/eat.22698

Slof-Op't Landt, M. T., Bartels, M., Middeldorp, C. M., van Beijsterveldt, C. M., Slagboom, P. E., Boomsma, D. I., … Meulenbelt, I. (2013). Genetic variation at the TPH2 gene influences impulsivity in addition to eating disorders. *Behavior Genetics, 43*(1), 24–33. doi:10.1007/s10519-012-9569-3

Sonneville, K. R., Calzo, J. P., Horton, N. J., Field, A. E., Crosby, R. D., Solmi, F., & Micali, N. (2015). Childhood hyperactivity/inattention and eating disturbances predict binge eating in adolescence. *Psychological Medicine, 45*(12), 2511–2520. doi: 10.1017/S0033291715000148

Spyrou, S. (2014). *Exploring men's experiences and understanding of binge eating disorder: An interpretative phenomenological analysis.* Unpublished PhD Thesis. London Metropolitan University, UK.

Sree, I. V. (2013). *Biological basis in eating disorders.* Retrieved from https://www.slideshare.net/vidyairdala/biological-basis-in-eating-disorders

Statistics Canada. (2013). *Immigration and ethnocultural diversity in Canada: National Household Survey 2011.* Ottawa, ON: Minister of Industry.

Retrieved from http://www.hireimmigrants.ca/resources-tools/news/statistics-canada-immigration-and-ethnocultural-diversity-in-canada/

Statistics Canada. (2015). *Section D—Eating disorders.* Retrieved from http://www.statcan.gc.ca/pub/82-619-m/2012004/sections/sectiond-eng.htm

Steiger, H. (2017). Evidence-informed practices in the real-world treatment of people with eating disorders. *Eating Disorders, 25*(2), 173–181. doi:10.1080/10640266.2016.1269558

Stheneur, C., Bergeron, S., & Lapeyraque, A. L. (2014). Renal complications in anorexia nervosa. *Eating and Weight Disorders, 19*, 455–460. doi:10.1007/s40519-014-0138-z

Stice, E., Marti, C., & Rohde, P. (2013). Prevalence, incidence, impairment, and course of the proposed DSM-5 eating disorder diagnoses in an 8-year prospective community study of young women. *Journal of Abnormal Psychology, 122*(2), 445–457.

Stoll, M., Bitterlich, N., & Cornelli, U. (2017). Randomised, double-blind, clinical investigation to compare orlistat 60 milligram and a customized polyglucosamine, two treatment methods for the management of overweight and obesity. *BMC Obesity, 4*, 1–9. doi:10.1186/s40608-016-0130-4

Strenger, A. M., Schnitker, S. A., & Felke, T. J. (2016). Attachment to God moderates the relation between sociocultural pressure and eating disorder symptoms as mediated by emotional eating. *Mental Health, Religion and Culture, 19*(1), 23–36. doi:10.1080/13674676.2015.108632

Stunkard, A. J., & Messick, S. (1985). The three-factor eating questionnaire to measure dietary restraint and hunger. *Journal of Psychosomatic Research, 29*, 71–83.

Su, X., Liang, H., Yuan, W., Olsen, J., Cnattingius, S., & Li, J. (2016). Prenatal and early life stress and risk of eating disorders in adolescent girls and young women. *European Child and Adolescent Psychiatry, 25*(11), 1245–1253. doi:10.1007/s00787-016-0848-z

Sue, D., Wing Sue, D., Sue, D. M. & Sue, S. (2016). Eating disorders. Chapter 10. In *Understanding abnormal behavior* (11th ed., pp. 297–326). Stamford, CT: Cengage Learning.

Sutin, A. R., & Terracciano, A. (2013) Perceived weight discrimination and obesity. *PLoS One, 8*(7), e70048. https://doi.org/10.1371/journal.pone.0070048

Svensson, E., Nilsson, K., Levi, R., & Suarez, N. C. (2013). Parents' experiences of having and caring for a child with an eating disorder. *Eating Disorders, 21*, 395–407. doi:10.1080/10640266.2013.827537

Tasca, G. A., Compare, A., Zarbo, C., & Brugnera, A. (2016). Therapeutic alliance and binge-eating outcomes in a group therapy context. *Journal of Counseling Psychology, 63*(4), 443–451. doi:10.1037/cou0000159

Tatham, M., Athanasia, E., Dodd, J., & Waller, G. (2016). The effect of pre-treatment psychoeducation on eating disorder pathology among patients with anorexia nervosa and bulimia nervosa. *Advances in Eating Disorders, 4*(2), 167–175. doi:10.1080/21662630.2016.1172975

Tetyana. (2013). *Avoiding refeeding syndrome in anorexia nervosa. Science of eating disorders: Making sense of the latest findings in eating disorders research.* Retrieved from www.scienceofeds.org/2013/03/12/avoiding-refeeding-syndrome-in-anorexia-nervosa/

Thaler, L., Israel, M., Antunes, J. M., Sarin, S., Zuroff, D. C., & Steiger, H. (2016). An examination of the role of autonomous versus controlled motivation in predicting inpatient treatment outcome for Anorexia Nervosa. *International Journal of Eating Disorders, 49*(6), 626–629.

Thompson-Brenner, H., Thompson, D. R., Boisseau, C. L., Richards, L. K., Bulik, C. M., Devlin, M. J., … Wilson, G. (2013). Race/ethnicity, education, and treatment parameters as moderators and predictors of outcome in binge eating disorder. *Journal of Consulting and Clinical Psychology, 81*(4), 710–721.

Trace, S. E., Baker, J. H., Peñas-Lledó, E., & Bulik, C. M. (2013). The genetics of eating disorders. *Annual Review of Clinical Psychology, 9*, 589–620. doi:10.1146/annurev-clinpsy-050212-185546

Treasure, J., & Cardi, V. (2017). Anorexia nervosa, theory and treatment: Where are we 35 years on from Hilde Bruch's foundation lecture? *European Eating Disorders Review, 25*(3), 139–147. doi:10.1002/erv.2511

Tseng, M.-C. M., Chang, C.-H., Liao, S.-C., & Chen, H.-C. (2017). Comparison of associated features and drug treatment between co-occurring unipolar and bipolar disorders in depressed eating disorder patients. *BMC Psychiatry, 17*, 81. doi:10.1186/s12888-017-1243-0

Ty, M., & Francis, A. J. P. (2013). Insecure attachment and disordered eating in women: The mediating processes of social comparison and emotion dysregulation. *Eating Disorders, 21*(2), 154–174.

Ulfvebrand, S., Birgegård, A., Norring, C., Högdahl, L., & von Hausswolff-Juhlin, Y. (2015). Psychiatric comorbidity in women and men with eating disorders results from a large clinical database. *Psychiatry Research, 230*(2), 294–299. doi:10.1016/j.psychres.2015.09.008

Valente, S. (2016). The hysterical anorexia epidemic in the French nineteenth-century. *Dialogues in Philosophy, Mental and Neuro Sciences, 9*(1), 22–23. Crossing Dialogues Association 20160601

Vall, E., & Wade, T. D. (2015). Predictors of treatment outcome in individuals with eating disorders: A systematic review and meta-analysis.

International Journal of Eating Disorders, 48(7), 946–971. doi:10.1002/eat.22411

van Amsterdam, N. (2013). Big fat inequalities, thin privilege: An intersectional perspective on 'body size'. *European Journal of Women's Studies*, 20, 155–169. http://dx.doi.org/10.1177/1350506812456461

Vandereycken, W., & van Deth, R. (1994). *From fasting saints to anorexic girls: The history of self-starvation.* New York, NY: New York University Press.

Vanderlinden, J., Claes, L., De Cuyper, K., & Vrieze, E. (2015). Dissociation and dissociative disorders. *Springer Science & Business Media Singapore Tracey Wade Encyclopedia of Feeding and Eating Disorders.* 10.1007/978-981-287-087-2_33-1. Retrieved from https://lirias.kuleuven.be/bitstream/123456789/530325/1/Dissociation+and+dissociative+disorders+encyclopedia+of+feeding+and+eating+disorders+(002).pdf

Vázquez, I. A., & Rodríguez, C. F. (2013). The role of the clinical psychologist in the treatment of overweight and obesity. *Papeles del Psicólogo*, 34(1), 49–56. http://www.papelesdelpsicologo.es

Vella-Zarb, R. A., Mills, J. S., Westra, H. A., Carter, J. C., & Keating, L. (2015). A randomized controlled trial of motivational interviewing + self-help versus psychoeducation + self-help for binge eating. *International Journal of Eating Disorders*, 48(3), 328–332. doi:10.1002/eat.22242

Wade, T. D., & Tiggemann, M. (2013). The role of perfectionism in body dissatisfaction. *Journal of Eating Disorders*, 1, 2. doi: 10.1186/2050-2974-1-2

Wade, T. D., Wilksch, S. M., Paxton, S. J., Byrne, S. M., & Austin, S. B. (2015). How perfectionism and ineffectiveness influence growth of eating disorder risk in young adolescent girls. *Behaviour Research and Therapy*, 66, 56–63. doi:10.1016/j.brat.2015.01.007

Walsh, T. (2017). *Anorexia nervosa in adults: Pharmacotherapy.* Retrieved from http://www.uptodate.com/contents/anorexia-nervosa-in-adults-pharmacotherapy

Watson, R. J., Adjei, J., Saewyc, E., Homma, Y., & Goodenow, C. (2017), Trends and disparities in disordered eating among heterosexual and sexual minority adolescents. *International Journal of Eating Disorders*, 50, 22–31. doi:10.1002/eat.22576

Weaver, K., Martin-McDonald, K., & Spiers, J. (2016). Lost alongside my daughter living with an eating disorder. *GSTF Journal of Nursing and Health Care (JNHC)*, 3(2). doi:10.5176/2345-718X_3.2.122. http://dl6.globalstf.org/index.php/jnhc/article/view/1591/1619

Webb, R. (2014). Roll up, roll up, to see a man talking about feminism. What could possibly go wrong? *New Statesman*, 143(5221), 20.

Webb, H. J., & Zimmer-Gembeck, M. J. (2014). The role of friends and peers in adolescent body dissatisfaction: A review and critique of 15 years of research. *Journal of Research on Adolescence*, 24(4), 564–590. doi:10.1111/jora.12084

Weinberger-Litman, S. L., Rabin, L. A., Fogel, J., Mensinger, J. L., & Litman, L. (2016). Psychosocial mediators of the relationship between religious orientation and eating disorder risk factors in young Jewish women. *Psychology of Religion and Spirituality*, 8(4), 265–276. doi:10.1037/a0040293

Williams, D. (2014). Lithium toxicity: Risk factors, monitoring, and management. *US Pharmacist.* Retrieved from https://www.uspharmacist.com/ce/lithium-toxicity-risk-factors-monitoring

Witt, A. A., & Lowe, M. R. (2014). Hedonic hunger and binge eating among women with eating disorders. *International Journal of Eating Disorders*, 47(3), 273–280. doi:10.1002/eat.22171

Woodside, B. (2013). Genetic contributions to eating disorders. In A. S. Kaplan & P. E. Garfinkel (Eds.), *Medical issues and the eating disorders: The interface.* New York, NY: Routledge

Woodside, B., Twose, R. M., Olteanu, A., & Sathi, C. (2016). Hospital admissions in severe and enduring anorexia nervosa: When to admit, when not to admit, and when to stop admitting. In S. Touyz, D. Le Grange, J. Hubert Lacey, & P. Hay (Eds.), *Managing severe and enduring anorexia nervosa: A clinician's guide* (pp. 171–184). New York, NY: Routledge.

Yu, J., Agras, W. S., & Bryson, S. (2013). Defining recovery in adult bulimia nervosa. *Eating Disorders*, 21(5), 379–394. doi:10.1080/10640266.2013.827536

Zaitsoff, S., Pullmer, R., Cyr, M., & Aime, H. (2015). The role of the therapeutic alliance in eating disorder treatment outcomes: A systematic review. *Eating Disorders*, 23(2), 99–114. doi:10.1080/10640266.2014.964623

Zeller, M. H., Inge, T. H., Modi, A. C., Jenkins, T. M., Michalsky, M. P., Helmrath, M., … Buncher, R. (2015). Severe obesity and comorbid condition impact on the weight-related quality of life of the adolescent patient. *Journal of Pediatrics*, 166(3), 651–659.e4. doi:10.1016/j.jpeds.2014.11.022

Zerwas, S., Lund, B. C., Von Holle, A., Thornton, L. M., Berrettini, W. H., Brandt, H., … Bulik, C. M. (2013). Factors associated with recovery from anorexia nervosa. *Journal of Psychiatric Research*, 47(7), 972–979. https://doi.org/10.1016/j.jpsychires.2013.02.011

Zhang, K. (2013). What I look like: College women, body image, and spirituality. *Journal of Religion and Health*, 52(4), 1240–1252. doi:10.1007/s10943-012-9566-0

Zugai, J., Stein-Parbury, J., & Roche, M. (2013). Effective nursing care of adolescents with anorexia nervosa: A consumer perspective. *Journal of Clinical Nursing*, 22(13–14), 2020–2029. doi: 10.1111/jocn.12182

Zwickert, K., & Rieger, E. (2013). Stigmatizing attitudes towards individuals with anorexia nervosa: An investigation of attribution theory. *Journal of Eating Disorders*, 1, 5. doi:10.1186/2050-2974-1-5

26 Substance-Related and Addictive Disorders

Diane Kunyk
and Charl Els

LEARNING OBJECTIVES

After studying this chapter, you will be able to:

- Conceptualize "addiction" as a prevalent, chronic, relapsing, and treatable medical disorder.
- Describe the features of the bio/psycho/social/spiritual theories for understanding addiction in Canadian settings.
- Describe the principles of safe and effective treatment of substance-related and addictive disorders.
- Outline essential components of screening, comprehensive assessment, matching patients with appropriate multimodal treatment interventions, as well as monitoring progress and effectiveness of treatment.
- Formulate an individualized nursing care plan.
- Contemplate the role of the nurse in advocating for patients with addiction.

KEY TERMS

- addiction • addictive substances • alcohol • ambivalence
- brief intervention • caffeine • cannabinoids • cannabis
- contemporaneous • craving • delirium tremens
- detoxification • gambling disorder • hallucinogens
- harm reduction • inhalants • intoxication • motivational interviewing • opioids • relapse • screening • therapeutic alliance • withdrawal

KEY CONCEPTS

- addiction

Addiction is recognized by both major disease classification systems as a bona fide, chronic, and relapsing medical condition (American Psychiatric Association [APA], 2013; World Health Organization [WHO], 2007). Advances in brain imaging and other research methods have demonstrated that repeated exposure to alcohol, tobacco, and/or other psychoactive substances over time may alter brain structure, chemistry, and function in susceptible individuals, leading to potential loss of control over the use of one or more substances and continued use despite harm or the knowledge of risk of harm. This conceptualization, along with emerging theories and understandings, has made advances in safe and effective treatment possible and provided increasingly optimistic outcomes for individuals and families affected by addiction.

Addiction may be expressed in individuals regardless of their age, gender, sexual orientation, socioeconomic status, education, culture, occupation, or other characteristics. Addiction is the most prevalent of all mental conditions, the leading preventable cause of death and disease globally, and the single greatest contributor to excess health care spending. For these reasons, it has been argued that addiction continues to be the most important illness of our time (Els, 2007). The future burden of addiction on Canadian society is uncertain

given the current unparalleled opioid epidemic and also the potential for increased risk of increased consumption and addiction given the Government of Canada's expressed intention to legalize marijuana.

Despite its importance, addiction is often neglected and undertreated in Canadian society. Conceptualizations of addiction as resulting from moral failure continue to be expressed in our public policies and popular media (Kunyk, Milner, & Overend, 2016). Individuals affected with addiction are often alienated and isolated from their families, workplaces, and communities. There are significant barriers (e.g., stigma and resources) for persons with addiction to overcome in order to access the treatment they need, and these systemic barriers may be as intractable as the disease of addiction itself.

Nurses encounter patients and their families who are struggling with addiction in their everyday practices and are favourably situated to help. With the necessary knowledge, skills, and attitudes conducive to health promotion and disease intervention, nurses are able to safely and effectively work with individuals, families, and communities experiencing the effects of addiction and thereby effectively reduce this care deficit.

This chapter reviews the categories of substance-related and addictive disorders, current theories regarding the

617

aetiology of substance use disorders (SUDs), and evidence-based treatment interventions. The role of the nurse is discussed in terms of early identification, assessment, and intervention planning with the purpose of helping to meet the needs of individuals, their families, and our broader society and to satisfy nurses' ethical duty of patient advocacy.

KEY CONCEPT

Addiction, a chronic, relapsing, and treatable medical condition, is the leading preventable cause of death, disability, and disease globally. It is a disease of the brain and not an expression of moral character.

IN-A-LIFE

Robert Munsch (June 11, 1945)

CANADIAN AUTHOR

Public Persona

Robert Munsch is a well-known and highly revered author of children's literature. He has published 54 children's books and continues to publish approximately two books every year. One of his books, *Love You Forever*, was written after Munsch and his wife lost two stillborn babies. This story chronicles the unconditional love between a mother and son throughout the cycle of life. It has sold more than 30 million copies and has been translated into French and Spanish. In 1999, Munsch was made a Member of the Order of Canada for his body of work. Amongst many accomplishments, Munsch is proud to be the most popular author whose books are borrowed but never returned from the Toronto Public Library saying, "I am happy to see that thieves like my books and will continue to try to serve the needs of the reading underworld" (Robinson, 2015, p. 7).

Personal Realities

Robert Munsch studied for 7 years to become a Jesuit priest only to decide that he was "lousy priest material." He subsequently earned a Master of Education in Child Studies from Tufts University. In a note to parents on his Web site, Munsch writes that he has struggled with addiction and has attended twelve-step recovery meetings for over 25 years. He has also revealed that he has been diagnosed with obsessive–compulsive and manic-depressive disorders.

Sources: www.robertmunsch.com; Robinson, M. (July 15, 2015). *Gone but not forgotten: 100,000 Toronto library books outstanding. The Star.* Retrieved from https://www.thestar.com/news/gta/2015/07/15/gone-but-not-forgotten-100000-toronto-library-books-outstanding.html.

■ DEFINITION

The American Society of Addiction Medicine (ASAM, 2011) provides the following definition:

> Addiction is a primary, chronic disease of brain reward, motivation, memory and related circuitry. Dysfunction in these circuits leads to characteristic biological, psychological, social and spiritual manifestations. This is reflected in an individual pathologically pursuing reward and/or relief by substance use and other behaviors.

> Addiction is characterized by inability to consistently abstain, impairment in behavioral control, craving, diminished recognition of significant problems with one's behaviors and interpersonal relationships, and a dysfunctional emotional response. Like other chronic diseases, addiction often involves cycles of relapse and remission. Without treatment or engagement in recovery activities, addiction is progressive and can result in disability or premature death (para.1 and 2).

■ NEUROBIOLOGY

Addictive substances, regardless of their legal classifications of licit and illicit, are used and misused for many reasons. These may include for their pleasurable effects, to alter mental status, to improve performance, to relieve boredom, or to self-medicate a mental disorder. These substances, when taken in excess, have in common the direct activation of the brain reward system. Stimulation of the reward pathway occurs, in part, through increasing extracellular dopamine concentrations in the limbic regions of the brain. Dopamine, a neurotransmitter, is involved in many aspects of reward and pleasure and is involved in the production of memories and behavioural reinforcement. Given their activation of the reward pathways of the brain, the taking of substances can be considered a reinforced behaviour. Chronic exposure to addictive substances may lead to pervasive changes in brain function at structural (molecular and cellular) and neurophysiologic levels, undermining the individual's voluntary control over its use. These underlying changes in brain circuits may persist beyond withdrawal, and the behavioural effects of these changes may be exhibited in the repeated experiences of craving and relapse of individuals exposed to drug-related stimuli (APA, 2013). From a neurobiologic perspective, addiction can be conceptualized as a *chronic, relapsing disease* of the brain, and the associated abnormal behaviour is the result of dysfunction of brain tissue (Volkow & Warren, 2014).

Given equal exposure to psychoactive substances, not all individuals who are exposed to addictive substances will develop addiction. Addiction comes to expression in individuals who may be considered potentially susceptible on any one or more of the following levels: biologic, psychological, social, or spiritual. For example, individuals who start using substances in adolescence are at higher risk of developing addiction than are those who start later in life. It has also been estimated that 40% to 60% of the vulnerability to addiction is attributable to genetic factors (Volkow & Warren, 2014). Gender differences have been established, with the prevalence among males consistently demonstrating higher rates of addiction (Crum, 2014). Women who regularly use or abuse substances are considered more vulnerable for developing addiction and at higher risk of health consequences from their use (Agabio, Campresi, Pisanu, Gess, & Franconi, 2016). Regardless of putative vulnerabilities, the manifestation of addiction has been described as "a cluster of cognitive, behavioural, and physiologic symptoms indicating that the individual continues using the substance despite significant substance-related problems" (APA, 2013, p. 483).

■ DIAGNOSTIC CRITERIA

The APA's (2013) *Diagnostic and Statistical Manual of Mental Disorders*, 5th ed. (*DSM-5*) classification of substance-related and addictive disorders refers to disorders related to taking of substances of abuse and includes two categories: SUDs and substance-induced disorders (substance intoxication, substance withdrawal, and other substance/medication-induced mental disorders).

The diagnosis of SUD is substance specific (e.g., alcohol, opioid, or tobacco use disorder). It is based on a pathologic pattern of 11 behaviours (Criteria) grouped into (1) impaired control, (2) social impairment, (3) risky use, and (4) pharmacologic categories. SUDs occur in a range of severity from mild to severe. Changes in severity may be observed across time (APA, 2013). For details of the eleven criteria, please consult the *DSM-5*.

The substance-induced disorder of **intoxication** is described as the development of a reversible substance-specific syndrome due to the recent ingestion of (or exposure to) a substance. The maladaptive behaviours associated with intoxication (e.g., belligerence, mood lability, cognitive impairment, impaired judgment, impaired social or occupational functioning) are due to the direct physiologic effects of the substance on the central nervous system (APA, 2013). These behaviours place the individual at significant risk for adverse effects (e.g., accidents, general medical complications, disruption in social and family relationships, vocational or financial difficulties, and legal problems).

Substance **withdrawal** is the development of a substance-specific maladaptive behavioural change that is due to the cessation, or reduction, of heavy and prolonged substance use. This may cause clinically significant distress or impairment in social, occupational, or other important areas of functioning, and as a result, most individuals will experience craving to readminister the substance to reduce the discomforting symptoms

(APA, 2013). Some withdrawal syndromes are life threatening, others are uncomfortable, and some are even less pronounced.

Classes of Substances

Although not fully distinct, there are 10 described classes of substances referred to in the *DSM-5*. The classification system includes **alcohol**; **caffeine**; **cannabis** (marijuana); **hallucinogens** (with separate categories for phencyclidine [PCP] [or similarly acting arylcyclohexylamines] and other hallucinogens); **inhalants**; **opioids**; sedatives, hypnotics, and anxiolytics; stimulants; tobacco (nicotine); and other (or unknown) substances (APA, 2013, p. 481). This last classification is for newer designer drugs that appear to regularly be entering the market. The diagnosis of SUD can be applied to all 10 classes of substances except for caffeine. The pharmacologic mechanisms by which each of these drugs produces reward to the brain are different, but what is common to these classes of drugs is that when they are taken in excess, the brain reward system is intensely activated (APA, 2013).

Clinical Course

Addiction is described as a *chronic disease*, specifically a chronic mental disorder—one that potentially threatens the health and well-being of individuals with the disorder as well as their family, friends, colleagues, community, and economy. There is considerable heterogeneity among people with SUD, but it is often observed that there are periods of sustained substance use that are interrupted by periods of partial or complete remission (a period when symptoms have abated). In some individuals, addiction to a single substance may lead to the **contemporaneous** use of (and possible addiction to) other psychoactive substances. Of particular note in this regard is the use of tobacco and caffeine, as these are often contemporaneously encountered with other substances but may be uncertainly addressed in many hospitals and addiction treatment facilities.

What is well acknowledged, however, is that when addiction is neglected and untreated, the course of the disease often typically progresses in severity and may even result in premature death (Kleber et al., 2006). Substance-related and addictive disorders are widely considered to be amenable to treatment. The outcomes to evidence-based interventions are similar to those for other chronic disease conditions, including hypertension, asthma, and type 2 diabetes (McLellan, Lewis, O'Brien, & Kleber, 2000). Most persons with substance-related disorders (SRDs) will have one or more **relapses** (a return to substance use after a drug-free period) during their process of recovery. Some of the most commonly cited precursors to relapse include substance-related reminder cues (e.g., sights, sounds, smells, or thoughts), negative mood states, positive mood states, and sampling the drug itself (even in small doses). Current **craving** (the experience of a strong desire or urge to take the substance) is often used as an outcome measure because it may be a signal of impending relapse (APA, 2013).

Non–Substance-Related Disorders

Ranges of other repetitive behaviours have been postulated to form part of the addiction-related disorder spectrum. These include behaviours such as "Internet gaming addiction," "sex addiction," "exercise addiction," "shopping addiction," and others. More research is needed for the non-SRDs and related conditions to reach the necessary internal consistency of criteria or the diagnostic stability for inclusion in the *DSM-5* classification system.

The *DSM-5* (APA, 2013) includes **gambling disorder** in its classification system due to the body of evidence indicating that gambling behaviours activate reward systems similar to those activated by substances of abuse and appear to produce some behavioural symptoms comparable to those of SUD. Please refer to the DSM-5 for diagnostic criteria.

■ EPIDEMIOLOGY

Nurses should be open to the possibility that patients are unlikely ever too young or old, too healthy or ill, or too educated or wealthy to have problems with substance use. In their practices, nurses are well positioned to detect areas of potential or actual need for patients and their families in regard to substance use in all of the settings in which nursing is practiced (e.g., home, community, ambulatory, inpatient, and long-term settings). The following section addresses the most commonly used substances in Canadian society.

Alcohol

Over 70% of youth (aged 15 to 24) and 80% of adults (aged 25+) reported using alcohol in the past year (Canadian Centre on Substance Abuse, 2014). This rate is more than 50% above the global average (Shield, Rylett, Gmel, Kehoe-Chan, & Rehm, 2013). In most instances, alcohol is used in moderation but, in general, for both men and women, the frequency of drinking alcohol *increases* with age, income, and education just as smoking and illicit drug use *decreases* across these variables. Alcohol is second only to tobacco in its prevalence of addiction in Canada. The prevalence rate of 12-month and lifetime alcohol use disorders are 13.9% and 29.1%, respectively, with only 19.8% with lifetime AUD ever treated (Grant et al., 2015).

Caffeine

Caffeine is the most widely used substance globally. Coffee, tea, and soft drinks are the major dietary sources of caffeine, while energy drink consumption continues to sharply increase each year (Verster, 2014). Caffeine is generally considered a functional or beneficial drug because it can improve mood and alertness at low doses. However, caffeine use can become disordered or problematic; among caffeine consumers who attempt to permanently stop using caffeine, more than 70% report withdrawal symptoms and 24% report headache plus other symptoms that interfered with functioning (APA, 2013).

Cannabis

Cannabis (commonly referred to as marijuana [MJ]) is in the process of becoming legalized and regulated in Canada. After a century of prohibition, marijuana remains the most commonly used illicit substance in Canada, and the single most commonly encountered substance in workplace drug testing, and second to alcohol in cases of driving under the influence of alcohol or other drugs. While the possession of MJ in Canada remains unlawful under the controlled Drugs and Substances Act, its medical use is permitted under the Regulations to the Act. Canadians have access to cannabis for medical purposes when authorized (not prescribed) by a medical practitioner. In 2016, the previously announced accessed regulations gave way to Health Canada's new Access to Cannabis for Medical Purposes Regulations (ACMPR).

Canadians are among the highest past-year users of cannabis globally; a series of national surveys have found past year use ranging from 10% to 14% (Health Canada, 2014). It is the most commonly used illicit substance in Canada, and the fourth most used substance after caffeine, alcohol, and tobacco. The prevalences of 12-month and lifetime cannabis use disorder are 2.5% and 6.3%. Only 13.2% with lifetime cannabis use disorder have participated in professional treatment or 12-step programs (Hasin et al., 2016).

Opioids

It has been established that Canada has the world's second-highest per capita levels of prescription **opioid** consumption globally, second in usage only to the United States. Canada's rate of use has sharply increased by 203% between 2000 and 2010 (International Narcotics Control Board, 2011). Opioid analgesics are widely diverted and improperly used, and their widespread use has resulted in a national epidemic of opioid overdose deaths and addictions. In Canada, the past-year prevalence of nonmedical prescription opioid use was 15.5% for students and 5.9% for adults (Fischer et al., 2013). Given its increasing and high consumption levels, it has been estimated that prescription opioids now constitute the third highest level of substance use burden of disease (after alcohol and tobacco) in Canada (Fischer & Argento, 2012).

Tobacco

The use of tobacco products remains the most important preventable cause of death and disease globally. With around 6 million lives lost annually, tobacco-related diseases claim more lives than do HIV, AIDS, malaria, and tuberculosis combined (WHO, 2015, p. 20). The deaths of 28% of males and 23% of females in Canada are attributable to the use of tobacco products (Manuel et al., 2016). Tobacco is a risk factor for six of the eight leading causes of mortality, and tobacco smoking remains the dominant risk factor for cancer in Canada (Krueger, Andres, Koot, & Reilly, 2016). With 18.4% of the population smoking daily or occasionally in the last year, with an average use of 13.9 cigarettes per day, tobacco continues to have the highest rates of addiction of any substance in Canada (Reid, Hammond, Rynard, & Burkhalter, 2015).

Societal Costs

Alcohol, tobacco, and other substances use exact a heavy toll on the health of individuals, their families, and communities. Taken together, substances are implicated in over 12% of mortality worldwide, and their use constitutes the leading cause of preventable death globally (WHO, 2009). In 2002, the costs incurred to Canadian society were estimated at nearly $40 billion when health care (e.g., hospitalization, treatment services), the workplace (e.g., employee assistance programs, toxicologic drug testing), transfer payments (e.g., social welfare, workers' compensation), crime and law enforcement (e.g., police, courts), and lost productivity (e.g., reduced output, sick time) were considered (Rehm et al., 2006).

■ AETIOLOGIC THEORIES

Addiction (used synonymously with the *DSM-5* designation of SUD) can be conceptualized as a disorder with a multifactorial pathogenesis and predisposing, precipitating, and modulating factors that encompass the body, the mind (psyche), and the spirit. It is further shaped and impacted by social, environmental, cultural, economic, and political influences in the development and expression of the disease, which may impact on conceptualizing and formulating safe and effective treatment. Addiction is not all-or-none but rather a matter of degree (West, 2006, p. 3). This disease typically develops, and comes to expression, in behavioural ways with varying degrees of embedded biologic, psychological, social, and spiritual aspects that cannot be explained in isolation or with any reductive theory. Environmental or conditioned cues—of which there may be tens of thousands that individuals associate with their substance use—also become a part of the addiction, and these are experienced within a complex environment where a range of dynamic factors likely influence the course of the disease.

Biologic Theories

When considering processes that increase the risk for addiction, the interplay between stressors in the environment and genes (the field of epigenetics) is a burgeoning field. Factors such as trauma, prenatal and postnatal stress, and adverse childhood experiences have the potential to change gene expression. These alternations may dysregulate the hypothalamic–pituitary axis (HPA), which may result in an increased sensitivity to stress. In turn, this may increase the risk of the individual in using substances to relieve this stress. At the same time, the use of substances can dysregulate the HPA, leading to a vicious cycle of worsening sensitivity to stress and substance use (Simkin, 2014).

There is large body of evidence examining the influence of addictive substances on the brain, including sophisticated brain imaging techniques that demonstrate structural and functional changes. The addicted brain has been demonstrated to be fundamentally different from the nonaddicted brain, and this is manifested by changes in gene expression, receptor availability, metabolic activity, and responsiveness to environmental cues (Volkow & Warren, 2014). These pervasive changes in brain function may persist on molecular, cellular, structural, and functional levels long after the individual stops consuming the substance. The demonstrated changes to brain structure and function form the foundation and evidence for addiction to be classified as a disease of the brain and a mental disorder.

The use of addictive substances has been found to increase extracellular levels of dopamine. The dopamine-related "high" (euphoria) becomes a reinforcement mechanism in the brain. The brain, in essence, remembers this pleasure and wants it repeated. But the neurochemical status in the brain readjusts to these increased levels of dopamine as being the "normal" neurochemical state; the individual then requires increased amounts of substances to produce the same dopamine-related effects (Volkow & Warren, 2014). Just as food is linked to daily survival, once the brain has become addicted to a substance, it attaches the same level of salience or significance to consuming the substance as it does to the level of life-sustaining functions or behaviours. The substance is no longer sought only for pleasure but for the need to relieve distress or withdrawal; on a subconscious level, it may be enjoyed at the same level of salience as life-sustaining elements of behaviour. Eventually, the drive to obtain and use the substance becomes one of the most important priorities despite adverse (and at times devastating) consequences.

Psychological Theories

The psychological theories refer to the relative contribution of psychological and psychiatric factors that reflect the individual's preferences, experiences, or problems. It is postulated that these factors influence the likelihood that addictive substances will be used initially or that the individual will develop an addiction. These theories suggest that some individuals are born with certain temperaments and subsequently develop particular personality traits, vulnerabilities, or even personality disorders that may make them more susceptible to addiction. From this theoretical perspective, addiction is considered a behavioural disorder occurring in a vulnerable phenotype, in which an intrinsic predisposed state determines the neuroplasticity that is induced (Swendsen & Le Moal, 2011).

Research increasingly focuses on the possibility that vulnerabilities acquired early in life may predispose individuals to psychiatric conditions (including addiction). Children of mothers who experience stress during pregnancy or children who have experienced disrupted maternal care during infancy and other early adverse experiences are considered important factors associated with substance initiation and addiction. It is postulated that the disrupted development and stress from such adverse childhood events (often defined by social and economic disadvantages) contribute to subsequent vulnerability to addiction (Swendsen & Le Moal, 2011).

There is a large body of literature demonstrating that SUDs are strongly associated with other mental disorders. Individuals with SUD often have mood, anxiety, or other psychiatric conditions. Self-medication, whereby substances are used (at least in part) as a means for reducing anxiety, depression, or other symptoms, is one explanation for this finding. The reverse causal association has also been proposed, whereby the use of substances may induce anxiety or other psychiatric conditions. By contrast, shared aetiologic models suggest that there may be specific factors that increase the risk of individuals developing more than one condition (Swendsen & Le Moal, 2011).

Social Theories

The WHO has determined that there are significant differences between some countries in their prevalence of alcohol, tobacco, and other substance addictions (WHO, 2009). These differences exist even between countries of similar income and geographic region. These findings may be attributable, in part, to differences in substance availability, legislation, and other health policies.

Culture is considered to be another factor influencing addiction prevalence rates. Migration studies have compared rates of addiction for homogeneous ethnic groups in the country of origin with those of the host country possessing a different culture. For example, studies of Mexican families migrating to the United States generally indicate lower rates of addiction in their country of origin than among corresponding groups in the United States (Grant et al., 2004). It has been hypothesized that the protective aspects of the country of origin may diminish over time and over generations, as a function of acculturation (Merikangas et al., 2009).

Spiritual Theories

Spirituality has a close relationship with the field of addiction treatment; individuals who have recovered from addiction often mention spiritual experiences or motivation as a major contributory factor in their recovery. Spirituality can be defined as the relationship between an individual and the sacred (numinous), perhaps represented by a transcendent higher being (or higher power) or force (or mind of the universe). This relationship is personal to the individual and does not require affiliation with any organized religion; religion is *not* necessary for an individual to develop his or her spirituality or, for that matter, to recover from addiction. Spirituality is an integral dimension of the Twelve Step tradition of Alcoholics Anonymous (AA). The 12 steps, formulated by William Wilson or "Bill W.," were derived from his experiences of living with alcohol addiction. These reference "a power greater than us," "God," "Higher Power," and "a spiritual experience" (refer to Box 26.1).

■ PREVENTION

Epidemiologic research has demonstrated that the onset of substance use typically begins during the adolescent years. Given this pattern, and the potential progression from experimental use to addiction, prevention initiatives often target children and adolescents. Knowledge-based programs in schools have *not* been shown to be effective, and those that target social competence and social influence have shown a *small* effect (Faggiano, Minozzi, Versino, & Buscemi, 2014). Effective interventions imbed school programs within a comprehensive approach that includes programs that teach parents and others ways to monitor their children and the skills to communicate with them effectively; community-based programs, such as mass media campaigns; and public policies, such as minimum purchasing age for tobacco (Griffin & Brown, 2014). Future research is needed to find ways to effectively disseminate the most promising prevention programs into our schools, families, and communities.

■ INTERDISCIPLINARY TREATMENT

The adaptation in the brain that results from chronic substance exposure is long lasting; therefore, addiction interventions must also reflect its chronic (and relapsing) nature. This model is similar to those for other chronic conditions (such as asthma, diabetes, and hypertension). Not surprisingly, the rates of recovery for addiction are comparable to those chronic conditions, and discontinuation of treatment is likely to result in similar rates of relapse (McLellan et al., 2000). As with other chronic diseases, effective addiction interventions require the involvement of multiple brain circuits

---

BOX 26.1 The Twelve Steps of Alcoholics Anonymous

1. We admitted we were powerless over alcohol—that our lives had become unmanageable
2. Came to believe that a Power greater than ourselves could restore us to sanity
3. Made a decision to turn our will and our lives over to the care of God *as we understood Him*
4. Made a searching and fearless moral inventory of ourselves
5. Admitted to God, to ourselves, and to another human being the exact nature of our wrongs
6. Were entirely ready to have God remove all these defects of character
7. Humbly asked Him to remove our shortcomings
8. Made a list of all persons we had harmed and became willing to make amends to them all
9. Made direct amends to such people wherever possible, except when to do so would injure them or others
10. Continued to take personal inventory and, when we were wrong, promptly admitted it
11. Sought through prayer and meditation to improve our conscious contact with God as we understood Him, praying only for knowledge of His will for us and the power to carry that out
12. Having had a spiritual awakening as a result of these steps, we tried to carry this message to alcoholics and to practise these principles in all our affairs

Source: The Twelve Steps are reprinted with permission of Alcoholics Anonymous World Services, Inc. (AAWS). Permission to reprint the Twelve Steps does not mean that the AAWS has reviewed or approved the contents of this publication or that the AAWS necessarily agrees with the views expressed herein. A.A. is a program of recovery from alcoholism *only*—use of the Twelve Steps in connection with programs and activities, which are patterned after A.A., but which address other problems, or in any other non-A.A. context, does not imply otherwise.

(reward, motivation, learning, inhibitory control, and executive function), and their associated disruption of behaviour indicates the need for a multimodal approach in its treatment. Within this paradigm, relapse is not interpreted as failure but rather as a temporary setback, and recovery is conceptualized as a "process" and not as an event.

To reflect treatment concepts and recommendations, the National Institute on Drug Abuse (NIDA) updated their seminal document *Principles of Drug Addiction Treatment* in 2012. These principles are intended to address addiction to alcohol, tobacco, and other drugs and are based on the existing body of scientific evidence. They provide a critical starting point for any discussion about the treatment of addiction (Box 26.2).

Goals of Addiction Treatment

Addiction treatment programs have as their goal not simply stabilizing the patient's condition but altering the course of the SRD as well as the patient's overall functioning. Safe and effective treatment for individuals with SRD requires the completion of screening, a comprehensive assessment, matching treatment to include the evidence-based modalities available for the particular disorder and comorbidities, monitoring of outcomes, and follow-up on a longitudinal basis. Treatment ought to be culturally sensitive and appropriate, taking into account the specific needs and preferences of the patient. Issues related to gender-related variables (e.g., lesbian, gay, queer or questioning, bisexual, two-spirited, asexual, and transgender individuals); pregnant women; ethnic minorities; age; and medical needs

are to be considered as well in the treatment provision. Box 26.3 outlines specific goals of addiction treatment.

The multimodal treatment of addiction typically involves a combination of psychosocial interventions as well as pharmacotherapy where (and if) available for a particular condition. A longitudinal approach for management of this chronic disease is ideal, and in general, the iterative approach to treatment is first to screen, engage, assess, motivate, and help to retain the patient in a safe and effective evidence-based treatment setting. Treatment retention and adherence to mutually agreed-upon goals generally maximize the potential benefits of treatment and improve outcomes.

Treatment further seeks to help educate patients, family members, caregivers, and significant others about addiction as a bona fide disease including its causes, consequences, longitudinal approaches to, and the options for, interdisciplinary treatment. In some cases and situations, **harm reduction** may be an interim step toward abstinence, and these philosophies are not considered to be mutually exclusive or incompatible. Understanding the complementary nature of these approaches is vital, and this may mean initially using harm reduction and thereby initially working toward reducing harm as a first step toward abstinence.

The **therapeutic alliance** (or the "helping alliance") between the nurse and the patient is a key ingredient for treatment success. This therapeutic alliance ideally builds a foundation of empathy, mutual respect, and trust; provides hope for recovery; and begins at the very first meeting with the patient. Nurses should aim to establish rapport and create a positive alliance with the

BOX 26.2 Principles of Addiction Treatment

1. Addiction is a complex but treatable disease that affects brain function and behaviour. Drugs of abuse alter the brain's structure and function, resulting in changes that persist long after drug use has ceased. This may explain why drug abusers are at risk for relapse even after long periods of abstinence and despite the potentially devastating consequences.

2. No single treatment is appropriate for everyone. Treatment varies depending on the type of drug and the characteristics of the patients. Matching treatment settings, interventions, and services to an individual's particular problems and needs is critical to his or her ultimate success in returning to productive functioning in the family, workplace, and society.

3. Treatment needs to be readily available. Because drug-addicted individuals may be uncertain about entering treatment, taking advantage of available services the moment people are ready for treatment is critical. Potential patients can be lost if treatment is not immediately available or readily accessible. As with other chronic diseases, the earlier treatment is offered in the disease process, the greater the likelihood of positive outcomes.

4. Effective treatment attends to multiple needs of the individual, not just his or her drug abuse. To be effective, treatment must address the individual's drug abuse and any associated medical, psychological, social, vocational, and legal problems. It is also important that treatment be appropriate to the individual's age, gender, ethnicity, and culture.

5. Remaining in treatment for an adequate period of time is critical. The appropriate duration for an individual depends on the type and degree of his or her problems and needs. Research indicates that most addicted individuals need at least 3 months in treatment to significantly reduce or stop their drug use and that the best outcomes occur with longer durations of treatment. Recovery from drug addiction is a long-term process and frequently requires multiple episodes of treatment. As with other chronic illnesses, relapses to drug abuse can occur and should signal a need for treatment to be reinstated or adjusted. Because individuals often leave treatment prematurely, programs should include strategies to engage and keep patients in treatment.

6. Behavioural therapies—including individual, family, or group counselling—are the most commonly used forms of drug abuse treatment. Behavioural therapies vary in their focus and may involve addressing a patient's motivation to change, providing incentives for abstinence, building skills to resist drug use, replacing drug-using activities with constructive and rewarding activities, improving problem-solving skills, and facilitating better interpersonal relationships. Also, participation in group therapy and other peer support programs during and following treatment can help maintain abstinence.

7. Medications are an important element of treatment for many patients, especially when combined with counselling and other behavioural therapies. For example, methadone, buprenorphine, and naltrexone (including a new long-acting formulation) are effective in helping individuals addicted to heroin or other opioids stabilize their lives and reduce their illicit drug use. Acamprosate, disulfiram, and naltrexone are medications approved for treating alcohol dependence. For persons addicted to nicotine, a nicotine replacement product (available as patches, gum, lozenges, or nasal spray) or an oral medication (such as bupropion or varenicline) can be an effective component of treatment when part of a comprehensive behavioural treatment program.

8. An individual's treatment and services plan must be assessed continually and modified as necessary, to ensure that it meets his or her changing needs. A patient may require varying combinations of services and treatment components during the course of treatment and recovery. In addition to counselling or psychotherapy, a patient may require medication, medical services, family therapy, parenting instruction, vocational rehabilitation, and/or social and legal services. For many patients, a continuing care approach provides the best results, with the treatment intensity varying according to a person's changing needs.

9. Many drug-addicted individuals also have other mental disorders. Because drug abuse and addiction—both of which are mental disorders—often co-occur with other mental illnesses, patients presenting with one condition should be assessed for the other(s), and when these problems co-occur, treatment should address both (or all), including the use of medications as appropriate.

10. Medically assisted detoxification is only the first stage of addiction treatment and by itself does little to change long-term drug abuse. Although medically assisted detoxification can safely manage the acute physical symptoms of withdrawal and, for some, can pave the way for effective long-term addiction treatment, detoxification alone is rarely sufficient to help addicted individuals achieve

BOX 26.2 Principles of Addiction Treatment (Continued)

long-term abstinence. Thus, patients should be encouraged to continue drug treatment following detoxification. Motivational enhancement and incentive strategies, begun at initial patient intake, can improve treatment engagement.

11. Treatment does not need to be voluntary to be effective. Sanctions or enticements from family, employment settings, and/or the criminal justice system can significantly increase treatment entry, retention rates, and the ultimate success of drug treatment interventions.

12. Drug use during treatment must be monitored continuously, as lapses during treatment do occur. Knowing their drug use is being monitored can be a powerful incentive for patients and can help them withstand urges to use drugs. Monitoring also provides an early indication of a return to drug use, signalling a possible need to adjust an individual's treatment plan to better meet his or her needs.

13. Treatment programs should assess patients for the presence of HIV/AIDS, hepatitis B and C, tuberculosis, and other infectious diseases as well as provide targeted risk reduction counselling, linking

patients to treatment if necessary. Typically, drug abuse treatment addresses some of the drug-related behaviours that put people at risk of infectious diseases. Targeted counselling specifically focused on reducing infectious disease risk can help patients further reduce or avoid substance-related and other high-risk behaviours. Counselling can also help those who are already infected to manage their illness. Moreover, engaging in substance abuse treatment can facilitate adherence to other medical treatments. Substance abuse treatment facilities should provide on-site, rapid HIV testing rather than referrals to off-site testing as research shows that doing so increases the likelihood that patients will be tested and receive their test results. Those providing treatment should also inform patients that highly active antiretroviral therapy (HAART) has proven effective in combating HIV, including among drug-abusing populations, and link them to HIV treatment if they test positive.

From the U.S. Government's National Institute on Drug Abuse. (Revised December 2012). Retrieved from http://www.drugabuse.gov/sites/default/files/podat_1.pdf

---

patient. This is the foundation for establishing the trusting relationship within which change can be negotiated. A healthy treatment relationship generally facilitates treatment, improves adherence with treatment, and ultimately improves outcomes.

In order to establish a therapeutic alliance, the nurse should aim to minimize or avoid premature and inappropriate confrontations, judgment, negative interactions,

BOX 26.3 Goals of Addiction Treatment

The *goals* of addiction treatment include the following:

- Treatment retention
- Reduction in severity and frequency of substance use episodes
- Reducing harm caused by substances, with the ultimate goal of total abstinence
- Management of comorbid psychiatric and medical conditions
- Improving the patient's quality of life
- Improving all areas of life affected by addiction (e.g., employment, interpersonal relationships, interface with the law/criminal justice system, physical health)
- Improving all levels of adaptive functioning
- Preventing relapse to substance use

advice without permission, and other approaches not congruent with motivation-based techniques. Some health professionals may experience an element of negative bias and stereotyping of people, perhaps stemming from their own particular background, psychodynamics, or their own losses or experiences with addiction. For the ethical professional, it is important to make the effort of processing any unresolved conflicts and losses in her/his own life and to successfully work through any related issues.

The evidence clearly suggests that a confrontational interpersonal style is generally not helpful for achieving goals in addiction treatment and can lead to the patient being more defensive, displaying increased levels of denial, decreased levels of treatment acceptance, and even disengagement in treatment. Among the most important and valuable skills and attitudes translating into treatment success for the patient are the nurse's appropriate empathy, boundary setting, confidence, instillation of hope, and the provision of support and encouragement.

Principles of Matching Treatment

As an overarching principle, treatment should be offered on the least restrictive level of care that is proven to be safe and likely to be effective. Patients are matched to the most appropriate level of care based on availability along with the assessment of their condition and comorbidities and with respect to the individuals' preferences. Refer to Box 26.4 for a description

BOX 26.4 Levels of Care for Adolescent and Adult Services

LEVEL 0.5: EARLY INTERVENTION

This level of service is for individuals who are at risk for developing substance-related problems or a service for those for whom there is not yet sufficient information to document a diagnosable substance use disorder.

LEVEL 1: OUTPATIENT SERVICES

This level of care typically consists of less than 9 hours of service/week for adults or less than 6 hours/week for adolescents for recovery or motivational enhancement therapies and strategies. This level encompasses organized services that can be delivered in a wide variety of settings.

LEVEL 2.1: INTENSIVE OUTPATIENT SERVICES

This level of care typically consists of 9 or more hours of service a week or 6 or more hours for adults and adolescents, respectively, to treat multidimensional instability. Level 2 encompasses services that are capable of meeting the complex needs of people with addiction and co-occurring conditions. It is an organized outpatient service that delivers treatment services during the day, before or after work or school, in the evening, and/or on weekends.

LEVEL 2.5: PARTIAL HOSPITALIZATION SERVICES

This level of care typically provides 20 or more hours of service a week for multidimensional instability that does not require 24-hour care. This level encompasses services that are capable of meeting the complex needs of people with addiction and co-occurring conditions. It is an organized outpatient service that delivers treatment services usually during the day as treatment or partial hospitalization services.

LEVEL 3.1: CLINICALLY MANAGED LOW-INTENSITY RESIDENTIAL SERVICES

This level of care typically provides a 24-hour living support and structure with available trained personnel and offers at least 5 hours of clinical service a week. It encompasses residential services that are described as co-occurring capable, co-occurring enhanced, and complexity-capable services, which are staffed by designated addition treatment, mental health, and general medical personnel who provide a range of services in a 24-hour living support setting.

LEVEL 3.3: CLINICALLY MANAGED POPULATION-SPECIFIC HIGH-INTENSITY RESIDENTIAL SERVICES

This adult-only level of care typically offers 24-hour care with trained counsellors to stabilize multidimensional imminent danger along with less intense milieu and group treatment for those with cognitive or other impairments unable to use full active milieu or therapeutic community. This level encompasses residential services that are described as co-occurring capable, co-occurring enhanced, and complexity-capable services, which are staffed by designated addiction treatment, mental health, and general medical personnel who provide a range of services in a 24-hour treatment setting.

LEVEL 3.5: CLINICALLY MANAGED MEDIUM-INTENSITY RESIDENTIAL SERVICES

For adolescents and adults, the purpose of this 24-hour care with trained counsellors to stabilize multidimensional imminent danger and prepare for outpatient treatment. Patients are able to tolerate and use full active milieu or therapeutic communities. This level encompasses residential services that are described as co-occurring capable, co-occurring enhanced, and complexity-capable services, which are staffed by designated addiction treatment, mental health, and general medical personnel who provide a range of services in a 24-hour setting.

LEVEL 3.7: CLINICALLY MANAGED MEDIUM-INTENSITY RESIDENTIAL SERVICES FOR ADOLESCENTS AND CLINICALLY MANAGED HIGH-INTENSITY RESIDENTIAL SERVICES FOR ADULTS

This level of care provides 24-hour care with trained counsellors to stabilize multidimensional imminent danger and prepare for outpatient treatment. Patients in this level are able to tolerate and use full active milieu or therapeutic communities. This level encompasses residential services that are describes as co-occurring capable, co-occurring enhanced, and complexity-capable services, which are staffed by designated addiction treatment, mental health, and general medical personnel who provide a range of services in a 24-hour treatment setting.

LEVEL 4: MEDICALLY MANAGED INTENSIVE INPATIENT TREATMENT

For adolescents and adults, this level of care offers 24-hour nursing care and daily physician care for severe, unstable problems in ASAM Dimensions 1, 2, or 3. Counselling is available to engage patients in treatment.

Source: American Society of Addiction Medicine. (2015). *What are the ASAM levels of care?* Retrieved from http://asamcontinuum.org/knowledgebase/what-are-the-asam-levels-of-care

of the levels of care that have been described by the American Society of Addiction Medicine (ASAM, 2015).

Screening, Brief Intervention, and Referral

It has been estimated that about one in five adults accessing primary care services reports problems related to substance use. Screening (*Ask*), brief intervention (*Advice and Assess*) and, when appropriate, referral (*Assist*), and follow-up (*Arrange*) are considered mainstays of early identification and intervention for substance-related and addictive disorders. However, the identification of SUD is often missed because of a lack of **screening**. A number of valid and reliable screening tools exist and are readily accessible. Screening for alcohol and drug use disorders, brief intervention, and referral for treatment are feasible and effective strategies in primary care settings provided that brief interventions and treatment facilities to which patients can be referred and treated promptly are available.

Screening is used to identify patients who are likely to have an SUD as determined by their responses to certain key questions. An example of a preliminary question about alcohol use is, "Do you sometimes drink beer, wine, or other alcoholic beverages?" If a positive response, screening would occur with options such as the CAGE (Ewing, 1984). If the screen is negative, this should be followed with individually tailored advice to maintain consumption below the "at-risk" drinking limits (Box 26.5). Concentration of alcohol in a standard drink can be found in Box 26.6. If the screen is positive, the patient may be advised to undergo more detailed diagnostic testing to confirm or rule out the disorder and/or to arrange for clinical follow-up. Only one single item has been validated in primary care settings to screen for drug use: "How many times in the past year have you used an illegal drug or used a prescription medication for nonmedical reasons?" Answering "one or more" represents a positive screen (Zgierska & Fleming, 2011).

Brief interventions can be defined as time-limited (i.e., 5 to 20 minutes), patient-centred counselling designed to reduce substance use. There is good evidence, for example, that patients who do not meet the diagnostic criteria for alcohol use disorders but are exceeding safe drinking limits can be supported and helped through brief intervention. Similarly, the *Canadian Best Practice Guidelines for Smoking Cessation* recommend that the assessment of tobacco use status should be updated for all patients by health providers on a regular basis (CAN-ADAPTT, 2011). The Canadian Nurses Association (2011) agrees that all nurses ought to be involved in tobacco cessation through assessing and documenting all forms of tobacco use, willingness to quit, and risk of exposure to second-hand smoke.

BOX 26.5 Canada's Low-Risk Alcohol Drinking Guidelines

Reduction of long-term health risks can be achieved by drinking no more than:

- 10 drinks a week for women, with no more than 2 drinks a day most days
- 15 drinks a week for men, with no more than 3 drinks a day most days.

Drinking is not advised when:

- Driving a vehicle or using machinery and tools
- Pregnant or planning to get pregnant
- Taking medicine or other drugs that interact with alcohol
- Doing any kind of dangerous physical activity
- Responsible for the safety of others (including work)
- Living with mental or physical health problems
- Making important decisions

Source: Butt, P., Beirness, D., Gliksman, L., Paradias, C., & Stockwell, T. (2011). *Alcohol and health in Canada: A summary of evidence and guidelines for low risk drinking.* Ottawa, ON: Canadian Centre of Substance Use.

Screening must also include identifying women who are pregnant or considering pregnancy and providing advice on abstention from substance use. Alcohol, tobacco, and other substances can have harmful effects on the foetus and can be responsible for lifelong consequences such as foetal alcohol spectrum disorder (FASD). Substances are transmitted into breast milk, and the nursing mother can expose the breast-fed baby to harmful chemicals, with a range of adverse outcomes and risks. It is important for nurses to note that due to stigma and fear, many women may underreport their consumption of alcohol (Zgierska & Fleming, 2011).

BOX 26.6 Conversion into a Standard Drink

Alcohol consumption is measured in terms of the numbers of "standard drink," each of which contains 13.6 g of alcohol. Different beverages contain different concentrations, and conversion into a "standard drink" is described as the following:

- 43 mL (1.5 oz) spirit (40% alcohol)
- 142 mL (5 oz) table wine (12% alcohol)
- 341 mL (12 oz) regular beer (5% alcohol)
- 85 mL (3 oz) fortified wine (18% alcohol)

Screening and brief interventions are promising interventions, but further evidence is required regarding their use.

Multidimensional Assessment

Assessment serves as an early mechanism to engage, motivate, and retain the patient in treatment, and to assess for any imminent risk of harm. It further aims to guide ongoing management while allowing for the measurement of progress and outcomes. This assessment process aims to gather information from many different sources that are relevant to the life of the patient affected by SUD. Such assessment involves evaluation of the following domains:

A comprehensive *substance use* assessment, including

- Onset of use or change of pattern of use
- Quantity per day or per week
- Frequency of use and periods of abstinence
- Route of use (e.g., injection, smoke, snort, oral ingestion)
- Prior treatment received (e.g., 12 steps, residential care)
- Sources of substances (e.g., black market, double doctoring, borrowing others' medication)

A comprehensive *psychiatric assessment*, including

- Obtaining a family and social history
- Details of any emotional and behavioural condition, or complications (psychiatric, emotional, behavioural status, including any potential for imminent and substantial risk of harm to self or to others; e.g., risk of suicide or risk of aggression, including homicide)

A comprehensive *physical assessment*, including

- Screening for infectious diseases (e.g., HIV, STDs, TB, hepatitis)
- The assessment of biomedical conditions and complications associated with substance use
- Focus on the risk for acute intoxication and/or withdrawal potential in the patient
- Laboratory testing (e.g., liver function testing)

Collateral information from others (with necessary consent):

- Assessment of the patient's level of *treatment acceptance* and elements of resistance, including
- Assessment of risk for relapse (relapse potential) and recovery environment
- The use of structured rating scales to help quantify clinical features and provide baseline for serial monitoring of progress

Management of Intoxication and Withdrawal

Intoxication is the result of being under the influence of, and responding to, the acute effects of alcohol and/or other substances of abuse. In the clinical setting, it is important to determine the substance(s) involved, the quantity of the ingested substance(s), and the patient's level of consciousness. Life-threatening intoxication is of immediate concern, and the first priority is for supportive care. Symptoms of intoxication and withdrawal specific to each class of substances are identified in the *DSM-5*.

In general, the signs and symptoms of withdrawal are the opposite of a substance's direct pharmacologic effects. **Detoxification** is a process by which, under care of a health provider, individuals are systematically withdrawn from addictive substances in either an inpatient or outpatient setting. The goal of detoxification is to provide withdrawal from substance use in a way that is compassionate and protects the patient's dignity and to prepare the patient for ongoing treatment of his or her SUD. It is important to recognize that detoxification is not the treatment of the SUD. Rather, it is only the management of withdrawal symptoms.

Harm Reduction

Countless examples of harm reduction exist, with varying levels of evidence to support its benefits and the most appropriate application in the context of SRD. Harm reduction is a pragmatic community health intervention designed to reduce the consequences of substance use to the individual, the family, and society and differs from moral or criminal approaches to substance abuse and addiction. The purpose of harm reduction is to *reduce the risk* for harm adverse consequences arising from substance use, and this approach works with the individual regardless of his or her commitment SUD. Harm reduction forms a part of the continuum of care and should not be viewed as exclusive of an overarching goal of abstinence. Fischer (2005, p. 13) suggests five general principles of harm reduction:

- Harm reduction focuses on the consequences of substance use, not on the use itself, requiring decisions about which harms to be targeted and in what order based on what is known about patient's welfare, public health, and the severity of the problem.
- Harm reduction focuses on the pragmatic and effective minimization of use-related harms.
- Meaningful and realistic efforts must be made to actively understand and consider the social and environmental context in which substance use occurs.

- Education, knowledge, and informed decision-making by substance users and potential users are key pillars of harm reduction.
- Misinformed or ineffective interventions or policy can be considered sources of substance-related harms and must also be targeted for harm reduction interventions.

As examples, interventions for alcohol-related harm reduction include education about the safe use of alcohol, provision of food at bars to reduce the incidence of rapid intoxication, and encouragement of the use of a "designated driver." (Box 26.7 addresses impaired driving.) Some examples of interventions for illicit drug-related hard reduction include naloxone distribution, supervised consumption sites, and needle exchange

---

BOX 2.7 Impaired Driving

Operating a motor vehicle while impaired by alcohol, cannabis, or other substance is the largest cause of criminal death and one of the leading criminal causes of injury in Canada. The level of impairment resulting from the use of *alcohol* is determined by measuring breath or blood alcohol levels (BALs), and the level at which a person is considered to be legally impaired varies with jurisdiction. Under the Criminal Code of Canada, the operator of a vehicle could be charged for driving with a BAL over 0.08%. Some provinces have passed legislation allowing for progressive administrative penalties for drivers with lower BALs (i.e., between 0.03% and 0.08%). These penalties do not include criminal charges; rather, they may include vehicle seizure, licence suspension, and fines.

The standard to determine impairment by *cannabis* has not yet been established. The presence of THC, the major psychoactive component in the plant, can be detected by roadside saliva testing. The level of THC must be measured through a blood test. Determining the level of THC by which someone is impaired by cannabis is complex. The individual's tolerance to THC can affect the degree of impairment. Furthermore, as it dissipates rapidly, the THC level may have dropped by the time the blood is collected from the suspected driver. In addition, frequent users can exhibit persistent levels long after use, while THC levels can decline more rapidly among occasional users. Resolving this issue is a pressing problem given the increased use of cannabis for medical treatment and recreation.

BOX 26.8 Supervised Consumption Facilities

Injection drug use (IDU) is when one or more psychoactive substance is injected directly into the body using a hypodermic needle and syringe for nonmedical reasons. As this is an illegal activity, and many do not have a stable address, accurate data on the prevalence and profile of IDU are difficult to obtain.

IDU places the individual at high risk for contracting blood-borne infections (e.g., HIV, hepatitis C) through the sharing of contaminated needles or injection equipment. Serious health complications may also arise such as overdoses, adverse drug reactions, and abscesses.

In this context of risk, the supervised injection facility "Insite" was implemented by the local health authority in Vancouver's Downtown Eastside in 2003. A comprehensive evaluation program has demonstrated largely positive outcomes in the facility's target population, including reduced injection risk behaviours, overdose rates and public disorder, and increased treatment service utilization.

Source: Vancouver Coastal Health Authority. (n.d.). Retrieved from http://www.vch.ca/your-health/health-topics/supervised-injection

---

programs. (Box 26.8 discusses supervised injection facilities.)

Psychosocial Interventions

Effective psychosocial treatment exists for the addictive disorders and includes **motivational interviewing** (MI); cognitive–behavioural therapy (CBT); other behavioural therapies (contingency management, community reinforcement, cue exposure and relaxation training, and aversion therapy); self-help groups and 12-step facilitation; relapse prevention; psychodynamic and interpersonal therapy; group therapy and family therapy; brief therapies; self-guided therapies; and hypnotherapy. The more common interventions are discussed in the following narrative.

Motivational Interviewing

Motivational interviewing (MI) is a directive, patient-centred style of counselling that helps patients to explore and resolve their **ambivalence** (the presence of both positive and negative feelings) about changing (Miller & Rollnick, 2002). Although it has wide application in practice for behavioural change, MI enjoys substantive uptake within the field of addiction. Some of the techniques in MI involve listening reflectively, eliciting motivational statements, and examining ambivalence. Those using this form of counselling avoid nontherapeutic responses such as directing and giving advice without patient permission, threatening with consequences, being coercive, and inappropriately raising concern without permission because these place the patient in an unhelpful, passive role. This model allows for the process of change to be viewed along a continuum where concrete steps can be taken to help individuals increase readiness for changing behaviour (see Chapter 6 for further discussion of MI).

Cognitive–Behavioural Therapy

Cognitive approaches to addiction hypothesize that if an individual can change the way he or she thinks about a situation, both the emotional reaction to it and the behavioural response will change. Psychoeducational materials, groups, and one-on-one interactions with nurses also impart information to reduce knowledge deficits related to alcohol, tobacco, and other substance dependence. For additional discussion on CBT, refer to Chapter 13.

Twelve-Step Programs

Twelve-step programs emphasize the conceptualization of addiction as an incurable, progressive disease that has spiritual, cognitive, and behavioural components. AA was the first 12-step self-help group and has become a worldwide fellowship of people with problems (current or past) related to alcohol, which provides support, individually and at meetings, to others who seek help. The only criterion for entry into AA is the "desire to quit drinking." Many treatment programs discuss concepts from AA, hold meetings at treatment facilities, and encourage patients to attend community meetings when appropriate. They also encourage continuing use of AA and other self-help groups as part of an ongoing plan for continued abstinence.

Twelve-step programs firmly endorse the need for abstinence and are considered by followers as lifelong programs of recovery with success attained one day at a time. The importance of recognizing and relying on a "higher power," or a power greater than the individual, is a central element of these programs. Members of 12-step groups can attend meetings on a self-determined or prescribed schedule that, if necessary, may be every day or even twice a day. Periods associated with high risk of relapse (e.g., holidays, weekends, family functions) are considered particularly appropriate times for attending meetings. A sponsor who is compatible with the patient can be particularly supportive and offer guidance through the recovery process, particularly during periods of high stress or increased craving.

The benefits from 12-step groups occur through the interplay of social interactions, prescribed behaviours, and mobilized psychological process. Meeting attendance, engagement in the program, and being a sponsor have been found to be supportive elements for abstinence. The evidence is mixed about the relative importance of spiritual/religious changes for explaining increased abstinence (Cavacuiti, Vasic, McCrady, & Tonigan, 2011). Inclusion in 12-step groups is considered a routine part of addiction treatment in most settings. However, an individual's refusal to participate in a self-help group is nonsynonymous with his or her resistance to treatment in general. Self-help groups are not beneficial for all people, and some persons may not embrace the spiritual dimension of the program. Alternative programs for sobriety, although not as widely available, have been developed to address this problem, such as Women for Sobriety and Secular Organizations for Sobriety. There are now more than 60 different 12-step fellowships available worldwide, including Alcoholic Anonymous, Cocaine Anonymous, Narcotics Anonymous, Dual Recovery Anonymous, among others.

Group Therapy

An integral and valuable component of the treatment regimen for many with an SUD is group therapy, and advantages of this approach include the following:

- The presence of others with an addiction may provide comfort.
- Other group members who are further along in their recovery may act as role models.
- Group members may offer a wide menu of coping strategies.
- The public nature of group settings can act as a deterrent for relapse. It has been noted that individuals recovering from SUDs may be highly skilled at detecting each other's concealed substance use or early relapse.

The efficacy of group therapy is similar to individual therapy, and it can be a successful component of a combined treatment program. For more detailed information about group therapy, refer to Chapter 14.

Family Therapy

Long-term family therapy is often beneficial following the initial stages of detoxification and stabilization. Families can often unwittingly enable addiction by, for instance, continuing to supply money to the individual, allowing adult children to live at home while continuing their substance use, and "bailing out" (rescuing) individuals from legal and other difficulties that result from substance use. Family therapy can bring these behaviours to light and assist family members to adopt alternative, more helpful ways of support. More detailed information is available in Chapter 15.

Pharmacotherapy

Pharmacotherapy, when available and appropriate, is routinely combined with psychosocial treatment and is not recommended for use in isolation from psychosocial interventions. Medications for SRD are generally utilized to treat intoxication and withdrawal, to reduce the reinforcing effects of drugs, to prevent relapse, and to treat comorbid medical or psychiatric conditions. For most of the SRDs, there is insufficient evidence for the use of pharmacotherapy. However, for the disorders related to alcohol, opioids, and tobacco, the empirical evidence supports the use of pharmacotherapy, and these will be specifically addressed by substance in the following section on nursing interventions for specific SRDs.

Relapse Prevention

Recovery from SUD can, for some, be defined as a long-term and ongoing process rather than a singular event. Ten interventions have been identified for the purposes of reducing relapse risk (Douaihy, Daley, Marlatt, & Spotts, 2011). These include helping patients to

- Understand relapse as a possible part of the recovery process and to learn how to identify warning signs
- Identify their own high-risk situations for relapse and develop effective cognitive and behavioural coping
- Enhance their communication skills and interpersonal relationships and to develop a recovery social network
- Reduce, identify, and manage negative emotional states (i.e., the acronym **HALT** warns not to become too Hungry, too Angry, too Lonely, or too Tired)
- Identify and manage cravings and any cues that may precede cravings
- Identify and challenge cognitive distortions
- Work toward a more balanced lifestyle
- Consider the use of medications in combination with psychosocial treatments
- Facilitate the transition between the levels of care between residential or hospital-based treatment programs and structured partial hospital or intensive outpatients programs
- Incorporate strategies to improve adherence to treatment and medications

Toxicology Testing/Drug Screening

Toxicology testing/drug screening can be a critical tool in the multimodal approach to addiction treatment. These tests can detect the presence of a substance (or its metabolite) in the body for a specified window period. These may be done to contribute to the confirmation of a diagnosis of SUD, to support recovery through frequent, random testing, and (more increasingly) are used in the workplace (i.e., pre-employment, periodic, or postaccident testing). The most commonly used matrices for drug testing are urine and serum, but other body fluids may be utilized under certain circumstances. Specific protocols (e.g., chain of custody) are followed to ensure

integrity of the specimens, and a medical review officer typically interprets results. With the exception of alcohol, the level of the substance detectable does not provide any reliable indication of the amount used or the level of impairment at the time of use or the time of testing. Drug testing does not have the technologic sophistication to distinguish between recreational use, drug abuse, drug misuse, accidental exposure, or addiction.

NURSING INTERVENTIONS FOR SPECIFIC SUBSTANCE-RELATED DISORDERS

There is no standardized intervention that will work for all individuals with an SRD because they may differ greatly with respect to severity, substance of abuse, and their own unique biologic, psychological, social, and spiritual considerations. Often, several approaches can work together; others may be deemed inappropriate. Treatment programs usually combine psychosocial interventions with other approaches to provide a comprehensive plan based on the individual's needs. Nursing interventions vary depending on the nature of the current problems, the status and severity of the illness, and the individual's situation. For an individual who is being detoxified, physical interventions (e.g., monitoring vital signs and neurologic functioning) are necessary. When the SUD is secondary to other physical or psychiatric problems, it may be a priority to address these concurrently rather than sequentially.

The following section is organized by the classes of substances and addresses some of their unique features. Greater level of detail has been provided to the substances most frequently abused in Canadian society: alcohol, cannabis, caffeine, opioids, and tobacco. These are the ones nurses are more likely to encounter in everyday practice including mental health and other settings (i.e., community health, hospital, and primary care).

Alcohol-Related Disorders

The effects of alcohol are dependent on a multitude of physiologic factors that include, among many others, dose, genetic factors, the level of tolerance, gender, body mass, body fat, liver mass, and metabolic rate. The acute effects of alcohol are usually characterized by feelings of warmth, relaxation, mild sedation, and a sense of social disinhibition. In alcohol-naïve individuals, a blood alcohol concentration of 160 mg% is associated with obvious intoxication symptoms and signs, which may not be evident in persons who have developed tolerance on physiologic or behavioural levels. In progressively higher concentrations, there is a greater depressant effect on inhibition and behavioural control, producing heightened emotions, emotional lability (or mood swings), impulsivity, and impaired motor and cognitive functioning (including impairment in memory, concentration, attention span, and judgment).

In increasingly higher concentrations, it also leads to more severe impairment of motor functions and speech, blackouts, confusion, delirium, respiratory failure, stupor, coma (at about 400 to 560 mg%), and death. Although sedating, alcohol impairs the quality of sleep by disturbing the normal sleep architecture.

Alcohol use is associated with worsening of certain psychiatric conditions and their symptoms, may increase the risk of depression, and may increase the risk of harm to self or others. Alcohol induces the liver enzyme system, which in turn leads to more rapid metabolism of therapeutic (and other) compounds, with an anticipated potential for lower therapeutic effects. Excessive or long-term use of alcohol can adversely affect any or all body systems, some of which could be serious, disabling, and irreversible even if alcohol use is discontinued. These include varying degrees of cognitive impairment, amnestic disorder, dementia, and other neurologic complications (e.g., neuropathies, cerebellar degeneration, and brain atrophy). In the category of alcohol-induced cognitive disorders, there are the conditions of Wernicke's syndrome and Korsakoff's syndrome. The former develops as a result of thiamine deficiency and manifests with oculomotor dysfunction, ataxia, and confusion, while the latter is characterized by retrograde and anterograde amnesia with confabulation (fabricated, distorted, or misinterpreted memories without any intention to deceive) as a key feature.

Alcohol Withdrawal

Reduction of consumption, or abstinence, may lead to withdrawal symptoms from alcohol that may even progress into life-threatening complications. Symptoms of withdrawal typically start hours after the last consumption of alcohol and may include nausea and vomiting, tactile disturbances, tremor, auditory disturbances, paroxysmal sweats, visual disturbances, anxiety, headaches (or sensations of fullness in the head), agitation, and disturbances in orientation and clouding of the sensorium. It may also include autonomic disturbances, for example, blood pressure increases, tachycardia, and diaphoresis, and in severe cases, withdrawal may progress to seizures (tonic–clonic), delirium (**delirium tremens**), or death. (Box 26.9 discusses the clinical features of withdrawal.)

Alcohol detoxification treatment consists of achieving safe withdrawal from alcohol followed by psychosocial interventions and the option of pharmacotherapy. Management of intoxication and withdrawal requires a safe environment, and hospitalization may be indicated if there is a history of seizures, delirium, or comorbid medical or psychiatric conditions. The level of withdrawal is used to determine the most appropriate dose of pharmacotherapy-assisted symptom-triggered detoxification management and is measured by conducting a brief rating scale, the Clinical Institute Withdrawal Assessment

---

BOX 26.9 Clinical Features of Alcohol Withdrawal

Minor Withdrawal: Patients are anxious and may experience nausea and vomiting, coarse tremor, sweating, tachycardia, and hypertension. Symptoms typically appear 6 to 12 hours after the last drink, or shortly after the BAL reaches 0, and are usually resolved within 48 to 72 hours.

Intermediate Withdrawal: Patients experience the symptoms of minor withdrawal in addition to seizures, dysrhythmias, and/or hallucinosis. Within 12 to 72 hours after cessation of drinking, grand mal and nonfocal seizures typically occur. Dysrhythmias range in severity from occasional ectopic beats to atrial fibrillation and supraventricular or ventricular tachycardia. Patients are aware of the unreal nature of their auditory or visual hallucinations and remain oriented and alert.

Major Withdrawal (Delirium Tremens): Patients experience severe agitation, gross tremulousness, marked psychomotor and autonomic hyperactivity, global confusion, disorientation, and auditory, visual, or tactile hallucinations. They tend to occur 5 or 6 days after severe, untreated withdrawal. Symptoms fluctuate and are often more severe at night. These may include severe diaphoresis and vomiting, tachycardia, hypertension, and fever. Sudden death can occur.

Source: Brands, B., Kahan, M., Selby, P., & Wilson, L. (2000). *Medical management of alcohol and drug-related problems: A physician's manual* (2nd ed.). Toronto, ON: Centre for Addiction and Mental Health.

---

for Alcohol (CIWA-R found in Appendix F). Medication (e.g., benzodiazepines) administered early in the course of withdrawal (and in sufficient dosages) can prevent the development of delirium tremens. The nursing care plan in this chapter provides an example of patient at risk for symptoms of alcohol withdrawal and medication management (please see Nursing Care Plan 26.1).

Poor nutrition and vitamin deficiencies are often symptoms of alcohol addiction. Thiamine (vitamin B_1) may be needed when a patient is in withdrawal to decrease ataxia (loss of control of body movements) and other symptoms of deficiency. It is usually given orally, 100 mg four times daily, but can be given intramuscularly or by intravenous infusion with glucose. Folic acid deficiency is corrected with administration of 1 mg orally, four times daily. The use of benzodiazepines, multivitamins, and thiamine, as well as fluid balance should be monitored, and supportive treatment provided.

NURSING CARE PLAN 26.1

PATIENT WITH ALCOHOL USE DISORDER

Kenneth W. is a 55-year-old lawyer with a 25-year history of alcohol use disorder. He is the youngest of three children born and raised on a farm. His mother is still living with his older sister, but his father died of cirrhosis, a complication of years of alcohol use. Kenneth is married and has two children who he rarely sees. Kenneth started binge drinking on weekends when he was in university, and this developed into a regular pattern once he started his law practice. His drinking has escalated after he started having difficulties with his partners at work, and he reports consuming up to 2 L of vodka a day. He began smoking in his early teens and continues to smoke a pack a day of cigarettes.

Recently, Kenneth was involved in a car accident and has been charged with operating a vehicle with a BAC over 0.08%. He was admitted to the hospital through the emergency department following the collision, with a gash above his right eye. Kenneth began to have symptoms of alcohol withdrawal and became anxious shortly after admission. He requested hospital admission for alcohol detoxification and was transferred to a detoxification and brief treatment unit.

Setting: Inpatient Detoxification Unit, Psychiatric Hospital

Baseline Assessment: First admission, last drink and cigarette at 7 PM. Admission vital signs: T 37.3°C, HR 98, R 20, and BP 140/88 on admission to the ER. He has a history of withdrawal seizures and hallucinations (likely delirium tremens during past withdrawal). He had a BAL of 0.15 mg%, becoming increasingly anxious and restless over the next hour. His CIWA score was 17, and he was given diazepam, 20 mg PO, as ordered, at that time. Decision to conduct CIWA 4-hourly.

Five hours after admission, vital signs were T 37.8°C, HR 110, R 22, and BP 152/100. He continued to be anxious and was tremulous, diaphoretic, and nauseous. CIWA score had increased to 22, and diazepam 20 mg PO stat was given. The decision was made to conduct CIWA scores hourly. The next CIWA score was 15, and 4 hours later, it was 10.

Associated Psychiatric Diagnosis	Medications
Alcohol use disorder (severe)	Deferred until detoxification is complete, after which consideration will be given to acamprosate, naltrexone, or disulfiram.
Alcohol withdrawal	Thiamine Folic acid Multivitamins Diazepam, 20 mg stat, followed by CIWA score, based on elevated BP, HR, and tremors Haloperidol, 5.0 mg IM PRN, for hallucinations or agitation
Tobacco withdrawal	Transdermal nicotine patch 21 mg QD PRN Nicotine inhaler 10 mg, puff on cartridge for 45 minutes, as directed PRN
Tobacco use disorder	Deferred, but continuation of nicotine replacement is offered post detoxification

Nursing Diagnosis 1: Risk Related to Alcohol Withdrawal

Defining Characteristics	Related Factors
Altered vital signs Altered cerebral function secondary to alcohol withdrawal Altered mood states	Withdrawal is common among patients consuming more than 40 drinks per week or in those with other risk factors. Symptoms of detoxification include fever, high blood pressure, tachycardia, tremor or sweating, confusion, and dehydration. Level of consciousness, orientation, perceptual disturbances (hallucinations or illusions), mood, and thought processes including suicide ideation and cognitive deficits

(Continued)

NURSING CARE PLAN 26.1 *(Continued)*

Outcomes

Initial	Discharge
1. Detoxification from alcohol will be monitored, based on CIWA score, and management implemented to treat symptoms and to prevent complications.	2. Bridging from inpatient from level IV care for detoxification to a regimen that is acceptable to KW and keeps him engaged in ongoing treatment

Interventions

Interventions	Rationale	Ongoing Assessment
Welcome to treatment and assure Kenneth that he is in a safe place. Inform of what he may expect during withdrawal. Start with engagement for treatment.	Begin to establish relationship, a therapeutic alliance, with the patient.	See Box 26.10.
Monitor vital signs, orientation, and identify stage of alcohol withdrawal and severity of symptoms.	The more severe the reactions, the more likely that anxiety, disorientation, confusion, and restlessness increase.	Administer (symptom triggered, CIWA) diazepam (for elevated BP, HR, and tremors) and haloperidol (for hallucinations or tremors) prn and report symptoms.
Institute seizure precautions (bed in low position, padded side rails).	Withdrawal seizures usually occur within 48 hours after last drink.	Monitor for seizure activity.
Orient the patient to surroundings and call light, and maintain consistent physical environment.	Disorientation often occurs as BAL drops. These symptoms can last several days.	Determine Kenneth's level of orientation to surroundings and whether he can use call light.
Avoid sudden moves, loud noises, discussion of the patient at bedside, and lighting that casts shadows downward.	Decreased environmental stimulation helps calm the patient, which in turn promotes optimal CNS responses.	Observe reactions to loud noises and monitor room environment.

Evaluation

Outcomes (at 3 days)	Revised Outcomes	Interventions
Orientated, hydrated, and no seizure activity	Engage in the development of a recovery plan.	Continue to monitor for any signs of disorientation.

Nursing Diagnosis 2: Discomfort Related to Tobacco Withdrawal

Defining Characteristics	Related Factors
Symptoms of tobacco withdrawal include irritability, restlessness, anxiety, insomnia, and fatigue.	Discomfort related to tobacco withdrawal may be difficult to distinguish from alcohol withdrawal.

Outcomes

Initial	Discharge
1. Will be comfortable without smoking during hospitalization period	2. Will be provided additional resources and supports to extend tobacco abstinence into a cessation attempt, if desired

NURSING CARE PLAN 26.1 *(Continued)*

Interventions

Intervention	Rationale	Ongoing Assessment
Explain that the hospital has a nonsmoking policy. This is to protect patients, visitors, and staff from the harmful effects of second-hand smoke. The purpose of the policy is not to "force" Kenneth to quit smoking or to "make his life difficult."	There are direct causes and linkages between exposure to second-hand smoke and serious health effects among nonsmokers.	Monitor Kenneth's level of comfort and assess for breakthrough cravings. Assess for sleep disruption; if present, may remove patch at bedtime.
Discuss prevention of discomfort related to tobacco withdrawal. Assess whether Kenneth's wife is a current smoker and the influence this may have on his ability to abstain.	The blood level of nicotine begins to drop immediately following smoking a cigarette. Smell off of clothing, and cigarette products, may provide potent cues to smoke.	
Offer a 21-mg transdermal nicotine patch qd to prevent tobacco withdrawal. This can be combined with other forms of NRT.	The higher dose 21-mg nicotine patch recommended for pack-per-day smoker; may not be of sufficient dosage to prevent breakthrough cravings. Side effects may include sleep disruption.	

Evaluation

Outcomes (Day 2)	Revised Outcomes	Interventions
Refused nicotine patch and becomes increasingly anxious to leave the unit to smoke.	Remain abstinent and engaged in the treatment regimen on the unit.	Offer prn nicotine inhaler to provide some immediate relief, and reoffer nicotine patch for longer-term effects.

Alcohol Use Disorder

The goal of treatment depends on the nature, extent, and severity of the alcohol use disorder. Coexisting conditions are also important determinants of the therapeutic approach and methods used. The best way to match the type and intensity of treatment to the individual needs of the patient remains unclear as no superior systematic outcomes have been demonstrated for residential or intensive day program treatment compared with once- or twice-weekly outpatient treatment (Willembring, 2011). Psychosocial interventions, as described earlier, should be offered at all stages of treatment in combination with pharmacotherapy and at the appropriate level of care. The suggestion to include attendance at AA is routinely offered. The outcome monitoring for alcohol use disorder treatment includes reporting on sobriety and abstinence. Serial monitoring of liver function tests, ethyl glucuronide, ethyl sulfate, carbohydrate-deficient transferrin, and early detection of alcohol consumption (EDAC) testing can provide valuable information on the course of the condition, success of treatment, and supplement the self-reported abstinence and sobriety.

Following detoxification (when necessary), there are several medication options to support the treatment of alcohol addiction. These include the following:

- *Disulfiram* is a medication that blocks the effects of aldehyde dehydrogenase and leads to a severely unpleasant reaction (including flushing, nausea, vomiting, and diarrhoea) when the person consumes alcohol. It is suitable only for reliable and motivated patients. This is an adjunct therapy that deters drinking while the individual learns new coping skills and alters abuse behaviours through other treatment approaches. Disulfiram's potential adverse effects include hepatotoxicity and neuropathy, which, along with potentially severe interactions with alcohol, limit its widespread use.
- *Naltrexone*, originally used as a treatment for opioid-related disorders, targets alcohol's effects on the brain and requires relatively normal liver functions. The use of this opioid antagonist medication cannot be in conjunction with any opioid medication as it will trigger an opioid withdrawal syndrome. It is further contraindicated in pregnancy and suicidal patients. Naltrexone may be particularly useful in

patients who continue to drink heavily. Targeted use of naltrexone also may be effective for decreasing alcohol consumption levels among problem drinkers who do not suffer from addiction.

- *Acamprosate* has the ability to curb cravings for alcohol and may be an effective adjunct treatment in motivated persons who are also receiving psychosocial interventions.
- *Topiramate*, not yet approved for this use, may represent a useful first-line treatment option for the management of AUD. It has been shown to have a greater beneficial effect in patients with a typology of craving characterized by drinking obsessions and automaticity of drinking (Guglielmo et al., 2015).

Caffeine-Related Disorders

Caffeine is a mild CNS stimulant that is found in many drinks (e.g., coffee, tea, cocoa, soft drinks, and energy drinks), chocolate, and in many over-the-counter medications (e.g., analgesics, stimulants, appetite suppressants, and cold relief preparations). A typical cup of brewed coffee contains 100 mg caffeine, but the content may vary greatly depending on the type of product or beverage.

Caffeine is not associated with any life-threatening illnesses, and typical daily dietary doses can be consumed under many circumstances. Caffeine has valuable therapeutic effects; it curbs fatigue and increases mental acuity, exerts stimulating effects on both mental and motor performance, and is subjectively viewed as beneficial by some in alleviating mood. It may, however, cause or exacerbate tremors; impair motor performance; and lead to anxiety, dysphoria, and insomnia. Higher doses increase the heart rate; stimulate respiratory, vasomotor, and vagal centres and cardiac muscles, resulting in increased heart contractibility; dilate pulmonary and coronary blood vessels; and constrict blood flow to the cerebral vascular system. The pervasive use of caffeine, and its integration into daily customs and routines, makes the recognition and treatment of caffeine-associated problems challenging.

Caffeine Intoxication

Symptoms of caffeine intoxication include restlessness, nervousness, excitement, insomnia, flushed face, diuresis, and gastrointestinal complaints. Symptoms that generally appear at levels of more than 1 g per day include muscle twitching, rambling flow of thought and speech, tachycardia or cardiac arrhythmia, periods of inexhaustibility, and psychomotor agitation (APA, 2013). The symptoms usually remit within the first day or so and do not have any known long-lasting consequences. Caffeine intoxication has been observed among young individuals after consumption of highly caffeinated products, including energy drinks. Individuals who have consumed very high doses of caffeine may require immediate medical attention as such doses may be lethal (APA, 2013).

Caffeine Withdrawal

When used in high doses over the course of time, caffeine can be associated with unpleasant withdrawal symptoms when abruptly tapered or discontinued. Withdrawal symptoms may include headache, insomnia, abnormal dreams, drowsiness, fatigue, impaired psychomotor performance, difficulty concentrating, craving, yawning, and nausea. Preferentially, caffeine should be reduced gradually in those considered to be consuming in excess, and this may occur over the course of days or weeks. Psychoeducation can help individuals learn about the caffeine contents of beverages and medication, providing the ability to gradually switch to decaffeinated beverages.

Cannabis-Related Disorders

There are more than 100 cannabinoids in marijuana. Although occasionally classified as a hallucinogenic drug, the effects of **cannabinoids** are less intense than that of other hallucinogens. Depending on the dose and route of administration, its effects begin shortly after administration (when smoked) and typically last from 1 to 3 hours (or longer when swallowed). Cannabis' effects include relaxation, euphoria, at times dyscoria (abnormal pupillary reaction or shape), distortion of senses, conjunctival injection, spatial misperception, time distortion (time standing still), tachycardia, hypotension, and increased appetite/food cravings ("the munchies"). Cannabis use and cannabis use disorders are associated with adverse consequences including impaired driving ability, cognitive decline, impaired education or occupational attainment, emergency room visits, psychiatric symptoms, and other drug use (Hasin et al., 2016). Cannabinoids are also synthetically produced and commercially available for the treatment of selected medical conditions/symptoms (e.g., appetite stimulation related to medical illness in HIV/AIDS, to remedy pain in some conditions, and for the treatment of nausea).

In the short term, cannabis can result in motor impairment, loss of coordination and balance, and slowing of reaction time. This translates into the potential for significant impairment in the ability to work in safety-sensitive positions (such as nursing) and safely operate machinery or a vehicle. When smoked, cannabis delivers to the body toxic chemicals similar to tobacco, and exposure during pregnancy may result in cognitive problems in offspring. Long-term use may impair consolidation of memory, recall ability, and cognition, hence interfering with academic functioning. Weight gain can also occur as a result of chronic appetite stimulation. Persons consuming high-potency cannabis, or heavy doses, may develop psychotic symptoms, and the use of cannabis is recognized as an independent risk factor in the development of schizophrenia and psychosis.

The mainstay for the treatment of cannabis use disorders is psychosocial treatment. This includes motivational enhancement, psychodynamic and interpersonal therapy, and relapse prevention. There is no medication proven to be superior to placebo in the treatment of this condition.

Hallucinogen-Related Disorders

The **hallucinogens** (the psychedelics) represent a broad classification encompassing agents with varied chemical structures that can elicit varied pharmacologic effects but produce similar alterations of perception, mood, and cognition in users. Some of these include a class of drugs, termed "entheogens," that are ingested to produce a nonordinary state of consciousness for religious or spiritual purposes. There are more than 100 different hallucinogens with substantially different molecular structures and unique features. They fall into two different chemical groups: serotonin or tryptamine related and phenylethylamine or amphetamine related. In addition, miscellaneous ethnobotanical compounds are within this classification (e.g., *Salvia divinorum*), but cannabis is not. Some of these substances (i.e., LSD) have a long half life and extended duration to the extent that the user may spend a day using and/or recovering from their effects, and others are short acting (APA, 2013). This classification also includes the "designer drugs" that sometime emerge on the market. Box 26.10 describes one of these designer drugs: "bath salts."

The hallucinogens have salient effects in changing the senses (e.g., visual, auditory, gustatory, tactile, and olfactory) and may induce euphoria or dysphoria, altered body image, distorted sensory perceptions, confusion, incoordination, and impaired judgment and memory. Hallucinogens typically affect the autonomic and regulatory nervous systems first, increasing heart rate and body temperature, and slightly elevating blood pressure. The individual may experience dry mouth, dizziness, and subjective feelings of being hot or cold. Intense mood and sexual behaviour changes may occur, and the subject may feel unusually close to others or distant and isolated. In severe cases, individuals have reported paranoia, depersonalization, illusions, delusions, and hallucinations.

Phencyclidine (PCP or angel dust), not a true hallucinogen, can affect many neurotransmitter systems; it interferes with the functioning of the glutamate but also enhances dopamine release. At low to moderate doses, PCP causes altered perception of body image but rarely produces visual hallucinations. PCP can also cause effects that mimic the primary symptoms of schizophrenia, such as delusions and mental turmoil. People who use PCP for long periods of time have memory loss and speech difficulties.

Ketamine ("Special-K"), an anaesthetic drug, follows the characteristics of PCP, albeit less potent on an equivalent mass basis. Ketamine has legitimate medical utility in both human and veterinary medicine, with specific value in emergency medicine. In illicit settings, it is often injected, insufflated (i.e., blown into a body cavity), smoked, or taken orally, and it has a similar physical appearance to cocaine (pure). Ketamine has been reported as a drug frequently used in "date rape" cases.

The mechanism of action on the brain is similar for both PCP and ketamine, namely, to block a specific subset of protein molecules (NMDA [*N*-methyl-D-aspartic acid] receptors) involved in memory functions of the brain. Upon administration, a state of acute mental decompensation can occur, characterized by diminished ability to think and carry on daily activities, and typically includes loss of memory (both long term and short term). A sense of detachment from the external world or from their own body occurs, and in these dissociative states, certain thoughts, emotions, sensations, and/or memories may not be integrated in the usual fashion when compared to a drug-free state. In sufficient doses, the appearance of disorganization can occur, possibly followed by the appearance of stupor.

> **BOX 26.10** Synthetic Cathinones ("Bath Salts")
>
> The term "bath salts" refers to an emerging family of drugs containing one or more synthetic chemicals related to cathinone, an amphetamine-like stimulant found naturally in the Khat plant. Their use can produce euphoria, increased sociability, and increased sex drive. Paranoia, agitation, hallucinations, psychotic and violent behaviour, and death have also been reported with its use. "Bath salts" take the form of a white or brown crystalline powder and can be taken orally, inhaled, or injected. Early indications are that synthetic cathinones have high abuse and addictive potential. Another danger is that these products may contain other unknown ingredients that may have their own harmful effects.
>
> Source: National Institute on Drug Abuse (NIDA). (2016a). *DrugFacts: Synthetic cathinones ("bath salts")*. Retrieved from https://www.drugabuse.gov/publications/drugfacts/synthetic-cathinones-bath-salts

---

Inhalant-Related Disorders

Inhalants refer to a group of chemical vapours or gasses, including organic solvents or *volatile substances*, that are inhaled, causing a high. These substances are not intended for human consumption, and although the effects may vary, several are considered CNS depressants. Inhalants typically are used by younger individuals in lower socioeconomic settings where they are often available, accessible, and generally affordable. Inhalants, particularly solvents, are a particular challenge in some

Indigenous communities of Canada. The inhalants are divided into four classes, but there are hundreds of different chemicals belonging to each class:

1. Volatile solvents (benzene, toluene, xylene, acetone, hexane, felt-tip markers, hobby glue, airplane glue, polyvinyl chloride cement, rubber cement, dry cleaning fluid, spot removers, degreasers, computer cleaners, paint and nail polish removers, paint thinners, correction fluids, lighter fluid)
2. Aerosols or spray cans (whipped cream and cooking oil sprays, hair spray, fluorocarbon, butane [pressurized liquids or gasses], asthma sprays, deodorants, air fresheners)
3. Gasses (oxide [laughing gas], chloroform, halothane, ether, butane, propane, enflurane, isoflurane, ethyl chloride)
4. Nitrates (amyl, butyl, isopropyl nitrate)

As a class, the inhalants are known to cause euphoria, sedation, emotional lability, and/or impaired judgment. In some cases, intoxication can result in respiratory depression, stupor, and coma. The chemical structure of the various types of inhalants is diverse, making it difficult to generalize about their effects. However, serious health consequences may ensue, including hearing loss, damage to the liver, kidney, lungs, and heart, as well as bone marrow suppression. Magnetic resonance imaging scans of users demonstrate severe changes in cerebral white matter, including atrophy, and a foetal solvent syndrome has been described (NIDA, 2005a). Fatalities may occur even on the first exposure and are not thought to be dose related.

Opioid-Related Disorders

The **opioids** represent a broad category of psychoactive substances, consisting of both licit and illicit substances that act by attaching to the endogenous opioid receptors in the brain. The opioid family of substances include:

1. Pure opioid agonists:
   a. Naturally occurring alkaloids: opium, morphine, and codeine
   b. Semisynthetic substances (e.g., heroin [diacetylmorphine])
   c. Synthetic substances (e.g., oxycodone, methadone, fentanyl, meperidine, hydrocodone, propoxyphene, tramadol)
2. Mixed agonist–antagonists (e.g., pentazocine, butorphanol)
3. Partial agonists: buprenorphine (combined with naloxone)

Opioids cause CNS depression, sleep or stupor, and analgesia and possess strong reinforcing properties that can quickly trigger addiction when used improperly. Opiates elicit their effects by binding to opioid receptors that are widely distributed throughout the brain and body. Two important effects produced by opioids are pleasure (or reward) and pain relief (analgesia). The brain itself also produces substances known as endorphins that activate the opiate receptors. Research indicates that endorphins are involved in many functions, including respiration, nausea, vomiting, pain modulation, and hormonal regulation (NIDA, 2005b).

Opioids may cause tolerance and physical dependence (sometimes rapidly) that appear to be specific for each receptor subtype. In the early stages, the use of opioids may be associated with euphoria in some cases. Tolerance develops particularly to the analgesic, respiratory depression, and sedative actions of the opioids. The common physical effects associated with the use of the opioids include sweating, nausea, constipation (which can progress to narcotic bowel syndrome), and dose-dependent sedation, fatigue, confusion, cognitive impairment, respiratory depression, as well as reproductive and endocrine effects (e.g., suppression of testosterone in men and menstrual irregularities in women). In some cases, opioids are used concurrently with other sedative substances (e.g., benzodiazepines, alcohol, barbiturates, or sedating antidepressants). In these cases, the risk of CNS and respiratory depression may be especially salient, thus warranting an even higher level of vigilance in their assessment and management. There is further a phenomenon called medication-induced headaches, for example, with the chronic use of analgesics, where the analgesic drug is causally linked to the exacerbation of the headache, and improvement is noticed when the analgesic is discontinued.

The demonstrated effectiveness of opioid analgesics for the management of acute pain and the limited therapeutic alternatives for chronic pain have combined to produce an overreliance on opioid medications (Fischer & Argento, 2012). The resultant increased usage of opioid prescribing has resulted in alarming increases in diversion, overdose, and addiction in Canada. It was first believed that pain protected against the development of addiction to opioid medications. However, the *iatrogenic* (caused by medical treatment) introduction of opioid addiction has now been well established with rates estimated from 15% to 24% (Volkow & McLennan, 2016).

Many Canadians initiate their misuse of opioids through a prescription for therapeutic purposes. In a study of opioid-dependent patients, 37% reported receiving opioids from physician prescriptions, 26% from both a prescription and "the street," and 21% from the street (Sproule, Brands, Li, & Catz-Biro, 2009). Inquiry into the patterns of abuse of opioids should occur if individuals report or are found to be "double doctoring," "borrowing pain medications from others," and "buying black market medications," when individuals run out of their medication early, or if triplicate prescriptions are reported to be lost or stolen.

Opioid Intoxication

Opioid intoxication typically does not require treatment except in cases where CNS or respiratory depression is a risk or where it is combined with other depressants (e.g., alcohol, barbiturates, or benzodiazepines). The use of an opioid receptor blocker, for example, naloxone or naltrexone, may be indicated in such cases, along with supportive treatment and monitoring of vital signs.

High doses of opioids, especially potent opioids such as fentanyl, can cause breathing to stop completely, which can lead to death (NIDA, 2016b). This is because opioid receptors are also found in the areas of the brain that control breathing rate. Fentanyl has emerged as a drug of misuse and is increasingly being reported as an accidental cause of death in Canada. Pharmaceutical-grade fentanyl is 50 to 100 times more potent than morphine, and street versions of the drug are often mixed with heroin and can be even more potent. As fentanyl is such a strong opiate, the chances of overdose occurring are greater than in the less-potent opioid medications. A fentanyl overdose can cause serious short-term and long-term health consequences, and in many cases, fentanyl misuse can be fatal. It is important that people understand the symptoms of overdose so that action can be taken as soon as possible to reduce the likelihood of a negative and potentially fatal outcome. (Box 26.11 discusses fentanyl overdose in the community setting.)

Opioid Withdrawal

When opioid use is discontinued or rapidly tapered after a period of continuous use, a rebound hyperexcitability withdrawal syndrome may occur. Withdrawal may be associated with severe cravings and mimics a "bad case of the flu," involving both the respiratory and GI systems. It may include symptoms of anxiety, dysphoria, nausea, vomiting, muscle aches, lacrimation or rhinorrhoea, papillary dilation, piloerection, sweating, diarrhoea, yawning, fever, and insomnia. These withdrawal symptoms are not typically life threatening but can be particularly uncomfortable and may lead to significant distress. Medically ill, pregnant, very young, and very old individuals at risk of opioid withdrawal may be more prone to developing medical complications during withdrawal from opioids or combination substances.

General supportive measure for managing withdrawal includes providing a safe and supportive environment with close monitoring. Detoxification management is usually not associated with medical complications and serves only as the first stage of ongoing treatment for addiction to opioids. Detoxification is conducted with the use of medication options, for example, methadone, buprenorphine (combined with naloxone in Canada), and Suboxone, or by the use of a tapering regimen of the existing opioid. Clonidine is also useful in curbing withdrawal symptoms during abrupt discontinuation of opioids and can be combined with naltrexone. Care must be taken to avoid the development of orthostatic hypotension during detoxification using clonidine (Tetrault & O'Connor, 2014).

Opioid Use Disorder

For the treatment of opioid use disorders in individuals who have not achieved abstinence through psychosocial interventions, there may be the option of opioid maintenance treatment (OMT, e.g., methadone maintenance treatment [MMT]). The pharmacologic options available in Canada include methadone, heroin, buprenorphine

---

BOX 26.11 Fentanyl Overdose Management in Community Settings

Background: The increased recreational use of fentanyl has seen a corresponding increase in fatal and nonfatal opioid poisonings in Canada. Severe opioid intoxication and overdose is a medical emergency that may cause preventable deaths and thus requires immediate attention.

Symptoms: The characteristic signs of opioid toxicity may include the following: varying degrees of clouded consciousness (e.g., confusion, drowsiness, unresponsive coma); respiratory problems (e.g., severe respiratory depression, respiratory arrest); markedly constricted (pinpoint) pupils; seizures, bradycardia; and hypotension.

Immediate Management: Once fentanyl overdose symptoms begin, it is important to get the individual help as soon as possible to reduce long-term or even fatal consequences. Calls to 911 or seeking emergency services as soon as possible are critical first steps.

Starting CPR if the person stops breathing or has no pulse is fundamental. Another step is to take any remaining pills from the person's mouth or patches from his or her skin so the person does not absorb more of the opioid.

Pharmacologic Therapy: Naloxone is given for acute opioid overdose. An opioid agonist, it is available as a nasal spray and in injectable form. Efforts are being made to increase the availability of naloxone in the community setting. These measures include take-home naloxone programs, permitting the administration of naloxone by first responders (e.g., firefighters, law enforcement officers), and through relaxed prescribing, dispensing, and reimbursement programs.

Source: National Institute on Drug Abuse. (2016b). *DrugFacts—Fentanyl*. Retrieved from https://www.drugabuse.gov/publications/drugfacts/fentanyl

(Suboxone, i.e., with naloxone), and naltrexone. For the first three options, the prescribing physician is required to have completed special training and to have been granted exemption and be registered at the provincial professional regulatory body.

In a person with opioid use disorder, discontinuation of the opioid will rapidly reverse tolerance and dependence within days or weeks. However, the underlying clinical changes will persist for months or longer, leaving the person particularly vulnerable to overdose. The intense drive to take the drug persists, but the tolerance that previously protected the individual from overdosing is no longer present. This phenomenon draws attention to the vulnerability of individuals to overdose in the postrehabilitation period.

Sedative, Hypnotic, and Anxiolytic-Related Disorders

Sedative, hypnotic, and anxiolytic-related (antianxiety) agents are synthetic medications that are sedating, induce sleep, and reduce anxiety. Barbiturates were the first class of drugs used to treat sleep disturbances and anxiety and have largely been replaced by benzodiazepines because of their comparative safety with regard to potential toxicity and addictive qualities. Benzodiazepines are often used to sedate individuals preoperatively, to treat seizures and alcohol withdrawal, and as muscle relaxants. The effects of benzodiazepines and other sedative–hypnotics include decreased anxiety, increased sedation, muscle relaxation, and increase seizure threshold.

The abuse of sedative, hypnotic, and anxiolytic-related agents is common and complex, especially among people who abuse other drugs to enhance their effects (e.g., opioids and alcohol) or to ease the agitation of drugs that have stimulant effects, such as ecstasy or cocaine. This is extremely dangerous and can put individuals at risk for overdose, causing coma or death. The combination of benzodiazepines and alcohol also complicates withdrawal treatment because the individual may seem to improve after the alcohol withdrawal symptoms subsides, only to have similar symptoms emerge as the benzodiazepine withdrawal syndrome appears. The severity of symptoms during benzodiazepine withdrawal depends on the duration and dosage of regular use as well as host factors such as psychiatric comorbidity, concurrent use of other substances, concurrent medical conditions, age, and gender (Dickenson & Eickelberg, 2014).

Stimulant-Related Disorders

This category of substances includes amphetamine and amphetamine-type stimulants, substances that are structurally different but have similar effects, such as methylphenidate, and cocaine. Amphetamines and other stimulants may be obtained by prescription for the treatment of obesity, attention deficit hyperactivity disorder,

and narcolepsy. These prescribed stimulants may be diverted to the black market.

Cocaine is a powerful and addictive stimulant that is snorted (powder), smoked (crack), or injected. Cocaine is highly addictive and is often coadministered with other addictive substances like alcohol or tobacco. When snorted, injected, or smoked, cocaine rapidly crosses the blood–brain barrier and peak intoxication occurs within seconds after intravenous injection or crack smoking. Injecting releases the substance directly into the bloodstream and heightens the intensity of its effects. Smoking entails the inhalation of cocaine vapour or smoke into the lungs, where absorption into the bloodstream is as rapid as by injection (NIDA, 2009). Cocaine use causes tachycardia, hypertension, dilated pupils, and rises in body temperature. It may contribute to seizures, myocardial infarcts, and cerebrovascular accidents and crosses the placenta.

When cocaine is used concomitantly with alcohol, a potentially dangerous interaction may develop. Taken in combination, the two drugs are converted by the body to cocaethylene, which has a longer duration of action in the brain and is more cardiotoxic than is either drug alone. Notably, this mixture of cocaine and alcohol is the most common two-drug combination that results in drug-related death (NIDA, 2009).

Shortly after cocaine is snorted, smoked, or injected, the individual experiences a sudden burst of alertness and energy ("cocaine rush"), euphoria, and increased feelings of self-confidence, being in control, and sociability. There is an increase in sense awareness (e.g., sexuality is heightened, and sound, touch, and sight are more acute). There is also a decreased need for sleep and a lowering of appetite. Along with this, anxiety and restlessness as well as agitation may occur. With the use of higher doses, there may also occur panic, mania, psychosis (hallucinations, disorganization, and delusions), and erratic and bizarre behaviours, potentially leading up to violence and potential risk of harm. In an individual with a vulnerability to depression, mania, or psychosis, the use of cocaine may experience exacerbation of symptoms of related psychiatric conditions.

The high is followed by a significant and intense depressive phase (letdown effect or "cocaine crash") in which the subject feels irritable, depressed, and tired and displays increased appetite and powerful cravings for the drug. The individual may desperately seek cocaine or even other drugs, to self-medicate some of the unpleasant side effects of the crash phase. Similar to the severe anxiety, restlessness, and agitation of intoxication, these symptoms may also appear during withdrawal. These, along with drug-seeking behaviour, may last for weeks, contributing to the extremely high relapse rates observed in these persons.

Long-term cocaine use depletes norepinephrine and, when the drug is discontinued, results in a "crash" causing the user to sleep 12 to 18 hours. Upon awakening, withdrawal symptoms may occur that are characterized by sleep disturbances with rebound rapid eye movement (REM) sleep, anergia (lack of energy), decreased libido, depression with possible suicidality, anhedonia, poor concentration, and cocaine craving. Depression typically resolves, and unless an underlying major depressive disorder is demonstrated, the use of antidepressants is not indicated.

Stimulant Withdrawal

Withdrawal from cocaine is usually relatively uncomplicated. There is a high risk of relapse, and the challenge is often to establish a recovery environment in which this risk is minimized. Cocaine detoxification is not typically associated with medical complications and usually requires only supportive care. However, if a patient develops psychotic symptoms (e.g., hallucinations, delusions, or paranoia) during intoxication phases, specific treatments to remedy them may be required, such as the use of atypical antipsychotics. Amphetamine withdrawal symptoms are not as pronounced as those of cocaine withdrawal and are treated similarly. Evidence in support of treatment for addiction using pharmacologic agents is limited and is similar to that used for cocaine.

Stimulant Use Disorder

Treatment is complex and involves assessing the psychobiologic, social, and pharmacologic aspects of abuse. Psychosocial interventions form the mainstay of treatment for cocaine addiction treatment, and residential care may be required in cases where relapse risk cannot be adequately managed on an outpatient basis. Stabilization of the patient's recovery environment is pivotal in achieving lasting abstinence from cocaine, and inclusion in a 12-step program is recommended (e.g., Narcotics Anonymous). Patients using cocaine should be advised to abstain from alcohol as well and, if applicable, offered opportunities to quit smoking. To date, there is no medication proven to be superior to placebo in regard to cocaine addiction treatment. However, there are promising options, for example, topiramate, disulfiram, or modafinil, which may be considered in cases where psychosocial treatment alone has failed to yield optimal results (DeLima, de Olivera Soceres, Reisser, & Farrell, 2002).

Tobacco-Related Disorders

If tobacco were introduced to the market today, it could not become a legal product because of its high lethality index. Tobacco smoke contains over 7,000 chemicals, of which there are at least 172 toxic substances, 33 hazardous air pollutants, 47 chemicals restricted as hazardous waste, and 67 known human or animal carcinogens (U.S. Department of Health and Human Services, 2010). These exist whether tobacco smoke is inhaled in the act of smoking or by nonsmokers out of the air indoors or outdoors. Nicotine is an addictive substance found within the tobacco plant, has both stimulant and depressant

effects, and is considered as the fundamental chemical "driver" of the process of addiction in the brain. The use of tobacco products without nicotine would not be addictive, but paradoxically, nicotine is not the harmful chemical found within tobacco products, and pharmaceutical-grade (and dosage) nicotine is generally considered to be safe. It is the tar and other substances and additives in tobacco products that threaten health.

A cigarette provides approximately 10 puffs, and a person who smokes 20 cigarettes per day (one pack) is taking 200 doses of nicotine daily. No other drug—not even cocaine—is dosed that frequently, and conditioned cues to smoke become established. As a result, desiring a cigarette becomes associated with everyday events such as getting up in the morning, drinking coffee or alcohol, taking a break, and having a conversation. The quantity and power of this conditioning are unique to cigarette smoking, and it is one of the reasons that smoking is so difficult to quit. Most Canadians initiate the use of tobacco between the ages of 11 and 15; for this reason, tobacco addiction is described as a paediatric disease that in most cases continues into adulthood unless successfully managed in childhood and adolescence. Signs of tobacco use disorder include the urge to smoke within minutes of waking, smoking at regular intervals throughout the day, and continuing to smoke despite wanting to quit. People who are addicted may become tolerant to the desired effects and may no longer experience pleasure from smoking but continue to smoke in order to avoid nicotine withdrawal.

Tobacco Withdrawal

Symptoms of tobacco withdrawal vary but may include cravings, irritability, restlessness, difficulty concentrating, depression, frustration, anxiety, insomnia, fatigue, and increased appetite. Most symptoms reach maximum intensity at 24 to 48 hours and are relieved within a few weeks, but some individuals may be unable to concentrate and have strong cravings to smoke for weeks or months after quitting smoking. In recognition of the harmful effects of second-hand smoke for the patients, staff, visitors, and others, most hospitals and health care facilities are smoke free. Some patients are often placed into involuntary tobacco withdrawal as a result of protections from secondhand smoke policies.

Detoxification interventions are safe and reliable and minimize the suffering from tobacco withdrawal. Detoxification is not considered cessation intervention and, by itself, does not contribute to long-term abstinence. Detoxification is achieved through identifying patients who smoke, offering nicotine replacement therapy (NRT) at sufficient doses, and not expecting a commitment to quit smoking. Effective detoxification requires repeated opportunities to receive NRT and provision of a supportive environment that includes omission of cues to smoke. Systematic measures that are required to ensure rapid treatment delivery include standing orders for NRT, ward stock for quick access, and supplies of a broad spectrum of NRT on hospital formulary (Els, Kunyk, Barak, Thomas, & Scharf, 2014).

Tobacco Use Disorder

There are individuals who are able to stop using tobacco independently (unassisted cessation), but others require formal assistance to achieve long-term abstinence. For some, quitting can be a complex process spanning months and/or years that requires support, medication, and multiple attempts. The optimal treatment design for tobacco use disorder treatment requires a comprehensive and multimodal approach that may include psychosocial and pharmacologic interventions. Clinical practice guidelines that can serve as a suitable template for the delivery of smoking cessation treatments by nurses can be found in Box 26.12.

There are many opportunities for nurses to positively intervene with patients who smoke, as over 70% want to quit, almost half have tried to quit at least once in the past year, and fully one third report that they want to quit in the next month (Reid et al., 2015). In a Cochrane review of nursing interventions, Rice, Hartmann-Boyd, and Stead (2013) concluded that smoking cessation and/or counselling given by nurses is effective. One nursing challenge is the incorporation of smoking behavioural monitoring and smoking cessation interventions as part of their daily practice. All patients should be asked about their tobacco use and provided with information and/or counselling to quit along with reinforcement and follow-up. To enhance the likelihood of a successful quit attempt, clinical findings support the offer, and provision, of simple and strategic behavioural counselling and pharmacotherapy to every person interested in quitting. Those who are not ready to make an attempt at cessation should be offered empathetic counselling designed to permit a reassessment of their reasons for continued smoking and an invitation to seek assistance with at any time. Several levels of evidence support the use of the following modalities.

Psychosocial Interventions

Psychosocial interventions, such as group, individual, telephone, office, or Web-based counselling, should be routinely offered in combination with medication for increased successful cessation rates (Cohen, Dragonetti, Herie, & Barker, 2014). The provision of simple advice regarding the avoidance of high-risk relapse situations,

---

BOX 26.12 CAN-ADAPTT Summary Statements for Counselling and Psychosocial Approaches

Ask: Tobacco use status should be updated for all patients/clients, by all health care providers on a regular basis.

Advise: Health care providers should clearly advise patients/clients to quit.

Assess: Health care providers should assess the willingness of patients/clients to begin treatment to achieve abstinence (quitting).

Assist: Every tobacco user who expresses the willingness to begin treatment to quit should be offered assistance.

a. Minimal intervention, of 1 to 3 minutes, is effective and should be offered to every tobacco user. However, there is a strong dose–response relationship between the session length and successful treatment, and so intensive interventions should be used whenever possible.

b. Counselling by a variety or combination of delivery formats (self-help, individual, group, helpline, Web-based) is effective and should be used to assist patients/clients who express a willingness to quit.

c. Because multiple counselling sessions increase the chances of prolonged abstinence, health care providers should provide four or more counselling sessions where possible.

d. Combining counselling and smoking cessation medication is more effective than either alone; therefore, both should be provided to patients/clients trying to stop smoking where feasible.

e. Motivational interviewing is encouraged to support patients/clients willingness to engage in treatment now and in the future.

f. Two types of counselling and behavioural therapies yield significantly higher abstinence rates and should be included in smoking cessation treatment: (1) providing practical counselling on problem-solving skills or skill training and (2) providing support as a part of treatment.

Arrange follow-up: Health care providers:

a. Should conduct regular follow-up to assess response, provide support, and modify treatment as necessary.

b. Are encouraged to refer patients/clients to relevant resources as part of the provision of treatment, where appropriate.

Reprinted with permission from CAN-ADAPTT. (2011). *Canadian smoking cessation clinical practice guideline*. Toronto, ON: Canadian Action Network for the Advancement, Dissemination and Adoption of Practice-informed Tobacco Treatment, Centre for Addiction and Mental Health. Retrieved from www.nicotinedependenceclinic.com

recognition of settings or circumstances where smoking has been particularly common, management of acute cravings, and development of smoke-free guidelines for home and vehicles are all important in accentuating the likelihood of cessation success. Although the evidence suggests that interventions are effective across a broad range of populations, tailored interventions may be advised for selected subpopulations (e.g., individuals with mental illness, women who are pregnant, and smokeless tobacco users).

Pharmacologic Interventions

Nicotine replacement therapy (NRT) is available in five forms: transdermal patch, chewing "gum," inhaler/vapourizer, lozenge, and spray. Individuals who smoke seek to maintain a certain individualized level of nicotine, and when their nicotine levels fall, distinct and significant discomfort usually occurs (withdrawal symptoms). NRT stimulates nicotine receptors and relieves withdrawal symptoms, and its appropriate use roughly doubles success rates of quit attempts. Combinations of NRT (e.g., patch and a short-acting version concurrently) have the advantage of allowing patients to titrate their nicotine intake to meet their unique needs and are associated with increased levels of success.

Bupropion is an antidepressant that was serendipitously found to be effective in tobacco cessation. Bupropion inhibits the reuptake of dopamine in the reward centres of the brain, as well as norepinephrine, a chemical associated with withdrawal symptoms. Its use has been shown to double success rates in those attempting to quit smoking.

Varenicline, a third-generation smoking cessation pharmacotherapy, directly and distinctly binds to $\alpha_4\beta_2$ nicotinic receptors. These receptor sites are completely blocked but only partially stimulated reducing the transmission of neurologic impulses and causing a reduced amount of dopamine to be released in the reward centres of the brain. Consequently, the patient experiences little to no withdrawal symptoms and no pleasurable sensation if a cigarette is smoked. Varenicline has been shown to more than double the chances of quitting when compared with placebo and helps about 50% more people to quit when compared to NRT. Combining two types of NRT has been shown to be as effective as varenicline (Cahill, Stevens, Perera, & Lancaster, 2013).

The Canadian labelling of NRT, bupropion, and varenicline is required to have a warning to heighten the level of awareness of adverse events and mitigate potential risks in patients taking cessation medications. These warnings note the potential risk of serious mental health events including changes in behaviour, depressed mood, hostility, and suicidal thoughts when quitting smoking. It is not conclusive whether these risks are due to the medications or to the effects of quitting smoking. The tobacco plant contains a class of chemicals, the β-carbolines, which are monoamine oxidase inhibitors (like certain antidepressants). Quitting smoking stops the ingestion of these naturally found antidepressants, and for this reason, depressive symptoms may be triggered in some individuals who are quitting smoking. Risks while taking tobacco cessation medications must always be weighed against the significant health benefits of quitting smoking, and the awareness that this symptomatology may also be expressed in response to tobacco cessation. Despite the absence of evidence for a causal link between cessation medications and neuropsychiatric adverse effects, prudence suggests screening for mood issues in patients who consume tobacco products as well as those going through the quitting process (Els, 2014). Current labelling also suggests that patients should be offered NRT prior to considering the use of varenicline.

Gambling Disorder

Gambling is the activity of risk taking for the purposes of gaining an advantage or benefit and produces vast revenue for investors as well as for government. Gambling disorder typically develops over the course of years, and most individuals with the disorder gradually increase their frequency of gambling and amount of wagering. The past-year prevalence of gambling disorder is 0.2% to 0.3% in the general population. Males are more likely to have a gambling disorder (although this gap appears to be narrowing); the lifetime prevalence for males is about 0.6% (APA, 2013). More recently, the Internet has expanded the range and accessibility of gambling to younger people (Tupperman & Wanner, 2012).

The mainstay of treatment for gambling disorder is psychotherapy, specifically cognitive and behavioural modalities. Brief interventions and motivational enhancement have also shown to have benefit in improving outcomes. There are no registered pharmacotherapeutic options, although some benefits have been demonstrated with the use of opioid antagonists (e.g., naltrexone), bupropion, lithium, and selective serotonin reuptake inhibitors (e.g., paroxetine and fluvoxamine). Individuals report benefit from attendance at Gamblers Anonymous (12-step based), and in some situations, voluntary self-exclusion programs may offer some degree of protection. Due to the high rates of co-occurrence of other psychiatric conditions, assessment and treatment of comorbid symptoms and syndromes are deemed prudent. The high rates of suicide in gambling addiction warrant special attention to prevention.

▎ SPECIAL POPULATIONS AND SITUATIONS

Youth

Adolescence constitutes the life stage with the greatest vulnerability to developing SUDs. Adolescence is a transition period that is characterized by considerable neurobiologic changes and an associated increased propensity for substance use, and it is also a time of increased sensitivity to stress. It is a time of life when self-regulatory executive functions are still maturing, associated with the enhanced neuroplasticity of their brains and their underdeveloped frontal cortex. This period is characterized by pronounced changes in behaviour, including loss of self-control, increased risk taking, novelty and sensation seeking, social interactions, and high activity. At the same time, there may be low levels of anxiety regarding the risk of harm, strong emotional states, and mood instability. During this age, the prefrontal cortex and limbic systems are undergoing prominent reorganization in myelination, neuronal plasticity, and structural rearrangements, and drug exposure might result in different neuroadaptations than those that occur during adulthood. Substance use during this critical period of cortical development may lead to increased vulnerability to addiction and to lifelong changes of executive function. In general, the younger individuals start using substances, the more likely they are to progress and exceed occasional experimentation and to move into frequent abuse, with a higher chance of developing addiction (Swendsen & Le Moal, 2011).

Not all young people who experiment with substances proceed to levels that bring health problems. The serious risks of substances to youth are physical (e.g., liver and heart damage, impaired brain function, impaired reproductive organ development), psychological (e.g., depression, sleep disorders, conduct disorders) and social (e.g., academic performance, relationships with family/friends, and increased exposure to risk situations). It is important to address a developing substance problem in young people as early as possible, with a recognition that they are different from adults in many ways: their unique developmental (e.g., difficulty comprehending future consequences) and psychiatric issues, differences in values and belief systems, and environmental considerations (such as strong peer influence). Family involvement plays a critical role in an adolescent's treatment and recovery.

Postsecondary Education Students

Peak lifetime alcohol use generally occurs in an individual's late teens and early 20s. The prevalence of heavy episodic (or binge) drinking (defined as reaching a BAL of 0.08 or higher, usually by consuming five or more drinks for men, four or more for women, in a 24-hour period) and the detrimental consequences resulting from this type of drinking have led to the classification of college binge drinking as a major public health problem (Larimer, Kilmer, & Whiteside, 2011).

Advances are being made in identifying effective strategies to reduce alcohol (and other substance) consumption and its consequences among this population. These interventions include developing CBT skills (such as identifying and planning for or avoiding risky situations

using protective strategies such as drink spacing, counting drinks, and limit setting), norm clarification (correcting misperceptions about drinking norms), using MI to reduce resistance and promote change, and challenging expectations. Environmental interventions are emerging as important components of an overall prevention strategy. These include strategies such as promoting alcohol-free options, creating an environment that supports health-promoting norms, limiting alcohol availability, restricting alcohol promotion, and developing policies/laws about consumption (Larimer et al., 2011).

Pregnancy and Lactation

Alcohol, tobacco, and other drug use during pregnancy can have serious detrimental effects on the course of pregnancy, as well as on the physiologic status of the foetus and newborn. Some women are able to stop using substances when they learn they are pregnant, but others may have difficulty stopping due to the severity of the addiction or withdrawal. Nurses should be aware that the use of substances is more stigmatized in pregnancy, so that women may minimize or deny their use, its harmful effects, and the need to seek care. The nurse should be aware of special social, emotional, and legal issues involving the treatment of pregnant women and be sensitive to their special needs. For example, women may fear that, by seeking prenatal care, their drug use will be detected by urine toxicology tests and cause them to lose custody of their children. Screening for intimate partner violence should be routine in this population as 34% of substance-abusing pregnant women report physical abuse (Wunsch & Weaver, 2011).

In most cases, providing information alone is insufficient to achieve sobriety/abstinence. A comprehensive approach to treatment in the perinatal period, including prenatal and perinatal care; pharmacologic interventions such as methadone maintenance programs; life skills training, such as relapse prevention and social skills training; mother–infant development assessment; and early childhood development programs and social work services, as required, is recommended. The newborn will require evaluation for neonatal intoxication and abstinence syndromes, as well as for foetal effects of psychoactive substance use. Substances are transmitted into breast milk, and the nursing mother can expose the breast-fed baby to harmful chemicals, with a range of adverse outcomes and risks. However, women actively engaged in addiction treatment should be encouraged to breastfeed as long as drug screens are clear (Wunsch & Weaver, 2011).

HIV/AIDS

Some individuals who abuse drugs and alcohol may be at high risk for sexual transmission of HIV/AIDS because they may be unable to take adequate precautions and use preventive methods while intoxicated or may engage in risky sexual encounters to obtain money or drugs.

Intravenous drug users may be considered particularly at risk for HIV/AIDS infection, because some may be placed in situations where hypodermic needles, syringes, and other supplies used to inject drugs are shared.

The concurrence of an SUD and HIV/AIDS infection requires exceedingly careful assessment and intervention planning. Continued alcohol and substance use can interfere with the medical treatment of HIV/AIDS; for example, alcohol, marijuana, cocaine, and amphetamines are immunosuppressants that further impair the seriously compromised immune system of individuals with HIV/AIDS. Addicted persons infected with HIV/AIDS may have difficulty adhering to medication schedules, and some would not benefit fully from antiviral medications because of this. Other complicating factors include the financial, social, and emotional stressors (including stigma) experienced by individuals with SUDs who must also cope with the devastating diagnosis of HIV/AIDS disease.

Addiction treatment programs have an important role for individuals with HIV/AIDS disease, SUDs, and concurrent mental health problems. Because the issues facing these individuals are so complex, planning treatment and priority setting are essential. Addiction treatment is nearly always necessary for the individual to follow with other HIV-/AIDS-related health and mental health interventions. At the initial diagnosis of HIV/AIDS infection, SUD issues therefore need to be evaluated and addressed.

Concurrent Substance Use and Other Mental Disorders

The risk for addiction in individuals with mental illness is significantly higher than for the general population, and many individuals with addiction also have concurrent mental disorders. Also known as dual diagnosis, comorbid substance use mental disorders, or concurrent mental disorders, these can be defined as the coexistence of at least one mental disorder and at least one other SUD as defined by the *DSM-5*. Some mental disorders are in part a by-product of long-term SUDs; some mental disorders predispose the individual to alcohol, tobacco, or other drug use. Nurses need to remember that individuals do not compartmentalize their problems, so health professionals should not either. Concurrent disorders are discussed in detail in Chapter 33.

Nurses With Substance Use Disorders

Nurses, similar to other health professionals, may also develop SUD. Rather than being protected by any special knowledge, skills, or insights they may have due to education or professional experiences, there is research indicating that nurses may be at particular risk for SUD because of high job strain, disruption, and fatigue related to shift work, ease of access to medications in the workplace, and their knowledge of the benefits of

medications. The evidence suggests that the prevalence of SUD among nurses is similar to, or greater than, the general population (Kunyk, 2015). When nurses abuse or become addicted to substances, more than their own health and welfare are placed at risk. There are also patient safety concerns due to the risk associated of impaired nursing practice, and when drugs are accessed from the workplace, patients may suffer from undermedication. To reduce these risks, and improve the recovery of the impaired nurse, the focus must be on prevention, early identification, multimodal treatment, and return to practice with long-term supports.

The issue of SUDs among nurses is sensitive and challenging to address. Nurses with SUD may not be able to recognize their illness or be constrained from seeking help because of stigma, risk of professional discipline or job loss, and loss of status (Kunyk, Inness, Reisdorfer, Morris, & Chambers, 2016). Refer further to Box 26.13. This inability places some responsibility on others to intervene. Nurses have a responsibility in this situation to ensure patient safety and to assist their nurse colleague in accessing appropriate care and supports (e.g., confidential employee assistance programs are available in many workplaces throughout Canada), with the goal of successful return to practice. Evidence does not support the use of discipline as an effective remedy in reducing the risks of nurses practicing while impaired by the use of substances (Kunyk, 2015). However, aftercare programs for health care professionals have been established as an effective mechanism for early intervention, supporting long-term recovery and detecting a relapse upon return to work. These programs monitor for continued engagement in evidence-based treatment programs that include random drug testing. A number of studies have followed physicians in these programs and demonstrated outcomes of approximately 80% practicing after 5 years (Brewster, Kaufman, Hutchinson, & MacWilliam, 2008; McLellann, Skipper, Campbell, & DuPont, 2008). The recognition of addiction as a treatable medical illness (as opposed to a moral weakness or lifestyle choice) places a "duty to accommodate" on the employer, and this is increasingly being reflected in employee wellness programs. For further information, see Chapter 16.

■ NURSES AS HEALTH ADVOCATES

The Code of Ethics for Registered Nurses (Canadian Nurses Association [CNA], 2017) serves as a foundation for nurses' ethical practice, and this includes endeavours that nurses may undertake to address social inequities. Nurses are expected to uphold principles of justice by safeguarding human rights, equity, and fairness and by promoting the public good. Individuals with addiction are among the more marginalized and impoverished members of Canadian society. The challenges associated

BOX 26.13 **Research for Best Practice**

HELP-SEEKING BY HEALTH PROFESSIONALS FOR ADDICTION

From Kunyk, D., Inness, M., Reisdorfer, E., Morris, H., & Chambers, T. (2016). Help seeking by health professionals for addiction: A mixed review study. International Journal of Nursing Studies, *60, 200–215. doi:10.1016/j/ijnurstu.2016.05.001*

Background: Facilitating help seeking by health professionals with addiction is a priority for reducing associated risks to their health and to patient safety.

Purpose: The purpose of this study was to identify the process by which health professionals seek help for addiction and the factors that facilitate or deter help seeking.

Method: We first conducted a meta-synthesis of the qualitative literature to garner an understanding of the help-seeking process for health professionals with addiction. We then conducted a narrative synthesis of the quantitative studies to generalize these findings through examination of convergent, complementary, and divergent findings.

Findings: The professionals and experiential context of health care compromises the health professional's readiness to seek help for addiction. Typically, a pivotal event initiates the help-seeking process. Help seeking most often results from reports of adverse events to formal organizations such as employers and regulatory bodies and oftentimes results in mandated treatment. This process is not sufficient for reaching most health professionals with addiction. Colleagues and families, often aware of the addiction earlier, would prefer to refer to voluntary and confidential treatment programs.

Implications: There is a large gap between health professionals requiring and receiving treatment for addiction, and this poses a substantive safety risk. Access to confidential, compassionate, and supportive alternative treatment programs offer potential for closing this gap.

---

with their illness are often exacerbated by the experience of stigma, placing an additional burden for overcoming barriers to accessing care. Stigma includes having fixed ideas and judgments—such as thinking that people with substance use and mental health problems are not normal, that they caused their own problems, or that they could simply get over their problems if they wanted to do so. The stigma and shame associated with SUD can, in effect, isolate those with addiction from the rest of society.

The use of substances threatens to affect the overall welfare of our nation and our health care system and poses a massive economic burden. Nurses are well positioned on the frontlines of the health care system to be provided opportunities to understand the needs and vulnerabilities of those with SUDs, to be aware of available services and resources, and to note the existing deficits. It is well within the role of the nurse to seek opportunities to reduce the stigma and misunderstanding associated with addiction, as well as to collaborate and advocate for broader societal changes through policy, legislation, and other mechanisms to improve conditions for preventing and treating addiction at a population level. In these times of health care reform, nurses may have to proactively advocate for health care systems that ensure accessibility, universality, and comprehensiveness of services in order to meet the needs of individuals with addictions and their families.

 SUMMARY OF KEY POINTS

- Addiction is recognized by the major global disease classification systems as a chronic medical disorder characterized by periods of remission and relapse. Substances of abuse alter the brain's structure and function, resulting in changes that persist long after their use has discontinued. Addiction is amenable to evidence-based treatment, yet it remains largely untreated.

- The *DSM-5* classification of substance-related and addictive disorders includes SUDs (ranging in severity from mild to severe) and substance-induced disorders (including substance intoxication and substance withdrawal). These are classified according to the class of substance: alcohol; caffeine; cannabis (marijuana); hallucinogens; inhalants; opioids; sedatives, hypnotics, and anxiolytics; stimulants; tobacco (nicotine); and other (or unknown) substances.

- The bio/psycho/social/spiritual model conceptualizes addiction as a disorder with multifactorial pathogenesis, including predisposing, precipitating, and modulating factors, that encompasses the body, the mind (psyche), and the spirit, as well as social and environmental influences.

- Accurate and comprehensive assessment is crucial in planning addiction treatment interventions.

Assessment should consider all substances for pattern of use, including factors of tolerance; withdrawal symptoms; consequences of use; loss of control over amount, frequency, or duration of use; desire or efforts to cease or control use; social, vocational, and recreational activities affected by use; and history of previous addiction treatment. It also includes investigating family and social support systems. Treatment plans must be assessed continually and modified as necessary to ensure that they meet the changing needs of the patient.

- In some individuals, reducing consumption or abstaining from substances may lead to withdrawal symptoms that may progress into life-threatening complications.
- Substance withdrawal can be assisted through symptom-triggered detoxification. It is important to recognize that detoxification is not the treatment of the SUD. Rather, it is only the management of withdrawal symptoms.
- The use of tobacco products remains the leading preventable cause of death and disease globally. Tobacco addiction is vastly undertreated; most individuals who smoke want to quit, but few are helped in doing so. Nurses can effectively intervene and, as a minimum, should incorporate the 5As (Ask, Advise, Assess, Assist, and Arrange follow-up) into their daily practice.
- The purpose of harm reduction is to reduce the risk for adverse consequences arising from substance use and works with the individual to achieve this goal regardless of his or her commitment to reduce use. Harm reduction forms only one part of a continuum of care and is not viewed as exclusive of the overarching goal of abstinence.
- Many individuals with SUDs also have other mental disorders, and patients presenting with one condition should be assessed for others. When these conditions co-occur, treatment should address both (or all) at the same time (integrated or parallel treatment).
- Stigma can be a massive barrier for individuals with SUDs, and the nurse is well placed to reduce this stigma and misunderstanding. It is within the nursing role to collaborate and advocate for broader societal changes through policy, legislation, and other mechanisms to improve conditions for preventing and treating addiction.

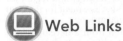 Web Links

http://www.aa.org This is the official site for the program of AA. Information about this program, access to resources, and locations are available.

http://www.al-anon.org The purpose of Al-Anon is to help families and friends recover from the effects of living with the problem drinking of a relative or friend.

www.camh.net The Centre for Addiction and Mental Health (CAMH) is Canada's largest addiction and mental health teaching hospital, as well as one of the world's leading research centres in the area of addiction and mental health.

www.ccsa.ca The Canadian Centre on Substance Abuse is a national agency that promotes informed debate on substance abuse; disseminates information on the nature, extent, and consequences of substance abuse; and supports and assists organizations involved in substance abuse treatment, prevention, and educational programming.

www.cfdp.ca The Canadian Foundation for Drug Policy is a nonprofit organization that recommends effective and humane drug laws and policies in Canada.

www.afmc.ca/etools/chec-cesc The Canadian Healthcare Education Commons' Virtual Library provides learners with access to educational materials including slides, study guides, videos, virtual patients, and electronic cases.

www.drugabuse.gov The National Institute on Drug Abuse Web site has research and treatment reports, news, and educational materials.

www.healthycanadians.gc.ca/anti-drug-antidrogue/index-eng.php The National Anti-Drug Strategy in Canada provides a focused approach aimed at reducing the supply of, and demand for, illicit drugs, addressing prescription drug abuse and addressing the crime associated with illicit drugs.

www.rnao.org The Registered Nurses of Ontario have developed clinical best practice guidelines for engaging clients who use substances, integrating smoking cessation into daily nursing practice, and supporting clients on methadone maintenance treatment.

References

Agabio, R., Campesi, I., Pisanu, C., Gessa, G., & Franconi, F. (2016). Sex differences in substance use disorders: Focus on side effects. *Addiction Biology, 21*, 1030–1042.

American Psychiatric Association. (2013). *Diagnostic and statistical manual of mental disorders* (5th ed.). Arlington, VA: Author.

American Society of Addiction Medicine. (2011). *Short definition of addiction.* Retrieved from www.asam.org/quality-practice/definition-of-addiction

American Society of Addiction Medicine. (2015). *What are the ASAM levels of care?* Retrieved from http://asamcontinuum.org/knowledgebase/what-are-the-asam-levels-of-care

Brands, B., Kahan, M., Selby, P., & Wilson, L. (2000). *Medical management of alcohol and drug-related problems: A physician's manual* (2nd ed.). Toronto, ON: Centre for Addiction and Mental Health.

Brewster, J., Kaufmann, M., Hutchinson, S., & MacWilliam, C. (2008). Characteristics and outcomes of a dependence monitoring programme in Canada: Prospective descriptive study. *BMJ, 337*, a2098.

Butt, P., Beirness, D., Gliksman, L., Paradias, C., & Stockwell, T. (2011). *Alcohol and health in Canada: A summary of evidence and guidelines for low risk drinking.* Ottawa, ON: Canadian Centre of Substance Use.

Cahill, K., Stevens, S., Perera, R., & Lancaster, T. (2013). Pharmacological interventions for smoking cessation: An overview and network meta-analysis. *Cochrane Database of Systematic Reviews,* (5), CD009329. doi:10.1002/14651858.CD009329.pub2

CAN-ADAPTT. (2011). *Canadian smoking cessation clinical practice guideline.* Toronto, ON: Canadian Action Network for the Advancement, Dissemination and Adoption of Practice-informed Tobacco Treatment, Centre for Addiction and Mental Health.

Canadian Centre of Substance Abuse. (2014). *Alcohol. Canadian Drug Summary.* Retrieved from http://www.ccsa.ca/Resource%20Library/CCSA-Canadian-Drug-Summary-Alcohol-2014-en.pdf

Canadian Nurses Association. (2011). *Joint position statement: The role of health professionals in tobacco cessation.* Retrieved from http://www2.cna-aiic.ca/CNA/documents/pdf/publications/JPS_Tobacco_Cessation_2011_e.pdf

Canadian Nurses Association. (2017). *Code of ethics for registered nurses.* Ottawa, ON: Author.

Cavacuiti, C. A., Vasic, A., McCrady, B. S., & Tonigan, J. S. (2011). Recent research into twelve-step programs. In C. Cavacuiti (Ed.), *Principles of addiction medicine: The essentials* (pp. 355–361). Philadelphia, PA: Lippincott Williams & Wilkins.

Cohen, S., Dragonetti, R., Herie, M., & Barker, M. (2014). Psychosocial interventions. In C. Els, D. Kunyk, & P. Selby (Eds.), *Disease interrupted: Tobacco reduction and cessation* (pp. 127–156). Quebec, Canada: Les Presses de L'Université Laval.

Crum, R. M. (2014). The epidemiology of substance use disorders. In R. K. Ries, D. A. Fiellin, S. C. Miller, & R. Saitz (Eds.), *The ASAM principles of addiction medicine* (5th ed., pp. 19–35). Philadelphia, PA: Wolters Kluwer.

DeLima, M. S., de Olivera Soceres, B. G., Reisser, A. A., & Farrell, M. (2002). Pharmacological treatment of cocaine dependence: A systematic review. *Addiction, 97*(8), 931–949.

Dickinson, W. E., & Eickelberg, S. J. (2014). Management of sedative-hypnotic intoxication and withdrawal. In R. K. Ries, D. A. Fiellin, S. C. Miller, & R. Saitz (Eds.), *The ASAM principles of addiction medicine* (5th ed., pp. 652–684). Philadelphia, PA: Wolters Kluwer.

Douaihy, A., Daley, D. C., Marlatt, G. A., & Spotts, C. E. (2011). Relapse prevention: Clinical models and intervention strategies. In C. Cavacuiti (Ed.), *Principles of addiction medicine: The essentials* (pp. 340–344). Philadelphia, PA: Lippincott Williams & Wilkins.

Els, C. (2007). Addiction is a mental disorder, best managed in a (public) mental health setting—But our system is failing us. *Canadian Journal of Psychiatry, 52*(3), 167–169.

Els, C. (2014). Neuropsychiatric considerations. In C. Els, D. Kunyk, & P. Selby (Eds.), *Disease interrupted: Tobacco reduction and cessation* (pp. 215–218). Quebec, Canada: Les Presses de L'Université Laval.

Els, C., Kunyk, D., Barak, Y., Scharf, D., & Thomas, E. (2014). Detoxification: Treatment of the 'other' tobacco use disorder. In C. Els, D. Kunyk, & P. Selby (Eds.), *Disease interrupted: Tobacco reduction and cessation* (pp. 245–248). Quebec, Canada: Les Presses de L'Université Laval.

Ewing, J. A. (1984). Detecting alcoholism: The CAGE questionnaire. *Journal of the American Medical Association, 252*, 1905–1907.

Faggiano, F., Minozzi, S., Versino, E., & Buscemi, D. (2014). Universal school-based prevention for illicit drug use. *Cochrane Database of Systematic Reviews, 12*, CD003020.

Fischer, B. (2005). Harm reduction. In Canadian Centre on Substance Abuse (Ed.), *Substance abuse in Canada: Current challenges and choices* (pp. 11–15). Ottawa, ON: Canadian Centre on Substance Abuse.

Fischer, B., & Argento, E. (2012). Prescription opioid related misuse, harms, diversion and interventions in Canada: A review. *Pain Physician, 15*, ES191–ES203.

Fischer, B., Ialomiteanu, A., Boak, A., Adlaf, E., Rehm, J., & Mann, R. E. (2013). Prevalence and key covariates of non-medical prescription opioid use among the general secondary student and adult populations in Ontario, Canada. *Drug and Alcohol Review, 32*, 266–887.

Grant, B. F., Goldstein, R. B., Saha, T. D., Chou, P., Jung, J., Zhang, H., ... Hasin, D. S. (2015). Epidemiology of DSM-5 alcohol use disorder results from the national epidemiologic survey on alcohol and related conditions III. *JAMA Psychiatry, 72*, 757–766. doi:10.1001/jamapsychiatry.2015.0584

Grant, B. F., Stinson, F. S., Hasin, D. S., Dawson, D. A., Chow, S. P., & Anderson, K. (2004). Immigration and lifetime prevalence of DSM-IV psychiatric disorders among Mexican Americans and non-Hispanic whites in the United States: Results from the National Epidemiologic Survey on Alcohol and Related Conditions. *Archives of General Psychiatry, 61*(12), 1226–1233.

Griffin, K. W., & Brown, G. J. (2014). Preventing substance use among children and adolescents. In R. K. Ries, D. A. Fiellin, S. C. Miller, & R. Saitz (Eds.), *The ASAM principles of addiction medicine* (5th ed., pp. 1572–1579). Philadelphia, PA: Wolters Kluwer.

Guglielmo, R., Martinotti, G., Quatrale, M., Ioime, L., Kadilli, I., Di Nicola, M., & Janiri, L. (2015). Topiramate in alcohol use disorders: Review and update. *CNS Drugs, 29*(5), 385–395. doi:10.1007/s40263-015-0244-0

Hasin, D. S., Kerridge, B. T., Saha, T. D., Huang, B., Pickering, R., Smith, S. M., ... Grant, B. G. (2016). Prevalence and correlates of DSM-5 cannabis use disorders, 2012–2013: Finding from the national epidemiologic survey on alcohol and related conditions-III. *American Journal of Psychiatry, 173*(6), 588–599. doi:10.1176/appi.jp.2015.15070907

Health Canada. (2014). *Canadian alcohol and drug use monitoring survey: Summary of results for 2012—detailed tables*. Retrieved from http://www.hc-sc.gc.ca/hc-ps/drugs-drogues/stat/_2012/summary-sommaire-eng.php

International Narcotics Control Board. (2011). Narcotic drugs technical report. In *Estimated world requirements for 2012—Statistics for 2010*. New York, NY: United Nations. Retrieved from https://www.incb.org/incb/en/narcotic-drugs/Technical_Reports/2011/narcotic-drugs-technical-report_2011.html

Kleber, H., Weiss, R., Anton, R., George, T., Greenfield, S., Kosten, T., ... Connery, H. S. (2006). *Practice guidelines for the treatment of patients with substance use disorders* (2nd ed.). Arlington, VA: American Psychiatric Association.

Kruegar, H., Andres, E. N., Doot, J. M., & Resilly, B. S. (2016). The economic burden of cancers attributable to tobacco smoking, excess weight, alcohol use, and physical inactivity in Canada. *Current Oncology, 23*(4), 241–249. doi:10.3747/co.23.2942

Kunyk, D. (2015). Substance use disorders among registered nurses: Prevalence, risks and perceptions in a disciplinary jurisdiction. *Journal of Nursing Management, 23*, 54–64. doi:10.1111/jonm.12081

Kunyk, D., Inness, M., Reisdorfere, E., Morris, H., & Chambers, T. (2016). Help seeking by health professionals for addiction: A mixed studies review. *International Journal of Nursing Studies, 60*, 200–215. doi:10.1016/j.inurstu.2016.05.001

Kunyk, D., Milner, M., & Overend, A. (2016). Disciplining virtue: Investigating the discourses of opioid addiction in nursing. *Nursing Inquiry, 23*(4), 315–326. doi:10.1111/nin.121444

Larimer, M. E., Kilmer, J. R., & Whiteside, U. (2011). College student drinking. In C. Cavacuiti (Ed.), *Principles of addiction medicine: The essentials* (pp. 177–180). Philadelphia, PA: Lippincott Williams & Wilkins.

Manuel, D. G., Perez, R., Sanmartin, C., Taljaard, M., Hennessy, D., Wilson, K., ... Rosella, L. C. (2016). Measuring burden of unhealthy behaviours using a multivariable predictive approach: Life expectancy lost in Canada attributable to smoking, alcohol, physical inactivity, and diet. *PLoS Medicine, 13*(8), 31002082. doi:10.1371/journal.ped.1002082

McLellan, A. T., Lewis, D., O'Brien, C., & Kleber, H. (2000). Drug dependence, a chronic medical illness: Implications for treatment, insurance, and outcomes evaluation. *Journal of the American Medical Association, 284*(13), 1689–1695.

McLellann, A. T., Skipper, G. S., Campbell, M., & DuPont, R. L. (2008). Five year outcomes in a cohort study of physicians treated for substance use disorders in the United States. *BMJ, 337*, a2038.

Merikangas, K. R., Conway, K. P., Swendsen, J., Febo, J., Dierker, L., Brunetto, W., ... Canino, G. (2009). Substance use and behaviour disorders in Puerto Rican youth: A migrant family study. *Journal of Epidemiology and Community Health, 63*(4), 310–316.

Miller, W. R., & Rollnick, S. (2002). *Motivational interviewing: Preparing people for change*. New York, NY: Guilford Press.

National Institute on Drug Abuse (NIDA). (2005a). *Research report series: Inhalant abuse*. Publication Number 05–3818. Bethesda, MD: Author.

National Institute on Drug Abuse (NIDA). (2005b). *Research report: Heroin: Abuse and addiction*. NIH Publication Number 05–4165. Bethesda, MD: Author.

National Institute on Drug Abuse (NIDA). (2009). *Research report: Cocaine: Abuse and addiction*. NIH Publication Number 09–4166. Bethesda, MD: Author.

National Institute on Drug Abuse (NIDA). (2012). *Principles of drug addiction treatment: A research-based guide* (3rd ed.). Rockville, MD: Author.

National Institute on Drug Abuse (NIDA). (2016a). *Drug facts: Synthetic cathinones ("bath salts")*. Retrieved from www.drugabuse.ov/publications/drugfacts/synthetic-cathinones-bath-salts

National Institute on Drug Abuse (NIDA). (2016b). *Drug facts—Fentanyl*. Retrieved from https://www.drugabuse.gov/publications/drugfacts/fentanyl

Rehm, J., Ballunas, D., Brochu, S., Fischer, B., Gnam, W., Patra, J., ... Taylor, B. (2006). *The costs of substance abuse in Canada 2002*. Ottawa, ON: Canadian Centre on Substance Abuse.

Reid, J. L., Hammond, D., Rynard, V. L., & Burkhalter, R. (2015). *Tobacco use in Canada: Patterns and trends, 2015 edition*. Waterloo, ON: Propel Centre for Population Health Impact, University of Waterloo.

Rice, V. H., Hartmann-Boyce, J., & Stead, L. F. (2013). Nursing interventions for smoking cessation. *Cochrane Database of Systematic Reviews, 8*, CD001188. doi:10.1002/14651858.pub4

Robinson, M. (July 15, 2015). *Gone but not forgotten: 100,000 Toronto library books outstanding*. The Star. Retrieved from https://www.thestar.com/news/gta/2015/07/15/gone-but-not-forgotten-100000-toronto-library-books-outstanding.html

Shield, K. D., Rylett, M., Gmel, G., Keho-Chan, G., & Rehm, J. (2013). Global alcohol exposure estimates by country, territory and region for 2005—A contribution to the Comparative Risk Assessment for the 2010 Global Burden of Disease study. *Addiction, 108*, 912–922.

Simkin, D. R. (2014). Neurobiology of addiction from a developmental perspective. In R. K. Ries, D. A. Fiellin, S. C. Miller, & R. Saitz (Eds.), *The ASAM principles of addiction medicine* (5th ed., pp. 1580–1600). Philadelphia, PA: Wolters Kluwer.

Sproule, B., Brands, B., Li, S., & Catz-Biro, L. (2009). Changing patterns in opioid addiction. *Canadian Family Physician, 55*(1), 68–69.

Swendsen, J., & Le Moal, M. (2011). Individual vulnerability to addiction. *Annals of the New York Academy of Sciences, 1216*, 73–85.

Tetrault, J. M., & O'Connor, P. G. (2014). Management of opioids intoxication and withdrawal. In R. K. Ries, D. A. Fiellin, S. C. Miller, & R. Saitz

(Eds.), *The ASAM principles of addiction medicine* (5th ed., pp. 668–684). Philadelphia, PA: Wolters Kluwer.

Tupperman, L., & Wanner, K. (2012). *Problem gambling in Canada.* Don Mills, ON: Oxford University Press.

U.S. Department of Health and Human Services. (2010). *How tobacco smoke causes disease: The biology and behavioral basis for smoking-attributable disease: A report of the Surgeon General.* Atlanta, GA: U.S. Department of Health and Human Services, Centers for Disease Control and Prevention, National Center for Chronic Disease Prevention and Health Promotions, Office on Smoking and Health.

Verster, J. C. (2014). Caffeine consumption in children, adolescents and adults. *Current Drug Abuse Reviews, 7*(3), 133–134.

Volkow, N., & McLellan, T. (2016). Opioid abuse in chronic pain—Misconceptions and mitigation strategies. *New England Journal of Medicine, 374*(13), 1253–1264. doi:10.1056/NEJMra1507771

Volkow, N. D., & Warren, K. R. (2014). Drug addiction: The neurobiology of behavior gone awry. In R. K. Ries, D. A. Fiellin, S. C. Miller, & R. Saitz (Eds.), *The ASAM principles of addiction medicine* (5th ed., pp. 3–18). Philadelphia, PA: Wolters Kluwer.

West, R. (2006). *Theory of addiction.* Oxford, UK: Blackwell Publishing/Addiction Press.

Willembring, M. J. (2011). Treatment of heavy drinking and alcohol use disorders. In C. Cavacuiti (Ed.), *Principles of addiction medicine: The essentials* (pp. 105–109). Philadelphia, PA: Lippincott Williams & Wilkins.

World Health Organization. (2007). *International statistical classification of disease and related health problems* (10th ed.). Geneva, IL: WHO Press.

World Health Organization. (2009). *Global health risks. Morality and burden of diseases attributable to selected major risks.* Geneva, IL: WHO Press.

World Health Organization. (2015). *WHO report on the global tobacco epidemic, 2015. Raising taxes on tobacco.* Geneva, IL: WHO Press.

Wunsch, M. J., & Weaver, M. F. (2011). Alcohol and other drug use during pregnancy: Management of mother and child. In C. Cavacuiti (Ed.), *Principles of addiction medicine: The essentials* (pp. 448–453). Philadelphia, PA: Lippincott Williams & Wilkins.

Zgierska, A., & Fleming, M. F. (2011). Screening and brief intervention. In C. Cavacuiti (Ed.), *Principles of addiction medicine: The essentials* (pp. 81–86). Philadelphia, PA: Lippincott Williams & Wilkins.

27 Personality Disorders and Disruptive, Impulse-Control, and Conduct Disorders

Wendy Austin

Adapted from chapters "Personality and Impulse Control Disorders" by Stephen Van Slyke and by Barbara, J. Limandri, and Mary Ann Boyd

LEARNING OBJECTIVES

After studying this chapter, you will be able to:

- Discuss the concepts of personality and personality trait.
- Describe what is known about the aetiology of personality disorders.
- Identify the common features of personality disorders.
- Name components of (mal)adaptive personality functioning that can be used to describe the severity of a personality disorder.
- Distinguish among the three clusters of personality disorders.
- Formulate nursing assessment and interventions for clients with specific personality disorders.
- Apply the nursing process to clients with borderline personality disorder.
- Identify concerns within the nurse–client relationship common to caring for clients with personality disorders.
- Name the disruptive, impulse control, and conduct disorders and describe intermittent explosive disorder, pyromania, and kleptomania.

KEY TERMS

- affective instability • attachment • communication triad • dialectical behaviour therapy (DBT) • dichotomous thinking • dissociation • emotional dysregulation • emotional vulnerability • emotions • identity diffusion • impulsivity • invalidating environment • kleptomania • metacognition • parasuicidal behaviour • projective identification • pyromania • reframing • self-identity • separation–individuation • skills groups • temperament • thought stopping • traits • trichotillomania

KEY CONCEPTS

- personality • personality disorder • personality traits

The concept of personality appears simple but is very complex. Historically, the term personality was derived from the Greek *persona*, the theatrical mask used by dramatic players. Originally, the term had the connotation of a projected pretense or illusion. With time, the connotation changed from being an external surface representation to the internal traits of an individual.

Today, personality is conceptualized as a complex pattern of psychological characteristics that, while not easily altered, can change and evolve across the lifespan as inherited attributes interact with environmental factors and experience (Newton-Howes, Clark, & Chanen, 2015). They are largely outside the person's awareness. Such characteristics include the individual's specific style of perceiving, thinking, and feeling about self, others, and the environment. These styles, known as **traits**, are similar and coherent across many different social or personal situations and are expressed in almost every facet of functioning. Intrinsic and pervasive, they emerge from a complicated interaction of genetics, neurobiologic dispositions, psychosocial experiences, and environmental situations that ultimately

make up the individual's distinctive personality (Widiger, 2012).

Psychologists are exploring personality from biologic, cognitive, and social perspectives (Maruszewski, Fajkowska, & Eysenck, 2010). While various theories about personality have evolved, the approach to understanding human personality through analyzing traits, as the attributes of individuals that consistently shape their ideas and actions, has been taken since Hippocrates' description of **temperament**. Hippocrates defined four types of temperament, each due to the dominance of one of four bodily humours: sanguine (blood), melancholic (black bile), choleric (yellow bile), and phlegmatic (phlegm) (Friedman & Schustack, 2012). In contemporary times, temperament is considered as the recognizable, distinctive, and relatively stable pattern of individual differences that are evident early in life. The empirically developed Big Five or five-factor model identifies key traits as **O**penness (to experience), **C**onscientiousness, **E**xtraversion, **A**greeableness, and **N**euroticism (emotional instability) (Friedman & Schustack, 2012). (Hint: Use the mnemonic **OCEAN** to

BOX 27.1 Personality and Video Game Playing Style

Researchers used the Big Five Inventory (BFI), which measures personality traits based on the five-factor model (FFM), to examine the personality dimensions of 1,210 World of Warcraft (WoW) players, all 18 years of age. WoW is the longest running multiplayer online role-playing video game involving a virtual world in which players have the choice of abilities for their character avatar (e.g., race, specialization) and of faction (Horde or Alliance). The researchers' hypothesis was that players choose their character based in part on their own personality. Using multivariate statistical analysis, they found a connection between BFI personality characteristics and participants' style of play (player versus environment, player versus player, role-play, or player versus player role-play) and the traits of extraversion, conscientiousness, neuroticism, and openness. No support was found for antisocial behaviour or aggressiveness when the personality scores of WoW players were compared with markers of antisocial personality factors. There were gender differences found among the factors of agreeableness, openness, and neuroticism with females scoring higher than males on these traits.

Bean, A., & Groth-Marnat, G. (2016). Video gamers and personality: A five-factor model to understand game playing style. *Psychology of Popular Media Culture, 5*(1), 27–38.

remember them.) A person who rates high in openness, for instance, is curious, actively seeks experiences, and is open to new ideas; one who is high in conscientiousness is organized, self-directed, and persevering. Extraversion is about the amount and intensity of an individual's need for activity, stimulation, and social interaction, while agreeableness is about levels of helpfulness, altruism, and empathy. Neuroticism refers to the level of emotional adjustment; someone with a high level of neuroticism is vulnerable to stress and shows instability in emotional responses, such as anger or depressiveness (Widiger & Costa, 2013). See Box 27.1, *Personality and Video Game Playing Style.*

KEY CONCEPT

Personality is a complex pattern of characteristics, largely outside the person's awareness, that compose the individual's distinctive and enduring pattern of perceiving, feeling, thinking, coping, and behaving. The personality emerges from a complicated interaction of biologic dispositions, psychological experiences, and environmental situations.

KEY CONCEPT

Personality traits are persistent patterns of perceiving, thinking, feeling, and behaving that shape the way in which a person responds to the world. Key traits have been identified as openness to experience, conscientiousness, extraversion, agreeableness, and neuroticism.

■ PERSONALITY DISORDERS

No sharp division exists between normal and abnormal personality functioning. Instead, personalities may be viewed on a continuum from normal at one end to abnormal at the other. Many of the same processes involved in the development of a "normal" personality are responsible for the development of a personality disorder (PD). "Normality" involves being able to function autonomously and with competence, to be adaptive in relation to one's social environment, as well as being able to self-develop and experience contentment. Deficits in these are potential signs of psychopathology and may appear as among the core features of personality disorders: adaptive inflexibility, self-defeating pattern of behaviour, and lack of resilience under subjective stress (Millon, 2016). To receive a DSM-5 diagnosis of PD, an individual must demonstrate the criteria behaviours persistently and to such an extent that they impair the ability to function socially and occupationally (American Psychiatric Association [APA], 2013). In some people, the underlying thoughts, feelings, and behaviours may be intermittent and interfere interpersonally without obvious impairment. Instead of having a PD, the individual is said to have traits of the disorder. For immigrants who may be having difficulty learning new social and cultural behaviour patterns and adjusting to a new culture, the diagnosis of a PD is often delayed to after this adjustment period. It is highly unusual for children to be diagnosed with a PD. This was previously true for adolescents, as well. As there is evidence that persons with borderline personality disorder (BPD) can reveal significant signs of the disorder in adolescence and may be helped with early intervention, the diagnosis of BPD can be given to an adolescent (Ronningstam et al., 2014). Recognition of PDs in the older adult is important as a means of finding ways to improve the health of this age group. A lifespan approach to PDs is increasingly seen as necessary (Newton-Howes et al., 2015).

KEY CONCEPT

A **personality disorder** is diagnosed when the perceptions, emotion, cognition, and behaviour of an individual substantially deviates from cultural expectations in a persistent and inflexible way, causing distress or impairment (APA, 2013).

BOX 27.2 **Research for Best Practice**

MENTAL HEALTH NURSES' ATTITUDES, BEHAVIOUR, EXPERIENCE, AND KNOWLEDGE REGARDING ADULTS WITH BPD

Dickens, G. L., Lamont, E., & Gray, S. (2016). Mental health nurses' attitudes, behaviour, experience and knowledge regarding adults with a diagnosis of borderline personality disorder: Systematic, integrative literature review. Journal of Clinical Nursing, 25, 1848–1875. doi:10.1111/jocn.13202

Question: Are mental health (MH) nurses' responses to individuals with BPD problematic? If so, what are potential solutions that support change?

Method: Systematic, integrative review. Databases were searched for papers (including dissertations, theses, conference presentations, and government reports), describing mental health nurses' attitudes, behaviour, experience, and knowledge toward adults with BPD. From 279 studies, 40 studies (published 1989–2015 with 1/3 of studies in the last 5 years; conducted in 10 countries) met inclusion criteria. Analysis of qualitative ($n = 11$) and mixed method ($n = 3$) studies involved metasynthesis; quantitative studies ($n = 25$) analysis was informed by the theory of planned behaviour (predicts behaviour based on experience, emotional and cognitive attitudes,

and perceived self-efficacy). There was only one direct observation study.

Results: Knowledge and experiences varied widely, but clients with BPD are regarded by MH nurses as highly challenging. Relative to other professions, MH nurses' attitudes were more negative; relative to other diagnostic groups, attitudes were more negative toward clients with BPD and responses to them could be countertherapeutic. Consistent across studies was a desire for knowledge, training, and development opportunities in relation to BPD. A therapeutic framework to guide practice was regarded as important.

Implications for Practice: Solutions to nurses' issues regarding caring for individuals with BPD need to be developed and implemented. Promising solutions are theoretical and skill-related education regarding BPD for nurses, as well as an interdisciplinary team approach that includes an evidence-based therapeutic framework, clinical supervision, and peer support.

Changing lifelong personality patterns is difficult and requires much understanding and support. Other people, however, including health care professionals, can become impatient with persons who have a PD or traits of a PD, expecting them to have control over their behaviour and change a way of being in the world that is less than optimal (see Box 27.2). Lack of knowledge about PDs, as well as the associated stigma, can affect both treatment-seeking behaviour and referrals for help (Sheehan, Nieweglowsik, & Corrigan, 2016).

Most individuals do not seek treatment for a PD; nurses will encounter these clients when they require treatment for other health problems or want help for symptoms such as hopelessness, anxiety, or relationship problems (Leahy & McGinn, 2012). Persons with BPD, however, may be frequent users of health services, comprising up to 20% of hospital admissions and outpatient referrals (Bateman, Gunderson, & Mulder, 2015), as they can require urgent care for self-harm and suicidal behaviours, as well as ongoing therapy for **emotional dysregulation** and interpersonal and behavioural problems. As BPD and avoidant personality disorder (AVPD) have a high comorbidity with depression and substance-related and anxiety disorders, individuals with these PDs seek treatment for these disorders (Ronningstam et al., 2014).

Understanding PDs is necessary to health care practice: it is not uncommon, significantly affects quality of life and overall health, can lead to premature mortality, affects the client–health professional relationship, and adds to the economic costs of health services. Unfortunately, within health care, the label of PD may be used to describe clients without their symptoms meeting diagnostic criteria, and it is too often used in a disparaging way, "more a term of abuse than a diagnosis" (Tyrer, Reed, & Crawford, 2015, p. 717). Research indicates that the presence of PD can predict the occurrence of later anxiety and depression, an indication of the need to include PDs in global studies of mental health (Moran et al., 2016). The contribution of personality disorders as contributors to ill health in a population and to the global burden of disease remains, however, insufficiently recognized.

When negative attitudes exist within health care services toward the diagnosis of PD, it can affect facilitation of clients' recovery and the very concept of recovery in terms of a PD. Recovery involves having hope, understanding one's capabilities and challenges, achieving a positive sense of self, connecting meaningfully with others, and engaging in life (see Chapter 2). Research exploring the experience of recovery for persons with a PD found that facilitators of recovery for them are also their core vulnerabilities: interpersonal relationships and social interaction. Participants described tensions between an alienating outside world and an isolating, but safe, inner world. Researchers concluded that the process of recovering involved discovering a sense of self that could exist in both worlds. Health care services can play a role in supporting this recovery process (Gillard, Turner, & Heffgen, 2015).

Common Features of Personality Disorders

The PD diagnosis is based on pervasive, maladaptive perceiving, thinking, feeling, and behaviour that have manifested in an individual's functioning across situations since adolescence or early adulthood (APA, 2013). Maladaptation in metacognition, or ways of perceiving and interpreting self, others, and events, of emotional responses, of interpersonal functioning, and of impulse control, is described below.

Impaired Metacognition

A significant, defining ability of the human mind is the capacity to take account of one's own and other's mental states in order to understand and predict behaviour (Fonagy, 1991). In personality disorders, there is evidence that this capacity, termed metacognition, is impaired (Dimaggio & Brüne, 2016; Fonagy, 1991). **Metacognition** (also termed "mentalizing" or "mindreading") is the ability to consider and identify one's own state of mind and that of others, reflect upon these mental states, deliberate upon their accuracy, and then apply this knowledge to problem solving. It allows us to form coherent and stable understandings of ourselves and others, to separate facts from fiction, to consider other persons' points of view, and to question our own. If we have problems in doing this, then we may respond to others and events in dysfunctional ways. Imagine an emergency nurse returning home after her team has tried and failed to save the lives of a young couple in an automobile collision. Her new roommate greets her with a cheery, "How's it going?" and she responds, "Okay, I guess." in a tired, tearful tone. A reply from the roommate, "Great! You can cook tonight. I know it's my turn but I am not in the mood," may reveal that the roommate has problems in recognizing complex emotions in others. Other individuals may have difficulty in being aware of their own mental states or in their ability to question their beliefs about others. In different PDs, different aspects of metacognition can be impaired (Moroni et al., 2016).

Maladaptive Emotional Response

Emotions are psychophysiologic reactions that define a person's mood and can be categorized as negative (e.g., anger, fright, anxiety, guilt, shame, sadness, envy, jealousy, disgust), positive (e.g., happiness, pride, relief, love), and neutral (e.g., hope, compassion, empathy, sympathy, contentment). Emotions can affect one's ability to learn and function by affecting one's memory and how one accesses and stores information; it can

affect one's ability to accurately perceive the environment. Dysfunction in emotional regulation (over or under emotional arousal or both) is characteristic of some PDs. For instance, individuals with BPD have been found to react to a sense of social rejection with greater than normal emotional intensity (McMain, Boritz, & Leybman, 2015), while the affect of individuals with AVPD appears inhibited as they have difficulty recognizing and communicating their emotions (Moroni et al., 2016). Individuals with narcissistic personality disorder (NPD) may appear unaffected by losses that would cause deep grief in others. If the loss, however, is of a person or situation that is important to the self-esteem of the individual with NPD, then a strong emotional distress can occur (Ronningstam, 2017).

Impaired Self-Identity and Interpersonal Functioning

Self-identity is central to the normal development of personality. **Self-identity** includes an integration of social and occupational roles and affiliations, self-attributed personality traits, attitudes about gender roles, beliefs about sexuality and intimacy, long-term goals, political ideologies, and religious beliefs. Without an adequately formed identity, an individual's goal-directed behaviour is impaired, and interpersonal relationships are disrupted. Abilities, limitations, and goals are shaped by one's identity. In personality disorders, self-identity is often impaired or incomplete.

Impulsivity and Destructive Behaviour

Individuals with PDs may come to the attention of mental health clinicians because their impulsive behaviour results in negative consequences to others or themselves. They seem unable to consider the consequences of their actions before acting on their impulses. For example, an individual may feel rage towards another and lack skills to resist the impulse to attack that person physically, even though this action may be punished. Nurses working in psychiatric inpatient settings associate **impulsivity** with unpredictability and thus with challenges in the provision of a safe milieu.

Severity of Disorder

Five reliable, clinically relevant components of (mal) adaptive personality functioning have been identified in a series of research studies (Verheul et al., 2008). These components and their facets are as follows:

- Self-control (stable self-image, self-reflective, emotional and aggressive regulation)
- Identity integration (enjoyment, purposefulness, self-respect, frustration tolerance)
- Relational capacities (intimacy, enduring relationships, feeling recognized)
- Responsibility (trustworthiness, responsible industry)
- Social concordance (respect, cooperation)

The components are associated with the severity of the personality pathology, and using the measure that evolved from the research, the Severity Indices of Personality Problems (SIPP-118), long-term changes in the functioning of a client can be determined (Verheul et al., 2008).

Diagnosis of Personality Disorders

Personality disorders are delineated in the American Psychological Association's (APA) *Diagnostic and Statistical Manual of Mental Disorders (DSM)* (APA, 2013). There are 10 PDs recognized as psychiatric diagnoses in the *DSM-5*, organized into three clusters (APA):

- Cluster A: paranoid (PPD), schizoid (SZPD), and schizotypal (STPD)
- Cluster B: antisocial (ASPD), borderline (BPD), narcissistic (NPD), and histrionic (HPD)
- Cluster C: avoidant (AVPD), dependent (DPD), and obsessive–compulsive (OCPD)

These PDs are discussed in this chapter. The disorders within a cluster have some similarities. Cluster A disorders, for instance, have social aversion in common; those in cluster B, dysregulation in emotion and behaviour; and in cluster C, fearfulness. BPD is highlighted in the chapter because it is severely incapacitating; its treatment is challenging, and its symptoms may provoke in the clinician negative reactions that interfere with the ability to provide effective care. Disruptive, impulse control, and conduct disorders, which commonly coexist with other mental disorders, are summarized at the end of the chapter. For the official APA diagnostic criteria of disorders in this chapter, please refer to the DSM-5.

An alternative approach to the diagnosis of personality disorders was developed during the work for the *DSM-5*. This alternative dimensional approach characterizes PDs by impairments in personality functioning (self [i.e., identity, self-direction] and interpersonal [i.e., empathy and intimacy]) and by pathologic traits (negative affectivity, detachment, antagonism, disinhibition, psychoticism). It is available in Section III of the *DSM-5*. This alternative model for PDs is regarded by many as innovative and is being explored through research studies (Waugh et al., 2017).

Epidemiology

While Canadian prevalence data are lacking for PDs, the reported prevalence of PDs is very similar across studies. In Statistics Canada's *Health State Descriptions for Canadians* (Langlois, Samokhvalov, Rehm, Spence, & Gorber, 2012, modified 2013), it is estimated that 6% to 15% of the population are affected by PDs. Among the most common PDs are OCPD (7.7%), AVPD (6.6%), PPD (5.6%), BPD (5.4%), and STPD (5.2%). Comorbidity between PDs is common. There is some consensus across studies of clinical populations that BPD is among the most frequent PD seen. Among persons in substance abuse clinics, prisons, or other forensic settings, up to 70% are reported to have ASPD (APA, 2013).

Gender does not appear to affect the prevalence of PD as a whole. Men, however, are much more likely to be diagnosed with ASPD than are women (Oltmanns & Powers, 2012). ASPD maybe underdiagnosed in women for such reasons as the emphasis on aggression against people or animals in conduct disorder (and evidence of conduct disorder before age 15 is required for an ASPD diagnosis), or that ASPD manifests differently in women, who are more likely to receive diagnoses of somatization (see Chapter 24) or histrionic disorders (discussed later in this chapter). It has been commonly assumed that BPD is more common in women, but higher prevalence rates among women are considered an artifact of sampling in clinical settings: women are more likely to seek treatment. The prevalence of disorders for which the affected individual rarely seeks help, such as pyromania, is particularly difficult to estimate.

Aetiology

The aetiology of PDs and of the disruptive, impulse control, and conduct disorders remains to some extent undetermined. A basic assumption underlying this category of mental disorders is that they evolve within the development of an individual's personality. What changes a normal personality to a disordered one might be genetic, epigenetic, neurobiologic, trauma and stress induced, environmental, or an interaction of such factors. Research is indicating that personality traits, evident in childhood, are about 50% inheritable, with the expression of an individual's genotype through interaction with the environment and unique life experiences (phenotype) composing the remainder. This indicates that personality traits are more plastic (i.e., changeable) than once believed and supports the potential effectiveness of clinical interventions (Newton-Howes et al., 2015).

Temperament is believed to be shaped by physiologic, neurobehavioural, genetic, epigenetic, and cultural influences. As temperament is considered at the core of personality, research regarding differences in temperament primarily utilizes the five-factor model of personality (Putnam & Gartstein, 2017). See Box 27.3 for research on test testing and temperament.

The influence of temperament and environment on the development of PDs is being explored. For example, a prospective, longitudinal study with adolescents explored temperament and maltreatment in predicting the emergence of BPD and ASPD. Measures of temperament, maltreatment, BPD, and ASPD symptoms were completed by 11- to 13-year-old participants (*n* = 245), most of whom (*n* = 206) were assessed again in 2 years. Childhood neglect was found to be a significant predictor of an increase in BPD symptoms, while childhood abuse predicted an increase in ASPD symptoms. As well, findings suggested that high capacity for interpersonal affiliation and self-regulation may protect children from

BOX 27.3 Research for Best Practice

TEMPERAMENT AND TEST ANXIETY

Liewa, J. Lench, H. C., Kao, G., Yeh, Y. C., & Kwoka, O. (2014). Avoidance temperament and social-evaluative threat in college students' math performance: A mediation model of math and test anxiety. Anxiety, Stress, & Coping, 27(6), 650–661. doi:http://dx.doi.org/10.1080/10615806.2014.910303

Objectives: To examine the role of avoidance temperament (i.e., fear and behavioural inhibition) and social-evaluative threat (i.e., fear of academic failure) on standardized test performance in university students.

Method: Undergraduate university students (*n* = 184) were assessed on temperamental fear and behavioural inhibition and then given 15 minutes to complete a standardized math test. After the test, students provided data on evaluative threat and their math performance

(scores on standardized college entrance exam and average grades in college math courses).

Results: Avoidance temperament was positively correlated with social-evaluative threat and low standardized math test scores, but not with grades in math courses.

Implications: Interventions targeting emotion regulation, stress management, and appropriate threat assessment for students at risk for test anxiety (and thus underperformance) may be useful in assisting those students to achieve better on standardized tests. More accurate assessment of such students' knowledge could be achieved if their behavioural inhibition in test taking is addressed. These results have implications for nursing students' preparation for the NCLEX.

---

developing such psychopathology in the presence of an adverse environment (Jovev et al., 2013). A challenge in determining the aetiology of PDs is their potential overlap with other mental disorders. For example, AVPD can overlap with social anxiety disorder (social phobia), and clients with diagnoses of social phobia may also met the criteria for AVPD.

Emotional and behavioural self-control problems characterize the disruptive, impulse control, and conduct disorders, but the underlying causes of these problems vary greatly, even among individuals with the same diagnosis (APA, 2013). The risk factors for them may be temperamental, genetic, epigenetic, physiologic, environmental, or an interaction among such factors. Further research is necessary to add clarity regarding the aetiologies of these and PDs.

Treatment of Personality Disorders

Psychological and psychosocial interventions are the primary approaches to the treatment of PDs, with psychopharmacology used adjunctively and usually on a short-term basis for specific symptoms. The overall goal is not to change an individual's fundamental personality but to help them build on their strengths and minimize problematic effects of their disorder (Lyness, 2016). The aims of treatment can include the reduction of life-threatening symptoms, the improvement of distressing mental state symptoms, greater social and interpersonal adjustment, and the acquisition of life skills (Bateman et al., 2015). Factors outside of therapy such as the client's circumstances, resources, life events, and cultural background can have strong effects on recovery;

it is important for therapists to recognize and ally with such factors (Pederson, 2015; Stone, 2016). It needs to be acknowledged that "the evidence-base for effective treatment of personality disorders is insufficient" (Bateman et al., 2015, p. 735) and that obtaining access to such treatment can be very difficult (Ronningstam et al., 2014). Selected approaches to psychotherapy used in the treatment of PDs are described below. Research supports the utility of each approach, but no evidence exists to date to determine one as superior to the others (Stone, 2016).

Dialectical Behaviour Therapy

Dialectical behaviour therapy (DBT), developed by Marsha Linehan (1993a) to treat individuals experiencing suicidality and self-injury, uses cognitive–behavioural therapy (CBT) strategies but also draws on Zen principles, dialectical philosophy, and behavioural science. DBT consists of four treatment components: individual therapy, group skills training, telephone coaching, and therapist consultation teams (i.e., therapy for the therapist). A variety of interventions including "mindfulness practice, skills training, relationship strategies, cognitive and behavioural techniques, and environmental interventions" are used (Pederson, 2015, p. 2). (See Chapter 13 for information on cognitive–behavioural techniques and mindfulness.)

For DBT to be effective, therapists and coaches must work with clients as partners and be willing to focus on interconnected behaviours (e.g., parasuicidal and substance abuse) and not a single diagnosis. Clients actively participate in treatment by collecting information about their own behaviours to recognize patterns, identifying behaviours to change, and working with the therapists to change them. Problem-solving, exposure techniques (i.e., gradual exposure to cues that set off aversive emotions), skill training, contingency management (i.e., reinforcement of positive behaviour), and cognitive modification are core procedures.

Skills groups are an integral part of DBT in which members practice emotional regulation, interpersonal effectiveness, mindfulness skills, and distress tolerance. Skills taught to manage intense, labile moods involve helping the client to label and analyze the context of the emotion and to use strategies to reduce emotional vulnerability. Learning to observe and describe emotions without judging or blocking them allows the individual to experience emotions without stimulating secondary feelings that cause more distress. For example, describing the emotion of anger without judging it as being "bad" can eliminate feelings of guilt that lead to self-injury.

Interpersonal effectiveness skills include the development of assertiveness and problem-solving skills within an interpersonal context. Clients are given strategies to meet their goals in a particular situation while at the same time maintaining relationships with others and sustaining their self-respect. Distress tolerance skills involve learning to tolerate and accept distress as a part of normal life. Self-management skills focus on learning how to control, manage, or change behaviours, thoughts, or emotional responses to events.

Cognitive–Behavioural Therapy

The principles and techniques of CBT are addressed in Chapter 13 of this text. In application to the treatment of PDs, CBT focuses on "clinical assessment," "cognitive conceptualization," "technical interventions," and "the therapeutic relationship" (David & Freeman, 2015, p. 16). For some PDs, such a ASPD, clinical assessment will involve not only a clinical interview and self-report psychological tests but also psychological tests based on clinicians' or relevant others' assessments and data. The relationship with the client will be a key component that includes modelling for change, as well as collaboration and empathy (David & Freeman).

Mentalization-Based Treatment

Mentalization-based treatment (MBT) originally was developed to treat clients with BPD in day hospital settings, but MBT is now used to treat a range of PDs, including ASPD. Mentalization is the necessary, everyday human ability to recognize and interpret one's own and others' thoughts, feelings, and intensions. It influences how one acts and reacts in the world. The importance of our ability to infer the meaning of our own and others' mental states needs to be recognized, as is the reality that it is not difficult to be mistaken. This ability requires a capacity to be inquisitive, to separate fact from fiction, and to learn from others' perspectives and behaviour. The capacity to mentalize evolves within one's early, childhood relationships and is affected by caregivers' ability to validate the child's mental states and to convey understanding, as well as by the quality

of the child's social environment (Bateman & Fonagy, 2016). An experimental study of the mentalization ability of individuals with BPD found that while they were equal to control group members on simple mentalization tasks, deficits became apparent as the complexity of the tasks increased. Childhood experiences of punishment were negatively correlated to mentalization ability (i.e., as the level of trauma increased, mentalization skills decreased) for both the BPD and control groups (Petersen, Brakoulias, & Langdon, 2016). The term, "mentalization," is sometimes used interchangeably with "metacognition"; there is, however, an emphasis on the role of early attachments in the work on mentalization (Dimaggio & Brüne, 2016; Fonagy, 1991).

The focus of MBT is assisting clients through a therapeutic process to learn about their mental states and then to explore how errors may lead to difficulties. Treatment involves engaging the client in the treatment process from assessment and diagnosis to treatment termination. It includes the identification of problems that might affect treatment, formulation of a hierarchy of therapeutic aims, the addressing of social and behavioural problems, planning for crisis, and monitoring of outcomes. Psychoeducation is important to the MBT process, as is the combination of individual and group therapy (Bateman & Fonagy, 2016).

Metacognitive Interpersonal Therapy

In this approach, as in most other psychotherapies, the therapeutic relationship is seen as the ground for validating clients' experiences and facilitating positive change. Initially, the therapist will assess clients' capacity for sharing a narrative of their life experience and their metacognitive abilities and then use the assessment to modulate each client's metacognitive interpersonal therapy (MIT) experience. Autobiographical details from clients focuses therapy on their specific problems in emotional and cognitive awareness, revealing the way beliefs triggered in specific life episodes have led to particular responses. Maladaptive interpersonal schema can then be explored and changed. Clients practice new behaviours and gain a sense of control over their actions (Dimaggio et al., 2017). There is some nongeneralizable evidence that MIT can be effective. For example, a case study of three non-BPD, non-ASPD clients who completed 2 years of weekly MIT found that at 3 months post therapy, each showed overall improvement in symptoms and emotional regulation (Dimaggio et al., 2017).

■ SPECIFIC PERSONALITY DISORDERS

Cluster A Disorders

Paranoid Personality Disorder

The most prominent features of paranoid personality disorder (PPD) are mistrust of others and the desire to avoid relationships in which one is not in control. Individuals with PPD are suspicious and guarded. They are consistently mistrustful of others' motives, even those of relatives and close friends. Actions of others are often misinterpreted as deception, deprecation, and betrayal, especially regarding fidelity or trustworthiness of a spouse or friend (Millon, Millon, Meagher, Grossman, & Ramnath, 2004). Minor innocuous incidents are often misinterpreted as having sinister or hidden meaning, and suspicions are magnified into major distortions of reality. People with paranoid personalities distance themselves from others and can be outwardly argumentative and abrasive; internally, they may hold private hopes of being understood and feel powerless, fearful, and vulnerable (Hayward, 2007). Imagine living with the belief that you can trust no one and that there are some persons or organizations actively "out to get you?" (Note: the PPD diagnosis excludes psychotic symptoms, like paranoid delusions and hallucinations.)

Other hallmark features of PPD are persistent ideas of self-importance (i.e., important enough to be the target of the harmful intentions of others) and the tendency to be rigid and controlled. The individual wants to appear controlled and objective, yet often reacts emotionally, displaying signs of nervousness, anger, envy, and jealousy. Fearful, the person will be hypervigilant to any environmental changes. Essentially, PPD is "a stable pattern of nonpsychotic paranoid behaviour" (Hopwood & Thomas, 2012, p. 582). If help is sought, it is unlikely that it will be from mental health professionals but rather from a resource, such as the police, that the person with PPD believes could stop the harm others are doing.

Demographically, PPD is associated with low income and disadvantaged populations; stress, trauma, and neglect appear to be causative factors. In clinical populations, PPD is a predictor of aggressive behaviour; in the forensic field, it is associated with excessive litigation, stalking, and violent behaviour (Lee, 2017). Narcissistic, avoidant, and obsessive–compulsive PDs can coexist with PPD, as can generalized anxiety disorder, mood disorders, and schizophrenia (Millon et al., 2004). Paranoid ideas can develop following a brain injury and in Alzheimer's dementia (Lee, 2017). Research on PPD is scarce, with the reluctance of persons with PPD to participate in studies a likely factor. PPD is difficult to treat; it is primarily psychotherapy, but the ongoing suspicion and mistrust experienced by the client can severely hamper therapeutic alliance and process. Cognitive analytic therapy (CAT) has been shown to be an effective, structured intervention in a single case study of a client with PPD, reported in depth by Kellett and Hardy (2014).

There remains controversy regarding PPD as a unique diagnostic construct. It is questioned whether or not paranoid symptoms are unique; they may be fully explained by normal personality traits or psychotic disorders (Hopwood & Thomas, 2012). Mistrust in persons (e.g., refugees and migrants) whose experiences have created mistrust should not be confused with that seen in PPD.

Nursing Care

Nurses are most likely to see these clients for other health problems but will need to formulate nursing diagnoses based on the client's underlying suspiciousness. An assessment of individuals with PPD reveals disturbed or illogical thoughts that demonstrate the misinterpretation of environmental stimuli. When making a nursing diagnosis of disturbed thought processes, it needs to be supported by assessment data. For example, an individual with PPD might become convinced that his or her partner was having an affair with a neighbour based on the observation that they both left for work at the same time each morning. Even if following them never revealed any sign of them together, the person may continue to believe, without question, that they were having an affair.

Because of their difficulty with developing relationships, individuals with PPD are often socially isolated and lack social support systems. The nursing diagnosis of social isolation, however, is not appropriate for the person with PPD because the defining characteristics of feelings of aloneness, rejection, desire for contact with people, and insecurity in social situations are not met.

Nursing interventions based on the establishment of a nurse–client relationship are difficult to implement because of the person's mistrust. A professional, matter-of-fact approach and the creation of a nonthreatening environment in which the client can feel as secure as possible are helpful. Nurses must ensure that their own response to a client who does not readily accept them as trustworthy does not further impede relationship building. If a trusting relationship is established, the nurse helps the individual identify specific problematic areas, such as getting along with particular others or improving workplace behaviour. Through therapeutic techniques such as acceptance and reflection, as well as recognition by the nurse of the ramifications for client of his or her view of the world (e.g., what it feels like to believe one's spouse is having an affair), the nurse and the client can examine a problematic area to gain another view of the situation. Changing thought patterns takes time. Client outcomes are evaluated in terms of small changes in thinking and behaviour. Although antipsychotics might be considered in its treatment, such as when there is escalating paranoia (Lyness, 2016), no medications have been found to be specifically effective in treating PPD (Silk & Feurino, 2012).

Schizoid Personality Disorder

Individuals with schizoid personality disorder (SZPD) are expressively impassive and interpersonally unengaged (Millon et al., 2004). They tend to be unable to experience the joyful and pleasurable aspects of life. They are introverted and reclusive, and clinically they appear distant, aloof, apathetic, and emotionally detached. They have difficulties making friends, seem uninterested in social activities, and appear to gain little satisfaction in personal relationships. In fact, they appear to be incapable of forming social relationships. Interests are directed at objects, things, and abstractions. As children, they engaged primarily in solitary activities, such as stamp collecting, computer games, electronic equipment, or academic pursuits such as mathematics or engineering. In addition, there seems to be a cognitive deficit characterized by obscure thought processes, particularly about social matters. Communication with others is confused and lacks focus. These individuals reveal minimum introspection and self-awareness, and interpersonal experiences are described in a very mechanical way. The low incidence of SZPD diagnoses without a comorbid diagnosis of another PD has raised questions about the usefulness of SZPD as a PD diagnostic category; it is argued that it should be omitted from future classifications of PDs (Hummelen, Pedersen, Wilberg, & Karterud, 2015).

Nursing Care

Impaired social interactions and chronic low self-esteem are typical diagnoses of individuals with SZPD. Major treatment goals are to enhance the experience of pleasure, prevent social isolation, and increase emotional responsiveness to others. Because these individuals often lack customary social skills, social skills training is useful in enhancing their ability to relate in interpersonal situations. The primary focus is to increase the person's ability to experience enjoyment. The nurse balances interventions between encouraging enough social activity that prevents the individual from retreating to a fantasy world and too much social activity that becomes intolerable. Because persons with SZPD typically shy away from interactions, establishing a therapeutic relationship can be challenging; patience in achieving a sense of relatedness is required (Hess, 2016). The evaluation of outcomes should be in terms of increasing the client's feelings of satisfaction with solitary activities.

Schizotypal Personality Disorder

People with the schizotypal personality disorder (STPD) are characterized by a pattern of social and interpersonal deficits. They do not form friendships easily and may be close only to first-degree relatives. Their beliefs about their world are often inconsistent with their cultural norms and appear odd to others. Ideas of reference (i.e., incorrect interpretations of events as having special, personal meaning) are often present, as are unusual perceptual delusions and odd, circumstantial, and metaphorical thinking and speech. Mood is constricted or inappropriate, and there are excessive social anxieties of a paranoid character that do not diminish with familiarity. Appearance and behaviour can be characterized as eccentric, or peculiar. An avoidant behaviour pattern is usually exhibited. The requirement that five of nine *DSM* criteria need to be met for an STPD diagnosis

means that two individuals with STPD may share only one diagnostic feature (Kwapil & Barrantes-Vidal, 2012).

In the International Classification of Diseases, the schizotypal category is not classified as a PD, but as part of the spectrum of schizophrenia. A study of individuals with SZPD and STPD using structural magnetic resonance imaging found that, when compared with healthy individuals in a control group, persons with either SZPD or STPD had greater white matter volume in the superior area of the corona radiata, which may relate to the cognitive and motor changes seen in these schizophrenia-related PDs (Via et al., 2016; Waldeck & Miller, 2000). If an individual with STPD becomes psychotic, they will seem highly disoriented and confused and may exhibit posturing, grimacing, inappropriate giggling, rambling speech, and peculiar mannerisms. Fantasy, hallucinations, and bizarre, fragmented delusions may be present. Regressive acts such as enuresis and encopresis may occur. These individuals may consume food in an infantile or ravenous manner. Symptoms mirror but fall short of features that would justify the diagnosis of schizophrenia. Individuals with STPD may be unable to engage in social interaction that can keep them functional.

Nursing Care

Depending on the amount of decompensation (i.e., deterioration of functioning and exacerbation of symptoms), the assessment of a client with an STPD can generate a range of nursing diagnoses. If a person has severe symptoms, such as delusional thinking or perceptual disturbances, the nursing diagnoses are similar to those for a person with schizophrenia (see Chapter 20). If symptoms are mild, the typical nursing diagnoses include social isolation, ineffective coping, low self-esteem, and impaired social interactions.

People with STPD need help in increasing their sense of self-worth and recognizing their positive attributes. Limiting dependency and supporting self-directed activities appropriately are focuses of care. Individuals with this PD can benefit from interventions (e.g., social skills training; environmental management) that increase psychosocial functioning. As eccentric thoughts and behaviours alienate others, reinforcing and modelling socially appropriate dress and behaviour for a person with STPD can help to improve overall appearance and ability to relate (Hayward, 2007). A challenge for the person with STPD will be to generalize from one situation to another, so attention to cognitive skills is important (Waldeck & Miller, 2000).

Continuum of Care

Persons with cluster A personality disorders are rarely seen in mental health treatment unless their daily activities are seriously affected or symptoms of depression or anxiety appear. Improvement in quality of life for persons with these PDs is possible through psychotherapy, although symptoms such as suspiciousness, lack of trust, and impaired social interactions can make it difficult to establish a therapeutic relationship (Hayward, 2007). Engaging therapeutically with individuals with cluster A disorders can be at variance with the standard approach used with other clients, given the difficulty these clients have in forming emotional connections. In order to reduce the extreme anxiety that interpersonal engagement can cause, nurses will need to carefully judge appropriate therapeutic distance (Hayward, 2007). Brief interventions, including self-care assistance, reality orientation, and role enhancement, can be helpful (Bulechek, Butcher, & McCloskey Dochterman, 2008). Nurses encountering clients with cluster A PDs in non–mental health settings may need to consult with a psychiatric mental health nursing specialist.

Cluster B Disorders

Borderline Personality Disorder

Clinical Course of Disorder

In 1938, the term *borderline* was first used to refer to a group of disorders that did not quite fit the definition of either neurosis or psychosis (Stern, 1938). The term evolved from the psychoanalytic conceptualization of the disorder as a dysfunctional personality structure. In 1980, BPD was formally recognized as a distinct disorder in the *DSM-III*. Today, in the *DSM-5*, the essential feature of BPD is "a pervasive pattern of instability of interpersonal relationships, self-image, and affects, and marked impulsivity that begins by early adulthood and is present in a variety of contexts" (APA, 2013, p. 663). Instability is a core component of this disorder. A meta-analysis of the prevalence of BPD in university students, across 43 studies with a total of 26,343 participants from six countries, indicated a range from 0.5% to 32.1% with a lifetime prevalence of 9.7% (Meaney, Hasking, & Reupert, 2016).

Individuals with BPD have difficulty with interpersonal relationships in that they experience them as intensive, alternately idealize and devalue others, and become frantic if they feel that they may be abandoned. They have problems with unstable, highly reactive moods, with developing a sense of self, with feelings of emptiness, and with maintaining reality-based cognitive processes. Intense, inappropriate anger and its control can be a problem for them. Impulsive or destructive behaviour, such as suicidal or self-mutilating acts, is an ongoing possibility. Persons with BPD may appear more competent than they actually are and often set unrealistically high expectations for themselves. When these expectations are not met, they experience intense shame, self-hate, and self-directed anger. They seem to live from one crisis to another. Some of the crises are caused by the individual's dysfunctional lifestyle or inadequate social milieu, but many are simply challenging human experiences, like the death of a spouse or

diagnosis of an illness, to which they react emotionally with minimal coping skills. The intensity of their dysregulation often frightens themselves and others. Friends, family members, and coworkers may come to limit their contact with them, which furthers their sense of aloneness, abandonment, and self-hatred. It also diminishes opportunities for learning self-corrective measures.

Affective Instability

Affective instability (i.e., rapid and extreme shift in mood) is a core characteristic of BPD and is evidenced by erratic emotional responses to situations and intense sensitivity to criticism or perceived slights. For example, a person may greet a casual acquaintance with intense affection, yet later be aloof with the same acquaintance. Friends describe individuals with BPD as moody, irresponsible, or intense. These individuals fail to recognize their own emotional responses, thoughts, beliefs, and behaviours. Clinically, when a stressful situation is encountered, the person with BPD reacts with shifts in emotions, appearing to have limited success in developing emotional buffers to stressful situations. Regulating anger, anxiety, and sadness is particularly problematic. Difficulty with the intensity and regulation of emotion negatively affects social behaviours and relationships, including relations with health professionals. These affective symptoms are a central component of the disorder (Zanarini et al., 2007).

Research does suggest that emotional dysregulation may play a central role in the development and maintenance of BPD (Stepp et al., 2014). When individuals with innate biologic propensity for intense emotional reactivity develop in an environment that is unsupportive of learning ways to regulate one's emotions, such a deficit will contribute to increased **affective instability** and dysregulated cognitions, behaviours, and interpersonal relationships. If this is so, helping the individual with BPD to develop emotional awareness and clarity and to improve their ability to cope with negative emotions may be effective in improving other BPD symptoms, as well (Stepp et al., 2014).

Identity Disturbances

Identity diffusion occurs when a person lacks aspects of personal identity or when personal identity is poorly developed (Erikson, 1968). Four factors of identity are most commonly disturbed: role absorption (i.e., narrowly defining self within a single role), painful incoherence (i.e., distressed sense of internal disharmony), inconsistency (i.e., lack of coherence in thoughts, feelings, and actions), and lack of normative commitment (Weston, Beton, & Defife, 2011). Other factors of personality identity (e.g., religious ideologies, moral value systems, and sexual attitudes) appear to be less important in identity diffusion. Clinically, these clients appear to have little sense of their own identity and direction; this becomes a source of great distress to them and is often manifested by chronic feelings of emptiness and boredom. It is not unusual for persons with BPD to direct their actions in accord with the wishes of other people.

Unstable Interpersonal Relationships

Individuals with BPD have an extreme fear of abandonment as well as a history of unstable, insecure attachments. Such a history is significant as **attachment** has been considered within psychology (since the time of Freud) to be an essential aspect in early human development. An infant needs to experience a secure physical and emotional bond to at least one primary caregiver to successfully develop a coherent sense of self and the ability to connect with others. Contemporary theorists, such as Schore (2017), propose that attachment is a psychobiologic mechanism that supports early development of abilities to regulate the emotional self. A fear of abandonment may stem from difficulties in early childhood attachment with the primary caregiver. Most persons with BPD have never experienced a consistently secure, nurturing relationship and thus are constantly seeking reassurance and validation. In an attempt to meet their interpersonal needs, they idealize others and establish intense relationships that violate others' interpersonal boundaries, which ultimately leads to rejection (Bartholomew & Horowitz, 1991). When these relationships do not live up to their expectations, the person with BPD tends to devalue the other person. Continually disappointed in relationships, this individual can feel estranged from others and inadequate in the face of perceived social standards. Intense shame and self-hate will follow. These feelings often result in self-injurious behaviours, such as cutting the wrist, self-inflicted burns, or head banging.

In social situations, persons with BPD can use elaborate strategies to structure interactions. That is, they restrict their relationships to ones in which they feel in control. They distance themselves from groups when feeling anxious (which is most of the time) and rarely use their social support system. Even if they are married or have a supportive extended family, they can be reluctant to share their feelings (Krause, Mendelson, & Lynch, 2003). They do not want to burden anyone, fear rejection, and assume that others are tired of hearing them repeat the same issues.

Cognitive Dysfunctions

An aspect of BPD is dichotomous thinking. Individuals with BPD will evaluate experiences, people, and objects in terms of mutually exclusive categories (e.g., good or bad, success or failure, trustworthy or deceitful); this informs extreme interpretations of events that would normally be viewed as including both positive and negative aspects. There are also times when thinking becomes disorganized. Irrelevant, bizarre notions and vague or scattered thought connections can be present, as well as delusions and hallucinations.

Another cognitive dysfunction common in BPD is dissociation, in which thoughts and ideas can be split off from consciousness. **Dissociation** can be conceptualized as lying on a continuum from minor dissociations of daily life, such as daydreaming, to a breakdown in the usually integrated functions of consciousness, memory, perception of self or the environment, and sensorimotor behaviours. For example, in driving familiar roads, people often get lost in their thoughts or dissociate and suddenly do not remember what happened during that part of the trip. Environmental stimuli are ignored, and there are changes in the perception of reality. The individual is physically present but mentally in another place. Dissociation can be a coping strategy for avoiding disturbing events. In dissociating, the person does not have to be aware of or remember traumatic events. There is a strong correlation between dissociation and self-injurious behaviour (Zanarini, Ruser, Frankenburg, & Hennen, 2000).

Dysfunctional Behaviours

Impaired Problem-Solving. In BPD, there is often a failure to engage in active problem-solving. Instead, problem-solving is attempted by soliciting help from others in a helpless, hopeless manner (Linehan, 1993a). Suggestions are rarely taken.

Impulsivity. Impulsivity is also characteristic of the individual living with BPD. When impulse driven, individuals will have difficulty delaying gratification or thinking through the consequences before acting on their feelings; their actions are often unpredictable. Essentially, they act in the moment and then must face the consequences afterwards. Gambling, spending money irresponsibly, binge eating, engaging in unsafe sex, and abusing substances are examples of such impulsive acts. Job losses, interrupted education, and unsuccessful relationships are common to the history of persons with BPD.

Self-Injurious Behaviours. Unsuccessful interpersonal relationships and turmoil in social experiences may lead the person with BPD to undermine himself or herself when a goal is about to be reached. The most serious consequences are suicide attempts or parasuicidal behaviours (i.e., deliberate self-injury with intent to harm oneself; see Chapter 19). Individuals who self-injure show a higher threshold and greater tolerance for pain and report less pain intensity compared to healthy controls with no history of self-injury. It remains unknown if this is a risk factor in the development of such behaviour or a consequence of repeated episodes of self-injury (Koenig, Thayer, & Kaess, 2016). In a systematic review and meta-analysis, the prevalence of nonsuicidal self-injury behaviour was determined as 17.2% for adolescents, 13.4% for young adults, and 5.5% for adults (Swannell, Martin, Page, Hasking, & St John, 2014).

The prevalence of self-injurious behaviour is estimated to be 65% to 80% of people with BPD (Brickman et al., 2014). In a sample of adults with nonsuicidal self-injury, with and without BPD, it was found that the self-injury of those with BPD was more frequent and severe than of those without a BPD diagnosis. Those with BPD had higher rates of skin carving, head banging, self-punching, and self-scratching and reported more severe symptoms, suicidal ideation, and emotional dysregulation. They did not differ from the non-BPD individuals in rates of mood, substance use, nor psychotic disorders, but had greater incidence of anxiety disorders (Turner et al., 2015).

Self-injurious behaviour can be compulsive, episodic, or repetitive and is more likely to occur when the individual with BPD is depressed; has highly unstable interpersonal relationships, especially problems with intimacy and sociability; and is hypervigilant (i.e., alert, watchful) and resentful (Paris, 2007; Yeomans, Hull, & Clarkin, 1994). Self-injurious behaviours associated with BPD are listed below.

- *Compulsive self-injurious behaviours* that may occur many times daily and are repetitive and ritualistic. For example, hair pulling, which can be a separate disorder (**trichotillomania**) or behaviour associated with other personality disorders, involves pulling out hair, especially from the scalp, eyebrows, and eyelashes. Hair is plucked, examined, and sometimes eaten. Hair-pulling sessions may take several hours. Most of those afflicted do not seek help unless the symptoms are severe and then they usually consult dermatologists or family practitioners.
- *Episodic self-injurious behaviours* are especially common in people with BPD and develop into habitual coping behavioural patterns during periods when stress (i.e., progressive tension manifested by feelings of anger, depression, or anxiety) rises to an intolerable level. The individual reports being numb or empty and ends this dissociated state with a self-injurious behaviour that elicits feeling. As noted previously, some individuals with BPD who self-injure experience little or no associated pain (Koenig et al., 2016); rather, tension is relieved and a sense of calmness or even pleasure may follow. These feelings are believed to be reinforcing, and the person learns to relieve stress and anxiety by self-mutilation. The individuals harm themselves to feel better, get rapid relief from distressing thoughts and emotions, and gain a sense of control.
- *Repetitive self-mutilation* occurs when occasional self-injury turns into an overwhelming preoccupation. Persons can be labelled as "cutters" or "burners," for example, and describe themselves as being addicted to self-harm. In an interpretive

phenomenologic study of people with BPD, Nehls (1999) described the emotional conflict when efforts to comfort oneself are interpreted by others as manipulation, resulting in care being denied.

Risk for Suicide. Sometimes, clients and the health care team determine the risk for suicide by whether the intended outcome of an episode is death or injury. The underlying assumption is that those who attempt to kill themselves are at higher risk than those who self-injure. In reality, all self-injurious behaviours should be considered potentially life threatening and taken seriously. Indicators of increased suicide risk for persons with BPD include changes in the type or pattern of self-harm, increase in the use of substances, significant changes in the individual's mental state, recent adverse life events, and recent discharge from hospital or treatment (National Health and Medical Research Council, 2012). For individuals with BPD who attempt suicide, the mortality rate is 8% to 10%, much higher than in the general population (Leichsenring, Leibing, Kruse, New, & Leweke, 2011).

Aetiology

The answer to what causes BPD is becoming clearer but remains undetermined. BPD appears to be caused by the interaction of genetic and biologic vulnerabilities and environmental factors. These play a further role in the creation of psychological risk factors. This is a "highly individualized disorder" so the diagnosis of BPD likely reflects many "unique influences and developmental trajectories" (Hooley, Cole, & Gironde, 2012, p. 415). A brief overview of the existing knowledge related to the aetiology of BPD follows.

Neurobiologic and Genetic Factors

Connections between genetic factors and neurobiology may increase the risk of BPD. There is evidence that genetic factors are involved in the development of BPD: it is five times more common among "first-degree biologic relatives" of individuals with BPD than among the general population (APA, 2013, p. 665). Empirical studies of the neurobiology of BPD have involved neuroendocrinology and biologic specimens, and structural and functional neuroimaging (Ruocco & Carcone, 2016). A systematic and integrative review of these studies found that endogenous stress hormones, neurometabolism, and brain structure and circuits (white matter pathways, gray matter volume) appear to be involved but that the casual interconnections among them and their association with emotion, cognition, and sense of self in persons with BPD need to be clarified, as does the role of the amygdala in coordinating the relevance of emotional stimuli for the individual (Ruocco & Carcone, 2016). There has been speculation that individuals with BPD have reduced volume in the amygdala, but the evidence for this remains inconsistent. Persons with BPD appear to have abnormal serotonergic function, associated with impulsive aggressive symptoms, and such a defect might be related to genetic factors (Leichsenring et al., 2011).

BPD may be related to "stress-induced compromises" in the neural circuits underlying regulatory processes (Hooley et al., 2012, p. 428). Genetic and environmental factors (e.g., childhood trauma) may together be affecting the response of the hypothalamus–pituitary–adrenal (HPA) axis, which plays a main role in the stress response, in persons with BPD. The genetic variants in the HPA axis were found to be a contributor to the pathogenesis of BPD with childhood trauma having a modulating effect when investigated in a large sample of individuals with BPD and healthy controls (Martin-Blanco et al., 2016). PET studies support the hypothesis that persons with BPD have abnormalities in the prefrontal brain regions (associated with emotion control); functional MRI studies add support to the hypothesis that persons with BPD have a dysfunctional frontolimbic network.

Psychosocial Risk Factors

Various studies show that childhood maltreatment appears to be a significant risk factor for BPD: 55% to 80% of individuals with BPD have reported a history of childhood sexual abuse and/or physical abuse (Jordan, 2004). Childhood neglect has been correlated with increase in BPD symptoms (Jovev et al., 2013). Clearly, more studies are needed to identify risk factors for the development of BPD.

Psychological Theories

Psychoanalytic Theories. The psychoanalytic views of BPD focus on two important psychoanalytic concepts: **separation–individuation** and projective identification. According to this theory, a person with BPD has not achieved the normal and healthy developmental stage of separation–individuation, during which a child develops a sense of self, a permanent sense of significant others (object constancy), and integration of seeing both bad and good components of self (Mahler, Pine, & Bergman, 1975). Object relations theory explains how "objects" (i.e., real and internalized relationships with significant people) contribute to personality and are expressed through defenses and interpersonal interactions (Clarkin, Yeomans, & Kernberg, 2006; Magnavita, 2004). Within this theory, individuals with BPD are viewed as lacking the ability to separate from the primary caregiver and develop a separate and distinct personality or self-identity. Psychoanalytic theory suggests that these separation difficulties occur because the primary caregivers' behaviours have been inconsistent or insensitive to the needs of the child. The child develops ambivalent feelings regarding interpersonal relationships and therefore has no basis for establishing trusting and secure relationships in the future. Children experience feelings of intense fear and anger in separating themselves from others. This problem continues into adulthood, and they continue to experience difficulties in maintaining personal boundaries and in interpersonal interactions and relationships. These individuals may falsely attribute to others their own unacceptable feelings, impulses, or thoughts, termed projective identification. In this theory, **projective identification** is believed to play an important role in the development of BPD and is a defense mechanism by which people with BPD protect their fragile self-image. For example, when overwhelmed by anxiety or anger at being disregarded by another, they defend against the intensity of these feelings by unconsciously blaming others for what happens to them. They project their feelings onto a significant other with the unconscious hope that the other knows how to deal with it. Projective identification becomes a defensive way of interacting with the world, which leads to more rejection.

Maladaptive Cognitive Processes. Individuals with personality disorders develop maladaptive cognitive schemas leading them to misinterpret environmental stimuli continuously, which in turn leads to rigid and inflexible behaviour patterns in response to new situations and people. Because those with BPD have been conditioned to anticipate rejection and disappointment in the past, they become entrenched in a pattern of fear and anxiety regarding encountering new people or situations. They have fears that a disaster is going to strike any minute. Early in life, individuals with BPD and other personality disorders develop maladaptive schemas or dysfunctional ways of interpreting people and events. Table 27.1 explains 18 major maladaptive schemas at work in those with personality disorders. The work of cognitive therapists is to challenge these distortions in thinking patterns and replace them with realistic ones. Therapists, too, have personal schemas regarding themselves and others; they need to identify their own schemas and ensure that therapeutic progress is not impeded by an unrecognized conflict with the schema of their clients (Leahy & McGinn, 2012).

Biosocial Theories

The biosocial learning theory was developed by Theodore Millon, who viewed BPD as a distinct disorder that develops as a result of both biologic and psychological factors (Millon & Davis, 1999). While he supported the biologic determination of personality, he believed that a child's interaction with the environment and learning and experience could greatly affect his or her biologic predisposition. He argued that individuals possess biologically based patterns of sensitivities and behavioural dispositions that shapes their experiences, including active–passive behaviour or a tendency to take initiative versus reacting to events, sensitivity to pleasure or pain, and sensitivity behaviour to self and others.

Table 27.1 Maladaptive Schemas	
Domain	Schemas With Definitions
I. Disconnection and rejection	1. *Abandonment/instability* Important people will not be there 2. *Mistrust/abuse* Other people will use the client for own selfish ends 3. *Emotional deprivation* Emotional connection will not be fulfilled 4. *Defectiveness/scheme* One is flawed, bad, or worthless 5. *Social isolation/alienation* Being different from or not fitting in
II. Impaired autonomy and performance	1. *Dependence/incompetence* Belief that one is unable to function on one's own 2. *Vulnerability to harm and illness* Fear that disaster is about to strike 3. *Enmeshment/undeveloped self* Excessive emotional involvement at the expense of normal social development 4. *Failure* Belief that one has failed
III. Impaired limits	1. *Entitlement/grandiosity* Belief that one is superior to other; entitled to special rights 2. *Insufficient self-control/self-discipline* Difficulty or refusal to exercise sufficient self-control
IV. Other directedness	1. *Subjugation* Excessive surrendering of control to others because of feeling coerced 2. *Self-sacrifice* Excessive focus on voluntarily meeting the needs of others at the expense of one's own gratification 3. *Approval seeking/recognition seeking* Excessive emphasis on gaining approval, recognition, or attention
V. Over-vigilance and inhibition	1. *Negativity/pessimism* Lifelong focus on the negative aspects of life 2. *Emotional inhibition* Excessive inhibition of spontaneous action, feeling, or communication 3. *Unrelenting standard/hypercriticalness* Belief that one must meet very high standards; perfectionistic, rigid 4. *Punitiveness* Belief that people should be harshly punished

Young, J. E. (1999). *Cognitive therapy for personality disorders: A schema-focused approach.* Sarasota, FL: Professional Resource Press.

Millon believed that BPD is a particular cycloid personality pattern representing a moderately dysfunctional dependent or ambivalent orientation, often expressed in intense endogenous moods, described as patterns of recurring dejection and apathy interspersed with spells of anger, anxiety, or euphoria.

A further elaboration of Millon's multidimensional model incorporates biologic explanations into the behaviour. Cloninger, Bayon, and Svrakic (1998) described personality disorder behaviours based on temperament and character dimensions derived from a factor analysis design. Cluster A disorders are associated with low-reward dependence and social attachment mediated by norepinephrine and serotonin. Cluster B disorders are associated with high novelty seeking mediated by dopamine. Novelty-seeking behaviour includes exhilaration, exploration, impulsivity, extravagance, and irritability. Cluster C disorders are associated with high harm avoidance mediated by γ-aminobutyric acid (GABA) and serotonin.

A biosocial theory of BPD proposed by Marsha Linehan and colleagues is similar to Millon's theory, with a focus on the interaction of both biologic and social learning influences. Their primary focus is on the particular behavioural patterns observed in BPD, including emotional vulnerability, self-invalidation, unrelenting crises, inhibited grieving, active passivity, and apparent competence (Linehan, 1993a; Box 27.4).

This biosocial viewpoint presents BPD as a multifaceted problem, a combination of a person's innate **emotional vulnerability** and his or her inability to control that emotion in social interactions (emotional dysregulation) and the environment (Linehan, 1993a). The emotional dysregulation and aggressive impulsivity entail both social learning and biologic regulation. Much of the neurobiologic research is directed at neurotransmitter functions (Silk, 2000) and neural firing between the limbic system and the frontal and prefrontal cortex. When these pathways are functional, the person has a

BOX 27.4 Behavioural Patterns in BPD

1. Emotional vulnerability. Person experiences a pattern of pervasive difficulties in regulating negative emotions, including a high sensitivity to negative emotional stimuli, high emotional intensity, and slow return to emotional baseline.
2. *Self-invalidation*. Person fails to recognize one's own emotional responses, thoughts, beliefs, and behaviours and sets unrealistically high standards and expectations for self. This may include intense shame, self-hate, and self-directed anger. Person has no personal awareness and tends to blame social environment for unrealistic expectations and demands.
3. *Unrelenting crises*. Person experiences a pattern of frequent, stressful, negative environmental events, disruptions, and roadblocks—some caused by the individual's dysfunctional lifestyle, others by an inadequate social milieu, and many by fate or chance.
4. Inhibited grieving. Person tries to inhibit and over-control negative emotional responses, especially those associated with grief and loss, including sadness, anger, guilt, shame, anxiety, and panic.
5. *Active passivity*. Person fails to engage actively in solving own life problems but will actively seek problem-solving from others in the environment; learned helplessness and hopelessness.
6. *Apparent competence*. Tendency for individuals to appear deceptively more competent than they actually are; it is usually due to failure of competencies to generalize across expected moods, situations, and time and failure to display adequate nonverbal cues of emotional distress.

From Linehan, M. (1993a). *Cognitive-behavioral treatment of borderline personality disorder* (p. 10). New York, NY: Guilford Press.

---

greater capacity to think about his or her emotions and modulate behaviours more responsibly.

The biosocial viewpoint supports the notion that the ability to control one's emotion is in part a learning process, learned from one's private experiences and encounters with the social environment. A risk factor associated with BPD is believed to develop when emotionally vulnerable individuals interact with an **invalidating environment**, a social situation that negates the individual's private emotional responses and communication. That is, when others whom the person respects or values are continuously insensitive to the person's core emotional responses, respond irrationally and inappropriately, or trivialize his or her painful experiences, the person receives confused messages about expressing feelings. Further, the message from significant others may be that negative emotions, in particular, are not to be expressed. Invalidation occurs as the individual's emotions are continuously dismissed, trivialized, devalued, punished, and discredited.

The most severe form of invalidation occurs in situations of child sexual abuse. Often, the abusing adult has told the child that this is a "special secret" between them, that the child should feel guilty if he or she tells anyone, and that telling someone would end their trust and special relationship. The child experiences feelings of fear, pain, and sadness, yet this trusted adult continuously dismisses the child's true feelings and tells the child what he or she should feel. Children often learn to endure sexual abuse for years, suppressing their true feelings. In disclosing the secret to a nonoffending adult, the child risks not being believed or attended to and possible punishment.

All children, not just those who are emotionally vulnerable, must learn to trust their own feelings and learn when and how to express them by interacting with their environments, including parents, families, friends, and social situations. If they constantly meet with an invalidating environment, they cannot learn to trust their own feelings—when to be angry, sad, or happy—they become emotionally dysregulated. This emotional dysregulation leads to further difficulties in identity disturbances, interpersonal relationships, and the development of impulsive, parasuicidal behaviours.

Interdisciplinary Treatment

BPD is a very complex disorder that requires the involvement of the entire health care team in its treatment. BPD often involves not only ongoing treatment but also urgent intervention for self-harm and suicidal behaviours. Although psychotherapy has not been shown to lead to remission of BPD (i.e., the diagnostic criteria are no longer met), it can help the individual better manage symptoms of the disorder (Leichsenring et al., 2011), such as dysfunctional moods, impulsive behaviours, and self-injurious behaviours. Evidence-based psychotherapy has been found to be more effective and less expensive to health care systems than other approaches (Meuldijk, McCarthy, Bourke, & Grenyer, 2017). Characteristics of evidence-based treatment for BPD include manual-directed (structured) approach, encouragement of a sense of agency (i.e., self-control), and therapists who are active, are validating, and assist with the connection of emotion to actions and events (Bateman et al., 2015). Specially trained therapists, representing a variety of mental health disciplines, including psychology, social work, and advanced practice nursing are often involved. This can be a lifelong disorder requiring ongoing treatment as the individual copes with multiple interpersonal crises.

Dialectical behaviour therapy is used to treat BPD as it has demonstrated effectiveness in decreasing self-harm behaviour and suicidality in BPD (Lyness, 2016). (See the DBT entry in the section on treatment of PDs in this chapter.) Behaviour patterns of BPD are perceived in this treatment approach as based in a dysfunctional emotional regulation system that evolved from biologic vulnerabilities and an invalidating environment. There are three facets: sensitivity to both positive and negative emotional stimuli, emotional intensity, and slow return to emotion baseline (Lynch & Cuper, 2012, p. 786).

When used on an inpatient basis, DBT requires staff commitment and reinforcement; significant improvement in depression, anxiety, and dissociation symptoms and a highly significant decrease in **parasuicidal behaviour** have been shown (Bohus et al., 2000). DBT is more often incorporated into a long-term outpatient treatment approach because the greatest effectiveness occurs when skills are learned over time and practiced in a variety of daily living settings (Feigenbaum, 2007). Members of the treatment team maintain a positive skills-coaching role with clients.

Psychopharmacotherapy

Although individuals with BPD are treated with medication, the efficacy of such treatments appears to be symptomatic at best. There is evidence that BPD symptoms can be alleviated in the short term by mood stabilizers (e.g., topiramate; for emotional dysregulation and impulsive-aggressive symptoms) and some second-generation antipsychotics (e.g., olanzapine; for cognitive–perceptual and impulsive–aggressive symptoms) (Bateman et al., 2015). Evidence does not support medication as treatment for overall reduction of severity of the disorder (National Health and Medical Research Council [Australia], 2012). Some medications used to treat BPD symptoms have side effects that are potentially harmful (e.g., valproate semisodium for women of child-bearing age) or are neurologic or metabolic in nature (e.g., antipsychotics; Leichsenring et al., 2011). Risks/benefits must be carefully considered in the symptomatic treatment of BPD.

Family Response to Disorder

The family of clients with BPD may feel captive to the symptoms of the disorder. Family members can be afraid to disagree with them or refuse to meet their multiple needs, fearing that self-destructive behaviours will follow. During the course of the disorder, family members can get "burned out" and withdraw from the individual, only adding to the person's fear of abandonment (Hoffman, Fruzzetti, & Buteau, 2007). They can experience stress, distress, and hopelessness, as well as the significant burden and the loss of their own social support. Psychoeducation for family members and friends can be effective in offering them knowledge regarding the disorder, problem-solving skills, family relationship skills, and a social network (Pearce et al., 2017). When a psychoeducation group intervention for family and friends of youth with BPD was evaluated, participants reported subjective burden was significantly decreased and knowledge of BPD increased; objective burden and distress, however, were unchanged. Longer follow-up after the conclusion of such groups may be required for behavioural change to be practiced and established (Pearce et al., 2017). DBT treatment that includes the involvement of family and friends has been developed (Van Wel et al., 2006). Refer further to Chapter 15.

Nursing Care

It is important to recognize that BPD is a devastating disorder that involves much emotional pain and distress and, too often, it is stigmatized (Hooley et al., 2012). Individuals living with BPD experience instability in a variety of areas, including mood, interpersonal relationships, self-esteem, and self-identity, and they can exhibit behavioural and cognitive dysregulations. These manifest in a number of ways, the most prominent of which are listed in Box 27.5. Due to their patterns of response, clients may have problems in daily living: maintaining intimate relationships, keeping a job, and living within the law (Box 27.6).

Individuals with BPD may enter the mental health system early (young adulthood or before), but because of their chaotic lifestyle, they typically do not receive consistent treatment. They drop in and out of treatment

---

BOX 27.5 Response Patterns of Individuals with BPD

Affective (mood) dysregulation
Mood lability
Problems with anger
Interpersonal dysregulation
Chaotic relationships
Fears of abandonment
Self-dysregulation
Identity disturbance or difficulties with sense of self
Sense of emptiness
Behavioural dysregulation
Parasuicidal behaviour or threats
Impulsive behaviour
Cognitive dysregulation
Dissociative responses
Paranoid ideation

Courtesy of M. Linehan, Department of Psychology, Box 351525, University of Washington, Seattle, WA 98195-1525.

BOX 27.6 CLINICAL VIGNETTE

BORDERLINE PERSONALITY DISORDER

JS is a 22-year-old single woman who was recently fired from her job as a data entry clerk. She is living with her mother and stepfather, who brought her to the emergency room after finding her crouched in a foetal position in the bathroom, her wrists bleeding. She seemed to be in a daze. This is her first psychiatric admission, although her mother and stepfather have suspected that she has "needed help" for a long time. In high school, she received brief treatment for a potential eating disorder. She remains very thin but is able to eat at least one meal per day. During periods of stress, however, she will go for days without eating.

JS is the second of three children. Her parents divorced when she was 3 years old. She has not seen her father since he left. Although she has pleasant memories of her father, her mother has told her that he beat JS and her sisters when he was drinking. When JS was 6 years old, her older sister died following an automobile accident. JS was in the car but was uninjured. As a child, JS was seen as a potential singing star. Her natural musical talent attracted her teachers' support, which encouraged her to develop her talent. She received singing lessons and entered provincial competitions in high school. Although she enjoyed the attention, she was never really comfortable in the limelight and felt "guilty" about having a talent that she sometimes resented. She was able to make friends but found that she was unable to keep them. They described her as "too intense" and emotional. She had one boyfriend in high school, but she was very uncomfortable with any physical closeness. After ending the relationship with the boyfriend, she concentrated on dieting to have a "perfect body." When her dieting attracted her parents' attention, she vowed to eat just enough to keep them "off her back about it." She spent much of her leisure time with her grandmother. She attended university briefly but was unable to concentrate. It was during her time at university and after her grandmother's death that JS began cutting her wrists during periods of stress. It seemed to calm her.

After leaving university, JS returned home. She had several jobs and short-lived friendships. She was usually fired from her job because of "moodiness," and it would take her several months before she would again find another. She would spend days in her room listening to music. Her recent episode followed being fired from work and spending 3 days in her bedroom.

What Do You Think?

- How would you describe JS's mood?
- Are JS's losses (father, sister, grandmother) really severe enough to affect her ability to relate to others now? Do the losses seem to relate to the self-injury?
- What behaviours indicate that there are problems with self-esteem and self-identity?

and usually do not remain with one clinician for long-term treatment. Persons with BPD usually seek help from health care workers because of consequences of life crises, medical conditions, or other psychiatric disorders (e.g., depression) or for physical treatment of self-injury. Thus, other problems may need attention before the client's underlying personality disorder can be addressed; at times, the nurse will not know that the person has BPD. During an assessment, however, it usually becomes clear that the client is affected by things more intensely than the average person or has an inflexible view of the world. The great difficulty the client has in changing behaviour, no matter the consequences, will also become apparent. He or she faces difficulty in successfully relating to other people and struggles to live a satisfying life.

Biologic Domain

Biologic Assessment

The client with BPD is usually able to maintain personal hygiene and physical functioning. Because of the comorbidity of BPD and eating disorders and substance abuse, a nutritional assessment may be needed. The assessment should also include the use of caffeinated beverages (e.g., coffee, tea, soft drinks) and alcohol. With individuals who engage in binging or purging, an assessment should include examining the teeth for pitting and discolouration, as well as the hands and fingers for redness and calluses caused by inducing vomiting. The client should be queried about physiologic responses of emotion. Sleep patterns also should be assessed because sleep alterations may suggest coexisting depression or mania.

Physical Indicators of Self-Injurious Behaviours. Clients with BPD should be assessed for self-injurious behaviours or suicide attempts. It is important to ask the individual about specific self-abusive behaviours, such as cutting, scratching, or overdosing. Clients frequently wear long sleeves to hide an injury on the arms. Specifically asking about thoughts of hurting oneself when experiencing a major upset provides an opportunity for prevention and for coaching the client towards alternative self-soothing measures.

Pharmacologic Assessment. The medications that clients with BPD are taking need to be identified and assessed. Initially, individuals may be reluctant to disclose all their medications as they may be concerned that some or all of their medication may be stopped. The development of rapport with special attention to a nonjudgemental approach is especially important when eliciting current medication practices. The client will play an important role in determining the efficacy of a medication in relieving targeted symptoms. The use of alcohol and street drugs should also be carefully assessed to determine drug interactions.

Nursing Diagnoses for the Biologic Domain

Nursing diagnoses focusing on the biologic domain include disturbed sleep pattern, imbalanced nutrition, self-mutilation or risk for self-mutilation, and ineffective therapeutic regimen management.

Interventions for the Biologic Domain

The interventions for the biologic domain may address a whole spectrum of problems. Usually, the individuals are managing hydration, self-care, and pain well. This section focuses on those areas most likely to be problematic.

Sleep Enhancement. The facilitation of regular sleep–wake cycles may be needed because of disturbed sleep patterns. Conservative approaches should be exhausted before recommending medication (see Chapter 28). Establishing a regular bedtime routine, monitoring bedtime snacks and drinks, and avoiding foods and drinks that interfere with sleep should be tried. If relaxation exercises are used, they should be adapted to the tolerance of the individual. Moderate exercises (e.g., brisk walking) 3 to 4 hours before bedtime activate both serotonin and endorphins, thereby enhancing calmness and a sense of well-being before bedtime. For individuals who have difficulty falling asleep and experience interrupted sleep, it helps to establish some basic sleeping routines. The bedroom should be reserved for sleep and intimacy, so it is best to keep items such as televisions, computers, and exercise equipment elsewhere. If the individual is not asleep within 15 minutes, he or she should get out of bed and go to another room to read, watch television, or listen to soft music. The client should return to bed when sleepy. If the person is not asleep in 15 minutes, the same process should be repeated.

Special consideration must be made for individuals who have been physically and sexually abused and who may be unable to put themselves in a vulnerable position (e.g., lying down in a room with other people or closing their eyes). These clients may need additional safeguards to help them sleep, such as a night light or repositioning of furniture to afford easy exit.

Nutritional Balance. The nutritional status of the person with BPD can quickly become a priority, particularly if the individual has coexisting eating disorders or substance abuse. Eating is often a response to stress, and clients can quickly become overweight. This is especially a problem when the individual has also been taking medications that can promote weight gain, such as antipsychotics, antidepressants, or mood stabilizers. Helping the client to learn the basics of nutrition, make reasonable choices, and develop other coping strategies is a useful intervention. If individuals are engaging in purging or severe dieting practices, teaching them about the dangers of both of these practices is important (see Chapter 25). Referral to an eating disorders specialist may be needed.

Prevention and Treatment of Self-Injury. Within inpatient settings, nurses may need to help clients with BPD (and other cluster B disorders) set limits on their behaviour. Limit setting should be accomplished in such a way that clients recognize that it is the behaviour that is unacceptable, and not them. This is key to the prevention of self-injury, which is frequently a major factor in the hospitalization of persons with BPD. Observing for antecedents of self-injurious behaviour and intervening before an episode is an important to the client's safety. Clients can learn to identify situations leading to self-destructive behaviour and develop preventive strategies. Because individuals with BPD are impulsive and may respond to stress by harming themselves, observation of the person's interactions and assessment of mood, level of distress, and agitation are important in determining the threat of self-injury.

Remembering that self-injury is an effort to self-soothe by activating endogenous endorphins, the nurse can assist the individual to find more productive and enduring ways to find comfort. Linehan (1993b) suggests using a self-soothing exercise and focusing on each of the five senses. For example, a client may try focusing in such ways as follows:

- Vision (e.g., look at photos of places one finds peaceful)
- Hearing (e.g., listen to beautiful music or the sounds of nature)

- Smell (e.g., use a drop of lavender oil on a pillow or handkerchief)
- Taste (e.g., drink a soothing, nonalcoholic, warm beverage)
- Touch (e.g., have a warm bath, pet a dog)

Pharmacologic Interventions. There is no specific drug available for the treatment of BPD, but medications for target symptoms may be used: selective serotonin reuptake inhibitors (SSRIs) for affective problems and aggressive impulses and low doses of an antipsychotic for symptoms related to cognitive–perceptive issues (Bateman et al., 2015). These should be on a short-term basis. Clients with BPD may be taking medications for a comorbid disorder, such as a mood disorder or a substance-related disorder.

TEACHING POINTS

Clients should be educated about any medications and their interactions with other drugs and substances. Interventions include teaching individuals about the medication and how and where it acts in the brain and body, helping establish a routine for taking prescribed medication, reporting side effects, and facilitating the development of positive coping strategies to deal with daily stresses, rather than relying on medications. Eliciting the client's partnership in care improves adherence and, thereby, outcomes.

Psychological Domain

Psychological Assessment

People with BPD have usually experienced significant losses in their lives that shape their view of the world. They experience inhibited grieving, "a pattern of repetitive, significant trauma and loss, together with an inability to fully experience and personally integrate or resolve these events" (Linehan, 1993a, p. 89). They may have unresolved grief that began years ago and avoid situations that evoke related feelings of separation and loss. During the assessment, the nurse can identify the losses (real or perceived) and explore the client's experience during these losses, paying particular attention to whether the individual has reached resolution. A history of physical or sexual abuse and an early separation from significant caregivers may provide important clues to the severity of the disturbances.

Mood fluctuations are common and can be assessed by any number of the depression and anxiety screening scales or by asking the following questions:

- What things or events bother you and make you feel happy, sad, and angry?
- Do these things or events trouble you more than they trouble other people?

- Do friends and family tell you that you are moody?
- Do you get angry easily?
- Do you have trouble with your temper?
- Do you think you were born with these feelings, or did something happen to make you feel this way?

Appearance and activity level generally reflect the person's mood and psychomotor activity. Many of those with BPD have been physically or sexually abused and thus should be assessed for depression. A dishevelled appearance can reflect depression or an agitated state. When feeling good, these individuals can be very engaging; they tend to be dramatic in their style of dress and attract attention, such as by wearing an unusual hairstyle or heavy makeup. Because physical appearance reflects identity, clients may experiment with their appearance and seek affirmation and acceptance from others. Body piercings, tattoos, and other adornments provide a mechanism to define self.

Impulsivity

Impulsivity can be identified by asking clients if they do things impulsively or on the spur of the moment (e.g., "Have there been times when you were hurt by your actions or were sorry later that you acted in the way you did?"). Direct questions about gambling, choices in sexual partners, sexual activities, fights, arguments, arrests, and alcohol drinking habits can also help in identifying areas of impulsive behaviour. Teaching the client strategies to slow down automatic responses (e.g., deep breathing, counting to 10) allows time to think before acting.

Cognitive Disturbances

The mental status examination of those with BPD usually reveals normal thought processes that are not disorganized or confused, except during periods of stress. Those with BPD usually exhibit dichotomous thinking, or a tendency to view things as absolute—either black or white, good or bad—with no perception of compromise. **Dichotomous thinking** can be assessed by asking clients how they view other people. Evidence of dichotomous thinking is indicated with responses of "good" or "bad," "wonderful" or "terrible."

Dissociation and Transient Psychotic Episodes

Individuals with BPD may experience periods of dissociation and of transient psychotic episodes. Dissociation can be assessed by asking if there are times when they do not remember events or have the feeling of being separate from their body. Some individuals refer to this as "spacing out." By asking specific information about how often, how long, and when dissociation first was used, the nurse can get an idea of how important dissociation is as a coping skill. It is important to ask the person what is happening in the environment when dissociation occurs. Frequent dissociation indicates a highly habitual coping mechanism that will be difficult to change.

Because transient psychotic states occur, it is also important to elicit data regarding the presence of hallucinations or delusions along with their frequency and circumstances. Terms such as "pseudopsychotic" or "quasipsychotic" are misleading and should not be used (Schroeder, Fisher, & Schäfer, 2013).

Risk Assessment: Suicide or Self-Injury

It is critical that individuals with BPD be assessed for suicidal and self-damaging behaviours, including alcohol and drug abuse. Further information regarding suicide assessment is found in Chapter 19; substance use in Chapter 26. Suicide is a real risk; it is estimated that about 10% of clients with BPD will die of suicide, many before the age of 40 years (Hooley et al., 2012). An assessment should include direct questions, asking if the person thinks about or engages in self-injurious behaviours. If so, the nurse should continue to explore the behaviours: what is done, how it is done, its frequency, and the circumstances surrounding the self-injurious behaviour. It is helpful to explain briefly to the client that sometimes people cut, scratch, or pick at themselves as a way of bringing some relief and comfort. Although the behaviour brings temporary relief, it also places the person at risk for infection.

Approaching the assessment in this way conveys a sense of understanding and is more likely to invite the individual to disclose honestly. This is important as revealed when men ($n = 15$) with a recent history of suicidal behaviour as well as substance use and antisocial or borderline behaviour described their experiences with treatment services while living in Toronto. In this qualitative study, these participants noted that they were unable to express their emotions and to navigate the health care system. They felt mislabelled, as complete assessments (including contextual factors) were not carried out; that they were treated disrespectfully; and that they felt compelled to lie or to attempt suicide to have their needs met. They desired connection with the staff but perceived them as disinterested or hostile (Strike, Rhodes, Bergmans, & Links, 2006).

Monitoring changes in the stress levels of a client with BPD is important, as increased stress (or distress) can be a trigger for self-harming behaviours, including a suicide attempt. Common risk factors for suicide attempts remain true for clients with BPD: history of recent attempts and hospitalizations and a history of childhood sexual abuse (Links, Kolia, Guimond, & McMain, 2013).

Nursing Diagnoses for the Psychological Domain

One of the first diagnoses to consider is the risk for self-mutilation because protection of the individual from self-injury is always a priority. If cognitive changes are present (dissociation and transient psychosis), two other diagnoses may be appropriate: disturbed thought process and ineffective coping. The disturbed thought process diagnosis is used if dissociative and psychotic episodes actually interfere with daily living. For example, a secretary could not complete processing letters because she was unable to differentiate whether the voices on the dictating machine were being transmitted by the machine or by her hallucinations. The nurse helped her learn to differentiate the hallucinations from dictation. The client learned to take her headset off, take a deep breath, and listen to her external environment. When she recognized "the voice" as her partner criticizing her, she was able to use her cognitive **reframing** strategies to refocus on reality.

If the individual copes with stressful situations by dissociating or hallucinating, the diagnosis of ineffective coping is used. The outcome in this instance would be the substitution of positive coping skills for the dissociations or hallucinations.

Other nursing diagnoses that are typically supported by assessment data include personal identity disturbance, anxiety, grieving, low self-esteem, powerlessness, posttrauma response, defensive coping, and spiritual distress. The identification of outcomes depends on the nursing diagnoses (see Fig. 27.1).

Interventions for the Psychological Domain

The greatest challenge of working with clients with BPD is engaging the individual in a therapeutic relationship that will survive its emotional ups and downs. Clients need to understand that the nurse is there to coach them to develop self-modulation skills. A relationship based on mutual respect and consistency is crucial for helping the person with those skills. Self-awareness skills, along with access to supervision and collaboration, are needed by the nurse. Research reveals, however, that nurses may struggle with negative attitudes towards clients with BPD and respond to them countertherapeutic ways (see Box 27.7).

Because individuals with BPD are frequently hospitalized, even nurses in acute care settings have an opportunity to develop a long-term relationship (Fig. 27.2). A recovery-focused approach to change can be successful, including for persons with BPD who exhibit suicidal behaviours, if clients feel supported and that their experience of what it means to live with BPD is understood (Holm & Severinsson, 2011).

A further challenge that may face nurses within this nurse–client relationship is maladaptive coping behaviour that persons with BPD may use that involves regarding a particular person as being all good or all bad, rather than seeing the person as a complex human being. This seeing others in terms of black and white, rather than in shades of gray, can create problems for individuals with BPD in maintaining their relationships. If this happens within the nurse–client relationship and/or affects the team approach to the client, it is important to respond professionally and appropriately, with understanding of the relationship dynamics.

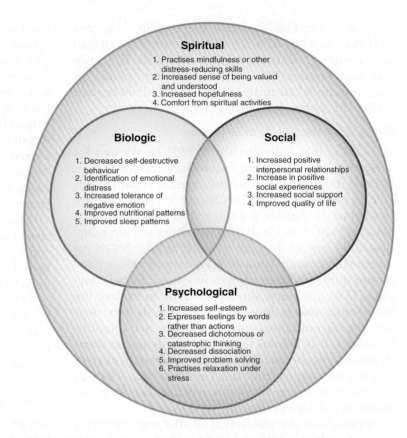

Figure 27.1. Bio/psycho/social/spiritual outcomes for individuals with BPD.

BOX **27.7**

THERAPEUTIC DIALOGUE

Borderline Personality Disorder

Ineffective Approach

Client: Hey, you know what? You are my favourite nurse. That night nurse sure doesn't understand me the way you do.

Nurse: Oh, I'm glad you are comfortable with me. Which night nurse?

Client: You know, Sue.

Nurse: Did you have problems with her?

Client: She is terrible. She sleeps all night or she is on the telephone.

Nurse: Oh, that doesn't sound very professional to me. Anything else?

Client: Yeah, she said that you didn't know what you were doing. She said that you couldn't nurse your way out of a paper bag (smiling).

Nurse: She did, did she. (Getting angry.) She should talk.

Client: Well, I gotta go to group. Where will you be? I feel so much better if I know where you are. I don't know how I can possibly be discharged tomorrow.

Effective Approach

Client: Hey, you know what? You are my favourite nurse. That night nurse sure doesn't understand me the way you do.

Nurse: like you, Sara. Tomorrow, you will be discharged, and I'm glad that you will be able to return home. (The

nurse avoided responding to "favourite nurse" statement. Redirected the interaction to impending discharge.)

Client: That night nurse slept all night.

Nurse: What was your night like? (Redirecting the interaction to Sara's experience.)

Client: It was terrible. Couldn't sleep all night. I'm not sure that I'm ready to go home.

Nurse: Oh, so you are not quite sure about discharge? (Reflection.)

Client: I get so, so lonely. Then, I want to hurt myself.

Nurse: Lonely feelings have started that chain of events that led to cutting, haven't they? (Validation.)

Client: Yes, I'm very scared. I haven't cut myself for 1 week now.

Nurse: Do you have a plan for dealing with your lonely feelings when they occur?

Client: I'm supposed to start thinking about something that is pleasant—like spring flowers in the meadow.

Nurse: Does that work for you?

Client: Yes, sometimes.

Critical Thinking Questions

- How did the nurse in the first scenario get sidetracked?
- How was the nurse in the second scenario able to keep the client focused on herself and her impending discharge?

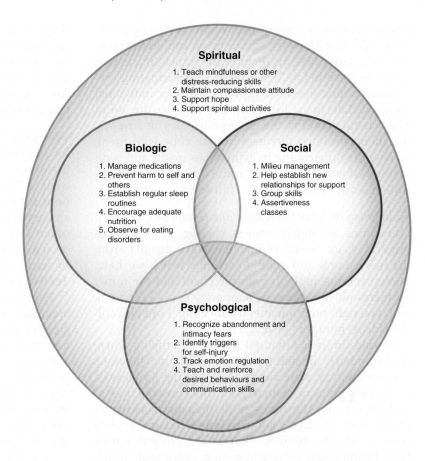

Figure 27.2. Bio/psycho/social/spiritual interventions for individuals with BPD.

Generalist nurses, including psychiatric and mental health nurses, do not function as the client's primary therapists, but they do need to establish a therapeutic relationship that strengthens the client's coping skills and self-esteem and supports individual psychotherapy. The therapeutic relationship helps the client to experience a model of healthy interaction with consistency, limit setting, caring, and respect for others (both self-respect and respect for the person). Clients who have low self-esteem need help in recognizing genuine respect from others and reciprocating with respect for others. In the therapeutic relationship, the nurse models self-respect by observing personal limits, being assertive, and clearly communicating expectations. Consistency is critical in building self-esteem (see Box 27.8).

Responding to Abandonment and Intimacy Fears. A key to helping individuals with BPD is recognizing their fears of both abandonment and intimacy. Informing the client of the length of the relationship as much as possible allows the individual to engage in and prepare for termination with the least pain of abandonment. If the client's hospitalization is time limited, the nurse overtly acknowledges the limit and reminds the person with each contact how many sessions remain.

In day treatment and outpatient settings, the duration of treatment may be indeterminate, but the nurse may not be available that entire time. The termination

---

BOX 27.8 Challenging Dysfunctional Thinking

Ms. S had worked for the same company for 20 years with a good job record. Following an accident, she made some minor mistakes in her work that she quickly corrected. She informed her company's nurse that her work was "really slipping" and that she was fearful of her coworkers' disapproval and getting fired from her job. The nurse asked her to keep a journal of coworkers' comments for the next week. At the next visit, the following dialogue occurred:

Nurse: I noticed that you received several compliments on your work. Even a close friend of your boss expressed appreciation for your work.

Ms. S: It was a light week at work. I really don't believe they meant what they said.

Nurse: I can see how you can believe that one or two comments are not genuine, but how do you account for four and five good reports on your work?

Ms. S: Well, I don't know.

Nurse: It looks like your beliefs are not supported by your journal entries. Now, what makes you think that your boss wants to fire you after 20 years of service?

process cannot be casual; this would stimulate abandonment fears. However, some clients end prematurely when the nurse informs them of the impending end as a way to leave before being rejected. Anticipating premature closure, the nurse explores with the individual anticipated feelings, including the wish to run away. After careful planning, the nurse anticipates, in advance, the client's feelings, discusses how to cope with them, reviews the progress the individual has made, and summarizes what the person has learned from the relationship that can be generalized to future encounters.

Establishing Personal Boundaries and Limitations. Personal boundaries are highly context specific. Our personal physical space needs (boundaries) are distinct from the behavioural and emotional limits which we have. These concepts apply to both the client and the nurse. Furthermore, limits may be temporary (e.g., "I can't talk with you right now, but after my meeting, I can be available for 30 minutes.") (see Chapter 6).

Testing limits is a natural way of identifying where the boundaries are and how strong they are. Therefore, it is necessary to state clearly the enduring limits (e.g., the written rules or contract) and the consequences of violating them. The limits must then be consistently maintained. Clarifying limits requires making explicit what is usually implicit. Despite the clinical setting (e.g., hospital, day treatment setting, outpatient clinic), the nurse must clearly state the day, time, and duration of each contact with the client and remain consistent in those expectations. This may mean having a standing appointment in day treatment or a mental health clinic or noting the time during each shift that the nurse will talk individually with the hospitalized client. The nurse should refrain from offering personal information, which is frequently confusing to the person with BPD. At times, the person may present in a somewhat arrogant and entitled way. It is important for the nurse to recognize such a presentation as reflective of internal confusion and dissonance. Responding in a very neutral manner avoids confrontation and a power struggle, which might also unwittingly reinforce the client's internal sense of inferiority.

Some additional strategies for establishing the boundaries of the relationship include the following:

- Documenting in the client chart the agreed-on appointment expectations
- Sharing the treatment plan with the client
- Confronting violations of the agreement in a nonpunitive way
- Discussing the purpose of limits in the therapeutic relationship and applicability to other relationships

When individuals violate boundaries, it is important to respond right away but without taking the behaviour personally. For example, if a client is flirtatious, simply say something like, "I feel uncomfortable with your overly friendly behaviour. It is out of place within our professional relationship. It is important that we maintain a professional relationship so that I may help you. We cannot and will not have a different kind of relationship."

Management of Dissociative States. The desired outcome for someone who dissociates is to reduce or eliminate the dissociative experiences. The natural tendency is to want to "fix it." Unfortunately, there are limited medications for dissociation, but because the SSRIs, dopamine antagonists, and serotonin–dopamine antagonists affect other target symptoms, the dissociative experiences decrease. Because dissociation occurs during periods of stress, the best approach is to help the individual develop other strategies to deal with stress.

The nurse can teach clients how to identify when they are dissociating and then to use some grounding strategies in the moment. Basic to grounding is planting both feet firmly on the floor or ground, then taking a deep abdominal breath to the count of four, holding it to the count of 4, exhaling to the count of 4, and then holding it to the count of 4. This is called the four-square method of breathing. The benefit of this approach is to bring about a deep, slow breath that activates the calming mechanisms of the parasympathetic system.

After the grounding exercise, the client uses one or more senses to make contact with the environment, such as touching the fabric of a nearby chair or listening to the traffic noise. As the client improves in self-esteem and the ability to relate to others, the frequency of dissociation should decrease.

The Use of Behavioural Interventions. The goal of behavioural interventions is to replace dysfunctional behaviours with positive ones. The nurse has an important role in helping individuals control emotions and behaviours by acknowledging and validating desired behaviours and by ignoring or confronting undesired behaviours. Clients often test the nurse for a response, and nurses must decide how to respond to particular behaviours. This can be challenging because even negative responses can be viewed as positive reinforcement for the client. In some instances, if the behaviour is irritating but not harmful or demeaning, it is best to ignore rather than focus on it. However, grossly inappropriate and disrespectful behaviours require confrontation and appropriate consequences which may include an apology to those disrespected and changes in client privileges.

Such incidences can be used to help the client understand why the behaviour is inappropriate and how it can be changed. The nurse should explore with the client what happened, what events led up to the behaviour, what were the consequences, and what feelings were aroused. Advanced practice nurses or other therapists will explore the origins of the client's behaviours and responses, but the generalist nurse needs to help the person explore ways to change behaviours involved in the current situation. The laboriousness of this analytical process may be a sufficient incentive for the client to abandon the dysfunctional behaviour.

Addressing Emotional Regulation. A major goal of cognitive therapeutic interventions is emotional regulation—recognizing and controlling the expression of feelings. Clients often fail even to recognize their feelings; instead, they respond quickly without thinking about the consequences. Remember, the time needed for taking action is shorter than the time needed for thinking before acting. Pausing makes up for the momentary lag between the limbic and autonomic response and the prefrontal response.

The nurse can help the client identify feelings and gain control over expressions such as anger, disappointment, or frustration. The goal is for individuals to tolerate their feelings without feeling compelled to act out those feelings on another person or on themselves.

A helpful technique for managing feelings is known as the **communication triad**. The triad provides a specific syntax and order for clients to identify and express their feelings and seek relief. The "sentence" consists of three parts:

- An "I" statement to identify the prevailing feeling
- A nonjudgemental statement of the emotional trigger
- What the individual would like differently or what would restore comfort to the situation

The nurse must emphasize with clients that they begin with the "I" statement and the identification of feelings, although many want to begin with the condition. If the person begins with the condition, the statement becomes accusatory and likely to evoke defensiveness (e.g., "When you interrupt me, I get mad."). Beginning with "I" allows the client to identify and express the feeling first and take full ownership. For example, the individual who is angry with another client in the group might say, "Joe, I feel angry ('I' statement with ownership of feeling) when you interrupt me (the trigger), and I would like you to apologize and try not to do that with me (what the individual wants and the remedy)." This simple skill is easy to teach, is easy to reinforce and to encourage others to reinforce, and is a surprisingly effective way of moderating the emotional tone.

Another element of emotional regulation is learning to delay gratification. When clients want something that is not immediately available, the nurse can teach individuals to distract themselves, find alternate ways of meeting the need, and think about what would happen if they have to wait to meet the need.

The practice of **thought stopping** might also help the person to control the inappropriate expression of feelings. In thought stopping, the client identifies what feelings and thoughts exist together. For example, when the person is ruminating about a perceived hurt, the individual might say "Stop that" (referring to the ruminative thought) and engage in a distracting activity. Three activities associated with thought stopping are effective:

- Taking a quick deep breath when the behaviour is noted (this also stimulates relaxation)
- Visualizing a stop sign or saying "stop" when possible (this allows the person to hear externally and internally)
- Deliberately replacing the undesired behaviour with a positive alternative (e.g., instead of ruminating about an angry situation, thinking about a neutral or positive self-affirmation)

The sequencing and combining of the steps puts the person back in control.

Addressing Dysfunctional Thinking. The nurse can help the individual address his or her problematic, dysfunctional ways of thinking by encouraging the person to think about the event in a different way. This is termed reframing. The client learns to take a more positive, yet realistic, perspective on a situation or issue. When a client engages in catastrophic thinking, the nurse can address such thinking by asking, "What is the worst that could happen?" and "How likely would that be to occur?" For dichotomous thinking, as when the client fixates on one extreme perception or alternates between the extremes only, the nurse can ask the person to think about any examples of exceptions to the extreme. The point of the challenge is not to debate or argue with the individual but to provide different perspectives to consider. Encouraging clients to keep journals of real interactions to process with the nurse or therapist is another effective way of testing the reality of their thinking and anticipations, affording more choices and flexibility (Box 27.9).

In problem-solving, the nurse might encourage the individual to debate both sides of the problem and then search for common ground. Practicing communication and negotiation skills through role-playing helps clients make mistakes and correct them without harm to their self-esteem. The nurse also encourages clients to use these skills in their everyday lives and report back on the results, asking individuals how they feel applying the skills and how doing so affects their self-perceptions. Success, even partial success, builds a sense of competence and self-esteem.

Management of Transient Psychotic Episodes. During psychotic episodes with auditory hallucinations, clients should be protected from harming themselves or others. In an inpatient setting, the client should be monitored closely and a determination made as to whether

BOX 27.9 Thought Distortions and Corrective Statements

Thought Distortion	Corrective Statement
Catastrophizing	
"This is the most awful thing that has ever happened to me."	"This is a sad thing, but not the most awful."
"If I fail this course, my life is over."	"If you fail the course, you can take the course again. You can change your major."
Dichotomizing	
"No one ever listens to me."	"Your husband listened to you last night when you told him…"
"I never get what I want."	"You didn't get the promotion this year, but you did get a merit raise."
"I can't understand why everyone is so kind at first and then always dumps me when I need them the most."	"It is hard to remember those kind things and times when your friends have stayed with you when you needed them."
Self-Attribution Errors	
"If I had just found the right thing to say, she wouldn't have left me."	"There is not a single right thing to say; and she left you because she chose to."
"If I had not made him mad, he wouldn't have hit me."	"He has a lot of choices in how to respond, and he chose hitting. You are responsible for your feelings and actions."

the voices are telling the person to engage in self-harm (command hallucinations). The client may be observed more closely and begin taking antipsychotic medications. In the community setting, the nurse should help the client develop a plan for managing the voices. For example, if the voices return, the individual contacts the clinic and returns for evaluation. There may be a friend or relative who should be contacted or a case manager who can help the person get the necessary protection if it is needed. In some instances, hearing the voices is a prelude to self-injury. Another person may be able to help the individual resist the voices. Once other aspects of the disorder are managed, the episodes of psychosis decrease or disappear.

Teaching and practicing distress tolerance skills help the individual have power over the voices and control intense emotions. When not experiencing hallucinations, the client can practice deep abdominal breathing, which calms the autonomic nervous system. Using brainstorming techniques, the individual identifies early internal cues of rising distress while the nurse writes them on an index card for the client to refer to later. Next, the nurse teaches some skills for tolerating painful feelings or events. To help the client, suggest the mnemonic "Wise Mind ACCEPTS" with the following actions:

- Activities to distract from stress
- Contributing to others, such as volunteering or visiting a sick neighbour
- Comparing yourself to people less fortunate than you
- Emotions that are opposite to what you are experiencing

- Pushing away from the situation for awhile
- Thoughts other than those you are currently experiencing
- Sensations that are intense, such as holding ice in your hand (Linehan, 1993b, pp. 165–166)

Client Education

Client education within the context of a therapeutic relationship is one of the most important, empowering interventions for the nurse to use. Teaching individuals skills to resist parasuicidal urges and self-harming behaviours, improve emotional regulation, enhance interpersonal relationships, tolerate stress, and enhance overall quality of life provides the foundation for long-term behavioural changes. These skills can be taught in any treatment setting as a part of the overall facility program (see Box 27.10). If nurses are practicing in a facility where DBT is the treatment model, they can be trained in DBT and can serve as group skills leaders.

Social Domain

Social Assessment

Some individuals with BPD can function very well except during periods when symptoms erupt. They hold jobs, are active in communities, and can perform well. During periods of stress, symptoms often appear. On the other hand, some individuals with severe BPD function poorly; they are always in a crisis, which they have often created.

Social Support Systems. The identification of social supports, such as family, friends, and religious organizations, is the purpose in assessing resources. Knowing how the

---

BOX 27.10 Psychoeducation Checklist: Borderline Personality Disorder

When caring for the client with BPD, be sure to include the following topic areas in the teaching plan:

- Management of medication, if used, including drug action, dosage, frequency, and possible adverse effects
- Regular sleep routines
- Nutrition
- Safety measures
- Functional versus dysfunctional behaviours
- Cognitive strategies (distraction, communication skills, thought stopping)
- Structure and limit setting
- Social relationships
- Community resources

---

person obtains social support is important in understanding the quality of interpersonal relationships. For example, some individuals consider their "best friends" to be their nurses, physicians, and other health care personnel. Because this is a false friendship (i.e., not reciprocal), it inevitably leads to frustration and disappointment. Helping the individual find ways to meet other people and encouraging the client's efforts are more realistic.

Interpersonal Skills. An assessment of the person's ability to relate to others is important because interpersonal problems are linked to dissociation and self-injurious behaviour. Information about friendships, frequency of contact, and intimate relationships will provide data about the person's ability to relate to others. Clients with BPD often are sexually active and may have numerous sexual partners. Their need for closeness clouds their judgement about sexual partners, and it is not unusual to find these individuals in abusive, destructive relationships with people with antisocial personality disorder (discussed later in this chapter). During assessment, nurses should use their own self-awareness skills to examine their personal response to the client. How the nurse responds to the individual can often be a clue to how others perceive and respond to this person. For example, if the nurse feels irritated or impatient during the interview, that is a sign that others respond to this person in the same way; on the other hand, if the nurse feels empathy or closeness, chances are this individual can evoke these same feelings in others.

Self-Esteem and Coping Skills. Coping with stressful situations is one of the major problems for people with BPD. An assessment of their coping skills and their ability to deal with stressful situations is important. Because the individual's self-esteem is usually very low, an assessment of self-esteem can

be done with a self-esteem assessment or by interviewing the client and analyzing the assessment data for evidence of personal self-worth and confidence. Clients with BPD perceive their families and friends as being weary of their numerous crises and their seeming unwillingness to break the cycle of self-destructiveness. Feeling rejected by their natural support system, these individuals may attempt to create one within the health care system. During periods of crisis or affective instability, especially during the late evening, early morning, or on weekends, they may call or visit the hospital, asking to speak to specific personnel who formerly cared for them. Sometimes, they bring gifts to nurses or call them at home. Because this attempt at a new social support system must fail as it cannot provide the desired support, the person continues to feel rejected. One of the goals of the treatment is to help the individual establish a natural support network.

Family Assessment. Family members may or may not be involved with the client. Individuals with BPD are often estranged from their families. In other instances, they are dependent on them, which is also a source of stress. If childhood abuse has occurred, the perpetrator may be a family member. Ideally, family members are interviewed for their perspectives on the client's problem. An assessment of any mental disorder in the client's family and of the current level of functioning is useful in understanding the client and identifying potential resources for support.

Nursing Diagnoses for the Social Domain

Defensive coping, chronic low self-esteem, and impaired social interaction are nursing diagnoses that address the social problems faced by clients with BPD.

Interventions for the Social Domain: Modifying Coping Behaviours

Environmental management becomes critical in caring for a person with BPD. Because the unit can be structured to represent a microcosm of the individual's community, clients have an opportunity to identify relationship problems, boundary violations, and stressful situations. When these situations occur, the nurse can help the individual cope by finding alternative explanations for the situation and practicing new skills. Individual sessions help the client try out some skills, such as putting feelings into words without actions. Role-playing may help individuals experience different degrees of effectively relating feelings without the burden of hurting someone they care about. Day treatment and group settings are excellent places for clients to learn more effective feeling management and to practice these techniques with each other. The group helps members develop empathy and diffuses attachment to any one person or therapist.

Building Social Skills and Self-Esteem. Many women with a diagnosis of BPD are involved in abusive relationships and lack the ability to resolve these relationships because of their extreme anxiety regarding separating from those they love and their extreme need to feel connected. These women verbalize desires to leave, but they do not have the strength and self-confidence needed to leave. Exposing them to a different style of interaction as well as validation from other people increases their self-esteem and ability to separate from negative influences.

Exploring Social Supports. Dependency on family members is a problem for many people with BPD. In some families, a client's positive progress may be met with negative responses, and individuals in these situations need help in maintaining a separate identity while staying connected to family members for social support. Family support groups sometimes help. Usually, the nurse helps the person explore new relationships that can provide additional social contacts.

Teaching Effective Ways to Communicate. An important area of client education is teaching communication skills. Clients lack interpersonal skills in relating because they often had inadequate modelling and few opportunities to practice. The goals of relationship skill development are to identify problematic behaviours that interfere with relationships and to use appropriate behaviours in improving relationships. The starting point is with communication. The nurse teaches the individual basic communication approaches, such as making "I" statements, paraphrasing what the other party says before responding, checking the accuracy of perceptions with others, compromising and seeking common ground, listening actively, and offering and accepting reactions. Besides modelling the behaviours, the nurse guides clients in practicing a variety of communication approaches for common situations. When role-playing, the nurse needs to discuss not only what the skills are and how to perform them but also the feelings clients have before, during, and after the role-play.

In day treatment and outpatient settings, the nurse can give the client homework, such as keeping a journal, applying role-playing skills to actual situations, and observing behaviours in others. In the hospital, the individual can experience the same process, and the nurse is available to offer immediate feedback. Whatever the setting, or even the specific problems addressed, the nurse must keep in mind and remind the client that change occurs slowly. Thus, working on the problems occurs gradually, with severity of symptoms as the guide to deciding how fast and how much change to expect.

Spiritual Domain

In addressing the spiritual domain, the qualities of the nurse that have been identified as important include receptivity (e.g., being genuinely available to the client as a person), humanity (e.g., taking time for the "little things" when giving care), competency (e.g., demonstrating safe practice), and positivity (e.g., having

a hopeful attitude and fostering a positive spirit) (Carr, 2008; see Chapter 11). In nursing clients with BPD, enacting these qualities may be challenging, as characteristics of BPD involving self-dysregulation and interpersonal dysregulation can sometimes promote a negative response to the person in the nurse. If the nurse does not grasp that the client's personality patterns do comprise a mental disorder, she or he may become frustrated with the lack of client behaviour change and progress. As well, trying to understand the worldview of the client with BPD can be difficult. Spiritual care is particularly important for such clients as they struggle with issues of self and connection, purpose and meaning. A review of the research on spirituality and persons with PDs, in fact, indicates that spiritual well-being may remain high for persons with borderline personality traits, even though general well-being is low (Bennett, Shepherd, & Janca, 2013). Nurses can play an important role in helping clients sustain such well-being through respectful, knowledgeable, and supportive connection within a therapeutic relationship.

Evaluation and Outcomes

Evaluation and outcomes vary depending on the severity of the disorder, the presence of comorbid disorders, and the availability of resources. For a client with severe symptoms or continual self-injury, keeping the individual safe and alive may be a realistic outcome. Helping the person resist parasuicidal urges may take years. In contrast, individuals who rarely need hospitalization and have adequate resources can expect to recover from the self-destructive impulses and learn positive interaction skills that promote a fulfilling lifestyle. Most clients fall somewhere in between, with periods of symptom exacerbation and remission. In these individuals, increasing the symptom-free time may be the best indicator of outcomes.

Continuum of Care

Treatment of BPD is long term. Hospitalization is sometimes necessary during acute episodes involving parasuicidal or suicidal behaviour. Brief psychiatric hospitalization as an intervention has be found to be effective in preventing such behaviour and in facilitating quick return to the community. Such brief admission is goal directed (e.g., prevention of self-harm), with potential interventions and conditions for premature (i.e., forced) discharge identified on admission. As an intervention, it permits nurses to support the individual with BPD to actively cope with symptoms (Helleman, Goossens, Kaasenbrood, & van Achterberg, 2014). Ongoing treatment in the outpatient or day treatment setting is important as individuals with BPD often appear more competent and in control than they are. They need continued follow-up and therapy, including individual therapy, psychoeducation, and positive role models (see Nursing Care Plan 27.1).

NURSING CARE PLAN 27.1

CLIENT WITH BPD

E.L. is a 26-year-old woman, admitted to the hospital's psychiatric unit via the emergency department. The manager of E.L.'s apartment building found her lying on floor of its entrance way, sobbing loudly and surrounded by her scattered mail. She had bleeding lacerations on both arms; the manager noticed faint scars on E.L.'s arms, as well. When her attempts to assist E.L. to her apartment were met with physical resistance and cursing, the manager called the police. E.L. cooperated when the police wanted to transport her to the hospital. Assessment of E.L. by an emergency physician and a psychiatric resident determined that she had a history of self-harm, as well as one psychiatric admission for suicidal behaviour from which she was discharged with a diagnosis of BPD and a referral for psychotherapy. E.L. states that she went for psychotherapy, but quit after a few months as it was not helpful. The therapist disliked her. Her current distress appears related to her new boyfriend's departure on a business trip. Despite her pleas, he refused to allow her to accompany him. E.L. works part-time as an office "temp." She has a married, younger brother living in another province. E.L.'s mother died suddenly of an aneurysm when E.L. was 7 years old; she refuses to speak of her father, saying only that she has had nothing to do with him since she left home at 16 years of age. E.L.'s lacerations were treated in the emergency department, and she was voluntarily admitted to the hospital's psychiatric unit.

Once on the psychiatric unit, E.L. is assigned a primary nurse, J.K. During her unit admission and nursing assessment, E.L. begins to cry. Through tears, she laughs and tells J.K., "I am just so relieved to be here and to have such a nice nurse like you. When I was here before, my primary nurse was so cold and critical of me." J.K. asks her to agree not to cut or harm herself in any way for the next 24 hours. E.L. shouts, "No! I can't promise that! If I could do that I wouldn't be here!" Observing E.L.'s level of distress during her assessment and her inability to agree not to self-harm, J.K. decides that E.L. requires close observation. J.K. orients E.L. to the unit facilities. In the lounge area, E.L. smiles at other clients sitting there and readily joins in conversation with them.

Setting: Inpatient Psychiatric Unit in a General Hospital

Baseline Assessment: E.L. is a 26-year-old woman, admitted to the psychiatric unit through the emergency department where she was treated for self-inflicted lacerations on both forearms. She is distressed and angry that her new boyfriend refused to allow her to accompany him on a business trip. She appears to understand this as a lack of commitment to their relationship and is fearful that he may connect with other women on his trip and that he is intending to "dump" her. Her behaviour since being found by her apartment manager has fluctuated between being distressed, angry, and resistant to assistance to being cooperative and relieved at receiving help.

Psychiatric Diagnosis	Medications
Borderline Personality Disorder	Sertraline (Zoloft) 150 mg qd for anxiety.

Nursing Diagnosis 1: Self-Mutilation

Defining Characteristics	Related Factors
Lacerations on forearms	Fears of abandonment secondary to boyfriend's departure on a business trip
Self-inflicted wounds	Inability to handle stress

Outcomes

Initial	Discharge
1. Remain safe and not harm herself.	4. Identify ways to respond to self-harming impulses if they return.
2. Identify feelings before and after cutting herself.	5. Verbalize alternate thinking with more realistic base.
3. Consider alternative response to self-harm to deal with feelings.	6. Identify community resources to provide structure and support.

NURSING CARE PLAN 27.1 *(Continued)*

Interventions

Interventions	Rationale	Ongoing Assessment
Monitor the client for changes in mood or behaviour that might lead to self-injurious behaviour.	Close observation establishes safety and protection of the client from self-harm and impulsive behaviours.	Document according to policy. Continue to observe for mood and behaviour changes.
Monitor for suicidal ideation.	Will indicate increased risk for suicide.	Document according to policy. Continue to observe for suicide risk.
Discuss with the client the need for close observation and rationale to keep her safe.	Explanation to the client for the purpose of nursing interventions helps her cooperate with the nursing activity.	Assess her response to the increasing level of observation.
Administer medications as prescribed and evaluate medication effectiveness in reducing anxiety and cognitive disorganization.	Allows for adjustment of medication dosage based on target behaviours and outcomes.	Observe for side effects.
Communicate information about the client's risk for self-harm and potential risk for suicide to other nursing staff.	The close observation should be continued throughout all shifts until the risk for self-harm has abated. Risk assessment includes distress level and presence of suicidal ideation.	Review the documentation of close observation for all shifts.
Teach relaxation techniques.	Provides an alternative way to deal with tension.	Support practice of techniques. Document.

Evaluation

Outcomes	Revised Outcomes	Interventions
Remained safe without further harming self. Identified fears of abandonment before cutting herself and relief of anxiety afterwards.	Will record her fears in a journal to gain further understanding of them.	Offer her a notebook to use as a journal.
Identified friends to call when fears return and hotlines to use if necessary.	Use hotlines or call friends if self-harm fears return.	Give the client hotline number. Advise her to record this number and her friends' contact numbers in an easily accessible place.
Notified staff when desire to self-harm occurred; discussed her feelings; used relaxation techniques to deal with tension.	Does not harm self for 3 days.	Remind her to call someone if urges return.
Enrolled in a day hospital program for 4 weeks.	Attend the day hospital program.	Follow-up on enrolment.

Nursing Diagnosis 2: Readiness for Enhanced Hope

Defining Characteristics	Related Factors
Wants to stop self-harming.	Desires a good relationship with boyfriend. Believes self-harming will negatively impact it.

NURSING CARE PLAN 27.1 *(Continued)*

Outcomes

Initial	Discharge
Discuss her hopes for change.	Identify two strategies to enhance hope for change.
Identify desired positive changes.	Select one positive change as a goal. Record the goal in journal.

Interventions

Interventions	Rationale	Ongoing Assessment
Develop a therapeutic relationship.	Individuals with BPD are able to consider positive change within the structure of a therapeutic relationship.	Assess her ability to relate and the nurse's response to the relationship.
Discuss her past experience with making a positive change in behaviour.	By identifying barriers to change and elements of success, she can identify a realistic goal.	Assess her ability to accept challenges related to change.
Acknowledge that change takes time and that it is usual for setbacks to occur.	Acknowledging that making changes in one's life is possible even when setbacks occur and progress is slow will support hope for realistic change.	Assess whether she is accepting of the time and effort to make a behavioural change.
Teach her cognitive behavioural techniques.	Learning about ways of identifying and assessing negative thoughts will help the client recognize those which detract from sustaining hope for change.	Review understanding of the techniques. Encourage questions about it.

Evaluation

Outcomes	Revised Outcomes	Interventions
E.L. is able to express realistic hope for change of self-harming behaviour and wants to seek new opportunities for support, such as the day treatment program.	None	Continue to identify ways to enhance hope through resources such as those at Hope Studies Central at the University of Alberta (https://sites.google.com/a/ualberta.ca/hope-studies/). Use journal to record ideas and strategies.

Carpenito, L. J. (2017). *Handbook of nursing diagnoses* (15th ed.). Philadelphia, PA: Lippincott Williams & Wilkins.

Antisocial Personality Disorder

Clinical Course of Disorder

In the *DSM-5*, the essential feature of ASPD is "a pervasive pattern of disregard for, and violation of, the rights of others that begins in childhood or early adolescence and continues into adulthood" (APA, 2013, p. 659). Because of its association with conduct disorders, ASPD is listed there as well as with PDs in the *DSM-5*. A diagnosis of ASPD cannot be given until an individual is 18 years of age; however, there must be a history of symptoms of conduct disorder before the age of 15 years (APA). Features of ASPD are discussed below, but for the official APA diagnostic criteria, see the DSM-5.

ASPD is related to, but not synonymous with, the older, broader term "psychopath." The work of Cleckley (1941), author of *The Mask of Sanity*, remains the greatest influence on contemporary understanding of psychopathy, but Cleckley's criteria have evolved by researchers such as Hare who has developed measures of psychopathy (e.g., Crego & Widiger, 2016; Psychopathy Checklist-Revised; Hare, 1991). While the DSM-5 criteria for ASPD include features essential to the psychopathy construct, these features are not required for an ASPD diagnosis to be given; most individuals with ASPD are not psychopathic, but most of those who are psychopathic meet ASPD diagnostic criteria (Hare & Neumann, 2009).

Individuals with ASPD fail to conform to the ethical and social standards of their community (e.g., deceitful, exploitive, callous). Although they can be superficially charming and facile communicators, in reality, they lack empathy and compassion. Easily irritated, they often act out aggressively without concerns for consequences and may end up in the correctional system. Although it has been suggested that, in forensic environments, an ASPD diagnosis indicates a higher risk for being a serious threat to others, research to date gives no credence to that claim (Edens, Kelley, Lilienfeld, Skeem, & Douglas, 2015). Most individuals with ASPD, however, will not come in conflict with the law; some find a niche in society, such as in business, the military, or politics, which rewards their competitive, tough behaviour (Millon et al., 2004). Given that ASPD is associated with low economic status in urban settings, the diagnosis may be misapplied when antisocial behaviour is an aspect of survival and protective strategies (APA, 2013, p. 662); criminal behaviour for gain without the personality features of ASPD does not meet ASPD diagnostic criteria.

Prevalence and Comorbidity

A national study in the United States found the lifetime prevalence of ASPD to be 3.6% (Compton, Conway, Stinson, Colliver, & Grant, 2005); the prevalence among individuals with severe alcohol use disorder and/or in clinical and forensic settings is much higher, over 70% (APA, 2013).

Aetiology

There appears to be both genetic and environmental influences (shared and nonshared) involved in the a etiology of ASPD, but the weight of these influences and whether these influences act independently or together has yet to be concluded. Through behavioural genetics studies, particularly with twins, knowledge of the aetiology of ASPD is evolving. In an overview of the behavioural genetics of ASPD and psychopathy, Werner, Few, and Bucholz (2015) note that studies indicate both psychopathic personality traits and ASPD are influenced by additive genetic factors and nonshared environmental factors (i.e., factors not in common with siblings, such as friends, independent activities) without there being a significant contribution of shared environment (i.e., same home with its elements of culture, parenting). Rosenström and colleagues (2017) used structured interview data (i.e., DSM interview for PDs) and a population-based twin sample ($n = 2,794$) to investigate genetic and environmental factors associated with ASPD criteria. Both independent and common pathway biometric models were compared. These researchers concluded that there is "a single, highly heritable common factor" liability for ASPD that may account for correlations among the ASPD criteria (Rosenström et al., 2017, p. 272). This finding challenges the results of other studies in this area.

Other research, which contributes to our understanding of the influences of nature (genetics) and nurture (environment) in ASPD, is a study of callous and unemotional behaviour in children (at 27 months of age) by Hyde and colleagues (2016). They used an adoption cohort of 561 families and assessed biologic mothers for a history of severe antisocial behaviour and observed the positive reinforcement behaviours of the adoptive mothers. Antisocial behaviour of biologic mothers predicted early callous–unemotional behaviours in their offspring, despite limited or no contact between them. High levels of adoptive mother positive reinforcement, however, appeared to buffer the effects of heritable risk. This finding has implications for prevention of ASPD, especially given that, for adults with severe antisocial behaviours, these behaviours begin in childhood (Hyde et al., 2016).

Individuals with antisocial and violent histories of offending behaviour have been found to have social cognition problems. Compared with members of a control group, offenders with ASPD had greater difficulty with mentalizing, such that mentalization scores predicted ASPD status. Specific impairments in "perspective taking, social cognition, and social sensitivity, as well as tendencies towards hypomentalizing and nonmentalizing" were greater in those with ASPD (Newbury-Helps, Feigenbaum, & Fonagy, 2017, p. 232). Such findings point to mentalization-focused interventions as a potential means of helping persons with such histories in overcoming social cognitive impairment (see section on MBT in this chapter).

Nursing Care

Persons with ASPD rarely seek mental health care for their disorder itself; they may, rather, seek treatment for depression, substance abuse, or uncontrolled anger or be hospitalized in forensic psychiatric settings for evaluation. Key areas of assessment are determining the quality of relationships, impulsivity, and the extent of irritability and aggression. The characteristics of ASPD mean that individuals with a diagnosis of ASPD will be indifferent to rules and norms and the rights and well-being of others and will use manipulation, including lying, to get what they want. They may, however, make good first impressions and be socially adept. It may be said that this is a disorder where the distress is felt by others. Attention to the protection of other clients and staff from manipulative and sometimes abusive behaviour is necessary. Self-awareness is especially important for the nurse because of the charming quality of many of these individuals. A matter-of-fact approach to such clients is appropriate; vigilance regarding manipulation in terms of bending hospital rules (e.g., regarding smoking, visitors, use of street drugs) or providing unnecessary information about other clients, staff, or oneself is important. At the same time, nurses' determination against being manipulated should not translate into unfair treatment of clients with ASPD. Nursing diagnoses for clients with ASPD are related to their interpersonal detachment, lack of awareness of others, avoidance of feelings, impulsiveness, and discrepancy between their perception of themselves and others' perception of them. Typical diagnoses are ineffective role performance (unemployment), ineffective individual coping, impaired communication, impaired social interactions, low self-esteem, and risk for violence. Outcomes should be short term and relevant to a specific problem. For example, if a person has been chronically unemployed, a reasonable short-term outcome would be to set up job interviews, rather than obtain a job.

Therapeutic relationships are difficult to establish with an individual with ASPD; an alliance may be formed, however, that allows the objectives of care and treatment to move forward. The ability to make genuine commitments is not typical for the individual with ASPD and this should be expected. The goal of the therapeutic relationship is to assist the client in identifying dysfunctional thinking patterns and developing healthier problem-solving behaviours.

Self-responsibility facilitation (encouraging a person to assume more responsibility for personal behaviour) is useful with clients with ASPD (Bulechek et al., 2008). The nursing activities that are particularly helpful include holding clients responsible for their behaviours, monitoring the extent to which self-responsibility is assumed, and discussing the consequences of not dealing with responsibilities. The nurse needs to refrain from arguing or bargaining about the unit rules, such as time for meals, use of the television room, and smoking. Instead, positive feedback is given to the individual for accepting additional responsibility or changing behaviour.

Self-awareness enhancement (exploring and understanding personal thoughts, feelings, motivation, and behaviours) is another nursing intervention that is important in helping these individuals develop a sense of understanding about relating positively to the rest of the world (Bulechek et al., 2008). Encouraging clients to recognize and discuss thoughts and feelings helps the nurse understand how the person views the world. Bear in mind, however, that individuals with ASPD may be telling the nurse what they believe the nurse wants to hear. Communication techniques discussed in the section on BPD are also helpful with these clients. In teaching the client about positive health care practices, impulse control, and anger management, the best approach is to engage the individual in a discussion about the specific challenges faced and then to direct the topic to the major teaching points and avoid being sidetracked (Box 27.11).

BOX 27.11 Psychoeducation Checklist: Antisocial Personality Disorder

When caring for the client with ASPD, be sure to include the following topic areas in the teaching plan:

* Positive health care practices, including substance abuse control
* Effective communication and interaction skills
* Impulse control
* Anger management
* Group experience to help develop self-awareness and impact of behaviour on others
* Analyzing an issue from the other person's viewpoint
* Maintenance of employment
* Interpersonal relationships and social interactions

In an inpatient unit, interventions can be used to assist the individual in developing positive interaction skills and to experience a consistent environment. For example, the focus of nursing interventions may be the client's continual disregard of the rights of others. On one unit, a client continually placed orders for pizzas in the name of another person on the unit. This individual was genuinely afraid of the person with ASPD. The victimized person always paid for the pizza and gave it to the other client. When the nursing staff realized what was happening, they confronted the client with ASPD about the behaviour and revoked his unit privileges.

Group interventions typically are more effective than individual modalities for persons with ASPD. Problem-solving groups that focus on identifying a problem and developing a variety of alternative solutions can be particularly helpful, as can groups with a focus on the development of empathy. Within group therapy, clients are able to confront each other with dysfunctional schemas or thinking patterns.

Milieu interventions, such as providing a structured environment with rules that are consistently applied to clients who are responsible for their own behaviour, are important. While living in close proximity to others, the individual with ASPD will demonstrate dysfunctional social patterns that can be identified and targeted for correction, such as the violation of unit rules.

Aggressive behaviour is often a problem for these individuals and their family members. Anger control assistance (helping to express anger in an adaptive, nonviolent manner) becomes a priority intervention; anger management techniques can be beneficial.

Social support for individuals with ASPD is often minimal as they have taken advantage of friends and relatives who no longer trust them. For new friendships to be developed and sustained and for re-engagement with family members to occur, new ways of interaction must be learned by the person with ASPD. As these ways of interaction need to include empathy and attachment, such goals may never become reality.

The outcomes of interventions for individuals with ASPD need to be evaluated in terms of management of specific problems, such as maintaining employment or developing a meaningful interpersonal relationship, as well as adherence to treatment recommendations and the development of health care practices for other health care issues (e.g., reduce smoking and alcohol consumption).

IN-A-LIFE

Ferdinand Waldo Demara (1921–1982)

THE GREAT IMPOSTOR

Public Persona

Ferdinand Waldo Demara spent much of his adult life using forged, stolen, or nonexistent credentials to gain employment in numerous and varied vocations. He became most famous for his masquerade as a commissioned Surgeon–Lieutenant in the Royal Canadian Navy in 1951, having stolen the identity of the Canadian physician Dr. Joseph Cyr. Demara was apparently competent in his role as a physician, relying on medical texts and a medical assistant. Demara had similar success in other branches of the military, as a psychologist in a college, as a prison warden, and as a well-respected schoolteacher.

Personal Realities

Demara's life was patterned by the establishment of personal connections with individuals (often in the context of a religious order), theft of this person's identity, and subsequent employment using these false credentials. Once caught, he would disappear, only to reappear claiming a new identity. It was a sense of emptiness and boredom that would kindle Demara's dreams and his need to act as an impostor to fulfill his seemingly well-intentioned passions.

Source: Crichton, R. (1959). *The great impostor.* New York, NY: Random House.

Histrionic Personality Disorder

"Hysteria" (a term derived from the Greek for "uterus") is one of the oldest mental disorders. It was described by early Egyptian and Greek physicians as a female illness in which the womb "wandered," producing symptoms wherever it was in the body. The term's influence reached modern psychiatry: conversion hysteria, somatization disorder, and hysterical personality disorder. The latter became histrionic personality disorder (HPD) in the DSM-III. Currently, the argument is being made that HPD should be deleted from the Diagnostic and Statistical Manual system as it is infrequently seen in clinical practice (Novais, Araújo, & Godinho, 2015) and research regarding its treatment is lacking (Paris, 2015).

Despite its roots in hysteria, HPD is not a female disorder: although more females may be diagnosed with HPD in clinical settings, its prevalence is similar across genders (APA, 2013). "Attention seeking" and "emotional" describe people with HPD, who are lively and dramatic and draw attention to themselves by their enthusiasm, dress, and apparent openness; they can be the "life of the party." Their speech, too, is dramatic; strong opinions without supporting facts are often expressed and readily changed. (A further historical note: "histrione" was used in ancient Rome to name actors in farces representing characters who were false and theatrical (Novais et al., 2015).) Persistent need for attention and approval is an aspect of this PD.

The person with HPD may be moody and experience a sense of helplessness when others are disinterested in them. Although they may be hypersensitive to the moods and thoughts of those they hope to please, individuals with HPD have difficulty achieving genuine intimacy in interpersonal relationships (Sadock, Sadock, & Ruiz, 2015). Their need for constant attention can quickly alienate others; without such attention they may become depressed.

As culture affects the norms for physical appearance, interpersonal behaviour, and emotional expressiveness, the traits expressed by an individual must be evaluated in context as to whether clinically significant impairment or distress exists before a diagnosis of HPD is made (APA, 2013). This disorder may co-occur with BPD, DPD (discussed later in this chapter), and ASPD, as well as anxiety disorders, substance abuse, and mood disorders (Millon et al., 2004).

Nursing Care

The ultimate treatment goal for individuals with HPD is to help them change the tendency to fulfill all their needs by focusing on others to the exclusion of themselves. In the nursing assessment, the nurse focuses on understanding the quality of the individual's interpersonal relationships. Those with HPD can be dissatisfied with spouses, partners, and friends as insufficiently supportive. During the assessment, the client may make statements that indicate low self-esteem. Because these individuals assume that they are incapable of handling life's demands and that they need a truly competent person to take care of them, they have not developed a positive self-concept or adequate problem-solving abilities.

Nursing diagnoses that are usually generated include chronic low self-esteem, ineffective individual coping, and ineffective sexual patterns. Outcomes focus on helping the individual develop autonomy, a positive self-concept, and mature problem-solving and coping skills.

A variety of interventions support the outcomes. A nurse–client relationship that allows the client to explore positive personality characteristics and develop independent decision-making skills forms the basis of the interventions. Reinforcing personal strengths, conveying confidence in the person's ability to handle situations, and examining negative perceptions of self can be done within the therapeutic relationship. Encouraging the client to act autonomously can also improve the individual's sense of self-worth. Assertiveness training may help increase the individual's self-confidence and improve self-esteem.

Narcissistic Personality Disorder

The use of the term "narcissism" for excessive self-love came from an ancient Greek myth. A young man, Narcissus, upon seeing his own reflection in a forest pool, fell in love and died pining for his own image: "Unwitting youth, himself/He wants;—at once beloving, and belov'd" (Ovid, 1807/2009, p. 949). Individuals with NPD seem to possess a form of self-love that causes problems for themselves and affects their relationships with others. They present as having an inexhaustible need for admiration, a grandiose sense of their own importance, and a lack of empathy (Sadock et al., 2015). The latter symptom is being challenged, as analysis of clinical cases suggests that empathy is not absent in individuals but dysfunctional and can fluctuate in terms of motivational disengagement or affective experience (Baskin-Sommers, Krusemark, & Ronningstam, 2014). Persons with NPD have a sense of being very special, which leads them to be preoccupied with fantasies of unlimited success, power, beauty, or ideal love. Their benign arrogance is associated with a strong sense of entitlement. Behavioural features associated with NPD include "vulnerable self-esteem, feelings of shame, sensitivity, and intense reactions of humiliation, emptiness or disdain to criticism or defeat, and vocational irregularities due to difficulties tolerating criticism or competition" (Ronningstam, 2012, p. 536). Others' perceptions of a person with NPD may be very different from that individual's self-perception. Behind grandiose notions of self-importance, for example, there may be a sense of insecurity (Ronningstam, 2012).

The aetiology of NPD is believed to include inheritance, temperament, and psychological trauma (e.g., neglect, deeply humiliating or fearful experiences, sudden loss of relationships); reactivation of such trauma can be a factor in seeking treatment. As well, change and unexpected life events can threaten the individual's self-esteem, stimulate emotional reactions, and severely impact his or her functioning (Ronningstam, 2017). Treatment for NPD is usually some form of psychotherapy, community based.

Nursing Care

The nurse usually encounters persons with NPD in clinical settings due to another medical condition, perhaps a coexisting psychiatric disorder. Within the nurse–client relationship, it is important to listen carefully and attempt to understand the person's own perceptions of experiences, bearing in mind that the person may not readily self-disclose. Understanding their sense of self-agency is helpful as it reflects self-awareness, self-esteem, and self-regulation; it allows for some differentiation regarding real competence and accomplishments from grandiose or self-devaluated ones (Ronningstam, 2012, 2017). Individuals with NPD tend to have a sense of entitlement and expect special consideration and "service"; a therapeutic response to such demands may be required. Nurses must pay close attention to their own reaction to the client: it will give clues as to the way others may respond to the client, as well as indicate any issues with therapeutic use of self that need to be addressed.

Cluster C Disorders

Avoidant Personality Disorder

AVPD is characterized by a desire for affiliation that is affected by a sense of personal inadequacy and intense fear of social rejection (Sanislow, da Cruz, Gianol, & Reagan, 2012). The person with AVPD thus avoids social situations, including occupational activities, in which there is interpersonal contact with others. They engage in interpersonal relationships only when they are certain that they will receive approval and be liked. They appear timid, shy, and hesitant. They perceive themselves as socially inept and inadequate and avoid new activities as they may be a new source of embarrassment (Sadock et al., 2015). Fantasy may become a means to gratify needs and to feel confident; withdrawing into fantasies can be a means of dealing with frustration and anger. Persons with AVPD experience feelings of tension, sadness, and anger that vacillate between desire for affection, fear of rebuff, embarrassment, and numbness of feeling (APA, 2013; Millon et al., 2004). They may have a fulfilling family life with their relationships restricted primarily to family members (Sadock et al., 2015).

Nursing Care

An assessment of these individuals reveals a lack of social contacts, a fear of being criticized, and evidence of chronic low self-esteem. The nursing diagnoses of chronic low self-esteem, social isolation, and ineffective coping can be used. The establishment of a therapeutic relationship is necessary to be able to help the client meet treatment outcomes. The nurse should expect the nurse–client relationship to take time to develop, as the individual is usually inexperienced in positive interpersonal relationships and will need time to trust that the nurse will not be critical and demeaning. Interventions should focus on assisting the client to identify positive responses from others, exploring previous achievements of success, and exploring reasons for self-criticism. The person's social dimension should be examined for activities that increase self-esteem and interventions focused on multiplying such activities. Social skills training may help reduce symptoms.

Dependent Personality Disorder

Individuals with dependent personality disorder (DPD) are desperate to keep others close and will be over willing to do anything to maintain closeness, including being submissive and without regard for self. Decision-making is difficult for persons with DPD, who adapt their behaviour to please those to whom they lean upon for guidance. Ingratiating to others but self-denigrating, the person with DPD's self-esteem is other determined. Behaviourally, they are fearful of adult responsibilities and seek nurturance and support from others. In interpersonal relationships, they need excessive advice and reassurance. They are compliant, conciliatory, and placating. They rarely disagree with others and are easily persuaded. Friends describe them as gullible. They are warm, tender, and noncompetitive. They timidly avoid social tension and interpersonal conflicts (APA, 2013; Sadock et al., 2015). DPD bears resemblance to HPD; individuals with DPD demonstrate high levels of self-attributed dependency needs, while those with HPD have a greater implicit dependency and will even argue against needing others (Bornstein, 1998).

Nursing Care

Nurses can determine the extent of dependency by an assessment of self-worth, interpersonal relationships, and social behaviours. They should determine whether there is currently someone on whom the person relies (e.g., parent, spouse) or if there has been a separation from a significant relationship by death or divorce.

Nursing diagnoses that are usually generated from the assessment data are ineffective individual coping, low self-esteem, impaired social interaction, and impaired home maintenance management. Home management may be a problem if the client does not have the necessary skills and has to make decisions related to finances, shopping, cooking, and cleaning. The challenge of caring for these individuals is to help them recognize their dependent patterns, motivate them to want to change, and teach them adult skills that have not been developed, such as balancing a cheque book, planning a weekly menu, and paying bills. Occasionally, if a client is extremely fatigued, lethargic, or anxious and the disorder interferes with efforts at developing more independence, antidepressants or antianxiety agents may be used.

These individuals readily engage in a nurse–client relationship and initially will look to the nurse to make all decisions. The nurse can support these individuals to make their own decisions by resisting the urge to tell them what to do. Ideally, these clients are in individual psychotherapy and working towards long-term personality changes. The nurse can encourage clients to stay in therapy and to practice the new skills that are being learned. Assertiveness training is helpful therapy. Persons with chronic illness may be more susceptible than others to developing this disorder (Sadock et al., 2015).

Obsessive–Compulsive Personality Disorder

OCPD bears a close resemblance to obsessive–compulsive disorder (OCD). A distinguishing difference is that those with OCD tend to have obsessive thoughts and compulsions when anxious but less so when anxiety decreases. With OCPD, the person does not demonstrate obsessions and compulsions as much as an overall inflexibility, perfectionism, and need to be in mental and interpersonal control. In an attempt to maintain control, the individual is preoccupied with orderliness, details, rules, organization, schedules, and lists; they have difficulty delegating tasks and working with others who may not do things exactly as they do (APA, 2013; Sadock et al., 2015). Their perfectionism can interfere with completion of tasks. As they have difficulty adapting to change, they strive to maintain a highly structured, organized life. They may have difficulty accepting new ideas and customs and react to them with rigidity and stubbornness. Nevertheless, persons with OCPD can do well in occupations requiring routine and attention to detail (Sadock et al., 2015). Some individuals with OCPD have difficulty discarding useless objects, even those without sentimental value (APA, 2013).

Nursing Care

These individuals seek mental health care when they have attacks of anxiety, spells of immobilization, sexual impotence, and excessive fatigue. To change the compulsive pattern, psychotherapy is needed. There may be a short-term adjunct pharmacologic intervention with an antidepressant or anxiolytic.

The nursing assessment focuses on the client's physical symptoms (sleep, eating, sexual), interpersonal relationships, and social problems. Typical nursing diagnoses include anxiety, risk for loneliness, decisional conflict, sexual dysfunction, disturbed sleep pattern, and impaired social interactions. People with OCPD realize that they can improve their quality of life, but they will find it extremely anxiety provoking to make the necessary changes. A supportive nurse–client relationship based on acceptance of the individual's need for order and rigidity will help the person have enough confidence to try new behaviours. Examining the person's belief that underlies the dysfunctional behaviours can set the stage for changing them through alterations in thinking patterns. The course of OCPD is typically fluctuating; when it begins in childhood, it tends to be more severe (Gorman & Abi-Jaoude, 2014).

Continuum of Care

Persons with cluster C PDs are typically treated with psychotherapy in the community, unless a coexisting disorder, such as depression, requires short-term hospitalization. Group and behaviour therapy can be helpful to augment positive changes.

■ OTHER PERSONALITY DISORDERS

Other PDs identified in the *DSM-5* but not addressed in this chapter are *General Personality Disorder, Personality Change Due to Another Medical Condition, Other Specified Personality Disorder* (does not meet full criteria for a PD), and *Unspecified Personality Disorder* (does not meet full criteria due to insufficient information or clinician's choice) (APA, 2013). See the DSM-5 for information about these PDs.

DISRUPTIVE, IMPULSE CONTROL, AND CONDUCT DISORDERS

Disruptive, impulse control, and conduct disorders are combined in the *DSM-5*. They are characterized by emotional and behavioural self-control problems that lead to violation of the rights of others or bring the person into conflict with societal norms or the authority figures (APA, 2013). These disorders, which often coexist with other disorders, are identified by the APA as follows:

- Oppositional defiant disorder
- Intermittent explosive disorder
- Conduct disorder
- Kleptomania
- Pyromania

Of these disorders, intermittent explosive disorder, pyromania, and **kleptomania** are considered in this chapter. Oppositional defiant disorder and conduct disorder are discussed in Chapter 30, "Psychiatric Disorders in Children and Adolescents." As previously noted, ASPD is listed in the *DSM-5* with the disruptive, impulse control, and conduct disorders as well as with the PDs. For official APA criteria of the disruptive, impulse control, and conduct disorders, please see the DSM-5.

Intermittent Explosive Disorder

Individuals with intermittent explosive disorder (IED) have outbursts of verbal and/or physical aggressiveness, out of proportion to provocation, that result in an assault of persons or animals or in the destruction of property. These episodes are over in minutes or hours

with the individual usually experiencing remorse. Such behaviour not only affects interpersonal relationships, but can have serious psychosocial consequences, such as job loss, school expulsion, automobile collisions, legal fines, or imprisonment. This diagnosis is given only after all other disorders with aggressive components (e.g., delirium, dementia, head injury, BPD, ASPD, substance abuse) have been excluded. Risk for suicide can be high. In a study of individuals with posttraumatic stress disorder (PTSD), IED, or comorbid PTSD and IED, it was found that those with both PTSD and IED had a high rate of suicide attempts, as well as aggressive behaviour (Fanning, Lee, & Coccaro, 2016). There is some evidence that IED is associated with childhood exposure to interpersonal traumatic events (Nickerson, Aderka, Bryant, & Hofmann, 2012).

CBT, addressing cognitive reframing, coping skills, and relaxation, has been used with some success, including via video conferencing (Osma, Crespo, & Castellano, 2016). Psychopharmacologic agents, such as fluoxetine, have been used as an adjunct to psychotherapy, but such treatment requires further research (Grant & Leppink, 2015).

Kleptomania

In **kleptomania**, individuals cannot resist the urge to steal, and they independently steal items that they could easily afford and/or that are not particularly useful or wanted (APA, 2013). The underlying issue is the act of stealing. The term kleptomania was first used in 1838 to describe the behaviour of several kings who stole worthless objects (Goldman, 1992). Individuals with this disorder experience an increase in tension and then gain pleasure and relief with the theft; they usually experience much guilt and shame afterwards. It is a rare condition (0.3% to 0.6% of general population) and occurs in about 4% to 24% of arrested shoplifters (APA, 2013). In clinical settings, approximately two thirds of clients with kleptomania are female; it is concurrent with a range of other mental disorders, including a 24% concurrency rate with bulimia (Grant & Potenza, 2008). The rate of suicide attempts found in a study of persons with kleptomania was high (24.3%), with the majority attributing their suicidality specifically to their kleptomania (Odlaug, Grant, & Kim, 2012). Researchers (Kim et al., 2017) who examined the incidence of addictive disorders among individuals with kleptomania ($n = 53$) found that approximately 21% ($n = 11$) met the criteria for an addictive disorder (four for substance use disorder; four for behavioural addiction [e.g., sex addiction, Internet addiction]; three for both). This suggests that assessment of kleptomania should include assessment for addictive disorder, as well as the need for further research in this area.

Kleptomania, which seems to have an early onset and a chronic trajectory, is difficult to detect (individuals with this disorder actively hide it from family and friends) and to treat. There is inconsistent success with various individual, group, and behavioural therapies; CBT is recommended but this approach, too, awaits further research (Aboujaoude, Gamel, & Koran, 2004).

Pyromania

Although **pyromania** has been recognized as a mental disorder for about 200 years, its inclusion in the DSM-5 did not occur without debate, as some believe that there is insufficient evidence that it is a distinct disorder; its incidence appears to be less than 1%. It was first defined as a distinct pathologic disorder in 1833 by Marc and viewed as an uncontrollable impulse to set fires (Nanayakkara, Ogloff, & Thomas, 2015); this understanding is similar to that of today. To be regarded as a disorder, and thus noncriminal behaviour, this intentional fire setting must be motiveless, except to achieve the arousal or relief it brings to the individual who is fascinated with fire. The frequency of fire setting for persons with pyromania fluctuates over time; there may be comorbidity with other disorders in this category, as well as with substance use, gambling disorders, and depressive and bipolar disorders (APA, 2013). (See the DSM-5 for specific criteria for pyromania.) CBT is used to treat this disorder (Burton, McNiel, & Binder, 2012), as are social skills training and the prescribing of SSRIs, but evidence for treatment efficacy is lacking (Nanayakkara et al., 2015).

Continuum of Care

Hospitalization for disruptive, impulse control, and conduct disorders is rare, except when there are comorbid psychiatric or medical disorders.

SUMMARY OF KEY POINTS

- Personality is a complex pattern of characteristics, largely outside of the person's awareness, that compose the individual's distinctive pattern of perceiving, feeling, thinking, coping, and behaving. The personality emerges from a complicated interaction of biologic dispositions, psychological experiences, and environmental situations.
- Personality disorder is an enduring pattern of inner experience and behaviour that deviates markedly from the expectations of the individual's culture, is pervasive and inflexible, has an onset in adolescence or early adulthood, is stable over time, and leads to distress or impairment.
- In the *DSM-5*, personality disorders are organized around three clusters: A, B, and C.
- In cluster A, paranoid personality disorder is characterized by a suspicious pattern, schizoid personality disorder by an asocial pattern, and schizotypal personality disorder by an eccentric pattern.

- People with cluster A personality disorders, whose odd, eccentric behaviours often alienate them from others, can benefit from interventions such as social skills training, environmental management, and cognitive skill building. Changing the patterns of thinking and behaving is difficult and takes time; client outcomes must therefore be evaluated in terms of small changes in thinking and behaviour. People with BPD (cluster B) have difficulties regulating emotion and have extreme fears of abandonment, leading to dysfunctional relationships; they often engage in self-injury.
- ASPD (cluster B) includes people who have no regard for and refuse to conform to social rules, including the law.
- Individuals with cluster B personality disorders often have difficulties with emotional regulation or being able to recognize and control the expression of feelings such as anger, disappointment, and frustration. The nurse can help these clients identify feelings and gain control over their feelings and actions by teaching communication skills and techniques, thought-stopping techniques, distraction, or problem-solving techniques.
- Cluster C personality disorders are characterized by anxieties and fears and include avoidant, dependent, and obsessive–compulsive disorders. The obsessive–compulsive personality disorder differs from the obsessive–compulsive anxiety disorder because the individual demonstrates an overall rigidity, perfectionism, and a need for control.
- For many persons with personality disorders, maintaining a therapeutic nurse–client relationship can be one of the most helpful interventions. Through this therapeutic relationship, the individual experiences a model of healthy interaction, establishing trust, consistency, caring, boundaries, and limitations that help to build the client's self-esteem and respect for self and others. In some personality disorders, nurses will find it more difficult to engage the individual in a true therapeutic relationship because of the person's avoidance of interpersonal and emotional attachment (e.g., ASPD or PPD).
- Individuals with personality disorders rarely receive inpatient treatment, except during periods of destructive behaviour or self-injury. Treatment is delivered in the community and over time. Continuity of care is important in helping the individual change lifelong personality patterns.
- Although not classified as personality disorders, the impulse control disorders share one of the primary characteristics of impulsivity, which leads to inappropriate social behaviours that are considered harmful to self or others and that give the individual excitement or gratification at the time the act is committed.

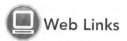 Web Links

borderlinepersonalitydisorder.com/consumer-recovery-resources This site provides information about recovering from borderline personality disorder, reviewed by a committee of people who have had the diagnosis and who are family members of a loved one with the diagnosis and two dedicated professionals who work with individuals diagnosed with BPD.

bpdcentral.com The site of BPD Central provides consumer, family, and professional information and resources.

bpdworld.org This British website provides information, advice, and support for those affected by personality disorders and other related conditions. This includes carers and professionals, as well as persons with BPD.

camh.ca/en/hospital/health_information/a_z_mental_health_and_addiction_information/Personality-Disorder/Pages/default.aspx This is the site of the Centre for Mental Health and Addiction in Toronto that provides information about personality disorders and their treatment.

References

Aboujaoude, E., Gamel, N., & Koran, L. M. (2004). Overview of kleptomania and phenomenological description of 40 patients. *Primary Care Companion to the Journal of Clinical Psychiatry, 6*(6), 244–247.

American Psychiatric Association (APA). (2013). *Diagnostic and statistical manual of mental disorders* (5th ed.). Washington, DC: Author.

Bartholomew, K., & Horowitz, L. (1991). Attachment styles among young adults: A test of a four-category model. *Journal of Personality and Social Psychology, 61*, 226–244.

Baskin-Sommers, A., Krusemark, E., & Ronningstam, E. (2014). Empathy in narcissistic personality disorder: From clinical and empirical perspectives. *Personality Disorders: Theory, Research, and Treatment, 5*(3), 323–333. doi:10.1037/per000006.1

Bateman, A., & Fonagy, P. (2016). *Mentalization-based treatment for personality disorders: A practical guide.* Oxford, UK: Oxford University Press.

Bateman, A. W., Gunderson, J., & Mulder, R. (2015). Treatment of personality disorder. *The Lancet, 385*, 735-743.

Bean, A., & Groth-Marnat, G. (2016). Video gamers and personality: A five-factor model to understand game playing style. *Psychology of Popular Media Culture, 5*(1), 27–38.

Bennett, K., Shepherd, J., & Janca, A. (2013). Personality disorders and spirituality. *Current Opinion in Psychiatry, 26*, 79–83.

Bohus, M., Haaf, B., Stiglmayr, C., Pohl, U., Böhme, R., & Linehan, M. (2000). Evaluation of inpatient dialectical-behavioral therapy for borderline personality disorder—A prospective study. *Behaviour Research and Therapy, 38*(9), 875–887.

Bornstein, R. F. (1998). Implicit and self-attributed dependency needs in dependent and histrionic personality disorders. *Journal of Personality Assessment, 71*(1), 1–14.

Brickman, L. J., Ammerman, B. A., Look, A. E., Mitchell E., Berman, M. E., & McCloskey, M. S. (2014). The relationship between non-suicidal self-injury and borderline personality disorder symptoms in a college sample. *Borderline Personality Disorder and Emotional Dysregulation, 1*(14), 1–8. doi:10.1186/2051-6673-1-14

Bulechek, G., Butcher, H., & McCloskey Dochterman, J. (Eds.). (2008). *Nursing interventions classification (NIC)* (5th ed.). St. Louis, MO: Mosby.

Burton, P. R. S., McNiel, D. E., & Binder, R. L. (2012). Firesetting, arson, pyromania, and the forensic mental health expert. *The Journal of the American Academy of Psychiatry and the Law, 40*, 355–365.

Carpenito, L. J. (2017). *Handbook of nursing diagnoses* (15th ed.). Philadelphia, PA: Lippincott Williams & Wilkins.

Carr, T. (2008). Mapping the processes and qualities of spiritual nursing care. *Qualitative Health Research, 18*(5), 686–700.

Clarkin, J. F., Yeomans, F. E., & Kernberg, O. F. (2006). *Psychotherapy for borderline personality: Focusing on object relations.* Washington, DC: American Psychiatric Press.

Cleckley, H. (1941). *The mask of sanity.* St. Louis, MO: Mosby.

Cloninger, C., Bayon, C., & Svrakic, D. (1998). Measurement of temperament and character in mood disorders: A model of fundamental states as personality types. *Journal of Affective Disorders, 51*(1), 21–32.

Compton, W. M., Conway, K. P., Stinson, F. S., Colliver, J. D., & Grant, B. F. (2005). Prevalence, correlates, and comorbidity of DSM-IV anti-social personality syndromes and alcohol and specific drug use disorders in the United States: Results from the National Epidemiologic Survey on Alcohol and Related Conditions. *Journal of Clinical Psychiatry, 66*(6), 677–685.

Crego, C., & Widiger, T. A. (2016). Cleckley's psychopaths: Revisited. *Journal of Abnormal Psychology, 125*(1), 75–87.

Crichton, R. (1959). *The great impostor.* New York, NY: Random House.

David, D. O., & Freeman, A. (2015). Overview of cognitive-behavioral therapy of personality disorders. In A. T. Beck, D. D. Davis, & A. Freeman (Eds.). *Cognitive therapy of personality disorders* (3rd ed., pp. 16–26). New York, NY: Guilford.

Dickens, G. L., Lamont, E., & Gray, S. (2016). Mental health nurses' attitudes, behavior, experience and knowledge regarding adults with a diagnosis of borderline personality disorder: Systematic, integrative literature review. *Journal of Clinical Nursing, 25*, 1848–1875. doi:10.1111/jocn.13202

Dimaggio, G., & Brüne, M. (2016). Dysfunctional understanding of mental states in personality disorders: What is the evidence? *Comprehensive Psychiatry, 64*(1), 1–3. doi:10.1016/j.comppsych.2015.09.014

Dimaggio, G., Salvatore, G., MacBeth, A., Ottavi, P., Buonocore, L., & Popolo, R. (2017). Metacognition interpersonal therapy for personality disorders: A cases study series. *Journal of Contemporary Psychotherapy, 47*, 11–21. doi:10.1007/s10879-016-9342-7

Edens, J. F., Kelley, S. E., Lilienfeld, S. O., Skeem, J. L., & Douglas, K. S. (2015). Predictive validity in a prison. *Law and Human Behavior, 39*(2), 123–129.

Erikson, E. (1968). *Identity: Youth and crisis.* New York, NY: Norton.

Fanning, J. R., Lee, R., & Coccaro, E. F. (2016). Comorbid intermittent explosive disorder and posttraumatic stress disorder: Clinical correlates and relationship to suicidal behavior. *Comprehensive Psychiatry, 70*, 125–133. doi:doi.org/10.1016/j.comppsych.2016.05.018

Feigenbaum, J. (2007). Dialectical behaviour therapy: An increasing evidence base. *Journal of Mental Health, 16*(1), 51–68.

Fonagy, P. (1991). Thinking about thinking: Some clinical and theoretical considerations in the treatment of a borderline patient. *International Journal of Psycho-Analysis, 72*(4), 639–656.

Friedman, H. S., & Schustack, M. W. (2012). *Personality: Classic theories and modern research.* Boston, MA: Allyn & Bacon.

Gillard, S., Turner, K., & Heffgen, M. (2015). Understanding recovery in the context of lived experience of personality disorders: A collaborative, qualitative study. *BMC Psychiatry, 15*(183), 1–13. doi:10.1186/s12888-015-0572-0

Goldman, M. (1992). Kleptomania: An overview. *Psychiatric Annals, 22*(2), 68–71.

Gorman, D. A., & Abi-Jaoude, E. (2014). Obsessive-compulsive disorder. *Canadian Medical Association Journal, 186*(11), E435. Appendix 1. Retrieved from www.cmaj.ca/lookup/suppl/doi:10.1503/cmaj.131257/-/DC1

Grant, J. E., & Leppink, E. W. (2015). Choosing a treatment for disruptive, impulse-control, and conduct disorders: Limited evidence, no approved drugs to guide treatment. *Current Psychiatry, 14*(1), 29–36.

Grant, J. E., & Potenza, M. N. (2008). Gender-related differences in individuals seeking treatment for kleptomania. *CNS Spectrums, 13*(3), 235–245.

Hare, R. D. (1991). *The Hare Psychopathy Checklist-Revised.* Toronto, ON: Multi-Health Systems.

Hare, R. D., & Neumann, C. S. (2009). Psychopathy: Assessment and forensic implications. *Canadian Journal of Psychiatry, 54*(12), 791–802.

Hayward, B. A. (2007). Cluster A personality disorders: Considering the "odd-eccentric" in psychiatric nursing. *International Journal of Mental Health Nursing, 16*(1), 15–21.

Helleman, M., Goossens, P. J. J., Kaasenbrood, A., & van Achterberg, T. (2014). Evidence base and components of brief admission as an intervention for patients with borderline personality disorder: A review of the literature. *Perspectives in Psychiatric Care, 50*, 65–75.

Hess, N. (2016). On making emotional contact with a schizoid patient. *British Journal of Psychotherapy, 32*(1), 53–64. doi:10.111/bjp.12193

Hoffman, P. D., Fruzzetti, A. E., & Buteau, E. (2007). Understanding and engaging families: An education, skills and support program for relatives impacted by borderline personality disorder. *Journal of Mental Health, 16*(1), 69–82.

Holm, A. L., & Severinsson, E. (2011). Struggling to recover by changing suicidal behaviour: Narratives from women with borderline personality disorder. *International Journal of Mental Health Nursing, 20*(3), 165–173.

Hooley, J. M., Cole, S. H., & Gironde, S. (2012). Borderline personality disorder. In T. A. Widiger (Ed.), *The Oxford handbook of personality disorders* (pp. 409–436). Oxford, UK: Oxford University Press.

Hopwood, C. J., & Thomas, K. M. (2012). Paranoid and schizoid personality disorders. In T. Widiger (Ed.), *The Oxford handbook of personality disorders* (pp. 582–602). Oxford, UK: Oxford University Press.

Hummelen, B., Pedersen, G., Wilberg, T., & Karterud, S. (2015). Poor validity of the DSM-IV Schizoid personality disorder construct as a diagnostic category. *Journal of personality disorders, 29*(3), 334–346.

Hyde, L. W., Waller, R., Trenacosta, C. J., Shaw, D. S., Neiderhiser, J. M., Ganiban, J. M., ... Leve, L. D. (2016). Heritable and nonheritable pathways to early callous-unemotional behaviors. *American Journal of Psychiatry, 173*(9), 903–909. doi:10.1176/appi.ajp.2016.15111381

Jordan, J. V. (2004). Personality disorder or relational disconnection. In J. J. Magnavita (Ed.), *Handbook of personality disorders* (pp. 120–134). Hoboken, NJ: John Wiley.

Jovev, M., McKenzie, T., Whittle, S., Simmons, J. G., Allen, N. B., & Chanen, A. M. (2013). Temperament and maltreatment in the emergence of borderline and antisocial personality pathology during early adolescence. *Journal of the Canadian Academy of Child and Adolescent Psychiatry, 22*(3), 220–229.

Kellett, S. & Hardy, G. (2014). Treatment of paranoid personality disorder with cognitive analytic therapy: A mixed methods single case experimental design. *Clinical Psychology and Psychotherapy, 21*, 452–464. doi:10.1002/cpp.1845

Kim, H. S., Christianini, A. R., Bertoni, D., Medeiros de Oliveira, M. C., Hodgins, D. C., & Tavares, H. (2017). Kleptomania and co-morbid addictive disorders. *Psychiatry Research, 250*, 35–37. doi.org/10.1016/j.psychres.2017.01.048

Koenig, J., Thayer, J. F., & Kaess, M. (2016). Pain sensitivity in self-injury: A meta-analysis on pain. *Psychological Medicine, 46*, 1597–1612. doi:10.1017/S0033291716000301

Krause, E. D., Mendelson, T., & Lynch, T. R. (2003). Childhood emotional invalidation and adult psychological distress: The mediating role of emotional inhibition. *Child Abuse and Neglect, 27*, 199–213.

Kwapil, T. R., & Barrantes-Vidal, N. (2012). Schizotypal personality disorder: An integrative review. In T. A. Widiger (Ed.), *The Oxford handbook of personality disorders* (pp. 437–477). Oxford, UK: Oxford University Press.

Langlois, K. A., Samokhvalov, A. V., Rehm, J., Spence, S. T., & Gorber, S. C. (2012, modified 2013). *Health state descriptions for Canadians*. Ottawa, ON: Statistics Canada.

Leahy, R. L., & McGinn, L. K. (2012). Cognitive therapy for personality disorders. In T. A. Widiger (Ed.), *The Oxford handbook of personality disorders* (pp. 727–750). Oxford, UK: Oxford University Press.

Lee, J. L. (2017). Mistrustful and misunderstood: a review of paranoid personality disorder. *Current Behavioral Neuroscience Reports, 4*, 151–165. doi:10.1007/s40473-017-0116-7

Leichsenring, F., Leibing, E., Kruse, J., New, A. S., Leweke, F. (2011). Borderline personality disorder. *The Lancet, 377*, 74–84.

Liewa, J. Lench, H. C., Kao, G., Yeh, Y. C., & Kwoka, O. (2014). Avoidance temperament and social-evaluative threat in college students' math performance: A mediation model of math and test anxiety. *Anxiety, Stress, & Coping, 27*(6), 650–661. Retrieved from http://dx.doi.org/10.1080/10615806.2014.910303

Linehan, M. (1993a). *Cognitive-behavioral treatment of borderline personality disorder*. New York, NY: Guilford.

Linehan, M. (1993b). *Skills training manual for treating borderline personality disorder*. New York, NY: Guilford.

Links, P. S., Kolia, N. J., Guimond, T., & McMain, S. (2013). Prospective risk factors for suicide attempts in a treated sample of patients with borderline personality disorder. *Canadian Journal of Psychiatry, 58*(2), 99–106.

Lynch, T. R., & Cuper, P. F. (2012). Dialectical behavior therapy of borderline and other personality disorders. In T. A. Widiger (Ed.), *The Oxford handbook of personality disorders* (pp. 785–793). Oxford, UK: Oxford University Press.

Lyness, J. M. (2016). Psychiatric disorders in medical practice. In L. Goldman & A. I. Schafer (Eds.), *Goldman-Cecil medicine* (25th ed., Vol. II, pp. 2346–2356, e2). Philadelphia, PA: Elsevier Saunders.

Magnavita, J. J. (Ed.). (2004). The relevance of theory in treating personality dysfunction. In *Handbook of personality disorders: Theory and practice* (pp. 56–77). Hoboken, NJ: John Wiley & Sons.

Mahler, M., Pine, F., & Bergman, A. (1975). *The psychological birth of human infant: Symbiosis and individuation*. New York, NY: Basic Books.

Martin-Blanco, A., Ferrer, M., Soler, J., Arranz, M. J., Vega, D., Calvo N., ... Pascual, J. C. (2016). Role of the hypothalamus-pituitary-adrenal genes and childhood trauma in borderline personality disorder. *European Archives of Psychiatry Clinical Neuroscience, 266*(4), 307–316.

Maruszewski, T., Fajkowska, M., & Eysenck, M. W. (2010). An integrative view of personality. In T. Maruszewski, M. Fajkowska, & M. W. Eysenck (Ed.), *Warsaw lectures in personality and social psychology, Vol. 1: Personality from biological, cognitive, and social perspectives* (pp. 1–9). Clinton Corners, NY: Eliot Werner Publications, Inc.

McMain, S. F., Boritz, T. Z., & Leybman, M. J. (2015). Common strategies for cultivating a positive therapy relationship in the treatment of personality disorders. *Journal of Psychotherapy Integration, 25*(1), 20–29.

Meaney, R., Hasking, P., & Reupert, A. (2016). Prevalence of borderline personality disorder in university samples: Systematic review, meta-analysis and meta-regression. *PLoS One, 11*(5), e0155439. doi:doi.org/10.1371/journal.pone.0155439

Meuldijk, D., McCarthy, A., Bourke, M. E., & Grenyer, B. F. S. (2017). The value of treatment for borderline personality disorder: Systematic review and cost-effectiveness analysis of economic evaluations. *PLoS One, 12*(3), e0171592. doi:10.1371/journal.pone.0171592

Millon, T. (2016). What is a personality disorder? *Journal of Personality Disorders, 30*(3), 289–306.

Millon, T., & Davis, R. (1999). *Personality disorders in modern life*. New York, NY: John Wiley.

Millon, T., Millon, C., Meagher, S., Grossman, S., & Ramnath, R. (2004). *Personality disorders in modern life* (2nd ed.). New York, NY: John Wiley.

Moran, P., Romaniuk, H., Coffey, C., Chanen, A., Degenhardt, L., Borschmann, R., & Patton, G. C. (2016). The influence of personality disorder on the future mental health and social adjustment of young adults: a population-based, longitudinal cohort study. *Lancet Psychiatry, 3*, 636–645. doi:doi.org/10.1016/S2215-0366(16)30029-3

Moroni, F., Procacci, M., Pellecchia, G., Semerari, A., Nicolò, G., Carcione, A., ... Colle, L. (2016). Mindreading dysfunction in avoidant personality disorder compared with other personality disorders. *The Journal of Nervous and Mental Disease, 204*(10), 752–757.

Nanayakkara, V., Ogloff, J. R. P., & Thomas, S. D. M. (2015). From haystacks to hospitals: An evolving understanding of mental disorder and firesetting. *International Journal of Forensic Mental Health, 14*(1), 66–75. doi:10.1080/14999013.2014.974086

National Health and Medical Research Council. (2012). *Clinical practice guidelines for the management of borderline personality disorder*. Melbourne, Australia: National Health and Medical Research Council.

Nehls, N. (1999). Borderline personality disorder: The voice of patients. *Research in Nursing and Health, 22*(4), 285–293.

Newbury-Helps, J., Feigenbaum, J., & Fonagy, P. (2017). Offenders with antisocial personality disorder display more impairments in mentalizing. *Journal of Personality Disorders, 31*(2), 232–255.

Newton-Howes, G., Clark, L. A., & Chanen, A. (2015). Personality disorder across the lifespan. *The Lancet, 385*, 727–734.

Nickerson A., Aderka, I. M., Bryant, R. A., & Hofmann, S. G. (2012). The relationship between childhood exposure to trauma and intermittent explosive disorder. *Psychiatry Research, 197*, 128–134. doi:10.1016/j.psychres.2012.01.012

Novais, F., Araújo, A., & Godinho, P. (2015). Historical roots of histrionic personality disorder. *Frontiers in Psychology, 6*(1463), 1–5. doi:10.3389/fpsyg.2015.01463

Odlaug, B. L., Grant, J. E., & Kim, S. W. (2012). Suicide attempts in 107 adolescents and adults with kleptomania. *Archives of Suicide Research, 16*, 348–359.

Oltmanns, T. F., & Powers, A. D. (2012). Gender and personality disorders. In T. A. Widiger (Ed.). *The Oxford handbook of personality disorders* (pp. 206–218). Oxford, UK: Oxford University Press.

Osma, J., Crespo, E., & Castellano, C. (2016). Multicomponent cognitive-behavioral therapy for intermittent explosive disorder by videoconferencing: A case study. *Anales de psiologia, 32*(2), 424–432.

Ovid. (1807/2009). *The metamorphoses of Publius Ovidus Naso in English blank verse, Vols. I & II*. J. J. Howard (Trans.). London, UK: Project Gutenberg EBook. Retrieved from http://www.gutenberg.org/files/28621/28621-h/28621-h.htm

Paris, J. (2007). *Half in love with death: Managing the chronically suicidal patient*. Mahwah, NJ: Lawrence Erlbaum.

Paris, J. (2015). *A concise guide to personality disorders*. Washington, DC: American Psychological Association. doi:doi.org/10.1037/14642-009

Pearce, J. M., Hulbert, C., McKechnie, B., McCutcheon, L., & Betts, J., & Chanen, A. M. (2017). Evaluation of a psychoeducational group intervention for family and friends of youth with borderline personality disorder. *Personality Disorder and Emotion Dysregulation, 4*(5), 1–7. doi:10.1186/s40479-017-0056-6

Pederson L. D. (2015). *Dialectical behavior therapy: A contemporary guide for practitioners*. Chichester, West Sussex, UK: John Wiley & Sons.

Petersen, R., Brakoulias, V., & Langdon, R. (2016). An experimental investigation of mentalization ability in BPD. *Comprehensive Psychiatry, 64*, 12–21. doi:http://dx.doi.org/10.1016/jcomppsych.2015.10.004

Putnam, S. P., & Gartstein, M. A. (2017). Aggregate temperament scores from multiple countries: Associations with aggregate personality traits, cultural dimensions, and allelic frequency. *Journal of Research in Personality, 67*, 157–170.

Ronningstam, E. (2012). Narcissistic personality disorder: The diagnostic process. In T. A. Widiger (Ed.), *The Oxford handbook of personality disorders* (pp. 527–549). Oxford, UK: Oxford University Press.

Ronningstam, E. (2017). Intersect between self-esteem and emotion regulation in narcissistic personality disorder—Implications for alliance building and treatment. *Borderline Personality Disorder and Emotion Dysregulation, 4*(3), 1–13. doi:10.1186/s40479-017-0054-8

Ronningstam, E., Simonsen, E., Oldham, J. M., Maffei, C., Gunderson, J., Chanen, A. M., & Millon, T. (2014). Studies of personality disorder: Past, present, and future in recognition of ISSPD's 25th anniversary. *Journal of Personality Disorders, 28*(5), 611–628.

Rosenström, T., Ystrom, E., Torvik, F. A., Czajkowski, N. O., Gillespie, G. A., Aggen, S. H., … Reichborn-Klennerud, T. (2017). Genetic and environmental structure of DSM-IV criteria for antisocial personality disorder: A twin study. *Behavioral Genetics, 47,* 265–277. doi:10.1007/s10519-016-9833-z

Ruocco, A., & Carcone, D. (2016). A neurobiological model of BPD: Systematic and integrative review. *Harvard Review of Psychiatry, 24*(5), 311–329.

Sadock, B. J., Sadock, V. A. & Ruiz, P. (2015). *Kaplan & Sadock's synopsis of psychiatry: Behavioral sciences/clinical psychiatry* (11th ed.). Philadelphia, PA: Wolters Kluwer.

Sanislow, C. A., da Cruz, K. L., Gianol, M. O., & Reagan, E. M. (2012). Avoidant personality disorder, traits, and types. In T. A. Widiger (Ed.), *The Oxford handbook of personality disorders* (pp. 549–565). Oxford, UK: Oxford University Press.

Schroeder, K., Fisher, H. L., & Schäfer, I. (2013). Psychotic symptoms in patients with borderline personality disorder: Prevalence and clinical management. *Current Opinion in Psychiatry, 26,* 113–119.

Schore, A. N. (2017). Modern attachment theory. In S. N. Gold (Ed.), *APA Handbook of trauma psychology, Vol. 1 Foundations in Knowledge* (pp. 398–406). Washington, DC: American Psychology Association.

Sheehan, L., Nieweglowski, K., & Corrigan, P. (2016). The stigma of personality disorders. *Current Psychiatry Reports, 18*(11), 1–7. doi:10.1007/s11920-015-0654-1

Silk, K. R. (2000). Borderline personality disorder. Overview of biologic factors. *Psychiatric Clinical North America, 23*(1), 61–75.

Silk, K. R., & Feurino III, L. (2012). Psychopharmacology of personality disorders. In T. Widiger (Ed.), *The Oxford handbook of personality disorders* (pp. 713–726). Oxford, UK: Oxford University Press.

Stepp, S. D., Scott, L. N., Morse, J. Q., Nolf, K. A., Hallquist, M. N., & Pilkonis, P. A. (2014). Emotion dysregulation as a maintenance factor of borderline personality disorder features. *Comprehensive Psychiatry, 55*(3),657–666. doi:10.1016/j.comppsych.2013.11.006

Stern, A. (1938). A psychoanalytic investigation and therapy in the borderline group of neuroses. *Psychoanalytic Quarterly, 7,* 467–489.

Stone, M. (2016). Borderline personality disorder: Therapeutic factors. *Psychodynamic Psychiatry, 44*(4), 505–540.

Strike, C., Rhodes, A. E., Bergmans, Y., & Links, P. (2006). Fragmented pathways to care: The experiences of suicidal men. *Crisis, 27*(1), 31–38.

Swannell, S. V., Martin, G. E., Page, A., Hasking, P., & St John, N. J. (2014). Prevalence of nonsuicidal self-injury in nonclinical samples: Systematic review, meta-analysis and meta-regression. *Suicide and Life-Threatening Behavior, 44*(3), 273–303. doi:10.1111/sltb.12070

Turner B. J., Dixon-Gordon, K. L., Austin, S. B., Rodriguez, M. A., Zachary Rosenthal, M., Chapman, A. L. (2015). Non-suicidal self-injury with and without borderline personality disorder: Differences in self-injury and diagnostic comorbidity. *Psychiatric Research, 230*(1), 28–35. doi:10.1016/j.psychres.2015.07.058

Tyrer, P., Reed, G. M., & Crawford, M. J. (2015). Classification, assessment, prevalence, and effect of personality disorder. *The Lancet, 385,* 717–725.

Van Wel, B., Kockmann, I., Blum, N., Pfohl, B., Black, D., & Heesterman, W. (2006). STEPPS group treatment for borderline personality disorder in the Netherlands. *Annals of Clinical Psychiatry, 18*(1), 63–67.

Verheul, R., Berghout, C. D., Busschbach, J. J. V., Bateman, A. W., Andrea, H., Dolan, C., … Fonagy, P. (2008). Severity indices of personality problems (SIPP-118): Development, factor structure, reliability, and validity. *Psychological Assessment, 20*(1), 23–34.

Via, E., Orfila, C., Pedreño, C., Rovira, A., Menchón, J. M., Cardoner, N., … Obiols J. E. (2016). Structural alterations of the pyramidal pathway in schizoid and schizotypal cluster A personality disorders. *International Journal of Psychophysiology, 110,* 163–170. doi:doi.org/10.1016/j.ijpsycho.2016.08.006

Waldeck, T. L., & Miller, L. S. (2000). Social skills deficits in schizotypal personality disorder. *Psychiatry Research, 93*(3), 237–246.

Waugh, M. H., Hopwood, C. J., Krueger, R. F., Morey, L. C., Pincus, A. L., & Wright, A. G. C. (2017). Psychological assessment with the *DSM-5* alternative model for personality disorders: Tradition and innovation. *Professional Psychology: Research and Practice, 48*(2), 79–89.

Werner, K. B., Few, L. R., & Bucholz, K. K. (2015). Epidemiology, comorbidity, and behavioral genetics of antisocial personality disorder and psychopathy. *Psychiatric Annals, 45*(4), 195–199. doi:10.3928/00485713-20150401-08

Weston, D. Beton, E., & Defife, J. A. (2011). Identity disturbance in adolescence: Associations with borderline personality disorder. *Development and Psychopathology, 23*(1), 305–313.

Widiger, T. A. (Ed.). (2012). *The Oxford handbook of personality disorders.* Oxford, UK: Oxford University Press.

Widiger, T. A., & Costa Jr, P. T. (2013). Personality disorders and the five-factor model of personality: Rationale for the 3rd edition. In T. A. Widiger & P. T. Costa Jr (Eds.), *Personality disorders and the five-factor model of personality* (3rd ed., pp. 3–11). Washington, DC: American Psychological Association.

Yeomans, F., Hull, J., & Clarkin, J. (1994). Risk factors for self-damaging acts in a borderline population. *Journal of Personality Disorders, 8*(1), 10–16.

Young, J. E. (1999). *Cognitive therapy for personality disorders: A schema-focused approach* (3rd ed.). Sarasota, FL: Professional Resource Press.

Zanarini, M. C., Frankenburg, F. R., Reich, D. B., Silk, K. R., Hudson, J. I., & McSweeney, L. B. (2007). The subsyndromal phenomenology of borderline personality disorder: A 10-year follow-up study. *American Journal of Psychiatry, 164*(6), 929–935.

Zanarini, M. C., Ruser, T., Frankenburg, F. R., & Hennen, J. (2000). The dissociative experiences of borderline patients. *Comprehensive Psychiatry, 41*(3), 223–227.

28 Sleep–Wake Disorders

Anne Marie Creamer

LEARNING OBJECTIVES

After studying this chapter, you will be able to:

- Describe the phases of sleep and physiologic changes that occur during sleep.
- Discuss the bio/psycho/social/spiritual factors that impact sleep.
- Identify strategies used to assess sleep and sleep disturbances.
- Name the sleep–wake diagnoses currently in use in North America.
- Explain the impact of medications and other substances on the stages of sleep.
- Discuss the interaction between mental illness and sleep.
- Describe the role nurses play in the assessment and management of sleep problems and sleep disorders.

KEY TERMS

- circadian • electroencephalogram (EEG)
- electromyogram (EMG) • electrooculogram (EOG)
- obstructive sleep apnea • polysomnography • sleep architecture • sleep efficiency • sleep hygiene
- sleep hypnogram • sleep latency • phases of sleep
- zeitgeber

KEY CONCEPTS

- insomnia • sleep

Nurses need to understand sleep. Knowledge of sleep and of the role sleep plays in healthy living is necessary across all areas of nursing practice. It is necessary to nurses' own health, given that the majority of nurses are shift workers. Poor sleep is associated with higher death rates; even when health status, age, gender, alcohol use, social network size, smoking, and obesity are considered, death rates remain higher (Motivala, 2011). Chronic insomnia symptoms are associated with hypertension and cardiovascular disease, including myocardial infarction. Sleep duration and quality are intimately linked with metabolic functions through a number of factors including insulin sensitivity and secretion, inflammatory processes, hormones such as ghrelin and leptin that impact satiety, and appetite and energy homeostasis (Morselli, Guyon, & Spiegel, 2012). Obesity is linked with **obstructive sleep apnea** (OSA), and those who are obese without apnea experience more waking in the night and daytime sleepiness. Short or long (≥9 hours) sleep duration and poor sleep quality predict higher incidence of diabetes. In Canada alone, financial losses due to workers not getting enough sleep amount to about twelve billion dollars a year (Hafner, Stepanek, Taylor, Troxel, & van Stolk, 2017). In this chapter, the question "What is sleep?" is answered, the phases of sleep

are explained, and sleep patterns over the lifespan are described. Sleep–wake disorders and ways to assess them are identified and common circadian rhythm disorders discussed. A bio/psycho/social/spiritual approach to nursing interventions for the disorders of insomnia and OSA is delineated.

HISTORICAL PERSPECTIVES ON SLEEP AND DREAMS

Over time, beliefs about the roles and importance of sleep and dreams have changed. In ancient times, the Egyptians and Mesopotamians thought that dreams were the means by which the gods communicated their wishes to mortals (Palagini & Rosenlicht, 2011). Joseph, the most famous dream interpreter in the Bible, impacted the decisions of the Pharaoh by his explanations. In fact, the earliest known document of dream interpretation was written by the Egyptians around 1275 BCE; this papyrus is found in the British Museum. In Greek mythology, Oneiros, the god of dreams, and Hypnos, the god of sleep, helped reduce human suffering. The Greek philosopher Plato ascribed the site of dream prophecy to the liver and felt that humans express their bestial desires while dreaming. However, Aristotle rejected the idea that dreams were prophecies and posited that dreams were residual perceptions travelling through the bloodstream and activating the heart. In the second century, an Asian "diviner" named Artemidorus Daldianus described more than 30,000 different types of dreams.

The 18th-century German philosopher Leibniz posited that dreams were a product of the mind. This concept was developed further in the late 19th century when Freud described dreams as expressions of man's emotions and attempts by the unconscious to reconcile psychological conflicts. Freud also hypothesized a mind/brain model that included neurobiologic aspects of psychological activities (Palagini & Rosenlicht, 2011).

When Hans Berger, a German psychiatrist, recorded electrical activity in the human brain in 1928, he demonstrated that different rhythms occurred during sleep and waking times (Roehrs, 2011). These brain signal recordings were called **electroencephalograms (EEG)**, and they allowed scientists to conduct more detailed studies of sleep without waking the person. By the late 1930s, all the major elements of sleep brain wave patterns were described. However, it was not until the 1950s that the cyclical variation of EEG patterns during sleep was identified. With the discovery of the rapid eye movement (REM) stage and its characteristic features, it became clear that sleep consists of two very different states: REM and non-REM or NREM. These states are as different from each other as each is from the wake state. Since then, a tremendous amount of research has explained much of what happens during sleep; among the many important questions that remain is *why* we sleep.

■ WHAT IS SLEEP?

Until recently, it was thought that sleep was a resting period for the brain; with the decrease of sensory input, brain activities diminished and sleep occurred (Roehrs, 2011). However, several other theories have been suggested (Harrison, 2012). For example, sleep is thought to have an important relationship with visual processes. Compared with the other senses, vision requires a very large amount of processing capacity in the brain; with sleep, visual input to the brain is reduced. Another theory is that sleep is necessary for the maintenance and enhancement of memory, with its two stages playing different roles. However, it is known that because humans can go for extended periods of time without REM sleep, as is seen when individuals take different medications like tricyclic antidepressants, NREM can play a role, albeit less efficiently, in memory processing. Animal studies have found that during critical periods in life, sleep is required for plastic processes that support the maturation of certain brain circuits. Considering that we spend about one third of our lives sleeping, it

is dumbfounding that so much about sleep remains unclear!

Sleep has two distinct phases, REM and non–rapid eye movement (NREM). The NREM stage is further subdivided into three stages according to depth:

- Intermediate stage 1 (drowsiness and sleep onset).
- Light stage 2.
- Deep stage 3 or slow-wave sleep (SWS). Until recently, there were four stages of NREM sleep, but stages 3 and 4 have been consolidated.

The amount and distribution of the sleep stages is called **sleep architecture**. In healthy young people, sleep progresses fairly consistently each night through stages NREM 1 to 3 within 45 to 60 minutes. NREM sleep always precedes REM sleep unless there are certain pathologies (e.g., narcolepsy). **Sleep latency** is the length of time it takes to fall asleep once the person tries to sleep. Although differences in individual sleepers exist, when asked how long it takes them to fall asleep, normal sleepers will report 15 to 30 minutes. This suggests that stage 2 is related to when the person believes he or she fell asleep. The first REM sleep episode occurs during the second hour of sleep; more rapid onset of REM sleep may suggest a problem like depression or narcolepsy. It normally takes 70 to 100 minutes for a young healthy person to move from stage 1 through to REM sleep. The sleeper may complete up to five cycles in a regular 8-hour night. A **sleep hypnogram** is a graphic display of the individual's experience of moving through the stages of sleep during a sleep period (Fig. 28.1). Another measure, **sleep efficiency**, is the ratio of the time spent sleeping to the total amount of time spent in bed.

The duration of the NREM–REM cycle usually stays the same, but as the night progresses, the REM episodes become longer and the NREM episodes become shorter. The SWS phase that occupied much of NREM during the first third of the night occupies less time as the night progresses. During the period of drowsiness as the person transitions from wakefulness to sleep, things that happen within the few minutes before dropping into phase 1 are often forgotten. The first REM cycle of the night is usually very short, lasting 1 to 5 minutes. These differences are thought to be related to different processes at work. The circadian oscillator (see below) is thought to influence REM sleep so that there is more REM sleep later in the night while more SWS at the beginning of the night is related to the homeostatic sleep system (see below). A good sleeper may return to wakefulness several times a night, with many of these occurrences taking place when the brain is moving between REM and NREM sleep and with changes in body position. However, these awakenings are usually only 30 to 60 seconds long and are not remembered in the morning. When asked, the sleeper may report waking one to three times in the night.

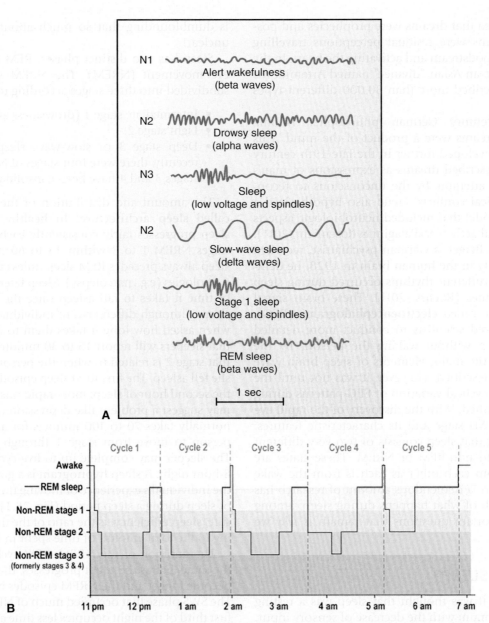

N1
Alert wakefulness
(beta waves)

N2
Drowsy sleep
(alpha waves)

N3
Sleep
(low voltage and spindles)

N2
Slow-wave sleep
(delta waves)

Stage 1 sleep
(low voltage and spindles)

REM sleep
(beta waves)

1 sec

A

Cycle 1   Cycle 2   Cycle 3   Cycle 4   Cycle 5

Awake
REM sleep
Non-REM stage 1
Non-REM stage 2
Non-REM stage 3
(formerly stages 3 & 4)

11 pm   12 pm   1 am   2 am   3 am   4 am   5 am   6 am   7 am

B

Figure 28.1. A: Brain wave patterns during a normal sleep cycle. Sleep cycles are divided into REM (rapid eye movement) and NREM (non–rapid eye movement) sleep. NREM is further divided into three stages: N1, N2, and N3. **B:** Normal hypnogram: The various stages of sleep are represented by levels on the vertical axis; time of night is shown on the horizontal axis. In this patient, there were four sleep cycles, each composed of a segment of NREM sleep followed by REM sleep. The length of REM sleep increased towards morning. Conversely, most of the stage N3 sleep was in the early portion of the night. In recent research, stages 3 and 4 have been consolidated. (Sources: Carney, P. R., Berry, R. B., & Geyer, J. D. (2012). *Clinical sleep disorders* (2nd ed.). Philadelphia, PA: Lippincott Williams & Wilkins; Rhoades, R. A., & Bell, D. R. (Eds.). (2012). *Medical physiology: Principles for clinical medicine* (4th ed.). Philadelphia, PA: Lippincott Williams & Wilkins.)

A person's usual length of sleep is dependent on several factors including personal choice, genetics, and the length of time one has been awake since the last sleep. Most young adults report sleeping about 7.5 hours on a weekday night and 8.5 hours on a weekend night. Several changes in sleep patterns occur over the person's lifetime (see below, special populations). Some people are "short sleepers." They may require less than the usual amount of sleep. In comparison with those with insomnia, they have no difficulty falling or staying asleep and are not troubled by daytime symptoms of insufficient sleep. Similarly, some individuals require longer than usual sleep time.

Different things are occurring in the body during the NREM and REM phases (see Table 28.1). For example, during NREM sleep, the body can move and mental activity is usually associated with little or fragmented activity.

Table 28.1	Stages of Sleep		
Stage	Percentage of Sleep Time During the Night	Physical Signs	Behavioural and Brain Activity
N1	2%–5%	Decrease in muscular activity; slow eye movement; pupils become smaller	Begin to fail to respond to auditory stimuli but easily awakened Awakened person reports not having been asleep
N2 Light NREM sleep	45%–55%	Eye movements stop; heart rate and respiration slow; body temperature, cerebral blood flow, and metabolism decrease.	Less likely to react to light or noise unless it is very bright or loud
N3 Slow-wave sleep (SWS); deepest stage of NREM sleep	13%–23%	Brain's temperature at its lowest; heart rate, respiration, and blood pressure decrease.	Harder to wake; possible confusion or disorientation after waking Will wake if the stimulus has strong personal meaning (e.g., mother hears her baby crying)
REM sleep	20%–25%	Rapid eye movements; general muscle tone is very low or absent; increased variability in pulse rate, blood pressure, and respiration Upper respiratory airway resistance increases; muscle tone in muscles associated with breathing is more flaccid. Body temperature is not regulated, no shivering or sweating Partial or full penile erection	EEG waves look similar to waves seen in wakefulness. Waking is more likely to occur towards the end of REM sleep period. Cerebral blood flow and metabolism are restored to waking-state level. Dreaming occurs. High level of brain activity

In contrast, during REM sleep, the body is almost paralyzed, except for episodes of REM and muscle twitches, and the brain is activated (Fig. 28.2). Therefore, someone walking about while dreaming is a sign of altered brain function.

KEY CONCEPT

Sleep is a behavioural and physiologic state of temporary disconnection from the environment, characterized by:
- Physical stillness characterized by no or few movements
- Stereotypical body postures (closed eyes, usually lying down)
- Reduced responsiveness to external stimulation
- Rapid reversibility between states, as compared with other states of altered vigilance like coma, hypothermia, or being anaesthetized (Landis, 2011; Peigneux, Urbain, & Schmitz, 2012)

■ DREAMING

Initially, it was believed that dreaming occurred only during REM sleep, but now, it is believed that about 20% of dreams occur during NREM sleep (Ropper & Samuels, 2009). The purpose of dreams is not yet known, but several theories have been suggested, some significantly different from others (Dubuc, n.d.). For example, Freud thought that our dreams are manifestations of our desires and motivation. In the 1970s, Hobson and McCarley (1977) proposed a model suggesting that the cortex is subjected to random stimulation by meaningless signals from the pons. However, we know that people who have injuries to two areas of the brain that are not involved in REM sleep report not dreaming. One area is where the occipital, temporal, and parietal cortices meet; this area is involved in spatial imagery (Fig. 28.3). The other area is located in the frontal cortex, which receives neural pathways from the mesolimbic system. This system is involved in positive reinforcement and motivation. Dream therapy is practiced today as a form of psychotherapy that helps the dreamer increase self-awareness. However, "dream symbols" found in popular books do not have a scientific basis.

■ BIOLOGIC PROCESSES

Process C and Process S

A two-process model provides a broad perspective on the sleep–wake cycle. These two processes oppose each other, enabling us to be awake during the daylight hours and sleep during the night. Process S, or homeostatic factor, represents sleep need. It drives how intensely we sleep, rising over the wake period and declining during sleep; the longer a person is awake, the stronger the drive to sleep. Additionally, loss of a specific phase of sleep results in a stronger drive to recover the lost phase. Adenosine may be a sleep-promoting substance that

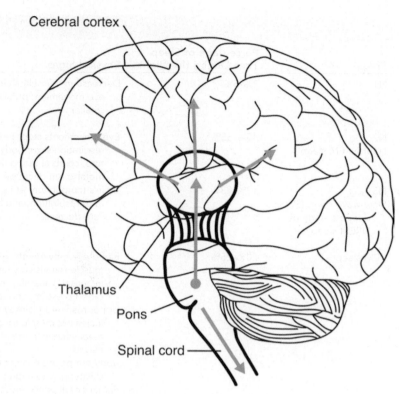

Figure 28.2. Pathways of brain activity during REM sleep. (Source: BSCS. (2003). *Sleep, sleep disorders, & biological rhythms*. NIH publication No. 04–4984. Bethesda, MD: National Institutes of Health. Copyright © 2003 by BSCS. All rights reserved. Used with permission.)

affects process S. Caffeine and theophylline, which is found in tea, act as antagonists at adenosine receptors and counter the effects of sleep deprivation.

Process C denotes circadian timing of the sleep–wake cycles in the day; the word "**circadian**" means "about the day." Circadian rhythms are biochemical, physiologic, and behavioural cycles in the body, lasting between 24.2 and 25.5 hours. While the difference between a 24-hour day and 24.2- to 25.5-hour day does

not seem significant, if the brain is unable to keep a consistent schedule, over a 3-week period, things that were done in the daytime would end up being done at night. Therefore, the body's ability to make adjustments to suit the environment is essential.

Circadian rhythms are thought to be coordinated by the molecular oscillations of neurons in the suprachiasmatic nuclei (SCN), two small areas in the left and right hypothalamus. Each SCN consists of a ventral SCN and

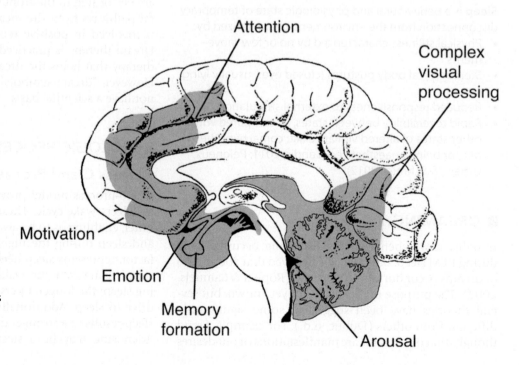

Figure 28.3. Areas of the brain active during REM sleep. (Source: BSCS. (2003). *Sleep, sleep disorders, & biological rhythms*. NIH publication No. 04–4984. Bethesda, MD: National Institutes of Health. Copyright © 2003 by BSCS. All rights reserved. Used with permission.)

a dorsal SCN. The neurons of the ventral SCN are now believed to receive and respond to external inputs, while the neurons of the dorsal SCN are believed to be the actual "clock." GABA excites the cells of the dorsal SCN but inhibits those of the ventral SCN. When a person feels jet lag, it is these opposing actions that are thought to explain what is happening. In order to maintain accuracy, these molecular oscillations are synchronized every day with external cues, also called **zeitgebers**. Examples of these cues include ambient temperature and noise, meal consumption, and the body's activity level. The strongest cue is the intensity of ambient light. These SCN neurons receive stimuli from specialized light-sensitive ganglion cells in the retina. Timing information from the SCN is transmitted to the sleep–wake centres in the brain, including the pineal gland (Fig. 28.4). The neurons in the SCN also seem to release vasopressin in a cyclical pattern. This vasopressin acts only in the brain, impacting wakefulness, in contrast to pituitary vasopressin, which affects water metabolism all over the body. Also, there are other oscillators located throughout the body, working at local levels.

The sleep–wake cycle is divided into two shorter cycles, each about 12 hours long. The longest period of sleepiness occurs when we normally go to bed in the evening and is deepest between 3:00 and 6:00 AM. This is also when body temperature is at its lowest. A second period of sleepiness usually occurs between 2:00 and 4:00 PM. Of note, if a person is exposed to bright light in the hours prior to the occurrence of minimum temperature, the internal clock is reset to a later time. Alternatively, exposure to bright light after the body's lowest temperature is reached will move the clock earlier.

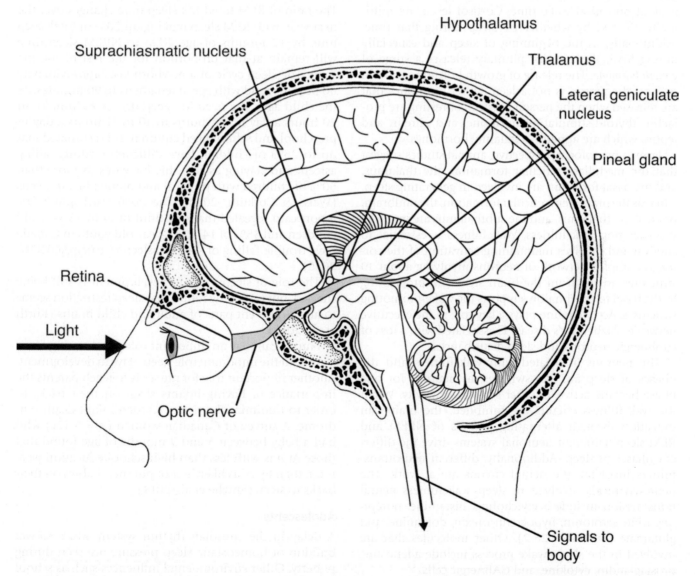

Figure 28.4. The biologic clock is located within the suprachiasmatic nucleus of the brain. (Source: BSCS. (2003). *Sleep, sleep disorders, & biological rhythms.* NIH publication No. 04–4984. Bethesda, MD: National Institutes of Health. Copyright © 2003 by BSCS. All rights reserved. Used with permission.)

Several hormones fluctuate over the day, including melatonin, cortisol, and growth hormone. Melatonin is produced in the pineal gland under the control of signals from the SCN. A smaller pineal gland has been noted in individuals with insomnia (Bumb et al., 2014). Melatonin is released into the bloodstream, beginning in the midevening, 1 to 2 hours before the usual bedtime, and peaks between 2:00 and 4:00 AM. The melatonin level begins to fall in the early morning because daylight inhibits the pineal gland's activity. As the level of melatonin rises, the need for sleep increases. Melatonin is thought to mediate dark signals and to stabilize and reinforce circadian rhythms. While melatonin has a hypnotic effect, it is more involved in the circadian rhythm of sleep–wake regulation.

The hormone *cortisol* is synthesized and released by the adrenal gland. Its levels are very low at evening bedtime but will rise while we are asleep, reaching the peak at our usual wake time. Cortisol levels are minimally affected by whether we sleep during that time. Additionally, at the beginning of sleep and especially during SWS, the anterior pituitary releases a surge of *growth hormone*. The release of growth hormone will not occur if the person is not asleep. Other hormones that are released when the person is asleep or resting are prolactin, thyroid-stimulating hormone, and ghrelin and leptin, which are appetite-regulating hormones.

From a neurologic perspective, animal studies suggest that the medullary reticular formation, the thalamus, and the basal forebrain are involved in generating sleep, whereas the brain stem reticular formation, the midbrain, brain stem, thalamus, and the subthalamus are involved in generating wakefulness. Wakefulness is essential to survival and involves maintaining activation of the cortex. A complex network of neurons involving about 10 structures arising from the brain stem and progressing to the basal telencephalon supports the wake-promoting structures. Acetylcholine plays a key role in the executive networks. Alzheimer's disease is associated with a loss of cholinergic neurons and sleep disturbances.

The neurons associated with wakefulness and the phases of sleep are like switches: as neurons for one phase become active, another set ceases activity. When the wakefulness circuits are inhibited, the brain can transition through alternating periods of NREM and REM sleep. Different neuronal systems drive the different phases of sleep. Additionally, different neurotransmitters involving the neural circuits are at work. The neurochemicals involved in sleep–wakefulness neural transmission include acetylcholine, histamine, norepinephrine, serotonin, hypocretin/orexin, dopamine, and glutamate (see Table 28.2). Other molecules that are involved in the sleep–wake process include adenosine, prostaglandin, cytokine, and GABAergic cells.

Normal sleep and several sleep disorders have been found to have genetic underpinnings, but a specific "sleep gene" has not been identified. Genome-wide association studies (see Epigenetics section in Chapter 9) have found 14 different areas linked with sleep disorders such as narcolepsy and night terrors (Sehgal & Mignot, 2011).

Sleep Pattern Changes Across the Life Span

Children

In the developing foetus, electrical patterns that can be associated with different sleep phases are seen at about 28-week gestation (Graven & Browne, 2008). REM sleep, which takes up most of the sleep cycle at this early phase, is thought to be associated with the development of sensory systems, including touch, motion, position, smell, taste, and hearing. At full term, the REM and NREM phases comprise equal parts of sleep (50:50). The ratio of REM to NREM sleep time changes over the next year, with REM sleep making up 20% of total sleep time by 12 months of age. REM to NREM sleep time will remain at that proportion for the rest of the life span. The sleep cycle of a newborn lasts approximately 60 minutes, and with age, it lengthens to 90 minutes. As the child ages, the need for sleep decreases from 16 to 20 hours a day in newborns to 10 to 11 hours a day in preschool and school-aged children. It is estimated that up to 25% of children have difficulty settling, falling asleep, and staying asleep; this increases to more than 50% of children with physical and mental health needs (Weiss & Corkum, 2012). The 2016 ParticipACTION report card revealed that one third of 5- to 13-year-old children and 45% of 14- to 17-year-old youth in Canada have trouble falling or staying asleep (ParticipACTION, 2016).

The role of sleep in brain development is still being studied, but one study found that sleep restriction seems to affect different parts of adult and child brains (Kurth et al., 2016).

Nurses can play an important role in educating families about the important role sleep plays in development. Another important role for nurses is to teach parents the importance of having infants sleep on their backs in order to minimize the risk of sudden infant death syndrome. A survey of Canadian women ($n = 6,421$) who had a baby between 5 and 9 months of age found that those moms with less than high school education were more than twice as likely to not put their babies on their backs to sleep (Smylie et al., 2014).

Adolescents

A delay in the circadian rhythm system and a slower buildup of homeostatic sleep pressure are seen during puberty. Other environmental influences such as school and homework, social and extracurricular activities, employment, and increased electronic media exposure

Table 28.2 Neurobiology of Sleep

Neurochemical	Site of Synthesis	Wake (+) or Sleep (−)	Action
Acetylcholine (ACh)	Brain stem and anterior hypothalamus of the basal forebrain	+	ACh has high activity during wakefulness (especially the basal forebrain) and REM sleep and significantly lower activity during NREM sleep. Specific Ach-releasing neurons in the brain stem are selectively active during REM sleep to decrease muscle tone, thereby preventing motor activity during sleep. Basal forebrain Ach cells are involved in promoting wakefulness behaviours, especially attention, sensory processing, and learning.
Histamine (HA)	HA cells in the posterior hypothalamus project into wake-promoting areas in the brain stem and basal forebrain.	+	Neurons from this region are most active, and HA release is highest during periods of wakefulness; less so during NREM sleep and least so during REM sleep. HA improves attention and psychomotor performance. Lesions in this area of the brain produce a coma-like sleepiness.
Norepinephrine (NE)	Locus caeruleus of the pons. NE-producing neurons extend into the cerebral cortex, hippocampus, and amygdala.	+	NE neurons fire regularly during wakefulness, slow down during SWS, and are inactive during REM sleep. During REM sleep, their inactivity seems to be related to loss of muscle tone. NE may be in promoting arousal in stressful situations, while excess NE may contribute to insomnia.
Serotonin (5-HT)	The raphe nuclei in the brain stem	+ (?)	There are many sources of 5-HT in the body, with at least 15 different receptors to bind to, influencing various behaviours in the body. Its impact on brain arousal is unclear, but it is thought that 5-HT cells are very active during wakefulness and decreased in SWS. 5-HT is not active during, and may even suppress, REM sleep. 5-HT may play a role in regulating muscle tone during sleep.
Hypocretin/orexin	Lateral hypothalamus between sleep-initiating GABA cells in the anterior hypothalamus and the wake-initiating histamine cells in the posterior hypothalamus	+	Wakefulness is sustained by projections of these neurons into many of the primary wake-promoting systems in the brain. Loss of these cells is associated with narcolepsy. Orexin also increases arousal in motivating situations such as seeking food.
Dopamine	Substantia nigra compacta and ventral tegmental area in the midbrain	+	Extracellular concentrations of dopamine are increased during wake periods.
Glutamate	Mesencephalic reticular formation in the midbrain	+	Imaging techniques have shown that these cells are more active during wakefulness, supporting the proposal that they are important in maintaining wakefulness. Lesions in this region may cause a coma-like state of sleepiness.
GABA	Hypothalamus	−	GABA neurons are most active during NREM sleep, less so during REM sleep and least so during wake periods. They are the most powerful sleep promoters in the brain. Bursts of GABA blocks transmission of signals into the cortex by inhibiting the histamine and cholinergic systems and serotonin and norepinephrine activity in the brain stem. Growth hormone–releasing hormone facilitates GABA.
Ghrelin and neuropeptide Y (NPY)	Hypothalamus	+	A hypothalamic NPY–orexin–ghrelin network is involved in integrating circadian, visual, and metabolic signals. The effects of ghrelin are less well understood. Sleep restriction to 4 hours a night is associated with increased plasma ghrelin levels and increased hunger.

Adapted from Peigneux, P., Urbain, C., & Schmitz, R. (2012). Sleep and the brain. In C. Morin & C. Espie (Eds.), *The Oxford handbook of sleep and sleep disorders* (pp. 11–37). New York, NY: Oxford University Press.

(screen time) impact the total sleep time adolescents are getting. Healthy adolescents need 8 to 10 hours of sleep in a 24-hour day (ParticipAction, 2016). Recent studies have shown that the more time adolescents spend in computer use and television viewing, the shorter the sleep duration and later the sleep times (Nuutinen, Ray, & Roos, 2013). Consequences of poor or insufficient sleep in adolescents include increased risk of anxiety, depression, suicidal ideation, school absence, and decreased cognitive function and problematic school behaviour (Colrain & Baker, 2011). Other increased risks associated with poor sleep include obesity, alcohol, cigarette and other substance use, and motor vehicle accidents caused by driving while drowsy.

Women

Compared with men, women generally have more difficulty getting to sleep and staying asleep (Driver, 2012). Women tend to sleep 15 to 20 minutes longer than men (7 vs. 6 hours and 42 minutes); they may awaken more easily and have more difficulty falling back to sleep. Additionally, women tend to use hypnotics more frequently than men, especially among the elderly. Hormonal changes seen with the menstrual cycle, pregnancy, and menopause can all negatively affect sleep. Some menopausal women find that hormone replacement therapy can help sleep problems. Insomnia symptoms are a known predictor for depression, especially among women.

Older Adults

It is recommended that older adults get 7 to 8 hours of sleep a night. However, sleep gradually changes as we age. Sleep becomes lighter; there is less slow-wave and REM sleep and more superficial sleep. The older person awakens more frequently in the night, especially in the latter part of the night, and the awakenings last longer. The circadian rhythm may shift an hour earlier, resulting in earlier bedtimes and morning awakenings (Bishop, Simons, King, & Pigeon, 2016). Also, the older brain finds it more difficult to adjust to challenges to circadian rhythm such as jet lag. The decrease in SWS is thought to reflect age-related neuronal loss in the brain. However, compared with younger adults, tests of alertness and attention in older adults who have been sleep-deprived found that the older adults did better.

Compared with matched controls, older people with sleep disorders have more problems with memory encoding and retrieval and attention span. Some describe visuoperceptual and orientation difficulties. The prevalence of some sleep disorders, such as OSA, periodic leg movement, REM sleep behaviour disorder, and advanced sleep phase disorder, starts to increase from about the age of 40 years. As many as 50% of older adults report difficulty initiating or maintaining sleep (Bishop et al., 2016).

The most common primary sleep disorders in older adults are insomnia, sleep disordered breathing, REM sleep behaviour disorder, and restless legs syndrome/periodic limb movements during sleep. Other causes include medical or psychiatric illnesses, psychosocial factors, and medications. The number of medications used by older adults correlates well with the severity of sleep problems; however, older adults are more vulnerable to sleeping medications because of slower drug absorption and elimination. In fact, many of the medications used for insomnia are on the BEERs list, a list of potentially inappropriate medications due to serious adverse effects when used in older adults, published by the American Geriatric Society (2015).

Cultural and Racial Factors

Much of what is discussed in the literature about racial and cultural differences comes from American sources. Research into the impact race plays on sleep is in the early phases. Researchers have looked at several aspects of sleep, including sleep duration, sleep architecture, and specific sleep disorders among people of different races. However, for nurse researchers, areas that may be of particular interest include how sleep and sleep disorders are perceived, which sleep measurement tools are culturally and linguistically appropriate, and what sleep health promotion interventions are effective.

Consequences of Inadequate Sleep

Inadequate sleep can result in a number of cognitive and psychological deficits (Caruso & Hitchcock, 2010). These include impaired performance of tasks requiring intense or prolonged attention, as well as cognitive slowing. Inadequate sleep impairs information processing and learning, cognitive flexibility, and imagination. Further, it decreases insight and ability to assess risks. Mood may be impaired; the person may experience depression, irritability, and anxiety. Chronically disturbed sleep both increases the risk for developing a mental illness and impedes recovery from one. For example, alcohol is linked with poor sleep quality, and insomnia is associated with an increased risk for alcohol dependence. Sleep loss is linked with increased risk of motor vehicle accidents and non–motor vehicle accidents; errors associated with sleep loss were linked with the *Exxon Valdez* oil tanker spill in 1989 (*Exxon Valdez* Oil Spill Trustee Council, 1990) and the Chernobyl nuclear reactor disaster in 1986 (Mitler et al., 1988).

▌ EPIDEMIOLOGY: CANADIAN SLEEP HABITS

A 2005 survey of Canadians found that men sleep on average 11 minutes less than women, but women experience more disturbed sleep because they wake more easily (Hurst, 2008). Women also have more trouble falling asleep. Men who work full time sleep on average 14 minutes less each night than do women who work full time. Those 14 minutes a night translate to approximately 85 hours less sleep per year. Those not in the labour force have about 24 minutes more sleep each night than those who work full time. Canadians who sleep with a partner sleep about 24 minutes less each night than those who sleep alone; those with two or more children get about 25 minutes less sleep each night. Another survey of 2,000 Canadians between 18 and 99 years of age found that 19.8% were dissatisfied with their sleep and 40.2% had one insomnia symptom at least three nights a week (Morin et al., 2011). More than a third of those surveyed did not feel rested after sleeping.

OVERVIEW OF SLEEP–WAKE DISORDERS

It is important to remember that occasionally having a disturbed sleep is a normal life experience, especially during times of stress. For a mental disorder diagnosis to be applied, the sleep issue must cause clinically significant disturbances in a number of areas, and these disturbances must be attributed to dysfunctional processes that underlie mental functioning (American Psychiatric Association [APA], 2013). The *Diagnostic and Statistical Manual of Mental Disorders* (5th ed.) (APA,

2013) lists 10 sleep–wake disorders. In addition to sleep problems, sleep–wake disorders include problems with staying awake when required. The 10 disorders include insomnia disorder, hypersomnolence disorder, narcolepsy, breathing-related sleep disorders, circadian rhythm sleep–wake disorders, NREM sleep arousal disorders, REM sleep behaviour disorder, restless legs syndrome, and substance/medication-induced disorder. Detailed diagnostic criteria for each of these sleep disorders is beyond the scope of this chapter; readers are encouraged to consult the *DSM-5*.

Sleep–wake disorders accompany mental disorders such as anxiety and depression, but, as previously noted, persistent sleep disturbances are also risk factors for the development of substance use and mental disorders. Furthermore, they may represent an early expression of an episode of a mental illness. For example, a person with bipolar disorder may identify changes in sleep patterns as something that precedes an episode of mania. The nurse who is aware of this and intervenes early may prevent this person's hospitalization, in addition to many other consequences of a manic episode. A recent study of 250 Canadians with a psychiatric diagnosis for at least 1 year found that 27.6% of the participants had trouble going to, or staying asleep "all the time," compared with 6.8% of the general population (Schofield et al. 2016). Figure 28.5 demonstrates the links between impaired sleep substance use, morbidity, and impaired function (Fleming, 2013).

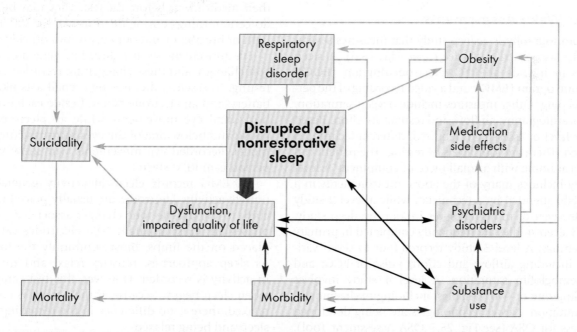

The primary effect of acute insomnia is daytime dysfunction, but when it is chronic, it is associated with psychiatric disorders that have a bidirectional relationship (coloured arrows) with sleep disturbance, substance use, dysfunction, and morbidity. Sleep deprivation, psychiatric disorders, and medication side effects can cause obesity that may cause or worsen a respiratory sleep disorder and directly or indirectly affect morbidity.

Figure 28.5. Interrelationship between disturbed sleep and dysfunction. (Source: Fleming, J. (2013). Psychiatric disorders and insomnia: Managing the vicious cycle. *Insomnia Rounds*, *2*(1). Retrieved from https://css-scs.ca/files/resources/insomnia-rounds/150-007_Eng.pdf. Copyright © 2013 by the Canadian Sleep Society. Used with permission.)

Other clinical disorders are seen very commonly with sleep–wake disorders, in particular, breathing-related sleep disorders, heart and lung disorders, neurodegenerative disorders (e.g., Alzheimer's disease), and musculoskeletal disorders (e.g., osteoarthritis). How a person sleeps can affect how they are able to manage their other conditions. For example, people who sleep poorly have more difficulty coping with pain (Smith, Nasir, Campbell, & Okonkwo, 2011). For this reason, it is essential to rule out and address contributors to sleep disturbances before assuming the issue can be addressed by a treatment for sleep complaints alone. Nurses can play an important role in identifying factors that affect sleep behaviours. Assessment based on a bio/psycho/social/spiritual framework will provide a systematic approach.

As with most mental disorder diagnoses, many of the sleep–wake disorders are further categorized in the *DSM-5* by how long the symptoms have been present, the degree of severity, and whether another disorder or factor is playing a prominent role. In some cases, the diagnosis of a sleep disorder is based on the symptoms the person has (e.g., insomnia), and specific testing may or may not be a component of diagnosis. Additionally, the *DSM-5* has "Other Specified" and "Unspecified" categories that allow for diagnoses of conditions that have symptoms characteristic of a particular sleep–wake disorder but do not meet full criteria for the condition. Refer to the *DSM-5* for a full description of sleep disorders.

Sleep–Wake Assessments

Polysomnography is a sleep study that measures several variables associated with sleep (see Fig. 28.6). A sleep study can include an EEG, **electrooculogram (EOG)**, **electromyogram (EMG)**, and a video recording of the person sleeping. Other measures include oxygen saturation, electrocardiography, air flow, and respiratory effort. Based on the level of assessment required, different techniques are used. There are four levels of testing. The patient can do this at home with a small piece of equipment. A level 1 study includes many of the above measurements in a sleep lab, attended by a technician while a level 2 study records seven or more measures in a home sleep study. Level 3 sleep studies are frequently completed in primary care settings. A level 3 study records four to seven variables, including airflow and effort, pulse or ECG, and oxyhaemoglobin saturation. A level 4 study involves recording one or two variables, including oxyhaemoglobin saturation. Newer technologies are being developed to assess for OSA (see Fig. 28.7 OSA Assessment Tool). Several factors can impact the results of these tests, including fever, drugs, electrolyte imbalance, and hypoxemia.

EEGs measure electrical activity in the brain and record brain wave patterns. Electrodes are stuck to the scalp using a paste and pick up and record electrical signals produced by postsynaptic potentials in brain neurons. The signals are amplified, digitalized, and filtered. The artifact is removed, and then, the result is examined for rhythms and transient events. The EEG plays a vital role in capturing the state of vigilance in the brain. In some settings, a cap with electrodes is worn instead and other, newer technologies such as the ear—EEG sensors are being developed and tested in an effort to make EEG studies less cumbersome and costly, more user-friendly, and portable (Looney, Goverdovsky, Rosenzweig, Morrell, & Mandic, 2016).

EEG patterns show waveforms that are specific to brain activity (Dubuc, n.d.). For example, delta waves are seen in deep sleep and coma. Theta waves are seen when limbic system activity is noted; this would suggest that the emotions and memory are involved. Alpha waves occur when persons are alert, but the eyes are closed and they are not actively processing information. Beta waves are seen when the person is alert and actively processing information; gamma waves may be related to communication between various parts of the brain when concepts are being formed. In NREM sleep, other waveforms called sleep spindles, K complexes, and high voltage waves are seen. Paradoxically, the EEG waves of REM sleep are similar to those seen in someone who is awake.

Patients who are scheduled for an EEG should wash their hair with shampoo the night before the test but refrain from using other hair products like conditioners and gels. They should not eat or drink anything containing caffeine for 8 hours prior to the test. Depending on the test's requirements, patients may or may not take their medications before the test. They may be asked to do certain things during the test, like look at a flashing light or breathe in and out deeply and quickly.

Eye movement in any direction generates electrical volt changes, and these changes are recorded with EOG testing. In essence, the moving eyeball acts like a small battery, and an electrode placed beside each eye records horizontal eye movements while an electrode placed above and below one of the eyes records vertical movements. Recorded eye movements will show when the person is in REM sleep.

An EMG records electrical activity generated with muscle activity. Electrodes are usually placed under the chin, where muscle tone changes associated with sleep phases are most apparent. The electrodes can also be placed on the limbs, most commonly the lower legs. As sleep approaches, muscles relax, and this change in activity is recorded. However, this test cannot show when sleep begins because, if the person is completely relaxed, there is no difference in the recording between sleep and being relaxed.

Respiratory and Cardiac Assessment

The person's efforts to breathe, and whether air is getting into the body, are assessed by different methods. Sensors pick up electrical or pressure changes and measure and record abdominal and/or chest movements. A sensor is placed in front of the person's nose and mouth to pick up

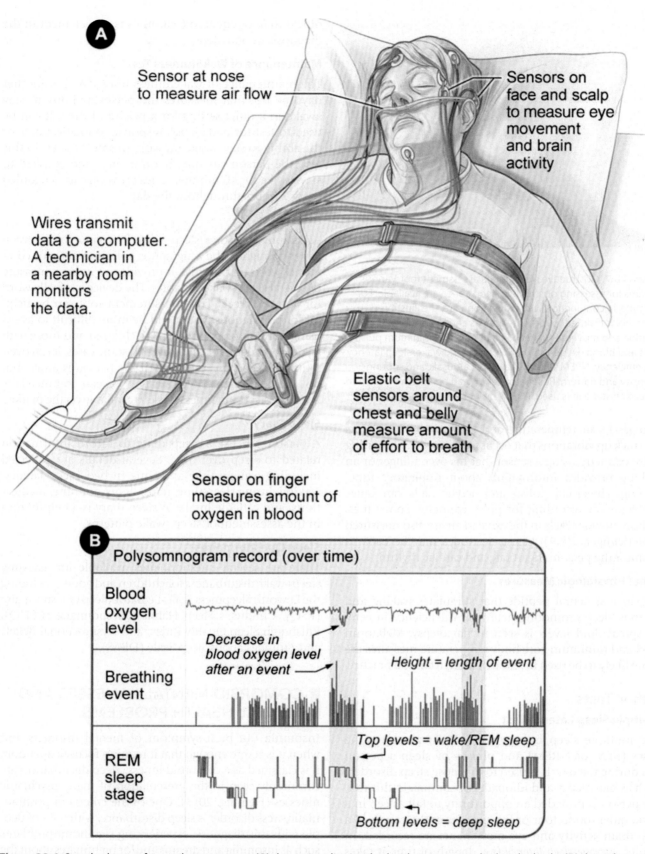

Figure 28.6. Standard setup for a polysomnogram: **(A)** the patient lies in a bed with sensors attached to the body; **(B)** the polysomnogram recording shows blood oxygen level, breathing event, and REM sleep stage over time. (Source: National Heart, Lung, and Blood Institute, U.S. Department of Health & Human Services. (2012). *What to expect during a sleep study*. www.nhlbi.nih.gov/. Used with permission.)

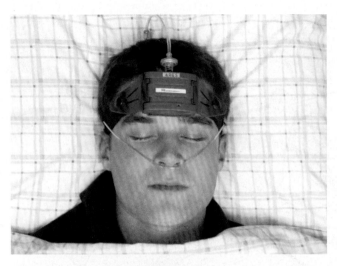

Figure 28.7. Obstructive sleep apnea assessment tool. Various systems for assessing obstructive sleep apnea are available. For example, in conjunction with a questionnaire, the illustrated ARES tool is claimed to measure apneas and hypopnoeas; head position and movement; mean, maximum, and minimum pulse rates and blood oxygen saturation; sleep and wake; sleep latency and efficiency; NREM/REM; behavioural arousals; and snoring intensity and pattern. Respiratory effort can be determined when a piezo crystal belt is used. ARES™ by Watermark Medical, Inc.

changes in air temperature and pressure. Some sensors also pick up vibrations that occur with snoring. Measuring pulse oximetry using a sensor that fits over a finger or an earlobe provides information about respiratory functioning. Fingernail polish and acrylic nails can cause problems for recording for pulse oximetry. Sometimes, carbon dioxide levels in the exhaled air are also measured (Dondelinger, 2009). Chest electrodes may be used to monitor the person's heart rate and cardiac rhythm.

Other Physiologic Measures

Orexin is a neural peptide that stimulates waking and inhibits sleep-promoting neurons. A deficiency in cerebrospinal fluid levels is seen in narcolepsy. Melatonin level and minimum core body temperature measures are more likely to be used in research than in clinical practice.

Other Tests

Multiple Sleep Latency Test

The multiple sleep latency test (MSLT) measures the types (REM or NREM) and **phases of sleep** a person has during the day. It is used to diagnose sleep disorders such as narcolepsy and idiopathic insomnia. In this test, the person is provided an opportunity to fall asleep in a dark, quiet room, four or five times over the course of a day. Brain activity and eye movements are recorded. In adults, average *sleep latency* (i.e., length of time it takes to fall asleep) is calculated. An average latency of less than 5 minutes indicates pathologic daytime sleepiness. An average latency of more than 10 minutes is normal. An MSLT demonstrating average sleep latency

of less than or equal to 8 minutes is one element in the diagnosis of narcolepsy.

Maintenance of Wakefulness Test

The maintenance of wakefulness test (MWT) is another daytime test that measures the person's ability to stay awake in a quiet setting for a period of time. It can be used to test for narcolepsy, response to medications, or the ability to stay awake for work or safety issues. In this test, the person sits quietly on a chair and is asked to stay awake for 40 minutes. These sessions are scheduled every 2 hours throughout the day.

Actigraphy

Actigraphy measures sleep–wake behaviour over several days and nights. The actigraph is a motion detector commonly worn on the wrist. It provides an indirect measure of several sleep–wake variables. The device is usually worn for about 1 week. This measurement tool can be helpful for populations that would be more difficult to assess using polysomnography, such as children and those with agitation or dementia. However, in some cases, it can overestimate sleep time, especially if the person is awake but not moving much. There are now several commercially available sleep and fitness trackers available on the market.

Sleep Diary

A person can use a sleep diary to record information related to sleep over time. Several details are collected including waking time and time in bed, sleep latency, waking during sleep time, naps, lights-out time, medications, and caffeine intake. A sleep diary is a helpful tool in the assessment of sleep–wake patterns.

Sleep Questionnaires

There are several questionnaires available for assessing sleep–wake disturbances for children and adults, including the Epworth Sleepiness Scale, Pediatric Sleep Questionnaire (PSQ), Children's Sleep Habits Questionnaire (CSHQ), Pittsburgh Sleep Quality Index, and Dysfunctional Beliefs and Attitudes about Sleep Scale (DBAS).

COMORBID MENTAL ILLNESSES AND MENTAL HEALTH PROBLEMS

Insomnia can be a symptom of mental disorders, but when it is severe enough that it requires focused attention, it is classified as a comorbid illness. Sleep disturbances are commonly seen in the presentation of many psychiatric illnesses (Fleming, 2013). One of the criteria of posttraumatic stress disorder is sleep disturbance, with 65% of people with this diagnosis experiencing significant problems such as insomnia and dreams and/or nightmares about the trauma. Those with generalized anxiety disorder (GAD) frequently experience difficulty falling or staying asleep, as well as a restless, unsatisfying sleep. In depression, the length of time to REM sleep is often shortened, but it remains normal in those diagnosed with GAD alone. Up to 70% of those with panic disorder can be awakened from sleep with a panic attack. Individuals with schizophrenia experience decreased latency to REM sleep onset, more wake time in the night, less total sleep time, and less SWS sleep, and it takes longer to fall asleep. Disturbances noted in mood disorders include disruptions in sleep continuity,

deficits in SWS, and REM sleep changes (Fleming, 2013). Approximately 80% of those with depression have insufficient sleep, while the other 20% sleep too much (Saleh, Ahmadi, & Shapiro, 2010). Many of the medications commonly used to treat psychiatric illnesses also affect sleep. See Table 28.3 for a list of medications used to treat other mental disorders and their impact on sleep.

Table 28.3 Effects of Commonly Used Psychiatric Drugs on Sleep and Waking

Drug Type	Examples	Pharmacologic Effect	Clinical Effects
Selective serotonin reuptake inhibitors (SSRIs)	Fluoxetine Fluvoxamine Citalopram	Increases extracellular levels of 5-HT, which inhibit REM sleep–producing cells	Decreased REM sleep Several SSRIs decrease sleep continuity and increase dreaming, nightmares, and sexual dreams.
Norepinephrine–dopamine reuptake inhibitors (NDRIs)	Bupropion	Inhibits reuptake of NE and DA into presynaptic neurons	Decreased REM latency and increased REM sleep; decreased slow-wave sleep
Serotonin–norepinephrine reuptake inhibitors (SNRIs)	Venlafaxine Duloxetine	Inhibits 5-HT and NE	Decreased sleep continuity and the percentage of REM sleep, vivid nightmares
Tricyclic antidepressants (TCAs)	Amitriptyline Nortriptyline Clomipramine Desipramine	Increases extracellular levels of 5-HT and NE, thereby inhibiting REM sleep–producing cells	Decreased REM sleep Some TCAs will increase slow-wave sleep.
Traditional amphetamine-like stimulants	Amphetamine Dextroamphetamine Methylphenidate	Increases extracellular levels of DA and NE	Increased wakefulness
Wake-promoting, nontraditional stimulants	Modafinil Armodafinil	Increases extracellular levels of DA	Increased wakefulness
Benzodiazepines	Diazepam Clonazepam Lorazepam Triazolam	Enhance GABA signalling via GABA_A receptors	Shortened sleep latency, decreased nocturnal wake times, increased total sleep; decreased REM possible
Nonbenzodiazepine sedative–hypnotics	Zolpidem Zopiclone	Enhance GABA signalling via GABA_A receptors, inhibiting the arousal systems	Improved sleep onset
Classic antihistamines	Diphenhydramine Triprolidine	Block HA H_1 receptors, reducing HA signalling	Increased NREM and REM sleep
Typical antipsychotics	Haloperidol Chlorpromazine	Block DA receptors, reducing DA signalling	Data inconclusive and inconsistent
Atypical antipsychotics	Clozapine Olanzapine Quetiapine Risperidone	See Chapter 12 for description of receptor-binding profile	Shortening of sleep onset latency (SOL), increases in sleep efficiency and total sleep time Olanzapine enhances slow-wave sleep and REM sleep
Mood stabilizers	Lithium	Exact mechanism unknown but may strengthen GABA inhibitory and reinforce serotonergic neurotransmission	Slowed circadian rhythms, increased slow-wave sleep and wake time after sleep onset, decreased REM sleep, increased sleep continuity
	Carbamazepine	Reinforces GABA and blocks excitatory glutamatergic neurotransmission	Increased sleep efficiency, decreased SOL, decreased wake time after sleep onset, increased slow-wave sleep
	Valproic acid	Similar to carbamazepine	Increased total sleep time and slow-wave sleep
	Lamotrigine	Similar to carbamazepine	Less well studied
Other mechanisms of action	Clonidine	Via α2-agonists, norepinephrine inactivates neurons in the locus caeruleus.	Increased NREM sleep
	Mirtazapine		Increased sleep continuity
	Trazodone		Increased slow-wave sleep and sleep continuity, suppressed REM sleep

Sources: España, R., & Scammell, T. (2011). Sleep neurobiology from a clinical perspective. *Sleep, 34,* 845–858; Mayers, A., & Baldwin, D. (2005). Antidepressants and their effect on sleep. *Human Psychopharmacology, 20,* 533–559; Riemann, D., & Nissen, C. (2012). Sleep and psychotropic drugs. In C. Morin & C. Espie (Eds.), *The Oxford handbook of sleep and sleep disorders* (pp. 190–220). New York, NY: Oxford University Press.

■ INSOMNIA

The fundamental characteristics of insomnia are being dissatisfied with sleep quantity or quality and having difficulty initiating and/or maintaining sleep. The *DSM-5* identifies several specific features of insomnia in addition to time and severity descriptors. Insomnia is more common among women and middle-aged and older people (Morin et al., 2011). Approximately 40% of people with insomnia also have a mental illness. Insomnia carries significant psychosocial, occupational, economic, and safety risks (Morin, 2012), and it has a profound impact on the economy: in Québec, for instance, the annual cost to the province has been estimated at $6.5 billion (Daley, Morin, LeBlanc, Grégoire, & Savard, 2009). Numerous studies have demonstrated that nondepressed individuals with insomnia have double the risk of developing depression compared with those without insomnia. Nurses can play an important role in assessing and supporting treatment. Additionally, they can play critical roles as educators and participate in research and policy development.

Several factors and conditions are linked with insomnia. Medical conditions include psychiatric disorders, other sleep disorders, chronic pain, and cardiovascular, respiratory, neurologic, and urinary problems, to name a few. Treating insomnia in individuals with hypertension has been found to decrease the person's blood pressure (Li et al., 2017). Frequently prescribed medications such as corticosteroids (e.g., prednisone), calcium channel blockers and beta-blockers (which are common antihypertensive medications), and decongestants are associated with insomnia. Examples of psychosocial stressors that are associated with insomnia include grief, job pressures, and the birth of a child.

Some behaviours perpetuate insomnia, such as drinking alcohol before bed, using the bed for tasks other than sleep and intimacy (e.g., eating, watching television), and having dysfunctional beliefs, such as focusing on potential catastrophic outcomes of insomnia (being fired, having an accident). **Sleep hygiene** is a term used to describe behaviours that promote healthy sleep habits. Box 28.1 reviews elements of sleep hygiene that nurses can include in educational programs.

KEY CONCEPT

Insomnia is "a subjective complaint of difficulty falling or staying asleep or poor sleep quality" (APA, 2013, p. 823).

BOX 28.1 Sleep Hygiene

Identify and break habits that disturb sleep:

- Have a set bedtime and waking time. The brain will adapt to a fixed sleeping and waking time.
- Avoid daytime napping. Sleeping during the day will disrupt nighttime sleep. If a nap is necessary, limit it to 30 to 45 minutes.
- Avoid alcohol 4 to 6 hours prior to bedtime. While alcohol will induce sleep in the immediate term, sleep will be disrupted as the blood alcohol level decreases.
- Develop a bedtime routine. This may include a warm bath or shower, or consuming warm milk, which contains tryptophan, a protein thought to promote relaxation.
- Set aside time to relax prior to bedtime. This can consist of a formal activity, such as breathing or deep relaxation exercises, or more informal activities, such as listening to calming music or reading.
- Relaxation techniques can be helpful (see Box 28.3 for an example).
- Maintain a healthy diet. Eat moderately and at regular times throughout the day rather than eating a large meal in the evening. A light carbohydrate snack at bedtime might be helpful. Avoid greasy foods.
- Caffeine consumed later in the day or in the evening may disturb sleep.
- For those who wake hungry in the early morning, adding a snack at bedtime may promote a later sleep. Avoid sugary snacks and greasy foods at bedtime; consume food containing tryptophan or high in protein, which will take some time to digest and therefore maintain a more constant blood sugar level.
- Exercise regularly. Those who exercise vigorously in the morning sleep best.
- Go to bed and get up the same time every day, regardless of how much sleep is obtained. This will help set the biologic clock.
- Keep the bed only for sleep and intimacy time. Maintaining that space as an exclusive place strengthens the association between lying on the bed and sleeping. Using the bed for other daily activities, such as eating or surfing the Internet, weakens the association between the bed and sleep.
- Keep a notepad and pen at the bedside to write down worries, thoughts, and plans that come to mind once in bed.
- Do not "try" to fall asleep or watch the clock if unable to sleep. This may make the problem worse. If unable to go to sleep, get up, leave the room, and do something boring.
- Ensure that the bedroom is comfortable (e.g., temperature, level of darkness, noise).
- Limit exposure to electronics before bedtime, and consider eliminating electronics from the bedroom.

IN-A-LIFE

Charles Dickens (1812–1870)

PUBLIC PERSONA

Charles Dickens experienced significant episodes of insomnia during his lifetime (Horne, 2008). When he couldn't sleep, he walked the streets of London, drawing inspiration from what he encountered for many of his 15 major novels. He would return home to sleep exactly in the middle of his northward-pointed bed with his arms out and his hands equidistant from the bed's edges.

REALITIES

The term "insomniac" did not appear until 38 years after Dickens' time (Horne, 2008). In Victorian Britain, the usual remedies for sleeplessness were either alcohol (whiskey or brandy for the more affluent, and gin for the poor) or opium. Laudanum, a solution of alcohol and morphine, was the most common form of opium consumed. It could be purchased easily and was so popular that Britain went to war with China to secure the free trade of opium. Another Victorian treatment for insomnia included embedding pillows with pieces of iron ore with magnetic polarity (called lodestones).

Nursing Management: Insomnia

Nursing diagnoses specific to sleep–wake disorders include insomnia and disturbed sleep pattern. When making a nursing diagnosis, several questions will help develop an understanding of what "normal" is for the patient and identify aspects of his or her sleep problem. The BEARS framework is a mnemonic that is helpful in guiding questions involved in assessing sleep (see Table 28.4). The person's medical and psychiatric history and collateral information from bed partners and family members need to be included in a comprehensive sleep assessment. See Figure 28.8 for the bio/psycho/social/spiritual outcomes of sleep loss.

Hospital inpatient units are often guided by rigid routines that are directed by care providers' schedules. Someone who normally eats a snack, takes a shower, and then reads quietly in bed until he or she is tired enough to fall asleep will struggle settling to sleep when the routine is disrupted by being on a noisy, active unit with lights being turned on and off, doors opening and closing, and alarms and phones ringing. Quieter, personalized settings are more conducive to promoting healthy sleep patterns. Patient education about sleep is a very important role for nurses. One study that provided sleep aids including an eye mask, ear plugs, and a white noise machine to patients on a nonintensive care unit and then compared the effect of providing education on how to use the aids with those who were not educated on how to use them found that patients who had the education used the aids more and had significantly less fatigue (Farrehi, Clore, Scott, Vanini, & Clauw, 2016). Simply educating the patient about the importance of sleep but not on how to use the aids did not make a difference. See Box 28.2 for nursing management strategies for hospitalized and institutionalized individuals.

Biologic Domain

Insomnia is thought to be the result of an imbalance in the sleep–wake-promoting systems of the brain, which causes a state of hyperarousal. The consequence is an increase in body and brain metabolism, manifested by an increased heart rate and temperature and elevated cortisol, norepinephrine, and epinephrine levels. Factors that predispose an individual to chronic insomnia include genetic factors and biologic traits such as hyperactivity, hypervigilance, increased metabolic rate, and chronically elevated cortisol or reduced melatonin levels. Not only are sleep disorders linked to an increased risk of developing other physical illnesses, but physical illnesses such as congestive heart failure, neurologic diseases, breathing problems, and diabetes can precipitate or worsen insomnia.

Table 28.4 BEARS Sleep Screening Questionnaire

Bedtime problems	Do you have any problems going to bed or falling asleep?
Excessive daytime sleepiness	Do you feel sleepy during the day? At work or school? Driving? Do you take naps during the day? When and for how long?
Awakenings during the night	Do you wake up during the night? What wakes you up? Do you have trouble getting back to sleep?
Regularity and duration of sleep	What time do you usually go to bed during the week? On weekends? How much sleep do you typically get?
Snoring and sleep-related breathing problems	Have you ever been told that you snore or seem to stop breathing in your sleep?

Adapted from *BEARS sleep screening questionnaire: Examples of developmentally appropriate trigger questions.* See Weiss, S., & Corkum, P. (2012). Pediatric behavioural insomnia—"Good night, sleep tight" for child and parent. *Insomnia Rounds*, 1(5). Retrieved from https://css-scs.ca/files/resources/insomnia-rounds/150-005_Eng.pdf

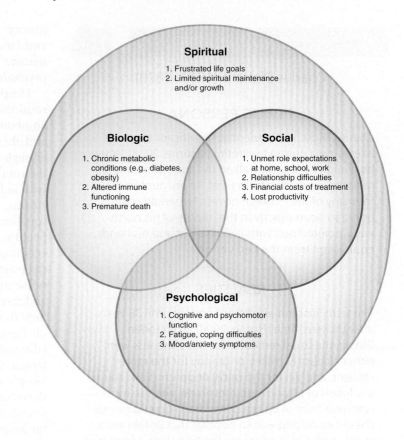

Figure 28.8. Bio/psycho/social/spiritual outcomes of sleep loss.

BOX 28.2 Nursing Management Strategies for Hospitalized and Institutionalized Patients

- Nursing and medical staff need to work together to minimize interruptions to patients' sleep at night.
- Nursing stations are usually not soundproofed; nurses need to protect patient privacy and sleep.
- Identify the patient's normal sleep routines and facilitate maintaining them where possible.
- Examine the medications the patient is taking to see if any might be affecting sleep; assess to see if any usual home medications have not been provided since admission.
- Identify and manage barriers to sleep (e.g., pain, excessive fluid and caffeine intake) where possible.
- Examine the environment for sources of possible disturbances: reduce alarm levels on equipment where possible; offer earplugs or headphones.
- Offer light therapy, relaxation techniques, sleep education, back rubs, bedtime snacks, eye masks, and ear plugs.

Adapted from Gilsenan, I. (2012). Nursing interventions to alleviate insomnia. *Nursing Older People, 24,* 14–18.

Many nonpharmacologic approaches are very helpful in the treatment of insomnia. These include acupuncture, exercise (including tai chi and yoga), massage, heat (sauna and hot tub), cooling (in hot environments), music and art therapy, and body and skin manipulations. Transcranial magnetic stimulation (TMS), which involves application of an electromagnetic field to the brain, thereby impacting nerve function, has been used to treat depression. The use of this treatment for insomnia is being investigated.

Pharmacologic Approaches to Insomnia

Historical Perspective

Over the ages, many different substances have been used to improve sleep (Riemann & Nissen, 2012). Alcohol and opium products have long been used by some people to promote sleep. However, these substances are known to have highs risks of abuse, dependence, and overdose. Bromides were used in the early 20th century, but these medications carried the risk of poisoning, nausea, rash, ataxia, and psychotic symptoms. Barbiturates began to be used in 1903 and were initially thought to be harmless, but they too were found to have a high risk of abuse, dependence, and overdose. Thalidomide was used mainly in Germany as an over-the-counter (OTC) product for sleep, but it was found to be highly teratogenic, and many babies were born with malformed limbs. In the 1960s, benzodiazepines were introduced.

Initially, they were thought to be effective and without risk of abuse, but mounting evidence suggests that there is a risk of developing tolerance, rebound insomnia, and falls during the night. When zopiclone was introduced to Canada, it was claimed to carry less risk of falls, tolerance, and abuse. However, it has been found to have some risk of abuse and dependence. Recently, zolpidem has been approved for use in Canada. Future medical treatments may include products aimed at orexin receptors.

Present-Day Pharmacotherapy

Sometimes, we overestimate the benefit of sleeping medication. A 2016 medical review of these medications found that evidence for important sleep outcomes was very limited (Wilt et al., 2016). Studies that compared effectiveness of the medications and how well they work in the long term are missing. Nurses need to keep in mind that not only can these medications cause cognitive and behavioural changes, but, infrequently, they have been linked with serious harms. A review of sleep preparations follows.

Herbal drugs sold OTC for sleep include humulus, passiflora, melissa, extractum cava, and valerian. Research on these products has not been comprehensive. Valerenic acid, thought to be the active ingredient of valerian, may be related to benzodiazepine-like activity on the GABA receptors. The use of this product is not recommended near conception, during pregnancy, or during lactation, because of possible mutagenic effects. Overall, no clear evidence supports the use of herbal products for insomnia (Riemann & Nissen, 2012).

A list of commonly used medications, their dosages, onset of action, and half-life elimination is found in Table 28.5. First-generation antihistamines such as diphenhydramine and hydroxyzine are commonly used in OTC products for insomnia. These medications have a 3- to 9-hour half-life, and CNS effects include sedation, decreased alertness, and slowed reaction times. Most drugs of this class also have some anticholinergic effects. The effects of these drugs on sleep have not been well studied and long-term use is not recommended. Besides sleepiness and grogginess, other side effects include psychomotor impairment, dizziness, tinnitus, decreased appetite, nausea and vomiting, constipation, and weight gain.

Chloral hydrate has been used in the past for insomnia but is no longer recommended. It is converted in the liver to trichloroethanol, which acts on the barbiturate binding site on GABA$_A$ receptors in the CNS. It has been found to reduce sleep latency and improve sleep continuity without significant effect on REM or SWS. However, a serious potential side effect is a liver lesion. Because the range between therapeutic and toxic effect is narrow, overdosing can be fatal. Difficulties with tolerance, loss of effectiveness, and severe withdrawal syndromes on discontinuation have been reported.

Melatonin has been found to help with the symptoms of jet lag and have a mild reduction on sleep latency, particularly in those with delayed sleep-phase syndrome. In the short term (less than 4 weeks), the side effect profile is low, but caution is needed for those with liver impairment. There is minimal risk of abuse or tolerance. The recommended dose for OTC melatonin is 3 to 5 mg. L-Tryptophan, an essential amino acid in the human diet, is a precursor of serotonin and is thought to be metabolized to serotonin in the brain. It has been found to decrease sleep latency without affecting SWS or REM sleep. The recommended dose is 500 to 1,000 mg, and the half-life is 1 to 2 hours.

Benzodiazepines (BZ), such as lorazepam, and benzodiazepine receptor agonists (BZRAs) like zopiclone are probably the most commonly used medications for the treatment of insomnia (Riemann & Nissen, 2012). These medications work by binding to the GABA receptor site, thereby enhancing the flow of negatively charged chloride ions into the neuron and decreasing the postsynaptic neuron's capacity to generate an action potential.

Table 28.5 Commonly Used Medications, Dosages, and Onset of Action and Half-Life Elimination			
Medication	**Dosage**	**Onset of Action**	**Half-life Elimination***
Diphenhydramine (Benadryl)	12.5–50 mg	15–60 minutes 0–80 minutes	2.4–7 hours
Doxepin (Silenor)	3–6 mg	30 minutes	15 hours
Flurazepam (Dalmane)	15–30 mg	15 minutes or less	40–114 hours
Hydroxyzine (Atarax)	50–100 mg	15–30 minutes	20–37 hours
Ramelteon (Rozerem)	8 mg	45 minutes	1–2.6 hours Metabolite MII: 2–5 hours
Suvorexant (Belsomra)	10–20 mg	30 minutes	12 hours
Temazepam (Restoril)	7.5–30 mg	30–60 minutes	9.5–12.5 hours
Trazodone (Desyrel)	25–100 mg	1–3 hours	7–10 hours
Triazolam (Halcion)	0.125–0.25 mg	15–30 minutes	1.5–5.5 hours
Zolpidem (Ambien)	5–10 mg	30 minutes	1.5–4.5 hours
Zopiclone (Imovane)	5.0–7.5 mg (lower in older adults)	30 minutes	5–12 hours

*Elimination can be affected by age and metabolic function.

This effect is very powerful because GABA$_A$ receptors are the most widespread receptors in the inhibitory synapses, which constitute up to 30% of all synapses in the CNS. There are two types of GABA$_A$ receptors: type 1 is found in most parts of the brain, and type 2 is primarily located in the spinal cord motor nerves and hippocampus parental neurons. BZ medications bind to both type 1 and 2 receptors, while the BZRAs bind more specifically with type 1 receptors. This may explain why BZs have muscle relaxant, anxiolytic, and anticonvulsant effects and can cause nighttime falls that result from muscle relaxation. Other side effects of both the BZs and BZRAs include next-morning hangovers, next-day performance deficits, amnesia, sleepwalking, and nocturnal eating. Difficulty driving a car, attention problems, and hangover effects occur primarily with longer-acting BZs. Some researchers advise that the risks outweigh the benefits of using these hypnotics in persons over 60 years of age (Glass, Lanctôt, Herrmann, Sproule, & Busto, 2005).

The use of other psychotropic medications such as antidepressants and atypical antipsychotics as first-line treatment for insomnia has not been thoroughly studied, and most cannot be recommended for general use. The serious side effect profile for many of these medications will place patients at risk. However, other medications used to treat specific psychiatric conditions can impact sleep as a side effect; and indeed, this side effect should be considered when selecting a drug. For example, a side effect of mirtazapine, which is an antidepressant, is somnolence. This medication may be used for someone who has depression and insomnia.

Caffeine taken orally is absorbed rapidly; peak blood levels are reached after 30 to 75 minutes. The half-life of one dose of caffeine is 3 to 7 hours. With increasing amounts of caffeine intake, the duration of action is longer because the renal clearance of caffeine is delayed and paraxanthine, one of its metabolites, accumulates. Caffeine blocks adenosine receptors, which are found throughout the brain, blood vessels, kidneys, heart, and gastrointestinal tract. Adenosine is thought to promote sleep by inhibiting cholinergic neurons in the basal forebrain that normally mediate arousal. Anxiety, insomnia, and mood changes can occur with high doses of caffeine in addition to high blood pressure, cardiac arrhythmias, and gastrointestinal effects. Taken 1 hour before sleep time, 77 to 322 mg of caffeine delays sleep onset, reduces total sleep time, and decreases SWS. No effect on REM sleep has been observed. Caffeine content in Tim Horton's coffee in Canada can range from 140 to 330 mg per cup (Tim Hortons Research and Development, 2015). Caffeine has been found to improve vigilance, attention, reaction times, and several aspects of memory.

Psychological Domain

Cognitive–behavioural models of insomnia posit that insomnia results from conditioning. Individuals with insomnia develop misperceptions and dysfunctional

ideas about their sleep that affect their ability to initiate and maintain sleep. For example, a person can develop and retain an idea that they "will never sleep well," thereby perpetuating poor sleep. Some people with insomnia will complain of not sleeping at all, but polysomnography testing may show that they do sleep. This is called a "sleep-state misperception"; it is thought to be caused by high-frequency EEG activity at sleep onset that may alter the person's perceptions of sleep and wake (Jungquist, 2011).

Several psychological and behavioural approaches can be used to treat insomnia and other sleep–wake disorders. These include sleep hygiene education, stimulus control therapy, sleep restriction, cognitive–behavioural therapy, and relaxation training. Nurses have been involved in education for implementing several of these therapies.

Stimulus Control Therapy

Stimulus control therapy involves implementing several behavioural strategies that promote conditioning the brain to associate the sleep environment with sleepiness. Strategies include using the bed for sleep and intimacy only (not watching TV or eating), maintaining a regular wake-up time and bedtime, and avoiding napping.

Sleep Restriction Therapy

Some people who are awake for long periods in the night will try to deal with poor sleep by sleeping later into the morning. This may lead to more difficulty falling asleep and, subsequently, later sleep-ins. Sleep restriction helps to reset the sleep–wake cycle. It involves restricting the total time in bed at night to the average amount of time the person would sleep, as long as it is not less than 4 hours. The person is advised to maintain a consistent bedtime and waking schedule and avoid daytime naps. This will cause a partial sleep deprivation, making it easier to fall asleep the next night. Increasing daytime activity will help deal with any daytime sleepiness.

Relaxation Training

Relaxation training involves learning and practicing several relaxation techniques that counteract muscle tension and cognitive arousal. Examples of these include guided imagery, progressive muscle relaxation, and mindfulness. The 5-4-3-2-1 exercise is an example of a relaxation strategy that nurses can teach (see Box 28.3).

Social Domain

Social factors that predispose someone to chronic insomnia may include societal or bed partner demands that disrupt the person's sleep schedule. Low income, inadequate family support, and family and/or work stressors are all associated with insomnia. The estimated $6.5 billion attributed to the cost of insomnia in Québec are accounted for by health care visits ($191.2 million), prescription medications ($16.5 million), alcohol used as a sleep aid ($339.8 million), insomnia-related

---

BOX 28.3 The 5-4-3-2-1 Relaxation Technique

While lying in bed with eyes closed:

- Think of 5 things that you could see in your bedroom if your eyes were open. Then, listen for 5 things that you can hear. Once you have heard 5 things, identify 5 things that you can physically feel (e.g., your head on the pillow, one leg touching the other).
- Next, think of 4 things you can see, 4 you can hear, 4 you can feel.
- Then, think of 3 things…
- Then 2…
- 1…
- If you are still awake, begin again at 5.

Adapted from O'Brien, D. (2017). *Self hypnosis: The Betty Erickson special.* Retrieved from http://ericksonian.info/therapeutic_scripts/self-hypnosis-the-betty-erickson-special/

---

absenteeism ($970.6 million), and insomnia-related productivity losses ($5.0 billion) (Daley et al., 2009).

Spiritual Domain

For some, spiritual distress can lead to insomnia. Conversely, insomnia can affect a person's capacity to address their personal spirituality. One research study in Saskatchewan showed that Aboriginal individuals who engage in traditional spirituality sessions with healing elders as an approach to reduce domestic violence experienced a significant reduction in the incidence of violence, sleep problems, and other symptoms of distress by the end of their sessions (Puchala, Paul, Kennedy, & Mehl-Madrona, 2010). A nursing study in Thailand, which examined the effectiveness of using Buddhist doctrine–based programs to enhance spiritual well-being, coping, and sleep quality among Thai seniors, found that practicing either meditation or chanting resulted in significant improvements in sleep quality (Wiriyasombat, Pothiban, Panuthai, Sucamvang, & Saengthong, 2011).

■ OBSTRUCTIVE SLEEP APNEA

Obstructive sleep apnea (OSA) is the most common sleep-related breathing disorder. A 2009 survey of Canadians by Statistics Canada found that approximately 3% of Canadian adults have been told by a health professional that they have sleep apnea; three quarters of these were 45 years of age and older, and men were almost twice as likely as women to have the disorder (Public Health Agency of Canada, 2010). However, the incidence of OSA is thought to be much higher; almost half of middle-aged men are thought to have OSA with up to 82% of them being undiagnosed

(Lang et al., 2017). Nurses can play an important role in helping identify people at risk for OSA in addition to educating about and advocating for assessment and treatment. Also, nurses can help individuals identify factors that promote adherence to treatment and intercede.

Signs and symptoms of untreated OSA include snoring, witnessed apneas, and restless sleep. A physical assessment may reveal an overweight or obese person (although not always) and specific oronasopharyngeal characteristics such as a large tongue with or without a scalloping pattern on the lateral aspects and/or crowding in the posterior aspect of the pharynx, which may be erythematous and/or oedematous. Nurses can identify patients at risk for OSA by asking questions using the STOP and BANG mnemonics (see Table 28.6). Positive responses to at least three of the eight questions suggest the need for a sleep assessment. Polysomnography is the best tool for assessing OSA but is not always available; portable home sleep studies are also used.

Nursing Management: Obstructive Sleep Apnea

Biologic Domain

In OSA, the person has partial and/or complete upper pharyngeal airway closure accompanied by ongoing efforts to breathe, resulting in sporadic oxyhaemoglobin desaturation and broken sleep. Mixed apneas, which are apneas associated with and without respiratory efforts, are also common. Respiratory events are seen more frequently during phases 1 and 2 of NREM sleep and REM sleep as opposed to SWS. When the person has a respiratory event, he or she will arouse from sleep, thereby ending the respiratory event. A diagnosis is applied when there are more than five episodes in an hour of partial and/or complete airway obstruction, each resulting in at least 10 seconds of hypopnoea or apnea. Daytime symptoms include sleepiness and fatigue, impaired cognition and daily function, and significant morbidity and mortality.

Table 28.6 BANG and STOP Mnemonics for Assessment of Sleep Apnea

BANG	STOP
Body mass index greater than 35	Do you Snore?
Age greater than 50	Do you feel Tired, fatigued, or sleepy during the day?
Neck size greater than 40 cm	Has anyone Observed your stopping breathing in your sleep?
Gender is male	Do you have high blood Pressure?

Adapted from Driver, H., Gottschalk, R., Hussain, M., Morin, C., Shapiro, C., & Van Zyl, L. (2012). *Insomnia in adults and children* (pp. 35). Retrieved from https://css-scs.ca/files/resources/brochures/Insomnia_Adult_Child.pdf

Risk factors for developing OSA include increased body mass index (BMI), genetics, race, and age (Sawyer, Deatrick, Kuna, & Weaver, 2010). Other risk factors include smoking cigarettes, consuming alcohol, and sedative and hypnotic medication use. Links have been found between OSA and specific medical conditions such as diabetes, polycystic ovary syndrome, hypertension, coronary artery disease, heart failure, and stroke. However, it is not known if the conditions are caused by OSA or contribute to its development.

Treatments for OSA include continuous positive airway pressure therapy (CPAP), surgical treatments, oral appliances, and weight loss. CPAP is most commonly used for treating OSA. It involves delivering a positive pressure into the person's airway through a nasal or full face mask. This pressure will help maintain the patency of the airway. The use of CPAP therapy has been shown to reduce respiratory events and oxyhaemoglobin desaturation, but its impact on daytime outcomes is not consistent. Improvements have been found in subjective sleepiness (especially among those with severe OSA), blood pressure, vigilance, OSA symptoms (e.g., snoring, dry mouth, morning headaches), and productivity after instituting CPAP treatment. Improvements in quality of life and neurobehavioural function have not been found consistently. However, adherence to CPAP is a significant limitation to effective treatment; rates of adherence range from 30% to 60% (Sawyer et al., 2010). Early experiences with CPAP, the individual's perceptions and beliefs about CPAP and OSA, and social and situational variables can negatively impact adherence. Newer technologies are being developed to deliver CPAP and promote adherence (see Fig. 28.9). Also, in Canada, it can be difficult for some individuals, including certain First Nations groups, to access CPAP therapy because of federal and provincial government policies (Marchildon et al., 2015). Nurses can play a role in advocating for access to this treatment.

Psychological Domain

Two of the main consequences of OSA are impaired cognitive performance and mood disturbance. Impaired executive function, including memory, mental flexibility, planning, organization, behavioural inhibition, and problem-solving can negatively impact work, school, and everyday life. The relationship between depression and OSA is complex; it varies depending on age, gender, and other health characteristics. The risk of depression depends on the severity of the OSA and excessive daytime sleepiness; as these become more serious, the risk of depression rises. Being aware of these links, nurses may need to screen for depression when they see individuals who have OSA and excessive daytime sleepiness. Social cognitive theory has been used as a framework for understanding adherence to CPAP treatment (Sawyer et al., 2010). Commitment to long-term use of CPAP has been found to be determined by the person's

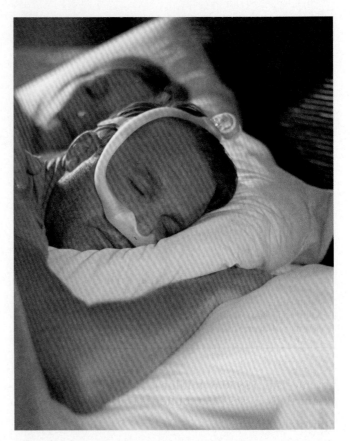

Figure 28.9. A variety of facial and nasal masks are used to treat obstructive sleep apnea. For an example, see the Philips Respironics DreamWear under the nose nasal mask.

experience with the treatment within the first week of starting treatment; a positive experience correlated with commitment to using CPAP. Understanding that specific signs and symptoms are because of OSA is an important motivator for seeking assessment and treatment. Other beliefs and perceptions that affected commitment to CPAP included outcome expectations, treatment goals, self-efficacy, and treatment barriers/facilitators.

Social Domain

OSA has been associated with decreased work productivity, marital problems, and motor vehicle and work incidents. The risk of a motor vehicle incident for those with untreated OSA is twice as likely as for those without. Nurses should ask individuals being assessed for OSA about their driving habits and occupational requirements. Questions should include the number of hours and days the person drives, history of vehicle incidents and near misses caused by sleepiness, and history of single-vehicle incidents. Those suspected to have severe OSA should avoid driving or operating heavy equipment until their OSA is treated. Those who live alone and have had a recent traumatic life event have been shown to have decreased adherence to CPAP; attending support groups and having an immediate social support person are promoting factors.

Spiritual Domain

While research that looks at the link between spirituality and OSA was not found in the literature, OSA has been found to be associated with a decreased quality of life (Sampaio, Pereira, & Winck, 2012). Understandably, it would be difficult to develop and participate in spiritual experiences if the person is dealing with impaired executive functioning, mood disturbance, sleepiness, and other related physical complaints in addition to social difficulties.

COMMON CIRCADIAN RHYTHM SLEEP–WAKE DISORDERS

Shift Workers

Approximately 15% to 20% of workers in industrialized countries are engaged in shift work, and intolerance of being awake during the night hours is not uncommon (Stokowski, 2012). For those trying to sleep during the day, typically, the duration is shorter and the quality is less consolidated than nighttime sleep. For example, ICU nurses in three British Columbia hospitals were found to get an average of 5.68 hours of sleep between two night shifts and 6.79 hours between two day shifts (Hirsch Allen et al., 2014). Health and safety problems associated with managing shift work may include an increased risk of gastrointestinal and cardiovascular disorders, depression, some cancers, and accidents and injuries due to decreased alertness (Rosenberg & Doghramji, 2011).

Among nurses, nightshift work has been associated with more work-related injuries (Hopcia et al., 2012) and regret about decisions made while at work are more likely to be reported by nurses with poor sleep quality (Scott, Arslanian-Engoren, & Engoren, 2014). A national survey of 6,312 Canadian nurses found that more than 25% had observed unsafe practice related to health professional fatigue and had considered resigning because of feelings of fatigue (Canadian Nurses Association, 2010a). Several strategies can be used to help cope with sleepiness associated with shift work (see Box 28.4).

Driving while sleepy and falling asleep at the wheel, reported by 60% and 18% of drivers respectively, certainly place individuals at risks for collisions. Vehicle crashes caused by sleepiness or fatigue account for about 20% of all accidents (MacLean, n.d.). Caffeine, short breaks, and naps can provide temporary relief but there is no substitute for sleep.

In 2010, the Canadian Nurses Association (CNA) released a position statement on nurse fatigue, which they defined as a "subjective feeling of tiredness (experienced by nurses) that is physically and mentally penetrative" (Canadian Nurses Association, 2010b, p. 1). This fatigue could not be "slept off" and so it is more than sleep deprivation, but circadian rhythm disturbances, sleepiness, and sleep habits were identified as contributing factors. The CNA has identified several systemic, organizational, and individual responsibilities to manage nurse fatigue. See Box 28.5 for the individual responsibilities of nurses.

Jet Lag

Jet lag occurs when a person travels by air across several time zones in a short period of time, and the person's internal clock is out of phase with the light–dark cycle of the destination. It is not clear why this happens. One hypothesis is that the body's biologic clocks become desynchronized and they take varying amounts of times to resynchronize. Symptoms of jet lag include poor sleep at night and feeling groggy during the day. Additionally, some travellers experience gastrointestinal upset and general malaise. Flying westbound is generally less challenging to adapt to than flying eastward. Because our internal clocks are a little longer than 24 hours, a person can move his or her internal clock *later* by approximately

---

BOX 28.4 Behavioural Strategies to Manage Effects of Shift Work

- If working 8-hour rotating shifts, rotate the shifts clockwise, from days to evenings to nights.
- Avoid switching to different shifts rapidly within a short time period.
- Follow a regular sleep schedule regardless of the shift you are working.
- Keep your bedroom as dark as possible when you are sleeping.
- When awake, spend as much time as possible in brightly lit rooms.
- Wear sunglasses to block blue light on the way home from work in the morning.

- Avoid scheduling appointments during your daytime sleep hours.
- After the last night shift, sleep 4 hours and then get up.
- Avoid eating large meals within 4 hours of going to bed.
- Avoid caffeine and nicotine before sleep.

A short nap (15 to 20 minutes) during the night shift may reduce sleepiness and increase alertness.

Adapted from Rosenberg, R., & Doghramji, P. (2011). Is shift work making your patient sick? Emerging theories and therapies for treating shift work disorder. *Postgraduate Medicine, 123*(5), 106–115.

BOX 28.5 Canadian Nurses Association Position Statement: Taking Action on Nurse Fatigue

Individual-level responsibilities for nurses managing fatigue:

1. Nurses learn to be aware of and recognize signs, symptoms, and responses to personal fatigue.
2. Nurses understand and work within the policies related to safe patient care within their organizations and within professional practice expectations.
3. Nurses take responsibility for mitigating and managing fatigue while at work, including professional approaches to decline work assignments. When deciding to work extra shifts, nurses act on their ethical obligation to maintain fitness to practice.

4. Nurses act on their ethical obligation to maintain fitness to practice when planning non–work-related activities.
5. Nurses work through their professional associations and nursing unions to advocate for safe patient care through safe scheduling practices in the work environment.

Nurses support policies, procedures, and health promotion initiatives that manage fatigue in the workplace.

Source: Canadian Nurses Association. (2010). *Position statement: Taking action on nurse fatigue.* Retrieved from https://www.cna-aiic.ca/~/media/cna/page-content/pdf-en/ps112_nurse_fatigue_2010_e.pdf?la=en. Reprinted with permission.

---

2 hours a day but *earlier* by only 1 to 1½ hours a day. Other factors that can contribute to jet lag include sleep deprivation, the discomfort of airplane travel, and in-flight caffeine and/or alcohol intake.

Treating Circadian Rhythm Disorders

Treatments of circadian rhythm disorders include melatonin, strategic avoidance or exposure to light and napping, BZRA medications (e.g., zopiclone), strategically consumed stimulants such as caffeine and modafinil, and bright light therapy. Bright light therapy is used to treat circadian rhythm disorders, including jet lag and shift work. Its effectiveness is dependent on the part of the circadian cycle during which it is used. This therapy works through the action of the light on the eyes and retina; the person does not need to look directly at the light in order to benefit. The usual "dose" of light is 5,000 lux shortly after waking in the morning, typically obtained through exposure to a 10,000-lux light box for 30 minutes every day. A benefit can be felt within days. Eye damage due to this therapy has not been found, but nausea, headache, and nervousness can occur.

SUMMARY OF KEY POINTS

- The brain has three different naturally occurring states: wakefulness, REM sleep, and NREM sleep. Coma and anaesthesia are other physiologic brain states not discussed in this chapter.
- Physical, psychological, social, and/or spiritual disturbances can cause sleep problems and vice versa. Any assessment of sleep complaints needs to include a review of these possible influences.
- Sleep disorders are common comorbidities of many mental disorders. However, sleep disturbances can

be risk factors as well as early or prodromal symptoms for mental disorders.
- Nurses have an important role to play in assessing and helping people manage sleep difficulties.
- Many nurses are also at risk for sleep-related problems because of the nature of their work. It is important that nurses understand the risks and manifestations of these problems and develop strategies to prevent and manage the issues.

ACKNOWLEDGMENTS

Dr. Rachel Morehouse, Medical Director, Atlantic Sleep Centre, Saint John Regional Hospital, Saint John N.B., supported the development of this chapter; this sharing of her knowledge regarding sleep was much appreciated.

 Web Links

css-scs.ca/ The Canadian Sleep Society (CSS)/Société Canadienne du Sommeil (SCS) has a website for clinicians, scientists, and technologists that promotes the advancement and understanding of sleep and its disorders.

sleepfoundation.org This is an American organization that provides information on a variety of sleep-related topics.

thebrain.mcgill.ca/ The Brain from Top to Bottom is a website supported by McGill University. Refer to the module on sleep and dreams. It has several modules that provide information on the brain at beginner, intermediate, and advanced levels. The modules are organized for social, psychological, neurologic, cellular, and molecular content.

References

American Geriatric Society 2015 Beers Criteria Update Expert Panel. (2015). American Geriatrics Society 2015 updated beers criteria for potentially inappropriate medication use in older adults. *Journal of the American Geriatric Society, 63,* 2227–2246. Retrieved from http://onlinelibrary.wiley.com/doi/10.1111/jgs.13702/full

American Psychiatric Association (APA). (2013). *Diagnostic and statistical manual of mental disorders* (5th ed.). Washington, DC: Author.

Bishop, T., Simons, K., King, D., & Pigeon, W. (2016). Sleep and suicide in older adults: An opportunity for intervention. *Clinical Therapeutics, 38,* 2332–2339.

Bumb, J. M., Schilling, C., Enning, F., Haddad, L., Paul, F., Lederbogen, F., … Nolte, I. (2014). Pineal gland volume in primary insomnia and health controls: A magnetic resonance imaging study. *Journal of Sleep Research, 23*(3), 274–280. doi:10.1111/jsr.12125

Canadian Nurses Association. (2010a). *Nurse fatigue and patient safety: Research report.* Retrieved from http://www.cna-aiic.ca/sitecore-modules/web/on-the-issues/better-care/patient-safety/nurse-fatigue-and-patient-safety?sc_lang=en

Canadian Nurses Association. (2010b). *Position statement: Taking action on nurse fatigue.* Retrieved from http://www2.cna-aiic.ca/CNA/documents/pdf/publications/PS112_Nurse_Fatigue_2010_e.pdf

Carney, P. R., Berry, R. B., & Geyer, J. D. (2012). *Clinical sleep disorders* (2nd ed.). Philadelphia, PA: Lippincott Williams & Wilkins.

Caruso, C., & Hitchcock, E. (2010). Strategies for nurses to prevent sleep-related injuries and errors. *Rehabilitation Nursing, 35,* 192–197.

Colrain, I., & Baker, F. (2011). Changes in sleep as a function of adolescent development. *Neuropsychology Review, 21,* 5–21.

Daley, M., Morin, C., LeBlanc, M., Grégoire, J. P., & Savard, J. (2009). The economic burden of insomnia: Direct and indirect costs for individuals with insomnia syndrome, insomnia symptoms, and good sleepers. *Sleep, 32,* 55–64.

Dondelinger, R. (2009). Sleep studies. *Biomedical Instrumentation and Technology, 43,* 458–462.

Driver, H. (2012). Sleepless women: Insomnia from the female perspective. *Insomnia Rounds, 1*(6). Retrieved from https://css-scs.ca/files/resources/insomnia-rounds/150-006_Eng.pdf

Driver, H., Gottschalk, R., Hussain, M., Morin, C., Shapiro, C., & Van Zyl, L. (2012). *Insomnia in adults and children.* Retrieved from https://css-scs.ca/files/resources/insomnia-rounds/150-006_Eng.pdf

Dubuc, B. (n.d.). *The different types of sleep.* The Brain from Top to Bottom website. Retrieved from http://thebrain.mcgill.ca/flash/a/a_11/a_11_p/a_11_p_cyc/a_11_p_cyc.html

España, R., & Scammell, T. (2011). Sleep neurobiology from a clinical perspective. *Sleep, 34,* 845–858.

Exxon Valdez Oil Spill Trustee Council. (1990). *Details about the accident.* Retrieved from http://www.evostc.state.ak.us/index.cfm?FA=facts.details

Farrehi, P., Clore, K., Scott, J. R., Vanini, G., & Clauw, D. (2016). Efficacy of sleep tool education during hospitalization: A randomized controlled trial. *The American Journal of Medicine, 129,* 1329.e9–1329.e17.

Fleming, J. (2013). Psychiatric disorders and insomnia: Managing the vicious cycle. *Insomnia Rounds, 2*(1). Retrieved from https://css-scs.ca/files/resources/insomnia-rounds/150-007_Eng.pdf

Gilsenan, I. (2012). Nursing interventions to alleviate insomnia. *Nursing Older People, 24,* 14–18.

Glass, J., Lanctôt, K., Herrmann, N., Sproule, B., & Busto, U. (2005). Sedative hypnotics in older people with insomnia: Meta-analysis of risks and benefits. *British Medical Journal, 19,* 1169–1173.

Graven, S., & Browne, J. (2008). Sleep and brain development: The critical role of sleep in fetal and early neonatal brain development. *Newborn and Infant Nursing Reviews, 8,* 173–79.

Hafner, M., Stepanek, M., Taylor, J., Troxel, W., & van Stolk, C. (2017). *Why sleep matters: The economic costs of insufficient sleep.* RAND Europe. Retrieved from https://www.rand.org/content/dam/rand/pubs/research_briefs/RB9900/RB9962/RAND_RB9962.pdf

Harrison, Y. (2012). The functions of sleep. In C. Morin & C. Espie (Eds.), *The Oxford handbook of sleep and sleep disorders* (pp. 61–74). New York, NY: Oxford University Press.

Hirsch Allen, A. J., Park, J. E., Adhaminm, N., Sirounis, D., Dodek, P., Rogers, A. E., & Avas, N. (2014). Impact of work schedules on sleep duration of critical care nurses. *American Journal of Critical Care, 23*(4), 290–295. doi:10.4037/ajcc2014876

Hobson, A., & McCarley, R. W. (1977). Brain as a dream state generator: An activation-synthesis hypothesis of the dream process. *American Journal of Psychiatry, 134,* 1335–1348.

Hopcia, K., Dennerlein, J., Hashimoto, D., Stoddard, A., Orechia, T., & Sorensen, G. (2012). A case–control study of occupational injuries for consecutive and cumulative shifts in hospital registered nurses and patient care associates. *Workplace Health and Safety, 60*(11), 437–444.

Horne, J. (2008). Insomnia—Victorian style. *The Psychologist, 21*(10), 910–911.

Hurst, M. (2008). *Who gets any sleep these days? Sleep patterns of Canadians.* Statistics Canada Catalogue No. 11-008-X Canadian Social Trends.

Retrieved from http://www.statcan.gc.ca/pub/11-008-x/2008001/article/10553-eng.htm

Jungquist, C. (2011). Insomnia. In N. Redeker & G. McEnany (Eds.), *Sleep disorders and sleep promotion in nursing practice* (pp. 71–93). New York, NY: Springer.

Kurth, S., Dean, D., Achermann, P., O'Muircheartaigh, J., Huber, R., Deoni, S., & LeBourgeois, M. (2016). Increased sleep depth in developing neural networks: New insights from sleep restriction in children. *Frontiers in Human Neuroscience, 10,* 456. https://doi.org/10.3389/fnhum.2016.00456

Landis, C. (2011). Physiological and behavioral aspects of sleep. In N. Redeker & G. McEnany (Eds.), *Sleep disorders and sleep promotion in nursing practice* (pp. 1–18). New York, NY: Springer.

Lang, C., Appleton, S., Vakulin, A., McEnvoy, D., Vincent, A., Wittert, G., … Adams, R. (2017). Associations of undiagnosed obstructive sleep apnea and excessive daytime sleepiness with depression: An Australian population study. *The Journal of Clinical Sleep Medicine, 13,* 575–582. doi:10.5664/jcsm.6546

Li, Y., Yang, Y., Li, Q., Yand, X., Wang, Y., Ku, W., & Li, H. (2017). The impact of the improvement of insomnia on blood pressure in hypertensive patients. *Journal of Sleep Research, 26,* 105–114.

Looney, D., Goverdovsky, V., Rosenzweig, I., Morrell, M., & Mandic, D. (2016). Wearable in-ear encephalography sensor for monitoring sleep: Preliminary observations from nap studies. *Annals of the American Thoracic Society, 13,* 2229–2233.

MacLean, A. (n.d.). *Commercial motor vehicles driver fatigue, long-term health, and highway safety: Research needs.* Retrieved from https://rsc-src.ca/en/report-from-abroad/commercial-motor-vehicles-driver-fatigue-long-term-health-and-highway-safety

Marchildon, G., Katapally, T., Beck, C., Abonyi, S., Episkenew, J., Pahwa, P., & Dosman, J. (2015). Exploring policy driven systemic inequities leading to differential access to care among indigenous populations with obstructive sleep apnea in Canada. *International Journal for Equity in Health, 14,* 148. doi:10.1186/s12939-015-0279-3

Mayers, A., & Baldwin, D. (2005). Antidepressants and their effect on sleep. *Human psychopharmacology, 20,* 533–559.

Mitler, M. M., Carskadon, M. A., Czeisler, C. A., Dement, W. C., Dinges, D. F., & Graeber, R. C. (1988). Catastrophes, sleep, and public policy: Consensus report. *Sleep, 11*(1), 100–109.

Morin, C. (2012). Insomnia: Prevalence, burden, and consequences. *Insomnia Rounds, 1*(1). Retrieved from https://css-scs.ca/files/resources/insomnia-rounds/150-001_Eng.pdf

Morin, C., LeBlanc, M., Bélanger, L., Ivers, H., Mérette, C., & Savard, J. (2011). Prevalence of insomnia and its treatment in Canada. *Canadian Journal of Psychiatry, 56,* 540–548.

Morselli, L., Guyon, A., & Spiegel, K. (2012). Sleep and metabolic function. *Pflügers Archiv: European Journal of Physiology, 463,* 139–160.

Motivala, S. (2011). Sleep and inflammation: Psychoneuroimmunology in the context of cardiovascular disease. *Annals of Behavioral Medicine, 42,* 141–152.

Nuutinen, T., Ray, C., & Roos, E. (2013). Do computer use, TV viewing, and the presence of the media in the bedroom predict school-aged children's sleep habits in a longitudinal study? *BMC Public Health, 13,* 684. doi:10.1186/1471-2458-13-684

O'Brien, D. (2017). *Self hypnosis: The Betty Erickson special.* Retrieved from http://ericksonian.info/therapeutic_scripts/self-hypnosis-the-betty-erickson-special/

Palagini, L., & Rosenlicht, N. (2011). Sleep, dreaming, and mental health: A review of historical and neurobiological perspectives. *Sleep Medicine Reviews, 15,* 179–186.

ParticipACTION. (2016). *Are Canadian kids too tired to move? The 2016 ParticipACTION report card on physical activity for children and youth.* Toronto, ON: ParticipACTION. Retrieved from https://www.participaction.com/sites/default/files/downloads/2016%20ParticipACTION%20Report%20Card%20-%20Full%20Report.pdf

Peigneux, P., Urbain, C., & Schmitz, R. (2012). Sleep and the brain. In C. Morin & C. Espie (Eds.), *The Oxford handbook of sleep and sleep disorders* (pp. 11–37). New York, NY: Oxford University Press.

Public Health Agency of Canada. (2010). *What is the impact of sleep apnea on Canadians?* Retrieved from http://www.phac-aspc.gc.ca/cd-mc/sleepapnea-apneesommeil/pdf/sleep-apnea.pdf

Puchala, C., Paul, S., Kennedy, C., & Mehl-Madrona, L. (2010). Using traditional spirituality to reduce domestic violence within aboriginal communities. *The Journal of Alternative and Complementary Medicine, 16,* 89–96.

Rhoades, R. A., & Bell, D. R. (Eds.). (2012). *Medical physiology: Principles for clinical medicine* (4th ed.). Philadelphia, PA: Lippincott Williams & Wilkins.

Riemann, D., & Nissen, C. (2012). Sleep and psychotropic drugs. In C. Morin & C. Espie (Eds.), *The Oxford handbook of sleep and sleep disorders* (pp. 190–220). New York, NY: Oxford University Press.

Roehrs, T. (2011). Normal sleep and its variations. In M. Kryger, T. Roth, & W. Dement. (Eds.), *Principles and practice of sleep medicine* (5th ed., pp. 1–100). St. Louis, MO: Elsevier Saunders.

Ropper, A. H., & Samuels, M. A. (2009). Sleep and its abnormalities. In A. H. Ropper & M. A. Samuels (Eds.), *Adams and Victor's principles of neurology* (9th ed.). Retrieved from http://www.accessmedicine.com/content.aspx?aID=3633173

Rosenberg, R., & Doghramji, P. (2011). Is shift work making your patient sick? Emerging theories and therapies for treating shift work disorder. *Postgraduate Medicine, 123*(5), 106–115.

Saleh, P., Ahmadi, N., & Shapiro, C. (2010). Sleep and psychiatric disease. In M. Kryger (Ed.), *Atlas of clinical sleep medicine* (pp. 254–260). Philadelphia, PA: Saunders Elsevier.

Sampaio, R., Pereira, M. G., & Winck, J. C. (2012). Psychological morbidity, illness representations, and quality of life in female and male patients with obstructive sleep apnea syndrome. *Psychology, Health and Medicine, 17*, 136–149.

Sawyer, A., Deatrick, J., Kuna, S., & Weaver, T. (2010). Differences in perceptions of the diagnosis and treatment of obstructive sleep apnea and continuous positive airway pressure therapy among adherers and non-adherers. *Qualitative Health Research, 20*(7), 873–892.

Schofield, R., Forchuk, C., Montgomery, P., Rudnick, A., Edwards, B., Meier, A., & Speechley, M. (2016). Comparing health practices: Individuals with mental illness and the general Canadian population. *Canadian Nurse, 112*(5), 23–27.

Scott, L., Arslanian-Engoren, C., & Engoren, M. (2014). Association of sleep and fatigue with decision regret among critical care nurses. *American Journal of Critical Care, 23*(1), 13–23. doi:http://dx.doi.org/10.4037/ajcc2014191

Sehgal, A., & Mignot, E. (2011). Genetics of sleep and sleep disorders. *Cell, 146*, 194–207.

Smith, M., Nasir, A., Campbell, C., & Okonkwo, R. (2011). Sleep disturbance and chronic pain: Behavioral interactions. In C. Morin & C. Espie (Eds.), *The Oxford handbook of sleep and sleep disorders* (pp. 846–863). New York, NY: Oxford University Press.

Smylie, J., Fell, D., Chambers, B., Sauve, R., Royle, C., Allan, B., & O'Campo, P. (2014). Socioeconomic position and factors associated with use of a nonsupine infant sleep position: Findings from the Canadian Maternity Experiences Survey. *American Journal of Public Health, 104*, 539–547.

Stokowski, L. (2012). Help me make it through the night (shift). *Ohio Nurses Review, 87*, 12–16.

Tim Hortons Research and Development. (2015). *Tim Hortons caffeine content.* Retrieved from https://www.timhortons.com/ca/en/pdf/CAFFEINE_CONTENT_-_Canada.pdf

Weiss, S., & Corkum, P. (2012). Pediatric behavioral insomnia—"Good night, sleep tight" for child and parent. *Insomnia Rounds, 1*(5), 1–6. Retrieved from https://css-scs.ca/files/resources/insomnia-rounds/150-005_Eng.pdf

Wilt, T., MacDonald, R., Brasure, M., Olson, C., Carlyle, M., Fuchs, E., … Kane, R. (2016). Pharmacologic treatment of insomnia disorder: An evidence report for a clinical practice guideline by the American College of Physicians. *Annals of Internal Medicine, 165*, 103–112. doi:10.7326/M15-1781

Wiriyasombat, R., Pothiban, L., Panuthai, S., Sucamvang, K., & Saengthong, S. (2011). Effectiveness of Buddhist doctrine practice-based programs in enhancing spiritual well-being, coping and sleep quality of Thai elders. *Pacific Rim International Journal of Nursing Research, 15*, 203–219.

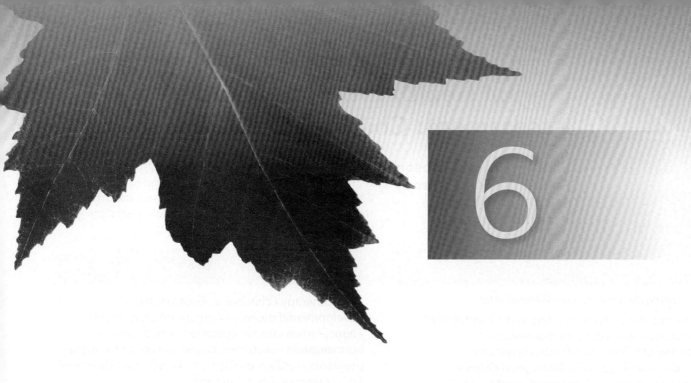

6

Mental Health
Across the
Lifespan

29 Mental Health Promotion and Assessment: Children and Adolescents

Lorelei Faulkner-Gibson, Kimberly Wong, Wendy Austin, and Cindy Peternelj-Taylor

Adapted from the chapters "Mental Health Promotion With Children and Adolescents" by Lorelei Faulkner-Gibson, Kimberly Wong, and Wendy Austin and "Mental Health Assessment of Children and Adolescents" by Lorelei Faulkner-Gibson and Kimberly Wong

LEARNING OBJECTIVES

After reading this chapter, you will be able to:

- Describe the protective factors in the mental health promotion of children and adolescents.
- Identify the risk factors for the development of psychopathology in childhood and adolescence.
- Analyze the role of the nurse in mental health promotion with children and families.
- Define the assessment process for children and adolescents.
- Discuss the techniques of assessment data collection used with children and adolescents.
- Discuss the synthesis of bio/psycho/social/spiritual assessment data for children and adolescents.
- Identify the responsibilities of nurses to recognize and assess the effects of maltreatment in children.

KEY TERMS

- bibliotherapy • childhood abuse/neglect • developmental delays • disorganized attachment • egocentrism • formal operations • maturation • normalization • protective factors • psychoeducational programs • resilience • risk factors • self-concept • social skills training • support groups

KEY CONCEPTS

- attachment • grief • personal fable

In this chapter, the importance of childhood and adolescent mental health is examined, the core prevention strategies and childhood stressors are identified, and guidelines for mental health promotion and risk reduction are provided. Assessment of the mental health of children and adolescents is outlined, including its components and the techniques required for an accurate, meaningful, and holistic result. By virtue of their close contact with families in health care settings and their role as educators, nurses are in a key position to identify and intervene with children and adolescents at risk for psychopathology. Knowing the difference between normal child development and psychopathology is crucial in helping parents to view their children's behaviour realistically and respond appropriately. The assessment of child abuse is addressed, as is the legal responsibility of Canadian nurses to report maltreatment of the most vulnerable members of society.

CHILDHOOD AND ADOLESCENT MENTAL HEALTH

The Child and Youth Advisory Committee of the Mental Health Commission of Canada (2016) has identified strategic directions for promotion, prevention, intervention and ongoing care, research, and evaluation to address the mental health needs of children and youth in their document, *The Mental Health Strategy for Canada: A Youth Perspective*. The committee's *Evergreen* framework (Kutcher & McLuckie, 2010) upholds the values of human rights; dignity, respect, and diversity; best available evidence; choice, opportunity, and responsibility; collaboration, continuity, and community; and access to information, programs, and services for all children, youth, and families. The framework is available to guide service providers, policy makers, and officials in creating mental health programs and services for children, youth, and families.

In *The Health of Canada's Young People: A Mental Health Focus*, Freeman and associates (2010) reported on views of youth about health and well-being, as well as the health behaviours of young people aged 11 to 15 years. The report indicated that there are mental health issues specific to age and gender and that positive adult relationships; supportive home, school, and community environments; and general health in the form of nutrition, safety, and security are all critical in the mental health of youth. Supportive social networks and positive childhood and adolescent experiences maximize the mental health of children and adolescents.

Children are more likely to be mentally healthy if they have normal physical and psychosocial development and a secure attachment at an early age. A secure, warm, responsive, and predictable attachment relationship between infants and their caregivers is critical to positive well-being and healthy development (Clinton, Feller, & Williams, 2016). **Attachment** is the emotional bond between a child and parent (or parental figure) that begins in infancy; a secure attachment helps the child explore the world without fear of rejection. Parents play a critical role in preventing adverse outcomes in their children and, if needed, can be assisted to learn ways of being optimally responsive to their children.

KEY CONCEPT

Attachment is the bond between a child and a parent (or parental figure) that begins in infancy and, when secure, allows the child to explore the world without fear of rejection.

Families play a highly significant role in the lives of children and adolescents as protectors, nurturers, mediators, and mentors for surviving and thriving in the world. Values are transmitted and interpreted within families. Children need to explore their world, to play, and to learn how to speak and listen to others: it is the family's role to provide the opportunities for doing so. Communal conditions and efforts are important, too (Siddiqi, Irwin & Hertzman, 2007). As the Nigerian proverb advises, "It takes a whole village to raise a child." When children enter the world, there will be both protective and risk factors that shape their health and well-being. Nurses and other health care professionals are there to assist and guide them in growing up to be as healthy as possible.

■ COMMON CHILDHOOD STRESSORS

Stress is an inevitable part of life and may occur in one or a number of spheres of influence in a child's life (Siddiqi et al., 2007). Stressors in each sphere of influence can include the following:

- Child: Difficult temperament, birth difficulties (e.g., genetic anomalies, prematurity, developmental delay, failure to thrive), extreme sensitivity to sensory experiences, suspected abuse/neglect, loss of a significant caregiver, withdrawal, extreme activity level, aggressive behaviour and emotional dysregulation/reactivity, substance abuse.
- Family: Primary caregivers may lack parenting knowledge, skills, and education. They may be

experiencing unresolved loss/trauma, developmental delay, financial and marital stress, chronic health problems, mental health problems, and/ or substance abuse resulting in negative attributions to the child. They may show insensitivity or responses of rejection, angry or harsh discipline, frightening behaviour, and a failure to protect the child. Ultimately, parent–child attachment may be negatively affected (Infant Mental Health Promotion, 2005, p. 2).
- Residential community: Neighbourhoods with a lower socioeconomic status may be exposed to toxic or hazardous wastes, residential overcrowding, and poor housing quality. They may also have limited access to services such as facilities for learning and recreation, child care, medical facilities, access to transportation, and opportunities for employment.

Regardless of the origin, stress often causes conflict and difficulty within family relationships. These responses to stress can disrupt parenting as well as the interactions between the parent and the child and can lead to short-term or long-term poor outcomes. The earlier these events begin, and the longer that the disruption lasts, the worse the outcomes.

Grief and Loss

Nurses need to recognize that grief and loss are universally experienced by children and among the most common stresses they encounter. Children respond to loss and grief based on their developmental stage and not as adults do. The most common losses experienced are death of a grandparent, parental divorce, family separation (parents who work away or are ill for periods of time), death of a pet, and loss of friends through moving or changing schools. Learning to mourn losses can lead to a renewed appreciation of the precious value of life and close relationships. Vast research shows that both children and adults who experience major losses are at risk for mental health problems, particularly if the natural grieving process is impeded. The grieving process differs somewhat between children and adults (see Table 29.1).

KEY CONCEPT

Grief is the subjective experience (i.e., the thoughts, feelings, body sensations, and behaviours) that accompanies the perception of a loss. Children grieve in stages, as do adults, but children's grief is shaped by developmental stages as well as experiences.

Children's responses to loss reflect their developmental level, as well as their previous experience. As early as age 3 years, children can have some concept of death.

Table 29.1 Grieving in Childhood, Adolescence, and Adulthood		
Children	Adolescents	Adults
• View death as reversible: do not understand that death is permanent until about age 7 years	• Understand that death is permanent but may flirt with death (e.g., reckless driving, unprotected sex) due to omnipotent feelings	• Understand that death is permanent: may struggle with spiritual beliefs about death
• Experiment with ideas about death by killing bugs, staging funerals, acting out death in play	• May be fascinated by death, enjoy morbid books and movies, listen to rock music about death and suicide	• May try not to think about death, depending on cultural background
• Mourn through activities (e.g., mock funerals, playing with things owned by the loved one); may not cry	• Mourn by talking about the loss, crying, and reflecting on it, sometimes becoming dramatic (e.g., overidentifying with the lost person, developing poetic or romantic ideas about death)	• Mourn through talking about the loss, crying, reviewing memories, and thinking privately about it
• May not discuss the loss openly, but express grief through regression, somatic complaints, behaviour problems, or withdrawal	• Often withdraw when mourning or seek comfort through peer groups; may feel parents do not understand their feelings	• Usually discuss loss openly, depending on the level of support available; may feel there is a "time limit" on how long it is socially acceptable to grieve
• Need repeated explanations to fully understand the loss; it may be helpful to read children's books that explain death	• Need permission to grieve openly because they may believe they should act strong or take care of the adults involved; need acceptance of their sometimes extreme reactions	• Need friends, family, and other supportive people to listen and allow them to mourn for however long it takes; need opportunities to review their feelings and memories

For example, the death of a pet goldfish provides an opportunity for the child to grasp the idea that the fish will never swim again. However, it is not until about age seven that most children understand the permanence of death. Before this age, they may verbalize that someone has "died" but in the next sentence ask when the dead person will be "coming back." Even though the finality of death is understood by early adolescence (Brown, 2009), adolescents sometimes flirt with death by engaging in risky behaviours, such as driving dangerously, as if they believe that they are immune to death. This phenomenon is a result of the *personal fable* (Elkind, 1967) whereby adolescents view themselves in an egocentric way and as unique and invulnerable to the consequences experienced by others. See Box 29.1 for research on children's perceptions of death.

The concept of death is difficult to grasp, and adults should be sensitive to the child's struggle to understand and cope with it. Research suggests that children want to be included in the rituals related to a death in the family (e.g., funerals, memorials) and thus to be recognized as mourners alongside adults. It allows them to participate in "saying good-bye" (Søfting, Dyregro, & Dyregrov, 2016). Most children closely watch their parents' response to grief and loss and use fantasy to fill the gaps in their understanding. In many cases, family members take turns grieving, and some children may sense that their parents are so overwhelmed by their own emotional pain that they cannot bear the children's grief. Adults may attribute certain responses or reactions to the child that may not be accurate. It is important for the nurse to be aware of this when working with families, and with differing familial and cultural norms, and to be able to assess and respond to their needs accordingly.

Children and adolescents may experience complicated grief. *Complicated grief* is a form of bereavement-related distress that can include such symptoms as being preoccupied with thoughts of the deceased, including difficulty accepting the death, and numbness, bitterness, or a sense of futility (Dillen, Fontaine, & Verhofstadt-Denève, 2009; Melhem, Moritz, Walker, Shear, & Brent, 2007). An indication that bereaved children may need mental health services is related to such things as level of functioning (e.g., grief responses), coping, self-esteem, and aspects of their family environment (e.g., stressors, parenting) (Brown, Sandler, Tein, Liu, & Haine, 2007).

Grief in childhood is shaped by developmental stages and life experiences (Pfund, 2006). As with adults, children's grief is experienced in stages. Children's grief usually begins without understanding the full effects of the loss, and they experience some numbness or dulling of emotional pain. This stage progresses to a greater acceptance of the reality of the loss, which leads to more intense psychological pain. Finally, they undergo a reorganization of identity to incorporate the loved person, which may involve engaging in new activities and interests.

KEY CONCEPT

Personal fable is an aspect of egocentric thinking in adolescence, characterized by the belief that one is unique and invulnerable to harm. This belief often leads to risk-taking behaviours such as unprotected sex, fast driving, and substance abuse.

Death of a parent in childhood or adolescence is a risk factor for mental health problems, traumatic grief,

BOX 29.1 Research for Best Practice

PERCEPTIONS OF DEATH OF CHILDREN AGES 5 AND 6 YEARS

Yang, S., & Park, S. (2017). A sociocultural approach to children's perceptions of death and loss. Omega—Journal of Death and Dying, 76(1), 53–77.

Question: What is the cognitive understanding of and emotional responses to death and bereavement of children aged 5 and 6 years?

Method: A phenomenographic method, aimed at obtaining description, analysis, and understanding of the children's concept, impressions, and feelings about death was used. Participating in the study were 84 Korean, Chinese, and Chinese American boys and girls (average age 5.7 years). None had experienced the death of a parent or sibling; a few had experienced the death of a grandparent or a pet. They were given blank paper, crayons, coloured pens, and pencils and asked to draw "whatever the word death brought to mind" (p. 58). After they completed their drawing, they were asked to describe it, with individual children being asked further about emotions associated with the drawing. Analysis involved categorizing as to form (realistic, metaphorical, irrelevant) and a "reading" of the drawing, including details of the who, what, where, when, why, and how of the picture.

Findings: The core themes of the drawings were "causes for death," "attempts to stop the dying," and "situations after death" (p. 61). Those who had cognitively acquired the concept of causality attributed death to internal factors (age, illness); the majority attributed it to external factors, usually violent ones such as accidents (car accidents, disasters), crimes (murder, robbery, kidnapping), or wars (bombs, tanks). Two children mentioned suicide. Stopping the dying to make the person live again was a prevalent theme (e.g., "a thief killed the bakery shop lady and people wearing a mask are dragging her to the operating room to make her alive" [p. 64]). These children have not yet grasped the concept of the irreversibility of death. Situations after death were in three categories: discovery and descriptions of a corpse, funeral or grave visit, and ascension or afterlife. The children understood rituals (from direct or indirect experience) as commemorating the departure of the deceased. Only 6% drew the afterlife, but several described it (e.g., "when people die, they have a good time in heaven" [p. 68]). When asked if they knew anyone who had died, most answered that they had seen it on TV.

Implications: As they had limited experience with death and as death is not spoken about commonly in Korean and Chinese cultures, the children's medium for learning about death was primarily through audiovisual means such as TV dramas, games, movies, and animation. The researchers conclude that this shaped their perspectives on death as mostly negative and argue that age-appropriate death education for young children is important.

---

lower self-esteem, and difficulties in school performance. When the death is by suicide, the bereavement is particularly difficult with children fearing further abandonment. They may struggle with a sense of responsibility and guilt that they were somehow responsible. Such a death can "disenfranchise" a family from the community, causing isolation and a grief experience for a child significantly different from that experienced by a child whose parent died from natural causes (Schreiber, Sands, & Jordan, 2017). Adults have difficulty knowing how to respond to a bereaved child, especially when the death was by suicide. Good communication with the surviving parent and age-appropriate support, such as with a support group, can be protective factors for children coping with such loss (Schreiber et al., 2017). The book and DVD, *Red Chocolate Elephants,* developed by Dr. Diana Sands (2010), Director of the Bereaved by Suicide Service, Sydney, Australia, is a particularly helpful resource for children and caring adults.

Loss and Preschool-Aged Children

The preschool-aged child may react more to a parent's distress about a death than to the death itself. Young children who depend totally on their parents may be frightened when they see their parents upset. Anything the parent can do to alleviate children's anxiety, such as reassuring them that the parent will be okay while maintaining their normal routines (e.g., regular bedtimes, snacks, play times), will help the bereaved child to feel secure. Because preschool-aged children have limited ability to verbalize their feelings, they may need to express them through fantasy play and activities, such as mock funerals. Books that explain death, such as *Charlotte's Web* by E. B. White (1952), may also be helpful. Parents should take care not to use euphemisms that could fuel misconceptions of death, such as "He went to sleep" or "Jesus took him." Young children may interpret these messages literally and fear going to sleep (because they might die) or focus their natural, grief-related anger on the irrational idea that the person deliberately has not returned. The best approach is to explain honestly that the person has died and is not coming back, to elicit the child's understanding and questions about what has happened, and then to repeat this process continually as the child gradually begins to grasp the reality of the situation. The decision whether to take a small child to a funeral depends on factors such as the child's preference and availability of adult support; inclusiveness with the family, however, can be a positive element in coping with a death.

Loss and School-Aged Children

School-aged children understand the permanence of death more clearly than do preschoolers, but they may be unable to express their feelings, not unlike many adults. Children in this age group may express their grief through somatic complaints; finding comfort in behaviours engaged in during earlier developmental stages, also known as regression; behavioural reactions; withdrawal; and even hostility toward parents. They may think that others expect them to cry and react with immediate emotional intensity to the death; when they do not react this way, they may feel guilty.

Loss and Adolescents

Adolescents who are in Piaget's stage of formal operations can better understand death as an abstract concept. **Formal operations** are the period of cognitive development characterized by the ability to use abstract reasoning to conceptualize and solve problems. Because adolescents tend to be idealistic and to think in extremes, they may even have poetic or romantic notions about death. Some teenagers may become fascinated with morbid rock music, movies, and books. Although they may be able to express their thoughts and feelings about death more clearly than younger children, they often are reluctant to do so for fear of being viewed as childish. Some adolescents assume a parental role in the family after a death, denying their own needs. School settings may be particularly helpful in providing group and individual support for grieving adolescents, particularly as a preventive intervention (Van Epps, Oppie, & Goodwin, 1997).

Families

The diversity of Canadian families is a reflection of the people who comprise them. There are families consisting of mother and father, those in same-sex marriages, others living in common-law relationships, and those embracing co-parenting relationships. It is important for the nurse to clarify with the child/youth and care provider who the *family* of reference is, and any unique circumstances. There are also families where parents may not cohabitate but co-parent children together. For example, a separated or divorced couple may continue to cohabitate (with one partner sleeping in a separate bedroom or living in a basement suite, in order to provide parental consistency and/or financial support), while others continue to co-parent but live separately.

Separation and/or Divorce

Separation and/or divorce can be particularly stress inducing for families and children alike.

Separation

Separation of families occurs for many reasons: marital/partner discord, parental mental/physical illness, work circumstances, ill extended family, or immigration. Many Canadian couples live in a variety of complex situations to cope with financial, professional, and life circumstances. This can include "living apart together," that is, being in an intimate relationship with someone living in another dwelling. It is estimated that in 2011, about 1.9 million Canadians aged 20 years and over were in a "living apart together" relationship (Statistics Canada, 2011a). According to this national census, the reasons individuals gave for living apart were due to studying for school (26%) and financial circumstances (25%), primarily for those under age 30. Individuals aged 40 to 49 identified "work circumstances" (32%). Regardless of the reason, many couples are living separately yet *together*. As this becomes more common in our society, the impact on children and youth must be addressed for them to feel safe and secure regardless of the circumstances.

One agency that is much attuned to this phenomenon is the Canadian Armed Forces. There are many support resources available for families in which parents are deployed away from home (see Web Links). The developmental age of children in military families will need to be taken into consideration regarding their understanding of where and what the parent may experience or how they may be upon return from a military mission. The child may also need support if there are critical events publicized in the media.

Divorce

Divorce can be one of the most stressful life events for both children and parents. Predivorce disruption and conflict may contribute to the overall functioning of the child/youth, so that when the actual divorce or separation occurs, it may or may not be perceived as a negative event (Strohschein, 2012). During times of stress, the child's/youth's ability to cope is determined by factors of resilience and overall family/parental coping and support.

In Canada, married couples are still the predominant family structure, with an increase of 5.5% from 2006 to 2011 (Statistics Canada, 2011b). Married couples with children account for 43% of Canadian families and common-law couples with children 9% of families. Married-couple families accounted for 67.0% of all census families in 2011, down from 70.5% in 2001. The number of common-law families increased 13.9% in 2011. Stepfamilies consisted of 12.7% of couples with children. The number of lone-parent families rose from 15.7% to 16.3%. About 8 in 10 lone-parent families were female lone-parent families.

In Canada, there are approximately 70,000 divorces a year; more than 40% of marriages do not make it to their 30th year (Government of Canada, 2008). Although many families adapt to separation and divorce without long-term negative effects for the children, there are often temporary difficulties dealing with this significant family change. Parental separation and divorce create changes in the family structure, which can result in a substantial reduction in the contact that children have with one of their parents. The child's response to divorce can be similar to the response to death. In some ways, divorce may be harder for the child to understand because the noncustodial parent is gone but still alive, and the parents have made a conscious choice to separate.

Analysis of data from Canada's Longitudinal Survey of Children and Youth shows that children who grow up in a married biologic-parent household do not have better short-term behavioural outcomes than those who do not (Wu, Hou, & Schimmele, 2008). Rather, behavioural outcomes are related to such things as income, family dysfunction, and parental nurturance. The response to the loss that divorce imposes varies depending on the child's predivorce experience (Kelly, 2003); the child's temperament; the parents' interventions; and the level of stress, change, and conflict surrounding the divorce (Hetherington & Kelly, 2002). Major changes in socioeconomic status, such as moving from a dual-earner status to a single-parent family status, and changing place of residence may account for variation in levels of distress among divorcing families.

The first 2 or 3 years after the couple's breakup tend to be the most difficult. Typical childhood reactions include confusion, guilt, depression, regression, somatic symptoms, acting-out behaviours (e.g., stealing, disobedience), fantasies that the parents will reunite, fear of losing the custodial parent, and alignment with one parent against the other. After an initial adjustment period, children usually accept the reality of the situation and begin coping adaptively. If the divorced parents remarry new partners, this often imposes another period of coping difficulties for the children. Children with stepparents and stepsiblings are at renewed risk for emotional and behavioural problems as they struggle to cope with the new relationships.

Protective factors against emotional and behavioural problems in children of divorce include parental nurturance, parents' mental health, joint custody, and low parental conflict (Kelly, 2003). For children of divorce and remarriage, protective factors also include a structured home and school environment with reasonable and consistent limit setting and a warm and support-

ive relationship with stepparents (Hetherington & Kelly, 2002). Helpful interventions for children of divorce include education regarding children's reactions; promotion of regular and predictable visitation; reduction of conflict between the parents through counselling, mediation, and clear visitation policies; continuance of usual routines; and family counselling to facilitate adjustment after remarriage (Table 29.2). It may not be the divorce itself but rather the continuing conflict between the parents that is most damaging to the child. Conflict and discord affects parenting skills (Chang & Kier, 2016); parents need to remember that children identify with both parents and need to view both positively. Therefore, it is helpful for parents to reinforce each other's good qualities and focus on evidence of their former partner's love and respect for the child.

Sibling Relationships

The family often consists of various constellations of parents, children, and others. The family is whoever they define themselves to be. Within many families, siblings are an integral part of that constellation. Some parents prefer not to have the siblings present if they have brought one child in for a mental health assessment. It is important for the nurse to encourage the parents/care providers to include the siblings in the process, as they often add information of which the parents may be unaware. Nurses also need to be aware of siblings who may also be mentally unwell or experiencing distress due to an unwell sibling or parent. Wright and Leahey (2013) encourage nurses to consider the sibling "rank order—the position of children in the family in respect to age and gender" (p. 60). Depending on parental functioning (e.g., mental or physical illness), or cultural and ethnic background, sibling position may have a positive or negative effect on children's functioning. For example, older children may be put in the position of care provider if both parents work outside the home. This may create added stress with respect to their ability to manage sibling care, domestic chores, and school work (or employment in the case of an adolescent).

The role of siblings in a child's development tends to be underemphasized, but there are several theoretical perspectives regarding relational development between siblings. Whiteman, McHale, and Soli (2011) present four perspectives within sibling research literature: psychoanalytic–evolutionary, social psychological, social learning, family–ecologic systems. No one theory is emphasized; however, because families function as a system and within the context of relationships, it would stand to reason that sibling relationships would be multidimensional and affected by numerous variables based on the context of their development. A growing body of research shows that sibling relationships significantly influence personality development. Positive sibling relationships can be protective factors against the development of psychopathology, particularly in troubled

Table 29.2   Play Therapy With a 4-Year-Old Child Whose Parents Are Divorcing

Child Statement	Nurse Response	Analysis and Rationale
(The child smashes two cars together and makes loud, crashing sound.)	That's a loud crash. They really hit hard.	The child may be expressing anger and frustration nonverbally through play. The nurse attempts to establish rapport with the child by relating at the child's level, using age-appropriate vocabulary.
Crrrash!	I know a boy who gets so mad sometimes that he feels like smashing something.	The child is engrossed in fantasy play, typical of preschoolers. Children often use toys as symbols of human figures. The nurse uses an indirect method of eliciting the child's feelings, because preschoolers often do not express feelings directly. Reference to another child's anger helps to normalize this child's feelings.
Yeah!	Sounds like you feel angry too sometimes … the same way the other boy feels.	The child is beginning to relate to the nurse and senses her empathy. The nurse reflects the child's feelings to facilitate further communication.
Yeah, when my mom and dad fight.	It's tough to listen to parents fighting. Sometimes, it's scary. You wonder what's going to happen.	The child is experiencing frustration and helplessness related to family conflict. The nurse expresses empathy and attempts to articulate the child's feelings, because preschool children have a limited ability to identify and label feelings.
My mom and dad are getting a divorce.	That's too bad. Children often feel mixed up when their parents get divorced. What's going to happen when they get the divorce?	The child has a basic awareness of the reality of the parents' divorce but may not understand this concept. The nurse expresses empathy and attempts to assess the child's level of understanding of the divorce.
Dad's not going to live in our house.	Oh, I guess you'll miss having him there all the time. It would be nice if you all could live together, but I guess that's not going to happen.	The preschool child focuses on the effects the divorce will have on him (egocentrism). The child seems to have a clear understanding of the consequences of the divorce. The nurse articulates the child's perspective and reinforces the reality of the divorce to avoid fuelling the child's possible denial and reconciliation fantasies.
(Silently moves cars across the floor.)	What do you think is the reason your parents decided to get a divorce?	The child expresses sadness nonverbally. The nurse further attempts to assess the child's understanding of the circumstances surrounding the divorce.
Because I did it.	What do you mean—you did it? How?	The child provides a clue that he may be feeling responsible. The nurse uses clarification to fully assess the child's understanding.
I made them mad because I left my bike in the driveway and Dad ran over it.	Do you think that's why they're getting the divorce?	The child uses egocentric thinking to draw a conclusion that his actions caused the divorce. The nurse continues to clarify the child's thinking. The goal is to elicit the child's perceptions so that misperceptions can be corrected.
Yeah, they had a big fight.	They may have been upset about the bike, but I don't think that's why they're getting a divorce.	The nurse goes on to explain why parents get divorced and to provide opportunities for the child to ask questions.
Why?	Because parents get divorced when they're upset with *each other*—when they can't get along—not when they're upset with their children.	

families in which the parents are emotionally unavailable. A Canadian longitudinal study revealed that sibling affection moderated the effects of stressful life events on "internalized symptomatology" (e.g., being anxious, depressive, overcontrolled) (Gass, Jenkis, & Dunn, 2007).

Nurses working with families need to pay attention not only to the parent–child dynamic but also to the sibling dynamic with regard to whether positive or negative behaviours are being modelled. "Children learn social competencies in their interactions with parents and siblings and by observing their family members' interactions with others" (Whiteman et al., 2011,

p. 9). Parents should be supported in modelling effective problem-solving and engage with their children in the same process to minimize sibling rivalry and maximize cooperative behaviour benefiting their children's social and emotional development throughout life. Sibling rivalry can begin with the birth of the second child. It is a natural experience, and some sibling rivalry is inevitable. The birth of a sibling can be a surprise for the first child who, up until then, was the sole focus of the parents' attention. The older sibling may react with anger and reveal not-so-subtle fantasies of getting rid of the new sibling (e.g., "I dreamed that the new baby died"). Parents should pay attention to these comments and observe behaviours while also recognizing that these reactions are natural. The child should be allowed to express feelings, both positive and negative, about the baby while being reassured of his or her special place in the family. Allowing the older child opportunities to care for the baby and reinforcing any nurturing or affectionate behaviour will promote positive bonding.

Physical Illness

Many children experience a major physical illness or injury at some point during their development. The experience of hospitalization and intrusive medical procedures can have a lasting and possibly acutely traumatic impact on many children. The likelihood of lasting psychological problems resulting from physical illness depends on the child's experiences during hospitalization; the child's developmental level and coping mechanisms; the family's level of functioning before, during, and after the illness; and the nature and severity of the illness. As with any major stressor, the perception of the event (i.e., meaning of the illness) will influence the family's ability to cope. Mental health effects from being physically compromised can begin at birth. For instance, extremely preterm children (born at 23 to 25 weeks' gestation), with or without neurodevelopmental disabilities, have been found to be at risk for anxiety and attention, social, and thought problems (Samuelsson et al., 2017). Common childhood reactions to physical illness include developmental regression (e.g., in toilet training, social maturity, autonomous behaviour), sleep and feeding difficulties, behavioural reactions (e.g., negativism, tantrums, withdrawal), somatic complaints that mask attempts at emotional expression (e.g., headaches, stomachaches), and depression. Infants and children younger than school age are particularly vulnerable to separation anxiety during illness and may regress to earlier levels of anxiety about strangers, becoming fearful of health care providers. Young children often have magical thinking about the illness, and their tendency to process information in concrete terms may lead to misperceptions about the illness and treatment procedures (e.g., dye = die; stretcher = stretch her) (Deering & Cody, 2002). Adolescents may be concerned about their body image and maintaining their sense of independence and control.

Nurses must remember that parents are the primary resource to the child and the experts who know the child's needs and reactions. Thus, nurses must maintain a collaborative approach in working with parents of both physically and mentally ill children. If the child is a sick infant, nurses should take care to allow the normal attachment process between parents and the infant to unfold, despite the health care professionals' efforts to assume some parenting functions. Parents who view their children as physically and emotionally fragile will feel disempowered in decision-making and boundary setting and may develop helpless or overprotective styles of dealing with their children.

Many parents react with fear and anxiety that can lead to feelings of guilt about their child's illness or injury, especially if the illness is genetically based or partially the result of their own behaviour (e.g., drug or alcohol abuse during pregnancy). Parents may project their feelings onto each other or onto health care professionals, lashing out in anger and blame. Nurses should view these responses as part of the grieving process and help parents to move forward confidently in caring for their children. Teaching parents how to care for their children's health needs and reinforcing their successes in doing so will help. For example, rather than reacting to what may appear to be an abdication of parenting responsibilities, nurses can instead use empathy to acknowledge the parent's feelings and discuss ways to help the parent regain a sense of control with comments such as the following:

> It's pretty confusing to know how best to respond to your child's behaviour. Before receiving her diagnosis, you felt comfortable setting reasonable limits on her behaviour, but now that seems to have changed. Sometimes parents feel reluctant and are even afraid of setting limits because they know how sick their child is.... It may seem odd, but children actually feel safer and more secure when their parents let them know what the boundaries for their behaviour are.... Let's talk about some of the boundaries that you might feel most comfortable setting up for Sophie to help her feel safe and secure while she is so ill?

Chronic physical illness in childhood presents a unique set of challenges, with survival rates of previously fatal diseases at an all-time high (Martinez & Ercikan, 2009). Although studies show that most children with chronic illnesses and their families are remarkably resilient and adjust to the stressors and regimens involved in their care (LeBlanc, Goldsmith, & Patel, 2003), research shows that children with chronic health conditions are at higher risk for developing anxiety-related disorders, academic problems, and learning disabilities (Martinez & Ercikan, 2009). Conditions that affect the central nervous system (CNS) (e.g., infections, metabolic diseases, CNS malformations, brain and spinal cord trauma) are particularly likely to result in psychiatric difficulties. Nurses who understand pathophysiologic processes are in a unique position to assess the interaction between biologic and psychological factors that contribute to mental health problems in chronically ill children (e.g., lethargy from high blood sugar levels or respiratory problems; mood swings from steroid use). Inactivity and a lack of sensory stimulation from hospitalization or bed rest may contribute to neurologic deficits and developmental delays.

The major challenge for a chronically ill child is to remain active despite the limitations of the illness and to become fully integrated into school and social activities. Children who view themselves as different or defective will experience low self-esteem and be more at risk for depression, anxiety, and behaviour problems. Studies show that parental perceptions of the child's vulnerability predict greater adjustment problems, even after controlling for age and disease severity (Anthony, Gil, & Schanberg, 2003). Educating parents about these facts and helping them to foster maximum independence within the limitations of the child's health problem is the key. For example, nurses might comment,

> Having kidney disease is no fun … and it must make you want to protect your son as much as possible. But too much protection will be a different sort of harm. Noah might feel he does not have possibilities in life like other children. We know he does. Even with all the limitations, what are the best things your son has going for him?

Physical and Developmental Challenges in Adolescence

Adolescence is a time of growing independence and, consequently, experimentation. Emotional extremes prevail. To adolescents, the world seems great one day and terrible the next; people are either for them or against them. Adolescents are struggling to consolidate their abilities to control their impulses and react to the many "crises" that may seem trivial to adults but are very important to teens. Biologic changes (e.g., the onset of puberty, height and weight changes, hormonal changes), psychological changes (e.g., increased ability for abstract thinking), and social changes (e.g., dating, driving, increased autonomy) are all significant. The primary developmental task of identity formation leads teenagers to test different roles and struggle to define who they are. This process may include testing various peer groups to find one that fits their unfolding self-image (see Box 29.2).

In addition to the typical challenges associated with adolescence regarding sexuality and gender development, adolescents who identify as lesbian, gay, bisexual, transgender, and queer or questioning, generally referred to as LGBTQ+ youth, face additional challenges of stigma, exclusion, and anxiety in finding suitable partners as a sexual minority. They are overrepresented in the homeless youth population as they may have left home to avoid conflict with their families. They experience violence at a higher rate than do their heterosexual

---

BOX 29.2 Research for Best Practice

THE MEANING OF VIDEO GAMES IN ADOLESCENT LIVES

Forsyth, S. R., Chesla, C. A., Rehm, R. S., & Malone, R. E. (2017). "It feels more real": An interpretive phenomenological study of the meaning of video games in adolescent lives. Advances in Nursing Science, 40(4), E1–E17.

Question: What are the effects of video gaming on adolescent identity formation?

Method: In this interpretive phenomenologic study (used in seeking deep understanding of everyday experiences), the researchers interviewed 20 adolescents (13 to 21 years; mean age = 17.7 years) in an American metropolitan location, who gamed for at least 2 hours on most days during the past year. These participants were asked to describe their experiences with school, friends, and family, favorite video games, and instances of play that stood out and "to reflect on what gaming meant to them" (p. 4).

Findings: Gaming offers a virtual social arena to adolescents that allows them to develop and test potential identities. A player can be transported and immersed in a game world where they can take risks, try out new social skills, and take on a new self (including gender).

Character creation appears to be part of the gaming experience, with one's avatar taking on an aspirational identity (i.e., better looking, stronger, good, a leader) or a shadow self ("I kind of look like a demon"; "I am in training to become a Sith"). Some participants described trying in real life to be more like their avatar (e.g., an extremely shy gamer created a more outspoken, joking avatar and eventually used the social skills developed to make friends). Girls sometimes played as a male; boys rarely tried on being female. Gaming provided a sense of freedom, control, competence, and confidence while real life was seen as constricted by schedules, rules, and expectations. Forms of interaction are limited in popular video games as violence tends to be a staple of play. Players stating that they disliked the violence accepted it as part of gaming.

Implications: Adolescents can use video games to develop virtual selves in tension with their real selves as they safely try on new ways of being and acting. Understanding of the role of popular gaming in the lives of adolescents is important for nurses who are helping adolescents meet their developmental challenges.

peers. As a result of these challenges, LGBTQ+ youth may experience higher rates of mental health issues such as problematic substance use, anxiety, depression, and suicidal ideation and attempts (Schwartz, Waddell, Andres, Yung, & Gray-Grant, 2017). Positive supportive environments are essential to mental health promotion for all children and youth; however, the mental health needs of LGBTQ+ youth can differ significantly from their heterosexual peers; addressing their mental health needs must also be understood within the context of the youth's gender, ethnic, cultural, and religious identities. Unfortunately, significant gaps remain regarding evidence-based models for promoting mental health and reducing mental health problems within this sexual minority group (Russell & Fish, 2016).

Adolescence often is a time of exploring social and personal boundaries. This can involve experimentation, which can increase the risk of poor physical health, mental health problems, substance use including tobacco, high-risk behaviours including driving at excessive speeds, high-intensity sports, and exploration of sexuality that may lead to unsafe sexual behaviours and psychological distress. According to the Sexual Information and Education Council of Canada, the overall Canadian teen pregnancy rate decreased by 20.3% from 2001 to 2010 (McKay, 2013). However, from 2006 to 2010, the national teen pregnancy rate increased by 1.1%; and in four provinces, the rate increased by 15.1% or more (New Brunswick, Newfoundland, Nova Scotia, Manitoba). Trends in teen pregnancy reflect sexual and reproductive health and overall well-being of young women in Canada, which is important for educators, policy makers, and especially nurses to pay attention to, as nurses are often the first contact many young women have in relation to their pregnancy.

Nurses will also be in the position to provide assessments, education, and, in some circumstances, intervention in relation to sexually transmitted infections (STIs). According to the Public Health Agency of Canada (2010b), the most common infections are chlamydia (15- to 24-year-old women, slightly older for young men); gonorrhoea (same age groups); infectious syphilis (older HIV-positive men and sex trade workers); human papillomavirus, which is more common at 70% of adult population (true numbers unknown); genital herpes (HSV1 and HSV2) (exact numbers unknown); and HIV (exact numbers unknown).

Among youth in later adolescence, approximately one in five reports symptoms associated with a major mental disorder and nearly 1 in 10 reports substance dependence (Centre for Addiction and Mental Health, 2012). Although most youths eventually become more conventional in their behaviour, some develop harmful behaviour patterns and addictions that endanger their mental and physical health. Adolescents whose psychiatric problems are developing are particularly vulnerable

to engaging in risky behaviours because they may have limited coping skills, may attempt to self-medicate their symptoms, and may feel an increased pressure to fit in with other teens. Moreover, high-risk behaviours tend to be interrelated (Eggert, Thompson, Randell, & Pike, 2002).

Adolescence is also a time when youth begin experimenting with drugs such as cannabis—one of the most commonly used illicit drugs worldwide. The Canadian Paediatric Association has expressed grave concern regarding the legalization of cannabis in Canada. Scientific research conducted over the past 15 years has demonstrated that cannabis use during adolescence can cause functional and structural changes to the developing brain. Cannabis use has been associated with cannabis use disorder, cannabis withdrawal syndrome, depression and anxiety, and psychotic disorders and schizophrenia (accumulating evidence is pointing toward a causal relationship with heavy use) and can impact school performance and cognitive decline (Grant & Bélanger, 2017).

Enhanced life skills and supportive school and family environments can mediate the effect of stressful life events (Burns, Andrews, & Szabo, 2002). Programs that enhance the school environment are associated with improved behaviour and well-being. Interventions that teach cognitive skills are associated with a reduction in one of the most prevalent mental health problems affecting adolescents—depression (Korczak, 2012; Puskar, Sereika, & Tusaie-Mumford, 2003). Current evidence suggests that for an intervention to be sustainable, it must encompass multiple components across several levels, including the classroom, curriculum, whole school, and school–community boundaries. Several approaches to mental health promotion with adolescents are recommended. First, intervening at the peer group level through educational programs, alternative recreational activities, and peer counselling is most successful. Adolescents are skeptical of authority figures and tend to take cues from one another. Nurses working with teenagers find it helpful to use a discussion approach that encourages questioning and argument, as opposed to talking down to them or "talking at" them.

Second, training in values clarification, decision-making, problem-solving, social skills, and assertiveness helps give adolescents the skills to cope with situations in which they are pressured by their peers (Botvin, 2000). Social psychological research shows that if just one person can find the strength to express an unpopular viewpoint in a group and decline to participate in a destructive activity, others will quickly follow. It takes enormous courage, as well as concrete knowledge and practice with assertiveness, to speak up in these situations.

A third type of intervention is a program that uses team efforts by teachers, parents, community leaders, and teen role models. These programs help at-risk youth by building self-esteem, setting positive examples, and working to involve the youth in community activities. It is important to note that teaching interpersonal skills, including cognitive and problem-solving skills, should be coupled with the promotion of positive school and family environments to prevent mental health problems in young people, notably depression (Burns et al., 2002).

It is also important to consider the use of social media and other digital forms of communication by which to reach adolescents. Program staff and youth perceive these forms of communication as credible and essential methods of communication in the context of public health programs. Public health interventions must continue to evolve and integrate new technologies in order to reach young people (Vyas, Landry, Schnider, Rojas, & Wood, 2012).

Approaches that have not proved effective include more education and information about dangerous activities without the supplemental behaviour training, as well as programs that provide inadequate training and support for the professionals implementing them.

DEVELOPMENT OF CHILD PSYCHOPATHOLOGY

The factors that affect the development of child psychopathology are also the factors that protect children. The issues presented are not independent components but are intertwined and interdependent, thus indicating that the care provided must be collaborative, holistic, and socially and culturally relevant to those involved. Creating a structure to describe the context in which child psychopathology develops is difficult, and one must remember that this is not a black and white process but that all aspects are systemically interwoven and affect the whole.

Protective Factors

Protective factors are attributes or conditions in individuals, families, communities, and society that allow stress and stressful occurrences to be addressed in more effective ways, risk to be mitigated, and harm to be diminished. Identified for several decades, they focus on children and adolescents' ability to develop self-confidence, positive relationships, competencies (skills/strengths), self-regulation, and community involvement (Blaustein & Kinniburgh, 2010; Brendtro, 2004; Canadian Council on Learning, 2008; Eriksson, Cater, Andershed, & Andershed, 2010; Foster, O'Brien, & Korhonen, 2012; Unger, 2013; Waddell, McEwan, Sheperd, Offord, & Hua, 2005; Zolkoski & Bullock, 2012). In the family, low stress, stable employment, adequate child care resources, and higher socioeconomic status can serve as protective factors. In the community, protective factors include positive and cohesive families, schools, and neighbourhoods. All of the protective factors intertwine to create a context in which the child/youth thrives. The research on resilience provides insight and direction to focus attention and care when working with children/youth and families (Eriksson et al., 2010).

Protective factors identified include the following:

- Individual attributes, such as problem-solving skills, sense of self-efficacy, accurate processing of interpersonal cues, positive social orientation, and self-regulation
- A supportive family environment, including attachment with adults in the family, low family conflict, and supportive relationships
- Environmental supports, including those that reinforce and support coping efforts and recognize and reward competence

Resilience

Nurses will work with a variety of children and youth and their families throughout their careers, but the majority will not have psychopathology. Many however will have experienced life circumstances that often lead to severe consequences, yet they function at or above what would be expected. These individuals have what is referred to as resilience. **Resilience** is the ability to overcome or rise above adversity, learn from the experience, and apply strategies and cope with other life events even when the situation dictates otherwise. Resilience refers to achieving positive outcomes despite challenging or threatening circumstances, coping successfully with traumatic experiences, and avoiding negative paths linked with risks (Zolkoski & Bullock, 2012). Resilience is commonly conceived as a state, depending on environmental and familial factors. "In the context of exposure to significant adversity, resilience is both the capacity of individuals to navigate their way to the psychological, social, cultural, and physical resources that sustain their wellbeing, and their capacity individually and collectively to negotiate for these resources to be provided in culturally meaningful ways" (Unger, 2013, p. 1). Therefore, resilience is not limited to the individual but can apply to a group, or to society's ability to move beyond negative circumstances.

Risk Factors

A **risk factor** is genetic, environmental, behavioural, or other influence that increases the probability of a disease, disorder, or trauma happening. Risk factors inhibit resilience while protective factors promote it. The number of stresses that children experience, the supports that they have in place, and their developmental stage influence their ability to cope with stressors.

Biologic and environmental risk factors include congenital defects, low birth weights, poverty, education level of parents, negative life experiences such as abuse or neglect, minority status, and racial discrimination (Clinton et al., 2016; Zolkoski & Bullock, 2012).

Impact of Social Determinants of Health

The World Health Organization (see, e.g., Currie et al., 2011) has brought attention to the broad social factors that influence the health and well-being of children. The health of young people and their families is generally determined less by lifestyle choices or application of medical knowledge than by the complex interaction of living conditions that often transcend the capacities of the individual, such as income and distribution of wealth; employment and working conditions; quality of food and housing and of health care and other social services; and equitable access to education. In short, communities and institutions, and economic and social circumstances, shape much of a child's development, pose as greater risk factors in his or her well-being, and have health impacts with short- and long-term implications for individuals and society.

Poverty

According to the United Nations Children's Fund (2012), an estimated 14% of children in Canada live in poverty, a rate higher than that of the general population (12%). The low-income rates for children vary significantly according to their type of family. For instance, in 2008, 6.5% of children in two-parent families were in a low-income environment, while almost one in four children (23.4%) in female lone-parent families faced this reality. Children in certain populations can be more at risk of low income. For example, it is known that in 2005, recent immigrant families had a low-income rate of 39.3% (Canada Parliament, 2010). Children/youth and families living in poverty are at increased risk of exposure to additional factors that will contribute to childhood psychopathology.

The effects of poverty on child development and family functioning are numerous and pervasive. The obstacles to overcoming the effects of poverty can seem insurmountable to young people. Lack of proper nutrition and lack of access to prenatal and mother–infant care can place children from impoverished families at risk for physical and mental health problems. Children from impoverished rural areas often lack access to educational and other community support resources. Children living in poverty-stricken inner-city neighbourhoods are vulnerable to violent crimes, crowded living conditions, and an increased access to drugs (Leventhal & Brooks-Gunn, 2000). Although crime, drug abuse, gang activity, and teenage pregnancy are seen in adolescents from all socioeconomic backgrounds, children living in poverty are more vulnerable to these problems because they may have limited opportunities for change (Kelly & Caputo, 2007).

A major focus of preventive nursing interventions for disadvantaged families involves simply forming a relationship that conveys respect and willingness to work as an advocate to assist clients' seeking out and accessing resources. In terms of Maslow's need hierarchy, families living in poverty may be more focused on survival needs (e.g., food, shelter) than on self-actualization needs (e.g., insight-oriented psychotherapy for themselves or their children). Unless the nurse can work as a partner with the family and address the issues most pressing for the family with an active problem-solving approach, other types of intervention may be fruitless. At the same time, it is inappropriate to assume that poor families will be resistant to or unable to benefit from psychotherapies or other mental health interventions.

Homelessness

Homelessness is a very complex phenomenon that reveals the failure of a society to ensure that systems and support are in place so that everyone has access to housing (Gaetz, Donaldson, Richter, & Gulliver, 2013). Persons who are homeless make up a heterogeneous population that includes women, children, youth, families, new immigrants, people with mental illness, ethnic minorities, and Indigenous peoples. The number of children staying in shelters in Canada increased by over 50% between 2005 (6,205) and 2009 (9,459) (Segaert, 2012). A national study found that, in 2009, an estimated 29,964 youth (ages 16 to 24 years) and 9,459 children (under the age of 16 years) stayed in emergency shelters across the country (Employment and Social Development Canada, 2012). Youth homelessness refers to youth who are homeless, at risk of homelessness, or caught in a cycle of homelessness for whatever reason. This includes the many homeless youth (some say as high as 80%) who don't live on the street and who are among the hidden homeless, living in temporary shelters or unsafe or crowded conditions (Hulchanski, Campsie, Chau, Hwang, & Paradis, 2009). Youth may cite parental drug and alcohol use as a reason for leaving home, as it is often associated with parental abandonment, family violence (sexual, physical, and psychological abuse), and neglect. Particularly, at-risk populations for becoming homeless or street involved are youth in foster care and lesbian, gay, bisexual, and transgender youth (Edidin, Ganim, Hunter, & Karnik, 2012).

There is an increased risk for physical health problems (e.g., nutritional deficiencies, infections, chronic illnesses, injuries as a result of violence, STIs), mental health problems (particularly **developmental delays** in language, fine or gross motor coordination, and social development; depression, anxiety, posttraumatic stress disorder, and psychotic symptoms; disruptive behaviour disorders; substance abuse), and educational underachievement in homeless youth. Many homeless youth have been physically or sexually abused, leading to elevated rates of externalizing disorders for boys and internalizing disorders for girls (Cauce et al., 2000).

Though a heterogeneous population, youth living on the street have typically experienced extreme stress in the course of their lives even before they ran away, with most fleeing temporary living arrangements (e.g., foster homes, friends, relatives) (Kelly & Caputo, 2007). Their runaway experience thus serves only to compound an already chronic history of trauma and disruption. The key is to prevent the conditions that preceded the runaway behaviour.

Unfortunately, responses to homelessness too often result only in greater social control measures (e.g., rendering panhandling illegal, excluding the homeless from the community) rather than the development of strategies to address underlying causes. Street nurses are often one of the few resources available to marginalized populations who face a variety of barriers to accessing traditional health care services. Not only do they experience mental health problems and criminal involvement, they lack knowledge of specialized providers, transportation to said providers, and the ability to pay for prescriptions, worse yet, they also encounter provider discrimination (Self & Peters, 2005). Street services are effective because they are delivered wherever the person feels comfortable: a school, youth centre, drop-in centre, mall, or simply the street.

The living conditions of many shelters place children at risk for irregular patterns of sleep, feeding, play, and bathing, all of which are important for normal development. Nurses working with homeless youth and families need to be aware of the effects of this lifestyle on children, because they have a limited ability to speak for themselves and because their needs are often overlooked. Transition services for women and children who are victims of abuse are available across the country; however, depending on the community and the ability of the women to access these resources, support may be limited. Nurturing one's children while living in homeless shelters is highly challenging.

While there is no evidence that Canada's efforts to date to reduce homelessness have had an overall positive effect, there are reasons to be optimistic. Meaningful collaboration at the national, provincial, municipal, and community levels to address this major social problem is occurring (e.g., Homeless Partnering Strategy; Housing First) (see Chapter 2).

Child Abuse and Neglect

Childhood abuse/neglect and maltreatment affects the overall growth and development of the individual and impacts health and well-being, even when the individual is resilient (Blaustein & Kinniburgh, 2010). One in three Canadians state that they experienced abuse before the age of 15 years (Public Health Agency of Canada, 2016). There are some characteristics associated with childhood abuse: male, Aboriginal identity, and having been under legal responsibility of the government at some time in childhood (Hango, 2017). A parent is the main perpetrator of physical abuse of children in Canada (Hango, 2017). Children and youth are far more likely to be victims of sexual offences than are adults, with police-reported rates five times higher than among adults (207 victims per 100,000 vs. 41 victims per 100,000). This was true for all types of sexual assaults, as well as other sexual offences. Rates of family violence toward girls were 56% higher, and they were four times as likely to be sexually assaulted (Sinha, 2011). Table 29.3 lists types and rates of abuse of children in Canada.

Childhood adversities, such as neglect and emotional, physical, and sexual abuse, have significant and long-term negative effects on the health and well-being of a child or adolescent. Physical abuse is associated with lower levels of social integration, trust, and physical and mental health among young adults. Such adverse experiences are a major predictor of troubled sleep in adulthood (Baiden, Fallon, den Dunnen, & Boateng, 2015); a risk factor for diabetes (Shields et al., 2016); a risk factor for a higher probability, as an adult, of not being involved in education, training, or employment in the past year and for being victimized (Hango, 2017); and, as the number of adversities multiply, a risk factor for becoming a serious, violent, and chronic juvenile offender (Fox, Perez, Cass, Baglivio, & Epps, 2015). Severe physical abuse can cause health conditions that continue in adulthood to limit, at least at times, daily living activities (Statistics Canada, 2017).

All types of child abuse exposure have been found to be associated with increased odds of suicidal ideation, plans, and attempts (Afifi et al., 2016). Adults with mental illness are more likely than not to have a trauma history of abuse and/or neglect—upward of 95% (McKenna, 2007). A Canadian study of child abuse exposure in the Canadian Armed Forces compared to the general population (Alfifi et al., 2016) found that individuals with a history of child abuse were more likely to join the military; additive effects for past year suicide ideation and plans were noted between deployment-related trauma and child abuse exposure. The importance of recognizing the impact of trauma in children and families and the subsequent long-term effects is well established. A foundational study, the Adverse Childhood Experiences study (Feletti et al., 1998), has demonstrated that abusive and traumatic events in childhood are associated with depression, cardiovascular disease, cancer, alcoholism, and substance misuse and abuse in adulthood, as well as encounters with the criminal justice system, and risk-taking behaviours in adolescence and adulthood. Prevention, early detection, and intervention in the maltreatment of children are warranted.

Table 29.3	Types and Rates of Abuse in Canada	
Type	Description	Rate
Neglect	Is often chronic and usually involves repeated incidents of failing to provide what a child needs for his or her physical, psychological, or emotional development and well-being	4.81 confirmed cases per 1,000 children
Physical abuse	May consist of just one incident or happen repeatedly. It involves deliberately using force against a child in such a way that the child either is injured or is at risk for being injured. Injuries may include bruises, lacerations, burns, and fractures caused by another person or object (e.g., belt, cords, cigarette). *Note:* Many injuries do not represent child abuse; therefore, when abuse is suspected, bruising must be assessed in the context of medical, social, and developmental histories; the explanation given; and the patterns of nonabusive bruising (Maguire, Mann, Sibert, & Kemp, 2005)	2.86 confirmed cases per 1,000 children
Emotional abuse	Involves harming a child's sense of self. It includes acts (or omissions) that result in, or place a child at risk for, serious behavioural, cognitive, emotional, or mental health problems.	1.23 confirmed cases per 1,000 children
Sexual abuse and exploitation	Involves using a child for sexual purposes, resulting in physical wounds such as bruises or bleeding of the genitals or rectum, STIs, sore throat, enuresis/encopresis, pregnancy, and foreign objects in the vagina or rectum. The child may also display sophisticated knowledge/behaviour/ preoccupation with sexual activities, withdrawal, hypervigilance, or sleep difficulties.	0.43 confirmed cases per 1,000 children

From Public Health Agency of Canada. (2010a). *Canadian Incidence Study of reported child abuse and neglect—2008: Major findings.* Ottawa, ON: Author.

Children in Care

The adjustment to an out-of-home placement can be viewed through the conceptual framework of Bowlby's stages of coping with parental separation. According to Bowlby (1960), the child initially responds to separation from parents with protest (crying, kicking, screaming, pleading, and attempting to elicit the parent's return). The child then moves to a state of despair (listlessness, apathy, and withdrawal, which lead to some acceptance of caregiving by others, but with reluctance to reattach fully). Finally, the child experiences detachment if the child and the new parent cannot manage to form an emotional bond. Because children often experience multiple placements, the potential for a disrupted attachment may be great by the time the child faces the prospect of a permanent family. After repeatedly undergoing separation and mourning, the child learns that rejection is inevitable and may automatically maintain distance from a new caregiver.

The trauma elicited, not only from the reason for children's placement but from their being exposed to multiple placements, can include detachment, diffuse rage, chronic depression, low self-esteem, and emotional dependency or insatiable need for nurturing and support. Sometimes, these symptoms develop into attachment disorders that can be challenging to treat (O'Connor, Bredenkamp, & Rutter, 1999) (see Box 29.3). It takes knowledgeable, committed, and resilient care providers to work with a child who is challenged by these significant emotional and behavioural problems and struggles to reciprocate caring.

It is estimated that, in 2007, there were 67,000 children in out-of-home care across Canada (Mulcahy & Trocmé, 2010). The difficulty with identifying and tracking the numbers of children in care is that child welfare services fall under the jurisdiction of provincial and territorial authorities. The various provincial legislation directives make it difficult to compare rates of children in out-of-home care across provinces.

The National Household Survey indicates that, of the approximately 30,000 children in care in Canada in 2011, 14,225 were Aboriginal. Overall, 4% of Aboriginal (First Nations, Métis, and Inuit) children were in care, compared with 0.3% of non-Aboriginal children, or 15,345 children (Statistics Canada, 2011b). The overrepresentation of Aboriginal children in care is of significant concern; however, research-based explanations for its occurrence are lacking (Fluke, Chabot, Fallon, MacLaurin, & Blackstock, 2010). There are several studies from the United States, Australia, and Canada that imply worker ethnicity, education, gender, political ideology, worker age, and agency policies play a role, yet there is limited information to this effect. Overall, Aboriginal children "receive less funding per child for federal child welfare services, and families living on reserve have been found to receive minor support from the voluntary sector" (Fluke et al., 2010, p. 67). Intergenerational trauma and the legacy of the residential school system continue to have an impact on the lives of Indigenous Canadians. The inherent "social, economic, and cultural risk factors" (Fluke et al., 2010, p. 67) need to be addressed by community leaders, in collaboration with governments and health care providers.

BOX 29.3 CLINICAL VIGNETTE

PREVENTIVE INTERVENTIONS WITH AN ADOLESCENT IN CRISIS

- Having been removed from their mother's care when she relapsed on cocaine and left them unattended, Aiden and Jenna have now been transferred to a second foster home. The plan is for the two children to return to their mother's home after she completes a 30-day drug treatment program. Aiden, who is in the 10th grade, is in the school nurse's office asking for aspirin for another headache.

- The nurse notices that Aiden's nose looks inflamed, he is sniffling, and he seems more "hyper" than usual. In a concerned tone of voice, she asks him if he has been using cocaine. "Just because my mother's a cokehead," he snaps, "doesn't give you the right to suspect me!" When the nurse gently says, "I'm sorry, I had no idea. Would you like to tell me about what's been happening with your mother?" Aiden responds less defensively and explains the situation about the foster home and his mother's drug problem. He says that if it were not for Jenna, his younger sister, he would have run away by now. His foster parents are "making him" go to school, but he is going to drop out as soon as he returns to live with his mother. The only thing he likes about school is playing basketball; the basketball coach, who is his gym teacher, wants him on the team.

- After a lengthy talk with Aiden, the nurse finishes the assessment interview and concludes that he is at risk for drug abuse, running away, and dropping out of school. He is also showing symptoms of depression, which he may be attempting to medicate with cocaine. Protective factors for Aiden include his strong attachment to his sister, his ability and willingness to express his thoughts and feelings, his interest in basketball, and a positive relationship with the basketball coach.

- The nurse discusses with Aiden what to do next. Using motivational interviewing strategies over several weeks, the nurse develops a plan with Aiden to attend the school's weekly drug and alcohol discussion group, so that he can talk with other teens from substance-abusing families and learn coping skills to prevent addiction. The nurse contacts the basketball coach, who agrees to find a student mentor who can shoot hoops with Aiden and help him come up with a plan to stay in school, maybe find a part-time job, and join the basketball team. Aiden agrees to check in regularly with the nurse to report how the plan is working, and they can revise it if needed. The nurse feels optimistic that with support from his peers, coach, mentor, and herself, Aiden can reduce his risk for depression and addiction. Aiden shows signs of resilience. He is motivated to "keep his act together for Jenna," capable of forming positive attachments, and willing to seek help when he knows where to find it.

IN-A-LIFE

Evelyn Lau (1971–)

Evelyn Lau is a noted poet, novelist, and short story writer. She was born in Vancouver, British Columbia, and wanted to pursue a career in the arts; however, this was not the desire of her traditional Chinese parents. Evelyn challenged her traditional family upbringing and left home when she was 14 years old. She spent much of the next 2 years living on the streets as a sex trade worker abusing addictive substances, resulting in suicide attempts. She has portrayed her experiences through her art, creating *Runaway: Diary of a Street Kid* (1989), which was later made into a CBC movie called *The Diary of Evelyn Lau*. Subsequently, her first collection of poetry, *You Are Not Who You Claim* (1990), reflected much of that same time, and Evelyn was the recipient of the Milton Acorn People's Poetry Award. A second memoir, *Inside Out*, was published in 2001.

She was the youngest poet to receive a nomination for the Governor General's Award for *Oedipal Dreams*. She won the Air Canada Award in 1990 for Most Promising Writer under 30 and the Vantage Woman of Originality Award in 1999. *Living Under Plastic*, her most recent work, won the Pat Lowther Award for best book of poetry by a woman in Canada. Evelyn Lau is Vancouver's Poet Laureate.

Evelyn has spoken and written about her experiences and how this has created the work and person she has become. She does not make excuses for her choices and shares openly her feelings on various topics. Her story is one of how rigid traditional values can clash with youths' desires and dreams and of how she was fortunate that, for her, it resulted in a successful career. Unfortunately, this is not the case for many youth who find themselves living on the street in a life of drugs and prostitution.

Parent With Mental Illness

A parent with mental illness can have a number of profound effects on a child, directly through genetics, the intrauterine environment and antenatal stressors, and experience of the illness itself or indirectly due to socioeconomic issues such as poverty, marital conflict, or addiction (Manning & Gregoire, 2006). Approximately 10% of pregnant women will develop postpartum depression, with a 50% to 62% chance of future depressions (Bernard-Bonnin, 2004; Public Health Agency of Canada, 2012). Postpartum depression can affect the mother–child bond and impact the attachment process for children. Therefore, it is important for nurses to assess the child presented to them and to gather a parental history of stressors and physical and mental illness throughout the pregnancy and during the child's development.

Many children know that something is wrong when a parent has a mental illness, but they may not be able to identify the problem specifically (Gladstone, Boydell, Seeman, & McKeever, 2011). They feel alone, left out, distanced, and powerless to participate in decisions. They report feeling angry, sad, and that somehow they are to blame for their parent's illness. They also worry that they will in turn become ill, and they fear the stigma that surrounds mental illness. Fortunately, the likelihood or severity of these problems can be reduced or eliminated when families have the knowledge and support they need. Children need age-appropriate information, their questions answered, an opportunity to talk about how they feel, and routine childhood experiences. As with other family stressors, it is important to keep children informed, in manageable ways and doses, and at times that the children determine (Gladstone et al., 2011). Nurses can help parents get started by modelling. For example, "Mommy isn't feeling well. She feels sad. It's because of an illness and it's not her fault. It is a sad time for all of us, but I'm here to talk with you about it when you need to do so."

Given the ethnic diversity of Canada, and the Canadian government's commitment in particular to the resettlement of refugees from the Middle East, nurses will inevitably come into contact with refugee families in their practice. Parental histories of pre- and postmigration trauma, anxiety, and depression, coupled with the stressors of learning a new language, seeking employment, and managing a household with limited resources and social networks, can weigh heavily on their ability to be responsive and nurturing parents, which may lead to inconsistencies in attachment with younger children and strained relationships with older children. Nurses need to be cautious that they do not prematurely judge parents' capabilities to parent, especially when older children have assumed many navigational roles (e.g., education system, health care system) as a result of their ease with communicating in a new language (Minhas et al., 2017).

Children with a mentally ill parent will usually need supportive relationships outside the home with someone (e.g., a teacher, coach, neighbour) who can provide a listening ear, extra support, and a measure of respite for the family. Children need to know that their routine in life will continue, including the fun times, and that their relationship with both parents is valued by the parents. Parents worry about how their mental illness will affect their child. Support and education need to be provided to all during these challenging times (Costea, 2011; Gladstone et al., 2011). Evidence shows that when children and their families are given information about the affected parent's mental illness, they show improved knowledge and long-standing positive effects in how they problem solve (a resilience-related quality) around parental illness (Beardslee, Gladstone, Wright, & Cooper, 2003; Gladstone et al., 2011).

Parent With a Substance Abuse Problem

Exposure to parental addiction in childhood is fairly common in Canada, with reported prevalence higher for women (20%) than for men (16%) (Langlois & Garner, 2013). Children whose parents are dependent on alcohol live in an unpredictable family environment and are more likely to experience abuse, and their efforts to cope with stress may disrupt their ability to perform in school and lead to other emotional problems (Casa-Gil & Navarro-Guzman, 2002). A study that examined the course of psychological distress among a nationally representative sample of Canadians (aged 18 to 74) revealed that those who experienced parental addictions had consistently higher distress scores than those who did not (Langlois & Garner, 2013).

Such experience appears associated, as well, with other childhood adversities, parental comorbidities, and a negative family environment; thus, understanding the effects of exposure to parental addiction on children requires further study (Langlois & Garner, 2013). The integrated role of biologic–genetic mechanisms and environmental mechanisms in creating an increased risk for psychological problems among children of those who abuse substances must be considered (see Chapter 26).

Biologic factors affecting children of those who abuse substances include fetal alcohol spectrum disorder, nutritional deficits stemming from neglect, and neuropsychiatric dysfunction. Genetic factors are at least partly responsible for the well-documented increased risk for substance abuse. Studies are beginning to link a family history of mental disorders and alcoholism with genetically transmitted mental disorders, which may be a precursor to alcohol abuse. The precise mechanism of family transmission of alcoholism remains unknown. Children of those who abuse substances may inherit a predisposition to a nonspecific form of biologic dysregulation that may be expressed phenotypically, either as alcoholism or as some other psychiatric disorder (e.g., hyperactivity, conduct disorder, depression), depending on the individual's developmental history.

Children of persons who abuse substances are at high risk for both substance abuse and behaviour disorders

(Mylant, Ide, Cuevas, & Meehan, 2002). Moreover, some evidence shows that other factors related to addiction, such as family stress, violence, divorce, dysfunction, and other concurrent parental psychiatric disorders (e.g., depression, anxiety), are as important as the alcoholism itself in increasing this risk (Ritter, Stewart, Bernet, Coe, & Brown, 2002). The experience of growing up in a substance-abusing family is marked by unpredictability, fear, and helplessness because of the cyclic nature of addictive patterns.

The literature on children of parents who have alcoholism has described several typical roles that children assume, including the "hero" (overly responsible children who may ignore their own needs to take care of parents and other children), "scapegoat" (problem children who divert the attention away from the parent), "mascot" (family clowns who relieve tension and mask feelings through joking), and "lost child" (children who suffer in silence but may exhibit difficulties at school or in later life) (Veronie & Freuhstorfer, 2001). These roles, combined with the enabling behaviours of other family members who attempt to cover up and minimize the effects of the addiction, may become so rigid and effective in masking the problem that children of substance abusers may not come to the attention of mental health professionals until after the parent stops drinking and family roles are disrupted.

The experience of growing up in a substance-abusing family can lead to poor self-concept if children feel responsible for their parents' behaviour. The child becomes isolated and learns to mistrust his or her own perceptions as the family denies the reality of the addiction. There is, however, no uniform pattern of outcomes, and many children demonstrate resilience (Harter, 2000). Resilience, as noted previously, is the phenomenon by which some children at risk for psychopathology—because of genetic or experiential circumstances—attain good mental health, maintain hope, and achieve healthy outcomes (Masten, 2001). Again, individual protective factors and preventive interventions are paramount.

MENTAL ILLNESS AMONG CHILDREN AND ADOLESCENTS

The Mental Health Commission of Canada (MHCC) estimates that 1.2 million children and youth are affected by mental illness in our country. Over 800,000 Canadian children and youth experience significant mental health issues (School-Based Mental Health and Substance Abuse [SBMHSA] Consortium, 2013). For Canadians aged between 15 and 34, suicide is the leading nonaccidental cause of death (Statistics Canada, 2017). It is highly relevant that two thirds of adults living with mental illness report experiencing first symptoms in their youth (SBMHSA Consortium, 2013). Most children and youth will not receive appropriate treatment, due to factors such as social stigma and problems with access and availability (SBMHSA Consortium,

2013). Fortunately, strategies endorsed by the MHCC, such as those of the Evergreen Framework (Kutcher & McLuckie, 2010), are allowing such service challenges to be addressed and, hopefully, overcome.

ADDRESSING RISKS AND CHALLENGES TO CHILDREN'S AND ADOLESCENTS' MENTAL HEALTH

Nurses and other healthcare professionals need to become aware of and use strategies to address negative alternations in the trajectory of children's overall functioning. Professional nursing emphasizes an interdisciplinary approach in which the nurse acts as the collaborator, coordinator, case manager, and advocate to establish linkages with physicians and nurse practitioners, teachers, speech and language specialists, social workers, and other professionals to develop and implement comprehensive preventative interventions (see Box 29.3). A view of parents as partners should be foremost. In the past, parents have been too often viewed as the culprits in creating children's mental health problems. Recent insights into the biologic and genetic origins of psychiatric disorders have contributed to a shift from blaming parents to seeking their collaboration in treatment.

Trauma-Informed Care for Children and Adolescents

The neurodevelopment of children exposed to traumatic events affects their cognitive and emotional development (Glaser, 2000; Hodas, 2004; Kinniburgh et al., 2005; McEwen, 2004, 2007; Porges, 2004; van der Kolk, 2006, 2009). "These children may demonstrate hypervigilance, intrusive thoughts, nightmares, bed-wetting, excessive clinginess, inconsolable crying, and severe tantrums" (Arvidson et al., 2011, p. 41). Programs that emphasize establishing self-regulation strategies and attachment attunement and that work toward development or repair of cognitive skills have been shown to shift affected children toward better success and reduced psychopathology (Arvidson et al., 2011; Blaustein & Kinniburgh, 2010; Mulvihill, 2005; Murphy & Bennington-Davis, 2005, 2006; Kinniburgh et al., 2005; van der Kolk, 2009). An example is the Attachment, Self-Regulation, and Competency program that works toward teaching both the health care provider and parent how to modulate their own emotional responses, attune to the child, and assist with their self-regulation. "Caregivers and clinicians play an essential role in restoring a sense of safety and security to traumatized children by developing predictable routines and rituals in their lives" (Arvidson et al., 2011, p. 42). Once the child is better able to self-regulate, they are more open to learning and experiencing the world from a safer perspective (Blaustein & Kinniburgh, 2010). A trauma-informed approach has been shown to benefit children attending inpatient settings and outpatient settings, as well as schools and residential care homes (Arvidson et al., 2011). Resources for such an approach are increasingly available. For instance, in British Columbia, the Child and Youth Mental Health and Substance Use Collaborative offers a "Trauma Informed Practice and Trauma Informed Services Resources List" (2017) for accessing provincial, national, and international resources. Most of the information is available online, but contact e-mail and the organization's name is included when this is not so.

At the individual level, such factors as secure attachment, good parenting, friendship and social support, meaningful employment and social roles, adequate income, and physical activity will strengthen mental health and, indirectly, reduce the impact or incidence of some mental health problems. At a system level, strategies that create supportive environments, strengthen community actions, develop personal skills, and orient health services can help to ensure that the population has some control over the psychological and social determinants of mental health.

Promotion and Prevention Programs

Promotion and prevention programs incorporate a range of techniques to provide reassurance and education, skills training, or direct intervention. The programs may use face-to-face techniques (e.g., home visits, educational groups), literature (e.g., pamphlets, books), phone (e.g., crisis lines), or electronic mechanisms (e.g., Internet, telehealth).

Psychoeducational Programs

Psychoeducational programs are a particularly effective form of mental health promotion and intervention. These programs are designed to teach parents and children basic coping skills for dealing with various stressors. Among other techniques, they use the process of **normalization** (i.e., teaching families what are typical behaviours and expected responses) and provide families with information about normal child development and expected reactions to various stressors so that the families will feel less isolated, know what to expect, and put their reactions into perspective. For example, if families learn that anger is a natural part of grieving, they will be less likely to view it as abnormal and more likely to accept and cope with it constructively.

An excellent example is *Transitions* (2013), a downloadable resource for teenagers and their families that is one aspect of the Teen Mental Health Web site developed by a Canadian expert in adolescent mental health, Stanley Kutcher at Dalhousie University, and his colleagues. *Transitions* is focused on helping youth make the transition from high school to university and covers topics ranging from study tips, time management, and exams to sexuality and dating to mental illness, unhealthy behaviours (e.g., violence), substance use, and suicide. Psychoeducational approaches that utilize parallel curricula, established with concurrent psychoeducational groups for adults and children, are helpful. Most foster care agencies now provide a program of education and training for prospective foster parents to help them know what to expect and how to help the child adjust to placement.

Social Skills Training

Social skills training is one psychoeducational approach that has been useful with youth who have low self-esteem, aggressive behaviour, or a high risk for substance abuse (Cavell, Ennett, & Meehan, 2001). **Social skills training** involves instruction, feedback, support, and practice with learning behaviours that help children to interact more effectively with peers and adults. When combined with assertiveness training, social skills training can be particularly helpful in providing children with coping skills to resist engaging in addictive or antisocial behaviours and to prevent social withdrawal under stress. Social skills training may be particularly helpful for children dealing with peer rejection or who are bullying others.

Bibliotherapy

Bibliotherapy is the therapeutic use of books, stories, and other reading materials. It can be used to help children, adolescents, and families to gain information and understanding about life stressors, illness, and recovery. It is a particularly potent form of intervention because it empowers families to learn and develop coping mechanisms on their own. A wide variety of books are available to help children understand issues such as death, divorce, chronic illness, stepfamilies, adoption, and the birth of a sibling. For instance, Baker (2007) describes the way stories about being in foster care can help foster children, parents, and caseworkers in discussing their own situation. By using eight stories to reveal the themes found in accounts of foster care (e.g., the fear of foster children in developing attachments; the way siblings can play a powerfully supportive role; the importance of recognizing the humanity of the biologic parents), Baker highlights the benefits of this therapeutic approach. Children and adolescents can find comfort and increased understanding through stories that reflect their own experience. Parents can use stories as a way to learn about their children's concerns: the adventures and/or tribulations of a story's characters can be a means to discover their child's thoughts and feelings about an experience. Some health centres and hospitals have patient library services available. Many mental health organizations such as the Canadian Mental Health Association, public health agencies, and Health Canada have pamphlets or Web site information designed for parents or children and youth about various physical and psychological problems. In addition to providing concrete information and advice, these reading materials help to reduce anxiety by pointing out common reactions to the various stressors so that families do not feel alone.

Support Groups

Support groups, groups composed of people with a similar experience or problem who meet regularly to sustain and support one another, are available for just about every kind of stressor that a family can experience, including substance abuse, death, divorce, and coping with a chronic illness. Both parents and children in groups can experience Yalom's (1985) healing effects of group therapy, including group cohesiveness, universality (awareness of the normalcy and commonality of one's reactions), catharsis, hope, and altruism (being able to help others; see Chapter 14).

Early Intervention Programs

Early intervention programs, possibly the most important form of primary prevention available to children and families, offer regular home visits, support, education, and concrete services to those in need. Research supports the effectiveness of these programs, which may be the key to preventing the placement of children outside the home (Gimpel & Holland, 2003; Tomlin & Viehweg, 2003). The assumption underlying these programs is that parents are the most consistent and important figures in children's lives, and they should be afforded the opportunity to define their own needs and priorities. With support and education, parents will be empowered to respond more effectively to their children.

Canada invests in early intervention to promote healthy child development by enhancing such programs as paid parental leave (1 year), child care, family resource centres, and early learning (Waddell et al., 2005). A number of jurisdictions have introduced promotion and prevention programs around the birth of a newborn, for example, Healthy Beginnings Postpartum Program in Alberta in which mothers and babies are visited by a nurse following discharge from a hospital birth and Healthy Beginnings: Enhanced Home Visiting in Nova Scotia where a home visitor shares information about child development to support families in making healthy choices. Intensive postpartum support (more than antenatal support) provided by a health care professional can help prevent postpartum depression (Dennis, 2005); early interventions can be effective in preventing child abuse, particularly when it is initiated prenatally, have developmental benefits in terms of cognition and problem behaviours, and reduce health problems in older children (Peacock, Konrad, Watson, Nickel, & Muhajarine, 2013). Population-based early intervention initiatives aimed at socioeconomically disadvantaged communities are directed toward the child (e.g., classroom enrichment, quality child care), parent (e.g., home visiting, parent help/information/crisis phone lines, parent–child play groups), and neighbourhood (information that engages families and connects them to community supports), with an emphasis on providing intensive services to children directly. They have demonstrated improvements in children's emotional problems, behavioural problems, social skills, and a decreased need for special education during the early years (ages 4 to 8) (Peters, Petrunka, & Arnold, 2003).

Programs designed for adolescent mental health should support and educate youth (e.g., through peer mentoring in community organizations and schools); enhance self-help and self-responsibility, coping skills, self-esteem, and skill development in ways that foster mental health; and teach youth when and how to seek assistance for problems (Federal-Provincial-Territorial Advisory Committee on Population Health, 2000). Particular emphasis has been given to ways of creating healthy images related to gender, body image, and empowerment.

Historically, nurses have been underused in school-based mental health efforts, although schools are good locations for other early intervention programs because they are physically near the families they serve and are less intimidating than mental health centres. Programs can be targeted for very young children before symptoms have time to develop. In numerous schools throughout Canada, Youth Health Centres have become familiar resources.

Electronic Media Services

The number of promotion and early intervention mental health services provided through electronic media (e.g., Internet, telehealth) is growing. Targeted support groups are increasingly available through the Internet. Dedicated Web sites providing both universal mental health information and confidential intervention services by e-mail are also available through some school systems. Similar services around specific mental health issues are also being tested with high-risk populations. Telehealth, which involves telephone and video support to rural and remote Canada (see Chapter 6), is increasingly offered both to practitioners and to children or their parents (Urness, Hailey, Delday, Callanan, & Orlik, 2004). The full capacity of these approaches is largely unknown, and contrary to professional fears, the users are generally more than satisfied with the services (Williams, May, & Esmail, 2001). Some users even prefer the anonymity of electronic media.

Comprehensive Approaches

Although a number of children's mental health promotion and prevention programs have proven effective on their own, less understood are the effects of programs that include an array of comprehensive health care services, parent education, and support on the mental health of children and youth (Breton, 1999; Peters et al., 2003). Best thinking to date suggests that the most effective strategies for reducing the burden of suffering from child psychiatric disorders are those that consist of a number of concurrent steps (Offord, Kraemer, Kazdin, Jensen, & Harrington, 1998). First, effective universal programs should be in place. Targeted programs should follow for those not helped sufficiently by the universal programs. Finally, for those unaffected by the targeted programs, clinical services should be available. To be effective, prevention programs need to start early, continue long term, and involve multiple domains in a child's life (Offord & Bennett, 2002).

Undertaking interventions to promote the mental health of children and adolescents is time and effort well spent. Many adult mental health problems can be prevented, coped with more effectively, or at least reduced in their scope and severity through focused intervention with children, youth, and families. Children and youth lack the power and voice to fight for their own needs, making them one of the most vulnerable groups in society. By virtue of their close interaction with families, nurses are in a key position to identify the mental health needs of children and youth and to intervene, particularly in times of crisis.

Community-Based Mental Health Promotion

Mental health promotion with children and youth can occur at individual, familial, community, and global levels. Multiple factors affect mental well-being; mental health does not equate to a lack of mental illness and is affected by the social determinants of health. Mental health promotion initiatives need to be individualized to the circumstances of the children and youth with whom nurses work (including their familial and social resources), must be sensitive to context (e.g., rural setting or urban multicultural setting), and must incorporate the latest empirical and theoretical developments. Among children and youth, in addition to the health and social services systems, the education system can be among the sites where mental health promotion initiatives take place.

▌ MENTAL HEALTH ASSESSMENT OF CHILDREN AND ADOLESCENTS

The assessment of children and adolescents generally follows the same format as that for adults (see Chapter 10), but there are significant differences. In working with children, adolescents, and families, we must recognize that the perspective of each person involved, including the nurse, will be particular to that individual. Children think in more concrete terms; the nurse therefore needs to ask more specific and fewer open-ended questions than would typically be asked of adults. Simple phrasing should be used because children have a narrower vocabulary than do adults. Examples include saying "sad" instead of "depressed" or "nervous" or "worried" instead of "anxious." Corroborate information that children offer with more sources (e.g., parents, teachers) than might be needed with adults. Artistic and play media (e.g., puppets, family drawings) can be used to engage children and evaluate their perceptions, inner worlds, fine motor skills, and intellectual functions. Children have a less specific sense of time and a less developed memory than do adults. When children are asked about a sequence of events or specific times when events occurred, they may not be able to provide accurate information.

Adolescents must be assessed within their cognitive and developmental range of functioning. Adolescents may or may not be willing participants in the assessment process, depending on why they have been referred and who has referred them. It is always important to meet with clients separately from their care providers, and this is especially true with adolescents. It is critical to ensure what level of confidentiality can be provided to the youth in the context of an individual interview. For example, issues of safety, such as suicidality, would need to be revealed to care providers, whereas issues of sexual identity are less immediately urgent. There is usually time to determine when or if this issue should be shared collaboratively with the child's/youth's care providers. Mental health assessment involves much more than completing assessment tools and considers far more than the individual. A conceptual framework used as a guide can assist in planning the goals of the assessment, as well as identifying the factors, types of information and sources, and the elements within the environment to be considered. Frameworks that shape the mental health assessment of children and youth in Canada are identified and described below.

The Canadian Mental Health Association's (CMHA) Framework for Support

The CMHA's Framework for Support (Trainor, Pomeroy, & Pape, 2004) identifies three resource bases important to mental health assessment: the Person Resource Base, the Knowledge Resource Base, and the Community Resource Base. This framework helps focus assessment on outcomes and, in particular, on those outcomes that play a critical role in recovery from mental illness. Specifically, it supports assessment of whether a child has access to the social determinants of good mental health (housing, school, family, friends, a sense of purpose), feels well and has a sense of personal control, and has various personal resources in place and ways to connect with the formal service system if needed. Finally, the framework assesses how the individual's age (child or youth) and life circumstances (e.g., breakup or death in family, being cut from a sport team) have challenged the child.

By focusing on the *Person Resource Base*, it is acknowledged that the child/youth is far more than a repository of illness and symptoms and that positive change builds on existing strengths. Hence, when approaching assessment, their understanding of their mental health problem/illness and their self-esteem, sense of belonging (within their family and community), and sense of purpose and meaning in the world are considered. The child's/youth's skills and capacities (sense of personal control, confidence, resilience, hope) to confront illness are assessed.

By focusing on the *Knowledge Resource Base*, consideration is given, not only to medical–clinical and social science knowledge but also to experiential (first-hand experience) and traditional knowledge (cultural ways). How children experience mental illness and how the family and community (public attitudes and conventional wisdom) accept it are noted. A critical analysis of such information assists in building a rich understanding of children and guards against drawing inaccurate assumptions. It can also identify inaccuracies and misconceptions that may be held within the family or community about mental illness.

By focusing on the *Community Resource Base*, an understanding of the many factors and social determinants (housing, education, income, meaningful work) that affect the everyday life of children and youth is gained (Trainor et al., 2004, pp. 8–10). The Community Resource Base also acknowledges the importance of both formal services (mental health services, generic community services) and the network of natural supports (family and friends, self-help, and consumer organizations) available to promote mental health and recovery. Equally important, it recognizes the person (child or youth) as having the power (age appropriate) to make choices about resources to use, if any, and to participate fully in decision-making.

Evergreen: A Child and Youth Mental Health Framework for Canada

The Mental Health Commission of Canada's (MHCC) Evergreen Framework provides values and strategic directions for child and youth mental health care in Canada (Kutcher & McLuckie for MHCC, 2010). The values identified are:

- Human rights
- Dignity, respect, and diversity
- Best available evidence
- Choice, opportunity, and responsibility
- Collaboration, continuity, and community
- Access to information, programs, and services

Health professionals should be cognizant of human rights documents in a way that informs their practice. These documents include United Nation's (UN) *Convention on the Rights of the Child* and the *Convention on the Rights of Persons with Disabilities*, as well as *A Canada Fit for Children* that is Canada's response to the UN's *A World Fit for Child*ren. Valuing dignity, respect, and diversity involves striving for equal access to services and programs for all children and their families in Canada. Ongoing commitment is necessary for best evidence-based programs to evolve; children and families need to be able to make informed choices about what best fits their needs. Collaboration among all those who have a significant role in a child's life allows for meaningful networks of support. Publically accessible mental health information, along with the promotion of access to programs and services, is crucial to an equitable health care system. These explicitly stated values contribute to a common vision for the evolution of child and adolescent mental health in Canada.

Four categories of strategic directions are identified in the Evergreen Framework, envisioned as separate but overlapping categories: *promotion*, *prevention*, *intervention and ongoing care*, and *research and evaluation*. The first three categories are part of the continuum of mental health care (see Chapter 4), while the fourth, research and evaluation, is an essential component to each of them, as well as being a component in itself. Within the Evergreen Framework, specific strategies for each category are identified.

The Bio/Psycho/Social/Spiritual Model

The holistic, integrated approach of the bio/psycho/social/spiritual model of health that is used to frame nursing practice in this textbook is applicable to child and adolescent care. Thus, a comprehensive evaluation includes a bio/psycho/social/spiritual history, mental status examination, additional testing (e.g., cognitive or neuropsychological), and, if necessary, records of the child's school performance and medical–physical history and information from other agencies that may be providing services (e.g., department of child and family services, juvenile court). Various assessment tools, including the Child Attention Profile and the Devereux Early Childhood Assessment (DECA), the Behaviour Assessment System for Children (BASC), the Child Behaviour Checklist (CBCL), or the Children's Depression Inventory (CDI), may be used.

■ COLLECTION OF ASSESSMENT DATA

Comprehensive collection of meaningful data is crucial to an accurate, holistic assessment of the mental health of a child or youth. Components of assessment data and the nursing skills necessary to them are addressed here. (Note: where appropriate, "child" will be the term used to refer to both children and adolescents).

The Clinical Interview

The clinical interview is the primary assessment tool used in child and adolescent psychiatry. A unique set of skills is necessary for interviewing children and adolescents. How the nurse obtains mental health information depends on the developmental level of each child, specifically considering the child's language and cognitive, social, and emotional skills. For example, the nurse should simplify questions for young children or children with developmental delays or communication issues (e.g., autism spectrum disorder, hearing impairment, English as a second language) so that these children can understand and respond accordingly.

The assessment interview may be the initial contact between the child and parent/guardian and the nurse. The first step is to establish a connection and rapport to build a relationship, and the second is to assess the interactions between the child and his or her caregivers. It is important to understand that children cannot be considered apart from their caregivers and the context in which they live. However, defining the caregiving context is sometimes a challenge. The nurse needs to identify the child's primary caregivers, the patterns of current caregiving relationships (e.g., how often the child goes to other caregivers), and the history of these relationships (e.g., multiple transitions, abrupt losses) (Carter et al., 2004). The nurse should also explore the family's definition of *family* and identify those included in the family constellation (Carter et al., 2004, pp. 114–115). This would include biologic, psychosocial, and spiritual relationships (e.g., uncle, Big Brother/Big Sister volunteer, friends, neighbours, godmother).

Building Rapport

To reduce anxiety and establish trust during the assessment, the nurse strives to develop rapport with the family members. The nurse can establish the relationship with the child/youth and family by recognizing the child's individuality and showing respect and concern for that child. The nurse should demonstrate sensitivity, objectivity, and confidentiality. Children will be more forthcoming if they believe that the nurse is listening carefully and is interested in what they have to say. Establishing rapport can be facilitated by making and maintaining eye contact (as culturally relevant); speaking slowly, clearly, and calmly, with friendliness and acceptance; using a warm and expressive tone; reacting to communications objectively; showing interest in what families are saying; and making the interview a joint undertaking (Sattler, 1998).

Building rapport, which can be challenging, is fundamental to any mental health assessment. The developmental transitions throughout childhood and adolescence are rapid, and there are few guidelines about how information from many sectors should be integrated, how impairment levels should be determined, or how assessing function that may be specific to context (relational or cultural) or caregiver (e.g., parents, relatives, day care staff, teachers) can be achieved practically (Carter et al., 2004).

The information in Box 29.4 can serve as a guide to asking specific questions during a comprehensive

---

BOX 29.4 Semistructured Interview With School-Aged Children

This guide identifies a range of areas and sample questions that can be addressed during an interview with a school-aged or adolescent child. The nurse should note that children generally prefer to be engaged in a conversation rather than peppered with questions. The interview should be tailored in a way that is comfortable and relevant for the child. Although some direct questions are inevitable, open-ended questions are preferable. Similarly, phrasing questions to get at what a child is thinking (e.g., "I can see you are trying to tell me something" or "tell me more") is preferable to asking "why" questions that tend to put people on the defensive. Note that in the guide, "Explain" means to explore an explanation; it does not indicate giving the command "explain" to the child or adolescent. Finally, trying to match the child's emotional state (unless hostile) helps people feel understood (Forgatch & Patterson, 1989). The interview can begin with a simple greeting, such as the following: "Hi, I am (your name and title). You must be Tom Brown. Come in."

FOR ALL SCHOOL-AGED CHILDREN

Presenting Concern

Thank you for coming to talk with me today. To begin, it would help me if I knew what, if anything, you have been told about why you are here or what will go on today.... Can you tell me *your* story of how you came to be here today? (If necessary, probe with specific questions below. Let the child take the lead and explore issues as he or she raises them. If the child raises a problem, explore it in detail).

Demographic Information

I'd like to know you better. Could you tell me about yourself?

Probes

1. How old are you?
2. When is your birthday?
3. Where do you live? (address)
4. And your telephone number is…?

School

Tell me about your school.

Probes

5. Which school do you go to? Is it close to your home? How do you get there each day?
6. Where do you go after school (home, sitter, etc.)… and who is there (parent/relative, sitter, no one)?
7. What do most kids think about your school? … What is it like for you?
8. What grade are you in? What do most kids think about it? … What is it like for you?
9. What subjects do you like the best? … Like least?
10. What subjects give you the least trouble? … Most trouble?
11. How well do you do in school—about the same as, better than, or not as well as other kids in your class?
12. On the whole, would you say that you are doing better or worse than last year?

(Continued)

BOX 29.4 **Semistructured Interview With School-Aged Children** *(Continued)*

13. What activities do you participate in at school?
14. How well do you get along with your classmates?
15. How well do you get along with your teachers?
16. Tell me how you spend a usual day at school.

HOME AND FAMILY

To help me understand your family, can you name each of the people who live with you … and then other important family members who live somewhere else … and I'll put them into a picture…. Now, using the picture, tell me a little about your family.

A genogram provides a useful diagram of family relationships. It resembles a family tree but includes additional relationships among individuals. It permits the nurse and the child to quickly see patterns in family history. It maps relationships and traits that may otherwise be missed and includes basic information about number of families, number of children in each family, birth order, and deaths. Some genograms include information on disorders running in the family such as alcoholism, depression, diseases, alliances, and living situations. Older children can provide additional information (e.g., about separation/divorce, death) for understanding family dynamics. (See Chapter 15 for detailed information regarding creating a genogram.)

Probes

17. Tell me a little about each of them.
    * Who makes you happy and who makes you sad/angry/worried? Explain.
    * Do you have a favourite photo of you and your family? Tell me about it … and why you like it.
18. What does your father do during the day—does he work? (Other activities at home/with friends?)
19. What does your mother do during the day—does she work? (Other activities at home/with friends?)
20. Tell me what your home is like.
21. Tell me about your room at home.
22. What chores do you do at home?
23. How do you get along with your father?
24. What does he do that you like? … Don't like?
25. How do you get along with your mother?
26. What does she do that you like? … Don't like?
27. (Where relevant) Some brothers and sisters get along well, whereas others don't get along at all … How do you get along with your brothers and sisters?
28. What do (does) they (he/she) do that you like? … That you don't like?
29. Who handles the discipline at home?
30. Tell me about how they (he/she) handle (handles) it.
    * When you do something good, what happens and who is involved?

* When you get in trouble, what happens and who is involved?
* If you want to do something different from the rest of your family, would that be okay? Explain … Who would support you?
* If you need help, what would you do? Would someone support you? Explain.
* Are there other relatives who are important to you? Tell me about who they are and how they connect with you (if not already discussed with the genogram).
* Would you say that your family is like most other families in your school/neighbourhood or different? Explain. Does that make it easy or difficult for you/your family … and in what ways and in what types of situations? This question gets at culture (ethnicity, socioeconomic status, language, beliefs/values, etc.) in a broad way.

INTERESTS

Now let's talk about the things you like to do.

Probes

31. What hobbies and interests do you have?
32. What do you do in the afternoons/evenings after school?
33. Tell me what you usually do on Saturdays and Sundays.
    * What do you do on special holidays? Tell me about the best holiday you ever had.
    * When you are having fun, what are you doing, who are you with? Tell me about a time when you were really having a good time.

Friends

Tell me about your friends.

Probes

34. What do you like to do with your friends?
    * Any best friends?
    * If you needed help, could you count on them to support you? Give an example.
    * If you wanted to do something different from them, would that be okay?

MOODS AND FEELINGS

Probes

35. Everybody feels happy at times. What things make you feel happiest?
36. What are you most likely to get sad about?
37. What do you do when you are sad?
38. Everybody gets angry at times. What things make you angriest?
39. What do you do when you are angry?

BOX 29.4 Semistructured Interview With School-Aged Children (Continued)

FEARS AND WORRIES

Probes

40. All children get scared sometimes about some things. What things make you feel scared?
41. What do you do when you are scared? … What takes away the fear?
    - How well does that work?
42. Tell me what you worry about … What takes away the worry?
    - How well does that work?
43. Any other things?

SELF-CONCERNS

Probes

44. What do you like best about yourself? … Anything else?
45. What do you like least about yourself? … Anything else?
46. Tell me about the best thing that ever happened to you.
47. Tell me about the worst thing that ever happened to you.
    - What did you do about this situation?
    - How well does that work?
    - Overall, how much would you say you believe in yourself?

SOMATIC CONCERNS

Probes

48. Do you ever get headaches?
49. (If yes) Tell me about them. (How often? What do you usually do?)
50. Do you get stomachaches?
51. (If yes) Tell me about them. (How often? What do you usually do?)
52. Do you get any other kinds of body pains?
53. (If yes) Tell me about them.
    - What do you do to ease these problems?
      - How well does that work?

THOUGHT DISORDER

Probes

54. Do you ever hear things that seem funny or unusual?
55. (If yes) Tell me about them. (How often? How do you feel about them? What do you usually do?)
56. Do you ever see things that seem funny or unreal?
57. (If yes) Tell me about them. (How often? How do you feel about them? What do you usually do?)

HELP-SEEKING

Probes

58. Tell me about a time when you have needed help. What did you do? Whom did you ask for help? What kind of help did you get? How did things work out?
59. Have you ever gone to see a counsellor before? Explain. Did it help?

MEMORIES AND FANTASY

Probes

60. What is the first thing you can remember from the time when you were a very little baby?
61. Tell me about your dreams.
62. Which dreams come back again?
63. Who are your favourite television characters?
64. Tell me about them.
65. What animals do you like best?
66. Tell me about these animals.
67. What animals do you like least?
68. Tell me about these animals.
69. What is your happiest memory?
70. What is your saddest memory?
71. If you could change places with anyone in the whole world, who would it be?
72. Tell me about that.
73. If you could go anywhere you wanted to right now, where would you go?
74. Tell me about that.
75. If you could have three wishes, what would they be?
76. What things do you think you might need to take with you if you were to go to the moon and stay there for 6 months?

ASPIRATIONS

77. What do you plan on doing when you become an adult?
78. What things will help you be successful? Is there anything standing in the way of you being successful?
    - How hopeful are you that you might be successful? (Suggestion—using a visual analogue with a series of faces on a line [sad face to very happy face], ask child to choose the face that best describes their hopefulness.)
79. If you could do anything you wanted when you become an adult, what would it be?

CONCLUDING QUESTIONS

80. Do you have anything else that you would like to tell me about yourself?
81. Do you have any questions that you would like to ask me?
    - What are you hoping will happen as a result of our talking today?

(Continued)

BOX 29.4 Semistructured Interview With School-Aged Children *(Continued)*

FOR ADOLESCENTS

These questions can be inserted after number 57 and prior to the "Help-Seeking" section.

SEXUAL RELATIONS

Adolescence is a very confusing time emotionally. Our bodies change as we begin to look more like adults. Our relationships also change. While our sexual relationships are new and exciting, they can also be puzzling, frustrating, or even frightening.

1. Do you have any romantic feelings or relationship(s) with guys or girls? Do you feel comfortable talking about them? With girls/guys/or both?
2. What makes you feel good about it/them?
3. What makes you feel not so good about them?
4. Do you have any special girlfriend or boyfriend?
5. (If yes) Tell me about her (him). Most people have lots of questions about their sexual relationships and yet are not sure whom to trust to talk openly.
6. What kind of sexual concerns do you have?
7. (If present) Tell me about them.
8. (If applicable) What do you think might be helpful to do about your concerns? (getting information, talking to someone, getting a checkup/some medication)

9. Are you interested in getting help? Would you like me to help you make the right connections?

DRUG AND ALCOHOL USE

10. Do your parents/sister/brothers drink?
11. (If yes) Tell me about their drinking. (How much, how frequently, and where?)
12. Do your friends drink alcohol?
13. (If yes) Tell me about their drinking.
14. Do you drink alcohol?
15. (If yes) Tell me about your drinking.
16. Do your parents use drugs?
17. (If yes) Tell me about the drugs they use. (How much, how frequently, and for what reasons?)
18. Do your friends use drugs?
19. (If yes) Tell me about the drugs they use.
20. Do you use drugs?
21. (If yes) Tell me about the drugs you use (Sattler, 1998).
22. Are you worried about the way your parents/siblings/friends use alcohol or drugs?
23. Are you worried about the way you use alcohol/drugs?
24. (If yes) Are you interested in getting help?
25. (If applicable) What do you think might be helpful to do regarding your concerns?

---

assessment of the child. The Community Resource Base of the Framework for Support (Trainor et al., 2004) provides a useful guide for identifying a range of stakeholders from the child's daily living activities (e.g., parent, school, day care, recreation, arts) as well as services (formal or informal) that might be consulted (with family permission) for related information about the various contexts in which the child interacts. These stakeholders can provide complementary information (formal or informal) about how the child is functioning in critical developmental domains (language and literacy, physical, cognitive, social, and emotional). They also provide an understanding of how the child is treated within, and copes with, various peer environments involving diverse cultures (e.g., ethnic, socioeconomic, language) and activities (e.g., scholastic, recreational, artistic). This information can assist the nurse in formulating a well-balanced and integrated mental health assessment (strengths and limitations from multiple contexts) of the child.

Child and Parent Observation

Because the child's primary environment is most often with the parent, child–parent interactions provide important data about the child–parent attachment and

parenting practices. As discussed earlier, attachment is the term used to name the emotional bonds between a child and parent (or parental figure) that begin in infancy (see the section below "Attachment: The Caregiving Context"). The nurse's observations focus on both the child alone and the child within the family. The nurse can make some of these observations while the family is in the waiting area, noting behaviours (Barnard, 1994):

- Sensitivity/clarity/responsiveness to cues
- How the child and parent get each other's attention
- How parent and child interact with and talk to each other (clarity of cues)
- How frequently each initiates conversation and how promptly each responds
- How the child and parent separate
- Whether the parent and child play together
- How responsive the parent is to the child's attention-seeking initiatives
- How the parent and child show affection to each other
- How attached the parent and the child appear
- Response to distress
- Whether the parent starts/stops/notes the distress/changes in activity

- How the parent consoles the child
- How the parent disciplines the child (clear directive voice, yells, hits)
- Social–emotional growth fostering
- Use of talking, smiling, laughing, singing, touching (praising or criticizing)
- Cognitive growth fostering
- Parent talks about/describes objects/ideas using developmentally appropriate and stimulating language
- Parent provides child with/points out objects of interest
- Parent encourages and/or allows the child to explore

Interview Techniques

To get an accurate picture of the child, the nurse should interview the child and parent individually for some part of the session because each can provide unique, meaningful information. Often, disagreement between child and parent regarding signs and symptoms relevant to diagnostic criteria emerges in separate interviews. Generally, children provide better information about internalizing symptoms (e.g., mood, sleep, suicide ideation), and parents provide better information about externalizing symptoms (e.g., behaviour disturbances, oppositionality, relationship with parents).

Discussion With the Child

After talking with the parent and child together, the nurse should ask to speak with the child alone for a while. Young children may fear separating from their parents. The nurse can reassure children by showing them where the waiting area is and telling them, "Mommy and Daddy are going to be waiting right here for you. You and I are going to be in a room close by. But if you get worried, we can come back out here to check on them." Introducing a toy or game or giving the child a transitional object to hold may help. For example, young children often like holding the family house or car keys, knowing that their parents cannot go anywhere without them. Remember that observing how the child separates from the parent is part of the data needed to complete the assessment.

Adolescents may act indifferent or even hostile when the nurse asks to speak with them alone. Remember that this can be a pose to cover anxiety and fear. Teens tend to be skeptical that adults can really understand their experience, suspicious that they will be blamed for their problems, and fearful that their thoughts and feelings are abnormal. The nurse should be patient with adolescents and show empathy for their concerns through comments such as, "I can see that you're pretty angry about being here. There might be a way that I can help…. But to help, I need to know from *you* what is going on that is making you so angry. I want to assure you that I am not here to judge or blame. I can also promise you that if

you tell me anything that I think needs to be shared with your parents, then I will tell you first." If the youth is particularly silent, the nurse might comment, "You've been pretty quiet during the last few minutes…. I'm not sure if that means you're having trouble expressing yourself…." The nurse should allow the adolescent time to respond and then offer other prompts. "That can be really frustrating. If that is the case, then, maybe if you just start talking, we can try to find some words together to express your ideas…." "You may be wondering if it is safe to tell me what you're thinking. It can be frightening to trust a stranger with your most private thoughts…." "You may be wondering whether I really meant what I said about confidentiality/keeping things private…. or about not judging you…. I guess the dilemma/problem is whether it is safer to keep troubling thoughts and feelings to oneself or to take a chance that someone might be able to help."

The initial assessment of a child begins with an introduction by the nurse, including a brief explanation of what the nurse and the child will be doing together. For children younger than 11 years of age, an additional explanation that the nurse helps worried or upset children by talking, playing, and getting together with their parents to think of ways to make things better is helpful. It is important to determine the child's understanding of the reason why the child is there. This helps to identify children's misconceptions (e.g., believing the nurse is going to give them an injection, thinking that they have done something bad) that could create barriers to working with them.

The nurse will require several releases of information from the child's guardian to obtain corroborating reports, such as the child's physical assessment from the paediatrician or paediatric nurse practitioner; the school's report about the child's academic (report card) and behavioural performance (interactions with peers and adults); and records of diagnosis and treatment from any previous psychiatric provider. Adolescents are often very sensitive when reports are requested from school. They worry about repercussions if they have had prior difficulties (e.g., disciplinary problems). It is important that the nurse explain how these reports will be used, whether the school will be involved in the development of treatment plans, and how the youth and family will participate.

Communication needs to be adapted to the child's age level (Box 29.5). The challenge is to avoid using overly complex vocabulary or talking down to children. Young children often express themselves more easily in the context of play than through adult-like conversation. For example, a child may use puppets to re-enact a conversation that he or she had with a sibling or parent. Children respond well to third-person conversation prompts, such as "Some kids don't like being compared to their brothers and sisters" or "I know a kid who was so sad when he lost his dog that he thought he would never be happy again."

Early in the interview, the goal is to explain the nurse's purpose, elicit any concerns the child may have about

BOX 29.5 Strategies for Interviewing Children

- Use a simple vocabulary and short sentences tailored to the child's developmental and cognitive levels.
- Be sure that the child understands the questions and that you do not lead the child to give a particular response. Presenting polar opposite choices (never … or all the time) or scaled questions (1 to 10) is helpful. For example, "Some people feel angry all the time, some only feel angry at certain times, and others don't seem to feel angry at all. On a scale of 1 to 10, where 1 means never and 10 means all the time, how often do you feel angry?" If the child chooses a number greater than 1, she can be asked to describe times when she is angry.
- Select the questions for your interview on an individual basis, using judgment and discretion and considering the child's age and developmental level.
- Be sure that the manner and tone of your voice do not reveal any personal biases.
- Speak slowly and quietly, and try to allow the interview to unfold, using the child's verbalizations and behaviour as guides.
- Use simple terms (e.g., "sad" for "depressed") in exploring affective reactions, and ask the child to give examples of how he or she behaves or how other people behave when emotionally aroused.
- Assume an accepting and neutral attitude toward the child's communications.
- Learn about children's current interests (e.g., by looking at Saturday morning television programs, talking with parents, visiting toy stores) (Sattler, 1998).

what is happening, and establish rapport with the child by engaging in unthreatening discussion. Many adults rarely ask children about things that truly interest them but expect children to respond readily to adult conversation. The nurse can establish a high degree of credibility simply by taking note of and asking about things that are obviously important to children (e.g., a sport that they participate in, a rock group displayed on a shirt, a toy they have brought with them). However, children have uncanny natural "radar" for dishonest adult behaviour. Attempts to establish rapport work only when the nurse is genuinely interested in the child's life.

Discussion With the Parents

After meeting alone with the child, the nurse lets the child know that it is the parents' turn to meet with the nurse. It needs to be emphasized that no one is being judged and that these meetings are about helping. The child should have a safe place to wait and be given age-appropriate activities. With the parents, the expectations should be reviewed and reassurances around confidentiality, building trust, and being nonjudgmental provided.

Parents should be asked to describe their view of the problem. When alone, parents often feel more comfortable discussing their children in depth and sharing their frustrations. Parents need this opportunity to speak freely, without being constrained by concern for the child's feelings. Although children often have a pretty good sense about their parents' reactions, it may not be constructive for them to hear the full force of the parents' complaints and feelings, such as their sense of helplessness, anger, or disappointment. Parents sometimes feel guilty and need permission to express their negative feelings without feeling judged. This session is an opportunity to enlist the help of parents as partners in understanding and addressing the child's problem. This time is also good for filling in any gaps in the history and clarifying the data obtained from the interview with the child.

Parents need the chance to describe the presenting problem in their own words. They can be encouraged by the asking of general questions, such as, "It is not easy for parents to recognize that childhood is sometimes unhappy and that their child needs help. A child's emotions and behaviour can be pretty confusing, even frightening, and many parents hope that, with time, the problems will disappear on their own. Unfortunately, that is sometimes not the case; and if left unattended over time, the problems can worsen. It takes great courage to seek help, and you took a big step in coming here today. I hope that by working together with your child, we will find some ways of assisting. I am interested in *your* story. Tell me what brings *you* here *today*." The nurse should then reflect an understanding of the problem, showing empathy and respect for both parent and child.

If the parents have very different perspectives about the problem, it can be helpful to ask each of them to provide a viewpoint. Asking other family members about their view of the problem is a way to clarify discrepancies, obtain additional data, and communicate awareness that different family members experience the same problem in different ways.

Child and Adolescent Rating Scales

There are a number of instruments available for conducting bio/psycho/social/spiritual assessments. They vary according to age and target areas of interest as well as purpose. Observational assessment and parent-report questionnaires are generally used for screening, whereas in-depth surveys and interviews help formulate diagnoses of psychopathology. Screening for early problems is both feasible and effective in improving rates of referral for mental health services. Screening can be administered in stages starting with short screens of groups of children (e.g., in clinics, day care, school) followed by more in-depth screens involving parents and observations of those identified to be at elevated risk. See Box 29.6 for screening tools for children and adolescent mental health.

Most effective screening methods involve brief standardized measures that are easy to administer, score, and interpret (Carter et al., 2004). It is important to remember that screening measures have proved most effective in evaluating the level of risk for children with socio-emotional problems within a population (e.g., a community, school) and are less effective in identifying with certainty an individual at risk (Costello, Egger, & Angold, 2005). This means that the nurse should not rely on one source of evidence but, instead, use multiple sources of data to understand a child's emotional well-being.

Several scales are useful for diagnosing specific problems in children and adolescents. Assessments performed for *diagnostic* purposes most often require trained, credentialed administrators and interpreters; they take more time to complete and score and are more

rigorous to administer than screens. However, evidence shows that they are very useful because they highlight both positive and negative aspects of the child and identify delays, evaluate the relative degree of impairment associated with extant problem behaviours, and facilitate the design of interventions that capitalize on children's strengths (Carter et al., 2004).

Assessment Within Age Groups

Assessment techniques vary with the age and developmental stage of the child.

Preschool-Aged Children

Preschool-aged children may have difficulty putting feelings into words and provide assistance (e.g., "When I see your face all wrinkled up, it tells me that you are mixed up—confused"). They think in very concrete terms. For example, when talking to a young boy (3 to 6 years)

BOX 29.6 Screening and Assessment Tools for Children and Adolescents

MEASURES OF ATTITUDES AND BEHAVIOURS

- The BASC, developed by Reynolds and Kamphouse (1998), is a tool to measure behaviours and emotions in children aged 2 to 18 years. The scales include a teacher rating scale, parent rating scale, and 180-item self-report of personality. The scale evaluates several dimensions, including attitude toward school, attitude toward teachers, sensation seeking, atypicality, locus of control, somatization, social stress, anxiety, depression, sense of inadequacy, relations with parents, interpersonal relations, self-esteem, and self-reliance.
- The Ages and Stages Questionnaire: Social–Emotional Version (Squires, Bricker, & Twombly, 2002) is a parent-report screen for measuring social–emotional and behavioural problems and competencies from birth to 5 years.
- The CBCL developed by Achenbach and Edelbrock (1983) is a 113-item self-report tool to identify forms of psychopathology and competencies that occur in children ages 4 to 16 years. This instrument provides scores on internalizing and externalizing behaviours.

SPECIFIC MEASURES FOR ANXIETY, OBSESSIVE–COMPULSIVE BEHAVIOURS, CONDUCT, DEPRESSION

- The Multidimensional Anxiety Scale for Children developed by March (1997) is a 39-item self-rating scale that assesses severity of anxiety in children and adolescents.
- The paediatric anxiety rating scale developed by the RUPP Anxiety Study Group (2002) is a

clinician-administered, 50-item semistructured interview to assess the severity of anxiety in children aged 6 to 17 years.
- The Kutcher Generalized Social Anxiety Disorder Scale for Adolescents has four subscale scores (fear and anxiety, avoidance, affective distress, and somatic distress) plus a total score (Brooks & Kutcher, 2004).
- The CDI developed by Kovacs (1982) is a 27-item self-rated symptom orientation scale for children aged 7 to 17 years that is useful for diagnosing physical symptoms, harm avoidance, social anxiety, and separation or panic disorder.
- The Children's Yale-Brown Obsessive–Compulsive Scale developed by Goodman et al. (1989) is a 19-item scale that can help diagnose childhood obsessive–compulsive disorder in children aged 6 to 17 years.
- The SNAP-IV developed by Swanson (1983) is a 90-item teacher and parent rating scale containing items from the Conners' questionnaire for measuring inattention and overactivity; it is useful for diagnosing attention deficit hyperactivity disorder (ADHD—inattentive and impulsive types) and oppositional defiant disorder.
- The 6-item Kutcher Adolescent Depression Scale (KADS) is a screening tool for youth at risk for depression that can be used in such institutional settings as schools. It evolved from the 11-item KADS that can be used for monitoring an adolescent's response to (psychopharmacologic) treatment (Brooks, 2004).

about the death of his father, it is important to recognize that, although children can acknowledge physical death, depending on their age, they can consider it as temporary or gradual and not fully separate from life. The young boy may believe that his father continues to live (in the ground where he was buried) and ask questions about his activities (e.g., how is Dad eating, going to the toilet, breathing, playing?) (National Cancer Institute, 2005). The child may also believe that something the child thought or did actually caused the father's illness and subsequent death. In response to death, children younger than 5 years will often exhibit disturbances in eating, sleeping, and bladder or bowel control that may result in a parent's seeking help (Grollman, 1990). Language should be kept simple and tailored to the child's developmental level. Any discussion about death should include concrete terms (e.g., cancer, died, death) and avoid euphemisms (e.g., "he passed away," "he is sleeping," "we lost him"), because they can confuse children and lead to misinterpretations.

Rapport with preschool-aged children can be achieved by joining their world of play. Play is an activity by which the child transforms an experience from real life into a symbolic, nonliteral representation. Play encourages verbalizations, promotes manual strength, teaches rules and problem-solving, and helps children master control over their environment (Taylor, Menarchek-Fetkovich, & Day, 2000). With children younger than 5 years of age, assessments may be conducted in a playroom. Useful materials are paper, pencils, crayons, paints, paintbrushes, easels, clay, blocks, balls, dolls, dollhouses, puppets, animals, dress-up clothes, and a water supply. Preschool-aged children should be informed about any rules for the play. For example, the child is told that so everyone is safe, there is no running or jumping in the playroom.

When observing the child in a free play setting, attention needs to be paid to initiation of play, energy level, manipulative actions, tempo, body movements, tone, integration, creativity, products, age appropriateness, and attitudes toward adults. In addition, themes of play, expression of emotions, and temperament are important to observe. The nurse must allow children to direct and initiate these themes. When evaluating the young child's peer relationships through play therapy in a play group or school setting, observe play settings and themes, initiation of play, response to peer initiations of play, integration of affect and action during play, resolution of conflicts, responses to suggestions of others during play, and the ability to engage in role taking and role reversals (Howes & Matheson, 1992).

The nurse's roles are to be a good listener; to use appropriate vocabulary; to tolerate a child's anxious, angry, or sad behaviour; and to use reflective comments about the child's play. Through play, the nurse can assess the child's sensorimotor skills, cognitive style, adaptability, language functioning, emotional and behavioural responsiveness, social level, moral development, cop-

ing styles, problem-solving techniques, and approaches to perceiving and interpreting the surrounding world. For example, when assessing a child's problem-solving skills, the nurse might say to a preschooler, "I can see that you've noticed the tent in the corner and would like to check it out. Yes, the tent does look interesting … but I can also see that the tent looks a little scary to you … and you do not want to check it out alone. Hmm … can you think of someone whom you would like to take with you?" Then, in response to the child's answer, the nurse says, "Mr. Bear … because he protects you …. Oh, then, Mr. Bear is a great choice. You chose a friend who would be sure to keep you safe …. You made a good decision."

In any assessment, both strengths and limitations need to be addressed, with strengths then built upon to address the child's problem areas. For example, the nurse might engage a preschooler with the comment, "Sara, you are a great storyteller; I wonder if you could tell me a story about this doll, Jane, who is afraid at day care just like you."

Lidz (2003) developed a tool that the clinician can use to assess preschoolers' play (Box 29.7). Analyzing children's perceptions of fairy tales can provide the clinician with clues to culture, problems, solutions, and elements of mental functioning (LeBuffe & Naglieri, 1999; Trad, 1989).

Drawings are also used in child assessment to illuminate the child's intellect, creative talents, neuropsychological deficits, body image difficulties, and perceptions of

---

BOX 29.7 Lidz Assessment Tool

Child's Name: _____ Birth Date: ____ Age: ____
Assessor: _____ Date of Assessment: ____

Describe typical play style/sequence.

Describe range of levels of play from lowest to highest level with age estimates and within contexts of independent/facilitated, familiar/unfamiliar, single/multiple toys.

Describe language and evidence of self-talk and internalized speech.

Describe interpersonal interactions with assessor and facilitator (if not assessor).

Describe content of any play themes.

What held the child's attention the longest? (For how long?) And what were the child's toy/play preferences?

Describe the child's affective state during play.

Implications of above for intervention: _____

From Lidz, C. S. (2003). *Early childhood assessment.* Hoboken, NJ: Wiley & Sons, Inc., Copyright 2003, John Wiley & Sons. Used with permission.

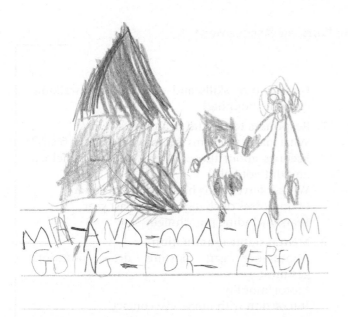

Figure 29.1. Me and my mom going for ice cream. Drawing and writing by a 5-year-old girl.

family life (Fig. 29.1). Types of drawings used in child assessments are free drawings; self-portraits; the kinetic family drawing; tree, person, house drawing; and a picture of someone of the opposite sex (Cepeda, 2000). The DECA (LeBuffe & Naglieri, 2003) screening instrument measures protective factors of attachment, self-control, and initiative in children 2 to 5 years of age. The DECA tool is used in the preschool classroom setting with the goal of promoting positive resilience in children.

School-Aged Children

Unlike preschool-aged children, school-aged (5 to 11 years) children can use more constructs, provide longer descriptions and make better inferences of others, and acquire more complete conceptions of various social roles. Children in middle school are more capable of verbal exchange and can tolerate limited periods of direct questioning. The nurse can establish rapport with school-aged children by using competitive board games, such as checkers and playing cards, or by colouring a picture or poster together with felt pens. A therapeutic game helpful in assessing the child's perceptions, cognition, and emotions and in establishing rapport between clinician and child is the thinking–feeling–doing game. In this game, the clinician and the child take turns drawing cards that pose hypothetical situations and ask what a person might think, feel, or do in such scenarios. For example, one card might say, "A boy has something on his mind that he is afraid to tell his father. What is he scared to talk about?" Another might read, "A girl heard her parents fighting. What were they fighting about? What was the girl thinking while she listened to her parents?"

Adolescents

Adolescents have an increased command of language concepts and have developed the capacity for abstract

and formal operations thinking. Their social world is also more complex. "Identity" is a core psychosocial developmental task of this phase of life (Erikson, 1968). Some early adolescents may assume that their subjective experiences are real and congruent with objective reality, which can lead to egocentrism (Shave & Shave, 1989). **Egocentrism** is a preoccupation with one's own appearance, behaviour, thoughts, and feelings. For example, a preteen may think that he caused his parents to divorce because he fought with his father the day before the parents announced their decision to separate. Because teenagers have a new, heightened sense of self-consciousness, they may be preoccupied during the interview with applying makeup or other self-grooming tasks.

During early adolescence, cognitive changes include increased self-consciousness, fear of being shamed, and demands for privacy and secrecy. An adolescent's willingness to talk to a nurse will depend partly on his or her perception of the degree of rapport between them. The nurse's ability to communicate respect, cooperation, honesty, and genuineness is important. Rejection by the adolescent, even outright hostility, during the first few interactions is not uncommon, especially if the teen is having behaviour problems at home, at school, or in the community. The nurse should be patient and avoid jumping to conclusions. Hostility or defiance may be a test of how much the teen can trust the nurse, a defense against anxiety, or a transference phenomenon (see Chapter 8).

Adolescents are likely to be defensive in front of their parents and concerned with confidentiality. At the start of the interview, the nurse should clearly convey to the adolescent what information will and will not be shared with parents. Adolescents generally prefer a straightforward, candid approach to the interview because they often distrust those in authority. Making a commitment to adolescents that they do not have to discuss anything they are not ready to reveal is important so that they will feel in control while they gradually build trust.

BIO/PSYCHO/SOCIAL/SPIRITUAL PSYCHIATRIC NURSING ASSESSMENT OF CHILDREN AND ADOLESCENTS

As discussed, the comprehensive assessment of the child or adolescent includes interviews with the child and parents, child alone, and parents alone. After completing these components, the child and parents are brought back together to receive a summary of the assessment and to respond as to whether it fits with their perceptions. The family must have a chance to share additional information and ask questions. They should be then thanked for their willingness to talk; an indication of the next steps should be given. The use of an assessment tool is helpful in organizing data for mental health planning and intervention (see Box 29.8). Feedback on the

BOX 29.8 Bio/Psycho/Social/Spiritual Psychiatric Nursing Assessment of Children and Adolescents

1. **Identifying information**
   Name
   Sex
   Date of birth
   Age
   Birth order
   Grade
   Ethnic background
   Religious preference
   List of others living in household

2. **Major reason for seeking help**
   Description of presenting problems or symptoms
   When did the problems (symptoms) start?
   Describe both the child's and the parent's perspectives.

3. **Psychiatric history**
   Previous mental health contacts (inpatient and outpatient)
   Other mental health problems or psychiatric diagnosis (besides those described currently)
   Previous medications and compliance
   Family history of depression, substance abuse, psychosis, etc., and treatment

4. **Current and past health status**
   Medical problems
   Current medications
   Surgery and hospitalizations
   Allergies
   Diet and eating habits
   Sleeping habits
   Height and weight
   Hearing and vision
   Menstrual history
   Immunizations
   If sexually active, birth control method used
   Date of last physical examination
   Paediatrician or nurse practitioner's name and telephone number

5. **Medications**
   Prescription (dosage, side effects)
   OTC drugs

6. **Neurologic history**
   Right handed, left handed, or ambidextrous
   Headaches, dizziness, fainting
   Seizures
   Unusual movement (tics, tremors)
   Hyperactivity
   Episodes of weakness or paralysis
   Slurred speech, pronunciation problems
   Fine motor skills (eating with utensils, using crayon or pencil, fastening buttons and zippers, tying shoes)

   Gross motor skills and coordination (walking, running, hopping)

7. **Responses to mental health problems**
   What makes problems (symptoms) worse or better?
   Feelings about those experiences (what helped and did not help)
   What interventions have been tried so far?
   Major losses or changes in the past year
   Fears, including punishment

8. **Mental status examination**
   Appearance, gait, posture, dress, nutrition, gestures
   Motor/motility
   Interaction with nurse, eye contact
   Psychosis, hallucinations, delusions
   Mood, affect, anxiety
   Speech (clarity, speed, volume), language (articulation, tone, modulation, coherence)
   Writing/reading (comprehension), content
   Thought patterns (organization, thought content)
   Intellectual ability, judgment, insight, general knowledge, orientation to date, time, person
   Activity level, stereotypes, mannerisms, obsessions or compulsions, attention, phobia

9. **Developmental assessment**
   Mother's pregnancy, delivery
   Child's Apgar score, whether preterm or full-term, weight at birth
   Physical maturation
   Psychosocial
   Language
   Developmental milestones: walking, talking, toileting

10. **Attachment, temperament/significant behaviour patterns**
    Attachment
    Concentration, distractibility
    Eating and sleeping patterns
    Ability to adjust to new situations and changes in routine
    Usual mood and fluctuations
    Excitability
    Ability to wait, tendency to interrupt
    Responses to discipline
    Lying, stealing, fighting, cruelty to animals, fire setting

11. **Self-concept**
    Beliefs about self
    Body image
    Self-esteem
    Personal identity

BOX 29.8 Bio/Psycho/Social/Spiritual Psychiatric Nursing Assessment of Children and Adolescents (Continued)

12. **Risk assessment**
    History of suicidal thoughts, previous attempts
    Suicide ideation, plan, lethality of plan, accessibility of plan
    History of violent, aggressive behaviour
    Homicidal ideation

13. **Family relationships**
    Relationship with parents
    Deaths/losses
    Family strengths and conflicts (nature and content)
    Nurturing and disciplinary methods
    Quality of sibling relationship
    Sleeping arrangements
    Who does the child relate to or trust in the family?
    Relationships with extended family

14. **School and peer adjustment**
    Learning difficulties and strengths
    Behaviour problems and strengths at school

School attendance
Relationship with teachers
Special classes
Best friend
Relationships with peers
Dating
Drug and alcohol use
Participation in sports, clubs, other activities
After-school routine

15. **Community resources**
    Professionals or agencies working with child or family
    Day care resources

16. **Functional status**
    See Functional Status section of this chapter.

17. **Stresses and coping behaviours**
    Psychosocial stresses
    Coping behaviours (strengths)

18. **Summary of significant data**

suggested next steps should be requested of both child and parents and any areas of disagreement discussed. A plan with which all can live is the goal.

When interviewing both child and parents, directly asking the child as many questions as possible is generally the best way for the nurse to get accurate, firsthand information and to reinforce interest in the child's viewpoint. Asking the child questions about the history of the current problem, previous psychiatric experiences (both good and bad), family psychiatric history, medical problems, developmental history (to get an idea of what the child has been told), school adjustment, peer relationships, and family functioning is particularly important. Adolescents, particularly in Western societies, are often preoccupied with love and romance. Although it tends to be considered "puppy love" by adults, unrequited love or a romantic relationship with a peer may be an important aspect of the adolescent's life and needs to be gently explored along with other peer relationships (Austin, 2003).

If necessary, the nurse can ask some or all of these same questions of the parents to get consensus or another opinion about the matter, attain supplemental information, or both. Keep in mind that developmental research shows moderate to low correlation between parent and child reports of family behaviour. It is helpful to discuss openly with the family the fact that different perspectives exist and to note that the nurse's role is not to judge or side with one view but rather to understand

the different perspectives and how they might be affecting the family.

Biologic Domain

Nurses should include a thorough history of psychiatric and medical problems in any comprehensive assessment. A physical assessment is necessary to rule out any medical problems that could be mistaken for psychiatric symptoms (e.g., weight loss resulting from diabetes, not depression; drug-induced psychosis). Pharmacologic assessment should include prescription and over-the-counter (OTC) medications. Nurses should ask about any allergies to food, medications, or environmental triggers.

Genetic Vulnerability

Research increasingly shows that major psychiatric disorders (e.g., depression, anxiety disorder, schizophrenia, bipolar disorder, substance abuse) can run in families. Thus, having a parent or sibling with a psychiatric disorder may indicate an increased risk for the same or another closely related disorder in a child or adolescent. In addition, many psychiatric disorders appearing in childhood, such as autism spectrum disorder, intellectual developmental disorder, some language disorders, attention deficit hyperactivity disorder (ADHD), Tourette's syndrome, enuresis (see Chapter 30), and trisomy disorders (e.g., Down syndrome), have genetic factors associated with their aetiology (American

Psychiatric Association, 2013). Certain disorders (e.g., ADHD, enuresis, stuttering) are more common in boys than in girls.

Neurologic Examination

A full neurologic evaluation is beyond the scope of practice for a baccalaureate-level or master's-level nurse without specific neuropsychiatric training. However, a screening of neurologic soft signs can help establish a database that will clarify the need for further neurologic consultation. The nurse should ask the child directly the brief neurologic screening questions suggested in Box 29.8 and also should note any soft signs of neurologic dysfunction, such as slurred speech, unusual movements (e.g., tics, tremors), hyperactivity, and coordination problems. The nurse can ask young children to hop on one foot, skip, or walk from toe to heel to assess their gross motor coordination and to draw with a crayon or pencil or to play pickup sticks or jacks to assess their fine motor coordination.

Psychological Domain

Children can usually identify and discuss what improves or worsens their problems. The assessment may be the first time that someone has asked the child to explain his or her view of the problem. It is also a perfect opportunity to discuss any life changes or losses (e.g., death of grandparents or pets, parental divorce) and fears.

Mental Status Examination

The mental status examination combines observation and a clinical interview (Chapter 10). The exam is conducted taking into account the child or youth's age and developmental level and presenting problems. The establishment of therapeutic rapport and the nurse's observational skills are the foundations of the assessment. The nurse should note the child's general appearance, including age (actual and apparent), self-care/hygiene, and dress. The nurse also should note the child's nonverbal behaviour, including posture, tone of voice, eye contact, and affect. What is the child or youth's attitude toward the interviewer, others involved, and the interview process itself? How active is the child? Does the child seem to have difficulty focusing on the interview, sitting still, refraining from impulsive behaviour, and listening without interrupting? Does the child seem underactive, lethargic, distant, or hopeless?

The child's sentence structure and vocabulary needs to be observed for a general sense of his or her intellectual functioning. Speech patterns, such as rate (overly fast or slow), clarity, and volume, and any speech dysfluencies (e.g., stuttering, halting) are important in screening for mood disorders (e.g., depression, mania), language disorders, psychotic processes, and anxiety disorders.

Asking children general questions about their everyday lives and observing the content and process of their play (e.g., ability to focus on an activity, play themes, boundaries between themselves and others) help to reveal the level of organization and content of their thinking. The level of speech organization should be noted. Young children normally shift subjects rather abruptly, but adolescents should continue with one train of thought before moving to another. Any morbid or eccentric thoughts, violent fantasies, and self-deprecating statements that could reflect a poor self-concept should also be noted. Assessment of preteens and adolescents should address substance use and sexual activity, because responses may provide useful information about high-risk behaviour or harmful substance use. In addition, the nurse should inquire about any obsessions or compulsions (e.g., worries about germs, severe handwashing).

Developmental Assessment

A developmental assessment is one of the core components of any psychiatric evaluation. Determining psychopathology involves evaluating the extent to which behaviours and experiences are appropriate for a child's age and stage of development. Developmental disorders are commonly associated with psychiatric and behavioural disorders.

Disorders characterized by intellectual disabilities (mild, moderate, severe, and profound forms) are distinguished from disorders that affect specific functional domains (communication disorders, specific learning disorders, attention deficit hyperactivity disorder, or motor disorders), as well as from an autism spectrum disorder that exhibits a distinctive pattern of deviation from the normal developmental trajectory. The conditions are not mutually exclusive, and comorbidity is common. Therefore, it is necessary to evaluate both the extent to which development is progressing at the right rate and the extent to which it is following the correct path.

It is best to obtain information from a variety of sources (parents, teachers, other professionals) and to use a number of different methods of gauging progress (developmental history, current functioning by report and on specific tests) to ensure an accurate developmental picture. A comprehensive assessment may require input from a range of professionals (psychiatrists, psychologists, speech/language and occupational therapists, physiotherapists) and entail some form of multidisciplinary evaluation (Bolton, 2001). The key areas for assessment include maturation, psychosocial development, and language.

Maturation

Healthy development of the brain and nervous system during childhood and adolescence provides the foundation for successful functioning throughout life. Such development, called **maturation**, unfolds through sequential and orderly growth processes. These processes are biologically and genetically based but depend on constant interactions with a stimulating and nurturing environment.

If trauma impairs the process of normal biologic maturation, developmental delays and disorders that may not be fully reversible can result. Trauma is defined as experiences that overwhelm an individual's capacity to cope. Trauma early in life, including child abuse, neglect, witnessing violence, and disrupted attachment, as well as later traumatic experiences such as violence, accidents, natural disaster, war, sudden unexpected loss, and other life events that are out of one's control can be devastating. There are a number of dimensions of trauma, including magnitude, complexity, frequency, duration, and whether it occurs from an interpersonal or external source (BC Provincial Mental Health and Substance Use Planning Council, 2013).

The nurse can assess for developmental delays by asking questions from specific sections of the mental status examination:

- *Intellectual functioning*: Evaluate the child's creativity, spontaneity, ability to count money and tell time, academic performance, memory, attention, frustration tolerance, and organization.
- *Gross motor functioning*: Ask the child to hop on one foot, throw a ball, walk up and down the hall, and run.
- *Fine motor functioning*: Ask the child to draw a picture or play pick-up sticks.
- *Cognition*: Evaluate the child's general level of cognition by assessing the child's vocabulary, level of comprehension, drawing ability, and responsiveness to questions. Testing, such as the Wechsler Intelligence Scale for Children (WISC-III), provides measures of intelligence quotient. A psychologist usually performs such tests. Request cognitive testing if there are concerns about developmental delays or learning disabilities.
- *Thinking and perception*: Evaluate level of consciousness; orientation to date, time, and person; thought content; thought process; and judgment.
- *Social interactions and play*: Assess the child's organization, creativity, drawing capacity, and ability to follow rules. Children experiencing developmental delays may remain engaged solely in parallel play instead of moving to reciprocal play. They may consistently play with toys designed for younger children, draw crude body pictures, or display receptive (understanding) or expressive (communicative) language problems.

Psychosocial Development

Assessment of psychosocial development is very important for children with mental health problems. Various theoretical models are available from which to choose; the most commonly used model is Erikson's stages of development (see Chapter 8). When considering this model, the child's gender identity and cultural background may be variables.

Language

At birth, infants can emit sounds of all languages. Maturation of language skills begins with babbling, or the utterance of simple, spontaneous sounds. By the end of the 1st year, children can make one-word statements, usually naming objects or people in the environment. By age 2 years, they should speak in short, telegraphic sentences consisting of a verb and noun (e.g., "want cookie"). Between ages 2 and 4, vocabulary and sentence structure develop rapidly. In fact, the preschooler's ability to produce language often surpasses motor development, sometimes causing temporary stuttering when the child's mind literally works faster than the mouth.

Language development depends on the complex interaction of physical maturation of the nerves, development of head and neck musculature, hearing abilities, cognitive abilities, exposure to language, educational stimulation, and emotional well-being. Social needs create a natural inclination toward communication, but the child needs reinforcement to develop correct pronunciation, vocabulary, and grammar.

Before a diagnosis of a communication disorder (i.e., impairment in language expression, comprehension, or both) can be made, the child must be tested to rule out hearing, visual, or other neurologic problems. Brain damage, especially to the left hemisphere (dominant for language in most individuals), can seriously impair the development of communication abilities in children. Any child who has experienced brain damage from anoxia at birth, congenital trauma, head injury, infection, tumour, or drug exposure should be closely monitored for signs of a communication disorder. Before the age of 5 years, the brain has amazing plasticity; and sometimes, other intact areas of the brain can take over functions of damaged areas, especially with immediate speech therapy. Genetically based disorders such as autism can cause language delays that are sometimes permanent and severe. Children with language delays need particular encouragement to communicate in a way that others can understand, because they tend to compensate by using nonverbal signals (Tanguay, 2000).

The nurse must recognize normal variations in child development and assess lags in the development of vocabulary and sentence structure during the critical preschool years (Table 29.4). Delays in this area can seriously affect other areas, such as cognitive, educational, and social development. Many children who receive psychiatric treatment have speech and language disorders that are sometimes undetected, either leading to or compounding their emotional problems.

By the time a child is 4 to 5 years old, he or she will have a vocabulary of approximately 2,000 words and will be able to listen well, and 90% to 100% of his or her speech will be understandable. Most English-speaking children will have mastered all English speech sounds by the age of 7 or 8. By school age, a child should be able

Table 29.4 Milestones for Normal Language Development in the Preschool Years

Age	Milestones
Birth to 3 months	Makes cooing sounds Has different cries for different needs Startles to loud sounds Soothed by calm, gentle voices
4–6 months	Babbles and makes different sounds Makes sounds back when you talk Turns his/her eyes toward a sound source Responds to music or toys that make noise
7–12 months	Waves hi/bye Responds to his/her name Lets you know what he/she wants using sounds and/or actions like pointing Begins to follow simple directions (e.g., Where is your nose?) Localizes correctly to sound by turning his/her head toward it Pays attention when spoken to
By 12–18 months	Uses common words and starts to put words together Enjoys listening to storybooks Points to body parts or pictures in a book when asked Looks at your face when talking to you
By 18–24 months	Understands more words than he/she can say Says two words together (e.g., More juice) Asks simple questions (e.g., What's that?) Takes turns in a conversation
2–3 years	Uses sentences of three or more words most of the time Understands different concepts (e.g., in/on, up/down) Follows two-part directions (e.g., Take the book and put it on the table) Answers simple questions (e.g., Where is the car?) Participates in short conversations
3–4 years	Tells a short story or talks about daily activities Talks in sentences with adult-like grammar Generally speaks clearly so people understand Hears you when you call from another room Listens to TV at the same volume as others Answers a variety of questions

Source: Speech-Language & Audiology Canada. (2014). *Speech, language and hearing milestones.* Retrieved from www.sac-oac.ca

to speak in complete sentences with minor grammatical errors. A child's language skills continue to develop through the school years. From about age 9 to 19, most growth occurs in the area of written language (Canadian Association of Speech-Language Pathologists and Audiologists, 2000).

Attachment: The Caregiving Context

Researchers and clinicians who assess early emerging social–emotional and behavioural problems tend to believe that children must be evaluated in relation to their primary caregivers (Carter et al., 2004). Although parents usually serve as the primary caregivers, in today's world, other family members (biologically or psychologically related), babysitters, day care, and club activity

staff, to name a few, often play a significant role in the development of child attachment and should be assessed. In addition, recognizing that children respond differently in different situations, the routine environments in which the child interacts need to be evaluated. Finally, the nurse considers the contexts of culture, class, ethnicity, language, stigma, and social exclusion on the therapeutic process and negotiates care that is sensitive to these influences as suggested by the Canadian Federation of Mental Health Nurses (2014), in the *Standards of Psychiatric-Mental Health Nursing.*

Secure Attachment

Secure attachments in early childhood produce cooperative, harmonious parent–child relationships in which the child is responsive to the parents' socialization efforts and likely to adopt the parents' viewpoints, values, and goals. Securely attached young children tend to socialize competently, be popular with well-acquainted peers during the preschool years, and have warm relationships with important adults in their lives. They see themselves and others constructively and have relatively sophisticated emotional and moral understanding (Thompson, 2002).

Mothers and fathers foster security of attachment and exploration and thus provide psychological security for the child. Security of attachment involves tender loving care, comfort and consolation, and external help with emotion regulation. Security of exploration, based on sensitive support from both mother and father, allows a child to explore to gain knowledge and skills (Grossman, Grossman, Kindler, & Zimmerman, 2008). The quality of the emotional bond between the infant and parental or caregiver figures provides the groundwork for future relationships.

The need to touch and be close to a parental figure appears biologically driven and has been demonstrated in classic studies of monkeys who bonded with a terrycloth surrogate mother (Harlow, Harlow, & Suomi, 1971). A secure attachment is based on the caretaker's consistent, appropriate response to the infant's attachment behaviours (e.g., crying, clinging, calling, following, protesting). Children who have developed a secure attachment protest when their parents leave them (beginning at about age 6 to 8 months), seek comfort from their parents in unfamiliar situations, and playfully explore the environment in the parent's presence. If the child develops an insecure attachment, perhaps due to unresponsiveness or mixed responses to a child's attachment behaviours on the part of parents, it is evidenced by clinging and lack of exploratory play when the parent is present and intense protest when the parent leaves (Thompson, 2002).

Disrupted Attachments

Disrupted attachments resulting from deficits in infant attachment behaviours, lack of responsiveness by caregivers to the child's cues, or both may lead to a diagnosis of reactive attachment disorder, feeding disorder, failure to thrive, or anxiety disorder. A reactive attachment disorder may exist when a child, before the age of 5 years, demonstrates a pattern of markedly disturbed and developmentally inappropriate attachment behaviours in which he or she rarely or minimally turns preferentially to an attachment figure for comfort, support, protection, and nurturance (APA, 2013). Infants with **disorganized attachment** appear to be unable to maintain the strategic adjustments in attachment behaviour, represented by organized avoidant or ambivalent attachment strategies, with the result that an alteration in both behavioural and physiologic behaviour occurs. Preschoolers with disorganized attachment manifest behaviours of fear, contradictory behaviour, or disorientation or disassociation in the caregivers' presence. Research findings indicate that attachment disorder behaviours correlate with attention and conduct problems (O'Connor & Rutter, 2000).

Attachment Theory

Attachment theory describes a disorganized attachment as a consequence of extreme insecurity that results from a disrupted attachment from the primary caregiver (Solomon & George, 1999). Emotional or physical separation can result from parental mental health problems, such as substance use or depression, or from frequently changing caregivers such as may be experienced by a child in foster care.

Bowlby's early studies (Bowlby, 1969) of maternal deprivation formed the initial framework for attachment theory, based on the notion that the infant tends to bond to one primary parental figure, usually the mother. Contemporary nursing theories, such as Barnard's parent–child interaction model (1994), have stressed the importance of the interaction between the child's spontaneous behaviour and biologic rhythms and the mother's ability to respond to cues that signal distress (Baker et al., 1998). The model provides the foundation for the development of several scales measuring dimensions of attachment. These standardized, observational assessment scales use routine parent–child interaction activities involving feeding (the Nursing Child Assessment of Feeding Scale, or NCAFS—76 items, birth to 1 year) and teaching (NCATS scale—73 items, birth to 3 years) to assess a dyad's strengths and limitations during the early years. Areas assessed include contingency (reciprocal communication patterns between caregiver and child), positioning (caregiver's sensitivity to child developmental stage and needs), verbalness (ability to stimulate language development), sensitivity (psychological availability and responsivity to the child), affect (positive or negative quality of communication patterns), and attention regulation (engaging and disengaging behaviours). Such measures can provide informed assessments to nurses in a variety of settings, such as postpartum hospital care, the home (e.g., public health newborn visits), or primary care settings (e.g., mental health nurse in community health centre).

Self-Concept

Self-concept is a child's knowledge about self. For young children, eliciting their view of themselves and the world through projective techniques is helpful. For example, the answers to "What would you wish for if you had three wishes?" can be revealing. An inability to wish for anything beyond a nice meal or place to live may reflect hopelessness, whereas wishes to conquer the world or put one's teacher in jail may indicate feelings of grandiosity. Another technique is to tell a story and ask the child to make up an ending for it. For example, a baby bird fell out of a nest—"What happened to it?" Or a little girl went to the mall with her mother but got lost—"What happened to her?" The nurse may design stories to elicit particular fears or concerns that based on what may be relevant for the individual child.

Drawings also provide an excellent window into the child's internal world (Fig. 29.2). Asking the child to draw a picture of a person can provide data about the child's self-concept, sexual identity, body image, and developmental level. By age 3 years, children should be able to draw some facial features and limbs, but their drawings may have an "x-ray" quality, in which clothing is transparent and the body can be seen underneath. Older children should produce more sophisticated drawings, unless they are resistant to the task. After the child has finished the

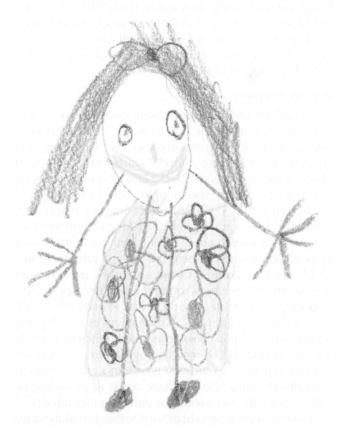

Figure 29.2. Self-portrait of a girl, age 5.

drawing, the nurse can ask what the person in the drawing is thinking and feeling, using this device to assess the child's mental processes. For example, one adolescent with school phobia drew a person fully dressed, in great detail, but with no feet. When asked about the drawing, he said that the boy could not go anywhere because his mother was afraid to let him leave home.

Other ways to assess children's self-concepts include asking them what they want to do when they grow up, what their best subjects are in school, what things they are really good at, and how well-liked they are at school. Before concluding an individual interview with a child, it is important to ask whether the child has any other information to share and whether he or she has any questions.

Nurses need to recognize the difference between self-concept and self-esteem. Self-esteem is a child's general attitude about himself. Self-concept and self-esteem have a lot in common and can be similarly assessed. Both are reflective processes that are also influenced by comparison with others around you and how others respond to you. The main difference in self-esteem is the addition of feelings.

Although relatively rare, some children's sense of self is affected by gender dysphoria; that is, they strongly feel that there is a discrepancy between the sex they were assigned at birth and their own sense of gender. For instance, a girl may feel she is a boy, even though her body is female. This gender confusion can occur at a young age and may or may not be temporary. If it causes significant distress for the child or youth, parents may wish for an assessment from a paediatric endocrinologist or from a nurse clinician, psychiatrist, or psychologist with expertise in this area.

Risk Assessment

The child should be asked about any suicidal or violent thoughts. The best way to assess these areas is to ask straightforward questions, such as, "Have you ever thought about hurting yourself? Have you ever thought about hurting someone else? Have you ever acted on these thoughts? Have you thought about how you would do it? What did you think would happen if you hurt yourself? Have you ever done anything to hurt yourself before?" Contrary to popular belief, talking about suicide with someone who can help can provide great relief to a child or youth. Further, no age should be exempt from assessment because even young children attempt suicide, and they are capable of violent acts toward other children, adults, and animals. An assessment of lethality and access to means must also be assessed to determine risk. Questions such as "Do you have a plan to hurt yourself (or others)? How would you go about hurting yourself (or others)?" and "Do you have access to guns, knives, pills ... (or whatever means the child has identified)?"

The Tool for Assessment of Suicide Risk for Adolescents (TASR-A) is a clinical tool that assists in the evaluation of adolescents at imminent risk for suicide. A semistructured measure, it helps clinicians ensure that in their evaluation of an adolescent, the most common risks factors are assessed. It was derived from the adult TASR that was developed for use in emergency room, hospitals, and outpatient settings (Chehil & Kutcher, 2012).

When a child shares the intent to commit a suicidal or violent act, the nurse must inform the child that the nurse will have to discuss this concern with the parent to keep the child and others safe. It is helpful to ask the child if there is anything in particular to be said to the parent and the child wants to be present when the nurse talks with the parents. Although painful, such conversations can serve as an abrupt halt to the charade of happiness that the child may feel forced to portray to the outside world and often open honest dialogue within a family in which none has occurred for some time. Alternatively, the conversation can sometimes give words to what the family feared but were without the skills or courage to break the silence. The nurse provides a safe environment for the family to begin to face the issues.

Substance use disorders across the lifespan account for more deaths, illness, and disabilities than any other preventable health condition. Screening for potential use and abuse of substances is becoming a priority in mental health assessment of adolescents. An interview guide has been adapted from questions on substance use developed by Adlaf (Adlaf & Zdanowicz, 1999) to serve as a useful screen for identifying substance use problems in youth. Other screening tools for clinicians include the SACS: Substances and Choices Scale (Christie et al., 2010) and the CAGE questionnaire for alcohol use (Ewing, 1984). Given that many younger children engage in substance use (see Chapter 26), assessing younger children should be considered, as well (Box 29.9). Inhalant abuse, also known as sniffing, huffing, or bagging, is the deliberate inhalation of a volatile substance in order to achieve an altered mental state. Although a worldwide phenomenon, in Canada, it often affects younger children when compared to other forms of substance misuse, likely due to the ease of availability. It is also more common in minority groups; higher rates have been found in some aboriginal communities. Nurses, together with other health professionals working in collaboration with families and communities, need to advocate for appropriate education to prevent inhalant abuse, consider appropriate treatment strategies, and contribute to increased understanding of this issue through research, as long-term chronic use has been shown to cause irreversible neurologic and neuropsychological effects (Baydala, 2010).

Social Domain

Nurses addressing the social domain when working with children and youth are particularly concerned with family relationships, school functioning, and community involvement.

BOX 29.9 Practice Note 0.1: An Interview Protocol for Reviewing Chemical Use in Youths

As with other topics, questions about substance use are interactive—the answers given determine, to some extent, the subsequent questions. The questions can be used for investigating the use of tobacco, alcohol, and drugs.

TOBACCO

- Many youth smoke, do you?
- Do you ever feel you should smoke less?
- Do you wish you could smoke less than you do now?
- Have others bothered you by complaining about your smoking?
- Have you felt bad or guilty because of your smoking?
- Have you thought you had a problem because of your smoking?
- Have you ever had a medical problem as a result of your smoking?
- Have you been in hospital because of your smoking?
- Have you gone to anyone for help for a smoking problem?
- How many of your friends smoke occasionally/regularly?
- How many of your family smoke occasionally/regularly?

ALCOHOL

- Many youth drink, do you?
- Are you always able to stop drinking when you want?
- Have you felt you should drink less?
- Have others bothered you by complaining about your drinking?
- Have you felt bad or guilty because of your drinking?
- Have you been arrested or warned by police because of your drinking?
- Have you ever had "blackouts" or "flashbacks" due to your drinking?

- Have you drunk in the early morning or drunk to get rid of a hangover?
- Have you ever had any medical problem as a result of your drinking?
- Have you been in hospital because of your drinking?
- Have you gone to anyone for help for a drinking problem?
- How many of your friends drink occasionally/regularly?
- How many of your family drink occasionally/regularly?

DRUGS

- Many youth use drugs; do you?
- Do you ever feel concerned about your drug use?
- Are you always able to stop using drugs when you want?
- Have you been arrested or warned by police because of your drug use?
- Have you ever had "blackouts" or "flashbacks" due to your drug use?
- Do you wish you could use fewer drugs than you do now?
- Have you ever had any medical problems as a result of your drug use?
- Have you gone to anyone for help for a drug problem?
- Have you ever seen a doctor or been in the hospital because of your drug use?
- How many of your friends use drugs occasionally/regularly?
- How many of your family use drugs occasionally/regularly?

Adapted from Adlaf, E. M., & Zdanowicz, Y. M. (1999). A cluster-analytic study of substance problems and mental health among street youths. *American Journal of Drug and Alcohol Abuse, 25*(4), 639–660.

Family Relationship

Children depend on adults to create a safe, nurturing, and appropriate environment to support their development. The quality of the home in terms of its ability to provide appropriate physical space (living space, sleeping arrangements, safety, cleanliness), child care arrangements (age-appropriate supervision), and stimulation (activities or resources) should be assessed, either through a home visit or by discussing these issues with the family. The Home Observation for Measurement of the Environment scale (Caldwell & Bradley, 1984) is a widely used standardized measure to assess the quality of the home environment for fostering child development at any age according to cognitive, social, and emotional growth. It is a 45-item binary (yes/no) scale and best administered in the home through parent interview and observation. The scale addresses six areas: emotional and verbal responsivity of caregiver, avoidance of restriction and punishment, organization of the environment, provision of appropriate play material, caretaker involvement with child, and opportunities for variety in daily stimulation.

When gathering a family history, a genogram and timeline are also useful tools to map family members according to birth order and medical and psychiatric histories; family roles, norms, boundaries, strengths, and subgroups; birth dates, deaths, and relationships; stage in the family cycle; and critical events. To understand fully the family's values, goals, and beliefs, the nurse must consider the family's ethnic, cultural, and economic background throughout the assessment (Wright & Leahey, 2013). A comprehensive family assessment should be considered (see Chapter 15 for assessment guidelines and how to create a genogram).

School Functioning

The child's adjustment to school is also significant. Often, children are referred for a mental health assessment as a result of changes in behaviour at school. Falling grades, loss of interest in normal activities, decreased concentration, or withdrawal from or aggression toward peers may indicate that the child is experiencing emotional problems. It is very important to obtain signed permission from the parents to talk to the child's teacher about observations of the child. The nurse may want to observe the child in school, if feasible, to see how the child functions there. The parent can request a treatment planning conference in which the teacher, parent, and nurse discuss the child's school performance and plan ways to promote the child's emotional, cognitive, and social functioning in school. For older children, and in particular adolescents, the nurse should include the child, if even for only a portion of the meeting. It is critically important that children feel that they are consulted and have an opportunity to participate in the planning processes. Although such involvement is not always comfortable or even desired by all parties, it provides formal recognition of each participant involved in the change process. Suggestions emanating from such planning sessions may range from having the child tested (e.g., for learning disabilities) to designing strategies for addressing predictable situations that routinely dissolve into chaos, in which rewards result for each party (e.g., extra computer time for the child, quiet time for the parent) for improved functioning.

Community

Assessing the child's economic status, access (psychologically, geographically, economically) to health and other services, housing and home environment, exposure to environmental toxins (e.g., lead), neighbourhood safety, and exposure to violence is important in understanding the social context of children and families. Such assessment is also important given the evidence from large, longitudinal population-based studies that have demonstrated the links between social disadvantage (socioeconomic, residential stability, community efficacy, and willingness to help neighbours) and mental illness in children (Xue, Levanthal, Brooks-Gunn, & Earls, 2005) and adults (Fryers, Melzer, Jenkins, & Brugha, 2005).

Children and adolescents function better if they are linked to community supports, such as churches, recreational programs, park district programming, and after-school programming. A number of voluntary organizations such as the YWCA or Big Brothers and Big Sisters offer mentoring relationship programs for children in communities. Before making a commitment, a family should visit the organization and talk with staff to ensure that the programs are well organized and monitored by trained staff. The mentor may perform a wide range of services, from taking a child to community events, helping with homework, or talking about how the child can achieve his or her dreams and goals. Some towns offer community-based juvenile justice programs to rehabilitate children who have had an altercation with the legal system. Juvenile justice programs provide support, such as individual and family counselling and prosocial recreational activities; teach children how to make positive choices about spending free time; and closely monitor their behaviours.

Functional Status

Functional status can be evaluated in children and adolescents using various scales. The American Psychiatric Association (2013) recommends the use of the World Health Organization Disability Assessment Scale Version 2.0 (WHODAS 2.0; WHO, 2011). The WHODAS 2.0 is a generic assessment instrument for health and disability used across all diseases, including mental, neurologic, and addictive disorders. It is a 36-item self-reporting scale that is applicable in both clinical and general population settings. It produces standardized disability levels and profiles and is applicable across cultures, in all *adult* populations. There is a direct conceptual link to the International Classification of Functioning, Disability and Health. The WHODAS 2.0 covers six domains: cognition, mobility, self-care, getting along, life activities, and participation. The WHODAS for Children and Adolescents has been developed (Canino, Fisher, Alegria, & Bird, 2013).

Stresses and Coping Behaviours

Biologic, behavioural, and personality predispositions, family, and community environment may affect a child's ability to cope with stressful life events. Stressful experiences for children include the death of a loved person or pet, parental divorce, violence, physical illness (especially chronic illness), mental illness, social isolation, racial discrimination, neglect, and physical and sexual abuse. The Difficult Life Circumstances scale (Barnard, 1989) is a 28-item self-report measure, administered in interview format to a parent, to identify the existence of chronic family problems in a variety of activities of daily life (e.g., partner in jail, financial problems, partner or child abuse).

Spiritual Domain

Spiritual assessment is an important aspect of the assessment of children and adolescents. Although adult spiritual assessment tools exist, to date no validated instrument exists for use with children and adolescents. Rubin and colleagues (2009) assessed the applicability of two adult scales (the Spiritual Involvement and Beliefs Scale, the Spirituality Well-Being Scale) with chronically ill and healthy adolescents and their parents. The conclusion made was that there is a need to develop a specific spirituality scale for adolescents, as less than half of the adolescents in the study considered either scale as an effective measure of their spiritual well-being. Parents, too, did not feel the scales to be adequate measures of their own spirituality. Measuring spirituality, even with adults, continues to have its challenges and limits.

Spiritual beliefs (the way spirituality is understood by an individual) are shaped by experience, family, friends, community, culture, and religious affiliation. With children and adolescents, in particular, developmental level is a significant factor. This can be seen in children's response to loss, for instance. In addressing the spiritual domain with children and adolescents, openness and receptivity to their questions and concerns, as well as sensitivity to their level of understanding, are important. Nurses can use stories to open discussion about the way a child or an adolescent understands and gives meaning to their experiences. There is a wide range of classic and contemporary literatures (across levels of development) that address spiritual concerns such as loneliness, illness, injury, disability, and death. For instance, *The Ten Good Things About Barney* by Viorst (1972) is a story about the death of a beloved animal that can help young children to express themselves about death and dying. Adolescents may be particularly hesitant to raise their spiritual concerns unless they feel safe and comfortable. Importantly, paediatric nurses describe approaching the spiritual domain primarily at the family level (Whitehead, 2008). There is recognition that establishing a relationship with the family, as well as the child, is foundational to understanding spiritual beliefs, values, and needs (see Chapter 15).

Spiritual assessment, including the expressed values and beliefs of children, youth, and families, should be appropriately documented so that other health professionals can be involved in spiritual care. Pastoral care services are a resource in many health services, and representatives of the family's religious or cultural community may be utilized as a resource under the family's direction. For example, Aboriginal elders and/or cultural workers have been described by paediatric nurses as being very helpful in the provision of spiritual care to Aboriginal families (Whitehead, 2008).

Evaluation of Child Abuse

The CFMHN's (2014) *Standards of Psychiatric-Mental Health Nursing* identifies nurses' roles in the assessment of clients at risk for violence and abuse. There are Canadian children who suffer maltreatment (intentional physical or emotional abuse, neglect, or sexual exploitation) each year as the result of their parents' action or inaction. The harmful psychiatric and behavioural effects of children's maltreatment are broad and similar across types of abuse, with treatment having the potential for comprehensive psychological benefit (Vachon, Krueger, Rogosch, & Cicchetti, 2015).

The 2008 Canadian Incidence Study of Reported Child Abuse and Neglect (Trocmé et al., 2010), the first national report on this issue, revealed an incidence rate of 16.19 substantiated investigations per 1,000 children. The three most common categories of substantiated maltreatment were exposure to domestic violence (31%), neglect (28%), and physical abuse (15%). Emotional maltreatment accounted for another 6% of cases, whereas sexual abuse cases represented only 2% of all substantiated investigations. Most referrals (68%) came from professionals (e.g., police and school). The Ontario Incidence Study of Reported Child Abuse and Neglect 2013 notes that 78% (97, 951) of the investigations were for concerns of abuse or neglect with 22% (27, 330) related to concerns for future maltreatment. Thirty-four percent of all maltreatment investigations were substantiated. There were differences in substantiation based on subtype of sexual abuse: those involving noncontact (e.g., sex talk, voyeurism, exploitation) had the highest rate; the least involved children referred to a child protection agency due to their behaviour or contact with a known perpetrator (Fallon et al., 2017).

Despite the need for vigilance regarding child maltreatment on the part of frontline health care practitioner, barriers to the identification of maltreated children exist: lack of confidence and certainty, inadequate training, concerns regarding communicating with parents, and complicated disclosure processes (Eniola & Evarts, 2017; Kraft, Rahm & Erikkson, 2017). There is less confidence in identifying and reporting abuse that is less overt in nature, such as emotional abuse or neglect; apprehension regarding institutional support (or its lack) is also a barrier (McTavish, MacMillan, & Wathen, 2016). All health practitioners require adequate preparation to recognize potential signs of child maltreatment and knowledge of how to appropriately follow up. Those in emergency departments need to follow an established clinical pathway for the evaluation of nonaccidental injuries in children: early recognition can prevent further injury and even death (Tiyyagura, Beucher, & Bechtel, 2017).

Assessment of child abuse needs to take into consideration the child's current developmental level and understands that compromises to early development may continue in various ways through all the developmental stages that follow. It is child centred (child welfare is critical) and family focused (most child abuse occurs within the family), has a community context (forms a key part of the child's environment), and is culturally sensitive (the nurse must be culturally competent). It also involves gathering information from a number of stakeholders and ensures that information is gathered in a coordinated way to maximize the integrity of the data collection.

Three general areas should be addressed in any assessment (English, 1996):

1. Are the child's immediate circumstances unsafe? Does the child have to be taken into care or removed to a safe place?
2. For current cases, what is the assessed risk of repeat abuse? What are the issues that merit intervention on a priority basis?
3. For ongoing cases, to what extent are interventions working? What is the current situation of the child, the family, and any substitute care arrangement?

In a review of the literature focused on physical, sexual, and psychological abuse and neglect of children, Hoft and Haddad (2017) concluded that a comprehensive screening tool or protocol for capturing all forms of child abuse and neglect has yet to be developed. No screening tool for psychological abuse was found; the one tool to identify neglect was without empirical support. Scales to assess physical abuse were noted, but for use in specific environments: the "Escape Form" (for all ages in the emergency room) and the "TEN-4 Bruising Clinical Decision Rule (children under 48 months in paediatric intensive care; Hoft & Haddad, 2017).

Nurses must understand the forensic implications of an assessment of a child for abuse. The information gathered needs to be such that it will have validity in court, if necessary. Language and vocabulary that are age-appropriate (e.g., anatomical terms) and nonleading questions must be used. Immediate referral to or consultation with a nurse or physician trained in this area, including the use of anatomically correct dolls in obtaining information, is recommended.

Nurses are ethically and legally responsible for reporting abuse to the appropriate provincial and child protection systems. Mandated reporting laws are designed to allow the provinces and territories and child protection systems to investigate the possibility of abuse, provide protection to children, and link families with the support and services that they need to reduce the risk for further abuse (see Web Links re: information on such provincial and territorial legislation).

Nurses working with traumatized children should resist the temptation to view the child as the only victim. It will help the nurse maintain empathy toward the parents if it is acknowledged that most parents were themselves traumatized as children and may therefore have limited coping mechanisms or little access to positive parental role models. Once agencies intervene to establish the child's safety, a family system approach that is supportive of the whole family unit is most effective.

Experts recommend that, when possible, nurses report abuse in the presence of the parents, preferably with the parent initiating the telephone call, and that

the professional should explain the reporting as necessary to provide safety for the child and to obtain services for the family. If the parents cannot be present when the report is made, the nurse should, at minimum, notify the family that the report was made and explain the reasons. A major protective factor against psychopathology stemming from abuse and neglect is the establishment of a supportive relationship with at least one adult who can provide empathy, consistency, and caring for the child.

The decision to report abuse sometimes poses an ethical dilemma for nurses as they try to balance the need to maintain the family's trust against the need to protect the child. This decision is further complicated by the knowledge that, if temporary out-of-home placement is necessary, the effect of the placement may also contribute to the child's and family's suffering. However, with interventions that support and attend to the parents with physical, financial, mental health (with respect to parents' own trauma history), and medical resources that will reduce stress within the family system, further distress, harm, and abuse can be prevented. See Chapter 34 for further understanding of caring for abused persons.

 SUMMARY OF KEY POINTS

- Nurses working with children and adolescents are in a key position to identify risk and protective factors for psychopathology and to intervene to reduce risk.
- Nurses who are aware of normal developmental processes can educate parents about their children's behaviours, help them better understand their children's reactions to stress, and decide when intervention may be warranted.
- If the process of normal biologic maturation in childhood is disrupted through trauma or neglect, developmental delays and disorders can occur, some of which may have irreversible effects.
- From early infancy, children exhibit different kinds of temperaments that are at least partially biologically determined.
- Studies of attachment show that the quality of the emotional bond between the child and the parental figure is an important determinant of the success of later relationships.
- Research shows that children who experience major losses, such as death or divorce, are at risk for developing mental health problems.
- Sibling relationships have significant effects on personality development. Positive sibling relationships can be protective factors against the development of mental health problems.
- Medical problems in childhood and adolescence may cause psychological problems when illness leads to behaviours common to an earlier

developmental stage (regression) or lack of full participation in family, school, and social activities.

- Striving for identity and independence may lead adolescents to participate in high-risk activities (e.g., substance use, including tobacco; unprotected sex; delinquent behaviours) that may lead to mental health problems.
- Poverty, homelessness, abuse, neglect, and parental alcoholism all create conditions that undermine a child's ability to make normal developmental gains and contribute to the child's vulnerability for various emotional and behavioural problems.
- Children who experience disrupted attachments because of out-of-home placements may have difficulty forming close relationships with their new parents and trusting others.
- Family support services and early intervention programs are designed to prevent the removal of the child from the family as a result of abuse or neglect and to maintain a strong, nurturing family system.
- Mental health assessment of children and adolescents includes evaluating the child's biologic, psychological, social, and spiritual factors.
- Assessment of children and adolescents differs from assessment of adults in that the nurse must consider the child's developmental level, specifically addressing the child's language, cognitive, social, and emotional skills. Establishing a treatment alliance and building rapport are essential to obtaining a good mental health history.
- The mental status examination includes observations and questions about the child's appearance, speech, language, vocabulary, orientation, knowledge base (including reading, writing, and math skills), attention level, activity level, memory, social skills, peer relationships, relationship to interviewer, mood, affect, suicidal or homicidal tendencies, thinking (presence or absence of hallucinations or delusions), substance use, and behaviours.
- Assessment of the child and caregiver together provides important information regarding child–parent attachment and parenting practices.
- A child's self-concept can be evaluated using tools such as play, stories, asking three wishes, and asking the child to draw a picture of himself or herself.
- If a child reveals suicidal ideation in the interview, the nurse must determine whether the child has a plan, let the parent know the child is suicidal, and make a plan to keep the child safe, including consideration of inpatient hospitalization.
- If a child reports to the nurse neglect or physical or sexual abuse, the nurse must by law report the child's disclosure to Child Protection Services.
- Protective factors that promote resiliency in children are active coping and the ability to solve problems, a sense of self-efficacy, self-esteem, accurate processing of social cues, supportive family environment, peer acceptance, and environmental supports that promote coping efforts and recognize and reward competence.

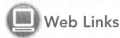 Web Links

canada.ca/en/public-health/services/reports-publications/canadian-incidence-study-reported-child-abuse-neglect.html The 2008 Canadian Incidence Study of Reported Child Abuse and Neglect can be found here.

Cwrp.ca/infosheets Information sheets about provincial reporting legislation on reporting child abuse and neglect are available at this site.

forces.gc.ca/en/caf-community-health-services-r2mr-deployment/deployment-resources-family-members.page Deployment resources for family members of the Canadian military.

youtube.com/watch?v=MuXvG9tbUMs How to make a genogram using the Skywalker Family can be found at this YouTube site.

medicine.usask.ca/documents/psychiatry/WHODAS2_20150123-1.pdf The WHODAS2 assessment form can be found at this site.

https://www.rainbowhealthontario.ca/ Rainbow Health Ontario (RHO) is a province-wide program working to improve access to services and promote the health of lesbian, gay, bisexual, trans, and queer (LGBTQ) communities. RHO is a valuable resource for a number of stakeholders, including community groups, service providers, researchers, policy makers, and educators.

https://www.cdc.gov/lgbthealth/youth-resources.htm The Centers for Disease Control and Prevention (CDC) hosts LGBT Youth Resources. Here, readers will find particularly relevant resources from the CDC, other government agencies, and community organizations that support positive environments for LGBT youth, their friends, educators, parents, and family members.

http://iacapap.org/iacapap-textbook-of-child-and-adolescent-mental-health "Promoting the mental health and development of children and adolescents through policy, practice and research" is the mandate of the International Association for Child and Adolescent Psychiatry and Allied Professionals (IACAPAP). Here, readers will find *The IACAPAP Textbook of Child and Adolescent Mental Health*, a comprehensive and innovative open access publication, complete with relevant pictures, graphics, video links, and PowerPoints for teaching purposes.

https://www.youthmentalhealth.ca/ Youth Mental Health Canada is a grassroot youth-driven and youth-led nonprofit organization that advocates for "greater funding of publicly funded, culturally sensitive, needs-based, innovative supports and services in healthcare and education."

http://www.caringforkids.cps.ca/ This easily accessible reliable parenting resource, developed by the Canadian Paediatric Society, is an excellent resource for parents and health care professionals alike. The site features resources related to growth and development, news to use (timely current events), helpful tips (e.g., communicating with teens), and an informative video library with many relevant titles specific to child and adolescent mental health.

http://www.kidsnewtocanada.ca/ Caring for Kids New to Canada is an excellent resource for health professionals working with immigrant and refugee families including resources dedicated to assessment and screening, mental health and development, and culture and health.

References

Achenbach, T. M., & Edelbrock, C. (1983). *The child behavior checklist: Manual for the child behavior checklist and revised child behavior profile.* Burlington, VT: Queen City Printers.

Adlaf, E. M., & Zdanowicz, Y. M. (1999). A cluster-analytic study of substance problems and mental health among street youths. *American Journal of Drug and Alcohol Abuse, 25*(4), 639–660.

Afifi, T. O., Taillieu, T., Zamorski, M. A., Turner, S., Cheung, K., & Sareen, J. (2016). Association of child abuse exposure with suicidal ideation, suicide plans, and suicide attempts in military personnel and the general population in Canada. *JAMA Psychiatry, 73*(3), 229–238. doi: 10.10.1001/jamapsychiatry.2015.2732

American Psychiatric Association. (2013). *Diagnostic and statistical manual of mental disorders* (5th ed.). Washington, DC: Author.

Anthony, K. K., Gil, K. M., & Schanberg, L. E. (2003). Parental perceptions of child vulnerability in children with chronic illness. *Journal of Pediatric Psychology, 28*(3), 185–190.

Arvidson, J., Kinniburgh, K., Howard, K., Spinazzola, J., Strothers, H., Evans, M., ... Blaustein, M. (2011). Treatment of complex trauma in young children: Developmental and cultural considerations in application of the ARC intervention model. *Journal of Child and Adolescent Trauma, 4*, 34–51.

Austin, W. (2003). *First love: The adolescent experience of amour.* New York, NY: Peter Lang Publishing Inc.

Baiden, P., Fallon, B., den Dunnen, W., & Boateng, G. O. (2015). The enduring effects of early childhood adversities and troubled sleep among Canadian adults: A population-based study. *Sleep Medicine, 16,* 760–767. doi.org.10.1016/j.sleep.2015.02.527

Baker, A. (2007). Fostering stories: Why caseworkers, foster parents, and foster children should read stories about being in foster care. *American Journal of Family Therapy, 35*, 151–165.

Baker J. K., Borchers, D. A., Cochran, D. T., Kaltofen, K. G., Orcutt, N., Peacock, J. A., et al. (1998). Kathryn E. Barnard: Parent–child interaction model. In A. Marriner-Tomey (Ed.), *Nursing theorists and their work* (4th ed., pp. 423–438). St. Louis, MO: Mosby.

Barnard, K. E. (1989). *Difficult life circumstances manual.* Seattle, WA: NCAST Publications, University of Washington, School of Nursing.

Barnard, K. E. (1994). The Barnard model. In G. Sumner & A. Spitz (Eds.), *NCAST caregiver/parent-child interaction feeding manual* (pp. 6–14). Seattle, WA: NCAST Publications, University of Washington, School of Nursing.

Baydala, L. (2010). Inhalant abuse. *Paediatrics & Child Health, 15*(7), 443–448.

BC Provincial Mental Health and Substance Use Planning Council. (2013). *Trauma-informed practice guide.* Retrieved from http://bccewh.bc.ca/publications-resources/documents/TIP-Guide-May2013.pdfdivorce

Beardslee, W. R., Gladstone T. R., Wright, E. J., & Cooper, A. B. (2003). A family-based approach to the prevention of depressive symptoms in children at risk: Evidence of parental and child change. *Pediatrics, 112*(2), e119–e131.

Bernard-Bonnin, A. C. (2004). Maternal depression and child development. *Pediatric Child Health, 9*(8), 575–583.

Blaustein, M. E., & Kinniburgh, K. M. (2010). *Treating traumatic stress in children and adolescents: How to foster resilience through attachment, self-regulation, and competency.* New York, NY: Guilford Press.

Bolton, P. (2001). Developmental assessment. *Advances in Psychiatric Treatment, 7*, 32–40.

Botvin, G. J. (2000). Preventing drug abuse in schools: Social and competence enhancement approaches targeting individual-level etiologic factors. *Addictive Behaviors, 25*(6), 887–897.

Bowlby, J. (1960). Grief and mourning in infancy and early childhood. *Psychoanalytic Study of the Child, 15*, 9–52.

Bowlby, J. (1969). *Attachment (Vol. 1 of Attachment and loss).* New York, NY: Basic Books.

Brendtro, L. (2009). Developmental audit. *Reclaiming Youth: Circle of Courage workshop series.* Victoria, BC.

Breton, J. J. (1999). Complementary development of prevention and mental health promotion programs for Canadian children based on contemporary scientific paradigms. *Canadian Journal of Psychiatry, 44*(3), 227–234.

Brooks, S. (2004). The Kutcher adolescent depression scale. *Child and Adolescent Psychopharmacology News, 9*(5), 4–6.

Brooks, S., & Kutcher, S. (2004). The Kutcher generalized anxiety disorder scale for adolescents: Assessment of its evaluative properties over the course of a 16-week pediatric psychopharmacotherapy trial. *Journal of Child and Adolescent Psychopharmacology, 14*(2), 273–286.

Brown, E. (2009). Helping bereaved children and young people. *British Journal of School Nursing, 4*(2), 69–73.

Brown, A., Sandler, I., Tein, J., Liu, X., & Haine, R. (2007). Implications of parental suicide and violent death for promotion of resilience of parentally-bereaved children. *Death Studies, 31*, 301–335.

Burns, J. M., Andrews, G., & Szabo, M. (2002). Depression in young people: What causes it and can we prevent it? *Medical Journal of Australia, 177*(Suppl.), S93–S96.

Caldwell, B., & Bradley, R. (1984). *Home observation for measurement of the environment.* Little Rock, AK: University of Little Rock at Arkansas.

Canada Parliament. House of Commons. Standing Committee on Human Resources, Skills and Social Development and the Status of Persons with Disabilities. (2010). *Federal poverty reduction plan: Working in partnership towards reducing poverty in Canada.* Report of the Standing Committee on Human Resources, Skills and Social Development and the Status of Persons with Disabilities, 40th Parliament, 3rd Session. Retrieved from http://www.parl.gc.ca/HousePublications/Publication.aspx?DocId=4770921&File=27&Mode=1&Parl=40&Ses=3&Language=E

Canadian Association of Speech-Language Pathologists and Audiologists. (2000). *School age speech & language development fact sheet.* Retrieved from http://www.saslpa.ca/school_age_speech_and_language.pdf

Canadian Council on Learning. (2008). *Evaluation of the Ontario Ministry of Education's Student Success/Learning to 18 strategy—Final report.* Toronto, ON: Ontario Ministry of Education.

Canadian Federation of Mental Health Nurses. (2014). *The Canadian standards for psychiatric-mental health nursing* (4th ed.). Toronto, ON: Author.

Canino, G. J., Fisher, P. W., Alegria, M., & Bird, H. R. (2013). Assessing child impairment in functioning in different contexts: Implications for use of services and the classification of psychiatric disorders. *Open Journal of Medical Psychology, 2*, 29–34.

Carter, A. S., Briggs-Gowan, M. J., & Davis, N. O. (2004). Assessment of young children's social-emotional development and psychopathology: Recent advances and recommendations for practice. *Journal of Child Psychology and Psychiatry, 45*(1), 109–134.

Casa-Gil, M. J., & Navarro-Guzman, J. I. (2002). School characteristics among children of alcoholic parents. *Psychological Reports, 90*(1), 341–348.

Cauce, A. M., Paradise, M., Ginzler, J. A., Embry, L., Morgan, C. J., Lohr, Y., & Theofelis, J. (2000). The characteristics and mental health of homeless adolescents: Age and gender differences. *Journal of Emotional and Behavioral Disorders, 8*(4), 230–239.

Cavell, T., Ennett, S. T., & Meehan, B. T. (2001). Preventing alcohol and substance abuse. In J. N. Hughes, A. M. LaGreca, & J. C. Conoley (Eds.), *Handbook of psychological services for children and adolescents* (pp. 133–160). Oxford, UK: Oxford University Press.

Centre for Addiction and Mental Health. (2012). *Mental health and addiction statistics.* Retrieved from http://www.camh.ca/en/hospital/about_camh/newsroom/for_reporters/Pages/addictionmentalhealthstatistics.aspx

Cepeda, C. (2000). *The concise guide to the psychiatric interview of children and adolescents.* Washington, DC: American Psychiatric Press.

Chang, J., & Kier, C. A. (2016). Introduction to the special issue: Divorce in the Canadian context—Interventions and family processes. *Canadian Journal of Counselling and Psychotherapy, 50*(3S), S1–S4.

Chehil, S., & Kutcher, S. (2012). *Suicide risk management: A manual for health professionals* (2nd ed.). Oxford, MS: Wiley-Blackwell.

Child and Youth Mental Health and Substance Use Collaborative. (2017, April). Trauma Informed Practice and Trauma Informed Services Resources List. Government of British Columbia and Doctors of BC. Retrieved from file:///C:/Users/drwen/Downloads/Trauma%20Informed%20and%20Trauma%20Specific%20Resources%20Guide%20April%202017.pdf

Christie, G., Marsh, R., Sheridan, J., Wheeler, A., Suaalii-Sauni, T., Black, S., & Butler, R. (2010). *The substances and choices scale manual.* Retrieved from http://www.sacsinfo.com/docs/SACSusermanual2010.pdf

Clinton, J., Feller, A. F., & Williams, R. C. (2016). The importance of infant mental health. *Paediatrics & Child Health, 21*(5), 239–241.

Costea, G. O. (2011). Considering the children of parents with mental illness: Impact on behavioral and social functioning. *Brown University Child and Adolescent Behavior Letter, 27*(4), 1–6.

Costello, E. J., Egger, H., & Angold, A. (2005). Ten-year research update review: The epidemiology of child and adolescent psychiatric disorders.

I. Methods and public health burden. *Journal of American Academy of Child and Adolescent Psychiatry*, 44(10), 972–986.

Currie, C., Zanotti, C., Morgan, A., Currie, D., de Looze, M., Roberts, C., ... Barkenow, V. (Eds.) (2011). *Social determinants of health and well-being among young people. Health Behaviour in School-aged Children (HBSC) study: International report from the 2009/2010 survey.* Copenhagen, Denmark: World Health Organization Regional Office for Europe.

Deering, C. G., & Cody, D. J. (2002). Communicating effectively with children and adults. *American Journal of Nursing*, 102(3), 34–42.

Dennis, C. L. (2005). Psychosocial and psychological interventions for prevention of postnatal depression: Systematic review. *British Medical Journal*, 331(7507), 15–24.

Dillen, L., Fontaine, J., & Verhofstadt-Denève, L. (2009). Confirming the distinctiveness of complicated grief from depression and anxiety among adolescents. *Death Studies*, 33, 437–461.

Edidin, J. P., Ganim, Z., Hunter, S. J., & Karnik, N. S. (2012). The mental and physical health of homeless youth: A literature review. *Child Psychiatry and Human Development*, 43(3), 354–375.

Eggert, L. L., Thompson, E. A., Randell, B. P., & Pike, K. (2002). Preliminary effects of brief school-based prevention approaches for reducing youth suicide: Risk behaviors, depression, and drug involvement. *Journal of Child and Adolescent Psychiatric Nursing*, 15(2), 48–64.

Elkind, D. (1967). Egocentrism in adolescence. *Child Development*, 38, 1025–1034.

Employment and Social Development Canada. (2012). *The National Shelter Study 2009–2009.* Retrieved from http://www.hrsdc.gc.ca/eng/communities/homelessness/reports/shelter_study.html

English, D. T. (1996). *The promise and reality of risk assessment: Protecting children.* Ottawa, ON: Public Health Agency of Canada. Retrieved from http://www.phac-aspc.gc.ca/ncfv-cnivf/familyviolence/html/nfntsptprevention_e.html

Eniola, K., & Evarts, L. (2017). Diagnosis of child maltreatment: A family medicine physician's dilemma. *Southern Medical Journal*, 110(5), 330–336.

Erikson, E. (1968). *Identity, youth and crisis.* New York, NY: Norton.

Eriksson, I., Cater, A., Andershed, A.-K., & Andershed, H. (2010). *Protection against externalizing and internalizing behavior among children at risk.* Paper presented at the annual meeting of the ASC Annual Meeting, San Francisco, CA.

Ewing, J. A. (1984). Detecting alcoholism: The CAGE questionnaire. *Journal of the American Medical Association*, 252(14), 1905–1907.

Fallon, B., Collin-Vézina, D., King, B., Houston, E., Joh-Carnella, N., & Black, T. (2017). *Sexual abuse substantiation by sub-types and outcomes of sexual abuse investigations by gender. CWRP Information Sheet # 188E.* Toronto, ON: Canadian Child Welfare Research Portal.

Federal-Provincial-Territorial Advisory Committee on Population Health. (2000). *The opportunity of adolescence: The health sector contribution.* Cat. N(o): H39–548/200E. Ottawa, ON: Author.

Federal-Provincial-Territorial Council of Ministers on Social Policy Renewal. (2000). *Public report: Dialogue on the national children's agenda—Developing a shared vision.* Ottawa, ON: Author.

Felitti, V. J., Anda, R. F., Nordenberg, D., Williamson, D. F., Spitz, A. M., Edwards, V., Koss, M. P., & Marks, J. S. (1998). Relationship of childhood abuse and household dysfunction to many of the leading causes of death in adults. The Adverse Childhood Experiences (ACE) Study. *American Journal of Preventive Medicine*, 14(4), 245–258.

Fluke, J., Chabot, M., Fallon, B., MacLaurin, B., & Blackstock, C. (2010). Placement decisions and disparities among Aboriginal groups: An application of the decision-making ecology through multi-level analysis. *Child Abuse and Neglect*, 34(1), 57–69.

Forgatch, M., & Patterson, G. (1989). *Parents and adolescents: Living together (Part 2: Family problem-solving).* Eugene, OR: Castalia Publishing Company.

Foster, K., O'Brien, L., & Korhonen, T. (2012). Developing resilient children and families when parents have mental illness: A family-focused approach. *International Journal of Mental Health Nursing*, 21(1), 3–11.

Fox, B. H., Perez, N., Cass, E., Baglivio, M. T., & Epps, N. (2015). Trauma changes everything: Examining the relationship between adverse childhood experiences and serious, violent and chronic juvenile offenders. *Child Abuse & Neglect*, 46, 163–173. doi.org/10.1016/j.chiabu.2015.01.011

Freeman, J. G., King, M., Pickett, W., Craig, W., Elgar, F., Janssen, I., & Klinger, D. (2010). *The health of Canada's young people: A Mental health focus.* Retrieved from http://www.phac-aspc.gc.ca/hp-ps/dca-dea/publications/hbsc-mental-mentale/assets/pdf/hbsc-mental-mentale-eng.pdf

Fryers, T., Melzer, D., Jenkins, R., & Brugha T. (2005). The distribution of the common mental disorders: Social inequalities in Europe. *Clinical Practice in Epidemiology and Mental Health*, 1, 14.

Gaetz, S., Donaldson, J., Richter, T., & Gulliver, T. (2013). *The state of homelessness in Canada.* Toronto, ON: Canadian Homelessness Research Network Press.

Gass, K., Jenkins, J., & Dunn, J. (2007). Are sibling relationships protective? A longitudinal study. *Journal of Child Psychology and Psychiatry*, 48(2), 167–175.

Gimpel, G., & Holland, M. (2003). *Emotional and behavioral problems of young children: Effective interventions in the preschool and kindergarten years.* New York, NY: Guilford Press.

Gladstone, B. M., Boydell, K. M., Seeman, M. V., & McKeever, P. D. (2011). Children's experiences of parental mental illness: A literature review. *Early Intervention in Psychiatry*, 5(4), 271–289.

Glaser, D. (2000). Child abuse and neglect and the brain: A review. *Journal of Child Psychology and Psychiatry*, 41(1), 97–116.

Goodman, W. K., Price, L. H., Rasmussen, S. A., Mazure, J. C., Fleischmann, R. L., Hill, C. L., ... Charney, D. S. (1989). The Children's Yale-Brown Obsessive Compulsive Scale (CYBOCS). I. Development, use, and reliability. *Archives of General Psychiatry*, 46, 1006–1011.

Government of Canada. (2008). *Family life—Divorce.* Retrieved from http://well-being.esdc.gc.ca/misme-iowh/.3ndic.1t.4r@-eng.jsp?iid=76

Grant, C. N., & Bélanger, R. E. (2017). Position Statement: Cannabis and Canada's children and youth. *Paediatrics & Child Health*, 22(2), 98–102.

Grollman, E. A. (1990). *Talking about death: A dialogue between parent and child* (3rd ed.). Boston, MA: Beacon Press.

Grossman, K., Grossman, K. E., Kindler, H., & Zimmerman, P. (2008). A wider view of attachment and exploration: The influence of mothers and fathers on the development of psychological security from infancy to young adulthood. In J. Cassidy & P. Shaver (Eds.), *Handbook of attachment: Theory, research, and clinical applications* (2nd ed., pp. 857–879). New York, NY: Guilford Press.

Hango, D, (2017, September). *Childhood physical abuse: Difference by birth cohort.* Insights on Canadian society. Statistics Canada Catalogue no. 75-006-X.

Harlow, H. F., Harlow, M. K., & Suomi, S. J. (1971). From thought to therapy: Lessons from a private laboratory. *American Scientist*, 59(5), 538–549.

Harter, S. (2000). Psychosocial adjustment of adult children of alcoholics: A review of recent empirical literature. *Clinical Psychology Review*, 20(3), 311–337.

Hetherington, E. M., & Kelly, J. (2002). *For better or for worse: Divorce reconsidered.* New York, NY: WW Norton.

Hodas, G. (2004). Restraint and seclusion are therapeutic failures. *Residential Group Care Quarterly*, 1, 12–13.

Hoft, M., & Haddad, L. (2017). Screening children for abuse and neglect: A review of the literature. *Journal of Forensic Nursing*, 13(1), 26–32. doi:10.1097/JFN.0000000000000136

Howes, C., & Matheson, C. (1992). Sequences in the development of competent play with peers: Social and social pretend play. *Developmental Psychology*, 28(5), 961–974.

Hulchanski, J. D., Campsie, P., Chau, S. B. Y., Hwang, S. H., & Paradis, E. (Eds.) (2009). *Finding home: Policy options for addressing homelessness in Canada.* Retrieved from http://www.homelesshub.ca/library/finding-home-policy-options-for-addressing-homelessness-in-canada-45761.aspx

Infant Mental Health Promotion. (2005). *Core prevention and intervention for the early years.* Retrieved from http://www.imhpromotion.ca/Portals/0/IMHP%20PDFs/Core%20Prevention_Supporting%20References.pdf

Kelly, J. (2003). Changing perspectives on children's adjustment following divorce: A view from the United States. *Childhood*, 10(3), 237–254.

Kelly, K., & Caputo, T. (2007). Health and street/homeless youth. *Journal of Health Psychology*, 12(5), 726–736.

Kinniburgh, K. J., Blaustein, M., & Spinazzola, J. (2005). Attachment, self-regulation, and competency: A comprehensive intervention framework for children with complex trauma. *Psychiatric Annals*, 35(5), 424–430.

Korczak, D. (2012). Identifying depression in childhood: Symptoms, signs and significance. *Pediatrics & Child Health*, 17(1), 572.

Kovacs, M. (1982). *Children's depression inventory.* North Tonawanda, NY: Multi-Health Systems.

Kraft, L. E., Rahm, G., & Erikkson, U. (2017). The school nurse's ability to detect and support abused children: A trust-creating process. *The Journal of School Nursing*, 33(2), 133–142.

Kutcher, S., & McLuckie, A. (2010). *Evergreen: A child and youth mental health framework for Canada.* Calgary, AB: Mental Health Commission of Canada.

Kutcher, S. & McLuckie, A.; for the Child and Youth Advisory Committee, Mental Health Commission of Canada. (2010). *Evergreen: A child and youth mental health framework for Canada.* Calgary, AB: Mental Health Commission of Canada.

Langlois, K. A., & Garner, R. (2013). Trajectories of psychological distress among Canadian adults who experienced parental addiction in childhood. *Health Reports*, 24(3), 14–21.

LeBlanc, L. A., Goldsmith, T., & Patel, D. R. (2003). Behavioral aspects of chronic illness in children and adolescents. *Pediatric Clinics of North America*, 50(4), 859–878.

LeBuffe, P. A., & Naglieri, J. A. (1999). *Devereux early childhood assessment. The Devereux Foundation.* Lewisville, NC: Kaplan Press.

LeBuffe, P. A., & Naglieri, J. A. (2003). *The Devereux early childhood assessment clinical form (DECA).* Lewisville, NC: Kaplan Press.

Leventhal, T., & Brooks-Gunn, J. (2000). The neighborhoods they live in: The effects of neighborhood residence on child and adolescent outcomes. *Psychological Bulletin, 126,* 309–337.

Lidz, C. S. (2003). *Early childhood assessment.* Hoboken, NJ: Wiley & Sons.

Maguire, S., Mann, M. K., Sibert, J., & Kemp, A. (2005). Are there patterns of bruising in childhood which are diagnostic or suggestive of abuse? A systematic review. *Archives of Disease in Childhood, 90*(2), 182–186.

Manning, C., & Gregoire, A. (2006). Effects of parental mental illness on children. *Psychiatry, 8*(1) 7–9.

March, J. (1997). *Multidimensional anxiety scale for children.* North Tonawanda, NY: Multi-Health Systems.

Martinez, Y., & Ercikan, K. (2009). Chronic illnesses in Canadian children: What is the effect of illness on academic achievement, and anxiety and emotional disorders? *Child: Care, Health and Development, 35*(3), 391–401.

Masten, A. S. (2001). Ordinary magic: Resilience processes in development. *American Psychologist, 56*(3), 227–238.

McEwen, B. S. (2004). Protection and damage from acute and chronic stress: Allostasis and allostatic overload and relevance to the pathophysiology of psychiatric disorders. *Annals of the New York Academy of Sciences, 1032,* 1–7.

McEwen, B. S. (2007). Physiology and neurobiology of stress and adaptation: Central role of the brain. *Physiological Review, 87,* 873–904.

McKay, A. (2013). *Trends in Canadian national and provincial/territorial teen pregnancy rates: 2001–2010.* Retrieved from http://www.sieccan.org/pdf/TeenPregancy.pdf

McKenna, K. (2007). *Training 'who' to do 'what': Reappraising the role function and purpose of training in the management of aggression and violence within clinical settings.* 5th European Congress on Clinical Violence in Psychiatry, October 25–27, Amsterdam, the Netherlands.

McTavish, J. R., MacMillan, H. L., & Wathen, C. N. (2016). *Briefing note: Mandatory reporting of child maltreatment.* VEGA Project and PreVAIL Research Network.

Melhem, N., Moritz, G., Walker, M., Shear, M. K., & Brent, D. (2007). Phenomenology and correlates of complicated grief in children and adolescents. *Journal of the American Academy of Child and Adolescent Psychiatry, 46*(4), 493–499.

Mental Health Commission of Canada. (2016). *The mental health strategy for Canada: A youth perspective.* Ottawa, ON: Author. Retrieved from https://www.mentalhealthcommission.ca/sites/default/files/2016-07/Youth_Strategy_Eng_2016.pdf

Minhas, R. S., Graham, H., Jegathesan, T., Huber, J., Young, E., & Barozzino, T. (2017). Supporting the development health of refugee children and youth. *Paediatrics & Child Health, 22*(2), 68–71.

Mulcahy, M., & Trocmé, N. (2010). *Children and youth in out-of-home care in Canada.* Retrieved from http://cwrp.ca/sites/default/files/publications/en/ChildrenInCare78E.pdf

Mulvihill, D. (2005). The health impact of childhood trauma: An interdisciplinary review, 1997–2003. *Issues in Comprehensive Pediatric Nursing, 28*(2), 115–136.

Murphy, T., & Bennington-Davis, M. (2005). *Restraint and seclusion: The model for eliminating their use in health care.* Marblehead, MA: HCPro, Inc.

Murphy, T. & Bennington-Davis, M. (2006). *Engagement model and trauma-informed care.* Presentation to Child and Youth Mental Health Programs, University of British Columbia, Vancouver, BC.

Mylant, M. L., Ide, B., Cuevas, E., & Meehan, M. (2002). Adolescent children of alcoholics: Vulnerable or resilient? *Journal of the American Psychiatric Nurses Association, 8*(2), 57–64.

National Cancer Institute, US National Institutes of Health. (2005). *Grief, bereavement, and coping with loss.* Retrieved from http://www.cancer.gov/cancertopics/pdq/supportivecare/bereavement/Patient/page1/AllPages

O'Connor, T. G., Bredenkamp, D., & Rutter, M. (1999). Attachment disturbances and disorders in children exposed to early severe deprivation. *Infant Mental Health Journal, 20*(1), 10–29.

O'Connor, T., & Rutter, M. (2000). Attachment disorder behavior following early severe deprivation: Extension and longitudinal follow-up. *Journal of the American Academy of Child and Adolescent Psychiatry, 39*(6), 709–712.

Offord, D. R., & Bennett, K. J. (2002). Prevention. In M. Rutter & E. Taylor (Eds.), *Child and adolescent psychiatry* (4th ed.). Oxford, UK: Blackwell Science.

Offord, D. R., Kraemer, H. C., Kazdin, A. E., Jensen, P. S., & Harrington, R. (1998). Lowering the burden of suffering from child psychiatric disorder: Trade-offs among clinical, targeted, and universal interventions. *Journal of the American Academy of Child and Adolescent Psychiatry, 37*(7), 686–694.

Peacock, S. Konrad, S., Watson, E., Nickel, D., & Muhajarine, N. (2013) Effectiveness of home visiting programs on child outcomes: A systematic review. *BMC Public Health, 13*(17). doi.org/10.1186/1471-2458-13-17

Peters, R., Petrunka, K., & Arnold, R. (2003). The Better Beginnings, Brighter Futures Project: A universal, comprehensive, community-based prevention approach for primary school children and their families. *Journal of Clinical Child and Adolescent Psychology, 32,* 215–227.

Pfund, R. (2006). *Palliative care nursing for children and young people.* Oxford, UK: Radcliffe.

Porges, S. (2004). Neuroception: A subconscious system for detecting threats and safety. *Zero to Three,* 19–24.

Public Health Agency of Canada. (2010a). *Canadian incidence study of reported child abuse and neglect—2008: Major findings.* Ottawa, ON: Author.

Public Health Agency of Canada. (2010b). *Canadian guidelines on sexually transmitted infections.* Retrieved from http://www.phac-aspc.gc.ca/std-mts/sti-its/cgsti-ldcits/section-5-1-eng.php

Public Health Agency of Canada. (2012). *Depression in pregnancy.* Retrieved from http://www.phac-aspc.gc.ca/mh-sm/preg_dep-eng.php

Public Health Agency of Canada. (2016). *Chief Public Health Officer's report on the state of public health in Canada: A focus on family violence in Canada.* Ottawa ON: Author. Cat: HP2-1DE-PDF. https://www.canada.ca/content/dam/canada/public-health/migration/publications/department-ministere/state-public-health-family-violence-2016-etat-sante-publique-violence-familiale/alt/pdf-eng.pdf

Puskar, K. R., Sereika, S., & Tusaie-Mumford, K. (2003). Effect of the Teaching Kids to Cope (TKC) program on outcomes of depression and coping among rural adolescents. *Journal of Child and Adolescent Psychiatric Nursing, 16*(2), 71–80.

Research Unit on Pediatric Psychopharmacology (RUPP) Anxiety Study Group. (2002). The pediatric anxiety rating scale (PARS): Development and psychometric properties. *Journal of the American Academy of Child and Adolescent Psychiatry, 41,* 1061–1069.

Reynolds, C. R., & Kamphouse, R. W. (1998). *Behavior assessment system for children (BASC).* Circle Pines, MN: American Guidance Service.

Ritter, J., Stewart, M., Bernet, C., Coe, M., & Brown, S. A. (2002). Effects of childhood exposure to familial alcoholism and family violence on adolescent substance use, conduct problems, and self-esteem. *Journal of Traumatic Stress, 15*(2), 113–122.

Rubin, D., Dodd, M., Desai, N., Pollock, B., & Graham-Pole, J. (2009). Spirituality in well and ill adolescents and their parents: The use of two assessment scales. *Pediatric Nursing, 35*(1), 37–42.

Russell, S. T., & Fish, J. N. (2016). Mental health in lesbian, gay, bisexual, and transgender (LGBT) youth. *Annual Review of Clinical Psychology, 12,* 465–487. http://doi.org/10.1146/annurev-clinpsy-021815-093153

Samuelsson, M., Holsti, A., Adamsson, M., Serenius, F., Häggöi, B., & Farooqi, A. (2017). Behavioral patterns in adolescents born at 23 to 25 weeks of gestation. *Pediatrics, 140*(1), e20170199. doi.org/10.1542/peds.2017-0199f

Sands, D. C. (2010). *Red chocolate elephants: For children bereaved by suicide.* Perth, Australia: Karrindale Pty, Limited.

Sattler, J. (1998). *Clinical and forensic interviewing of children and families.* San Diego, CA: Jerome Sattler Publisher.

School-Based Mental Health and Substance Abuse (SBMHSA) Consortium. (2013). *School-based mental health in Canada: A final report. Mental Health Commission of Canada.* Calgary, AB: Author. Retrieved from http://www.mentalhealthcommission.ca/sites/default/files/SubstanceAbuse_SBMHSA_Scan_ENG_0_1.pdf

Schreiber, J. K., Sands, D. C., & Jordan, J. R. (2017). The perceived experience of children bereaved by parental suicide. *Omega: Journal of Death & Dying (OMEGA), 75*(2), 184–206.

Schwartz, C., Waddell, C., Andres, C., Yung, D., & Gray-Grant, D. (2017). *Supporting LGBTQ+ youth. Children's Mental Health Research Quarterly, 11*(2), 1–16. Vancouver, BC: Children's Health Policy Centre, Faculty of Health Sciences, Simon Fraser University.

Segaert, A. (2012). *The national shelter study: Emergency shelter use in Canada 2004–2009.* Ottawa, ON: Homelessness Partnering Secretariat, Human Resources and Skills Development Canada.

Self, B., & Peters, H. (2005). Street outreach with no streets. *Canadian Nurse, 101*(1), 20–24.

Shields, M. E., Hovdestad, W. E., Pelletier, C., Dykxhoorn, J. L., O'Donnell, S. C., & Tonmyr, L. (2016). Childhood maltreatment as a risk factor for diabetes: Findings from a population-based survey of Canadian adults. *BMC Public Health, 16*(879), 1–12. doi:10.1186/s12889-016-3491-1

Siddiqi, A., Irwin, L. G., & Hertzman, C. (2007). *Total environment assessment model for early child development: Evidence report for the World Health Organization's Commission on the Social Determinants of Health.* Retrieved from http://www.who.int/social_determinants/resources/ecd_kn_evidence_report_2007.pdf

Sinha, M. (Ed.) (2011). *Measuring violence against women: Statistical trends.* Retrieved from http://www.statcan.gc.ca/pub/85-002-x/2013001/article/11766-eng.pdf

Søfting, G. H., Dyregro, A., & Dyregrov, K. (2016). Because I'm also part of the family, children's participation in rituals after the loss of a parent or sibling: A qualitative study from the children's perspective. *OMEGA—Journal of Death and Dying, 73*(2), 141–158.

Statistics Canada. (2011a). *Living apart together.* Retrieved from http://www.statcan.gc.ca/pub/75-006-x/2013001/article/11771-eng.htm

Statistics Canada. (2011b). *National household survey.* Retrieved from http://www5.statcan.gc.ca/researchers-chercheurs/result-resultat

Statistics Canada. (2017). *Health at a glance: Suicide rates on overview.* Statistics Canada catalogue n. 82-624-X. Retrieved from http://www.statcan.gc.ca/pub/82-624-x/2012001/article/11696-eng.htm

Strohschein, L. (2012). Parental divorce and child mental health: Understanding predisruption effects. *Journal of Divorce and Remarriage, 53*(6), 489–502.

Shave, D., & Shave, B. (1989). *Early adolescence and search for self: A developmental perspective.* New York, NY: Praeger Publishers.

Solomon, J., & George, C. (1999). *Attachment disorganization.* New York, NY: Guilford Press.

Speech-Language & Audiology Canada. (2014). *Speech, language and hearing milestones.* Retrieved from www.sac-oac.ca

Squires, J., Bricker, D., & Twombly, E. (2002). *The ASQ: SE user's guide.* Baltimore, MD: Paul H. Brookes Publishing.

Steinhausen, H. C. (2006). Developmental psychopathology in adolescence: Findings from a Swiss study–The NAPE Lecture 2005. *Acta Psychiatrica Scandinavica, 113*(1), 6–12.

Stiffman, A. R., Hadley-Ives, E., Dore, P., Polgar, M., Horvath, V. E., Striley, C., & Elze, D. (2000). Youths' access to mental health services: The role of providers' training, resource connectivity, and assessment of need. *Mental Health Services Research, 2*(3), 141–154.

Sturm, R., Ringel, J. S., & Andreyeva, T. (2003). Geographic disparities in children's mental health care. *Pediatrics, 112*(4), e308.

Swanson, J. M. (1983). *The SNAP-IV.* Irvine, CA: University of California, Irvine.

Tanguay, P. (2000). Pervasive developmental disorders: A 10-year review. *Journal of the American Academy of Child and Adolescent Psychiatry, 39*, 1079–1095.

Taylor, K. M., Menarchek-Fetkovich, M., & Day, C. (2000). The play history interview. In K. Gitlin-Weiner, A. Sandgrund, & C. Scafer (Eds.), *Play diagnosis and assessment* (2nd ed.). New York, NY: Wiley.

Thompson, R. (2002). Attachment theory and research. In M. Lewis (Ed.), *Child and adolescent psychiatry: A comprehensive textbook* (3rd ed.). Philadelphia, PA: Lippincott Williams & Wilkins.

Tiyyagura, G., Beucher, M., & Bechtel, K. (2017). Nonaccidental injury in pediatric patients: Detection, evaluation, and treatment. *Pediatric Emergency Medicine Practice, 14*(7), 1–20.

Tomlin, A. M., & Viehweg, S. A. (2003). Infant mental health: Making a difference. *Professional Psychology: Research and Practice, 34*(6), 617–625.

Trad, P. (1989). *The pre-school child assessment, diagnosis and treatment.* New York, NY: Wiley.

Trainor, J., Pomeroy, E., & Pape, B. (2004). *A framework for support* (3rd ed.). Toronto, ON: Canadian Mental Health Association.

Trocmé, N., Fallon, B., MacLaurin, B., Sinha, V., Black, T., Fast, E., … Holroyd, J. (2010). *Canadian Incidence Study of reported child abuse and neglect—2008: Major findings.* Ottawa, ON: Public Health Agency of Canada.

Unger, A. (2013). Children's health in slum settings. *Archives of Disease in Childhood, 98*(10), 799–805.

United Nations Children's Fund. (2012). *UNICEF report card 10.* Retrieved from http://www.unicef.ca/en/discover/article/unicef-report-card-10#Report%20Card

Urness, D., Hailey, D., Delday, L., Callanan, T., & Orlik, H. (2004). The status of telepsychiatry services in Canada: A national survey. *Journal of Telemedicine and Telecare, 10*(3), 160–164.

Vachon, D. D., Krueger, R. F., Rogosch, F. A., & Cicchetti, D. (2015). Assessment of the harmful psychiatric and behavioral effects of different forms of child maltreatment. *JAMA Psychiatry, 72*(11), 1135–1142. doi:10.1001/jamapsychiatry.2015.1792

van der Kolk, B. (2006). Clinical implications for neuroscience in research in PTSD. *Annals of the New York Academy of Sciences, 1071*, 277–293.

van der Kolk, B. (2009). *New frontiers in trauma treatment.* Presentation at Coquitlam, BC.

Van Epps, J., Opie, N. D., & Goodwin, T. (1997). Themes in the bereavement experience of inner city adolescents. *Journal of Child and Adolescent Psychiatric Nursing, 10*, 25–36.

Veronie, L., & Freuhstorfer, D. B. (2001). Gender, birth order and family role identification among children of alcoholics. *Current Psychology: Developmental, Learning, Personality, Social, 20*(1), 53–67.

Viorst, J. (1972). *The ten good things about Barney.* New York, NY: Simon & Schuster.

Vyas, A., Landry, M., Schnider, M., Rojas, A. M., & Wood, S. F. (2012). Public health interventions: Reaching Latino adolescents via short message service and social media. *Journal of Medical Internet Research, 14*(4), 31–40.

Waddell, C., McEwan, K., Shepherd, C. A., Offord, D. R., & Hua, J. M. (2005). A public health strategy to improve the mental health of Canadian children. *Canadian Journal of Psychiatry, 50*(4), 226–233.

White, E. B. (1952). *Charlotte's web.* New York, NY: HarperCollins.

Whitehead, M. (2008). *Pediatric nurses' perspectives of spirituality and spiritual care within nurse-patient relationships: An interpretive description.* Unpublished Master Thesis. University of Alberta, Canada.

Whiteman, S. D., McHale, S. M., & Soli, A. (2011). Theoretical perspectives on sibling relationships. *Journal of Family Theory and Review, 3*, 124–139.

Williams, T. L., May, C. R., & Esmail, A. (2001). Limitations of patient satisfaction studies in telehealthcare: A systematic review of the literature. *Telemedicine Journal and E-Health, 7*(4), 293–316.

World Health Organization. (2011). *WHO disability assessment schedule 2.0.* Retrieved from http://www.who.int/classifications/icf/whodasii/en/index.html

Wright, L. M., & Leahey, M. (2013). *Nurses and families: A guide to family assessment and intervention* (6th ed.). Philadelphia, PA: F. A. Davis.

Wu, Z., Hou, F., & Schimmele, C. (2008). Family structure and children's psychosocial outcomes. *Journal of Family Issues, 29*(12), 1600–1624.

Xue, Y., Leventhal, T., Brooks-Gunn, J., & Earls, F. J. (2005). Neighborhood residence and mental health problems of 5- to 11-year-olds. *Archives of General Psychiatry, 62*(5), 554–563.

Yalom, I. D. (1985). *The theory and practice of group psychotherapy* (2nd ed.). New York, NY: Basic Books.

Yang, S., & Park, S. (2017). A sociocultural approach to children's perceptions of death and loss. *Omega—Journal of Death and Dying, 76*(1), 53–77.

Zolkoski, S. M., & Bullock, L. M. (2012). Resilience in children and youth: A review. *Children and Youth Services Review, 34*(12), 2295–2303.

30 Psychiatric Disorders in Children and Adolescents

Lorelei Faulkner-Gibson and Kimberly Wong

Adapted from the chapter "Psychiatric Disorders Diagnosed in Children and Adolescents" by Lorelei Faulkner-Gibson, Kimberly Wong, and Wendy Austin

LEARNING OBJECTIVES

After studying this chapter, you will be able to:

- Identify the common psychiatric disorders usually first diagnosed in infancy, childhood, or adolescence.
- Describe aspects of the nursing care of psychotic, bipolar, depressive, anxiety, and obsessive–compulsive disorders.
- Discuss the prevalence, possible causes, and nursing interventions for trauma- and stressor-related disorders.
- Identify the bio/psycho/social/spiritual nursing domains in the care of children with neurodevelopmental disorders, particularly autism spectrum disorder.
- Relate the assessment data of children with attention deficit hyperactivity disorder to the development of nursing diagnoses, interventions, and evaluation of outcomes.
- Compare the disruptive, impulse control, and conduct disorders.
- Using Tourette's syndrome as an example, explain the challenges facing children and adolescents with motor disorders.
- Discuss the behavioural intervention strategies for the treatment of enuresis and encopresis.

KEY TERMS

- communication disorders • compulsions • concordant • encopresis • enuresis • externalizing disorders • habit reversal therapy • internalizing disorders • learning disorders • obsessions • school phobia • stereotypic behaviour • tic

KEY CONCEPTS

- attention • autism spectrum disorder • developmental delay • hyperactivity • impulsiveness

---

Child and adolescent mental health is a relatively new phenomenon in the field of psychiatry. As research into the neurobiology and genetics of human development advances, the various categories and diagnoses identified will evolve. The understanding of child psychiatric disorders has benefited from advances in several fields, including developmental biology, neuroanatomy, psychopharmacology, genetics, and epidemiology.

The most recent version of the *Diagnostic and Statistical Manual of Mental Disorders* (5th ed.; *DSM-5*; American Psychiatric Association [APA], 2013) integrates current evidence relevant to nurses' practice with children and families, in a way that will not only guide their practice but also impact future research. The classifications of child and adolescent psychiatric disorders discussed in this chapter include schizophrenia spectrum and other psychotic disorders; bipolar and related disorders; depressive disorders; anxiety disorders;

obsessive–compulsive disorder (OCD); trauma- and stressor-related disorders; neurodevelopment disorders of childhood; disruptive, impulse control, and conduct disorders; motor disorders; and elimination disorders.

The prevalence of child psychiatric disorders varies. For example, although childhood schizophrenia is rare, first onset of psychosis is typically in mid–late adolescence. Attention deficit hyperactivity disorder (ADHD) is a relatively common diagnosis in children; however, over the last 20 years, there has been recognition that ADHD continues into adulthood (Canadian ADHD Resource Alliance [CADDRA], 2013a). Prevalence is impacted by changes to diagnostic classification and will evolve over time. Gender ratios may also vary with some disorders according to age and genetics. For example, ADHD is more prevalent in boys than girls in childhood (3:1); however, that difference is not evident in adulthood (CADDRA, 2013a).

BOX 30.1 History and Hallmarks of Childhood and Adolescent Disorders

- Maternal age and health status during pregnancy
- Exposure to medication, alcohol, or other substances during pregnancy
- Course of pregnancy, labour, and delivery
- Infant's health at birth
- Eating, sleeping, and growth in first year
- Health status in first year
- Interest in others in first 2 years
- Motor development
- Mastery of bowel and bladder control
- Speech and language development
- Activity level
- Response to separation (e.g., school entry)
- Regulation of mood and anxiety
- Medical history in early childhood
- Social development
- Interests

Approximately one in five Canadians lives with a mental illness (Mental Health Commission of Canada, 2011). In 2011, there were 6.7 million people living with mental illness; 1 million were children and adolescents between 9 and 19 years of age. Based on predications regarding demographic changes, it is expected that over 8.9 million people in Canada will be living with mental illness in 2041; thus, approximately 1.25 million will be children and adolescents.

It is recognized that only about 25% of Canadian children and adolescents experiencing mental disorders are likely to receive specialized treatment (Waddell, McEwan, Shepard, Offord, & Hua, 2005). This discrepancy appears to be the result of limited access to treatment and appropriate mental health services, as well as the reality that psychiatric problems are less easily diagnosed in children than they are in adults. One factor contributing to this difference is that sometimes the symptoms of disorders are difficult to distinguish from the turbulence of normal growth and development. For example, a 4-year-old child who has an invisible imaginary friend is normal; however, an adolescent with an invisible friend might be experiencing a hallucination. Current estimates for the frequency of the various psychiatric disorders are also inconsistent, partly because of changing definitions of these disorders.

An overview of the psychiatric disorders diagnosed in children and adolescents that a nurse may encounter in practice, and the bio/psycho/social/spiritual domains of nursing care for this population experiencing these mental health challenges, is presented. The spiritual domain of nursing care for child and adolescent psychiatric disorders is presented separately. All of the psychiatric disorders of childhood and adolescence should be viewed within the context of growth and development models (Box 30.1). Safety and self-esteem are priority considerations. A more in-depth look at ADHD with respect to assessment, management, and follow-up is provided. The various aspects of family dynamics are incorporated within this overview.

SCHIZOPHRENIA SPECTRUM AND OTHER PSYCHOTIC DISORDERS

The symptoms of psychotic disorders cluster into five common domains, often referred to as positive symptoms: delusions, hallucinations, disorganized thinking (speech), grossly disorganized or abnormal motor behaviour (including catatonia), and negative symptoms. Negative symptoms typically are deficits of normal emotional responses or of other thought processes and commonly include flat or blunted affect and emotion, poverty of speech (alogia), inability to experience pleasure (anhedonia), lack of desire to form relationships (asociality), and lack of motivation (avolition). Research suggests that negative symptoms may contribute to a poorer quality of life, functional disability, and burden on others when compared to positive symptoms, and unfortunately, they respond less well to antipsychotic medication (see Chapter 20).

Brief Psychotic Disorder

In children and youth, what is commonly observed and diagnosed is either "brief psychotic disorder" or "substance-/medication-induced psychotic disorder," prior to a confirmed diagnosis of schizophrenia or other related psychotic disorder. Although psychosis can occur in children under 13 years, it is rare (Loth, 2012).

Treatment Interventions

Most psychoses, including schizophrenia, are treated with antipsychotic medications. These medications often cause unpleasant side effects that contribute to clients stopping or being inconsistent in adhering to their medication regimen. This affects the duration and prognosis of the illness. For example, with the advent of the second-generation antipsychotic medications, the increase in metabolic illnesses has increased. Many adolescents experience a substantial weight gain, which can further contribute to stigma and illness (Panagiotopoulos, Ronsley, Kuzeljevic, & Davidson, 2012). Nurses working with clients need to provide support and work to mitigate these side effects while supporting medication adherence. Reducing the duration of untreated psychosis is critical to remission and recovery.

Nursing Care

The nursing care priority for a child or adolescent with a diagnosis of psychosis is to ensure safety. Altered perceptions affect the individual's organization and thus affect adequate intake, output, and general hygiene and health. Education of the child or adolescent experiencing psychosis and the family as to signs and symptoms of relapse is important. Encouragement of daily exercise, healthy nutrition, and the maintenance of social connections will assist in the promotion of recovery and the prevention of an illness relapse. Monitoring of medication adherence and follow-up is critical. Engaging families in support programs also alleviates the stigma associated with psychotic illnesses.

Biologic Domain

It is well established that schizophrenia spectrum disorders typically have a neurologic basis with some linkages to genetics. No definitive cause has been identified to date. There is strong evidence that first-degree relatives of individuals with schizophrenia are at higher risk in developing the disorder. In relation to brief psychotic disorder, there may be evidence of a marked stressor, or postpartum onset, or it may be related to catatonia (APA, 2013). The incidence is approximately 9% of first-onset psychosis. The symptoms typically dissipate within 1 month; however, if the duration is longer, the diagnosis may be altered. See Box 30.2 for early warning signs of psychosis.

BOX 30.2 Early Warning Signs of Psychosis

Withdrawal from activities and social contacts
Irrational, angry, or fearful responses to friends and family
Sleep disturbances
Deterioration in studies or work
Inappropriate use of language—words that do not make sense
Sudden excesses, such as extreme religiosity and extreme activity
Deterioration in personal hygiene
Difficulty controlling thoughts and difficulty concentrating
Hearing voices or sounds others don't hear
Seeing people or things others don't see
A constant feeling of being watched
Inability to turn off the imagination, delusions, and off-the-wall ideas
Mood swings and increased anxiety
Somatic symptoms: weakness, pains, and bizarre body sensations

---

Psychosocial Domain

A lack of insight is often experienced by those with a psychotic disorder, and children and adolescents often do not recognize that they are ill, or if they do, they often do not tell their families or friends out of fear of stigma. Many families may not be aware of symptoms until they become overtly severe. The earlier the symptoms are identified and treated, the more likely the illness will move into remission. The better the medical and psychosocial management are, the better chance of remission and recovery. Family education and support are critical to prognosis and remission. Early psychosis intervention (EPI) programs are available in most provinces to provide support, education, and group or individual support (see Web Links).

■ BIPOLAR AND RELATED DISORDERS

Bipolar disorder often first presents during adolescence. Symptoms include periods of mania (extreme optimism, euphoria, and feelings of grandeur; rapid, racing thoughts and hyperactivity; a decreased need for sleep; increased irritability; impulsiveness and possibly reckless behaviour; and alternate periods of depression) (CMHA, 2013a). This can be a very difficult experience for both adolescents and their family, as the youth may engage in behaviours that contribute to ongoing stigma about mental illness (Leibenluft, 2011). Bipolar disorder is rare in children, and the observed symptoms may fall into a diagnosis of ADHD, oppositional defiant disorder (ODD), or disruptive mood regulation disorder (see section "Disruptive Mood Regulation Disorder").

Treatment Intervention

Caution should be taken in initiating biologic treatment for bipolar disorders in children and adolescents to ensure that, in fact, it is bipolar illness being treated. In children, medications are not typically used unless the symptoms observed are interfering with social functioning and are unresponsive or limited in response to other therapeutic interventions. Lithium carbonate is the common treatment; however, long-term use can have effects on liver, kidney, and thyroid functioning. Blood levels must be drawn to ensure a stable and effective level of lithium. See Chapter 12 for an overview of lithium.

Nursing Care
Biologic Domain

A family history of bipolar disorder is correlated with a "10-fold increased risk among adult relatives" (APA, 2013, p. 130). Females tend to have an increased incidence of rapid cycling phases in this disorder (National Institute of Mental Health, 2013). Various mood stabilizer medications are used, with most clients requiring daily or weekly blood tests to assess for therapeutic levels until stable.

Psychosocial Domain

The risk of suicide among the population of individuals with bipolar disorder is 15 times the general population. With suicide being the leading cause of nonaccidental death in individuals 15 to 24 years of age (CMHA, 2013b; Statistics Canada, 2012), it is critical to assess for risk and intent with this group. Bipolar illness can affect various relationships in the individual's life. Education for friends and school assists the youth. (See Web Links for an online educational resource.)

■ DEPRESSIVE DISORDERS

As noted in Chapter 29, many children and adolescents have lived experience of mental illness. Children and youth are often challenged by disturbances in mood. Approximately 3.5% of youth suffer from a depressive disorder (Canadian Mental Health Association [CMHA], 2014a). Treatment for depressive disorders is multimodal, depending on the child's age and symptom presentation (Public Health Canada, 2016).

Assessing children and adolescents for depression can be especially challenging for nurses and other mental health clinicians. Children may not be able to tell the clinician how they feel, and some adolescents may simply be reluctant to talk about how they are feeling.

As a result, some clinicians purport that depressive disorders in children and adolescents are among the most underdiagnosed mental health disorders. Children and adolescents with a depressive disorder may demonstrate physical symptoms of headaches and stomachaches or avoid situations in which they are feeling overwhelmed or begin to slowly withdraw from social activities (CMHA, 2014b, 2014c). They should be screened for suicidal ideation as early as ten years of age (see Chapter 29). A diagnosis of a depressive disorder in adolescence is a risk factor for other concurrent disorders such as anxiety disorders, disruptive behaviour, and substance abuse disorders. Unfortunately, these latter diagnoses may persist even when the depression is resolved (Stanford Children's Health, 2017).

Major Depressive Disorder

Depressive disorders have prevalence rates of up to 3% in children and 8% in adolescents, with a lifetime prevalence of 25% by the end of adolescence (Zinck, Bagnell, Bond, & Newton, 2009). According to Statistics Canada (2012), in 2009, 202 Canadian individuals aged 15 to 19 committed suicide. Suicide is second only to accidental death as the leading cause of death in this age group (Statistics Canada, 2012). In 2013, 35 individuals aged 10 to 14 years died by suicide; this is a rate of 1.9/100,000 (Statistics Canada, 2017).

Disruptive Mood Dysregulation Disorder

This diagnostic category is new for the *DSM-5* and especially for the assessment of children. The category was developed to better distinguish bipolar disorder in children from other related disorders. The incidence of this disorder is estimated to be 2% to 5% of children, who demonstrate a chronically irritable temperament, and the majority of whom are male (APA, 2013; Axelrod, 2013). "In severe mood dysregulation, irritability is defined as having two components: (1) temper outbursts that are developmentally inappropriate, frequent, and extreme; and (2) negatively balanced mood (anger or sadness) between outbursts" (Leibenluft, 2011, p. 4). According to a study review by Shanahan and colleagues (2014), there appears to be an overlap with childhood diagnoses of depression and/or ODD. As this new category for children unfolds, it will be important that nurses work closely with children and families to ensure they access the best and most appropriate interventions.

Treatment Interventions

Cognitive–behavioural therapy (CBT) is the treatment of choice for most children and youth experiencing depression, which requires training for most individuals to implement. The use of mindfulness, for a variety of circumstances, is also an easily accessible treatment for most children, adolescents, and their families. See Chapter 13 for cognitive–behavioural techniques and mindfulness, as well as Web Links for a link to the Centre for Addiction and Mental Health's information on CBT. Pharmaceutical intervention is not typically used unless the symptoms observed are interfering with social functioning and are unresponsive or limited in response to other therapeutic interventions.

Nursing Care

Nurses will need to ensure that they are assessing levels of mood in a developmentally conducive manner and that risk assessments have been conducted to rule out concerns of suicidality. The child's functioning will be impacted by numerous factors, including knowledge and support of the education system, family capacity for coping and seeking treatment, and the child's or adolescent's understanding and motivation to participate in treatment.

Nurses need to develop comfort and confidence in assessing children and youth regarding suicidal thoughts and intention. Various age-appropriate tools are available to assist the nurse with those assessments. Education and support are needed for parents and caregivers to understand that asking about suicide does not increase the risk of suicide.

Biologic Domain

Depression has been demonstrated to have a familial or genetic link. Depression can also be caused by stressful events or experiences, medical illness, or medications. Regardless of the cause, depression can look very different in children and youth than it does in adults. Young children may become withdrawn, have trouble sleeping, regress in certain behaviours (e.g., bed wetting), or become irritable. Older children may start to report headaches and stomachaches or withdraw from activities and friends. Adolescents may be better able to articulate what is happening for them, but they may not necessarily report directly to parents. They may experience sadness and become withdrawn and may exhibit increases or decreases in sleep and appetite (HealthLinkBC, 2017).

Psychosocial Domain

Depression has been linked with life stressors (Box 30.3). Stressors for children can include the death or loss of a pet, parental separation or divorce, or household relocation. There is also evidence that depression (and anxiety) is higher in children who have suffered maltreatment and demonstrated poor coping skills or other life stressors such as "substance abuse, emotional maltreatment, primary caregivers' mental illness, sexual abuse, and numerous moves in a year" (Tonmyr, Williams, Hovdestad, & Draca, 2011, p. 497). The most

serious concern regarding children and youth with depression is their risk of suicide. Suicide screening and assessment need to start with children as young as 10 years and increase over adolescence (see Chapter 29). Children often report feeling relieved when finally asked about their feelings.

■ ANXIETY DISORDERS

Anxiety disorders are the most prevalent mental illness in Canadian children between 4 and 17 years of age. Approximately 4 in 100 children have severe problems with worries and fears warranting a clinical diagnosis (Waddell, Shepherd Schwartz, & Barican, 2014). Many childhood fears are developmentally normal: it is common for toddlers to fear the dark, for school-aged children to fear animals, and for teenagers to worry about relationships with peers. These typical anxiety experiences do not usually interfere with the child's development and functioning (Children's Health Policy Centre, Simon Fraser University, 2007). Children with anxiety disorders, however, experience excessive, prolonged, or recurrent fears or symptoms of anxiety, with accompanying impairment in age-appropriate functioning at home, at school, and with peers (Manassis, 2004). Mood and anxiety disorders often coexist; therefore, it is important to assess for both especially in children.

BOX 30.3 Questions, Choices, and Outcomes

Mrs. S has just returned with her son Jared to the child psychiatric inpatient services following an overnight pass. She reports that the visit did not go well due to Jared's anger and defiance. She remarked that this behaviour was distressingly similar to his behaviour before the hospitalization. She expressed additional concern because of the upcoming discharge from the hospital. After saying goodbye to Jared, she pulled the nurse aside and stated that she had decided to file for divorce.

Mrs. S indicated that she had not told her husband or the family therapist. When asked whether Jared knew about her decision, Mrs. S suddenly realized that he may have overheard her discussing the matter with her sister on the telephone during this home visit.

How should the nurse approach this situation?

Choice	Possible Outcomes
Discuss her hypothesis about Jared's behaviour and his uncertainty.	Mother can see the relationship between Jared's behaviour and her plan for divorce.
	Mother ignores the nurse.
	Mother is interested but does not see the connection.
Ignore the statement.	Child and family did not learn about the connection between Jared's behaviour and the events at home.
Encourage mother to sort out her problems.	The focus is then on mother's problems.

Analysis

The best response is focusing on the possible relationship between Jared's recent behavioural deterioration and his uncertainty of his family's future. If the nurse ignores the statement or focuses on the mother's interpretation of Jared's behaviour, the mother is less likely to appreciate the connection between pending divorce and Jared's behaviour. The nurse should also emphasize the importance of discussing the matter in family therapy.

To screen quickly for one or more anxiety disorders in children, the following questions may be useful:

- Does the child worry or ask for parental reassurance every day?
- Does the child consistently avoid age-appropriate situations or activities or avoid doing them without a parent?
- Does the child have frequent episodes of stomachaches, headaches, or hyperventilation?
- Does the child have daily repetitive rituals?

These four questions address the main thoughts, behaviours, and feelings related to anxiety seen in children (Manassis, 2004).

The following are the main types of anxiety disorders: generalized anxiety disorder (GAD), specific phobias, posttraumatic stress disorders. (PTSDs), panic disorder, and agoraphobia, which are more common in females and usually develop in childhood through early adulthood (Public Health Agency of Canada, 2016). The focus in this chapter will be on the more common childhood diagnoses. Separation anxiety, a disorder diagnosed in childhood, as well as GAD, which occur in both adults and children (see Chapter 23), will be discussed.

Generalized Anxiety Disorder

GAD is characterized by excessive anxiety and worry about many events or activities. The intensity, duration, or frequency of the anxiety and worry is out of proportion to the actual likelihood or impact of the anticipated event. Children tend to worry excessively about their competence or the quality of their performance, such as academic performance or athletic prowess on sports teams. However, the focus of the worry can change over time. In addition to the excessive and debilitating anxiety and worry, the child may experience feeling on edge and being easily fatigued, have difficulty concentrating, and experience irritability, muscle tension, and disturbed sleep (American Psychological Association [APA], 2013). For the full criteria of GAD, see the DSM-5 (APA, 2013).

GAD affects an estimated 1 out of 150 school-aged children in Canada (Tonmyr et al., 2011; Waddell et al., 2014). Risk for developing GAD includes a genetic predisposition as evidenced by a family history of anxiety and environmental factors including experiencing stressful or traumatic events. Many individuals with GAD report that they have felt anxious and nervous all of their lives (APA, 2013). Clinicians may be of two schools of thought as how GAD develops in an individual. Psychodynamic theory explains anxiety to be a result of conflict between the id and ego, while cognitive–behavioural theory explains that the behaviours of anxiety are a method of coping with the individual's imaginings of worst-case scenarios (Bhatt, 2017).

Treatment Interventions

In the Child/Adolescent Anxiety Multimodal Treatment Study (CAMS), participants (youth ages 7 to 17; 50.4% male) were randomly assigned to experimental groups: CBT (Coping Cat program), pharmacotherapy (sertraline), CBT and pharmacotherapy, or pill placebo (Walkup et al., 2008). Those children rated as much or very much improved did best with combination therapy. CBT was slightly more effective than sertraline, and the children experienced less insomnia, fatigue, sedation, and restlessness. All therapies were superior to placebo. In this CAMS research, an examination of coping efficacy and self-talk as mediators to anxiety management with the youth found that treatment assignment was not associated with a reduction in anxious self-talk but that improvements in coping were a mediator of treatment gains (Kendall et al., 2016, p. 2). The implication of these findings indicates that although the child's/youth's self-talk did not necessarily alter, the impact of the treatments focusing on the child's ability to cope with symptoms did.

Separation Anxiety Disorder

Separation anxiety disorder is excessive anxiety on separation from home or a major attachment figure before adulthood (taken as the age of 18 years). It is manifested by acute distress, frequent nightmares about separation, and reluctance or refusal to separate. It causes clinically significant impairment in social or academic functioning. (See the DSM-5 for the APA (2013) diagnostic criteria.) Separation anxiety disorder may be the childhood equivalent of panic disorder in adults. Although many children experience some discomfort on separation from their mothers or major attachment figures, children with separation anxiety disorder suffer great distress when faced with ordinary separations, such as going to school. In most cases, the mother is the focus of the child's concern, but this may not be so, especially if the mother is not the primary caregiver. The child may exhibit extraordinary reluctance or even refusal to separate from the primary caregiver. When asked, most children with separation anxiety disorder will express worry about harm or permanent loss of their major attachment figure. Other children may express worry about their own safety.

Epidemiology and Aetiology

The prevalence of separation anxiety disorder is estimated at 4% of school-aged children; thus, it is relatively common. Anxiety disorders run in families, and it appears that both environmental and genetic factors affect the risk for separation anxiety disorder. For example, it may emerge after a move, change to a new school, or death of a family member or pet. Traits such as shyness and behavioural inhibition (reluctance in new situations) are believed to be inherited (Rapee & Spence, 2004). Furthermore, not only are children with an enduring "inhibited" temperament at greater risk for anxiety disorders but also their immediate family members are at greater risk for anxiety disorders, when compared with a psychiatric control group. Others have argued in favour of environmental determinants of separation anxiety, contending that anxious parents communicate to the child that the world is inhospitable and menacing in order to keep the child near. Available data suggest that the long-term outcome of childhood disorders is favourable in many cases but may evolve and take other forms in adulthood. For example, separation anxiety in childhood may reemerge as panic disorder in adults, or children may present with sleep difficulties and/or oppositional symptoms when in fact they are anxious (Shanahan et al., 2014; Koda, Charney, & Pine, 2003).

Treatment Interventions

Specific to school phobia, most clinicians agree that the child should return to school as soon as possible because resistance to attending school invariably mounts the longer the child remains absent. Several therapeutic approaches are used in treating separation anxiety disorder, including individual psychotherapy, behavioural treatment, and pharmacotherapy (Public Health Agency of Canada, 2016). Several programs are available to support families and children to address issues of anxiety and/or school phobia. While individual psychotherapy has not traditionally been successful, depending on the cause, it may be a supportive process with family engagement (Garland, Clark, & Earle, 2009; Kahn, Nursten, & Carroll, 2014). To be successful, these techniques require close collaboration with the family and the school and may also include medication (Labellarte & Ginsberg, 2003). In rare cases, school phobia can be a side effect of antipsychotic medication (Scahill, Leckman, Schultz, Katsovich, & Peterson, 2003). When another disorder such as depression is identified, it becomes the focus of treatment. In some cases, the school phobia may resolve when the primary disorder is successfully treated.

Nursing Care

The child's developmental history and response to new situations and prior separations provide essential background information for understanding the child's current separation anxiety. The assessment should also include a review of recent life events and the methods the family has used to promote the child's return to school. Finally, the family history with respect to anxiety, panic attacks, or phobias is also informative.

A common manifestation of anxiety is **school phobia**, in which the child refuses to attend school, preferring to stay at home with the primary attachment figure. However, it should be noted that school phobia is a common presenting complaint in child psychiatric clinics and may be part of separation anxiety disorder, general anxiety disorder, social phobia, OCD, depression, or conduct disorder (Shanahan et al., 2014).

School phobia or avoidance is often what prompts the family to seek consultation for the child. The onset of school refusal may be gradual or acute. Because school phobia can be a behavioural manifestation of several different child psychiatric disorders, it requires careful assessment. Issues to consider are whether the parents have been aware that the child is avoiding school (separation vs. truancy), what efforts the family has made to return the child to school, the presence of significant subjective distress in the child with anticipation of going to school, sleep problems contributing, and whether school refusal occurs in the context of other behavioural, social, or emotional problems (Shanahan et al., 2014; Fox-Lopp & McLaughlin, 2015).

■ OBSESSIVE–COMPULSIVE DISORDER

As with anxiety disorders, obsessive-compulsive disorder (OCD) occurs in both adults and children. OCD is characterized by intrusive thoughts that are difficult to dislodge (**obsessions**, i.e., unwanted persistent, intrusive thoughts, impulses, or images related to anxiety) or by ritualized behaviours that the child feels driven to perform (**compulsions**, i.e., unwanted behavioural acts or patterns) to prevent or reduce anxiety. The most common obsessions in children are fears of contamination. Worries about personal and family safety are also frequent. The most common compulsions are excessive washing, cleaning, and checking actions. In earlier editions of the DSM, OCD was classified as an anxiety disorder; however, in 2013, OCD was classified as a distinct disorder within the classification of OCD and Related Disorders (see Chapter 23). Left undiagnosed and untreated OCD can affect the child's or adolescent's physical, psychological, social, and emotional well-being.

Epidemiology and Aetiology

Historically, OCD was regarded as a neurosis, and the primary symptoms were viewed as the expression of unresolved sexual and aggressive impulses. Recent evidence from family genetic studies, pharmacologic trials, and neuroimaging studies has dramatically shifted the conceptualization of OCD. OCD was once considered uncommon in adults and even rarer in children, but research over the last two decades has identified OCD as one of the most common psychiatric illnesses in both children and adults. The estimated prevalence of OCD in children ages 4 to 17 years is approximately 0.4% (Waddell et al., 2014).

Family studies and twin studies indicate that genetic determinants play a significant role in the aetiology of OCD, as well as anxiety disorders, and recur with a greater than expected frequency in the families of clients with OCD or Tourette's disorder (Van Grootheest, Cath, Beekman, & Boomsma, 2005). Many biologic theories of OCD hypothesize that abnormalities in serotonin metabolism and frontal–striatal circuitry operation is responsible for the creation of OCD symptomatology. The serotonin hypothesis is based on the observation that, in most cases, individuals with OCD respond to SSRIs as opposed to nonserotonergic medications or placebos (Cameron, 2007). Neuroimaging studies and neurosurgical evidence suggest that OCD is associated with hyperactive operation in the frontal–striatal circuitry of the brain, which includes the orbital–frontal cortex, anterior cingulated cortex, caudate nucleus, and thalamus (Leonard, Ale, & Freeman, 2005). Despite advances in the genetics, diagnosis, and treatment of OCD in children and adolescents, little is known about the disorder's long-term outcome (Stewart et al., 2017).

Treatment Interventions

Treatment goals focus on reducing the obsessions and compulsions and their effects on the child's development. CBT, particularly exposure and response prevention (ERP), was found to be an effective intervention in children with OCD (Bolton & Perrin, 2008). Exposure consists of gradual confrontation with events or situations that trigger obsessions and cause the urge to ritualize. According to the theory behind ERP therapy, repeated exposure works because the client learns that the immediate anxiety will subside even if he or she does not complete the ritual. Response prevention complements exposure and consists of instructing the client to delay the execution of the ritual. When ERP are combined, the client is confronted with a triggering stimulus such as dirt (exposure) but agrees not to do the handwashing for a brief period (response prevention) and tracks the anxiety level during the exercise.

Successful CBT of children with OCD includes parents, both to include them in the treatment plan and to reduce their involvement in the ritualized behaviour. For example, the child may demand that the parent participate in a washing and checking ritual (Bolton & Perrin, 2008). Because of the dynamic impact OCD in children and adolescents has on families, they should be involved in psychosocial interventions whenever possible (Cameron, 2007; Freeman et al., 2014).

Nursing Care

Recurrent worries and ritualistic behaviour can occur normally in children at stages of development. The first step in the assessment of OCD in children is to distinguish between normal childhood rituals and worries and pathologic rituals and obsessional thoughts (Cameron, 2007). Obsessional thoughts are recurrent, nagging, and bothersome. Although children may describe obsessions as occurring "out of the blue," external events may trigger obsessions. For example, a child may fear contamination whenever he or she is in contact with a certain person or object. Likewise, compulsions waste time, cause distress, and interfere with daily living (Box 30.4).

BOX 30.4 CLINICAL VIGNETTE

KIMBERLY AND OCD

Kimberly, an 11-year-old fifth grader, comes for an evaluation because her mother and teacher have become increasingly concerned about her repetitive behaviours. In retrospect, Kim's mother recalls first noticing repetitive rituals about 2 years ago, but she did not become alarmed about these behaviours until recently when they began to interfere with daily living. At the time of referral, Kim exhibits complicated jumping rituals that involve a specific number of jumps and a particular manner of jumping. She also turns light switches off and on and performs complex movements, such as blinking in patterns and thrusting her arms back and forth a certain number of times. Her mother also reports Kim's near-constant request for reassurance about her own safety. In recent months, her incessant demands for reassurance have been more frequent and elaborate. For example, Kim's mother has to answer three times that everything is all right and then say, "I swear to it."

At the evaluation, Kim expresses fears that some ill fate, such as catastrophic illness or injury, will befall her. This fear is triggered by contact with any individual who seems sick, chance exposures to foul smells or dirt, or minor scrapes or bumps. Once the fear is triggered, she becomes increasingly anxious and consumed with the fear that she will develop an illness and die. Sometimes, her fears are specific, such as cancer or AIDS; other times, her fears are more ambiguous, as evidenced by statements that "something bad will happen" if she doesn't complete the ritual. Kim acknowledges that the ritual is probably not related to the feared event, but she is reluctant to take a chance. If the ritual does not reduce her anxiety, she seeks reassurance from her mother.

Kim's medical history was negative for serious illness or injury; she was born after an uncomplicated pregnancy, labour, and delivery and achieved developmental milestones at appropriate times. Indeed, her mother could recall no unusual problems in the first few years of life except that Kim was typically anxious in new situations. Kim's mother reports a prior history of panic attacks, but the family history is otherwise negative for anxiety disorders, including OCD.

The severity of the child's and family's response to OCD will determine the appropriate nursing diagnoses. The amount of distress within the family context can be quite detrimental to overall family and individual functions (Stewart et al., 2017). When the obsessions and compulsions emerge, children or adolescents are in distress because of the disturbing and relentless nature of the symptoms. What distinguishes families experiencing OCD from families of children with other mental disorders is the inextricable way that they are brought into the illness. Parents may be pulled into the child's rituals. The term *family accommodation* is often used to refer to family responses that are direct (e.g., participation in or assistance with the ritual) or indirect (e.g., modification in the family's lifestyle around the OCD symptomatology) (Cameron, 2007). Ineffective coping, compromised family coping, and ineffective role performance are likely nursing diagnoses for these families.

TRAUMA- AND STRESSOR-RELATED DISORDERS

It is well documented that early chronic stress or trauma affects how the developing brain grows and evolves (Bellis & Zisk, 2014; Gunnar & Quevedo, 2007; National Scientific Council on the Developing Child, 2012; Perry, 2004; Porges, 2004; van der Kolk, 2009). Childhood trauma can be the result of a number of factors that can include physically or emotionally absent parent, erratic or inconsistent caregiving, abuse (verbal, sexual, or emotional), neglect, violence in the home or community, and war or disasters. Traumatic reactions may occur with unexpected events that may be a one-time incident, or ongoing, such as frequent hospitalizations for chronic illness contributing to a child experiencing traumatic effects (Afifi et al., 2015; Brave Heart et al., 2011; Saunders & Adams, 2014).

There is increasing awareness of the intergenerational transfer of stressor and traumatic effects onto children. A child may be affected by traumatic events that happened to a parent or to a community. Collective trauma, when a significant number of members of a social group are exposed to a traumatic event (e.g., a natural disaster, or a political event, or residential school Bombay, Matheson, & Anisman, 2014), or historical trauma, when cumulative psychosocial wounding occurs across generations due to mass group trauma experiences (e.g., the colonization of indigenous peoples; Brave heart, 2003), can have long-term effects on children born into such communities. Trauma-informed care in child and adolescent psychiatric settings is increasingly being recommended (see Chapter 17).

The brains of children and adolescents with trauma histories prepare them to live in a state of neurologic hyperarousal in order to be alert and safe in their environment (Mulvihill, 2005). Traumatized children often do not come out of this hyperaroused state and are "hypervigilant and focused on nonverbal cues" even when they are in a situation that is perceived to be "safe" (Mulvihill, 2005; Perry, 2002a, p. 6). Traumatized children often have difficulty with verbal interactions or therapy when memories evoke "trauma-related physical sensations and physiologic hyper- or hypoarousal, which evoke emotions" (van der Kolk, 2006, p. 284). There are many triggers—loud noises, tone of voice, nonverbal behaviours, gender, the environment, the gender, stance, intonation, or touch of other—that can initiate a hyperarousal response. The reactivity is in the form of automatic fight-or-flight system and can take the form of overt aggression or internal withdrawal and may impact the child's/youth's ability to reach their developmental milestones (Gunnar & Quevedo, 2007; Marusak, Martin, Etkin, & Thomason, 2015; Perry, 2001, 2002b, 2002c; van der Kolk, 2006). Adolescents may rely on less sophisticated coping strategies and engage in substance use, cutting, sensory-seeking behaviours, or sexual behaviours. Self-esteem and self-awareness are affected, leaving the individual without a positive sense of self-identity (Blaustein & Kinniburgh, 2010). When nurses work with children/youth or families in these circumstances, they need to be aware of what the triggers may be, how to mitigate them, and how to access the families' coping strategies when possible.

It is evident that preparation of children regarding planned hospitalization (e.g., surgery) is important, as is preparation for how to behave should a natural disaster occur. Such preparation increases a child's sense of self-efficacy and resilience, if it is carried out age-appropriately. For instance, comics about the escapades of "Silly Timmy" and his friends facing thunderstorms, an earthquake, and a tsunami were effective when used with kindergarten children (Sharpe & Izadkhah, 2014). Nurses can be a resource for such preparation.

Reactive Attachment Disorder

Attachment disorders are typically identified prior to the age of 5 years. Previously, Mary Ainsworth's (1979) work on attachment described four types: secure, insecure avoidant, insecure ambivalent/resistant, and disorganized. It is recognized that children without secure attachment will struggle with relationships throughout their lives if difficulties with attachment are not addressed early in development (Cornell & Hamrin, 2008). The *DSM* diagnosis of disinhibited social engagement disorder is similar to Ainsworth's insecure–ambivalent–resistive attachment style; it occurs in about 20% of severely neglected children. The behaviours seen with this disorder include a lack of social or cultural boundaries and overfamiliarity with strangers (APA, 2013). The *DSM* diagnosis of reactive attachment disorder (RAD) is most similar to Ainsworth's disorganized attachment style, the style most likely to develop into later psychopathology without early intervention (Holmes, 2004; Glowinski, 2011; Zeanah & Gleason, 2010). The focus here will be on RAD.

Epidemiology and Aetiology

The prevalence of RAD is unknown; however, it is thought to occur primarily in populations of severely neglected children with symptoms displaying between the ages of 9 months to 5 years. The incidence is thought to be about 10%. Prognosis is dependent on the caregiving environment following the severe neglect.

Treatment Intervention

Some of the interventions used for treating RAD are relevant for PTSD and acute traumatic stress response, depending on the context and situation.

Any pharmaceutical intervention would be limited to symptom management. Medications are not typically used unless the symptoms observed are interfering with social functioning and are unresponsive or limited in response to other therapeutic interventions.

The first component of intervention is to explore the rationale for the various behaviours being expressed by the child/youth and that the caregivers are experiencing. The nurse works with the caregivers to learn the child's language of emotional expression (verbal and nonverbal). The caregiver begins to attune to the child's expressions of need and reciprocate to meet that need; the pattern of coregulation begins. The caregiver then develops a consistent response to the child that is predictable. From this point, the caregiver and child learn self-regulation strategies to calm or arouse the child as reflective of the circumstance at hand. As the child and caregiver develop competence in these areas, the child will be increasingly free to develop and to learn new skills. This is not a "quick-fix" process and may take several months to years for some families. The nurse may determine that the parents may be struggling with their own issues of attachment and trauma histories. In order to work with the child, the care provider will need support and educate the parents regarding regulation and attunement of their own emotions as they attend to the child's. There are several programs that work with families on these issues, for example, Attachment, Self-Regulation and Competencies (Blaustein & Kinniburgh, 2010) and the CASA Trauma program (Ashton, O'Brien-Langer, & Silverstone, 2015).

Nursing Care

Care for a family with a child or adolescent with RAD is complex. The first component of intervention is the provision of psychoeducation about the disorder, context, and strategies of therapy. Interventions will depend on the age of the child/youth, symptoms being expressed, and severity of the attachment dysfunction at the time. Relational therapy between the therapist and child is paramount to establish trust and rapport, as well as with the

family. Some interventions will include specific behavioural management components such as the Incredible Years by Webster-Stratton and Reid (see, e.g., Webster-Stratton, 2011) or Parent–Child Interaction Therapy by Eyberg and Boggs (see Buckner, Lopez, Dunkel, & Joiner, 2008). The use of these programs will depend greatly on the caregivers' ability to participate and the overall issues facing the child. Family or individual therapy is recommended; pharmacotherapy is used only if required for a coexisting diagnosis (Mayo Clinic, 2017).

Biologic Domain

There do not appear to be specific biologic factors attributed to the development of RAD; however, parents who may be compromised neurologically or psychologically may create an environment in which RAD could develop.

Psychosocial Domain

RAD can also develop from unpredictable care providers who create a sense of fear in the child to the extent that they are unsure of where their safety net may be (Cornell & Hamrin, 2008). Children with RAD do not typically turn to their primary attachment figure for "comfort, support, protection, or nurturance" (American Psychiatric Association, 2013, p. 266). The nurse may suspect potential for attachment concerns if the primary caregiver is being seen because the child has nonorganic failure to thrive or if the primary caregiver has an active psychiatric illness such as postpartum depression (Cornell & Hamrin, 2008). Children placed in institutional care for extended periods of time are more likely to develop RAD than those in a consistent, reliable, and predictable care environment (Humphreys, Nelson, Fox, & Zeanah, 2017; Smyke et al., 2012)

Disinhibited Social Engagement Disorder

The child will demonstrate behaviours towards strangers or adults unfamiliar to the child that puts the child at increased risk of further exposure to abusive situations or abduction. The child appears to have a blatant disregard of social inhibition when approaching strangers both verbally and physically, may go with the stranger, and does not check back with primary caregiver before heading off. Understanding of this behaviour needs to be taken in context of other diagnoses such as developmental delay or impulsivity.

The prevalence of this disorder remains unknown; however, in high-risk populations, the incidence is about 20% of children. Causes are similar to RAD, and this may cause challenges with diagnosis. Contributing factors include repeated changes of primary care providers such as children in foster or institutional care or situations of sever neglect (Smyke et al., 2012). As with RAD, pharmacologic intervention is not used except for symptom management. See Nursing Care section of

RAD for guidance regarding care of disinhibited social engagement disorder.

Posttraumatic Stress Disorder and Acute Stress Disorder

Children's exposure to one or more traumatic events in their lives can lead to a trauma response or PTSD. The National Child Traumatic Stress Network (NCTSN, 2013) identifies that one in four children will be exposed to trauma prior to the age of 16 years. A child may have been exposed to domestic violence, community violence, war, natural disasters, or various forms of abuse and neglect. All of these events put a child/youth and family at risk of developing PTSD. Children experience and express their symptoms of PTSD differently from adults. For example, expression of recurrent involuntary distressing memories may manifest in repetitive play themes, as nightmares, or as reenactment of the event in a dissociative space or in play or in regression of otherwise acquired skills (e.g., bed wetting) (APA, 2013; NCTSN, 2013; Public Health Agency of Canada, 2011). The *DSM-5* criteria for PTSD apply to adults, adolescents, and children over 6 years, with notations regarding children's symptom expression (APA, 2013). There are separate PTSD criteria for children 6 years and younger. *DSM-5* criteria for acute stress disorder apply to adults, adolescents, and children, with notations regarding children's symptom expression (APA, 2013). See Chapters 17 and 34.

Treatment Intervention

CBT has been shown to be most effective in treating PTSD. Approaches include stress management and relaxation strategies, creating a story or narrative to assist with understanding events, correcting misinformation or distorted beliefs, deflecting self-blame, and engaging parents or primary care providers in the process (Kelty Mental Health Resource Centre, 2013; NCTSN, 2013) (see also Chapter 17). Pharmaceutical intervention is not typically used unless the symptoms observed are interfering with social functioning and are unresponsive or limited in response to other therapeutic interventions.

Nursing Care

Creating safety, support, guidance, and education for the child/youth and family, regardless of the cause of the trauma, will be the primary focus for the nurse.

Biologic Domain

Over the past 20 years, research regarding the neurodevelopmental effects of trauma and neglect on the developing brain has been evolving (Bellis & Zisk, 2014; Blaustein & Kinniburgh, 2010; Gunnar & Quevedo, 2007; Mulvihill, 2005; Perry, 1994, 2004; Porges, 2004; Siegel, 2001; van der Kolk, 2005, 2006). Although there may not be an overt genetic pathway, the environmental exposures that create a brain sensitive and receptive

to developing PTSD are clear. Gender plays a role: risk is increased for females. Risk negatively correlates with age: the younger the age of exposure, the greater the risk of developing PTSD (APA, 2013). Temperament and preexisting psychopathology may also increase the risk for anxiety or panic disorders and depression.

Psychosocial Domain

Children exposed to various life stressors, who live in communities where violence and/or war exists, and those who are deprived of the basic determinants of health (nutrition, housing, safety) are at risk. Resilience may be a protective factor; however, depending on the circumstance/event, it is not absolute.

In the event of a natural disaster where the family home may no longer exist, it will be important for the parent/primary caregivers to create an atmosphere of as much normalcy as possible. Supporting the child's/youth's and family's return to regular routines as much as possible will help with recovery and general wellness. Activities such as regular exercise, relaxation, a balanced diet, positive relationships, stress management, adequate sleep, community involvement, and social support are very important in managing anxiety in relation to PTSD or acute stress response and for general wellness (see Box 30.5). Children or youth may need the assistance of medication during this time; however, that is a collaborative conversation between the family, child/youth, and therapist and physician involved.

■ NEURODEVELOPMENTAL DISORDERS OF CHILDHOOD

Under the primary influences of genes and environment, development may be said to proceed along several pathways, such as attention, cognition, language, affect, and social and moral behaviours. The neurodevelopmental disorders' common feature is significant developmental delays or deficits in one or more areas. These deficits can be closely interwoven. For example, a language delay can interfere with a child's social development and contribute to behaviour problems (Russell & Grizzle, 2008). There are several categories of these childhood disorders in the *DSM-5* (APA, 2013): intellectual disability, communication disorders (e.g., childhood-onset fluency disorder [stuttering]), autism spectrum disorder (ASD), ADHD, specific learning disorder, and motor disorders (e.g., tic disorders; APA, 2013).

KEY CONCEPT

Developmental delay is the development of a child that is outside the norm, including delayed socialization, communication, peculiar mannerisms, and idiosyncratic interests.

BOX 30.5 Tips for Caregivers Managing a Child's Symptoms of PTSD

Maintain a calm, structured home environment (e.g., practice relaxation, develop routines).

Keep your routines the same (morning, school, homework, bedtime).

Provide clear expectations, limits, and consequences.

Help your child learn about and identify feelings.

Pay attention to your child's feelings.

Remain calm when your child is anxious.

Hold realistic expectations for your child's age—change them if you need to.

Plan for transitions (e.g., getting to school).

Focus on the here and now—use the sense to notice what is going on in the moment (e.g., your child describes what he or she hears, see). PTSD anxiety forces children to be focused on the future.

Show your child the way you identify and accept your feelings.

Show your child how to solve problems.

Take care of your own needs—parenting an anxious child can be challenging.

Talk to others for support, and ask for help when you need it.

Be aware of and manage your own reactions. Seek help if you are struggling with this.

Praise effort and provide rewards for effort.

Source: Kelty Mental Health Resource Centre. (2013). *Post-traumatic stress disorder*. Retrieved from http://keltymentalhealth.ca/mental-health/disorders/post-traumatic-stress-disorder

Autism Spectrum Disorder (ASD)

Autism has been a subject of considerable interest and research effort since its original description more than 70 years ago, when Leo Kanner (1943) described the profound isolation of these children and their extreme desire for sameness. The impairment in communication can be severe and affect both verbal and nonverbal communication (APA, 2013). Children with autism manifest delayed and deviant language development, as evidenced by *echolalia* (repetition of words or phrases spoken by others), and a tendency to be extremely concrete in the interpretation of language. Pronoun reversals and abnormal intonation are also common. Other common features of severe autism categorized as **stereotypic behaviour** (i.e., behaviour patterns that are repetitive and unchanging) include repetitive rocking, hand flapping, and an extraordinary insistence on sameness. The child may also engage in self-injurious behaviour, such as hitting, head banging, or biting. For some children, their unusual interests may evolve into fascination with specific objects, such as fans or air conditioners, or a particular topic, such as Prime Ministers of Canada.

 KEY CONCEPT

An **autism spectrum disorder** is a neurodevelopmental disorder that is distinguished by a marked impairment of development in social interaction and communication with a restrictive repertoire of repetitive activity and interest.

Children with ASD may or may not have an intellectual disability, but they commonly show an uneven pattern of intellectual strengths and weaknesses. They can show a lifelong pattern of being rigid in style, being intolerant of change, and be prone to behavioural outbursts in response to environmental demands or changes in routine. ASD is diagnosed with a severity level requiring support (level 1), substantial support (level 2), or very substantial support (level 3) in the areas of social communication and restricted, repetitive behaviours. Children may or may not have accompanying intellectual impairment; language impairment; association with a known medical or genetic condition or environmental factor; association with another neurodevelopmental, mental, or behavioural disorder; and catatonia.

The literature quite clearly supports the need for early screening and referral programs to promote early diagnosis and treatment (Daniels & Mandell, 2014; Pinto-Martin, Souders, Giarelli, & Levy, 2005). Some early developmental indicators that suggest that a child should be referred for a full assessment include lack of babbling or gestures at 12 months, lack of single words by 16 months, lack of two-word combinations by 18 months, and any regression or loss of words or skills. Other developmental indicators include lack of joint attention (pointing to show), lack of response to name, and unusual or absent eye contact and use of facial expression (Perry & Condillac, 2003). Parents who report concerns about their child's development should be taken seriously. Early identification through screening followed by psychosocial support and education about the disorder and treatment options can help families to adjust and cope (Pinto-Martin et al., 2005). Nursing has a pivotal role to play in all these areas.

Epidemiology and Aetiology

There has been a dramatic rise in the incidence of ASD, from 6.4 per 1,000 children aged 8 years in 2002 to 11.4 per 1,000 in 2008 for the 13 sites that provided data for both surveillance years in the United States (Centers for Disease Control and Prevention, 2012). The use of broader diagnostic criteria, more systematic assessment practices, and increased awareness and attention by health care professionals are factors that may be contributing to this apparent increase (Persico & Bourgeron, 2006). ASD occurs more often in boys than in girls, with the ratio ranging from 2:1 to 5:1. However, when girls are affected, they are often diagnosed later than boys. Researchers attributed this to differences between the sexes in autism symptoms. They found that girls have less severe autistic mannerisms (Hiller, Young, & Weber, 2014). About half of children with ASD are intellectually disabled, and about 25% have seizure disorders.

The specific cause of ASD remains elusive, though research continues in the areas of genetics, neurology, and metabolic disorders. Numerous theories suggest various causes for autism, including genetics, perinatal insult, and impaired parent–child interactions (Volkmar, Klin, & Paul, 2004). Low IQ and autism recur at a higher than expected rate in the siblings of children with autism, and monozygotic twins are more likely to be **concordant** (mutually affected) than are dizygotic twins, suggesting that genetic factors play a role in the disorder. Other proposed causes include perinatal complications, such as exposure to infectious agents or medications during gestation, prematurity, and gestational bleeding. The role of environment in autistic disorders has been conclusively demonstrated only for prenatal or perinatal exposure to viral agents, such as rubella and cytomegalovirus, and prenatal exposure to thalidomide and valproic acid. Vaccinations, especially the MMR vaccine, have also drawn attention as a possible causative factor. However, recent epidemiologic studies and meta-analyses have excluded a widespread causal role for vaccines in autism (Taylor, Swerdfeger, & Eslick, 2014). The specific cause remains unknown and may result from multiple factors. Studies of genetic, epigenetic, and environmental factors are finally beginning to provide some insights into solving the complexities of autistic disorder (Anagnostou et al., 2014; Volkar et al., 2014). Structural and functional imaging studies also provide intriguing leads for future inquiry (Fig. 30.1).

Nursing Care

The nursing assessment is an ongoing process in which attention is given to establishing a positive relationship with the child and the family. The assessment should include a review of the child's capacity for self-care and maladaptive behaviours (Anagnostou et al., 2014; Pinto-Martin et al., 2005; Sherer & Schreibman, 2005). Self-injury and aggression are sometimes present, and children may need to be protected from hurting themselves and others. Inquiry should also include the presence of perseverative behaviours and preoccupation with restricted interests. These odd behaviours may not necessarily cause a problem, but they often interfere with the child's relationships.

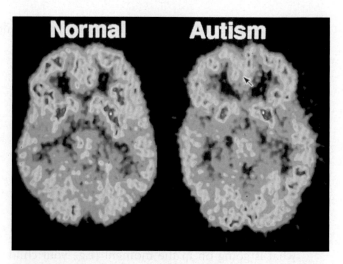

Figure 30.1. The client with autism (*right*) may have decreased metabolic rates in the cingulate gyrus and other associated areas; however, wide heterogeneity in brain metabolic patterns is seen in clients with autism. (Courtesy of Monte S. Buchsbaum, MD, Mount Sinai Medical Centre and School of Medicine, New York, NY.)

Assessment data generate a variety of potential nursing diagnoses, including social isolation. Because of the long-term nature of these disorders, the aims of treatment may change with time. However, throughout childhood, the focus should be on the development of age-appropriate adaptive and social skills. The family may be grieving the loss of a "normal" child it had expected and is trying to cope with the multitude of problems inherent in raising a child with a disability. Therefore, an important domain to consider in the nursing assessment is the effect of the child's developmental delays on the family. Having a child with ASD is bound to influence family interaction, and responding to the child's needs may adversely affect family functioning. For example, sleep disruption in family members who care for children with ASD may increase family stress.

Biopsychosocial Domain

Planning interventions for youngsters with severe developmental problems consider the child, family, and community supports, such as schools, rehabilitation centres, mental health centres, or group homes and available respite services. First and foremost, the various clinicians involved in the child's treatment should collaborate with the family to promote reaching the same general goals. As the number of clinicians and educators involved increases, the chance of fragmentation in treatment planning also increases. The nurse can serve as a case coordinator to ensure that the plan of care is both comprehensive and appropriate in meeting the needs of both the child and the family.

Continuum of Care

ASD is chronic and usually requires long-term care at various levels of intensity. Children and adolescents with autism are a heterogeneous group, and as such, they have diverse needs. It is essential that intervention treatment plans be based on individual patterns of strengths and limitations (Anagnostou et al., 2014; Perry & Condillac, 2003). Intervention treatment consists of designing academic, interpersonal, and social experiences that support the child's development. Children with autism, even those who are severely affected, may be able to live at home and attend a special school for children with autism that uses behaviour modification. Public schools are increasingly able to accommodate some children with autism, often with the support of an educational assistant. Other outpatient services may include family counselling, home care, and medication. As the child moves towards adulthood, living at home may become more difficult, given the appropriate need for greater independence. The level of structure required depends primarily on IQ and adaptive functioning. Ongoing support and respite for the family are critical and an essential part of the intervention treatment plan in which nursing plays an integral role. Autism services in some communities facilitate residential and supported living care.

Promoting Interaction

Many of the core deficits in ASD fall within the domain of social development, regardless of the level of cognitive functioning of the particular child or youth. The goal of intervention in the social domain is to increase meaningful relationships by teaching skills that support the development of social interest, social initiation, social responsiveness, empathy, and understanding of the other's perspective. It is critical that intervention treatment plans include strategies to enhance social understanding, social relating, and play skills and that these strategies take into account the individual's cognitive, learning, linguistic, and developmental abilities (Anagnostou et al., 2014; Perry & Condillac, 2003). Interventions fostering nonverbal social interactions may sometimes be more useful than those based on speech. For higher-functioning children, activities such as getting the mail, passing out snacks, or taking turns in the context of simple games can engage them in social activities without requiring the use of their limited language skills. Structuring social interactions so that the child has to share a task with another (e.g., carrying a load of books) may help to boost confidence in relating to others.

Ensuring Predictability and Safety

When children with ASD are hospitalized, milieu management—a consistent, structured environment with predictable routines for activities, mealtimes, and bedtimes—is necessary for successful treatment. Changes in routine may provoke disorganization in the child with ASD, leading to emotional disequilibrium and explosive behaviour. The safety of the inpatient unit offers an opportunity to try behavioural strategies, such as

rewards for managing transitions. Healthcare professionals can explore with family the strategies that have been successful for managing behaviours in the past and can also share new successful strategies with parents or primary caregivers.

Self-Care

In teaching self-care skills, the nurse needs to consider the child's current adaptive skills and language limitations. Developing a list of activities for children to post in their bedroom may be effective. Drawings or symbols may be useful for nonverbal children. Physical safety is an important concern for children who are cognitively delayed and may have impaired judgment.

Supporting Family

Autism and related disorders are chronic conditions that call for extraordinary patience and determination. Unfortunately, lack of integration of medical, psychiatric, social, and educational services can add to the family's burden. Family stress research has repeatedly demonstrated that parents (especially mothers) of children with ASDs experience greater stress, depression, and mental health difficulties than parents of children with other types of disability (Perry & Condillac, 2003). Parents may manifest feelings of denial, grief, guilt, anger, and sorrow at various points as they adjust to their child's disability. The nurse can offer parents the opportunity to express their frustrations and disappointments and can be alert for indications that parents are in need of additional assistance, such as parent support groups or respite care. Residential and respite care may be necessary in some cases. After making the decision to place a child into someone else's care, family members may experience guilt, loss, and a sense of failure concerning their inability to care for the child at home.

Family interventions include support, education, counselling, and referral to self-help groups. Whenever possible, the nurse provides education to help parents determine appropriate expectations for their child with ASD and to meet the child's special needs. The following are examples of potentially useful nursing interventions focusing on the family:

- Interpreting the treatment plan for parents and the child
- Modelling appropriate behaviour modification techniques
- Including the parents as cotherapists for the implementation of the care plan
- Assisting the family members in identifying and resolving their sense of loss related to the diagnosis
- Coordinating support systems for parents, siblings, and family members
- Maintaining interdisciplinary collaboration

- Facilitating access to and encouraging families to use formal support services such as respite care
- Assisting parents to advocate/lobby on behalf of their child and children with disabilities

There are a number of support services in Canada and throughout the provinces; however, it is best that parents access services through legitimate agencies and organizations. For examples of these, see Web Links.

Evaluation of client and family outcomes is an ongoing process. Short-term outcomes might consist of discrete behavioural improvements, such as reducing self-injurious behaviour by 50%. The long-term goal is for the client to achieve the highest level of functioning. The prognosis depends on the severity of the impairments, the interventions available, and the cognitive ability of the child. The use of standardized rating scales before and after the treatment can improve the precision of outcome measurement (Perry & Condillac, 2003).

IN-A-LIFE

Temple Grandin (1949–)

SCIENTIST AND A PERSON WITH AUTISM

Public Persona

Dr. Temple Grandin is a gifted scientist and world-renowned expert on cattle. Her book *Thinking in Pictures and Other Reports of My Life With Autism* (1996) is an astonishing examination of the profoundly different way in which a person with autism conceives and experiences the world. Her story shows the extraordinary way in which she uses her visual thinking ability to develop her field of animal science. It gives us a view of her world and helps us understand the reason she identifies with Data, the android in *Star Trek*. In 2010, her story appeared as a movie, *Temple Grandin*, starring Claire Danes.

Personal Realities

As a child, Temple experienced life as chaotic, full of engulfing sensations of sound, smell, and touch. She would scream, rock, or spin continually and shut the world out by fixing for hours on one object. At first thought to be deaf when she did not learn to speak, she was taken to a neurologist and labelled "brain damaged." Although she gained a sense of language and speech, connecting with others was affected by her inability to understand them or them, her. She dreamed of a magic machine that could give her safe "hugging." Her mother's dedication to her and the guidance of a gifted science teacher enabled her to create a life as a scientist.

Specific Learning Disorders

Specific **learning disorders** (also called learning disabilities) are among the most common neurodevelopmental disorders in children and are defined as difficulties in learning and using academic skills. They are important causes of poor school performance. For this diagnosis to be given, a child must have specific difficulties for over 6 months. These need to be significantly different from what is expected for their age and interfere with their performance in school or work. See the *DSM-5* for the APA (2013) diagnostic criteria.

Communication Disorders

Communication disorders involve deficits in speech, language, and communication. *Speech* refers to the motor aspects of making sounds and includes "articulation, fluency, voice, and resonance quality" (APA, 2013, p. 41). *Language* consists of higher-order aspects of formulating and comprehending a conventional system of symbols (e.g., spoken words, sign language, pictures) (APA). *Communication* involves verbal and/or nonverbal behaviour (whether or not intentional) that influences another person (APA). Communication disorder in the *DSM-5* includes "language disorder, speech sound disorder, childhood-onset fluency disorder (stuttering), social (pragmatic) communication disorder, and other specified and non-specified communication disorders" (APA, 2013, p. 41).

Nursing Care Related to Learning Disabilities and Communication Disorders

For children with learning disabilities, the negative effects of low achievement or failure may be manifested in low self-esteem and reduced academic effort. Some children and adolescents may also exhibit difficulties in age-appropriate social interactions. Postsecondary students with learning disabilities have been observed to exhibit poor self-concept, have difficulties with interpersonal skills, and have deficits in processing and study skills (Ransby & Swanson, 2003). Research also suggests that children and adolescents with **learning disorders** experience more feelings of loneliness, depression, stress, and suicidal ideations than their peers without learning disabilities (Buysse, Goldman, & Skinner, 2003). For the child/adolescent with learning disabilities, nurses can focus on building self-confidence and helping the family connect with guidance and educational resources that support his or her ongoing development.

Communication disorders are an area in which assessments must be absolutely relevant to the cultural and linguistic background of the individual, if they are to be valid. Speech pathologists conduct the diagnostic assessment. Services such as speech therapy (directed at the motor aspects of speaking) or social skills groups (directed at the social and interpersonal aspects of language) may be available in some school districts and can be obtained if a speech or language disorder has been identified. For some children with communication disorders, the services offered by the school may be insufficient. In such cases, the nurse can help the family locate resources that can provide these needed services.

For the child with a communication disorder, interventions focus on fostering social and communication skills, identifying and addressing low self-esteem, and making referrals for specific speech or language therapy. Modelling appropriate communication in spontaneous situations with the child can be a useful intervention for some children. As with other neurodevelopmental disorders, education and support of the parents are a key intervention.

Neurobehavioural Disorder Associated With Prenatal Alcohol Exposure (ND-PAE) and Foetal Alcohol Spectrum Disorder (FASD)

ND-PAE is identified by the APA as a condition needing further study (APA, 2013). It is intended as a classification that can include the range of developmental disabilities arising due to exposure to alcohol in utero (APA). Its broader criteria could increase treatment options for those affected by its symptoms (Cook et al., 2015). See the *DSM-5* for the symptoms of ND-PAE. FASD is a set of effects due to prenatal alcohol exposure. Its diagnosis requires physical and neurodevelopment assessments by an interprofessional team. For a diagnosis of FASD to be made, pervasive brain dysfunction needs to be indicated in at least three of these neurodevelopmental areas: "motor skills; neuroanatomy/neurophysiology; cognition; language; academic achievement; memory; attention; executive function, including impulse control and hyperactivity; affect regulation; and adaptive behaviour, social skills or social communication" (Canada FASD Network, 2016, p. 193). There are sentinel facial features that can warrant the diagnosis without confirmation of the mother's intake of alcohol during pregnancy due to their specific association with FASD. Good evidence of the mother's prenatal alcohol use is sufficient for an "at-risk" diagnosis for FASD (Canada FASD Network).

Epidemiology and Aetiology

The prevalence of ND-PAE is estimated to be between 2% and 5% in the United States (APA, 2013). The prevalence of FASD is approximately 1% in Canada. The amount of alcohol needed to have negative effects on the developing foetus is unknown. There is no safe amount or safe time in the gestational period for alcohol consumption recommended.

Treatment Interventions

There are no medications approved specifically to treat ND-PAE or FASD. However, several medications can help improve some of the symptoms. For example,

medication might help manage high energy levels, inability to focus, aggression, anxiety, or depression. Medications can affect each child differently. One medication might work well for one child, but not for another. To find the right treatment, a trial of different medications and doses may be explored. It is important for the nurse to work closely with the child and family to monitor both negative and positive effects of medication prescribed.

Nursing Care

The bio/psycho/social/spiritual care of the child with ND-PAE or FASD can be complex; therefore, each child or adolescent must be reviewed individually to determine what symptoms are causing dysfunction. Most interventions focus on providing support with executive functioning, social skills teaching and practice, self-regulation skills, and positive behavioural supports. The coexisting or predominant symptoms of the disorder will determine the intervention strategies employed. For example, if the child or adolescent has challenges of impulsiveness and hyperactivity, interventions similar to those used with a child with ADHD may be beneficial. Factors of cognitive processing may impact the effect of interventions used. Each child will need to be assessed and worked with individually to truly identify the best approach.

DISRUPTIVE, IMPULSE CONTROL, AND CONDUCT DISORDERS

The disruptive behaviour disorders within the *DSM-5* include ODD, conduct disorder, intermittent explosive disorder, kleptomania, and pyromania (APA, 2013). For purposes of this text, we will focus on ODD and conduct disorder, syndromes marked by significant problems of conduct. These **externalizing disorders** contrast with disorders of depressive and anxiety disorders, which are referred to as **internalizing disorders** because the symptoms tend to be within the child.

Oppositional Defiant Disorder

Unfortunately, some children are labelled oppositional if they challenge authority or have temper tantrums. To be a disorder, however, the argumentative, defiant, angry behaviour needs to be continual over a period of months and be present with more than family members. There cannot be another mental health disorder that accounts for it, such as substance use disorder or psychosis. There is some discourse that ODD may be a disorder of emotional dysregulation. Further research will need to be conducted to affirm this aspect of the diagnosis (Cavanagh, Quinn, Duncan, Graham, & Balbuena, 2017).

Treatment Interventions

The nurse will need to work with the child and family to attend to coexisting conditions such as ADHD, anxiety disorder, or depression. Specific interventions to support the child coping with anxiety may alleviate some of the oppositional traits. Similarly, if the ADHD is treated medically or structurally, the symptoms of ODD may be alleviated. The nurse will need to provide additional teaching and direction regarding ODD to support groups and agencies primarily focused on working with children with ADHD and depressive and anxiety disorders (Ollendick et al., 2016).

Nursing Care

Families of children who have ODD may be frustrated and focused on the negative behaviour challenges of the child. The nurse's task is to assist the family to refocus and find the child's strengths and skills, as well as learn to respond to negative behaviours in ways that promote positive change. Similar to working with the child with a trauma history, the caregivers work to develop strategies to attune to their child and understand the child's emotional triggers. The family is taught to work with the child to recognize those feelings and develop new coping skills that allow the child to socialize with others in a more positive manner (Boston Children's Hospital, 2013). Depending on the child's age and family circumstances, some programs take a behavioural modification approach. The evidence for successful outcomes with this approach is inconsistent. Mindfulness is being used in some programs as a strategy; others are incorporating technology, such as computer games, to teach children emotional regulation (Boston Children's Hospital, 2013).

Biologic Domain

The aetiology of ODD is complex; however, there is growing evidence that indicates both genetic and environmental components (Bornovalova, Hicks, Iacono, & McGue, 2010). Complicating a diagnosis of ODD is often a coexisting condition such as ADHD, a learning disability, internalizing disorder, and/or trauma disorder (Shanahan et al., 2014). If ODD persists into adulthood, the challenges the youth and adult face may be significant (Burke, Row, & Boylan, 2014).

Psychosocial Domain

Children with ODD that persists across their development struggle socially: they experience frequent conflicts with peers, teachers, siblings, and caregivers. The child may have experienced negative parenting (e.g., neglectful, punitive, erratic), perhaps due to parental frustration or a parent's own oppositional traits. The child may have experienced bullying or may be the bully. If the challenges are significant, the family will need to consider if the child's recovery will be better supported in a new school environment. The nurse will need to work closely with those involved with the child to create an environment where the child learns new communication strategies and others learn ways to respond to the child that are helpful and supportive of change. Evaluation for secondary contributing disorders such

as ADHD, anxiety, or depression will need to occur (Boylan, Vaillancourt, Boyle, & Szatmari, 2007).

Conduct Disorder

Conduct disorder has been identified as having three potential onsets: childhood before the age of 10 years, adolescence after 10 years, and unspecified, wherein no information is available to determine the age of onset. Childhood-onset conduct disorder may have a poorer prognosis than adolescent onset. The disorder typically occurs in males and may or may not have precursor conditions such as ODD, ADHD, or internalizing disorders. There is some indication that a traumatic childhood or poor attachment may also lead to the development of conduct disorder symptoms.

Nursing Care

Determining what the child/youth and family are ready to address is critical with this population. There are several family-based treatments that have demonstrated success over time. The challenge for the nurse is engaging the child/youth and family in the process (Box 30.6). For example, multisystem therapy is an intensive family-and community-based treatment program that focuses on addressing all environmental systems—home, school, neighbourhood—and works towards affecting change in all domains. The primary focus is developing the child's/youth's relationships, identifying and building on strengths, developing responsibility and accountability, and promoting success (Henggeler & Sheidow, 2012).

Biologic Domain

There is evidence of genetic contribution that is complicated by environmental factors. For instance, the risk for conduct disorder is increased in the offspring of individuals with conduct disorder. The effects of a traumatic home environment that includes family disruption, parental mental illness, poverty, community violence, and abuse also increase the risk for conduct disorder in biologic or adopted children (Bornovalova et al., 2010; Kim-Cohen et al., 2005). Recent studies have been examining the neurodevelopment of children with conduct disorder. There is exploratory research indicating some evidence that there may be a reduction in gray matter in the brain in areas that govern social–emotional functioning; the cause, however, remains unclear (Fairchild et al., 2011). Lower than average intelligence, verbal IQ in particular, may be contributory to the diagnosis. Males with conduct disorder often exhibit more overt aggression, whereas females tend to be more subversive in their aggression (APA, 2013).

Psychosocial Domain

Children/youth with conduct disorder are often in trouble with the law, school authorities, and family. They often experience rejection from caregivers, school, and their community. They may also be exposed to abusive home environments if parents also have conduct traits

BOX 30.6 CLINICAL VIGNETTE

LEON (CONDUCT DISORDER)

Leon, a 14-year-old boy, was admitted to the child psychiatric inpatient service from the emergency department after a fight with his mother. His mother reported that she and Leon had argued earlier in the evening and that he stormed out of the house screaming and vowing that he would never return. Several hours later, Leon came back, yelling and demanding entry into the apartment. Leon's father was working and not at home. While his mother was getting up to open the door, Leon continued to yell and scream, waking the neighbours. This led to further arguing between Leon and his mother. Before long, the police were called, and Leon was taken to the emergency department.

The admission interview revealed that Leon had run away on several occasions and had even stayed away overnight. Although he strongly denied drug use, he had gotten drunk on several occasions. He had also been in several fights, the latest of which resulted in an expulsion from school. Three months before admission, he was caught trying to steal a CD from a music store. More recently, he boasted that he and his friends had snatched a purse at an outdoor concert and had broken into a car to steal its contents. Leon's school performance has been declining; he was truant on several occasions and will probably have to repeat ninth grade.

Leon was born in Cape Breton, N.S., and is the oldest of three children. His family moved to Toronto shortly after his birth. His father is employed as a janitor and is illiterate. His mother works as a secretary and has recently completed a BA in English. There is much marital discord at home. Leon has received no treatment except for consultation with the school social worker.

WHAT DO YOU THINK?

- When conducting a nursing assessment, what would you want to learn about Leon's school performance?
- What information could you provide Leon's parents about pharmacotherapy? About behaviour management?
- How would you present the material so it meets the learning needs of both parents?

---

or there are environmental contributors such as poverty or violence. The context in which a diagnosis is applied needs to be taken into account if it is considered normative for the community and general survival. Coexisting disorders that are often associated with conduct disorder are ODD, ADHD, learning and/or communication disorders, as well as internalizing disorders such as anxiety, depression, and likely PTSD (see Box 30.7).

Attention Deficit Hyperactivity Disorder

All children have occasional experiences with inattention and high energy levels. For most children, these occurrences do not interfere with daily life. According to the Canadian ADHD Resource Alliance (CADDRA, 2011), ADHD is a neuropsychiatric developmental disorder affecting 5% to 12% of school-aged children, 8% to 10% of males under the age of 18, and 3% to 4% of females under 18 (CADDRA, 2013b; Ramtekkar, Reiersen, Todorov, & Todd, 2010). It is associated with functional impairments such as school challenges, peer problems, and family conflict. Parents and teachers describe children with ADHD as restless, always on the go, highly distractable, unable to wait for their turn,

heedless, and frequently disruptive. Often, it is their disruptive behaviour that brings these children into treatment. Children with inattentive ADHD often are missed and do not receive a diagnosis until later in life. Children and youth with ADHD can struggle in a multitude of domains at different times throughout their development. It is likely that, at some point in their career, nurses will work with children, adolescents, and adults with ADHD. See the *DSM-5* for APA diagnostic criteria for ADHD (APA, 2013).

Both clinical observations and laboratory studies support the conclusion that children with ADHD can be prone to impulsiveness and risk-taking behaviours (Biederman & Faraone, 2005). In behavioural terms, children with ADHD often fail to consider the consequences of their actions, exercise poor judgment, and tend to have more than the usual lumps, bumps, and bruises because of their risk-taking behaviour. They often require a high degree of structure and supervision. In many cases, it is the hyperactivity that prompts the search for treatment. Parents typically report that the child's hyperactivity started early in life and is evident in most situations. These behaviours, although challenging, often are not deemed problematic until the child

BOX 30.7 Research for Best Practice

CHANGE IN A FATHER'S PERCEPTIONS OF MENTAL HEALTH WHEN HIS CHILD IS DIAGNOSED WITH A MENTAL ILLNESS

Morris, M. (2014). Diagnosis in young children: How a father's perceptions of mental health change. Journal of Child and Adolescent Psychiatric Nursing, 27(2), 52–60.

Questions: How does diagnosing mental illness in a young child (less than 10 years) affect a parent's perception of mental health?

Methods: Case study method was used, guided by Denzin's interpretive interactionism, in which "epiphanies" or pivotal life experiences that deeply affect one's sense of self and the world are explored. "Joe," the father in this case study, has a son, "Billy," who struggled behaviourally when he attended kindergarten in a charter school. Joe was asked to come with Billy to help him adjust. When, on the advice of the school counsellor, this ended, Billy reacted violently, destroying part of his classroom and hurting teachers and classmates. Diagnoses proposed for Billy, now 7 years old, include attachment disorder, ADHD, mood disorder, bipolar disorder, and low-grade autism. Billy's parents have sought help for him from a play therapist with a specialty in attachment, an occupational therapist, a psychotherapist,

an alternative school psychologist, and a neurologist. Joe and his wife have reached out to other parents with similar experiences.

Findings: Themes that emerged for Joe were "alienation from peers, ambivalence, shifting orientation to mental illness, school system stigmatization/conflict with mental health care, and discovery of mental health care specialists and new peers." Joe stated, "It has been this progression of acceptance." "… I even started to see going to play therapy, it was partly just for me as much as for [Billy] … I actually was looking forward to going because … I was getting as much out of it as he was in a lot of ways. I wasn't exactly expecting that, I guess…."

Implications for Nursing Practice: The researcher notes that the loss of self-agency experienced by this parent in his interactions with school and health care systems was notable. This points to the need for active promotion of a meaningful sense of agency and hope in working with parents, in addition to offering medical and technologic interventions.

---

enters a more structured environment such as day care, kindergarten, or school.

The diagnosis of ADHD is based upon the ability to observe symptoms that seem to occur consistently in at least two different environments, such as home and school. For the diagnosis to be given, there must be at least some symptoms present before the age of 12 years and they must be present for at least 6 months. A physical exam should be performed, as well as a hearing and eyesight test, to rule out any physical reasons for the symptoms. A psychoeducational assessment is recommended to determine whether other learning disabilities coexist with the ADHD or cause the symptoms (CADDRA, 2013b).

Longitudinal studies that followed groups of children with ADHD into adulthood have shown the persistence of symptoms (Biederman & Faraone, 2005; Uchida, Spencer, Faraone, & Biederman, 2015). There is change in symptom presentation as an individual grows and develops and perhaps acquires compensatory strategies; however, even when symptoms are not prominent, they remain associated with clinically significant impairments (Centre for ADHD Awareness, Canada [CADDAC], 2013). Older adolescents and young adults with a history of ADHD may struggle with staying in school and keeping a job and maintaining relationships and have more

traffic violations and accidents than individuals without the diagnosis of ADHD (CADDAC, 2013).

KEY CONCEPT

Attention is a complex process that involves the ability to concentrate on one activity to the exclusion of others and the ability to sustain that focus.

KEY CONCEPT

Impulsiveness refers to acting in the moment without considering the consequences of the act, which may be potentially highly harmful, and without considering alternative actions.

KEY CONCEPT

Hyperactivity refers to excessive motor activity, movement, and/or utterances when it is not appropriate and may be purposeless (e.g., fidgeting, tapping, or talkativeness; APA, 2013).

Epidemiology and Aetiology Factors

ADHD emerged as the first psychiatric disorder to be diagnosed and treated in children, with studies of stimulant treatment beginning in 1937 and regulatory approval for it occurring in the 1960s (Doyle, 2004). ADHD has emerged from the 20th century with a good deal of scientific investigation of its validity and clarification of clinical controversies. Nevertheless, the aetiology of ADHD remains unclear. No one causal factor is necessary or sufficient to trigger the disorder, and risk factors are interchangeable. Risk factors can include prenatal exposure to nicotine, alcohol, and other substances. Maternal stress can have an impact on the developing foetus. The development of the disorder includes genetic predisposition and biologic, environmental, and psychosocial factors (Children's Health Policy Centre, 2017). What is critical is the total number of risk factors (Biederman & Faraone, 2005).

Numerous environmental exposures, including food sensitivity, food additives, and lead poisoning, have been examined as potential causes of ADHD and generally have been found to be false (Biederman & Faraone, 2005). A balanced diet and regular activity and exercise are a good strategy for everyone. There is increasing evidence, however, that a relative lack of omega-3 fatty acids may contribute in many psychiatric and neurodevelopmental disorders, including ADHD (Richardson, 2006). A positive correlation has been found between obstetrical complications and ADHD and learning disorders. A Quebec study of 64 children aged 6 to 12 diagnosed with ADHD was conducted to assess for a history of obstetrical complications using the Kinney Medical and Gynecological Questionnaire. Children with ADHD and a learning disability in mathematics or reading had a higher rate of neonatal complications than children with ADHD and no disability (Bhat, Grizenko, Ben-Amor, & Joober, 2005). These results further support what has already been shown for ADHD and learning disorders individually: that the events in the early life of a child are critical to brain development.

For many decades, studies have shown that ADHD has a genetic transmission among families (Faraone, 2004; Schachar, 2014). Recently, brain imaging studies have revealed that there is "atypical brain structure in ADHD, implicating multiple neural systems including attention, cognitive control, and working memory" (Dang et al., 2016). Through MRI research studies (not a common diagnostic process), there is demonstrated reduction in brain volume and changes with development. It is with this understanding that ADHD has been reclassified most recently in the *DSM-5* under neurodevelopmental disorders. Parents may request a brain scan based on this new literature; however, as mentioned, it is not a diagnostic process at this time.

Treatment Interventions

Treatment of ADHD typically is conducted in community clinic settings. Optimal treatment is multimodal (includes several types of interventions), encompassing five main areas: (1) psychoeducation for the child and family; (2) behavioural and/or occupational interventions for the child; (3) individual and family support, counselling, and therapy; (4) school accommodations; and (5) medication management.

A combined behavioural–psychosocial and pharmaceutical approach allows for significantly lower doses of medication than a medication-only approach in achieving treatment outcomes and decreasing the risk of side effects (Chronis, Jones, & Raggi, 2006). Medication can mitigate the symptoms of hyperactivity, impulsiveness, and inattention; therefore, teaching the parent, child, and school personnel about the importance of the medication in ADHD and the potential side effects is a place to begin. Explaining to the child that the medication improves concentration and the ability to sit still can help strengthen motivation and adherence to treatment; however, nonadherence is typically more a matter of forgetting than one of deliberate avoidance.

For more than 40 years, the primary treatment for ADHD has been stimulant medications. Although each of these medications has demonstrated efficacy in controlled studies, methylphenidate (Ritalin) has received considerably more research effort and has emerged as the first-line effective therapy to treat ADHD (Flapper & Schoemaker, 2008). It should be noted that stimulants are not effective in all cases; alternatives have been created such as norepinephrine reuptake inhibitor (atomoxetine). Many of the newer treatments for ADHD have been developed to treat symptoms for longer periods of time throughout the day. Occasionally, the use of antidepressants may be beneficial. The overuse of medication to treat ADHD is an ongoing concern of parents and others. Careful assessment and education for child/youth and family will determine the individual need and areas of concern. As with most mental health disorders in children, the aim of treatment for ADHD is to decrease symptoms, enhance functionality, and improve well-being for the child and his or her close contacts. The CADDRA Guide to ADHD Pharmacological Treatments is available in chart format, including coloured images of the medication. (See Web Links.)

Well-managed medication is an important intervention for the core symptoms of ADHD to facilitate the other areas of intervention (CADDRA, 2011). Parent training and social skills training also help diminish disruptive and defiant behaviours (see Nursing Care Plan 30.1). Treatment plans need regular upgrading to address important social, cognitive, psychological, and physical changes that occur as the child ages (Children's Health Policy Centre, Simon Fraser University, 2007).

Nursing Care

The primary focus of the assessment is the impact of ADHD symptoms on academic and social functioning. The nurse tries to determine the contribution of symptoms of ADHD with the acute psychiatric problem. Assessment data are collected through direct interview, observation of the child and parent, and teacher ratings. Because children with ADHD may have difficulty sitting through long sessions, interviews are typically brief or involve an activity to engage the child. Parents and teachers are extremely important sources for assessment data. To this end, the nurse can make use of several standardized instruments (Box 30.8) including those outlined in the *Canadian ADHD Practice Guidelines* (2011), available at the Canadian ADHD Resource Alliance (CADDRA) Web site.

The association of ADHD with other psychiatric disorders warrants a careful and fulsome assessment. Medical history is essential, consisting of perinatal course, childhood illnesses, hospital admissions, injuries, seizures, tics, physical growth, overall health status, and timing of the child's last physical examination. Family history is also an important part of assessment data.

Children with ADHD can be very active; they struggle to sit still and often fidget or bounce their leg to keep moving. They may be more active during sleep than children without the disorder. A functional assessment of eating, sleeping, and activity patterns is therefore essential. Assessing daily food intake, typical diet, and frequency of eating will help identify any nutrition problems. Caffeinated products can contribute to hyperactivity. Sleep is often disturbed for children with ADHD and, consequently, the family. A detailed sleep assessment can provide points for interventions and help the interpretation of drug effects.

With the severity of the responses, regarding family functioning and school environment, several nursing diagnoses could be generated from the assessment data, including self-care deficit, risk for imbalanced nutrition, risk for injury, and disturbed sleep pattern. The outcomes should be individualized to the child (see Fig. 30.2).

Psychosocial

ADHD often occurs in the context of psychosocial adversity. It is important to review the family situation, including parenting style, stability of household membership, consistency of rules and routines, and life events, such as divorce, moves, deaths, and job loss. Identification of these factors can be useful in shaping a care plan that builds on potential strengths and mitigates the effects of environmental factors that may perpetuate the child's disruptive behaviour. Data regarding school performance, behaviour at home, and comorbid psychiatric disorders are essential for developing school interventions and behaviour plans and establishing the baseline severity for medication.

Parents of children with ADHD report more frequent and severe interparental discord and child-rearing disagreements, more negative parenting practices, greater caregiver strain, and more psychopathology themselves. With the added burden that ADHD is highly heritable, one or both parents may also suffer from symptoms that can contribute to family dysfunction (Schachar, 2014). Children with ADHD (impulsive/hyperactive) can be bossy, intrusive, immature, boisterous, aggressive, and less aware of social cues. Such behaviours affect social function, making and keeping friends, and can

---

BOX 30.8 Standardized Tools for ADHD Diagnosis

The Conners Parent Questionnaire is a 48-item scale that a parent completes about his or her child. Each item is a statement that the parent rates on a four-point scale from 0 (not at all) to 3 (very much). The Conners Teacher Questionnaire is a 28-item questionnaire that the child's teacher completes according to the same four-point scale as the parent questionnaire. Both questionnaires have been standardized by age and gender for a mean of 50 and a standard deviation of 10 (Conners, 1989; Goyette, Conners, & Ulrich, 1978).

The ADHD Rating Scale asks parents or teachers to respond directly to 18 items (see Barkley, 1998, for a description of this scale). A similar scale called the SNAP-IV is available online for free at www.adhd.net. The SNAP-IV was used as the primary outcome measure in the MTA Cooperative Group Study (1999).

The Child Behaviour Checklist (CBCL) is a 118-item questionnaire that a parent completes. In addition to the 118 questions about specific behaviours and psychiatric symptoms, the CBCL also includes questions concerning the child's competence in social and academic spheres as well as age-appropriate activities. Normative data are available allowing the conversion of raw scores to standard scores for age and gender. There is also a teacher version of this scale.

Note that the diagnosis of ADHD is not made on the basis of questionnaires alone. Data from these rating scales augment the information gathered through interview and observation. These questionnaires can be especially useful before and after initiating a treatment plan to measure the change.

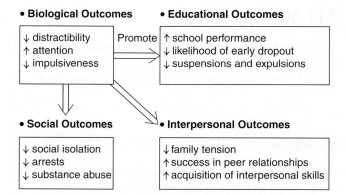

Figure 30.2. Long-term outcomes of optimal treatment for clients with attention deficit hyperactivity disorder.

contribute to parental unwillingness to take their ADHD child on social outings or vacations.

Behavioural programs should focus on creating success and achievement for the child or adolescent. The system should be based on acknowledgment for positive behaviour, such as waiting or completing chores. Interventions may also include specific cognitive-behavioural techniques in which the child learns to "stop, look, and listen" before doing. Depending on the severity of the child's symptoms, family situation, and school environment, several nursing diagnoses could be generated from the assessment data, including impaired social interaction, ineffective role performance, and compromised family coping. Short-term outcomes, such as decreasing the number of classroom ejections within a 2-week period, may be useful for one child, whereas reducing the frequency and amplitude of angry

outbursts at home may be relevant to another child. Building on the child's strengths and capacity, children with ADHD may function better in individualized sports or activities. Removal of these activities as consequences for unacceptable behaviour is not necessarily productive for changing behaviour.

Family treatment is nearly always a component of cognitive–behavioural treatment approaches with the child. This may involve parent education training that focuses on the principles of creating a home environment that has increased predictability and structure. This may prove to be a challenge for parents who have ADHD themselves. At times, the institution of a more formal behaviour management strategy may be required, such as boundary setting and the use of reward systems, as well as revised expectations about the child's behaviour. School programming often involves increasing structure in the child's school day to offset the child's tendency to act without forethought and to be easily distracted by extraneous stimuli. Specific remediation is required for the child with comorbid deficits in learning or language. Some children may require specialized self-contained classrooms; however, they typically have coexisting challenges such as learning disabilities and oppositional defiant or conduct disorder.

The planning of nursing interventions must be done within the context of the family, treatment setting, and school environment. With the parents, clinical team members, and school personnel, the nurse participates in designing a plan of care that fits the child's and family's needs. Resiliency support and focus on strength, for all members of the family, is important and the child moves through life stages.

NURSING CARE PLAN 30.1

ATTENTION DEFICIT HYPERACTIVITY DISORDER

Liam, age 6 years, comes to the mental health clinic with his mother, Avery, because of concerns raised by his teacher. Liam is distracted and disruptive in class and displays motor restlessness. Avery explains that Liam satisfactorily adjusted to kindergarten, but since his entry into first grade this year, his teacher has reported that he has problematic behaviours, such as not waiting his turn and interrupting his peers. On reflection, Avery recalls that kindergarten was an active, half-day program and notes that in first grade, Liam is now expected to sit quietly in his seat and pay attention for longer periods.

Liam's medical history is unremarkable. Avery's pregnancy with Liam was unplanned, her first, and without complications, although the labour was long and resulted in a caesarean section. Significant marital discord began during the pregnancy, culminating in divorce before Liam's first birthday. Liam was healthy at birth and grew

normally, without developmental delays. He genuinely wants to play with other children, but his intrusive style and inability to wait his turn can create frequent conflicts with them. The family history is positive for substance abuse in his father who, according to Avery, was disruptive in school, had trouble concentrating, and was highly impulsive, problems which continued into adulthood. Liam's father is inconsistent in his visits with his son.

During the two evaluation sessions, Liam is active but cooperative. His speech is fluent and normal in tone and tempo, if somewhat loud. His discourse is coherent, but at times, he makes rather abrupt changes in conversation without warning his listeners. Psychological testing at the school revealed average to above average intelligence. Parent and teacher questionnaires concurred that Liam was overactive, impulsive, inattentive, and quarrelsome, but not defiant.

(Continued)

NURSING CARE PLAN 30.1 *(Continued)*

Setting: Mental Health Centre, Child and Adolescent Services

Baseline Assessment: Liam is a 6-year-old boy with prominent hyperactivity and disruptive behaviour. These problems interfere with his interpersonal relationships and academic progress. He lives with Avery, his single mother. Avery is discouraged and feels unable to manage Liam's behaviour.

Associated Psychiatric Diagnosis	Medications
Attention deficit hyperactivity disorder Other issues of note: Parent–child relational problem (mother exhausted/ father absent) Educational problems (peer conflict) Low income (mother in entry-level job) Disruption of family by separation (father inconsistent in visitation routine) GAF = 52* *Although the *DSM-5* does not endorse the Global Assessment of Functioning Score, it may still be seen on a diagnostic report.	Methylphenidate 5 mg at breakfast and lunch (i.e., at 8 AM and 12 noon) and then adding 5 mg at 4 PM.

Nursing Diagnosis 1: Impaired Social Interaction (Liam)

Defining Characteristics	Related Factors
Cannot establish and maintain developmentally appropriate social relationships Has interpersonal difficulties at school Is not well accepted by peers Is easily distracted Interrupts others Cannot wait his turn in games Speaks out of turn in the classroom	Impulsive behaviour Overactive Inattentive Risk-taking behaviour (e.g., tried to climb out the window to get away from Avery) Failure to recognize the effects of his behaviour on others

Outcomes

Initial	Discharge
1. Decrease hyperactivity and disruptive behaviour.	4. Improve capacity to identify alternative responses in conflicts with peers.
2. Improve attention and decrease distractibility.	5. Improve capacity to interpret behaviour of age-mates.
3. Decrease the frequency of acting without forethought.	

NURSING CARE PLAN 30.1 *(Continued)*

Interventions

Interventions	Rationale	Ongoing Assessment
Educate the mother about ADHD and the use of stimulant medication. Provide written information about ADHD, which Avery may share with the teacher and school.	Better understanding helps to ensure adherence; parents and teachers often miscast children with ADHD as "troublemakers."	Determine the extent to which the parent or teacher "blames" Liam for his problems.
Monitor adherence to medication schedule.	Inconsistent use may contribute to a failed trial of medication.	Use of parent and teacher questionnaires; inquire regarding behaviour across the day.
Ensure that the medication is both effective and well tolerated.	Stimulants can affect appetite and sleep and can cause irritability when wearing off (called "rebound").	Administer parent and teacher questionnaires; check weight; ask about sleep and appetite.

Evaluation

Outcomes	Revised Outcomes	Interventions
Liam shows decreased hyperactivity and less disruption in the classroom.	Improve the ability to identify disruptive classroom behaviour.	Initiate a point system to reward appropriate behaviour.
Liam shows improved attention and decreased distractibility.	Improve school performance.	Move to the front of the classroom as an aid to attention.

Evaluation

Outcomes	Revised Outcomes	Interventions
Mother and teacher attest to Liam's decreased impulsive behaviour.	Increase Liam's capacity to recognize the effects of his behaviour on others.	Encourage participation in structured activities.
Liam identifies alternative responses such as walking away until it is his turn.	Increase the frequency of acting on these alternative approaches.	Inquire about small friendship groups (work on socialization strategies) at school, if available.
Liam improves interpretation of motives and behaviours of others.	Improve acceptance by peers.	Encourage participation in community activities.

Nursing Diagnosis 2: Parent–Child Relational Problem, Ineffective Coping (Avery)

Defining Characteristics	Related Factors
Verbalizes discouragement and inability to handle the situation with Liam	Chronicity of ADHD
Expresses frustration in her parenting abilities, admits to "giving in"	More than average child-rearing problems

(Continued)

NURSING CARE PLAN 30.1 *(Continued)*

Outcomes

Initial	Discharge
1. Verbalize frustration at trying to raise a child with ADHD alone.	3. Identify coping patterns that decrease the sense of frustration and increase parental competence.
2. Identify positive methods of interacting with and teaching Liam that will support the parent–child relationship as well as meet Liam's developmental needs.	4. Initiate a collaborative relationship with the teacher.
	5. Identify sources of support in the community and begin to access these resources.

Interventions

Interventions	Rationale	Ongoing Assessment
Assess the mother's discouragement and feelings about parenting, identifying specific problem areas.	Helping the mother verbalize her feelings and identify problem areas helps in formulating problem-solving strategies.	Assess the severity of the problems with which she is living.
Refer the mother to a community health centre for free parenting class.	Parent training based on clear directives and rewards can be effective for decreasing impulsive and disruptive behaviours.	Monitor the mother's level of confidence and perceived change in Liam's behaviour.
Refer the mother to a credible, supportive self-help organization.	Parent groups such as Children and Adults with Attention Deficit Disorder (CHADD) can be sources of support and information.	Determine whether contact was made and whether it was helpful.
Make contact with school to enhance collaboration with the mother and to address teachers' questions regarding ADHD.	Assess the effectiveness of medication and other interventions, based on feedback from teachers.	Determine whether the mother has been able to contact the teacher.

Evaluation

Outcomes	Revised Outcomes	Interventions
After four sessions, Avery expresses her frustrations, but she has begun to identify different ways of relating to Liam and his developmental needs.	None	None
Through attending the parenting class and joining a support group, Avery begins to change her coping patterns, decrease her frustrations, and increase parental competence.	Complete the parenting class; attend at least two support group meetings each month.	If necessary, refer for additional parent counselling.
Avery initiates a collaborative relationship with Liam's teacher.	Avery and Liam's teacher mutually develop and implement behaviour plans for home and school.	Have the mother observe in the classroom; have the mother visit highly structured classroom.

Reference for Nursing Diagnoses: Carpenito, L. J. (2017). *Nursing diagnosis: Application to clinical practice.* Philadelphia, PA: Wolters Kluwer.

MOTOR DISORDERS: TOURETTE'S DISORDER

Motor disorders include developmental coordination disorder, stereotypic movement disorder, and tic disorders (American Psychiatric Association, 2013). Tic disorders, specifically Tourette's disorder, will be the focus here. A **tic** is a sudden motor movement. Tics have different degrees of severity, and no two children have the same pattern (Singer, 2005). Tourette's disorder involves both motor (shrugs, blinks, grimaces to smelling, touching objects or people) and vocal (humming, yelling a word) tics and exhibits a waxing and waning course. Regarding prognosis, by late adolescence/early adulthood, the disorder will have disappeared for one third of those diagnosed with it, improved for another one third, and continue to fluctuate for the remaining third (Singer, 2013).

Tourette's disorder is undetectable in CAT, PET, and MRI scans (Murray, 2008), and there are no diagnostic laboratory tests for it. The Yale Global Tic Severity Scale has been found to be a reliable and valid instrument for the assessment of paediatric Tourette's syndrome (Storch et al., 2005).

Epidemiology and Aetiology

The prevalence of Tourette's disorder is estimated to be from 3 to 8 per 1,000 in school-aged children, with boys being affected more than girls at a 2:1 to 4:1 ratio (APA, 2013). Named after George Gilles de la Tourette, a French neurologist who described "maladie des tics" in the late 1880s, Tourette's syndrome was originally deemed psychological in origin—Freud considered it a form of hysteria—with treatment thus being psychoanalytic therapy and/or hypnosis (Bennett, Keller, & Walkup, 2013). In the 1960s, a biologic aetiology became the preferred causal explanation, supported by the efficacy (although limited) of treatment with antipsychotics (e.g., chlorpromazine and haloperidol). Today, innovations in neuroscience and genetics have moved understanding of this disorder further: it is viewed as the result of an interplay of brain, behaviour, and environment. The individual with tic disorder is seen as having a biologic (genetic) vulnerability that is affected by physiologic arousal related to stress (personal, environmental) (Bennett et al., 2013).

Treatment Interventions

A Canadian review of evidence-based treatment of tic disorders that made recommendations regarding pharmacotherapy concluded that behaviour therapy and the alpha-2-adrenergic antagonists are the first line of therapy for children with tic disorders (Pringsheim et al., 2012). A similar review but focused on behavioural and other therapies (e.g., brain stimulation) strongly recommended habit reversal therapy with accompanying psychoeducation, and with or without pharmacotherapy (Steeves et al., 2012).

Nursing Care

A major focus of the nursing care of a child or adolescent with Tourette's disorder is the careful exploration of the way that tics are affecting the individual's physical, psychological, social, and academic well-being. The way the family members are dealing with the symptoms is important information, as well. A completion of a family history of tic disorder may also provide critical assessment data.

To get a clear understanding of an individual child's manifestation of the disorder, a functional assessment is required. Specific information is needed regarding when tics occur and when their severity decreases (usually when the child is calm, asleep, concentrating, or focused on an activity) and when severity increases (usually when the child is excited, emotionally upset, fatigued) (Bennett et al., 2013). As the child can suppress the tics for brief periods, it is not uncommon to learn that the child has more frequent tics at home than at school. It is helpful to explore, however, the times in class that are associated with increased severity of the tics. For instance, is it when new material is being taught or when the child is called upon to speak? Older children and adults may describe a "premonitory urge" or a physical sensation before having a tic and a sense of tension reduction afterwards (APA, 2013). This cycle of tension–tic–tension reduction makes it possible to envision tics as goal-directed behaviours (Singer, 2013). This is an important perspective for treatment of the disorder.

Biologic Domain

The neurologic abnormality related to tic disorder likely involves several genes, but which ones remain unknown. Direct and indirect evidence has found that corticostriatal–thalamocortical pathways are involved in the expression of this disorder. The possibility of dopaminergic abnormality continues to receive attention because of the therapeutic response to neuroleptics in vocal and motor tics (Singer, 2005). Many approaches are being used to search for a genetic site, including cytogenetics, candidate gene studies, and molecular genetic studies. Linkage analyses have suggested several chromosomal locations, without a clear reproducible locus or convergence of findings (Singer, 2005, 2013). It is recognized that "Obstetrical complications, older parental age, lower birth weight, and maternal smoking during pregnancy are associated with worse tic severity" (APA, 2013, p. 83).

Psychosocial Domain

The *psychoeducation* component of addressing Tourette's syndrome is crucial. It involves providing the child and family general information about Tourette's disorder that includes its prevalence, course, and aetiology. The behavioural model of treatment should be explained. They will need to learn about the role context and consequences in the expression and maintenance of the child's tics. It is in the modification of these, targeting internal and external reinforcements of the tics, that forms the basis of the functional intervention. The *functional assessment*, described earlier, allows for the identification of tic triggers and consequences specific to the child and for *functional interventions* to reduce or eliminate them to be developed (Bennett et al., 2013). There is good-to-moderate efficacy for reduction of the expression and severity of tics with the use of behavioural interventions.

Teachers, guidance counsellors, and school nurses will need current information about Tourette's disorder and related problems. Discussions with school personnel often include issues such as how to deal with tic behaviours if they are disruptive in the classroom (Box 30.9), how to manage teasing from other children, and how to deal with medication side effects. In some situations, a brief presentation about Tourette's disorder to the class/school can reduce teasing and help both teachers and classmates tolerate the tic symptoms (Prestia, 2003). Psychoeducation about Tourette's syndrome may be necessary for some health professionals, as well. A qualitative study of parents' and caregivers' daily experiences and challenges revealed that they found little understanding or support from some health professionals

and suggested that more training was required (Ludlow, Brown, & Schulz, 2016).

There are videos and information pamphlets available to use as resources; see Tourette's Syndrome Foundation, in Web Links. Informative presentations foster openness and understanding and help students with this disorder feel included. Before initiating these interventions, it is essential to identify the child's needs and to pursue these strategies in collaboration with the family and other clinical team members. If evidence shows that Tourette's disorder is hindering academic progress, the nurse can help families negotiate with the school to obtain appropriate services.

Comprehensive Behavioural Intervention for Tics (CBIT) is a treatment whose efficacy has been measured in randomized control trials. This behavioural approach is based on the assumption that, while tics are neurologic in origin, their expression is determined by the interplay of biologic and environmental factors (Yang et al., 2016). It has three elements: psychoeducation, functional assessment and intervention, and **habit reversal therapy** (HRT) (Bennett et al., 2013). In CBIT, the child with Tourette's disorder is coached in HRT. This is based on the fact that a premonitory urge occurs prior to tic expression and then the expression of the tic relieves the tension. This positively reinforces the tic behaviour. HRT involves using a competing response (i.e., one that is incompatible with tic expression) to diminish the habitual undesired behaviour (tic). Deep breathing is one such competing behaviour (Bennett et al.,

---

BOX 30.9 Tics and Disruptive Behaviours

INEFFECTIVE APPROACH

Teacher: I see the tics. He jerks his head, makes faces, and flicks his hands.

Nurse: What do you do about them?

Teacher: What can I do? If he isn't disrupting the class, I leave him alone, even when he is throwing spitballs.

Nurse: Spitballs! He shouldn't be allowed to throw spitballs.

Teacher: Oh, I thought that was a part of his problem.

Nurse: Well, throwing spitballs has nothing to do with tics.

EFFECTIVE APPROACH

Teacher: I see the tics. He jerks his head, makes faces, and flicks his hands.

Nurse: He cannot help the tics that you are seeing. Tic disorders can exhibit a wide range of severity, from mild to severe and from simple to complex. Some complex tics may be difficult to distinguish from habits or rituals.

Teacher: What about things like throwing spitballs? When he does things like that, I try to ignore that behaviour.

Nurse: Sounds like you give him the benefit of the doubt. (Validation) However, throwing a spitball is not a tic behaviour.

Teacher: What should I do?

Nurse: How do you usually handle that type of behaviour? (A modification of reflection)

Teacher: I'd ask him to stop and sometimes to go into the hall.

Nurse: Disruptive behaviour that is voluntary in a student with a tic disorder should be handled as you would handle any other child.

CRITICAL THINKING CHALLENGE

• Compare the responses of the nurse in these scenarios. What made the difference in the teacher's responsiveness to the nurse?

2013). Children and adolescents can be taught how to deep breathe when they feel tic expression is imminent. Using HRT to manage symptoms and to maintain his or her everyday routine despite tic expression can bring rewards for the child (positive reinforcement) in the form of a sense of achievement and self-efficacy, as well as increased opportunities to stay active and engaged with others (Bennett et al., 2013).

CBIT also involves recognizing the positive consequences or secondary gains of tics for the child, such as no chores when tics occur, mom giving massages and sympathy, or teacher excusing homework. Such positive consequences reinforce the tic "behaviour," and thus, the severity and frequency of tics can increase (Bennett et al., 2013). It is important to ensure that parents do not misinterpret behavioural interventions as indicating that tics are voluntary; this could create inappropriate expectations of the child. Nurses need to be knowledgeable about CBIT in order to assist and support the child and family in enacting this treatment and to appropriately monitor changes in the frequency, intensity, complexity, and interference of the tics as they occur. They may serve as consultants with the child's school.

■ ELIMINATION DISORDERS

Enuresis

Enuresis means involuntary or intentional voiding of urine in inappropriate places. It may occur at night (nocturnal) or during the day (diurnal) or both. See the *DSM-5* (APA, 2013) for diagnostic criteria for enuresis. The behaviour cannot be attributed to a medication side effect or to another medical condition. Even without treatment, 50% of these children can achieve dryness by the age of 10 years.

Epidemiology and Aetiology

The prevalence of nocturnal enuresis varies with age and gender, being most common in young boys—an estimated 15% to 20% of 5-year-old boys, 7% of boys aged 7 to 9 years, and 1% of 14-year-old boys have nocturnal enuresis. The frequency in girls is about half that of boys in each age group. The aetiology of enuresis is unknown, with probably no single cause. Most children with nocturnal enuresis are urologically normal. The prevalence of nocturnal enuresis decreases from early childhood to adolescence, and time is the cure for bed wetting in most of or much of cases (Nield & Kamat, 2004).

Treatment Interventions

Treatment for enuresis encompasses both behavioural interventions and pharmacotherapy.

Simple behavioural interventions are undemanding strategies that the child may achieve with help from parents. They include reward for "staying dry" such as receiving a sticker on a chart, being wakened to urinate at night, retention control training to enlarge the bladder, and fluid restriction. A Cochrane systematic review of the literature found evidence that these simple interventions are superior to no active treatment, but inferior to more complex behavioural interventions such as alarms and to some pharmacotherapy (Caldwell, Nankivell, & Sureshkumar, 2013). Alarms are devices that children wear or lie upon while sleeping, which are activated by moisture. Imipramine (Tofranil) and amitriptyline (Elavil), tricyclic antidepressants, have shown efficacy in the treatment of nocturnal enuresis when given once daily an hour prior to bedtime. They have the multiple systemic side effects of anticholinergics (see Chapter 12). The majority of children will relapse once the medication is stopped (Nield & Kamat, 2004). This can cause recurrence of parental frustration and shame and humiliation in addition to feelings of failure in the child. A study of treatment response to outpatient training using such interventions found that after 4 months, 46% of children ($n = 66$) had a full response; 15%, good response; and 21%, only partial response. After 16 months, 53% of children ($n = 34$) had a full response; 6%, good response; and 25%, partial; use of pharmacotherapy declined over time (Cobussen-Boekhorst, van Genugten, Postma, Feitz, & Kortmann, 2012).

The most effective nonpharmacologic treatment is the bed wetting alarm. In this form of behavioural treatment, the bed is equipped with a pad that sets off a buzzer if the child wets. The buzzer then wakes up the child, thereby reminding the child to void. Six to sixteen weeks of alarm treatment may be necessary for the majority of children to experience two consecutive weeks of dry night.

Nursing Care

The nursing assessment should include the child's developmental history, the onset and course of enuresis, prior treatment, presence of emotional problems, medical history, and family history of enuresis, diabetes, or kidney disease. Psychosocial issues such as a change in living arrangements, a new child in the family, or a death should also be documented because stress can be a contributing factor to the problem (Nield & Kamat, 2004). Nurses should also explore the family's home environment and family attitudes about the child's enuresis. Routine laboratory tests such as urinalysis and a urine culture are used to determine the presence of infection; nurses should obtain baseline data regarding toileting habits, including daytime incontinence, urinary frequency, and constipation, and he or she should refer children with persistent daytime enuresis for consultation with a urologist (Reiner, 2003).

The nurse can explore and dispel myths and a misconception that parents may have about bed wetting, such as that the child is lazy, defiant, attention seeking, or misbehaving (Schlomer, Rodriguez, Weiss, & Copp, 2013). In addition, education about bed wetting and its causes may help to alleviate parents' feelings of frustration and the child's feelings of humiliation and shame. The nurse can also encourage parents to limit fluid intake in the evening and treat constipation (if present).

Encopresis

Encopresis involves soiling clothing with feces or depositing feces in inappropriate places, whether involuntarily or intentionally. See the *DSM-5* (APA, 2013) for the diagnostic criteria for encopresis. The soiling is not the result of a medical disorder, such as aganglionic megacolon (Hirschsprung's disease). The most common form of encopresis is faecal impaction accompanied by leakage around the hardened mass of stool. Because of the loss of muscle tone in the lower bowel, the child loses the usual urge to defecate and may not feel the leakage. Surprisingly, the child may not detect the smell of the stool because the olfactory apparatus becomes accustomed to the odour. If left untreated, this problem generally resolves independently by middle adolescence (North American Society for Pediatric Gastroenterology, Hepatology and Nutrition, 2006). Encopresis can affect the lives of children in the following areas: physical, psychological, educational, social, emotional, and in the area of self-esteem.

Epidemiology and Aetiology

The problem of encopresis has received less attention in paediatric literature compared with enuresis. As with enuresis, encopresis is more common in boys, and the frequency of the condition declines with age. Recorded prevalence of encopresis varied between studies from 1% to 4% in children older than 4 years of age, 1% to 2% in children 7 years of age, and 1.6% in those 10 to 11 years of age, with boys three to four times more likely to have encopresis than girls (Bongers, Tabbers, & Benninga, 2007). Faecal incontinence is reported to be responsible for 3% of referrals to healthcare professionals.

The diagnosis of encopresis includes both retentive faecal incontinence and nonretentive faecal incontinence, which present as a single symptom without any organic cause or signs of constipation (Bongers et al., 2007). The reasons for withholding stool and starting the cycle of faecal impaction are unclear but are usually not the result of physical causes. However, as noted, once the faecal impaction occurs, there is a loss of tone in the bowel and leakage.

Nursing Care

The assessment includes a detailed interview with the child and parent regarding the pattern of the encopresis. A calm, matter-of-fact approach can help to reduce the child's embarrassment. A physical examination is also necessary; collaboration with the child's family physician or consulting paediatrician is therefore essential. The presence of encopresis does not necessarily signal severe emotional or behavioural disturbances, but the nurse should inquire about other psychiatric disorders. The diagnosis of encopresis is presumed given a history of intermittent constipation and soiling. Collaboration with the family physician and paediatrician often is helpful to rule out rare medical conditions, such as Hirschsprung's disease.

TEACHING POINTS

Effective intervention begins with educating the parents and the child about normal bowel function and the self-perpetuating cycle of faecal impaction and leakage of stool around the hardened mass of feces. The short-term goal of this educational effort is to decrease the anger and recrimination that often complicate the picture in these families. It is important for parents to understand that soiling from overflow incontinence is not a willful and defiant manoeuvre. Parents are encouraged to maintain a consistent, positive, and supportive attitude in all aspects of treatment (North American Society for Pediatric Gastroenterology, Hepatology and Nutrition, 2006). Because encopresis often results in a loss of bowel tone, it may help to motivate children by emphasizing the need to strengthen their muscles. In many cases, cleaning out the bowel is necessary before initiating behavioural treatment. Disimpaction may be accomplished with the use of oral cathartics such as polyethylene glycol. Once the colon has been evacuated, long-term laxative use is often continued during the bowel retraining program. A high-fibre diet is also recommended.

The behavioural treatment program involves daily sitting on the toilet after each meal for a predetermined period (e.g., 5 to 10 minutes). The child and parents can measure the time with an ordinary kitchen timer, and the parents can encourage the child to read or look at picture books while sitting. They can give the child rewards in the form of stars, stickers, or points for complying with the retraining program and add bonuses for successful defecation. The family can tally stickers or points on a calendar, and the child can "cash in" collected points for small prizes (Reiner, 2003). Children with nonretentive faecal incontinence should not be treated with laxatives. After the exclusion of underlying organic diseases, the treatment is based on the following aspects: education, toilet training, a daily bowel diary with a reward system, and medication. Loperamide has been found effective in the short-term treatment of nonretentive faecal incontinence (Bongers et al., 2007).

SPIRITUAL DOMAIN OF NURSING CARE

Spirituality is a universal human phenomenon with an assumption of the wholeness of individuals and their connectedness to a higher being that integrates the quest for meaning and purpose in life. Religion is both the organized expressions of one's spirituality and the practice of worship. Spirituality supports a sense of hope, comfort, and strength and serves as a coping mechanism especially in times of illness (Elkins & Cavendish, 2004). Nurses recognize that those in their care, from the youngest child to the oldest adult, are integral beings with spiritual needs requiring the support of their families (Veloza-Gomez, Munoz de Rodriguez, Guevara-Armenta, & Mesa-Rodriguez, 2017).

Regardless of the child's or adolescent's psychiatric diagnosis, the nurse begins the plan of care with an assessment of the client and family's spirituality. The nurse must feel comfortable asking spiritual assessment questions and be nonjudgmental, open, and honest. The family's beliefs, practices, and spiritual needs are identified by asking open-ended questions that are not specific to the client's and family's religious background. The child's or youth's developmental stage, cognitive abilities, and social interactions are important components of an accurate assessment (Elkins & Cavendish, 2004). It is important to understand whether and how the family's and/or caregivers' spirituality is helping them make sense of the child's illness and its effect on their coping. Spiritual may influence the response of both the child and adolescent and the family to treatment, including acting as a barrier to it. This can occur, for instance, if psychiatric illness is not accepted as real, caused by sin, or a sign of bad faith. Children and adolescents may be fearful of repercussions of sharing information with family if they have experienced conflict between traditional belief systems and their own beliefs. If the child or adolescent has a history of trauma that involves a religious institution or an individual within such an institution, the spirituality assessment will be particularly important.

Based on the nurse's assessment of a child's or adolescent's spiritual needs, spiritual care is provided within the context of a therapeutic relationship. The nurse uses active listening to build rapport in addition to gathering information (Nash, Darby, & Nash, 2015), with the aim to build trust and to provide consistency in meeting the young client's need for safety and security. This need for safety and security is one of the first spiritual needs of children. Specifically, the nurse can help to minimize the separation of the child from family and try to ensure the same nurse cares for the child daily whenever possible. Developing and adhering to a routine with a child and family also help to provide predictability. Religious practices that are carried out at the same time every day can be scheduled into the plan of care. A referral to clergy or other spiritual support can be offered to the family (Elkins & Cavendish, 2004), as well as to an adolescent. Incorporating spiritual care into the plan of care is essential for optimal health and for positive outcomes when resolving crises.

The spiritual issues of a child or adolescent may be shaped by their psychiatric illness and/or the family's and community's response to it. For instance, children or adolescents experiencing suicidal ideation may be influenced by what they or their family believe will happen after death to those who commit suicide. Would they go to a better place, or find enlightenment, or be punished (Preet, 2007)? For those with a psychotic disorder, the beliefs about hallucinations and delusions of the family and community matter. Psychosis has been viewed as a sign of a spiritual inhabitation (positive or negative) or as a curse, a perspective that should be explored in the spiritual assessment. The therapeutic relationship with the family will be an asset in understanding the situation, protecting the child from any potential harm, and supporting the family. The ADHD symptoms of a child or adolescent may not be tolerated within the setting of the family's religious worship. This rejection has the potential to cut the child or adolescent and the family from important emotional and social support. Education for all those involved by a representative of the healthcare team, such as the nurse, can be a helpful intervention.

SUMMARY OF KEY POINTS

- Improved methods of assessing and defining psychiatric disorders have enhanced appreciation for the frequency of psychiatric disorders in children and adolescents.
- An estimated 14% of children 4 to 17 years of age (more than 800,000) in Canada experience mental disorders that cause significant distress and impairment at home, at school, and in the community.
- The developmental disorders include intellectual disability, ASDs, and specific developmental disorders. Assessment findings should guide nursing management. Specific developmental disorders include communication disorders and learning disorders. These disorders are fairly common in the general population, but they are more common in children with other primary psychiatric disorders.
- Child psychiatric disorders can be divided into externalizing and internalizing disorders. Externalizing disorders include the disruptive behaviour disorders: ODD and conduct disorder. Internalizing disorders include depression and anxiety disorders.
- ADHD is defined by the presence of inattention, impulsiveness, and, in most cases, hyperactivity.

This heterogeneous disorder affects boys more often than girls.

- Effective treatment of ADHD often involves multiple approaches, including medication and parent teaching.
- Assessment of children involves securing data from multiple sources, including the child, parents, and school personnel.
- Standardized rating instruments can assist data collection from multiple informants.
- Separation anxiety is a relatively common anxiety disorder in school-aged children. OCD is more common in adolescents.
- Treatment of separation anxiety and OCD may include medication, behavioural therapy, or a combination of these treatments.
- Major depression in children/youth is believed to be similar to major depression in adults; however, it may be expressed differently.
- The efficacy of antidepressant medications is less well established in children and adolescents than in adults.
- Childhood schizophrenia is a rare disorder.
- Elimination disorders include encopresis and enuresis. Behavioural therapy approaches are the most effective treatment for these disorders. Medication may also be used.

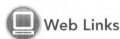 **Web Links**

autismcanada.org/ This site of Autism Canada has screening tools, educational videos, and ways to connect with interested others regarding autism.

autismspeaks.ca *Autism Speaks Canada*, along with the international *Autism Speaks*, supports research and services on autism spectrum disorder, including Asperger's syndrome. Information about this developmental brain disorder can be found at this site.

caddra.ca The *Canadian ADHD Resource Alliance* offers health care professionals of all disciplines resources such as practice guidelines, assessment toolkits, and training courses.

caddra.ca/pdfs/Medication Chart English CANADA. pdf The CADDRA Guide to ADHD Pharmacological Treatments is available at this site in chart format, including coloured images of the medication.

camh.ca/en/hospital/health information/a z mental health and addiction information/CBT/Pages/default. aspx This is where the Centre for Addiction and Mental Health's overview of cognitive–behaviour therapy is to be found.

cmha.ca/mental health/children-and-depression/#. WbL7JsiGPIU The Canadian Mental Health Association's site with information about children and depression.

canfasd.ca/2015/12/14/new-canadian-guideline/ The Canadian guidelines for diagnosing fetal alcohol spectrum disorder (FASD) are available at this Web site of the Canada FASD Research Network.

chadd.org Children and Adults with Attention-Deficit/ Hyperactivity Disorder is an American support and advocacy organization whose Web site features blogs and chat rooms as well as training and continuing education opportunities for parents, teachers, and health professionals.

keltymentalhealth.ca/mental-health/disorders/bipolar-disorder Information about bipolar disorder, including that of children, can be found at this site.

nctsnet.org The National Child Traumatic Stress Network provides information and resources for children and their families who have been exposed to traumatic events.

teenmentalhealth.org Based at Dalhousie University and developed by Dr. Stanley Kutcher, expert in adolescent mental health, and his colleagues, this site offers free downloadable learning modules on child and adolescent health designed for first contact health providers, such as family physicians. Although beyond the practice scope of preregistration nursing students, the modules on child anxiety disorders, adolescent anxiety disorders, child and adolescent depression (MDD), and ADHD are informative, overviewing identification, diagnosis, and treatment of the disorders.

tourette.ca The Tourette Syndrome Foundation is a Canadian advocacy and support network currently developing a "virtual community" for individuals and families living with Tourette disorder. The site offers resources such as videos and a book for the newly diagnosed.

References

Afifi, T. O., MacMillan, H. L., Taillieu, T., Cheung, K., Turner, S., Tonmyr, L., & Hovdestad, W. (2015). Relationship between child abuse exposure and reported contact with child protection organizations: Results from the Canadian Community Health Survey. *Child Abuse and Neglect, 46*, 198–206.

Ainsworth, M. D. S. (1979). Infant–mother attachment. *American Psychologist, 34*, 932–937.

American Psychiatric Association. (2013). *Diagnostic and statistical manual of mental disorders* (5th ed.) (DSM-5). Washington, DC: Author.

Anagnostou, E., Zwaigenbaum, L., Szatmari, P., Fombonne, E., Fernandez, B. A., Woodbury-Smith, M., … Scherer, S. W. (2014). Autism spectrum disorder: Advances in evidence-based practice. *Canadian Medical Association Journal, 186*(7), 509–519. doi: 10.1503/cmaj.121756

Ashton, C. K., O'Brien-Langer, A., & Silverstone, P. H. (2015). The CASA trauma and attachment group (TAG) program for children with have attachment issues following early developmental trauma. *Journal of the Canadian Academy of Child and Adolescent Psychiatry, 25*(1), 35–42.

Axelrod, D. (2013). Taking disruptive mood dysregulation disorder out for a test drive. *American Journal of Psychiatry, 170*(2), 136–139.

Barkley, R. A. (1998). *Attention deficit hyperactivity disorder: A handbook for diagnosis and treatment* (2nd ed.). New York, NY: Guilford.

Bellis, M. D., & Zisk, A. (2014). The biological effects of childhood trauma. *Child and Adolescent Psychiatric Clinics of North America, 23*, 185–222.

Bennett, S. M., Keller, A. E., & Walkup, J. T. (2013). The future of tic disorder treatment. *Annals of the New York Academy of Sciences, 1304*(1), 32–39.

Bhat, M., Grizenko, N., Ben-Amor, L., & Joober, R. (2005). Obstetric complications in children with attention deficit/hyperactivity disorder and learning disability. *McGill Journal of Medicine, 8*(2), 109–113.

Bhatt, N. V. (2017). Anxiety disorders. *Medscape Drugs & Diseases Online.* Retrieved from http://emedicine.medscape.com/article/286227-overview#a8

Biederman, J., & Faraone, S. (2005). Attention-deficit hyperactivity disorder. *Lancet, 366*(7), 237–248.

Blaustein, M., & Kinniburgh, K. (2010). *Treating traumatic stress in children and adolescents: How to foster resilience through attachment, self-regulation, and competency.* New York, NY: Guilford Press.

Bolton, D., & Perrin, S. (2008). Evaluation of exposure with response-prevention for obsessive compulsive disorder in children and adolescents. *Journal of Behavior Therapy and Experimental Psychiatry, 39*(1), 11–22.

Bombay, A., Matheson, K., & Anisman, H. (2014). The intergenerational effects of Indian Residential Schools: Implications for the concept of historical trauma. *Transcultural Psychiatry, 51*(3), 320–338.

Bongers, M., Tabbers, M., & Benninga, M. (2007). Functional nonretentive fecal incontinence in children. *Journal of Pediatric Gastroenterology and Nutrition, 44*(1), 5–13.

Bornovalova, M., Hicks, B., Iacono, W., & McGue, M. (2010). Familial transmission and heritability of childhood disruptive disorders. *American Journal of Psychiatry, 167*, 1066–1074.

Boston Children's Hospital. (2013). *Disruptive behavior disorders.* Retrieved from http://www.childrenshospital.org/health-topics/conditions/disruptive-behavior-disorders

Boylan, K., Vaillancourt, T., Boyle, M., & Szatmari, P. (2007). Comorbidity of internalizing disorders in children with oppositional defiant disorder. *European Child and Adolescent Psychiatry, 16*(8), 484–494.

Brave Heart, M. Y. H. (2003). The historical trauma response among natives and its relationship with substance abuse: A Lakota illustration. *Journal of Psychoactive Drugs, 35*(1), 7–13.

Brave Heart, M. Y. H., Chase, J., Elkins J, & Altschul, D. B. (2011). Historical trauma among Indigenous Peoples of the Americas: Concepts, research, and clinical considerations. *Journal of Psychoactive Drugs, 43*(4), 282–290.

Buckner, J., Lopez, C., Dunkel, S., & Joiner, T. (2008). Behaviour management training for the treatment of reactive attachment disorder. *Child Maltreatment, 13*(3), 289–297.

Burke, J. D., Rowe, R., & Boylan, K. (2014). Functional outcomes of child and adolescent oppositional defiant disorder symptoms in young adult men. *Journal of Child Psychology and Psychiatry, 55*(3), 263–272.

Buysse, V., Goldman, B. D., & Skinner, M. L. (2003). Seeing effects on friendship formation among young children with and without disabilities. *Exceptional Children, 68*(4), 503–517.

Caldwell, P. H., Nankivell, G., & Sureshkumar, P. (2013). Simple behavioral interventions for nocturnal enuresis in children (Review). *Cochrane Database of Systematic Reviews*, Art no. jCD003637. doi:10.1002/14651858.CD003637.pub3

Cameron, C. L. (2007). Obsessive-compulsive disorder in children and adolescents. *Journal of Psychiatric and Mental Health Nursing, 14*(7), 696–704.

Canada Fetal Alcohol Spectrum Disorder Research Network. (2016). Fetal alcohol spectrum disorder: A guideline for diagnosis. *Canadian Medical Association Journal, 188*(3), 191–197.

Canadian ADHD Resource Alliance. (2011). *Canadian ADHD practice guidelines (CAP-guidelines)* (3rd ed.). Toronto, ON: Author.

Canadian ADHD Resource Alliance. (2013a). *Adult ADHD.* Retrieved from http://www.caddra.ca/public-information/adults

Canadian ADHD Resource Alliance. (2013b). *Information for educators.* Retrieved from https://www.caddra.ca/public-information/educators/

Canadian Mental Health Association. (2014a). *Mental illness in children and youth.* Author. Retrieved from https://www.cmha.bc.ca/documents/mental-illnesses-in-children-and-youth-2/

Canadian Mental Health Association. (2014b). *Bipolar disorder.* Retrieved from http://www.cmha.ca/mental-health/understanding-mental-illness/bipolar-disorder/

Canadian Mental Health Association. (2014c). *Childhood depression.* Retrieved from http://www.cmha.ca/mental_health/children-and-depression/#.WbL7JsiGPIU

Carpenito, L. J. (2017). *Nursing diagnosis: Application to clinical practice.* Philadelphia, PA: Wolters Kluwer.

Cavanagh, M. Quinn, D., Duncan, D., Graham, T., & Balbuena, L. (2017). Oppositional defiant disorders is better conceptualized as a disorder of emotional dysregulation. *Journal of Attention Disorders, 21*(5), 381–389. Retrieved from http://journals.sagepub.com/doi/abs/doi:10.1177/1087054713520221

Centre for ADHD Awareness, Canada. (2013). *Adult attention deficit hyperactivity disorder.* Retrieved from http://www.caddac.ca/cms/page.php?82%29

Centers for Disease Control and Prevention. (2012). Prevalence of autism spectrum disorders—Autism and Developmental Disabilities Monitoring Network, 14 sites, United States, 2008. *MMWR Surveillance Summaries, 61*(SS03), 1–19.

Children's Health Policy Centre, Simon Fraser University. (2007). Addressing attention problems in children. *Children's Mental Health Research Quarterly, Fall.* Retrieved from http://www.childhealthpolicy.sfu.ca/research_quarterly_08/rq-pdf/RQ-4-07-Fall.pdf

Chronis, A. M., Jones, H., & Raggi, V. (2006). Evidence-based psychosocial treatments for children and adolescents with attention deficit/hyperactivity disorder. *Clinical Psychology Review, 26*(4), 486–502.

Cobussen-Boekhorst, H. J., van Genugten, L. J., Postma, J., Feitz, W. F., & Kortmann, B. B. (2012). Treatment responses of outpatient training for children with enuresis in a tertiary healthcare setting. *Journal of Pediatric Urology, 9*, 516–520.

Conners, C. K. (1989). *Conners' Rating Scales Manual.* North Tonawanda, NY: Multi-Health Systems.

Cook, J. Green, C., Lilley, C., Anderson, S., Baldwin, M., Chudley, A., ... Rosales, T. (2015). Fetal alcohol spectrum disorder: A guideline for diagnosis across the lifespan. *Canadian Medical Association Journal, 188*(3). Retrieved April 4, 2017 from http://www.cmaj.ca/content/188/3/191

Cornell, T., & Hamrin, V. (2008). Clinical interventions with children with attachment problems. *Journal of Child and Adolescent Psychiatric Nursing, 21*(1), 35–37.

Dang, L. C., Samanez-Larkin, G. R., Young, J. S., Cowan, R. L., Kessler, R. M., & Zald, D. H. (2016). Caudate asymmetry is related to attentional impulsivity and an objective measure of ADHD-like attentional problems in healthy adults. *Brain Structure and Function, 221*(1), 277–286.

Daniels, A. M., & Mandell, D. S. (2014). Explaining differences in age at autism spectrum disorder diagnoses: A critical review. *Autism, 18*(5), 583–597.

Doyle, R. (2004). The history of attention deficit/hyperactivity disorder. *Psychiatric Clinics of North America, 27*(2), 203–214.

Elkins, M. & Cavendish, R. (2004). Developing a plan for spiritual care. *Holistic Nursing Practice, 18*(4), 179–184; 185–186.

Fairchild, G., Passamonti, L., Hurford, G., Hagan, C. C., von dem Hagen, E. A., van Goozen, S., ... Calder, A. J. (2011). Brain structure abnormalities in early-onset and adolescent-onset conduct disorder. *American Journal of Psychiatry, 168*(6), 624–633.

Faraone, S. V. (2004), Genetics of adult attention deficit hyperactivity disorder. In T. Spencer (Ed.), *Psychiatric Clinics of North America, 27*(2), 303–321.

Flapper, B. & Schoemaker, M. (2008). Effects of methylphenidate on quality of life in children with both developmental coordination disorder and ADHD. *Developmental Medicine and Child Neurology, 50*(4), 294–299.

Fox-Lopp, J., & McLaughlin, T. (2015). The effects of classroom interventions on anxiety disorders in elementary school children: A brief review. *International Journal of Multidisciplinary Research and Development, 2*(1), 10–15.

Freeman, J., Sapyta, J., Garcia, A., Compton, S., Khanna, M., Flessner, C., ... Franklin, M. (2014). Family-based treatment of early childhood obsessive-compulsive disorder: The pediatric obsessive-compulsive disorder treatment study for young children (POTS Jr)—A randomized clinical trial. *JAMA Psychiatry, 71*(6), 689–698.

Garland, E. J., Clark, S. L., & Earle, V. (Illustrator). (2009). *Taming worry dragons: A manual for children, parents, and other coaches* (94th ed.). Vancouver, BC: Children's & Women's Health Centre of British Columbia.

Glowinski, A. L. (2011). Reactive attachment disorder: An evolving entity. *Journal of the American Academy of Child and Adolescent Psychiatry, 50*(3), 210–212.

Goyette, G. H., Conners, C. K., & Ulrich, R. F. (1978). Normative data on the revised Connors parent and teacher rating scales. *Journal of Abnormal Child Psychology, 6*, 221–236.

Gunnar, M., & Quevedo, K. (2007). The neurobiology of stress and development. *Annual Review of Psychology, 58*, 145–173.

HealthLinkBC. (2017). *Depression in children and teens.* Retrieved from http://www.healthlinkbc.ca/kb/content/major/ty4640.html

Henggeler, S. W., & Sheidow, A. J. (2012). Empirically supported family-based treatments for conduct disorder and delinquency in adolescents. *Journal of Marital and Family Therapy, 38*(1), 30–58.

Hiller, R. M., Young, R. L., & Weber, N. (2014). Sex differences in autism spectrum disorder based on DSM-5 criteria: Evidence from clinician and teacher reporting. *Journal of Abnormal Child Psychology, 42*(8), 1381–1393.

Holmes, J. (2004). Disorganized attachment and borderline personality disorder. A clinical perspective. *Attachment and Human Development, 6*, 181–190.

Humphreys, K. L., Nelson, C. A., Fox, N. A., & Zeanah, C. H. (2017). Signs of reactive attachment disorder and diminished social engagement disorder at age 12 years: Effects of institutional care history and high quality foster-care. *Developmental Psychopathology, 29*(2), 675–684.

Kahn, J., Nursten, J., & Carroll, H. (2014). *Unwilling to school: School phobia or school refusal: A psychosocial problem.* Toronto, ON: Pergamon of Canada.

Kanner, L. (1943). Autistic disturbances of affective contact. *Nervous Child, 2*, 217–250.

Kelty Mental Health Resource Centre. (2013). *Post-traumatic stress disorder.* Retrieved from http://keltymentalhealth.ca/mental-health/disorders/post-traumatic-stress-disorder

Kendall, P. C., Cummings, C. M., Villabø, M. A., Narayanana, M. K., Tredwell, K., Birmaher, B., ... Albano, A. M. (2016). Mediators of changes in the child/adolescent anxiety multimodal treatment study. *Journal of Consulting and Clinical Psychology, 84*(1), 1–14.

Kim-Cohen, J., Arsenault, L., Caspi, A., Tomás, M. P., Taylor, A., & Moffitt, T. (2005). Validity of DSM-IV conduct disorder in 4½-5-year-old children: A longitudinal epidemiological study. *American Journal of Psychiatry, 162*(6), 1108–1117.

Koda, V. H., Charney, D. S., & Pine, D. S. (2003). Neurobiology of early-onset anxiety disorders. In A. Martin, L. Scahill, D. S. Charney, & J. F. Leckman (Eds.), *Pediatric psychopharmacology: Principles and practice* (1st ed., pp. 138–149). New York, NY: Oxford University Press.

Labellarte, M. J., & Ginsberg, G. S. (2003). Anxiety disorders. In A. Martin, L. Scahill, D. S. Charney, & J. F. Leckman (Eds.), *Pediatric psychopharmacology: Principles and practice* (1st ed., pp. 497–510). New York, NY: Oxford University Press.

Leibenluft, E. (2011). Severe mood dysregulation, irritability, and the diagnostic boundaries of bipolar disorder in youths. *American Journal of Psychiatry, 162*(2), 129–142.

Leonard, H. L., Ale, C. M., & Freeman, J. B. (2005). Obsessive-compulsive disorder. *Child and Adolescent Psychiatric Clinics of North America, 14*, 727–743.

Loth, A. K. (2012, February 7). Childhood-onset schizophrenia. *Medscape.* Retrieved from http://emedicine.medscape.com/article/914840-overview

Ludlow, A., Brown, R., & Schulz, J. (2016). A qualitative exploration of the daily experiences and challenges faced by parents and caregivers of children with Tourette's syndrome. *Journal of Health Psychology.* doi: 10.1177/1359105316669878

Manassis, K. (2004). Childhood anxiety disorders: Approach to interventions. *Canadian Family Physician, 50*, 379–384.

Marusak, H. A., Martin, K. R., Etkin, A., & Thomason, M. E. (2015). Childhood trauma exposure disrupts the automatic regulation of emotional processing. *Neuropsychopharmacology, 40*, 1250–1258.

Mayo Clinic. (2017). *Reactive attachment disorder.* Retrieved from http://www.mayoclinic.org/diseases-conditions/reactive-attachment-disorder/home/ovc-20336559

Mental Health Commission of Canada. (2011). *Making the case for investing in mental health in Canada.* Retrieved from https://www.mentalhealthcommission.ca/sites/default/files/2016-06/Investing_in_Mental_Health_FINAL_Version_ENG.pdf

MTA Cooperative Group. (1999). A 14-month randomized clinical trial of treatment strategies for attention-deficit/hyperactivity disorder. Multimodal treatment study of children with ADHA. *Archives of General Psychiatry, 56*(12), 1073–1086.

Mulvihill, D. (2005). The health impact of childhood trauma: An interdisciplinary review, 1997–2003. *Issues in Comprehensive Pediatric Nursing, 28*(2), 115–136.

Murray, B. (2008). Disorders diagnosed in infancy, childhood or adolescence. In P. O'Brien, W. Kennedy, & K. Ballard (Eds.), *Psychiatric mental health nursing: An introduction to theory and practice* (pp. 207–234). Boston, MA: Jones and Bartlett Publishers.

Nash, P., Darby, K., & Nash, S. (2015). *Spiritual care with sick children and young People: A handbook for chaplains, paediatric health professionals, arts therapists, and youth workers.* London, UK: Jessica Kingsley Publishers.

National Child Traumatic Stress Network. (2013). *Effective treatments for youth trauma.* Retrieved from http://www.nctsn.org/resources/audiences/parents-caregivers/treatments-that-work

National Institute of Mental Health. (2013). *Bipolar disorder.* Retrieved from http://www.nimh.nih.gov/health/topics/bipolar-disorder/index.shtml

National Scientific Council on the Developing Child. (2012). *The science of neglect: The persistent absence of responsive care disrupts the developing brain: Working Paper 12.* Retrieved from https://developingchild.harvard.edu/resources/the-science-of-neglect-the-persistent-absence-of-responsive-care-disrupts-the-developing-brain/

Nield, L., & Kamat, D. (2004). Enuresis: How to evaluate and treat. *Clinical Pediatrics, 43*(5), 409–415.

North American Society for Pediatric Gastroenterology, Hepatology and Nutrition. (2006). Evaluation and treatment of constipation in infants: Clinical practice guidelines. *Journal of Pediatric Gastroenterology and Nutrition, 43*(3), 1–13.

Ollendick, T. H., Greene, R. W., Austin, K. E., Fraire, M. G., Halldorsdottir, T., Benoit Allen, K., ... Wolff, J. C. (2016). Parent management training and collaborative & proactive solutions: A randomized control trial for oppositional youth. *Journal of Clinical Child & Adolescent Psychology, 45*(5), 591–604.

Panagiotopoulos, C., Ronsley, R., Kuzeljevic, B., & Davidson, J. (2012). Waist circumference is a sensitive screening tool for assessment of metabolic syndrome risk in children treated with second-generation antipsychotics. *Canadian Journal of Psychiatry, 57*(1), 34–44.

Perry, B. D. (1994). Neurobiological sequelae of childhood trauma: Post traumatic stress disorders in children. In M. Murburg (Ed.), *Catecholamine function in post-traumatic stress disorder: Emerging concepts.* Washington, DC: American Psychiatric Press.

Perry, B. D. (2001). The neurodevelopmental impact of violence in childhood. In D. Schekty & E. Benedek (Eds.), *Textbook of child and adolescent forensic psychiatry* (pp. 221–238). Washington, DC: American Psychiatric Association.

Perry, B. D. (2002a). *The vortex of violence: How children adapt and survive in a violent world.* Retrieved from www.childtrauma.org

Perry, B. D. (2002b). *Brain structure and function I: Basics of organization.* Retrieved from http://www.childtrauma.org/ctamaterials/brain_I.asp

Perry, B. D. (2002c). *Brain structure and function II: Special topics information work with maltreated children.* Retrieved from http://www.childtrauma.org/ctamaterials/brain_II.asp

Perry, B. D. (2004). *Maltreatment and the developing child: How early childhood experience shapes child and culture.* Retrieved from http://www.lfcc.on.ca/mccain/perry.pdf

Perry, A. & Condillac, R. (2003). *Evidence-based practices for children and adolescents with autism spectrum disorders: Review of the literature and practice guide.* Toronto, ON: Children's Mental Health.

Persico, A. & Bourgeron, T. (2006). Searching for ways out of the autism maze: Genetic, epigenetic and environmental clues. *Trends in Neurosciences, 29*(7), 349–358.

Pinto-Martin, J., Souders, M., Giarelli, E., & Levy, S. (2005). The role of the nurse in screening for autistic spectrum disorder in pediatric primary care. *Journal of Pediatric Nursing, 20*(3), 163–169.

Porges, S. (2004). Neuroception: A subconscious system for detecting threats and safety. *Zero to Three, 24*(5), 19–24.

Preet, J. (2007). Suicide and spirituality: A clinical perspective. *Southern Medical Journal, 100*(7), 752–755.

Prestia, K. (2003). Tourette's syndrome: Characteristics and interventions. *Intervention in School and Clinic, 39*(2), 67–71.

Pringsheim, T., Doja, A., Gorman, D., McKinlay, D., Day, L., Billinghurst, L., ... Sandor, P. (2012). Canadian Guidelines for evidence-based treatment of tic disorders: Pharmacotherapy. *Canadian Journal of Psychiatry, 57*(3), 133–143.

Public Health Agency of Canada (PHAC). (2011). *Responding to stressful events: Helping children cope.* Ottawa, ON: Author. Retrieved from https://www.canada.ca/content/dam/phac-aspc/migration/phac-aspc/publicat/oes-bsu-02/pdf/helping-child-cope_e.pdf

Public Health Agency of Canada. (2016). *Report from the Canadian chronic disease surveillance system: Mood and anxiety disorders in Canada 2016.* Retrieved from https://www.canada.ca/content/dam/canada/health-canada/migration/healthy-canadians/publications/diseases-conditions-maladies-affections/mood-anxiety-disorders-2016-troubles-anxieux-humeur/alt/mood-anxiety-disorders-2016-troubles-anxieux-humeur-eng.pdf

Ramtekkar, U. P., Reiersen, A. M., Todorov, A. A., & Todd, R. D. (2010). Sex and age differences in attention-deficit/hyperactivity disorder symptoms and diagnoses: Implications for DSM-V and ICD-11. *Journal of the American Academy of Child and Adolescent Psychiatry, 49*(3), 217–228.

Ransby, M., & Swanson, H. L. (2003). Reading comprehension skills of young adults with childhood diagnosis of dyslexia. *Journal of Learning Disabilities, 36*(6), 538–555.

Rapee, R., & Spence, S. (2004). The etiology of social phobia: Empirical Evidence and an initial model. *Clinical Psychology Review, 24*, 737–767.

Reiner, W. G. (2003). Elimination disorders: Enuresis and encopresis. In A. Martin, L. Scahill, D. S. Charney, & J. F. Leckman (Eds.), *Pediatric psychopharmacology: Principles and practice* (1st ed., pp. 686–698). New York, NY: Oxford University Press.

Richardson, A. J. (2006). Omega-3 fatty acids in ADHD and related neurodevelopmental disorders. *International Review of Psychiatry, 18*(2), 155–172.

Russell, R., & Grizzle, K. (2008). Assessing child and adolescent pragmatic language competencies: Toward evidence based-assessments. *Clinical Child and Family Psychology Review, 11*(1), 59–73.

Saunders, B. E., & Adams, Z. W. (2014). Epidemiology of traumatic experiences in childhood. *Child & Adolescent Psychiatric Clinics of North America, 23*, 167–184.

Scahill, L., Leckman, J. F., Schultz, R. T., Katsovich, L., & Peterson, B. S. (2003). A placebo-controlled trial of risperidone in Tourette syndrome. *Neurology, 60*, 1130–1135.

Schachar, R. (2014). Genetics of attention deficit hyperactivity disorder (ADHD): Recent updates and future prospects. *Current Developmental Disorders Report, 1*, 41–49.

Schlomer, B., Rodriguez, E., Weiss, D., & Copp, H. (2013). Parents' beliefs about nocturnal enuresis causes, treatments, and the need to seek professional medical care. *Journal of Pediatric Urology, 9*, 1043–1048.

Shanahan, L., Copeland, W. E., Angold, A., Bondy C. L & Cosello, J. (2014). Sleep problems predict and are predicted by generalized anxiety/depression and oppositional defiant disorder. *Journal of the American Academy of Child and Adolescent Psychiatry, 53*(5), 550–558. Retrieved January 15, 2017 from http://dx.doi.org/10.1016/j.jaac.2013.12.029

Sharpe, J., & Izadkhah, Y. O. (2014). Use of comic strips in teaching earthquakes to kindergarten children. *Disaster Prevention and Management, 23*(2), 138–156. doi:10.1108/DPM-05-2013-0083

Sherer, M. R., & Schreibman, L. (2005). Individual behavioral profiles and predictors of treatment effectiveness for children with autism. *Journal of Consulting and Clinical Psychology, 75*, 525–538.

Siegel, D. (2001). Toward an interpersonal neurobiology of the developing mind: Attachment relationships, "mindset," and neural integration. *Infant Mental Health Journal, 22*(1–2), 67–94.

Singer, H. S. (2005). Tourette's syndrome: From behaviour to biology. *Lancet Neurology, 4*(3), 149–159.

Singer, H. S. (2013). Motor control, habits, complex motor stereotypies, and Tourette syndrome. *Annals of the New York Academy of Sciences, 1304*(1), 22–31.

Smyke, A. T., Seanah, C. H., Gleason, M. M., Drury, S. S., Fox, N. A., Nelson, C. A., & Guthrie, D. (2012). A randomized controlled trail comparing foster care and institutional care for children with signs of reactive attachment disorder. *American Journal of Psychiatry, 169*, 508–514.

Stanford Children's Health. (2017). *Overview of mood disorders in children and adolescents.* Retrieved from http://www.stanfordchildrens.org/en/topic/default?id=overview-of-mood-disorders-in-children-and-adolescents-90-P01634

Statistics Canada. (2012). *Suicide rates: An overview.* Retrieved from http://www.statcan.gc.ca/pub/82-624-x/2012001/article/11696-eng.htm

Statistics Canada. (2017). *Death and mortality rate, by selected grouped causes, age grouped and cause, Canada, annual [CARSIM (October)].* Retrieved October 1, 2017 from http://www5.statcan.gc.ca/casim/a26?lang=eng&ID=1020551

Steeves, T, McKinlay, B. D., Gorman, D., Billinghurst, L., Day, L., Carroll, A., ... Pringsheim, T. (2012). Canadian guidelines for evidence-based treatment of tic disorders: Behavioural therapy, deep brain stimulation, and transcranial magnetic stimulation. *Canadian Journal of Psychiatry, 57*(3), 144–151.

Stewart, S. E., Hu, Y., Leung, A., Chan, E., Hezel, D. M., Lin, S. Y., ... Pauls, D. L. (2017). A multisite study of family functioning impairment in pediatric obsessive-compulsive disorder. *Journal of the American Academy of Child and Adolescent Psychiatry, 56*(3).

Storch, E. A., Murphy, T. K., Geffken, G. R., Sajid, M., Allen, P., Roberti, J. W., & Goodman, W. K. (2005). Reliability and validity of the Yale Global Tic Severity Scale. *Psychological Assessment, 17*(4), 486–491.

Taylor, L. E., Swerdfeger, A. L., & Eslick, G. D. (2014). Vaccines are not associated with autism: An evidence-based meta-analysis of case-control and cohort studies. *Vaccine, 32*(29), 3623–3629.

Tonmyr, L., Williams, G., Hovdestad, W., & Draca, J. (2011). Anxiety and/or depression in 10–15-year-olds investigated by child welfare. *Canadian Journal of Adolescent Health, 48*, 493–498.

Uchida, M., Spencer, T., Faraone, S., & Biederman, J. (2015). Adult outcome of ADHD: An overview of results from the MGH longitudinal family studies of pediatrically and psychiatrically referred youth with and without ADHD of both sexes. *Journal of Attention Disorders,* 1–12. doi:10.1177/1087054715604360

van der Kolk, B. (2005). Developmental trauma disorder. *Psychiatric Annals, 35*(5), 401–408.

van der Kolk, B. (2006). Clinical implications for neuroscience in research in PTSD. *Annals of the New York Academy of Sciences, 1071*, 277–293.

van der Kolk, B. (2009). *New frontiers in trauma treatment.* Presentation at Coquitlam, BC.

Van Grootheest, D., Cath, D., Beekman, A., & Boomsma, D. (2005). Twin studies on obsessive compulsive disorder: A review. *Twin Research and Human Genetics, 8*(5), 450–458.

Veloza-Gomez, M., Munoz de Rodriguez, L., Guevara-Armenta, C., & Mesa-Rodriguez, S. (2017). The importance of spiritual care in nursing practice. *Journal of Holistic Nursing, 35*(2), 118–131.

Volkmar, F. R., Klin, A., & Paul, R. (2004). *Handbook of autism and pervasive developmental disorders* (3rd ed.). New York, NY: Wiley.

Volkar, F. R., Siegel, M., Woodbury-Smith, M., King, B., McCracken, J., & State, M. (2014). Practice parameter for the assessment and treatment of children and adolescents with autism spectrum disorder. *Journal of the American Academy of Child and Adolescent Psychiatry, 53*(2), 237–257.

Waddell, C., McEwan, K., Shepherd, C., Offord, D., & Hua, J. M. (2005). A public health strategy to improve the mental health of Canadian children. *Canadian Journal of Psychiatry, 50*(4), 226–233.

Waddell, C., Shepherd, C. A., Schwartz, C., & Barican J. (2014). *Child and youth mental disorders: Prevalence and evidence-based interventions.* Vancouver, BC: Children's Health Policy Centre, Simon Fraser University. Retrieved from http://childhealthpolicy.ca/wp-content/uploads/2014/06/14-06-17-Waddell-Report-2014.06.16.pdf

Walkup, J. T., Albanao, A. M., Piacentini, J., Birmaher, B., Compton, S. N., Sheril, J. T., ... Kendall, P. C. (2008). Cognitive behavioural therapy, sertraline, or a combination in childhood anxiety. *New England Journal of Medicine, 359*, 2753–2766.

Webster-Stratton, C. (2011). *The incredible years: Parents, teachers and children's training series. Program content, methods, research and dissemination 1980–2011.* Seattle, WA: Incredible Years, Inc.

Yang, C., Hao, Z., Zhu, C., Guo, Q., Mu, D., & Zhang, L. (2016). Interventions for tic disorders: An overview of systematic reviews and meta-analyses. *Neuroscience and Biobehavioral Reviews, 63*, 239–255. Retrieved from doi.org/10.1016/j.neurobiorev.2015.12.0.013

Zeanah, C. H., & Gleason, M. M. (2010). *Reactive attachment disorder: A review for DSM-V* (pp. 1–54). Washington, DC: American Psychiatric Association.

Zinck, S., Bagnell, A., Bond, K., & Newton, A. S. (2009). The Cochrane library and the treatment of major depression in children and youth: An overview of reviews. *Evidence-Based Child Health: A Cochrane Review Journal, 4*(4), 1336–1350.

Mental Health of Older Adults: Promotion and Assessment

Sharon L. Moore

Adapted, in part, from the chapter "Mental Health Assessment of the Older Adult" by Mary Ann Boyd, Mickey Stanley, and Annette M. Lane

LEARNING OBJECTIVES

After studying this chapter, you will be able to:

- Identify important bio/psycho/social/spiritual factors occurring in late adulthood.
- Identify risk factors related to geriatric psychopathology.
- Analyze the nurse's role in mental health promotion with older adults and their families.
- Discuss mental health promotion and illness prevention interventions that are especially effective with older adults.
- Compare changes in normal aging with those associated with mental health problems in older adults.
- Select various techniques in assessing older adults who have mental health problems.
- Delineate the important areas of assessment for the biologic, psychological, social, and spiritual domains in completing the geriatric mental health nursing assessment.

KEY TERMS

- apraxia • dysphagia • functional status • gerotranscendence
- insomnia • middle-old • old-old • polypharmacy
- young-old

KEY CONCEPTS

- aging in place • bio/psycho/social/spiritual geriatric mental health nursing assessment • late adulthood • normal aging

---

Global aging is occurring at an unprecedented rate, and Canada, like many other countries, is experiencing a boom in population growth of seniors. On July 1, 2016, the population of Canada was 36.3 million; it is estimated to reach almost 48 million by 2036. Over the 5-year period from 2006 to 2011, the number of people aged 60 to 64 rose by 29.1%; the number of people aged 65 or older rose by 14.1%, and the number of people aged 100 or older rose by 25.7% (CIHR, 2013). In 2016, persons over the age of 65 accounted for 16.5% of the population (Statistics Canada, 2016), a proportion predicted to rise to 25% by 2036 (Public Health Agency of Canada [PHAC], 2010). A demographic milestone was met in 2015 when the number of adults 65 years and older became larger than the number of children under 15 years, a trend that has continued in 2016, with 16.5% of the population 65 years of age and older compared to 16.1% of the population 14 years of age and younger (Statistics Canada, 2016).

Many recent initiatives in Canada are being directed towards improving health and quality of life for older persons. Age-friendly cities, with the encouragement

of the Public Health Agency of Canada (2016), have been growing across the country since the World Health Organization launched the *Global Age-Friendly Cities Project* in 2000, to better support and enable people to "age actively" and foster physical and mental health.

In 1920, the average life span in Canada was 60 years (Statistics Canada, 2005). By 2009, this life span increased to 79 years for men and 83 years for women (Statistics Canada, 2012a). Health care providers are facing new and increased challenges as the generation known as "the baby boomers" (born 1946–1964) moves into the rank of older adults. By the year 2036, projections are that there will be almost 10.4 million adults 65 years of age and older, comprising 25% of the Canadian population. The fastest growing segment of the older population is the group 85 years of age and older (CIHR, 2013).

Although Canadians are living longer—and healthier—lives with the increase in aging population, there is a concomitant increase in the number of older adults with mental health issues. One in four seniors lives with a mental health problem or illness (Mental Health Commission of Canada [MHCC], 2011). Mental disorders can substantially impair functioning and can result in unnecessary hospitalizations and nursing home placement, poorer health outcomes, and increased rates of mortality. For example, older persons who suffer from depression have worse outcomes after medical events such as hip fractures, heart attacks, or cancer. For older adults, it takes less alcohol to exacerbate medical and mental health problems, and in turn, medical and emotional problems may contribute to further alcohol use (Alberta Health Services, 2014). In Canada, the rate of suicide for males aged 85 to 89 is 34.0 per 100,000, nearly double that of the suicide rate among all Canadian males at 17.4 deaths/100,000 (Statistics Canada, 2017a). Persons with severe mental illness have a life expectancy reduced by about 25 years largely due to other medical conditions; this close link between mental and physical health needs to be recognized in the care of older adults with multimorbidity (Gallo, 2017). A way to meet such health challenges is to take a comprehensive, life course approach to aging (CIHR, 2013). Key to this is enacting steps to promote mental health and to recognize and address mental health issues early on and take action to mitigate negative outcomes.

This chapter explores mental health promotion strategies with older adults as well as identifies common mental health challenges and disorders. A bio/psycho/social/spiritual model for comprehensive geriatric mental health nursing assessment that serves as the basis of care for older adults is presented.

Nurses need to understand and respond well to the unique needs of this population. Older adults have attributes and mental health needs that are not readily met within generic treatment programs (MHCC, 2011). Mental health promotion and mental illness prevention efforts, targeted at older adults' needs, are key to helping older adults live healthy lives with purpose and meaning. Healthy aging has become a mantra for living well in the 21st century (Bryant et al., 2012; Lezwijn, Vaandrager, Naaldenberg, Wagemakers, & van Woerkum, 2011). Research on aging is focused not only on the examination of life span (number of years in an individual's life) but also the health span (number of years of good health and functioning) (National Institute on Aging [NIA], 2011). While many nurses believe they are not practicing gerontologic nursing, given the aging landscape of society, the majority of nurses will frequently encounter older adults in their practice. An important role for nurses with this population is to promote wellness, optimal functioning, and quality of life in healthy aging to life's end (Deveraux Melillo, 2017).

MENTAL HEALTH PROMOTION OF THE OLDER ADULT

Late adulthood can be divided into **young-old** (65 to 74 years), **middle-old** (75 to 84 years), and **old-old**

(85 years and older). The transition across these chronologic periods is more than a series of birthdays; it is a gradual bio/psycho/social/spiritual process that may be viewed as both positive and negative. From a positive perspective, the later years provide time for personal growth and development, providing an opportunity to do all the things that were impossible when work and family responsibilities took precedence. Travelling, visiting friends, and engaging in neglected hobbies enhance quality of life and improve well-being.

In late adulthood, changes in health status can also lead to negative outcomes. A loss in physical functioning can lead to a loss in independence, which can result in an unplanned change in residence. Family relationships change, as once dependent children grow into adulthood and become parents themselves. Friendships change, and losses occur. Many older adults retire from meaningful lifelong work and are faced with establishing new meaning in life. To have a sense of hope and meaning and purpose is a critical factor in older adults' mental health and is one of the factors that serves as a protection against suicide and despair in later life (Moore, 2005; Moore, Metcalf, & Schow, 2000). In all health care settings, communication is an integral factor in nursing care. Research shows the importance of nurse–client interactions in helping older adults have hope and meaning in life (Haugan, 2013). Communication with older adults requires special attention to verbal interactions and environmental influences. Box 31.1 highlights some necessary considerations.

KEY CONCEPT

Late adulthood can be divided into three chronologic groups: *young-old* (ages 65 to 74 years), *middle-old* (ages 75 to 84 years), and *old-old* (age 85 years and older).

Biologic Domain

The human life span encompasses the stages of embryogenesis, growth and development, and senescence or growing old (Panno, 2010). During senescence, there is a natural, gradual deterioration of the body: aging affects the cells of every major bodily organ (NIA, 2011/2013). During aging, arteries will become more rigid; body fat will increase; some brain neurons will be lost without affecting basic functioning; ventricular walls of the heart will thicken; high-frequency sounds will not be easily heard; some hormones (e.g., oestrogen, testosterone) will decrease, while others (e.g., insulin, vasopressin) increase; night vision will decline; mild arthritis will affect joints; and vital capacity of the lungs will decline (Panno, 2010). Immunosenescence occurs (i.e., the immune system's effectiveness in defending the body from pathogens decreases), leaving the body

BOX 31.1 Communicating With Older Adults

- Greet the older person by name.
- Invest time in a caring and respectful interaction.
- Focus the person's attention on the exchange of communication; the older adult may need extra time to begin to process information.
- Face the person when speaking to him or her.
- Minimize distractions in the room, including other people, objects in your hands, noise, and other activities.
- Reduce glare from room lighting by dimming too-bright lights. Conversely, avoid sitting in shadows.
- Speak slowly and clearly. Older adults may depend on lip reading, so ensure that the individual can see you. Speak loudly, but do not shout. It is not necessary to over enunciate with exaggerated lip movements.

- Use short, simple sentences and be prepared to repeat or revise what you have said.
- Limit the number of topics discussed at one time to prevent information overload.
- Ask one question at a time to minimize confusion. Allow plenty of time for the person to answer and express ideas.
- Frequently summarize the important points of the conversation to improve understanding and comprehension.
- Avoid the urge to finish sentences.
- If the communication exchange is going poorly, postpone it for another time.
- Encourage connectedness with like-minded persons.

more vulnerable and the older adult less responsive to vaccines (NIA, 2011/2013). The metabolic activities that sustain human life also create stress that ultimately damages the body. For example, when oxygen is used by cells to convert food into energy, there are by-products created called *free radicals*. These are also created by environmental factors, like tobacco smoke and sun exposure. Some free radicals cause damage to components of cells, including DNA. The role of such oxidation (free radical) damage in aging is being explored.

The complex role genetics plays in aging is a key area of study. For instance, in the New England Centenarian Study, researchers found 281 genetic markers that were 61% accurate in predicting who was 100 years old, 73% accurate in predicting who was 102 years old or older, and 85% accurate in predicting who was 105 years old or older. The genetic component of longevity seems to increase with exceptional age (Sebastiani et al., 2012). Exceptionally long-lived individuals appear to delay health problems until late in life (NIA, 2011/2013). Senescence occurs, of course, at the cellular as well as the organism level. Epigenetic studies are finding that senescent cells undergo changes in their chromatin (see Chapter 9); similar changes are found in prematurely aging cells (Berger, 2013).

Human aging is increasingly viewed as modifiable with delaying specific biologic aspects of aging being targeted (Kennedy, 2016). There is a shift, too, from a deficit approach to aging (i.e., focused on decreases in functioning) to an approach that centres on the idea of resilience, adapting well to life's losses and adversities (Stephens, Breheny, & Mansvelt, 2015). As is true across the life span, the biologic domain of the older adult is shaped and influenced by each of the other domains, from having a positive attitude towards aging to possessing sufficient social support to sustaining a sense that one's life is meaningful.

Psychological Domain

Cognitive Function

Changes in cognition are most likely accounted for by structural and functional changes in the brain (Rosenzweig & Barnes, 2003). These alterations are probably highly specific because aspects of cognitive decline are very specific (e.g., secondary memory), and many abilities are preserved. Moreover, external factors, including activity levels, socioeconomic status, education, and personality, may modify the development or the expression of age-related changes in cognition (see Chapter 34). Normal aging does not impair consciousness. Alertness is required for attention, but the alert client may not necessarily be able to attend. Attention has two aspects: sustained attention (vigilance) and selective attention (ability to extract relevant from irrelevant information). Numerous studies indicate that older adults perform well on tests of sustained and selective attention (Ebersole, Touhy, Hess, & Jett, 2007; Yevchak, Loeb, & Fick, 2008). Earlier findings of poor performance on tests of selective attention have been attributed to lack of control for perceptual difficulties (e.g., vision and hearing deficits).

Slower reaction time may affect how quickly an older adult responds to questions. Hurrying older adults to answer questions may interfere with their ability to provide the correct answer. This has been labelled the *speed–accuracy shift*, by which the older adult focuses more on accuracy than on speed in responding. Caution tends to increase, whereas risk-taking behaviour tends to decrease; older adults are more likely to make errors of omission (leaving the answer out) than errors of commission (making a guess) (Zimprich, 2002).

Recent studies have shown that there are several factors that contribute to cognitive health in later years (Evers, Klusmann, Schwarzer, & Heuser, 2011; Lee & Hung, 2011; Newberg, 2011). Meditation, prayer, and other spiritual practices have a positive effect on the aging brain such that memory, mood and cognition, and overall mental health are improved (Newberg, 2011). Lifestyle interventions have been found to enhance cognitive functioning and brain reserve (Lam & Cheng, 2012). Reminiscence is recognized as a key strategy to "foster identity and self-continuity, and to achieve a sense of coherence and meaning in life" for older persons (O'Rourke, Cappeliez, & Claxton, 2011, p. 272) with autobiographical memory appearing "to exert both direct and indirect effects on well-being" (p. 279). Alternately, health care professionals can use a "life story toolkit" that focuses on the use of life review to develop life storybooks with older adults (Moya & Arnold, 2012).

A key psychosocial resource for older adults' physical and mental health is hope (Duggleby et al., 2012; Hammer, Mogensen, & Hall, 2009; Moore, 2012). While there are many definitions of hope, its positive role in living and facilitating meaning and life is well documented (Duggleby et al., 2012; Hammer et al., 2009; Haugan, 2013; Moore, 2012). Hope provides a reason to live and allows one to see the smallest ray of light when the world looks dark. Hope allows the older person to go on in the face of adverse circumstances and to be "okay" regardless of the outcome.

Learning

Intelligence and personality are stable across the life span in the absence of disease; however, the learning abilities of older adults may be more selective, requiring motivation ("How important is this information?"), meaningful content ("Why do I need to know this?"), and familiarity with the idea or content. Although age causes no differences in the ability to process knowledge to learn a skill, younger people are more likely to employ strategies to learn tasks. Level of education needs to be considered in evaluating responses on mental status examinations because responses may reflect socioeconomic status and occupation.

Memory

Other than overall intelligence, age-related memory alterations have been more widely studied than any other aspect of cognition. Contrary to popular belief, memory loss is not a normal part of aging. To remember events, individuals must first attend to information and process it. Older adults may well dismiss information that is not important to them. Memory problems in later life are believed to result from encoding problems or "getting" the information in the first place. This problem may be related to sensory problems, not paying attention, or a general failure to link the "to-be-remembered" information to existing knowledge through association or to strengthen the memory through repetition. However, it is important not to confuse decline with

deficit. Although a decline in memory ability may be frustrating for the older individual, it does not necessarily hamper his or her ability to function daily. Threats to memory include medications, depression (impairs concentration and attention), poor nutrition, infection, heart and lung disease (lack of oxygen), thyroid problems (can cause symptoms of depression or confusion that mimic memory loss), alcohol use, and sensory loss (interferes with perception).

Development

The psychologist Erik Erikson identified "integrity versus despair" as a developmental task specific to late adulthood. An extension of his theory published by Joan Serson Erikson, his wife, included old age as a ninth stage, gerotranscendence (Erikson & Erikson, 1997). **Gerotranscendence**, developed further by Tornstam (1989), is a psychosocial theory that regards aging as the final stage in a "possible natural progression towards maturation and wisdom" (Tornstam, 2005, p. 1), which generally results in increased satisfaction and meaning in life. Rather than emphasizing decrements in physical capacity for function, gerotranscendence theory provides for continued growth in dimensions such as spirituality and inner strength (Wadensten & Carlsson, 2007a, b). It has been applied, for example, in support groups for institutionalized older adults focused on the promotion of mental health and well-being (Wang, Lin, & Hsieh, 2011). Duggleby and colleagues (2012), in their meta-synthesis of hope, older adults, and chronic illness, found that transcendence beyond current difficulties was a major theme in how older persons coped and hoped. They described transcendence as "a process that involved the subprocesses of reaching inwardly and outwardly finding meaning and purpose" (p. 1218). This process of transcending occurred through positive reappraisal and "included the subprocesses of reevaluating hope and seeing positive possibilities" (p. 1218).

The concept of gerotranscendence may be used in establishing health promotion interventions. The following guidelines may help the nurses support older adults in their process towards gerotranscendence:

- Accept the possibility that behaviours resembling the signs of gerotranscendence are normal signs of aging.
- Foster strategies to find and maintain hope.
- Foster the older persons' ability to imagine other perspectives.
- Respond to the older person's thoughts and conversation about death.
- Introduce topics of conversation that may facilitate older adults' personal growth.
- Accept, create, and introduce new types of activities, recognizing that each person is unique in their likes and dislikes.

- Create opportunities for older persons to connect with one another and to engage in conversations that facilitate reminiscence and life review.
- Facilitate opportunities for older persons to come together and talk about existential issues such as hope, spirituality, and transcending.

Relationship Strains

As family relationships change, interpersonal relationship strains can develop. Disappointments with lifestyles of adult children and changes in caregiving responsibilities may affect the quality of a longtime family relationship. In some instances, young-old adults assume caregiving responsibilities for their old-old relatives. It is also common for grandparents to assume some caregiving responsibilities for their grandchildren. A change in work status of grandparents (the fact that many of them work today) has drastically changed the "face" of grandparenting in Canada.

With Canadians living longer and healthier lives, grandparents are playing a larger part in the lives of their families. A century ago, grandparents could expect to have only 10 years with their grandchildren; that statistic has doubled to 20 years today. As most Canadian women can expect to live to be at least 83 years of age, many will spend nearly half of their lives as grandmothers. As well, many more Canadians can expect to become great-grandparents than those in the past and healthy grandparents and great-grandparents may have more rewarding opportunities for interactions with younger kin. Margolis and Iciaszczyk (2015) found that improved health of older Canadians may be related to individuals choosing more health-promoting behaviours throughout the life course, due in large part to education. While relationship strains can occur, "families are our most valuable resources, providing not only caregiving but also a sense of worth, emotional ties, and human dignity in approaching life's end" (Walsh, 2012, p. 170). Irrespective of the varied family structures, "what remains constant is the centrality of relatedness" (Walsh, 2012, p. 170). Nurses must strive to understand and support families and to encourage the development of meaning and purpose not just individually, but collectively. They must recognize the potential for aging adults to achieve personal, relational, and spiritual growth and possibility.

Social Domain

Functional Status

Functional status is the extent to which a person can independently carry out personal care, home management, and social functions in everyday life in a way that has meaning and purpose; something that often changes during the later years. Estimates of the prevalence of functional dependency vary, but in general,

studies show that difficulty in performing activities of daily livings (ADLs) increases with advancing age and that rates of dependency are significantly higher for women than for men, particularly for women who live alone (von Strauss, Aguero-Torres, Kareholt, Winblad, & Fratiglioni, 2003).

Although older women and men have similar paths to life satisfaction, a Canadian study conducted by Bourque, Pushkar, Bonneville, and Beland (2005) reported that there are important differences. Men's greater independence allows them to be less dependent on environmental and social factors for life satisfaction; women's greater social embeddedness enables them to be as satisfied as men with life in general, even though their life circumstances may be poorer.

Research has demonstrated the importance of physical activity (particularly aerobic activity) in middle-aged and older adults in reducing functional limitations and disability in later years (Paterson & Warburton, 2010). This is a prime opportunity for nurses to promote not only physical well-being but mental well-being as well.

Retirement

While, in previous years, there has been a trend towards early retirement in Canada, legislated changes in the Canada Pension Plan provide incentives for workers to delay their retirement (Sheets & Gallagher, 2013). Canadians, regardless of their education, are working later and delaying retirement (Statistics Canada, 2012b). The transition from a paid work role to a potentially less structured and purposeful pattern of living can lead to alterations in self-concept. While retirement is often chosen, it is frequently characterized as a stressful life event that may bring psychological, social, and economic uncertainty. It affects social roles, income, use of health services, and participation in leisure activities. In retirement, leisure takes on a different kind of meaning. Retirement can signal a loss of socialization, self-esteem and meaning for men in particular making them more vulnerable to mental health problems. Although these changes are often associated with negative myths and stereotypes, most people do very well in retirement.

Cultural Impact

As the population ages in Canadian society, it is also becoming more culturally diverse, and diversity is changing the landscape of aging populations. The senior population of Canada is heterogenous, composed of many groups whose similarities and differences intersect (e.g., First Nations, lesbian gay bisexual transgendered [LGBT], employed, immigrants, refugees, ethnocultural and racialized groups) (MHCC, 2011). North American communities are increasingly a reflection of multiple ethnic histories and values. Before the 1960s, immigrants to

Canada were mostly from Europe; since the late 1980s, immigrants are increasingly from Asia, Central and South America, and Africa (Tam, Fletcher, & Chi, 2004). Wide cultural variations exist in family expectations of and responsibilities for the older adult. Some groups, such as First Nations and Asian cultures, tend to value highly the experience and wisdom of their older family members, and younger family members feel a responsibility for their care. This cultural belief can create additional pressures for younger family members who may not have the resources to fulfill these expectations.

First Nations peoples in Canada have articulated a description of mental wellness that is meaningful across the life span and that focuses on strengths and resilience rather than deficits. As per the *First Nations Mental Wellness Continuum Framework*, mental wellness is described as:

> a balance of the mental, physical, spiritual, and emotional. This balance is enriched as individuals have: **purpose** in their daily lives whether it is through education, employment, care giving activities, or cultural ways of being and doing; **hope** for their future and those of their families that is grounded in a sense of identity, unique indigenous values, and having a belief in spirit; a sense of **belonging** and connectedness within their families, to community, and to culture; and finally a sense of **meaning** and an understanding of how their lives and those of their families and communities are part of creation and a rich history. (Health Canada and Assembly of First Nations, 2015, p. 1)

The Framework represents a call for nurses and all health care professionals to recognize that "cultural values, sacred knowledge, language and practices of First Nations are essential determinants of individual, family, and community health and wellness" (Health Canada and Assembly of First Nations, 2015, p. 22).

Canada welcomes thousands of immigrants and refugees each year. Those displaced by conflict in their home country, such as refugees from Syria, have often been severely traumatized. Nurses and other health care professionals can play a significant role in promoting immigrant and refugee mental health, identifying challenges to it, and connecting individuals and families to settlement resources (see Chapter 3). Immigrants and refugees who come to Canada frequently experience loneliness and uprootedness. Older adults, in addition to facing such problems, often do not speak the language, become further isolated, and have difficulty expressing mental health needs. A study of older adult refugees fleeing Syria to Lebanon found that two thirds of them had poor or very poor health status and believed that they were a burden to their families. Their nutritional status was poor as they limited their food intake to allow more for younger members. For older refugees, mobility is often a problem and, upon leaving their homes, they lose their social networks and perhaps the esteem in which they were held. The researchers

noted that older refugees need targeted assistance but are often overlooked as a vulnerable group (Strong, Varady, Chahda, Doocy, & Burnham, 2015). Nurses working with immigrants and refugees need to ensure that the mental health needs of the older adults do not go unnoticed.

Further research is needed to understand and address the relationships between cultural issues related to aging, health, and health care delivery. We do know that treatment and intervention are most effective when clients, families, and the health care team can work together to integrate clients' beliefs and cultural values into the plan of care.

Social Activities

While the majority of older adults acknowledge that their health is good, there are health conditions that may prevent participation in home maintenance and leisure activities such as walking, gardening, and active sports. However, there has been increasing support for the importance of physical and social activity in successful aging. In a study of older adults volunteering for Habitat for Humanity, it was found that these volunteers were not physically healthier than their community counterparts but were mentally healthier (Brown, Mefford, Chen, & Brown, 2009). Positive attitudes around notions of "everyone contributes" and "adjusting to limitations" were displayed.

Social connectedness is "a subjective evaluation of the extent to which one has meaningful, close, and constructive relationships with others (i.e., individuals, groups, and/or society)" (O'Rourke & Sidani, 2017, p. 43) and is the opposite of social isolation and loneliness. Social isolation poses serious health risks for older persons; it can put them at risk for suicide, depression, alcohol abuse, and other mental health issues (Alberta Health Services, 2014). In fact, a report on senior cohousing in Canada suggests that while social isolation is a greater threat to an older adult's life than smoking, social connection is central to a flourishing life (Critchlow, 2014). In 2016, the Government of Canada convened a nationwide Working Group on Social Isolation and Social Innovation to address this issue, acknowledging that "the social and economic contributions of seniors will likely be increasingly connected to the success of the entire country" (Government of Canada, 2017, p. 4). Nurses have key roles to play in minimizing social isolation for seniors using "upstream solutions" involving primary intervention strategies to address this problem (Wilson, Harris, Hollis, & Mohankumar, 2011). Nurses can identify the potential for social isolation and build strategies to mitigate against this.

Impacts of Aging on Housing and Communities

The aging of the Canadian population is requiring a reshaping of the pattern of housing needs, the demand

IN-A-LIFE

Lynne Mitchell-Pedersen, Outstanding Canadian Nurse

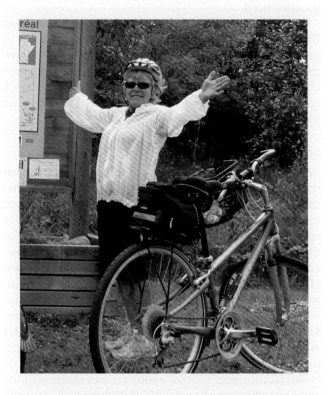

LYNNE MITCHELL-PEDERSEN

Lynne is a trail blazer in Canadian Gerontological Nursing. As the founding president of the Canadian Gerontological Nursing Association (CGNA) in 1983, Lynne has profoundly influenced and shaped the history of Gerontological nursing in Canada, an achievement noted when she was selected as a keynote speaker for the 2017 CGNA biennial conference. She, along with Dr. Colin Powell and her nursing colleagues were instrumental in orchestrating the diminution of the use of physical restraints in the care of older people. Lynne brought a world of compassion and caring to understanding and problem-solving around "vocalizing" behaviour of residents in personal care, facilitating more responsive staff caring to the so-called "difficult" behaviour. Lynne did the Ascent for Alzheimer's, a climb of Mount Kilimanjaro in Africa, the highest free-standing mountain in the world. Lynne loves the great outdoors and, at the age of 75 years, completed a 1,400 km bike trip on the Trans Canada Trail across Manitoba. Lynne continues to inspire nurses, colleagues, family, and friends as she continues to make a difference in the world.

for services, and the ways in which communities are being structured to make them more responsive to older adults. The majority of Canadian seniors in 2011 lived in private dwellings with the remainder (7.9%) living in collective dwellings, including special care facilities (Canadian Mortgage and Housing Corporation [CMHC], 2013). Most older adults prefer to "age in place" in surroundings that are familiar to them until their health prohibits them from doing so. Reasons besides health status for moving to special care facilities include availability of care in the home and access to home care; moving was more likely with increased age, low income and education, and living alone (CMHC, 2013). Factors influencing a move to supportive housing include changes in health or financial status, need for care, availability of help, and marital status (CMHC, 2016). The fact that a negative change in health status is a primary barrier to older adults' capacity to "age in place" has implications for health promotion. Nurses need to be vigilant in their assessment skills, providing ongoing support and facilitating early intervention when needed.

The rapid growth in numbers of older seniors who live alone, are frail, or have disabilities will necessitate considerable expansion of supportive housing choices that enable them to stay in the community. Exciting new initiatives using senior cohousing are occurring in Canada. This innovative cohousing approach fosters social connection, affordability, shared energy consumption, active participation, and collective responsibility, all of which can contribute to a sense of meaning and purpose in life. Exemplars of these communities are Wolf Willow in Saskatchewan and Harbourside Cohousing in Sooke, British Columbia. Such innovative opportunities for Canada's aging population are prime examples of how housing can allow seniors to sustain a fulfilling life (Critchlow, 2014).

Residential Care

The various residential care models that are in place in Canada are in part a response to the medical model emphasized in most long-term care facilities and the need to develop alternatives to nursing home care. Residential care models include a spectrum of residential living environments, such as foster care homes, family homes, personal care homes, residential care facilities, and assisted living arrangements.

Approximately 7% of seniors live in nursing homes and health care facilities, and "the proportion of seniors who enter those facilities rises steadily with age, to 13% of those 75 and older" (CMHC, 2008, p. 5). In 2011, 7.9% of older adults over the age of 65 lived in residential care and that number increased to 43.5% of persons in their nineties (Statistics Canada, 2015). Residential facilities are seeing increased numbers of older adults with mental and physical health challenges, presenting both opportunities and challenges to supporting these individuals. As the population ages, it stands to reason that more older people will be living in long-term care environments.

Assisted Living

The assisted living concept has emerged as an important long-term care alternative for older adults who are mentally and physically frail. Assisted living provides community-based residential services for older adults and adults with physical disabilities who need help with ADLs. Assisted living services combine housing, personal services, and light medical or nursing care. Perhaps the most important feature of these assisted living facilities is the orientation towards the older resident that empowers the frail older adult by sharing responsibilities for care and ADLs, enhancing their choices, and managing risks.

It is important to recognize the role that transcendence plays as a developmental resource in old age. Research investigating living with chronic illness into old age found themes based on strengths of adaptation and adjusting; many older persons demonstrated inner strength despite age and physical or mental challenges (Moe, Hellzen, Ekker, & Enmarker, 2013). Even though the oldest old women and men were vulnerable, they had inner strength. The researchers concluded that "encouraging participation using the inner strength of even the oldest old can contribute to strengthen their experiences of independence, integrity, and enjoying life" (Moe et al., 2013, p. 189). Regardless of one's age or where they live, older adults always want to feel a sense of meaning and purpose in life and that they are making a contribution (Welsh, Moore, & Getzlaf, 2012).

Spiritual Domain

Humanists suggest that the main purpose of life is to find meaning and that this can be accomplished through creations (or accomplishments), experiences in the world, and attitude towards suffering (Frankl, 1963). Successful aging is broadening our understanding of what constitutes spirituality. In nursing, spirituality is recognized as a basic quality, inherent in all humans. The spiritual perspective includes critical attributes such as:

- Connectedness (with other humans, nature, universal forces, or God)
- Beliefs in powers or forces beyond the self and a faith that affirms life
- A creative energy
- Hope

"Spirituality, when understood as an intimate relation with a transcendent force, placing a high value on social relations and stressing respect and value for oneself" (Tomás, Sancho, Galiana, & Oliver, 2016, p. 1385), provides a means for dealing with difficult life situations and finding a sense of meaning and purpose in life.

HEALTHY AGING: THE EXAMPLE OF SEXUAL HEALTH

Cross-cultural research confirms that healthy aging is an ongoing process of adaptation across the four primary bio/psycho/social/spiritual domains (Scharlach & Hoshino, 2013). Sexual health, an important aspect of overall well-being at any age, serves as a good illustration of this necessary adaptation. As one ages, the desire for intimacy does not go away. Many older adults continue to have an active and fulfilling sex life (Mayo Clinic, 2011). Research shows that sexually transmitted infections among the older population are rising, emphasizing that practicing safe sex is as important for older persons as for younger persons (Brandon, 2016). There are physical changes that can affect one's ability to have and enjoy sex (e.g., vaginal dryness in women, often relieved by using a lubricant, and impotence or erectile dysfunction in men, often relieved by medication) (NIA, 2009). In both these instances, encouraging consultation with a family physician may be useful, while the nurse reassures that these issues are common and can most often be remedied. There are some physical illnesses, disabilities, and medications that can cause sexual problems (NIA, 2009). Conditions such as arthritis, chronic pain, dementia, diabetes, heart disease, incontinence, surgery, mastectomy, prostatectomy, and certain medications can affect sexual desire and performance. There are some strategies for each of these conditions that may help alleviate worrisome symptoms and increase pleasure, performance, and desire. Communication with one's partner is a key strategy. Problems in the relationship can create problems in the bedroom (NIA, 2009).

The sustaining of sexual health in older adulthood illustrates well the developmental tasks of healthy aging. These have been identified across sociocultural contexts (United States, Japan, and Sweden) as continuity (maintenance of roles and activities), compensation (accommodation and social support), connection (meaningful relationships), contribution (generativity and engagement), and challenge (stimulation and growth) (Scharlach & Hoshino, 2013).

In recent years, the needs of lesbian, gay, bisexual, and transgender older adults has come to the fore as a neglected area of health care. Although research shows that "LBG individuals mostly adjust well to ageing identities" (McParland & Camic, 2016, p. 3433), they are often marginalized within the mainstream health care contexts, lack accesses to services and frequently experience social isolation. Research still shows evidence of societal stigma attached to LGBT communities but also of the resilience they possess. Nurses are well suited to drawing on this resilience and helping to transform prior negative experiences into supportive and helpful care practices. It could be as simple as finding an older adult member of the community to "plant the seeds of engagement, trust and hope" (Hoy-Ellis, Ator, Kerr, & Milford, 2016, p. 62) where they feel accepted and welcome. This could be a seniors' centre, community group, a church or a café. Innovative programs such as Seniors Preparing for Rainbow Years (SPRY) in which the Montrose Centre in Houston, Texas (an agency offering a range of services tailored to LGBTQ adults over 60) partnered with Legacy Community Health (a federally funded health centre) to provide mental health services to the aging LGBTQ community demonstrate that innovative programming is possible and it works.

RISK FACTORS FOR GERIATRIC PSYCHOPATHOLOGY

Chronic Illnesses

Although the frequency of acute conditions declines with advancing age, about 90% of older adults have chronic medical conditions that can adversely affect function. Poor physical health is a well-established risk factor for mental disorders. The major chronic conditions experienced by older adults are ischemic heart disease, hypertension, vision impairment, hearing impairment, osteo- and rheumatoid arthritis, dementia, cerebrovascular disease, chronic obstructive pulmonary disease, and depression (World Health Organization, 2012). More than 120,000 older Canadians die of cancer, cardiovascular disease, or respiratory distress every year (Statistics Canada, 2010). Chronic illnesses can reduce physiologic capacity and consequently increase functional dependency. In addition, during acute episodes of illness, many older adults lose functional ability because they have limited reserves or cannot mobilize reserves to regain their premorbid performance levels.

Polypharmacy

Polypharmacy, the use of several medications, is often associated with chronic illness and long-term drug therapy. While there can be some positive benefits to medications such as drug therapy to manage diseases affecting the cardiovascular, musculoskeletal, and cerebrovascular systems (Hubbard et al., 2015), many times, polypharmacy contributes to negative health outcomes. According to Kaufman (2015) almost 17% of people over the age of 65 are taking ten or more drugs. The bodily changes that occur with aging means that many drugs are associated with increased sensitivity and potential harm. This can in turn lead to undesirable side effects such as confusion, hypertension, falls, blurred vision, constipation, urinary retention, cognitive impairment,

and adverse reactions. Often, adverse reactions can suggest other problems for which more drugs are added (Chu, 2017). Older people can then develop a growing toxicity to numerous drugs. Adverse drug reactions can cause depression, cognitive impairment, falls and fractures, and other problems as noted above. Such adverse effects can lead to disability and death in older people (Kaufman, 2015).

The Beers Criteria is an internationally recognized list of drugs, developed by Dr. Mark Beers, that identifies potentially inappropriate drugs to prescribe to seniors due to a heightened risk of adverse effects. Updated in 2012 and again in 2015 by a panel of experts of the American Geriatric Society (AGS), the Beers Criteria aid prescribers in avoiding the use of inappropriate and high-risk drugs (American Geriatrics Society, 2015). Such avoidance reduces drug-related complications in older persons. In using the Beers Criteria, it is important to understand the reason a medication is included on the list. The risk/benefit ratio for a particular individual may mean that the medication is the appropriate intervention but that it needs to be used with caution. An alternative to a medication on the list is often not an alternative medication, but rather a nonpharmacologic strategy, such as a lifestyle change (Steinman, Beizer, DuBeau, Laird, Lundebjerg, & Mulhausen, 2015).

Serious problems result when coordination of the care delivery and treatment regimen specific to prescribed medications is lacking. These problems are compounded when the client uses over-the-counter drugs, herbal remedies, and home or folk remedies without considering their potential interaction with prescribed drugs. Nurses can follow the principles delineated in Box 31.2 to improve drug therapy with older adults.

Bereavement and Loss

Older adults experience many losses—friends and family members die, physical health is compromised, and social status diminishes. Loss of one's spouse, particularly when the relationship has been long and satisfying, constitutes a major life event. Women are more likely to lose their spouses and tend to be widowed at a younger age than are men. Consequently, women have more time to adjust and develop substitute social relationships to replace the spouse. Conversely, men tend to lose their wives at an older age, have fewer social networks to replace the spouse, and express feelings of loneliness and abandonment. Because of differences in longevity, men and women usually experience life events at different ages.

Regardless of gender differences, survivors are at higher risk for depression and may face financial issues after the death of a loved one. Health care professionals should work closely with grieving survivors to help them understand that their lives will be displaced for some time. Support sessions on the grief process, facilitating

---

BOX 31.2 Drug Therapy Interventions

- Administer priority/life essential medications first.
- Minimize the number of drugs that the person uses, keeping only those drugs that are essential.
- Always consider alternatives among different drug classifications or dosage forms that are more suitable for older adults. Monitor the claim trends for Beers drugs.
- Implement preventive measures to reduce the need for certain medications. Such prevention includes health promotion through proper nutrition, exercise, and stress reduction.
- Most age-dependent pharmacokinetic changes lead to potential accumulation of the drug; therefore, medication dosage should start low and go slow.
- Exercise caution when administering medication with a long half-life or in an older adult with impaired renal or liver function. Under these conditions, the time may be extended between doses.
- Be knowledgeable of each drug's properties, including such factors as half-life, excretion, and adverse effects. For example, venlafaxine HCl (Effexor), a structurally novel antidepressant that inhibits

the reuptake of serotonin and norepinephrine, requires regular monitoring of the older person's blood pressure.

- Assess the individual's clinical history for physical problems that may affect excretion of medications to assess for orthostatic hypotension and the potential for falls.
- Monitor laboratory values (e.g., creatinine clearance) and urinary output in clients receiving medications eliminated by the kidneys.
- Monitor plasma albumin levels in clients receiving drugs that have high binding affinity to protein.
- Regularly monitor the older person's reaction to all medications to ensure a therapeutic response.
- Look for potential drug interactions that may complicate therapy. Antacids lower gastric acidity and may decrease the rate at which other medications are dissolved and absorbed.
- Remind older adults to consult with their health care provider before taking any over-the-counter medications.

---

meaningful engagement and connectedness, can help older persons feel supported and understand that they are not alone.

Poverty

Poverty among seniors is on the rise again in Canada based on the 2013 census information (Madden, 2016). According to the Broadbent Institute, the highest rates are among older single women living alone, aboriginal and immigrant older adults, persons with disabilities, and older gay and lesbians. In Canada, "the seniors' poverty rate has increased from a low of 3.9% in 1995 to 11.1%, or one in nine, in 2013. Fully 28% of single women and 24% of single male seniors are living in poverty in this country." Factors contributing to this issue are government assistance programs that have not kept pace with household incomes of Canadians; many of these individuals have not had employer pension plans, and many more Canadians will not have enough savings to live into retirement years (Shillington, 2016). Poverty has significant effects on this population, including higher mortality rates, poorer health, lower health-related quality of life, lower likelihood of participating in health screening programs, and higher likelihood of using the emergency department for acute illness (Fleming, Evans, & Chutka, 2003).

Suicide and the Lack of Social Support

Suicide is a leading cause of preventable death in Canada and worldwide. The Canadian Association for

Suicide Prevention (CASP, n.d.) reports that more than 10 older adults over the age of 60 die by suicide every week in Canada and "approximately 1,000 are admitted to Canadian hospitals each year as a consequence of intentional self-harm" (p. 4). Older adults tend to use more lethal methods than younger people in their suicide attempts (Heisel, Neufeld, & Flett, 2016). Hanging and firearms are the most common method of suicide for men, while women tend to use self-poisoning or suffocation (see Chapter 19). The general population engages in suicidal behaviour approximately 20 times for every death to suicide; older adults, in contrast, may do so fewer than four times (Canadian Coalition for Seniors' Mental Health, 2006). The loss of friends and family, debilitating illnesses, loss of independence, and social isolation can contribute to feelings of overwhelming sadness, depression, and loneliness. Depression is the most common mental health problem in older adults, and it is a serious risk factor for suicide (CASP, 2015). Suicide in older adults is most often not related to one single event but multiple factors that accumulate (Stanley, Hom, Rogers, Hagan, & Joiner, 2016).

■ MENTAL ILLNESS PREVENTION

It is projected that by 2041, adults between 70 and 89 years of age will have higher rates of mental illness (including dementia) than any other age group (MHCC, 2012). This fact alone calls for urgent action to look for ways to promote mental health and to prevent mental health issues. There is growing evidence of the cumulative benefits of regular physical activity when sustained over time (Evers et al., 2011; Lee & Hung, 2011; MHCC, 2009). An improvement in mental health and psychological well-being has been noted, and there is some early, promising evidence that links participation in regular physical activity with a decreased likelihood of developing dementia (Larson et al., 2006; Wang, Larson, Bowen, & van Belle, 2006). While these benefits are widely known, there are also a large number of older Canadians who do not participate in enough activity to maintain or promote their health and well-being. Further, there is growing evidence about the relationship between attitudes, aging, and physical and mental health. As successful aging is gaining further prominence, research studies are pointing to powerful effects of attitudes and beliefs in relation to overall well-being (Bryant et al., 2012).

Preventing Depression and Suicide

Mental illness prevention is aimed at addressing the risk factors associated with mental illness and enhances protective factors, thereby impeding illness onset and/or limiting its duration (MHCC, 2012). Depression is one of the most common mental disorders in older adults (see Chapter 22). Recognition and early intervention are the keys to preventing ongoing depressive episodes. Early indications of symptomatology can be identified in primary care settings. Several preventive interventions, such as grief counselling for widows and widowers, self-help groups, and social activities, are helpful. Community-based projects have been effective in significantly reducing suicide rates in older adults (Heisel & Meaning Centered Men's Group [MCMG], 2016). By assessing and addressing cognitive and social–cognitive vulnerability factors and by focusing on the promotion of life satisfaction, nurses can help not only to prevent suicide but also to assist the older adult in achieving a healthier and more meaningful life (Heisel & MCMG, 2016). Increasingly, studies are exploring concepts such as meaning and hope and the role that these play in helping older adults live well (Moore, 2012; Moore, Hall, & Jackson, 2014).

Reducing the Stigma of Mental Health Treatment

The stigma of mental illness continues to interfere with the willingness of older adults to seek treatment. Today's older Canadians grew up during a time when institutionalization in asylums, electroconvulsive treatments, and other treatment approaches were regarded with fear. This fear can lead to denial of problems. The work of the MHCC has recognized the critical importance of combating stigma and discrimination. The commission has launched a 10-year antistigma campaign, recognizing that combating stigma requires a multipronged effort sustained over a long period of time and includes ongoing community-based education

and action, media campaigns, and forums of exchange between affected individuals and other Canadians to enhance public awareness, and professional awareness campaigns to reduce structural discrimination in the health care system and in the mental health system itself (MHCC, 2012).

Nurses are in a primary position to participate in these initiatives at local and national levels. They can also assist older adults in understanding mental health concerns when they arise and encourage them to access appropriate services. They can reassure older adults that many of the issues they experience are common and very amenable to intervention. Nurses must realize that the therapeutic nurse–client interaction is a key strategy that they can develop and, by so doing, foster hope, transcendence, and meaning in life in the older adults they work with (Haugan, 2013; Wiechula, Conroy, Kitson, Marshall, Whitaker, & Rasmussen, 2016) (see Box 31.3).

Use of Medications

With the approval of new medications, older adults will be able to treat health problems with pharmacologic agents that were not previously available. Side effects and drug interactions should be carefully monitored to detect untoward symptoms and delirium (see Chapter 32).

Education of older adults and their families regarding a medication regimen is crucial to ensure adherence and to minimize untoward effects. Basic principles regarding neurobiologic changes in normal aging (as previously discussed) should be applied when designing teaching strategies. The nurse must consider the older adult's pace of learning as well as any visual and hearing deficits. Education should include the reason for administering the drug and important side effects of the drug. The nurse should provide instructional aids, large-print labelling, and devices such as medication calendars that encourage adherence to the treatment plan. Clients should be aware that they can reject childproof containers for their medications if they have trouble opening them.

Avoiding Premature Institutionalization

In Canada, as in many countries around the world, health care reform has drastically affected how health care is delivered. Such reform has focused on a move from institutional care to home care. Research has demonstrated that there is significant potential for home care to support the mental health and well-being of seniors in the community (Ontario Home Care Association, 2010). Supportive community-based services can help to avoid premature institutionalization in seniors. There is evidence that governments are increasingly recognizing the impacts of population aging and looking to make necessary changes. These include appropriate adaptations, including issues related to mobility, safety and security, and facilitation of ADL; improved access to transportation and to location of services; proper housing management practices; and newer housing and

BOX 31.3 Research for Best Practice

WHAT FACTORS INFLUENCE THE CARING RELATIONSHIP BETWEEN A NURSE AND PATIENT?

Wiechula, R., Conroy, T., Kitson, A., Marshall, R. J., Whitaker, N., & Rasmussen, P. (2016). Umbrella review of the evidence. What factors influence the caring relationship between a nurse and patient? Journal of Advanced Nursing, 72(4), 723–724.

The Question: What factors influence the caring relationship between a nurse and patient?

Methods: Umbrella review methodology (informed by Joanna Briggs Institute guidelines) was used to guide systematic reviews. An extensive search of several databases was conducted (Psych Info, PubMed, CINAHL, Scopu, WoS, Embase) using key words nurse, patient, and relationship. Data were critically appraised, extracted, and synthesized.

Findings: Effective nursing is based on relationships and the ability of the nurse to establish a relationship with the patient. Caring relationships occur around six areas: expectations, values, knowledge and skills, communications, context, and the impact of the relationship.

Implications for Nursing: The importance of the therapeutic relationship is frequently overlooked. Therapeutic relationship can help to provide caring, compassion, and hope. Compassion and technical skills should go hand in hand. Nurses and patients benefit from a positive care relationship. Trust provides a foundation for care and is a powerful and meaningful component that shapes the illness experience. Understand that *caring* makes a difference.

---

infrastructures that include a wider range of housing choices, accessible community facilities, and opportunities for active living and volunteer involvement (CMHC, 2008). There are housing initiatives across Canada with alternate levels of care to facilitate increased access to health services for seniors. There are innovative trends in housing design that combine assisted living with programs such as active living and creative arts. Other programs across Canada (e.g., The Meanderthals hiking groups and elder hostels) are also directed at promoting active lifestyles and the physical and mental well-being of seniors.

Vital to mental health promotion is identifying and addressing mental health challenges. A strengths-based approach to addressing mental health concerns that identifies individuals' strengths and resources rather than only their deficits allows strategies to be identified that promote mental health and well-being (Hirst, Lane, & Stares, 2015). The MHCC (2016) predicts that by 2041, older adults will have the highest rate of mental illness in Canada. They suggest that one in four older adults currently lives with mental health problems or a mental illness and with the aging population the need for mental health services and health professionals will increase.

MENTAL HEALTH ASSESSMENT OF THE OLDER ADULT

As noted previously, normal aging is associated with some physical decline, such as decreased sensory abilities and decreased pulmonary and immune functions, but many important functions do not change. Intellectual function, capacity for change, and productive engagement with life remain stable. Many myths exist about normal aging. In fact, agism as a social prejudice is tolerated in Canadian society more than prejudice related to gender or race, most often—according to seniors— taking the form of ignoring older adults or assuming that they are incompetent with nothing to contribute to society (Sheridan Centre for Elder Research, 2016). Some people believe that "senility" is normal or that depression or hopelessness is natural for older individuals. If older adults and family members believe these myths, they will be less likely to seek treatment for themselves or their elders with real problems. Even if they seek help for themselves or their older adults, health care providers may fail to identify depression or simply attribute symptoms to normal aging. A survey of over 1,500 Canadians found that 78% of older adults surveyed had experienced their complaints dismissed by health care professionals as simply part of aging (Sheridan Centre for Elder Research, 2016).

As the population ages, there will be increased numbers of seniors with mental health illnesses and problems. Older adults with mental health problems comprise different population groups. One group consists of those with long-term mental illnesses who have reached the ranks of the older adult population. These individuals usually understand their disorders and treatments. Unfortunately, the changes associated with aging can affect a client's control of his or her chronic mental illness. Symptoms may reappear, and medications may need to be adjusted. Another group includes individuals who are relatively free of mental health problems until their later years. These individuals, who may already have other health problems, develop late-onset mental disorders, such as depression, psychotic symptoms, or dementia. For these individuals and their family members, the development of a mental disorder can be very traumatic. Research that examined the relationship between age and depression in older adults in Canada found that "there is a linear increase in depressive symptoms after age 65, but this occurs in the context of medical comorbidity and is not an independent effect of aging" (Wu, Schimmele, & Chappell, 2012, p. 3).

Mental health problems in older adults can be especially complex because of coexisting medical problems and treatments. Many symptoms of somatic disorders mimic or mask psychiatric disorders. For example, fatigue may be related to anaemia, but it also may be symptomatic of depression. In addition, older individuals are more likely to report somatic symptoms than psychological ones, making identification of a mental disorder even more difficult.

A mental health assessment is necessary when psychiatric or mental health issues are identified or when clients with mental illnesses reach their later years (usually about age 65 years). The assessment generally follows the same format as described in Chapter 10. However, the overall health care issues for older adults can be very complex, so it follows that certain components of the geriatric mental health nursing assessment are unique. The geriatric assessment emphasizes some areas that are less critical to the standard adult assessment.

KEY CONCEPT

Normal aging is associated with some physical decline, such as decreased sensory abilities and decreased pulmonary and immune functions, but many important functions do not change.

▉ TECHNIQUES OF DATA COLLECTION

The nurse assesses whether or not the older client understands the nature and purpose of the assessment (Sadock, Sadock, & Ruiz, 2015) and uses an interview format that may take a few sessions to complete. Self-report standardized tests, such as depression and cognitive functioning tools, may be used. A wide variety of physiologic disorders may cause changes in mental status for older adults; thus, results of laboratory tests often are significant. For example, urinalysis can detect a urinary tract infection that has affected a client's cognitive status. Box 31.4 contains a representative listing of common physiologic causes of changes in mental status. In addition, medical records from other health care

---

BOX 31.4 Changes That Affect Mental Status

- Acid–base imbalance
- Dehydration
- Drugs (prescribed and over the counter)
- Electrolyte changes
- Hypothyroidism
- Hypothermia and hyperthermia
- Hypoxia
- Infection and sepsis

---

providers are useful in developing a complete picture of the client's health status.

An important source of client data is family members, who often notice changes that the older individual overlooks or fails to recognize. A client with memory impairment may be unable to give an accurate history. By interviewing family members, the nurse expands the scope of the client assessment. Moreover, the nurse has an opportunity to evaluate the caregivers themselves to determine whether they can care for the older individual adequately and how they are coping with the situation. For example, a husband may be unable to care for his wife but is unwilling to admit it. If the nurse can establish rapport with the husband, the nurse may use the assessment interview as an opportunity to help the husband to examine his wife's care requirements realistically. The nurse may be able to explain to the husband the impact of caregiving on his health. For instance, it is not uncommon for the caregiving spouse to experience significant physical and mental health decline because of extreme and prolonged stresses. While family members can make significant contributions to the assessment, it is important to see the client alone, as well. Aspects of the assessment, such as concerns regarding sexual health and intimate relationships, are best discussed with the individual. There may be concerns involving suicidal thoughts or paranoid ideation that the client will be reluctant to share in front of family members (Sadock et al., 2015). If the nurse suspects neglect or abuse of the client is occurring, exploring this possibility with the client can take place at this time.

▉ BIO/PSYCHO/SOCIAL/SPIRITUAL GERIATRIC MENTAL HEALTH NURSING ASSESSMENT

At the beginning of the assessment, the nurse should determine the client's ability to participate. For example, if a client is using a wheelchair, he or she may have physical limitations that prevent full participation in the assessment. The older client must be able to hear the nurse. For a client with compromised hearing, the nurse must attend to voice projection and volume. Shouting at the older individual is unnecessary. Nurses should remember to lower the pitch of their voice because higher-pitched sounds are often lost with presbycusis (loss of hearing sensitivity associated with aging). The nurse should eliminate distracting noises, such as from a television or radio, and ensure that the client's hearing aid is in place and turned on. Facing the client and using distinct enunciation will help lipreading clients understand what is being said. Sometimes, deafness is mistaken for cognitive dysfunction. If a client's hearing is questionable, the nurse should examine the client for buildup of cerumen. If this is not believed to be contributing to hearing loss, the nurse can enlist the help of a speech and language specialist. Generally, the pace of the interview should mirror the older adult's ability to move through the assessment. Usually, the pace will be slower than the pace used with younger populations.

KEY CONCEPT

A **bio/psycho/social/spiritual geriatric mental health nursing assessment** is the comprehensive, deliberate, and systematic collection and interpretation of bio/psycho/social/spiritual data that are based on the special needs and problems of older adults to determine current and past health, functional status, and human responses to mental health problems, both actual and potential (Box 31.5).

Biologic Domain

Collecting and analyzing data for the assessment of the biologic domain include areas similar to those discussed in Chapter 10. The assessment components include present and past health status, physical examination results, physical functioning, and a pharmacology review. When focusing on the biologic domain, the nurse pays special attention to the client's general physical appearance as well as any observable manifestations of illness. The nurse should assess how all physical problems affect the client's mental well-being. For example, pain and immobility are physical problems that can negatively affect mental health. Low-energy level may be immediately apparent. Women with obvious osteoporosis are experiencing pain most of the time. Men undergoing radiation for prostate cancer worry about sexual functioning and urinary incontinence.

Present and Past Health Status

A review of the older adult's current health status includes examining health records and collecting information from the client and family members. The nurse must identify chronic health problems that could affect mental health care. For example, the client's management of diabetes mellitus could provide clues to the

likelihood of complications such as retinopathy or neuropathy, which in turn will affect the individual's ability to follow a mental health treatment regimen. A history of psychiatric treatment should be documented.

Physical Examination

The nurse reviews the physical examination findings, paying special attention to recent laboratory values, such as urinalysis, white and red blood cell counts, and fasting blood glucose data (see Chapter 10). Results of neurologic tests could indicate compromise of the neuromuscular systems. Many psychiatric medications lower the seizure threshold, making a history of seizures, which can cause behavioural changes, an important assessment component. The nurse should note any evidence of movement disorders, such as tremors, abnormal movements, or shuffling. If a client has been taking conventional antipsychotics, assessment for symptoms of tardive dyskinesia, using one of the appropriate assessment tools should be considered (see Chapter 12 for additional discussion of tardive dyskinesia).

The nurse should take routine vital signs during the assessment. Any abnormalities in blood pressure (i.e., hypertension or hypotension) should be noted because many psychiatric medications affect blood pressure. Generally, these medications may cause orthostatic hypotension, which can lead to dizziness, unsteady gait, and falls. A baseline blood pressure is needed for future monitoring of medication side effects. Lying, sitting, and standing blood pressures are especially useful in assessing for orthostatic hypotension.

Physical Functions

The older client's physical functioning within the context of the normal changes that accompany aging and the presence of any chronic disorders should be assessed, taking note of the client's use of any personal devices, such as canes, walkers, wheelchairs, or oxygen, or environmental devices, such as grab bars, shower benches, or hospital beds. Specific areas to consider are nutrition and eating, elimination, and sleep patterns.

Nutrition and Eating

Nutrition and physical activity are important in fostering successful aging (Wilcox, 2012). An assessment of the type, amount, and frequency of food eaten is standard in any assessment of the older adult. Any unintentional weight loss of more than 4.5 kg should be noted. Nutrition changes need to be evaluated in light of mental health problems. For example, is a client's weight loss related to an underlying physical problem or to the client's belief that she is being poisoned, which makes her afraid to eat? Or, is the older adult not eating because of an active wish to die?

Eating is often difficult for older adults, who may experience a lack of appetite. Eating and appetite patterns should be assessed because many psychiatric medications

BOX 31.5 Biopsychosocial–Spiritual Geriatric Mental Health Nursing Assessment

I.   Major reason for seeking help _____

II. Initial information
     Name_____
     Age _____ Current marital status _____
     Gender _____ Caregiver's name _____
     Living arrangements _____

III. Level of independence:
     High (needs no help) _____
     Moderate (lives independently, but needs some help with instrumental activities) _____
     Low (relies on others for help in meeting functional and instrumental activities) _____
     Physical limitations _____
     Level of education completed _____

	Normal	Treated	Untreated
Physical functions: system review	☐	☐	☐
Activity/exercise	☐	☐	☐
Sleep patterns	☐	☐	☐
Appetite and nutrition	☐	☐	☐
Hydration	☐	☐	☐
Elimination	☐	☐	☐
Existing physical illnesses	☐	☐	☐

List any chronic illnesses
Presence of pain (Use standardized instrument if pain is present.) No _____ Yes _____
Score _____ Treatment of pain _____

Medication (prescription and over the counter)	Dosage	Side Effects	Frequency of Side Effects

Significant Laboratory Tests	Values	Normal Range

IV. Responses to mental health problems
     Major concerns regarding mental health problem _____
     Major loss/change in past year: No _____ Yes _____
     Fear of violence: No _____ Yes _____
     If yes, type of violence _____
     Strategies for managing problems/disorder _____

V.   Mental status examination _____
     General observation (appearance, psychomotor activity, attitude) _____
     Orientation (time, place, person)
     Mood, affect, emotions (Geriatric Depression Scale should be used if evidence of depression) _____
     Speech (verbal ability, speed, use of words correctly) _____

BOX 31.5 Biopsychosocial–Spiritual Geriatric Mental Health Nursing Assessment (*Continued*)

Thought processes (hallucinations, delusions, tangential, logic, repetition, rhyming of words, loose connections, disorganized) (*Describe the content of hallucinations, delusions.*)
Cognition and intellectual performance (*Use standardized test scores as well as observations.*)
Attention and concentration _____
Abstract reasoning and concentration _____
Memory (recall, short term, long term) _____
Judgment and insight _____
(MMSE, CASI scores) _____

VI. Significant behaviours (psychomotor, agitation, aggression, withdrawn) (*Use standardized test if behaviours are problematic.*) _____
When did problem behaviour begin? Has it gotten worse?

VII. Self-concept (beliefs about self: body image, self-esteem, personal identity)

VIII. Risk assessment
Suicide: High _____ Moderate _____ Low _____
Assault/homicide: High _____ Low _____
Suicide thoughts or ideation: No _____ Yes _____
Current thoughts of harming self _____ Plan _____
Means _____
Means available
Assault/homicide thoughts: No _____ Yes _____
What do you do when angry with a stranger? _____
What do you do when angry with family or partner? _____
Have you ever hit or pushed anyone? No _____ Yes _____
Have you ever been arrested for assault? No _____ Yes _____
Current thoughts of harming others _____

IX. Functional status (*Use standardized test such as FAQ.*) _____

X. Cultural assessment
Cultural group _____
Cultural group's view of health and mental illness _____
By what cultural rules do you try to live? _____
Special, cultural foods that are important to you _____

XI. Stresses and coping behaviours
Social support _____
Family members _____
Which members are important to you? _____
On whom can you rely? _____
Community resources _____

XII. Spiritual assessment _____
XIII. Economic status _____
XIV. Legal status _____
XV. Quality of life _____

Summary of significant data that can be used in formulating a nursing diagnosis:

SIGNATURE/TITLE _____ Date _____

can affect digestion and may impair an already compromised gastrointestinal tract. A common problem of older individuals who live in long-term care facilities is **dysphagia,** or difficulty swallowing. Dysphagia can lead to dehydration, malnutrition, pneumonia, or asphyxiation. People who have been exposed to conventional antipsychotics (e.g., haloperidol, chlorpromazine) may have symptoms of tardive dyskinesia, which can make swallowing difficult.

Xerostomia, or dry mouth, which is common in older adults, also may impair eating. This may be the case for clients who are currently receiving treatment for a mental disorder, particularly with medications that have anticholinergic properties. Dry mouth is also a side effect of many other anticholinergic medications, such as cimetidine, digoxin, and furosemide. Frequent rinsing with a non–alcohol-based mouthwash will help to correct the dry condition. Decreased taste or smell is common among older adults and may reduce the pleasure of eating so that the client may eat less. Making meal times social and relaxing experiences can help the older individual compensate for some of the loss of pleasure associated with decreased taste or smell. Preparing favourite foods will also enhance the quality of meals and meal times.

Alcohol or substance use needs to be assessed. Its effects on older adults vary related to age, physical and mental health problems, and use of other medications. The Canadian Community Health Survey of 2015 reported that, among Canadian 65 years and older, 10% of males and 4% of females met the definition of "heavy drinker": five or more drinks (if male; four or more if female) on one occasion at least once a month over the past year (Statistics Canada, 2017b). Even low consumption of alcohol can be dangerous when taken with some medications, and older adults are more likely to be taking multiple medications. Older adults may use alcohol as a means of managing pain (Brennan & Soohoo, 2013) or as a way to deal with stresses such as health issues, retirement, loss of independence, death of friends and life partners, and moving from home to supportive care environments. Physiological vulnerability and the incompatibility of alcohol with many medications taken by older adults, however, increase the health risks of excessive drinking (Alberta Health Services, 2014). The use of the CAGE questionnaire (see Chapter 26, Box 26.6) or the SMAST-G (Short Michigan Alcoholism Screening Test—Geriatric Version) (University of Michigan Alcohol Research Centre, 1991) may be helpful in this area. If an older adult screens negatively for problem drinking using one of these scales, yet the nurse believes that the client may have an alcohol problem, using the other instrument, as well, is indicated. The instruments can target different facets of problem drinking.

Elimination

The client's urinary and bowel functions should also be assessed. Older individuals are more likely to experience constipation because the peristaltic movement of the bowel slows down with aging. Medications with anticholinergic properties can cause constipation, leading to faecal impaction. Abuse of laxatives is common among older adults and requires evaluation. Although the addition of fibre is recommended for constipation, such measures may cause bloating and excessive gas production. Older clients are also more likely to experience urinary frequency because the strength of the sphincter muscle decreases. Because many older adults drink fewer fluids to manage urinary incontinence, fluid intake also becomes

an important factor in assessing urinary functioning and constipation. Urinary incontinence is a symptom of a disorder that requires follow-up and treatment.

Sleep

As part of normal aging processes, sleep patterns change, and clients often sleep less than they did when younger. Any recent changes in sleep patterns should be evaluated as to whether they are related to normal aging or are symptomatic of an underlying disorder (see Chapter 28). **Insomnia**, the inability to fall or remain asleep throughout the night, can be related to depression and lead to the regular use of sleep medications. Clients with insomnia report that they cannot sleep at night and do not feel rested in the morning. Approximately 57% of older adults complain of sleep disturbances of some kind (e.g., insomnia, early morning wakening, or the inability to fall asleep) (Brandt & Piechocki, 2013). Sleep problems may be linked to the use of alcohol or other drugs, so if the client reports sleep problems, the nurse should ask about his or her use of alcohol, over-the-counter medications, and prescription drugs.

Pain

Older adults are more likely to experience pain than younger adults because they are at increased risk for chronic illness and may be suffering from the consequences of a lifetime of injuries. For a number of older individuals, pain is a constant companion. The experience of chronic pain may be a contributing factor to unexplained behaviour and personality changes. There are several pain assessment instruments. One of the most popular instruments is the Wong-Baker FACES Pain Rating Scale, initially developed for children but now used for all age groups (Wong & Baker, 1988). It is important to use the scale correctly by having clients point to the face that shows their level of pain; research has shown that many nurses use it incorrectly by selecting the face they believe indicates the client's level of pain (Jastrzab, Kerr, & Fairbrother, 2009). The assessment of pain is especially critical for those older adults who are cognitively impaired and living in long-term care institutions. Pain is an underrecognized, underassessed, and undertreated phenomenon in this population (Kassalainen, Agarwal, Dolovich, Brazil, & Papaioannou, 2015). Kaasalainen and her colleagues found that physicians and nurses expressed uncertainty about assessing pain in cognitively impaired individuals, admitted reluctance to administer opioids, and voiced concerns about overmedicating these residents. They also found that nurses rely on clients requesting medication for pain even though it is known that many clients hesitate to ask.

Pharmacologic Assessment

One of the most important areas of the biologic domain is the pharmacologic assessment. Polypharmacy, the concurrent use of several different medications, is common in older individuals. The client and family should be asked to list all medications and times that the client takes them. Information regarding medication, which clients have been taking until recently, is also important as, for example, they may have been using a monoamine oxidase inhibitor or suddenly stopped taking a prescribed medication such as a benzodiazepine or a selective serotonin reuptake inhibitor (see Chapter 12). Asking family members to bring in all the medications that the client is taking, including over-the-counter medications, vitamins, and herbal supplements, is a good idea. Because older adults are more sensitive than younger people to medications, the possibility of drug–drug interactions is greater. Adverse drug interactions may cause delirium in older adults and constitute a medical emergency that may result in death (see Chapter 32). Also, when considering potential drug interactions, the nurse should ask the older individual about his or her consumption of grapefruit juice, which contains naringin, a compound that inhibits the CYP3A4 enzyme involved in the metabolism of many medications (e.g., antidepressants, antiarrhythmics, erythromycin, several statins). The American Geriatrics Society (AGS) updated the Beers Criteria, the most highly used information source for prescribing medications in older adults, which may provide a useful resource when examining pharmacologic interventions (American Geriatrics Society, 2015). Comprehensive geriatric assessment has proven effective for addressing many problems associated with polypharmacy.

Psychological Domain

The assessment of the psychological domain provides the nurse with the opportunity to identify limitations, behavioural symptoms, and reactions to illness. The nurse assesses many of the same areas as in other adult assessments, but again, the emphasis may be different. The following discussion focuses on the responses of older adults to mental health problems, mental status examinations, behavioural changes, stress and coping patterns, and risk assessments.

Responses to Mental Health Problems

Many older clients are reluctant to admit that they have psychiatric symptoms, particularly if their culture stigmatizes mental illness and may deny having mental or emotional problems. They may also fear that if they admit to any symptoms, they may be placed outside their home. Clients who do not recognize or admit to having psychiatric symptoms are increasingly vulnerable to being taken advantage of or injured.

Throughout the assessment, the nurse evaluates the client's verbal reports, obvious symptoms, and family reports. If a client flatly denies any psychiatric symptoms (e.g., depression, mood swings, outbursts of anger, memory problems), the nurse should respectfully accept the older adult's answer and avoid arguments or confrontation (Box 31.6). If the client's family members

contradict the client's report or symptoms are obvious during the interview, the nurse can approach the issue while planning care. Nurses may need to use conflict resolution strategies in helping families and clients obtain appropriate care despite disagreement about symptoms experienced by the older adults.

Mental Status Examination

The areas of special interest in the mental status examination are mood and affect, thought processes, and cognitive functioning. The nurse should interpret the results in light of any accompanying physical problems, such as chronic pain, or life changes, such as loss of a spouse.

Mood and Affect

Depression is not a normal part of aging, yet it is the most common mental disorder in older adults (Centers for Disease Control and Prevention [CDC], 2017; Skoog, 2011) and associated with the following risk factors: loss of spouse, physical illness, education below high school, impaired functional status, and heavy alcohol consumption. In older people, other disorders may mask depression. When symptoms are present, they may be attributed to normal aging or atherosclerosis or other age-related problems. Older clients are less likely to report feeling sad or worthless than are younger clients. As a result, family members and primary care providers may overlook depression in older adults. Depressive symptoms are much more common than a full-fledged depressive disorder, as characterized by the *Diagnostic and Statistical Manual of Mental Disorders-5* (American Psychiatric Association, 2013). Between 10% and 15% of older adults living in the community experience depressive symptoms, with approximately 50% of older adults living in long-term care facilities showing signs of depression (MHCC, 2012). Untreated depression in older adults may result in the overuse of health care services, longer hospital stays, decreased treatment compliance, and increased morbidity and mortality.

The CDC (2017) states that "Someone who is depressed has feelings of sadness or anxiety that last for weeks at a time. He or she may also experience–

- Feelings of hopelessness and/or pessimism
- Feelings of guilt, worthlessness and/or helplessness
- Irritability, restlessness
- Loss of interest in activities or hobbies once pleasurable
- Fatigue and decreased energy
- Difficulty concentrating, remembering details and making decisions
- Insomnia, early–morning wakefulness, or excessive sleeping
- Overeating or appetite loss
- Thoughts of suicide, suicide attempts
- Persistent aches or pains, headaches, cramps, or digestive problems that do not get better, even with treatment" (CDC, 2017, p. 3).

BOX 31.6

THERAPEUTIC DIALOGUE

Assessment Interview

Tom, 79 years old, is being seen for the first time in a geriatric mental health clinic because of recent changes in his behaviour and his accusations that family members are trying to steal his house and car. He locked his wife out of the house, accusing her of being unfaithful. When Susan, the nurse assigned to his case, is conducting the assessment interview, Tom cooperates and is very pleasant until the nurse begins to assess the psychological domain.

Ineffective Approach

Nurse: Have there been times when you have had problems with any members of your family?
Client: No. (Silence)
Nurse: Have you noticed that lately you have been getting more upset than usual?
Client: No. Who has been talking to you?
Nurse: Your wife seems to think that you may be getting a little more upset than usual.
Client: You are just like her. She keeps telling me something is wrong with me. (Getting very agitated)
Nurse: Please, I'm trying to help you. I understand that you locked your wife out of the house last week.
Client: Leave me alone. (Gets up and leaves.)

Effective Approach

Nurse: How have things been going at home?
Client: All right.
Nurse: (Silence)
Client: Well, my wife and I sometimes argue.

Nurse: Oh. Most husbands and wives argue. Any special arguments?
Client: No. Just the usual. I don't pick up after myself enough. I don't dress right to suit her. But, lately, she's gone a lot.
Nurse: She is gone a lot?
Client: Yeah! A lot.
Nurse: The way you say that, it sounds like you have some feelings about her being gone.
Client: You're damned right I do—and you would, too.
Nurse: I'm missing something.
Client: Well, if you must know, I think she's having an affair with the man next door.
Nurse: Really? That must upset you to think your wife is having an affair.
Client: I am devastated. I feel so bad.
Nurse: Would you say that you are depressed?
Client: Well, wouldn't you be? Yes, I'm feeling pretty low.

Critical Thinking Challenge

- How do the very first questions differ in the two interviews?
- What therapeutic techniques did the nurse use in the second interview to avoid the pitfalls the nurse encountered in the first scenario?
- How did the nurse in the second scenario elicit the client's delusion about his wife's affair?
- From the data that the second nurse gathered, how many of the client's problems can be identified?

The Geriatric Depression Scale (GDS) is a useful screening tool with demonstrated validity and reliability (Hyer & Blount, 1984). The GDS was designed as a self-administered test, although it also has been used in observer-administered formats. One advantage of the test is its "yes/no" format, which may be easier for older adults than the Hamilton Rating Scale for Depression, which uses a scale from 0 to 4 (see Appendix E). This tool is easy to administer and provides valuable information about the possibility of depression (Box 31.7). If results are positive, the nurse should refer the client to a psychiatrist or advanced practice nurse for further evaluation.

Among residents in long-term care facilities, the usefulness of the GDS depends on the degree of cognitive impairment. Residents who are mildly impaired may be able to answer yes/no questions; however, moderately to severely impaired older adults will be unable to do the same. A well-validated scale for individuals with dementia is the Cornell Scale for Depression in Dementia

[CSDD] (Alexopoulos, Abrams, Young, & Shamoian, 1988). The CSDD is an interview-administered scale that uses information from both the client and an outside informant.

Anxiety is another important mood for nurses to assess in older adults because it can interfere with normal functioning. In dementia, anxiety is common (Skoog, 2011). The rating anxiety in dementia (RAID) scale was developed as a global scale to assess anxiety in clients with dementia (Shankar, Walker, Frost, & Orrell, 1999). The domains that the RAID scale assesses include worry, apprehension and vigilance, motor tension, autonomic hyperactivity, and phobias and panic attacks.

Thought Processes

Thought processes and content are critical in the assessment of older adults. Can the client express ideas and thoughts logically? Can the client understand questions and follow the conversation of others? If the older adult

---

BOX 31.7 Geriatric Depression Scale (Short Form)

1. Are you basically satisfied with your life?	Yes	No
2. Have you dropped many of your activities and interests?	Yes	No
3. Do you feel that your life is empty?	Yes	No
4. Do you often get bored?	Yes	No
5. Are you in good spirits most of the time?	Yes	No
6. Are you afraid that something bad is going to happen to you?	Yes	No
7. Do you feel happy most of the time?	Yes	No
8. Do you often feel helpless?	Yes	No
9. Do you prefer to stay at home rather than go out and do new things?	Yes	No
10. Do you feel you have more problems with memory than most?	Yes	No
11. Do you think it is wonderful to be alive now?	Yes	No
12. Do you feel pretty worthless the way you are now?	Yes	No
13. Do you feel full of energy?	Yes	No
14. Do you feel that your situation is hopeless?	Yes	No
15. Do you think that most people are better off than you are?	Yes	No

Score: ___/15 One point for "No" to questions 1, 5, 7, 11, 13

One point for "Yes" to other questions

Normal	3 ± 2
Mildly depressed	7 ± 3
Very depressed	12 ± 2

Adapted from Sheikh, J. I., & Yesavage, J. A. (1986). Geriatric Depression Scale (GDS): Recent evidence and development of a shorter version. In T. L. Brink (Ed.), *Clinical gerontology: A guide to assessment and intervention* (pp. 165–173). Binghamton, NY: Haworth Press. © By the Haworth Press, Inc. All rights reserved. Reprinted with permission.

---

shows any indication of hallucinations or delusions, the nurse should explore the content of the hallucination or delusion. If the client has a history of mental illness, such as schizophrenia, these symptoms may be familiar to family members, who can validate whether they are old or new problems. If this is the first time the client has experienced these abnormal thought processes, the nurse should further evaluate the content. Suspicious and delusional thoughts that characterize dementia often include some of the following beliefs:

- People are stealing my things.
- My spouse is having an affair.
- My relative is an impostor.

If a client shares any such thoughts, the nurse can complete further assessment by using the Behavioural Pathology in Alzheimer's Disease (BEHAVE-AD) Rating Scale. This 25-item scale is based on caregivers' reports within the previous 2 weeks (Reisberg & Ferris, 1985). The BEHAVE-AD measures thought and behavioural disturbances in seven major categories, with each item scored on a four-point scale of severity (0 to 3), including delusions, hallucinations, activity disturbances, aggressiveness, diurnal rhythm disturbances, mood disturbances, and anxieties and phobias. The BEHAVE-AD also contains a four-point global assessment of the overall magnitude of the behaviour symptoms in terms of disturbance to the caregiver, dangerousness to the client, or both. The reliability of the BEHAVE-AD (0.95 and 0.96; $p < 0.01$) is comparable to that of the Mini-Mental State Examination (MMSE) (Reisberg, Auer, & Monteiro, 1997).

Cognition and Intellectual Performance

Cognitive functioning includes such parameters as orientation, attention, short- and long-term memories, consciousness, and executive functioning. Intellectual functioning, also considered a cognitive measure, is rarely formally assessed with a standardized intelligence test in older adults. Considerable variability among individuals depends on lifestyle and psychosocial factors. Some changes in cognitive capacity accompany aging, but important functions are spared. Normal cognitive changes during aging include a slowing of information processing and memory retrieval. Abnormalities of consciousness, orientation, judgment, speech, or language are not related to age but to underlying neuropathologic changes. Cognitive changes in older adults are associated with delirium or dementia or with schizophrenia.

An assessment of cognition should include the number of years of education. When assessing cognitive functioning, nurses should use standardized instruments in combination with their assessment skills to assess for cognitive impairment in older adults residing in hospitals and long-term care facilities. Of such instruments, the MMSE, discussed in Chapter 10, is recommended for use in screening for cognitive functioning related to dementia (Leifer, 2009). Various studies suggest that an MMSE score below 24 of 30 has a reasonable sensitivity (80% to 90%) and specificity (80%) for discriminating between those with dementia and those without. Studies suggest that education has a protective effect against cognitive decline in early-stage mild cognitive impairment but that this effect disappears in late-stage mild cognitive impairment (Ye et al., 2013). Assessment should always take into account not only an individual's educational background but also his/her cultural background as these can influence scores.

Severe cognitive deterioration may occur in older individuals with schizophrenia. In assessing the cognitive status of this population, the Cognitive Abilities Screening Instrument (CASI) demonstrates greater specificity than does the MMSE (Sherrell, Buckwalter, Bode, & Strozdas, 1999). The CASI is a 25-item test developed as a research instrument and piloted in Japan and the United States (Teng et al., 1994). The total score ranges from 0 (poor) to 100 (good), with a suggested cutoff of 74 for classifying dementia. The CASI provides quantitative assessment of nine domains: attention, concentration, orientation, long-term memory, short-term memory, language, visual construction (copying pentagons), fluency (naming four-legged animals), and abstraction and judgment. Because it determines the level of cognitive impairment, the CASI could be used in establishing individualized care plans.

In 2012, the diagnostic approach to Alzheimer's disease was revised at the fourth Canadian Consensus Conference on the Diagnosis and Treatment of Dementia, based in part on recommendations by the International Working Group and workgroups of the National Institute on Aging/Alzheimer Association. These recommendations can be found in Gauthier et al. (2012) (see Chapter 32).

Behaviour Changes

Behaviour changes in older adults can indicate neuropathologic processes and thus require nursing assessment. If such changes occur, it is most likely that family members will notice them before the client does. **Apraxia** (the inability to execute a voluntary movement despite normal muscle function) is not attributed to age but indicates an underlying disease process, such as Alzheimer's disease, Parkinson's disease, or other disorders. Various other behaviour problems are associated with psychiatric disorders in older individuals, including irritability, agitation, apathy, and euphoria. Other behaviours in older adults who are experiencing psychiatric problems include wandering and aggressive behaviours. The BEHAVE-AD Rating Scale identifies these behaviours.

The neuropsychiatric inventory (NPI) was developed in 1994 to assess behaviour problems associated with dementia. The scale assesses 10 behaviour problems: delusions, hallucinations, dysphoria, anxiety, agitation/aggression, euphoria, disinhibition, irritability/lability, apathy, and aberrant motor behaviour (Cummings et al., 1994). The NPI was subsequently refined to include two more behavioural problems: nighttime behavioural disturbances such as difficulties with sleep and changes in eating patterns. The NPI also added a component to assess for caregiver distress (Cummings, 1997). This very popular tool is used in many medication clinical trials. There are two versions. The standard version is used when the client is still at home, whereas a different version is used when the client is in a long-term care facility.

Stress and Coping Patterns

Identifying stresses and coping patterns is just as important for older individuals as it is for younger adults. Unique stresses for older clients include living on a fixed income, handling declining health, losing partners and friends, and ultimately confronting death. Coping ability varies, depending on clients' unique circumstances. As is true for adults of all ages, some older adults respond to stressful events with amazing adaptability, whereas others become depressed and suicidal.

Loss of a spouse is common in late life, especially for women in older age groups. Forty-five percent of women and 15% of men over the age of 65 have lost a spouse (Itzhar-Nabarro & Smoski, 2012). Bereavement, a natural response to the death of a loved one, includes crying and sorrow, anxiety and agitation, insomnia, and loss of appetite. These symptoms of grief may cause much suffering, but they do not lead to a major depressive disorder except, perhaps, when the person is vulnerable to depressive disorders (APA, 2013). Although bereavement is a normal response, the nurse must identify it and develop interventions to help the individual successfully resolve the loss. Bereavement is an important and well-established risk factor for depression. Factors such as previous mental or physical health conditions in the surviving spouse, high levels of caregiver strain before the death of the spouse, and a lack of social support increase the likelihood of depression post bereavement (Itzhar-Nabarro & Smoski, 2012; Stahl & Schulz, 2013).

Loneliness is another concern in older adults that significantly impacts health and well-being. It is also an issue that nurses can positively influence by assessing for it. "Similar to pain and suffering, loneliness is part of human beings' embodied condition … and what it means to be human" (Smith, 2012, p. 52). Events such as bereavement and loss put individuals at increased risk for feeling lonely. Older adulthood is a time when such events become more frequent, thus experiences of loneliness can increase, as well.

Risk Assessment

Suicide is a major mental health risk for older adults. Men 85 years of age and older have the highest suicide rate of all age groupings in Canada (Government of Canada, 2006). Most older individuals who die by suicide have visited their family physician within the month of their death (Gregg, Fiske, & Gatz, 2013).

When caring for the older client with mental health problems, the nurse always should consider the individual's potential to die by suicide. Depression is the greatest risk factor for suicide. In assessing an older client, the nurse should consider the following characteristics as indications of high risk for committing suicide:

- Depression
- Previous suicide attempts
- Family history of suicide
- Firearms in the home
- Abuse of alcohol or other substances
- Unusual stress
- Chronic medical condition (e.g., cancer, neuromuscular disorders)
- Feelings of helplessness and hopelessness
- Feelings of being a burden to others
- Social isolation

KEY CONCEPT

Current mental health policies focus on **aging in place** and community-based care; integration aims at moving away from older, more stigmatizing approaches of long-term institutionalization and custodial care.

Social Domain

An assessment of the social domain includes determining the client's interactions with others in his or her family and community. The nurse targets social support because it is so important to the well-being of older adults, functional status because of the potential physical changes that can affect this area, and social systems, which encompass all community resources.

Social Support

Remaining active throughout one's life is one of the best predictors of mental health and wellness in an older individual. People obtain their sense of self-worth through their interactions with others in their environment. A sense of "who one is" is closely tied to the roles that a person plays in life. When older adults relinquish such roles because of physical disabilities, become isolated from friends and family, or begin to sense that they are a burden to those around them rather than contributing members of society, a sense of hopelessness and helplessness may follow.

The role of social support is critical to assess in this age group. Social support is a reciprocal concept, meaning that simply receiving assistance increases the person's sense of being a burden. Those older individuals who also believe that they contribute to the welfare of others are most likely to remain mentally healthy. For this reason, pets are often "lifesavers" for older adults who live alone. Nothing can be more understanding and accepting of an older adult's behaviour or disabilities than a beloved pet.

Robotic animals (e.g., dogs, cats, rabbits, and seals) have been designed to respond with gestures and sounds to interact with older adults, including those with cognitive impairment. Pet robots can have a positive effect (e.g., reduce feelings of loneliness and stress and improve quality of life) on older adults living in nursing homes when compared with control groups without actual animal pets. Sensors can be included in the robotic pet that permit the assessment of the older adult, including an alarm system when deterioration is noted (Preu & Legal, 2017). Nevertheless, although robotic pets do not require the care that live pets do, their cost can be prohibitive, and essentially, their engagement with an older adult is not genuinely intimate. It is worthwhile to consider ways to enable a living pet to be with an older adult, such that the pet's optimal welfare is ensured. Further exploration of both pet options, real and robotic, as means to improve the quality of life of older adults need to be explored (Preuß & Legal, 2017).

In assessing clients' social support, the nurse should assess the range of formal and informal social contacts. The frequency of contacts with others (in person and through telephone calls, letters, and cards) should be noted. Research has shown that social support and the quality of relationships are significant in contributing to quality of life for older persons (Merz & Huxhold, 2010). The amount of social support currently experienced should be compared with the amount and kinds of support the client received in the past, as well as clients' perspective on their support. Determining whether these contacts are actually satisfying and supporting to the client is essential. For some individuals, knowing that a son who is living in another city can be contacted and will come to them if necessary is sufficient support. For others, a daily visit from an adult child is viewed as lacking in caring and support. If family members are important to the client's well-being, the nurse should complete a more in-depth family assessment (see Chapter 15).

The nurse can use the following questions to focus on social support:

- Do you have a special person you can call or contact if you need help? Who would that be?
- Do you have a neighbour with whom you are comfortable in asking for assistance?
- In the past 2 weeks, how often has someone provided you with help, such as giving you a ride somewhere or helping around the house?
- In general, other than your children, are there close friends or relatives with whom you are in contact at least once a month?

Other important questions for assessing social support include questions regarding the quality of relationships with family and others. For older clients who are isolated with few social contacts, the nurse can develop interventions to improve social support.

Functional Status

As part of a complete assessment, the nurse will need to assess the older adult's functional status. Functional activities or ADLs are the activities necessary for self-care (i.e., bathing, toileting, dressing, transferring). Instrumental ADLs (IADLs) include those that facilitate or enhance the performance of ADLs (i.e., shopping, using the telephone, using transportation). These aspects are critical to consider for any older adult living alone. When possible, the older adult should be observed for his or her ability to complete ADLs, rather than relying on self-report or report of the family. Common tools used to assess functional status include the Index of Independence in ADLs and the IADLs (Katz & Akpom, 1976). The Functional Activities Questionnaire (FAQ) measures an adult's functional abilities based on the information from family members and caregivers. The older person is rated on 10 complex, higher-order activities, such as writing cheques, assembling tax records, and driving (Pfeffer, Kursaki, Harrah, Chance, & Filos, 1982). The Functional Autonomy Measuring System (Hebert, Guilbeault, & Pinsonnault, 2002; McKye, Naglie, Tierney, & Jaglal, 2009) is designed for use in a community setting and measures a person's actual performance on a task (e.g., performs task alone; with cueing or help; total help needed). Client and family reports can be used in completing it.

Social Systems

Community resources are essential to an older adult's ability to maintain mental health and wellness, as well as to his or her ability to remain at home throughout the later years. Senior centres are federally or provincially funded community resources that provide a wide array of services to Canada's older population. They may provide daily balanced meals at a nominal cost. In addition, they provide opportunities for socialization, which is key to combating loneliness and social isolation. Many senior centres provide annual influenza and pneumonia vaccination clinics and education on such topics as fall prevention and the recognition and prevention of elder abuse. Additional community resources that are specific to older individuals include geriatric assessment clinics and adult day programs.

During the assessment, the nurse must determine which community resources are available and if the older client uses them. Lack of transportation to and from these community resources may be a barrier to use. Most communities have buses available for older or disabled individuals. As more communities are recognizing the importance of being "age friendly," more resources are being made available and accessible for older persons. Nurses may need to assist the older adult in accessing these important resources.

While Canada does fairly well with respect to poverty rates among seniors (6.7%) in comparison with other countries, the poverty rates for older adults rose between the mid-1990s and late 2000s; there are still many seniors who are classified as low income (Conference Board of Canada, 2013). A number of older adults rely on Canada Pension Plan (or for older adults living in Quebec, the Quebec Pension Plan), Old Age Security, and Guaranteed Income Supplement for their monthly income. For these older individuals, this financial support, although less than adequate in most instances, is their only source of income. The nurse should assess a client's sources of financial support. Nurses are sometimes uncomfortable asking for financial information, fearing that they are invading the client's privacy. However, such data are important for the nurse to determine whether an older individual's resources adequately meet his or her needs, and this purpose may be explained to the client. The source of financial support is also important. For example, a client whose income is adequate and comes from personal resources is more likely to be independent than is a client who depends on family members for income.

The nurse should ask the client about accessible health care facilities; available transportation to and from health care facilities; formal supports such as physicians, nurses, and other health care professionals; and the client's ability to pay for medications and health aids. Information about available health care resources beyond standard provincial health care (e.g., plans to pay for additional services such as medications or foot care) will alert the nurse to what services the client currently can and cannot access. In urban areas that are likely to have adequate health care resources, cultural and language barriers may prohibit access. People who live in rural areas where health care resources are limited are less likely to enjoy the full range of health care resources than are those in urban areas. For instance, older adults in Canadian rural settings are likely to have greater difficulty accessing geriatric mental health services than those in urban sites. Even where geriatric mental health services are available, there can be reluctance on the part of older adults and/or their families to access them due to lack of information regarding the services and resources, stigma, or cultural beliefs regarding seeking help outside of one's family. Initiatives of the Mental Health Commission of Canada (MHCC) and its Seniors Advisory Committee involve strategies aimed at reducing the stigma of mental illness and aging (MHCC, 2011, 2012).

Legal Status

A growing trend in Canada and the United States is to view older adults as a special population whose rights deserve increased attention. Instances of elder abuse are far too common. Nurses are client advocates and need to be vigilant in recognizing the signs of neglect or abuse, such as unexplained injuries (see Chapter 34). At times, abuse can take the form of another individual (sometimes an adult child) usurping the rights of the older person. Unless the older person is medically and legally determined to be incompetent, he or she has the same rights to personal decision-making as any other adult, including the right to refuse treatment.

Social Support Transitions

Older adults may compensate for loss of family by expanding friendship networks, and employment may become an important method of establishing a network in later life. The older adult can be prepared for the transition by receiving information about internal developmental processes, sources of social support, and opportunities for personal growth. Older adults who are single, widowed, or divorced may wish to find new relationships.

Online dating sites are increasingly popular for this purpose. Use of an online environment increases the number of potential mates, friends, or casual companions available to the individual. It allows meeting others who may be compatible prior to connecting in person. Dating sites used by Canadians older adults include Zoosk, Elite Single, Match, eHarmony and OurTime with many of these sites with filters to enable searching for faith-based or gay and lesbian choices; there are, as well, specific, focused dating sites. Making online connections, however, is not without its dangers. These dangers include the compromising of personal information, becoming a target for online predators, and financial scams. These scams, typically international in scope, involve establishing a relationship over months and then asking for money for an emergency or for trip expenses to meet the person (Wion & Loeb, 2015).

Nursing assessment of the single older adult should include a simple question regarding whether the person is dating or interested in dating. Once a dialogue is opened, the nurse can offer information, including ways of staying safe, such as using an email address that may be easily discarded and does not reveal personal information and using a public place for a first meeting with someone met online (Wion & Loeb, 2015). Nurses need to reflect on their own biases regarding dating and romance for seniors to ensure that they are not acting in a judgmental way. There are opportunities for nurses to support connectedness among older adults and initiate strategies to foster hope and meaning in life through life transitions.

Lifestyle Support

There is increasing evidence that healthy lifestyles can promote physical and mental health and reduce the length of time individuals are affected by disability (Boggatz & Meinhart, 2017). Some studies have found that self perceptions of health and aging are amenable to interventions and when older adults were encouraged to develop more positive views of their health their physical activity

increased and they achieved more active and healthy life styles (Beyer, Wolff, Warner, Schuz, & Wurm, 2015). For instance, a randomized-controlled study found that an 8-week physical exercise program significantly increased the happiness of older adults when compared with a control group. There was no difference in happiness scores on the Oxford Happiness Inventory between the groups prior to the exercise intervention (Khazaee-Pooli, Sadeghi, & Majlessi, 2015). Lifestyle interventions, such as exercise promotion and nutrition counselling, are particularly important in later life because a tendency to slow down and to become more sedentary usually accompanies aging. For many, retirement provides an opportunity to restructure the time that was previously spent working. Developing regular exercise habits can help maintain physical and psychological well-being. Self-help programs generally include components of exercise, nutrition, health screening, and health habits.

Community Services

More emphasis should be placed on community care options, services that provide both sustenance and growth. Examples of supportive services that foster independent community living include information and referral services; transportation and nutrition services; legal and protective services; comprehensive senior centres; homemaker and handyman services; matching of older with younger individuals to share housing; and use of the supports available through churches, community groups, or mental health and other community agencies (e.g., area agencies on aging) to maintain elderly individuals in the community for as long as possible. The availability and accessibility of these services vary greatly, and eligibility requirements may exist. A Canadian Mental Health Association project, funded by Population Health in Canada, examined seniors' mental health and home care using mental health promotion principles. A variety of methods grounded in the principle of participation explored the perspectives of seniors, family caregivers, and home care providers. A policy guide was developed (in 2004 and updated in 2008 and still in use today in 2017 across Canada) as an outcome of the project to provide direction for a holistic model of care, incorporating both medical and psychosocial supports to meet the needs of seniors (MacCourt, 2008).

Spiritual Domain

Spiritual needs are basic for all age groups and are requirements for establishing meaning and purpose, love and relatedness, and forgiveness. There is growing evidence of the significance that spirituality plays in successful aging (Harrington, 2016; Haugan, 2013; Lavretsky, 2010). Spirituality is sometimes expressed through commitment to organized religion, while other times, it is expressed differently. Aging is a process that can bring individuals closer to understanding the finite nature of existence and evokes an awareness of their spiritual needs. With advanced age, many people begin to reflect on their successes and failures. During such reflection, many seek out God or a higher being to make sense of the past and establish hope for the future.

The process of spiritual assessment involves active listening, thoughtful observing, and sensitive questioning. The nurse may simply ask if the older adult would find comfort from a visit from a minister or a spiritual leader. Many forms of religion use various rituals that are important to the older individual's daily routine. The nurse should explore and honour these aspects to the extent possible.

A sense of quality of life is closely tied to values and beliefs about life's meaning. For many older individuals, quality of life is not reflected in material possessions or physical health but more by contentment over how the person has lived life and the extent to which his or her life has had meaning and purpose. Keeping close personal contacts with friends and family and having the opportunity to share stories of lifetime experiences are important to mental health and spiritual well-being. For older individuals, physical illnesses may affect the quality of life more than psychiatric disorders. The assessment of quality of life becomes especially important when assessing a client living in a continuing care facility or isolated in his or her own home.

The nurse can support a client's spiritual growth by exploring the meanings that a particular life change has for the elder. In later life, existential issues, such as experiencing losses, redefining meanings in existence, and finding and nurturing hope, replace, on the whole, the performance and future orientation that characterize earlier adulthood.

SUMMARY OF KEY POINTS

- The aging of the Canadian population is a significant force shaping our society.
- Late adulthood is conceived as having three chronologic groups: young-old (65 to 74 years), middle-old (75 to 84 years), and old-old (85 years and older).
- Normal aging is associated with some physical decline, but most functions do not change. Intellectual functioning, capacity for change, and productive engagement with life remain.
- Cognitive changes with aging are, for the most part, accounted for by structural and functional changes in the brain, with external factors (e.g., activity levels, socioeconomic status) also having an effect.
- Threats to memory in older persons include medications, depression, poor nutrition, infection,

heart and lung disease, thyroid problems, alcohol use, and sensory loss.

- Nurses need to recognize that older persons may need more time to process information and that they tend to focus on accuracy in their answers rather than on giving a prompt reply.
- Aging affects pharmacokinetics, including drug absorption, distribution, metabolism, and excretion, and nurses need to know the drug therapy implications of such changes.
- Gerotranscendence is a concept related to aging in which spiritual growth and the development of inner strength is emphasized over decrements in functioning.
- The majority of Canadian seniors wish to "age in place" and need adequate support to do so.
- Risks to health during this phase of the life span include chronic illness, polypharmacy, loss and bereavement, poverty, and social isolation. The latter has been associated with suicide.
- Older persons experience many physical changes, but they can remain sexually active.
- Mental health assessments are necessary when older clients face psychiatric or mental health issues. The bio/psycho/social/spiritual geriatric mental health nursing assessment examines many sources of data, including self-reports, laboratory test results, and reports from family members.
- Mental health assessments are necessary when older clients face psychiatric or mental health issues. The bio/psycho/social/spiritual geriatric mental health nursing assessment examines many sources of data, including self-reports, laboratory test results, and reports from family members.
- The bio/psycho/social/spiritual geriatric mental health nursing assessment is based on the special needs and problems of older individuals. This assessment examines current and past health, functional status, and human responses to mental health problems taking into account social support, spiritual needs, legal issues, and quality of life.
- The assessment of the biologic domain involves collecting data about the past and present health status, physical examination findings, physical functions (i.e., nutrition and eating, elimination patterns, sleep), pain, exercise, and pharmacologic information.
- The assessment of the psychological domain includes the client's responses to mental health problems, mental status examination, behavioural changes, stress and coping patterns, and risk assessment.
- There are a number of screening tools that nurses can use to complement a comprehensive assessment (for activities of daily living and cognitive and mental health issues).

- Coping with stresses and transitions vary among older adults. Determining stresses and coping skills along with the meaning of these stresses is important.
- Assessing and intervening with older adults should always occur within a climate of respect and recognition for his/her life history and experience and ability to be part of the process.
- Nurses can play a significant role in the mental health promotion of older persons and in supporting them and their families in living meaningful, hopeful lives.

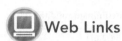 Web Links

Alzheimer Society of Canada website includes information about the society, Alzheimer's disease (AD), how to care for someone with AD, and research updates.

AgeIsMore.com: The Revera reports on agism and other resources are found at this site.

Canadian Coalition for Seniors' Mental Health, established in 2002, has as its goal supporting collaborative initiatives that will facilitate positive mental health for seniors through innovation and dissemination of best practices. National evidence-informed guidelines can be downloaded (Depression, Suicide, Delirium, and Mental Health Issues in Long-term Care).

Canadian Gerontological Nursing Association represents nurses who work with and for older adults in a wide variety of settings. Its interests include education, research, and clinical practice. It encourages and supports members through research grants, scholarships, conference funding, and certification study sessions.

Government of Canada website provides information on government financial plans for older adults (e.g., CPP).

Mental Health Commission of Canada's excellent website contains a multitude of current information, publications, and what's new in Canada. The Mental Health Strategy for Canada and the Guidelines for Seniors Mental Health can be downloaded.

National Seniors Council: This is the website of the National Seniors Council in Canada (formerly the National Advisory Council on Aging). It advises the Canadian Government on all matters related to well-being and quality of life for seniors.

Canadian Academy of Geriatric Society: Dedicated to promoting mental health in the Canadian elderly population through the clinical, educational, and research activities of its members.

Canada Mortgage and Housing Corporation (CMHC) website provides information about how older adults can adapt their homes for increasing disabilities and financial assistance programs for housing for older adults.

National Institute on Aging has a website dedicated to the scientific effort to understand the nature of aging and to extend healthy, active years of life.

National Initiative for the Care of the Elderly (NICE), an international network of researchers, practitioners, and students dedicated to improving the care of older adults in Canada and abroad.

Public Health Agency of Canada: Mental health promotion website for the Public Health Agency of Canada.

Seniors Mental Health Policy Lens (SMHPL) was developed as part of a national project, "Psychosocial Approaches to the Mental Health Challenges of Late Life," awarded to the BC Psychogeriatric Association by Health Canada, Population Health Fund. This site contains the SMHPL toolkit.

Wongbakerfaces.org: Information regarding the Wong-Baker FACES Pain Rating Scale and its use can be found at this site.

References

Alberta Health Services. (2014). *Alcohol and health: Alcohol and seniors*. Edmonton, AB: Author. Retrieved from http://www.albertahealthservices.ca/assets/info/hp/edu/if-hp-edu-amh-alcohol-and-seniors.pdf

Alexopoulos, G. S., Abrams, R. C., Young, R. C., & Shamoian, C. (1988). Cornell scale for depression in dementia. *Biological Psychiatry, 23*, 271–284.

American Geriatrics Society. (2015). Updated Beers Criteria for potentially inappropriate medication use in older adults. *Journal of the American Geriatrics Society, 63*(11), 2227–2246. doi:10.1111/jgs.13702

American Psychiatric Association. (2013). *Diagnostic and statistical manual of mental disorders* (5th ed.). Washington, DC: Author.

Berger, S. (2013). Balancing act: Cell senescence, aging related to epigenetic changes: Penn study links epigenetics, aging, mutations in nuclear proteins to better understand cancer, rare disorders. *Penn Medicine News Release*. Retrieved from http://www.uphs.upenn.edu/news/News_Releases/2013/08/berger/

Beyer, A. K., Wolff, J. K., Warner, L. M., Schuz, B., & Wurm, S. (2015). The role of physical activity in the relationship between self perceptions of ageing and self-related health in older adults. *Psychology and Health, 30*(6), 671–685. doi.org/10.1080/08870446.2015.1014370

Boggatz, T., & Meinhart, C. M. (2017). Health promotion among older adults in Austria: A qualitative study. *Journal of Clinical Nursing, 23*, 1106–1118. doi:10.1111/jocn.13603

Bourque, P., Pushkar, D., Bonneville, L., & Beland, F. (2005). Contextual effects on life satisfaction of older men and women. *Canadian Journal on Aging, 24*(1), 31–44.

Brandon, M. (2016). Psychosocial aspects of sexuality with aging. *Geriatric Rehabilitation, 32*(3), 151–155. doi:10.1097/TGR.0000000000000116

Brandt, N. J., & Piechocki, J. M. (2013). Treatment of insomnia in older adults. Re-evaluating the benefits and risks of sedative hypnotics. *Journal of Gerontological Nursing, 39*(4), 48–54.

Brennan, P. L., & Soohoo, S. (2013). Pain and use of alcohol in later life: Prospective evidence from the health and retirement study. *Journal of Aging and Health, 25*(4), 656–677.

Brown, J. W., Mefford, L., Chen, S., & Brown, A. (2009). Health and function of older persons volunteering for Habitat for Humanity. *Southern Online Journal of Nursing Research, 9*(3). Retrieved from https://www.snrs.org/sites/default/files/SOJNR/2009/Vol09Num03Art02.pdf

Bryant, C., Bei, B., Gilson, K., Komiti, A., Jackson, H., & Judd, F. (2012). The relationship between attitudes to aging and physical and mental health in older adults. *International Psychogeriatrics, 24*(10), 1674–1683. doi:10.1017/S1041610212000774

Canada Mortgage and Housing Corporation. (2008). *Impacts of the aging of the Canadian population on housing and communities: Research highlights*. Retrieved from http://www.cmhc-schl.gc.ca/odpub/pdf/65913.pdf

Canada Mortgage and Housing Corporation. (2013, October). Environment scan on Canadian Seniors' transitions to special care facilities (socioeconomic series). *Research Highlight*. Retrieved from https://www.cmhc-schl.gc.ca/odpub/pdf/67899.pdf

Canada Mortgage and Housing Corporation. (2016, May). Analysis of housing choices and changing housing needs of seniors and pre-seniors by age group (socio-economic series). *Research Highlight*. Retrieved from https://www.cmhc-schl.gc.ca/odpub/pdf/68656.pdf

Canadian Association for Suicide Prevention (CASP). (n.d.). *Suicide risk in the aging population*. Retrieved from http://suicideprevention.ca/suicide-risk-in-the-aging-population/

Canadian Broadcasting Corporation. (2015). More Canadians are 65 and over than under age 15, StatsCan says. *CBC Newscast*. Retrieved from http://www.cbc.ca/news/business/statistics-canada-seniors-1.3248295

Canadian Coalition for Seniors' Mental Health. (2006). *National guidelines for seniors' mental health: The assessment and treatment of depression*. Retrieved from www.ccsmh.ca

Canadian Coalition for Seniors' Mental Health. (2009). *Suicide prevention among older adults: A guide for family members*. Toronto, ON: Author. Retrieved from https://suicideprevention.ca/wp-content/uploads/2014/06/ccsmh_suicideBooklet.pdf

Canadian Institutes of Health Research (CIHR). (2013). *Living longer, living better: Canadian Institutes of Health Research Institute of Aging 2013–18 strategic plan.* Ottawa, ON: Author. Retrieved from http://www.cihr-irsc. gc.ca/e/47179.html

Centers for Disease Control and Prevention. (2017). *Depression is not part of growing older.* Retrieved from https://www.cdc.gov/aging/mentalhealth/ depression.htm

Chu, R. (2017). Preventing in-patient falls: The nurse's pivotal role. *Nursing, 47*(3), 24–30. doi:10.1097/01.NURSE.0000512872.83762.69

Conference Board of Canada. (2013). *Elderly poverty.* Retrieved from http:// www.conferenceboard.ca/hcp/details/society/elderly-poverty.aspx

Conn, D. K. (2003). Oral presentation to the Standing Senate Committee on Social Affairs, Science and Technology. *Bulletin of the Canadian Academy of Geriatric Psychiatry, 10*(3), 5–8.

Critchlow, M. (2014). *Canadian senior cohousing: Housing alternatives for an aging population.* Vancouver, BC: Presentation to the Canadian Senior Cohousing panel at SFU Friesen Conference. Retrieved from http:// canadianseniorcohousing.com/?page_id=1363

Cummings, J. L. (1997). The neuropsychiatric inventory: Assessing psycho-pathology in dementia patients. *Neurology, 48*(5 Suppl 6), S10–S16.

Cummings, J. L., Mega, M., Gray, K., Rosenberg-Thompson, S., Carusi, D. A., & Gornbein, J. (1994). The Neuropsychiatric inventory: Comprehensive assessment of psychopathology in dementia. *Neurology, 44*(12), 2308–2314.

Deverau Melillo, K. (2017). Geropsychiatric nursing: What's in your toolkit? *Journal of Gerontological Nursing, 43*(1), 3–6. doi:10.3928/00989134-20161215-01

Duggleby, W., Hicks, D., Nekolaichuk, C., Holtslander, L., Williams, A., Chambers, T., & Eby, J. (2012). Hope, older adults, and chronic illness: A metasynthesis of qualitative research. *Journal of Advanced Nursing, 68*(6), 1211–1223. doi:10.1111/j.1365-2648.2011.05919.x

Ebersole, P., Touhy, T. A., Hess, P., & Jett, K. (2007). *Toward healthy aging: Human needs and nursing response.* Philadelphia, PA: Mosby.

Erikson, E. H., & Erikson, J. M. (1997). *The lifecycle completed, extended version.* New York, NY: WW Norton.

Evers, A., Klusmann, V., Schwarzer, R., & Heuser, I. (2011). Improving cognition by adherence to physical or mental exercise: A moderated mediation analysis. *Aging and Mental Health, 15*(4), 446–455. doi:10.1080/13607863.2010.543657

Fleming, K. C., Evans, J. M., & Chutka, D. S. (2003). A cultural and economic history of old age in America. *Mayo Clinic Proceedings, 78*(7), 914–921. Retrieved from http://0-search.proquest.com.aupac.lib.atha-bascau.ca/docview/216864158?accountid=8408

Frankl, V. (1963). *Man's search for meaning: An introduction to logotherapy.* New York, NY: Pocket Books.

Gallo, J. (2017). Multimorbidity and mental health. *American Journal of Geriatric Psychiatry, 25*(5), 520. doi.org/10.1016/j.jagp2017.02.007

Gauthier, S., Patterson, C., Chertkow, H., Gordon, M., Herrmann, N., Rockwood, K., … Soucy, J. P. (2012). Recommendations of the 4th Canadian consensus conference on the diagnosis and treatment of dementia (CCCDTD4). *Canadian Geriatrics Journal, 15*(4), 120–126.

Gregg, J. J., Fiske, A., & Gatz, M. (2013). Physician's detection of late-life depression: The roles of dysphoria and cognitive impairment. *Aging and Mental Health, 13*(45), 1–11.

Government of Canada. (2006). *The human face of mental health and mental illness in Canada-2006 (Cat. No. HP5-19/2006E).* Ottawa, ON: Minister of Public Works and Government Services Canada.

Government of Canada. (2017). *Social isolation of seniors—Volume 1: Understanding the issue and finding solutions.* Ottawa, ON: Author. Retrieved from https://www.canada.ca/en/employment-social-development/ corporate/partners/seniors-forum/social-isolation-toolkit-vol2.html

Hammer, K., Mogensen, O., & Hall, E. O. C. (2009). The meaning of hope in nursing research: A metasynthesis. *Scandinavian Journal of Caring Sciences, 23*, 549–557. doi:10.1111/j.1471-6712.2008.00635.x

Harrington, A. (2016). The importance of spiritual assessment when caring for older adults. *Ageing and Society, 36*(1), 1–16. doi:10.1017/ S0144686X14001007

Haugan, G. (2013). Nurse–patient interaction is a resource for hope, meaning in life and self-transcendence in nursing home patients. *Scandinavian Journal of Caring Sciences,* 1–15. doi:10.1111/scs.12028

Health Canada and Assembly of First Nations. (2015). *First Nations mental wellness continuum framework.* Ottawa, ON: Author. Retrieved from http://publications.gc.ca/collections/collection_2015/sc-hc/H34-278-1-2014-eng.pdf

Hebert, R., Guilbeault, J., & Pinsonnault, E. (2002). *Functional autonomy measuring system user guide.* Sherbrooke, QC: Centre d'expertise de l'Institut universitaire de geriatrie de Sherbrooke.

Heisel, M. J., & The MCMG. (2016). Enhancing psychological resiliency in older men facing retirement with meaning-centered men's groups.

In A. Batthyany (Ed.), *Logotherapy and existential analysis. Logotherapy and Existential Analysis: Proceedings of the Viktor Frankl Institute Vienna 1.* Switzerland: Springer Publishing. doi:10.1007/978-3-319-29424-715

Heisel, M. J., Neufeld, E., & Flett, G. L. (2016). Reasons for living, meaning in life, and suicide ideation: Investigating the roles of key positive psychological factors in reducing suicide risk in community-residing older adults. *Aging and Mental Health, 20*(2), 195–207. doi:10.1080/13607863.2015.1078279

Hirst, S., Lane, A., & Stares, R. (2015). Health promotion with older adults experiencing mental health challenges: A literature review of strength-based approaches. *Clinical Gerontologist, 36*, 329–355. doi:10.1080/07317115.2013.788118

Hoy-Ellis, C. P., Ator, M., Kerr, C., & Milford, J. (2016). Innovative approaches address aging and mental health needs in LGBTQ communities. *Generations: Journal of the American Geriatric Society on Aging, 40*(2), 56–62.

Hubbard, R. E., Peel, N. M., Scott, I. A., Martin, J. H., Smith, A., Pillans, P. I., Poudel, A., & Gray, L. C. (2015). Polypharmacy among inpatients aged 70 years or older in Australia. *Medical Journal of Australia, 202*(7), 373–377. doi:10.5694/mja13.00172

Hyer, L., & Blount, J. (1984). Concurrent and discriminant validities of the geriatric depression scale with older psychiatric inpatients. *Psychological Reports, 54*, 611–616. doi:10.2466/pr0.1984.54.2.611

Itzhar-Nabarro, Z., & Smoski, M. J. (2012). A review of theoretical and empirical perspectives on marital satisfaction and bereavement outcomes: Implications for working with older adults. *Clinical Gerontologist, 35*, 257–269. doi:10.1080/07317115.2012.657604

Jastrzab, G., Kerr, S., & Fairbrother, G. (2009). Misinterpretation of the Faces Pain Scale-Revised in adult clinical practice. *Acute Pain, 11*, 51–55.

Kaasalainen, S., Agarwal, G., Dolovich, L., Brazil, K., & Papaioannou, A. (2015). Managing pain medications in long-term care: Nurses' views. *British Journal of Nursing, 24*(9), 484–489.

Katz, S. & Akpom, C. A. (1976). A measure of primary sociobiological functions. *International Journal of Health Service, 6*(3), 493–508.

Kaufman, G. (2015). Multiple medicines: The issues surrounding polypharmacy. *Nursing and Residential Care, 17*(4), 198–203.

Kennedy, B. (2016). Advances in biological theories of aging. In V. L. Bergtson & B. K. Kennedy. *Handbook of theories of aging* (3rd ed., pp. 107–111). New York, NY: Springer Publishing Company.

Khazaee-Pooli, M., Sadeghi, R., & Majlessi, F. (2015). Effects of physical exercise programme on happiness among older people. *Journal of Psychiatric and Mental Health Nursing, 22*, 47–57. doi:10.1111/jpm.12168

Lam, L. C., & Cheng, S. T. (2012). Maintaining long-term adherence to lifestyle interventions for cognitive health in late life. *International Psychogeriatrics, 25*(2), 171–73. doi:10.1017/S1041610212001603

Larson, E. B., Wang, L., Bowen, J. D., McCormick, W. C., Teri, L., Crane, P., & Kukull, W. (2006). Exercise is associated with reduced risk for incident dementia among persons 65 years of age and older. *Annals of Internal Medicine, 144*(2), 73–81.

Lavretsky, H. (2010). Spirituality and aging. *Aging Health, 6*(6), 749–769.

Lee, Y. J., & Hung, W. L. (2011). The relationship between exercise participation and well-being of the retired elderly. *Aging and Mental Health, 15*(7), 873–881. http://0-dx.doi.org.aupac.lib.athabascau. ca/10.1080/13607863.2011.569486

Leifer, B. (2009). Alzheimer's disease: Seeing the signs early. *Journal of the Academy of Nurse Practitioners, 21*(11), 588–595. doi:10.1111/j.1745-7599.2009.00436.x

Lezwijn, J., Vaandrager, L., Naaldenberg, J., Wagemakers, A., & van Woerkum, C. (2011). Healthy ageing in a salutogenic way: Building the HP 2.0 framework. *Health and Social Care in the Community, 19*(1), 43–51. doi:10.1111/j.1365-2524.2010.00947.x

MacCourt, P. (2008). *Promoting seniors' well-being: A seniors' mental health policy lens toolkit.* Victoria, BC: British Columbia Psychogeriatric Association. Retrieved from http://seniorspolicylens.ca/

MacCourt, P. (2017). *Social isolation of seniors; Volume 1: Understanding the issue and finding solutions. Federal, Provincial, and Territorial (F/P/T) Forum of Ministers Responsible for Seniors.* Retrieved from https://www. canada.ca/en/employment-social-development/corporate/partners/ seniors-forum/social-isolation-toolkit-vol1.html

Madden, T. (2016). *Seniors poverty rates on the rise in Canada.* London, UK: London Poverty Research Centre at Kings. Retrieved from http://pover-tyresearch.ca/blog/seniors-poverty-rates-on-the-rise-in-canada/

Margolis, R., & Iciaszczyk, N. (2015). The changing health of Canadian grandparents. *Canadian Studies in Population, 42*(3–4), 63–76.

Mayo Clinic. (2011). *Sexual health and aging: Keep the passion alive.* Rochester, NY: Author. Retrieved from http://www.mayoclinic.com/ health/sexual-health/HA00035

McKye, K. A., Naglie, G., Tierney, M., & Jaglal, S. (2009). Comparison of older adults' and occupational therapists' awareness of functional abilities at discharge from rehabilitation with actual performance in the home. *Physical and Occupational Therapy in Geriatrics, 27*(3), 229–244.

McParland, J., & Camic, P. M. (2016). Psychosocial factors and ageing in older lesbian, gay, and bisexual people: A systematic review of the literature. *Journal of Clinical Nursing, 25,* 3425–3437. doi:10.1111/jocn.13251

Mental Health Commission of Canada. (2009). *Toward recovery and well-being. A framework for a mental health strategy for Canada.* Ottawa, ON: Author. Retrieved from https://www.mentalhealthcommission.ca/sites/default/files/FNIM_Toward_Recovery_and_Well_Being_ENG_0_1.pdf

Mental Health Commission of Canada. (2011). *Guidelines for comprehensive mental health services for older adults in Canada.* Ottawa, ON: Author. Retrieved from https://www.mentalhealthcommission.ca/sites/default/files/mhcc_seniors_guidelines_1.pdf

Mental Health Commission of Canada. (2012). *Changing directions: Changing lives: The mental health strategy for Canada.* Ottawa, ON: Author. Retrieved from http://www.mentalhealthcommission.ca/English/node/721

Mental Health Commission of Canada (MHCC). (2016). *Advancing the mental health strategy for Canada: A framework for action.* Ottawa, ON: Author. Retrieved from https://www.mentalhealthcommission.ca/English/media/3746

Merz, E. M., & Huxhold, O. (2010). Wellbeing depends on social relationship characteristics: Comparing different types and providers of support to older adults. *Aging and Society, 30*(5), 843–857.

Ministry of Healthy Living and Support. (2008). *Seniors in British Columbia: A healthy living framework.* Retrieved from http://www.hls.gov.bc.ca/seniors/PDFs/seniors_framework_web.pdf

Moe, A., Hellzen, O., Ekker, K., & Enmarker, I. (2013). Inner strength in relation to perceived physical and mental health among the oldest old people with chronic illness. *Aging and Mental Health, 17*(2), 189–196. doi:10.1080/13607863.2012.717257

Montgomery, P., & Shepard, L. D. (2010). Insomnia in older people. *Reviews in Clinical Gerontology, 20*(3), 205–218. doi:https://doi.org/10.1017/S095925981000016X

Moore, S. L. (2005). Hope makes a difference. *Journal of Psychiatric and Mental Health Nursing, 12*(1), 100–105. doi:10.1111/j.1365-2850.2004.00802.x

Moore, S. L. (2012). The experience of hope and aging: A hermeneutic photography study. *Journal of Gerontological Nursing, 38*(10), 28–36. doi:http://0-dx.doi.org.aupac.lib.athabascau.ca/10.3928/00989134-20120906-93

Moore, S. L., Hall, S. E., & Jackson, J. (2014). Exploring the experience of nursing home residents' participation in a hope-focused group. *Nursing Research and Practice, Article ID 623082,* 1–9.

Moore, S. L., Metcalf, B., & Schow, E. (2000). Meaning in life: Examining the concept. *Geriatric Nursing, 21*(1), 27–29. doi:10.1067/mgn.2000.105790

Moya, H., & Arnold, P. (2012). A life story toolkit to support recovery from mental distress. *Mental Health Practice, 16*(1), 14–18.

National Institute on Aging. (2009). *Sexuality in later life.* UAS: U.S. Department of Health and Human Services. Retrieved from http://www.nia.nih.gov/health/publicaiton/sexuality-later-life

National Institute on Aging. (2011/2013). *Biology of aging: Research today for a better tomorrow.* US Department of Health and Human Services. Retrieved from http://www.nia.nih.gov/health/publication/biology-aging

Newberg, A. B. (2011). Spirituality and the aging brain. *Generations: Journal of the American Society on Aging, 35*(2), 83–91.

Ontario Home Care Association. (2010). *Home care in 2010—Essential for an aging population.* Retrieved from http://www.homecareontario.ca/public/docs/publications/position%20papers/2010/home-care-essential-for-an-aging-population.pdf

O'Rourke, N., Cappeliez, P., & Claxton, A. (2011). Functions of reminiscence and the psychological well-being of young-old and older adults over time. *Aging and Mental Health, 15*(2), 272–281.

O'Rourke, H., & Sidani, S. (2017). Definition, determinants, and outcomes of social connectedness for older adults: A scoping review. *Journal of Gerontological Nursing, 43*(7), 43–52. doi:10.3928/00989134-20170223-03

Panno, J. (2010). *Aging: Modern theories and therapies* (2nd ed.). New York, NY: Facts on File.

Paterson, D. H., & Warburton, E. R. (2010). Physical activity and functional limitations in older adults: A systematic review related to Canada's physical activity guidelines. *International Journal of Behavioral and Nutrition and Physical Activity, 7*(38). doi:10.1186/1479-5868-7-38

Pfeffer, R., Kurosaki, T., Harrah, C., Chance, J., & Filos, S. (1982). Measurement of functional activities in older adults in the community. *Journal of Gerontology, 37*(3), 323–329.

Preuß, D., & Legal, F. (2017). Living with the animals: Animal or robotic companions for the elderly in smart homes. *Medical Ethics, 43,* 407–410. doi:10.1136/medethics-2016-103603.

Public Health Agency of Canada. (2016). *Age-friendly communities in Canada: Community implementation guide.* Ottawa, ON: Author. Retrieved from https://www.canada.ca/en/public-health/services/publications/healthy-living/age-friendly-communities-canada-community-implementation-guide.html

Public Health Agency of Canada (PHAC). (2010). *The Chief Public Health Officer's report on the state of public health in Canada 2010.* Ottawa, ON: Author.

Reisberg, B., Auer, S., & Monteiro, I. (1997). Behavioural pathology in Alzheimer's disease (BEHAVE-AD) rating scale. *International Psychogeriatrics, 8*(3), 301–308. doi:https://doi.org/10.1017/S1041610297003967

Reisberg, B., & Ferris, S. (1985). A clinical rating scale for symptoms of psychosis in Alzheimer's disease. *Psychopharmacology Bulletin, 21,* 101–104.

Rosenzweig, E. S., & Barnes, C. A. (2003). Impact of aging on hippocampal function: Plasticity, network dynamics and cognition. *Progress in Neurobiology, 69*(3), 143–179. doi:10.1016/S0301-0082(02)00126-0

Sadock, B. J., Sadock, V. A., & Ruiz, P. (2015). *Kaplan & Sadock's synopsis of psychiatry: Behavioral sciences/clinical psychiatry* (11th ed.). Philadelphia, PA: Wolters Kluwer.

Scharlach, A. E., & Hoshino, K. (2013). Conclusion. In Scharlach, A. E. & Hoshino, K. (Eds.), *Healthy aging in sociocultural context* (pp. 97–105). New York, NY: Routledge.

Sebastiani, P., Solovieff, N., De Wan, A., Walsh, K. M., Puce, A., Hartley, S. W., & Perls, T. T. (2012). Genetic signatures of exceptional longevity in humans. *PLoS One, 7*(1), e29848. doi:10.1371/journalpone.00229848

Shankar, K. K., Walker, M., Frost, D., & Orrell, M. W. (1999). The development of a valid and reliable scale for rating anxiety in dementia (RAID). *Aging and Mental Health, 3*(1), 39–49. doi:10.1080/13607869956424

Sheets, D. J., & Gallagher, E. M. (2013). Aging in Canada: State of the art and science. *Gerontologist, 53*(1), 1–8. doi:10.1093/geront/gns150

Sheikh, J. I., & Yesavage, J. A. (1986). Geriatric Depression Scale (GDS): Recent evidence and development of a shorter version. In T. L. Brink (Ed.), *Clinical gerontology: A guide to assessment and intervention* (pp. 165–173). Binghamton, NY: Haworth Press. © By the Haworth Press, Inc.

Sherrell, K., Buckwalter, K., Bode, R., & Strozdas, L. (1999). Use of the cognitive abilities screen instrument to assess elderly persons with schizophrenia in long-term care settings. *Issues in Mental Health Nursing, 20,* 541–558.

Sheridan Centre for Elder Research. (2016). *Revera report on ageism: Independence and choice as we age.* Mississauga, ON: Revera. Retrieved from www.ageismore.com

Shillington, R. (2016). *An analysis of the economic circumstances of Canadian seniors.* Ottawa, ON: Broadbent Institute. Retrieved from https://d3n8a8pro7vhmx.cloudfront.net/broadbent/pages/4904/attachments/original/1455216659/An_Analysis_of_the_Economic_Circumstances_of_Canadian_Seniors.pdf?1455216659

Skoog, I. (2011). Psychiatric disorders in the elderly. *Canadian Journal of Psychiatry, 56*(7), 387–397.

Smith, J. M. (2012). Loneliness in older adults: An embodied experience. *Journal of Gerontological Nursing, 38*(8), 45–53.

Stahl, S. T., & Schulz, R. (2013). Changes in routine health behaviors following late-life bereavement: A systematic review. *Journal of Behavioral Medicine, 37*(4), 736–755. doi:10.1007/s10865-013-9524-7

Stanley, I. H., Hom, M. A., Rogers, M. L., Hagan, C. R., & Joiner, T. E. (2016). Understanding suicide among older adults: A review of psychological and sociological theories. *Aging and Mental Health, 20*(2), 113–122. http://dx.doi.org/10.1080/13607863.2015.1012045

Statistics Canada. (2005). *Life expectancy at birth, by sex, by provinces.* Ottawa, ON: Author. Retrieved from http://www.40.statscan.ca/101/cst01/health26.htm

Statistics Canada. (2010). *Statistics Canada population estimates 1971–2010.* Ottawa, ON: Author. Retrieved from http://www.statcan.gc.ca/daily-quotidien/100628/dq100628a-eng.htm

Statistics Canada. (2012a). *Summary tables: Life expectancy at birth, by sex, by provinces.* Ottawa, ON: Author. Retrieved from http://www.statcan.gc.ca/tables-tableaux/sum-som/101/cst01/healh26-eng.htm

Statistics Canada. (2012b). *Years to retirement, 1998 to 2009. Insights on Canadian Society (75-006-X).* Ottawa, ON: Author. Retrieved from http://www.statcan.gc.ca/daily-quotidien/121204/dq121204b-eng.pdf

Statistics Canada. (2015). *Living arrangements of seniors.* Ottawa, ON: Author. Retrieved from http://www12.statcan.gc.ca/census-recensement/2011/as-sa/98-312-x/98-312-x2011003_4-eng.cfm

Statistics Canada. (2016). *Annual demographic estimates: Canada, provinces & territories.* Ottawa, ON: Author. Retrieved from http://www.statcan.gc.ca/pub/91-215-x/91-215-x2016000-eng.pdf

Statistics Canada. (2017a). *Suicides and suicide rate, by sex and by age group (both sexes, males, females, rates).* Retrieved from http://www.statcan.gc.ca/tables-tableaux/sum-som/l01/cst01/hlth66d-eng.htm

Statistics Canada. (2017b). *Heavy drinking 2015.* Ottawa, ON: Author. Retrieved from http://www.statcan.gc.ca/pub/82-625-x/2017001/article/14765-eng.htm

Steinman, M. A., Beizer, J. L., DuBeau, C. E., Laird, R. D., Lundebjerg, M. E., & Mulhausen, P. (2015). Geriatrics Society 2015 Beers Criteria—A guide for patients, clinicians, health systems, and payors. *Journal of the American Geriatrics Society, 65*(11), e1–e7. doi:10.1111/jgs.13701

Stephens, C., Breheny, M., & Mansvelt, J. (2015). Healthy ageing from the perspective of older people: A capability approach to resilience. *Psychology and Health, 30*(6), 715–731. doi:org/10.1080/08870446.2014.904862

Strong, J., Varady, C., Chahda, N., Doocy, S., & Burnham, G. (2015). Health status and health needs of older refugees from Syria in Lebanon. *Conflict and Health, 1*, 1–10. doi:10.1186/s/3031-014-0029-y

Tam, E. Y., Fletcher, P. C., & Chi, I. (2004). Cultural and gender diversity in health. *STRIDE, 1*. Retrieved from http://www.stridemagazine.com

Teng, E., Kazuo Hasegawa, K., Homma, A., Imai, Y., Larson, E., Graves, A., ... White, L. R. (1994). The cognitive abilities screen instrument (CASI): A practical test for cross-cultural epidemiological studies of dementia. *International Psychogeriatrics, 6*(1), 45–58.

Tomás, J. M., Sancho, P., Galiana, L., & Oliver, A. (2016). A double test on the importance of spirituality, the "forgotten factor", in successful aging. *Social Indicators Research, 127*, 1377–1389. doi:10.1007/s11205-015-1014-6

Tornstam, L. (1989). Gero-transcendence: A theoretical and empirical reformulation of the disengagement theory. *Aging Clinical and Experimental Research, 1*, 55–63. doi:10.1007/BF03323876

Tornstam, L. (2005). *Gerotranscendence: A developmental theory of positive aging.* New York, NY: Springer.

University of Michigan Alcohol Research Centre. (1991). *Short Michigan Alcoholism Screening Test—Geriatric Version (SMAST-G).* Retrieved from http://www.hartfordign.org/publications/trythis/issue17.pdf

von Strauss, E., Aguero-Torres, H., Kareholt, I., Winblad, B., & Fratiglioni, L. (2003). Women are more disabled in basic activities of daily living than men only in very advanced ages: A study on disability, morbidity, and mortality from the Kungsholmen Project. *Journal of Clinical Epidemiology, 56*(7), 669–677. http://doi.org/10.1016/S0895-4356(03)00089-1

Wadensten, B., & Carlsson, M. (2007a). Adoption of an innovation based on the theory of gerotranscendence by staff in a nursing home—Part III. *International Journal of Older People Nursing, 2*, 302–314. doi:10.1111/j.1748-3743.2007a.00087.x

Wadensten, B., & Carlsson, M. (2007b). The theory of gerotranscendence in practice: Guidelines for nursing—Part II. *International Journal of Older People Nursing, 2*, 295–301. doi:10.1111/j.1748-3743.2007b.00085.x

Walsh, F. (2012). Successful aging and family resilience. *Annual Review of Gerontology and Geriatrics, 32*(1), 151–172. doi:10.1891/0198-8794.32.153

Wang, J. J., Lin, Y. H., & Hsieh, L. Y. (2011). Effects of gerotranscendence support group on gerotranscendence perspective, depression, and life satisfaction of institutionalized elders. *Aging and Mental Health, 15*(5), 580–586. doi:10.1080/13607863.2010.543663

Wang, L., Larson, E. B., Bowen, J. D., & van Belle, G. (2006). Performance-based physical function and future dementia in older people. *Archives of Internal Medicine, 166*, 1115–1120.

Welsh, D., Moore, S. L., & Getzlaf, B. A. (2012). Meaning in life: The perspectives of long-term care residents. *Research in Gerontological Nursing, 5*(3), 185–194. doi:10.3928/19404921-20120605-05

Wiechula, R., Conroy, T., Kitson, A., Marshall, R. J., Whitaker, N., & Rasmussen, P. (2016). Umbrella review of the evidence. What factors influence the caring relationship between a nurse and patient? *Journal of Advanced Nursing, 72*(4), 723–724. doi:10.1111/jan.12862

Wilcox, B. (2012). Successful aging: Is there hope? *Canadian Medical Association Journal, 184*(18), 1973–1974. doi:10.1177/070674371105600702

Wilson, D. M., Harris, A., Hollis, V., & Mohankumar, D. (2011). Upstream thinking and health promotion planning for older adults at risk of social isolation. *International Journal of Older People Nursing, 6*(4), 282–288. doi:10.1111/j.1748-3743.2010.00259.x

Wion, R. K., & Loeb, S. J. (2015). Older adults engaging in online dating: What gerontological nurses should know. *Journal of Gerontological Nursing, 41*(10), 25–25. doi:10.3928/00989134-20150826-67

Wong, D., & Baker, C. (1988). Pain in children: Comparison of assessment scales. *Pediatric Nursing, 14*(1), 9–17.

World Health Organization. (2012). *Good health adds years to life. Global brief for World Health Day 2012.* Geneva, Switzerland: Author. Retrieved from http://apps.who.int/iris/bitstream/10665/70853/1/WHO_DCO_WHD_2012.2_eng.pdf

World Health Organization. (2013). *Mental health action plan 2013–2020.* Geneva, Switzerland: Author. Retrieved from http://www.who.int/mental_health/action_plan_2013/en/

Wu, Z., Schimmele, C. M., & Chappell, N. L. (2012). Aging and late-life depression. *Journal of Aging and Health, 24*(1), 3–28.

Ye, B. S., Seo, S. W., Cho, H., Kim, S. Y., Lee, J. S., Kim, E. J., ... Na, D. L. (2013). Effects of education on the progression of early versus late-stage mild cognitive impairment. *International Psychogeriatrics, 25*(4), 597–606. doi:10.1017/S1041610212002001

Yevchak, A. M., Loeb, S. J., & Fick, D. M. (2008). Promoting cognitive health and vitality: A review of clinical implications. *Geriatric Nursing, 29*(5), 302–310. doi:10.1016/j.gerinurse.2007.10.017

Zimprich, D. (2002). Cross-sectionally and longitudinally balanced effects of processing speed on intellectual abilities. *Experimental Aging Research, 28*(3), 231–251. doi:10.1080/03610730290080290

Dorothy Forbes and
Wendy Austin

LEARNING OBJECTIVES

After studying this chapter, you will be able to:

- Distinguish the clinical characteristics, onset, and course of the neurocognitive disorders (NCDs), delirium, and dementia.
- Describe the biologic, psychological, social, and spiritual factors that relate to NCDs in older adults.
- Discuss the emotional impact of dementia for the patient, family, and caregiver.
- Formulate nursing diagnoses based on a bio/psycho/social/spiritual assessment of patients with impaired cognitive function.
- Identify the expected outcomes and nursing interventions and provide an evaluation for patients with impaired cognition.

KEY TERMS

- agnosia • aphasia • apraxia • beta-amyloid plaques • bradykinesia • catastrophic reactions • cortical dementias • delirium superimposed on dementia • disinhibition • hyperactive delirium • hypoactive delirium • illusions • mixed delirium • neurofibrillary tangles • oxidative stress • postoperative delirium • subcortical dementia

KEY CONCEPTS

- cognition • delirium • dementia • memory

Cognition and memory are important in many psychiatric disorders, but in this chapter on neurocognitive disorders (NCDs), they are the key concepts (American Psychiatric Association [APA], 2013). Cognition is the ability to think and know. The definition is further refined to be understood as a relatively high level of intellectual processing in which perceptions and information are acquired, used, or manipulated.

Specific functions include the acquisition and use of language, the ability to be oriented in time and space, judgment, reasoning, attention, comprehension, concept formation, planning, and the use of symbols, such as numbers and letters used in mathematics and writing. Cognition and behaviour are so closely linked that even mild cognitive impairment (MCI) can affect a person's daily functioning (Wadley, Okonkwo, Crowe, & Ross-Meadows, 2008). MCI is the name given to subjective cognitive decline paired with objective cognitive impairment, but without substantial functional impairment being present. It is viewed as a stage between normal aging and dementia, but further research is required for MCI to be predictive of dementia (Brodaty et al., 2017).

Memory, a facet of cognition, refers to the ability to recall or reproduce what has been learned or experienced. It is more than simple storage and retrieval; it is a complex cognitive mental function that includes most areas of the brain, especially the hippocampus, which

is believed to be essential to the transfer of some memories from short-term to long-term storage. Defects of memory are an essential feature of many cognitive disorders, particularly dementia. In relation to cognition, it is important to note that memory loss increases with age, and this reality poses challenges to the older adult.

The NCDs discussed in this chapter, delirium and dementia, are characterized by deficits in cognition or memory that represent a clear-cut deterioration from a previous level of functioning. Delirium is a disorder of acute cognitive impairment and can be caused by a medical condition (e.g., infection) or substance abuse, or it may have multiple aetiologies. Dementia is characterized by chronic cognitive impairments and is differentiated by the underlying cause, not by symptom patterns, which are often similar. Some dementias are irreversible and progressive. Some organic compounds and chemicals, such as lead, manganese, and toluene (one of the toxins in glue and paint), may produce the symptoms of dementia. Once a person with chemically induced symptoms is evaluated and treated, the symptoms of dementia may resolve.

Delirium's essential features are fluctuating alterations in attention or awareness along with a change in baseline cognition that cannot be explained by a preexisting or evolving NCD (APA, 2013, p. 599). Predisposing factors include advanced age, previous delirium, dementia, and sensory impairments; precipitating factors can be alcohol or drug withdrawal, surgery and anaesthesia, infection, intracranial insults or fluid–electrolyte imbalances (Canadian Coalition for Seniors' Mental Health, 2006; Luetz, Weiss, Boettcher, Burmeister, Wernecke, & Spies, 2016). (For delirium tremens, the delirium that occurs following untreated withdrawal from a substance such as alcohol, see Chapter 26.)

Cortical dementias such as Alzheimer's disease (AD) and prion disease result from a disease process that globally afflicts the cortex. **Subcortical dementia** is caused by dysfunction or deterioration of deep grey- or white-matter structures inside the brain and brain stem. Symptoms of subcortical dementia may be more localized and tend to disrupt arousal, attention, and motivation, but they can produce a variety of clinical behavioural manifestations. Examples of subcortical dementias include those due to Huntington's disease, Parkinson's disease, and HIV infection. In this chapter, AD is highlighted because it is the most prevalent form of dementia in Canada.

KEY CONCEPT

Cognition involves multiple brain processes that enable an individual to perceive, learn, and recall specific information for the purpose of reasoning or problem-solving. It is based on a system of complex interrelated abilities, such as perception, reasoning, judgment, intuition, and memory, which allow one to be aware of oneself and one's surroundings. Impairments in these abilities can result in a failure of the afflicted person to recognize that he or she is not well and is in need of treatment.

KEY CONCEPT

Memory is a facet of cognition concerned with retaining and recalling past experiences, whether they occurred in the physical environment or internally as cognitive events.

KEY CONCEPT

Delirium is a temporary disorder of physical origin with an abrupt onset characterized by fluctuating consciousness and attention.

KEY CONCEPT

Dementia is characterized by chronic, progressive neurocognitive impairment and is differentiated by affected areas in the brain, by underlying cause, and by symptom patterns.

■ DELIRIUM

Clinical Course of the Disorder

Delirium is an acute disorder of physical origin that develops over a short period of time, and it is characterized by fluctuating consciousness and attention. The individual with delirium has reduced ability to focus, sustain, or shift attention, which is marked by a decline in cognitive function (memory, orientation, speech, thinking), perceptual abnormalities, circadian disruption, and psychomotor disturbances. Delirium is usually reversible if treated promptly, but it is a serious disorder associated with high morbidity and mortality. Delirium occurs across all care settings, but the highest prevalence occurs with critically ill patients (Rivosecchi, Smithburger, Svec, Campbell, & Kane-Gill, 2015). Delirium is associated with longer duration of hospitalization and increased mortality (Pendlebury et al., 2015). The pathophysiologic mechanisms leading to delirium remain largely unknown in spite of its immense impact and life-threatening nature.

EMERGENCY

Delirium is a neuropsychiatric disorder that develops rapidly and has potentially severe consequences, including brain damage and death, if it goes unrecognized and without appropriate intervention.

Diagnostic Criteria

Impaired consciousness is the key diagnostic criterion of delirium (Sadock, Sadock, & Ruiz, 2015). Patients become less aware of their environment and lose the ability to focus, sustain, and shift attention. Associated cognitive changes typically include problems in memory, orientation, and language. Patients may not know where they are, may not recognize familiar objects, or may be unable to carry on a conversation. Hypoactive delirium in which the person's cognitive and motor responses are slowed and reduced is not uncommon but may be overlooked (RNAO, 2016). Delirium may be confused with dementia, which can also present with impaired memory and disorientation (Candy et al., 2012). It is possible to have a **delirium superimposed on a dementia (DSD)**.

An important diagnostic indicator is that delirium develops rapidly, usually over hours or days. There can be rapid improvement when its underlying cause is identified and removed (Sadock et al., 2015). Nurses are in a unique position to plan, implement, and evaluate care for these patients. Despite this key role, nurses too often do not recognize delirium in their patients. Factors that contribute to such underrecognition include the fluctuating nature of delirium, lack of knowledge regarding delirium, inadequate use of delirium assessment tools, and the challenge of distinguishing among delirium, dementia, and **delirium superimposed on dementia** (El Hussein,

Hirst, & Salyers, 2015). (For the American Psychological Association criteria for delirium, please see the DSM-5.)

Delirium in Special Populations

Children

Delirium can occur in infants, children, and adolescents and may be related to medications (anticholinergic agents) or fever. It is also associated with sepsis, endocrine–metabolic disturbances, and complex medical challenges with close monitoring necessary to ensure early detection (Grover et al., 2012; Porter, Holly, & Echevarria, 2016). Delirium in the young can be challenging to diagnose, especially if the child is at a preverbal developmental stage, and symptoms may be mistaken for uncooperative behaviour. Those with a prolonged stay in hospital, especially in an intensive care unit and/or with severe illness, are at an increased risk for delirium (Porter et al., 2016). Care of paediatric patients needs to include delirium hygiene (e.g., limiting changes and noise; monitoring medication response), alertness to indicators of delirium, and timely intervention if it occurs.

Older Adults

Although delirium may occur in any age group, it is most common among older adults, although it may go unrecognized, especially in those over 85 years of age (Voyer et al., 2012). Early diagnosis and resolution are critical to achieving favourable outcomes. Older adults often present with multiple medical comorbidities and higher risk for postoperative complications. **Postoperative delirium** in the older adult is associated with increased length of hospital stay, rise in morbidity rates, decline in function, and greater risk of death. Screening for delirium should be considered as part of the clinical routine for older adults in their first postoperative days. Delirium in older adults is associated with poor outcomes, including increased length of stay, greater use of physical restraints, continuous sedation, increased unintended removal of catheters, and higher mortality rates (Balas et al., 2012). Nurses must be vigilant in assessment for delirium, recognizing that delirium, dementia, and depression present with overlapping clinical features and may coexist in the older adult (RNAO, 2016).

Epidemiology and Risk Factors

Statistics concerning the prevalence of delirium are based primarily on older individuals in acute care settings. Estimated prevalence rates range from 10% to 30% of patients. In nursing homes, the prevalence is much higher, approaching 60% of those older than the age of 75 years. The use of opioid analgesics in the management of postoperative pain has been found to correlate with the development of respiratory depression and postoperative delirium (Leung et al., 2009). Mechanical ventilation has been identified as the strongest risk factor for delirium in critically ill patients (Von Rueden et al., 2017). Delirium occurs in as many as 30% of patients hospitalized for cancer and in 30% to 40% of those hospitalized with acquired immunodeficiency syndrome (AIDS). Delirium is common in terminally ill patients nearing death.

The most powerful risks for developing delirium, however, are present before admission: for example, old age, severe illness, dementia, visual/hearing impairments, polypharmacy, alcohol abuse, fracture, infection, pain, and renal impairment. Any drug being taken by the patient presenting with delirium may be relevant to it (Sadock et al., 2015). Table 32.1 identifies delirium risk factors and related interventions. Box 32.1 presents a vignette of an individual who experienced delirium after using an over-the-counter (OTC) sleeping medication.

Aetiology

The aetiology of delirium is complex and usually multifaceted. A lack of generally accepted theories of causation has resulted in considerable variability in the research. Integrating the research and applying it to practice have been difficult. To date, studies focus almost exclusively on biologic causes of delirium, with psychosocial factors viewed as contributing or facilitating. Genetic studies and methods for brain research in humans offer new possibilities for studies related to delirium; however, lumbar punctures and brain scans for research are considered unethical in patients with impaired mental capacity, because they are unable to provide informed consent (van Munster, de Rooij, & Korevaar, 2009). Because environmental and psychosocial factors have been explored only in small, uncontrolled studies, conclusions cannot be drawn about these factors. For this reason, the following discussion of aetiology covers biologic theories of cause.

The most commonly identified causes of delirium, in order of frequency, are the following:

- Medications.
- Infections (particularly urinary tract and upper respiratory).
- Fluid and electrolyte imbalance; metabolic disturbances.
- The probability of the syndrome's developing increases with the presence of predisposing factors such as advanced age, brain damage, or dementia. Sensory overload or underload, immobilization, sleep deprivation, and psychosocial stress also contribute to delirium.

Because delirium has multiple causes, a wide variety of brain alterations may also be responsible for its development. In certain cases, delirium may be the only manifestation of an underlying medical problem needing immediate attention, as seen in cases of sepsis or myocardial infarction (Voyer et al., 2012). Even though the most widely propagated theory centres on the neurotransmitter system, several theories have identified that the causes relate to brain disturbances such as inflammation, physiologic stress, oxygen supply, and sleep–wake cycle. The burden of proof for such diverse hypotheses

Table 32.1 Delirium Risk Factors and Interventions

Risk Factor	Sample Intervention

Cognitive impairment, dementia, disorientation	Cognitive orientation/reorientation
	Environmental aids:
	  • Adequate lighting
	  • Clear signage
	  • Clock
	  • Calendar
	Avoid unnecessary room changes
	Use clear communication

Sensory deprivation, isolation	Therapeutic or cognitively stimulating activities:
	  • Personally valued activities and familiar background stimulation
	  • Reminiscence
	  • Family/friend visits
	Note: Avoid unnecessary isolation, sensory deprivation, and sensory overload.

Sensory impairment (e.g., hearing or vision impairment)	Optimize sensory function by:
	  • Ensuring hearing and visual aids are available and working
	  • Ensuring adequate lighting
	  • Resolving reversible causes of impairment (e.g., impacted ear wax)

Infection, fever	Look for and treat infection
Presence of urinary catheter	Avoid unnecessary catheterization Screen for and treat urinary tract infection Remove indwelling catheters ASAP Consider in-and-out catheterization over indwelling catheterization
Dehydration and/or constipation	Monitor nutrition, hydration, and bladder/bowel function

Electrolyte abnormalities (hyper- or hyponatremia)	Prevent electrolyte disturbance/dehydration by:
	  • Ensuring adequate fluid intake
	  • Considering offering subcutaneous or intravenous fluids if necessary
	  • Restoring serum sodium, potassium, and glucose levels to normal limits

Sodium and/or potassium and/or calcium abnormalities	Pay attention to those who are at increased risk for dehydration (i.e., taking diuretics, diarrhoea, pneumonia, UTI, etc.)
Poor nutrition	Follow nutrition support advice Maintain adequate intake of nutrients and glucose Ensure proper fit of dentures Take time to open food packaging/set up tray Encourage families to be present at mealtimes to assist with feeding
Anaemia	Identify and manage treatable causes of anaemia
Hypoxia	Optimize oxygenation and monitor oxygen saturation levels
Inadequately controlled pain	Assess, monitor, and control pain
Sleep deprivation or disturbance	Promote high-quality sleep Use nonpharmaceutical sleep enhancement methods Avoid nursing or medical procedures during sleeping hours, and schedule medication rounds to avoid disturbing sleep if possible Reduce noise and light to a minimum during sleeping hours

Immobilization or limited mobility
  • Use of restraints
  • Prolonged bed rest or sedation, immobility after surgery
Poor functional status/functional impairment
	Avoid use of restraints
	Minimize use of medical devices (e.g., IV lines, catheters) that may restrict mobility or function
	Encourage mobilization, including:
	  • Walking, if possible
	  • Getting out of bed
	  • Range-of-motion exercises
	  • Self-care activities
	Provide appropriate walking aids if needed
	Encourage mobilization soon after surgery
	Physical and occupational therapy as needed (after surgery)

Polypharmacy and use of high-risk medications (e.g., psychoactive medications, sedative–hypnotics, benzodiazepines, anticholinergics, antihistamines, meperidine)	Carry out medication reviews for people taking multiple drugs, and modify dosage or discontinue drugs that increase the risk of delirium when possible

Adapted with permission from Registered Nurses' Association of Ontario. (2016). *Delirium, dementia, and depression in older adults: Assessment and care* (2nd ed.). Toronto, ON: Registered Nurses' Association of Ontario.

BOX 32.1 CLINICAL VIGNETTE

Delirium

Mrs. Campbell, a widowed 72-year-old woman living in her own home, has been having trouble sleeping. Her daughter visits her and suggests that she try an OTC sleeping medication. Mrs. Campbell has also been taking antihistamines for allergies and the antidepressant amitriptyline. Three nights later, a neighbour calls the daughter, concerned because she encountered Mrs. Campbell wandering the streets, unable to find her home. When the neighbour approached Mrs. Campbell to help her home, she began to scream and strike out at the neighbour.

The daughter visits immediately and discovers that her mother does not know who she is, does not know what time it is, appears dishevelled, and is suspicious that people have been in her home stealing the things she cannot find. Mrs. Campbell does not recall taking any medication, but when her daughter investigates, she finds that 10 pills of the new sleeping aid have already been used. Mrs. Campbell is irritable and refuses to go to the hospital, but over the course of a few hours, she appears to calm down, and the following morning her daughter is able to take her to see her physician. After hearing the history, the physician hospitalizes Mrs. Campbell, withholds all medication, and provides intravenous hydration. Within 3 days, she is again able to recognize her daughter, and her mental status appears to be greatly improved.

What Do You Think?

- Identify risk factors that may have contributed to Mrs. Campbell's experiencing delirium.
- How could the addition of an OTC sleeping medication interact with the antihistamine and antidepressant to be responsible for her delirium?

---

varies from the role of melatonin to imbalance between dopamine and acetylcholine activity in the brain (van Munster et al., 2009). Major theories of causation are

- A general reduction in brain functioning, which can result from a decrease in the supply, uptake, or use of substances for metabolic activity
- Damage of enzyme systems, the blood–brain barrier, or cell membranes
- Reduced brain metabolism resulting in decreased acetylcholine synthesis
- Imbalance of neurotransmitters such as acetylcholine, norepinephrine, and dopamine
- Increased plasma cortisol level in response to acute stress, which affects attention and information processing
- Involvement of the white matter, especially in the thalamocortical projections (Tune, 2000)
- Direct brain insults that reflect dysfunction or damage of the brain, resulting from mainly indiscriminate effects such as hypoxia or metabolic disturbance (Maclullich, Ferguson, Miller, de Rooij, & Cunningham, 2008)

Interprofessional Treatment and Priority Care

The interprofessional team needs to act promptly to identify and intervene in delirium. Its management involves four key steps: (1) elimination or correction of the underlying cause(s), (2) management of behavioural disturbances, (3) anticipation and prevention of complications of delirium, and (4) support and restoration of functional needs (White & Bayer, 2007). A current challenge to the potential use of nondrug therapy interventions is the lack of controlled trials that evaluate drug therapy, dosing schedules, or combination regimens (Candy et al., 2012).

When developing a treatment plan for a patient in whom delirium is suspected, close attention must be paid to correcting any organic or disease-related factors. Initially, life-threatening illnesses must be ruled out or corrected, such as cerebral hypoxia, hypertensive encephalopathy, intracranial haemorrhage, meningitis, severe electrolyte and metabolic imbalances, hypoglycaemia, and intoxication. If possible, the use of all suspected medications should be stopped and vital signs monitored at least every 2 hours. Many patients with delirium are seriously ill, thus necessitating close or constant nursing care. The plan of care requires close observation for changes in vital signs, behaviour, and mental status. Patients are monitored until the delirium subsides. If the delirium still exists at discharge, it is critical that referrals be implemented for postdischarge follow-up assessment and care.

Nursing Management: Human Response to Delirium

By definition, a biologic insult must be present for delirium to occur, but psychological and environmental factors are often involved. Because delirium develops in a matter of hours or days and has been associated with increased mortality, nurses should be particularly vigilant in assessing patients who are at increased risk for this syndrome. (If the patient is a child, the assessment process presented in Chapter 29 should be used.) If the patient is an older person, the assessment that follows will serve as a guide. Special efforts should be made to include family members in the nursing process.

Biologic Domain

Biologic Assessment

The onset of symptoms is typically signalled by a rapid or acute change in behaviour. To assess the symptoms, the nurse needs to know what is normal for the individual. Caregivers, family members, or significant others may be the only resource for accurate information and should be interviewed.

Current and Past Health Status

History should include a description of the onset, duration, range, and intensity of associated symptoms. Chronic physical illness, dementia, depression, other psychiatric illnesses, referrals, and any past hospitalizations should be identified. Sorting out historical information may be particularly problematic when delirium accompanies acute illness, recent surgery, or infection.

Physical Examination and Review of Systems

In an attempt to discover the underlying cause of suspected delirium, monitoring of vital signs is crucial. An examination of body systems needs to be conducted. Laboratory data are gathered, including complete blood count, blood/urine glucose, blood urea nitrogen, creatinine, serum electrolyte analyses, liver function, and oxygen saturation levels. Fluid balance and bowel action disturbances relating to constipation or a recent history of diarrhoea should be assessed.

Physical Functions

A functional assessment includes physical functional status (activities of daily living [ADL]), the use of sensory aids (eyeglasses, contact lenses, and hearing aids), mobility aids, dentures/braces, sleep pattern, usual activity level and any recent changes, and pain assessment. Sleep disturbances are a symptom of delirium and may precipitate confusion. Often, the sleep–wake cycle of the patient becomes reversed, with the individual attempting to sleep during the day and be awake at night. Restoration of a normal sleep cycle is extremely important.

Pharmacologic Assessment

A substance use history (including alcohol intake and tobacco use) should be obtained (see Chapters 26 and 33). Information regarding medication use must be obtained, with particular attention given to new medications or changes in the dose or strength of current medications. Table 32.2 lists some of the drugs that can cause an acute change in mental status. Special attention should be given to combinations of medications because drug interactions can cause delirium.

Information regarding OTC medications should be included in this assessment. OTC medications are often

---

Table 32.2   Categories of Drugs That Can Cause "Acute Change in Mental Status"*

Mnemonic: ACUTE CHANGE IN MS

Drug Category	Examples of Drugs
Antiparkinsonian drugs	trihexyphenidyl, benztropine, bromocriptine, levodopa, selegiline (deprenyl)
Corticosteroids	prednisolone
Urinary incontinence drugs	oxybutynin (Ditropan), flavoxate (Urispas)
Theophylline	theophylline
Emptying drugs (motility drugs)	metoclopramide (Reglan), cisapride (Propulsid)
Cardiovascular drugs (including antihypertensives)	digoxin, quinidine, methyldopa, reserpine, beta-blockers (propranolol to a less amount), diuretics, ACE inhibitors (captopril, enalapril), calcium channel antagonists (nifedipine, verapamil, diltiazem)
H₂ blockers	cimetidine (uncommon on its own but increased risk with renal impairment)
Antimicrobials	cephalosporins, penicillin, quinolones, others
NSAIDs	indomethacin, ibuprofen, naproxen, salicylate compounds
Geropsychiatry drugs	1. Tricyclic antidepressants (e.g., amitriptyline, desipramine to a lesser extent, imipramine, nortriptyline) 2. SSRIs—safer but watch if hyponatremia present 3. Benzodiazepines (e.g., diazepam) 4. Antipsychotics (e.g., haloperidol [Haldol], chlorpromazine, risperidone)
ENT drugs	Antihistamines, decongestants, cough syrups in OTC preparations
Insomnia	nitrazepam, flurazepam, diazepam, temazepam
Narcotics	meperidine, pentazocine (risky)
Muscle relaxants	cyclobenzaprine (Flexeril), methocarbamol (Robaxin)
Seizure drugs	phenytoin, primidone

*This table notes some examples of possible medications that can contribute to delirium. It is the physiologic status of the older adult and the combination of medications, among other factors, that increase risk. Therefore, "Watch and Beware."

Reprinted from Flaherty, J. H. (1998). Commonly prescribed and over the counter medications: Causes of confusion. *Clinics in Geriatric Medicine, 14*(1), 101–125, copyright (1998), with permission from Elsevier.

thought of as harmless, but several medications, such as cold medications, taken in sufficient quantities may produce restlessness and confusion, especially in children and older individuals.

Findings from the medication and physical assessments are integrated and analyzed with a focus on improving health outcomes. Chronic pain may lead an individual to use more medication than has been intended. The increase in medication then results in delirium. Careful monitoring of the effectiveness of pain medications may be supportive in the order of a more effective medication that results in less potential misuse. Because many classes of medications have been associated with delirium, the focus is on changes in the type and number of medications and how medications relate to other findings in the history and physical assessment.

Nursing Diagnoses for the Biologic Domain

The nursing diagnoses typically generated from assessment data are acute confusion, impaired memory, disturbed thought processes, impaired environmental interpretation syndrome, or disturbed sensory perception (visual or auditory) (North American Nursing Diagnosis Association [NANDA], 2012). However, astute nurses will also use nursing diagnoses based on their observations linked to indicators such as hyperthermia, dehydration, cyanosis, acute pain, risk for infection, and disturbed sleep pattern. Observation skills are most needful in critically ill/lethargic patients who are voiceless due to the effects of intubation and mechanical ventilation.

Interventions for the Biologic Domain

Important interventions for a patient experiencing acute confusional state include providing a safe, calm, and therapeutic environment; removing the stressor (if possible); and maintaining fluid and electrolyte balance. Nurses are often involved in the assessment of vital signs, blood glucose levels, pulse oximetry monitoring, and interpretation of laboratory or diagnostic profiles related to chemistry studies, drug levels, urinalysis, and arterial blood gas analysis. Other interventions include ensuring adequate nutrition, preventing aspiration and decubitus ulcers, and those related to a particular nursing diagnosis that focus on individual symptoms and underlying causes—for example, for patients with disturbed sleep patterns. Protocols to enhance sleep with an emphasis on noise reduction and appropriate timing of laboratory and/or X-ray tests (if any) have been delineated (Cmiel, Karr, Gasser, Oliphant, & Neveau, 2004; Humphries, 2008) (see Chapter 28). Interventions to prevent delirium can reduce the length of stay in health facilities.

Safety Interventions

Behaviours exhibited by the delirious patient, such as hallucinations, delusions, illusions, aggression, or agitation (restlessness or excitability), may pose safety problems. The patient must be protected from physical harm through the use of low beds, padded guardrails (use with caution when putting up both bedrails, as a confused person may try to climb over the rail), bed alarms, and careful supervision. Risk for injury is a high-priority diagnosis because individuals with delirium are more likely to fall or injure themselves during a confused state (Carpenito-Moyet, 2017). "Prevention of Falls and Fall Injuries in the Older Adult" (RNAO, 2005, updated 2011) is a good resource to use for assessment and response to risk for falls.

Pharmacologic Interventions

There is a lack of research to support the use of drugs in the management of delirium; in fact, they may worsen symptoms (White & Bayer, 2007). Pharmacologic treatment of delirium, however, is commonly directed at decreasing agitation and related psychotic symptoms (Balas et al., 2012). The goal of psychopharmacologic management is typically focused on treatment of the behaviours associated with delirium, such as agitation, inattention, sleep disorder, and psychosis, with the aim of making the patient comfortable. The decision to use medications should be based on the specific symptoms. Dosages are usually kept very low. Medications should be chosen with reference to potential side effects (particularly anticholinergic effects, oversedative effects, hypotension, and respiratory suppression) (see Box 32.2 for research on best practices with respect to use of sedatives). The use of antipsychotic agents in older individuals is discussed in greater detail later in the chapter. To avoid worsening the patient's condition, benzodiazepines should be used only when the delirium is related to alcohol withdrawal, but polypharmacy is not encouraged at this point. In some patients, the sedation effect may further impair cognition or a paradoxic agitation may.

Administering and Monitoring Medications

Patients experiencing delirium may resist taking medications because of their confusion. If a medication is given, ideally, it should be oral. Medications should *not* be hidden in food.

Monitoring and Managing Side Effects. Monitoring drug action and side effects is especially important because the cause of the delirium may not be known, and the patient may inadvertently be affected by the medication. Both aripiprazole and haloperidol have been shown to be effective in providing relief from delirium symptoms, but aripiprazole was found to be more tolerable due to lack of extrapyramidal side effects (Boettger, Friedlander, Breitbart, & Passik, 2011, p. 481). Patients should be monitored for sedation, hypotension, or extrapyramidal symptoms such as dystonia; repetitive, involuntary muscle movements (e.g., lip smacking); and/or an extreme urge to be moving constantly. Although mental status often fluctuates during delirium, it may also be influenced by these medications, and any changes or

BOX 32.2 Research for Best Practice

SEDATING MEDICATIONS AND DELIRIUM IN OLDER INPATIENTS

From Rothberg, M., Herzig, S., Pekow, P., Avrunin, J. Lagu, T., & Lindauer, P. (2013). Association between sedating medications and delirium in older inpatients. Journal of the American Geriatrics Society, 61(6), 923–930.

The Objective: To examine the association between sedative medication, identified in the Beers criteria of potentially inappropriate medications (PIM) for older adults, and delirium in a large cohort of hospitalized older patients with common medical conditions.

Methods: A retrospective cohort study was conducted that involved patients at 374 American hospitals (N = 225,028) who were 65+ years of age and admitted over a 22-month period with one of six diagnoses: acute myocardial infarction, chronic pulmonary disease, community-acquired pneumonia, congestive heart failure, ischemic stroke, or urinary tract infection. Hospital-acquired delirium was defined as initiation of an antipsychotic medication or restraints on hospital day 3 or later. Chi-square and *t*-tests were carried out to assess associations between delirium, participant characteristics, and sedative use. Regression analysis was used to model the association between sedation and delirium. A second "nested case–control" study was conducted with matched controls (matched on hospital, primary diagnosis, sex, and age within 3 years) identified for each delirium case. The controls had a length of stay at least as long as the time when treatment for delirium began in their matched case. Cases and controls were assessed for treatment with the sedatives of interest to the study (i.e., identified in Beers criteria).

Findings: The median age of the sample was 82 years with 17% (38,883 patients) receiving one or more sedative medications. Four percent of participants were identified as having hospitalized delirium. In the cohort study, diphenhydramine and short-acting benzodiazepines were associated with a greater risk of subsequent delirium. In the case–control study, both short- and long-acting benzodiazepines, diphenhydramine, and promethazine were associated with delirium. Amitriptyline and muscle relaxants were not associated with delirium in either study. Patients with delirium had longer length of stay, higher costs, and higher mortality than did patients who did not experience delirium.

Implications for Nursing: The prevalence of sedation use in older hospitalized adults and the associated risk for delirium warrants a high level of vigilance by nurses. It appears that sedative medications identified as PIM are commonly prescribed and that some are associated with more risk for delirium than others are. Further investigation is needed.

---

worsening of mental status after the administration of the medication should be reported immediately to the prescriber. Some side effects may also be confused with the symptoms of delirium. For example, akathisia (see Chapter 12) may appear to be agitation or restlessness. The patient's physical condition and concurrent medication regimen may also influence the bioavailability, metabolism, distribution, and elimination of these medications. Adequate hydration and nutrition must be maintained. When using antipsychotic medications, closely monitor the patient for symptoms of neuroleptic malignant syndrome (see Chapter 12). The appearance of these symptoms may be confused with those related to delirium and therefore missed.

The use of medications for treating symptoms related to delirium should be discontinued as soon as possible, but these medications should be withdrawn gradually during a period of several days or weeks.

Identifying Drug Interactions. The aetiology of delirium is often a drug–drug interaction. OTC sleeping, cold, or allergy medication may be the cause. It is the nurse's responsibility to critically review each patient's medication record and discuss findings with the attending physician/nurse practitioner to avoid drug overdosage and intoxication, which can worsen symptoms. If medication is the underlying cause, it is important to identify accurately which medications are involved before administering any other drugs. Consultation with a clinical pharmacist may also be helpful, but exploring a patient's medication history in a physical assessment allows access to relevant data for guiding the care plan. Many of the medications used to treat symptoms of delirium (e.g., restlessness, altered sleep cycle) may in fact have potential side effects that worsen symptoms (Balas et al., 2012).

Teaching Points

To prevent future occurrences, the nurse needs to educate the patient, family, and caregivers about the underlying causes and predisposing factors related to delirium. If the delirium is not resolved before discharge, caregivers need to know how to care for the patient at home and offer information on where to receive additional community or social welfare support.

Psychological Domain

Assessment

The psychological assessment of the individual with delirium focuses on cognitive changes revealed through the mental status examination as well as the resulting behavioural manifestations. Since nurses are with patients around the clock, they are often the key interprofessional team members who first notice that the patient is experiencing a change in mental status or other indications of distress such as pain, anxiety, and behavioural changes. A needs-based care plan can then be implemented to promote the patient's comfort and safety. Changes in mental status must be monitored frequently for an early detection of delirium, especially in older individuals. In addition, other factors such as stressors and environmental changes may contribute to the symptoms.

Mental Status

Rapid onset of global cognitive impairment that affects multiple aspects of intellectual functioning is the hallmark of delirium. An essential nonpharmacologic nursing intervention for a patient experiencing delirium is to identify and help correct any unstable physiologic and haemodynamic conditions that evoke an acute change in mental status, such as sepsis, poisoning, or drug intoxication. Mental status evaluation usually reveals several changes such as the following:

- Fluctuations in the level of consciousness with a reduced awareness of the environment
- Difficulty focusing and sustaining or shifting attention
- Severely impaired memory, especially immediate and recent memory

Patients may be disoriented to time and place but rarely to person. Environmental perceptions are often disturbed. The patient may believe that shadows in the room are really people. Thought content is often illogical, and speech may be incoherent or inappropriate to context. Each variation in mental status tends to fluctuate over the course of the day. On any given day, an individual with delirium may appear confused and uncooperative but later may be lucid and able to follow instructions. Nurses must assess and document the cognitive status of the individual throughout the day so that interventions can be modified accordingly.

Calculations, orientation (especially to time), and recall are most affected in delirium, whereas naming and registration are relatively preserved. Several rating scales are available for use in assessing the cognitive and behavioural fluctuations of delirium (Box 32.3).

Behaviour

Delirious patients exhibit a wide range of behaviours, complicating the process of making a diagnosis and planning interventions. At times, the individual may be

---

> ### BOX 32.3 Rating Scales for Use with Delirium
>
> #### THE CONFUSION ASSESSMENT METHOD (CAM)
>
> Inouye, S. K., van Dyck, C. H., Alessi, C. A., Balkin, S., Siegal, A. P., & Horwitz, R. I. (1990). Clarifying confusion: The confusion assessment method. *Annals of Internal Medicine, 113*, 941–948.
>
> #### DELIRIUM RATING SCALE (DRS)-R-98
>
> Trzepacz, P. T., Mittal D., Torres, R., Kanary, K., Norton, J., & Jimerson, N. (2001). Validation of the Delirium Rating Scale-revised-98: Comparison with the delirium rating scale and the cognitive test for delirium. *Journal of Neuropsychiatry and Clinical Neurosciences, 13*, 229–242.
>
> #### NEECHAM CONFUSION SCALE
>
> Miller, J., Neelon, V., Champagne, M., Bailey, D., Ng'andu, N., Belyea, M., et al. (1997). The assessment of acute confusion as part of nursing care. *Applied Nursing Research, 10*(3), 143–151.

---

restless or agitated and at other times lethargic and slow to respond. Precautions to prevent falls, aspiration, and accidental self-inflicted injuries should be established to ensure patient safety. Delirium can be categorized into three types:

- **Hyperactive delirium** involves behaviours such as being overly alert, exhibiting disturbing episodes of psychomotor hyperactivity, and marked excitability (may hallucinate). The patient may scream out in fear, describe hallucinations, pull at tubes, attempt to climb out of bed, and may attempt to hit staff (Balas et al., 2012).
- **Hypoactive delirium** is marked by lethargy, sleepiness, apathy, and psychomotor slowing; this is the "quiet" patient for whom the diagnosis of delirium often is missed (especially in seriously ill patients), as such patients often remain withdrawn or lie quietly in bed.
- **Mixed delirium** involves behaviour that fluctuates between the hyperactive and the hypoactive states over brief or long periods.

Nursing Diagnoses for the Psychological Domain

The nursing diagnosis of acute confusion is also associated with impaired cognitive functioning. Although the underlying cause of confusion is physiologic, nursing care should focus on the psychological domain, as well as the physical. Other typical nursing diagnoses related to the psychological domain include risk for acute confusion, disturbed thought process, ineffective coping, disturbed personal identity, and deficient knowledge (specify).

Interventions for the Psychological Domain

Staff members should have frequent interactions with patients and support them with institutional and community resources if they are confused, experiencing illusions, or hallucinating. Patients should be encouraged to express their fears and discomforts that result from frightening or disconcerting psychotic experiences. Adequate lighting, easy-to-read calendars and clocks, a quiet noise level, and frequent verbal orientation may reduce this frightening experience. If the patient wears eyeglasses or uses a hearing aid, these devices should be used. Including familiar personal possessions such as favourite clothing and footwear, or wall paintings in the environment, may also help. Interventions that may be useful for these individuals are discussed in detail later in the chapter (see the section on dementia).

Social Domain

Assessment

Discussions should be initiated with the family to determine whether the patient's behaviours are new. An assessment of living arrangements may provide information about sensory stimulation or social isolation. Cultural and educational background must be considered when the patient's mental capacity is evaluated. New immigrants and individuals from certain ethnic backgrounds may not be familiar with the information used in tests of general knowledge (e.g., names of prime ministers, geographic knowledge), or in testing memory (e.g., date of birth in cultures that do not routinely celebrate birthdays), or orientation (e.g., sense of placement and location may be conceptualized differently in some cultures). Some cultural practices may involve using substances such as elixirs that contain chemicals that may exacerbate delirium. The assessment should be language-specific and address such practices, as well as include exploring other relevant culture-specific practices.

Family Roles

Delirium is a burden not only for the patient but also for the patient's family caregivers (Balas et al., 2012). Family support for the individual and understanding of the disorder must therefore be assessed. The behaviours exhibited by the person experiencing delirium may be frightening or at least confusing for family members and significant others. Some family members may actually contribute to the patient's increased agitation. Observing and assessing family interactions and family members' ability to understand delirium is important. If feasible, family presence may help to calm and reassure the patient.

Nursing Diagnoses for the Social Domain

Among the several nursing diagnoses associated with the social domain, the most typical are interrupted family processes, ineffective protection, ineffective role performance, ineffective community coping, and risk for injury.

Interventions for the Social Domain

The environment needs to be safe to protect the patient from injuries. A predictable, orienting environment will help to reestablish order to the patient's life. That is, a calendar, clock, music, and other items may be provided to help orient the patient to time, place, and person. If the patient is agitated, de-escalation techniques should be used (see Chapter 11). Physical restraint should be avoided as much as possible.

Support for Families

Families can be encouraged to work with staff members to reorient the patient and provide a supportive environment. Families need to understand that important decisions requiring the patient's input should be delayed if possible until the patient has fully recovered. Although patients may be able to participate in decision-making, they may not remember the decision later; it is therefore important to have several witnesses present and to document and keep record of any images and information in an ethical manner.

Spiritual Domain

Because delirium involves global cognitive impairment, including fluctuations in the level of consciousness and severely impaired memory, and may include agitation or lethargy, persons with delirium are very dependent on others for their comfort, dignity, and spiritual well-being. Communication and connection with others is often seriously affected, and the nurse will need to enact well the critical qualities of spiritual care: receptivity, humanity, competency, and positivity (see Chapter 11). Patients experiencing hallucinations, delusions, and/or illusions in delirium may understand them as having a spiritual cause or ancestral connection or purpose. This can make them more or less frightening at the time, depending on the meaning attributed to them, particularly if a family member had undergone a similar experience ending in a poor outcome. The patient may benefit from a visit offered by his or her spiritual leader. Once the delirium passes, the person may want to discuss such experiences (if remembered). The confusion of delirium necessitates, for the most part, that spiritual care of the patient is intensively "in the moment," as the nurse strives to sustain the person through the episode with family and religious support.

Evaluation and Treatment Outcomes

The primary treatment goal is the prevention or resolution of the delirious episode with return to previous cognitive status. Outcome measures include

- Correction of the underlying physiologic alteration
- Resolution of confusion

- Family member verbalization of understanding of confusion
- Prevention of injury

Resolution of confusion is the primary goal; however, the nurse makes important contributions to all four of these outcomes. The end result of delirium can be full recovery, incomplete recovery, incomplete recovery with some residual cognitive impairment, or a downward course leading to death.

Continuum of Care

The nurse may encounter patients with delirium in a number of management settings (e.g., home, nursing home, ambulatory care, day treatment, outpatient setting, hospital). Patients usually are admitted to an acute care setting for rapid evaluation and treatment of the underlying aetiology. An abrupt change in cognitive status can also occur while the patient is hospitalized for another reason. Delirium often persists beyond discharge from the hospital. Discharge planning should routinely include family education and referrals to community health care providers and social welfare facilities. If the patient will return to a residential long-term care setting, communication with facility staff about the patient's hospital stay, family support, and treatment regimen is crucial. Education of family members of persons with delirium (reversible or irreversible) in palliative care settings is also important (Irwin, Pirrello, Hirst, Buckholz, & Ferris, 2013). For a checklist of psychoeducational topics to guide teaching of caregivers of individuals with delirium, see Box 32.4.

Delirium superimposed on dementia (DSD) occurs when a patient with dementia develops a delirium (Fick, Hodo, Lawrence, & Inouye, 2007). The co-occurrence of delirium and dementia (overlap syndrome) substantially impairs functional recovery from acute illness and hospitalization, as compared with those affected by

---

BOX 32.4 Psychoeducation Checklist: Delirium

When caring for the patient with delirium, be sure to include the caregivers, as appropriate, and address the following topic areas in the teaching plan:

- Psychopharmacologic agents, if used, including drug action, dosage, frequency, and possible adverse effects
- Underlying cause of delirium
- Mental status changes
- Safety measures
- Hydration and nutrition
- Avoidance of restraints
- Decision-making guidelines

---

depression or delirium alone. This suggests that depression and delirium act in an additive and independent fashion to produce higher rates of adverse outcomes. Analysis of data from a Delirium Prevention Trial found that patients (aged 70+) with the overlap syndrome of delirium and dementia had resided in a nursing home prior to hospitalization and had experienced cognitive/functional impairment, depression, and higher levels of medical comorbidity than had all other patients (Givens, Jones, & Inouye, 2009). The overlap syndrome carries significant risk for functional decline.

DSD is often poorly identified or misdiagnosed. Fick et al. (2007) used case vignettes to assess experienced nurses' recognition of DSD. The researchers found that nurses were more able to recognize dementia and hyperactive delirium than dementia and hypoactive delirium (or hypoactive delirium alone). These case vignettes can be used as a learning tool for nurses.

■ DEMENTIA

Dementia is an irreversible syndrome characterized by ongoing decline in intellectual functioning sufficient to disrupt physical, social, and/or occupational functioning. Dementia falls within three categories: early-onset familial AD (FAD); rapidly progressive dementia such as Creutzfeldt-Jakob disease (CJD), which is a mandatory reportable condition in Canada; and later-onset dementia, which includes four primary types of dementia: AD, vascular dementia, dementia with Lewy bodies (DLB), and frontotemporal dementia (FTD).

■ ALZHEIMER'S DISEASE

In 1901, Alois Alzheimer observed Auguste Deter, a 51-year-old patient at the Frankfurt Asylum who exhibited strange behavioural symptoms and memory disturbance. The patient died 5 years later, but the neuropathology results revealed neuritic plaques and neurofibrillary tangles; over the years, this discovery became consistent and was named AD (Kaiser et al., 2012).

Clinical Course of Disorder

AD is a progressive neurodegenerative disorder characterized by memory loss, irreversible cognitive deficits, and behavioural changes (Carter, Resnick, Mallampalli, & Kalbarczyk, 2012). The person's ability to function gradually declines, although physical status often remains intact until late in the disease. AD is a terminal illness.

Two subtypes of AD have been identified: the less common early-onset AD (familial symptoms of dementia starting before age 65) and late-onset AD (older than 65 years). AD is also routinely conceptualized in terms of three stages: early, middle, and late. Signs and symptoms of AD change as the person passes from one stage of the illness to another (Table 32.3). Persons living with AD tend to pass through a specific sequence of deterioration

Table 32.3 Stages of Dementia

Early Stages
Forgetfulness
Problems with orientation (e.g., cannot follow directions)
Communication difficulties
Limited attention span
Difficulty learning new things
Changes in mood and behaviour
May understand how they are changing and may wish to help plan and direct future care

Middle Stages
Memory problems are obvious (e.g., does not know address, own history).
Restlessness (e.g., wandering, pacing)
Spatial problems that may affect mobility
Confused, difficulty following a topic of conversation
Problems understanding verbal and written language
Changes in wake–sleep patterns; lack of appetite
Apprehensive and/or withdrawn
Uninhibited behaviour
Delusions and hallucinations

Late Stage
Severe cognitive impairment (memory, information processing, orientation)
Loses capacity for recognizable speech
Needs help with eating, toileting; may be incontinent
Loses ability to walk without assistance, to sit without support, to smile, hold head up
May have impaired swallowing and loss of weight

End of Life
Changes in blood circulation; skin breakdown
No longer accepting food and drink
Increased sleepiness; changes in breathing
Agitation
May have buildup of secretions; fever
Still experiences and senses emotion
Spiritual experience may be important.

Adapted from Alzheimer Society of Canada. (2016c). *Stages of Alzheimer's disease.* Retrieved from http://www.alzheimer.ca/en/About-dementia/Alzheimer-s-disease/Stages-of-Alzheimer-s-disease. Refer to this site to see strategies for responding to the symptoms of each stage.

and symptoms (Forbes et al., 2012). Staging (i.e., identifying the stage the person is experiencing) is a useful technique for determining the person's current cognitive status and provides a sound basis for decisions in clinical management. People with AD live an average of 8 years with the disease, but some people may survive up to 20 years. The course of the disease depends in part on age at diagnosis and whether a person has other health conditions (see Alzheimer's Association, 2016b).

Diagnostic Criteria

The Canadian diagnostic criteria for dementia were re-evaluated in 2012 by the fourth Canadian Consensus Conference on the Diagnosis and Treatment of Dementia (CCCDTD4). The new criteria are based on recommendations made at this conference and those of the National Institute on Aging (NIA) and the Alzheimer's Association, both based in the United States. The criteria for AD include cognitive and/or behavioural symptoms that (1) interfere with the ability to function at work or at usual activities; (2) represent a decline from previous levels of functioning and performing; and (3) are not related to delirium or a major psychiatric disorder. Cognitive impairment is detected and diagnosed through a combination of history taking from the person and a knowledgeable informant and an objective cognitive assessment, such as a mental status examination. Neuropsychological testing and neuroimaging should only be performed by a dementia specialist when the routine history and mental status examination cannot provide a confident diagnosis (Gauthier et al., 2012a, 2012b).

The cognitive and/or behavioural impairment must involve a minimum of two of the following domains: (1) impaired ability to acquire and remember new and retained information; (2) impaired reasoning and handling of complex tasks and poor judgment; (3) impaired visuospatial abilities; (4) impaired language functions (speaking, reading, writing); and (5) changes in personality, behaviour, or comportment (CDKTN, 2012). Table 32.4 lists the presenting symptoms related to each

Table 32.4 Key Diagnostic Characteristics of Alzheimer's Disease

Diagnostic Criteria	Symptoms
Impaired ability to acquire and remember information	Repetitive questions or conversations, misplacing personal belongings, forgetting events or appointments, getting lost on a familiar route
Impaired reasoning and handling of complex tasks, poor judgment	Poor understanding of safety risks, inability to manage finances, poor decision-making ability, inability to plan complex or sequential activities
Impaired visuospatial abilities	Inability to recognize faces or common objects or to find objects in direct view despite good visual acuity, inability to operate simple implements, or orient clothing to the body
Impaired language functions (speaking, reading, writing)	Difficulty thinking of common words while speaking, hesitations; speech, spelling, and writing errors
Changes in personality, behaviour, or comportment	Uncharacteristic mood fluctuations such as agitation; impaired motivation, initiative, apathy; loss of drive; social withdrawal; decreased interest in previous activities; loss of empathy; compulsive or obsessive behaviours; socially unacceptable behaviours

Source: Gauthier, S., Patterson, C., Chertkow, H., Gordon, M., Herrmann, N., Rockwood, K., ... Soucy, J. P. (2012a). Fourth Canadian Consensus Conference on the Diagnosis and Treatment of Dementia. *Canadian Journal of Neurological Sciences, 39*(Suppl. 5), S1–S8; Gauthier, S., Patterson, C., Chertkow, H., Gordon, M., Herrmann, N., Rockwood, K., ... Soucy, J. P. (2012b). Recommendations of the 4th Canadian Consensus Conference on the Diagnosis and Treatment of Dementia (CCCDTD4). *Canadian Geriatric Journal, 15*(4), 120–126.

BOX 32.5 Ten Warning Signs of Alzheimer's Disease

To help the public know the warning signs of AD, the Alzheimer Society of Canada lists the following:

1. Memory loss that affects day-to-day function
2. Difficulty performing familiar tasks
3. Problems with language
4. Disorientation of time and place
5. Poor or decreased judgment
6. Problems with abstract thinking
7. Misplacing things
8. Changes in mood and behaviour
9. Changes in personality
10. Loss of initiative

For more information, see http://www.alzheimer. ca/en/About-dementia/Alzheimer-s-disease/10-warning-signs (Alzheimer Society of Canada, 2016d).

of these criteria. Box 32.5 lists 10 warning signs of AD. Clinical diagnosis is therefore based on the person's detailed history, a comprehensive physical and neurologic examination, and the application of established diagnostic criteria that are reliable and valid. Diagnosis may be supported through neuropsychological testing and diagnostic investigations, such as neuroimaging of the brain to detect and monitor progressive atrophy. However, there are currently no validated biomarkers for Alzheimer's disease, but researchers are investigating several promising candidates, including brain imaging, proteins in cerebrospinal fluid, proteins in blood, and genetic risk profiling.

Mild Cognitive Impairment

According to the Alzheimer's Association (2016b), long-term studies suggest that 10% to 20% of those aged 65 years and older may have MCI. The diagnostic criteria for MCI include a change in cognition over time in comparison with the person's previous level of performance. In addition, the cognitive performance is lower than expected for the person's age and education level. This change can occur in a variety of cognitive domains, including memory, executive function, attention, language, and visuospatial skills. An impairment in episodic memory (i.e., the ability to learn and retain new information) is seen most commonly in MCI patients who subsequently progress to a diagnosis of AD dementia. Persons with MCI commonly have mild problems performing complex functional tasks such as paying bills, preparing a meal, or shopping. They may take more time, be less efficient, and make more errors at performing such activities

than in the past. Nevertheless, they generally maintain their independence of function in daily life, with minimal aids or assistance. It is not yet possible to tell for certain what the outcome of MCI will be for a specific person or to determine the underlying cause of MCI from a person's symptoms (Alzheimer's Association, 2016c).

Epidemiology and Risk Factors

Currently, 564,000 Canadians are living with dementia. In 15 years, this figure will increase to 937,000. The annual cost to Canadians to care for those living with dementia is $10.4 billion (Alzheimer Society of Canada, 2016a).

Age is the most acknowledged risk factor for developing AD. It is estimated that dementia affects 1 in 14 people over the age of 65 and 1 in 6 over the age of 80. Females are at higher risk, even discounting the fact that they tend to live longer. A gene called apolipoprotein E (ApoE) has been shown to play a small part in the development of AD and vascular dementia. Specifically, the ApoE4 variant somehow preferentially promotes the production of the A-beta protein, constituting a significant risk. It is also possible to inherit genes that cause dementia such as familial early-onset AD and Huntington's disease. Conditions that affect the heart, arteries, or blood circulation all significantly affect a person's chances of developing dementia, particularly vascular dementia. These conditions include diabetes, midlife high blood pressure, high blood cholesterol levels, midlife obesity, heart problems, and stroke. Indeed, a history of stroke doubles the risk of dementia in older adults. People who experience severe or repeated head injuries are at increased risk of dementia. On the other hand, there is evidence that lifestyle factors such as a Mediterranean diet, regular physical activity, zero to moderate (250 to 500 mL per day) amounts of alcohol, and social and mental activities may reduce the risk of dementia (Alzheimer's Society UK, 2016b; van den Berg & Splaine, 2012).

Aetiology

Researchers have yet to identify a definitive cause of AD. In the brain of a person with AD, the cortex shrivels up, damaging areas involved in thinking, planning, and remembering. Shrinkage is especially severe in the hippocampus that plays a key role in formation of new memories. Ventricles (fluid-filled spaces within the brain) grow larger (Fig. 32.1).

Magnetic resonance imaging and cerebrospinal fluid and/or amyloid positron emission tomography (see Chapter 9) have been found supportive in identifying or ruling out the presence of AD pathology; these potentially offer opportunities for improving diagnostic sensitivity and specificity (Schott & Warren, 2012).

Beta-Amyloid Plaques

Following Alois Alzheimer's discovery of neuritic plaques and neurofibrillary tangles, accumulations of two

Healthy brain | Advanced alzheimer's

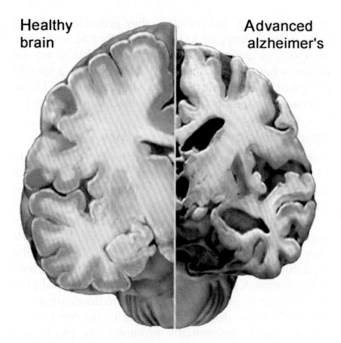

Figure 32.1. Healthy brain and advanced AD brain. (Courtesy of National Institute on Aging.)

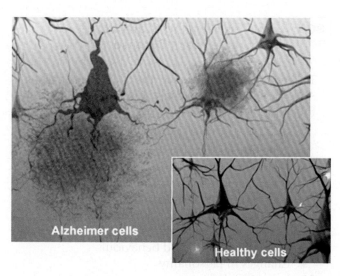

Alzheimer cells

Healthy cells

Figure 32.2. Plaques and tangles. (Courtesy of National Institute on Aging.)

separate proteins in the brain—beta-amyloid peptide and tau proteins—have been associated with AD (Casey, 2012). Diamond (2011), previous Scientific Director Emeritus of the Alzheimer Society of Canada, explains that plaques are made largely of a protein called beta amyloid (A-beta). In low concentrations, A-beta may be part of the body's defenses against invading bacteria and other microbes. However, in AD, A-beta accumulates in the brain to a level that overwhelms the enzymes and other molecules that clear away A-beta and the plaques. Both the production of A-beta and, especially, the processes that clear it away appear to be defective, at least in part because the impaired blood vessels in the brain cannot adequately pick up and remove the A-beta. There is evidence that these fine blood vessels proliferate and become leaky, possibly allowing hazardous substances to get into the brain. The accumulating individual A-beta molecules begin to clump together to form small aggregates called oligomers. Their continuing aggregation eventually leads to the formation of the amyloid plaques. However, it is the oligomers, not the plaques, that are the real problem; they appear to be toxic to the brain's nerve cells and, by the time enough A-beta molecules have stuck together to form the plaques, the damage has already been done (Fig. 32.2).

Alpha-synuclein, a protein found in neurons, is thought to play a key role in the remodelling of synapses and in microtubule transport and has been found to be associated with **beta-amyloid plaques** in AD (Casey, 2012). Antibodies to beta amyloid, such as bapineuzumab and solanezumab, were thought to reduce the number of beta-amyloid plaques in the brain (Casey, 2012), However, more recent evidence from trials of bapineuzumab and solanezumab have revealed negative results (Laske, 2014). Ongoing trials with new drugs that appear to reduce the production of amyloid in people with Alzheimer's disease continue (Alzheimer's Society UK, 2016a).

IN-A-LIFE 🏠

Dame Iris Murdoch (1919–1999)

PUBLIC PERSONA

Born in Dublin, Ireland, Dame Iris Murdoch became a much-loved philosopher and writer, the author of 36 novels, several plays, essays, and philosophical works, and engaged in a critical study of Jean-Paul Sartre. Over her life, she filled 95 diaries with her aspirations and analysis of her own shortcomings. Her book, *The Sea, The Sea* won the Booker Prize in 1978. Iris Murdoch was elected as a fellow to St. Anne's College, Oxford, in 1948 and remained a tutor there until 1963.

PERSONAL REALITIES

Iris Murdoch married John Bayley in 1956. In the mid-1990s, she began to show signs of AD. Her extensive vocabulary became diminished; she had difficulty answering questions, and there was a noticeable decline in the quality of her last book, *Jackson's Dilemma*. She died of AD in 1999. Her husband's book about her life, an *Elegy for Iris* (1999), was made into a movie, *Iris*, in 2001.

Neurofibrillary Tangles

Neurofibrillary tangles are made of a protein called tau (Diamond, 2011). Tau is present in normal nerve cells, but in AD, it becomes chemically altered (phosphorylated) and tends to pile up as threadlike tangles, preventing its normal functions. A critical function is to provide a kind of railroad track system inside the nerve cells and along the nerve fibres that are spun off from the cell body. The tau pathways are inside the nerve cells and fibres. Their main role in fibres is to convey essential nutrient and instructional chemicals and tiny organelles (structures) up and down the fibres in both directions. Interruption in this internal transport does not stop the nerve messages, but the tangles choke the cells to death. The first casualties of the compromised internal transport system are the distant nerve endings, which are especially vulnerable. The synapses deteriorate, impairing the transmission of messages to the next cell. The first symptoms of AD appear. Synapses are now a prime focus of researchers to find curative therapies. Another important function of the tau protein, which suffers in AD, is its role in nerve sprouting. Sprouting of new branches leads to new connections between nerve cells; not only do more connections help the nerve cells keep communicating with one another as the disease progresses but new sprouts can also help compensate for lost connections. Consequently, a new interest in the cure for AD is toward developing therapies that promote nerve sprouting, including ways to normalize the altered tau protein.

Inflammation

An inflammatory response is normal whenever and wherever the body suffers trauma or is attacked by some kind of potentially threatening influence, such as an infection or a toxin. Neuroinflammation is the inflammatory response that occurs in the brain of the person with AD. Unfortunately, with AD, this inflammatory immune response can become excessive; the brain's immune cells (microglia) become overactive, and instead of helping, they actually worsen the situation by overproducing substances that can promote the death of cells and possibly also contribute the formation of tangles. As well, although not yet proven to result from the inflammation, AD appears to cause both proliferation and impairments of the brain's blood vessels, changes that exacerbate the progression of the disease (Diamond, 2011).

Oxidative Stress and the Role of Antioxidants

Oxidative stress refers to the threatening situation created when reactive oxygen species (ROS) begin to accumulate faster than the body can get rid of them. ROS are normal products of metabolism. However, if ROS are allowed to build up, they become damaging, poisoning the cells of the body, including those of the brain. Normally, this is prevented by the body's antioxidants. Natural antioxidants also occur in food, such as vitamins C and E.

Unfortunately, as AD progresses, the production of ROS increases to levels that overwhelm the available antioxidants, which themselves are reduced by a number of factors, including stress. Probably most of the risk factors for AD contribute to this stress, as does the accumulating A-beta protein. Somewhat paradoxically, in the earlier stages, before the accumulation reaches toxic levels, the A-beta acts as an antioxidant and could represent the body's early protective response to the disease. Oxidative stress is becoming one of the key targets of AD treatments (Diamond, 2011).

Many scientists now believe that oxidative stress is the primary event in AD responsible for the impairment of both mitochondria and calcium regulation. Mitochondria are tiny organelles found in all cells, and their role is critically important in satisfying the cell's energy needs. Mitochondrial impairment in AD is a key factor contributing to the impairment of the brain's nerve cells and the glial cells. There are about 10 glial cells for every nerve cell in the brain, and they have a huge caregiving role in maintaining the health and connectivity of the brain cells. It seems highly likely that many or most of the features of AD are primarily due to direct actions of the disease, not on the nerve cells but on the glial cells. Sick glial cells lose their ability to maintain the normal healthy functioning of the nerve cells (Diamond, 2011).

In nerve cells, calcium is involved in the creation of nerve messages and their transfer across the synapses to other nerve cells. The concentrations of calcium inside cells have to be rigorously regulated. In AD, calcium regulation is disturbed and nerve cell functions are impaired, eventually affecting cognition and memory storage. One player in the dysregulation of calcium in AD is a gene that has mutated over time; the abnormal genes, and in this instance the consequent impaired calcium regulation, enhance the accumulation of the threatening A-beta protein (Diamond, 2011).

Genetic Factors

The rare FAD is almost totally attributable to genes that have mutated to an extent that makes them function abnormally, and the abnormal functions are responsible for the disease. This form of AD can result from mutations in one of three genes, *APP, PSEN1, or PSEN2* (Genetica Home Reference, 2013). The abnormal genes are passed from generation to generation (Ringman, 2011). Genetic mutations account for only 5% of Alzheimer's cases where the onset is early middle age (Casey, 2012). Genetic forms of AD, including trisomy 21, typically involve mutations related to beta-amyloid (Casey, 2012).

Interprofessional Treatment

In designing services and interventions, the interprofessional team must keep in mind that AD has a progressively deteriorating clinical course and that the anatomic and neurochemical changes that occur in the brain are accompanied by impairments in cognition, affect, behaviour, and psychosocial functioning. The nature and range of information and services needed by persons living with dementia and families throughout their journey with dementia can vary dramatically at different stages. Pharmacologic intervention modestly improves cognitive symptoms and may subsequently decrease the rate of disease progression, typically at the early stage of AD (Forbes et al., 2012).

For a variety of reasons (e.g., stigma, reluctance of family physicians to make a diagnosis as they believe little can be done), many persons living with dementia never receive a diagnosis of dementia, which limits their ability to receive appropriate treatment and services. Heightening awareness of the importance of receiving an informed diagnosis, possibly from a neurologist or geriatrician, is strongly recommended. Initial assessment of the person suspected of having dementia has three main objectives: (1) confirmation of the diagnosis through neuropsychological testing and diagnostic investigations, such as neuroimaging of the brain type and severity of dementia; (2) establishment of baseline levels in a number of functional spheres; and (3) establishment of a therapeutic relationship with the patient and family that will continue through subsequent phases of the disease. Treatment efforts currently focus on managing the cognitive symptoms, delaying the cognitive decline (e.g., memory loss, confusion, and problems with learning, speech, and reasoning), treating the noncognitive symptoms (e.g., psychosis, mood symptoms, agitation), and supporting the caregivers as a means of improving the quality of life for both persons living with dementia and their family and friend caregivers.

Priority Care Issues

The priority of care for AD will change throughout its course. There appears to be four phases of health care experience for persons living with dementia and their caregivers, each with health service implications, a meta-analysis of studies has determined (Prorok, Horgan, & Seitz, 2013). In the first phase, *seeking information and understanding*, there is distress regarding the changes in the individual and uncertainty about what is happening, a situation that public awareness and education could, at least in part, relieve. *Identifying the problem* comes with the formal diagnosis of dementia, bringing anxiety but also relief as understanding of the changes is achieved. The *role transition* phase includes both the person living with dementia and his or her caregivers beginning to prepare for coping with the illness. It is important that informed support is available to them and goals and potential treatments are discussed. The final phase, *living with change*, evolves as current and future care needs are focused upon (Prorok et al., 2013).

What may living with such changes be like? Persons with dementia usually experience difficulties remembering the last meal taken or how to use a knife and fork and confuse names of even close relations, house addresses, or significant dates. Impaired self-care (loss of ability to perform routine household chores, bathing, dressing, and eating) becomes prominent as the disease progresses. Often, they may ask the same questions repetitively, despite answers being previously given. The disease places the person at an increased risk of getting lost, even inside the home. Close observation is necessary outside the home. As the disease progresses, the person becomes highly dependent due to deterioration in physiologic functions (e.g., enuresis) added to the existing cognitive challenges. Initially, the priority is delaying cognitive decline and supporting family members. Later, the priority changes to protecting the person from injury. Near the end, the physical and emotional needs of the person living with dementia are the focus of care.

Family Response to Disorder

Families are often the first to be aware of the cognitive problems of a loved one. The person living with dementia may be unaware of the extent of memory impairment. A diagnosis of AD means long-term care responsibilities, while the essence of the person living with dementia diminishes day by day. Nurses need to support them and their families with education about treatment and choices (Casey, 2012) as well as healthy coping strategies. Most families wish to keep their relative at home as long as possible to maintain contact and to avoid costly nursing home placement. The symptoms that often result in placement are incontinence that cannot be managed and behavioural problems, such as wandering, especially at night, and aggression.

The needs of family members should also be considered. Caring for a family member with dementia takes its toll. Caregivers' health is often compromised, and normal family functioning is threatened. Caregiver distress is a major health risk for the family, and "caregiver burnout" is a common cause of the institutionalization of persons living with dementia.

Nursing Management: Human Response to Alzheimer's Disease

The development and implementation of appropriate, effective, and safe nursing care and services that support persons living with dementia and their families are a particular challenge because of the complex nature of the illness. Although AD is caused by biologic changes, the psychological and social domains are seriously affected by this disorder (see Box 32.5). The assessment of the person with AD needs to follow the geriatric mental health nursing assessment found in Chapter 31.

Biologic Domain
Assessment

Nursing assessment provides a foundation for the creation of a needs-specific patient care plan since the gathered data serve as evidence for appropriate interventions. Beta-amyloid protein "plaques" in the brain are one of the defining features of AD. However, the effects of beta amyloid on a person's brain and cognitive abilities are not straightforward. Research has shown that up to a third of older people without cognitive problems also have beta-amyloid accumulation in their brains (Rowe et al., 2010). The beta amyloid can be present for years before symptoms of dementia become apparent (Villemagne et al., 2011), and the proportion of those with beta amyloid in their brains who go on to develop AD remains unknown. Thus, at the CCCDTD4, it was recommended that if amyloid imaging technology becomes available in Canada, amyloid imaging must only ever be used in conjunction with a thorough and detailed clinical exam and in consultation with specialists (Gauthier et al., 2012a, 2012b). Further, since it is unknown what proportion of people with positive amyloid scans will go on to develop AD, amyloid imaging should not be used for screening people without symptoms of dementia, as the potential harms outweigh the benefits (Alzheimer Society of Canada, 2014; Canadian Dementia Knowledge Translation Network [CDKTN], 2012).

The nursing assessment should include a medical history, current medication profile (prescription and OTC medications), home and traditional remedies, substance use history (including alcohol intake and smoking history), chronic physical or psychiatric illness, and a description of the onset, duration, range, and intensity of symptoms associated with dementia. Past history of hospitalization and the respective reasons must be noted. The onset of AD symptoms is typically gradual, with insidious changes in behaviour. To conduct a thorough assessment of the patient, the nurse needs to know what is typical for the individual; therefore, caregivers, family members, and significant others can be sources of valuable information.

Physical Examination and a Review of Body Systems

A review of body systems must be conducted on each person suspected of experiencing AD. Specific biologic assessment parameters include vital signs, neuromuscular status, nutritional and weight status, bladder and bowel function, hygiene, skin integrity, rest and activity level, sleep patterns, and fluid and electrolyte balance. The neurologic function is usually preserved through the early and middle stages of AD, although seizures, gait disturbances, and tremors may occur at any time. In the later stages of the disease, neurologic signs such as flexion contractures and primitive reflexes are prominent features.

Physical Functions

At first, limitations may primarily involve instrumental activities, such as shopping, preparing meals, and performing other household chores. Later in the disease process, basic physical dysfunctions occur, such as incontinence, ataxia, dysphagia, and contractures. Incontinence can be a major source of stress and a considerable burden to family caregivers.

Assessment of physical functions includes ADL, recent changes in functional abilities (dressing, toileting, and feeding), use of sensory aids (eyeglasses and hearing aids), activity level, and assessment of pain.

Self-Care

Alterations in the central nervous system (CNS) associated with AD impair the person living with dementia's ability to retrieve information from the environment and from memories, retain new information, and give meaning to current situations. Therefore, persons living with dementia often neglect self-care activities such as bathing, eating, and oral and skin care.

Sleep–Wake Disturbances

About one quarter to a half of older adults with AD and other dementias experience some form of sleep disruption. The sleep–wake disturbances that commonly occur in persons with dementia are hypersomnia, insomnia, and reversal of the sleep–wake cycle. The disruptions in sleep at night are particularly difficult for family caregivers. The neurobiologic basis of these sleep disorders is related to degenerative changes in the suprachiasmatic nucleus of the hypothalamus that result in the loss of the expression of vasopressin (AVP) mRNA (Liu et al., 2000).

Persons with dementia may nap frequently in the daytime. Their nighttime periods of wakefulness mean that they have reduced rapid eye movement sleep. Sleep disturbances often increase as dementia advances. Where the person is unable to provide a reliable sleep history, the nurse must obtain the information from the person's caregiver. Such history usually encompasses sleep hygiene measures, use of sleep-promoting medications, and history of any sleep difficulties or underlying medical conditions. Increasing daylight exposure, engaging in daytime activities and exercises, and adhering to basic sleep hygiene measures can enhance nighttime sleep.

Activity and Exercise

Despite being physically capable, a person in the early phase of AD will often withdraw from normal activities due to the developing symptoms of memory loss, decrease in self-motivation, and, possibly, depression.

Nutrition

Eating can become a problem for persons with dementia as they may have difficulty chewing and swallowing. As the disease progresses, they may lose the ability to feed themselves or recognize what is offered as food. The hyperactive patient requires frequent feedings of a high-protein, high-carbohydrate diet in the form of finger foods (which they can carry while on the go). Most persons with dementia prefer to feed themselves with their fingers when appropriate rather than have someone feed them. Weight loss is a common consequence. It is important to monitor persons with altered appetites for hydration and electrolyte imbalances.

Pain

Assessment and documentation of any physical discomfort or pain the person living with dementia may be experiencing should be included in the psychogeriatric nursing assessment (see Chapter 31). Although AD is not usually thought of as a physically painful disorder, patients often have other comorbid physical diseases. In the early stages of AD, the patient can usually respond to verbal questions regarding pain. Later, it may be difficult to assess the comfort level objectively, especially if the person cannot communicate. However, pain should be assessed through physical examination and use of a pain assessment scale (see Web Link on managing pain).

Nursing Diagnoses for the Biologic Domain

The unique and changing needs of persons with dementia present a challenge for nurses in all settings. A sample of common nursing diagnoses includes imbalanced nutrition: less (or more) than body requirements, feeding self-care deficit, impaired swallowing, bathing/hygiene self-care deficit, dressing/grooming self-care deficit, toileting self-care deficit, constipation (or perceived constipation), bowel incontinence, impaired urinary elimination, functional incontinence, total incontinence, deficient fluid volume, risk for impaired skin integrity, impaired physical mobility, activity intolerance, fatigue, disturbed sleep pattern, pain, chronic pain, ineffective health maintenance, and impaired home maintenance.

Interventions for the Biologic Domain

The numerous interventions for the biologic domain vary throughout the course of the disease. Initially, the person with dementia requires simple directions for self-care activities and initiation of psychopharmacologic treatment. At the end of the disorder, total care is required.

Self-Care Interventions

Promotion of self-care supports cognitive functioning and a sense of independence. In the early stages, the nurse (and family members) should maximize normal perceptual experiences by ensuring that the person with dementia has appropriate eyeglasses and working hearing aids. If eyeglasses and hearing aids are needed, but not used, persons with dementia are more likely to have false perceptual experiences. Ongoing monitoring of self-care is necessary throughout the course of AD. Oral hygiene can be a problem and, although this may be difficult, requires excellent basic nursing care. Aging and many medications reduce salivary flow, leading to a painfully dry and cracking oral mucosa. Drugs that have xerostomia (dry mouth) as a side effect and are commonly prescribed for persons with progressive dementia include antidepressant, antispasmodic, antihypertensive, bronchodilator, and some antipsychotic agents. For persons experiencing xerostomia, hard candy or chewing gum may stimulate salivary flow, or modification of the drug regimen may be necessary. Glycerol mouthwash may also provide some relief from xerostomia.

Nutritional Interventions

Maintenance of nutrition and hydration are essential nursing interventions. The person's weight, oral intake, and hydration status should be monitored carefully. They need to eat well-balanced meals that are appropriate to their activity level and eating abilities, with special attention given to electrolyte balance and fluid intake.

The dining environment should be calm and food presentation appealing. If the person eats only a small portion of food at one meal, reduce the presentation of food in terms of the amount and number of choices. One-dish meals (e.g., a casserole) are ideal. If the person is distressed, delay feeding because eating, chewing, and swallowing difficulties are accentuated and choking becomes a risk.

Persons living with dementia should be presented food that is appropriate for their individual needs. When swallowing is a problem, thick liquids or semisoft foods are more effective than are traditionally prepared foods. If the patient is likely to choke or aspirate food, semisolid foods should be offered, because liquids flow into the pharyngeal cavity more quickly and may cause choking. In the later stages, some patients hoard food in their mouths; others swallow too rapidly or fail to chew their food sufficiently before attempting to swallow. The nurse needs to watch for swallowing difficulties that place the person at risk for aspiration and asphyxiation. Swallowing difficulties may result from changes in oesophageal motility and decreased secretion of saliva.

As dementia progresses, and food intake is low, oral assisted feedings are encouraged and vitamin and mineral supplements may be indicated. Percutaneous feeding tubes in persons with advanced dementia are not recommended. Careful hand-feeding is at least as good as tube feeding for the outcomes of death, aspiration pneumonia, functional status, and patient comfort. Tube feeding is associated with agitation, increased use of physical and chemical restraints, and worsening pressure ulcers (see Web Link on *Meal Times* for additional information).

Supporting Bowel and Bladder Function

Urinary or bowel incontinence affects many persons with dementia. During middle stage of the disease, incontinence may be caused by the person's apathy or inability to communicate the need to use the toilet or locate a toilet quickly, undress appropriately to use the toilet, or recognize the sensation of fullness signalling the need to urinate or defecate.

For the person who is incontinent because of an inability to locate the toilet, reorientation may be helpful. Displaying pictures or signs on bathroom doors provides visual cues while verbal prompts promote reorientation to the environment.

Getting to know the person's habits and moods can help the nurse identify signals that indicate a need to void. The person can then be assisted to reach the bathroom in time. Positioning the person near the toilet or placing a portable commode nearby may help if the person cannot reach a toilet quickly. If the person demonstrates dressing **apraxia** (cannot undress appropriately), clothing can be modified with easy-to-open fasteners in place of zippers or buttons. For nocturnal incontinence, limiting the amount of fluid consumed after the evening meal and taking the person to the toilet just before going to bed or upon awakening during the night should reduce or eliminate nocturia.

Indwelling urinary catheters are contraindicated in persons with dementia, because they are generally not well tolerated and because hand restraints are often needed to prevent them from removing the catheter. Indwelling urinary catheters foster the development of urinary tract infections and may compromise the person's dignity and comfort. Urinary incontinence can be managed with the use of disposable incontinent products.

Persons with dementia often experience constipation, although they may not be able to report this change. Therefore, subtle signs such as lethargy, reduced appetite, and abdominal distension need to be assessed frequently. Medications, decreased food and liquid intake, lack of motor activity, and decreased intestinal motility contribute to developing constipation. The person's diet should be rich in fibre, including bran or whole grains, vegetables, and fruit. Adequate oral intake (minimum of 1,500 to 2,000 mL per day) helps to prevent constipation. A gentle laxative such as milk of magnesia (1 to 2 tablespoons every other evening) is commonly used to promote bowel elimination. Enemas and harsher chemical cathartics should be avoided because they may increase pain or discomfort.

Sleep Interventions

Disturbed sleep cycles are particularly stressful to the person with dementia, family, caregivers, and nursing staff. Disturbed sleep is difficult to manage from a behavioural perspective, and the person's overall level of health may suffer because sleep serves a restorative function. Bright light therapy such as Brite-light boxes and ceiling-mounted light fixtures have shown promise in improving sleep in persons with dementia by regulating the sleep–wake cycle (Forbes, Blake, Thiessen, Peacock, & Hawranik, 2014). However, the best source of bright light is natural daylight. Physical activity such as walking and socializing outdoors has been shown to improve nighttime sleep (Brown et al., 2013).

Other sleep hygiene interventions that are helpful include having a fixed bedtime and awakening time that are the same every day; having certain activities that are always associated with going to bed (e.g., a particular piece of music or putting on a specific body lotion); avoiding napping during the day; avoiding alcohol 4 to 6 hours before bedtime; and having lots of fluids during the day but not a few hours before going to bed (Brown et al., 2013). In addition, rest periods (in reclining chairs) in the morning and afternoon may help to eliminate late-day confusion (sundowning) and nighttime awakenings.

Benzodiazepines or other sedative–hypnotics should be the last choice for insomnia (American Geriatrics Society, 2013). These may be prescribed for a short time for restlessness or insomnia, but they may also cause a paradoxic reaction of agitation and insomnia.

Activity and Exercise Interventions

Activity and exercise programs appear to have a significant impact on improving cognitive functioning and ability to perform ADL (Forbes et al., 2015). To promote a feeling of success, any activity or exercise plan must be culturally sensitive and adapted to the person's functional ability and interests. The activity or exercise must be designed to prevent excess stress (both physical and psychological). If the program of rest, activity, and exercise is truly individualized, the resultant feelings of value and competency may enhance the person's functional ability, cognition, and sleep pattern.

Pain and Comfort Management

Nursing care of noncommunicative persons with dementia and pain can be challenging. Common behaviours associated with pain may be difficult to interpret or absent. Signs to watch for that may indicate pain include body language and nonverbal signs that may indicate the person is uncomfortable; changes in behaviour (especially anxiety, agitation, shouting, and sleep disturbances); pale or flushed skin tone; dry, pale gums; mouth sores; vomiting; feverish skin; and swelling of any part of the body. Because of the difficulty in identifying and monitoring pain, persons with dementia are often undertreated. Undertreatment of pain may result in further cognitive and behavioural problems.

Relaxation

Approaching the person living with dementia in a calm, confident, unhurried manner; maintaining a soothing, quiet environment; avoiding unnecessary noise or chatter around them and lowering vocal tone and rate when addressing them; maintaining eye contact; and using touch judiciously are likely to promote a sense of security conducive to relaxation and comfort. Simple relaxation exercises can be used by the person to reduce stress.

Administering and Monitoring Medications

In the last two decades, the discovery of successful dementia medications has been abysmally low. The main challenges include (1) the significant gaps of knowledge in the classification of dementias and complexity of the underpinning biologic mechanisms of the most common forms of late-onset dementias; (2) low signal to noise ratio and the lack of validated biomarkers as entry and/or end-point criteria; and (3) poor recruitment and retention rates in drug trials, particularly in the asymptomatic and early disease stages (Gauthier et al., 2016). Thus, because no medication can cure AD, psychopharmacologic interventions have two goals: maintenance of cognitive function and treatment of related psychiatric and behavioural disturbances that cause discomfort for the individual, interfere with treatment, or worsen the individual's functional and/or cognitive status. Medications for AD must be used with caution. Doses must be kept extremely low, and individuals should be monitored closely for any side effects or worsening of cognitive status. "Start low and go slow" is the principle guiding the administration of psychopharmacologic agents to older adults.

Often, convincing the person living with dementia to take the medication is one of the biggest nursing challenges. They may be unwilling, even though they previously agreed to take the drugs. The nurse will need to investigate and hypothesize the reason(s) for their reluctance to take medication. It may be because of difficulty swallowing pills, paranoid ideas, or lack of understanding. The underlying reason(s) for medication refusal will determine the strategy. If the person has difficulty swallowing, most medications come in concentrate liquid form and can be easily swallowed. Medications should never be mixed in food without the person being made aware. If suspicion or paranoia is the reason, the nurse will need to try to identify the conditions under which the person feels safe to take the medication, such as in the presence of a favourite nurse or relative.

Cholinesterase Inhibitors. In Canada, three cholinesterase inhibitors (CIs) are approved: Aricept (donepezil), Exelon (rivastigmine), and Reminyl (galantamine). They help preserve the ability of sick nerve endings in the brain to transmit the nerve messages to the next cell in the chain. However, over time (usually 2 to 3 years or more), the sick nerve endings degenerate to the point where no transmitter is released at all, and the drugs are then totally ineffective. All three CIs are recommended as a treatment option for mild to severe AD with cerebrovascular disease and for dementia associated with Parkinson's disease. The research is inconsistent related to the use of CIs for the treatment of vascular dementia.

Some people are affected by the side effects from CIs, which include diarrhoea, insomnia, nausea, infection, and bladder problems. To avoid side effects, CIs are now contained in a skin patch, allowing the drug to be absorbed directly into the body.

N-Methyl-D-Aspartate Antagonists. Overstimulation of the N-methyl-D-aspartate receptor by glutamate (excitatory neurotransmitter) is considered to have a role in AD. When cells get sick, especially nerve cells, glutamate leaks out, and its concentrations outside the sick nerve cells can be so high that the increased amount taken back by way of the glutamate receptors is toxic and leads to the death of the nerve cells. The drug Ebixa (memantine hydrochloride) acts by blocking the glutamate receptors and preventing the reuptake of toxic amounts of the glutamate into the nerve endings. Since the glutamate threat develops late in AD, memantine is effective at moderate to advanced stages of the disease

(Diamond, 2011). Insufficient research evidence exists to recommend for or against combining memantine with CIs (Gauthier et al., 2012a, 2012b).

Antipsychotic Agents. Antipsychotic drugs have historically been used to treat the severe distortions in thought, perception, and emotion that characterize psychosis and have increasingly been used to treat the behavioural and psychological symptoms (e.g., delusion, aggression, and agitation) in persons with dementia. The adverse effects include sedation, higher risks of falls and hip fractures, Parkinson's disease–type symptoms, cardiovascular events (stroke and heart attack), and the greater risk of death. Thus, judicious use of antipsychotics has been recommended and a guideline with 15 specific recommendations regarding antipsychotic use to treat agitation or psychosis in persons living with dementia was developed (American Psychiatric Association, 2016). The CCCDTD4 recommended that risperidone, olanzapine, and aripiprazole be used for severe agitation, aggression, and psychosis associated with dementia where there is risk to the person and/or others (Gauthier et al., 2012a, 2016b). However, identifying and addressing the causes of behaviour change can make drug treatment unnecessary.

Antidepressant Agents and Mood Stabilizers. A depressed mood is common in persons living with dementia. However, they often respond with improved mood to physical activity such as a walk outdoors, engagement in a group activity, and psychotherapeutic intervention (individual or group therapy), and if necessary, in combination with pharmacotherapy. Low doses of selective serotonin reuptake inhibitors (SSRIs) are often used for people with Alzheimer's disease and depression because they have a lower risk than do some other antidepressants of causing interactions with other medications (Alzheimer's & Dementia Caregiver Centre, 2016).

Antianxiety Medications (Sedative–Hypnotics). Antianxiety medications, also known as benzodiazepines, should only be used as a last resort for insomnia, agitation, or delirium (American Geriatrics Society, 2013). Large-scale studies consistently show that the risk of motor vehicle accidents, falls, and hip fractures leading to hospitalization and death can more than double in older adults taking benzodiazepines and other sedative–hypnotics. Sedative–hypnotic agents may be prescribed for a short time for restlessness or insomnia, but they may also cause a paradoxical reaction of agitation and insomnia (especially in older adults).

Other Medications. Clinical observations indicate that persons with dementia are more vulnerable to the effects of anticholinergic drugs that can cause confusion and amnesia. Anticholinergic medications should be avoided for them if at all possible due to the CNS effects. In addition, there is some evidence that higher cumulative anticholinergic use is associated with an increased risk for dementia (Gray et al., 2015). See Box 32.6 for

BOX 32.6 Medications to be Avoided With Persons Living With Dementia

Antispasmodic medications	• Atropine • Belladonna alkaloids • dicyclomine (Bentyl) • hyoscyamine (Levsinex) • Oxybutynin (Ditropan) • scopolamine • tolterodine (Detrol)
Antihistamines	• brompheniramine (Dimetane) • carbinoxamine, chlorpheniramine (Chlor-Trimeton) • clemastine (Tavist) • cyproheptadine (Periactin) • dexchlorpheniramine (Polaramine) • diphenhydramine (Benadryl or Sominex) • hydroxyzine (Atarax) • phenindamine (Nolahist) • meclizine • triprolidine (Actifed/Myidyl)
Antiparkinson agents	• benztropine mesylate (Cogentin) • trihexyphenidyl HCL (Artane)
Barbiturates	• phenobarbital (Luminal Sodium)
Benzodiazepines	• Short-acting benzodiazepines: triazolam (Halcion) and midazolam (Versed) • Intermediate-acting benzodiazepines: lorazepam (Ativan), temazepam (Restoril), alprazolam (Xanax), oxazepam (Serax), estazolam (ProSom) • Longer-acting benzodiazepines: diazepam (Valium), chlordiazepoxide (Librium), clorazepate (Tranxene), halazepam (Paxipam), prazepam (Centrax), quazepam (Doral) and clonazepam (Klonopin), flurazepam (Dalmane)
CNS stimulants	• amitriptyline (Limbitrol or Limbitrol DS): used to treat symptoms of depression • fluoxetine (Prozac, Prozac Weekly): used to treat depression, obsessive–compulsive disorder, some eating disorders, and panic attacks
Antimuscarinics	• oxybutynin • tolterodine • trospium
Tricyclic antidepressants	• amitriptyline (Elavil) • clomipramine (Anafranil) • desipramine (Norpramin or Pertofrane) • doxepin (Sinequan) • imipramine (Tofranil) • protriptyline (Vivactil) • trimipramine (Surmontil)

Sources: American Geriatrics Society 2015 Beers Criteria Update Expert Panel (2015). American Geriatrics Society 2015 updated Beers criteria for potentially inappropriate medication use in older adults. *Journal of the American Geriatrics Society*, 63(11), 2227–2246. doi:10.1111/jags.13702; Green, A. R., Segal, J., Tian, J., Oh, E., Roth, D. L., Hilson, L. ... Boyd, C.M. (2017). Use of bladder antimuscarinics in older adults with impaired cognition. *Journal of the American Geriatrics Society*, 65(2), 390–394. doi:10.1111/jags.14498; Healthcare Provider's Guide To Alzheimer's Disease (AD): Diagnosis, pharmacologic management, non-pharmacologic management, and other considerations This material is provided by UCSF Weill Institute for Neurosciences as an educational resource for health care providers. Retrieved from http://memory.ucsf.edu/sites/memory.ucsf.edu/files/wysiwyg/UCSF_Alzheimer%27s_Providers7-13-17.pdf5; Starr, J. M. (2016). Diagnosis and management of dementia in older people. *Medicine in Older Adults*, 45(1), 51–54.

examples of medications that should not be taken by persons living with dementia if at all possible.

Psychological Domain

Psychological Assessment

As the disease progresses, personality changes can take the form of either an accentuation or a marked alteration from a person's previous lifelong character traits. The neural substrates underlying personality change in AD are not understood, but researchers have identified two contrasting patterns. One is marked by apathy, lack of spontaneity, and passivity. The other involves growing irritability, sarcasm, self-preoccupation, and intolerance of and lack of concern for others.

Cognitive Status

Cognitive disturbance is the clinical hallmark of dementia. The most commonly used cognitive assessment instrument is the Mini-Mental State Examination (MMSE; Box 32.7). If cognitive deterioration occurs rapidly, delirium should be suspected. The patient should be quickly evaluated by a physician because delirium calls for immediate attention to diagnose and treat the underlying cause.

Memory. The most dramatic and consistent cognitive impairment is in memory. Persons with early-stage dementia appear mildly forgetful and repetitive in conversation. They misplace objects, miss appointments,

---

BOX 32.7 Cognitive Assessment Tools for Use With Persons Living With Dementia

MENTAL STATUS QUESTIONNAIRES

Mini-Mental State Examination

Folstein, M. F., Folstein, S. E., & McHugh, P. R. (1975). Mini-mental state: A practical method for grading the cognitive state of patients for the clinician. *Journal of Psychiatric Research, 12,* 189–198. See Chapter 10 for components of the mental status examination.

Cognitive Abilities Screening Instrument

Teng, E. L., Hasegawa, K., Homma, A., Imai, Y., Larson, E., Graves, A., ... Chiu, D. (1994). The Cognitive Abilities Screening Instrument (CASI): A practical test for cross-cultural epidemiological studies of dementia. *International Psychogeriatrics, 6,* 45–58.

Montreal Cognitive Assessment

Nasreddine, Z. S., Phillips, N. A., Bedirian, V., Charbonneau, S., Whitehead, V., Collin, I., ... Chertkow, H. (2005). The Montreal Cognitive Assessment, MoCA: A brief screening tool for mild cognitive impairment. *Journal of the American Geriatrics Society, 53*(4), 695–699. See www.mocatest.org for more details.

COMBINATION OF COGNITIVE AND FUNCTIONAL ASSESSMENT

Brief Cognitive Rating Scale

Reisberg, B., Schneck, M. K., & Ferris, S. H. (1983). The Brief Cognitive Rating Scale (BCRS): Findings in primary degenerative dementia. *Psychopharmacology Bulletin, 19,* 47–50.

   Includes five scales: concentration, recent memory, remote memory, orientation, and functioning and self-care.

Agitation Scale

Rosen, J., Burgio, L., Kollar, M., Cain, M., Allison, M., Fogleman, M., ... Zubenko, G. S. (1994). The Pittsburgh agitation scale: User-friendly instrument for rating agitation in dementia patients. *The American Journal of Geriatric Psychiatry, 2*(1), 52–59.

RATING SCALES OF ACTIVITIES OF DAILY LIVING

Progressive Deterioration Scale

DeJong, R., Osterlund, O. W., & Roy, G. W. (1989). Measurement of quality-of-life changes in patients with Alzheimer's disease. *Clinical Therapeutics, 11,* 545–554.

Dependence Scale

Stern, Y., Albert, S. M., Sano, M., Richards, M., Miller, L., Folstein, M., ... Lafleche, G. (1994). Assessing patient dependence in Alzheimer's disease. *Journal of Gerontology, 49,* M216–M222.

RATING SCALE OF QUALITY OF LIFE

Quality of Life–Alzheimer's Disease

Thorgrimsen, L., Selwood, A., Spector, A., Royan, L., de Madariaga Lopez, M., Woods, R. T., & Orrell, M. (2003). Whose quality of life is it anyway?: The validity and reliability of the Quality of Life-Alzheimer's Disease (QoL-AD) scale. *Alzheimer Disease and Associated Disorders, 17*(4), 201–208.

RATINGS SCALES FOR RELATIVES

Geriatric Evaluation by Relatives Rating Scale Instrument

Schwartz, G. E. (1983). Development and validation of the Geriatric Evaluation by Relatives Rating Instrument (GERRI). *Psychological Reports, 53,* 478–488.

and forget what they were just doing. They may lose track of a conversation or television story. Initially, they may complain of memory problems, but in the course of the illness, insight is lost and they become unaware of what is lost. Sometimes, they may confabulate, making what appears to be an appropriate explanation of why the information or object is missing. Eventually, all aspects of memory are impaired. Short-term memory loss is usually readily evident by the person's inability to recall three or four words given to him or her at the beginning of an assessment. Often, the earliest symptom of AD is the inability to retain new information.

Language. Language is progressively impaired. Individuals with AD may initially have **agnosia**, difficulty finding a word in a sentence or in naming an object. They may be able to talk around it, but the loss is noticeable. Later, fluent **aphasia** develops, comprehension diminishes, and, finally, they become mute and unresponsive to directions or information.

Visuospatial Impairment. Deficits in visuospatial tasks that require sensory and motor coordination develop early; drawing is abnormal, and the ability to write may change. Inaccurate drawings on the MMSE or clock drawings are diagnostic of impairment. Sequencing tasks, such as cooking or other self-care skills, become impaired. The individual becomes unable to complete complex tasks that require calculations, such as balancing a chequebook.

Executive Functioning. Judgment, reasoning, and the ability to problem solve or make decisions are also impaired in the late stage of AD. It is hypothesized that as the disease progresses, the degeneration of neurons is spread diffusely throughout the neocortex.

Psychotic Symptoms

Suspiciousness, Delusion, and Illusions. During the early and middle stages of dementia, many persons are aware of their cognitive losses and compensate with hyperalertness. In a hyperalert state, one becomes aware of many environmental stimuli one does not readily understand. **Illusions** (mistaken perceptions) are common with dementia. These experiences can be very frightening for the person living with dementia and their family. A kind, caring approach is needed.

As the disease progresses, delusions develop in 34% to 50% of people with dementia. These characteristic delusions are different from those discussed in the psychotic disorders. Common delusional beliefs include the following:

- Belief that his or her partner is engaging in marital infidelity
- Belief that other patients or staff are trying to hurt him or her
- Belief that staff or family members are impersonators

- Belief that people are stealing his or her belongings
- Belief that strangers are living in his or her home
- Belief that people on television are real

Hallucinations. Hallucinations occur frequently in dementia and are usually visual or tactile (they can also be auditory, gustatory, or olfactory). A frequent concern is that children, adults, or strange creatures are entering the house or the person's room. These hallucinations may not seem unusual to the person. If possible, the content and form of hallucination should be ascertained because this information may suggest a treatable disorder. For example, an auditory hallucination commanding the person to commit suicide may be caused by a treatable depression, not dementia.

Mood Changes

Recognition of coexisting (and often treatable) psychiatric disorders in persons with dementia is often missed. One of the challenges of caring for them is when there is the coexistence of depression. Depression is characterized by alterations in sleep, lack of eye contact, feelings of sadness, expression of somatic concerns, and decrease in self-care. A recent meta-analysis (Graham, 2013) revealed a correlation between depression and subsequent vascular dementia and AD, as depressed older adults were more than twice as likely to develop vascular dementia and 65% more likely to develop AD compared with older adults who were not depressed. A person with dementia may experience one or more depressive episodes with symptoms such as psychomotor retardation, anxiety, feelings of guilt and worthlessness, sadness, frequent crying, insomnia, loss of appetite, weight loss, and suicidal rumination. Depressive symptoms are most prevalent in the early stages of dementia, which may be attributed to the person's awareness of cognitive changes, memory loss, and functional decline. However, dysphoric symptoms can occur at any stage, even in the most disoriented older person. In more advanced stages of dementia, an assessment of depression depends more on changes in behaviour than on the verbal expression of concerns.

Anxiety. It is common to observe symptoms of anxiety with depression; therefore, it is important to assess for depression when signs of anxiety appear. Moderate anxiety is a natural reaction to the fear engendered by gradual deterioration of intellectual function and the realization of impending loss of control over one's life. Becoming unsure of one's surroundings and the expectations of others and failing to complete a task once regarded as simple creates a source of anxiety in a person. It is thought that anxious behaviour occurs when the person is pressed to perform beyond his or her ability.

Catastrophic Reactions. **Catastrophic reactions** are overreactions or extreme anxiety reactions to everyday situations. Catastrophic responses occur when environmental stressors are allowed to continue or increase beyond the person's threshold of stress tolerance. Behaviours indicative of catastrophic reactions typically include verbal or physical aggression, violence, agitated or anxious behaviour, emotional outbursts, noisy behaviour, compulsive or repetitive behaviour, agitated night awakening, and other behaviours in which the person is cognitively or socially inaccessible. Factors that contribute to catastrophic responses in persons with progressive cognitive decline include fatigue, change in routine (pace or caregiver), demands beyond the person's ability, overwhelming sensory stimuli, and physical stressors, such as pain or hunger.

Behavioural Responses

Apathy and Withdrawal. Apathy, the inability or unwillingness to become involved with one's environment, is common in AD, especially in moderate to late stages. Apathy leads to withdrawal from the environment and a gradual loss of empathy for others. The lack of empathy is very difficult for families and friends to understand.

Restlessness, Agitation, and Aggression. Restlessness, agitation, and aggression become more prominent in the middle to late stages of dementia. Restlessness should be further evaluated to determine its underlying cause. If the restlessness occurs during medication change or adjustment, side effects should be suspected.

Agitation and aggressive physical contacts are among the most dangerous behaviour management problems encountered in any setting. They often result in the placement of the person with dementia in a nursing home. Careful evaluation of the antecedents of the behaviour enables the nurse to plan nursing care that prevents future occurrences.

Aberrant Motor Behaviour. Symptoms such as fidgeting, picking at clothing, wringing hands, loud vocalizations, and wandering may all be signs of underlying conditions such as dehydration, medication reaction, pain, or infection (suggesting delirium). One of the most difficult behaviours for which to determine an underlying cause is hypervocalization: the screams, curses, moans, groans, and verbal repetitiveness that are common in the later stages of dementia. In the assessment of these hypervocalizations, it is important to identify when the behaviour is occurring and any antecedents to the behaviour.

Disinhibition. One of the most frustrating symptoms of AD is disinhibition, acting on thoughts and feelings without exercising appropriate social judgment. The person living with dementia may decide that he or she is more comfortable naked than with clothes. Or the person may not be able to find his or her clothes and may walk into a room of people without any clothes on. This behaviour is extremely disconcerting to family.

Hypersexuality. A closely related symptom is hypersexuality, inappropriate and socially unacceptable sexual behaviour. The person may begin talking and behaving in ways that are uncharacteristic of premorbid behaviour.

Stress and Coping Skills. Persons living with dementia seem extremely sensitive to stressful situations and often do not have the coping abilities to deal with the situation. A careful assessment of the triggers that precede stressful situations will help in understanding and preventing a future event.

Nursing Diagnoses for the Psychological Domain

A multitude of potential nursing diagnoses can be identified for the psychological domain of this population. A sample of common nursing diagnoses can include chronic confusion, impaired environmental interpretation syndrome, risk for violence (self-directed or directed at others), risk for loneliness, risk for caregiver role strain, ineffective individual coping, hopelessness, and powerlessness (Carpenito-Moyet, 2017).

Interventions for the Psychological Domain

The therapeutic relationship is the basis for assessing and recommending interventions for the person living with dementia and their family members. Care entails a long-term relationship, much support, and expert nursing care.

Cognitive Impairment

Validation Therapy. Validation therapy emerged in the 1970s as a method for communicating with persons with AD. It was developed as a contrast to reality therapy, which attempted to provide a here-and-now, factual focus to the interaction. Validation therapy focuses on the emotions and subjective reality of the persons using an empathic approach. In validation therapy, individuals with cognitive impairment are viewed on one of four stages of a continuum: malorientation, time confusion, repetitive motion, and vegetation. The benefits of validation therapy are reported as restoration of self-worth, less withdrawal from the outside world, communication and interaction with other people, reduction of stress and anxiety, help in resolving unfinished life tasks, and facilitation of independent living for as long as possible. These outcomes are highly desirable; however, the research is inconclusive regarding the effectiveness of validation therapy (Heerema, 2017). Validation therapy is a useful model for nursing care of persons with dementia. The nurse does not try to reorient the person but rather respects the individual's sense of reality.

Memory Enhancement. Interventions for progressive memory impairment should always be a part of the treatment plan. The sooner the persons living with dementia begin taking a CI, the slower the cognitive decline. However, pharmacologic agents are only a small part of the intervention picture. The nursing goal is to maintain memory functioning as long as possible. The nurse should make a concerted effort to reinforce short- and long-term memory. For example, reminding persons with dementia what they had for breakfast, which activity was just completed, or who their visitors were a few hours ago will reinforce short-term memory. Encouraging individuals to tell the stories of their earlier years will help bring long-term memories into focus. In the earlier stages of AD, there is considerable frustration when the person realizes that he or she has short-term memory loss. In a matter-of-fact manner, the nurse should "fill in the blanks" and then redirect to another activity. Pictures of familiar people, places, and activities are also important tools in memory retrieval. Using scents (perfume, shaving lotions, spices, different foods) to stimulate memory retrieval and asking persons with dementia to relate memories are also useful. Formalized

reminiscence groups also help them relive their earlier experiences and support long-term memories.

Orientation Interventions. To enhance cognitive functioning, attempts should be made to remind persons with dementia of the day, time, and location. However, if the person begins to argue that he or she is really at home or that it is really 1992, the person need not be confronted by facts. Any confrontation could easily escalate into an argument. Instead, the nurse should either redirect the person or focus on the topic at hand (see Box 32.8).

Maintaining Language. Losing the ability to name an object (agnosia) is frustrating. For example, the person living with dementia may describe a flower in terms of

---

BOX 32.8

THERAPEUTIC DIALOGUE

The Person With Alzheimer's Disease

Lois's daughter has told the home care nurse that on several occasions, Lois has been found cowering and fearful under the kitchen table, saying she was hiding from voices. The nurse also knows that Lois denies having any difficulty with her memory or her ability to care for herself.

Ineffective Approach

Nurse: I'm here to see you about your health problems.

Patient: I have no problems. Why are you here?

Nurse: I'm here to help you.

Patient: I do not need any help. I think there is a mistake.

Nurse: Oh, there is no mistake. Your name is Ms. W, isn't it?

Patient: Yes, but I don't know who you are or why you are here. I'm very tired, please excuse me.

Nurse: OK. I will return another day.

Effective Approach

Nurse: Hello, my name is Susan Miller. I'm the home health nurse and I will be spending some time with you.

Person with dementia (PWD): Oh, alright. Come in. Sit here.

Nurse: Thank you.

PWD: There is nothing wrong with me, you know.

Nurse: Are you wondering why I am here? Tell me what is on your mind (open-ended statement).

PWD: I know why you are here. My children think that I cannot take care of myself.

Nurse: You're feeling concerned and perhaps a little worried your family seems to think you need more help at home?

PWD: Of course I can care for myself. When people get older, they slow down. I'm just a little slower now and that upsets my children.

Nurse: You are a little slower, and that's what you think is concerning your children.

PWD: I sometimes forget things.

Nurse: Such as… (open-ended statement)

PWD: Sometimes, I cannot remember a telephone number or a name of a food.

Nurse: … and that causes problems.

PWD: According to my children, it does!

Nurse: What about you? What causes problems for you?

PWD: Sometimes the radio says terrible things to me.

Nurse: That must be frightening to experience while listening to the radio.

PWD: It's terrifying. Then, my daughter looks at me as if I am crazy. Am I?

Nurse: Some people, when they become older, experience challenges with their memory. Also for some people, the daily living tasks that used to be carried out easily become more challenging. For you, it seems doubly scary because you doubt yourself and you're afraid your daughter doesn't understand.

PWD: Oh, OK. Will you tell my daughter that I am not crazy?

Nurse: Sure, I would be happy to meet with both you and your daughter if you would like (acceptance).

Critical Thinking Challenge

- How did the nurse's underlying assumption that the person living with dementia would welcome the nurse in the first scenario lead to the nurse's rejection by the person?
- What communication techniques did the nurse use in the second scenario to open communication and set the stage for the development of a sense of trust?

colour, size, and fragrance but never be able to name it a flower. When this happens, the nurse should immediately say the name of the item. This reinforces cognitive functioning and prevents disruption in the interaction. Referral to speech therapists may also be useful if the language impairment impedes communication.

Supporting Visuospatial Functioning. The person living with dementia with visuospatial impairments loses the ability to sequence automatic behaviours, such as getting dressed or eating with silverware. For example, persons living with dementia often put their clothes on backward, inside out, or with undergarments over outer garments. Once dressed, they become confused as to how they arrived at their current state. If this happens, the nurse should begin to place clothes for dressing in a sequence so that the person can move from one article to the next in the correct sequence. This same technique can be used in other situations, such as eating, bathing, and toileting.

Managing Suspicions, Illusions, and Delusions. Persons' suspiciousness and delusional thinking must be addressed to be certain that they do not endanger themselves or others. Often, delusions are verbalized when persons living with dementia are placed in a situation they cannot master cognitively. The principle of nonconfrontation is most important in dealing with suspiciousness and delusion formation. No efforts should be made to ease the person's suspicions directly or to correct delusions. Efforts should be directed at determining the circumstances that trigger suspicion or delusion formation and creating a means of avoiding these situations.

Frequent causes of suspicion are changes in daily routine and strangers. The common accusations that "Someone has entered my room," or "Someone has changed my room," can be managed by asking, "Do you want to see if anything is missing?" Such accusations usually arise when the person cannot remember what the room looked like or when the room was rearranged or cleaned.

Persons with dementia often hide or misplace their belongings and later complain that the item is missing. It is helpful if the nurse and other caregivers pay attention to the person's favourite hiding places and communicate this so that objects can be more easily retrieved. An outburst of delusional accusations after a social outing or other activity may indicate that the activity was too long, the setting was too stimulating, there was too much activity, or the pace was too fast for the person. All these elements can be modified, or it may be necessary to engage the person in quieter activities.

Persons with dementia may have delusions that a spouse, child, or other significant person is an impostor. If this situation occurs, it is important to assert in a matter-of-fact manner, "This is your wife Barbara" or "I am your daughter Jenny." More vigorous assertions, such as offering various types of proof, tend to increase puzzlement as to why a person would go so far to impersonate the spouse or child.

When persons experience illusions, the nurse needs to find the source of the illusion and remove it from the environment if possible. For example, if the person is watching a television program featuring animals and then verbalizes that the animal is in the room, switch the channel and redirect the conversation. Some persons living with dementia may no longer recognize the reflection in the mirror as self and become agitated, thinking that a stranger is staring at them. Potentially misleading or disturbing stimuli, such as mirrors or artwork, can be easily covered or removed from the environment.

Managing Hallucinations. Reassurance and distraction may be helpful for the person living with dementia who is hallucinating. For example, an 89-year-old person with AD in a residential care facility would get up each night, walk to the nursing station, and whisper to the nurses, "There's a man in my bed who won't let me sleep. You should patrol this place better!" If the hallucination is not too disturbing for the person, it can often be dismissed calmly with diversion or distraction. Because this person did not seem too concerned by the man in her bed, the nurse may gently respond by saying, "I'm sorry you have to put up with so much. Just wait here (or come with me) and I'll make sure your room is ready for you." The nurse should then take the person back to her room and help her into bed.

Frightening hallucinations and delusions should be first dealt with by decreasing the perceptual cues (cover mirrors or turn off the television) and by encouraging the person living with dementia to stay physically close to their caregivers. For example, one person complained to her nurse that she was being poisoned by deadly bugs that crawled up and down her arms and legs while she tried to sleep at night. Reassurance and protection should be provided. Persons often benefit if nurses give them a specific distracting intervention to alleviate anxiety and to help diminish the hallucination, such as applying moisturizing lotion to her legs and arms to repel the bugs at night. The nurse does not agree with the person's hallucination or delusion but lets the person know that the feelings are justified based on his or her perception of the threat. If these strategies are not effective, as a last resort, antipsychotic medication may help this person sleep at night.

Interventions for Mood Changes

Managing Depression. Psychotherapeutic nursing interventions for depression that accompanies dementia are similar to interventions for any depression. It is important to spend time alone with the person living with dementia and to personalize their care as a way of communicating the person's value. Encouraging the expression of negative emotions is helpful because they can talk honestly to a nonjudgmental person about their feelings. Depressed persons, especially in the early stage of dementia, may attempt and commit suicide. It is wise to remove potentially harmful objects from the environment.

Do not force depressed persons to interact with others or participate in activities, but encourage activity and exercise. One of the psychogenic aspects of depression is a sense of lowered worth related to the person's actual decreased competence to work and to deal with the problems of daily living. Therefore, it may be helpful to involve the person in a simple repetitive task or project (such as folding linens or setting the table), especially one that involves helping someone else. Assist the person to meet self-care needs while encouraging independence when possible.

Managing Anxiety. Cognitively impaired persons are particularly vulnerable to anxiety. As persons with dementia become increasingly unsure of their surroundings or what is expected of them, they tend to react with fear and distress. They may feel lost, insecure, and left out. Failure to complete a task once regarded as simple creates anxiety and agitation. Often, they cannot explain the source of their anxiety. The difficulty in developing interventions for the anxious person living with dementia is that the symptoms may also be a sign of underlying illnesses, such as depression, pain, infection, or other physical illnesses.

In many cases, lowering the demands, or perceived demands, on the person will be conducive to promoting comfort. Although maintaining autonomy in any remaining function is a high priority in nursing care, it may decrease persons' anxieties or stress levels to have things done for them at certain points along the illness continuum. Frequently, as the day progresses and they become more fatigued, their ability to cope with stressors is increasingly challenged. Many persons living with dementia experience "sundowning" where they have an increased restlessness and agitation as the day draws to a close. In addition, being sensitive to the pronounced startle reflexes and potential hypersensitivity to touch also helps reduce stress.

The threshold for stress is progressively lowered in AD and other progressive dementias. A healthy person frequently uses cognitive coping strategies when under stress, whereas the person with dementia can no longer use many of these strategies. Effective nursing interventions include simplifying routines, making routines as consistent and predictable as possible, reducing the number of choices the person must make, identifying areas in which control can be maintained, and creating an environment in which the person feels safe. With any of the therapeutic interventions discussed, the nurse is reminded that each person has relative strengths and weaknesses and that sound nursing judgment must be used in each situation.

Commonly used therapeutic approaches may exacerbate anxiety in a person living with dementia. For example, reality orientation is contraindicated in the later stages of dementia because it is possible that the person's disoriented behaviour or language has inherent meaning. If the disoriented behaviour or language is continuously neglected or corrected by the nurse, the person's sense of isolation and anxiety may increase.

Another therapeutic intervention that may (or may not) be contraindicated in persons with dementia is providing the person with information before a difficult or painful procedure. Anticipatory preparation for nonroutine events may produce anxiety because the person is unable to retain information, use reasoning skills, or make sound judgments. Telling persons with dementia that they are scheduled for an upcoming diagnostic test only communicates, on an emotional level, that something distressing is about to happen. A simple explanation immediately before the event may be more helpful.

Managing Catastrophic Reactions. If persons living with dementia react catastrophically, the nurse needs to remain calm, minimize environmental distractions (quiet the environment), get their attention, and softly assure them that they are safe. Give information slowly, clearly, and simply, one step at a time. Let the person know that you understand the fear or other emotional response, such as anger or anxiety.

As the nurse becomes skilled at identifying antecedents to the person's catastrophic reactions, it becomes possible to avoid situations that provoke such reactions. Persons living with AD respond poorly to change and respond well to structure. Attempts to argue or reason with them only escalate their dysfunctional responses.

Interventions for Behaviour Problems

Managing Apathy and Withdrawal. As the person living with dementia withdraws and becomes more apathetic, the nurse is challenged to engage the person in meaningful activities and interactions. To provide this level of care, the nurse must know the premorbid functioning of the person. Close contact with family helps give the nurse ideas about meaningful activities. For example, the use of a multisensory room known as Snoezelen therapy has been shown to have significant improvements in behaviours for short periods after the therapy (Bauer et al., 2015) and involvement with music, art therapy, and a psychomotor activity (Lancioni et al., 2016) have been shown to reduce apathy.

Managing Restlessness and Wandering. Restlessness and wandering are major concerns for family caregivers in the home setting and for staff in long-term care settings. The principal means of dealing with restless persons with dementia who wander into other patients' rooms or out the door in a long-term care setting is to have an adequate number of staff to provide supervision. Electronic security systems and bed occupancy sensors are other strategies that can be used in homes and long-term care settings. An easy strategy is hanging bells on an exit door handle.

Wandering behaviour may be interrupted in more cognitively intact persons by distracting them verbally or visually. Persons who are beyond verbal distraction may be distracted by physically joining them on their walk and then interrupting their course of action and gently redirecting them back to the house or facility. In a long-term care setting, colour and structure of the setting can serve as cues and window boxes that contain photographs of family, personal mementoes, or pieces of art may cue a person living with dementia to identify their room.

Managing Aberrant Behaviour. When persons living with dementia are picking in the air or wringing their hands, simple distraction may work. Hypervocalizations have meaning to the person. The nurse should develop strategies to try to reduce the frequency of vocalizations such as offering comfort measures (change of position, a snack or drink, or warm facecloth to refresh the person's hands and face). Gotell, Brown, and Ekman (2009) revealed that caregiver singing and background music can enable the hypervocal person with dementia to express positive emotions and moods.

Managing Agitated Behaviour. The Alzheimer's Association (2016a) suggests the following strategies when dealing with an agitated person with dementia:

- Find out what may be causing the agitation, and try to understand.

- Provide reassurance: Use calming phrases such as "You're safe here," "I'm sorry that you are upset," and "I will stay until you feel better."
- Involve the person in activities: Try using art, music, or other activities to help engage the person and divert attention away from the anxiety.
- Modify the environment: Decrease noise and distractions, or relocate.
- Find outlets for the person's energy: The person may be looking for something to do. Take a walk or go for a car ride.
- Check yourself: Do not raise your voice, show alarm or offense, or corner, crowd, restrain, criticize, ignore, or argue with the person.

See Clinical Vignette, Box 32.9.

Reducing Disinhibition. Anticipation of disinhibiting behaviour is the key to nursing interventions for this problem. **Disinhibition** can take many forms, from undressing in a public setting to touching someone inappropriately to making cruel statements. With keen behavioural assessment of the person with dementia, the nurse should be able to anticipate the likely socially inappropriate behaviour and redirect the person or change the context of the situation. If the person starts undressing in the dining room, offering a robe and gently escorting him or her to another part of the room might be all that is needed. If the person is trying to fondle a staff member or another patient, having the person

---

BOX 32.9 CLINICAL VIGNETTE

A NURSE'S DILEMMA

It is 8 AM and you are working as a nurse on an inpatient general medical unit of a large urban hospital. A 72-year-old man is admitted to your unit with symptoms of disorientation to time and place, and he is intermittently exhibiting signs of agitation. He thinks you are his child, and he falls asleep while you ask him questions about his symptoms. When you ask him to sign a consent form and hand him a pen, he looks at you as if he didn't understand your request.

The patient's wife tells you that he has had trouble with his memory for the past 3 or 4 years but that her husband has been "acting strange for the past 4 days." The patient's wife denies any history of substance abuse or head injury but states that her husband has been recently diagnosed as having dementia of the Alzheimer's type.

The patient's physician gives a verbal order to restrain the patient "as needed" while writing orders for lab work.

What Do You Think?

- What assessment techniques would you use to determine whether this patient has dementia, delirium, or both?
- What nursing diagnosis would be included in the patient's plan of care?
- What nursing interventions would promote comfort and safety for this patient?
- Is this patient able to give consent?
- What would be the possible outcomes of physically restraining this patient (e.g., would restraints be helpful or harmful for the patient)?

leave the immediate area or redirecting the patient may alleviate the situation.

Social Domain

Social Assessment

Dementia interferes with a person's ability to interact socially as much as it disrupts intellectual functioning. The social domain assessment should include those areas explained in Chapter 31, including functional status, social systems, legal status, and quality of life.

The person's whole social network is affected by dementia, and the needs of the primary caregiver also need to be considered. It is important to assess family caregiver's health status and willingness to use supportive resources to maintain their own health throughout the dementia journey.

The extent of primary caregiver's personal, informal, and formal support systems must also be assessed, as well as personal resources, skills, and stressors. The assessment of the social domain provides objective data on the person's social circumstances and impressions of his or her family structure, sociocultural beliefs, attitudes toward health and disease, myths about dementia, patterns of communication, and degree of psychopathology (such as potential for abuse). When persons with dementia reside in the community, home visits will prove useful because it gives the nurse information about the person in their own environment. From this assessment, the nurse can identify the situational and psychosocial stressors that affect the family and patient and can begin to develop relationships and interventions to strengthen coping strategies.

Nursing Diagnoses for the Social Domain

Typical nursing diagnoses for the social domain are deficient diversional activity, impaired social interaction, social isolation, risk for loneliness, caregiver role strain, ineffective coping, hopelessness, and powerlessness (Carpenito-Moyet, 2017). Outcomes are determined according to nursing diagnoses.

Interventions for the Social Domain

Safety Interventions

One of the primary concerns of the nurse should be safety for the patient. In the early stages of the illness, safety may not seem to be a prime concern. However, early behaviours suggesting dementia are often related to safety, such as the person getting lost while driving or going the wrong way on a highway. Determining the ability of persons with dementia to drive and taking away their drivers' licenses are recognized as challenges for family caregivers and health care providers. Safety may be an issue in the home when the person engages in unsupervised cooking, cleaning, or household tasks. (For resources and suggestions, see Web Links). Day care centres provide a safe and structured environment for these individuals. Family members should be encouraged to continually assess the abilities of the person to live at home safely and to implement appropriate responses and safety strategies.

In hospital and long-term care settings, the safety issues are different. By the time persons with dementia are admitted to a facility, they are in the middle to late stage of their illness. Cognitive impairments are more pronounced, and safety is of greater concern. Most psychogeriatric units are locked, and in a dementia unit, there often is an electronic alarm system to alert the staff of persons attempting to leave the secured floor. Staff and visitors need to be vigilant of unsafe situations.

Environmental Interventions

The need for stimulation varies from individual to individual and can change, depending on many factors, including cognitive intactness, alertness, emotional state, and physical state. The amount of stimulation received also influences each person's behaviour. Lack of stimulation or intense stimulation may cause emotional distress and aggression. Generally speaking, the more severe the dementia, the less stimulation can be integrated. The nurse should attempt to determine each person's optimal level of stimulation at various times of the day. Music and hand massage are effective in reducing agitation in patients with dementia (Hicks-Moore & Robinson, 2008).

Socialization Activities

Overlearned social skills are rarely lost with having dementia. It is not unusual for the person to respond appropriately to a handshake or smile well into the disease process. Even persons who are no longer able to communicate coherently will carry on long discussions with people who are willing to listen and respond. There is a strong risk for social isolation because of communication difficulties. Reinforcing social remarks and gestures, such as eye contact, smiling, greetings, and farewells, can promote a sense of competency and self-esteem (Box 32.10). Pet therapy may enhance social interaction in cognitively impaired individuals. It is important to remember that the ability to laugh and play is not lost, and the psychosocial benefits of humour are well known.

The nurse who engages a person with dementia in an activity is encouraged to (1) avoid confrontation, (2) allow the level of autonomy best tolerated by the person, (3) simplify activities and directions to the point that they can be mastered, (4) provide adequate structure, and (5) recognize that instructions may not be carried out correctly. It is important to monitor the length of time, crowding, and noise level when the person participates in a group activity because all these factors may increase his or her stress level.

Activities that elicit pleasant memories from an earlier time in the person's life (reminiscence) may produce a soothing effect. Eliciting pleasant memories may be

---

BOX 32.10 Psychoeducation Checklist: Tips for Caregivers of Persons With Dementia

When caring for the person living with dementia, be sure to include the caregivers, as appropriate, and address the following topic areas in the teaching plan:

- Psychopharmacologic agents, if used, including drug action, dosage, frequency, and possible adverse effects
- Rest and activity
- Consistency in routines
- Nutrition and hydration
- Sleep and comfort measures
- Protective environment
- Communication and social interaction
- Diversional measures
- Community resources

---

enhanced by gentle stimulation of the person's senses, for example, viewing and discussing photo albums, looking at personal memorabilia, providing a favourite food item, playing a musical instrument, or listening to music the person preferred in younger years.

It may be useful to incorporate movement or dance along with a singing exercise. If the person with dementia resists structured exercise, it may be because of a fear of falling or injury or of demonstrating to others that their health is failing. Persons often forget how to move or how to coordinate their movements in relation to objects. Therefore, exercise should be light and enjoyable. Encourage the person to participate and to take rest periods at intervals throughout the activity in an effort to minimize stress (see Web Link on Power of Music).

Home Visits

Recognizing the importance of supporting persons with dementia to remain at home for as long as possible and support their family caregivers in sustaining their role, cost-effective in-home and community-based long-term care services are expanding. Their goals are to maintain such persons in a self-determining environment that provides the most homelike atmosphere possible, to allow maximum personal choice for care recipients and caregivers, and to encourage optimal family caregiving involvement without overwhelming the resources of the family network. All services for these persons and their families are provided within a context of continuity of care, a concept that mandates access to a variety of health and supportive services over an unpredictable and changing clinical course.

Community Actions

Home care nurses and community public health nurses working with persons with dementia are especially knowledgeable about all aspect of the illness and care. These nurses often consult with local organizations, such as the Alzheimer Society of Canada, and participate on interprofessional teams. Issues of care, safety, and access to services often require professional expertise and influence.

Family Interventions

Family caregivers are faced with extreme challenges. Caregivers are either spouses of the person or children, usually a daughter, who may also have other responsibilities, such as children and a job. The caregiver often feels isolated, frustrated, and trapped. The potential for abuse of the person with dementia is significant, especially if agitated and aggressive behaviours are present. The use of home care services may assist in decreasing the burden and depression in family caregivers.

In 2012, more than 8 million Canadians, or 28% of people aged 15 and over, provided help or care to a relative or friend with a chronic health problem. Family caregivers are more likely to be women (30%) in comparison to men (26%) (Turcotte, 2016). It is important that the nurse recognize and assess the needs of the caregivers for support and relief from the 24-hour responsibility. Determining the availability of family members or friends to assist with personal care of the person with dementia should be included in the assessment (see Box 32.10). Home care may assist with personal care needs of the person and provide respite for the caregiver. Caregivers should be encouraged to attend support groups and carve out personal time. Educational and training programs may help in understanding the complex nature of dementia. Community resources, such as day care centres, home care agencies, and other community services, can be an important aspect of nursing care for the person and their family caregivers (see Box 32.11).

Spiritual Domain

The changes in cognition and ability to communicate that occur in dementia may discourage some nurses from attempting to provide individualized spiritual care. Yet despite communication impairment, the need to be respected, to have hope, and to connect with others and, perhaps, a higher power does not diminish. If the spiritual domain is neglected in care, the person with dementia may be denied important comforting and supportive measures. It is important to understand the person's spiritual beliefs as early as possible in the progression of dementia when they may be better able to explain what has spiritual importance for them. Their religious beliefs, rituals, and their participation in a religious community can be explored at this time. The diagnosis of dementia may have brought despair that

BOX 32.11 Research for Best Practice

EMERGENCE OF DEMENTIA AS A FIRST NATIONS' HEALTH CONCERN

From Jacklin, K., Walker, J., & Shawande, M. (2013). The emergence of dementia as a health concern among First Nations populations in Alberta, Canada. Canadian Journal of Public Health, *104(1), e39–e44.*

The Questions: Dementia is predicted to increase as a health challenge for Canadian health care systems, yet there are few data available concerning the prevalence of dementia in First Nations communities. The questions asked in this study were as follows: Are rates for dementia increasing more rapidly among First Nations (FN) populations than non–First Nation (NFN) populations? Are FN populations experiencing dementia at a younger age than NFN populations? Does the sex distribution of dementia differ between these populations?

Methods: Population-level data from Alberta Health and Wellness were analyzed. Physician-treated prevalence rates for dementia were calculated for FN and NFN populations seeking treatment between 1998 and 2009. Using linear regression models, trends in age-adjusted rates over time were compared; age and sex effects were examined.

Findings: The age-standardized prevalence of dementia rose higher for FN populations (7.5/1,000) than NFN populations (5.6/1,000). The prevalence also rose more quickly for FNs ($p = 0.032$). Dementia appears to disproportionately affect younger age groups (60 to 69; 70 to 79) and males in FN populations when FN and NFN data are compared. The researchers note that the increase in prevalence may be driven by trends among FN populations, such as demographic transitions (the rate

of FN population increase; the number of those over 60 is predicted to increase 3.4 times by 2031), factors related to social determinants of health (e.g., lower income and lower educational attainment), and higher rates of conditions/factors associated with dementia (e.g., diabetes, heart disease, smoking, and obesity). Research associating increased risk of dementia with posttraumatic stress disorder may also play a role, given the traumatic legacy of residential school experiences.

Implications for Nursing: Nurses need to be cognizant of the increased risk for dementia among FN populations and to work to identify and help address preventable factors contributing to it. As well, population-level health databases need to have data elements that allow identification of disease prevalence among First Nations, Inuit, and Métis populations.

Update: February 27, 2017: As this 2013 research indicated, the rate for dementia in Canada among indigenous peoples is cause for concern. It is higher than that of the nonindigenous population. The Government of Canada, as part of its Dementia Research Strategy, has invested $1 million in research that addresses the needs of indigenous peoples with, or at risk of developing, dementia. One project focuses on the validation of a Canadian Indigenous Cognitive Assessment Tool and another explores a community approach to care of indigenous peoples with dementia. Source: www.canada.ca/en/institutes-health-research/news/2017/02/ government _of_ Canada invests in dementiaresearchaboutindigenouspeop.html

---

challenged the person's existing spiritual beliefs. This needs to be recognized, and opportunities for the person to express spiritual distress should be created.

For persons with dementia, Procedural and Emotional Religious Activity Therapy (PERAT) is an approach that may provide some spiritual support (Vance, Moore, Farr, & Struzick, 2008). Based on matching the cognitive ability of the person with the cognitive demands of an emotionally meaningful activity, such as a religious or spiritual activity, PERAT involves an assessment of the person's religious and spiritual history and of their cognitive status. Tasks are selected for their procedural memory capability and emotional salience to the person. Materials (i.e., items that have an emotional attachment) for the activities are obtained, usually from family members. Making family photographs, religious

pictures, and books available within the person's setting can be helpful and soothing. Activities can include reciting favourite scripture, engaging in prayer, holding a religious icon, or maintaining a shrine. This is a counterproductive approach if the activities are not spirituality appropriate to the individual person, and more research is required to develop this approach (Vance et al., 2008).

Evaluation and Treatment Outcomes

The objectives of nursing interventions are to help the person living with dementia remain as independent as possible and to function at the highest cognitive, physical, emotional, spiritual, and social levels. The maximum level of functional ability can be promoted when nursing care is related to and based on the remaining abilities of the person. Those who receive diagnoses of AD or other types of dementia still have a wide and varying range of functional abilities. As cognitive decline progresses, there is a tendency for caregivers to perform more and more tasks for the person. It is essential to assess for strengths and to assist in the maintenance of existing skills. Adaptive and appropriate behaviours continue to some degree, even in the presence of increasing cognitive decline. It is important for nursing interventions to focus on more than the maintenance of optimal physical functional ability; interventions also must focus on meeting psychological, social, and spiritual needs of the person.

Nurses can maintain quality of life if they protect a person's overall well-being by balancing physical, mental, social, and spiritual health. Figure 32.3 illustrates the truly bio/psycho/social/spiritual aspects of the treatment of individuals with dementia by summarizing potential outcomes of nursing care.

Forbes et al. (2008) and Jansen et al. (2009) studied the role of home care and other agencies in meeting the needs of Canadians with dementia and their family and friend caregivers. Service *availability* and *acceptability* were the overarching themes of the study findings. Family caregivers desired an integrated continuing care model that includes the person with dementia and

family as partners in care, addresses all the determinants of health, and encompasses sensitivity, flexibility, and diversity. Home care providers described challenges to service availability as including service waitlists, lack of home care provider training, lack of community-based dementia care, lack of service infrastructure, and sociocultural and geographical barriers. Agency partnerships, however, facilitated availability. Key to the acceptability of services was comprehensive personal care with adequate service time for such care, as well as for support of the family caregivers. A difficulty family caregivers specifically identified was navigating the health care system. This type of research, focused on the voices of those directly affected by and involved with dementia care, has direct implications for the evolution of services.

Continuum of Care

Community Care

In 2012, 2.2 million Canadians 15 years of age and older received help or care at home because of a long-term health condition, a disability, or problems related to aging. However, nearly half a million Canadians did not receive the needed help or care in the 12 previous months for a chronic health condition. Of the 2.2 million Canadians who did receive home care,

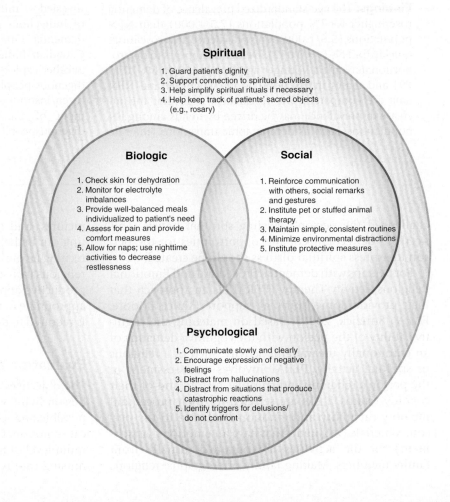

Figure 32.3. Bio/psycho/social/spiritual interventions for persons with dementia.

15% (331,000) did not receive all the help they needed (Turcotte, 2014). These estimates illustrate the need for greater investment in Canadian home care services.

Service delivery models vary across the country, with services provided through the public sector and/ or contracted with private sector providers. Most home care programs provide case management, nursing, and personal care. There is a wide variation in the provision of therapies such as physiotherapy, occupational therapy, speech and language pathology, respiratory therapy, dietetic care, and social work. Similarly, home care programs vary in the range of and access to homemaking services such as cleaning, laundry, meal preparation, and, very rarely, assistance with transportation, shopping, and banking (Canadian Home Care Association, 2013). Collaboration among health care providers of different disciplines and in various settings is needed to meet the highly individualized needs of persons living with dementia and their family caregivers (Forbes et al., 2012). For more information on caring for the person with dementia, see Nursing Care Plan 32.1.

NURSING CARE PLAN 32.1

PERSON LIVING WITH DEMENTIA

LW is a 76-year-old widow who lives with her oldest son. He is with her during the evening and night. Recently, her children have noticed that she is becoming more forgetful and seems to have periods of confusion. LW refuses to see a health care provider but did agree to go in for a routine checkup. Her daughter helped her get dressed and took her to the primary health care clinic.

Setting: Primary Health Care Clinic

Baseline Assessment: A well-groomed woman is accompanied by her daughter. LW says there is nothing wrong, but her daughter disagrees. A review of body systems reveals poor hearing and vision but is otherwise unremarkable. MMSE score is 19. Daughter reports that LW has become very suspicious of neighbours and has changed her locks several times.

Associated Diagnoses	Medications
Probable dementia of the Alzheimer's type (some memory problems)	galantamine (Reminyl) 4 mg bid, titrate to 8 mg bid over 4 wk.
History of breast cancer, unilateral mastectomy, arthritis	
Other relevant factors:	
Social problems (suspiciousness)	

Nursing Diagnosis 1: Impaired Memory

Defining Characteristics	Related Factors
Inability to recall information	Neurocognitive changes associated with dementia
Inability to recall past events	
Observed instances of forgetfulness	
Forgets to perform daily activities—grooming	

Outcomes

Initial	Long Term
Maintain or improve current memory.	Delay cognitive decline associated with dementia.

(Continued)

NURSING CARE PLAN 32.1 *(Continued)*

Interventions	Rationale	Ongoing Assessment
Develop memory cues in home. Have clocks and calendars well displayed. Make lists for person living with dementia.	Maintaining current level of memory involves providing cues that will help person recall information.	Contact family members for the person's ability to use memory cues.
Teach the person and family about taking an acetylcholinesterase inhibitor. Review expected effects, side effects, and adverse effects. Develop a titration schedule with family to decrease the appearance of side effects.	Confidence and self-esteem improve when a person feels better.	Monitor response to medications and suggestions.
Observe the person for visuospatial impairment. If present, sequence habitual activities, such as eating, dressing, bathing, etc.	Visuospatial impairment is one of the symptoms of dementia.	Observe for appropriate dress, bathing, eating, etc.

Evaluation

Outcomes	Revised Outcomes	Interventions
LW did have some improvement in memory. Suspiciousness and grooming improved.	Continue maintaining memory.	Continue with memory cues and galantamine.

Acute Care Setting

Although admission to an acute care setting is not likely related to dementia, older adults with other conditions may have symptoms of dementia. A comprehensive admission assessment that encompasses dementia, followed by the development of an individualized (and constantly updated) care plan that involves the patient, significant others, and a variety of health care professionals, is the foundation of an effective and efficient predischarge plan. Attention to all aspects of this process is necessary for continuity of care. The hospital-based nurse may initiate family education and counselling as part of discharge planning.

Nursing Home Care

As dementia progresses, most family members can no longer manage the symptoms, such as wandering at night and incontinence. A nursing care home may be necessary where care is usually provided by nurses' aides, who need support and direction from other health care professionals. Persons with dementia require complex nursing care, yet the skill level of people providing the direct care is often minimal, making education and support of the care providers a significant focus for nursing homes.

■ OTHER MAJOR NCDS (DEMENTIAS)

Dementia symptoms may occur as a result of a number of NCDs and underlying aetiologies. The subsequent sections provide a brief description of some of the aetiologic subtypes identified in the *Diagnostic and Statistical Manual of Mental Disorders* (5th edition) (APA, 2013). In each case, significant cognitive decline must be evident in one or more cognitive domains (e.g., language, learning and memory, social cognition); the cognitive deficits affect independence in everyday life, and they do not occur exclusively with delirium (APA, 2013, p. 602). Nursing interventions for the subtypes of major NCDs are similar to those described for individuals with AD.

Vascular Neurocognitive Disorder

Vascular dementia, also called multi-infarct dementia, is the second most common form of dementia following AD. More than 20% of all those who have dementia have vascular dementia. When AD and vascular dementia occur at the same time, the condition is called mixed dementia. Vascular dementia occurs from multiple cerebral infarctions (transient ischemic attacks [TIAs]) or a stroke. These occur when blood flow in the brain is blocked or a blood vessel bleeds, preventing the blood from flowing properly through the vessel. Certain medical conditions such as type II diabetes, high blood pressure, and an unhealthy lifestyle are all contributory factors to developing vascular dementia. It is essential that anyone who demonstrates symptoms of dementia or who has a history of stroke should have a complete physical examination that includes diet, smoking, medication history, review of recent stressors, and an array of laboratory tests.

The behaviour changes that result from vascular dementia are similar to those found in AD, such as loss of memory, judgment and reasoning, depression, emotional lability, wandering or getting lost in familiar places, bladder or bowel incontinence, difficulty in following instructions, gait changes, and problems handling daily activities. However, these symptoms usually begin more suddenly, rather than developing slowly, as is the case in AD. Often, the neurologic symptoms associated with a TIA are minimal (slight weakness in an extremity, dizziness, or slurred speech) and may last only a few days. Thus, the clinical progression is often described as steplike deterioration, with the person's cognitive and functional status plateauing for a period of time, followed by a rapid decline in function after another series of small strokes. Treatment aims to reduce the primary risk factors for vascular dementia, including hypertension, diabetes, and additional strokes. Interventions that reduce the tendency of the blood to clot and of platelets to aggregate include lifestyle changes (diet, exercise, and smoking cessation) and using appropriate medications. Increasingly, physicians are recommending anticoagulants and medication to control hypertension, elevated levels of cholesterol, and glucose. There is insufficient and inconsistent evidence on which to make a recommendation either for or against the use of the currently available CIs for the treatment of vascular dementia (Gauthier et al., 2012a, 2012b).

NCD (Dementia) With Lewy Bodies

The clinical features of DLB and Parkinson's disease dementia (PDD; see below) often overlap. DLB should be diagnosed when this pattern of dementia occurs before or concurrently with PDD. In addition, AD and DLB frequently coexist. Persons with DLB may have symptoms much like those of both Parkinson's disease and AD, making it impossible to offer guidelines that could separate the diagnoses with a high specificity (CDKTN, 2012).

DLB usually progresses quickly. Symptoms include a progressive loss of memory, language, reasoning, and other higher mental functions, and occasionally, depression, anxiety, and apathy. Obvious changes in alertness may also happen. The person may be sleepy during the day but wide awake at night, unable to sleep. Visual hallucinations are common and can be worse during times of increased confusion. The visual hallucinations often come back repeatedly and typically are of people, children, or animals. People with the disease may also make errors in perception, for example, seeing faces in a carpet pattern. Some features of DLB that resemble those in Parkinson's disease include rigidity (stiffness of muscles), tremors (shaking), stooped posture, and slow, shuffling movements.

NCD (Dementia) With Parkinson's Disease

PDD can be diagnosed when there is well-established Parkinson's disease followed by gradual onset of cognitive decline. Parkinson's disease is a neurodegenerative disease. The most common symptoms affect movement such as **bradykinesia** (the slowing of body movements), rigidity, resting tremor, and postural changes. The person's gait is unstable, resulting in frequent falls. Approximately 20% of people with Parkinson's disease will develop PDD, usually 10 to 15 years following a diagnosis of Parkinson's disease. The hallmark abnormality in Parkinson's disease is Lewy bodies, deposits of a protein called alpha-synuclein, in a specific brain region critical for control of movement. People can live with Parkinson's for years, although currently there is no cure. Medical treatment of Parkinson's disease typically is with anticholinergics and dopamine agonists. However, anticholinergic medications may cause adverse mental effects (e.g., confusion, memory problems, restlessness, and hallucinations) (Katzenschlager, Sampaio, Costa, & Lees, 2003).

Frontotemporal NCD (Dementia)

FTD tends to occur at a younger age than AD, accounting for approximately 2% to 5% of all dementia. FTD is an umbrella term for a group of rare disorders that primarily affect the frontal and temporal lobes of the brain, the areas generally associated with personality and behaviour. With this form of dementia, a person may have symptoms such as sudden onset of memory loss, behaviour changes, or difficulties with speech and movement. In some cases, brain cells in these areas shrink or die. In other cases, the brain cells in these areas get larger, containing round, silver "Pick's bodies." Pick's disease refers to a subtype of FTD that has these specific abnormalities.

Since the frontal and temporal areas of the brain are affected, early symptoms of FTD often involve behaviour and/or speech. Changes in behaviour may include becoming either withdrawn and apathetic or disinhibited and impulsive. The person may lose interest in personal hygiene, become easily distracted, or repeat the same action over and over again. Overeating or compulsively putting objects in the mouth may occur. Sometimes incontinence is an early symptom of FTD. There may be significant decline in language ability (e.g., speech production, word finding, object naming, grammar, or word comprehension) (APA, 2013).

A person with FTD may have changes in personality but continue to manage the running of a home and manage all the psychomotor and spatial skills needed to maintain employment. However, the person often loses his or her position due to changes in personality. The individual may become easily irritated, loud, and argumentative. This is particularly distressing to a family if they do not understand that these are symptoms of FTD.

Dementia Caused by Other General Medical Conditions

People of any age, race, or gender are at risk for dementia caused by a medical condition known to cause cerebral pathology. Older adults are particularly vulnerable to the development of dementia caused by general medical conditions because so many are affected by one or more of these illnesses. Strong relationships have been reported between the following chronic medical illness and the development of dementia.

NCD (Dementia) Caused by HIV Infection

The noncommunicable disease (NCD) of dementia associated with HIV infection is known as AIDS dementia complex (ADC). ADC has been observed in nearly two thirds of all persons with AIDS. AIDS is caused by human immunodeficiency virus 1 (HIV-1), which infects and destroys T lymphocytes as well as the CNS. HIV-1 directly invades the CNS and allows opportunistic infections of the CNS and other organ systems. Although there has been a proportional increase in ADC at AIDS diagnosis, survival has improved markedly in the era of highly active antiretroviral therapy (HAART) (Dore et al., 2003). The essential features of ADC are disabling cognitive impairment accompanied by motor dysfunction, speech problems, and behavioural change. Dementia only exists when neurocognitive impairment in the person is severe enough to interfere markedly with day-to-day function.

NCD (Dementia) Due to Traumatic Brain Injury

When head trauma occurs in the context of a single traumatic injury, the resulting dementia is usually not progressive, but repeated head injury (e.g., from the sport of boxing) may lead to a progressive dementia. When the nurse observes progressive decline in intellectual functioning after a single incident of head trauma, the possibility of another superimposed process must be considered. Head injury associated with a prolonged loss of consciousness (days to months) may be followed by delirium, dementia, or a profound alteration in personality. Falls are a common cause of head injury in the older adult. Subarachnoid haemorrhage is often a result of an unwitnessed fall and often gets missed, leading to the potential for permanent brain damage and/or death. Subarachnoid haemorrhage is treatable if caught early.

The degree and type of cognitive impairment or behavioural disturbances demonstrated by a person with head trauma depend on the location and extent of the brain injury (as with other forms of dementia). Repeated head injuries, such as those sustained by young, healthy boxers, may lead to *dementia pugilistica* or "punchdrunk syndrome." Symptoms and signs of dementia pugilistica develop progressively over a long latent period sometimes amounting to decades, with the average time of onset being about 12 to 16 years after the start of a career in boxing. The condition is thought to affect around 15% to 20% of professional boxers. Additionally, chronic traumatic encephalopathy has been reported in athletes who engage in contact sports and experience repeated head injuries and concussions over the course of their careers (Omalu, Fitzsimmons, Hammers, & Bailes, 2010; Omalu, Hamilton, Kamboh, DeKosky, & Bailes, 2010).

NCD (Dementia) Due to Huntington's Disease

Huntington's disease is a progressive, genetically transmitted autosomal dominant disorder. Anyone with a parent with Huntington's has a 50% chance of inheriting the gene. People are born with the defective gene, but symptoms usually do not appear until middle age. Symptoms include the following: involuntary movements such as twitches and muscle spasms; balance problems; personality changes such as irritability, depression, and mood swings; difficulties with memory, concentration, learning new things, or making decisions; and, in late stage, difficulty concentrating, eating independently, or swallowing. Medications can help manage symptoms, but cannot slow down or stop the disease, and there is currently no cure for Huntington's disease. However, there are several drug trials under way, which may discover new treatment approaches (Alzheimer Society of Canada, 2016a).

NCD (Dementia) Due to Prion Disease

Prion disease is a rare form of deadly dementia that is caused by infectious proteins known as *prions*. When prions are abnormally shaped, they can attack the brain, kill cells, and create gaps or holes in brain tissue. Prion diseases affect both humans and animals. The best-known prion disease in humans is CJD. It affects about one to two persons per million worldwide each year, with about 35 new cases being diagnosed in Canada every year (Alzheimer Society of Canada, 2016b).

There are two types of CJD: classic CJD and variant CJD (vCJD). Classic CJD is primarily composed of the sporadic type of CJD, which accounts for 90% of cases in Canada. It affects people between 45 and 75 years old. The cause of sporadic CJD is not known. The disease appears without warning and most people die within 1 year. vCJD affects younger people with an average age of 28 years. This form of CJD can develop from eating beef or game meat (e.g., such as elk, deer, moose) that was infected with bovine spongiform encephalopathy (BSE), and a recent case was reported to be transmitted by a blood transfusion from a person with vCJD in the United Kingdom.

At present, there is no effective treatment for the disease, and nothing has been found to slow progression of the illness. Because of its rapid clinical course, an important nursing role is assisting family members to understand and come to terms with the illness and to make decisions related to treatment setting and life-sustaining treatments.

Substance-/Medication-Induced NCD (Dementia)

If dementia results from the persisting effects of a substance (e.g., abuse of drugs, a medication, or exposure to toxins), the person is diagnosed with substance-/medication-induced NCD (dementia). Other causes of dementia (e.g., dementia caused by a general medical condition) must always be considered, even in a person with a dependence on or exposure to a substance. For example, head injuries often result from substance use and may be the underlying cause of the NCD.

Drugs of abuse are the most common toxins in young adults, and prescription drugs are the most common toxins in older people. In older persons, dementia results from the use of long-acting benzodiazepines, barbiturates, meprobamate, and a host of other drugs, depending on their dose and the length of time they have been used. Drugs such as flurazepam (Dalmane), with a half-life of more than 120 hours, accumulate rapidly in a person's body. Other drugs accumulate more slowly or require relatively high doses for toxicity to develop. A toxic aetiology should be suspected in every person with a probable diagnosis of dementia. The nurse should inquire about exposure to drugs and toxins (exposure to toxins at work sites, medication use, and recreational drug use), and any substances known to be potentially injurious to the nervous system should be withdrawn if possible.

Most of the dementias in this category are related to chronic alcohol abuse. Understanding the cognitive deficits associated with chronic alcohol consumption is complicated. Alcoholic dementia is directly related to the toxic effects of alcohol, although the vitamin deficiencies associated with alcoholism (thiamine and niacin) are also known to be aetiologically related to dementia. Individuals with alcoholism also have a high incidence of systemic illnesses that can affect cognition (e.g., cirrhosis, cardiomyopathy), and they are susceptible to repeated head injuries, which carry cognitive consequences of their own.

Chemicals and organic compounds that impair functioning of the CNS usually have their primary effects on other body systems: the gastrointestinal, renal, hepatic, blood-forming, and peripheral nervous systems. For example, metal poisonings generally produce gastrointestinal symptoms and peripheral neuropathy. Cognitive changes with poisoning tend to be more characteristic of delirium than dementia, with altered levels

of consciousness a prominent feature. Many adolescents and indigent adults engage in the act of "huffing" because the cost of purchasing spray paint, hair spray, glue, and other aerosol products is relatively inexpensive (compared with illicit street drugs). The nurse is reminded to evaluate people who abuse drugs for signs of cognitive impairment because neural and cognitive symptoms tend to appear before permanent brain damage occurs. It is also important to realize that the person's cognitive status may not immediately improve after discontinuation of use of the offending agent. The effects of drugs taken for a long period may be long lasting, and improvement may be slow following discontinuation of drug use. For example, in dementia associated with chronic alcoholism, cognition may improve only after many months of abstinence.

 SUMMARY OF KEY POINTS

- NCDs, such as delirium and dementia, are characterized clinically by significant deficits in cognition or memory that represent a clear-cut change from a previous level of functioning. In some disorders, the loss of cognitive function is progressive, such as in AD.
- Two major syndromes of cognitive impairment in older adults are delirium and chronic cognitive impairments, such as dementia. It is crucial to recognize the differences because the interventions and expected outcomes of the two syndromes differ.
- The symptoms of depression can overlap with the symptoms of both delirium and dementia. One individual may have one, two, or three of the conditions in the triad of delirium, dementia, and depression simultaneously.
- Delirium is characterized by a disturbance in attention (e.g., ability to focus) and awareness (reduced orientation to environment) that develops over a short period of time. It requires rapid detection and treatment because in 25% of cases, it is a sign of impending death.
- Usually, delirium is caused by a combination of precipitating factors. The most commonly identified causes are medications, infections (particularly urinary tract and upper respiratory tract infections), fluid and electrolyte imbalance, and metabolic disturbances such as electrolyte imbalance or poor nutrition. Other important predisposing factors include advanced age, brain damage, pre-existing dementia, and bio/psycho/social/spiritual stressors.
- The primary goal of treatment of delirium is prevention or resolution of the acute confusional episode with return to previous cognitive status and interventions focusing on (1) elimination or

correction of the underlying cause and (2) symptomatic, safety, and supportive measures.

- Dementia is characterized by the gradual onset of decline in cognitive function, especially memory, usually accompanied by changes in behaviour and personality. Neurologic changes and damage in the brain may be present for many years before symptoms present. Although there are many proposed reasons for these changes, they are not entirely understood. Thus, cures for specific types of dementia have not been discovered.

- AD is an example of a progressive, degenerative dementia. Treatment efforts currently focus on the reduction of cognitive symptoms (e.g., memory loss, confusion, and problems with learning, speech, and reasoning) in attempts to improve the quality of life for both the person living with dementia and their family caregivers.

- Several potential explanations for the presentation of AD symptoms are currently being explored: the buildup of beta-amyloid plaques, neurofibrillary tangles that become chemically altered, excessive neuroinflammatory responses, and oxidative stress that many researchers believe may be the primary event in AD as oxidative stress are responsible for the impairment of both mitochondria and calcium regulation. In addition, there is a rare FAD that is almost totally attributable to genes that have mutated to an extent that makes them function abnormally resulting in a form of AD.

- Symptoms of NCD (dementia) may occur as a result of a number of other types of NCDs including vascular dementia, DLB, PDD, and FTD. Symptoms of dementia may also be related to other conditions such as HIV infection, traumatic brain injury, Huntington's disease, and prion disease.

- Educating families and caregivers about what to expect related to the progressive cognitive decline and behaviour changes, safety issues, and available community resources is essential to ensuring appropriate and adequate care.

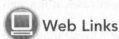 Web Links

the4at.com A brief clinical instrument for delirium detection, developed in the United Kingdom, can be found at this site. It is free to download and use. A link to references regarding its validation is provided.

alzheimer.ca The Alzheimer Society of Canada website provides information and resources related to AD.

alzheimer.ca/en/Living-with-dementia/Caring-for-someone/End-of-life-care/Managing-pain This site provides detail and a rating scale for managing pain in persons with AD.

alzheimer.ca/~/media/Files/national/brochures-day-to-day/day_to_day_meal_times_e.pdf A person-centred approach including strategies for dealing with mealtimes for persons with AD is addressed at this site.

alzheimer.ca/en/We-can-help/Resources/Power-of-music This is the link to the Power of Music video discussed in this chapter.

alz.org The Alzheimer's Association Web site provides information, resources, and consumer and caregiver support. This a US-based organization.

alzheimers.org.uk/caring The Alzheimer's Society, UK, Web site provides information about dementia, symptoms and diagnosis of dementia, living with dementia, caring for a person with dementia, and the latest research on dementia.

brainxchange.ca/public/home.aspx This Web site describes the latest resources and upcoming knowledge exchange opportunities. Topics of interest can be discussed by connecting with others in the network or through support from brainXchange staff.

livingwithdementia.uwaterloo.ca/caresupport/index.html This site addresses strategies and support for persons living with dementia.

radar.fsi.ulaval.ca/documents/Formulaire_RADAR_en_2014-Autv4.pdf RADAR stands for *Recognize Active Delirium As part of Routine* and is a 3-step process to identify delirium in older adults developed at Laval University.

rnao.ca/bpg/guidelines/assessment-and-care-older-adults-delirium-dementia-and-depression A best practice guideline on the assessment of care of delirium, dementia, and depression in older adults can be found at this site.

References

Alzheimer Society of Canada. (2014). *Amyloid imaging.* Retrieved from http://www.alzheimer.ca/en/News-and-Events/feature-stories/amyloid-imaging

Alzheimer Society of Canada. (2016a). *Dementia numbers.* Retrieved from http://www.alzheimer.ca/en/About-dementia/What-is-dementia/Dementia-numbers

Alzheimer Society of Canada. (2016b). Mild cognitive impairment. Retrieved from http://www.alzheimer.ca/~/media/Files/national/Other-dementias/other_dementias_MCI_e.pdf

Alzheimer Society of Canada. (2016c). *Stages of Alzheimer's disease (what happens).* Retrieved from http://www.alzheimer.ca/en/About-dementia/Alzheimer-s-disease/Stages-of-Alzheimer-s-disease

Alzheimer Society of Canada. (2016d). *Ten warning signs of AD.* Retrieved from http://www.alzheimer.ca/en/About-dementia/Alzheimer-s-disease/10-warning-signs

Alzheimer's & Dementia Caregiver Centre. (2016). *Depression and Alzheimer's.* Retrieved from https://www.alz.org/care/alzheimers-dementia-depression.asp

Alzheimer's Association. (2016a). *Anxiety and agitation.* Retrieved from https://www.alz.org/care/alzheimers-dementia-agitation-anxiety.asp

Alzheimer's Association. (2016b). *Inside the brain: Alzheimer's brain tour.* Retrieved from http://www.alz.org/research/science/alzheimers_brain_tour.asp

Alzheimer's Association. (2016c). *Mild cognitive impairment.* Retrieved from http://www.alz.org/dementia/mild-cognitive-impairment-mci.asp

Alzheimer's Society UK. (2016a). *New drug found to safely reduce amyloid beta production in people with Alzheimer's disease.* Retrieved from https://www.alzheimers.org.uk/site/scripts/news_article.php?newsID=2688

Alzheimer's Society UK. (2016b). *Risk factors for dementia.* Retrieved from https://www.alzheimers.org.uk/site/scripts/documents_info.php?documentID=102

American Geriatrics Society. (2013). *Choosing wisely: Five things that physicians and patients should question.* Retrieved from http://www.americangeriatrics.org/files/documents/jgs12226.pdf

American Geriatrics Society 2015 Beers Criteria Update Expert Panel (2015). American Geriatrics Society 2015 updated Beers criteria for potentially inappropriate medication use in older adults. *Journal of the American Geriatrics Society, 63*(11), 2227–2246. doi:10.1111/jags.13702

American Psychiatric Association. (2013). *Diagnostic and statistical manual of mental disorders* (5th ed.). Washington, DC: Author.

American Psychiatric Association. (2016). *New practice guidelines on antipsychotic use in dementia*. Retrieved from http://www.medscape.com/viewarticle/862795

Balas, M. C., Rice, M., Chaperon, C., Smith, H., Disbot, M., & Fuchs, B. (2012). Management of delirium in critically ill older adults. *Critical Care Nurse, 32*(4), 15–26.

Bauer, M., Rayner, J. A., Tang, J., Koch, S., While, C., & O'Keefe, F. (2015). An evaluation of Snoezelen(®) compared to 'common best practice' for allaying the symptoms of wandering and restlessness among residents with dementia in aged care facilities. *Geriatric Nursing, 36*(6), 462–6. doi:10.1016/j.gerinurse.2015.07.005

Boettger, S., Friedlander, M., Breitbart, W., & Passik, S. (2011). Aripiprazole and haloperidol in the treatment of delirium. *Australian and New Zealand Journal of Psychiatry, 45*(6), 477–482.

Brodaty, H., Aerts, L. Crawford, J. D., Hefferman, M., Kochan, N. A., Reppermund, S., ... Sachdev, P. S. (2017). Operationalizing the diagnostic criteria for mild cognitive impairment: The salience of objective measures in predicting incident dementia. *American Journal of Geriatric Psychiatry 25*(5):485–497. doi:10.1016/j.jagp.2016.12.012

Brown, C. A., Berry, R., Tan, M., Khoshia, A., Turlapati, L., & Swedlove, F. (2013). A critique of the evidence base for non-pharmacological sleep interventions for persons with dementia. *Dementia, 12*(2), 174–201.

Canadian Coalition for Seniors' Mental Health. (2006). *National guidelines for seniors' mental health: Assessment and treatment of delirium*. Toronto, ON: Authors.

Canadian Dementia Knowledge Translation Network (CDKTN). (2012). *Recommendations for the diagnosis and treatment of dementia 2012: Based on the Canadian Consensus Conference on the Diagnosis and Treatment of Dementia 2012 (CCCDTD4)*. Retrieved from http://www.slideboom.com/presentations/702016/Canadian-Consensus-Conference-2012-Dementia-Diagnosis-and-Treatment-Recommendations

Canadian Home Care Association (CHCA). (2013). *Portraits of home care in Canada*. Ottawa, ON: Author.

Candy, B., Jackson, K. C., Jones, L., Leurent, B., Tookman, A., & King, M. (2012). Drug therapy for delirium in terminally ill adult patients. *Cochrane Database of Systematic Reviews, 11*, CD004770. doi:10.1002/14651858.CD004770.pub2

Carpenito-Moyet, L. (2017). *Handbook of nursing diagnoses* (15th ed.). Philadelphia, PA: Wolters Kluwer.

Carter, C. L., Resnick, E. M., Mallampalli, M., & Kalbarczyk, A. (2012). Sex and gender differences in Alzheimer's disease: Recommendations for future research. *Journal of Women's Health, 21*(10), 1018–1023.

Casey, G. (2012). Alzheimer's and other dementias. *Kai Tiaki Nursing New Zealand, 18*(6), 20–24.

Cmiel, C. A., Karr, D. M., Gasser, D. M., Oliphant, L. M., & Neveau, A. J. (2004). Noise control: A nursing team's approach to sleep promotion. *American Journal of Nursing, 104*(2), 40–48.

DeJong, R., Osterlund, O. W., & Roy, G. W. (1989). Measurement of quality-of-life changes in patients with Alzheimer's disease. *Clinical Therapeutics, 11*, 545–554.

Diamond, J. (2011). *Alzheimer's disease: What's it all about? Where do we stand in the search for a cure? Hope, courage, progress*. Toronto, ON: Alzheimer Society of Canada. Retrieved from http://www.alzheimer.ca/~/media/Files/national/Research/Research_Lay_Report_2011_e.ashx

Dore, G. J., McDonald, A., Li, Y., Kaldor, J. M., Brew, B. J.; National HIV Surveillance Committee. (2003). Marked improvement in survival following AIDS dementia complex in the era of highly active antiretroviral therapy. *AIDS, 17*(10), 1539–1545.

El Hussein, M., Hirst, S., & Salyers, V. (2015). Factors that contribute to underrecognition of delirium by registered nurses in acute care settings: A scoping review of the literature to explain this phenomenon. *Journal of Clinical Nursing, 24*(7/8), 906–915. doi:10.1111/jocn.12693

Fick, D. M., Hodo, D. M., Lawrence, F., & Inouye, S. K. (2007). Recognizing delirium superimposed on dementia. *Journal of Gerontological Nursing, 33*(2), 40–47.

Flaherty, J. H. (1998). Commonly prescribed and over the counter medications: Causes of confusion. *Clinics in Geriatric Medicine, 14*(1), 101–125.

Folstein, M. F., Folstein, S. E., & McHugh, P. R. (1975). Mini-mental state: A practical method for grading the cognitive state of patients for the clinician. *Journal of Psychiatric Research, 12*, 189–198.

Forbes, D., Blake, C., Thiessen, E. J., Peacock, S., & Hawranik, P. (2014). Light therapy for improving cognition, activities of daily living, sleep, challenging behaviour, and psychiatric disturbances in dementia. *Cochrane Database of Systematic Reviews, 2*, CD003946.

Forbes, D. A., Finkelstein, S., Blake, C., Gibson, M., Morgan, D. G., Markle-Reid, M., ... Thiessen, E. J. (2012). Knowledge exchange throughout the dementia care journey by rural community-based health care practitioners, persons with dementia, and their care partners: A qualitative interpretive descriptive study. *Journal of Rural and Remote Health, 12*, 2201.

Forbes, D. A., Forbes, S. C., Blake, C. M., Thiessen, E. J., & Forbes, S. (2015). Exercise programs for people with dementia. *The Cochrane Database of Systematic Reviews, 4*, CD006489.

Forbes, D. A., Markle-Reid, M., Hawranik, P., Peacock, S., Kingston, D., Morgan, D., ... Jansen, S. L. (2008). Availability and acceptability of Canadian home and community-based services: Perspectives of family caregivers of persons with dementia. *Home Health Care Services Quarterly, 27*(2), 75–99.

Gauthier, S., Albert, M., Fox, N., Goedert, M., Kivipelto, M., Mestre-Ferrandiz, J., & Middleton, L. T. (2016). Why has therapy development failed in the last two decades? *Alzheimer's & Dementia 12*, 60–64.

Gauthier, S., Patterson, C., Chertkow, H., Gordon, M., Herrmann, N., Rockwood, K., ... Soucy, J. P. (2012a). Fourth Canadian Consensus Conference on the Diagnosis and Treatment of Dementia. *Canadian Journal of Neurological Sciences, 39*(Suppl. 5), S1–S8.

Gauthier, S., Patterson, C., Chertkow, H., Gordon, M., Herrmann, N., Rockwood, K., ... Soucy, J. P. (2012b). Recommendations of the 4th Canadian Consensus Conference on the Diagnosis and Treatment of Dementia (CCCDTD4). *Canadian Geriatric Journal, 15*(4), 120–126.

Genetica Home Reference. (2013). *Alzheimer disease*. Retrieved from http://ghr.nlm.nih.gov/condition/alzheimer-disease

Givens, J., Jones, R., & Inouye, S. (2009). The overlap syndrome of depression and delirium in older hospitalized patients. *Journal of the American Geriatrics Society, 57*(8), 1347–1353.

Gotell, E., Brown, S., & Ekman, S.-L. (2009). The influence of caregiver singing and background music on vocally expressed emotions and moods in dementia care: A qualitative analysis. *International Journal of Nursing Studies, 46*(4), 422–430.

Graham, J. (2013). Does depression contribute to dementia? In *New York Times, Old Age: Caring and Coping*. Retrieved from http://newoldage.blogs.nytimes.com/2013/05/01/does-depression-contribute-to-dementia/

Gray, S. L., Anderson, M. L., Dublin, S., Hanlon, J. T., Hubbard, R., Walker, R., ... Larson, E. B. (2015). Cumulative use of strong anticholinergics and incident dementia: A prospective cohort study. *American Medical Association Internal Medicine, 175*(3), 401–407. doi:10.1001/jamainternmed.2014.7663

Green, A. R., Segal, J., Tian, J., Oh, E., Roth, D. L., Hilson, L. ... Boyd, C. M. (2017). Use of bladder antimuscarinics in older adults with impaired cognition. *Journal of the American Geriatrics Society, 65*(2), 390–394. doi:10.1111/jags.14498

Grover, S., Kate, N., Malhotra, S., Chakrabarti, S., Mattoo, S., & Avasthi, A. (2012). Symptom profile of delirium in children and adolescents—Does it differ from adults and elderly? *General Hospital Psychiatry, 34*(6), 626–632.

Healthcare Provider's Guide To Alzheimer's Disease (AD): Diagnosis, pharmacologic management, non-pharmacologic management, and other considerations. UCSF Weill Institute for Neurosciences. Retrieved from http://memory.ucsf.edu/sites/memory.ucsf.edu/files/wysiwyg/UCSF_Alzheimer%27s_Providers7-13-17.pdf5

Heerema, E. (2017). *Using validation therapy for people with dementia*. Retrieved from https://www.verywell.com/using-validation-therapy-for-people-with-dementia-98683

Hicks-Moore, S. L., & Robinson, B. A. (2008). Favorite music and hand massage: Two interventions to decrease agitation in residents with dementia. *Dementia, 7*(1), 95–108.

Humphries, J. D. (2008). Sleep disruption in hospitalized adults. *Nursing, 17*(6), 391–395.

Inouye, S. K., van Dyck, C. H., Alessi, C. A., Balkin, S., Siegal, A. P., & Horwitz, R. I. (1990). Clarifying confusion: The confusion assessment method. *Annals of Internal Medicine, 113*, 941–948.

Irwin, S. A., Pirrello, R. D., Hirst, J. M., Buckholz, G. T., & Ferris, F. D. (2013). Clarifying delirium management: Practical, evidence-based, expert recommendations for clinical practice. *Journal of Palliative Care Medicine, 16*(4), 423–435.

Jacklin, K., Walker, J., & Shawande, M. (2013). The emergence of dementia as a health concern among First Nations populations in Alberta, Canada. *Canadian Journal of Public Health, 104*(1), e39–e44.

Jansen, L., Forbes, D. A., Markle-Reid, M., Hawranik, P., Kingston, D., Peacock, S., ... Leipert, B. (2009). Formal care providers' perceptions of home and community-based services: Informing dementia care quality. *Home Health Care Services Quarterly, 28*(1), 1–23.

Kaiser, N. C., Melrose, R. J., Liu, C., Sultzer, D. L., Jiminez, E., Su, M., ... Mendez, M. F. (2012). Neuropsychological and neuroimaging markers in early versus late-onset Alzheimer's disease. *American Journal of Alzheimer's Disease and Other Dementias, 27*(7), 520–529.

Katzenschlager, R., Sampaio, C., Costa, J., & Lees, A. (2003). Anticholinergics for symptomatic management of Parkinson's disease. *Cochrane Database of Systematic Reviews, (2)*, CD003735.

Lancioni, G. E., Singh, N. N., O'Reilly, M. F., Sigafoos, J., D'Amico, F., Renna, C., & Pinto, K. (2016). Technology-aided programs to support positive verbal and physical engagement in persons with moderate or severe

Alzheimer's disease. *Frontiers in Aging Neuroscience, 8*, 87. doi:10.3389/fnagi.2016.00087

Laske, C. (2014). Phase 3 trials of solanezumab and bapineuzumab for Alzheimer's disease. *New England Journal of Medicine, 370*, 1459–1460. doi:10.1056/NEJMc1402193

Leung, M. J., Sands, P. L., Paul, S., Joseph, T., Kinjo, S., & Tsai, T. (2009). Does postoperative delirium limit the use of patient-controlled analgesia in older surgical patients? *Anesthesiology, 111*(3), 625–631.

Liu, R. Y., Zhou, J. N., Hoogendijk, W. J. G., van Heerikhuize, J., Kamphorst, W., Unmehopa, U. A., ... Swaab, D. F. (2000). Decreased vasopressin gene expression in the biological clock of Alzheimer disease patients with and without depression. *Journal of Neuropathology and Experimental Neurology, 59*(4), 314–322.

Luetz, A., Weiss, B., Boettcher, S., Burmeister, J., Wernecke, K.-D., & Spies, C. (2016). Routine delirium monitoring is independently associated with a reduction of hospital mortality in critically ill surgery patients. *Journal of Critical Care, 35*, 168–173.

Maclullich, A. M., Ferguson, K. J., Miller, T., de Rooij, S. E., & Cunningham, C. (2008). Unravelling the pathophysiology of delirium: A focus on the role of aberrant stress responses. *Journal of Psychosomatic Research, 65*(3), 229–238.

Nasreddine, Z. S., Phillips, N. A., Bedirian, V., Charbonneau, S., Whitehead, V., Collin, I., ... Chertkow, H. (2005). The Montreal Cognitive Assessment, MoCA: A brief screening tool for mild cognitive impairment. *Journal of the American Geriatrics Society, 53*(4), 695–699.

North American Nursing Diagnosis Association (NANDA). (2012). *Nursing diagnoses: Definition and classification 2012–2014.* Philadelphia, PA: NANDA International.

Omalu, B. I., Hamilton, R. L., Kamboh, I. M., DeKosky, S. T., & Bailes, J. (2010). Chronic traumatic encephalopathy (CTE) in a National Football League player: Case report and emerging medicolegal practice questions. *Journal of Forensic Nursing, 6*(1), 40–46.

Omalu, B. I., Fitzsimmons, R. P., Hammers, J., & Bailes, J. (2010). Chronic traumatic encephalopathy in a professional wrestler. *Journal of Forensic Nursing, 6*(3), 130–136.

Pendlebury, S. T., Lovett, N. G., Smith, S. C., Dutta, N., Bendon, C., Lloyd-Lavery, A., ... Rothwell, P. M. (2015). Observational, longitudinal study of delirium in consecutive, unselected acute medical admissions: Age-specific rates and associated factors, mortality and re-admission. *BMJ Open, 5*(11):e007808. doi:10.113b/bmjopen-2015-007808

Porter, S., Holly, C., & Echevarria, M. (2016). Infants with delirium: A primer on prevention, recognition, and management. *Pediatric Nursing, 42*(5), 223–229.

Prorok, J. C., Horgan, S., & Seitz, D. P. (2013). Health care experiences of people with dementia and their caregivers: A meta-ethnographic analysis of qualitative studies. *Canadian Medical Association Journal, 185*(14), E669–E680.

Registered Nurses Association of Ontario. (2005, updated 2011). *Prevention of falls and fall injuries in the older adult.* Toronto, ON: Author.

Registered Nurses Association of Ontario. (2016). *Delirium, dementia and depression in older adults: Assessment and care.* Toronto, ON: Author.

Reisberg, B., Schneck, M. K., & Ferris, S. H. (1983). The Brief Cognitive Rating Scale (BCRS): Findings in primary degenerative dementia. *Psychopharmacology Bulletin, 19*, 47.

Ringman, J. M., (2011). Setting the stage for prevention of familial Alzheimer's disease. *Lancet Neurology, 10*(3), 200–201.

Rivosecchi, R. M., Smithburger, P. L., Svec, S., Campbell, S., & Kane-Gill, S. L. (2015). Nonpharmacological interventions to prevent delirium: An evidence-based systematic review. *Critical Care Nurse, 35*(1), 39–48.

Rosen, J., Burgio, L., Kollar, M., Cain, M., Allison, M., Fogleman, M., ... Zubenko, G. S. (1994). The Pittsburgh agitation scale: User-friendly instrument for rating agitation in dementia patients. *The American Journal of Geriatric Psychiatry, 2*(1), 52–59.

Rothberg, M., Herzig, S., Pekow, P., Avrunin, J. Lagu, T., & Lindauer, P. (2013). Association between sedating medications and delirium in older inpatients. *Journal of the American Geriatrics Society, 61*(6), 923–930.

Rowe, C. C., Ellis, K. A., Rimajova, M., Bourgeat, P., Pike, K., Jones, G., ... Villemagne, V. L. (2010). Amyloid imaging results from the Australian Imaging, Biomarkers and Lifestyle (AIBL) study of aging. *Neurobiology of Aging 31*(8), 1275–1283.

Sadock, B. J., Sadock, V. A., & Ruiz, P. (2015). *Kaplan's and Sadock's synopsis of psychiatry* (11th ed.). Philadelphia, PA: Wolters Kluwer.

Schott, J. M., & Warren, J. D. (2012). Alzheimer's disease: Mimics and chameleons. *Practical Neurology, 12*(6), 358–366.

Schwartz, G. E. (1983). Development and validation of the Geriatric Evaluation by Relatives Rating Instrument (GERRI). *Psychological Reports, 53*, 478–488.

Starr, J. M. (2016). Diagnosis and management of dementia in older people. *Medicine in Older Adults, 45*(1), 51–54.

Stern, Y., Albert, S. M., Sano, M., Richards, M., Miller, L., Folstein, M., ... Lafleche, G. (1994). Assessing patient dependence in Alzheimer's disease. *Journal of Gerontology, 49*, M216–M222.

Teng, E. L., Hasegawa, K., Homma, A., Imai, Y., Larson, E., Graves, A., ... Chiu, D. (1994). The Cognitive Abilities Screening Instrument (CASI): A practical test for cross-cultural epidemiological studies of dementia. *International Psychogeriatrics, 6*, 45–58.

The Regents of the University of California. (2016). *Medications to be avoided.* Retrieved from http://memory.ucsf.edu/ftd/medical/treatment/avoid/single

Thorgrimsen, L., Selwood, A., Spector, A., Royan, L., de Madariaga Lopez, M., Woods, R. T., & Orrell, M. (2003). Whose quality of life is it anyway?: The validity and reliability of the Quality of Life-Alzheimer's Disease (QoL-AD) scale. *Alzheimer Disease and Associated Disorders, 17*(4), 201–208.

Trzepacz, P. T., Mittal, D., Torres, R., Kanary, K., Norton, J., & Jimerson, N. (2001). Validation of the Delirium Rating Scale-revised-98: Comparison with the delirium rating scale and the cognitive test for delirium. *Journal of Neuropsychiatry and Clinical Neurosciences, 13*, 229–242.

Tune, L. (2000). Delirium. In C. E. Coffey & J. L. Cummings (Eds.), *American Psychiatric Press textbook of geriatric neuropsychiatry* (2nd ed., pp. 441–462). Washington, DC: American Psychiatric Press.

Turcotte, M. (2014). Insights on Canadian Society: Canadians with unmet home care needs. *Statistics Canada.* Catalogue no. 75-006-X. ISSN 2291-0859.

Turcotte, M. (2016). *Family caregiving: What are the consequences?* Retrieved from http://www.statcan.gc.ca/pub/75-006-x/2013001/article/11858-eng.htm

van den Berg, S., & Splaine, M. (2012). Policy brief: Risk factors for dementia. In *Policy recommendations by Alzheimer's Disease International.* Retrieved from http://www.alz.co.uk/sites/default/files/policy-brief-risk-factors-for-dementia.pdf

van Munster, B. C., de Rooij, S. E., & Korevaar, J. C. (2009). The role of genetics in delirium in the elderly patient. *Dementia and Geriatric Cognitive Disorders, 28*(3), 187–195.

Vance, D., Moore, B., Farr, K., & Struzick, T. (2008). Procedural memory and emotional attachment in Alzheimer disease: Implications for meaningful and engaging activities. *Journal of Neuroscience Nursing, 40*(2), 96–102.

Villemagne, V. L., Pike, K. E., Chetelat, G., Ellis, K. A., Mulligan, R. S., Bourgeat, P., ... Rowe, C. C. (2011). Longitudinal assessment of Aβ and cognition in aging and Alzheimer disease. *Annals of Neurology, 69*(1), 181–192.

Von Rueden, K.T., Wallizer, B., Thurman, P., McQuillan, K., Andrews, T., Merenda, J., & Son, H. (2017). Delirium in trauma patients: Prevalence and predictors. *Critical Care Nurse, 37*(1), 40–47.

Voyer, P., Richard, S., McCusker, J., Cole, M. G., Monette, J., Champoux, N., ... Belzile, E. (2012). Detection of delirium and its symptoms by nurses working in a long-term care facility. *Journal of the American Medical Directors Association, 13*(3), 264–271.

Wadley, V. G., Okonkwo, O., Crowe, M., & Ross-Meadows, L. A. (2008). Mild cognitive impairment and everyday function: Evidence of reduced speed in performing instrumental activities of daily living. *American Journal of Geriatric Psychiatry, 16*, 416–424.

White, S., & Bayer, A. (2007). Delirium—A clinical overview. *Reviews in Clinical Gerontology, 17*, 45–62.

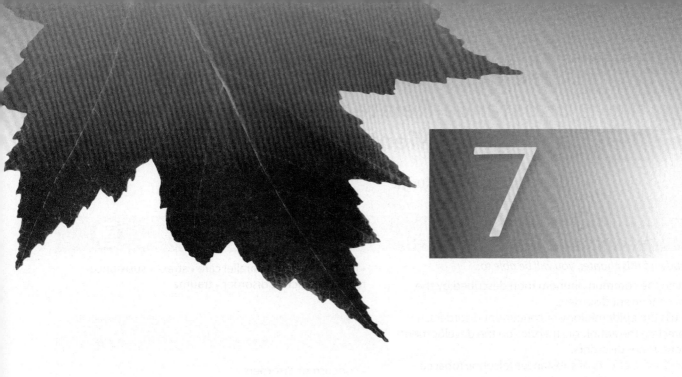

Care of Persons
With
Additional
Vulnerabilities

33 Care of Persons With Concurrent Substance-Related, Addictive, and Other Mental Disorders

Charl Els and Diane Kunyk

LEARNING OBJECTIVES

After studying this chapter, you will be able to:

- Explain the common phenomenon described by the term concurrent disorders.
- Discuss the epidemiology of concurrent disorders.
- Appreciate the aetiologic theories on the development of concurrent disorders.
- Describe the effects of substances (alcohol, tobacco, and other drugs) on mental status.
- Describe the most common concurrent disorders.
- Outline assessment approaches to concurrent disorders.
- Outline care and treatment approaches specific to concurrent disorders.
- Appreciate the opportunities and challenges in the care and treatment of concurrent disorders.
- Identify some future directions for research and care in the field of concurrent disorders.

KEY TERMS

- integrated care • parallel care • stress • substance-related/addictive disorder • trauma

KEY CONCEPT

- concurrent disorders

Numerous epidemiologic and clinical studies report the co-occurrence of **substance-related/addictive disorders** with psychiatric (mental) disorders—a common phenomenon referred to as concurrent disorders. The 5th edition of the *Diagnostic and Statistical Manual of Mental Disorders (DSM-5)* (American Psychiatric Association [APA], 2013) lists the symptoms of more than 300 psychiatric conditions, and it divides substances into ten categories. The number of possible combinations of concurrent disorders is enormous and tend to be heterogeneous. The most salient examples of combinations of substance-related/addictive disorders with other mental disorders in the literature, which will be discussed in detail in this chapter, include the following:

- Co-occurring addictive and mood disorders
- Co-occurring addictive and anxiety disorders
- Co-occurring addictive and posttraumatic stress disorder (PTSD)
- Co-occurring addictive attention deficit hyperactivity disorders
- Co-occurring addictive and psychotic disorders
- Co-occurring addictive and personality disorders

It is important to note that in addition to intoxication with, and withdrawal from, substances may mimic a range of bona fide psychiatric conditions, called the substance-induced mental disorders, which *are not synonymous* with the co-occurrence of psychiatric and substance-related/addictive disorders. Examples include the following nine conditions (the first three of which were previously referred to as "organic brain syndrome"): substance-induced delirium, substance-induced persisting dementia, substance-induced amnestic disorder, substance-induced psychotic disorder, substance-induced mood disorder, substance-induced anxiety disorder, substance-induced persisting perceptual disorder, substance-induced sexual dysfunction, and substance-induced sleep disorder (Yuodelis-Flores, Goldsmith, & Ries, 2014). Substance-associated suicidal behaviour may also occur, which may incur serious risk. Although these conditions frequently dissipate in the absence of ongoing substance use, suicidal behaviour may persist beyond the substance intoxication or withdrawal period. Distinguishing symptoms of substance-induced disorder from bona fide psychiatric disorders is often difficult and represents a pivotal challenge for clinicians. For further information on the diagnoses associated with different classes of substances, please refer to the DSM-5 (APA, 2013, p. 482).

Concurrent disorders have also been called *dual disorders, comorbidity, co-occurring substance use and mental health problems, mentally ill chemical abuser,* and *dual diagnosis.* In many jurisdictions, however, the term dual diagnosis is reserved for persons with an intellectual disability and a mental health problem. The term *trimorbidity* has been utilized in the context of the co-occurrence of PTSD, traumatic brain injury, and a substance-related/addictive disorder.

The co-occurrence of mental and substance-related/addictive disorders represents a prevalent, pervasive, and urgent health issue. Given that concurrent disorders are associated with more severe adverse outcomes than either condition alone, identifying and treating individuals with concurrent disorders are high priorities. These negative outcomes include, among others, increased rates of rehospitalization and incarceration, disruption of family and social relationships, homelessness, depression, suicide, comorbid medical problems, relapse, and treatment dropout (McKee, 2017). As patients, these individuals are among the most complex, intractable, and difficult clinical scenarios in health care. One ubiquitous problem concerning this heterogeneous and complex population is that "these patients typically have many disorders and severe life problems in addition to mental illness and substance use disorders" (Drake & Green, 2013, p. 105).

A pervasive problem in Canada is that the disease burden associated with concurrent mental health and addictive disorders is insufficiently matched by the allocation of health care resources.

Further, one of the most salient challenges has been that health care systems have tended to be organized for the care and treatment delivery of single disorders, for example, either for mental disorders or for substance-related/addictive disorders, but not for both simultaneously. Despite the integration of mental health and addiction services in many of Canada's care systems, service provision may remain compartmentalized. This has often resulted in persons with concurrent disorders not fitting well into either the mental health or the addiction treatment systems, and hence "falling through the cracks," thus precluding access to safe and effective care and treatment. In the report by the Mental Health Commission of Canada (MHCC, 2016), *Advancing the Mental Health Strategy for Canada: A Framework for Action (2017–2022),* it is acknowledged that integration of addiction and mental health services continues to present challenges to Canadians. One recommendation from this document is to improve collaboration in the delivery of services to people with concurrent disorders (MHCC, 2016).

The knowledge and practice related to the care and treatment of concurrent disorders is a dynamic, complex, challenging, and evolving area in health care. Despite systemic challenges, increased knowledge and enhanced skills in caring for persons with concurrent disorders have the potential to improve outcomes for this vulnerable population. It is important for nurses to recognize that, despite the challenges associated with concurrent disorders, treatment is effective, harm can be reduced, and many patients have the potential to recover and live normal lives. Excess health care costs to society can also be curbed.

This chapter outlines the concept of concurrent disorders and the aetiologic models for concurrent substance-related, addictive, and other mental disorders. The general principles of care and treatment are outlined and nursing strategies and interventions specific to this population are recommended. Given the vast number of possible combinations of mental illness and addiction, only the most prevalent and clinically meaningful examples of such disorders are discussed. This chapter focuses on an integrated approach to care and treatment, in contrast to sequential or parallel models, aimed at the prevention of these disorders and reduction of the severity and progression of existing concurrent conditions. See Chapter 26 for a comprehensive presentation of substance-related and addictive disorders.

EPIDEMIOLOGY OF CONCURRENT DISORDERS

It is estimated that approximately 50% of persons seeking help for addiction also suffer from a mental disorder, while 15% to 20% of persons with mental illness also suffer from an addictive disorder (Mueser & Gingrich, 2013; United States Department of Health and Human Services, Substance Abuse and Mental Health Services Administration, 2015). In persons with severe and persistent mental illness, the rates of addiction tend to be much higher. Lifetime substance use is particularly high in persons suffering from psychotic disorders (Margolese et al., 2004). Almost one half (51.7%) of individuals presenting with first episode psychosis meet criteria for any lifetime alcohol or drug use disorder (Brunette et al., 2017), echoing international estimates of lifetime prevalence for individuals with schizophrenia, which is around 50% (Mueser, Bennet, & Kushner, 1995). Substance use and addictive disorders are some of the most commonly comorbid conditions for individuals with serious mental illness (Mueser & Gingrich, 2013).

Canada's first (and most recent) national assessment of the prevalence of concurrent disorders (Rush et al., 2008) suggests that Canadian rates may be at the lower end of the range reported internationally. In a secondary analysis of data from the 2002 Canadian Community Health Survey (*n* = 36,984), Rush and colleagues (2008) report the 12-month prevalence to be 1.7%, with no significant gender and age differences found. Rates were highest in British Columbia and lowest in Quebec. The actual numbers, however, may be much higher as the Canadian studies excluded certain populations who are known to be at high risk for concurrent disorders (e.g., PTSD and personality disorders).

Another Canadian study (Rush & Koegl, 2008) examined the prevalence and profile of people with concurrent disorders, collecting data on 9,839 cases from specialty tertiary inpatient, specialty outpatient, and community-based mental health programs. Their findings suggest that the overall prevalence of concurrent disorders is 8.9% and that rates are highest in the inpatient settings and within selected populations (i.e., younger adults, persons with personality disorders).

The high prevalence rates of mental disorders among incarcerated individuals, when compared with the general population, have been well established. Newly admitted male offenders entering the federal correctional system in Canada were examined for prevalence rates of major mental disorders. The study findings revealed that most (73%) met the criteria for any current mental disorder, and 38% of all admissions met the criteria for both a current mental disorder and one of the substance use disorders (Beaudette & Stewart, 2016).

When compared with their heterosexual counterparts, lesbian, gay, and bisexual individuals have been found to experience poorer mental health and higher rates of substance misuse. In a study examining pooled data from the 2007–2012 cycles of the Canadian Community Health Survey, researchers concluded that this was also the case for co-occurrence of anxiety or mood disorders and heavy drinking. Their findings indicate that gay or lesbian respondents had a 2.0-fold higher adjusted odds ratio, and bisexual respondents had a 3.3-fold increase in odds ratio, than did heterosexual respondents of reporting co-occurring anxiety or mood disorders and heavy drinking (Pakula, Shoveller, Ratner, & Carpiano, 2016).

KEY CONCEPT

The term **concurrent disorders** is used when an individual has at least one substance-related or addictive disorder co-occurring with at least one other mental disorder. Other than detecting the presence of a substance-induced disorder, nurses must be attentive to the possibility that patients presenting with either an addictive disorder or another mental illness may have more than one condition, that is, a concurrent disorder. It is established that about half the number of persons presenting with a substance-related/addictive disorder also experience a mental disorder; one in five persons presenting with a mental disorder also suffers from a substance-related/addictive disorder. Screening for a concurrent mental illness or substance-related/addictive disorder is recommended with the presentation of either condition.

AETIOLOGIC THEORIES: DEVELOPMENT OF CONCURRENT DISORDERS

Despite its high prevalence and established negative consequences, an explanation for the aetiology of co-occurrence of substance-related/addictive disorders and other mental disorders remains largely unclear. Four general models have emerged with varying degrees of empirical support for each model's validity: (1) common factor models, (2) secondary substance use disorder models (including supersensitivity and self-medication models), (3) secondary psychiatric disorder models, and (4) bidirectional models (Mueser, Drake, & Wallach, 1998).

The *common factor model* suggests that the same set of variables may contribute to an increased risk for the development of substance-related/addictive and other mental health problems. The cited risk factors may be biologic, psychological (including temperamental), social, or environmental. There is some degree of support for this theory in that the current evidence suggests that individuals with co-occurring disorders are likely to differ from those with either substance use disorders or psychiatric disorders alone on various neurobiologic aspects (Balhara, Kuppili, & Gupta, 2017).

The *secondary substance use disorder model* proposes that mental health conditions increase the relative risks of developing a substance use disorder. This model includes the *supersensitivity model*, which proposes that there is an existing vulnerability in persons suffering from psychiatric disorders that results in their sensitivity to even small amounts of substances. There is also the *self-medication* model, which suggests that people use substances to relieve subjective distress related to their mental illness. Despite its intuitive appeal, there is minimal empirical support for this theory; it may be more applicable to anxiety and mood disorders than to psychotic disorders. It has, however, been suggested that the accumulation of multiple risk factors related to mental illness, including subjective distress, may indeed increase the relative risk of a substance-related/addictive disorder.

The *secondary psychiatric disorder model* suggests that the use of substances may precipitate mental health conditions in persons who would not otherwise have developed them. It should be noted that substance use is associated with the development of certain psychiatric symptoms. For example, amphetamines can cause psychotic symptoms and alcohol may cause depressive symptoms. However, the evidence to suggest that substance use is causally linked to the development of a bona fide psychiatric disorder is limited. One early study examined the link between cannabis (smoking marijuana) and schizophrenia. Andréasson, Engström, Allebeck, and Rydberg (1987) studied the association between cannabis and the development of schizophrenia during a 15-year follow-up in a cohort of 45,570 Swedish conscripts and concluded that cannabis is an independent risk factor for schizophrenia. Since this time, an overview of five systematic reviews concluded that cannabis use is likely to increase the risk of developing schizophrenia and other psychoses; the higher the use, the greater the risk (National Academies of Sciences, Engineering, and Medicine, 2017). There is also emerging evidence that regular cannabis is associated with increase in the risk for developing social anxiety (Kedzior & Laeber, 2014).

The *bidirectional model* posits a two-way aetiologic process whereby addictive disorders and other mental illnesses increase the risk for the development of the other condition. Although both conditions should be considered primary, the temporal onset for alcohol-related concurrent disorders suggests that the alcohol use disorder is more commonly the primary condition (Fergusson, Boden, & Horwood, 2009; Flensborg-Madsen et al., 2009).

The link between **stress** and/or **trauma** and the development of addictive disorders have also been empirically validated. Individuals who have been exposed to traumatic events may increase substance use, which can in turn lead to new traumatic exposures, which may perpetuate the stress–substance use cycle. Both acute stress and chronic stress lead to changes in the natural neurochemical homeostasis, modulated by numerous factors, which may increase the risk of the development of substance-related/addictive disorders. Impulsivity, which may be a feature of some psychiatric conditions, has also been linked with an increased risk of developing substance-related/addictive disorders.

IN-A-LIFE

Clara Hughes (1972–)

PUBLIC PERSONA

Clara Hughes is a six-time Olympic medalist in cycling and speed skating. In 2006, when she stepped onto the Olympic podium in Torino, Italy, she became the first athlete to win multiple medals in both the Summer and Winter Games. Four years later, she proudly carried the national flag at the head of the Canadian team during the opening ceremony of the Vancouver Olympic Winter Games. Among others, her awards include Officer of the Order of Canada; Member of the Order of Manitoba; Inductee Canada Sports Hall of Fame; Star on Canada's Walk of Fame; Honorary Doctorate of Law, University of Manitoba; Honorary Doctorate of Law, University of British Columbia; and Honorary Doctorate of Letters, University of New Brunswick (http://clara-hughes.com/about-clara/awards).

PERSONAL REALITIES

In her book, *Open Heart, Open Mind*, Hughes chronicles spending her teenage years misusing alcohol, tobacco, and other drugs. After years of intense competition, she shares her realization that her physical extremes, emotional setbacks, and partying habits were masking a severe depression. She has also shared that she struggled with an eating disorder (Arsenault, 2015). After winning the bronze in the last speed-skating race of her career, Hughes decided to retire, determined to transform her depression into something positive. She has since advocated for a variety of social causes, and in 2010, Hughes became national spokesperson for Bell Canada's Let's Talk campaign, which is dedicated to breaking down the stigma of mental illness.

Sources: Arsenault, A. (2015, September 6). Olympian Clara Hughes reveals doping infraction. *CBC News*. Retrieved from http://www.cbc.ca/news/canada/olympian-clara-hughes-reveals-doping-infraction-1.3215617 Hughes, C. (2015). *Open heart, open mind*. New York, NY: Simon & Schuster.

ASSESSMENT APPROACHES SPECIFIC TO CONCURRENT DISORDERS

Assessment of persons with concurrent disorders follows the principles of assessment for each category of the mental disorder encountered, as well as for substance use patterns and complications. The protocols for screening for tobacco use, illicit substance use, substance use disorders, at-risk drinking, and alcohol use disorders are discussed in Chapter 26.

Treatment planning for persons with concurrent disorders is based on the principle of treatment matching, that is, utilizing the least restrictive level of care that is proven to be safe and likely to be effective. The criteria for placement of a person on a certain level of care are predominantly based on consensus best practices of care and treatment. To allow for adequate treatment planning and appropriate utilization of resources in persons with concurrent disorders, assessment of the following six domains is recommended: (1) acute intoxication and/or withdrawal potential, (2) biomedical conditions and complications, (3) emotional/behavioural/cognitive conditions and complications, (4) readiness to change, (5) relapse/continued use/continued problem potential, and (6) recovery environment.

CARE AND TREATMENT APPROACHES SPECIFIC TO CONCURRENT DISORDERS

Care and treatment for concurrent disorders should include screening and comprehensive assessment for both substance-related/addictive disorders and other mental health disorders, psychosocial and pharmacologic interventions, and a plan for coordinated care. As this population is highly heterogeneous, there is no single approach or set of interventions that is proven to be effective for all persons with concurrent disorders (Kavanagh, Mueser, & Baker, 2003; McKee, 2017).

Different models of care and treatment exist for persons with concurrent disorders: sequential (serial) treatment (whereby care is received in sequential treatment episodes in separate systems of care), **parallel care** (accessed for all disorders simultaneously, but in different systems, with varying degrees of coordination), and **integrated care** (where care is provided for both disorders by the same cross-trained team members in the same program, resulting in an integration of services). Mueser, Noordsy, Drake, and Fox (2003) identified seven components of integrated care in their best practice guidelines:

- Integration of services (integrated care)
- Comprehensive approach to assessment and treatment
- Assertiveness (actively reaching out to persons with concurrent disorders)
- Reduction of negative consequences (e.g., harm reduction)
- Time-unlimited services (reflecting the chronic and severe nature of concurrent disorders)
- Adapting interventions to the person's stage of treatment
- Using multiple psychotherapeutic modalities

Improving care and treatment for persons suffering from concurrent disorders requires changes to the health care delivery system to allow for simultaneous and coordinated care or integrated care of conditions. Despite the obvious disadvantages of treating mental health disorders separately from addictions in those suffering from both disorders, it is not yet the rule for patients to have access to truly integrated care and treatment systems, at the right level of treatment matching (Canadian Institutes of Health Information, 2013). The optimal degree of integration should ensure that evidence-based safe and effective care is available, accessible, and affordable to each person suffering from a concurrent disorder. Early detection of the disorders, as well as primary, secondary, and tertiary prevention, warrants special attention. Box 33.1 outlines general treatment principles for individuals with concurrent disorders.

Treatment Matching

The overarching principle in matching persons to the right level of care is to provide treatment at the least restrictive level of care that will be effective and safe. The concept of treatment matching has been formalized and is guided by a set of placement criteria. These provide separate placement criteria for individualized treatment plans through a multidimensional assessment that evaluates

---

> **BOX 33.1 General Treatment Principles for Concurrent Disorders**
>
> 1. All good treatment proceeds from an empathic, hopeful nurse–patient relationship.
> 2. Consequently, the nurse should promote opportunities to initiate and maintain continuing empathic, hopeful relationships whenever possible.
> 3. Care should be taken to remove arbitrary barriers to initial assessment and evaluation including initial psychopharmacology evaluation (e.g., length of sobriety, alcohol level, etc.).
> 4. As a general principle, medication for a known serious mental illness should not be discontinued because a patient is using substances.
> 5. A substance disorder evaluation and/or treatment should not be denied because a patient is on a prescribed nonaddictive psychotropic medication.
> 6. When mental illness and substance disorder coexist, both disorders require specific and appropriately intensive primary treatment.
> 7. The specific content of dual primary treatment for each person must be individualized according to diagnosis, phase of treatment, level of functioning and/or disability, and assessment of level of care based on acuity, severity, medical safety, motivation, and availability of recovery support.
>
> Source: Minkoff, K. (2001). Developing standards of care for individuals with co-occurring psychiatric and substance disorders. *Psychiatric Services, 52*(5), 597–599.

---

acute intoxication/withdrawal; biomedical conditions/complications; emotional, behavioural, or cognitive conditions/complications; readiness to change; relapse, continued use, or continued problem potential; and recovery environment. Based on this multidimensional assessment, treatment placement on one of five levels is recommended: Level 0.5 (early intervention), Level I (outpatient services), Level II (intensive outpatient/partial hospitalization services), Level III (residential/inpatient services), or Level IV (medically managed intensive inpatient services).

Indications for Hospitalization

Substance use and mental illness are both risk factors for self-harm or suicide. Such risk has to be carefully and iteratively assessed and attention should be given to detecting other risk factors, which include previous attempts at self-harm, any history of violence and/or trauma, lack of social support systems, and physical illness. Those at imminent and substantial risk of harm to self should be hospitalized to ensure safety. Other indications for hospitalization may include complicated withdrawal syndromes, or where interventions on a less restrictive level of care have failed to yield the necessary outcomes. Individual approaches should incorporate engagement, persuasion, active treatment, and relapse prevention (RP). Psychoeducation and support for treatment adherence will be important. Multimodal and integrated pharmacotherapy and behavioural approaches are key treatment options.

IMPLEMENTING INTERVENTIONS FOR SPECIFIC CONCURRENT DISORDERS

There is no single intervention that will work for every individual with a concurrent disorder, because each person may differ greatly with respect to severity, substance of abuse, mental illness, and the individual's unique biologic, psychological, social, and spiritual considerations. Often several approaches can work together while others are deemed inappropriate. Treatment programs usually combine psychosocial interventions with other different approaches to provide a comprehensive plan based on the individual's needs. Nursing interventions vary depending on the nature of the current problems, the status and severity of the illnesses, and the individual's situation. Continuity of treatment is clearly important, but even more critical is the need to develop specific evidence-based treatments—pharmacologic and psychosocial interventions—for specific situations and specific individuals. A summary of evidence-based nursing approaches for patients with concurrent disorders is found in Box 33.2. The following section discusses the most salient examples of concurrent disorders that nurses will encounter during their practice.

Concurrent Addictive and Mood Disorders

Mood disorders (e.g., major depressive disorder, persistent depressive disorder) represent some of the most common psychiatric disorders in the general population, and approximately 15% to 50% of those entering treatment for a substance use disorder have a lifetime diagnosis of at least one depressive disorder (Nunes & Wiss, 2014). Although bipolar disorder is less common than other mood disorders, the likelihood of having a substance use disorder is significantly elevated, with a prevalence of 40% (Nunes & Wiss, 2014). Mood disorders and comorbid substance use represent an example of a common vulnerability as a result of genetic and/or environmental factors.

It is often challenging for clinicians to distinguish between substance-induced mood symptoms and those associated with a bona fide mood disorder. To distinguish, it is useful to examine the onset of the conditions and to determine which condition preceded which or to investigate the persistence of mood symptoms during periods of sobriety and abstinence. It is often necessary to wait for a period of 4 weeks of sobriety/abstinence before diagnosing an independent mood disorder versus a substance-induced mood disorder. This poses obvious clinical concerns in terms of having to wait for several weeks prior to intervening. Suffering from a mood

---

> **BOX 33.2** Summary of Evidence-Based Nursing Approaches for Patients With Concurrent Disorders
>
> 1. The focus of the intervention must be person-focused and aimed at enhancing engagement in treatment.
> 2. Assessment ought to include the presenting problems, substance use, mental health status, medications, family and other support, and issues specific to the patient's age, gender, culture, and other circumstances.
> 3. Negotiate realistic goals that are broken into small, achievable steps.
> 4. Interaction ought to be respectful, flexible, optimistic, understanding, and persevering.
> 5. The minimization of harm is a priority.
> 6. Explore warning signs of deteriorating mental health, and identify high-risk situations for drug use. Develop a plan of care in the event of a relapse of the mental illness or the substance use.
> 7. Encourage participation in self-help groups, psychosocial interventions, and other sources of support.
>
> Source: Cleary, M., Walter, G., Hunt, G. E., Clancy, R., & Horsfall, J. (2008). Promoting dual diagnosis awareness in everyday clinical practice. *Journal of Psychosocial Nursing, 46*(12), 43–49.

disorder and addiction may increase the risk of suicide and shorten life expectancy, and it may also adversely impact the clinical course of either or both disorders.

Treatment of co-occurring depression with suitably matched antidepressant medication is helpful in reducing both substance abuse and depressive symptomatology. It should, however, not be considered stand-alone treatment and will unlikely resolve the addictive disorder, hence necessitating integrated care and treatment of both conditions. Similar to other studies of mood disorders, the placebo response rate is high. The selective serotonin reuptake inhibitors (SSRIs) are among the most favourable first-line options due to their tolerability and safety profile. The tricyclic antidepressants may be problematic in this population due to the sedating effects, the risk of overdose, as well as the risk of seizures. If SSRIs fail, alternative options include compounds like duloxetine (although not in alcohol-abusing persons), mirtazapine, venlafaxine, desvenlafaxine (serotonin and norepinephrine reuptake inhibitor, or SNRI), or bupropion. Bupropion should not be used in persons with a history of seizures or those in alcohol withdrawal (see Chapters 12 and 26). Cognitive–behavioural therapy (CBT) and community reinforcement approaches have demonstrated benefits in depression and substance use, while integrated group therapy, which is based on CBT, has shown benefit in those with bipolar disorder and substance use (see Chapters 13 and 14). For comorbid bipolar disorder, the mainstay of treatment is medication, and acute mania is typically treated with both a mood stabilizer and a neuroleptic (e.g., an atypical antipsychotic) compound. For stabilization following acute care, a mood stabilizer is recommended. Lithium treatment may not yield the same favourable results in persons with concurrent disorders as in those without.

Concurrent Addictive and Anxiety Disorders

Persons with anxiety disorders are two to five times more likely to have an addiction problem when compared with the general population. In the short-term, it is reported that some substances may relieve symptoms of anxiety; but in the medium and long term, these very substances may worsen symptoms of anxiety. Of the range of anxiety disorders, panic disorder is the single anxiety disorder most closely associated with addiction to alcohol, while generalized anxiety disorder (GAD) is the one most closely associated with dependence on substances other than alcohol. The presence of GAD is also associated with a more rapid progression from first alcoholic beverage to addiction, as compared with individuals without anxiety disorder. For most persons with anxiety and an addictive disorder, it has been determined that the anxiety disorder generally preceded the development of the addictive disorder. The association between substance-related conditions and obsessive–compulsive disorder is considered the least robust of all the anxiety disorders.

CBT is considered the most effective treatment for anxiety co-occurring with an addictive disorder, and some benefits may be yielded from pharmacotherapy. In general, the use of benzodiazepines (or other substances with an abuse potential) should be avoided. There is a limited evidence to guide treatment, but in general, the SSRIs or SNRIs may be considered helpful, along with psychotherapy (see Chapter 23).

Concurrent Addictive and Posttraumatic Stress Disorder (PTSD)

Although PTSD affects fewer than 10% of the population, around 60% of persons who suffer from PTSD also suffer from an addictive disorder. Persons with PTSD are two to four times more likely to struggle with an addictive disorder, compared to those in the general population (McCauley, Killeen, Gros, Brady, & Back, 2012). The relationship between trauma, subsequent PTSD, and the development of addiction is complex and frequently complicates treatment. Persons suffering from PTSD may resort to self-medicating with substances to relieve or distract from the distressing emotions related to the symptoms of the illness. The use of marijuana for medical purposes ("medical marijuana") is not yet considered an evidence-based approach to the care and treatment

of PTSD (National Academies of Science, Engineering, Medicine, January 2017). Treatment is offered by combining a first-line medication for PTSD (e.g., SSRI) with one of three modalities: prolonged exposure therapy (PE), cognitive processing therapy (CPT), or EMDR (eye movement desensitization and reprocessing therapy).

Concurrent Addictive and Attention Deficit Hyperactivity Disorder

Attention deficit hyperactivity disorder (ADHD) is the most common behavioural disorder of childhood, and those with ADHD are more prone to develop addictive disorders, especially if ADHD remains untreated in the early stages. This is particularly the case for those with concurrent conduct disorder. The majority of children with ADHD continue to have symptoms in adulthood even though they may not meet the criteria for the disorder as an adult. The diagnosis of ADHD is complicated in persons who are already using substances as their use may mimic symptoms of ADHD and the latter is often underdiagnosed in clinical populations. Major depressive disorder, bipolar disorder, or psychotic disorders may also co-occur in those with ADHD and substance-related/addictive disorders, further complicating diagnostic uncertainty.

Attention placed on prevention, early identification, and care/treatment strategies can diminish the adverse consequences of ADHD. These include the trait of impulsivity and one of its most damaging consequences, namely, that of substance use and addiction. Stimulant medications (dextroamphetamine or methylphenidate) are the mainstay of treatment, and, despite the abuse potential of these drugs, clinical evidence suggests that such treatment can be conducted safely and effectively. Nonstimulant medications such as atomoxetine, clonidine, and modafinil are also considered reasonable options. Precautions should be taken to avoid abuse when using medications that are associated with risk of abuse. Psychosocial interventions that are proven to yield benefits include contingency management and CBT.

Concurrent Addictive and Psychotic Disorders

The rate of addiction is substantially elevated in those with psychotic disorder when compared with persons in the general population. Substance use may accelerate the onset of a psychotic disorder in a vulnerable individual, and cannabis has been determined to be an independent risk factor in the development of schizophrenia. Transient substance-induced psychotic features are not uncommon in persons intoxicated with substances (Ziedonis et al., 2014). The most obvious psychotic symptoms related to alcohol use occur during alcohol withdrawal. Symptoms typically emerge within 2 days from stopping consumption and often present with command hallucinations and/or agitation. Cannabis use may be associated with suspiciousness, confusion, and memory impairment, while the psychosis associated with cocaine use is typically associated with transient paranoia. Substance use may also worsen the symptoms and complicate the diagnostic certainty, course, and treatment of the illness.

A wide range of substances may mimic psychotic symptoms, during both intoxication and withdrawal. The first step in management is to ensure adequate safety and security. Following this, the concurrent treatment of psychotic symptoms and substance use is indicated. Special attention should be given to medication adherence, and the use of depot antipsychotics may have a special utility in ensuring such. The use of atypical antipsychotics appears to be superior to the use of typical/conventional antipsychotics in this regard, as the former appear to better target negative symptoms and are less prone to be associated with dysphoria. Atypical antipsychotics are also associated with greater success in smoking cessation in persons with schizophrenia. Psychosocial approaches that have demonstrated effectiveness are motivational enhancement therapy, RP, and 12-step facilitation.

Concurrent Addictive and Personality Disorders

Although antisocial personality disorder is the most commonly associated personality disorder with substance-related/addictive disorders, the most challenging is likely borderline personality disorder. Both the addiction and the personality disorder are likely to result in complex and serious behavioural problems, often with an associated risk of harm to self. It is also often associated with the co-occurrence of other mental disorders, for example, MDD, an eating disorder, or OCD. The category of concurrent personality disorders and substance-related/addictive disorders poses some of the most vexing problems in care of this population.

Attention should first be paid to ensuring safety to self and to others. General principles of treatment include offering pharmacotherapy for comorbid conditions like MDD, OCD, or an eating disorder. No medication is indicated for any specific personality disorder. Behavioural interventions form the mainstay of treatment, specifically dialectical behavioural therapy (DBT). Applying the principles of DBT for the population of concurrent disordered individuals has demonstrated significant benefit by teaching cognitive self-control techniques that allow for turning themselves to abstinence. Principles that have been found beneficial in this context include the following:

- Do not give lethal drugs to lethal people.
- Combine pharmacotherapy with a psychosocial treatment.
- Do not reinforce dysfunctional, ineffective behaviour.
- Catch the patient "being good" (e.g., acting skillfully).
- Validate appropriate behaviour (see Chapter 27).

■ NURSING MANAGEMENT: SUMMARY

Nurses working in nonpsychiatric inpatient and community settings may be the first health care contact made by a person with a concurrent disorder. It is important to recognize that the stigma associated with both substance use and mental disorders can affect the person's readiness to address these illnesses. A helpful, knowledgeable, and nonjudgmental approach to the person may open a "window of opportunity" for seeking care and treatment. As persons with concurrent disorders may have difficulty relating openly with others and with trusting those in positions of authority, engaging the person in a way that concretely addresses presenting issues (e.g., acquiring social services, getting relief from psychiatric symptoms) can be particularly helpful. Note that assessment procedures that are protracted, are complicated, and involve intimate personal questions may be discouraging to the individual. As well, it may take some time and further engagement for the individual to be willing and able to provide an accurate history of substance use, severity of symptoms, and problems in living. Denial to oneself regarding these issues is a common defensive mechanism for persons with addiction (and in concurrent disorders); it may therefore be particularly difficult for them to always offer a reliable history. Medical records, other health care professionals, family members, and significant others may be of assistance to the person and the nurse in developing an accurate health history.

Families of the individual with a concurrent disorder will need education about concurrent disorders and guidance as to the best way to support their family member in recovery. Developing and sustaining a healthy lifestyle is an important aspect of recovery, and families can be particularly helpful in this area. Nurses can provide information at a level appropriate to the family, as well as the individual, on diet, exercise, sleep routine, stress management, and leisure activities. These are essential to a lifestyle that supports sobriety and prevents relapse. At times, families of persons with a concurrent disorder are no longer involved in their lives or are also living with addiction and/or mental health problems. Nurses need to assess the existing support system of the individual, as finding alternative supports and/or social services may need to be an immediate goal.

Psychoeducation regarding goal setting can give the individual a core strategy for making positive change. Access to crisis counselling is important, as is housing that allows for a situation supportive of recovery. Opportunities for a social network that reinforces sobriety and the maintenance of treatment plans for psychiatric symptoms will be important. Nurses can assist by referrals to local groups (e.g., Alcoholics Anonymous, or reasonable alternative; mental health drop-in clubs; partnership with volunteers) that aim to facilitate the development of such social networks. At an appropriate

---

BOX 33.3 Psychoeducational Topics for Relapse Prevention

- Understanding addiction
- Effects and interaction of tobacco, alcohol, and other drugs in the body
- What is my relationship with tobacco, alcohol, and other drugs?
- How to live in a healthy way
- Leisure and relaxation
- Coping with stress
- Coping with anger
- Communicating with others
- Problem-solving strategies
- The relapse cycle
- Strategies for preventing relapse
- My plan for avoiding relapse
- My personal cues that relapse is imminent
- Dealing with crisis

---

point in recovery, referral to vocational and employment guidance will be a priority. Relapse prevention is crucial to the care of the person in recovery from a concurrent disorder; patient education, whether offered on a one-to-one basis or in a group setting, is a key strategy. See Box 33.3 for recommended psychoeducational topics.

■ WHERE DO WE GO FROM HERE?

In some settings, mental health and addiction systems continue to operate independently from each other and remain compartmentalized. As a result, the focus of treatment for people with concurrent disorders tends to be on one component of their concurrent disorder but not the other. This challenge is likely as intractable as concurrent disorders themselves. Apart from research into the effectiveness of different treatment approaches, research into systems' approaches is also direly needed (see Box 33.4 on research for best practice). Universal education and training are needed for the workforce responsible for the care and treatment of those with

---

BOX 33.4 Research for Best Practice

INTEGRATED CARE PATHWAY FOR CO-OCCURRING MAJOR DEPRESSIVE AND ALCOHOL USE DISORDERS: OUTCOMES OF THE FIRST TWO YEARS

Samokhvalov, A. V., Awan, A., George, T. P., Irving, J., Le Foll, B., Perrotta, S., ... Rehm, J. (2017). Integrated care pathway for co-occurring major depressive and alcohol use disorders: Outcomes of the first two years. American Journal on Addictions, 26(6), 602–609. doi:10.1111/ajad.12572

Background: Treatment as usual (TAU) for individuals with concurrent major depressive (MDD) and alcohol use disorder (AUD) typically involves management of each disorder consecutively by different health providers at different periods of time. Emerging clinical evidence suggests that a more ideal approach is to combine psychotherapy and pharmacotherapy and deliver treatment in a coordinated manner. An integrated care pathway (ICP) is a structured multidisciplinary care plan that details essential steps in the care of patients with a specific clinical problem. At the Centre for Addiction and Mental Health in Toronto, an ICP has been developed specifically for individuals experiencing concurrent MDD and AUD. The purpose of this study was to evaluate the clinical outcomes of the ICP and to compare these to TAU.

Method: In this retrospective chart review, two cohorts of patients were formed based on treatment received. ICP treatment included pharmacotherapy for AUD and MDD based on a defined algorithm and clinical scales in conjunction with 16 sessions of psychotherapy. TAU

included pharmacotherapy for MDD and/or AUD with the choice of medications and timing of visits at the health provider's discretion. Eighty-one patients met the inclusion criteria for the ICP group. Of the 126 patients meeting the inclusion criteria in the TAU cohort, 81 were matched with the ICP cohort by sex, age, alcohol consumptions, and severity of depression scores.

Findings: The structured care plan with the ICP yielded significantly better outcomes in drinking patterns and severity of depression symptoms when compared with the TAU cohort. The ICP cohort had a significantly lower dropout rate; both cohorts demonstrated significant reduction in the number of heavy drinking day and standard drinks per week, with a significantly higher reduction of both indicators over time in the ICP group. Although no data was available for the TAU cohort, a significant reduction in depressive symptom severity was observed in the ICP cohort.

Implications for Practice: Integrated care plans have been shown to be effective in a number of settings. What this study adds is demonstration of positive outcomes when transferring this approach into care planning for individuals with concurrent disorders. Nurses are a vital member of multidisciplinary teams responsible for planning and implementing integrated care plans.

concurrent disorders. The only reasonable solution to prevent those with concurrent disorders from "falling through the cracks" is to ensure integration of the national agendas for mental health and addiction. Unless we have a unified approach to all components of concurrent disorders, enjoying parity with regard to health care spending, our patients will not be able to reach their potential and thrive.

 SUMMARY OF KEY POINTS

- *Concurrent disorders* refers to the term used when individuals suffer from at least *one* substance-related or addictive disorder as well as one or more *other* mental disorders. When these conditions co-occur, treatment should address both (or all) at the same time (integrated or parallel treatment).
- Many individuals with co-occurring disorders, despite the associated challenges, do recover and live productive lives.
- An important reason why persons with addiction relapse to drug use is the presence of untreated mental illness. An important reason why persons with mental illness relapse is untreated addiction issues.
- When mental illness and addiction coexist, both disorders require specific and appropriate primary treatment.
- Both disorders should be considered "primary" and both should be treated at the same time.
- The specific content of primary treatment for each person with concurrent disorders must be individualized according to diagnosis, phase of treatment, level of functioning and/or disability, and assessment of level of care based on acuity, severity, medical safety, motivation, and availability of recovery support.
- The most effective approach for patients is integrated care whereby health care professionals, programs, and resources co-located and such services offered on a long-term basis with continuity of care across programs and time. Patients benefit from a longitudinal care approach rather than episodic care.
- Psychoeducation regarding the effects of tobacco, alcohol, and other drug use, a healthy lifestyle, and RP is another key element of nursing care for persons with concurrent disorders, in addition to health education regarding their co-occurring mental disorder.

 Web Links

https://www.porticonetwork.ca/web/knowledgex-archive/primary-care/resources-patients-families/resources-concurrent-disorders Portico: Canada's Mental Health & Addiction Network lists several resources of relevance to PMH nurses in Canada, including *Concurrent Substance Use and Mental Health Disorder: An Information Guide* (available in both English and French) and *A Family Guide to Concurrent Disorders.*

http://www.camh.ca/en/education/about/AZCourses/Pages/default.aspx The Centre for Addiction and Mental Heatlh (CAMH) is an excellent resource for individuals interested in learning more about concurrent disorders. In particular, CAMH offers a *Concurrent Disorders Core Online Course,* open to anyone, and a *Concurrent Disorder Certificate Program* designed for mental health and addictions' professionals.

References

American Psychiatric Association. (2013). *Diagnostic and statistical manual of mental disorders* (5th ed.). Washington, DC: Author.

Andréasson, S., Engström, A., Allebeck, P., & Rydberg, U. (1987). Cannabis and schizophrenia: A longitudinal study of Swedish conscripts. *Lancet,* 2(8574), 1483–1486.

Arsenault, A. (2015). Olympian Clara Hughes reveals doping infraction. *CBC News.* Retrieved from http://www.cbc.ca/news/canada/olympian-clara-hughes-reveals-doping-infraction-1.3215617

Balhara, Y. P. S., Kuppili, P. P., & Gupta, R. (2017). Neurobiology of comorbid substance use disorders and psychiatric disorders: Current state of the evidence. *Journal of Addictions Nursing,* 28(1), 11–26. doi:10.1097/JAN.0000000000000155

Beaudette, J. N., & Stewart, L. A. (2016). National prevalence of mental disorders among incoming Canadian male offenders. *Canadian Journal of Psychiatry,* 61(10), 624–632.

Brunette, M. F., Mueser, K. T., Babbin, S., Meyer-Kalos, P., Rosenheck, R., Correll, C. U., … Kane, J. M. (2017). Demographic and clinical correlates of substance use disorders in first episode psychosis. *Schizophrenia Research,* Advance online publication. doi:10.1016/j.schres.2017.06.039

Canadian Institutes of Health Information. (2013). *Hospital mental health services for concurrent mental illness and substance use disorders in Canada.* Retrieved from https://www.cihi.ca/en/hospital-mental-health-services-for-concurrent-mental-illness-and-substance-use-disorders-in-canada

Cleary, M., Walter, G., Hunt, G. E., Clancy, R., & Horsfall, J. (2008). Promoting dual diagnosis awareness in everyday clinical practice. *Journal of Psychosocial Nursing,* 46(12), 43–49.

Drake, R. E., & Green, A. I. (2013). The challenge of heterogeneity and complexity in dual diagnosis. *Journal of Dual Diagnosis,* 9(2), 105–106.

Fergusson, D. M., Boden, J. M., & Horwood, L. J. (2009). Tests of causal links between alcohol abuse or dependence and major depression. *Archives of General Psychiatry,* 66(3), 260–266.

Flensborg-Madsen, T., Mortensen, E. L., Knop, J., Becker, U., Sher, L., & Grøbaek, M. (2009). Comorbidity and temporal ordering of alcohol use disorders and other psychiatric disorders: Results from a Danish register-based study. *Comprehensive Psychiatry,* 50(4), 307–314.

Hughes, C. (2015). *Open heart, open mind.* New York, NY: Simon & Schuster Canada.

Kavanagh, D. J., Mueser, K. T., & Baker, A. (2003). Management of comorbidity. In M. Teesson & H. Proudfoot (Eds.), *Comorbid mental disorders and substance use disorders: Epidemiology, prevention and treatment* (pp. 78–120). Sydney, Australia: National Drug and Alcohol Research Centre.

Kedzior, K. K., & Laeber, L. T. (2014). A positive association between anxiety disorders and cannabis use or cannabis use disorders in the general population—A meta-analysis of 31 studies. *BMC Psychiatry,* 14, 136–158.

Margolese, H. C., Malchy, L., Carlos Negrete, J., Tempier, R., & Gill, K. (2004). Drug and alcohol use among patients with schizophrenia and related psychoses: Levels and consequences. *Schizophrenia Research,* 67, 157–166.

McCauley, J. L., Killeen, T., Gros, D. F., Brady, K. T., & Back, S. E. (2012). Posttraumatic stress disorder and co-occurring substance use disorders: Advances in assessment and treatment. *Clinical Psychology,* 19(3), 713–719. doi:10.1111/cpsp.12006

McKee, S. A. (2017). Concurrent substance use disorders and mental illness: Bridging the gap between research and treatment. *Canadian Psychology,* 58(1), 50–57. doi:10.1037/cap0000093

Mental Health Commission of Canada. (2016). *Advancing the mental health strategy for Canada: A framework for action (2017–2022).* Ottawa, ON: Author.

Minkoff, K. (2001). Developing standards of care for individuals with co-occurring psychiatric and substance disorders. *Psychiatric Services,* 52(5), 597–599.

Mueser, K. T., Bennet, M., & Kushner, M. G. (1995). Epidemiology of substance use disorders among persons with chronic mental illnesses. In A. F. Lehman & L. B. Dixon (Eds.), *Double-jeopardy: Chronic mental illness and substance use disorders* (Vol. 3, pp. 9–25). Langhorne, PA: Harwood Academic.

Mueser, K. T., Drake, R. E., & Wallach, M. A. (1998). Dual diagnosis: A review of etiological theories. *Addictive Behaviours, 23*(6), 717–734.

Mueser, K. T., & Gingrich, S. (2013). Treatment of co-occurring psychotic and substance use disorders. *Social Work in Public Health, 28*, 424–439. doi:10.1080/19371918.2013.774676

Mueser, K. T., Noordsy, D. L., Drake, R. E., & Fox, L. (2003). *Integrated treatment for dual disorders: A guide to effective practice.* New York, NY: Guildford Press.

National Academies of Sciences, Engineering, and Medicine. (2017). *The health effects of cannabis and cannabinoids: The current state of evidence and recommendations for research.* Washington, DC: The National Academies Press. doi:10.17226/24625

Nunes, E. V., & Wiss, R. D. (2014). Co-occurring addictive and mood disorders. In R. K. Ries, D. A. Fiellin, S. C. Miller, & R. Saitz (Eds.), *The ASAM principles of addiction medicine* (5th ed.). Philadelphia, PA: Wolters Kluwer.

Pakula, B., Shoveller, J., Ratner, P. A., & Carpiano, R. (2016). Prevalence and co-occurrence of heavy drinking and anxiety and mood disorders among gay, lesbian, bisexual, and heterosexual Canadians. *American Journal of Public Health, 106*(6), 1042–1048. doi:10.2105/AJPH.2016.303083

Rush, B., & Koegl, C. J. (2008). Prevalence and profile of people with co-occurring mental and substance use disorders within a comprehensive mental health system. *Canadian Journal of Psychiatry, 53*(12), 810–821.

Rush, B., Urbanoski, K., Bassani, D., Castel, S., Wild, T. C., Strike, C., & Somers, J. (2008). Prevalence of co-occurring substance use and other mental disorders in the Canadian population. *Canadian Journal of Psychiatry, 53*(12), 800–809.

Samokhvalov, A. V., Awan, A., George, T. P., Irving, J., Le Foll, B., Perrotta, S., … Rehm, J. (2017). Integrated care pathway for co-occurring major depressive and alcohol use disorders: Outcomes of the first two years. *American Journal on Addictions, 26*(6) 602–609. doi:10.1111/ajad.12572

United States Department of Health and Human Services, Substance Abuse and Mental Health Services Administration. (2015). *Receipt of services for behavioral health problems: Results from the 2014 National Survey on Drug Use and Health.* Rockville, MD: Author.

Yuodelis-Flores, C., Goldsmith, R. J., & Ries, R. K. (2014). Substance-induced mental disorders. In R. K. Ries, D. A. Fiellin, S. C. Miller, & R. Saitz (Eds.), *The ASAM principles of addiction medicine* (5th ed.; pp. 1287–1299). Philadelphia, PA: Wolters Kluwer.

Ziedonis, D. M., Fan, X., Bizamcer, A. N., Wyatt, S. A., Tonelli, M. E., Smelson, D. (2014). Co-occurring addiction and psychotic disorders. In R. K. Ries, D. A. Fiellin, S. C. Miller, & R. Saitz (Eds.), *The ASAM principles of addiction medicine* (5th ed.). Philadelphia, PA: Wolters Kluwer.

34 Care of Persons With a History of Abuse

Elizabeth A. McCay

Adapted from the chapter "Caring for Abused Persons" by Mary R. Boyd

LEARNING OBJECTIVES

After studying this chapter, you will be able to:

- Describe the biopsychosocial theories of abuse.
- Discuss theories explaining why some persons become abusive and why some persons remain in violent relationships.
- Describe the bio/psycho/social/spiritual consequences of abuse.
- Describe the diagnostic criteria for posttraumatic stress disorder (PTSD).
- Discuss the three major symptom categories found in PTSD and their associated aetiologic factors.
- Describe the diagnostic criteria for dissociative identity disorder (DID).
- Integrate bio/psycho/social/spiritual theories into the analysis of human responses to abuse.
- Formulate nursing care plans for survivors of abuse.

KEY TERMS

- abuse • acute stress disorder (ASD) • alexithymia
- behavioural sensitization • complex posttraumatic stress disorder (C-PTSD) • cycle of violence • dissociation
- dissociative identity disorder (DID) • emotional abuse
- extinction • fear conditioning • neglect • physical abuse • posttraumatic stress disorder (PTSD) • sexual abuse • traumatic bonding

KEY CONCEPTS

- resilience • self-esteem

Violence demonstrated in the **abuse** of women, men, children, and elders is a national health problem that causes significant harm in survivors. Abuse of any type permanently changes survivors constructions of reality and the meaning of their lives. It wounds deeply, endangering core beliefs about self, others, and the world. It usually devastates the survivor's self-esteem.

Nurses encounter survivors of abuse in all health care settings. For this reason, they must be knowledgeable about abuse. They must understand its indicators, causes, assessment techniques, and effective nursing interventions. The importance of assessing for abuse in health care settings is readily recognized (Gallop, McCay, Austin, Bayer, & Peternelji-Taylor, 1998; MacMillan et al., 2009), and intimate partner violence (IPV) is increasingly recognized as a serious public health issue (Mason & Rinn, 2014). It requires nurses to possess the necessary educational background to ask questions about abuse that will ultimately prevent further abuse (Beynon et al., 2012; Mason & O'Rinn, 2014) and facilitate recovery. Adopting the Routine Universal Comprehensive Screening Protocol was found to be an effective strategy that increased public health nurses' knowledge and comfort to enquire about domestic abuse within a maternal–child visiting programme (Vanderburg, Wright, Boston, & Zimmerman, 2010). Failure to assess for abuse communicates a powerfully disturbing message: that the most traumatic event of a patient's life is too upsetting for others to hear. Protection and recovery from abuse require survivors to remember and discuss terrible events. Secrecy and silence may protect perpetrators and seriously endangers survivors. If nurses do not allow and encourage survivors to tell their stories, the abuse experiences will continue to haunt patients as symptoms of mental disorders.

This chapter focuses on the nursing process with women, men, children, and elders who are survivors of abuse. It provides basic nursing information needed to address the multiple, complex problems of these patients.

KEY CONCEPT

Self-esteem is how one feels about oneself. Its components are self-acceptance, self-worth, self-love, and self-nurturing.

■ TYPES OF ABUSE

Most abuse that women, men, children, and elders experience is intimate violence; that is, the perpetrator is a loved and trusted partner or family member. As a result, the world and home may no longer be safe, people seem dangerous, and life may become a tortured existence of warding off ever-present threats. However, for some resilient individuals, healthy relationships across the life span appear to be protective, such that minimal psychological sequelae occur in adult life in spite of childhood abuse (Wingo, Ressler, & Bradley, 2014). For example, one Canadian study provides evidence that resilience offered protection for First Nation's youth who were exposed to emotional, physical, and/or sexual abuse; specifically, the presence of community and family resilience significantly reduced symptoms of posttraumatic stress disorder (PTSD) (Zahradnik et al., 2010).

KEY CONCEPT

Resilience is the capacity to overcome adversity in spite of extreme stress and involves the balancing of risk and protective factors.

Woman Abuse

Woman abuse, domestic violence, spousal abuse, partner abuse, and battered wives are terms used interchangeably to denote violence directed towards women. However, some of these terms do not specifically refer to the abuse of a woman by an intimate partner. For example, the term *domestic violence* may be used in cases in which one person directs abuse against an entire family. The terms *spouse abuse* and *partner abuse* could indicate the couple in whom abuse occurs, either heterosexual or homosexual, lives together but is unmarried. For these reasons, *woman abuse* has been chosen as the most appropriate term to use in this chapter in designating violence, including rape, directed towards a woman by an intimate partner.

Woman abuse is a significant health problem that crosses all ethnic, racial, and socioeconomic lines. In 2009, there were nearly 1.6 million self-reported incidents of woman abuse in Canada (Sinha, 2013). According to Statistics Canada, men account for 83% of violence that is committed against women (Canadian Centre for Justice Statistics, 2013). Specific rates of victimization were assessed in the 2014 General Social Survey on Victimization. Survey results indicated that women and men report similar levels of spousal violence; however, women are twice as likely as men to report the most severe types of abuse (Canadian Centre for Justice Statistics, 2016). It is possible that these figures may be conservative due to underreporting. Many women are afraid or reluctant to identify their abusers. In some cases, they fear retaliation against themselves or their children. In other cases, they continue to hold strong feelings for their partners, despite the abuse. On the other hand, men, given the societal expectation of male strength, may not want to admit to being victims of violence. A recent critique of the Canadian literature regarding violence against women underscores the importance of considering the context in which the violence occurs (Dragiewicz & DeKeseredy, 2012). For example, violent responses in women are frequently in self-defense (DeKeseredy, 2007; Sheehy, 2016), whereas men may use violence to exert control over their partner (DeKeseredy & Dragiewicz, 2007; Dragiewicz & DeKeseredy, 2012). An additional analysis of the 2004 Canadian General Social Survey on Victimization adds further evidence that IPV is more chronic and severe for women than for men (Ansara & Hindin, 2010, 2011).

It is important to recognize that women of all ages and sociocultural backgrounds may experience abuse. Regardless, certain factors have been found to be associated with increased risk for violence in women. Specifically, police-reported and self-reported victimization data indicate that women who are at higher risk of violence are younger (15 to 24 years of age), with the risk of victimization decreasing with age (Canadian Centre for Justice Statistics, 2013). Women living with disabilities, such as a physical or mental health challenge that restricts activity, or who are young and/or experience emotional and financial abuse may be at increased risk of spousal abuse (Canadian Centre for Justice Statistics, 2013). Further, evidence suggests that single, divorced, and separated women may be at greater risk for abuse than are married women (Brownridge et al., 2008; Romans, Forte, Cohen, Du Mont, & Hyman, 2007). Moreover, this group is at particularly high risk for severe violence. Danger assessments show that abusive ex-partners often exhibit obsessive threatening behaviour after their relationships end and pose significant dangers to women. Forty-three percent of women seen in emergency departments (EDs) attributed their abuse to a past partner. These findings emphasize that ending a relationship often does not end violence (Fishwick, Campbell, & Taylor, 2004; Stewart, MacMillan, & Wathen, 2013). This information is important for health care providers, who frequently pressure women to end abusive relationships. Rates of woman abuse vary among women of different racial backgrounds. Research supports that Indigenous women are at high risk for violence in their intimate relationships. Specifically, the results of the 2014 General Social Survey (GSS) data indicate that Aboriginal women in Canada are three times as likely to experience IPV by a male partner (Boyce, 2016). Even higher rates of woman abuse have been reported for Indigenous women by other studies. For example, a study in Ontario documents that 8 of 10 Indigenous women experienced violence in their intimate relationships (Health Canada, 2009), with 87% reporting physical abuse and 57% reporting sexual abuse. Further, physical abuse of women in northern Indigenous communities is thought to be pervasive, with estimates ranging from 75% to 90% (Health Canada, 2009) (see Box 34.1 on research in this field).

BOX 34.1 Research for Best Practice

RECLAIMING OUR SPIRITS: DEVELOPMENT AND PILOT TESTING OF A HEALTH PROMOTION INTERVENTION FOR INDIGENOUS WOMEN WHO HAVE EXPERIENCED INTIMATE PARTNER VIOLENCE

Varcoe, C., Browne, A. J., Ford-Gilboe, M., Dion Stout, M., McKenzie, H., Price, R., ... Merritt-Gray, M. (2017). Reclaiming our spirits: Development and pilot testing of a health promotion intervention for Indigenous women who have experienced intimate partner violence. Research in Nursing and Health, 40(3), 237–254.

The Question: What is the impact of a health promotion intervention to support indigenous women who have experienced intimate partner violence?

Method: An evidence-based health promotion intervention based on promising outcomes of prior feasibility studies was modified and piloted with urban indigenous women who had experienced IPV. Researchers used an indigenous lens to inform the adaption of the intervention situating it within decolonizing approaches aimed at reducing risks associated with colonial relationships and historical trauma.

A steering committee of Indigenous women leaders with expertise in IPV guided all aspects of the study. The approach used in the intervention was informed by qualitative interviews with Indigenous leaders, elders' wisdom and teachings, previous research, and strategies that addressed the women's needs in a safe way and supported their health. Such work resulted in a set of principles that centred on Indigenous identity as a strength and shaped the revision of the intervention. The revised intervention included nurses working one to one with women over a 6-month period. A key feature of the adapted intervention was a circle led by an elder who taught traditional practices to support women participants.

A pilot study was carried out to evaluate the feasibility of implementing the modified intervention with indigenous women, determine its acceptability to women and providers, and collect data prior to commencing a broader efficacy study. Pre- and postintervention measures included demographic information and experience of abuse as well as multiple measures to assess mental health, chronic pain, health and service use, quality of life, and social support. Qualitative interviews explored individual experiences of the intervention.

Twenty-one adult women who were identified as Indigenous, had experienced violence from an intimate partner, and lived in the study community were recruited and completed preintervention surveys. Twelve women completed both pre- and postintervention surveys and 16 participated in postintervention qualitative interviews. Thirteen women who completed individual interviews also participated in a focus group to solicit group feedback. Interviews were also carried out with elders and nurses involved in the study. The data provided a description of the characteristics and experiences of indigenous women who have experienced IPV.

Findings: Women participating in the pilot represented a diversity of Indigenous communities. All had experienced significant IPV, racism, and financial insecurity and more than half had unstable housing situations. Many women also experienced significant health issues, including HIV and substance abuse. Overall, women found the intervention to be acceptable. The weekly circle and traditional teaching and practices were particularly helpful as was access to nurses. Women who participated in the pilot reported increased confidence, trust, feeling of safety and hope, and connection to others. Women also described themselves as fighters working to improve their lives and heal. Challenges experienced by the women made participation difficult, most notably triggering of past trauma. The sample size precluded statistical testing, but a reduction in women's trauma symptoms and increased sense of agency were observed trends. Changes were made to the intervention that provided additional structure both to the approach used in the intervention group and for staff support and training in trauma-informed care. At the conclusion of the pilot, participants renamed the modified intervention to "Reclaiming Our Spirits."

Implications for Nursing: Nurses working with Indigenous women in urban areas who have experienced IPV need to take into account the multiple traumas to which such women have been exposed. Indigenous women's experiences of violence are situated within the historical context of economic hardship, racism, and neocolonization. Effectiveness in practice requires a comprehensive grasp of the context of Indigenous women's lives and complexity of issues facing women including health issues, loss, and challenges posed by triggering trauma. Recognizing the importance of indigenous healing practices and traditions is critical in building on the strengths and resilience in indigenous women. Nurses also need to attend to women's needs related to the social determinants of health such as acceptable housing and adequate income, supporting women in areas they regard as most important. Engaging and supporting women through not only listening and teaching but also offering practical assistance in navigating health care and services are paramount. The critical importance of nurse's role in advocating for system and structural changes to indigenous health care cannot be overstated.

The perpetuation of violence begins early in dating relationships. Data from the 2014 GSS indicate that dating violence constitutes approximately 52% of all IPV (Canadian Centre for Justice Statistics, 2016). The majority of victims are female, and those most at risk for dating violence are between the ages of 15 to 19 (Canadian Centre for Justice Statistics, 2016). Several recent Canadian studies have focused on the underlying factors that influence dating violence in youth populations. A qualitative study of 40 adolescent girls aged 15 and 16 years provides some insight into factors associated with high rates of dating violence (Banister, Jakubec, & Stein, 2003; Sears, Byers, & Price, 2007). Specifically, the study findings highlight the tremendous power imbalance that exists in dating relationships for adolescent girls, which frequently gives rise to a tolerance of violence simply to maintain the relationship (Banister et al., 2003). A related study demonstrates that higher levels of affiliation with deviant peers are associated with high-risk lifestyles, as well as increased levels of dating violence among a community sample of adolescent girls (N = 550) in Québec (Vézina et al., 2011). Further, peer group relational aggression was found to predict dating violence among both male and female adolescents (Ellis, Chung-Hall, & Dumas, 2013). The importance of familial factors for adolescent boys in dating violence is highlighted in a longitudinal study of dating violence in adolescent boys residing in Montreal (LaVoie et al., 2002). Specifically, harsh parenting and antisocial behaviour were found to be predictive of dating violence in 717 boys aged 16 to 17 years living in a less affluent area of Montreal (LaVoie et al., 2002). In the 2014 GSS, dating violence accounted for 15% of nonfamilial violence (Canadian Centre for Justice Statistics, 2016). It is also noteworthy that dating violence was found to be more prevalent than was spousal abuse (Canadian Centre for Justice Statistics, 2016). Research suggests that supporting youth in the context of early dating relationships is important since future patterns of violence and assault are frequently established in early relationships (Wolfe, 2006).

Battering

Battering is the single greatest cause of serious injury to women. Battering can be defined as repeated physical or sexual violence with the intent of coercive control (Humphreys & Campbell, 2011). Estimates of injury related to battering seen in emergency departments (EDs) range from 14% to 50% (Campbell, Torres, McKenna, Sheridan, & Landenburger, 2004). Overall, women are four times more likely to be victims of homicide by a spouse than are men (Canadian Centre for Justice Statistics, 2016). Further, in 2010, there were 593 shelters in Canada specifically for women who have experienced abuse (Burczycka & Cotter, 2011). Sixty-seven percent of women who were residing in shelters were seeking a secure setting away from an abusive partner (Burczycka & Cotter, 2011). Indeed, the realistic fear of being killed is one factor that keeps many women from leaving abusive partners, even after years of severe abuse. Intimate partner violence against women is more likely to be consistent with battering, such that it is severe, repetitive, and likely to result in injury and has been found to be associated with a wide range of poor mental health outcomes, such as increased anxiety and suicidal ideation (Afifi, Boman, Fleisher, & Sareen, 2009). Moreover, many women who experience abuse also live with PTSD (Stewart et al., 2013). In a study of 65 women receiving treatment from three Canadian urban mental health centres, women reporting early-onset sexual abuse were more likely to meet the criteria for complex PTSD than were women reporting late-onset PTSD (McLean & Gallop, 2003). In addition, based on an analysis of the Canadian Community Health Survey, PTSD was determined to be associated with severe physical health problems such as cardiovascular disease, chronic pain, and cancer among others, as well as increased suicide attempts, poor quality of life, and increased disability (Sareen et al., 2007). IPV has a significant negative effect on women's physical and mental health, and this impact continues after leaving a violent relationship (Ford-Gilboe et al., 2009).

Battering also poses a significant danger to unborn children. The literature suggests that there is an increased risk of violence for women who are pregnant, although this observation may be related to increased opportunities for detection of abuse at health clinics during pregnancy. Furthermore, violence during pregnancy is likely to contribute to postpartum depression (Brownridge et al., 2011; Cook & Dickens, 2009). According to a 2009 Canadian GSS, 11% of women who reported being victims of IPV also reported being pregnant (Sinha, 2013). Abuse during pregnancy is a significant risk factor for several fetal and maternal complications, including low birth weight, low maternal weight gain, infections, and anaemia (Sinha, 2013). Moreover, abuse of women often results in their use of alcohol and other drugs (AOD), which, in turn, may harm unborn children (Department of Justice, Canada, 2012; Parker, Bullock, Bohn, & Curry, 2004).

Rape and Sexual Assault

Rape and sexual assault are common in Canada. Sexual assault includes any form of nonconsenting sexual activity, ranging from fondling to penetration. According to the 2014 GSS, there were 633,000 incidents of sexual assault reported in the Canadian population aged 15 years and older (Perreault, 2015). Also, based on the 2014 GSS, rates of sexual victimization for women were found to be almost seven times higher than for men (Perreault, 2015). Overall, age is a risk for sexual assault with 47% of all sexual assault incidents reported being against women aged 15 to 24 (Conroy & Cotter, 2017). Most sexual assaults are underreported for the same reason that domestic violence is underreported—women may feel embarrassed and ashamed and fear being blamed for the assault (Ansara & Hindin, 2010).

Sex and Increased Risk for Human Immunodeficiency Virus

Woman abuse is also a risk factor for human immuno-deficiency virus (HIV) infection among women. In one study where screening for domestic violence was part of ongoing care for an HIV population in Alberta, a strong association was found between domestic violence victimization and HIV infection (Siemieniuk, Krentz, Gish, & Gill, 2010). Of those individuals with HIV who were screened, 34% reported having experienced abuse; and among these, more than half were abused as children (Siemieniuk et al., 2010). Further, women were 1.6 times more likely than men and over twice as likely as heterosexual men to have experienced IPV. An association was also found between a history of domestic violence and delayed access to care, missed appointments, and an increased use of clinic resources such as social work. An abusive partner may increase the risk for HIV infection in several ways. Women who have abusive partners may not be able to avoid sexual contact. Fear of a partner's violent behaviour may prevent women from insisting on the use of condoms. A woman's insistence on condom use can imply that either partner is being unfaithful and can result in abuse.

It is noteworthy that Indigenous peoples are over-represented among HIV and AIDS cases in Canada. Indigenous peoples made up 3.8% of the Canadian population in 2006 but accounted for 12.2% of all new infections and 8.9% of all prevalent infections by the end of 2011 (Public Health Agency of Canada, 2012). Therefore, the estimated infection rate among Indigenous persons is 3.5 times higher than among non-Indigenous persons (Public Health Agency of Canada, 2012). A study undertaken by the Cedar Project Partnership found that Indigenous people who are sexual abuse survivors were twice as likely to be HIV-positive compared to those who did not report any sexual abuse (Cedar Project Partnership, 2008). Further, Varcoe and Dick (2008) conducted an ethnographic study to explore the experiences of Indigenous rural women and the intersecting risks of violence and HIV infection. The study highlighted the challenges faced by Indigenous women within the context of Canadian society and the effects of colonization. Women's health was dramatically impacted by inequities of gender, poverty, and position in society. The participants were not injection drug users, yet all were concerned that they were or had been at risk of HIV. Further, high rates of sexual abuse documented among Indigenous youth (48% of 543 surveyed) are clearly linked to an increased risk for HIV infection through injection drug use and/or ongoing sexual contact (Cedar Project Partnership, 2008).

Stalking

Stalking is a crime of intimidation. In legal terms, stalking is referred to as criminal harassment and involves behaviour that occurs over a period of time and which causes individuals to experience significant distress or fear for their safety or that of someone they know (Department of Justice, Canada, 2003). Examples include following or communicating with another person, repeatedly watching someone's house or workplace, or directly threatening another person or their family member (Milligan, 2011). Criminal harassment legislation was introduced in 1993 to deal with harassment and prevent escalation into serious physical harm primarily against women. The legislation applies to all victims of harassment (Department of Justice, Canada, 2003). In 2009, however, females accounted for three quarters of all individuals experiencing criminal harassment with almost half of these incidents by a former intimate partner. Those who were stalked by an ex-spouse were pursued for well over a year (Canadian Centre for Justice Statistics, 2005). In contrast, males were more often harassed by a casual acquaintance (37%) than by a former (21%) or current (2%) intimate partner (Milligan, 2011). Probation was the most common sentence imposed for those found guilty of criminal harassment in 2008/2009 (Canadian Centre for Justice Statistics, 2011). Over the years, the criminal code has been amended to put in place procedural protections for the victim when an individual is accused and convicted of criminal harassment such as prohibiting possession of weapons (Department of Justice, Canada, 2012).

Abuse of Men

Although discussion around sexual assault and violence is typically focused on women, a review of the literature indicates that the rate of violence and sexual assault is higher in men than traditionally believed (Romans et al., 2007; Stermac, Del Bove, & Addison, 2004). In 2014, there were an equal number of men and women who reported being victims of spousal violence in the last 5 years (Canadian Centre for Justice Statistics, 2016). Although women reported severe violence more often than men, men were more than 3.5 times more likely to be the victim of kicking, biting, hitting, or being hit with something (Canadian Centre for Justice Statistics, 2016).

The consequences of violence and sexual assault can also be devastating for men. Hopton and Huta (2013) evaluated an intervention designed specifically for men who had experienced childhood abuse (sexual, physical, and/or emotional). Their findings suggest that male survivors who seek services are suffering from high rates of self-reported posttraumatic stress and symptoms of depression. Men are less likely than are women to seek help despite significant levels of functional distress. The authors suggest that factors such as stigma, underrecognition and underreporting of male sexual abuse, and the lack of services tailored to the needs of men are barriers to seeking treatment. In a secondary analysis of GSS data, Ansara and Hinden (2011) found that although men may experience the same physical abuse as women, they are less likely to report any negative reactions. A study examined 141 cases from a sexual assault database located in a large urban Ontario city (Stermac et al., 2004). The data suggest that male victims of sexual assault are more likely to be young, street involved, with an increased vulnerability such as either a cognitive or a physical disability (Stermac et al., 2004). The authors suggest that future research is needed to understand better this previously unrecognized vulnerable group.

Child Abuse

All forms of child abuse deprive children of the rights and protection to which they are entitled. These rights are clearly set out in the United Nations Convention of the Rights of the Child (United Nations, 1989) and include basic rights to the provision of an adequate standard of living, to be protected from harm and abuse, and to participate in children's programmes and services (Canadian Child Care Federation, 2012).

The prevalence of child abuse is far reaching. Specifically, in the data from the 2012 Canadian Community Health Survey, Afifi et al. (2014) found a strong association between child abuse and mental conditions including suicidal ideation. The 2008 Canadian Incidence Study of Reported Child Abuse and Neglect estimated that there were 235,842 child maltreatment investigations that year (Public Health Agency of Canada, 2010). Of course, this figure does not include cases that were unreported. The most common forms of child maltreatment included witnessing IPV (34%), neglect (34%), physical violence (20%), and emotional neglect (9%) (Public Health Agency of Canada, 2010). In 2012, 40% of those who were identified as Indigenous indicated that they had been abused in their childhood sexually, physically, or both (Canadian Centre for Justice Statistics, 2016). Indigenous people were also twice as likely as non-Indigenous people to report witnessing violence as a child (Canadian Centre for Justice Statistics, 2016). It is also extremely important to acknowledge the child abuse that occurred in the residential schools for Indigenous children within the last century (Truth and Reconciliation Commission of Canada, 2015). Nearly half (48.1%) of those who attended residential schools and reported that experience as negative also reported an abuse history (Elias et al., 2012). The Law Commission of Canada noted that Indigenous children were the only children who were designated to live in an institution, away from their families and communities, because of their race. Frequently, these children were prohibited from speaking their mother tongue and were deliberately deprived of all connections with their culture and identity, placing this group of children at high risk for abuse (Law Commission of Canada, 2000). The report acknowledges the profound level of harm to the children, families, and communities that occurred as a result of these children being displaced and mistreated.

A recent study by Bombay, Matheson, and Anisman (2011) examined the relationship between the intergenerational experience of residential schools and depressive symptomatology among First Nation adults. First Nation adults who had a parent who attended a residential school were compared with First Nation adults who had a parent who did not attend a residential school. Second-generation adults whose parents attended residential schools demonstrated significantly greater levels of depression than did those adults whose parents did not attend residential schools. The study results suggest that the residential school experience evoked intergenerational trauma most likely through experiences of childhood adversity, trauma, and perceived discrimination (Bombay et al., 2011). Elias et al. (2012) examined the impact of residential school system and found that direct or indirect exposure to residential schools was associated with histories of trauma and suicidal behaviours.

Child Neglect

Child neglect is one of the most common forms of child abuse reported (Fallon et al., 2015). Physical **neglect** occurs when a parent or guardian does not meet a child's needs such as food, clothing, shelter, cleanliness, health care, or emotional needs (Department of Justice, Canada, 2017). Neglect can be as harmful as physical abuse. In some instances, such as child abandonment, neglect is a crime in Canada (Department of Justice, Canada, 2017). Indicators of physical neglect may include diaper dermatitis, lice, scabies, dirty appearance, clothing inappropriate for the weather, and unclean and unsafe living environments. Just how to respond to neglected children and their families is relatively unknown. A systematic literature review highlights the dramatic need for effective interventions to neglected children and their families (Allin, Wathen, & MacMillan, 2005).

Physical Abuse

Physical abuse is the deliberate use of force against a child and may include hitting, slapping, punching, biting, burning, kicking, pushing, shoving, choking, or any other type of physical action directed towards the child that results in nonaccidental injury (Department of Justice, Canada, 2017). Injuries to children caused by physical abuse range from mild to severe and life threatening. Types of injuries include cutaneous injuries (e.g., contusions, abrasions, burns, bite marks), abusive head trauma (e.g., direct trauma, vigorous shaking), ocular injuries (e.g., retinal haemorrhage), ear injuries (e.g., contusions, swelling), and abdominal trauma (e.g., blunt abdominal trauma from punching or kicking) (Gary & Humphreys, 2004; Kelley, 2011). The leading cause of death in children who have been maltreated is head trauma, followed by abdominal trauma (Kelley, 2011). Often, clothing hides these injuries, and practitioners must look for other signs of abuse, such as fear, aggressive or withdrawn behaviour, poor social relations, learning problems, delinquent behaviour, and wearing clothing that is meant to cover injuries but is inappropriate for the weather. In addition, when treating a child with such injuries, professionals should suspect abuse when explanations are implausible and inconsistent with injuries, when involved parties give different versions of the incident, or when treatment seeking is delayed (Kelley, 2011).

Sexual Abuse

The general age of consent in Canada is 16 years old; therefore, any sexual behaviour towards a child under the age of 16 in Canada constitutes a crime (Department of Justice, Canada, 2017). The age of consent is 18 when the sexual activity takes place in a relationship of trust, dependency, or authority (Department of Justice, Canada, 2017). According to the criminal code, punishable sexual offenses against children include sexual touching, sexual exploitation, making or possessing child pornography, luring a child over the Internet, sexual exploitation, living off of or procuring prostitution, voyeurism, and intercourse (Cotter & Beaupré, 2014).

There are three categories of **sexual abuse**: incest, sexual abuse perpetrated by a nonfamily member, and paedophilia. Incest is defined in the Criminal Code of Canada (1985) in this way: everyone commits incest who, "Knowing that another person by blood relationship is his or her parent, child, brother, sister, grandparent, or grandchild, as the case may be, has sexual intercourse with that person" (5.155). This definition limits the illegal sexual activity to sexual intercourse; it does not include fondling, oral sex, and masturbation. These acts, when committed against children, are covered under other laws not restricted to blood relatives. Paedophilia describes those who have a sexual fixation on young children that usually translates into sexual acts with the victims. Police-reported data in Canada in 2012 indicated that 55% of sexual assault victims were under the age of 18, despite making up only 20% of the Canadian population (Cotter & Beaupré, 2014). Approximately 81% of victims were female and 97% of persons accused were male (Cotter & Beaupré, 2014). Further, police-reported data from 2012 reveal that the largest percentage (44%) of sexual assaults against children were committed by an acquaintance, while 38% of sexual assaults against children were committed by family members (Cotter & Beaupré, 2014). MacMillan and colleagues (2013) studied risk factors for both physical and sexual abuse in the Ontario Child Health Study and found living in poverty in childhood was associated with an increased risk of physical (and severe physical) and sexual abuse, particularly if the child was born to a young mother.

Several factors may mediate the effects of child sexual abuse. In general, younger children with a history of emotional difficulties may be more traumatized than older and more stable children. Repeated abuse for long periods with more violence and bodily penetration results in greater traumatization. Sexual abuse by someone whom the child knows and trusts causes more severe trauma. The child abused by a family member experiences a devastating breach of trust, loss of a safe home, and threats to fundamental survival requirements, which for some may last a lifetime (Draughon & Urbancic, 2011).

Emotional Abuse

Emotional abuse includes acts or omissions that psychologically damage the child (Kelley, 2011; Wekerle et al., 2009), such as humiliating a child, constantly yelling, and criticizing or threatening a child (Department of Justice, Canada, 2017). The emotionally abused child does not have visible injuries to alert others, but has a severely disturbed sense of security. Consequently, emotional abuse severely affects a child's self-esteem and often leaves permanent emotional scars, which can take a prolonged time to heal (Department of Justice, Canada, 2017). In Canada, various forms of emotional abuse against children constitute a crime and may include serious forms of harmful threats or threats to a child's personal property, such as a pet (Department of Justice, Canada, 2017). According to Canadian child welfare statistics, an estimated 4.06 children out of 1,000 experience emotional or psychological abuse, a figure that is readily acknowledged to be underestimated (Public Health Agency of Canada, 2010). It is also recognized that children who experience emotional abuse are more likely than are children who are not emotionally abused to have increased psychological difficulties, such as depression, and increased risk-taking behaviour (Chamberland, Laporte, Lavergne, & Baraldi, 2003; Wekerle et al., 2009). Children who witness domestic violence are also thought to be victims of emotional abuse, and they demonstrate increased anxiety and insecurity compared with children who do not witness domestic violence (Chamberland et al., 2003; Wolfe, Crooks, Lee, McIntyre-Smith, & Jaffe, 2003). Frequently, emotional abuse occurs within the context of other forms of abuse or maltreatment, underlining the complexity and urgent need for responsive and innovative interventions for this serious problem.

Factitious Disorder Imposed on Another

Factitious disorder imposed on another is also a form of child abuse (see Chapter 24). Previously known as factitious disorder by proxy, or Munchausen's syndrome by proxy, this disorder includes intentionally imposing physical or psychological signs or symptoms of an illness in another person, usually a child (Zaky, 2015), and is listed as factitious disorder imposed on another in the current *Diagnostic and Statistical Manual of Mental Disorders* (*DSM-5*) (American Psychiatric Association, 2013). The signs of this disorder include repeated hospitalizations and medical evaluations of the child without definitive diagnosis, symptoms or medical signs that are inappropriate or inconsistent, symptoms that disappear when the child is away from the parent, a parent who encourages medical tests for the child, parental uneasiness as the child recovers, and a parent who is less concerned with the child's health than with spending time with caregivers (Bass & Glaser, 2014). This disorder was once thought to be relatively rare; however, it is now recognized as more common and with serious outcomes, such as the death of a child (Flaherty & MacMillan, 2013).

Secondary Abuse: Children of Battered Women

Exposure to violence is a serious stressor for children (Berman, Hardesty, Lewis-O'Connor, & Humphreys, 2011; Zahradnik et al., 2010). Research on children of battered women has become more evident over the past 25 years (Clements, Oxtoby, & Ogle, 2008). Children growing up in an environment where their mother is being abused experience the effects of living in an unpredictable and frightening environment (Letourneau et al., 2013). Children who grow up in violent families frequently experience living with secrecy, relocations as the mother leaves home to seek safety, economic hardship, as well as maternal depression that may reduce her ability to nurture (Letourneau et al., 2013). According to the 2014 GSS, 51% of victims of spousal violence with children in the home believed their children had seen the violence (Canadian Centre for Justice Statistics, 2016). Children who witness violence in the home are more likely to be the victims of childhood abuse as well. Data from the 2014 GSS indicated that 70% of children who witnessed violence were also victims of physical or sexual abuse (Canadian Centre for Justice Statistics, 2016). Further, witnessing violence in the home is associated with an increased likelihood of being the victim of spousal violence later in life. According to the 2014 GSS, victims of spousal violence were almost twice as likely to report having witnessed abuse as a child (Canadian Centre for Justice Statistics, 2016). Research has substantiated the traumatic long-term effects of witnessing violence and indicates that children who witness violence are more likely to experience negative outcomes throughout childhood, such as dropping out of school, PTSD, and/or problems with alcohol or illicit drug use (Zahradnik et al., 2010). Emerging research has shed some light on the important role of resilience in moderating the relationship between youth exposure to violence and mental health for school age youth who had been exposed to violence (Zahradnik et al., 2010). For example, a Canadian study described the impact of IPV on the mother–child relationship and identified that both mothers and infants compensate for the effects of exposure to IPV, with infants providing clearer cues to the mothers and mothers demonstrating sensitivity and responsiveness (Letourneau et al., 2013).

Elder Abuse

The population aged 65 years and older now represents one of the fastest-growing cohorts of the population, increasing from 9% in 1981 to 16.6% in 2016 (Sinha, 2012; Statistics Canada, n.d.). It is the first time since confederation that there are more people aged 65 and older than children aged 0 to 14 (Statistics Canada, 2015). In the coming decades, it is projected that Canada's population will continue to age considerably, with the proportion of Canadians aged 55 years and older rising from 27% in 2011 to 35% in 2031 (Brennan, 2012). This is the result of the aging of baby boomers, decreasing fertility rates, and increase in life expectancy (Statistics Canada, 2016). Elder abuse, in the context of a growing aging population, is increasingly recognized as a serious problem in Canada and other countries. Despite this observation, it has been reported that seniors aged 65 years and older have the lowest risk of experiencing violence compared with any other age groups, regardless of whether the abuse was by a family member or not (Sinha, 2012). Adult children (34 per 100,000) have been identified most often as responsible for family violence against older adults, with women being particularly vulnerable (Sinha, 2012). Specifically, senior women have been found to be more vulnerable to family violence, at a rate of 34% higher than men (Sinha, 2012). Data from the 2014 GSS indicated that Canadians aged 65 or older accounted for 3% of all victims of police-reported crime (Canadian Centre for Justice Statistics, 2016). Risk factors for elder abuse include both risk within the environment such as a caregiver who is depressed and inadequate economic resources, as well as characteristics of the vulnerable elder individual, which predispose to abuse, such as cognitive impairment, lack of empowerment, or difficulty with activities of daily living (ADL) (Fulmer et al., 2011).

Same-Sex Intimate Partner Violence

Individuals in same-sex relationships are at an increased risk of experiencing spousal violence. Data from the 2014 GSS indicated that people who were identified as gay, lesbian, or bisexual were twice as likely as heterosexual individuals to be victims of spousal violence (Canadian Centre for Justice Statistics, 2016). Lesbian or bisexual women were particularly vulnerable to spousal violence when compared to heterosexual women (11% and 3%, respectively) (Canadian Centre for Justice Statistics, 2016). Although the prevalence of spousal violence is high in this population, access to same-sex specific resources is limited. A study of 280 individuals who were identified as gay, lesbian, and/or queer concluded that there was a lack of same-sex specific spousal violence resources in Canada (St. Pierre & Senn, 2010). Further, participants found mainstream services to be insensitive, judgmental, and poorly equipped with resources specific to same-sex spousal violence (St. Pierre & Senn, 2010). Individuals who were open about their sexual orientation were more likely to seek out support from police, medical professionals, or shelters (St. Pierre & Senn,

2010). Therefore, nurses should use gender-neutral language such as "partner" or "spouse" when assessing for spousal violence in order to give gay, lesbian, or queer individuals the opportunity to disclose (St. Pierre & Senn, 2010).

Human Trafficking

Human trafficking remains a poorly understood problem despite increased awareness in recent years on the part of policy makers and human rights advocates (Kaye, Winterdyk, & Quarterman, 2014). Human trafficking ".... involves the recruitment, transportation, harbouring and/or exercising control, direction or influence over the movements of a person in order to exploit that person, typically through sexual exploitation or forced labour" (Public Safety Canada, 2012).

The United Nations Education, Scientific and Cultural Organization (UNESCO, 2000) estimates that approximately two million people are victims of trafficking every year, although the full extent of trafficking is challenging to estimate due to victims' reluctance to report to authorities, and difficulties in identifying victims (Karam, 2014). Individuals may be exploited through force, coercion, or deception with individuals experiencing physical abuse and emotional trauma (Kaye et al., 2014). Human trafficking most commonly occurs through sexual exploitation of women and children, but it can also occur through forced labour (Public Safety Canada, 2012). Control of victims can be exercised through many forms such as taking away one's identity documents, through intimidation, physical violence, or threats of harm to one's self or family (Oxman-Martinez, Lacoirx, & Hanley, 2005). As such, human trafficking is seen as a violation against human rights (Kaye et al., 2014).

Human trafficking in Canada is a lucrative activity with well organized and extensive trafficking networks reaching across the country and international borders (Oxman-Martinez et al., 2005; Public Safety Canada, 2012). Most cases involve sexual exploitation in large urban areas although the reach can extend to smaller centres. The majority of victims of human trafficking in Canada are female, primarily Indigenous women and girls, and almost half are between the ages of 18 and 24 (Karam, 2014; Oxman-Martinez et al., 2005). It is difficult to estimate the extent of human trafficking because of the hidden nature of the crime and victims' reluctance to report. Human trafficking is estimated to account for less than 1% of all police-reported incidents in Canada although the rate has increased in recent years, possibly due to better reporting and detecting (Karam, 2014; Public Safety Canada, 2012).

Extreme poverty and deprivation, unemployment, and conflict situations in the world are among the factors contributing to human trafficking. Victims may also be lured into trafficking through the promise of financial reward and better quality of life. Persistent and difficult socioeconomic conditions are thought to contribute to the high prevalence of Indigenous women involved in trafficking. For those who have experienced trafficking, the need for protection and safety is paramount. Comprehensive services are required to support victims and ameliorate the deleterious effects of trafficking including health services including mental health services; housing, income support, and access to employment and skill development; and immigration status (Oxman-Martinez et al., 2005).

Canada was one of the first countries to sign the Protocol to Prevent, Suppress and Punish Trafficking in Persons, Especially Women and Children (Palermo Protocol, 2000). In 2012, the Government of Canada launched the National Action Plan to Combat Human Trafficking (Public Safety Canada, 2012) as part of its efforts to address this crime through prevention, protection, prosecution, and partnerships. The plan is considered to be a working document to identify trends, challenges, and priority areas that will inform federal efforts in an ongoing way. In spite of efforts to combat human trafficking, primarily through the criminal justice system, more needs to be done to support victims to ensure their safety and access to the requisite services (Kaye et al., 2014; Oxman-Martinez et al., 2005).

■ THEORIES OF ABUSE

Many theories have attempted to explain violence between intimate partners and in the family. The theories reviewed here have been categorized as biologic, psychological, and social. In all likelihood, family violence is truly a bio/psycho/social/spiritual phenomenon that no one theory can fully explain (Fig. 34.1). Violent or aggressive behaviour therefore needs to be regarded in a broader context as a complex multifactorial phenomenon (Lucea, Glass, & Laughon, 2011). Additional theories that are more specific to the phenomenon of woman abuse are also presented.

Biologic Theories
Neurologic Problems

Aggressive behaviour may be associated with several neurologic conditions, including traumatic brain injury, seizure disorder, and dementia (see Chapter 18). Neurodevelopmental factors and traumatic brain injury can produce seizure disorders, attentional dysfunction, or focal neurobehavioural syndromes, all of which are associated with aggressive behaviour. The most common association between seizures and aggressive behaviour occurs during the postictal period (the period immediately after the seizure), during which the individual may be confused.

Damage to the orbitofrontal cortex often causes impulsive, labile, irritable, and socially inappropriate

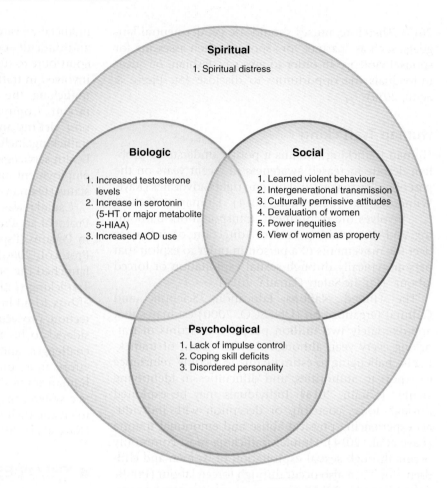

Figure 34.1. Bio/psycho/social/spiritual aetiologies for violent behaviour.

behaviour. Individuals with such damage often respond aggressively to trivial stimuli. In addition, damage to the neocortex, limbic system, and hypothalamus may result in aggressive behaviour. These systems have hierarchic control over one another. Damage to higher centres may disinhibit aggression from lower centres. Aggressive behaviour also may be related to disruptions in neurotransmitter systems. Those with mental disorders are at an increased risk for developing aggressive behaviour. Disruption in serotonin, dopamine, and gamma-aminobutyric acid systems has been linked with several psychiatric disorders, including depression, schizophrenia, impulsive behaviour, suicide, and aggression (Comai, Tau, & Gobbi, 2012). Complex interactions among neurotransmitter systems and their respective receptors are thought to play a role in aggressive behaviour. Psychopharmacologic agents (e.g., atypical antipsychotics, anticonvulsants, and lithium) have changed the course of treatment for aggressive behaviour by effecting change at an intracellular level (Comai et al., 2012).

Links With Substance Abuse

The use of AOD is commonly associated with violent incidents. Other factors, such as low family income, stress, and abuse in the family of origin, are often more important (Stewart et al., 2013). The relationship of AOD to violence may result from three factors:

(1) AOD-induced cognitive impairment, (2) the user's expectations that AOD increases the tendency towards aggression, and (3) socioculturally grounded beliefs that people are unaccountable for their behaviour while intoxicated (Abbey, Zawacki, Buck, Clinton, & McAuslan, 2003).

Studies have demonstrated that drinking alcohol may change perceptions about accountability for behaviour (Abbey et al., 2003). The belief that intoxicated behaviour will be judged less harshly may encourage and provide an excuse for those who abuse substances to engage in normally unacceptable behaviours. Research shows that people attempt to justify their criminal behaviour by blaming alcohol after the fact (Abbey et al., 2003), given the general belief that alcohol use is associated with aggression (Stewart et al., 2013). Alcohol use has also been associated with IPV both in terms of its occurrence and its severity through a biochemical effect that impacts cognitive and physical function and reduces self-control (Kelly, Gonzalez-Guarda, & Taylor, 2011; Stewart et al., 2013). For those individuals who are impulsive, alcohol use is a concern. There has been increasing concern about the growing number of drug-facilitated sexual assault. In particular, flunitrazepam has become known as the date rape drug (Du Mont et al., 2010). A recent Canadian study of primarily female sexual assault victims receiving care at hospital-based treatment centres found that 21% of the sample (*n* = 882) met the criteria for suspected drug-facilitated assault. The researchers conclude that treatment centres need to be prepared to respond to date rape victims, since it is a common problem (Du Mont et al., 2010).

Psychological Theories

Psychopathology theory seeks to understand violence by examining the psychological characteristics and mental health conditions that are associated with violent behaviour in individual men and women (Corvo & Johnson, 2013). Theorists from this perspective focus on personality traits, internal defense systems, and mental disorders. Outdated theories that have been particularly damaging attribute psychopathology to women, such as masochism or depression as reasons for victimization (Hoff, 2016). One underlying assumption of this labelling was that some women enjoy abuse and deliberately provoke attacks because they need to suffer.

Research on batterers has shown that there is not a common profile or a typical batterer; however, studies have found evidence of personality disorders, including antisocial, borderline, narcissistic, and dependent characteristics (Dutton, 2007).

Social Theories

Covering the many sociologic theories of violence is beyond the scope of this chapter. Sociologic theories posit that abuse occurs because of cultural norms that permit and even glamorize violent behaviour (Lucea, Glass, & Laughon, 2011). A study conducted by Ellis et al. (2013), among Canadian high school students, showed that aggressive adolescent peer groups influenced relationships and was predictive of later dating violence. In another study, dating violence was seen as unacceptable by adolescents; however, behaviours such as grabbing, hitting, and kicking within dating relationships were regarded as acceptable in certain situations such as when "joking around" (Sears, Byers, Whelan, & Saint-Pierre, 2006). In keeping with these findings, a qualitative study by Canadian researchers revealed that young adolescent girls (15 and 16 years of age) were so eager to have a male dating partner that they were willing to tolerate physical violence and verbal abuse, just to "keep the guy" (Banister et al., 2003).

Family violence is also related to qualities of the community in which the family is embedded. The relationship of poverty, social isolation, and child abuse has been well established (Coulton, Crampton, Irwin, Spilsbury, & Korbin, 2007; Leschied, Chiodo, Whitehead, Hurley, & Marshall, 2003; MacMillan, Tanaka, Duku, Vaillancourt, & Boyle, 2013). Economic disadvantage creates tremendous stress for families, increasing the risk for child abuse and maltreatment. It should be kept in mind that economically impoverished families may seek social services more frequently, and as such, the reporting of abuse may be increased in these families (MacMillan et al., 2013). However, not all poor families abuse their children. One difference between poor families who do and do not abuse their children lies in the degree of social cohesion and mutual caring found in their communities (Rothman, 2007). Neighbourhoods with high levels of child abuse frequently have severe social disorganization and lack of community identity. In addition, they have higher rates of juvenile delinquency, drug trafficking, and violent crime (O'Campo, Burke, Peak, McDonnell, & Gielen, 2005). Regardless, there is evidence that some neighbourhoods may provide a protective effect. For example, a Canadian study found that immigrant women who were living in low-income and high-immigrant neighbourhoods were less likely to experience abuse, notwithstanding the length of time that the women had spent in Canada (Daoud, O'Campo, Urquia, & Heaman, 2012).

Family Stress Theory

One of the most accepted theories of elder abuse is the family stress theory. The theory hypothesizes that providing care for an elder induces stress within the family. Family stress includes economic hardship, loss of sleep, and intrusions into family activities and routines. Moreover, caring for a dependent elder takes an enormous physical toll on the caregiver. If there is no relief, the caregiver may become overwhelmed, lose control, and abuse the elder (Norris, Fancey, Power, & Ross, 2013). With the aging of the Canadian population, the demands on family members to provide care are rising, as are the associated stress of caregiving and the increased risk for elder abuse (McCann-Beranger, 2010). Other characteristics of caregivers that may predispose them to abuse elderly parents include alcohol or drug abuse, dementia, restricted outside activities, unrealistic expectations, and a blaming, hypercritical personality.

Social Learning Theory

Violent families create an atmosphere of tension, fear, intimidation, and tremendous confusion about intimate relationships (Bancroft, Silverman, & Ritchie, 2011). Children in violent homes often learn violent behaviour as an approved and legitimate way to solve problems, especially within intimate relationships. Social learning theory posits that men who witness violence in their homes often perpetuate violent behaviour in their families as adults (Berman et al., 2011). Moreover, women who grow up in violent homes learn to accept violence and expect it in their own adult relationships (Berman et al., 2011). In a Canadian study of intergenerational violence, negative childhood experiences of family violence carried over into adolescence and intimate relationships (Laporte, Jiang, Pepler, & Chamberland, 2011). Further, female adolescents were found to be at greater risk for revictimization, whereas males who reported violence in childhood, particularly by their fathers, were more likely to be aggressive towards their girlfriends. It is also important to note that although violence in the home can have a serious and negative effect on children, it does not necessarily predict with certainty that violence will occur in future relationships. As Berman and colleagues (2011) point out, the relationship between exposure to violence and being violent towards others is a complex one associated with a range of factors.

Theoretic Dynamics Specific to Woman Abuse

Feminist Theories

Feminist theory focuses on issues of gender, inequality, power and privilege, patriarchy, and the subordination of women as explanations for woman abuse (Damant et al., 2008; Kelly et al., 2011). According to the feminist perspective, woman abuse results from a patriarchal society that perpetuates attitudes that support violence against women (Ford-Gilboe, Wuest, & Merritt-Gray, 2005; Kelly et al., 2011). Further, the concept of patriarchy is particularly germane, since it focuses on power inequalities and gender and offers explanations that go beyond individual conditions to examine the social conditions that support the abuse of woman (Hunnicutt, 2009).

Feminists also point to a power inequity in society as a contributing factor to woman abuse. Women have made many advances in recent years; however, men continue to control most institutions (Kelly et al., 2011). Women continue to earn less than do men for paid work and are less likely to advance to positions of authority and power (Singh & Peng, 2010). Moreover, marriage often victimizes women in ways other than through violence. Although men now contribute to household work, most women who hold jobs outside the home continue to perform most household and child care tasks (Lachance-Grzela & Bouchard, 2010). A Canadian qualitative study interviewed three ethnocultural groups and found that gender-neutral explanations rationalized the fact that women continue to do the majority of housework (Beagan, Chapman, D'Sylva, & Bassett, 2008). The authors make the case that subtle explanations, such as these regarding gender assignment of housework, are much more difficult to challenge. This power inequity is reflected in higher depression rates among married women than among married men (Nolen-Hoeksema, 2002). According to the Canadian Survey of Labour and Income Dynamics, one in five Canadian women experienced low income for at least a year following the breakup of their marriage, with women under the age of 40 being at higher risk of poverty (Gadalla, 2008). Further, findings from a feminist grounded theory study of 40 single mothers who recently left abusive partners in Ontario and New Brunswick reveal that the majority of participants continued to experience ongoing harassment, even though these single mothers had left their abusive partners (Ford-Gilboe et al., 2005). The central challenges faced by these women included decreased resources, persistent persecution, and ongoing chronic health problems that were, in fact, a consequence of leaving the abusive relationship (Ford-Gilboe et al., 2005).

Women are viewed as property in many parts of the world. As described in the seminal work of Kilbourne (1987, 1999), the entertainment and advertising industries perpetuate the image of women as property by depicting them as objects and often portraying the dismembering of women's bodies. Moreover, the explicit portrayal in the media of women in various states of undress and in seductive postures suggests that they are vulnerable and openly welcome sexual advances. Frequently, the message is, "Buy the product and get the woman" (Kilbourne, 1987).

The focus on women's body parts in advertising dehumanizes women and that dehumanization is often the first step in making women acceptable targets of violence. For example, a 3-month study of newspaper coverage of disabled men and women in Canada and Israel indicated that women received less media coverage than did men, yet the media coverage of women demonstrated a higher level of victimization and violence, overall (Gold & Auslander, 1999). In addition, Hassouneh and Curry (2011) cite a number of studies demonstrating that women with disabilities experience more IPV than do those without disabilities.

Theories of Why Women Stay in Violent Relationships

A more appropriate question than "Why do women stay in violent relationships?" is "How does she ever manage to leave given all the strikes against her?" (Anderson & Saunders, 2003). There are many reasons why women stay in violent relationships (Ford-Gilboe, Varcoe, Wuest, & Merrit-Gray, 2011). One of the strongest reasons is economic (Canadian Women's Foundation, 2013, November). Despite years of progress, women still earn less than do men for equal work (Drolet & Mumford, 2012). Many women lack the education or skills that would allow them to earn an adequate living outside the home. For these women, leaving their abusive partners means that they and their children would be homeless and without any source of support for even basic necessities. Furthermore, many shelters for battered women have long waiting lists and provide only temporary housing. Given the obstacles to leaving abusive relationships, it is not surprising that mortal fear was found to be the single strongest predictor of women's seeking help in response to IPV in a descriptive study of Canadian GSS data (Barrett & Pierre, 2011). On the other hand, women's fear for their lives and the lives of their children and other relatives may also keep women from attempting to leave abusive relationships (Anderson & Saunders, 2003).

The socialization of women to assume major responsibility for marriages and child-rearing is frequently another barrier to leaving abusive relationships (Jones & Vetere, 2017). Society teaches women that their proper place is at home and their primary responsibility is caring for their husbands and children, although this trend is beginning to shift as reflected in household division of labour (Marshall, 2006). Many women believe that making their marriage a success is their responsibility. Therefore, when they are abused, they assume that it is their fault and that their duty is to remain and try harder for their children's sake (Jones & Vetere, 2017). Moreover, many women who were abused in childhood or witnessed abuse of their mothers think that abuse is part of a normal relationship (Kelly, 2011). Women also face political and legal obstacles in leaving abusive partners. If a man is arrested for assault and no action is taken to prevent future violence, he may be released shortly and retaliate against his partner.

Research suggests that factors influencing women's decisions to stay or leave a relationship are complex and varied. Alhalal, Ford-Gilboe, Kerr, and Davies (2012) examined indicators of intrusion (i.e., unwanted interference in everyday life) that predicted whether women remained separated from an abusive partner. Levels of depression and symptoms of PTSD were associated with an increased risk of returning to an abusive partner and being less likely to remain separated. Furthermore, in a study of help-seeking behaviour focused on the power dynamic between partners of women experiencing IPV, Kaukinen, Meyer, and Akers (2013) observed that women were more likely to seek support to deal with IPV if status incompatibilities between partners favour women.

Even more difficult to understand is why some women stay in violent dating relationships. Straus (2004) found the prevalence of violence in dating relationships among university students in 16 countries to range from 17% to 45%. This is similar to Brownridge's (2006) report on a number of Canadian studies that estimated dating violence to range from 25% to 45%. Understanding the phenomenon of dating violence is critical to preventing long-term violence in relationships. One factor is that dating violence often does not occur until the relationship has been sustained for a long time. Research has shown that the length of the relationship, as well as the level of commitment, is positively correlated with physical and sexual abuse. Women with strong emotional commitments and who have invested in the relationship in terms of time, money, or children may be more reluctant to leave (Hendy, Eggen, Gustitus, McLeod, & Ng, 2003).

Survivors may go through a process consisting of several phases in leaving an abusive relationship (Anderson & Saunders, 2003). Women may leave and return several times as they are learning new coping skills. The phases may involve cognitive and emotional "leaving" before actually leaving the relationship. The phases may include (1) enduring and managing the violence while disconnecting from self and others; (2) acknowledging the abuse, reframing it, and counteracting it; and (3) disengaging and focusing on her own needs (Anderson & Saunders, 2003). The phase immediately following separation from an abusive partner is extremely important as the woman attempts to establish a new life (Ford-Gilboe et al., 2009). Based on the findings from a qualitative study of 15 women residing in eastern Canada, a four-stage process of "reclaiming the self" emerged as the main psychological process central to leaving an abusive partner (Wuest & Merritt-Gray, 2001), which is consistent with the stages described by Anderson and Saunders (2003).

Cycle of Violence

Many cases of woman abuse reflect a recognized cycle of violence (Walker, 1979, 1984).Walker's work is regarded as seminal and describes the cyclical nature of abusive relationships, as well as the behaviour of abused women within the context of the cycle (Kelly, Gonzalez-Guarda, & Taylor, 2011). This cycle consists of three recurring phases that often increase in frequency and severity (Walker, 1979, 1984) and is fully described in Figure 34.2.

Traumatic Bonding

The formation of strong emotional bonds under conditions of intermittent maltreatment has been reported in several studies with human and animal subjects. For example, people taken hostage may show positive regard for their captors. Abused children often show strong attachment to their abusing parents. Cult members show strong loyalty to malevolent cult leaders (Dutton, 2008, 2011). Therefore, the relationship between battered women and their partners may be just one example of **traumatic bonding**—the development of strong emotional ties between two people, one of whom intermittently abuses the other. Dutton and Painter put forth the theory of traumatic bonding to describe the bonds women develop for their abusers. Traumatic bonding suggests that a power imbalance and intermittent abuse help to form extremely strong emotional attachments. Traumatic bonding theory (Dutton, 2008, 2011; Dutton & Painter, 1993) explains why the cycle of violence is so powerful in entrapping a woman in a violent relationship.

The woman in a power imbalance perceives herself to be in a powerless position in relation to her partner, whom she perceives as extremely powerful. As the power imbalance intensifies, she feels increasingly worthless, less capable of fending for herself, and, therefore, more in need of her partner. This cycle of dependency and lowered self-esteem is continually repeated, eventually creating a strong affective bond to the partner (Dutton, 1995, 2008, 2011).

Intermittent reinforcement or punishment is one of the strongest learning paradigms in behavioural theory, especially in maintaining a particular behaviour (Dutton, 1995, 2008, 2011). An example that is often

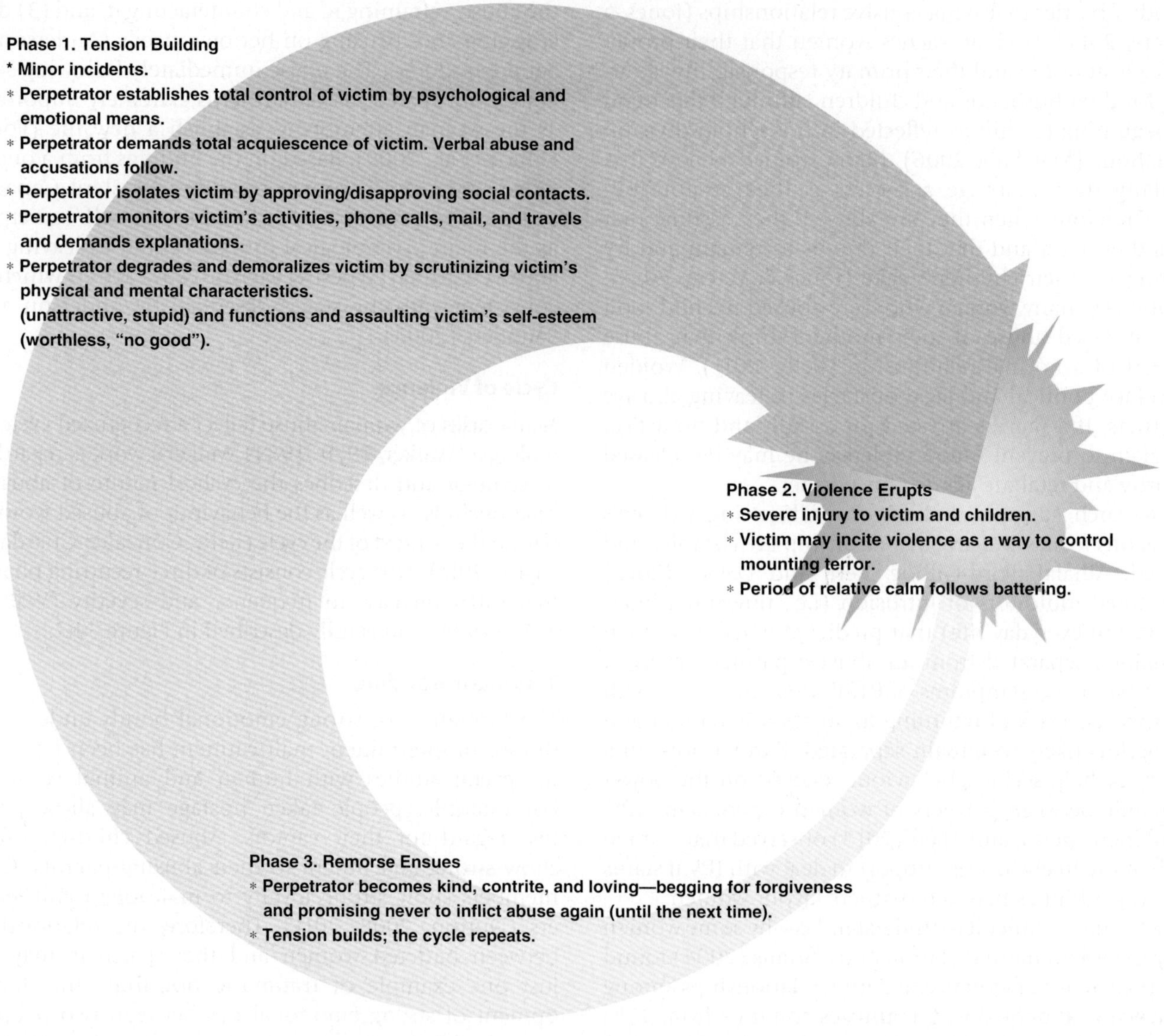

Phase 1. Tension Building
* Minor incidents.
* Perpetrator establishes total control of victim by psychological and emotional means.
* Perpetrator demands total acquiescence of victim. Verbal abuse and accusations follow.
* Perpetrator isolates victim by approving/disapproving social contacts.
* Perpetrator monitors victim's activities, phone calls, mail, and travels and demands explanations.
* Perpetrator degrades and demoralizes victim by scrutinizing victim's physical and mental characteristics.
(unattractive, stupid) and functions and assaulting victim's self-esteem (worthless, "no good").

Phase 2. Violence Erupts
* Severe injury to victim and children.
* Victim may incite violence as a way to control mounting terror.
* Period of relative calm follows battering.

Phase 3. Remorse Ensues
* Perpetrator becomes kind, contrite, and loving—begging for forgiveness and promising never to inflict abuse again (until the next time).
* Tension builds; the cycle repeats.

Figure 34.2. The cycle of violence. Adapted from Walker, 1979, 1984. (Adapted from Walker, L. (1979). *The battered woman*. New York, NY: Harper & Row;Walker, L. (1984). *The battered woman syndrome*. New York, NY: Springer Publishing Co.)

used to illustrate this concept is the gambler who persistently puts coins in a slot machine. Despite substantial losses, the gambler persists because the next time just might be the big payoff. Therefore, the gambler is not rewarded every time, but intermittently. To apply this to battered women, women may stay because this time the man may actually mean what he says and stop the abuse. After all, he has been kind and loving intermittently.

Research suggests that traumatic bonding is especially important when a woman attempts to leave her abusive partner (Dutton, 1995, 2008, 2011). When a woman leaves an abusive relationship, especially after a battering incident, she is emotionally drained and vulnerable. As time passes, her fear of her abuser diminishes, and needs supplied by the partner become evident. At this time, she is particularly susceptible to the abuser's attempts to persuade her to return to the relationship (Dutton & Painter, 1993).

SURVIVORS OF ABUSE: HUMAN RESPONSES TO TRAUMA

The experience of violence and abuse is overwhelming for most survivors and often has devastating long-term consequences. Victimization, such as IPV and childhood abuse, does not produce a single uniform syndrome or response. Research on the effects of abuse reflects the devastating long-term effects of trauma, which results in a range of responses that are characteristic for trauma survivors (Ansara & Hindin, 2011; Daigneault, Hébert, & McDuff, 2009; Hovsepian, Blais, Manseau, Otis, & Girard, 2010). Ansara and Hindin (2011) analyzed data from the 2004 Canadian GSS on Victimization to explore the consequences associated with different forms of abuse. The findings suggest that a pattern of violence is associated with negative psychosocial outcomes—particularly for women experiencing more severe and chronic abuse.

Biologic Responses

Victims of violence experience mild to severe physical consequences. Mild injuries may include bruises and abrasions of the head, neck, face, trunk, and extremities. Severe injuries include multiple traumas, major fractures, major lacerations, and internal injuries, including chest and abdominal injuries and subdural haematomas (Health Canada, 2002; Woods & Gill, 2011). Loss of vision and hearing can result from blows to the head. Physical or sexual violence may result in head injuries that can produce changes in cognition, affect, motivation, and behaviour. Victims of sexual abuse may have vaginal and perineal trauma that is sufficient to require surgical repair (Ford-Gilboe et al., 2011; Health Canada, 2002). Anorectal injuries may also be present, including the disruption of anal sphincters, retained foreign bodies, and mucosal lacerations. The most common responses to violence and abuse include:

- Major depressive disorder (MDD)
- Acute stress disorder (ASD)
- Posttraumatic stress disorder (PTSD)
- Dissociative identity disorder (DID)

Major Depressive Disorder

Major depressive disorder (MDD), one of the most common responses to abuse, is a biologically based disorder that can result from the effects of chronic stress on neurotransmitter and neuroendocrine systems. The body's response to stress is a complex, integrated system of reactions, encompassing the body and mind. Threat or stress engages the stress system, which consists of the hypothalamic–pituitary–adrenal (HPA) axis and the sympathetic nervous system (Miller, Chen, & Zhou, 2007). Engagement of the HPA axis is associated with the release of corticotropin-releasing hormone (CRH) from the pituitary gland. CRH stimulates the pituitary gland to secrete adrenocorticotropic hormone (corticotropin), which stimulates the adrenal cortex to secrete cortisol. Stress also engages the sympathetic nervous system, causing the locus caeruleus and the adrenal medulla to release norepinephrine.

The CRH and locus caeruleus and norepinephrine systems participate in a mutually reinforcing feedback loop. That is, increases in CRH stimulate increased firing of the locus caeruleus and increased release of norepinephrine. Similarly, stressors that activate norepinephrine neurons increase CRH concentrations in the locus caeruleus. These systems prepare the threatened person to respond to danger by enhancing the person's arousal, attention, perception, energy, and emotion and by suppressing the immune response (Wong & Yehuda, 2002).

The stress response is meant to be of limited duration. However, when resistance or escape is impossible, the human stress system becomes overwhelmed and disorganized (Herman, 1997; Zaleski, Johnson, & Klein, 2016). Exposure to severe stressors early in life has been shown to compromise the regulation of HPA activity for a lifetime and may have differential effects according to gender with women being twice more likely to experience depression (Carter-Snell & Hegadoren, 2003; Gobinath, Mahmoud, & Galea, 2015). Accordingly, Carter-Snell and Hegadoren (2003) theorize that the increased occurrence of sexual abuse in girls may contribute to the increased prevalence of stress disorders reported in women. Most types of abuse result in extreme forms of chronic stress. A protracted or dysregulated stress response has been associated with the development of MDD (American Psychiatric Association, 2013). Survivors of abuse report many of these symptoms. In a study examining the impact of IPV on women's mental health, women exposed to IPV had a higher incidence and severity of depression, anxiety, PTSD, as well as thoughts of suicide than did nonabused women, with no differences observed between those women who were psychologically abused versus those who were physically and psychologically abused (Pico-Alfonso et al., 2006). Further, a Toronto-based qualitative study of Latin American immigrant women found that these women experienced a profound link between IPV and depression (Godoy-Ruiz, Toner, Mason, Vidal, & McKenzie, 2015).

Acute Stress Disorder and Posttraumatic Stress Disorder

The experience of trauma exerts tremendous physical and psychological stress on survivors. The cluster of signs and symptoms that frequently occur after major trauma is now labelled **acute stress disorder** (ASD) and **posttraumatic stress disorder** (PTSD); for a comprehensive discussion of PTSD and ASD, see Chapter 17. Lasiuk and Hegadoren (2006), in their historical overview of the PTSD concept, describe the often-misunderstood link between the condition "hysteria" (as described in early 19th-century Europe), war trauma, and PTSD. Subsequent research has demonstrated that symptoms of ASD and PTSD occur not only after war but also after many types of severe trauma, including physical abuse, sexual abuse, and rape.

A review of research on the epidemiology of PTSD suggests several gender differences. For example, an analysis of prevalence data from 11 countries (including Canada) documented that women were twice as likely as men to develop PTSD (Dückers & Olff, 2017). Several factors may contribute to these differences. One factor is that men and women experience different types of traumatic events (Cyr et al., 2017). For example, men more frequently experience assaults, whereas women more frequently experience sexual assaults, according to Canadian victimization data (Ogrodnik, 2010). Other factors that may contribute to a higher prevalence of PTSD in women include higher rates of anxiety and depressive disorders and traumatic events before the age of 15 years (Carter-Snell & Hegadoren, 2003; Orsillo, Raja, & Hammond, 2002). One study of 1,698 urban young adults, focused on the impact of exposure to traumatic events, found that women's risk for PTSD varied according to the type of trauma (i.e., assaultive), as well as prior experience of trauma, whereas men's risk of PTSD was not related to the type of trauma or the experience of prior trauma (Breslau & Anthony, 2007). Women with PTSD frequently have comorbid anxiety, depressive disorders, or both, and the association among childhood abuse, PTSD, and substance abuse is also becoming well established (Boughner & Frewen, 2016; Walton et al., 2011).

Hyperarousal

After a traumatic experience, the stress system seems to go on permanent alert, as if the danger might return at any time (Lanius et al., 2017). In this state of physiologic hyperarousal, the traumatized person is hypervigilant for signs of danger, startles easily, reacts irritably to small annoyances, and sleeps poorly. These symptoms are characteristic of increased noradrenergic function (O'Donnell, Hegadoren, & Coupland, 2004), particularly in the locus caeruleus and limbic system (hypothalamus, hippocampus, and amygdala), and of increased dopamine activity, particularly in the prefrontal cortical dopamine system (Bandelow et al., 2017). Dopamine hyperactivity is associated with the hypervigilance seen in PTSD. Many people with PTSD do not return to their normal baseline level of alertness. Instead, they seem to have a new baseline of elevated arousal, as if their "thermostat" had been reset (Lanius et al., 2017). Based on advances in neuroscience, however, a sensorimotor approach to therapy is evolving that shows promise for helping persons with PTSD to restore normal arousal levels (Ogden, Minton, & Pain, 2006).

Behavioural sensitization may be one mechanism underlying the hyperarousal seen in PTSD. This phenomenon, sometimes referred to as *kindling*, occurs after an exposure to severe, uncontrollable stressors. The sensitized person reacts with a magnified stress response to later, milder stressors (Monroe & Harkness, 2005). Research has provided evidence that exposure to traumatic stress may led to neuroplastic changes in the brain, which result in increased sensitivity and reactivity to future stressors (Adamec, Hebert, & Blundell, 2011). Rabellino and colleagues (2016) found increased neural activities within the amygdala and periaqueductal gray, in individuals with PTSD as compared to individuals without PTSD, during subliminal processing of trauma-related words and fearful faces. Further, individuals who have been traumatized frequently react to environmental stimuli that activate regions in the brain linked to the expression of intense emotions and limit the brain's capacity to integrate and communicate experience, as well as modulate physiologic arousal (van der Kolk, 2006).

The state of hyperarousal causes other problems for survivors. The loss of neuromodulation leads to a loss of affect regulation and difficulties with engaging in present experience so that the survivor finds it difficult

to negotiate interpersonal relationships (van der Kolk, 2006). In addition, the continual arousal may desensitize the survivor to real threat and decrease the probability that he or she will respond to perceived danger (Messman-Moore & Long, 2003). This development may cause persons to miss clues of danger and place themselves in situations that can lead to revictimization.

Intrusion

Long after abuse has stopped, survivors relive it as though it were continually recurring. Flashbacks and nightmares, which the survivor experiences with terrifying immediacy, are vivid and often include fragments of traumatic events exactly as they happened (Courtois & Ford, 2014). Moreover, a wide variety of stimuli that may have been associated with the trauma can elicit flashbacks and dreams. Consequently, survivors avoid such stimuli (Shalev & Bremner, 2016). Three related but somewhat different explanations may account for the vivid, disturbing flashbacks and dreams that individuals with PTSD have: disturbances of memory, classic conditioning (fear conditioning), and extinction.

Memory function is altered in PTSD (van der Kolk, 2006). Memory deficits include short-term memory and potentiation of recall of traumatic experiences and dissociative flashbacks. Human beings are bombarded constantly by sensory stimuli yet attend to and remember only a fraction of it (Johnsen & Asbjørnsen, 2008). People seem to remember best those events that have emotional effects and occur when they are alert, aroused, and responsive to their internal and external environments. Because noradrenergic activity is elevated in individuals with PTSD when exposed to emotional and traumatic stimuli, memory encoding may be improved, leading to intrusive thoughts and memories (O'Donnell et al., 2004). Conversely, administration of an α_2-adrenoceptor agonist clonidine disrupts memory reconsolidation after retrieval, leading to improvements of PTSD symptoms (Gamache, Pitman, & Nader, 2012).

During stress, there is a massive release of neurotransmitters, particularly norepinephrine, epinephrine, and opioid peptides. This flood of "stress hormones" may lead to structural changes in the brain that potentiate long-term memory (Wolf, 2009). In most situations, this type of memory has survival value: remembering events that occur during danger may protect oneself during similar future situations. However, in PTSD, the memories occur when the individual is not in danger. Research supporting this hypothesis demonstrated that if norepinephrine is administered to animals immediately after training, long-term memory is enhanced. Epinephrine and endogenous opioids may influence memory consolidation (transforming short-term memory to long-term memory) by affecting norepinephrine (McGaugh, 2015; van Stegeren, 2008).

The hippocampus and amygdala are involved in memory consolidation. The hippocampus is involved in object memory and placement of memory traces in space and time (MacDonald, Lepage, Eden, & Eichenbaum, 2011; van Stegeren, 2008). High levels of stress have been shown to damage the hippocampus and decrease its volume, producing memory deficits such as amnesia and deficits in autobiographical memory (memory of one's life story) (Bremner, 2006). The amygdala integrates sensory information for storage in and retrieval from memory. The amygdala also attaches emotional significance to sensory information and transmits this information to all the other systems involved in the stress response. Overreactivity of the amygdala might explain the recurrent and intrusive traumatic memories and the excessive fear associated with traumatic reminders characteristic of PTSD (Rabellino et al., 2016).

Classic conditioning, or **fear conditioning**, occurs when a neutral stimulus (the conditioned stimulus [CS]) is paired with an aversive unconditioned stimulus that elicits an unconditioned fear response. After repeated pairing, the CS alone will elicit the fear response, which is now the conditioned response (CR). For example, certain sights, sounds, or smells that occurred in close proximity to the traumatic event may elicit a fear response in the future. The result of this process is that an individual becomes fearful and anxious in response to a wide variety of stimuli (Lissek & van Meurs, 2015; Shin, Rauch, & Pitman, 2006); therefore, a wide variety of stimuli can elicit symptoms of PTSD.

The amygdala and hippocampus also appear to be important players in fear conditioning (O'Donnell et al., 2004; Sanders, Wiltgen, & Fanselow, 2003; Shin et al., 2006). Other important brain sites in PTSD in addition to the hippocampus and amygdala include the thalamus, locus caeruleus, and medial prefrontal cortex. Interaction between the cortex and the amygdala may be necessary for specific stimuli to elicit traumatic memories. Cortisol and norepinephrine are two neurochemical systems associated with the stress response (Bremner, 2006).

Extinction is the loss of a learned conditioned emotional response after repeated presentations of the conditioned fear stimulus without a contiguous traumatic event. In other words, the individual no longer responds with fear to the CR. For example, many children are afraid of the dark; however, after many uneventful nights, children gradually lose their fear. Failure of the neuronal mechanisms involved in extinction also may explain the continued ability of conditioned stimuli to elicit traumatic memories and flashbacks in PTSD (Bremner, 2006; Etkin & Wager 2007; van Elzakker, Dahlgren, Davis, Dubois, & Shin, 2014). Further, research on brain dysfunction associated with PTSD resulting from childhood abuse of women has shown that damage to the medial prefrontal cortex interferes with extinguishing fear responses (Nemeroff et al., 2006). In addition, individuals with damage to the medial prefrontal cortex show emotional dysfunction and an inability to relate in social situations that require correct interpretation of the emotional expressions of others. These findings suggest that dysfunction of this area of the brain may play a role in pathologic emotions that follow exposure to extreme stressors, such as childhood sexual abuse (Lanius, Frewen, Vermetten, & Yehuda, 2010).

Avoidance and Numbing (Dissociative Symptoms)

Survivors try to avoid people or situations that might provoke memories of the trauma. This restriction in their activities may interfere with normal functioning. Survivors also report anhedonia (loss of ability to sense pleasure) and may report that they feel as if parts of themselves have died. These disturbing symptoms may lead them to engage in acts of self-mutilation to feel alive or ultimately to suicide (Dyer et al., 2009; Lanius et al., 2010).

Persons who are completely powerless may go into a state of surrender. In that state, they escape the situation by altering their state of consciousness, that is, by dissociating (Courtois, 2008; Herman, 2015). **Dissociation** is defined as a disruption in the normally occurring linkages between subjective awareness, feelings, thoughts, behaviours, and memories (APA, 2013). It refers to changes in awareness in light of traumatic experience (Bryant, 2007) and is conceptually recognized as a trauma-related altered state of consciousness (TRASC) (Lanius, 2015). Dissociation is a complex psychophysiologic process that produces alterations in sense of self, accessibility of memory and knowledge, and integration of behaviour (Briere, Weathers, & Runtz, 2005; Courtois, 2008). In simpler words, persons who dissociate are making themselves "disappear." That is, they have the feeling of leaving their bodies and observing what happens to them from a distance. During trauma, dissociation enables persons to observe the event while experiencing no pain, or only limited pain, and to protect themselves from awareness of the full impact of the traumatic event.

Following a review of relevant literature pertaining to the conceptualization and measurement of dissociation, Holmes and colleagues (2005) identify that dissociation consists of two domains: detachment (being an outside observer) and compartmentalization (phenomena such as amnesia), which offers promise regarding an improved understanding of dissociation and treatment choice. A study of Montreal school-aged girls indicates that sexual abuse was associated with eight times the level of dissociation and four times the level of PTSD in the girls who had been sexually abused compared with matched controls without sexual abuse (Collin-Vézina & Hebert, 2005). Examples of dissociation include (1) derealization and depersonalization (the experience of self or the environment as strange or unreal), (2) periods of disengagement from the immediate environment during stress, such as "spacing out", (3) alterations in bodily perceptions, (4) emotional numbing, (5) out-of-body experiences, and (6) amnesia for abuse-related memories

(Holmes et al., 2005). Fear activates the endogenous opioid system, producing stress-induced analgesia (SIA) (Gueze et al., 2007; van der Kolk, 2005). SIA may be associated with avoidance and numbing. The purpose of SIA is to protect against pain in dangerous situations so that the individual (animal or human) can defend itself (fight) or escape the situation (flight). In severely stressed animals, opiate withdrawal symptoms can be produced by removing the stressor or by injecting naloxone, an opiate antagonist. In people with PTSD, SIA can become conditioned to stimuli resembling the original trauma. Excessive opioid and norepinephrine secretion can interfere with memory. Freezing or numbing responses may prevent animals from remembering situations of overwhelming stress. Trauma-related dissociative reactions after prolonged exposure to severe, uncontrollable stress may be analogous to this effect in animals (Hopper et al., 2007; van der Kolk, 2005).

Dissociative PTSD is now recognized as a separate subtype distinct from PTSD with hyperarousal responses in the DSM-5 (APA, 2013). Research supports unique patterns of neural activity in individuals with dissociative subtype. For example, Harricharan and colleagues (2016) found higher functional connectivity in brain regions associated with passive coping in individuals with dissociative PTSD, as compared to individuals with hyperarousal PTSD through fMRI testing. Similarly, Daniels, Frewen, Theberge, and Lanius (2016) found differences in brain mass volume between the dissociative and nondissociative PTSD subtypes.

Dissociative Identity Disorder

Dissociation exists on a continuum, with most people experiencing short, situation-specific episodes, such as daydreaming (Holmes et al., 2005). Among survivors of abuse, dissociative symptoms may be part of the symptom picture of ASD and PTSD or they may be the predominant symptom (Lasiuk & Hegadoren, 2006). In such cases, the disorder is **dissociative identity disorder** (DID) (formerly multiple personality disorder) (Ross, 2009; Ross & Ness, 2010). The hallmarks of DID are two or more distinct identities with unique personality characteristics and an inability to recall important information about self or events that is too extensive to be explained by ordinary forgetfulness (APA, 2013). Other memory disturbances linked with dissociation include intermittent and disruptive intrusions of traumatic memories into awareness and difficulties in determining whether a given memory reflects an actual event or information acquired through another source (Putnam, 1994). Please refer to the American Psychiatric Association (2013) for the diagnostic criteria for DID.

Two other dimensions of dissociation that are associated with DID include passive influence experiences and hallucinatory experiences. A passive influence experience is a situation in which a person feels as if he or she were controlled by a force from within. These experiences may include a sense that one is being made to do something against one's will that may be distasteful or harmful to self and others (Vermetten, Schmahl, Lindner, Loewenstein, & Bremner, 2006).

Many survivors of abuse report dissociative perceptual disturbances, such as visual hallucinations, extrasensory perceptions, and peculiar time distortions (Holmes et al., 2005; Vermetten et al., 2006). The hallucinatory experiences in dissociative disorders are distinct in several ways from those that occur in psychotic disorders. They are often experienced as internalized, rather than externalized, voices and may be associated with specific experiences or people. The affected person hears the voices distinctly; the voices often have particular attributes such as gender, age, and affect. The voices may be supportive and comforting or berating. Hallucinatory experiences may also involve the appearance of "shadowy figures," ghosts or spirits, or rapidly moving objects. The person is generally aware that the voices or images are not real.

The overall prevalence of DID is unknown. Prevalence estimates suggest that the prevalence of DID can be as high as 1.5% of American adults across 12 months (American Psychiatric Association, 2013). The cause of DID is unknown. However, the patient history invariably includes pathologic levels of stress such as a traumatic event in childhood (American Psychiatric Association, 2013; Kihlstrom, 2005). Causative factors that have been identified include a traumatic event, a psychological or genetic vulnerability to develop the disorder, formative environmental factors, and the absence of external support (Korol, 2008). Examples of psychological vulnerability include being suggestible or easily hypnotized. Formative environmental events may include a lack of role models who demonstrate healthy problem-solving or practices to relieve anxiety or stress. Many who experience DID lack supportive others, such as parents, siblings, other relatives, and supportive people outside the family (e.g., teachers) (Korol, 2008).

Complex Trauma

In her landmark book and seminal work, *Trauma and Recovery*, Herman (1997, p. 119) proposed a diagnosis: **"complex posttraumatic stress disorder"** (C-PTSD). She noted that survivors of prolonged, repeated trauma experience characteristic personality changes, including problems of relatedness, identity, and vulnerability to repeated harm, inflicted by others or self. The symptoms of C-PTSD include impaired affect modulation (difficulty modulating anger or sexual behaviours; self-destructive and suicidal behaviours); impulsive/risk-taking behaviour; alterations in attention and consciousness (amnesia, dissociation); somatization; chronic characterologic changes, including alterations in relations with others (an inability to trust or maintain relationships, a tendency to be revictimized or to victimize others); and alterations in systems of meaning (e.g., despair, hopelessness, loss of previously sustaining beliefs) (Courtois & Ford, 2014; van der Kolk, 2005). Despite receiving considerable attention in the literature, C-PTSD is not included in the *DSM-5*, although, as noted above, there is now a dissociative subtype of PTSD, which enables some issues pertaining to C-PTSD to be addressed (American Psychiatric Association, 2013).

These symptoms are similar to those of borderline personality disorder (BPD). Many people with BPD were severely abused in childhood (Courtois & Ford, 2014). Splitting self and others into "all good" or "all bad" may result from a developmental arrest: a fragmentation of self, based on modes of organizing experience that were common in earlier developmental stages. Self-mutilation, often labelled as masochism or manipulative behaviour, may be a way of regulating psychological and biologic equilibrium when ordinary means of self-regulation have been disturbed by trauma. Psychotic episodes in patients with BPD are similar to flashbacks, intrusive recollections of traumatic memories that were stored on a somatosensory level (van der Kolk, 2005). Research findings demonstrate that the diagnoses of both BPD and C-PTSD were significantly higher in a group of women with early-onset sexual abuse compared with late-onset sexual abuse, suggesting that women with a history of childhood sexual abuse might be better understood within the rubric of C-PTSD (McLean & Gallop, 2003).

Substance Abuse and Dependence

Childhood abuse, PTSD, and substance abuse are known to be associated (Cross, Crow, Poweres, & Bradley, 2015). In a study to investigate the links between child abuse and IPV, child abuse was found to have a direct effect on PTSD symptoms and depression together with indirect effects on binge drinking (Machisa, Christofides, & Jewkes, 2017). Investigators have reported that in a sample of women drawn from substance abuse treatment centres in Ontario, Canada, 56% had experienced adult physical abuse (Mason & O'Rinn, 2014). Individuals who are injection drug users are more likely to experience violence. In a Canadian study of drug users in Vancouver, almost half the study participants had experienced at least one incident of physical or sexual violence over a median 5.5 years of follow-up (Kennedy, McNeil, Milloy, Dong, Kerr, & Hayashi, 2017).

Survivors who experience PTSD, depression, and other forms of emotional distress may abuse substances, including alcohol and other sedative drugs, in order to alleviate the symptoms of anxiety and distress (Flanagan, Korte, Kileen, & Back, 2016). Drug and alcohol help reduce a state of hyperarousal and function as a maladaptive coping strategy to deal with the abuse (Simmons, Knight, & Menard, 2015). A number of trauma-related responses can be seen in individuals with PTSD. These responses may include chronic interpersonal difficulties, somatization, and substance abuse. Since the outcomes of complex trauma can vary widely, a comprehensive assessment is essential (Courtois & Ford, 2014). In a review of global literature on mental health and risk factors among Indigenous women who experienced IPV, women's experiences of IPV were associated with poverty, discrimination, and substance abuse. Alcohol use was found to be a maladaptive coping mechanism for those who had experienced child abuse and revictimization

as adults (Chmielowska & Fuhr, 2017). Higher rates of IPV among Indigenous women were attributed to experiences of colonization (Chmielowska & Fuhr, 2017).

Psychological Responses

Low Self-Esteem

The consequences of abuse are devastating, and the term "low self-esteem" seems inadequate. Child abuse is associated with lower self-esteem, which in turn has been associated with an increased risk for alcohol abuse and IPV. Furthermore, a history of sexual abuse is associated with a range of mental health challenges including low self-esteem, depression, anxiety, substance misuse, and adult victimization (Mason & O'Rinn, 2014). In a scoping review of studies looking at IPV and mental health issues, living with an abusive partner was found to lead many women to experience depression, anxiety, and low self-esteem (Mason & O'Rinn, 2014). In a systematic review of studies looking at mental health outcomes in those who had experienced IPV, research findings showed that IPV has adverse effects on mental health and that the severity and extent of IPV can increase mental health symptoms. Psychological violence was found to have a particularly significant effect on those who experienced IPV and should be taken as serious form of violence because of its impact on mental health (Lagdon, Stringer, & Armour, 2014). Prolonged exposure to abuse including verbal and emotional abuse can be internalized and negatively affect feelings of self-worth (Ansara & Hindin, 2011; Jenney, 2009; Stark, 2009). In a study exploring IPV and depression in Latin American women in Canada, investigators found a strong connection between mental health problems and the lived experiences of IPV. Women described feelings of low self-esteem and worthlessness resulting from IPV along with constant fear, stress and worry, disrupted sleep, and sadness (Godoy-Ruiz et al., 2015).

Guilt and Shame

A history of abuse is often associated with guilt and shame (Ansara & Hindin, 2011; Stewart et al., 2013). In a study of women who experienced IPV, Beck and colleagues (2011) found an association of shame and guilt with PTSD among women in the sample seeking mental health services. The investigators observed that the findings support conclusions from the literature that feelings of shame and guilt are seen in those who have experienced trauma. In a study examining the psychosocial consequences associated with different forms of abuse, data from the 2004 Canadian GSS were analyzed. The investigators found that any pattern of violence was associated with negative psychosocial outcomes for both women and men. The psychosocial impact on women however was greater because of their experience of more severe and chronic abuse and control and included changes in interpersonal functioning, feelings of depression, anxiety, shame, guilt, feeling victimized, and lowered self-esteem

(Ansara & Hindin, 2011). The experience of being battered is so degrading and humiliating that women are often afraid to disclose it. Many women may be reluctant to disclose abuse because of fear for themselves, feelings of shame, or fear of being judged by others (Ansara & Hindin, 2010). A systematic review synthesizing research evidence concerning adults' disclosure of domestic violence when accessing health care services found that guilt, shame, and powerlessness were recurring themes, particularly for older women when accessing care (Robinson & Spilsbury, 2008).

Anger

Chronic irritability, unexpected or uncontrollable feelings of anger, and difficulties with the expression of anger are frequent experiences for survivors of abuse (Campbell et al., 2004). They may express anger towards the perpetrator and/or those who have been spared the suffering or someone whom the victim believes could have prevented the abuse (Barnett, Miller-Perrin, & Perrin, 1997). In a qualitative study of women survivors of IPV that used Kubler–Ross' model of the stages of grief, investigators explored how women came to terms with their experiences of violence. All women in the study reported feeling anger at some stage, sometimes associated with guilt, primarily related to the impact of IPV on children, and anger at their partner for what he had done (Messing, Mohr, & Durfee, 2015). However, some incest survivors have difficulty expressing anger and may demonstrate helplessness or numbness or mask it with compliance and perfectionism (Campbell et al., 2004). Anger may surface at a later time and play a role in recovery that enables women to protect themselves from further abuse and "advocate for their children" (Thomas, Bannister, & Hall, 2012).

Problems With Intimacy

The abused child experiences intrusion, abandonment, devaluation, or pain in the relationship with the abuser, instead of the closeness and nurturing that are normal for intimate relationships, such as those between the parent and the child (Draughon & Urbancic, 2011). As a result, many survivors have difficulty trusting and forming intimate relationships. Sexual problems are common among survivors of abuse. Among the most common and chronic problems are fear of intimate sexual relationships, feelings of repulsion towards sex, lack of enjoyment of sex, dysfunctions of desire and arousal, and failure to achieve orgasm. Some survivors engage in compulsive promiscuity and prostitution, reflecting their internalization of the message that the only thing that they are good for is sex (Draughton & Urbancic, 2011; Lemieux & Byers, 2008; Maniglio, 2009).

Revictimization

Many women who have been sexually abused as children are revictimized on multiple occasions later in life. Among women with a history of child sexual abuse, the risk of sexual revictimization is doubled or even tripled (Classen, Palesh, & Aggarwal, 2005; Filipas & Ullman, 2006). In a study of women receiving treatment from three Canadian urban mental health centres, women who had experienced previous trauma in childhood were more likely to experience PTSD following IPV (Wuest et al., 2009). Numerous factors have been related to revictimization, including PTSD symptoms, dissociation, affect dysregulation, the use of AOD, interpersonal problems, and sexual behaviours (Classen et al., 2005). Proneness to revictimization may result from a general vulnerability in dangerous situations that may be associated with dissociation. Dissociation makes women unaware of their environment and also may make them look confused or distracted. Shock and dissociation can also occur while the abuse is occurring and afterwards in order for the woman to avoid dealing with her immediate feelings (McCue, 2008). **Alexithymia** may also add to a woman's risk for revictimization. Difficulty in labelling and communicating feelings may make it difficult for a woman to set limits on sexual advances. Moreover, these women may not be able to read accurately the emotional cues of others, which diminishes their ability to respond effectively in interpersonally dangerous situations (Cloitre, Scarvalone, & Difede, 1997; Ogden et al., 2006).

Women with abuse histories frequently have difficulty with boundaries. During childhood abuse, they experienced boundary violations as normal and connected with their expectations of intimate relationships. Confusion over boundaries may result in confusion about appropriate behaviour in adult intimate relationships (Messman-Moore & Long, 2003). Further, the sexual behaviour pattern of survivors may place them at risk for revictimization. One effect of sexual victimization is that the child's sexuality is shaped by "traumatic sexualization." Traumatic sexualization occurs when a child is rewarded for sexual behaviour with affection, attention, privileges, and gifts. As a result, the child may learn that her self-worth is tied to her sexuality, and she may use sexual behaviour to manipulate others (Breitenbecher, 2001; Messman-Moore & Long, 2003).

NURSING MANAGEMENT: HUMAN RESPONSE TO ABUSE

Exposure to traumatic experiences such as abuse can have a deleterious effect on one's health. Approaches to working with women experiencing IPV should be informed by trauma-informed care, an approach grounded in a substantial body of research and practice knowledge. A trauma-informed approach is based on an understanding of the impact of violence on individual's lives (Ford-Gilboe et al., 2011) and as such can guide the nurse–client encounters.

Nurses encounter survivors of abuse in many health care settings. For example, it has been observed that in Ontario between 4.1% and 22% of adult women presenting to EDs, family medicine practices and women's health clinics report IPV (Beynon et al., 2012). In another

Canadian study exploring the extent to which women disclosed IPV in EDs, it was found that only 2% reported abuse to a health professional (Catallo, Jack, Ciliska, & MacMillan, 2013). The principal reason for nondisclosure was fear of "being found out." The women's fears centred around such consequences such as involvement of Children's Aid or violence associated with being exposed (Catallo et al., 2013).

These findings have implications for nurses who are in a position to support women to disclose IPV by, for example, conducting the assessment in a private setting and reducing the number of professionals who interact with the client. Barriers to asking about IPV by nurses and physicians including insufficient time, lack of understanding and knowledge of cultural practices, ensuring privacy for clients, and uncertainty regarding how to ask clients about IPV are among the main reasons (Beynon et al., 2012; Thurston et al., 2009). In addition, the importance of supporting a sense of efficacy for nurses working in EDs has been identified by Canadian researchers (Hollingsworth & Ford-Gilboe, 2006).

The paediatric ED provides a unique opportunity to identify and respond to child survivors, as well as battered mothers (Campbell et al., 2004). Brownridge and colleagues (2016) cite a number of studies that point to the cumulative risk of exposure to IPV and child maltreatment. Children exposed to IPV are more likely to be victims themselves. Black, Trocmé, Fallon, and Maclaurin (2008) found that over one third of the child mistreatment investigations in Canada, excluding Quebec, involved exposure to domestic violence. Identifying battered mothers may be the most important means of identifying child abuse. Conversely, when nurses suspect child abuse, they cannot ignore the possibility that the mother is also a victim. Recognizing children who are traumatized by witnessing the battering of their mothers is also essential. However, despite the opportunity the paediatric ED affords, disturbingly few battered women are identified there. Addressing the issue of family violence is critical given the potential for the cycle to continue across generations. Health care providers in paediatric EDs have reported several obstacles to identification, including lack of training, time constraints, powerlessness, lack of comfort, lack of control over the victim's circumstances, and fear of offending the patient (Beynon et al., 2012; Catallo et al., 2013; Thurston et al., 2009).

Identification of women who have experienced violence can also occur in settings where perinatal (antenatal and postpartum) care is provided. In a comprehensive scoping review, Jackson and Mantler (2017) note that IPV is common during antenatal periods and can result in PTSD. Significant stressors and limited social supports can pose risks and negative health outcomes for both mother and child.

Nurses may encounter elder abuse in virtually any setting. Examples include EDs, medical–surgical units, psychiatric units, and homes during home care visits. In addition, nurses may encounter elder abuse in nursing homes. Events such as unnecessary chemical (medications) or physical restraints used to control an elder's behaviour may be abusive and should be investigated.

Although some aspects of care are specific to adult, child, or elderly survivors of abuse, many elements are common in the nursing care of all survivors, regardless of age or setting. The goals of all nursing interventions in cases of abuse are to stop the violence and to ensure the survivor's safety. Victimization removes all power and control from a woman, child, or elder. Therefore, as appropriate for age and ability, all nursing interventions should empower survivors to act on their own behalf and must be done in a collaborative partnership. To that end, nurses must be willing to offer support and information and not impose their own values on survivors by encouraging them to leave abusive relationships. Assessments need to be carried out in a thoughtful manner to minimize the number of times a woman must share her experiences with multiple health providers (Catallo et al., 2013). Strong psychological and economic bonds tie many women to their perpetrators. Moreover, adult survivors who are capable of making decisions are the experts on their situations. They are the best judges of how to deal with the abuse, and their life choices need to be respected (Registered Nurses' Association of Ontario, 2005).

However, removing children and elders from their families or caregivers often is necessary to ensure immediate safety. If the home of an abused or neglected child or elder cannot be made safe, the nurse must support other professionals involved in placing the child or elder in a foster or nursing home (Gary & Humphreys, 2004). However, intervening in cases of elder abuse is not a clear-cut issue. Nurses must allow elders whose decision-making is not impaired an appropriate degree of autonomy in deciding how to manage the problem, even if they choose to remain in the abusive situation (Fulmer et al., 2011; Killick & Taylor, 2009). Forcing elders to do something against their wishes is itself a form of victimization.

Intervention strategies for elders depend on whether the elders accept or refuse assistance and whether they can make decisions. If the elder refuses treatment, the nurse must remain nonjudgemental and provide information about available services and emergency numbers. The Canadian approach to adult protection legislation, concerned with preventing abuse and neglect, has been guided by reforms in adult guardianship and substitute decision-making. There are four Canadian jurisdictions with adult protection legislation in place (Canadian Network for the Prevention of Elder Abuse, 2011).

Biologic Domain

Biologic Assessment

Research indicates that health care providers often fail to respond therapeutically to survivors of abuse. In many instances, they neglect to identify abuse as the cause of traumatic injuries or mental health problems (Ford-Gilboe et al., 2011; Gutmanis, Beynon, Tutty, Wathen, & MacMillan, 2007; Plichta, 2007). Even more damaging, health care professionals may treat abuse survivors derogatorily, blaming them for the abuse or for staying in abusive situations. Often, abuse survivors have been severely traumatized, and their behaviours are difficult and disruptive. In some cases, caregivers react negatively, labelling this behaviour as attention seeking and manipulative (Reeves, 2015). When nurses react to their patients in a negative, punitive manner, they retraumatize them (Gallop, McCay, Guha, & Khan, 1999). It is not uncommon to see this behaviour punished by staff avoidance, time in seclusion rooms, and overmedication. BPD symptoms or severe symptoms associated with trauma should be interpreted as ineffective coping strategies, developed in response to severe trauma, rather than as deliberate attempts to manipulate staff (Hattendorf & Tollerud, 1997; Huband & Tantam, 2000). Nurses may also make inaccurate assumptions about who experiences IPV (e.g., the poor) and may therefore respond in ways that not only do not help the woman but which contribute to victim blaming (Ford-Gilboe et al., 2011).

To improve providers' responses, the Canadian Nurses Association (CNA, 1992) has long recommended that students acquire the necessary knowledge and skill acquisition to prevent violence, as well as to detect and intervene with individuals who are survivors of abuse and violence. Nurses can play a significant role in addressing family violence because nurses are frequently the first professionals to interact with individuals affected by family violence. Nurses are particularly suited to support women who have experienced IPV. Jack and colleagues (2016) undertook a qualitative study of a nurse home visiting programme to assess and support women experiencing IPV. The study showed that women were open to disclosing IPV provided that the nurse client interaction was situated within a nonstructured discussion of health issues by knowledgeable nurses.

Nurses should assess everyone for violence—both women and men, no matter what age or presenting problem. An awareness of violence and a high index of suspicion are the most important elements in assessing the problem (Campbell et al., 2004). If suspected abuse is never assessed, it will never be uncovered. Establishing a trusting nurse–patient relationship is one of the most important steps in assessing any type of abuse. Survivors are unlikely to disclose sensitive information unless they perceive the nurse to be trustworthy and nonjudgemental. Important considerations in establishing open communication are ensuring confidentiality and providing a quiet, private place in which to conduct assessment. The law mandates that nurses report child abuse to the authorities, and nurses must make that responsibility clear before beginning the assessment. Child abuse is usually reported to the Children's Aid Society.

IN-A-LIFE

Sheldon Kennedy (1970–)

PROFESSIONAL HOCKEY PLAYER

Public Persona

Canadian-born Sheldon Kennedy played professional hockey in the National Hockey League. He was an outstanding and talented hockey player who began training in the Canadian Hockey League at a young age. As a junior-level hockey player in Winnipeg, he was coached by Graham James, one of the most nationally famous and highly respected coaches.

Personal Realities

In 1996, Kennedy came forward with sexual abuse allegations against his former coach. Kennedy said that the assaults took place between the ages of 14 and 19 and occurred on a weekly basis. On September 3, 1996, Kennedy reported the sexual abuse by James to the Calgary city police. In January 1997, Graham James was sentenced to 3½ years in prison for the sexual abuse. Kennedy then went public with his story, including the revelation of the many times he contemplated suicide. Shortly afterwards, the NHL sponsored Kennedy to enrol in a substance abuse programme for his drinking and drug problems.

Kennedy's courage has brought hope to many, and he has dedicated his career to prevention and education about child abuse. Together with his business partner Wayne McNeil, he founded Respect Group Inc., an organization that works in partnership with the Canadian Red Cross and that is devoted to the prevention of abuse, bullying, and harassment. In 2013, the Calgary Child Advocacy Centre was renamed the Sheldon Kennedy Child Advocacy Centre with Kennedy functioning as lead director. The centre works in partnership with organizations, community leaders, corporate and individual champions, and government to support children, youth, and families who have been traumatized by abuse and bring increase awareness of the issue. Kennedy has received numerous awards and honours for his work including the Queen Elizabeth II Diamond Jubilee Medal and the University of Guelph Lincoln Alexander Outstanding Leader Award. In 2014, he was named a Member of the Order of Canada.

www.sheldonkennedycac.ca/contact
respectgroupinc.com
www.lieutenantgovernor.ab.ca/aoe/community-service/sheldon-kennedy/index.html

Lethality Assessment

The most important assessment and the one to be done first is to assess safety and the level of risk (Ford-Gilboe et al., 2011). The nurse must ascertain whether survivors are in danger for their life, either from homicide or suicide, and, if children are in the home, whether they are in danger (Campbell et al., 2009). The nurse should take immediate steps to ensure the survivor's safety. In the case of suspected child abuse assessed in a health care agency, an interdisciplinary team consisting of physicians, psychologists, nurses, and social workers usually makes this decision. In other settings, the nurse may be the person to make that decision. Nurses do not have to obtain proof of abuse, only a reasonable suspicion. The Danger Assessment Screen developed by Jacquelyn Campbell and colleagues (1993) is a useful tool for assessing the risk that either the adult survivor or the perpetrator will commit homicide (Box 34.2).

Most survivors do not report abuse to health care workers without being asked specifically about it. Routine screening or asking about IPV by health care providers is low—approximately 5% to 25% in ED settings. Sprague et al. (2016) reporting on the results of a scoping review of IPV identification programmes in health care settings reported that between 38% and 59% of women have experienced IPV that are in contact with health care professionals. Even among women who present at EDs with injuries likely resulting from IPV, the rate of inquiry is less than 80% (Gutmanis et al., 2007). In a survey of 250 Canadian EDs (McClennan, Worster, & MacMillan, 2008), 31.9% reported having IPV policies and procedures in place. Remarkably, there had been no significant change over a 10-year period (1994–2004) in the existence of IPV polices in Canadian EDs, despite the call for recommendations for routine screening (Sprague et al., 2012).

Survivors may be reluctant to report abuse because of shame and fear of retaliation, especially if the victim depends on the abuser as caregiver. In addition, children may be afraid that they will not be believed. Care needs to be exercised in the use of language when assessing for IPV. For instance, a woman may not disclose her experiences as abusive, and a more useful approach may be to ask if she has experienced specific acts of abuse (Ford-Gilboe et al., 2011). The evidence to support routine screening is mixed. MacMillan and colleagues (2009) carried out a randomized control trial to determine the effectiveness of screening. The findings were not sufficiently conclusive to recommend routine screening. At this time, best practice is regarded as including routine universal screening, together

---

BOX 34.2 Danger Assessment

Several risk factors have been associated with homicides (murders) of both batterers and battered women in research that has been conducted after the killings have taken place. We cannot predict what will happen in your case, but we would like you to be aware of the danger of homicide in situations of severe battering and to see how many of the risk factors apply to your situation. (The "he" in the questions refers to your husband, partner, ex-husband, ex-partner, or whoever is currently physically hurting you.)

1. Has the physical violence increased in frequency during the past year?
2. Has the physical violence increased in severity during the past year, or has a weapon or threat with weapon been used?
3. Does he ever try to choke you?
4. Is there a gun in the house?
5. Has he ever forced you into sex when you did not wish to do so?
6. Does he use drugs? By drugs, I mean "uppers" or amphetamines, speed, angel dust, cocaine, "crack," street drugs, heroin, or mixtures.
7. Does he threaten to kill you, or do you believe he is capable of killing you?
8. Is he drunk every day or almost every day? (In terms of quantity of alcohol.)
9. Does he control most or all of your daily activities? For instance, does he tell you whom you can be friends with, how much money you can take with you shopping, or when you can take the car? (If he tries, but you do not let him, check here _____ .)
10. Has he ever beaten you while you were pregnant? (If never pregnant by him, check here _____ .)
11. Is he violently and constantly jealous of you? (For instance, does he say, "If I can't have you, no one can.")
12. Have you ever threatened or tried to commit suicide?
13. Has he ever threatened or tried to commit suicide?
14. Is he violent towards the children?
15. Is he violent outside the home?

TOTAL YES ANSWERS: _____ .

THANK YOU. PLEASE TALK TO YOUR NURSE, ADVOCATE, OR COUNSELLOR ABOUT WHAT THE DANGER ASSESSMENT MEANS IN TERMS OF YOUR SITUATION.

Adapted from Campbell, J. C., McKenna, L. S., Torres, S., Sheridan, D., & Landenburger, K. (1993). Nursing care of abused women. In J. C. Campbell & J. Humphreys (Eds.), *Nursing care of survivors of family violence* (p. 259). St. Louis, MO: Mosby.

with comprehensive staff education and ongoing agency and managerial support (Registered Nurses' Association of Ontario, 2005). Rather than simply focusing on screening, nurses should carry out an assessment in which the nurse seeks to identify and follow up with appropriate interventions in order to provide an effective and comprehensive response to IPV (Ford-Gilboe et al., 2011). For that reason, nurses must develop a repertoire of age appropriate, culturally sensitive abuse-related questions using an approach that is trauma informed (Ford-Gilboe et al., 2011).

Appropriate questions to ask in assessing abuse in women are found in the Abuse Assessment Screen in Box 34.3. Other questions that might be useful in eliciting disclosure are as follows: "When there are fights at home, have you ever been hurt or afraid?" "It looks like someone has hurt you. Tell me about it." "Some women have described problems like yours and have told me that their partner has hurt them. Is that happening to you?" (Campbell et al., 2004). Women vary in their decision to disclose abuse and to whom they disclose. There is great variation in help-seeking responses (Barrett & Pierre, 2011). Because many women may keep their experiences of IPV private and health care providers may not know if a woman is experiencing abuse, nurses should provide care that is trauma informed. A trauma-informed approach in dealing with all women creates a climate of trust and promotes a woman's safety and comfort. Ensuring privacy for women, attending to women's responses, and explaining procedures clearly are examples of approaches to support all women including those who disclose trauma (Ford-Gilboe et al., 2011).

BOX 34.3 Abuse Assessment Screen

1. Have you ever been emotionally or physically abused by your partner or someone important to you?
   YES _____
   NO _____
2. Within the past year, have you been hit, slapped, kicked, or otherwise physically hurt by someone?
   YES _____
   NO _____
   If YES, by whom: _____
   Number of times: _____
   Mark the area of injury on body map.
3. Within the past year, has anyone forced you to have sexual activities?
   If YES, who: _____
   Number of times: _____
4. Are you afraid of your partner or anyone you listed above?
   YES _____
   NO _____

Further, Ford-Gilboe and colleagues (2011) suggest the nurse use an approach that feels comfortable and respects the safety, privacy, and confidentiality of the woman. Should a woman disclose IPV, the following response on the part of the nurse can support the woman: (a) listen to her story in a nonjudgmental way, (b) affirm she is not to blame, (c) document what the woman reports in her own words, (d) assess her level of risk and discuss safety strategies, (e) conduct a comprehensive health assessment, (f) ask the woman what she needs, (g) discuss referral to services if the woman wishes (Ford-Gilboe et al., 2011).

Most survivors are not offended when health care workers ask about abuse directly, as long as they conduct the interview nonjudgementally. Survivors may perceive failure to ask about abuse as evidence of lack of concern, adding to the feelings of entrapment and helplessness. The high prevalence of abuse and the reluctance of survivors to volunteer information about it mandate routine screening of every patient for abuse by explicit questioning. Perhaps even more important, the nurse must complete such screening in privacy, away from the woman's partner, the child's parents or legal guardians, or the elderly person's relative or companion (Campbell et al., 2004; Ford-Gilboe et al., 2011; Fulmer, et al., 2011; Kelley, 2011). If a partner, parent, other relative, or companion accompanies the patient to the health care facility, protocols should be in place to separate the patient from these individuals until the assessment is completed. One approach is to ask the other person to wait in the reception area, explaining that assessments are always done in private.

After the assessment is completed in a health care agency, the nurse should offer the adult survivor use of the telephone. The agency appointment may be the only time that the survivor can make calls in private to family, who might offer support, or to the police, lawyers, or shelters. Scheduling future appointments may provide the survivor with a legitimate reason to leave the perpetrator temporarily and continue to explore her options.

History and Physical Examination

All survivors who report or for whom the nurse suspects abuse should receive a complete history and physical examination. For example, Wuest et al. (2009) in their study of chronic pain in a community sample of women who had left their abusive partner found that more than 35% of the women experienced significant pain and in particular joint pain. Throughout, the nurse must remain nonjudgemental and communicate openly and honestly in their interactions with persons who have experienced IPV (Ford-Gilboe et al., 2011).

A Canadian grounded theory study of woman survivors of child sexual abuse indicates that feeling safe with a health care provider who is sensitive and willing to listen can facilitate disclosure (Schachter, Radomsky, Stalker, & Teram, 2004). It is not the nurse's responsibility to judge any situation, whether the decision to remain in an abusive relationship, the abusive actions of children's parents, or abuse perpetrated by caregivers of the elderly. Therefore, nurses must continually monitor their own feelings towards the abuser and survivor, especially in cases of child abuse. Working with child survivors often causes distress and feelings of anger and inadequacy. A range of supports such as training, organizational support, and supervision can assist emergency room nurses in caring for survivors of IPV (van der Wath, van Wyk, & van Rensburg, 2013). Nurses should reflect on their beliefs and values and how these may shape their practice including their interactions with women (Ford-Gilboe et al., 2011; Gutmanis et al., 2007; Long & Smyth, 1998; Registered Nurses' Association of Ontario, 2005).

The history should include past and present medical histories, ADLs, and social and financial supports. The nurse should obtain a detailed history of how injuries occurred. As with any history, the nurse begins with the complaint that brought the patient to the health care agency. The nurse assesses whether the explanation for the injuries or symptoms is plausible, given their nature. Discrepancies between the history and the physical examination findings may suggest abuse or neglect. The nurse moves from safe to more sensitive topics, such as the nature of the injuries. Walker (1994) suggests using what she calls the "four-incident technique" to elicit a complete abuse history. The nurse asks survivors to describe four battering incidents: the first incident that they remember, the most recent incident, the worst incident, and a typical incident. This series of questions is designed to elicit a complete picture of the **cycle of violence** and its progression. If the child is too young or an elder is too impaired to give a history, the nurse should interview one or both parents of the child or the caregiver of the elder. If the survivor is a child or dependent elder who cannot describe what happened or make decisions about personal safety and care, the health care team may take steps to place the survivor in protective custody and defer additional assessment to the appropriate agency. The physical examination should include a neurologic examination, radiographs to identify any old or new fractures, and an examination for sexual abuse. Nurses assessing the elderly need to be familiar with normal aging and with the signs and symptoms of common illnesses in the elderly to distinguish those conditions from abuse (Fulmer et al., 2011). Similarly, nurses need to know healthy child development to detect deviations that abuse or neglect may cause. For children, assessing developmental milestones, school history, and relationships with siblings and friends is important (Kelley, 2011); any discrepancies between the history and the physical examination and implausible explanations for injuries and other symptoms should alert the nurse to the possibility of abuse. Box 34.4 lists indicators of actual or potential abuse that need to be thoroughly assessed for all survivors.

BOX 34.4 History and Physical Findings Suggestive of Abuse

PRESENTING PROBLEM

- Vague information about the cause of the problem
- Delay between occurrence of injury and seeking of treatment
- Inappropriate reactions of significant other or family
- Denial or minimizing of seriousness of injury
- Discrepancy between the history and the physical examination findings

FAMILY HISTORY

- Past family violence
- Physical punishment of children
- Children who are fearful of parent(s)
- Father and/or mother who demands unquestioning obedience
- Alcohol or drug abuse
- Violence outside the home
- Unemployment or underemployment
- Financial difficulties or poverty
- Use of elder's finances for other family members
- Finances rigidly controlled by one member

HEALTH AND PSYCHIATRIC HISTORY

- Fractures at various stages of healing
- Spontaneous abortions

- Injuries during pregnancy
- Multiple visits to the ED
- Elimination disturbances (e.g., constipation, diarrhoea)
- Multiple somatic complaints
- Eating disorders
- Substance abuse
- Depression
- PTSD
- Self-mutilation
- Suicide attempts
- Feelings of helplessness or hopelessness
- Low self-esteem
- Chronic fatigue
- Apathy
- Sleep disturbances (e.g., hypersomnia, hyposomnia)
- Psychiatric hospitalizations

PERSONAL AND SOCIAL HISTORY

- Feelings of powerlessness
- Feelings of being trapped
- Lack of trust
- Traditional values about home, partner, and children's behaviour
- Major decisions in family controlled by one person
- Few social supports (isolated from family, friends)

(Continued)

BOX 34.4 History and Physical Findings Suggestive of Abuse *(Continued)*

- Little activity outside the home
- Unwanted or unplanned pregnancy
- Dependency on caregivers
- Extreme jealousy by partner
- Difficulties at school or work
- Short attention span
- Running away
- Promiscuity
- Child who has knowledge of sexual matters beyond that appropriate for age
- Sexualized play with self, peers, dolls, toys
- Masturbation
- Excessive fears and clinging in children

NEUROLOGIC SYSTEM

- Difficulty with speech or swallowing
- Hyperactive reflexes
- Developmental delays
- Areas of numbness
- Tremors

MENTAL STATUS

- Anxiety, fear
- Depression
- Suicidal ideation
- Difficulty concentrating
- Memory loss
- Verbal aggression
- Themes of violence in artwork and schoolwork

DISTORTED BODY IMAGE

- History of chronic physical or psychological disability
- Inability to perform ADLs
- Delayed language development

PHYSICAL EXAMINATION FINDINGS

General Appearance

- Fearful, anxious, hyperactive, hypoactive
- Watching partner, parent, or caregiver for approval of answers to questions
- Poor grooming or inappropriate dress
- Malnourishment
- Signs of stress or fatigue
- Flinching when approached or touched
- Inappropriate or anxious nonverbal behaviour
- Wearing clothing inappropriate to the season or occasion to cover body parts

Vital Statistics

- Elevated pulse or blood pressure
- Other signs of autonomic arousal (exaggerated startle response, excessive sweating)
- Underweight or overweight

Skin

- Bruises, welts, oedema, scars
- Burns (cigarette, immersion, friction from ropes, a pattern like electric iron or stove)
- Subdural haematoma
- Missing hair
- Poor skin integrity: dehydration, decubitus ulcers, untreated wounds, urine burns, or excoriation

Eyes

- Orbital swelling
- Conjunctival haemorrhage
- Retinal haemorrhage
- Black eyes
- No glasses to accommodate poor eyesight

Ears

- Hearing loss
- No prosthetic device to accommodate poor hearing

Mouth

- Bruising
- Lacerations
- Missing or broken teeth
- Untreated dental problems

Abdomen

- Abdominal injuries during pregnancy
- Intra-abdominal injuries

Genitourinary System or Rectum

- Bruising, lacerations, bleeding, oedema, tenderness
- Untreated infections

Musculoskeletal System

- Fractures or old fractures in various stages of healing
- Dislocations
- Limited range of motion in extremities
- Contractures

Medications

- Medications not indicated by physical condition
- Overdose of drugs or medications (prescribed or over the counter)
- Medications not taken as prescribed

Communication Patterns/Relations

- Verbal hostility, arguments
- Negative nonverbal communication, lack of visible affection
- One person answers questions and looks to the other person for approval
- Extreme dependency of family members

The nurse should thoroughly document all findings. Injuries should be photographed if possible, but this can be done only with written permission from an adult survivor or one of the child's parents. If the survivor will not permit photographing, the nurse should document the injuries on a body map. Survivors may need assurance that their medical records will not be released to anyone without written permission and that documentation of injuries will be important if legal action is taken. If the survivor does not admit abuse, the nurse cannot note abuse in the record. However, the nurse can document that the description of injuries is inconsistent with the injury pattern.

Biologic indicators, such as elevated pulse and blood pressure, sleep and appetite disturbances, exaggerated startle responses, flashbacks, and nightmares, may suggest PTSD or depression. Signs and symptoms of dissociation include memory difficulties, a feeling of unreality about oneself or events, a feeling that a familiar place is strange and unfamiliar, auditory or visual hallucinations, and evidence of having done things without remembering them (Etkin & Wager, 2007; Laschinger & Nosko, 2015; Mason, Wolf, O'Rinn, & Ene, 2017). If any of these signs or symptoms is present, the survivor requires a thorough diagnostic workup for PTSD and DID. In a Canadian study of women survivors of IPV, only 7.1% of women had a formal diagnosis of PTSD although almost half met the diagnostic criteria for PTSD. Women who had experienced previous trauma in childhood such as severe abuse were more likely to demonstrate symptoms of PTSD following IPV (Wuest et al., 2009).

The nurse should assess every adult or adolescent who discloses victimization for substance abuse. The Michigan Alcoholism Screening Test (MAST; Selzer, 1971) and the Drug Abuse Screening Test (DAST; Skinner, 1982) are two screening instruments for use in any health assessment. An adolescent version of the MAST is also available (Snow, Thurber, & Hodgson, 2002). If the results of these tests or the answers to any alcohol-related or drug-related questions are positive, the nurse should evaluate the survivor further for an alcohol or drug disorder.

In a Canadian study of community home visiting (Jack et al., 2016), researchers observed that there was no one approach that should be used to ask about women's experience of abuse. Study findings showed that integration of questions within less structured discussion of parenting, safety, or relationships is a more promising approach to engaging women who may be experiencing IPV. The authors note that a strong therapeutic relationship in any health care setting is the foundation for assessment and use of case finding for IPV (Jack et al., 2016).

Nursing Diagnoses for the Biologic Domain

Selected nursing diagnoses focusing on the human responses that nurses manage in the biologic domain may include posttrauma syndrome, delayed growth and development, impaired memory, and rape trauma syndrome.

Interventions for the Biologic Domain

Restoring health is a primary concern for survivors of abuse. When injuries are severe and surgery is required, the survivor may require hospital admittance.

Treating Physical Symptoms

Treatment of trauma symptoms may include cleaning and dressing burns or other wounds and assisting with casting of broken bones (see Box 34.5 for more information). Malnourished and dehydrated children and elders may require nursing interventions such as intravenous therapy or nutritional supplements that alleviate the alteration in nutrition and fluid and electrolyte balance.

Promoting Healthy Daily Activity

Teaching sleep hygiene and promoting exercise, leisure time, and nutrition will help battered survivors regain a healthy physical state and learn self-care. Taking care of oneself may be difficult, yet important, for survivors who have spent years trying to separate themselves from their bodies (dissociate) to survive years of abuse (Collin-Vézina, Cyr, Pauzé, & McDuff, 2005; Walker, 1994). A history of IPV threatens the physical and mental health of women and children in many ways (Dillon, Hussein, Loxton, & Rahman, 2013; Ford-Gilboe et al., 2005, 2017; MacIntosh, Ford-Gilboe, & Varcoe, 2015; Varcoe et al., 2011). Techniques such as going to bed and rising at consistent times, avoiding naps and caffeine, and scheduling periods for relaxation just before retiring may be useful in promoting sleep. Aerobic exercise is a useful technique for relieving anxiety and depression and promoting sleep.

Administering and Monitoring Medications

Survivors with a comorbid mood or anxiety disorder including PTSD may require pharmacologic interventions. Although only nurses with advanced preparation and prescriptive authority may prescribe medications, all nurses must be familiar with medications used to treat mood and anxiety disorders and the side effects of these drugs. Medications may be contraindicated for young and elderly survivors.

The autonomic nervous system is involved in many of the symptoms of depression and PTSD. Therefore, the use of agents that decrease its activity can help treat these symptoms (Friedman, 2001; Sutherland & Davidson, 1999). Tricyclics and other antidepressants are effective in treating depression and some symptoms of PTSD, such as nightmares, sleep disorders, and startle reactions. They are less effective in treating other PTSD symptoms, such as numbing (Friedman, 2001). The benzodiazepines are useful in treating anxiety and sleep disturbances in PTSD, but because they can cause dependence, they are contraindicated in women who also have a substance abuse disorder.

Approved for treating PTSD, the selective serotonin reuptake inhibitor (SSRI) sertraline (Zoloft) has improved PTSD symptoms in women but not in men

---

BOX 34.5 Special Concerns for Victims of Sexual Assault

ASSESSMENT FOCUS

The history and physical examination of the survivor of sexual assault differ significantly from other assessment routines because the evidence obtained may be used in prosecuting the perpetrator (Sheridan, 2004). Therefore, the purpose is twofold:

- To assess the patient for injuries
- To collect evidence for forensic evaluation and proceedings

Usually, someone with special training, such as a nurse practitioner who has taken special courses, examines a rape or sexual assault victim. Generalist nurses may be involved in treating the injuries that result from the assault, including genital trauma, such as vaginal and anal lacerations, and extragenital trauma, such as injury to the mouth, throat, wrists, arms, breasts, and thighs (Sheridan, 2004).

KEY INTERVENTIONS

Nursing intervention to prevent short- or long-term psychopathology after sexual assault is crucial. Psychological trauma following rape and sexual assault includes immediate anxiety and distress and the development of

PTSD, depression, panic, and substance abuse (Resnick, Acierno, Holmes, Kilpatrick, & Jager, 1999).

Key interventions include:

- Early treatment because initial levels of distress are strongly related to later levels of PTSD, panic, and anxiety (Resnick et al., 1999).
- Supportive, caring, and nonjudgemental nursing interventions during the forensic rape examination are also crucial. This examination often increases survivors' immediate distress because they must recount the assault in detail and submit to an invasive pelvic or anal examination.
- Anxiety-reducing education, counselling, and emotional support, particularly in regard to unwanted pregnancies and sexually transmitted diseases, including HIV. All survivors should be tested for these possibilities. Treatment may include terminating a pregnancy; administering medications to treat gonorrhoea, *Chlamydia*, trichomoniasis, and syphilis; and administering medications that may decrease the likelihood of contracting HIV infection.
- Interventions that are helpful for survivors of domestic violence; these also apply to the survivors of sexual assault.

(Henney, 2000) (see Chapter 12 for information on monitoring medications and their side effects).

Managing Care of Patients With Comorbid Substance Abuse

Survivors who have a comorbid substance abuse disorder need referral to a treatment centre for alcohol and drug disorders. The treatment centre should have programmes that address the special needs of survivors. Alcohol-dependent and drug-dependent survivors frequently stop treatment and return to alcohol and drug abuse if their abuse-related problems are not addressed appropriately (Ouimette, Moos, & Brown, 2003). As might be expected, research findings suggest that attitudes such as self-blame and stigmatization seem to be important variables related to substance abuse for women with a history of childhood sexual abuse (Dufour & Nadeau, 2001). Child maltreatment has been associated with a number of long-term health consequences into adulthood including drug and alcohol misuse (Gilbert et al., 2009).

Devries et al. (2014) carried out a systematic review of studies looking at the association between IPV and alcohol use and found a clear relationship between IPV and alcohol use in women. Survivors, especially those with substance abuse problems, are at high risk for HIV infection and AIDS. If women do not know their HIV status, they should be encouraged to get tested. Those

with positive test results should receive counselling and begin taking appropriate medications. Those without HIV need to be taught about the high-risk behaviours for HIV infection and how to protect themselves from contracting HIV infection.

Psychological Domain

Psychological Assessment

A mental status evaluation should be part of every health assessment. Symptoms such as anhedonia, difficulties concentrating, feelings of worthlessness or guilt, and thoughts of death or suicide suggest depression or PTSD. A thorough assessment of suicidal intent is crucial.

Nursing Diagnoses for the Psychological Domain

Selected nursing diagnoses focusing on the human responses that nurses manage in the psychological domain may include ineffective coping, hopelessness, chronic low self-esteem, anxiety, risk for self-directed violence, and risk for other-directed violence.

Interventions for the Psychological Domain

Assisting With Psychotherapy for Counselling

Psychotherapy may include individual, group, family, or marital therapy. Only psychiatric nurse specialists at the master's or doctoral levels who have had training in these therapeutic methods may conduct psychotherapy. In addition, the nurse therapist should have training in conducting therapy specifically with survivors of abuse. That training should include care of PTSD, DID, depression, and substance abuse. Evidence-based cognitive therapies for individuals with PTSD such as cognitive processing therapy assist the individual to reevaluate their appraisal of negative cognitions that relate to the trauma memory (Peri et al., 2015; Stirman et al., 2017). Exposure to the trauma memory is the basis for most evidence-based interventions for PTSD.

The ultimate goal is for the survivor to integrate the trauma in memory as a past event that no longer has the power to terrorize. Hipolito et al. (2014) explored the role of spirituality and personal empowerment for its protective function for PTSD in a sample of more than 300 men and women. Researchers looked at the relationship between childhood abuse and IPV. Interestingly, spirituality indirectly positively impacted health/well-being through its effect on individuals' sense of empowerment.

Family or marital therapy may be unwise unless the perpetrator of abuse has obtained therapy for himself or herself and demonstrated change. Otherwise, survivors are placed in a very difficult situation. If they disclose abuse in family or marital therapy, perpetrators may retaliate with violence, but if they do not disclose the abuse, the crucial issue will not be addressed (Landenburger, Campbell & Rodriguez, 2004). Antunes-Alves and Stefano (2014) argue that a couples therapy approach to IPV may be effective under specific circumstances, given that the contributing factors to IPV are not the same in all situations. Standard couples therapy for IPV is not recommended (Stith & McCollum, 2011).

Several issues in nursing practice must be addressed for all survivors (Ford-Gilboe, Vacoe, Wuest, & Merritt-Gray, 2011). All nurses can implement these interventions, using skills appropriate to their educational level and training. Nurses must address the guilt, shame, and stigmatization that survivors experience. They can approach these issues in several ways. Assisting survivors to verbalize their experience in an accepting, nonjudgemental atmosphere is the first step. Nurses must challenge directly attributions of self-blame for the abuse and feelings of being dirty and different. Helping survivors to identify their strengths and validating thoughts and feelings may help to increase self-esteem. An anonymous case report by a nursing student describes the importance of therapy for nurses who have a history of childhood sexual abuse in promoting their own healing journey and ultimately their capacity to help others (Anonymous, 1998).

Working With Children

Children may need to learn a "violence vocabulary" that allows them to talk about their abuse and assign responsibility for abusive behaviour. Children also need to learn that violence is not okay and it is not their fault.

Allowing children to discuss their abuse in the safety of a supportive, caring relationship may alleviate anxiety and fear (Berman et al., 2011).

A range of therapies, both individualized and group approaches can help children work through their anxieties and express their feelings. A range of interventions, primary, secondary, and tertiary, can promote safety at many levels (Berman, Hardesty, Lewis-O'Connor, & Humphreys, 2011). Other techniques used with children to reduce fear include reading stories about recovery from abusive experiences (literal or metaphoric), using art or music to express feelings, and psychodrama. In addition, teaching strategies to manage fear and anxiety, such as relaxation techniques, coping skills, and imagery, may give the child an added sense of mastering his or her fear (Barnett et al., 1997; Draughon & Urbancic, 2011). In a comprehensive review of child maltreatment literature, MacMillan (2000) indicates that research supports the use of abuse-specific cognitive–behavioural therapy as a treatment to improve the outcome for school-aged children. In a review of treatment approaches for children exposed to traumatic events, Silverman et al. (2008) found that cognitive–behavioural therapy–related interventions were promising in helping children and adolescents.

Managing Anger

Anger and rage are part of the healing process for survivors (Walker, 1994). Expression of intense anger may be uncomfortable for many nurses. However, they should expect anger expression and develop comfortable ways to respond. Moreover, an important nursing intervention is teaching and modelling anger expression appropriately. Inappropriate expressions of anger might drive supportive people away. Anger management techniques include appropriately recognizing and labelling anger and expressing it assertively rather than aggressively or passive aggressively. Assertive ways of expressing anger include owning the feeling by using "I feel" statements and avoiding blaming others. Teaching anger management and conflict resolution may be especially important for children who have seen nothing but violence to resolve problems (Lowenthal, 2001). Howell, Miller, Barnes, and Graham-Bermann (2015) in reporting on a case study exploring resilience in young children conclude that interventions for children should take into account developmental level and focus on a strengths-based approach to help children impacted by IPV.

Teaching Skills and Clarifying Identity

Other nursing interventions include teaching self-protection skills, healthy relationship skills, and healthy sexuality. Again, this teaching may be especially important for children who have no role models for healthy relationships. Children also need to know what constitutes controlling and abusive behaviour and how to get help for abuse.

Children who have been sexually abused may become confused about their sexuality. They may regard sex as dirty and as something that can be used against other people. Discussions about healthy sexuality and feelings about sex may help these children regain a healthy perspective on sex-related matters (Kelley, 2011).

Group therapy with survivors offers a powerful method to counter self-denigrating beliefs and to confront issues of secrecy and stigmatization (Urbancic, 2004). Moreover, one of the therapeutic factors in group therapy—universality or the discovery that others have had similar experiences—may be a tremendous relief, especially to child survivors. Intervention programmes for children exposed to IPV have been demonstrated to have a positive impact (Graham-Bermann, Miller-Graff, Howell, & Grogan-Taylor, 2015). A recent study evaluating an intervention for women and children to address the effects of exposure to IPV found that children aged 4 to 6 who participated in the intervention experienced less symptomatology compared with those in the wait-list comparison group (Graham-Bermann et al., 2015).

Providing Education

Education is a key nursing intervention for survivors. As appropriate to age or condition, survivors must understand the cycle of violence and the danger of homicide that increases as violence escalates or the survivor attempts to leave the relationship. Survivors also need information about resources, such as shelters for battered women, legal services, government benefits, and support networks (Registered Nurses' Association of Ontario, 2005; Walker, 1994). Before giving the survivor any written material, the nurse must discuss the possibility that if the perpetrator were to find the information in the survivor's possession, he or she might use it as an excuse for battering.

Survivors also need education appropriate for age and cognitive ability about the symptoms of anxiety, depression, dissociation, and PTSD. They must understand that these symptoms are common in anyone who has sustained significant stressors and are not signs of being "crazy" or weak. If survivors require medications for these symptoms, they must know how to monitor symptoms so that the effectiveness of pharmacologic management can be determined (see Box 34.6).

One of the most important teaching goals is to help survivors develop a safety plan (Ford-Gilboe et al., 2011). The first step in developing such a plan is helping the survivor recognize the signs of danger. Changes in tone of voice, drinking and drug use, and increased criticism may indicate that the perpetrator is losing control. Detecting early warning signs helps survivors to escape before battering begins (Campbell et al., 2004; Urbancic, 2004).

The next step is to devise an escape route (Ford-Gilboe et al., 2011; Walker, 1994). This involves mapping the house and identifying where the battering usually occurs

---

BOX 34.6

Psychoeducation Checklist: Abuse

When caring for the patient who has been abused, be sure to address the following topics in the teaching plan:

✓ Cycle of violence
✓ Access to shelters
✓ Legal services
✓ Government benefits
✓ Support network
✓ Symptoms of anxiety, dissociation, and PTSD
✓ Safety or escape plan
✓ Relaxation
✓ Adequate nutrition and exercise
✓ Sleep hygiene
✓ HIV testing/counselling

---

and what exits are available. The survivor needs to have a bag packed and hidden, but readily accessible, that has what is needed to get away. Important things to pack are clothes, a set of car and house keys, bank account numbers, birth certificate, insurance policies and numbers, marriage license, valuable jewellery, important telephone numbers, and money (Ford-Gilboe et al., 2011; Walker, 1994). The survivor must carefully hide the bag so that the perpetrator cannot find it and use it as an excuse for assault. If children are involved, the adult survivor should make arrangements to get them out safely. That might include arranging a signal to indicate when it is safe for them to leave the house and to meet at a prearranged place (Walker, 1994). A safety plan for a child or dependent elder might include safe places to hide and important telephone numbers, including 911 and those of the police and fire departments and other family members and friends. Riddell, Ford-Gilboe, and Leipert (2009) highlight the particular challenges and barriers faced by rural women in escaping IPV. The researchers found that women's unique understanding of the rural context and their personal situations reflected their resilience and had a significant impact on their ability to leave abusive relationships.

Finding Strength and Hope

Providing hope and a sense of control is important for survivors of trauma (Campbell et al., 2004). Nurses can help survivors find hope and view themselves as survivors by assisting them to identify specific strengths and aspects of their lives that are under their control. This type of intervention may empower women to find options to remain in an abusive relationship. The research by Ford-Gilboe and colleagues (2005) indicates that women were able to promote the health of their families after leaving an abusive partner, offering hope and a means of understanding for nurses working with women who are struggling to find the strength to choose health. In a study looking at the family health and well-being following separation from an abusive partner, Broughton and Ford-Gilboe (2017) found that social support positively influenced family health through access to information, tangible resources, and emotional support.

Using Behavioural Interventions

Treatment for depression, anxiety, and PTSD symptoms can be divided into two categories: exposure therapy and anxiety management training (Rothbaum & Foa, 2007). Only professionals trained in exposure therapy techniques can use them; however, nurses need to be familiar with this approach. The goal of exposure therapy, which includes flooding and systematic desensitization, is to promote the processing of the traumatic memory by exposing the survivor to the traumatic event through memories or some cue that reactivates trauma memories. Through repeated exposure, the event loses its ability to cause intense anxiety (Morrison, Berenz, & Coffey, 2014; Paunović, 2011).

Coping With Anxiety

Anxiety management is a crucial intervention for all survivors. There is a high comorbidity among trauma, PTSD, and anxiety disorders (Hahn, Aldarondo, Silverman, McCormick, & Koenen, 2015; Lagdon, Armour, Stringer, 2014; Orsillo et al., 2002). During treatment, survivors will experience situations and memories that provoke intense anxiety and must know how to soothe themselves when they experience painful feelings. Moreover, most survivors struggle with control issues, especially involving their bodies.

Anxiety management training may include progressive relaxation, deep breathing, imagery techniques, and cognitive restructuring. Progressive relaxation entails systematically tensing and then relaxing the major muscle groups. Visualization consists of imagining a scene that is especially relaxing (e.g., spending a day at the beach) while practicing relaxation and deep breathing. Any interventions that reduce dysphoric symptoms can help survivors feel more in control of their situation.

Anxiety disorders, PTSD, and depression, are associated with cognitive distortions that cognitive therapy techniques can challenge (Monson & Shnaider, 2014). Self-defeating thoughts in anxiety disorders involve perceptions of threat and danger, and those in depression involve negative self-perceptions (Blackburn & Davidson, 1990). Nurses can teach survivors how to identify and challenge these self-defeating thought patterns. Cognitive therapy techniques have been shown to be an effective intervention for women who have experienced IPV (Arroyo, Lundahl, Butters, Vanderloo, & Woord, 2017).

Nurses must become accustomed to measuring gains in small steps when working with survivors. Making any changes in significant relationships has serious consequences, and it can be done only when the adult survivor is ready. Carter-Snell and Hegadoren (2003) point out that women are frequently primary caregivers and,

as such, may have limited resources to devote to therapy. Therefore, the context of each individual woman's life needs to be kept in mind. It is easy for nurses to become angry or discouraged, and they must be careful not to communicate these feelings to survivors (Campbell et al., 2004; Urbancic, 2004). Discussing such feelings with other staff provides a way of dealing with them appropriately. In such discussions with supervisors or other staff members, the nurse must protect the patient's confidentiality by discussing feelings around issues, not particular patients. The nurse should frame the discussion in such a way that individual patients cannot be identified.

Social Domain

Social Assessment

An evaluation of social networks and daily activities may provide additional clues of psychological abuse and controlling behaviour (Broughton & Ford-Gilboe, 2017; Ford-Gilboe et al., 2009). When a nurse assesses social isolation, evaluating the reasons behind it is crucial. Many perpetrators isolate their family from all social contacts, including other relatives. Some survivors isolate themselves because they are ashamed of the abuse or fear nonsupportive responses. An evaluation of social support is important for other reasons. Having supportive family or friends is crucial in short-term planning for developing a safety plan and is also important to long-term recovery. A survivor cannot leave an abusive situation if she has nowhere to go. Supportive family and friends may be willing to provide shelter and safety.

Nurses can assess restrictions on freedom that may suggest abuse and control by asking such questions as "Are you free to go where you want?" "Is staying home your choice?" and "Is there anything that you would like to do that you cannot?"

The degree of dependency on the relationship is another important variable to assess. Women who have young children and are economically dependent on the perpetrator may feel that they cannot leave the abusive relationship. Those who are emotionally dependent on the perpetrator may experience an intense grief reaction that further complicates their leaving (Campbell et al., 2004). Elders and children are often dependent on the abuser and cannot leave the abusive situation without alternatives.

Nursing Diagnoses for the Social Domain

Selected nursing diagnoses focusing on the human responses that nurses manage in the social domain may include hopelessness, powerlessness, and ineffective role performance.

Interventions for the Social Domain

Working With Abusive Families

Family interventions in cases of child abuse focus on behavioural approaches to improve parenting skills (Kelley, 2011). A behavioural approach has multiple components. *Child management skills* help parents manage maladaptive behaviours and reward appropriate behaviours. *Parenting skills* teach parents normal growth and development and how to be more effective and nurturing with their children. Using strength-based approaches can help parents develop effective parenting strategies (Kelley, 2011).

Anger control and stress management skills are important parts of behavioural programmes for families. Anger control programmes teach parents to identify events that increase anger and stress and to replace anger-producing thoughts with more appropriate ones. Parents learn self-control skills to reduce the expression of uncontrolled anger. Parenting programmes that teach strategies based on behavioural and social learning theories have been shown to help parents develop skills in managing their children's disruptive behaviour (Andrade, Browne, & Naber, 2015). Stress reduction techniques include relaxation techniques and methods for coping with stressful interactions with their children (Lowenthal, 2001). These skills may be especially important in families in which elder abuse is occurring. Both caregivers and abused elders may need to learn assertive ways to express their anger and healthy ways to manage their stress. Helping caregivers find ways to get some relief from their caregiving burdens may be crucial in reducing abuse that comes from exhaustion in trying to manage multiple roles. Examples might be to identify agencies that offer respite care or agencies that offer day care for elders and support groups in which caregivers can share experiences and gain support from others dealing with similar issues.

Working in the Community

Nurses may be involved in interventions to reduce violence at the community level. Many abusive parents and battered women are socially isolated. Assistance in developing support networks may help reduce stress and, therefore, reduce abuse. The nurse has an important role in helping a woman access the formal and informal networks and services that may be required (Ford-Gilboe et al., 2011; Kelley, 2011).

Community health nurses (CHNs) may play a vital role in assessing for and preventing abuse as well as health-promoting initiatives that help end violence. Malone (2012) identifies a number of strategies for CHNs to implement such as assessing for safety of the person, understanding the importance of and learning how to ask about abuse, making appropriate referrals for abused individuals, and working collaboratively with others to develop broad-based preventive approaches to family violence. Specifically, nurses may make home visits to abusive parents or to families whose children are at risk. Such home visiting programmes for prevention and early identification are regarded as being effective (Flemington & Fraser, 2016), although MacMillan et al. (2009) caution that many home visiting programmes have not

demonstrated a reduction in physical abuse and neglect when assessed using randomized controlled trials. The researchers point to two programmes shown to prevent child maltreatment—the Nurse–Family Partnership and Early Start. On the other hand, Ford-Gilboe et al. (2017) report on an intervention they developed and are testing for Canadian women experiencing IPV referred to as iCAN Plan 4 Safety—referred to as iCAN. In the double-blind randomized controlled trial, 450 Canadian women who had experienced IPV participated in either an interactive online safety and health intervention or usual care. The intervention is designed to help women in the community increase their awareness of safety risks, reflect on their priorities, and create a plan of strategies and for their safety and health concerns. Study findings will contribute to knowledge about the effectiveness of online safety and health interventions for women in a range of circumstances.

Olds (2006) reports on a long-term study looking at the impact of nurses' home visits to low-income mothers and their infants to improve health and life outcomes for mother and child. Results demonstrated positive outcomes including fewer injuries associated with child neglect and better maternal life outcomes such as workforce participation and fewer subsequent pregnancies. However, abuse of any kind is a volatile situation, and nurses may place themselves or the survivor in danger if they make home visits. Nurses should carefully assess this possibility before proceeding. If necessary, the nurse and the adult survivor may need to arrange a safe place to meet.

Spiritual Domain

Although abuse and violence can devastate one's understanding of life and one's relationship with the sacred, spirituality can be a source of great strength. It can be a significant personal coping resource (Humphreys, 2000). Spirituality can serve as a coping mechanism and strengthen resilience in women experiencing IPV (Drumm et al., 2014). A spiritual response to violence and abuse begins with a sense of connection to a higher power (or with an attempt to connect) that allows a healing journey to begin (Knapik, Martsolf, & Draucker, 2008). Some individuals find that the struggle to recover and rebuild after abuse has made them stronger; it has helped them to grow spiritually, to have greater self-acceptance, and to express greater compassion towards others (Wright, Crawford, & Sebastian, 2007). For many individuals, however, abuse shatters any sense of a just, benevolent, and meaningful world. It becomes incredibly challenging for them to evolve a new sense of personal spirituality.

When abuse is perpetrated by a religious leader, it can be particularly devastating. The person is violated spiritually as well as physically (Guido, 2008). Women sexually abused by members of the clergy have described their survival as involving a reorientation away from structured traditional religious practice towards a form of spirituality that is more relationally grounded (Flynn, 2008).

Nurses and other health professionals have, in the past, tended to focus primarily on the biopsychosocial domains of patients who have been abused. It is important to understand how spirituality affects both the impact of abuse and the healing from it (Pargament, Murray-Swank, & Mahoney, 2008). Such understanding can inform discussions with patients about spirituality and can point to ways of support for patients who want to explore spirituality as a means of healing (Knapik et al., 2008). Nurses can offer patients an environment in which spiritual concerns can be expressed and compassionate responses expected (Humphreys, 2000).

EVALUATION AND TREATMENT OUTCOMES

Evaluation and outcome criteria depend on the setting for interventions. For instance, if the nurse encounters a survivor in the ED, successful outcomes might be that injuries are appropriately managed and the patient's immediate safety is ensured. For long-term care, outcome criteria and evaluation might centre on ending abusive relationships. Examples of other outcome criteria that would indicate successful nursing intervention are recognizing that one is not to blame for the violence, demonstrating knowledge of strengths and coping skills, and reestablishing social networks.

The evaluation of nursing care for abused children depends on attaining goals mutually set with the parents. An end to all violence is the optimal outcome criterion; however, attainment of smaller goals indicates progress towards that end. Outcomes such as increased problem-solving and communication skills within the family, increased self-esteem in both children and parents, and increased use of nonphysical forms of discipline may all indicate progress towards the total elimination of child abuse.

Follow-up efforts are important in evaluating the outcomes of elder abuse. The optimal outcome is to end all abuse and keep elderly persons in their own living environments, if appropriate. Although the abuse may have been resolved temporarily, it may flare up again. Ongoing support for the caregiver and assistance with caregiving tasks may be necessary if the elder person is to remain at home. Nursing home or assisted living may be the most desirable option if the burden is too great for the family and the likelihood of ongoing abuse or neglect is high.

Another important outcome of nursing intervention with survivors is appropriate treatment of any disorder resulting from abuse (e.g., ASD, PTSD and other anxiety disorders, DID, major depression, substance abuse). Follow-up nursing assessments should monitor symptom reduction or exacerbation, adherence to any medication regimen, and side effects of medication. The ultimate outcome is to end violence and enable the survivor to return to a more productive, safe, and nurturing life without being continually haunted by memories of the abuse.

Treatment for the Batterer

Participants in programmes that treat batterers are usually there because the court has mandated the treatment. Programmes are often outpatient groups that meet weekly for an extended period of time, often 36 to 48 weeks. Some advocate longer programmes, believing that chronic offenders require 1 to 5 years of treatment to change abusive behaviour.

Risk factors for IPV including psychological conditions in the perpetrator such as trauma, mood symptoms, and addiction should inform the treatment used rather than adopt a one-size-fits-all approach (Crane & Eason, 2017). Psychological conditions, such as personality disorders, trauma or mood symptoms, as well as addiction, have been established as risk factors for IPV perpetration and factor prominently into a recovery-oriented treatment approach.

Intervention programmes often use feminist-based interventions, cognitive–behavioural techniques, or a psychoeducational, skill-building approach (Crane & Easton, 2017; Glancy & Saini, 2005; Roy, Chateauvert, Drouin, & Richard, 2014). This approach offers batterers tools that help them see that their violent acts are not uncontrollable outbursts but rather foreseeable behaviour patterns that they can learn to interrupt. Cognitive–behavioural interventions target three elements: (1) what the batterer thinks about just before a battering incident, (2) the batterer's physical and emotional responses to these thoughts, and (3) what the batterer does that progresses to violence (e.g., yelling, throwing things). The group teaches members to recognize and interrupt negative feelings about their partners and to reduce physiologic arousal through relaxation techniques. Juodis, Starzomski, Porter, and Woodworth (2014) note that many intervention programmes incorporate safety planning for women and children.

Psychoeducational topics are often similar to those covered by the Duluth Curriculum, which is a commonly used programme that holds the perpetrator to account and promotes egalitarian behaviours; however, it is not a treatment (Crane & Easton, 2017). Topics may include nonviolence, nonthreatening behaviour; respect; support and trust; honesty and accountability; sexual respect; and partnership, negotiation, and fairness. Other programmes also offer more in-depth counselling, arguing that psychoeducational approaches do not address the true problem (Healey, Smith, and O'Sullivan 1998; Pender, 2012). If the problem were simply a deficit in skills, the batterer would be dysfunctional in work or relationships outside the family. Batterers need resocialization that convinces them that they do not have the right to abuse their partners. Other programmes add a moral aspect by taking a value-laden approach against violence and confronting batterers' behaviours as unacceptable and illegal.

Accountability for violent acts is an important early goal in treating batterers (Morrsion & Davenne, 2016). Most batterers deny responsibility for their actions and refuse to look at battering as a choice. Therefore, it is important that batterers become accountable for their actions. Interventions aimed at getting batterers to acknowledge their violence across the full range of abusive acts that they have committed, for example, verbal abuse, intimidation, controlling behaviour, and sexual abuse. Batterers may use several tactics to avoid accountability, and all must be addressed. Those tactics include denying the abuse ever happened ("I never touched her"), minimizing the abuse by downplaying the violent acts or underestimating its effects ("It was just a slap" or "she bruises easily"), and blaming the abuse on the victim ("she pushed me too far"), alcohol or other drugs ("I was high"), or other life circumstances ("I had too many pressures at work").

Because batterers typically minimize or deny their violent behaviour, it is often necessary to interview the survivor to gain a complete picture of the batterer's behaviour. A trained victim advocate usually contacts partners. There are other reasons for contacting partners. This may be the first contact the partner has had with professionals, and she may benefit by telling her story. Many partners do not know that services are available to them, and this is an opportunity to tell her what is available. In addition, advocates often explain the batterer programme and emphasize that it takes a long time and requires batterer's to take responsibility for their violent behaviour. Partners need to hear that many batterers are not willing to change their behaviour. Another important point that partners need to know and discuss with professionals is that batterers often use entry into treatment as a justification for pressuring partners to remain in the relationship and seems to be a good indicator that abuse will continue. It is also noteworthy that women's perceptions of their risk of assault appears to be fairly accurate in predicting repeated assaults and should be taken into account when assessing risk factors (Heckert & Gondolf, 2004).

Batterer intervention must be culturally competent (Healey et al., 1998; Saunders, 2008). Many factors can affect violence against women, including socioeconomic status, racial or ethnic identity, country of origin, and sexual orientation, and those differences must be addressed. Another factor that must be addressed is AOD use. Intervention programmes may require batterers to undergo substance abuse treatment concurrently, and batterers are required to remain sober and submit to random drug testing.

Treatment programmes alone are not sufficient to stop many batterers (Crane & Easton, 2017; Healey et al., 1998; Lawson, 2003; Moe, 2007). To be effective, programmes must operate within a comprehensive intervention effort that includes criminal justice support. The criminal justice response includes arrest, incarceration, adjudication, and probation supervision that includes issuing a warrant if the batterer does not attend the batterer programme or supervision. The combination of criminal justice response and batterer treatment may convey a more powerful message to the batterer about the seriousness of his actions than a batterer programme alone. Unfortunately, many offenders never show up for batterer intervention, and arrests for violation of probation may be rare because of overload and staffing shortages. Involvement of the criminal justice system is important in terms of fairness (Lawson, 2003). Inaction by the criminal justice system is serious; it sends the message that there is little concern for violence against women and that batterers can get away with it.

Anger management attributes battering to out-of-control anger and teaches anger management techniques. There are several arguments against this approach. It does not address the real issue—batterers' desire to control their partners. Batterers are able to control their behaviour in other difficult situations but choose anger and intimidation to control their partners. Anger management may merely teach batterers nonviolent methods to exert control. Couples counselling may endanger the survivor. Women will not be free to disclose, and any disclosures may give the batterer reason to retaliate. Self-help groups modelled on Alcoholics Anonymous are inappropriate for initial intervention for several reasons. Without trained facilitators who will confront denial and excuses, batterers may never accept accountability for their violence. On the other hand, an untrained facilitator may use an excessively confrontational approach that is abusive and models antagonistic behaviour.

How effective is batterer treatment? Results from an extended follow-up of court-ordered batterer intervention programmes show that many men continue to be assaultive during or on completion of treatment. Most batterer intervention programmes are regarded as being mixed in their effectiveness. Radatz and Wright (2016) cite Gondolf's review of more than 40 evaluations of programmes and found that almost 50% of batterers engaged in IPV after a 4-year follow-up period. Further, a qualitative study captured characteristics of the engagement process from the perspective of men who had been violent and who were participating in groups aimed on reducing the recidivism rate for IPV. Typically, dropout rates in such groups are considered to be high. Twenty-seven men were involved in semistructured interviews and a second sample of 13 men participated in a focus group (Roy, Chateauvert, Drouin, & Richard, 2014). Findings of the study showed that men perceived engagement to be a process that occurred over time. The dimensions of engagement were centred on individual change and included attendance, contributing, relating to workers, relating with members, contracting, working on own problems, and working on others. Men found the attitudes of facilitators in building a working alliance to be of value. The researchers point to the importance of supporting men's engagement. Engagement is seen as a multidimensional concept that supports men in taking a more active role in making changes in their lives.

 SUMMARY OF KEY POINTS

- The abuse of women, men, children, and elders is a national health problem that requires awareness and sensitivity from nurses.
- The abuse of women may be physical, emotional and psychological, or social.
- Child abuse may be neglectful, physical, sexual, or emotional. Other forms of child abuse include factitious disorder imposed on another and witnessing abuse of their mothers or significant caregivers.
- The abuse of Indigenous children in residential schools was particularly harmful because these children were segregated from their families and communities, frequently for years at a time.
- Elder abuse may be physical, emotional, neglectful, or financial.
- Among the many theories that have been proposed to explain abuse are psychopathology, social learning, sociologic, feminist, neurobiologic, BPD, and substance abuse.
- A well-documented cycle of violence consists of three phases of increasing frequency and severity.
- Child abuse leaves many scars that can lead to such problems in adulthood as depression, anxiety, self-destructive behaviour, poor self-esteem, and lack of trust.
- Responses to abuse include depression, ASD, PTSD, and DID.
- Nurses need to be familiar with the signs and symptoms of abuse and be vigilant when assessing patients.
- Nurses can help victims of abuse to view themselves as survivors.

Web Links

phac-aspc.gc.ca/ncfv-cnivf/familyviolence/refer_e.html The Public Health Agency of Canada, Health Promotion section, is a resource for information about family violence including the Family Violence Initiative, which brings together government departments and agencies to address family violence in Canada. This website includes links to resources and programmes in provincial and territorial jurisdictions.

http://www.justice.gc.ca/eng/cj-jp/fv-vf/index.html The website of the Department of Justice provides information on violence in Canada, including forms and types of violence, resources within each jurisdiction, and the Family Violence Initiative that informs the public and legal community about family violence and funds projects to support long-term programmes. The site also includes information for the public in a variety of languages, publications for professionals, relevant research, Canadian legislation, and information targeted to children 10 years and up.

cnpea.ca The website of the Canadian Network for the Prevention of Elder Abuse provides information about issues related to abuse and neglect in later life and the strategies being used to address them.

http://cbpp-pcpe.phac-aspc.gc.ca/public-health-topics/violence-prevention/ Canadian Best Practices Portal of the Public Health Agency of Canada is a repository of resources on violence prevention for different age cohorts and groups. Information includes statistical data, government strategies (e.g., frameworks and action plans), discussion/position papers (e.g., recommendations; screening tools; fact sheets), and systematic reviews of the research.

http://www.prevnet.ca/partners/organizations/prevention-of-violence-canada Prevention of Violence Canada, PREVNet, is a national network of researchers and more than 60 organizations serving children and youth whose mission is to stop bullying in Canada and promote safe and healthy relationships for children and youth. PREVNet was launched in 2006 with the National Centres of Excellence to support education, research, training, and policy change in bullying prevention. The website includes a number of reports, tools, research summaries, and resources.

http://www.canadianwomen.org/our-approach-to-violence The Canadian Women's Foundation provides a number of resources including fact sheets on their website addressing violence against women.

http://www.redcross.ca/how-we-help/violence--bullying-and-abuse-prevention/child-and-youth-serving-organizations The Canadian Red Cross website includes a section on violence, bullying, and abuse prevention with resources, online course, links to protective legislation, and information targeted to the workplace, Indigenous peoples, parents, youth, and organizations.

References

Abbey, A., Zawacki, T., Buck, P., Clinton, A., & McAuslan, P. (2003). Sexual assault and alcohol consumption. What do we know about their relationship and what types of research are needed? *Aggression and Violent Behavior, 277,* 1–33.

Adamec, R., Hebert, M., & Blundell, J. (2011). Long lasting effects of predator stress on pCREB expression in brain regions involved in fearful and anxious behavior. *Behavioural Brain Research, 221*(1), 118–133. doi:10.1016/j.bbr.2011.03.008

Afifi, T. O., Boman, J., Fleisher, W., & Sareen, J. (2009). The relationship between child abuse, parental divorce, and lifetime mental disorders and suicidality in a nationally representative adult sample. *Child Abuse and Neglect, 33*(3), 139–147. doi:10.1016/j.chiabu.2008.12.009

Afifi, T. O., MacMillan, H. L., Boyle, M., Taillieu, T., Cheung, K., & Sareen, J. (2014). Child abuse and mental disorders in Canada. *Canadian Medical Association Journal, 186*(9), E324–E332. doi:10.1503/cmaj.131792

Alhalal, E. A., Ford-Gilboe, M., Kerr, M., & Davies, L. (2012). Identifying factors that predict women's inability to maintain separation from an abusive partner. *Issues in Mental Health Nursing, 33*(12), 838–850. doi:10.3109/01612840.2012.714054

Allin, H., Wathen, C. N., & MacMillan, H. (2005). Treatment of child neglect: A systematic review. *Canadian Journal of Psychiatry, 50*(8), 497.

American Psychiatric Association. (2013). *Diagnostic and statistical manual of mental disorders* (5th ed.). Washington, DC: Author.

Anderson, D. K., & Saunders, D. G. (2003). Leaving an abusive partner: An empirical review of predictors, the process of leaving, and psychological well-being. *Trauma, Violence and Abuse, 4*(2), 163–191.

Andrade, B. F., Browne, D. T., & Naber, A. R. (2015). Parenting skills and parent readiness for treatment are associated with child disruptive behavior and parent participation in treatment. *Behavior Therapy, 46*(3), 365–378. doi:10.1016/j.beth.2015.01.004

Anonymous. (1998). Battling back from childhood sexual abuse and surviving the journey. *Journal of Psychosocial Nursing and Mental Health Services, 36*(12), 13–17.

Ansara, D. L., & Hindin, M. J. (2010). Formal and informal help-seeking associated with women's and men's experiences of intimate partner violence in Canada. *Social Science and Medicine, 70*(7), 1011–1018. doi:10.1016/j.socscimed.2009.12.009

Ansara, D. L., & Hindin, M. J. (2011). Psychosocial consequences of intimate partner violence for women and men in Canada. *Journal of Interpersonal Violence, 26*(8), 1628–1645. doi:10.1177/0886260510370600

Antunes-Alves, S., & Stefano, J. D. (2014). Intimate partner violence: Making the case for joint couple treatment. *The Family Journal, 22*(1), 62–68. doi:10.1177/1066480713505056

Arroyo, K., Lundahl, B., Butters, R., Vanderloo, M., & Wood, D. S. (2017). Short-term interventions for survivors of intimate partner violence: A systematic review and meta-analysis. *Trauma, Violence and Abuse, 18*(2), 155–171. doi:10.1177/1524838015602736

Bancroft, L., Silverman, J. G., & Ritchie, D. (2011). *The batterer as parent: Addressing the impact of domestic violence on family dynamics.* Los Angeles, CA: Sage Publications.

Bandelow, B., Baldwin, D., Abelli, M., Bolea-Alamanac, B., Bourin, M., Chamberlain, S. R., …. Riederer, P. (2017). Biological markers for anxiety disorders, OCD and PTSD: A consensus statement. part II: Neurochemistry, neurophysiology and neurocognition. *The World Journal of Biological Psychiatry, 18*(3), 162–214. doi:10.1080/15622975.2016.1190867

Banister, E. M., Jakubec, S. L., & Stein, J. A. (2003). "Like what am I supposed to do?" Adolescent girls' health concerns in their dating relationships. *Canadian Journal of Nursing Research, 35*(2), 16–33.

Barnett, O. W., Miller-Perrin, C. L., & Perrin, R. D. (1997). *Family violence across the lifespan: An introduction.* Thousand Oaks, CA: Sage.

Barrett, B. J., & Pierre, M. S. (2011). Variations in women's help seeking in response to intimate partner violence: Findings from a Canadian population-based study. *Violence Against Women, 17*(1), 47–70. doi:10.1177/1077801210394273

Bass, C., & Glaser, D. (2014). Early recognition and management of fabricated or induced illness in children. *Lancet, 383*(9926), 1412–1421. doi:10.1016/S0140-6736(13)62183-2

Beagan, B., Chapman, G. E., D'Sylva, A., & Bassett, B. R. (2008). It's just easier for me to do it': Rationalizing the family division of foodwork. *Sociology, 42*(4), 653–671.

Beck, J. G., McNiff, J., Clapp, J. D., Olsen, S. A., Avery, M. L., & Hagewood, J. H. (2011). Exploring negative emotion in women experiencing intimate partner violence: Shame, guilt, and PTSD. *Behavior Therapy, 42*(4), 740–750. doi:10.1016/j.beth.2011.04.001

Berman, H., Hardesty, J., Lewis-O'Connor, A., & Humphreys, J. C. (2011). Childhood exposure to intimate partner violence. In J. Humphreys & J. C. Campbell (Eds.), *Family violence and nursing practice* (pp. 279–318). New York, NY: Springer.

Beynon, C. E., Gutmanis, I. A., Tutty, L. M., Wathen, C. N., & MacMillan, H. L. (2012). Why physicians and nurses ask (or don't) about partner violence: A qualitative analysis. *BMC Public Health, 12*(1), 473.

Black, T., Trocmé, N., Fallon, B., & Maclaurin, B. (2008). The Canadian child welfare system response to exposure to domestic violence investigations. *Child Abuse and Neglect, 32*(3), 393–404.

Blackburn, I., & Davidson, K. (1990). *Cognitive therapy for depression and anxiety.* Boston, MA: Blackwell Scientific Publications.

Bombay, A., Matheson, K., & Anisman, H. (2011). The impact of stressors on second generation Indian residential school survivors. *Transcultural Psychiatry, 48*(4), 367–391. doi:10.1177/1363461511410240

Boughner, E., & Frewen, P. (2016). Gender differences in perceived causal relations between trauma-related symptoms and substance use disorders in online and outpatient samples. *Traumatology, 22*(4), 288–298. doi:10.1037/trm0000071

Boyce, J. (2016). *Victimization of Aboriginal people in Canada, 2014.* Canadian Centre for Justice Statistics. Catalogue no. 85-002-X. Ottawa, ON: Statistics Canada.

Breitenbecher, K. H. (2001). Sexual victimization among women: A review of the literature focusing on empirical investigations. *Aggression and Violent Behavior, 6*, 415–432.

Bremner, J. D. (2006). Traumatic stress: Effects on the brain. *Dialogues in Clinical Neuroscience, 8*(4), 445–461.

Brennan, S. (2012). *Victimization of older Canadians, 2009.* Juristat article, Catalogue no. 85-002-x. Ottawa, ON: Statistics Canada.

Breslau, N., & Anthony, J. C. (2007). Gender differences in the sensitivity to posttraumatic stress disorder: An epidemiological study of urban young adults. *Journal of Abnormal Psychology, 116*(3), 607–611.

Briere, J., Weathers, F. W., & Runtz, M. (2005). Is dissociation a multidimensional construct? Data from the multiscale dissociation inventory. *Journal of Traumatic Stress, 18*(3), 221–231.

Broughton, S., & Ford-Gilboe, M. (2017). Predicting family health and well-being after separation from an abusive partner: Role of coercive control, mother's depression and social support. *Journal of Clinical Nursing, 26*(15–16), 2468–2481. doi:10.1111/jocn.13458

Brownridge, D. A. (2006). Intergenerational transmission and dating violence victimization: Evidence from a sample of female university students in Manitoba. *Canadian Journal of Community Mental Health, 25*(1), 75–93.

Brownridge, D. A., Chan, K. L., Hiebert-Murphy, D., Ristock, J., Tiwari, A., Leung, W., … Santos, S. C. (2008). The elevated risk for non-lethal post-separation violence in Canada. *Journal of Interpersonal Violence, 23*(1), 117–135. doi:10.1177/0886260507307914

Brownridge, D. A., Taillieu, T., Afifi, T., Chan, K. L., Emery, C., Lavoie, J., & Elgar, F. (2016). Child maltreatment and intimate partner violence among Indigenous and non-Indigenous Canadians. *Journal of Family Violence, 32*(6), 607–619.

Brownridge, D. A., Taillieu, T. L., Tyler, K. A., Tiwari, A., Chan, K. L., & Santos, S. C. (2011). Pregnancy and intimate partner violence: Risk factors, severity, and health effects. *Violence Against Women, 17*(7), 858–881. doi:10.1177/1077801211412547

Bryant, R. A. (2007). Does dissociation further our understanding of PTSD? *Journal of Anxiety Disorders, 21*(2), 183–191.

Burczycka, M., & Cotter, A. (2011). *Shelters for abused women in Canada, 2010.* Juristat article, Catalogue no. 85-002-x. Ottawa, ON: Statistics Canada.

Campbell, J. C., McKenna, L. S., Torres, S., Sheridan, D., & Landenburger, K. (1993). Nursing care of abused women. In J. C. Campbell & J. C. Humphreys (Eds.), *Nursing care of survivors of family violence* (pp. 248–289). St. Louis, MO: Mosby.

Campbell, J. C., Torres, S., McKenna, L. S., Sheridan, D. J., & Landenburger, K. (2004). Nursing care of survivors of intimate partner violence. In J. C. Campbell & J. C. Humphreys (Eds.), *Family violence and nursing practice* (pp. 307–360). Philadelphia, PA: Lippincott Williams & Wilkins.

Campbell, J. C., Webster, D. W., & Glass, N. (2009). The danger assessment: Validation of a lethality risk assessment instrument for intimate partner femicide. *Journal of Interpersonal Violence, 24*(4), 653–674.

Canadian Centre for Justice Statistics. (2005). *Family violence in Canada: A statistical profile 2005.* Ottawa, ON: Statistics Canada.

Canadian Centre for Justice Statistics. (2011). *Family violence in Canada: A statistical profile.* Ottawa, ON: Statistics Canada.

Canadian Centre for Justice Statistics. (2013). *Measuring violence against women: Statistical trends.* Catalogue no. 85-002-X. Ottawa, ON: Statistics Canada.

Canadian Centre for Justice Statistics. (2016). *Family violence in Canada: A statistical profile, 2014.* Catalogue no. 85-002-X. Ottawa, ON: Statistics Canada.

Canadian Child Care Federation. (2012). *Respecting children's rights at home.* Ottawa, ON: Author.

Canadian Network for the Prevention of Elder Abuse. (2011). *Canadian laws on abuse and neglect.* Retrieved from www.cnpea.ca/canadian_laws_on_abuse_and_neglect.htm

Canadian Nurses Association. (1992). *Family violence clinical guidelines for nurses.* Ottawa, ON: National Clearing House on Family Violence.

Canadian Women's Foundation. (2013, November). *Fact sheet: Moving women out of violence.* Retrieved from www.canadianwomen.org/sites/canadianwomen.org/files/FACT%20SHEET%20-%20Stop%20the%20Violence%20-%20June%2019%202012.pdf

Carter-Snell, C., & Hegadoren, K. (2003). Stress disorders and gender: Implications for theory and research. *Canadian Journal of Nursing Research, 35*(2), 34–55.

Catallo, C., Jack, S. M., Ciliska, D., & MacMillan, H. L. (2013). Minimizing the risk of intrusion: A grounded theory of intimate partner violence disclosure in emergency departments. *Journal of Advanced Nursing, 69*(6), 1366–1376. doi:10.1111/j.1365-2648.2012.06128.x

Cedar Project Partnership, Pearce, M. E., Christian, W. M., Patterson, K., Norris, K., Moniruzzaman, A., … Spittal, P. M. (2008). The Cedar Project: Historical trauma, sexual abuse and HIV risk among young Aboriginal people who use injection and non-injection drugs in two Canadian cities. *Social Science and Medicine, 66*(11), 2185–2194.

Chamberland, C., Laporte, L., Lavergne, C., & Baraldi, R. (2003). *Psychological abuse: Children's invisible suffering (CECW Information Sheet #5E).* Retrieved from Canadian Child Welfare Research Portal, Université de Montréal: http://cwrp.ca/sites/default/files/publications/en/PsycAbuse5E.pdf

Chmielowska, M., & Fuhr, D. C. (2017). *Intimate partner violence and mental ill health among global populations of Indigenous women: A systematic review.* Heidelberg, Germany: Springer Science & Business Media.

Classen, C. C., Palesh, O. G., & Aggarwal, R. (2005). Sexual revictimization: A review of the empirical literature. *Trauma, Violence and Abuse, 6*(2), 103–129.

Clements, M., Oxtoby, C., & Ogle, R. L. (2008). Methodological issues in assessing psychological adjustment in child witnesses of intimate partner violence. *Trauma, Violence and Abuse, 9*(2), 114–127.

Cloitre, M., Scarvalone, P., & Difede, J. (1997). Posttraumatic stress disorder, self and interpersonal dysfunction among sexually retraumatized women. *Journal of Traumatic Stress, 10*(3), 437–452.

Collin-Vézina, D., & Hebert, M. (2005). Comparing dissociation and PTSD in sexually abused school-aged girls. *Journal of Nervous and Mental Disease, 193*(1), 47–52.

Collin-Vézina, D., Cyr, M., Pauzé, R., & McDuff, P. (2005). The role of depression and dissociation in the link between childhood sexual abuse and later parental practices. *Journal of Trauma and Dissociation, 6*, 71–97.

Comai, S., Tau, M., & Gobbi, G. (2012). The psychopharmacology of aggressive behavior: A translational approach: Part 1: Neurobiology. *Journal of Clinical Psychopharmacology, 32*(1), 83–94. doi:10.1097/JCP.0b013e31823f8770

Conroy, S., & Cotter, A. (2017). *Self-reported sexual assault in Canada, 2014.* Juristat article, Catalogue no. 85-002-X. Ottawa, ON: Statistics Canada.

Cook, R., & Dickens, B. (2009). Dilemmas in intimate partner violence. *International Journal of Gynecology and Obstetrics, 106*(1), 72–75.

Corvo, K., & Johnson, P. (2013). Sharpening Ockham's Razor: The role of psychopathology and neuropsychopathology in the perpetration of domestic violence. *Aggression and Violent Behavior, 18*(1), 175–182. doi:10.1016/j.avb.2012.11.017

Cotter, A., & Beaupré, P. (2014). *Police-reported sexual offences against children and youth in Canada, 2012.* Juristat article, Catalogue no. 85-002-X. Ottawa, ON: Statistics Canada.

Coulton, C. J., Crampton, D. S., Irwin, M., Spilsbury, J. C., & Korbin, J. E. (2007). How neighborhoods influence child maltreatment: A review of the literature and alternative pathways. *Child Abuse and Neglect, 31* (11–12), 1117–1142.

Courtois, C. A. (2008). Complex trauma, complex reactions: Assessment and treatment. *Psychological Trauma: Theory, Research, Practice and Policy, S*(1), 86–100.

Courtois, C. A., & Ford, J. D. (2014). Defining and understanding complex trauma and complex traumatic stress disorders. In Courtois C. A. & Ford, J. D.(Eds.), *Treating complex traumatic stress disorders: Scientific foundations and therapeutic models* (pp. 13–30). New York, NY: Guilford Publications

Crane, C. A., & Easton, C. J. (2017). Integrated treatment options for male perpetrators of intimate partner violence. *Drug and Alcohol Review, 36*(1), 24–33. doi:10.1111/dar.12496

Criminal Code of Canada. (1985). *Criminal Code of Canada, Part V, Section 155.* Retrieved from http://laws-lois.justice.gc.ca/PDF/C-46.pdf

Cross, D., Crow, T., Powers, A., & Bradley, B. (2015). Childhood trauma, PTSD, and problematic alcohol and substance use in low-income, African-American men and women. *Child Abuse and Neglect, 44*, 26–35. doi:10.1016/j.chiabu.2015.01.007

Cyr, K., Chamberland, C., Clement, M. E., Wemmers, J. A., Collin-Vézina, D., Lessard, G., … Damant, D. (2017). The impact of lifetime victimization and polyvictimization on adolescents in Québec: Mental health symptoms and gender differences. *Violence and Victims, 32*(1), 3–21. doi:10.1891/0886-6708

Daigneault, I., Hébert, M., & McDuff, P. (2009). Men's and women's childhood sexual abuse and victimization in adult partner relationships: A study of risk factors. *Child Abuse and Neglect, 33*(9), 638–647.

Damant, D., Lapierre, S., Kouraga, A., Fortin, A., Hamelin-Brabant, L., Lavergne, C., … Lessard, G. (2008). Taking child abuse and mothering into account: Intersectional feminism as an alternative for the study of domestic violence. *Affilia, 23*(2), 123–133.

Daniels, J. K., Frewen, P., Theberge, J., & Lanius, R. A. (2016). Structural brain aberrations associated with the dissociative subtype of post-traumatic stress disorder. *Acta Psychiatrica Scandinavica, 133*(3), 232–240. doi:10.1111/acps.12464

Daoud, N., O'Campo, P., Urquia, M. L., & Heaman, M. (2012). Neighbourhood context and abuse among immigrant and non-immigrant women in Canada: Findings from the maternity experiences survey. *International Journal of Public Health, 57*(4), 679–689. doi:10.1007/s00038-012-0367-8

DeKeseredy, W. S. (2007). Factoids that challenge efforts to curb violence against women. *Domestic Violence Report, 12*, 81–82.

DeKeseredy, W. S., & Dragiewicz, M. (2007). Understanding the complexities of feminist perspectives on woman abuse. *Violence Against Women, 13*(8), 874–884.

Department of Justice, Canada. (2003). *Stalking is a crime called criminal harassment.* Ottawa, ON: Government of Canada.

Department of Justice, Canada. (2012). *A handbook for police and Crown prosecutors on criminal harassment.* Ottawa, ON: Government of Canada.

Department of Justice, Canada. (2017). *Family violence initiative: Child abuse is wrong: What can I do?* Ottawa, ON: Government of Canada.

Devries, K. M., Child, J. C., Bacchus, L. J., Mak, J., Falder, G., Graham, K., … Heise, L. (2014). Intimate partner violence victimization and alcohol consumption in women: A systematic review and meta-analysis. *Addiction, 109*(3), 379–391. doi:10.1111/add.12393

Dillon, G., Hussain, R., Loxton, D., & Rahman, S. (2013). Mental and physical health and intimate partner violence against women: A review of the literature. *International Journal of Family Medicine, 2013*, 313909. doi:10.1155/2013/313909

Dragiewicz, M., & DeKeseredy, W. S. (2012). Claims about women's use of non-fatal force in intimate relationships: A contextual review of Canadian research. *Violence Against Women, 18*(9), 1008–1026. doi:10.1177/1077801212460754

Draughon, J. E., & Urbancic, J. C. (2011). Childhood sexual abuse. In J. Humphreys & J. C. Campbell (Eds.), *Family violence and nursing practice* (pp. 319–346). New York, NY: Springer.

Drolet, M., & Mumford, K. (2012). The gender pay gap for private-sector employees in Canada and Britain. *British Journal of Industrial Relations, 50*(3), 529–553. doi:10.1111/j.1467-8543.2011.00868.x

Drumm, R., Popescu, M., Cooper, L., Trecartin, S., Siefert, M., Foster, T., & Kilcher, C. (2014). "God just brought me through it": Spiritual coping strategies for resilience among intimate partner violence survivors. *Clinical Social Work Journal, 42*, 385–394.

Du Mont, J., Macdonald, S., Rotbard, N., Bainbridge, D., Asllani, E., Smith, N., & Cohen, M. M. (2010). Drug-facilitated sexual assault in Ontario, Canada: Toxicological and DNA findings. *Journal of Forensic and Legal Medicine, 17*(6), 333–338. doi:10.1016/j.jflm.2010.05.004

Dückers, M. L., & Olff, M. (2017). Does the vulnerability paradox in PTSD apply to women and men? An exploratory study. *Journal of Traumatic Stress, 30*(2), 200–204. doi:10.1002/jts.22173

Dufour, M. H., & Nadeau, L. (2001). Sexual abuse: A comparison between resilient victims and drug-addicted victims. *Violence and Victim, 16*(6), 655–672.

Dutton, D. G. (1995). *The domestic assault of women.* Vancouver, BC: UBC Press.

Dutton, D. G. (2007). *The abusive personality: Violence and control in intimate relationships* (2nd ed.). New York, NY: Guilford Press.

Dutton, D. G. (2008). My back pages: Reflections on thirty years of domestic violence research. *Trauma, Violence and Abuse, 9*(3), 131–143.

Dutton, D. G. (2011). *The domestic assault of women: Psychological and criminal justice perspectives.* Vancouver, BC: UBC Press.

Dutton, D. G., & Painter, S. (1993). Emotional attachments in abusive relationships: A test of traumatic bonding theory. *Violence and Victims, 8*(2), 105–120.

Dyer, K. F., Dorahy, M. J., Hamilton, G., Corry, M., Shannon, M., MacSherry, A., … McElhill, B. (2009). Anger, aggression, and self-harm in PTSD and complex PTSD. *Journal of Clinical Psychology, 65*(10), 1099–1114. doi:10.1002/jclp.20619

Elias, B., Mignone, J., Hall, M., Hong, S.P., Hart, L., & Sareen, J. (2012). Trauma and suicide behaviour histories among a Canadian Indigenous population: An empirical exploration of the potential role of Canada's residential school system. *Social Science and Medicine, 74*(10), 1560–1569. doi:10.1016/j.socscimed.2012.01.026

Ellis, W. E., Chung-Hall, J., & Dumas, T. M. (2013). The role of peer group aggression in predicting adolescent dating violence and relationship quality. *Journal of Youth and Adolescence, 42*(4), 487–499. doi:10.1007/s10964-012-9797-0

Etkin, A., & Wager, T. D. (2007). Functional neuroimaging of anxiety: A meta-analysis of emotional processing in PTSD, social anxiety disorder, and specific phobia. *American Journal of Psychiatry, 164*(10), 1476–1488.

Fallon, B., Van Wert, M., Trocmé, N., MacLaurin, B., Sinha, V., Lefebvre, R., … Goel, S. (2015). *Ontario incidence study of reported child abuse and neglect-2013 (OIS-2013).* Toronto, ON: Child Welfare Research Portal.

Filipas, H. H., & Ullman, S. E. (2006). Child sexual abuse, coping responses, posttraumatic stress disorder, and adult sexual revictimization. *Journal of Interpersonal Violence 21*(5), 652–672.

Fishwick, N. J., Campbell, J. C., & Taylor, J. Y. (2004). Theories of intimate partner violence. In J. C. Campbell & J. C. Humphreys (Eds.), *Family violence and nursing practice* (pp. 29–57). Philadelphia, PA: Lippincott Williams & Wilkins.

Flaherty, E. G., MacMillan, H. L., & Committee on Child Abuse and Neglect. (2013). Caregiver-fabricated illness in a child: A manifestation of child maltreatment. *Pediatrics, 132*(3), 590–597. doi:10.1097/JFN.0000000000000066

Flanagan, J. C., Korte, K. J., Killeen, T. K., & Back, S. E. (2016). Concurrent treatment of substance use and PTSD. *Current Psychiatry Reports, 18*(8), 1–9. doi:10.1007/s11920-016-0709-y

Flemington, T., & Fraser, J. A. (2016). Maternal involvement in a nurse home visiting programme to prevent child maltreatment. *Journal of Children's Services, 11*(2), 124–140. doi:10.1108/JCS-02-2015-0003

Flynn, K. (2008). In their own voices: Women who were sexually abused by members of the clergy. *Journal of Child Sexual Abuse, 17*(3–4), 216–237.

Ford-Gilboe, M., Varcoe, C., Scott-Storey, K., Wuest, J., Case, J., Currie, L. M., …. Wathen, C. N. (2017). A tailored online safety and health intervention for women experiencing intimate partner violence: The iCAN plan 4 safety randomized controlled trial protocol. *BMC Public Health, 17,* 273. doi:10.1186/s12889-017-4143-9

Ford-Gilboe, M., Varcoe, C., Wuest, J., & Merritt-Gray, M. (2011). Intimate partner violence and nursing practice. In J. Humphreys & J. C. Campbell (Eds.), *Family violence and nursing practice* (pp. 115–154). New York, NY: Springer.

Ford-Gilboe, M., Wuest, J., & Merritt-Gray, M. (2005). Strengthening the capacity to limit intrusion: Theorizing family health promotion in the aftermath of women abuse. *Qualitative Health Research, 15*(4), 477–501.

Ford-Gilboe, M., Wuest, J., Varcoe, C., Davies, L., Merritt-Gray, M., Campbell, J., & Wilk, P. (2009). Modelling the effects of intimate partner violence and access to resources on women's health in the early years after leaving an abusive partner. *Social Science and Medicine, 68*(6), 1021–1029. doi:10.1016/j.socscimed.2009.01.003

Friedman, M. J. (2001). Allostatic versus empirical perspective in pharmacotherapy for PTSD. In J. P. Wilson, M. J. Friedman, & J. Lindy (Eds.), *Treating psychological trauma and PTSD* (pp. 94–124). New York, NY: Guilford.

Fulmer, T., Sengstock, M. C., Blankenship, J., Caceres, B., Chandracomar, A., Ng, N., & Wopat, H. (2011). Elder mistreatment. In J. Humphreys & J. C. Campbell (Eds.), *Family violence and nursing practice* (pp. 347–366). New York, NY: Springer.

Gadalla, T. M. (2008). Gender differences in poverty rates after marital dissolution: A longitudinal study. *Journal of Divorce and Remarriage, 49*(3–4), 225–238.

Gallop, R., McCay, E., Austin, W., Bayer, M., & Peternelji-Taylor, C. (1998). Working with psychiatric clients who have been sexually abused. *Journal of the American Psychiatric Nursing Association, 4,* 9–17.

Gallop, R., McCay, E., Guha, M., & Khan, P. (1999). The experience of hospitalization and restraint of women who have a history of childhood sexual abuse. *Health Care Women International, 20*(4), 401–416.

Gamache, K., Pitman, R. K., & Nader, K. (2012). Preclinical evaluation of reconsolidation blockade by clonidine as a potential novel treatment for posttraumatic stress disorder. *Neuropsychopharmacology, 37*(13), 2789–2796. doi:10.1038/npp.2012.145

Gary, F. A., & Humphreys, J. C. (2004). Nursing care of abused children. In J. C. Campbell & J. C. Humphreys (Eds.), *Family violence and nursing practice* (pp. 252–287). Philadelphia, PA: Lippincott Williams & Wilkins.

Gilbert, R., Widom, C. S., Browne, K., Fergusson, D., Webb, E., & Janson, S. (2009). Burden and consequences of child maltreatment in high-income countries. *The Lancet, 373*(9657), 68–81.

Glancy, G., & Saini, M. A. (2005). An evidenced-based review of psychological treatments of anger and aggression. *Brief Treatment and Crisis Intervention, 5*(2), 229–248.

Gobinath, A. R., Mahmoud, R., & Galea, L. A. M. (2015). Influence of sex and stress exposure across the lifespan on endophenotypes of depression: Focus on behavior, glucocorticoids, and hippocampus. *Frontiers in Neuroscience, 8,* 420. doi:10.3389/fnins.2014.00420

Godoy-Ruiz, P., Toner, B., Mason, R., Vidal, C., & McKenzie, K. (2015). Intimate partner violence and depression among Latin American women in Toronto. *Journal of Immigrant and Minority Health, 17*(6), 1771–1780. doi:10.1007/s10903-014-0145-1

Gold, N., & Auslander, G. (1999). Gender issues in newspaper coverage of people with disabilities: A Canada-Israel comparison. *Women and Health, 29*(4), 75–96.

Graham-Bermann, S. A., Miller-Graff, L. E., Howell, K. H., & Grogan-Kaylor, A. (2015). An efficacy trial of an intervention program for children exposed to intimate partner violence. *Child Psychiatry and Human Development, 46*(6), 928–939. doi:10.1007/s10578-015-0532-4

Gueze, E., Westenberg, H. G. M., Jochims, A., de Kloet, C. S., Bohus, M., Vermetten, E., & Schmahl, C. (2007). Altered pain processing in veterans with posttraumatic stress disorder. *Archives of General Psychiatry, 64,* 76–85.

Guido, J. (2008). A unique betrayal: Clergy sexual abuse in the context of the Catholic religious tradition. *Journal of Child Sexual Abuse, 17*(3–4), 255–269.

Gutmanis, I., Beynon, C., Tutty, L., Wathen, C. N., & MacMillan, H. L. (2007). Factors influencing identification of and response to intimate partner violence: A survey of physicians and nurses. *BMC Public Health, 7*(1), 12.

Hahn, J. W., Aldarondo, E., Silverman, J. G., McCormick, M. C., & Koenen, K. C. (2015). Examining the association between posttraumatic stress disorder and intimate partner violence perpetration. *Journal of Family Violence, 30*(6), 743–752. doi:10.1007/s10896-015-9710-1

Harricharan, S., Rabellino, D., Frewen, P. A., Densmore, M., Théberge, J., McKinnon, M. C., … Lanius, R. A. (2016). fMRI functional connectivity of the periaqueductal gray in PTSD and its dissociative subtype. *Brain and Behavior, 6*(12), e00579. doi:10.1002/brb3.579

Hassouneh, D., & Curry, M. A. (2011). Nursing care of women with disabilities who experience abuse. In J. Humphreys & J. C. Campbell (Eds.), *Family violence and nursing practice* (pp. 181–206). New York, NY: Springer.

Hattendorf, J., & Tollerud, T. R. (1997). Domestic violence: Counseling strategies that minimize the impact of secondary victimization. *Perspectives in Psychiatric Care, 33*(1), 14–23.

Healey, K., Smith, C., & O'Sullivan, C. (1998). *Batterer intervention: Program approaches and criminal justice strategies.* Washington, DC: U.S. Department of Justice, National Institute of Justice.

Health Canada. (2002). *Woman abuse: Information from the National Clearing House on family violence.* Ottawa, ON: Author.

Health Canada. (2009). *Woman abuse: Overview paper.* Ottawa, ON: Author.

Heckert, A. D., & Gondolf, E. W. (2004). Battered women's perceptions of risk versus risk factors and instruments in predicting repeat reassault. *Journal of Interpersonal Violence, 19*(7), 778–800.

Hendy, H. M., Eggen, D., Gustitus, C., McLeod, K. C., & Ng, P. (2003). Decision to leave scale: Perceived reasons to stay in or leave violent relationships. *Psychology of Women Quarterly, 27*(2), 162–173.

Henney, J. E. (2000). Sertraline approved for posttraumatic stress disorder. *Journal of the American Medical Association, 283*(5), 596.

Herman, J. (1997). *Trauma and recovery: The aftermath of violence—From domestic abuse to political terror.* New York, NY: Basic Books.

Herman, J. L. (2015). *Trauma and recovery: The aftermath of violence—From domestic abuse to political terror* (pp. 1099–1114). UK: Hachette.

Hipolito, E., Samuels-Dennis, J. A., Shanmuganandapala, B., Maddoux, J., Paulson, R., Saugh, D., & Carnahan, B. (2014). Trauma-informed care: Accounting for the interconnected role of spirituality and empowerment in mental health promotion. *Journal of Spirituality in Mental Health, 16*(3), 193–217. doi:10.1080/19349637.2014.925368

Hoff, L. A. (2016). *Battered women as survivors.* New York, NY: Routledge.

Hollingsworth, E., & Ford-Gilboe, M. (2006). Registered nurses' self-efficacy for assessing and responding to woman abuse in emergency department settings. *Canadian Journal of Nursing Research, 38*(4), 54–77.

Holmes, E. A., Brown, R. J., Mansell, W., Fearon, R. P., Hunter, E. C. M., Frasquilho, F., … Oakley, D. A. (2005). Are there two qualitatively distinct forms of dissociation? A review and some clinical implications. *Clinical Psychology Review, 25*(1), 1–23.

Hopper, L. M., Spiteri, A., Lambeth, S. P., Schapiro, S. J., Horner, V., & Whiten, A. (2007). Experimental studies of traditions and underlying transmission processes in chimpanzees. *Animal Behavior, 73,* 1021–1032.

Hopton, J. L., & Huta, V. (2013). Evaluation of an intervention designed for men who were abused in childhood and are experiencing symptoms of posttraumatic stress disorder. *Psychology of Men and Masculinity, 14*(3), 300–313. doi:10.1037/a0029705

Hovsepian, S. L., Blais, M., Manseau, H., Otis, J., & Girard, M. (2010). Prior victimization and sexual and contraceptive self-efficacy among adolescent females under child protective services care. *Health Education and Behavior, 37*(1), 65–83. doi:10.1177/1090198108327730

Howell, K. H., Miller, L. E., Barnes, S. E., & Graham-Bermann, S. A. (2015). Promoting resilience in children exposed to intimate partner violence through a developmentally informed intervention: A case study. *Clinical Case Studies, 14*(1), 31–46. doi:10.1177/1534650114535841

Huband, N., & Tantam, D. (2000). Attitudes to self-injury within a group of mental health staff. *British Journal of Medical Psychology, 73,* 495–504.

Humphreys, J. (2000). Spirituality and distress in sheltered battered women. *Journal of Nursing Scholarship, 32*(3), 273–278.

Humphreys, J., & Campbell, J. C. (2011). *Family violence and nursing practice.* New York, NY: Springer.

Hunnicutt, G. (2009). Varieties of patriarchy and violence against women: Resurrecting "patriarchy" as a theoretical tool. *Violence Against Women, 15*(5), 553–573. doi:10.1177/1077801208331246

Jack, S. M., Ford-Gilboe, M., Davidov, D., MacMillan, H. L., O'Brien, R., Gasbarro, M., … the NFP IPV Research Team. (2016). Identification and assessment of intimate partner violence in nurse home visitation. *Journal of Clinical Nursing, 26*(15–16), 2215–2228. doi:10.1111/jocn.13392

Jackson, K. T., & Mantler, T. (2017). Examining the impact of posttraumatic stress disorder related to intimate partner violence on antenatal, intrapartum and postpartum women: A scoping review. *Journal of Family Violence, 32*(1), 25–38.

Jenney, A. (2009). Coercive control: How men entrap women in personal life by Evan Stark, Oxford University Press, NY (2007) 452p. *Children and Youth Services Review, 31*(1), 169–170. doi:10.1016/j

Johnsen, G. E., & Asbjørnsen, A. E. (2008). Consistent impaired verbal memory in PTSD: A meta-analysis. *Journal of Affective Disorders, 111*(1), 74–82. doi:10.1016/j.jad.2008.02.007

Jones, A., & Vetere, A. (2017). 'You just deal with it. You have to when you've got a child': A narrative analysis of mothers' accounts of how they coped, both during an abusive relationship and after leaving. *Clinical Child Psychology and Psychiatry, 22*(1), 74–89. doi:10.1177/1359104515624131

Juodis, M., Starzomski, A., Porter, S., & Woodworth, M. (2014). What can be done about high-risk perpetrators of domestic violence? *Journal of Family Violence, 29*(4), 381–390. doi:10.1007/s10896-014-9597-2

Karam, M. (2014). *Trafficking in persons in Canada, 2014.* Juristat article, Catalogue no. 85-002-X. Ottawa, ON: Statistics Canada.

Kaukinen, C. E., Meyer, S., & Akers, C. (2013). Status compatibility and help-seeking behaviors among female intimate partner violence victims. *Journal of Interpersonal Violence, 28*(3), 577–601. doi:10.1177/0886260512455516

Kaye, J., Winterdyk, J., & Quarterman, L. (2014). Beyond criminal justice: A case study of responding to human trafficking in Canada. *Canadian Journal of Criminology and Criminal Justice, 56*(1), 23–48. doi:10.3138/cjccj.2012.E33

Kelley, S. J. (2011). Theories and research on child maltreatment. In J. Humphreys & J. C. Campbell (Eds.), *Family violence and nursing practice* (pp. 91–114). New York, NY: Springer.

Kelly, S. J. (2011). Theories and research on child maltreatment. In J. Humphreys & J. C. Campbell (Eds.), *Family violence and nursing practice* (pp. 279–318). New York, NY: Springer.

Kelly, U. A., Gonzalez-Guarda, R. M., & Taylor, J. (2011). Theories of intimate partner violence. In J. Humphreys & J. C. Campbell (Eds.), *Family violence and nursing practice* (pp. 51–90). New York, NY: Springer.

Kennedy, M. C., McNeil, R., Milloy, M. J., Dong, H., Kerr, T., & Hayashi, K. (2017). Residential eviction and exposure to violence among people who inject drugs in Vancouver, Canada. *International Journal of Drug Policy, 41*, 59–64. doi:10.1016/j.drugpo.2016.12.2017

Kihlstrom, J. F. (2005). Dissociative disorders. *Annual Review of Clinical Psychology, 1*(1), 227–253.

Kilbourne, J. (1987). *Still killing us softly.* Cambridge, MA: Cambridge Documentary Films.

Kilbourne, J. (1999). *Can't buy my love: How advertising changes the way we think and feel.* New York, NY: Simon & Schuster.

Killick, C., & Taylor, B. J. (2009). Professional decision-making on elder abuse: Systematic narrative review. *Journal of Elder Abuse and Neglect, 21*(3), 211–238. doi:10.1080/08946560902997421

Knapik, G., Martsolf, D., & Draucker, C. (2008). Being delivered: Spirituality in survivors of sexual violence. *Issues in Mental Health Nursing, 29*, 335–350.

Korol, S. (2008). Familial and social support as protective factors against the development of dissociative identity disorder. *Journal of Trauma & Dissociation, 9*(2), 249–267.

Lachance-Grzela, M., & Bouchard, G. (2010). Why do women do the lion's share of housework? A decade of research. *Sex Roles, 63*(11–12), 767–780.

Lagdon, S., Armour, C., & Stringer, M. (2014). Adult experience of mental health outcomes as a result of intimate partner violence victimisation: A systematic review. *European Journal of Psychotraumatology, 5*(1). doi:10.3402/ejpt.v5.24794

Landenburger, K., Campbell, D. W., & Rodriguez, R. (2004). Nursing care of families using violence. In J. C. Campbell & J. C. Humphreys (Eds.), *Family violence and nursing practice* (pp. 220–251). Philadelphia, PA: Lippincott, Williams & Wilkins.

Lanius, R. A. (2015). Trauma-related dissociation and altered states of consciousness: A call for clinical, treatment, and neuroscience research. *European Journal of Psychotraumatology, 6*(1), 27905–27909. doi:10.3402/ejpt.v6.27905

Lanius, R. A., Frewen, P. A., Vermetten, E., & Yehuda, R. (2010). Fear conditioning and early life vulnerabilities: Two distinct pathways of emotional dysregulation and brain dysfunction in PTSD. *European Journal of Psychotraumatology, 1*, 1–10. doi:0.3402/ejpt.v1i0.5467

Lanius, R. A., Rabellino, D., Boyd, J. E., Harricharan, S., Frewen, P. A., & McKinnon, M. C. (2017). The innate alarm system in PTSD: Conscious and subconscious processing of threat. *Current Opinion in Psychology, 14*, 109–115. doi:10.1016/j.copsyc.2016.11.006

Laporte, L., Jiang, D., Pepler, D. J., & Chamberland, C. (2011). The relationship between adolescents' experience of family violence and dating violence. *Youth and Society, 43*(1), 3–27.

Lasiuk, G., & Hegadoren, K. (2006). Posttraumatic stress disorder. Part 1: Historical development of the concept. *Perspectives in Psychiatric Care, 42*(1), 13–20.

LaVoie, F., Herbert, M., Tremblay, R., Vitaro, F., Vezina, L., & McDuff, P. (2002). History of family dysfunction and perpetuation of dating violence by adolescent boys: A longitudinal study. *Journal of Adolescent Health, 30*, 375–383.

Law Commission of Canada. (2000). *Restoring dignity: Responding to child abuse in Canadian institutions.* Ottawa, ON: Minister of Public Works and Government Services.

Lawson, D. M. (2003). Incidence, explanations, and treatment of partner violence. *Journal of Counseling and Development, 81*(1), 19–32.

Lemieux, S. R., & Byers, E. S. (2008). The sexual well-being of women who have experienced child sexual abuse. *Psychology of Women Quarterly, 32*, 126–144.

Leschied, A. W., Chiodo, D., Whitehead, P. C., Hurley, D., & Marshall, L. (2003). The empirical basis of risk assessment in child welfare: The accuracy of risk assessment and clinical judgment. *Child Welfare, 82*(5), 527–540.

Letourneau, N., Morris, C. Y., Secco, L., Stewart, M., Hughes, J., & Critchley, K. (2013). Social support needs identified by mothers affected by intimate partner violence. *Journal of Interpersonal Violence, 28*(4), 2873–2893. doi: 10.1177/0886260513488685

Lissek, S., & van Meurs, B. (2015). Learning models of PTSD: Theoretical accounts and psychobiological evidence. *International Journal of Psychophysiology, 98*(3), 594–605. doi:10.1016/j.ijpsycho.2014.11.006

Long, A., & Smyth, A. (1998). The role of mental health nursing in the prevention of child sexual abuse and the therapeutic care of survivors. *Journal of Psychiatric and Mental Health Nursing, 5*, 129–136.

Lowenthal, B. (2001). Teaching resilience to maltreated children. *Reclaiming Children and Youth, 3*, 169–173.

Lucea, M. B., Glass, N., & Laughon, K. (2011). Theories of aggression and family violence. In J. Humphreys & J. C. Campbell (Eds.), *Family violence and nursing practice* (pp. 1–28). New York, NY: Springer.

MacDonald, C. J., Lepage, K. Q., Eden, U. T., & Eichenbaum, H. (2011). Hippocampal "time cells" bridge the gap in memory for discontiguous events. *Neuron, 71*(4), 737–749. doi:10.1016/j.neuron.2011.07.012

Machisa, M. T., Christofides, N., & Jewkes, R. (2017). Mental ill health in structural pathways to women's experiences of intimate partner violence. *PLoS One, 12*(4). doi:10.1371/journal.pone.0175240

MacIntosh, J., Wuest, J., Ford-Gilboe, M., & Varcoe, C. (2015). Cumulative effects of multiple forms of violence and abuse on women. *Violence and Victims, 30*(3), 502–521.

MacMillan, R. (2000). Adolescent victimization and income deficits in adulthood: Rethinking the costs of criminal violence from a life-course perspective. *Criminology, 38*, 553–588. doi:10.1111/j.1745-9125.2000.tb00899.x

MacMillan, H. L., Tanaka, M., Duku, E., Vaillancourt, T., & Boyle, M. H. (2013). Child physical and sexual abuse in a community sample of young adults: Results from the Ontario child health study. *Child Abuse and Neglect, 37*(1), 14–21. doi:10.1016/j.chiabu.2012.06.005

MacMillan, H. L., Wathen, C. N., Jamieson, E., Boyle, M. H., Shannon, H. S., Ford-Gilboe, M., … McNutt, L. A. (2009). Screening for intimate partner violence in health care settings: A randomized trial. *Journal of the American Medical Association, 302*, 493–501. doi:10.1001/jama.2009.1089

Malone, M. (2012). Violence in society. In L. Stamler & L. Yiu (Eds.), *Community health nursing.* Toronto, ON: Pearson.

Maniglio, R. (2009). The impact of child sexual abuse on health: A systematic review of reviews. *Clinical Psychology Review, 29*(7), 647–657.

Marshall, K. (2006). *Converging gender roles.* Catalogue no. 75-001-XPE. Ottawa, ON: Statistics Canada.

Mason, R., & O'Rinn, S.E. (2014). Co-occurring intimate partner violence, mental health, and substance use problems: A scoping review. *Global Health Action, 9*(1), 24815. doi:10.3402/gha.v7.24815

Mason, R., Wolf, M., O'Rinn, S., & Ene, G. (2017). Making connections across silos: Intimate partner violence, mental health, and substance use. *BMC Women's Health, 17*, 29. doi:10.1186/s12905-017-0372-4

McCann-Beranger, J. (2010). *Exploring the role of elder mediation in the prevention of elder abuse.* Department of Justice, Canada. Family, Children and Youth Section.

McClennan, S., Worster, A., & MacMillan, H. (2008). Caring for victims of intimate partner violence: A survey of Canadian emergency departments. *Canadian Journal of Emergency Medicine, 10*(4), 325.

McCue, M. L. (2008). *Domestic violence: A reference handbook.* Santa Barbara, CA: ABC-CLIO.

McGaugh, J. L. (2015). Consolidating memories. *Annual Review of Psychology, 66*, 1–24. doi:0.1146/annerev-psycho-014954

McLean, L. M., & Gallop, R. (2003). Implications of childhood sexual abuse for adult borderline personality disorder and complex posttraumatic stress disorder. *American Journal of Psychiatry, 160*(2), 369–371.

Messing, J. T., Mohr, R., & Durfee, A. (2015). Intimate partner violence and women's experiences of grief. *Child and Family Social Work, 20*(1), 30–39. doi:10.1111/cfs.12051

Messman-Moore, T. L., & Long, P. J. (2003). The role of childhood sexual abuse sequelae in the sexual revictimization of women: An empirical review and theoretical reformulation. *Clinical Psychology Review, 23,* 537–571.

Miller, G. E., Chen, E., & Zhou, E. S. (2007). If it goes up, must it come down? Chronic stress and the hypothalamic-pituitary-adrenocortical axis in humans. *Psychological Bulletin, 133*(1), 25–45.

Milligan, S. (2011). *Criminal harassment in Canada, 2009.* Juristat Bulletin Catalogue no. 85-005-x. Ottawa, ON: Statistics Canada.

Moe, M. A. (2007). Silenced voices and structured survival: Battered women's help-seeking. *Violence Against Women, 13,* 676–699.

Monroe, S. M., & Harkness, K. L. (2005). Life stress, the "kindling" hypothesis, and the recurrence of depression: Considerations from a life stress perspective. *Psychological Review, 112*(2), 417–445.

Monson, C. M., & Shnaider, P. (2014). *Treating PTSD with cognitive-behavioral therapies: Interventions that work.* Washington, DC: American Psychological Association.

Morrison, J. A., Berenz, E. C., & Coffey, S. F. (2014). Exposure-based, trauma-focused treatment for comorbid PTSD-SUD. In P. Ouimette & P. J. Brown (Eds.), *Trauma and substance abuse: Causes, consequences, and treatment of comorbid disorders* (2nd ed., pp. 253–280). Washington, DC: American Psychological Association.

Morrison, B., & Davenne, J. (2016). Family violence perpetrators: Existing evidence and new directions. *Practice: The New Zealand Corrections Journal, 4*(1).

Nemeroff, C. B., Bremner, J. D., Foa, E. B., Mayberg, H. S., North, C. S., & Stein, M. B. (2006). Posttraumatic stress disorder: A state-of-the-science review. *Journal of Psychiatric Research, 40*(1), 1–21.

Nolen-Hoeksema, S. (2002). Gender differences in depression. In I. H. Gotlib & C. L. Hammen (Eds.), *Handbook of depression* (pp. 492–509). New York, NY: Guilford.

Norris, D., Fancey, P., Power, E., & Ross, P. (2013). The critical-ecological framework: Advancing knowledge, practice, and policy on older adult abuse. *Journal of Elder Abuse and Neglect, 25*(1), 40–55. doi:10.1080/08946566.2012.712852

O'Campo, P., Burke, J., Peak, G. L., McDonnell, K. A., & Gielen, A. C. (2005). Uncovering neighbourhood influences on intimate partner violence using concept mapping. *Journal of Epidemiology and Community Health, 59*(7), 603–608.

O'Donnell, T., Hegadoren, K., & Coupland, N. (2004). Noradrenergic mechanisms in the pathophysiology of post-traumatic stress disorder. *Neuropsychobiology, 50*(4), 273–283.

Ogden, P., Minton, K., & Pain, C. (2006). *Trauma and the body: A sensorimotor approach to psychotherapy.* New York, NY: W.W. Norton & Company.

Ogrodnik, L. (2010). *Child and youth victims of police-reported violent crime, 2008.* Ottawa, ON, Canada: Statistics Canada

Olds, D. L. (2006). The nurse–family partnership: An evidence-based preventive intervention. *Infant Mental Health Journal, 27*(1), 5–25.

Orsillo, S. M., Raja, S., & Hammond, C. (2002). Gender issues in PTSD with comorbid mental health disorders. In R. Kimerling, P. Ouimette, & J. Wolfe (Eds.), *Gender and PTSD* (pp. 207–231). New York, NY: Guilford.

Ouimette, P., Moos, R. H., & Brown, P. J. (2003). Substance use disorder—Posttraumatic stress disorder comorbidity: A survey of treatments and proposed practice guidelines. In P. Ouimette & P. J. Brown (Eds.), *Trauma and substance abuse: Causes, consequences, and treatment of comorbid disorders* (pp. 91–110). Washington, DC: American Psychological Association.

Oxman-Martinez, J., Lacroix, M., & Hanley, J. (2005). *Victims of trafficking in persons: Perspectives from the Canadian community sector.* Department of Justice, Research and Statistics Division. Retrieved from http://canada.justice.gc.ca/eng/rp-pr/cj-jp/tp/rr06_3/rr06_3.pdf

Palermo Protocol. (2000). *UN protocol to prevent. Suppress and Punish Trafficking in Persons.*

Pargament, K., Murray-Swank, N., & Mahoney, A. (2008). Problem and solution: The spiritual dimension of clergy sexual abuse and its impact on survivors. *Journal of Child Sexual Abuse, 17*(3-4), 397–420. doi:10.1080/10538710802330187

Parker, B., Bullock, L., Bohn, D., & Curry, M. A. (2004). In J. C. Campbell & J. C. Humphreys (Eds.), *Family violence and nursing practice* (pp. 77–96). Philadelphia, PA: Lippincott Williams & Wilkins.

Paunović, N. (2011). Exposure inhibition therapy as a treatment for chronic posttraumatic stress disorder: A controlled pilot study. *Psychology, 2*(6), 605–614. doi:10.4236/psych.2011.26093

Pender, R. L. (2012). ASGW best practice guidelines: An evaluation of the Duluth model. *Journal for Specialists in Group Work, 37*(3), 218–231. doi: 10.1080/01933922.2011.632813

Peri, T., Gofman, M., Tal, S., & Tuval-Mashiach, R. (2015). Embodied simulation in exposure-based therapies for posttraumatic stress disorder–a possible integration of cognitive behavioral theories, neuroscience, and psychoanalysis. *European Journal of Psychotraumatology, 6.* doi:10.3402/ejpt.v6.29301

Perreault, S. (2015). *Criminal victimization in Canada, 2014.* Juristat article, Catalogue no. 85-002-X. Ottawa, ON: Statistics Canada.

Pico-Alfonso, M. A., Garcia-Linares, M. I., Celda-Navarro, N., Blasco-Ros, C., Echeburúúa, E., & Martinez, M. (2006). The impact of physical, psychological, and sexual intimate male partner violence on women's mental health: Depressive symptoms, posttraumatic stress disorder, state anxiety, and suicide. *Journal of Women Health, 15*(5), 599–611. doi:10.1089/jwh.2006.15.599

Plichta, S. B. (2007). Interactions between victims of intimate partner violence against women and the health care system: Policy and practice implications. *Trauma, Violence and Abuse, 8*(2), 226–239.

Public Health Agency of Canada. (2010). *Canadian Incidence Study of Reported Child Abuse and Neglect 2008: Major findings.* Ottawa, ON: Author.

Public Health Agency of Canada. (2012). *Summary: Estimates of HIV prevalence and incidence in Canada, 2011.* Ottawa, ON: Author.

Public Safety Canada. (2012). *National action plan to combat human trafficking.*

Putnam, F. W. (1994). Dissociative disorders in children and adolescents. In S. J. Lynn & J. W. Rhue (Eds.), *Dissociation: Clinical and theoretical perspectives* (pp. 175–189). New York, NY: Guilford.

Rabellino, D., Densmore, M., Frewen, P. A., Théberge, J., McKinnon, M. C., & Lanius, R. A. (2016). Aberrant functional connectivity of the amygdala complexes in PTSD during conscious and subconscious processing of trauma-related stimuli. *PLoS One, 11*(9), e0163097.

Radatz, D. L., & Wright, E. M. (2016). Integrating the principles of effective intervention into batterer intervention programming: The case for moving toward more evidence-based programming. *Trauma, Violence and Abuse, 17*(1), 72–87

Reeves, E. (2015). A synthesis of the literature on trauma-informed care. *Issues in Mental Health Nursing, 36*(9), 698–709

Registered Nurses' Association of Ontario. (2005). *Woman abuse: Screening, identification and initial response.* Toronto, ON: Author.

Resnick, H., Acierno, R., Holmes, M., Kilpatrick, D. G., & Jager, N. (1999). Prevention of post-rape psychopathology: Preliminary findings of a controlled acute rate treatment study. *Journal of Anxiety Disorders, 13*(4), 359–370.

Riddell, T., Ford-Gilboe, M., & Leipert, B. (2009). Strategies used by rural women to stop, avoid or escape from intimate partner violence. *Health Care for Women International, 30*(1), 134–159.

Robinson, L., & Spilsbury, K. (2008). Systematic review of the perceptions and experiences of accessing health services by adult victims of domestic violence. *Health and Social Care in the Community, 16*(1), 16–30.

Romans, S., Forte, T., Cohen, M. M., Du Mont, J., & Hyman, I. (2007). Who is most at risk for intimate partner violence?: A Canadian population-based study. *Journal of Interpersonal Violence, 22*(12), 1495–1514.

Ross, C. A. (2009). Errors of logic and scholarship concerning dissociative identity disorder. *Journal of Child Sexual Abuse, 18*(2), 221–231.

Ross, C. A. & Ness, L. (2010). Symptom patterns in dissociative identity disorder patients and the general population. *Journal of Trauma and Dissociation, 11*(4), 458–468. doi:10.1080/15299732.2010.495939

Rothbaum, B. O., & Foa, E. B. (2007). Cognitive-behavioral therapy for posttraumatic stress disorder. In B. A. van der Kolk, A. C. McFarlane, & L. Weisaeth (Eds.), *Traumatic stress: The effects of overwhelming experience on mind, body, and society* (pp. 491–509). New York, NY: Guilford.

Rothman, L. (2007). Oh Canada! Too many children in poverty for too long. *Paediatrics and Child Health, 12*(8), 661–665.

Roy, V., Chateauvert, J., Drouin, M., & Richard, M. (2014). Building men's engagement in intimate partner violence groups. *Partner Abuse, 5*(4), 420–438. doi:10.1891/1946-6560.5.4.420

Sanders, M. J., Wiltgen, B. J., & Fanselow, M. S. (2003). The place of the hippocampus in fear conditioning. *European Journal of Pharmacology, 463*(1), 217–223.

Sareen, J., Cox, B. J., Stein, M. B., Afifi, T. O., Fleet, C., & Asmundson, G. J. G. (2007). Physical and mental comorbidity, disability, and suicidal behavior associated with posttraumatic stress disorder in a large community sample. *Psychosomatic Medicine, 69*(3), 242–248.

Saunders, D. G. (2008). Group interventions for men who batter: A summary of program descriptions and research. *Violence and Victims, 23*(2), 156–172.

Schachter, C. L., Radomsky, N. A., Stalker, C. A., & Teram, E. (2004). Women survivors of child sexual abuse. How can health professionals promote healing? *Canadian Family Physician, 50,* 405–412.

Sears, H. A., Byers, E. S., Whelan, J. J., & Saint-Pierre, M. (2006). If it hurts you, then it is not a joke: Adolescents' ideas about girls' and boys' use and experience of abusive behavior in dating relationships. *Journal of Interpersonal Violence, 21*(9), 1191–1207.

Sears, H. A., Byers, E. S., & Price, L. (2007). The co-occurrence of adolescent boys' and girls' use of psychologically, physically, and sexually abusive behaviours in their dating relationships. *Journal of Adolescence, 30,* 487–504.

Selzer, M. L. (1971). The Michigan Alcoholism Screening Test: The quest for a new diagnostic instrument. *American Journal of Psychiatry, 127,* 89–94.

Shalev, A. Y. & Bremner, D. (2016). Posttraumatic stress disorder: From neurobiology to clinical presentation. In Bremner, J. D. (Ed.), *Posttraumatic stress disorder: From neurobiology to treatment* (pp. 3–26). Hoboken, NJ: John Wiley & Sons.

Sheehy, E. (2016). Defending battered women in the public sphere. *International Journal for Crime, Justice and Social Democracy, 5*(2), 81–95. doi:10.5204/ijcjsd.v512.309

Sheridan, D. (2004). Legal and forensic nursing responses to family violence. In J. C. Campbell & J. C. Humphreys (Eds.), *Family violence and nursing practice* (pp. 386–406). Philadelphia, PA: Lippincott Williams & Wilkins.

Shin, L. M., Rauch, S. L., & Pitman, R. K. (2006). Amygdala, medial prefrontal cortex, and hippocampal function in PTSD. *Annals of the New York Academy of Sciences, 1071*(1), 67–79.

Siemieniuk, R. A. C., Krentz, H. B., Gish, J. A., & Gill, M. J. (2010). Domestic violence screening: Prevalence and outcomes in a Canadian HIV population. *AIDS Patient Care and STDs, 24*(12), 763–770. doi:10.1089/apc.2010.0235

Silverman, W. K., Ortiz, C. D., Viswesvaran, C., Kolko, D. J., Putnam, F. W., & Amaya-Jackson, L. (2008). Evidence-based psychosocial treatments for children and adolescents exposed to traumatic events. *Journal of Clinical Child & Adolescent Psychiatry, 37,* 156–183.

Simmons, S. B., Knight, K. E., & Menard, S. (2015). Consequences of intimate partner violence on substance use and depression for women and men. *Journal of Family Violence, 30*(3), 351–361. doi:10.1007/s10896-015-9691-0

Singh, P., & Peng, P. (2010). Canada's bold experiment with pay equity. *Gender in Management: An International Journal, 25*(7), 570–585. doi:10.1108/17542411011081374

Sinha, M. (2012). *Family violence in Canada: A statistical profile, 2010.* Juristat article, Catalogue no. 85-002-x. Ottawa, ON: Statistics Canada.

Sinha, M. (2013). *Family violence in Canada: A statistical profile, 2011.* Juristat article, Catalogue no. 85-002-x. Ottawa, ON: Statistics Canada.

Skinner, H. A. (1982). The drug abuse screening test. *Addictive Behavior, 7,* 363–371.

Snow, M., Thurber, S., & Hodgson, J. M. (2002). An adolescent version of the Michigan alcoholism screening test. *Adolescence, 37*(148), 835.

Spence Laschinger, H. K., & Nosko, A. (2015). Exposure to workplace bullying and post-traumatic stress disorder symptomology: The role of protective psychological resources. *Journal of Nursing Management, 23*(2), 252–262. doi:10.1111/jonm.12122

Sprague, S., Madden, K., Simunovic, N., Godin, K., Pham, N. K., Bhandari, M., & Goslings, J. C. (2012). Barriers to screening for intimate partner violence. *Women and Health, 52*(6), 587–605. doi:10.1080/03630242.2012.690840

Sprague, S., Slobogean, G. P., Spurr, H., McKay, P., Scott, T., Arseneau, E., ... Swaminathan, A. (2016). A scoping review of intimate partner violence screening programs for health care professionals. *PLoS One, 11*(12), 1–17. doi:10.1371/journal.pone.0168502

St. Pierre, M. & Senn, C. Y. (2010). External barriers to help-seeking encountered by Canadian gay and lesbian victims of intimate partner abuse: An application of the barriers model. *Violence and Victims, 25*(4), 536–552. doi:10.1891/0886-6708.25.4.536

Stark, E. (2009). Rethinking coercive control. *Violence Against Women, 15*(12), 1509–1525.

Statistics Canada. (2015). "Canada's population estimates: Age and sex". *The Daily.* September 29. Statistics Canada Catalogue no. 11-001-X. Retrieved from http://www.statcan.gc.ca/daily-quotidien/150929/dq150929b-eng.pdf. Accessed August 10, 2017.

Statistics Canada. (2016). *Canadian demographics at a glance.* Catalogue no. 91-003-X. Ottawa, ON: Author.

Statistics Canada. (n.d.). Table 051-0001. *Population by sex and age group (table).* CANSIM (database). Last updated September 28, 2016. Retrieved from http://www.statcan.gc.ca/tables-tableaux/sum-som/l01/cst01/demo10a-eng.htm. Accessed August 18, 2017.

Stermac, L., Del Bove, G., & Addison, M. (2004). Stranger and acquaintance sexual assault of adult males. *Journal of Interpersonal Violence, 19*(8), 901–915.

Stewart, D., MacMillan, H., & Wathen, N. (2013). Intimate partner violence/La violence entre partenaires intimes. *Canadian Journal of Psychiatry, 58*(6), S1–S15, SS1–SS17.

Stirman, S. W., Finley, E. P., Shields, N., Cook, J., Haine-Schlagel, R., Burgess, J. F., ... Monson, C. (2017). Improving and sustaining delivery of CPT for PTSD in mental health systems: A cluster randomized trial. *Implementation Science, 12*(1), 32. doi:10.1186/s13012-017-0544-5

Stith, S. M., & McCollum, E. E. (2011). Conjoint treatment of couples who have experienced intimate partner violence. *Aggression and Violent Behavior, 16*(4), 312–318. doi:10.1016/j.avb.2011.04.012

Straus, M. A. (2004). Prevalence of violence against dating partners by male and female university students worldwide. *Violence Against Women, 10*(7), 790–811.

Sutherland, S. M., & Davidson, J. T. (1999). Pharmacological treatment of posttraumatic stress disorder. In P. A. Saigh & J. D. Bremner (Eds.), *Posttraumatic stress disorder: A comprehensive text* (pp. 327–353). Boston, MA: Allyn & Bacon.

Thomas, S. P., Bannister, S. C., & Hall, J. M. (2012). Anger in the trajectory of healing from childhood maltreatment. *Archives of Psychiatric Nursing, 26*(3), 169–180. doi:10.1016/j.apnu.2011.09.003

Thurston, W. E., Tutty, L. M., Eisener, A. C., Lalonde, L., Belenky, C., & Osborne, B. (2009). Implementation of universal screening for domestic violence in an urgent care community health center. *Health Promotion Practice, 10*(4), 517–526. doi:10.1177/1524839907307994

Truth and Reconciliation Commission of Canada. (2015). *Honouring the truth, reconciling for the future.* Winnipeg, MB: Truth and Reconciliation Commission of Canada.

United Nations. (1989). *Convention on the rights of the child.* Retrieved from http://www.ohchr.org/EN/ProfessionalInterest/Pages/CRC.aspx

United Nations Educational, Scientific and Cultural Organization (UNESCO). (2000). *Report of the Special Rapporteur on violence against women, its causes and consequences.* UNESCO.

Urbancic, J. C. (2004). Sexual abuse in families. In J. C. Campbell & J. C. Humphreys (Eds.), *Family violence and nursing practice* (pp. 186–219). Philadelphia, PA: Lippincott Williams & Wilkins.

van der Kolk, B. A. (2005). Developmental trauma disorder. *Psychiatric Annals, 35*(5), 401.

van der Kolk, B. A. (2006). Clinical implications of neuroscience research in PTSD. *Annals of the New York Academy of Sciences, 1071*(1), 277–293.

van der Wath, A., van Wyk, N., & Janse van Rensburg, E. (2013). Emergency nurses' experiences of caring for survivors of intimate partner violence. *Journal of Advanced Nursing, 69*(10), 2242–2252. doi:10.1111/jan.12099

van Elzakker, M. B., Dahlgren, M. K., Davis, F. C., Dubois, S., & Shin, L. M. (2014). From Pavlov to PTSD: The extinction of conditioned fear in rodents, humans, and anxiety disorders. *Neurobiology of Learning and Memory, 113,* 3–18. doi:10.1016/j.nim.2013.11.014

van Stegeren, A. H. (2008). The role of the noradrenergic system in emotional memory. *Acta Psychologica, 127*(3), 532–541.

Vanderburg, S., Wright, L., Boston, S., & Zimmerman, G. (2010). Maternal child home visiting program involves nursing practice for screening of woman abuse. *Public Health Nursing, 27*(4), 347–352.

Varcoe, C., Browne, A. J., Ford-Gilboe, M., Dion Stout, M., McKenzie, H., Price, R., ... Merritt-Gray, M. (2017). Reclaiming our spirits: Development and pilot testing of a health promotion intervention for Indigenous women who have experienced intimate partner violence. *Research in Nursing and Health, 40*(3), 237–254.

Varcoe, C., & Dick, S. (2008). The intersecting risks of violence and HIV for rural Aboriginal women in a neo-colonial Canadian context. *Journal of Aboriginal Health, 4* (1), 42–2.

Varcoe, C., Hankivsky, O., Ford-Gilboe, M., Wuest, J., Wilk, P., Hammerton, J., & Campbell, J. (2011). Attributing selected costs to intimate partner violence in a sample of women who have left abusive partners: A social determinants of health approach. *Canadian Public Policy/Analyse De Politiques, 37*(3), 359–380.

Vermetten, E., Schmahl, C., Lindner, S., Loewenstein, R. J., & Bremner, J. D. (2006). Hippocampal and amygdalar volumes in dissociative identity disorder. *American Journal of Psychiatry, 163*(4), 630–636.

Vézina, J., Hébert, M., Poulin, F., Lavoie, F., Vitaro, F., & Tremblay, R. E. (2011). Risky lifestyle as a mediator of the relationship between deviant peer affiliation and dating violence victimization among adolescent girls. *Journal of Youth and Adolescence, 40*(7), 814–824. doi:10.1007/s10964-010-9602-x

Walker, L. (1979). *The battered woman.* New York, NY: Harper & Row.

Walker, L. (1984). *The battered woman syndrome.* New York, NY: Springer Publishing Co.

Walker, L. (1994). The abused women: A survivor therapy approach [Film]. Available from Newbridge Communications, Inc., 333 East Street, New York, NY 10016.

Walton, G, Co, S. J., Milloy, M. -J., Qi, J., Kerr, T., & Wood, E. (2011). High prevalence of childhood emotional, physical and sexual trauma among a Canadian cohort of HIV-seropositive illicit drug users. *AIDS Care, 23*(6), 714–721. doi:10.1080/09540121.2010.525618

Wekerle, C., Leung, E., Wall, A. M., MacMillan, H., Boyle, M., Trocme, N., & Waechter, R. (2009). The contribution of childhood emotional abuse to teen dating violence among child protective services-involved youth. *Child Abuse and Neglect, 33*(1), 45–58. doi:10.1016/j.chiabu.2008.12.006

Wingo, A. P., Ressler, K. J., & Bradley, B. (2014). Resilience characteristics mitigate tendency for harmful alcohol and illicit drug use in adults with a history of childhood abuse: A cross-sectional study of 2024 inner-city men and women. *Journal of Psychiatric Research, 51,* 93–99. doi:10.1016/j.jpsychires.2014.01.007

Wolf, O. T. (2009). Stress and memory in humans: Twelve years of progress? *Brain Research, 1293,* 142–154.

Wolfe, D. A. (2006). Preventing violence in relationships: Psychological science addressing complex social issues. *Canadian Psychology, 47,* 44–50.

Wolfe, D. A., Crooks, C. V., Lee, V., McIntyre-Smith, A., & Jaffe, P. G. (2003). The effects of children's exposure to domestic violence: A meta-analysis and critique. *Clinical Child and Family Psychology Review, 6*(3), 171–187.

Wong, C. M. & Yehuda, R. (2002). Sex differences in posttraumatic stress disorder. In F. Lewis-Hall, T. S. Williams, J. A. Panetta, & J. M. Herrera (Eds.), *Psychiatric illnesses in women* (pp. 57–96). Washington, DC: American Psychiatric Press.

Woods, S. J., & Gill, J. (2011). Family violence: Long-term health consequences of trauma. In J. Humphreys & J. C. Campbell (Eds.), *Family violence and nursing practice* (pp. 29–50). New York, NY: Springer.

Wright, M. O., Crawford, E., & Sebastian, K. (2007). Positive resolution of childhood sexual abuse experiences: The role of coping, benefit-finding and meaning-making. *Journal of Family Violence, 22,* 597–608. doi:10.1007/s10896-007-9111-1

Wuest, J., & Merritt-Gray, M. (2001). While leaving abusive male partners, women engaged in a 4 stage process of reclaiming self. *Canadian Journal of Nursing Research, 32,* 79–94.

Wuest, J., Ford-Gilboe, M., Merritt-Gray, M., Varcoe, C., Lent, B., Wilk, P., & Campbell, J. (2009). Abuse-related injury and symptoms of posttraumatic stress disorder as mechanisms of chronic pain in survivors of intimate partner violence. *Pain Medicine, 10*(4), 739. doi:10.1111/j.1526-4637.2009.00624.x

Zahradnik, M., Stewart, S. H., O'Connor, R. M., Stevens, D., Ungar, M., & Wekerle, C. (2010). Resilience moderates the relationship between exposure to violence and posttraumatic reexperiencing in Mi'kmaq youth. *International Journal of Mental Health and Addiction, 8*(2), 408–420.

Zaky, E. A. (2015). Factitious disorder imposed on another (Munchausen syndrome by proxy), potentially lethal form of child abuse. *Journal of Child and Adolescent Behavior, 3,* e106. doi:10.4172/2375-4494.1000e106

Zaleski, K. L., Johnson, D. K., & Klein, J. T. (2016). Grounding Judith Herman's trauma theory within interpersonal neuroscience and evidence-based practice modalities for trauma treatment. *Smith College Studies in Social Work, 86*(4), 377–393. doi:10.1080/00377317.2016.1222110

35 Care of Persons Under Forensic Purview

Cindy Peternelj-Taylor

LEARNING OBJECTIVES

After studying this chapter, you will be able to:

- Describe the complexity of mental health challenges experienced by persons under forensic purview.
- Examine the issues that are critical to the development of therapeutic relationships in forensic settings.
- Consider the challenges and opportunities that exist for nursing given the diversity of settings in which forensic nurses practise.
- Analyze the issues inherent in professional role development for nurses practising in the forensic milieu.
- Evaluate the societal norms that affect contemporary care and treatment of persons under forensic purview.
- Discuss the strategies for ongoing education, research, and practice development in forensic nursing.

KEY TERMS

- boundary violations • compassionate release
- dynamic security • forensic nursing • static security

KEY CONCEPTS

- criminalization of persons with mental illness • custody and caring • manipulation • othering • recovery
- vulnerable

In Canada, as in many Western countries, large numbers of vulnerable and at-risk individuals find themselves seeking mental health care under the auspices of the criminal justice system. This chapter focuses on persons under forensic purview: those who have violated the law in some way, including those remanded in custody while awaiting trial (charged but not yet sentenced); those who have been remanded in a secure forensic facility for psychiatric evaluation and/or treatment; those who are found unfit to stand trial (UST) or not criminally responsible on account of a mental disorder (NCRMD); as well as those individuals who have been charged, sentenced by the courts to community supervision, or incarcerated in provincial, territorial, or federal correctional facilities. Nurses practising where the domains of criminal justice and health care intersect are typically referred to as *forensic* nurses, and their ability to provide competent and ethical care is often compromised by social and political animosity toward crime, criminality, and mental disorder.

Forensic nurses are responsible for providing mental health care and treatment to persons under forensic purview in a variety of secure institutional facilities, including forensic psychiatric units within general hospitals, forensic mental health (FMH) hospitals, jails, prisons, correctional facilities, and institutions for youth in custody. They are also involved in community-based court

diversion schemes and community treatment orders (CTOs), and they assist forensic clients with recovery and reintegration into the community. Practising "at the interface of justice and mental health where the patient population does not fit neatly into either department" (Martin et al., 2013, p. 172) can be particularly challenging for nurses. A variety of terms are used to refer to this evolving specialty area, including forensic psychiatric nursing, FMH nursing, community FMH nursing, and correctional or prison nursing. For simplicity, **forensic nursing** is used throughout this chapter and refers to nurses who integrate psychiatric and mental health nursing "philosophy and practice within a sociocultural context that includes the criminal justice system to provide comprehensive care to clients, families, and communities" (Peternelj-Taylor & Hufft, 2006, p. 379).

CRIMINALIZATION OF THE MENTALLY ILL

Throughout Canada, jails, prisons, and custodial facilities for persons in conflict with the law have become, by default, repositories for individuals with mental illness. In the past decade alone, the number of individuals with significant mental health needs within the federal correctional system in Canada has more than doubled. When compared with the general Canadian population, mental health problems are up to three times more common among federal correctional populations. Mental health services within correctional facilities have not kept up with this dramatic increase, and in many facilities, treatment is often nonexistent or unsatisfactory when compared with the community standard (Dupuis, MacKay, & Nicol, 2013; Office of the Correctional Investigator [OCI], 2015). Unfortunately, for many individuals experiencing mental health problems and/or illness, correctional facilities have become "de facto psychiatric institutions" with "access to psychiatric care only [occurring] after they have been criminalized" (Chaimowitz, 2012, p. 5). The criminalization of persons with mental illness has frequently been attributed to the deinstitutionalization movement that occurred in the 1960s and the 1970s. Unfortunately, the ongoing failure of provincial, territorial, and federal governments to provide sufficient mental health funding to fully realize the goals of deinstitutionalization (e.g., independent living within the community) has resulted in a fragmented mental health system with woefully inadequate community-based services (Chaimowitz, 2012; Ormston, 2010). Individuals who experience chronic mental illness are often well known by the police, the courts, mental health services, emergency departments, jails, and correctional facilities. Critics conclude that for many individuals caught up in this web, their only crime is that they are "guilty of mental illness" (Kanapaux, 2004).

As outlined in the *Mental Health Strategy for Canada*, the overrepresentation of people with mental health problems and illnesses in the criminal justice system (whether on remand, in correctional custody, or in a forensic facility) needs to be reduced (Mental Health Commission of Canada [MHCC], 2012). Furthermore, those who are in the system need to be able to access appropriate services, treatments, and supports that are "consistent with professionally accepted standards" (MHCC, 2012, p. 47). In collaboration with the MHCC, a Correctional Service Canada Federal–Provincial/Territorial partnership developed the *Mental Health Strategy for Corrections in Canada* (Correctional Service Canada [CSC] Federal–Provincial/Territorial Partnership, 2012) to meet the needs of youth and adults with mental health problems and illnesses enmeshed with the criminal justice system. Seven key components of this strategy are highlighted in Box 35.1. Forensic nurses are critical to the adoption, implementation, and evaluation of this strategy.

KEY CONCEPT

Mental health care resource shortages and a fragmented mental health system have led to correctional facilities becoming psychiatric institutions by default. **Criminalization of persons with mental illness** occurs when persons with an untreated mental illness contravene the law and enter the justice system rather than the health care system.

BOX 35.1	Mental Health Strategy for Corrections in Canada: Key Elements

1. Mental Health Promotion
2. Screening and Assessment
3. Treatment, Services, and Supports
4. Suicide and Self-Injury Prevention and Management
5. Transitional Services and Supports
6. Staff Education, Training, and Support
7. Community Supports and Partnerships

From Correctional Service Canada, Federal–Provincial/Territorial Partnership. (2012). *Mental health strategy for corrections in Canada*. Retrieved from http://www.csc-scc.gc.ca/health/092/MH-strategy-eng.pdf

THE PARADOX OF CUSTODY AND CARING

Forensic settings are controversial. They arouse strong convictions from various sectors who debate their proper place in society. Nursing practice within this domain is particularly complex because it brings together the "coupling of two contradictory socioprofessional mandates: to punish and to provide care" (Holmes, 2005, p. 3). This paradox is disconcerting because a clear distinction between these two mandates is not always easily demarcated. Forensic settings provide society with two fundamental services: social necessities and social goods. Social necessities are considered essential to a community's existence; conversely, social goods are perceived as kindnesses, and although not necessarily essential, they are of benefit to the community nonetheless. Forensic settings meet their social necessity mandate through social control of those in their care. The protection of the community at large is perceived as a direct consequence of the processes of confinement and control. Forensic settings also provide social goods in the form of health care to those who are confined. In essence, forensic nurses are charged with the predicament of providing social good (e.g., health care) within institutions dedicated to the provision of social necessities (e.g., confinement) (Peternelj-Taylor, 2004; Peternelj-Taylor & Johnson, 1995).

This coexistence of social control and nursing care creates a paradox for nurses (Holmes, 2005, 2007), one that is laden with clinical issues and moral dilemmas not commonly encountered in more traditional health care settings. This paradox requires special attention and discernment because it permeates every aspect of forensic nursing. It is likely the single factor that differentiates forensic nursing from mental health nursing in a more general sense (Peternelj-Taylor, 2000). It is within this paradox, where the competing demands for custody and caring are embraced, that the moral climate of forensic institutions is shaped (Austin, 2001) (Fig. 35.1).

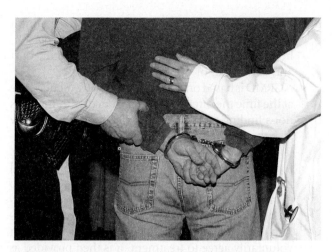

Figure 35.1. Custody and caring. (Courtesy of the Division of Media and Technology, University of Saskatchewan.)

KEY CONCEPT

Nurses in forensic settings must meet the competing demands of **custody** (confinement and security) **and caring** (nursing care).

FORENSIC NURSING: A MODEL FOR CARE

Nurses working with clients under forensic purview will find a familiar psychiatric and mental health nursing role, one that is "like 'stepping through the looking glass'—everything is the same, yet different" (Smith, 2005, p. 54). To illustrate the uniqueness of caring for this population, a model of care is presented. It highlights the contextual and clinical practice issues affecting the articulation of a professional nursing role with persons under forensic purview, regardless of setting. The five components of this model are the forensic client, nurse–client relationship, professional role development, treatment setting, and societal norms. Although each component of the model is discussed separately, in reality the components are dynamic and interactive in nature. Peternelj-Taylor and Hufft (2006) conclude that health care goals must be consistent with the reality of the client's life circumstances, as well as with the realities and the limitations of the setting in which nursing practice takes place. It may well be that not all forensic nurses will engage fully with each component of the model of care presented. However, the model as presented herein reflects the nature and scope of contemporary forensic nursing in Canada (Fig. 35.2).

Determinants of Health and the Forensic Client

As a group, persons under forensic purview present with a multitude of long-neglected physical and mental health care challenges, often complicated by

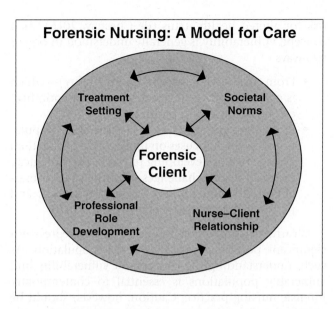

Figure 35.2. Forensic nursing: a model for care. (From Peternelj-Taylor, C. (2004). *NURS 486—Forensic nursing in secure environments [Course material]*. Saskatoon, SK: College of Nursing, University of Saskatchewan.)

significant substance abuse problems. The health and psychosocial issues that they experience are often complex and multifaceted, contributing to the challenges encountered in their attempts to engage in treatment, relapse prevention, recovery, and reintegration. Frequently, their lives have been marked by illiteracy, poverty, and homelessness. Cultural and ethnic minorities, in particular, are overrepresented in correctional institutions (Kouyoumdjian, Schuler, Matheson, & Hwang, 2016; OCI, 2015, 2016). Morbidity and mortality data suggest that those who are incarcerated experience higher rates of disease and disability when compared with nonincarcerated populations, which highlights the need for nursing leadership in primary, secondary, and tertiary levels of intervention. Persons under forensic purview frequently experience discrimination, stigmatization, and marginalization, and they often lack supportive relationships commonly associated with emotional and mental well-being (MHCC, 2012). Moreover, they are totally dependent on the system (whether it is the correctional system or the health care system) to meet their health care needs. Given the magnitude of these commingling issues, many forensic clients are at risk for dual, multiple, and overlapping sources of vulnerability. Yet, referring to those who have committed crimes against society as "vulnerable" seems somewhat contrary to conventional wisdom (Peternelj-Taylor, 2005).

Vulnerability and Vulnerable Populations

Broadly defined, vulnerability refers to a multifaceted concept that represents the commingling of resources, risk factors, and health status among a particular population or aggregate of people, which places them at risk for altered health status (de Chesnay, 2016). As a concept, vulnerability is generally understood in one of two ways:

- From an individual focus (vulnerability)—which is concerned with such notions as "susceptibility" or "at risk for health problems"
- From an aggregate view (vulnerable populations)—which focuses on those with a greater than average risk of developing physical, psychological, or social health challenges by virtue of their marginalized status, limited access to resources, and personal characteristics (de Chesnay, 2016)

Clearly, persons under forensic purview represent a significant portion of society's at-risk population. As such, understanding the concepts of vulnerability and vulnerable populations is essential to contemporary forensic nursing practice. Caution, however, should be exercised, as labelling someone as being a member of a vulnerable population can be perceived as patronizing by those receiving care, thereby further marginalizing those at risk. Nurses are positioned at the interface of vulnerability and as such are challenged to engage in partnerships that encourage growth in their clients. Students and nurses alike can best work with vulnerable populations within FMH settings by learning how to actualize respect, significant to the development and maintenance of therapeutic relationships, even with unlikable clients (Rose, Peter, Gallop, Angus, & Liaschenko, 2011).

KEY CONCEPT

Persons or populations are considered **vulnerable** when attributes, factors, or assigned status places them at greater risk for injury or poor health when compared with others.

Clients Experiencing Mental Illness

There is a great variation in the nature and severity of mental illnesses experienced by individuals who come into conflict with the law. In 1992, the Corrections and Conditional Release Act (Bill C-30) was proclaimed. This ended the Lieutenant Governor's Warrant system, whereby clients who were found "not guilty by reason of insanity" were held at the pleasure of the Lieutenant Governor for an unspecified period of time. It created review boards that are mandated to oversee the care and disposition of persons found UST or NCRMD (Statistics Canada, 2009). Under current Canadian law, an individual who comes into conflict with the law and is mentally ill can be found as follows:

- UST, when it is recognized that the accused is not fully capable of instructing legal counsel or not capable of understanding the nature and the consequences of a trial. In such situations, the judge

has one of two choices: disposition for detention in hospital or a conditional discharge (the person, however, can later be found "fit" and tried in court and convicted, or deemed NCRMD).
- NCRMD is based on the accused person's mental state at the time the offence was committed. Although it is not a finding of guilt, the court or review board may give the following dispositions: detention in hospital, conditional discharge, or an absolute discharge. Individuals detained in a hospital are not required to submit to treatment; the disposition is meant to detain the person and make care available. If treatment is required, owing to the individual's deteriorating mental status, and the individual does not voluntarily agree to treatment, it is then provided as per provincial or territorial mental health acts.
- In some jurisdictions, instead of going to trial, CTOs and court diversion schemes are options that may be exercised through community or provincial mechanisms (Dupuis et al., 2013; Miladinovic & Lukassen, 2014; Statistics Canada, 2009).

In all cases, the mentally disordered offender challenges the collective wisdom of both the health care system and the criminal justice system, creating a "crossover" of sorts, particularly when the individual has been found responsible for his or her crimes despite the mental illness. The incarceration experience represents a significant stressful life event, even for those who do not have a mental disorder; separation from family and friends, limitations on privacy, overcrowding, and fear of assault severely affect the individual's quality of life. For those with mental illness, prisons are dangerous places; they are often victimized by other offenders; they are at greater risk for engaging in self-harming behaviour and attempting suicide; and they are often confined to segregation for their own protection. Unfortunately, such experiences can completely overwhelm the resources of individuals with mental illness. When compared with individuals in the community, offenders experience greater rates of schizophrenia, depression, bipolar disorder, anxiety disorders, and substance abuse disorders (Dupuis et al., 2013; Kouyoumdjian et al., 2016). In a recent study on prevalence of mental disorders among incoming male federal offenders, Beaudette, Power, and Stewart (2015) found that 70% of male offenders met the diagnostic criteria for at least one mental disorder. Refer further to Box 35.2.

Suicide is the leading cause of death for persons under forensic purview, particularly those remanded or sentenced to a prison or correctional facility. A narrative review of related research studies has found that more than one in five persons in Canadian correctional facilities have attempted suicide (Kouyoumdjian et al., 2016). Withdrawal from drugs or alcohol and the reality of incarceration or commitment to an FMH facility, coupled with comorbid mental disorders, may exacerbate a client's risk for suicide and thus warrants ongoing

BOX 35.2 Prevalence of Mental Health Disorders Among Male Federal Offenders at Intake

Mental Health Disorder	Prevalence Rate %
Alcohol or Substance Use Disorders	49.6%
Antisocial Personality Disorder	44.1%
Anxiety Disorders	29.5%
Mood Disorders	16.9%
Borderline Personality Disorder	15.9%
Pathologic Gambling	5.9%
Primary Psychotic	3.3%

Source: Beaudette, J. N., Power, J., & Stewart, L. A. (2015). *National prevalence of mental disorders among federally-sentenced men offenders (Research Report, R-357)*. Ottawa, ON: Correctional Service Canada.

assessment, intervention, and evaluation by forensic nurses. Recognizing factors that may contribute to a client's vulnerability is critical. High-risk periods are considered those immediately following hospitalization, incarceration, release, or upon the receipt of bad news (Enggist, Møller, Galea, & Udesen, 2014; Olson, 2012).

Recovery

Recovery is a major tenet of the MHCC's (2012) *Mental Health Strategy for Canada*, one that can be particularly challenging for persons under forensic purview, especially

following a serious offence. Moreover, while detention, hospitalization, and/or incarceration are opportunities for recovery, the person has to be an active participant in the recovery journey, which can be especially trying when the person is not voluntarily seeking treatment (Drennan & Alred, 2012; McLoughlin, Geller, & Tolan, 2011). For persons under forensic purview, recovery is multifaceted and includes clinical recovery (symptom relief), functional recovery (life skills), social recovery (social inclusion), personal recovery (satisfying life living with illness), and offender recovery (redefinition of self). Of these, coming to terms with the offence clearly requires the active participation of the person (Drennan & Alred, 2012). Hope, empowerment, self-determination, and responsibility are considered the key principles of recovery (MHCC, 2012). In 2015, the MHCC released comprehensive guidelines for recovery-oriented practice; unfortunately, specific directions regarding how to adapt these guidelines to forensic or compulsory settings are not addressed. Forensic nurses can, however, foster recovery in a number of ways: through supporting hope, engaging in respectful dialogue, strengthening the working alliance, attending to personal strengths, bridging security and therapy, and supporting personal responsibility (Clarke, Lumbard, Sambrook, & Kerr, 2016; Drennan & Alred, 2012). Recovery is possible and needs to underpin the nursing care of persons under forensic purview. The concept of success in the FMH system, from the perspective of service users and service providers, was examined by Livingston (2016). Refer further to Box 35.3.

BOX 35.3 Research for Best Practice

WHAT DOES SUCCESS LOOK LIKE IN THE FORENSIC MENTAL HEALTH SYSTEM?

Livingston, J. D. (2016). What does success look like in the forensic mental health system? Perspectives of service users and service providers. International Journal of Offender Therapy and Comparative Criminology. *Published online March 21, 2016. doi:10.1177/0306624X16639973*

Purpose: The purpose of this study was to examine the concept of success in an FMH system as understood by FMH service users or providers.

Methods: Eighteen (18) FMH service users who received services after being found NCRMD and ten (10) FMH service providers who provided either hospital- or community-based services to persons found NCRMD consented to take part in the study. Participants were interviewed by the researcher, using open-ended questions following a semistructured interview schedule. Interview data were analyzed using a thematic analytical framework with an interpretive/constructivist approach.

Findings: In general, success was seen as a dynamic multidimensional holistic process that a person works toward, and not simply an end state. Six different themes emerged: (1) a normal life, (2) an independent life, (3) a compliant life, (4) a healthy life, (5) a meaningful life, and (6) a progressing life.

Implications for nursing: Understanding success as a holistic multidimensional concept may assist nurses in their practice with FMH service users. Although important and essential to FMH services, nurses need to be concerned with more than risk management and recidivism reduction. Linkages between these concepts and success as described by the participants are essential. This research contributes to our understanding of the process of recovery, and more importantly working *with* clients on their recovery journeys.

Recovery for persons under forensic purview includes clinical recovery through symptom relief, functional recovery through improving life skills, social recovery through community reintegration, personal recovery through achieving life satisfaction despite illness, and offender recovery through a redefinition of self.

Special Populations in the Forensic Setting

Although it could be argued that all persons under forensic purview have special mental health needs requiring the attention of special services and interventions by forensic nurses, groups more likely to require unique approaches include women, older adults, youth, cultural minorities, transgender offenders, and families.

The Female Forensic Client

The past decade has seen a marked increase in the number of women confined to forensic settings, and although they represent a small percentage of the overall forensic population, they currently account for the largest growth in Canada and other Western countries (Blanchette & Brown, 2006). The OCI (2016) reports that since 2006–2007 the number of women in custody under federal jurisdiction increased 35%, while the number of Indigenous women increased by 57%. Nationally, Indigenous women represent the fastest growing group under federal jurisdiction; more than one in three federally sentenced women is Aboriginal.

In general, women most likely to find themselves within forensic settings are those who have grown up in poverty, have limited education and job skills, and have been exposed to violence, victimization, and discrimination. Women are often the primary caregivers for dependent children; as such, the fear of losing custody of their children is ever present (Blanchard, 2004; Blanchette & Brown, 2006; OCI, 2015, 2016). Female forensic clients are frequently victims as well as perpetrators of crime, having experienced physical, emotional, and sexual abuse as children and as adults, at the hands of fathers, husbands, boyfriends, acquaintances, and strangers (Green, Miranda, Daroowalla, & Siddique, 2005).

Common health concerns include significant substance abuse problems; higher rates of blood-borne infections such as HIV/AIDS and hepatitis B and C viruses; significant mental health concerns including anxiety-related disorders (e.g., posttraumatic stress disorder), concerns related to personality disorders (e.g., poor interpersonal functioning and complex and self-injurious behaviours), and serious mental illness (including depression and schizophrenia); pregnancy and gynaecologic problems; obesity; and chronic disorders such as diabetes, hypertension, epilepsy, and respiratory diseases (Green et al., 2005; Kouyoumdjian et al., 2016; OCI, 2015, 2016).

The management of self-injurious behaviour among women under forensic purview is particularly challenging for forensic nurses. Mangnall and Yurkovich (2010), in a study of deliberate self-harm in incarcerated women, reported that the most common method for self-harm was cutting, followed by carving arms, burning with an iron or with cigarettes, as well as swallowing glass shards, snipping veins with fingernail clippers, and punching walls or head-banging. In addition, although such behaviours typically result in immediate relief for the women, in practice, it is not uncommon for forensic nurses and correctional staff alike to be at odds with each other as they grapple to provide appropriate care for this group. In such cases, nursing typically assumes a therapeutic response, while corrections adopts a more punitive or custodial stance (Mangnall & Yurkovich, 2010; OCI, 2015, 2016).

In a comprehensive Canadian study addressing nonsuicidal self-injury (NSSI) in federally incarcerated women, Power, Brown, and Usher (2013) engaged participants in semistructured interviews focused on (1) reasons for self-injuring, (2) precipitating events, and (3) emotions experienced prior to, and after, the self-injury. While some common themes emerged in the data in relation to reasons (affect regulation), precipitating events (interpersonal conflict), emotions experienced prior to NSSI (anger and frustration), and emotions experienced after NSSI (relief), the researchers concluded that NSSI needs to be understood from a heterogeneous perspective and that effective treatment approaches need to consider the unique experiences of each individual woman.

Finally, approaches to self-injurious behaviour ultimately need to address underlying motivations versus simply trying to stop the behaviour (as in the custodial response). Dialectical behavioural therapy has been found to be a useful approach when working with women who engage in NSSI, in both outpatient and inpatient settings (Power et al., 2013).

The Older Forensic Client

For an increasing number of older Canadians, growing old in a prison or in a forensic psychiatric facility is a harsh reality. Forensic clients are considered to be "older" if aged 50 or more years. The transformation to being "older" is thought to be accelerated by 10 to 15 years within this group of clients (Hayes, Burns, Turnbull, & Shaw, 2012; Human Rights Watch, 2012). Twenty-five percent of federally incarcerated offenders are over the age of 50 years, an increase of one third within the latter part of the last decade (OCI, 2016).

Depending on the nature of imprisonment or hospitalization, persons under forensic purview may experience stressors related to general survival (particularly those who are incarcerated), coping with financial pressures, and withdrawal from drugs or alcohol, as well as the cumulative impact of high-risk behaviours, negative lifestyle practices, and inadequate health care, coupled with psychosocial issues related to confinement and isolation (Beckett, Peternelj-Taylor, & Johnson, 2003; Human Rights Watch, 2012). Older forensic clients experience both physical and mental health care needs that set them apart from their younger counterparts, as well as those typical age-related problems experienced by their nonincarcerated peers. Common concerns evident in this population include cardiovascular diseases, pulmonary disorders, diabetes, arthritis, and cancer. Common mental health risks include stress, social isolation, major depressive disorder, alcohol use disorder, suicide, and, increasingly, neurocognitive disorders such as Alzheimer's and other dementias (Beckett et al., 2003; Enggist et al., 2014; Hayes et al., 2012; Human Rights Watch, 2012; OCI, 2015, 2016). In short, those 50 years and older generally present with a high burden of disease. The Alzheimer Society Canada (2010) predicts a "rising tide" of dementia within the general Canadian population in the coming years, which will be felt by forensic and correctional authorities alike.

The health care needs of those under forensic purview clearly challenge traditional forensic and correctional resources and budgets, and questions related to the ability of these facilities to adequately care for older forensic clients are real (Beckett et al., 2003; Human Rights Watch, 2012; OCI, 2015, 2016). For increasing numbers of older and infirm forensic clients, the fear of dying while confined is a terse reality. Although **compassionate release** to community-based long-term care facilities, known in Canada as *Royal Prerogative of Mercy*, is allowed under the Corrections and Conditional Release Act, ongoing fears about community safety, bed shortages in long-term care facilities, and the stigma surrounding the circumstances of the forensic client's hospitalization or incarceration are considered on an individual basis (Beckett et al., 2003; Human Rights Watch, 2012). This option, however, is available to only a very few long-term and infirm forensic clients. In 2014–2015, the Parole Board of Canada denied all 28 formal requests (OCI, 2016).

As a result, palliative care within forensic setting is a poignant reality. Meeting the needs of terminally ill forensic clients within secure environments is a time-consuming, resource-intensive, exhaustive effort fraught with perplexing moral dilemmas not commonly encountered in traditional health care settings (Stone, Papadopoulos, & Kelly, 2012). In many secure environments, in the United States in particular, the implementation of palliative care programming is accomplished through the use of prisoner/inmate caregivers under the supervision of forensic nurses (Loeb et al., 2013). To date, this approach to palliative care within correctional environments has not been adopted in Canada. Instead, nurses and other health care professionals grapple with the complex issues facing dying prisoners, in an effort to provide them with a "good death" (Burles, Peternelj-Taylor, & Holtslander, 2016).

Youth

The Youth Criminal Justice Act (YCJA), introduced in 2003, governs youth aged 12 to 17 who come into conflict with the law (Statistics Canada, 2016). As a group, youth under forensic purview are a vastly underserved population with greater than average health care needs, and because of this, they are particularly vulnerable to adverse outcomes. Studies consistently show that rates of anxiety disorders, attention deficit hyperactivity disorder (ADHD), depression, and substance abuse disorders are higher among youth in custody when compared with youth in the general population. Frequently, their behavioural problems associated with their criminal charges mask their overall health care needs and thwart treatment efforts. It is not uncommon for youth who find themselves in custody to experience symptoms consistent with a wide array of mental health disorders, even though they may not have a formal diagnosis as such. Additionally, youth frequently demonstrate health patterns related to their family environments, as families commonly struggle with mental and physical health problems and substance abuse issues, and present with criminal histories and records (Shelton & Pearson, 2005).

Since 2010–2011, the number of youth under correctional jurisdictions in Canada has declined by 31%. Approximately 90% of youth involved with the criminal justice system are currently engaged in community supervision, with the remainder detained in open or secure custody. However, Aboriginal youth continue to be disproportionately represented in the Canadian criminal justice system. During the 2014–2015 year, 44% of female youth and 29% of male youth admitted to custody were Aboriginal, which is particularly alarming when one considers that Aboriginal youth represent about 7% of the general Canadian youth population (Statistics Canada, 2016). The mental health care concerns of Aboriginal youth are equally alarming. High rates of foetal alcohol spectrum disorder (FASD), significant substance use issues, suicidal ideation, self-harm, histories of attempted suicide, and high rates of physical, sexual, and emotional abuse affect a large portion of the youth involved with a child protection agency at the time of their admission (Latimer & Foss, 2004). In a systematic literature review of FASD within correctional systems, Popova and colleagues (2011) concluded that individuals with FASD have 19 times greater risk of being incarcerated. Appropriate assessment and rehabilitative accommodations for this group are necessary, given the cognitive disabilities associated with FASD. Tragically, most forensic nurses will come into contact with youth through the criminal justice system because very few hospitals are set up to deal with the complexity of needs experienced by youth who come into conflict with the law. However, confinement in and of itself will not facilitate improvement in the mental health of this vulnerable group. Efforts targeting prevention of mental health problems through the provision of services, treatments, and supports in the community are emphasized by the MHCC (2012), particularly when working with youth. Such initiatives are seen as an investment for the future and may prevent at-risk youth from involvement with the criminal justice system. Finally, intersectoral approaches that bring together justice, law, social services, education, and health care are necessary to address the complexity of issues facing at-risk youth. Forensic nurses are ideally situated to meet the needs of this group through engagement in interprofessional and intersectoral collaborations.

Transgender Clients

Most recently, the OCI (2016) has expressed concern that correctional policies regarding the care of transgender clients not only are outdated but also place transgender persons at risk for sexual harassment and assault. Offenders who are transgender, who have not had sex reassignment surgery, are placed and held in correctional institutions that correspond to their biologic sex. Current policies dictate that offenders are eligible for surgery only after living as a transgender person in the community (and not prison) for 1 year. Forensic nurses working with transgender clients need to approach their work with respect, substantive knowledge, and sensitivity.

Culturally Diverse Clients

The ethnic diversity of Canada as a whole is reflected in the demographic profile of Canadian forensic facilities. However, as might be predicted, clients representing ethnic and racial minorities are disproportionately represented, particularly in correctional facilities. The population of federally sentenced visible minorities increased by 40% in the last 5 years, with new growth seen in Aboriginal, Black, Asian, and other ethnic minorities. Of note, 25% of this group is represented by those who are foreign-born, which contributes to further challenges related to institutional adjustment and programming as well as transition to the community. Unfortunately, comparable figures for hospitalization in forensic settings operated by the health care system are unavailable (OCI, 2013).

Aboriginal people make up approximately 4.3% of Canada's adult population, but they represent about 24.4% of the federal incarcerated population (OCI, 2015). Overrepresentation of Aboriginal people within the criminal justice system is attributed to a number of complex factors related to the effects of rapid culture change, cultural oppression, and marginalization (Kirmayer, Brass, & Tait, 2000), resulting in high rates of poverty, substance abuse, and victimization within families and communities of origin (Latimer & Foss, 2004). There has been a growing awareness among the health care and criminal justice systems of the need to provide culturally sensitive and appropriate programming.

In the past, programs were developed on the assumption of sameness; this approach not only negated the forensic client's ethnic identity and culture of origin but also created barriers in the formation of therapeutic relationships and treatment programs, which ultimately interfered with successful community rehabilitation.

Families

In recent years, the needs of family members, the "forgotten clients" (Goldkuhle, 1999), have necessitated expanded roles for forensic nurses and community-based partnerships. Incarceration is a "family affair," and family members, children, and friends represent a hidden forensic population; they are not accounted for and they are rarely discussed by policy makers or health service providers. Incarceration has unintended consequences on families: higher rates of female-headed households, family disruption, family breakup, forced kinship care, and foster care (Cooke, 2014; Freudenberg, Daniels, Crum, Perkins, & Richie, 2005). Women whose partners are incarcerated are often mothering children who are also at risk for early and repeated incarceration. The legacy of family violence is profound. Family members have often experienced various types of violence (e.g., child abuse, intimate partner violence, elder abuse), and children in particular are more likely to experience physical, emotional, and cognitive problems and engage in self-destructive patterns that increase their likelihood of spending time within the forensic system (i.e., prisons) when compared with children of nonincarcerated parents (Cooke, 2014).

All too often, forensic nurses assess their clients in isolation from their support systems, home environments, and daily routines, which is particularly problematic. Creating a forensic family genogram is helpful when working with forensic clients (Kent-Wilkinson, 1999). A genogram is both an assessment and an intervention tool, one that can assist nurses in identifying individual and family patterns (e.g., mental health history, criminal behaviour, substance abuse) and contribute to more comprehensive assessments, interventions, and appropriate community referrals for family members (see Chapter 15 for information regarding genograms).

Collaborating with family members is critical to the safe reintegration of the forensic client into the community. Gaining a more holistic understanding of the family may provide opportunities to enhance psychosocial interventions and contribute to family stability (Cooke, 2014). Working more closely with families is a role that is increasingly being embraced by forensic nurses, particularly those affiliated with community-based FMH programs. For instance, family caregivers can play a vital role in the provision of community care of older offenders with dementia (Encinares, 2007). Many factors affect the forensic client's care in, and readjustment to, the community, including family dynamics, stress, and the family's degree of involvement. Family members can be profoundly impacted by the offence. They receive little support and frequently experience shame and stigma (Pierce, 2011), in addition to guilt and remorse regarding the forensic client's criminal acts (Encinares & Lorbergs, 2001). In some cases, the behaviours of family members can sabotage treatment and reintegration plans, and nursing staff members often bear the brunt of sarcasm and hostility (Encinares & Golea, 2005).

Nurse–Client Relationship

Nursing by its very nature is relational; it is through the nurse–client relationship that nurses gain a deeper understanding and appreciation of the human condition. In fact, the ability to establish and maintain a therapeutic relationship with a forensic client is among the most important competencies required by forensic nurses (Peternelj-Taylor, 2002, 2004, 2012). In the forensic milieu, the emphasis of the therapeutic relationship as a primary intervention strategy is dependent on how the nurse's role is defined and on the context of the setting in which nursing practice takes place. For example, for forensic nurses practising in an inpatient forensic psychiatric unit, working in a sex offender treatment program, or counselling HIV-positive clients in a prison setting, the therapeutic relationship is fundamental to the identification and resolution of problems. In other areas of forensic nursing practice (e.g., an ambulatory care clinic in a correctional facility), the therapeutic relationship may be more in the background. Regardless of the setting or the nature of the relationship, it cannot be assumed that a therapeutic relationship will be present simply by virtue of one's nursing role (Peternelj-Taylor, 2004; Schafer & Peternelj-Taylor, 2003).

Engagement in a therapeutic relationship can be especially difficult for nurses when the client is accused (or convicted) of committing a morally reprehensible act; such a client may "evoke feelings of disgust, repulsion, and fear" (Jacob, Gagnon, & Holmes, 2009, p. 153). Clients may engage in threatening behaviours, break rules, and test boundaries, and they are unappreciative of nurses' efforts in providing health care. Nurses, as members of society, are not immune to prevailing attitudes, beliefs, and stereotypes, and these may negatively colour their perceptions, therapeutic responses, and professional roles with forensic clients. The belief that every client has the potential to change and the right to treatment is one not shared by all forensic nurses (Peternelj-Taylor & Johnson, 1995). Martin (2001) warns that nurses "need to be cautious that their approach to patients does not reinforce the stigma and discrimination of the wider community" (p. 29).

To be successful, forensic nurses need to explore honestly and candidly their own preconceived ideas, attitudes, feelings, beliefs, and stereotypes regarding the forensic client. All too often, nurses can get caught up in the sensationalism that surrounds a particular forensic client (often fuelled by media hype), or the setting in which practice takes place, and ultimately, they can lose sight of the person in need of care. Furthermore, it is not uncommon for nurses who are employed in forensic settings to experience additional stressors unique to their work, which ultimately affect their ability to establish and maintain therapeutic relationships with the clients in their care. Some examples are issues related to personal safety (i.e., threat of violence by forensic clients) (Jacob et al., 2009), ethical dilemmas (Peternelj-Taylor, 2004), understaffing (Cyr & Paradis, 2012), secondary trauma and related posttraumatic stress disorder (Happell, Pinikahana, & Martin, 2003), and competing and conflicting expectations held between health care and correctional authorities (Lazzaretto-Green et al., 2011).

Common Relationship Issues Experienced by Forensic Nurses

Although barriers to therapeutic relationships can be found in all areas of nursing, it is the "special circumstance" (Austin, 2001) of forensic settings, where the moral climate is shaped by the divergent and competing demands for custody and caring, that contributes to forensic settings being described as "hotbeds" for potential problems. This is in part due to the complexity of health care needs experienced by forensic clients, the seductive pull of helping and the intensity of relationships that can develop, the professional isolation experienced by forensic nurses, and the cultural and philosophical differences that exist between forensic clients, forensic nurses, and other members of the treatment team (Lazzaretto-Green et al., 2011; Peternelj-Taylor, 2002, 2005, 2012; Schafer & Peternelj-Taylor, 2003). Forensic nurses, like all nurses, are moral agents, and as such, they are responsible for practising ethically with the clients in their care, regardless of the setting in which care is provided.

Othering

It is within these habitats of special circumstance that nurses meet forensic clients, and how the client is perceived is often illustrated by the language in which nurses frame their care. For example, are the clients seen as inmates, cons, psychopaths, murderers, psychos, or borderlines? Such labels not only evoke stereotypical images but also, more importantly, cast the individual into the role of the "other" (Peternelj-Taylor, 2004). Mason, Hall, Caulfield, and Melling (2010) found that clients labelled personality disordered were perceived by forensic nurses as a management issue, as opposed to those labelled mentally ill who were considered from a clinical perspective. Such negative forms of engagement, known as *exclusionary othering*, can affect all aspects of nursing care and promote marginalization, stigmatization, and underinvolvement in a client's care. *Inclusionary othering*, on the other hand, is promoted as a way of learning about the other as an individual and not simply as a crime or a label. One way of coming to know the forensic client is through role-taking and trying to understand the world from the client's perspective. Although this may be a tall order when working with forensic clients, nurses can learn about othering by gaining an appreciation for what it means to be othered (Canales, 2000, 2010).

KEY CONCEPT

Othering is about the way one perceives and engages with another person. It can be exclusionary and negative (i.e., the other is different from and thus "less than" me) or inclusionary, tolerant, and accepting (i.e., the other is different from me, so I need to learn about his or her world view).

IN-A-LIFE

Sean Clifton (1968–)

MENTAL HEALTH ADVOCATE

Public Persona

Persons under forensic purview are highly stigmatized and often demonized as monsters by the media and public alike. Sean's story is featured in John Kastner's 2013 documentary *NCR: Not Criminally Responsible*. Sean agreed to take part in the documentary in hopes of showing another side of mental illness. Through his participation in the documentary, his personal journey of recovery is showcased. Now a mental health advocate, he frequently does presentations with the parents of his victim, who have forgiven him. He is the 2015 recipient of the Royal Ottawa Foundation for Mental Health's Inspiration Award (personal category) and states "I have been approached by people at screenings and things, who have found my story inspirational. If I have helped one person through the whole thing then it's worth it." A follow-up documentary *Not Criminally Responsible: Wedding Secrets* was released in 2016.

Personal Realities

Sean had a troubled upbringing, and after his parents split up, he lived with his mother who had her own mental health issues. It was during his early adolescence that he began to experience mental health problems; he was bullied at school and had relationship difficulties. Sean was well known to police in his hometown for his odd and sometimes eccentric behaviour, but he was never known to

be violent. This all changed in 1999, when, at the age of 31, he violently stabbed a young woman, who fortunately lived following surgery. Sean was arrested in a dazed state and thrust into the criminal justice system. He was jailed for 9 months before undergoing a psychiatric evaluation. Diagnosed with paranoid schizophrenia and obsessive compulsive disorder, Sean was found not criminally responsible on account of mental disorder (NCRMD). Afterwards, he finally began to receive the mental health care he desperately needed. He spent more than 10 years under the care of the Brockville Mental Health Centre and is now living independently in the community, has a part-time job, and is a volunteer promoting mental health awareness.

Boundary Violations

The complexities and uncertainties surrounding boundaries and **boundary violations** in practice can be difficult for forensic nurses to manage and lead to ongoing confusion in practice. The inability to differentiate the professional relationship from a social relationship by attempting to have one's personal needs met through the nurse–client relationship is consistently discussed as a precursor to boundary violations in the nursing literature (Peternelj-Taylor, 2012; Peternelj-Taylor & Schafer, 2008; Pilette, Berck, & Achber, 1995) (see Chapter 6). In forensic settings, nurses are often warned about getting "too close" to their patients while at the same time painted as "victims of circumstances" when boundaries are transgressed with a forensic client. However, it is important to remember that, from an ethical perspective, the nurse is the one responsible for managing boundaries within the nurse–client relationship, not the client. Mixed messages regarding treatment boundaries can be especially disconcerting for forensic clients, who frequently have problems with boundaries in general. Forensic health care professionals, including nurses, are most vulnerable to transgressing boundaries when they are experiencing major life stressors in their personal lives, such as changing life circumstances, relationship problems, bereavement, or personal caregiving responsibilities. During such times, they are also at risk of being "targeted" by forensic clients who are looking to exploit the therapeutic relationship for personal gain (Faulkner & Regehr, 2011; Peternelj-Taylor, 2012).

Manipulation

The potential for manipulation is a very real factor in secure environments, one that requires thoughtful consideration by nurses in the provision of nursing care. As Austin (2001) notes, "cautioning, scepticism, and the questioning of patients' motives and actions are part of the daily experience of forensic nurses" (p. 13). Forensic clients can be powerful, dominant, intimidating, needy, charming, good looking, and attentive, leading Gutheil and Brodsky (2008) to conclude that even the most ethical clinician can be tested by the manipulative behaviours of forensic clients. In some cases, individuals in forensic settings will attempt to manipulate health care services for some secondary gain (e.g., medication, escape from the prison environment, social diversion), and issues pertaining to safety cannot be ignored (Peternelj-Taylor, 2004; Schoenly, 2013).

Jacob (2014) notes that "the fact that patients are conceptualized as being con artists and manipulators inevitably affects the way care is delivered" (p. 50). When a forensic client is labelled a manipulator, nurses and others will generally respond more punitively and fail to engage the client in a therapeutic dialogue surrounding the meaning of his or her behaviours; in such cases, the opportunity for mutual problem-solving around the manipulative behaviours is lost in the relationship (Peternelj-Taylor, 2004). To be successful, forensic nurses need to be astutely aware that there exists the potential for manipulation in all interactions with forensic clients, while simultaneously adhering to their professional responsibilities embedded within the therapeutic nurse–client relationship. In short, they have to negotiate the path between assuming the worst and recognizing that it can always happen (Schoenly, 2013; Smith, 2005).

 KEY CONCEPT

Manipulation is a concern in secure environments because it can involve the use of deceit to reach a goal that could not be pursued openly (e.g., escape).

Professional Role Development

Historically, role development for forensic nurses has been difficult, owing to the myth that nurses who work with forensic clients are "second-class nurses" unable to secure employment elsewhere (Peternelj-Taylor & Johnson, 1995; Pullan & Lorbergs, 2001). In a recent study, Harris (2013) reported that the stigma experienced by FMH nurses impacted negatively on their adaptation to their professional roles. During this time of a global nursing shortage, recruitment and retention of forensic nurses can be particularly challenging for both mental health care and correctional administrators (Cyr & Paradis, 2012; Pullan & Lorbergs, 2001). Given the breadth and scope of forensic nursing as illustrated within this chapter, it should be evident that forensic nurses are highly skilled and knowledgeable professionals, committed to the health and well-being of the clients in their charge, as well as the community at large.

Professional Nursing Identity

The role of nurses as moral agents in their work with persons under forensic purview is one of the greatest challenges that nurses experience when working in forensic environments. Remaining true to their professional nursing roles and avoiding being seduced or co-opted into assuming custodial roles, where expectations and responsibilities seem more clearly defined, can be especially challenging (Holmes, 2007; Peternelj-Taylor & Johnson, 1995; Smith, 2005). Tensions that exist between custody and caring in forensic environments make it "difficult to maintain the therapeutic culture known to nurses" (Jacob, 2014, p. 48). In forensic settings operated by the criminal justice system, forensic nurses must have a strong nursing identity in order to maintain their professional authority and responsibility, without succumbing to the temptation to align themselves with the correctional staff. However, forensic nurses who work within the health care system should also heed this lesson, for they too can assume a more custodial stance, especially when they believe that CTOs or dispositions in hospital are lenient forms of punishment. Thus, even when the care of forensic clients is the responsibility of the health care system, incongruent attitudes among health care staff may prevail. Lawson (2005) states that when we "set ourselves up as judge and jury" (p. 149), we minimize our ability to be therapeutic.

Professional Development for Forensic Nurses

In 1981, Petryshen published a classic paper entitled "Nursing the Mentally Disordered Offender." Since then, forensic nursing in Canada has undergone significant transformations in education, research, and practice developments related to the provision of nursing care to forensic clients.

Education

Forensic nursing content is slowly finding its way into undergraduate and graduate nursing curricula across the country, primarily through existing courses in psychiatric mental health or community health nursing. For example, the College of Nursing, University of Saskatchewan, offers an online senior elective nursing course entitled *Forensic Nursing in Secure Environments* in its undergraduate baccalaureate program. Furthermore, continuing professional development for nurses who practise in forensic settings is also critical, as it reinforces the therapeutic identity of nurses, assists with nursing policy development (Smith, 2005), and contributes to recruitment and retention in this specialized area of practice (Thorpe, Moorhouse, & Antonello, 2009).

Research

Embracing a research agenda in forensic nursing will guide nursing practice in this highly specialized area; provide new insights into primary, secondary, and tertiary health care (including recovery and reintegration into the community); and contribute to nursing science through the advancement of nursing knowledge regarding vulnerable populations in general (Peternelj-Taylor, 2005). Two research developments in this specialized area of practice include (1) the University of Ottawa's Research Chair in Forensic Nursing, established in 2009 to foster the development and dissemination of forensic nursing research and promote graduate student training, and (2) the Centre for Behavioural Science and Justice Studies, an interdisciplinary collaboration between the University of Saskatchewan, the Correctional Service Canada, and the Saskatchewan Ministry of Justice–Corrections and Policing. Such developments are fundamental to the advancement of forensic nursing as a specialty and will contribute to evidence-based care for those under forensic purview.

Practice Developments

Forensic nurses may find guidance in the Canadian Federation of Mental Health Nurses' (2014) *Canadian Standards for Psychiatric–Mental Health Nursing*; however, standards to guide the unique needs of Canadian FMH nurses are nonexistent. Recognizing the need to build upon traditional mental health standards when working with persons under forensic purview, Martin and colleagues (2013) developed 16 standards to guide education, practice, and research in FMH nursing. Although written from an Australian perspective, these standards could easily cross international jurisdictions, as they capture the essence of FMH nursing in caring for clients under forensic purview.

In July 2007, the Forensic Nurses Society of Canada (FNSC) was approved as an emerging special interest group by the Canadian Nurses Association (CNA). The mission of the Society is "to promote evidence-based comprehensive health care across the spectrum of forensic nursing with an aim to prevent violence or reduce its consequences on the individual." Such acknowledgment by the CNA is a formal recognition of forensic nursing as a specialty area; however, certification as a designated specialty remains uncertain (see Chapter 7).

Treatment Setting

Unlike more traditional practice settings, the interpersonal climate, organizational culture, and social context of forensic settings result in forensic environments being identified among the most severe and extreme environments known to society. Power, control, and implicit authority are manifested in the physical and interpersonal environments of both correctional systems and health care systems and can be incompatible with the achievement of treatment goals (Austin, 2001; Holmes, 2005).

Security Awareness

When working with forensic clients, issues surrounding safety and security are considered critical competencies, and nurses often struggle to find the right balance between their caring and custodial roles. The therapeutic treatment needs of their clients must always be considered within the context of maintaining security. Forensic settings (apart from community-based programs) are typically highly controlled environments, with the whereabouts of clients constantly monitored through a variety of institutional routines, mechanisms, rules, and regulations (Austin, 2001; Peternelj-Taylor & Johnson, 1995). Surveillance of staff and clients is deemed critical to the safe operation of all forensic facilities. Because of this, however, nursing staff members often experience additional stressors because they too are subject to the judgment of others: those who watch over are watched over in turn (Holmes, 2005).

Forensic nurses quickly become aware of two forms of security awareness: **static security** and **dynamic security**. Static security awareness includes such things as the structural or environmental artifacts common to secure environments, for example, the use of two-way radios, personal protection alarms, video monitoring, electronic door locks, internal barriers, and perimeter fences or walls. Dynamic security awareness, on the other hand, is concerned with institutional policies, staffing patterns, methods of operation, and relational security. Finding the right balance between the security needs of the forensic setting (and the community at large) and the client's treatment needs is a balancing act at best. Practical points for competent and safe practice are found in Box 35.4.

In forensic settings operated under the jurisdiction of the health care system (e.g., forensic psychiatric hospitals and FMH units), forensic nurses assume broader roles in the maintenance of security. This can be particularly disconcerting because they may be expected to handcuff clients before a court visit or search them for contraband before and after personal visits (or absences from the unit) while at the same time engage them in a therapeutic nurse–client relationship. This overt attention to custodial roles can jeopardize the fragility of the developing therapeutic relationship, and systems often need to be in place that enable nurses from other units, or those not responsible for direct nursing care, to assist with these necessary custodial measures.

Risk Assessment and Management

Nurses practising in forensic settings work with clients with a proven capacity for violence. In recent years, risk assessment and management have become increasingly important competencies required of forensic nurses. Risk assessment is critical because it guides intervention and treatment. Simply stated, the greater the assessed risk, the higher the levels of intervention and supervision that are required; conversely, the lower the assessed risk, the lower the levels of intervention and supervision that are required, regardless of whether the forensic client is seeking treatment within a secure environment

---

BOX 35.4 Tips for Security Awareness in Forensic Settings

- When working in institutional settings, never bring anything in or take anything out for a client, regardless of how insignificant the request may seem.
- Let coworkers know your whereabouts at all times; interview clients in designated interview rooms or in places visible to other staff members. When working in the community, always leave your itinerary, the anticipated length of your visits, and how you can be reached.
- Observe policies and procedures related to security awareness specific to the forensic setting in which you are working. Ask questions in order to understand the rationale behind the policies.

- Do not share personal information about yourself, or other staff members, with clients.
- Clients will sometimes engage in sexually inappropriate banter or gestures. Report this immediately, no matter how embarrassed you may be.
- Be aware of the location of staff members in relation to clients. Use a buddy system (e.g., another staff member) when uncomfortable approaching a client, especially when entering the client's living space.
- In all cases, open communication is critical to safe and competent nursing practice. Report all suspicious behaviours as soon as possible.

---

or a community treatment program (Woods, 2013). Although a detailed discussion of risk assessment and management is beyond the scope of this chapter, it is mentioned here because increasingly, forensic nurses, with additional training and experience, are using actuarial (or statistical) tools and structured clinical judgment to formulate treatment plans that increasingly include risk assessment and management (Encinares & Golea, 2005; Encinares & Lorbergs, 2001; Encinares, McMaster, & McNamee, 2005). In a review of the literature, Woods and Lasiuk (2008) concluded that forensic nurses should integrate the use of empirically guided approaches to risk, including actuarial measures and structured clinical approaches, along with their own subjective qualitative clinical assessments. However, reliance on clinical judgment alone, as noted in some settings, warrants further education and training in practice (Woods, 2013).

■ SOCIETAL NORMS

Humane care is defined by society, including the public, politicians, and the media (Mason, Lovell, & Coyle, 2008). The continual expansion of correctional facilities, however, reveals society's failure to address complex health and social issues. The Canadian Association of Elizabeth Fry Societies has declared "Women don't belong in cages: Prisons are the real crime" (see Web Links). There is a societal expectation that imprisonment will deter others from committing crimes, as well as contribute to community safety. This can mean that prisons are more readily funded than other strategies to deal with poverty, homelessness, and mental illness. The impact of interpersonal violence and illicit drug-related activities on individuals and communities is not sufficiently addressed, nor is the lack of health care services available to vulnerable and marginalized groups.

Understanding the comprehensive needs of individuals whose lives have become enmeshed within the criminal justice system requires an understanding of both the individual and the social determinants of health that are associated with mental health, mental illness and delinquency, and criminal activity. Such an understanding provides for greater opportunities for the development of interventions and policies that may be effective at promoting mental health, preventing crime, and reducing the risk of repeat offending among those with a mental illness. Forensic nursing is uniquely positioned to intervene with the socially significant health issues associated with crime, incarceration, and release. Hospitalization and incarceration alike provide opportunities for effective mental health interventions that have the potential for secondary gains, such as improving public safety, decreasing health care costs, and decreasing recidivism (Kouyoumdjian et al., 2016). Such interventions must be grounded in the conviction that caring for forensic clients as vulnerable members of society is the appropriate and decent thing to do.

 SUMMARY OF KEY POINTS

- The provision of nursing care to persons under forensic purview is a challenging and rewarding psychiatric and mental health nursing experience, one that balances the conflicting convictions of custody and caring.
- Components of care in forensic nursing include the forensic client, nurse–client relationship, professional role development, treatment setting, and societal norms.
- The ability to engage the forensic client in a therapeutic relationship is critical to competent forensic nursing care. Relationship issues experienced by forensic nurses include othering, boundary violations, and manipulation.

- Forensic nurses are uniquely situated to provide nursing care to forensic clients in a variety of community- and institution-based treatment settings.
- Intersectoral and interprofessional approaches that bring together justice, law, social services, education, and health care are deemed necessary to address the multitude of issues facing forensic clients, their families, and their communities.

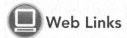 **Web Links**

www.caefs.ca The Canadian Association of Elizabeth Fry Societies (CAEFS) is made up of 26 self-governing community-based societies from across Canada that work with, and for, women and girls in the justice system, particularly those who are, or may be, criminalized.

www.csc-scc.gc.ca The Correctional Service Canada (CSC) contributes to the protection of society by actively assisting offenders (with sentences of over 2 years) to become law-abiding citizens while exercising safe, secure, and humane control. CSC's website is a resource for Canadian policy, legislation, and research.

www.forensicnurse.ca/about The Canadian Forensic Nurses Association, a special interest group of CNA, aims to provide a network for forensic nurses in Canada and a forum to discuss evidence-based practice unique to the diverse areas of forensic nursing in Canada.

www.forensicnurses.org The International Association of Forensic Nurses (IAFN) brings together nurses whose practice interfaces in some way with the law.

www.iafmhs.org The mandate of the International Association of Forensic Mental Health Services (IAFMHS) is to enhance the standards of FMH services within an international context and to promote an international dialogue about all aspects of FMH, including violence and family violence.

www.health.uottawa.ca/forensic-research The University of Ottawa's Research Chair in Forensic Nursing was established to foster the development and dissemination of forensic nursing research and promote graduate student training.

www.johnhoward.ca The John Howard Society of Canada is an organization of provincial and territorial societies aimed at understanding and responding to problems of crime and the criminal justice system.

www.oci-bec.gc.ca The Office of the Correctional Investigator has the authority to act as an ombudsman for federal offenders. The primary function of the office is to investigate and bring resolution to individual offender complaints.

www.prisonersofage.com This website features photographs, interviews, and documentaries with older inmates and correctional personnel and provides a glimpse into their lives, crimes, and the challenges they experience.

www.usask.ca/cfbsjs The Centre for Behavioural Science and Justice Studies at the University of Saskatchewan is an interdisciplinary collaboration with an aim to establish a prairie-based centre for enhanced research and training in the area of forensic behavioural science and justice.

www.usask.ca/nursing/custodycaring The College of Nursing, University of Saskatchewan, in collaboration with the Regional Psychiatric Centre, CSC, has hosted a biennial international nursing conference showcasing innovations in practice, education, research, administration, and policy development in the fields of correctional health and forensic mental health care in Canada and abroad.

References

Alzheimer Society of Canada. (2010). *Rising tide: The impact of dementia on Canadian society*. Retrieved from http://www.alzheimer.ca/en/Get-involved/Raise-your-voice/Rising-Tide

Austin, W. (2001). Relational ethics in forensic psychiatric settings. *Journal of Psychosocial Nursing and Mental Health Services, 39*(9), 12–17.

Beaudette, J. N., Power, J., & Stewart, L. A. (2015). *National prevalence of mental disorders among federally-sentenced men offenders (Research Report, R-357)*. Ottawa, ON: Correctional Service Canada.

Beckett, J., Peternelj-Taylor, C., & Johnson, R. (2003). Growing old in the correctional system. *Journal of Psychosocial Nursing and Mental Health Services, 41*(9), 12–18.

Blanchard, B. (2004). Incarcerated mothers and their children: A complex issue. *Forum on Correctional Research, 16*(1), 45–46.

Blanchette, K., & Brown, S. L. (2006). *The assessment and treatment of women offenders: An integrative perspective*. Chichester, UK: John Wiley & Sons.

Burles, M. C., Peternelj-Taylor, C., & Holtslander, L. (2016). A 'good death' for all? Examining issues for palliative care in correctional settings. *Mortality, 21*(2), 93–111. doi.org/10.1080/13576275.2015.1098602

Canadian Federation of Mental Health Nurses. (2014). *Canadian standards for psychiatric-mental health nursing* (4th ed.). Toronto, ON: Author.

Canales, M. K. (2000). Othering: Toward an understanding of difference. *Advances in Nursing Science, 22*(4), 16–31.

Canales, M. K. (2010). Othering: Difference understood? A 10-year analysis and critique of the nursing literature. *Advances in Nursing Science, 33*, 15–34.

Chaimowitz, G. (2012). Position paper: The criminalization of people with mental illness. *Canadian Journal of Psychiatry, 57*(2), 1–6.

Clarke, C., Lumbard, D., Sambrook, S., & Kerr, K. (2016). What does recovery mean to a forensic mental health patient? A systematic review and narrative synthesis of the qualitative literature. *Journal of Forensic Psychiatry and Psychology, 27*(1), 38–54. doi:10.3109/01612840.2013.87 310310.1080/14789949.2015.1102311

Cooke, C. L. (2014). Nearly invisible: The psychosocial and health needs of women with male partners in prison. *Issues in Mental Health Nursing, 35*, 979–982.

Correctional Service Canada, Federal–Provincial/Territorial Partnership. (2012). *Mental health strategy for corrections in Canada*. Retrieved from http://www.csc-scc.gc.ca/health/092/MH-strategy-eng.pdf

Cyr, J. J., & Paradis, J. (2012). The forensic float nurse: A new concept in the effective management of service delivery in a forensic program. *Journal of Forensic Nursing, 8*(4), 188–194.

de Chesnay, M. (2016). Vulnerable populations: Vulnerable people. In M. de Chesnay, & B. A. Anderson (Eds.), *Caring for the vulnerable: Perspectives in nursing theory, practice and research* (4th ed., pp. 3–18). Burlington, MA: Jones & Bartlett.

Drennan, G., & Alred, D. (2012). Recovery in forensic mental health settings. In G. Drennan, & D. Alred (Eds.), *Secure recovery: Approaches to recovery in forensic mental health settings* (pp. 1–22). Abingdon, UK: Routledge.

Dupuis, T., MacKay, R., & Nicol, J. (2013). Current issues in mental health in Canada: Mental health and the criminal justice system. *Background Paper* (Publication No. 2013-88-E). Ottawa, ON: Library of Parliament.

Encinares, M. (2007). Mental health forum: Community care of elderly offenders with dementia. *Journal of Chinese Clinical Medicine, 2*(1), 34–41.

Encinares, M., & Golea, G. (2005). Client centered-care for individuals with dual diagnoses in the justice system. *Journal of Psychosocial Nursing and Mental Health Services, 43*(9), 29–36.

Encinares, M., & Lorbergs, K. (2001). Framing nursing practice within a forensic outpatient service. *Journal of Psychosocial Nursing and Mental Health Services, 39*(9), 35–41.

Encinares, M., McMaster, J. J., & McNamee, J. (2005). Risk assessment of forensic patients: Nurses' role. *Journal of Psychosocial Nursing and Mental Health Services, 43*(3), 30–36.

Enggist, S., Møller, L., Galea, G., & Udesen, C. (2014). *Prisons and health*. World Health Organization. Retrieved from http://www.euro.who.int/__data/assets/pdf_file/0005/249188/Prisons-and-Health.pdf

Faulkner, C., & Regehr, C. (2011). Sexual boundary violations committed by female forensic workers. *Journal of the American Academy of Psychiatry and the Law, 39*, 154–163.

Freudenberg, N., Daniels, J., Crum, M., Perkins, T., & Ritchie, B. E. (2005). Coming home from jail: The social and health consequences of community reentry for women, male adolescents, and their families. *American Journal of Public Health, 95*(10), 1725–1726.

Goldkuhle, U. (1999). Professional education for correctional nurses: A community-based partnership model. *Journal of Psychosocial Nursing and Mental Health Services, 37*(9), 38–44.

Green, B. L., Miranda, J., Daroowalla, A., & Siddique, J. (2005). Trauma exposure, mental health functioning, and program needs of women in jail. *Crime and Delinquency, 51,* 133–151.

Gutheil, T. G., & Brodsky, A. (2008). *Preventing boundary violations in clinical practice.* New York, NY: Guilford Press.

Happell, B., Pinikahana, J., & Martin, T. (2003). Stress and burnout in forensic psychiatric nursing. *Stress and Health, 19*(2), 63–68.

Harris, D. M. (2013). Working in forensic mental health. In P. Callaghan, N. Oud, J. H. Bjørngaard, H. Nijman, T. Palmstierna, R. Almvik, & B. Thomas (Eds.), *Proceedings of the 8th European Congress on violence in clinical psychiatry* (pp. 395–398). Amsterdam, NL: Kavanah, Dwingeloo & Oud Consultancy.

Hayes, A. J., Burns, A., Turnbull, P., & Shaw, J. J. (2012). The health and social needs of older male prisoners. *International Journal of Geriatric Psychiatry, 27,* 1155–1162.

Holmes, D. (2005). Governing the captives: Forensic psychiatric nursing in corrections. *Perspectives in Psychiatric Care, 41*(1), 3–13.

Holmes, D. (2007). Nursing in corrections: Lessons from France. *Journal of Forensic Nursing, 3*(3–4), 126–131.

Human Rights Watch. (2012). *Old behind bars: The aging prison population in the United States.* Retrieved from http://www.hrw.org/reports/2012/01/27/old-behind-bars-0

Jacob, J. D. (2014). Understanding the domestic rupture in forensic psychiatric nursing practice. *Journal of Correctional Health Care, 20*(1), 45–58.

Jacob, J. D., Gagnon, M., & Holmes, D. (2009). Nursing so-called monsters: On the importance of abjection and fear in forensic psychiatric nursing. *Journal of Forensic Nursing, 5*(3), 153–161.

Kanapaux, W. (2004). Guilty of mental illness. *Psychiatric Times, XXI*(1). Retrieved from http://www.psychiatrictimes.com/p040101a.html

Kent-Wilkinson, A. (1999). Forensic family genogram: An assessment and intervention tool. *Journal of Psychosocial Nursing and Mental Health Services, 37*(9), 52–56.

Kirmayer, L. J., Brass, G. M., & Tait, C. L. (2000). The mental health of Aboriginal peoples: Transformations of identity and community. *Canadian Journal of Psychiatry, 45*(7), 607–616.

Kouyoumdjian, F., Schuler, A., Matheson, F., & Hwang, S. (2016). Health status of prisoners in Canada. *Canadian Family Physician, 62,* 215–222.

Latimer, J., & Foss, L. C. (2004). *A one-day snapshot of Aboriginal youth in custody across Canada: Phase II.* Ottawa, ON: Department of Justice Canada. Retrieved from http://www.justice.gc.ca/eng/rp-pr/cj-jp/yj-jj/yj2-jj2/index.html

Lawson, L. (2005). Furthering the search for truth and justice. *Journal of Forensic Nursing, 1*(4), 149–150.

Lazzaretto-Green, D., Austin, W., Goble, E., Buys, L., Gorman, T., & Rankel, M. (2011). Walking a fine line: Forensic mental health practitioners' experience of working with correctional officers. *Journal of Forensic Nursing, 7*(3), 109–119.

Livingston, J. D. (2016). What does success look like in the forensic mental health system? Perspectives of service users and service providers. *International Journal of Offender Therapy and Comparative Criminology,* 1–21. doi:10.1177/0306624X16639973

Loeb, S. J., Hollenbeak, C. S., Penrod, J., Smith, C. A., Kitt-Lewis, E., & Crouse, S. B. (2013). Care and companionship in an isolating environment: Inmates attending to dying peers. *Journal of Forensic Nursing, 6,* 35–44.

Mangnall, J., & Yurkovich, E. (2010). A grounded theory exploration of deliberate self-harm in incarcerated women. *Journal of Forensic Nursing, 6,* 88–95.

Martin, T. (2001). Something special: Forensic psychiatric nursing. *Journal of Psychiatric and Mental Health Nursing, 8,* 25–32.

Martin, T., Maguire, T., Quinn, C., Ryan, J., Bawden, L., & Summers, M. (2013). Standards of practice for forensic mental health nurses: Identifying contemporary practice. *Journal of Forensic Nursing, 9*(3), 171–178.

Mason, T., Hall, R., Caulfield, M., & Melling, K. (2010). Forensic nurses' perceptions of labels of mental illness and personality disorder: Clinical versus management issues. *Journal of Psychiatric and Mental Health Nursing, 17,* 131–140.

Mason, T., Lovell, A., & Coyle, D. (2008). Forensic psychiatric nursing: Skills and competencies: I. Role dimensions. *Journal of Psychiatric and Mental Health Nursing, 15,* 118–130.

McLoughlin, K. A., Geller, J. L., & Tolan, A. (2011). Is recovery possible in a forensic hospital setting? *Archives of Psychiatric Nursing, 25*(5), 390–391.

Mental Health Commission of Canada. (2012). *Changing directions, changing lives: The mental health strategy for Canada.* Retrieved from http://strategy.mentalhealthcommission.ca/pdf/strategy-text-en.pdf

Mental Health Commission of Canada. (2015). *Guidelines for recovery-oriented practice.* Ottawa, ON: Author.

Miladinovic, Z., & Lukassen, J. (2014). Verdicts of not criminally responsible on account of mental disorder in adult criminal courts, 2005/2006–2011/2012. *Juristat.* Retrieved from http://www.statcan.gc.ca/pub/85-002-x/2014001/article/14085-eng.htm

Office of the Correctional Investigator. (2013). *Annual report of the Office of the Correctional Investigator 2012–2013. (No. PS100-2013E-PDF).* Ottawa, ON: Her Majesty the Queen in Right of Canada. Retrieved from http://www.oci-bec.gc.ca/cnt/rpt/pdf/annrpt/annrpt20122013-eng.pdf

Office of the Correctional Investigator (OCI). (2015). *Annual report of the Office of the Correctional Investigator 2014–2015.* Retrieved from http://www.oci-bec.gc.ca/cnt/rpt/pdf/annrpt/annrpt20142015-eng.pdf

Office of the Correctional Investigator (OCI). (2016). *Annual report of the Office of the Correctional Investigator 2015–2016.* Retrieved from http://www.oci-bec.gc.ca/cnt/rpt/pdf/annrpt/annrpt20152016-eng.pdf

Olson, R. (2012). *Prison inmate suicide—Why it matters.* Centre for Suicide Prevention. Retrieved from http://suicideinfo.ca/Library/Resources/iEinfoExchange/iE8PrisonInmateSuicide.aspx

Ormston, E. F. (2010). The criminalization of the mentally ill. *Canadian Journal of Community Mental Health, 29*(2), 5–10.

Peternelj-Taylor, C. (2000). The role of the forensic nurse in Canada: An evolving specialty. In D. Robinson & A. Kettles (Eds.), *Forensic nursing and multidisciplinary care of the mentally disordered offender* (pp. 192–212). London, UK: Jessica Kingsley Publishers.

Peternelj-Taylor, C. (2002). Professional boundaries: A matter of therapeutic integrity. *Journal of Psychosocial Nursing and Mental Health Services, 40*(4), 22–29.

Peternelj-Taylor, C. (2004). An exploration of othering in forensic psychiatric and correctional nursing. *Canadian Journal of Nursing Research, 36*(4), 130–146.

Peternelj-Taylor, C. (2005). Conceptualizing nursing research with offenders: Another look at vulnerability. *International Journal of Law and Psychiatry, 28,* 348–359.

Peternelj-Taylor, C. (2012). Boundaries and desire in forensic mental health nursing. In A. Aiyegbusi & G. Kelly (Eds.), *Professional and therapeutic boundaries in forensic mental health practice* (pp. 124–136). London, UK: Jessica Kingsley Publishers.

Peternelj-Taylor, C. A., & Hufft, A. G. (2006). Forensic nursing. In W. K. Mohr (Ed.), *Psychiatric-mental health nursing* (6th ed., pp. 377–393). Philadelphia, PA: Lippincott Williams & Wilkins.

Peternelj-Taylor, C. & Johnson, R. (1995). Serving time: Psychiatric mental health nursing in corrections. *Journal of Psychosocial Nursing and Mental Health Services, 33*(8), 12–19.

Peternelj-Taylor, C., & Schafer, P. (2008). Management of therapeutic boundaries. In A. Kettles, P. Woods, & R. Byrt (Eds.), *Forensic mental health nursing: Capabilities, roles and responsibilities* (pp. 309–331). London, UK: Quay Books.

Petryshen, P. (1981). Nursing the mentally disordered offender. *Canadian Nurse, 77*(6), 26–28.

Pierce, S. (2011). The lived experience of parents of adolescents who have sexually offended: I am a survivor. *Journal of Forensic Nursing, 7,* 173–181.

Pilette, P. C., Berck, C. B., & Achber, L. C. (1995). Therapeutic management of helping boundaries. *Journal of Psychosocial Nursing and Mental Health Services, 33*(1), 40–47.

Popova, S., Lange, S., Bekmuradov, D., Mihic, A., & Rehm, J. (2011). Fetal alcohol spectrum disorder prevalence estimates in the correctional system: A systematic literature review. *Canadian Journal of Public Health, 102*(5), 336–340.

Power, J., Brown, S. L., & Usher, A. M. (2013). Non-suicidal self-injury in women offenders: Motivations, emotions, and precipitating events. *International Journal of Forensic Mental Health, 12,* 192–204.

Pullan, S. E., & Lorbergs, K. A. (2001). Recruitment and retention: A successful model in forensic psychiatric nursing. *Journal of Psychosocial Nursing and Mental Health Services, 39*(9), 18–25.

Rose, D. N., Peter, E., Gallop, R., Angus, J. E., & Liaschenko, J. (2011). Respect in forensic psychiatric nurse-patient relationships: A practical compromise. *Journal of Forensic Nursing, 7,* 3–16.

Schafer, P. E., & Peternelj-Taylor, C. (2003). Therapeutic relationships and boundary maintenance: The perspective of forensic patients enrolled in a treatment program for violent offenders. *Issues in Mental Health Nursing, 24,* 605–625.

Schoenly, L. (2013). Safety for the nurse and the patient. In L. Schoenly, & C. M. Knox (Eds.), *Essentials of correctional nursing* (pp. 55–79). New York, NY: Springer.

Shelton, D., & Pearson, G. (2005). ADHD in juvenile offenders: Treatment issues nurses need to know. *Journal of Psychosocial Nursing and Mental Health Services, 43*(9), 38–46.

Smith, S. (2005). Stepping through the looking glass: Professional autonomy in correctional nursing. *Corrections Today, 54–56,* 70.

Statistics Canada. (2009). *Section A—Overview of issues: Mental health and the criminal justice system.* Retrieved from http://www.statcan.gc.ca/pub/85-561-m/2009016/section-a-eng.htm

Statistics Canada. (2016). *Youth correctional statistics in Canada, 2014/2015.* Retrieved from http://www.statcan.gc.ca/pub/85-002-x/2016001/article/14317-eng.htm

Stone, K., Papadopoulos, I., & Kelly, D. (2012). Establishing hospice care for prison populations: An integrative review assessing the UK and the USA perspective. *Palliative Medicine, 26,* 969–978.

Thorpe, G., Moorhouse, P., & Antonello, C. (2009). Clinical coaching in forensic psychiatry: An innovative program to recruit and retain nurses. *Journal of Psychosocial Nursing and Mental Health Services, 47*(5), 43–47.

Woods, P. (2013). Risk assessment and management approaches on mental health units. *Journal of Psychiatric and Mental Health Nursing, 20,* 807–813.

Woods, P., & Lasiuk, G. (2008). Risk prediction: A review of the literature. *Journal of Forensic Nursing, 4*(1), 1–11.

Appendix A

Brief Psychiatric Rating Scale

Patient's name_____ Date _____ Interviewer's name_____

Hospital _____ Ward _____ Date of admission _____

Instructions: This form consists of 24 symptom constructs, each to be rated on a 7-point scale of severity ranging from "not present" to "extremely severe." If a specific symptom is not rated, mark "NA" (not assessed). Circle the number headed by the term that best describes the patient's present condition

NA		1	2	3	4	5	6	7
Not assessed		Not present	Very mild	Mild	Moderate	Moderately severe	Severe	Extremely severe

1.	Somatic concern	NA	1	2	3	4	5	6	7
2.	Anxiety	NA	1	2	3	4	5	6	7
3.	Depression	NA	1	2	3	4	5	6	7
4.	Guilt	NA	1	2	3	4	5	6	7
5.	Hostility	NA	1	2	3	4	5	6	7
6.	Suspiciousness	NA	1	2	3	4	5	6	7
7.	Unusual thought content	NA	1	2	3	4	5	6	7
8.	Grandiosity	NA	1	2	3	4	5	6	7
9.	Hallucinations	NA	1	2	3	4	5	6	7
10.	Disorientation	NA	1	2	3	4	5	6	7
11.	Conceptual disorganization	NA	1	2	3	4	5	6	7
12.	Excitement	NA	1	2	3	4	5	6	7
13.	Motor retardation	NA	1	2	3	4	5	6	7
14.	Blunted affect	NA	1	2	3	4	5	6	7
15.	Tension	NA	1	2	3	4	5	6	7
16.	Mannerisms and posturing	NA	1	2	3	4	5	6	7
17.	Uncooperativeness	NA	1	2	3	4	5	6	7
18.	Emotional withdrawal	NA	1	2	3	4	5	6	7
19.	Suicidality	NA	1	2	3	4	5	6	7
20.	Self-neglect	NA	1	2	3	4	5	6	7
21.	Bizarre behavior	NA	1	2	3	4	5	6	7
22.	Elated mood	NA	1	2	3	4	5	6	7
23.	Motor hyperactivity	NA	1	2	3	4	5	6	7
24.	Distractibility	NA	1	2	3	4	5	6	7

Reprinted with permission from Lukoff, D., Liberman, R. P., & Nuechterlein, K. H. (1986). Symptom monitoring in the rehabilitation of schizophrenic patients. *Schizophrenia Bulletin, 12*(4), 578–602.

Appendix B

Simpson-Angus Rating Scale

1. GAIT: The patient is examined as he or she walks into the examining room; the gait, the swing of the arms, and the general posture all form the basis for an overall score for this item. This is rated as follows:

   0 Normal
   1 Diminution in swing while the patient is walking
   2 Marked diminution in swing with obvious rigidity in the arm
   3 Stiff gait with arms held rigidly before the abdomen
   4 Stooped shuffling gait with propulsion and retropulsion

2. ARM DROPPING: The patient and the examiner both raise their arms to shoulder height and let them fall to their sides. In a normal subject, a stout slap is heard as the arms hit the sides. In the patient with extreme Parkinson's syndrome, the arms fall very slowly.

   0 Normal, free fall with loud slap and rebound
   1 Fall slowed slightly with less audible contact and little rebound
   2 Fall slowed, no rebound
   3 Marked slowing, no slap at all
   4 Arms fall as though against resistance, as though through glue

3. SHOULDER SHAKING: The subject's arms are bent at a right angle at the elbow and are taken one at a time by the examiner who grasps one hand and also clasps the other around the subject's elbow. The subject's upper arm is pushed to and fro, and the humerus is externally rotated. The degree of resistance from normal to extreme rigidity is scored as follows:

   0 Normal
   1 Slight stiffness and resistance
   2 Moderate stiffness and resistance
   3 Marked rigidity with difficulty in passive movement
   4 Extreme stiffness and rigidity with almost a frozen shoulder

4. ELBOW RIGIDITY: The elbow joints are separately bent at right angles and passively extended and flexed, with the subject's biceps observed and simultaneously palpated. The resistance to this procedure is rated. (The presence of cogwheel rigidity is noted separately.) Scoring is from 0 to 4, as in the Shoulder Shaking test.

   0 Normal
   1 Slight stiffness and resistance
   2 Moderate stiffness and resistance
   3 Marked rigidity with difficulty in passive movement
   4 Extreme stiffness and rigidity with almost a frozen shoulder

5. FIXATION OF POSITION OR WRIST RIGIDITY: The examiner holds the wrist in one hand and the fingers in the other hand, with the wrist moved to extension, flexion, and both ulnar and radial deviation. The resistance to this procedure is rated as in Items 3 and 4.

   0 Normal
   1 Slight stiffness and resistance
   2 Moderate stiffness and resistance
   3 Marked rigidity with difficulty in passive movement
   4 Extreme stiffness and rigidity with almost a frozen shoulder

6. LEG PENDULOUSNESS: The patient sits on a table with the legs hanging down and swinging free. The ankle is grasped by the examiner and raised until the knee is partially extended. It is then allowed to fall. The resistance to falling and the lack of swinging form the basis for the score on this item.

   0 The legs swing freely
   1 Slight diminution in the swing of the legs
   2 Moderate resistance to swing
   3 Marked resistance and damping of swing
   4 Complete absence of swing

7. HEAD DROPPING: The patient lies on a well-padded examining table, and the head is raised by

the examiner's hand. The hand is then withdrawn, and the head is allowed to drop. In the normal subject, the head will fall upon the table. The movement is delayed in extrapyramidal system disorder, and in extreme parkinsonism, it is absent. The neck muscles are rigid, and the head does not reach the examining table. Scoring is as follows:

0   The head falls completely, with a good thump as it hits the table
1   Slight slowing in fall, mainly noted by lack of slap as the head meets the table
2   Moderate slowing in the fall, quite noticeable to the eye
3   The head falls stiffly and slowly
4   The head does not reach the examining table

8. GLABELLA TAP: The subject is told to open the eyes wide and not to blink. The glabella region is tapped at a steady, rapid speed. The number of times the patient blinks in succession is noted:

0   0 to 5 blinks
1   6 to 10 blinks
2   11 to 15 blinks
3   16 to 20 blinks
4   21 or more blinks

9. TREMOR: The patient is observed walking into the examining room and then is reexamined for this item:

0   Normal
1   Mild finger tremor, obvious to sight and touch
2   Tremor of hand or arm occurring spasmodically
3   Persistent tremor of one or more limbs
4   Whole body tremor

10. SALIVATION: The patient is observed while talking and then asked to open the mouth and elevate the tongue. The following ratings are given:

0   Normal
1   Excess salivation to the extent that pooling takes place if the mouth is open and the tongue raised
2   When excess salivation is present and might occasionally result in difficulty in speaking
3   Speaking with difficulty because of excess salivation
4   Frank drooling

Scoring: Each item is rated on a five-point scale, with 0 meaning the complete absence of the condition and 4 meaning the presence of the condition in extreme form. The score is obtained by adding the items and dividing by 10.

Reprinted with permission from Simpson, G. M., & Angus, J. W. S. (1970). A rating scale for extrapyramidal side effects. *Acta Psychiatrica Scandinavica, 212*(Suppl.), 11–19.

Appendix C

Abnormal Involuntary Movement Scale (AIMS)

	None	Minimal	Mild	Moderate	Severe
Facial and Oral Movements					
1: Muscles of facial expression (e.g., movements of forehead, eyebrows, periorbital area, cheeks; include frowning, blinking, smiling, grimacing)	0	1	2	3	4
2: Lips and perioral area (e.g., puckering, pouting, smacking)	0	1	2	3	4
3: Jaw (e.g., biting, clenching, chewing, mouth opening, lateral movement)	0	1	2	3	4
4: Tongue Rate only increase in movement both in and out of the mouth, NOT inability to sustain movement	0	1	2	3	4
Extremity Movements					
5: Upper (arms, wrists, hands, fingers) Include choreic movements (i.e., rapid, objectively purposeless, irregular, spontaneous), athetoid movements (i.e., slow, irregular, complex, serpentine) Do NOT include tremor (i.e., repetitive, regular, rhythmic)	0	1	2	3	4
6: Lower (legs, knees, ankles, toes) (e.g., lateral knee movement, foot tapping, heel dropping, foot squirming, inversion and eversion of the foot)	0	1	2	3	4
Trunk Movements					
7: Neck, shoulders, hips (e.g., rocking, twisting, squirming, pelvic gyrations)	0	1	2	3	4
8: Severity of abnormal movements	0	1	2	3	4
Global Judgment					
9: Incapacitation due to abnormal movements	0	1	2	3	4

10: Patient's awareness of abnormal movements
Rate only the patient's report

No awareness	0
Aware, no distress	1
Aware, mild distress	2
Aware, moderate distress	3
Aware, severe distress	4

Global Judgment

11: Current problems with teeth and/or dentures

No	0
Yes	1

12: Does the patient usually wear dentures?

No	0
Yes	1

Examination Procedures for AIMS

Either before or after completing the examination procedure, observe the patient unobtrusively, at rest (e.g., in the waiting room). The chair to be used in this examination should be a hard, firm one without arms.

1: Ask the patient whether there is anything in his/her mouth (i.e., gum, candy, etc.) and if there is, to remove it.

2: Ask the patient about the *current* condition of his/her teeth. Ask the patient if he/she wears dentures. Do teeth or dentures bother the patient *now*?

3: Ask the patient whether he/she notices any movements in the mouth, face, hands, or feet. If yes, ask the patient to describe and to what extent they *currently* bother him/her or interfere with his/her activities.

4: Have the patient sit in the chair with hands on knees, legs slightly apart, and feet flat on the floor. (Look at the entire body for movements while in this position.)

5: Ask the patient to sit with his/her hands hanging unsupported. If male, between legs; if female and wearing a dress, hanging over knees. (Observe hands and other body areas.)

6: Ask the patient to open his/her mouth. (Observe tongue at rest within the mouth.) Do this twice.

7: Ask the patient to protrude the tongue. (Observe tongue at rest within the mouth.) Do this twice.

[a]8: Ask the patient to tap the thumb, with each finger, as rapidly as possible for 10–15 seconds; separately with right hand, then with left hand. (Observe facial and leg movements.)

9: Flex and extend the patient's left and right arms (one at a time). (Note any rigidity and rate on NOTES.)

10: Ask the patient to stand up. (Observe in profile. Observe all body areas again, hips included.)

[a]11: Ask the patient to extend both arms outstretched in front with palms down. (Observe trunk, legs, and mouth.)

[a]12: Have the patient walk a few paces, turn, and walk back to the chair. (Observe hand and gait.) Do this twice.

---

[a]Activated movements.

Source: Guy, W. (1976). *ECDEU: Assessment manual for psychopharmacology (DHEW Publication No. 76-338)*. Washington, DC: Department of Health, Education, and Welfare, Psychopharmacology Research Branch.

Appendix D

Simplified Diagnoses for Tardive Dyskinesia (SD-TD)

PREREQUISITES—The three prerequisites are as follows. Exceptions may occur.

1. A history of at least 3 months' total cumulative neuroleptic exposure. Include amoxapine and metoclopramide in all categories below as well.
2. **SCORING/INTENSITY LEVEL.** The presence of a **TOTAL SCORE OF FIVE OR ABOVE.** Also, be alert for any change from baseline or scores below five that have at least a "moderate" (3) or "severe" (4) movement on any item or at least two "mild" (2) movements on two items located in different body areas.
3. Other conditions are not responsible for the abnormal involuntary movements.

DIAGNOSES—The diagnosis is based upon the current exam and its relation to the last exam. The diagnosis can shift depending upon (a) whether movements are present or not, (b) whether movements are present for 3 months or more (6 months if on a semiannual assessment schedule), and (c) whether neuroleptic dosage changes occur and affect movements.

- **NO TD**—Movements **are not** present on this exam **or** movements are present, but some other condition is responsible for them. The last diagnosis must be NO TD, PROBABLE TD, or WITHDRAWAL TD.
- **PROBABLE TD**—Movements **are** present on this exam. This is the first time they are present, **or** they have never been present for 3 months or more. The last diagnosis must be NO TD or PROBABLE TD.

- **PERSISTENT TD**—Movements **are** present on this exam, **and** they have been present for 3 months or more with this exam or at some point in the past. The last diagnosis can be any except NO TD.
- **MASKED TD**—Movements **are not** present on this exam, **but** this is due to a neuroleptic dosage increase or reinstitution after a prior exam when movements were present. Also, use this conclusion if movements are not present due to the addition of a nonneuroleptic medication to treat TD. The last diagnosis must be PROBABLE TD, PERSISTENT TD, WITHDRAWAL TD, or MASKED TD.
- **REMITTED TD**—Movements **are not** present on this exam, **but** PERSISTENT TD has been diagnosed **and** neuroleptic dosage increase or reinstitution has occurred. The last diagnosis must be PERSISTENT TD or REMITTED TD. If movements reemerge, the diagnosis shifts back to PERSISTENT TD.
- **WITHDRAWAL TD**—Movements **are not seen while** receiving neuroleptics or at the last dosage level **but are seen within** 8 weeks following a neuroleptic reduction or discontinuation. The last diagnosis must be NO TD or WITHDRAWAL TD. If movements continue for 3 months or more after the neuroleptic dosage reduction or discontinuation, the diagnosis shifts to PERSISTENT TD. If movements do not continue for 3 months or more after the reduction or discontinuation, the diagnosis shifts to NO TD.

Instructions	Other Conditions (Partial List)
1. The rater completes the assessment according to the standardized exam procedure. If the rater also completes evaluation items 1–4, he or she must also sign the preparer box. The form is given to the physician. Alternatively, the physician may perform the assessment.	1. Age 2. Blind 3. Cerebral Palsy 4. Contact Lenses 5. Dentures/No Teeth 6. Down's Syndrome 7. Drug Intoxication (specify) 8. Encephalitis
2. The physician completes the Evaluation section. The physician is responsible for the entire Evaluation section and its accuracy.	9. Extrapyramidal Side Effects (specify) 10. Fahr's Syndrome 11. Heavy Metal Intoxication (specify) 12. Huntington's Chorea
3. It is recommended that the physician examines any individual who meets the three prerequisites or who has movements not explained by other factors. Neurologic assessments or differential diagnostic tests that may be necessary should be performed.	13. Hyperthyroidism 14. Hypoglycaemia 15. Hypoparathyroidism 16. Idiopathic Torsion Dystonia 17. Meige's Syndrome 18. Parkinson's Disease 19. Stereotypies
4. File form according to policy or procedure.	20. Sydenham's Chorea 21. Tourette's Syndrome 22. Wilson's Disease 23. Other (specify)

Source: Sprague, R. L., & Kalachnik, J. E. (1991). Reliability, validity, and a total score cutoff for the Dyskinesia Identification System Condensed User Scale (DISCUS) with mentally ill and mentally retarded populations. *Psychopharmacology Bulletin, 27*(1), 51–58.

Appendix E

Hamilton Rating Scale for Depression

Clinic No._____ Date_____ Rating No._____ Code Number_____
Sex_____ Age_____ Patient's Name_____
Patient's Address_____ Tel_____

Item	Range	Score
1. Depressed mood	0–4	
2. Guilt	0–4	
3. Suicide	0–4	
4. Insomnia initial	0–2	
5. Insomnia middle	0–2	
6. Insomnia delayed	0–2	
7. Work and interest	0–4	
8. Retardation	0–4	
9. Agitation	0–4	
10. Anxiety (psychic)	0–4	
11. Anxiety (somatic)	0–4	
12. Somatic gastrointestinal	0–2	
13. Somatic general	0–2	
14. Genital	0–2	
15. Hypochondriasis	0–2	
16. Insight	0–4	
17. Loss of weight	0–2	
	Total score	
Diurnal variation (M.A.E.)	0–2	
Depersonalization	0–4	
Paranoid symptoms	0–4	
Obsessional symptoms	0–4	

The scale is designed to measure the severity of illness of patients already diagnosed as suffering from depressive illness. It is obviously not a diagnostic instrument because that requires much more information (e.g., previous history, family history, precipitating factors).

As far as possible, the scale should be used in the manner of a clinical interview. The first time, the interview should be conducted in a relaxed, free, and easy manner, giving the patients time to unburden themselves and giving them the opportunity to speak of their problems and ask whatever questions they wish. It may then be necessary to obtain further information by asking them questions. At subsequent assessments, the interview can be briefer and more to the point.

An observer rating scale is not a checklist in which each item is strictly defined. The raters must have sufficient clinical experience and judgment to be able to interpret the patients' statements and reticence about some symptoms and to compare them with other patients. They should use all sources of information (e.g., from relatives and nurses).

The scale consists of 17 items, the scores of which are summed to give a total score. These are four other items, one of which (diurnal variation) is excluded on the grounds that it is not an additional burden on the patient. The last three are excluded from the total score because they occur infrequently, although information on them may be useful for other purposes.

The method of assessment is simple. For some symptoms, it is difficult to elicit such information as will permit full quantification. If present, score 2; if absent, score 0; and if doubtful or trivial, score 1. For those symptoms where more detailed information can be obtained, the score of 2 is expanded into 2 for mild, 3 for moderate, and 4 for severe. In case of difficulty, the raters should use their judgment as clinicians.

Source: Hamilton, M. (1960). A rating scale for depression. *Journal of Neurology, Neurosurgery and Psychiatry, 23,* 56.

Clinical Institute Withdrawal Assessment of Alcohol Scale, Revised (CIWA-Ar)

Patient: _____ Date: _____ Time: _____ (24 hour clock, midnight = 00:00)

Pulse or heart rate, taken for 1 minute: _____ Blood pressure: _____

NAUSEA AND VOMITING—Ask "Do you feel sick to your stomach? Have you vomited?" Observation.
- 0 no nausea and no vomiting
- 1 mild nausea with no vomiting
- 2
- 3
- 4 intermittent nausea with dry heaves
- 5
- 6
- 7 constant nausea; frequent dry heaves and vomiting

TREMOR—Arms extended and fingers spread apart. Observation.
- 0 no tremor
- 1 not visible, but can be felt fingertip to fingertip
- 2
- 3
- 4 moderate, with patient's arms extended
- 5
- 6
- 7 severe, even with arms not extended

PAROXYSMAL SWEATS—Observation.
- 0 no sweat visible
- 1 barely perceptible sweating, palms moist
- 2
- 3
- 4 beads of sweat obvious on forehead
- 5
- 6
- 7 drenching sweats

TACTILE DISTURBANCES—Ask "Have you any itching, pins and needles sensations, any burning, or any numbness, or do you feel bugs crawling on or under your skin?" Observation.
- 0 none
- 1 very mild itching, pins and needles, burning or numbness
- 2 mild itching, pins and needles, burning or numbness
- 3 moderate itching, pins and needles, burning or numbness
- 4 moderately severe hallucinations
- 5 severe hallucinations
- 6 extremely severe hallucinations
- 7 continuous hallucinations

AUDITORY DISTURBANCES—Ask "Are you more aware of sounds around you?" "Are they harsh?" "Do they frighten you?" "Are you hearing anything that is disturbing to you?" "Are you hearing things you know are not there?" Observation.
- 0 not present
- 1 very mild harshness or ability to frighten
- 2 mild harshness or ability to frighten
- 3 moderate harshness or ability to frighten
- 4 moderately severe hallucinations
- 5 severe hallucinations
- 6 extremely severe hallucinations
- 7 continuous hallucinations

VISUAL DISTURBANCES—Ask "Does the light appear to be too bright?" "Is its color different?" "Does it hurt your eyes?" "Are you seeing anything that is disturbing to you?" "Are you seeing things you know are not there?" Observation.
- 0 not present
- 1 very mild sensitivity
- 2 mild sensitivity
- 3 moderate sensitivity
- 4 moderately severe hallucinations
- 5 severe hallucinations
- 6 extremely severe hallucinations
- 7 continuous hallucinations

ANXIETY—Ask "Do you feel nervous?" Observation.

0 no anxiety, at ease
1 mild anxious
2
3
4 moderately anxious, or guarded, so anxiety is inferred
5
6
7 equivalent to acute panic states as seen in severe delirium or acute schizophrenic reactions

AGITATION—Observation.

0 normal activity
1 somewhat more than normal activity
2
3
4 moderately fidgety and restless
5
6
7 paces back and forth during most of the interview, or constantly thrashes about

HEADACHE, FULLNESS IN HEAD—Ask "Does your head feel different?" "Does it feel like there is a band around your head?" Do not rate for dizziness or light-headedness. Otherwise, rate severity.

0 not present
1 very mild
2 mild
3 moderate
4 moderately severe
5 severe
6 very severe
7 extremely severe

ORIENTATION AND CLOUDING OF SENSORIUM—Ask "What day is this?" "Where are you?" "Who am I?"

0 oriented and can do serial additions
1 cannot do serial additions or is uncertain about date
2 disoriented for date by no more than 2 calendar days
3 disoriented for date by more than 2 calendar days
4 disoriented for place/or person

Total **CIWA-Ar** Score _____
Rater's Initials _____
Maximum Possible Score 67

This assessment for monitoring withdrawal symptoms requires approximately 5 minutes to administer. The maximum score is 67 (see instrument). Patients scoring less than 10 do not usually need additional medication for withdrawal.

Source: Sullivan, J. T., Sykora, K., Schneiderman, J., Naranjo, C. A., & Sellers, E. M. (1989). Assessment of alcohol withdrawal: The revised Clinical Institute Withdrawal Assessment for Alcohol scale (CIWA-Ar). *British Journal of Addiction, 84*, 1353–1357.

Glossary

A

absorption: Movement of drug from the site of administration into plasma.

acetylcholine (ACh): An important neurotransmitter associated with cognitive functioning, and disruption of cholinergic mechanisms damages memory in animals and humans.

acetylcholinesterase (AChE): Key enzyme that inactivates the neurotransmitter acetylcholine. AChE is found in high concentrations in the brain and is one of two cholinesterase enzymes capable of breaking down ACh.

acetylcholinesterase inhibitors (AChEIs): Mainstay of pharmacologic treatment of dementia; these drugs inhibit AChE, resulting in an enhancement of cholinergic activity. AChEIs have been shown to delay the decline in cognitive functioning but generally do not improve cognitive function once it has declined; therefore, it is important that this medication be started as soon as the diagnosis is made.

active listening: Focusing on what the patient is saying in order to interpret and respond to the message in an objective manner, while using techniques such as open-ended statements, reflection, and questions that elicit additional responses from the patient.

acute stress disorder (ASD): A mental disorder characterized by persistent, distressing stress-related symptoms that last between 2 days and 1 month and that occur within 1 month after a traumatic experience.

adaptability: Capacity of a person to survive and flourish.

adaptive inflexibility: Rigidity in interactions with others, achievement of goals, and coping with stress.

addiction: A chronic, relapsing, and treatable brain disorder that results from the prolonged effects of exposure of the brain to drugs (substances or chemicals).

addictive substances: There are 10 classes of addictive substances referred to in the *DSM-5*: alcohol; caffeine; cannabis (marijuana); hallucinogens (with separate categories for phencyclidine [PCP] [or similarly acting arylcyclohexylamines] and other hallucinogens); inhalants; opioids; sedatives, hypnotics, and anxiolytics; stimulants; tobacco (nicotine); and other (or unknown) substances.

adherence: A patient's maintenance of the therapeutic regimen; includes self-administering medications as prescribed, keeping appointments, and following other treatment suggestions; it exists on a continuum and can be conceived of as full, partial, or nil.

adverse reactions: Unwanted medication effects that may have serious physiologic consequences.

affect: An expression of mood manifest in a pattern of observable behaviours.

affective blunting: Flat or blunted emotion.

affective instability: Rapid and extreme shifts in mood, erratic emotional responses to situations, and intense sensitivity to criticism or perceived slights; one of the core characteristics of borderline personality disorder.

affective lability: Abrupt, dramatic, unprovoked changes in the types of emotions expressed.

afferent: Toward the central nervous system or a particular structure.

affinity: Degree of attraction or strength of the bond between a drug and its receptor.

aggression: Behaviours or attitudes that reflect rage, hostility, and the potential for physical or verbal destructiveness; usually occurs if the person believes someone is going to do him or her harm.

agitation: Inability to sit still or attend to others, accompanied by heightened emotions and tension.

agnosia: Failure to recognize or identify objects despite intact sensory function, or a disturbance in executive functioning (ability to think abstractly, plan, initiate, sequence, monitor, and stop complex behaviour).

agonists: Chemicals producing the same biologic action as the neurotransmitter.

agoraphobia: Anxiety about being in places from which escape might be difficult or embarrassing, or about being in places in which help may not be readily available if a panic attack should occur.

akathisia: A medication-related, involuntary movement disorder characterized by the inability to sit still; may be experienced as "jitteriness" without obvious motor behaviour.

alexithymia: Inability to experience and communicate feelings consciously.

allodynia: Lowered pain threshold.

allostasis: Adaptive processes that maintain homeostasis through the production of various brain and peripheral stress-related chemicals and promote adaptation to perceived threat or stress.

alogia: Brief, empty verbal responses; often referred to as *poverty of speech*.

ambivalence: Presence and expression of two opposing forces, leading to inaction.

amino acids: Building blocks of proteins that have different roles. Amino acids function as neurotransmitters in as many as 60% to 70% of synaptic sites in the brain.

amygdala: A bulb-like structure attached to the tail of the caudate and often considered part of the limbic system.

anger: An affective state experienced as the motivation to act in ways that warn, intimidate, or attack those who are perceived as challenging or threatening.

anhedonia: Inability to gain pleasure from activities.

anorexia nervosa: A life-threatening eating disorder characterized by refusal to maintain body weight appropriate for age, intense fear of gaining weight or becoming fat, a severely distorted body image, and refusal to acknowledge the seriousness of weight loss.

antagonists: Chemicals blocking the biologic response at a given receptor site.

anticholinergic crisis: A potentially life-threatening medical emergency that occurs as a result of overdose or sensitivity to drugs with anticholinergic properties.

anxiety: Apprehension or dread in response to internal or external stimuli perceived to be a threat that can be experienced in physical, emotional, cognitive, and/or behavioural ways.

anxiolytics: Drugs that reverse or diminish anxiety.

apathy: Reactions to stimuli that are decreased, along with a diminished interest and desire.

aphasia: Alterations in language ability.

apraxia: Impaired ability to execute motor activities despite intact motor functioning.

assertiveness: A set of behaviours and a communication style that is open, honest, direct, and confident that enables the expression of emotions, including anger, in a manner that assumes responsibility.

assessment: A purposeful, systematic, and dynamic process in the nurse's relationship with individuals in his or her care. It involves the collection, validation, analysis, synthesis, organization, and documentation of client health–illness information.

attachment: Emotional bond between the infant and parental figure.

attention: A complex mental process that involves the ability to concentrate on one activity to the exclusion of others, as well as the ability to sustain focus.

attention deficit hyperactivity disorder (ADHD): Neurodevelopmental disorder of childhood. Core symptoms include inattention, hyperactivity and impulsivity.

autism spectrum disorder: A neurodevelopmental disorder that is distinguished by a marked impairment of development in social interaction and communication with a restrictive repertoire of repetitive activity and interest.

automatic thoughts: Spontaneous words and images generated in a particular situation that may be illogical and/or difficult to stop.

autonomic nervous system: Part of the nervous system that regulates involuntary vital functions including cardiac muscle, smooth muscles, and glands. It is composed of the sympathetic and parasympathetic systems.

autonomy: Concept that each person has the fundamental right of self-determination.

avolition: Inability to complete projects, assignments, or work.

B

basal ganglia: One set of structures in each hemisphere; areas of grey matter containing many cell bodies or nuclei.

behaviour modification: A specific, systematized behaviour therapy technique that can be applied to individuals, groups, or systems.

behaviour therapy: Interventions that reinforce or promote desirable behaviours or alter undesirable ones.

behaviourism: A paradigm shift in understanding human behaviour that was initiated by Watson, who theorized that human behaviour is developed through a stimulus–response process rather than through unconscious drives or instincts.

beneficence: The ethical principle of "try to do good"; promote benefit.

bereavement: The objective event or occurrence of having suffered a loss.

best practice guidelines (BPGs): Broad or specific recommendations for health care based on the best current evidence.

bibliotherapy: The use of books and other reading materials to help individuals cope with various life stressors.

binge eating: Episodes of uncontrollable, ravenous eating of large amounts of food within discrete periods of time, usually followed by feelings of guilt that result in purging.

binge eating disorder: Binge eating disorder is a clinical eating disorder characterized by frequent consumption of very large amounts of food, coupled with feelings of being out of control, ashamed and disgusted by the eating behaviour, and experiencing high body dissatisfaction. As an eating disorder, it is more common than anorexia nervosa and bulimia nervosa.

bioavailability: The amount of the drug that actually reaches systemic circulation; affected significantly by the route by which a drug is administered.

biogenic amines: Small molecules manufactured in the neuron that contain an amine group. These include dopamine, norepinephrine, and epinephrine (all synthesized from the amino acid tyrosine); serotonin (from tryptophan); and histamine (from histidine).

biologic markers: Physical indicators of disturbances within the central nervous system that differentiate one disease state from another.

bio/psycho/social/spiritual geriatric mental health nursing assessment: The comprehensive, deliberate, and systematic collection and interpretation of bio/psycho/social/spiritual data that are based on the special needs and problems of older adults to determine current and past health, functional status, and human responses to mental health problems, both actual and potential.

bio/psycho/social/spiritual model: Consists of separate but interacting domains that can be understood independently but that are mutually interdependent with the other domains.

biotransformation (metabolism): The process by which a drug is altered, often broken down into smaller substances known as *metabolites*.

body dissatisfaction: The belief that one's current body size differs from a highly valued ideal body size and that this difference deserves negative appraisal and may be expressed through comments including "I feel too fat/too gross."

body image: Self-perception of one's body. Extreme discrepancy between body image and others' perceptions of one's body indicates a *body image distortion*.

body image distortion: When the individual perceives his or her body disparately from how the world or society views it.

boundaries: The defining limits of individuals, objects, or relationships.

boundary violation: Behaviour by a professional that has violated the limits (what is and is not permitted) in a professional–client relationship.

bradykinesia: An extrapyramidal condition characterized by a slowness of voluntary movement and speech.

brainstem: Area of the brain containing the midbrain, pons, and medulla, which continues beneath the thalamus.

breach of confidentiality: Release of patient information without the patient's consent in the absence of legal compulsion or authorization to release information.

Broca's area: A section of the left frontal lobe of the brain thought to be responsible for the articulation of speech.

bulimia nervosa: An eating disorder in which the individual engages in recurrent episodes of binge eating and compensatory behaviour to avoid weight gain through purging methods such as self-induced vomiting or use of laxatives, diuretics, enemas, or emetics or through nonpurging methods such as fasting or excessive exercise.

bullying: Persistent physical or psychological harm that is intentionally inflicted on an individual who feels unable to avoid or stop the harm.

burnout: Psychological exhaustion, detachment, and loss of sense of accomplishment related to chronic work-related stress.

butyrylcholinesterase (BuChE): A nonspecific cholinesterase found in the brain and especially in the glial cells. Both acetylcholinesterase and BuChE work in the gastrointestinal tract. If these enzymes are inhibited, the breakdown of acetylcholine will be delayed, resulting in an increase in acetylcholine activity.

C

case management: Problem-solving and coordinating services for the patient to ensure continuity of services and overcome system rigidity, fragmentation of services, misuse of facilities, and inaccessibility.

catatonic excitement: Hyperactivity characterized by purposeless activity and abnormal movements like grimacing and posturing.

central sulcus: Posterior boundary of the frontal lobe that separates it from the parietal lobe.

cerebellum: Part of the brain that is responsible for controlling movement and postural adjustments; it receives information from all parts of the body.

cerebrospinal fluid: Cushioning fluid that circulates around the brain beneath the arachnoid layer in the subarachnoid space; it is colourless and contains sodium chloride and other salts.

chemical restraints: Use of medication to control patients or manage behaviour.

cholecystokinin: A neuropeptide found in high levels in the cerebral cortex, hypothalamus, and amygdala; it is also excreted by the gastrointestinal system in response to food intake, which is believed to play a role in the control of eating and satiety by controlling the release of dopamine.

chronobiology: Study and measure of time structures or biologic rhythms.

circadian rhythm (cycle): From the Latin *circa* and *dies*, meaning "about a day"; refers to a biologic system that fluctuates or oscillates in a pattern that repeats itself in about a day.

circumstantiality: Occurs when an individual takes a long time to make a point because his or her conversation is indirect and contains excessive and unnecessary detail.

clang association: Repetition of word phrases that are similar in sound but in no other way, for example, "right, light, sight, might."

classical conditioning: A learning situation in which an unconditioned stimulus initially produces an unconditioned response; over time, a conditioned response is elicited for a specific stimulus (Pavlov).

clearance: Total amount of blood, serum, or plasma from which a drug is completely removed per unit of time.

clinical domain outcome statements: Statements that indicate a reduction in symptoms of illness or cure of a specific mental illness.

closed group: A group in which all the members begin at one time. New members are not admitted after the first meeting.

cognition: A system of multiple brain processes, such as perception, reasoning, judgment, intuition, and memory, that allow one to be aware of oneself and one's surroundings.

cognitive restructuring: A process in which cognitions (automatic thoughts, intermediate and core beliefs) are identified, analyzed, and modified to effect positive change in mood and behaviour.

cognitive schema (core beliefs): Basic beliefs so fundamental that they are accepted as absolute truths; assist in evaluating and assigning meaning to events and influence subsequent affective and behavioural responses.

cognitive–behavioural model: A model of perception that includes emotion, cognition, environment, and physical and psychological factors.

cognitive–behavioural therapy: Psychotherapy focused on identifying, analyzing, and ultimately changing the habitually inflexible and negative cognitions about oneself, others, and the world that contribute to distress and problematic behaviours.

collaborative mental health care: Care that is provided from different specialties, disciplines, or sectors that work together to offer complementary services and mutual support.

collaboration: The process of working together toward common goals; client-centred care.

collective trauma: When a traumatic event is experienced by a significant proportion of a given social group; it can have long-term consequences for the social group beyond its additive effect on individuals such that social norms, dynamics, functioning, and structure of the group may be modified.

communication triad: A technique used to provide a specific syntax and order for patients to identify and express their feelings and seek relief. The "sentence" consists of three parts: (1) an "I" statement to identify the prevailing feeling, (2) a nonjudgmental statement of the emotional trigger, and (3) a statement of what the person would like differently or what would restore comfort to the situation.

community treatment orders (CTOs): A type of mandatory outpatient treatment, usually initiated by a physician, that can require an individual with a mental illness who does not meet provincial involuntary admission criteria to comply with stipulated treatment.

comorbidity (comorbid): Disease that coexists with the primary disease.

compassion fatigue: Disengagement on the part of caregiving professionals; frequently equated with burnout.

compassionate release: *Parole by exception* for incarcerated offenders, allowed under the Corrections and Conditional Release Act, and considered on an individual basis (e.g., for palliative care due to a terminal illness).

competence: The degree to which the patient is able to understand and appreciate the information given during the consent process; the patient's cognitive ability to process information at a specific time; the patient's ability to gather and interpret information and make reasonable judgments based on that information to participate fully as a partner in treatment.

competency: Capability of acting appropriately and effectively in a role. It involves the use of internal resources (e.g., knowledge, skills, attitudes) and external resources (e.g., policies, the interprofessional team, research).

comprehensive family assessment: Collection of all relevant data related to family health, psychological well-being, and social functioning to identify problems for which the nurse can generate solutions with the family and enhance family strengths.

compulsions: Behaviours that are performed repeatedly, in a ritualistic fashion, with the goal of preventing or relieving anxiety and distress caused by obsessions.

concordant: Used in genetics to indicate that both members of twins have the same trait.

concrete thinking: Lack of abstraction in thinking, in which people are unable to understand punch lines, metaphors, and analogies.

concurrent disorders: The term used when an individual has at least one substance-related or addictive disorder co-occurring with at least one other mental disorder.

confabulation: False memories, perceptions, or beliefs that are the consequence of neurologic dysfunction or damage.

confidentiality: An ethical duty of nondisclosure; the patient has the right to disclose personal information without fear of it being revealed to others.

conflict resolution: A specific type of counselling in which the nurse helps the patient resolve a disagreement or dispute.

content themes: Repetition of concerns or feelings that occur within the therapeutic relationship. Themes may emerge as symbolic representations of fears.

continuum of care: Is a comprehensive system of services and programs spanning the range from mental health promotion and illness prevention to very specialized services designed to match the needs of the individuals and populations with the appropriate care and treatment, which vary according to levels of service, structure, and intensity of care.

coping: An individual's constantly changing cognitive and behavioural efforts to manage specific external or internal demands that are appraised as taxing or exceeding the individual's resources.

corpus callosum: Functional link between the two hemispheres of the brain, made up of a thick band of fibres.

cortex: Outer surface of the mature brain.

cortical dementia: A type of dementia that is characterized by amnesia, aphasia, apraxia, and agnosia.

counselling interventions: Specific time-limited interactions between a nurse and a patient, family, or group experiencing intermediate or ongoing difficulties related to their health or well-being.

countertransference: The nurse's reactions to a patient that are based on the nurse's unconscious needs, conflicts, problems, and views of the world. It can significantly interfere with the nurse–patient relationship.

criminalization of persons with mental illness: When persons with an untreated mental illness contravene the law and enter the justice system rather than the health care system.

crisis: A severely stressful experience for which coping mechanisms fail to provide any adaptation, whether the experience is positive or negative.

crisis intervention: A specialized short-term (usually no longer than 6 hours) goal-directed therapy designed to assist patients in an immediate manner, after which they are usually transferred to an inpatient unit or an intensive outpatient setting.

crisis response: Occurs when an individual encounters an obstacle or problem important to life goals that cannot be solved by customary problem-solving methods; acute, time limited, and may be developmental, situational, or interpersonal in nature.

cultural brokering: Act of bridging, linking, or mediating between groups or individuals of different cultural systems for the purpose of reducing conflict or producing change.

cultural competence: The ability to give care and services appropriate to the cultural characteristics of the person, family, or community receiving them.

cultural safety: Composed of the components of cultural awareness, cultural sensitivity, and cultural competence, cultural safety grows from an analysis of power imbalances and institutional discrimination that are related to health and health care, in order that the root causes of health inequities can be addressed.

culture: A way of life that is the totality of learned values, beliefs, norms, and way of life that influence an individual's thinking, decisions, and actions in certain ways.

custody and caring: Nurses in forensic settings must meet the competing demands of custody (confinement and security) and caring (nursing care).

cycle of violence: A three-phase pattern of tension, abuse, and remorse in which the abuser experiences tension and engages first in abuse and then in seemingly sincere expressions of love, contrition, and remorse.

cyclothymic: A term used to describe periods of hypomanic and depressive episodes that do not meet full criteria for a major depressive episode.

D

de-escalation: An interactive process of calming and redirecting a patient who has an immediate potential for violence directed at others or self.

defence mechanisms: Coping styles; the automatic psychological process protecting the individual against anxiety and creating awareness of internal or external dangers or stressors.

defining characteristics: Key signs and symptoms that relate to each other and inform a nursing diagnosis.

deinstitutionalization: Downsizing or elimination of psychiatric hospitals with a new orientation to community-based services.

delirium: A temporary disorder of physical origin with an abrupt onset characterized by fluctuating consciousness and attention.

delirium tremens: An acute syndrome related to alcohol withdrawal that is characterized by gross tremulousness, disorientation, delusions, hallucinations (auditory, visual or tactile), tachycardia, sweating, hypertension, irregular tremor, and severely agitated behaviour.

delusion: A false, fixed belief, based on an incorrect inference about reality, not shared by others, inconsistent with the individual's intelligence or cultural background and which cannot be corrected by reasoning.

delusional disorder: A disorder in which there is the presence of nonbizarre delusions; includes several subtypes: erotomania, grandiose, jealous, somatic, mixed, and specified.

dementia: A state characterized by chronic, progressive neurocognitive impairment and is differentiated by affected areas in the brain, by underlying cause, and by symptom patterns.

denial: Refusal to acknowledge some painful aspect of external reality or subjective experience that would be apparent to others. *Psychotic denial* is when there is gross impairment in reality testing.

deontology: The approach to ethics that sets duty or obligation as the basis of doing right.

depersonalization: A nonspecific experience in which the individual loses a sense of personal identity and feels strange or unreal.

depressive episode: In a major depressive episode, either a depressed mood or a loss of interest or pleasure in nearly all activities must be present for at least 2 weeks. Four of seven additional symptoms must be present: disruption in sleep, appetite (or weight), concentration, energy; psychomotor agitation or retardation; excessive guilt or feelings of worthlessness; and suicidal ideation.

desensitization: A rapid decrease in drug effects that may develop within a few minutes or over a period of days, months, years, or lifetime of exposure to a drug.

detoxification: Process of safely and effectively withdrawing a person from an addictive substance, usually under medical supervision.

developmental delay: The development of a child that is outside the norm, including delayed socialization, communication, peculiar mannerisms, and idiosyncratic interests.

diagnosis-specific outcomes: Outcomes based on nursing diagnoses.

dialectical behaviour therapy (DBT): An important approach to treatment that combines numerous cognitive and behaviour therapy strategies. It requires patients to understand their disorder by actively participating in formulating treatment goals by collecting data about their own behaviour, identifying treatment targets in individual therapy, and working with the therapists in changing these target behaviours.

diathesis: Constitutional predisposition or vulnerability to a disorder.

dichotomous thinking: Tendency to view things as absolute, either black or white, good or bad, with no perception of compromise.

dietary restraint: A cognitive effort to restrict food intake for the purpose of weight loss or the prevention of weight gain.

disaster: A social phenomenon that occurs when a hazard, originating in the geophysical or biologic environment or as the result of unintentional or malicious human action, exceeds a community's ability to cope.

discrimination: The negative differential treatment of others because they are members of a particular group.

disinhibition: A concept borrowed from physics and biology and based on the idea of a dynamic, self-regulatory model of equilibrium in which equilibrium is defined (Piaget) as compensation for external disturbance; a mechanism for providing the self-regulation by which intelligence adapts to internal and external changes.

disordered water balance: A state of chronic fluid imbalance, vacillating between normal and hyponatraemic, that commonly occurs in psychiatric patients with chronic illnesses.

disorganized symptoms: Symptoms of schizophrenia that make it difficult for the person to understand and respond to the ordinary sights and sounds of daily living; include *confused speech and thinking* and *disorganized behaviour*.

dissociation: A disruption in the normally occurring linkages among subjective awareness, feelings, thoughts, behaviour, and memories.

dissociative identity disorder (DID): A mental disorder characterized by the existence of two or more distinct identities with unique personality characteristics and the inability to recall important information about oneself or events.

distraction: The purposeful focusing of attention away from undesirable sensations.

distribution: The amount of a drug that may be found in various tissues at the site of the drug action for which it is intended.

disturbances of executive functioning: Problems in the ability to think abstractly, plan, initiate, sequence, monitor, and stop complex behaviour.

diversity: The variation among people in terms of factors such as ethnicity, natural origin, race, gender identity, gender expression, ability, age, physical characteristics, religion, values and beliefs, sexual orientation, socioeconomic class or life experiences.

drive for thinness: An intense physical and emotional process that overrides all physiologic body cues.

dual diagnosis: Presence of both substance-related disorder and mental illness.

dyad: A group of only two people who are usually related, such as a married couple, siblings, or parent and child.

dynamic security: Security awareness that is concerned with institutional policies, staffing patterns, methods of operation, and relational security.

dysfunctional family: A family whose interactions, decisions, or behaviours interfere with the positive development of the family and its individual members.

dyslexia: Significantly lower score for mental age on standardized test in reading that is not due to low intelligence or inadequate schooling.

dysphagia: Difficulty swallowing.

dysthymic disorder: A milder but more chronic form of major depressive disorder.

dystonia: An impairment in muscle tone that is generally the first extrapyramidal symptom to occur, usually within a few days of initiating an antipsychotic. Dystonia is characterized by involuntary muscle spasms, especially of the head and neck muscles.

E

echolalia: Parrot-like repetition of another's words; inappropriate choice of topics.

echopraxia: Involuntary imitation of another person's movements and gestures; regressed behaviour that is child-like or immature.

efferent: Away from the central nervous system or other particular structure.

efficacy: Ability of a drug to produce a response as a result of the receptor or receptors being occupied.

egocentrism: Tendency to view the world as revolving around oneself.

emotion: The psychophysiologic reaction that shapes the individual's experience of a feeling state.

emotional circuit: The interrelationship between the emotional processes of the limbic system and the neurocognitive processes of the frontal lobe and other parts of the cortex. It is hypothesized that the functioning of this system determines the meaning a person gives to a particular situation.

emotional dysregulation: Inability to control emotion in social interactions.

emotional vulnerability: Sensitivity and reactivity to environmental stress.

emotion-focused coping: Coping strategies directed at managing one's emotional distress (e.g., through exercise, prayer/meditation, expressing emotions, talking to friends, etc.).

empathic linkage: Ability to feel in oneself the feelings being expressed by another person or persons.

empathy: The experience of putting oneself in another person's circumstances and imagining his or her feelings.

encopresis: Soiling clothing with faeces or depositing faeces in inappropriate places.

endorphins: Neurotransmitters that have opiate-like behaviour and produce an inhibitory effect at opiate receptor sites; probably responsible for pain tolerance.

enmeshment: An extreme form of intensity in family interactions.

enuresis: Involuntary excretion of urine after the age at which a child should have attained bladder control.

epidemiology: The study of patterns of disease distribution in time and space that focuses on the health status of population groups or aggregates, rather than on individuals, and involves quantitative analysis of the occurrence of illnesses in population groups; basic science of public health.

epigenesis: A concept borrowed from embryology theory regarding the development of a plant or animal. It is also used to refer to a change in genetic expression as a result of environment influences.

episode: A period of a minimal duration of 2 weeks during which an individual experiences symptoms that meet the diagnostic criteria for that disorder.

equilibration: Compensation for external disturbances; a mechanism for providing the self-regulation by which intelligence adapts to external and internal changes (Piaget).

erotomania: The belief that someone (often a public figure) is in love with one or involved with one in a relationship when, in reality, one is a stranger to him or her.

ethics: Consideration of the way a person should act to live a good life with and for others.

ethnocentrism: The notion that one's own culturally learned ideas and values are central and correct for everyone.

excretion: The elimination of drugs from the body either unchanged or as metabolites. *Clearance* refers to the total volume of blood, serum, or plasma from which a drug is completely removed per unit of time.

exhibitionism: A behaviour associated with paraphilias involving exposing one's genitals to strangers, with occasional masturbation.

existential anxiety: The foreboding that arises from an awareness of human mortality. Also referred to as *angst*.

exposure therapy: The treatment of choice for agoraphobia that puts the patient into contact with the feared situations until the stimuli no longer produce anxiety.

expressed emotion: Family members' responses that include one or more of the following dynamics: critical comments, hostility, or emotional overinvolvement.

extended family: Several nuclear families who may or may not live together and function as one group.

externalizing disorders: Disorders that are characterized by acting-out behaviour.

extinction: Elimination of a classically conditioned response by the repeated presentation of the conditioned stimulus without the unconditioned stimulus or elimination of an operantly conditioned response by no longer presenting the reward after the response.

extrapyramidal motor system: Collection of neuronal pathways that provides significant input in involuntary motor movements.

F

factitious disorder: A type of psychiatric disorder characterized by somatization, in which the person intentionally causes an illness for the purpose of becoming a patient.

factitious disorder by proxy: (Münchausen syndrome by proxy): The intentional production or feigning of physical or psychological signs or symptoms in one person by another who desires to indirectly assume the sick role.

family: A group of people who are committed to each other and involved relationally in a complex process where economics, emotion, context, and experiences are interwoven and multilayered.

family development: A broad term that refers to all the processes connected with the growth of a family, including changes associated with work, geographic location, migration, acculturation, and serious illness.

family dynamics: The patterned interpersonal and social interactions that occur within the family structure over the life of a family.

family life cycle: A process of expansion, contraction, and realignment of relationship systems to support the entry, exit, and development of family members.

family structure: According to Minuchin, the organized pattern within which family members interact.

15-minute family interview: An assessment/intervention framework that consists of five key components: manners, therapeutic conversations, genogram and ecomap therapeutic questions, and commending individual and family strengths.

first-pass effect: Loss of orally administered drugs prior to entering the systemic circulation due to metabolism in the gastrointestinal wall.

fissures: The grooves of the cerebrum.

flight of ideas: Repeated and rapid changes in the topic of conversation, generally within just one sentence or phrase.

flooding: A type of therapy for agoraphobia in which highly anxiety-provoking stimuli are presented to the patient in vivo or with imagery, with no relaxation until the anxiety dissipates.

foetal alcohol syndrome: A group of noncurable growth, mental, and physical problems that may occur in a baby when a mother ingests alcohol during pregnancy.

forensic nursing: Nursing practice in which psychiatric and mental health nursing philosophy and skills are integrated within a sociocultural context that includes the criminal justice system in order to provide comprehensive care to clients, families, and communities.

formal group roles: The designated leader and members of a group.

formal operations: The period of cognitive development, described by Piaget, characterized by the ability to use abstract reasoning to conceptualize and solve problems.

functional activities: Activities of daily living necessary for self-care (i.e., bathing, toileting, dressing, and transferring).

functional status: Extent to which a person has the ability to carry out independent personal care, home management, and social functions in everyday life that has meaning and purpose.

G

gate-control model: Pain response based on the model that pain perception involves pathways in the dorsal horn of the spinal column that relay noxious stimuli to the brain and that certain other nerve fibres function as an antagonistic "gate" to augment or dampen the subjective experience of pain.

gender role: How one functions and behaves as a male or a female in relation to others in society, also referred to as *sex role identity.*

genogram: A multigenerational schematic diagram that lists family members and their relationships.

genome: The complete set of human genes.

genomics: The study of the complete DNA structure or genome.

gerotranscendence: A psychosocial theory of aging that regards aging as the final stage in a natural progression toward maturation and wisdom that generally results in increased satisfaction and meaning in life.

glia (white matter): A fatty or lipid substance with a white appearance that surrounds the pathways of the cell body axons.

grey matter: The cortex, with its grey-brown colour due to the capillary blood vessels.

grief: The subjective experience (e.g., thoughts, feelings, behaviours, and body sensations) that accompanies the perception of a loss.

group: An open or closed social system with structures, norms, and customary ways of acting.

group cohesion: Forces that act on the members to stay in a group.

group dynamics: Interactions within groups.

group process: The "what is happening" in the group; how members are interacting and relating as individuals and as a whole group, including nonverbal communications.

groupthink: The tendency of many groups to avoid conflict and adopt a normative pattern of thinking that is often consistent with the group leader's ideas.

guided imagery: The purposeful use of imagination to achieve relaxation or direct attention away from undesirable sensations; especially useful in stress management.

gyri: Bumps and convolutions in the brain.

H

half-life: The time required for plasma concentrations of a drug to be reduced by 50%.

hallucinations: Perceptual experiences that occur in the absence of actual external sensory stimuli and may be auditory, visual, tactile, gustatory, or olfactory.

hallucinogen: A class of drug that produces euphoria or dysphoria, altered body image, distorted or sharpened visual and auditory perception, confusion, uncoordination, and impaired judgment and memory.

hallucinogen persisting perception disorder: A transient and intermittent disorder associated with the long-term use of hallucinogens; includes depression, prolonged psychosis, and flashbacks.

harm reduction: A community health intervention designed to reduce the harm (consequences) of substance use to the individual, the family, and society by reducing the risk for adverse consequences arising from substance use without necessarily reducing its use.

helplessness: The perception of having limited ability or ambition to change one's current life situation; characterized by a sense of being unable to help oneself and a sense that there is a lack of support or protection.

hippocampus: Subcortical grey matter embedded within each temporal lobe that may be involved in determining the best way to store information or memory; "time-dating" memory.

historical trauma: The process by which a social group is affected by the consequences of multiple, collectively experienced adversities across time that outweigh group resiliency factors, become cumulative, and are carried forward to subsequent generations such that the trauma may be considered as part of a single trajectory.

HIV-1-associated cognitive–motor complex: Neurologic complications that occur with HIV-1 that are directly attributable to infection of the brain and include impaired cognitive and motor function.

home visits: Delivery of nursing care in a patient's living environment.

homeostasis: The body's ability to maintain a stable internal environment despite changing environmental conditions.

hopelessness: A perception of having no hope that one's life situation or circumstance will change or improve; characterized by feelings of inadequacy and an inability to act on one's own behalf.

hyperactivity: Excessive motor activity, movement, and/or utterances that may be either purposeless or aimless.

hyperalgia: Increased nociceptor sensitivity.

hyperesthesia: Increased sensation of pain.

hypervigilance: Sustained attention to external stimuli as if expecting something important or frightening to happen.

hypofrontality: Reduced cerebral blood flow and glucose metabolism in the prefrontal cortex of people with schizophrenia.

hypomanic episode: Mildly dysphoric mood that meets the same criteria as for a manic episode except that it lasts at least 4 days rather than 1 week and no marked impairment in social or occupational functioning is present.

hyponatraemia: Decreased sodium concentration in the blood.

hypothalamic–pituitary–adrenal (HPA) axis: Neurotransmitters responsible for behavioural responses to fear and anxiety that are usually held in balance until information from the sensory processing areas in the thalamus and cortex alerts the amygdala. If events are interpreted as threatening, this axis is activated, initiating the stress response.

hypothalamus: Immediately ventral and slightly anterior to the thalamus, forming the floor and part of the walls of the third ventricle.

I

ideas of reference: False belief that other people, objects, and events are related to or have a special significance for oneself (e.g., a person on television is sending one signals).

identity: An integration of a person's social and occupational roles and affiliations, self-attributed personality traits, attitudes about gender roles, beliefs about sexuality and intimacy, long-term goals, political ideology, and religious beliefs.

identity diffusion: Occurs when parts of a person's identity are absent or poorly developed; a lack of consistent sense of identity.

illogical thinking: A thinking error that occurs when a person draws a faulty conclusion; for example, a university student equates failure on an examination with loss of future career.

illusions: Disorganized perceptions that create an oversensitivity to colours, shapes, and background activities, which occur when the person misperceives or exaggerates stimuli in the external environment.

impulsiveness: Acting in the moment without considering the consequences of the act, which may be potentially highly harmful, and without considering alternative actions.

incidence: A rate that includes only new cases that have occurred within a clearly defined time period.

indicators: Representation of the dimension of outcome; data or information to answer the question of how close the patient is coming toward an outcome.

individual roles: Group roles that either enhance or detract from the group's functioning but have nothing to do with either the group task or maintenance.

individual treatment plan: A plan of care that identifies the patient's problems, outcomes, interventions, the individuals assigned to implement interventions, and evaluation criteria.

informal group roles: Positions in the group with rights and duties directed toward other group members. These positions are not formally sanctioned.

informal support systems: Family members, friends, and neighbours who can provide care and support to the individual.

informed consent: Consent for treatment given by a competent adult after being provided the available information necessary for making an informed choice; based on the ethical principle of autonomy.

inhalants: Organic solvents, also known as volatile substances, that are central nervous system depressants and when inhaled cause euphoria, sedation, emotional lability, and impaired judgment.

inhibited grieving: Inability to fully experience and personally integrate or resolve significant traumatic events and loss.

insight: The ability of the individual to be aware of his or her own thoughts and feelings and to compare them with the thoughts and feelings of others.

interoceptive awareness: The sensory response to emotional and visceral cues, such as hunger.

insomnia: Inability to fall or remain asleep throughout the night.

instrumental activities: Activities that facilitate or enhance the performance of activities of daily living (e.g., shopping, using the telephone, transportation). These aspects are critical to consider for any older adult living alone.

interdisciplinary approach: Interventions from different disciplines integrated into the delivery of patient care.

interdisciplinary treatment plan: A plan of care that identifies the patient's problems, outcomes, interventions, members of different disciplines assigned to implement interventions, and evaluation criteria.

intermediate beliefs: Attitudes, rules or expectations, and assumptions that influence one's perceptions, affect, and behaviours; often take the form of "should" statements that are rigid and unrealistic.

internalizing disorders: Anxiety disorders and depression in which the symptoms tend to be within the individual.

interoceptive awareness: Term used to describe the sensory response to emotional and visceral cues, such as hunger.

intrinsic activity: The ability of a drug to produce a biologic response when it becomes attached to its receptor.

invalidating environment: A highly personal social situation that negates the individual's emotional responses and communication.

invincibility fable: The egocentric phenomenon seen in adolescence where the individual views his or herself as unique, invulnerable, and immune to death.

ischaemic cascade: Cell breakdown resulting from brain cell injury.

J

judgment: The ability to reach a logical decision about a situation and to choose a course after looking at and analyzing various possibilities.

K

kindling: Repetitive stimulation of certain tracts may facilitate conduction of impulses in the future and lead to enhancement of intense behaviours after even mild stimulation.

kleptomania: A disorder in which the patient is unable to resist the urge to steal and independently steals items that he or she could easily afford. These items are not particularly useful or wanted. The underlying issue is the act of stealing.

Korsakoff's syndrome: A chronic memory disorder caused by severe deficiency of thiamine. There is a profound deficit in the ability to form new memories; associated with a variable deficit in recall of old memories despite a clear sensorium. Confabulation is a key feature.

L

lability of mood: Rapid alternations of mood, usually between euphoria and irritability.

late adulthood: Three chronologic groups: *young-old* (ages 65 to 74 years), *middle-old* (ages 75 to 84 years), and *old-old* (age 85 years and older).

lateral ventricles: The horn-shaped first and second ventricles that are the largest of the brain's ventricles.

learning disorder: A discrepancy between actual achievement and expected achievement that is based on a person's age and intellectual ability.

least restrictive environment: The patient has the right to treatment in an environment that restricts the exercise of free will to the least extent; an individual cannot be restricted to an institution when he or she can be successfully treated in the community.

lethality: The probability that a person will complete suicide. Lethality is determined by the seriousness of the person's intent and the likelihood that the planned method will result in death.

level of consciousness: An individual's level of arousal or wakefulness.

limbic system (limbic lobe): Structures including the septum and the fornix, as well as the amygdala, hippocampus, cingulate, parahippocampal gyrus, epithalamus, portions of the basal ganglia, parolfactory area, and the anterior nucleus of the thalamus.

longitudinal fissure: The longest and deepest groove of the cerebrum, separating the right and left hemispheres.

loose associations: Absence of the normal connectedness of thoughts and ideas; sudden shifts without apparent relationship to preceding topic.

M

magical thinking: The belief that one's thought, words, or actions have the power to cause or prevent things happening; similar to Piaget's preoperational thinking in young children.

maintenance function: A term used to describe the informal role of group members that encourages the group to stay together.

malingering: The production of illness symptoms intentionally with an obvious self-serving goal such as being classified as disabled and avoiding work.

mandatory outpatient treatment (MOT): Legal provisions that can require an individual with a mental illness to comply with a treatment plan while living in the community.

mania: A state characterized by an abnormally and persistently elevated, expansive, or irritable mood and grandiose ideas of self-importance.

manic episode: A distinct period during which there is an abnormally and persistently elevated, expansive, or irritable mood.

manipulation: Influencing others or a situation for one's own benefit.

maturation: The process of completing a state of development; a ripening.

maturity fears: The feeling of being overwhelmed by adult responsibilities. Starvation is viewed as a response to these fears.

memory: A facet of cognition concerned with retaining and recalling past experiences, whether they occurred in the physical environment or internally as cognitive events.

meningeal layer: The inner layer of dura mater that becomes continuous with the spinal dura mater and sends extensions into the brain for support and protection of the different lobes or structures.

mental disorder: A health condition characterized by alterations in a variety of factors that include mood and affect, behaviour, thinking, and cognition.

mental health: A state of well-being in which the individual realizes self-potential, copes with life stresses, and is able to work productively and contribute to his or her society.

mental health act: A law that gives certain powers and sets the conditions (including time limits) for those powers, to stipulated health care professionals and designated institutions regarding the admission and treatment of individuals with a mental disorder.

mental health problem: A term used when signs and symptoms of mental illnesses occur but do not meet specified criteria for a disorder.

mental illness: A term used to mean all diagnosable mental disorders.

mental status examination: Systematic assessment of an individual's appearance, affect, behaviour, and cognitive processes, reflecting the examiner's observations and used in clinical settings to evaluate developmental, neurologic, and psychiatric disorders.

mesocortical: Medial aspects of the cortex.

metabolism: Biotransformation, or the process by which a drug is altered.

milieu therapy: An approach using the total environment to provide a therapeutic community; a therapeutic environment.

misidentification: Delusions in which the person believes that a familiar person is replaced by an impostor.

mixed episode: Irritability or excitement and depression occurring at the same time.

mobbing: Occurs when several people gang up and bully an individual.

mood: A pervasive, sustained emotion that influences one's perception of the world and can be described as *euthymic* (normal), *euphoric* (elated), or dysphoric (depressed, disquieted, restless). Normal variations in mood (e.g., sadness, euphoria, anxiety) occur as responses to specific life experiences, are time limited, and are not associated with significant functional impairment.

mood disorder: Recurrent disturbances or alterations in mood that cause psychological distress and behavioural impairment.

moral agent: A person engaged in determining or expressing a moral (ethical) choice.

moral dilemma: The need to make a morally relevant choice between conflicting options.

moral distress: An embodied response that occurs when one acknowledges an ethical obligation, makes a moral choice regarding fitting ethical action, but is then unable to act on this moral choice because of internal or external constraints.

moral treatment: An approach to curing mental illness, popular in the 1800s, which was built on the principles of kindness, compassion, and a pleasant environment.

motivational interviewing (MI; motivational enhancement therapy): A directive, client-centred style of psychotherapy that helps clients to explore and resolve their ambivalence about changing.

mourning: The external manifestation of grief, which is highly influenced by gender, ethnicity, culture, religion, and the cause of death.

multiaxial diagnostic system: A diagnostic structure that includes more than one domain of information, such as the psychiatric diagnoses of the *DSM-5*.

multidisciplinary approach: Several disciplines providing services to a patient at one time.

multigenerational transmission process: The transmission of emotional processes from one generation to the next.

music therapy: The controlled use of music to promote physiologic or psychological well-being.

myoclonus: Twitching or clonic spasms of a muscle group.

myoglobinuria: The presence of myohaemoglobin in the urine due to sustained muscular rigidity and necrosis.

N

negative symptoms: Symptoms of schizophrenia that reflect a lessening or loss of normal functions, such as restriction or flattening in the range and intensity of emotion (*affective flattening* or *blunting*); reduced fluency and productivity of thought and speech (*alogia*); withdrawal and inability to initiate and persist in goal-directed activity (*avolition*); and inability to experience pleasure (*anhedonia*).

neglect: Failure to protect from injury or to provide for the physical, psychological, and medical needs of a child or dependent elder.

neologisms: Words that are made up that have no common meaning and are not recognized.

neuritic plaques: Extracellular lesions consisting of β-amyloid protein and apolipoprotein A (apoA) cores that form in the nucleus basalis of Meynert, gradually increase in number, and are abnormally distributed throughout the cholinergic system.

neurocognitive impairment: Includes short- and long-term memory, vigilance or sustained attention, verbal fluency or the ability to generate new words, and executive functioning, which includes volition, planning, purposive action, and self-monitoring behaviour.

neurofibrillary tangles: Fibrous proteins, or *tau proteins*, that are chemically altered and twisted together and spread throughout the brain, interfering with nerve functioning in cholinergic neurons. It is hypothesized that formation of these neurofibrillary tangles are related to the apolipoprotein E_4 (apoE_4).

neurohormones: Hormones produced by cells within the nervous system, such as antidiuretic hormone (ADH).

neuroleptic malignant syndrome: A syndrome caused by neuroleptic medications that are dopamine receptor blockers. The classic signs and symptoms include hyperthermia, lead-pipe rigidity, changes in mental status, and autonomic nervous system changes.

neuropeptides: Short chains of amino acids that exist in the central nervous system and have a number of important roles, including as neurotransmitters, neuromodulators, or neurohormones.

neurotransmitters: Chemicals circulating in the synaptic areas of neurons that initiate, block, or modulate nerve signal transmission and ultimately control neural function.

nihilism: A psychiatric term for the belief that one is dead or nonexistent.

nociceptive: Pertaining to a neural receptor for painful stimuli.

nonmaleficence: A principle of bioethics asserting the obligation to inflict no harm.

nonverbal communication: The gestures, expressions, and body language used in communications between the nurse and the patient.

normal aging: A life stage associated with some physical decline, such as decreased sensory abilities and decreased pulmonary and immune functions, but many important functions do not change.

normalization: Teaching individuals and families about normal development, behaviours, and responses that can be expected (e.g., child development, the grieving process).

no-self-harm contract: Written or verbal agreement between the health care professional and the patient that the patient will not engage in suicidal or other self-harming behaviour for a specific period of time.

nuclear family: Two or more people related by blood, marriage, or adoption.

nurse–client relationship: A time-limited interpersonal process with definable phases during which the client is able to consider alternative behaviours, try new health care strategies, and discuss complex health problems.

nursing diagnosis: A clinical judgment about individual, family, or community responses to actual or potential problems/life processes and involves selecting provided nursing interventions to achieve desired outcomes.

nursing intervention: Treatments or activities, based upon clinical judgment and knowledge, that are used by nurses to enhance patient or client outcomes.

nursing process: Problem-solving method used by nurses that involves assessment, planning, implementation, and evaluation.

O

object relation: The psychological attachment to another person or object.

observation: Ongoing assessment of the patient's mental and health status to identify and subvert any potential problems.

obsessions: Unwanted, intrusive, and persistent thoughts, impulses, or images that are incongruent with the person's usual thought patterns and cause significant anxiety and distress.

obsessive–compulsive disorder (OCD): A disorder characterized by intrusive thoughts that are difficult to dislodge (obsessions) and ritualized behaviours that the person feels driven to perform (compulsions).

obstructive sleep apnea: Repetitive pauses in breathing during sleep due to collapse of the upper airway; symptoms include snoring and restless sleep.

oculogyric crisis: A medication side effect resulting from an imbalance of dopamine and acetylcholine, in which the muscles that control eye movements tense and pull the eyeball so that the patient is looking toward the ceiling; may be followed by torticollis or retrocollis.

open group: A group in which new members can join at any time.

operant behaviour: A type of learning that is a consequence of a particular behavioural response, not a specific stimulus.

opiate: Any substance that binds to an opiate receptor in the brain to produce an agonist action, causing central nervous system depression, sleep or stupor, and analgesia.

orientation: An individual's ability to perceive and grasp the significance of environmental information related to time, place, and person.

orientation phase: The first phase of the nurse–patient relationship in which the nurse and the patient get to know each other. During this phase, the patient develops a sense of trust.

othering: The way one perceives and engages with another person that can be exclusionary and negative (i.e., the other is different from and thus "less than" me) or inclusionary and tolerant or accepting (i.e., the other is different from me, so I need to learn about his or her world view).

outcomes: Patient response to nursing care at a given point in time consisting of the patient's state, behaviour, or perception that is variable and can be measured.

P

panic: A normal but extreme overwhelming form of anxiety often experienced when an individual is placed in a real or perceived life-threatening situation.

panic attacks: Discrete periods of intense fear or discomfort that are accompanied by significant somatic or cognitive symptoms.

panic control treatment: Systematic structured exposure to panic-invoking sensations such as dizziness, hyperventilation, tightness in chest, and sweating.

panicogenic: Substances that produce panic attacks.

paranoia: Suspiciousness and guardedness that is unrealistic and often accompanied by grandiosity.

parasomnia: Disorders of abnormal physiologic or behavioural events that occur in relationship to sleep, specific sleep stages, or during transition from sleep to wakefulness.

parasuicidal behaviours: Deliberate acts of self-injury.

parieto-occipital sulcus: Separates the occipital lobe from the parietal lobe.

passive listening: A nontherapeutic mode of interaction that involves sitting quietly and allowing the patient to talk without focusing on guiding the thought process; includes body language that communicates boredom, indifference, or hostility.

perceptions: The awareness reached as a result of sensory inputs of real stimuli that are usually altered.

persecutory delusions: Delusions in which the person believes that he or she is being conspired against, cheated, spied on, followed, poisoned, drugged, maligned, harassed, or obstructed in the pursuit of long-term goals.

person- and family-centred care: An approach to the planning, provision, and evaluation of health care that is focused on persons and their families and grounded in respect for their autonomy, recognition of their vulnerability, and support of their right to be partners in decision-making.

personal fable: Egocentric thinking in adolescence characterized by the belief that one is unique and invulnerable to harm, manifesting in risk-taking behaviours.

personality: A complex pattern of characteristics, predominately outside the person's awareness, that compose a person's distinctive pattern of perceiving, feeling, thinking, and behaving.

personality disorder: An enduring pattern of inner experience and behaviour that deviates markedly from the expectations of the individual's culture; is pervasive and inflexible; has an onset in adolescence or early adulthood; is stable over time; and leads to distress or impairment.

personality traits: Prominent aspects of personality that are exhibited in a wide range of important social and personal contexts.

person–environment relationship: The interaction between the individual and the environment that changes throughout the stress experience.

pet therapy: The therapeutic use of animals as pets to promote physical, psychological, or social well-being.

pharmacodynamics: The study of the biologic actions of drugs on living tissue and the human body in general.

pharmacogenomics: The science of pharmacology combined with genetic knowledge.

pharmacokinetics: The study of how the human body processes a drug, including absorption, distribution, metabolism, and elimination.

phobia: Persistent, unrealistic fear of situations, objects, or activities that often leads to avoidance behaviours.

phototherapy: Also known as *light therapy*; involves exposing the patient to an artificial light source during winter months to relieve seasonal depression.

physical restraints: The application of wrist, leg, and body straps made of leather or cloth for the purpose of controlling or managing behaviour.

pia mater: The third layer of the central nervous system, in Latin, "soft mother."

pineal body: Located in the epithalamus; contains secretory cells that emit the neurohormone melatonin (as well as other substances), which has been associated with sleep and emotional disorders and modulation of immune function.

plasticity: The ability of the brain to change its structure and function in response to internal and external pressures.

point prevalence: Basic measure that refers to the proportion of individuals in a population who have a particular disorder at a specified point in time.

polydipsia: Excessive thirst that can be chronic in patients with severe mental illness.

polypharmacy: Use of several different medications at one time.

polysomnography: A special procedure that involves the recording of the electroencephalogram throughout the night. This procedure is usually conducted in a sleep laboratory.

polyuria: Excessive excretion of urine.

positive self-talk: Countering fearful or negative thoughts by using preplanned and rehearsed positive coping statements.

positive symptoms: Symptoms of schizophrenia that reflect an excess or distortion of normal functions, including delusions and hallucinations.

posttraumatic stress disorder: A mental disorder characterized by persistent, distressing symptoms lasting longer than 1 month after exposure to an extreme traumatic stressor.

poverty: The state when sufficient income and access to essential goods and services, housing, and employment required to meet the necessities of life relative to one's society are missing.

powerlessness: The perception of having no power or control over one's life circumstance; feeling that the world will never be fair; feeling helpless and totally ineffectual; or feeling one lacks legal or other authority.

prejudice: The preconceived, unreasonable judgment of others, usually negative, based solely on their membership in a particular group.

pressured speech: A speech pattern in which the person is talkative due to a sense of pressure to speak; a symptom of manic episodes of bipolar disorder.

prevalence: The total number of people who have a particular disorder within a given population at a specific time.

prevention: Interventions used before the initial onset of a disorder that become distinct from the treatment.

principlism: The approach to ethics that uses common principles or ethical norms as the basis for ethical decision-making. In health ethics, the principles used include *nonmaleficence* (do no harm), *beneficence* (promote benefit), *respect for autonomy* (the right to make one's own decisions), and *justice* (fairness in the distribution of risks and benefits).

problem-focused coping: Coping composed of inner- or outer-directed coping strategies. Outer-directed strategies attempt to eliminate or alter a situation or another's behaviour, while inner-directed strategies aim at altering one's own beliefs, attitudes, skills, responses, etc.

process recording: A verbatim transcript of a verbal interaction usually organized according to the nurse–patient interaction. It often includes analysis of the interaction.

projective identification: A psychoanalytic term used to describe behaviour of people with borderline personality disorder when they falsely attribute to others their own unacceptable feelings, impulses, or thoughts.

pseudodementia: Memory difficulties in older adults with major depression (may be mistaken for early signs of dementia).

pseudologia fantastica: False stories of personal triumph that are a core symptom of factitious disorders.

pseudoneurologic symptoms: Somatic symptoms of conversion disorders that pertain to neurologic conditions affecting voluntary motor or sensory function (e.g., impaired balance, paralysis, blindness, deafness). The symptoms do not follow neurologic paths but rather follow the individual's conceptualization of the problem.

pseudoparkinsonism: Sometimes referred to as *drug-induced parkinsonism*; presents identically as Parkinson's disease without the same destruction of dopaminergic cells.

psychoanalytic movement: Freud's radical approach to psychiatric mental health care, which involved using a new technique called *psychoanalysis* based on unconscious motivations for behaviour, or drives.

psychodrama: A group role-playing technique used to encourage expression of emotion and exploration of problems.

psychoeducation: An educational approach used to enhance knowledge and shape behaviour so that coping skills are learned or enhanced.

psychoendocrinology: The study of the relationships among the nervous system, endocrine system, and behaviour.

psychoimmunology: The study of immunology as it relates to emotions and behaviour.

psychopathy: Refers to individuals who behave impulsively and are interpersonally irresponsible, act hastily and spontaneously, are shortsighted, and fail to plan ahead or consider alternatives. Equated with antisocial personality disorder.

psychopharmacology: A subspecialty of pharmacology that studies medications that affect behaviour through their actions in the CNS and that are used to treat psychiatric and neurodegenerative disorders.

psychosis: A state in which the individual is experiencing hallucinations, delusions, or disorganized thoughts, speech, or behaviour.

purging: A compensatory behaviour to rid oneself of food already eaten by means of self-induced vomiting or the use of laxatives, enemas, or diuretics.

pyromania: An irresistible impulse to start fires.

R

rapidly cycling bipolar disorder: The occurrence of four or more mood episodes during the past 12 months.

rapport: Interpersonal harmony characterized by understanding and respect.

rate: A proportion of the cases in the population compared to the total population.

reaction time: The lapse of time between stimulus and response.

receptor: Site where a substance can specifically interact with the cell membrane to produce a change; biologic action of a drug depends on how its structure interacts with a specific receptor.

recovery: When related to mental illness means gaining and retaining hope, understanding of one's abilities and disabilities, engagement in an active life, personal autonomy, social identity, meaning and purpose in life, and a positive sense of self.

recovery model: An approach that supports individual potential for recovery, focusing on the personal journey involved, the upholding of human rights, a positive culture of healing, and recovery-oriented services.

regressed behaviour: Behaving in the manner of a less mature life stage; childlike and immature.

relapse: Return of symptoms after a period of remission.

relational ethics: The approach to ethics that situates ethical action in relationship, recognizing that complexity, vulnerability, and the environment are important considerations.

relaxation: A mental health intervention that promotes comfort, reduces anxiety, alleviates stress, reduces pain, and prevents aggressive behaviour.

religiosity: A psychiatric symptom characterized by excessive or affected piety.

REM sleep: A sleep cycle state of rapid eye movement.

reminiscence: Thinking about or relating past experiences.

reminiscence therapy: The healing process of looking back on specific times or events in one's life.

remission: A period when the symptoms of a disease are abated.

resilience: The capacity to overcome adversity in spite of extreme stress; involves the balancing of risk and protective factors.

resolution phase: The termination phase of the nurse–patient relationship that lasts from the time the problems are resolved to the close of the relationship.

restraint: The use of any manual, physical, or mechanical device or material, which when attached to the patient's body (usually the arms and legs) restricts the patient's movements.

retrocollis: The neck muscles pull the head back.

risk factors: Characteristics that do not cause the disorder or problem and are not symptoms of the illness but rather are factors that have been shown to influence the likelihood of developing a disorder.

risk/rescue ratio: Refers to the lethality of means of suicide and the likelihood of rescue. Risk is lowest when intent is weak and the method used has low lethality. The likelihood of rescue is dependent on communication of intent and lower lethality of means.

role: An individual's social position and function within an environment.

ruminations: Repetitive thoughts that are forced into a patient's consciousness even when unwanted; when a person goes over and over the same ideas endlessly; part of an obsessive style of thinking.

S

satiety: Internal signals that indicate one has had enough to eat.

schema: A cognitive structure that screens, codes, and evaluates the incoming stimuli through which the individual interprets events.

schizoaffective disorder: An interrupted period of illness during which at some point there is a major depressive, manic, or mixed episode, along with two of the following symptoms of schizophrenia: delusions, hallucinations, disorganized speech, disorganized or catatonic behaviour, or negative symptoms (affective flattening, alogia, or avolition).

school phobia: Anxiety in which the child refuses to attend school in order to stay at home and with the primary attachment figure. School phobia is a common presenting complaint in child psychiatric clinics and may be part of separation anxiety, general anxiety, social phobia, obsessive–compulsive disorder, depression, or conduct disorder.

seclusion: The involuntary confinement of a person in a room that the person is physically prevented from leaving for the purposes of safety or behavioural management.

sedative–hypnotics: Medications that induce sleep and reduce anxiety.

selectivity: The ability of a drug to be specific for a particular receptor.

self-awareness: Being cognizant of one's own beliefs, thought motivations, biases, physical and emotional limitations, and the impact one may have on others.

self-concept: The sum of beliefs about oneself, which develops over time.

self-disclosure: The act of revealing personal information about oneself.

self-efficacy: Self-effectiveness.

self-esteem: The way one feels about oneself; components are self-acceptance, self-worth, self-love, and self-nurturing.

self-identity: Formed through the integration of social and occupational roles and affiliations, self-attributed personality traits, attitudes about gender roles, beliefs about sexuality and intimacy, long-term goals, political ideology, and religious beliefs. Without an adequately formed identity, goal-directed behaviour is impaired and interpersonal relationships are disrupted.

self-monitoring: Observing and recording one's own information, usually behaviour, thoughts, or feelings.

separation–individuation: A process during which the child develops a sense of self, a permanent sense of significant others (object constancy), and an integration of both bad and good as components of the self-concept.

serotonin: Centrally mediates the release of endorphins. Along with histamine and bradykinin, serotonin stimulates the pain receptors to generate experienced pain. Serotonin is involved in inhibiting gastric secretion, stimulating smooth muscle, and serving as a central neurotransmitter.

serotonin syndrome: A toxic side effect that occurs as a result of the newer serotonergic drugs; this syndrome is thought to be caused by hyperstimulation of the 5-HT receptor in the brain stem and spinal cord.

severe and persistent mental illness: Mental disorders that are long term and have recurring periods of exacerbation and remission.

sexual abuse: Sexual misconduct toward another person.

sexuality: Basic dimension of every individual's personality, undergoing periods of growth and development, and influenced by biologic and psychosocial factors.

sibling position: A child's place in the family based on birth order (e.g., first born, youngest).

side effects: Unwanted or untoward effects of medications.

sleep: A behavioural and physiologic state of temporary disconnection from the environment, characterized by physical stillness with no or few movements, stereotypical body postures, reduced responsiveness to external stimulation, and reversibility between states, as compared with other states of altered vigilance like coma, hypothermia, or being anaesthetized.

social change: The structural and cultural evolution of society; is constant and, at times, erratic.

social comparison: Evaluating oneself against idealized others, such as models or attractive peers, and is a major factor in body dissatisfaction, weight anxiety, and disturbed eating.

social distance: Degree to which the values of a formal organization and its primary group members differ.

social functioning: Performance of daily activities within the context of interpersonal relations and family and community roles.

social network: Linkages among a defined set of people, among whom there are personal contacts.

social skills training: A psychoeducational approach that involves instruction, feedback, support, and practice with learning behaviours, it helps people interact more effectively with peers and also children with adults.

social support: Resources provided to an individual by others that may moderate the adverse effects of stress.

somatization: When unexplained physical symptoms are present that are related to psychological distress or psychiatric illness.

somatic symptom disorder: One in which the patient experiences physical symptoms as a result of psychological stress, to the extent that daily living is disrupted.

speech: The motor aspects of speaking.

spinal cord: A long, cylindrical collection of neural fibres continuous with the brain stem, housed within the vertebral column.

spirituality: A complex, even mysterious, concept related to one's connection to the sacred and to the beliefs and values that give meaning to one's life.

splitting: A primitive defense mechanism involving the compartmentalization of opposite and conflicting affect states so that self, others, and events are understood as all one way or all another (e.g., viewing a particular person as being all good or all bad).

standards of practice: The explicit responsibilities and competencies of a profession.

static security: Security awareness focused on structural or environmental artefacts common to secure environments, for example, the use of two-way radios, personal protection alarms, video monitoring, electronic door locks, internal barriers, and perimeter fences or walls.

stereotypic behaviour: Repetitive, driven, nonfunctional, and potentially self-injurious behaviour, such as head banging, rocking, and hand flapping, seen in autistic disorder, with an extraordinary insistence on sameness.

stereotyping: The expectation that an individual will act in a characteristic manner that conforms to a perception, usually negative, of the individual's cultural group.

stereotypy: Repetitive, purposeless movements that are idiosyncratic to the individual and to some degree outside of the individual's control.

stigma: The negative, discriminatory, and rejecting attitudes and behaviour toward a characteristic or element exhibited by an individual or group. It can occur at three levels: self, public, and structural.

stigmatization: A process of assigning negative characteristics and identity to a person or group and causing that person or group to feel unaccepted, devalued, ostracized, and isolated from the larger society.

stress: The relationship between the person and the environment that is appraised as exceeding the person's resources and endangering his or her well-being.

stress–diathesis model: An explanation about the relationship between stress and mental illness that proposes that preexisting genetic, biologic, and psychological vulnerabilities interact with negative or stressful life events to cause illness; an inverse relationship between vulnerability and stress is predicted (i.e., the more vulnerable the individual, the less stress is required to cause illness).

stressors: Events that initiate a stress response; can be physical, psychological, or social; can be short term (acute) or long term (chronic).

structured interaction: Purposeful interaction that allows patients to interact with others in a way that is useful to them.

subcortical: Structures inside the hemispheres and beneath the cortex.

subcortical dementia: Dementia that is caused by dysfunction or deterioration of deep grey or white matter structures inside the brain and brainstem.

substance abuse: A maladaptive use of chemical substance(s) leading to clinically significant outcomes or distress (e.g., recurrent legal problems, failure to perform, engaging in physically hazardous behaviour). Criteria for abuse do not include tolerance, withdrawal, or compulsive use.

substance dependence: Continued use of a substance despite significant substance-related problems, along with a pattern of repeated self-administration that can result in tolerance, withdrawal, and compulsive drug-taking behaviour.

substance P: The most common nociceptive transmitter that is released and transported along the central and peripheral pain synapses in the presence of noxious stimuli.

substitute decision-maker: An individual appointed to make health care decisions on behalf of another who is unable to consent to treatment.

subsystems: A systems term used by family theorists to describe subgroups of family members who join together for various activities.

suicidal contagion: A social phenomenon seen among adolescents: when one teenager takes his or her life, others may follow.

suicidal ideation: Thinking about and planning one's own death without actually engaging in self-harm.

suicide: The act of killing oneself voluntarily.

symbolism: The use of a word or a phrase to represent an object, event, or feeling.

symptom expression: The behavioural symptoms of mental illness linked to their neurobiologic basis.

synapse: The region across which nerve impulses are transmitted through the action of a neurotransmitter.

systematic desensitization: A method used to desensitize patients to anxiety-provoking situations by exposing the patient to a hierarchy of feared situations. The patient is taught to use muscle relaxation as levels of anxiety increase through multisituational exposure.

T

tangentiality: When the topic of conversation changes to an entirely different topic that is within a logical progression but causes a permanent detour from the original focus.

tardive dyskinesia: A late-appearing extrapyramidal side effect of antipsychotic medication that includes abnormal involuntary movements of the mouth, tongue, and jaw such as lip smacking, sucking, puckering, tongue protrusion, the bonbon sign, athetoid (worm-like) movements of the tongue, and chewing.

target symptoms: Specific symptoms for which psychiatric medications are prescribed, such as hallucinations, delusions, paranoia, agitation, assaultive behaviour, bizarre ideation, social withdrawal, disorientation, catatonia, blunted affect, thought blocking, insomnia, and anorexia.

task function: The group role that focuses on the task of the group.

telehealth: The use of electronic information and communication technologies to support health care services over distance.

tenuous stability: Fragile personality patterns that lack resiliency under subjective stress.

thalamus: Thought to play a role in controlling electrical activity in the cortex; provides the relay mechanism for information to and from the cerebrum.

theory: An imaginative grouping of knowledge, ideas, and experience that are represented symbolically and seek to illuminate a given phenomenon.

therapeutic communication: The ongoing process of interaction, verbal and nonverbal, through which meaning emerges.

therapeutic index: A ratio of the maximum nontoxic dose to the minimum effective dose.

thought broadcasting: Belief that one's thoughts are open to others or are being broadcast to the world.

thought insertion: Belief that thoughts or ideas are being inserted into one's mind by someone or something external to one's self.

thought stopping: A practice in which a person identifies negative feelings and thoughts that exist together, says "stop," and then engages in a distracting activity.

thymoleptic: Mood stabilizing.

tidal model: A theory-based approach to mental health nursing that emphasizes empowering collaboration between the nurse and the person receiving nursing care.

token economy: Applies behaviour modification techniques to multiple behaviours; clients are rewarded with tokens for selected desired behaviours.

tolerance: Increased amounts of a substance are needed to achieve intoxication or desired effect, or there is diminished effect with the same amount of the substance.

torticollis: The neck muscles pull the head to the side.

toxicity: The point at which concentrations of a drug in the bloodstream become harmful or poisonous to the body.

transference: The unconscious assignment to others of feelings and attitudes that were originally associated with important figures such as parents or siblings.

transition times: A term used to describe times of addition, subtraction, or change in status of family members.

transitional object: A symbolic attachment figure, such as a blanket or a stuffed animal, that a child may cling to when a parent is not available.

trauma-informed care: An approach to all clients that is based on knowledge of trauma and its effects with policies and practices incorporating principles of safety, choice and control, as well as compassion, collaboration, and trustworthiness.

traumatic bonding: A strong emotional attachment between an abused person and his or her abuser, formed as a result of the cycle of violence.

traumatic stressor: Any event (or events) that may cause or threaten death, serious injury, or sexual violence to an individual, a close family member, or a close friend.

triad: A group consisting of three people.

trichotillomania: Chronic, self-destructive hair pulling that results in noticeable hair loss, usually in the crown, occipital, or parietal areas, though sometimes of the eyebrows and eyelashes.

U

unipolar: A term used to describe depression where the affected person has never experienced a manic episode. When a manic episode has been experienced, the depression is termed *bipolar*.

universal preventive interventions: Preventive interventions that are targeted to everyone within a general public or whole population group.

urine specific gravity: A measure of the degree of concentration of solutes in urine.

utilitarianism: The approach to ethics that sets what is right to do as being what gives the best consequences (happiness, pleasure, preference, satisfaction) for the greater number of people.

V

ventricles: The four cavities of the brain.

verbal communication: The use of the spoken word, including its underlying emotion, context, and connotation.

verbigeration: Purposeless repetition of words or phrases.

vicious circles of behaviour: A term used to describe the tendency to become trapped in rigid and inflexible patterns of behaviour that are self-defeating.

violence (violent behaviour): A physical act of force intended to cause harm to a person or an object and to convey the message that the perpetrator's, and not the victim's, point of view is correct.

voluntary admission: The legal status of a patient who has consented to being admitted to the hospital for treatment, during which time he or she maintains all civil rights and is free to leave at any time, even if it is against medical advice.

vulnerability: A multifaceted concept that represents the commingling of resources, risk factors, and health status among a particular population or aggregate of people, which places them at risk for altered health status.

W

waxy flexibility: Posture held in an odd or unusual fixed position for extended periods of time.

well-being: A state in which the individual realizes self-potential, copes with life stresses, and is able to work productively and contribute to society.

Wernicke's area: An area in the left superior temporal gyrus of the brain thought to be responsible for comprehension of speech.

Wernicke's syndrome: An alcohol-induced amnestic disorder caused by a thiamine-deficient diet and characterized by diplopia, hyperactivity, ataxia, and delirium.

withdrawal: The adverse physical and psychological symptoms that occur when a person ceases to use a substance.

word salad: A string of words that are not connected in any way.

work: The job, occupation, or task one performs as a means of providing a livelihood.

work–life balance: Achieved when an individual finds a satisfactory interaction among all the domains of his or her life.

working phase: The second phase of the nurse–patient relationship, in which patients can examine specific problems and learn new ways of approaching them.

workplace health: The promotion and maintenance of the health and well-being of workers through policies, programmes, and practices that promote safety, minimize risk, and create a positive, responsive, equitable workplace culture and a supportive workplace climate.

workplace violence: The intimidation, harassment, abuse, or assault of an individual in his or her place of employment.

X

xerostomia: Dry mouth.

Z

zeitgebers: Specific events or cues that function as time givers or synchronizers and that result in the setting of biologic rhythms.

Index

Page numbers followed by "b" indicate boxed materials; page numbers followed by "f" indicate figures; page numbers followed by "t" indicate tables.

CCS0218